PDR FOR HERBAL MEDICINES

SECOND EDITION

PDR

for Herbal Medicines™

MEDICAL ECONOMICS COMPANY

MONTVALE, NEW JERSEY

PDR

for Herbal Medicines™

ISBN: 1-56363-361-2

Contents

Foreword

With 150,000 copies of its first edition in print, *PDR for Herbal Medicines* has almost instantly become one of the nation's leading pharmacological references. The reasons for its phenomenal reception are evident. Hundreds of herbal remedies now fill the shelves in virtually every supermarket and pharmacy, and the popularity of self-medication with "natural" supplements continues to rise, making the benefits—and risks—of these preparations an ever more compelling concern.

Now, to better address the host of questions that still surround most herbal remedies, *Physicians' Desk Reference®* is proud to present this completely revised and updated second edition of *PDR for Herbal Medicines*. Significantly enhanced and expanded, this new edition extends both the range and depth of the original volume. Among the many improvements you'll find:

■ **Broader Coverage:** With some 100 new entries, the book now covers a total of 700 botanicals, including a wide selection of popular Chinese herbs.
■ **More Research Data:** Hundreds of entries have been augmented with additional information on safety and efficacy.
■ **Additional Adverse Effects:** The entries include new information on drug/herb interactions. The Side Effects and Interactions indices have been enriched and expanded
■ **Available Formulations:** Whenever applicable, the herbal monographs now list the names and suppliers of popular commercial preparations.
■ **New Indices:** The index section has been enhanced with four additional indices:
— Homeopathic Indications Index
— Asian Indications Index
— Safety Guide
— Manufacturers Index
■ **Better Organization:** In this edition, remedies appear under their more familiar common name, instead of their botanical designation. All monographs are cross-referenced by scientific name.

One important aspect of the first edition does, however, remain constant. Because it is still extremely hard to come by reliable information on the swarm of unregulated "dietary supplements" in today's marketplace, this new edition continues to provide you with the closest available analog to FDA-approved labeling—the findings of the German Regulatory Authority's herbal watchdog agency, commonly called "Commission E." This agency has conducted an intensive assessment of the peer-reviewed literature on some 300 common botanicals, weighing the quality of the clinical evidence and identifying the uses for which the herb can reasonably be considered effective. Its conclusions represent the best expert consensus on medicinal herbs currently available.

For the herbs not considered by Commission E, *PDR for Herbal Medicines* provides the results of an exhaustive literature review conducted by the respected PhytoPharm U.S. Institute of Phytopharmaceuticals under the direction of noted botanist, Dr. Joerg Gruenwald. These additional monographs, now some 400 in number, provide a detailed introduction to an array of exotic botanicals that you'll be hard pressed to find in any other source.

To make the information in the monographs as useful and accessible as possible, *PDR®* has echoed the structure of standard U.S. product labeling. Each monograph contains up to ten standard sections, covering considerations ranging from description to dosage. Here's a closer look at what you will find:

■ **Title:** Each monograph begins with the herb's generally accepted common name, followed by its scientific name. In addition, all monographs are cross-referenced by their botanical designation.

■ **Trade Names:** Listed here are common commercial preparations of the herb.

■ **Description:** This section provides a detailed botanical overview of the herb, including information on its medicinal parts; flower and fruit; leaves, stem, and root; unique characteristics, habitat, production, related plants, and additional common names and synonyms.

■ **Actions and Pharmacology:** Here you'll find data on the active compounds or heterogeneous mixtures found in the plant, followed by a summary of the herb's clinical effects. If various parts of the plant possess different pharmacological activity, the parts are discussed individually, here and throughout the remainder of the monograph.

■ Indications and Usage: Information on the uses of the herb is listed under five categories, as applicable:
— Approved by Commission E
— Unproven Uses
— Chinese Medicine
— Indian Medicine
— Homeopathic
Approved uses are presented in list fashion. Other uses are described with provisos as necessary regarding route and form of administration.

■ Contraindications: Although most natural remedies can be used under all medical circumstances, a few pharmacologically potent herbs must be avoided in the presence of certain medical conditions. If any such contraindications exist, they are summarized here.

■ Precautions and Adverse Reactions: Found in this section are any cautions or special considerations regarding safe use of the herb, including any restrictions on use in pregnancy or childhood. Although most herbal remedies are notably free of known side effects, any reported in the available literature are noted here.

■ Overdosage: As we all know, "natural" is not synonymous with "benign," and an overdose of many "healing" herbs can have serious—even fatal—consequences. Whenever adverse effects of overdose have been found in the literature, they are reported here, along with the appropriate medical interventions to be undertaken when an overdose occurs.

■ Dosage: Listed here are common modes of administration, forms and strengths of available commercial preparations, methods for preparing the natural herb, and representative dosage recommendations drawn from the literature. Note, however, that dosage recommendations can be used only as a general guide. The potency of individual preparations and extracts is subject to substantial variation, so the manufacturer's directions should be consulted whenever available.

■ Literature: This section provides you with a unique bibliography of the technical literature. Because German researchers have been particularly active in the herbal arena, you will find an unusual number of German-language citations. However, work in the English literature is included as well.

To assist you in quickly locating the information you require, the monographs have been indexed by name, therapeutic category, general indications, homeopathic indications, Asian indications, and side effects. To aid you in evaluating potential risk, a drug/herb interaction guide and a safety guide are also included. An index of manufacturers completes the set. Here's an overview of what each index provides:

■ Alphabetical Index: This index includes all scientific, common, and brand names found in the herbal monographs, together with appropriate page numbers.

■ Therapeutic Category Index: This index lists the monographs and their page numbers, alphabetically by accepted common name, under appropriate therapeutic category headings. Herbs deemed effective by Commission E are flagged with a (•) symbol at their left. To facilitate comparison with prescription and nonprescription drugs, *PDR's* standard therapeutic categories are used throughout.

■ Indications Index: This index lists herbs and their page numbers, alphabetically by accepted common name, under their various indications. Herbs deemed effective for the indication by Commission E are flagged with a (•) symbol at their left. To help you quickly identify conventional alternatives, the indication headings match those found in *PDR's* Indications Index, which appears in the *PDR Companion Guide™* and the *PDR Electronic Library ™* CD-ROM.

■ Homeopathic Indications Index: Included in this index are only the uses found in homeopathy. Herbs, which homeopaths typically prescribe by scientific name, are listed here in the same manner, followed by their accepted common name in parentheses. As in the main indications index, headings are chosen to match those in the *PDR Companion Guide*.

■ Asian Indications Index: Entries in this index are limited to uses found in Chinese and Indian medicine. (Chinese entries are signified with a "C;" Indian entries with an "I.") Herbs are listed by accepted common name. Once again, indication headings employ the nomenclature used in the *PDR Companion Guide*.

■ Side Effects Index: In this index, you'll find a list of all herbs associated with a given adverse reaction. Herbs are listed alphabetically by accepted common name, with the scientific name and page number appended. Nomenclature employed in the side effect headings matches that used in PDR's Side Effects Index, another feature of the *PDR Companion Guide* and the *PDR Electronic Library* CD-ROM.

■ **Drug/Herb Interactions Guide:** In this convenient reference, each potential interaction is listed under both the name of the drug and the name of the interacting herb. A brief description of the interaction's effect follows each item.

■ **Safety Guide:** This section lists botanicals in three precautionary categories:
— Not for use during pregnancy
— Not for use while nursing
— For use only under supervision
Here, the scientific, common, and brand names of all herbs in each category are listed alphabetically, together with the appropriate page number for further information.

■ **Manufacturers Index:** This index provides you with contact information for each supplier whose products appear in the herbal monographs. The names of the products, together with the page number of the monograph in which they appear, are included in each manufacturer's entry.

Following the indices, just as in *PDR* itself, you'll find an extensive full-color identification section. The first part of the section—the Herb Identification Guide—encompasses nearly 400 of the most widely used herbs. The second part—the Product Identification Guide—includes photos of some of the more popular commercial formulations. Together, these guides provide you with a truly unique reference unmatched in any other printed resource. We've also included a brief glossary of the unfamiliar terms found in the monographs.

PDR for Herbal Medicines is the product of one of the most thorough and inclusive examinations of the herbal literature ever undertaken. Nevertheless, it's important to remember that it merely summarizes and synthesizes key data from the underlying research reports, and of necessity includes neither every published report nor every recorded fact.

As in all scientific investigation, conclusions regarding the effectiveness of the herbs discussed in this compendium are based on the preponderance of current evidence and cannot be considered firm or final. The publisher does not warrant that any herb will unfailingly and uniformly exhibit the properties ascribed to it by Germany's Commission E or any other scientific authority.

In the United States, herbal products are marketed under the provisions of the Dietary Supplement and Health Education Act of 1994, which prohibits their sale for the diagnosis, treatment, cure, or prevention of any disease. Enumeration of specific commercial preparations within an herbal monograph should not be construed as a claim or warranty of their efficacy for any purpose, by either the manufacturer or the publisher. Furthermore, it should be understood that, just as omission of a product does not signify rejection, inclusion of a product does not imply endorsement, and that the publisher is not advocating the use of any product or substance described herein.

Please remember, too, that dosing of herbal preparations is highly dependent on a variety of factors, such as cultivation and harvesting conditions, the specific parts of the plant to be processed, the extraction methods employed, and the dosage form chosen by the manufacturer. Since there are no official standards governing the production of herbal medicines in the United States, and the potency and the purity of herbal products are subject to substantial variation, dosage ranges set forth in the herbal monographs must be employed only as general guidelines.

In addition, the publisher does not guarantee that every possible hazard, adverse effect, contraindication, precaution, or consequence of overdose is included in the summaries presented here. The publisher has performed no independent verification of the data reported herein, and expressly disclaims responsibility for any error, whether inherent in the underlying literature or resulting from erroneous translation, transcription, or typography.

When patients approach you—as they surely will—for advice on the latest herbal "discovery" to hit the nightly news, we hope that *PDR for Herbal Medicines* will provide you with all the facts you need to offer sound, rational guidance firmly grounded in fact. Certainly such counseling is the aim of every dedicated health care professional. And at *PDR*, we fully share that goal.

Alphabetical Index

Listed here are all scientific, common, and brand names to be found in the herbal monographs. Generally accepted common names that serve as monograph titles appear in bold type. Scientific names are shown in italic type. Brand names are followed by the supplier's name in parentheses. If an entry lists two page numbers, the first refers to a photograph of the plant or product in the Identification Guide, the second to the herbal monograph.

A

C

D

G

T

Therapeutic Category Index

Entries in this index are organized by prescribing category, enabling you to quickly identify botanicals with similar properties. Within each category, herbs are listed alphabetically by their accepted common name, with the scientific name shown in parentheses. Botanicals deemed effective by the German Regulatory Authority's "Commission E" are marked with a (•) symbol at their left. If an entry lists two page numbers, the first refers to a photograph of the plant in the Herb Identification Guide, the second to the herbal monograph. The index lists herbs by general category only. To locate botanicals considered appropriate for a specific indication, please consult the Indications Index.

• Denotes recommendation by Commission E.

ANTIARRHYTHMICS

ANTICONVULSANTS

ANTIDEPRESSANTS

• Denotes recommendation by Commission E.

• Denotes recommendation by Commission E.

ANTIEMETICS

• **Denotes recommendation by Commission E.**

ANTIFLATULENTS

ANTIFUNGALS

ANTIHYPERTENSIVE AGENTS

ANTI-INFECTIVES

ANTI-INFLAMMATORY AGENTS, SKIN AND MUCOUS MEMBRANE

• Denotes recommendation by Commission E.

• Denotes recommendation by Commission E.

• Denotes recommendation by Commission E.

ANTISEBORRHEIC AGENTS

ANTISPASMODICS

• Denotes recommendation by Commission E.

• Denotes recommendation by Commission E.

CENTRAL NERVOUS SYSTEM STIMULANTS

CHOLINESTERASE INHIBITORS

COGNITIVE ENHANCING AGENTS

COLD & COUGH PRODUCTS WITH ANALGESICS

CONTRACEPTIVES

(*See under* Oral contraceptives)

COUGH & COLD PRODUCTS

DIGESTIVE AIDS

• **Denotes recommendation by Commission E.**

DIGESTIVE ENZYMES

• Denotes recommendation by Commission E.

• Denotes recommendation by Commission E.

• Denotes recommendation by Commission E.

• Denotes recommendation by Commission E.

GASTROINTESTINAL STIMULANTS

GOUT PREPARATIONS

• Denotes recommendation by Commission E.

HAIR GROWTH STIMULANTS

HEMOSTATICS

INFECTION PROPHYLAXIS AGENTS

• Denotes recommendation by Commission E.

• Denotes recommendation by Commission E.

LIVER PRODUCTS

LOCAL ANESTHETICS

• Denotes recommendation by Commission E.

• Denotes recommendation by Commission E.

MUSCLE RELAXANTS

NARCOTIC ANTITUSSIVES

NARCOTICS

NON-NARCOTIC ANTITUSSIVES

• Denotes recommendation by Commission E.

• Denotes recommendation by Commission E.

• Denotes recommendation by Commission E.

• Denotes recommendation by Commission E.

REVITALIZING AGENTS

SALIVA PRODUCTS

SCABICIDES & PEDICULICIDES

SEDATIVES & HYPNOTICS

SKELETAL MUSCLE RELAXANTS

SKIN & MUCOUS MEMBRANE AGENTS

• Denotes recommendation by Commission E.

SMOKING CESSATION AIDS

SMOOTH MUSCLE RELAXANTS

STIMULANT LAXATIVES

SUNBURN PREPARATIONS

VAGINAL PREPARATIONS

VASOPROTECTIVE AGENTS

VENOUS INSUFFICIENCY PRODUCTS

• Denotes recommendation by Commission E.

• Denotes recommendation by Commission E.

• Denotes recommendation by Commission E.

Indications Index

Entries in this index are organized by specific indication, enabling you to quickly review the botanical alternatives for a particular diagnosis. For ease of comparison with prescription and over-the-counter medications, the index employs the same nomenclature found in the Indications Index of the PDR Companion Guide™. *Under each heading, herbs are listed alphabetically by accepted common name, with the scientific name shown in parentheses. Botanicals deemed effective by the German Regulatory Authority's "Commission E" are marked with a (•) symbol at their left. If an entry lists two page numbers, the first refers to a photograph of the plant in the Herb Identification Guide, the second to the herbal monograph. For more information on both proven and traditional remedies, be sure to check the appropriate underlying monograph.*

APPETITE, SUPPRESSION OF

APPREHENSION

ARRHYTHMIAS

ARTERIOSCLEROSIS

ARTERIOSCLEROSIS PROPHYLAXIS

BRONCHIAL CONGESTION

BRONCHITIS, ACUTE

• Denotes recommendation by Commission E.

• Denotes recommendation by Commission E.

• Denotes recommendation by Commission E.

• Denotes recommendation by Commission E.

• Denotes recommendation by Commission E.

DIET, SUPPLEMENTATION OF

DIGESTIVE DISORDERS, SYMPTOMATIC RELIEF OF

• **Denotes recommendation by Commission E.**

DIGESTIVE INSUFFICIENCIES, SYMPTOMATIC RELIEF OF

DROPSY

(*See under* Edema, idiopathic)

DYSENTERY

DYSMENORRHEA, UNSPECIFIED, SYMPTOMATIC RELIEF OF

• Denotes recommendation by Commission E.

FISSURE, ANAL

FLATULENCE, RELIEF OF

FLUID RETENTION

FROSTBITE, POSSIBLY EFFECTIVE IN

FUNGAL INFECTIONS, SKIN

(*See under* Infections, mycotic, cutaneous)

FURUNCULOSIS

FURUNCULOSIS, SYMPTOMATIC RELIEF OF

GALLSTONES

(*See under* Biliary calculi, chemical dissolution of)

GASTRIC ULCERS, ACTIVE, BENIGN, SHORT-TERM TREATMENT OF

GASTRITIS

• Denotes recommendation by Commission E.

• **Denotes recommendation by Commission E.**

• Denotes recommendation by Commission E.

• Denotes recommendation by Commission E.

• **Denotes recommendation by Commission E.**

• Denotes recommendation by Commission E.

• Denotes recommendation by Commission E.

• Denotes recommendation by Commission E.

• Denotes recommendation by Commission E.

RESPIRATORY TRACT DISORDERS

• Denotes recommendation by Commission E.

• **Denotes recommendation by Commission E.**

SKIN, IRRITATION, MINOR, PAIN ASSOCIATED WITH

SKIN, RADIATION DAMAGE, TREATMENT OF

SLEEP DISORDERS

SLEEP, INDUCTION OF

SMOKING CESSATION, TEMPORARY AID TO

SNAKEBITE

• Denotes recommendation by Commission E.

• Denotes recommendation by Commission E.

• Denotes recommendation by Commission E.

• Denotes recommendation by Commission E.

• Denotes recommendation by Commission E.

Homeopathic Indications Index

Entries in this index are organized by specific indication, enabling you to quickly review the botanicals used by homeopaths for a particular diagnosis. For ease of comparison with prescription and over-the-counter medications, the index employs the same nomenclature found in the Indications Index of the PDR Companion Guide™. *Under each heading, herbs are listed alphabetically by scientific name, with the accepted common name shown in parentheses. If an entry lists two page numbers, the first refers to a photograph of the plant in the Herb Identification Guide, the second to the herbal monograph. For more information on any of these botanicals, be sure to check the appropriate underlying monograph.*

Asian Indications Index

Entries in this index are organized by specific indication, enabling you to quickly review the botanicals used in Asian medicine for a particular diagnosis. For ease of comparison with prescription and over-the-counter medications, the index employs the same nomenclature found in the Indications Index of the PDR Companion Guide™. *Under each heading, herbs are listed alphabetically by accepted common name, with the scientific name shown in parentheses. An "I" in parentheses indicates Indian usage; a "C" denotes Chinese medical applications. If an entry lists two page numbers, the first refers to a photograph of the plant in the Herb Identification Guide, the second to the herbal monograph. For more information on any of these botanicals, be sure to check the appropriate underlying monograph.*

ABORTION
(*See under* Pregnancy, termination of)

ACHES, MUSCULAR
(*See under* Pain, muscular, temporary relief of)

ACID INDIGESTION
(*See under* Hyperacidity, gastric, symptomatic relief of)

ACNE, UNSPECIFIED
Duckweed (*Lemna minor*) (C) G-10, 258

AIRWAY OBSTRUCTION DISORDERS
(*See under* Bronchial asthma)

ALCOHOL DEPENDENCE
Betel Nut (*Piper betle*) (I) .. G-4, 74
Cayenne (*Capsicum annuum*) (I) .. G-8, 165

ALCOHOL INTOXICATION, MANAGEMENT OF
Coffee (*Coffea arabica*) (I) . G-9, 202
Quinine (*Cinchona pubescens*) (C) G-20, 626
Tamarind (*Tamarindus indica*) (I) 753

AMENORRHEA
Aloe (*Aloe barbadensis*; *Aloe capensis*; *Aloe vera*) (I) ... G-3, 16
Astragalus (*Astragalus species*) (C) 54
Bog Bean (*Menyanthes trifoliata*) (C) G-6, 110
Burning Bush (*Dictamnus albus*) (I) G-7, 130
Chinese Cinnamon (*Cinnamomum aromaticum*) (C) 182
Chinese Rhubarb (*Rheum palmatum*) (C) ... G-8, 185
Henna (*Lawsonia inermis*) (I) ... G-14, 391
Myrrh (*Commiphora molmol*) (C) G-18, 534
Red-Rooted Sage (*Salvia miltiorrhiza*) (C) 636
Safflower (*Carthamus tinctorius*) (C) ... 652
Saffron (*Crocus sativus*) (C) G-21, 653

AMENORRHEA, SECONDARY
(*See under* Menstrual disorders)

AMNESIA
Lemon-Wood (*Schisandra sphenanthera*) (C) 464

ANEMIA, UNSPECIFIED
Arjun Tree (*Terminalia arjuna*) (I) 39
Cassia (*Cassia angustifolia*) (I) 684
Chocolate Vine (*Akebia quinata*) (C) 189
Fennel (*Foeniculum vulgare*) (I) . G-11, 302
Henna (*Lawsonia inermis*) (I) .. G-14, 391
Lycium Berries (*Lycium barbarum*) (I,C) 487
Nux Vomica (*Strychnos nux vomica*) (I) G-18, 547
Plumbago (*Plumbago zeylanica*) (C) 599
Senna (*Cassia senna*) (I) ... G-22, 684

ANGINA
(*See under* Angina pectoris)

ANGINA PECTORIS
Ginkgo (*Ginkgo biloba*) (C) G-12, 342

(I) denotes use in Indian medicine. (C) denotes use in Chinese medicine.

(I) denotes use in Indian medicine. (C) denotes use in Chinese medicine.

DYSPNEA
Bog Bean (*Menyanthes trifoliata*) (C) G-6, 110
Ginger (*Zingiber officinale*) (C) G-12, 339
Jimson Weed (*Datura stramonium*) (C) G-15, 436
Lemon-Wood (*Schisandra sphenanthera*) (C) 464
Schisandra (*Schisandra chinensis*) (C) 669

DYSTOCIA
Saffron (*Crocus sativus*) (C) G-21, 653

DYSURIA, SYMPTOMATIC RELIEF OF
Black Nightshade (*Solanum nigrum*) (I) G-6, 101
Coconut Palm (*Cocos nucifera*) (I) G-9, 201
Coriander (*Coriandrum sativum*) (I) G-9, 221
Duckweed (*Lemna minor*) (C) G-10, 258
Grape (*Vitis vinifera*) (I) G-13, 362
Henna (*Lawsonia inermis*) (I) G-14, 391
Jambolan (*Syzygium cumini*) (I) 429
Plantain (*Musa paradisiaca*) (I) 597
Psyllium (*Plantago ovata*) (I) 612
Rauwolfia (*Rauwolfia serpentina*) (I) 631

ECZEMA, UNSPECIFIED
(*See under* Skin, inflammatory conditions)

EDEMA, ADJUNCTIVE THERAPY IN
Areca Nut (*Areca catechu*) (C) G-4, 38
Celandine (*Chelidonium majus*) (C) G-8, 169
Croton Seeds (*Croton tiglium*) (C) 234
Ma-Huang (*Ephedra sinica*) (C) G-16, 488
Scarlet Pimpernel (*Anagallis arvensis*) (C) G-22, 668

EDEMA, IDIOPATHIC
Alisma (*Alisma plantago-aquatica*) (C) G-3, 13
Bog Bean (*Menyanthes trifoliata*) (C) G-6, 110
Cayenne (*Capsicum annuum*) (I) G-8, 165
Chinese Rhubarb (*Rheum palmatum*) (C) G-8, 185
Coriander (*Coriandrum sativum*) (I) G-9, 221
Duckweed (*Lemna minor*) (C) G-10, 258
Indian Squill (*Urginea indica*) (I) 421
Japanese Atractylodes (*Atractylodes japonica*) (C) 430
Morning Glory (*Ipomoea hederacea*) (C) 523
Southern Tsangshu (*Atractylodes lancea*) (C) 706
Vervain (*Verbena officinalis*) (C) G-25, 788

ENTERITIS
Figs (*Ficus carica*) (C) G-11, 310
Schisandra (*Schisandra chinensis*) (C) 669
Southern Tsangshu (*Atractylodes lancea*) (C) 706

ENURESIS
Schisandra (*Schisandra chinensis*) (C) 669

EPILEPSY
Asa Foetida (*Ferula foetida*) (I) 47
Bistort (*Persicaria bistorta*) (C) G-5, 82
Calotropis (*Calotropis procera*) (I) 141
Cotton (*Gossypium hirsutum*) (I) 228
Duckweed (*Lemna minor*) (C) G-10, 258
Gotu Kola (*Centella asiatica*) (I) G-13, 359
Jatamansi (*Nardostachys jatamansi*) (I) 433
Picrorhiza (*Picrorhiza kurroa*) (C) 589
Storax (*Liquidambar orientalis*) (C) G-23, 734

ERECTILE DYSFUNCTION
Asiatic Dogwood (*Cornus officinalis*) (C) 51
Betel Nut (*Piper betle*) (I) G-4, 74
Fenugreek (*Trigonella foenum-graecum*) (C) G-11, 304
Nutmeg (*Myristica fragrans*) (I) G-18, 545
Siberian Ginseng (*Eleutherococcus senticosus*) (C) 693
Walnut (*Juglans regia*) (C) G-25, 793

ERYSIPELAS
Black Nightshade (*Solanum nigrum*) (C) G-6, 101
Duckweed (*Lemna minor*) (C) G-10, 258
Ground Ivy (*Glechoma hederacea*) (C) 372
Psyllium (*Plantago ovata*) (I) 612

EXHAUSTION
Arjun Tree (*Terminalia arjuna*) (I) 39
Chinese Cinnamon (*Cinnamomum aromaticum*) (C) 182
Japanese Atractylodes (*Atractylodes japonica*) (C) 430
Lotus (*Nelumbo nucifera*) (I) G-16, 481

EYE SIGHT IMPAIRMENT
Lycium Berries (*Lycium barbarum*) (C) 487

EYES, WATERY
(*See under* Lacrimation, symptomatic relief of)

FATIGUE, SYMPTOMATIC RELIEF OF
Green Tea (*Camellia sinensis*) (I) G-13, 369
Salep (*Orchis species*) (I) 657
Schisandra (*Schisandra chinensis*) (C) 669

FEVER, REDUCTION OF
Anemarrhena (*Anemarrhena asphodeloides*) (C) 31
Basil (*Ocimum basilicum*) (I) G-4, 64
Behen (*Moringa oleifera*) (I) 67
Bistort (*Persicaria bistorta*) (C) G-5, 82
Black Catnip (*Phyllanthus amarus*) (I) 91

(I) denotes use in Indian medicine. (C) denotes use in Chinese medicine.

FLATULENCE, RELIEF OF

FLU SYMPTOMS

(*See under* Influenza syndrome, symptomatic relief of)

FURUNCULOSIS

HEART FAILURE, CONGESTIVE
(*See under* Congestive heart failure, adjunct in)

HEARTBURN
(*See under* Hyperacidity, gastric, symptomatic relief of)

HEAT STROKE
Sandalwood (*Santalum album*) (I) 659
Turmeric (*Curcuma domestica*) (C) 775

HELMINTHIASIS
Agrimony (*Agrimonia eupatoria*) (C) . G-3, 10
Aloe (*Aloe barbadensis*; *Aloe capensis*; *Aloe vera*) (I) ... G-3, 16
Asa Foetida (*Ferula foetida*) (C) 47
Calamus (*Acorus calamus*) (I) G-7, 138
Calotropis (*Calotropis procera*) (I) 141
Croton Seeds (*Croton tiglium*) (I,C) 234
Dill (*Anethum graveolens*) (I) G-10, 252
Giant Milkweed (*Calotropis gigantea*) (I) 338
Indian Squill (*Urginea indica*) (I) 421
Kamala (*Mallotus philippinensis*) (I) 442
Knotweed (*Polygonum aviculare*) (C) G-15, 448
Lemongrass (*Cymbopogon citratus*) (I) G-16, 465
Lotus (*Nelumbo nucifera*) (I) G-16, 481
Morning Glory (*Ipomoea hederacea*) (I,C) 523
Neem (*Antelaea azadirachta*) (I) G-18, 539
Northern Prickly Ash (*Zanthoxylum americanum*) (I) 545
Onion (*Allium cepa*) (C) ... G-19, 557
Papaya (*Carica papaya*) (I) G-19, 565
Plantain (*Musa paradisiaca*) (I) 597
Plumbago (*Plumbago zeylanica*) (C) 599
Pomegranate (*Punica granatum*) (C) ... G-20, 605
Tropical Almond (*Terminalia chebula*) (I) 772
Turmeric (*Curcuma domestica*) (I) 775
Walnut (*Juglans regia*) (I) G-25, 793

HEMATEMESIS
Adrue (*Cyperus articulatus*) (C) ... G-3, 6
Henbane (*Hyoscyamus niger*) (I) .. G-14, 389
Lycium Bark (*Lycium chinense*) (C) 486
Pineapple (*Ananas comosus*) (I) 593
Red Sandalwood (*Pterocarpus santalinus*) (I) ... 635

HEMATURIA
Chocolate Vine (*Akebia quinata*) (C) 189
Cleavers (*Galium aparine*) (C) 193
Luffa (*Luffa aegyptica*) (I) G-16, 483
Oriental Arborvitae (*Thuja orientalis*) (C) 560

HEMOPTYSIS
Asparagus (*Asparagus officinalis*) (C) G-4, 52
Ginseng (*Panax ginseng*) (C) ... 346
Great Burnet (*Sanguisorba officinalis*) (C) G-13, 366
Oak Gall (*Quercus infectoria*) (I) 550
Oriental Arborvitae (*Thuja orientalis*) (C) 560
Pineapple (*Ananas comosus*) (I) 593
Turmeric (*Curcuma domestica*) (C) 775

HEMORRHAGE, NASAL
Coriander (*Coriandrum sativum*) (I) G-9, 221
Gotu Kola (*Centella asiatica*) (C) G-13, 359
Great Burnet (*Sanguisorba officinalis*) (C) G-13, 366
Henbane (*Hyoscyamus niger*) (I) .. G-14, 389
Lycium Bark (*Lycium chinense*) (C) 486
Oriental Arborvitae (*Thuja orientalis*) (C) 560
Rehmannia (*Rehmannia glutinosa*) (C) 640
Turmeric (*Curcuma domestica*) (C) 775

HEMORRHOIDS
Acacia (*Acacia arabica*) (I) 3
Black Pepper (*Piper nigrum*) (I) G-6, 103
Cabbage (*Brassica oleracea*) (I) ... G-7, 134
Carambola (*Averrhoa carambola*) (I) 148
Coriander (*Coriandrum sativum*) (I,C) G-9, 221
Garden Cress (*Lepidium sativum*) (I) G-12, 326
Grape (*Vitis vinifera*) (I) .. G-13, 362
Lycium Berries (*Lycium barbarum*) (I) 487
Oak Gall (*Quercus infectoria*) (I,C) 550
Oleander (*Nerium oleander*) (I) G-19, 555
Papaya (*Carica papaya*) (I) G-19, 565
Picrorhiza (*Picrorhiza kurroa*) (C) 589
Psyllium (*Plantago ovata*) (I) ... 612
Tamarind (*Tamarindus indica*) (I) 753
Tropical Almond (*Terminalia chebula*) (I) 772

HEMOSTASIS, AN AID IN
Agrimony (*Agrimonia eupatoria*) (C) . G-3, 10
Arjun Tree (*Terminalia arjuna*) (I) 39
Basil (*Ocimum basilicum*) (C) ... G-4, 64

HEPATITIS, CHRONIC
Areca Nut (*Areca catechu*) (C) G-4, 38

HEPATITIS, UNSPECIFIED
Black Nightshade (*Solanum nigrum*) (C) ... G-6, 101
Jasmine (*Jasminum officinale*) (C) G-15, 432

(I) denotes use in Indian medicine. (C) denotes use in Chinese medicine.

(I) denotes use in Indian medicine. (C) denotes use in Chinese medicine.

Northern Prickly Ash (*Zanthoxylum americanum*) (I) 545
Oleander (*Nerium oleander*) (I) G-19, 555
Red Sandalwood (*Pterocarpus santalinus*) (I) ... 635

ORCHITIS

Henbane (*Hyoscyamus niger*) (I) ... G-14, 389

PAIN, ABDOMINAL

Fennel (*Foeniculum vulgare*) (C) G-11, 302
Fenugreek (*Trigonella foenum-graecum*) (C) G-11, 304
Ground Ivy (*Glechoma hederacea*) (C) 372
Jasmine (*Jasminum officinale*) (C) G-15, 432
Lesser Galangal (*Alpinia officinarum*) (C) 467
Radish (*Raphanus sativus*) (C) ... G-20, 628

PAIN, BONE

False Schisandra (*Kadsura japonica*) (C) 301
Ma-Huang (*Ephedra sinica*) (C) G-16, 488

PAIN, EAR

Basil (*Ocimum basilicum*) (I) ... G-4, 64
Black Nightshade (*Solanum nigrum*) (I) G-6, 101
Bog Bean (*Menyanthes trifoliata*) (C) G-6, 110
Indian Nettle (*Acalypha indica*) (I) 419
Tobacco (*Nicotiana tabacum*) (I) .. G-24, 762

PAIN, EPIGASTRIC

Adrue (*Cyperus articulatus*) (C) ... G-3, 6
Bitter Orange (*Citrus aurantium*) (C) G-5, 86
Sandalwood (*Santalum album*) (C) 659

PAIN, JOINT

Asiatic Dogwood (*Cornus officinalis*) (C) 51
Birthwort (*Aristolochia clematitis*) (C) G-5, 80
Chinese Cinnamon (*Cinnamomum aromaticum*) (C) 182
Divi-Divi (*Caesalpinia bonducella*) (I) 253
Duckweed (*Lemna minor*) (C) G-10, 258
European Mistletoe (*Viscum album*) (C) G-11, 291
Henbane (*Hyoscyamus niger*) (C) G-14, 389
Japanese Mint (*Mentha arvensis piperascens*) (I) 431
Plumbago (*Plumbago zeylanica*) (C) 599
Red-Rooted Sage (*Salvia miltiorrhiza*) (C) 636
Scarlet Pimpernel (*Anagallis arvensis*) (C) .. G-22, 668
Soybean (*Glycine soja*) (C) G-22, 707

PAIN, LUMBAR

Asiatic Dogwood (*Cornus officinalis*) (C) 51
European Mistletoe (*Viscum album*) (C) G-11, 291
Nux Vomica (*Strychnos nux vomica*) (I) G-18, 547
Walnut (*Juglans regia*) (C) G-25, 793
White Nettle (*Lamium album*) (C) G-25, 806

PAIN, MENSTRUAL

False Schisandra (*Kadsura japonica*) (C) 301
Red-Rooted Sage (*Salvia miltiorrhiza*) (C) 636

PAIN, MUSCULAR, TEMPORARY RELIEF OF

Camphor Tree (*Cinnamomum camphora*) (I) G-7, 143
European Mistletoe (*Viscum album*) (C) G-11, 291

PAIN, NEUROGENIC

Peanut (*Arachis hypogaea*) (I) 575
Quinine (*Cinchona pubescens*) (I) G-20, 626
Radish (*Raphanus sativus*) (I) .. G-20, 628

PAIN, RENAL

Siberian Ginseng (*Eleutherococcus senticosus*) (C) 693

PAIN, STOMACH

Benzoin (*Styrax benzoin*) (C) 73
Croton Seeds (*Croton tiglium*) (C) 234
False Schisandra (*Kadsura japonica*) (C) 301
Henbane (*Hyoscyamus niger*) (C) .. G-14, 389
Jasmine (*Jasminum officinale*) (I) G-15, 432
Siam Benzoin (*Styrax tonkinesis*) (C) 692
Sumatra Benzoin (*Styrax paralleloneurum*) (C) 738

PAIN, TOOTH

Betel Nut (*Piper betle*) (I) .. G-4, 74
Calamus (*Acorus calamus*) (I) G-7, 138
Catechu (*Acacia catechu*) (I) ... 163
Cinnamon (*Cinnamomum verum*) (I) G-8, 190
Clove (*Syzygium aromaticum*) (I) G-8, 195
Henbane (*Hyoscyamus niger*) (I) G-14, 389
Japanese Mint (*Mentha arvensis piperascens*) (I,C) ... 431
Jasmine (*Jasminum officinale*) (I) G-15, 432
Lycium Berries (*Lycium barbarum*) (I) 487
Northern Prickly Ash (*Zanthoxylum americanum*) (I) 545
Pellitory (*Anacyclus pyrethrum*) (I) 577
Red Sandalwood (*Pterocarpus santalinus*) (I) ... 635
Tobacco (*Nicotiana tabacum*) (I) . G-24, 762
Wild Thyme (*Thymus serpyllum*) (C) . G-26, 815

PAIN, UNSPECIFIED

Henbane (*Hyoscyamus niger*) (I) ... G-14, 389
Lycium Bark (*Lycium chinense*) (C) 486

(I) denotes use in Indian medicine. (C) denotes use in Chinese medicine.

(I) denotes use in Indian medicine. (C) denotes use in Chinese medicine.

VOMITING

WARTS

WHEEZING, SYMPTOMATIC RELIEF OF

(*See under* Bronchial asthma)

WHOOPING COUGH

(*See under* Pertussis)

WOUND CARE, ADJUNCTIVE THERAPY IN

Side Effects Index

Presented here is an alphabetical list of every side effect cited in the herbal monographs. Under each heading, herbs associated with the reaction are listed alphabetically by accepted common name, with the scientific name shown in parentheses. For ease of comparison with prescription and over-the-counter medications, the index employs the same nomenclature found in the Side Effects Index of the PDR Companion Guide™. *If an entry lists two page numbers, the first refers to a photograph of the plant in the Herb Identification Guide, the second to the herbal monograph.*

Drug/Herb Interactions Guide

This section catalogs potentially adverse drug/herb combinations by both the generic name of the drug or drug category and the accepted common name of the herb. Under each bold-face drug entry you'll find a list of the herbs with which the agent may interact. Likewise, under a bold-face herb entry you'll find a list of potentially interactive drugs. A description of the interaction's effect follows each item in the list. Further information on each drug can be found in Physicians' Desk Reference®. *Information on each herb appears in the Herbal Monographs section of this book.*

ADONIS
Calcium
(Increases action of Adonis)
Digoxin
(Increases action of Adonis)
Glucocorticoids
(Increases action of Adonis)
Laxatives
(Increases action of Adonis)
Quinidine
(Increases action of Adonis)
Saluretics
(Increases action of Adonis)

ADONIS VERNALIS
(*See under* Adonis)

AESCULUS HIPPOCASTANUM
(*See under* Horse Chestnut)

ALCOHOL
German Chamomile
(May increase sedative effect)
Rauwolfia
(Increases impairment of motor skills)
Valerian
(Additive depressive effects with Valerian)
White Willow
(Enhances toxicity of salicylates)

ALKALINE DRUGS
Green Tea
(Decreased absorption of alkaline drugs due to tannin component in tea)
Oak
(Absorption of alkaline drugs may be reduced or inhibited)

ALKALOIDS
Oak
(Absorption of alkaloids may be reduced or inhibited)

ALOE
Antiarrhythmics
(Aloe-induced hypokalemia may affect cardiac rhythm)
Cardiac Glycosides
(Increases effect of cardiac glycosides)
Corticosteroids
(Increased potassium loss)
Licorice
(Increased potassium loss)
Thiazide Diuretics
(Increased potassium loss)

ALOE BARBADENSIS
(*See under* Aloe)

ALOE CAPENSIS
(*See under* Aloe)

ALOE VERA
(*See under* Aloe)

ALPHA ADRENERGIC BLOCKERS
Saw Palmetto
(Saw Palmetto has an additive alpha adrenergic blocking effect when given in combination with alpha blockers)

ALPINE CRANBERRY
Medication and Food that Increase Uric Acid Levels
(Decreases effect of Alpine Cranberry)

AMANTADINE HYDROCHLORIDE
Belladonna
(Increases anticholinergic effect of herb)
Henbane
(Increased anticholinergic action)
Scopolia
(Increased effect when given simultaneously with herb)

ANDROGENS
Saw Palmetto
(Saw Palmetto antagonizes the effect of androgens)

ANTIARRHYTHMICS
Aloe
(Aloe-induced hypokalemia may affect cardiac rhythm)

Buckthorn
(Increased effect due to potassium loss with chronic use of herb)
Cascara Sagrada
(Potentiates arrhythmias with prolonged use of Cascara)
Licorice
(Licorice-induced hypokalemia increases risk of arrhythmias)
Senna
(Senna-induced hypokalemia may increase risk of arrythmia)

ANTICHOLINERGICS
Jimson Weed
(Co-administration of Jimson Weed with other anticholinergic drugs may increase the frequency and/or severity of anticholinergic side effects such as dry mouth, constipation, drowsiness, and others)

ANTICOAGULANT DRUGS, UNSPECIFIED
Arnica
(Coumarin component in Arnica may increase anticoagulant effect)
Astragalus
(Astragalus may potentiate anticoagulant effects)
Horse Chestnut
(Horse Chestnut has a coumarin componant and may interact with warfarin, salicylates and other drugs with anticoagulant properties)

ANTICONVULSANTS
Evening Primrose
(Evening Primrose oil may lower seizure threshold and decrease effectiveness of anticonvulsant medications)

ANTIHISTAMINES
Henbane
(Increased anticholinergic action)

ANTIHYPERTENSIVE AGENTS, UNSPECIFIED
Yohimbe Bark
(May need to adjust antihypertensive medications due to hypertensive effect of Yohimbe)

ANTIPLATELET DRUGS
White Willow
(Additive effect with salicylates)

ANTITHROMBOLYTIC DRUGS
Ginkgo
(Increases effect of antithrombolytic drugs)

ARCTOSTAPHYLOS UVA-URSI
(*See under* Uva-Ursi)

ARNICA
Anticoagulant drugs, unspecified
(Coumarin component in Arnica may increase anticoagulant effect)
Warfarin Sodium
(Additive anticoagulant effect)

ARNICA MONTANA
(*See under* Arnica)

ARTEMISIA ABSINTHIUM
(*See under* Wormwood)

ASPIRIN
Cayenne
(Decreased bioavailability of aspirin)
Feverfew
(Increased antithrombotic effect)

ASTRAGALUS
Anticoagulant drugs, unspecified
(Astragalus may potentiate anticoagulant effects)
Immunosuppressants
(Decreased effectiveness of immunosuppressive effect due to immunostimulant effect of Astragalus)

ASTRAGALUS SPECIES
(*See under* Astragalus)

ATROPA BELLADONNA
(*See under* Belladonna)

BARBITURATES
Rauwolfia
(Synergistic effect)
White Willow
(Enhances toxicity of salicylates)

BELLADONNA
Amantadine Hydrochloride
(Increases anticholinergic effect of herb)
Quinidine
(Increases anticholinergic effect of herb)
Tricyclic Antidepressants
(Increases anticholinergic effect of herb)

BENZODIAZEPINES
German Chamomile
(May increase sedative effect)

BILBERRY
Salicylates
(Increases prothrombin time; caution should be observed when used concurrently)
Warfarin Sodium
(Increases prothrombin time; caution should be observed when used concurrently)

BLADDERWRACK
Hypoglycemic Drugs
(Herb may have an additive hypoglycemic effect when taken with other hypoglycemic drugs)

BREWER'S YEAST
MAO Inhibitors
(Increase in blood pressure)

BUCKTHORN
Antiarrhythmics
(Increased effect due to potassium loss with chronic use of herb)
Cardiac Glycosides
(Increased effect due to potassium loss with chronic use of herb)
Corticosteroids
(Increases hypokalemic effects)
Digoxin
(Herb may cause hypokalemia, which may increase digoxin toxicity)
Licorice Root
(Increases hypokalemic effects)
Thiazide Diuretics
(Increases hypokalemic effects)

BUGLEWEED
Diagnostic Procedures Using Radioactive Isotopes
(Herb interferes with these isotopes)
Thyroid Preparations
(Effect not specified)

CALCIUM

Adonis
(Increases action of Adonis)
Lily-of-the-Valley
(Increases the effect of Lily-of-the-Valley)
Squill
(Increases effectiveness and side effects of herb)

CALCIUM SALTS

Kombé Seed
(Increases effects and side effects of herb)
Oleander
(Increased efficacy and side effects when given simultaneously with herb)
Strophanthus
(Simultaneous administration with herb enhance both effects and side effects)
Strophanthus Gratus
(Simultaneous administration with herb enhance both effects and side effects)

CAMELLIA SINENSIS

(*See under* Green Tea)

CAPSICUM ANNUUM

(*See under* Cayenne)

CARBONIC ANHYDRASE INHIBITORS

White Willow
(Potentiates action of salicylates)

CARDIAC GLYCOSIDES

Aloe
(Increases effect of cardiac glycosides)
Buckthorn
(Increased effect due to potassium loss with chronic use of herb)
Cascara Sagrada
(Increased effect due to potassium loss with chronic use of herb)
Chinese Rhubarb
(Increased effect due to potassium loss with chronic use of herb)
Frangula
(Increased effect due to potassium loss with chronic use of herb)
Guarana
(Increased effect due to potassium loss with chronic use of herb)
Ma-Huang
(Disturbance of heart rhythm)

CARDIOACTIVE STEROIDS

Castor Oil Plant
(Increased effect due to potassium loss with chronic use of herb)

CARICA PAPAYA

(*See under* Papaya)

CASCARA SAGRADA

Antiarrhythmics
(Potentiates arrhythmias with prolonged use of Cascara)
Cardiac Glycosides
(Increased effect due to potassium loss with chronic use of herb)
Corticosteroids
(Increases hypokalemic effect)
Digoxin
(Herb may cause hypokalemia, which may increase digoxin toxicity)
Indomethacin
(Decreases therapeutic effect of Cascara)
Thiazide Diuretics
(Increases hypokalemic effect)

CASSIA SENNA

(*See under* Senna)

CASTOR OIL PLANT

Cardioactive Steroids
(Increased effect due to potassium loss with chronic use of herb)

CAYENNE

Aspirin
(Decreased bioavailability of aspirin)

CENTRAL NERVOUS SYSTEM STIMULANTS

Ma-Huang
(Ma-Huang has an additive effect on the CNS when combined with CNS stimulants)

CHASTE TREE

Dopamine Antagonists
(Decreased dopaminergic effect of herb)

CHINESE RHUBARB

Cardiac Glycosides
(Increased effect due to potassium loss with chronic use of herb)
Digoxin
(Herb may cause hypokalemia, which may increase digoxin toxicity)

CINCHONA PUBESCENS

(*See under* Quinine)

COFFEA ARABICA

(*See under* Coffee)

COFFEE

Drugs, unspecified
(Herb can hinder (or decrease) resorption of other drugs)

CONVALLARIA MAJALIS

(*See under* Lily-of-the-Valley)

CORTICOSTEROIDS

Aloe
(Increased potassium loss)
Buckthorn
(Increases hypokalemic effects)
Cascara Sagrada
(Increases hypokalemic effect)
Echinacea Angustifolia
(Echinacea may potentially interfere with the anti-cancer chemotherapeutic effect of corticosteroids)

CYCLOSPORINE

St. John's Wort
(The herb induces the cytochrome P450 enzyme system and will lower cyclosporine serum levels)

CYTISUS SCOPARIUS

(*See under* Scotch Broom)

DATURA STRAMONIUM

(*See under* Jimson Weed)

DIAGNOSTIC PROCEDURES USING RADIOACTIVE ISOTOPES

Bugleweed
(Herb interferes with these isotopes)

DIGITALIS

Methylxanthines
(Increases risk of cardiac arrhythmias)
Phosphodiesterase Inhibitors
(Increases risk of cardiac arrhythmias)

Quinidine
(Increases risk of cardiac arrhythmias)
Sympathomimetic Agents
(Increases risk of cardiac arrhythmias)

DIGITALIS GLYCOSIDE PREPARATIONS

Licorice
(Licorice-induced hypokalemia increases risk of digitalis toxicity)
Rauwolfia
(Severe bradycardia when used in combination with digitalis glycosides)
Senna
(Senna-induced hypokalemia may increase toxicity of digitalis preparations)

DIGITALIS LANATA

Methylxanthines
(Risk of cardiac arrhythmias)
Phosphodiesterase Inhibitors
(Risk of cardiac arrhythmias)
Quinidine
(Risk of cardiac arrhythmias)
Sympathomimetic Agents
(Risk of cardiac arrhythmias)

DIGITALIS PURPUREA

(*See under* Digitalis)

DIGOXIN

Adonis
(Increases action of Adonis)
Buckthorn
(Herb may cause hypokalemia, which may increase digoxin toxicity)
Cascara Sagrada
(Herb may cause hypokalemia, which may increase digoxin toxicity)
Chinese Rhubarb
(Herb may cause hypokalemia, which may increase digoxin toxicity)
Frangula
(Herb may cause hypokalemia, which may increase digoxin toxicity)
Guarana
(Herb may cause hypokalemia, which may increase digoxin toxicity)
Lily-of-the-Valley
(Increases the effect of Lily-of-the-Valley)
Squill
(Squill potentiates the positive inotropic and negative chronopic effects of digoxin)
St. John's Wort
(Co-administration of the herb with digoxin has resulted in a significant decrease in the digoxin area under the curve)
Uzara
(Herb contains cardiac glycosides and may have additive effect when taken with digoxin, possibly increasing digoxin toxicity)

DIOSCOREA VILLOSA

(*See under* Wild Yam)

DIURETICS

Kombé Seed
(Increases effects and side effects of herb)

DOPAMINE ANTAGONISTS

Chaste Tree
(Decreased dopaminergic effect of herb)

DRUGS THAT CAUSE THROMBOCYTOPENIA

Quinine
(Herb increases risk of thrombocytopenia)

DRUGS, UNSPECIFIED

Coffee
(Herb can hinder (or decrease) resorption of other drugs)
Flax
(Absorption of other drugs may be delayed when taken simultaneously)
Niauli
(Co-administration may result in decreased effect of drugs that undergo liver metabolism)
Psyllium
(Absorption of other drugs may be decreased if taken simultaneously with herb)
Psyllium Seed
(Absorption of other drugs may be decreased if taken simultaneously with herb)

ECHINACEA ANGUSTIFOLIA

Corticosteroids
(Echinacea may potentially interfere with the anti-cancer chemotherapeutic effect of corticosteroids)
Immunosuppressants
(The immune-stimulating effect of Echinacea may interfere with drugs that have immunosuppressant effects)

EPHEDRA SINICA

(*See under* Ma-Huang)

ESTROGEN

Senna
(Senna decreases estrogen levels when taken with estrogen supplements)
Wild Yam
(Additive effect)

ETHANOL

Yohimbe Bark
(Increased anxiogenic effects)

EVENING PRIMROSE

Anticonvulsants
(Evening Primrose oil may lower seizure threshold and decrease effectiveness of anticonvulsant medications)

FENUGREEK

Hypoglycemic Drugs
(Herb may have an additive hypoglycemic effect when taken with other hypoglycemic drugs)

FEVERFEW

Aspirin
(Increased antithrombotic effect)
Warfarin Sodium
(Increased antithrombotic effect)

FLAX

Drugs, unspecified
(Absorption of other drugs may be delayed when taken simultaneously)

FRANGULA

Cardiac Glycosides
(Increased effect due to potassium loss with chronic use of herb)

Digoxin
(Herb may cause hypokalemia, which may increase digoxin toxicity)

FUCUS VESICULOSUS
(*See under* Bladderwrack)

GALEGA OFFICINALIS
(*See under* Goat's Rue)

GERMAN CHAMOMILE
Alcohol
(May increase sedative effect)
Benzodiazepines
(May increase sedative effect)
Warfarin Sodium
(Hydroxycoumarin component in Chamomile may elevate prothrombin times)

GINKGO
Antithrombolytic Drugs
(Increases effect of antithrombolytic drugs)

GINKGO BILOBA
(*See under* Ginkgo)

GINSENG
Hypoglycemic Drugs
(Increases hypoglycemic effect)
Loop Diuretics
(Increases diuretic resistance)
MAO Inhibitors
(Combination increases chance for headache, tremors, mania)

GLUCOCORTICOIDS
Adonis
(Increases action of Adonis)
Kombé Seed
(Increases effects and side effects of herb)
Licorice
(Licorice potentiates effect of glucocorticoids)
Lily-of-the-Valley
(Increases the effect of Lily-of-the-Valley)
Oleander
(Increased efficacy and side effects when given simultaneously with herb)
Squill
(Increases effectiveness and side effects of herb)
Strophanthus
(Simultaneous administration with herb enhance both effects and side effects)
Strophanthus Gratus
(Simultaneous administration with herb enhance both effects and side effects)

GLYCYRRHIZA GLABRA
(*See under* Licorice)

GOAT'S RUE
Hypoglycemic Drugs
(Herb may have an additive hypoglycemic effect when taken with other hypoglycemic drugs)

GREEN TEA
Alkaline Drugs
(Decreased absorption of alkaline drugs due to tannin component in tea)

GUANETHIDINE
Ma-Huang
(Increased sympathomimetic effects)

GUARANA
Cardiac Glycosides
(Increased effect due to potassium loss with chronic use of herb)
Digoxin
(Herb may cause hypokalemia, which may increase digoxin toxicity)

HALOPERIDOL
Milk Thistle
(Silymarin in combination with haloperidol causes a decrease in lipid peroxidation)

HALOTHANE
Ma-Huang
(Disturbance of heart rhythm)

HENBANE
Amantadine Hydrochloride
(Increased anticholinergic action)
Antihistamines
(Increased anticholinergic action)
Phenothiazines
(Increased anticholinergic action)
Procainamide
(Increased anticholinergic action)
Quinidine
(Increased anticholinergic action)
Tricyclic Antidepressants
(Increased anticholinergic action)

HORSE CHESTNUT
Anticoagulant drugs, unspecified
(Horse Chestnut has a coumarin componant and may interact with warfarin, salicylates and other drugs with anticoagulant properties)

HYOSCYAMUS NIGER
(*See under* Henbane)

HYPERICUM PERFORATUM
(*See under* St. John's Wort)

HYPNOTICS
Valerian
(Additive effect when taken with Valerian)

HYPOGLYCEMIC DRUGS
Bladderwrack
(Herb may have an additive hypoglycemic effect when taken with other hypoglycemic drugs)
Fenugreek
(Herb may have an additive hypoglycemic effect when taken with other hypoglycemic drugs)
Ginseng
(Increases hypoglycemic effect)
Goat's Rue
(Herb may have an additive hypoglycemic effect when taken with other hypoglycemic drugs)

IMMUNOSUPPRESSANTS
Astragalus
(Decreased effectiveness of immunosuppressive effect due to immunostimulant effect of Astragalus)
Echinacea Angustifolia
(The immune-stimulating effect of Echinacea may interfere with drugs that have immunosuppressant effects)

INDIAN SQUILL
Methylxanthines
(Can increase the risk of cardic arrhythmias when given simultaneously with this herb)

Phosphodiesterase Inhibitors
(Can increase the risk of cardic arrhythmias when given simultaneously with this herb)
Quinidine
(Can increase the risk of cardic arrhythmias when given simultaneously with this herb)
Sympathomimetic Agents
(Can increase the risk of cardic arrhythmias when given simultaneously with this herb)

INDINAVIR SULFATE
St. John's Wort
(The herb induces the cytochrome P450 enzyme system and will lower indinavir serum levels)

INDOMETHACIN
Cascara Sagrada
(Decreases therapeutic effect of Cascara)
Senna
(Decreased therapeutic effect of Senna)
Wild Yam
(Wild Yam may decrease the anti-inflammatory effect of indomethacin)

INSULIN
Psyllium
(Effect unspecified; insulin dose should be decreased)

JIMSON WEED
Anticholinergics
(Co-administration of Jimson Weed with other anticholinergic drugs may increase the frequency and/or severity of anticholinergic side effects such as dry mouth, constipation, drowsiness, and others)

KOMBÉ SEED
Calcium Salts
(Increases effects and side effects of herb)
Diuretics
(Increases effects and side effects of herb)
Glucocorticoids
(Increases effects and side effects of herb)
Laxatives
(Increases effects and side effects of herb)
Quinidine
(Increases effects and side effects of herb)

LAXATIVES
Adonis
(Increases action of Adonis)
Kombé Seed
(Increases effects and side effects of herb)
Lily-of-the-Valley
(Increases the effect of Lily-of-the-Valley)
Oleander
(Increased efficacy and side effects when given simultaneously with herb)
Squill
(Increases effectiveness and side effects of herb)
Strophanthus
(Simultaneous administration with herb enhance both effects and side effects)
Strophanthus Gratus
(Simultaneous administration with herb enhance both effects and side effects)

LEVODOPA
Rauwolfia
(Decreased effect; increases in extra-pyramidal symptoms)

LICORICE
Aloe
(Increased potassium loss)
Antiarrhythmics
(Licorice-induced hypokalemia increases risk of arrhythmias)
Digitalis Glycoside Preparations
(Licorice-induced hypokalemia increases risk of digitalis toxicity)
Glucocorticoids
(Licorice potentiates effect of glucocorticoids)
Loop Diuretics
(Additive effect of hypokalemia)
Thiazide Diuretics
(Additive effect of hypokalemia)

LICORICE ROOT
Buckthorn
(Increases hypokalemic effects)

LILY-OF-THE-VALLEY
Calcium
(Increases the effect of Lily-of-the-Valley)
Digoxin
(Increases the effect of Lily-of-the-Valley)
Glucocorticoids
(Increases the effect of Lily-of-the-Valley)
Laxatives
(Increases the effect of Lily-of-the-Valley)
Quinidine
(Increases the effect of Lily-of-the-Valley)
Saluretics
(Increases the effect of Lily-of-the-Valley)

LINUM USITATISSIMUM
(*See under* Flax)

LOOP DIURETICS
Ginseng
(Increases diuretic resistance)
Licorice
(Additive effect of hypokalemia)
Uva-Ursi
(The sodium-sparing effect of Uva-Ursi may antagonize the diuretic effect of the loop diuretics)

LYCOPUS VIRGINICUS
(*See under* Bugleweed)

MA-HUANG
Cardiac Glycosides
(Disturbance of heart rhythm)
Central Nervous System Stimulants
(Ma-Huang has an additive effect on the CNS when combined with CNS stimulants)
Guanethidine
(Increased sympathomimetic effects)
Halothane
(Disturbance of heart rhythm)
MAO Inhibitors
(Increases sympathomimetic effects of ephedrine)

Oxytocin
(Development of high blood pressure)

MAO INHIBITORS

Brewer's Yeast
(Increase in blood pressure)

Ginseng
(Combination increases chance for headache, tremors, mania)

Ma-Huang
(Increases sympathomimetic effects of ephedrine)

Scotch Broom
(Increased risk of hypertensive crisis)

MATRICARIA RECUTITA

(*See under* German Chamomile)

MEDICATION AND FOOD THAT INCREASE URIC ACID LEVELS

Alpine Cranberry
(Decreases effect of Alpine Cranberry)

Uva-Ursi
(Decreases effect of herb)

MELALEUCEA VIRIDIFLORA

(*See under* Niauli)

METHYLXANTHINES

Digitalis
(Increases risk of cardiac arrhythmias)

Digitalis Lanata
(Risk of cardiac arrhythmias)

Indian Squill
(Can increase the risk of cardic arrhythmias when given simultaneously with this herb)

Squill
(Increases risk of cardiac arrhythmias)

MILK THISTLE

Haloperidol
(Silymarin in combination with haloperidol causes a decrease in lipid peroxidation)

Phenothiazines
(Silymarin in combination with phenothiazines causes a decrease in lipid peroxidation)

Phentolamine Mesylate
(Silymarin antagonizes the effect of phentolamine)

Yohimbine Hydrochloride
(Silymarin antagonizes the effect of yohimbine)

MORPHINE SULFATE

Yohimbe Bark
(Potentiates effects of morphine)

NALTREXONE HYDROCHLORIDE

Yohimbe Bark
(Potentiates Yohimbe side effects)

NERIUM OLEANDER

(*See under* Oleander)

NEUROLEPTICS

Rauwolfia
(Synergistic effect)

NIAULI

Drugs, unspecified
(Co-administration may result in decreased effect of drugs that undergo liver metabolism)

NIFEDIPINE

Senna
(Inhibits activity of Senna via calcium channel blockade)

NON-STEROIDAL ANTI-INFLAMMATORY DRUGS

Uva-Ursi
(Uva-Ursi may potentiate the gastrointestinal irritation caused by NSAIDs)

White Willow
(Use with caution; effect not specified)

OTC STIMULANTS

Yohimbe Bark
(Potentiates hypertensive effect)

OAK

Alkaline Drugs
(Absorption of alkaline drugs may be reduced or inhibited)

Alkaloids
(Absorption of alkaloids may be reduced or inhibited)

OENOTHERA BIENNIS

(*See under* Evening Primrose)

OLEANDER

Calcium Salts
(Increased efficacy and side effects when given simultaneously with herb)

Glucocorticoids
(Increased efficacy and side effects when given simultaneously with herb)

Laxatives
(Increased efficacy and side effects when given simultaneously with herb)

Quinidine
(Increased efficacy and side effects when given simultaneously with herb)

Saluretics
(Increased efficacy and side effects when given simultaneously with herb)

ORAL CONTRACEPTIVES

St. John's Wort
(Breakthrough bleeding has been reported with concomitant use of the herb with oral contraceptives)

OXYTOCIN

Ma-Huang
(Development of high blood pressure)

PANAX GINSENG

(*See under* Ginseng)

PAPAYA

Warfarin Sodium
(Increased INR levels)

PAULLINIA CUPANA

(*See under* Guarana)

PAUSINYSTALIA YOHIMBE

(*See under* Yohimbe Bark)

PHENOTHIAZINES

Henbane
(Increased anticholinergic action)

Milk Thistle
(Silymarin in combination with phenothiazines causes a decrease in lipid peroxidation)

Wormwood
(Wormwood preparations should not be administered with drugs known to lower the seizure threshold)

PHENTOLAMINE MESYLATE

Milk Thistle
(Silymarin antagonizes the effect of phentolamine)

PHOSPHODIESTERASE INHIBITORS

Digitalis
(Increases risk of cardiac arrhythmias)
Digitalis Lanata
(Risk of cardiac arrhythmias)
Indian Squill
(Can increase the risk of cardic arrhythmias when given simultaneously with this herb)
Squill
(Increases risk of cardiac arrhythmias)

PHOTOSENSITIZING AGENTS

St. John's Wort
(An additive photosensitizing effect is expected when the herb is used with photosensitizing drugs such as tetracyclines, sulfonamides, and thiazides)

PLANTAGO AFRA

(*See under* Psyllium Seed)

PLANTAGO OVATA

(*See under* Psyllium)

PROCAINAMIDE

Henbane
(Increased anticholinergic action)

PSYLLIUM

Drugs, unspecified
(Absorption of other drugs may be decreased if taken simultaneously with herb)
Insulin
(Effect unspecified; insulin dose should be decreased)

PSYLLIUM SEED

Drugs, unspecified
(Absorption of other drugs may be decreased if taken simultaneously with herb)

QUERCUS ROBUR

(*See under* Oak)

QUINIDINE

Adonis
(Increases action of Adonis)
Belladonna
(Increases anticholinergic effect of herb)
Digitalis
(Increases risk of cardiac arrhythmias)
Digitalis Lanata
(Risk of cardiac arrhythmias)
Henbane
(Increased anticholinergic action)
Indian Squill
(Can increase the risk of cardic arrhythmias when given simultaneously with this herb)
Kombé Seed
(Increases effects and side effects of herb)
Lily-of-the-Valley
(Increases the effect of Lily-of-the-Valley)
Oleander
(Increased efficacy and side effects when given simultaneously with herb)
Scopolia
(Increased effect when given simultaneously with herb)
Squill
(Increases risk of cardiac arrhythmias; increases effectiveness and side effects of herb)
Strophanthus
(Simultaneous administration with herb enhance both effects and side effects)
Strophanthus Gratus
(Simultaneous administration with herb enhance both effects and side effects)

QUININE

Drugs that Cause Thrombocytopenia
(Herb increases risk of thrombocytopenia)

RAUWOLFIA

Alcohol
(Increases impairment of motor skills)
Barbiturates
(Synergistic effect)
Digitalis Glycoside Preparations
(Severe bradycardia when used in combination with digitalis glycosides)
Levodopa
(Decreased effect; increases in extra-pyramidal symptoms)
Neuroleptics
(Synergistic effect)
Sympathomimetic Agents
(Increases blood pressure)

RAUWOLFIA SERPENTINA

(*See under* Rauwolfia)

RESERPINE

St. John's Wort
(Hypericum antagonizes the effect of reserpine)

RHAMNUS CATHARTICUS

(*See under* Buckthorn)

RHAMNUS FRANGULA

(*See under* Frangula)

RHAMNUS PURSHIANA

(*See under* Cascara Sagrada)

RHEUM PALMATUM

(*See under* Chinese Rhubarb)

RICINUS COMMUNIS

(*See under* Castor Oil Plant)

SACCHAROMYCES CEREVISIAE

(*See under* Brewer's Yeast)

SALICYLATES

Bilberry
(Increases prothrombin time; caution should be observed when used concurrently)
White Willow
(Use with caution; effect not specified)

SALIX SPECIES

(*See under* White Willow)

SALURETICS

Adonis
(Increases action of Adonis)
Lily-of-the-Valley
(Increases the effect of Lily-of-the-Valley)
Oleander
(Increased efficacy and side effects when given simultaneously with herb)
Squill
(Increases effectiveness and side effects of herb)

Strophanthus
(Simultaneous administration with herb enhance both effects and side effects)
Strophanthus Gratus
(Simultaneous administration with herb enhance both effects and side effects)

SAW PALMETTO

Alpha Adrenergic Blockers
(Saw Palmetto has an additive alpha adrenergic blocking effect when given in combination with alpha blockers)
Androgens
(Saw Palmetto antagonizes the effect of androgens)

SCOPOLIA

Amantadine Hydrochloride
(Increased effect when given simultaneously with herb)
Quinidine
(Increased effect when given simultaneously with herb)
Tricyclic Antidepressants
(Increased effect when given simultaneously with herb)

SCOPOLIA CARNIOLICA

(*See under* Scopolia)

SCOTCH BROOM

MAO Inhibitors
(Increased risk of hypertensive crisis)

SELECTIVE SEROTONIN REUPTAKE INHIBITORS

St. John's Wort
(Concomitant use with the herb will result in an additive serotonin effect and possible toxicity)

SENNA

Antiarrhythmics
(Senna-induced hypokalemia may increase risk of arrythmia)
Digitalis Glycoside Preparations
(Senna-induced hypokalemia may increase toxicity of digitalis preparations)
Estrogen
(Senna decreases estrogen levels when taken with estrogen supplements)
Indomethacin
(Decreased therapeutic effect of Senna)
Nifedipine
(Inhibits activity of Senna via calcium channel blockade)

SERENOA REPENS

(*See under* Saw Palmetto)

SILYBUM MARIANUM

(*See under* Milk Thistle)

SQUILL

Calcium
(Increases effectiveness and side effects of herb)
Digoxin
(Squill potentiates the positive inotropic and negative chronopic effects of digoxin)
Glucocorticoids
(Increases effectiveness and side effects of herb)
Laxatives
(Increases effectiveness and side effects of herb)
Methylxanthines
(Increases risk of cardiac arrhythmias)
Phosphodiesterase Inhibitors
(Increases risk of cardiac arrhythmias)
Quinidine
(Increases risk of cardiac arrhythmias; increases effectiveness and side effects of herb)
Saluretics
(Increases effectiveness and side effects of herb)
Sympathomimetic Agents
(Increases risk of cardiac arrhythmias)

ST. JOHN'S WORT

Cyclosporine
(The herb induces the cytochrome P450 enzyme system and will lower cyclosporine serum levels)
Digoxin
(Co-administration of the herb with digoxin has resulted in a significant decrease in the digoxin area under the curve)
Indinavir Sulfate
(The herb induces the cytochrome P450 enzyme system and will lower indinavir serum levels)
Oral Contraceptives
(Breakthrough bleeding has been reported with concomitant use of the herb with oral contraceptives)
Photosensitizing Agents
(An additive photosensitizing effect is expected when the herb is used with photosensitizing drugs such as tetracyclines, sulfonamides, and thiazides)
Reserpine
(Hypericum antagonizes the effect of reserpine)
Selective Serotonin Reuptake Inhibitors
(Concomitant use with the herb will result in an additive serotonin effect and possible toxicity)
Sympathomimetic Agents
(St. John's Wort may have MAO inhibitor properties and caution should be used with sympathomimetic agents)
Theophylline
(The herb induces the cytochrome P450 enzyme system and will lower theophylline serum levels)

STROPHANTHUS

Calcium Salts
(Simultaneous administration with herb enhance both effects and side effects)
Glucocorticoids
(Simultaneous administration with herb enhance both effects and side effects)
Laxatives
(Simultaneous administration with herb enhance both effects and side effects)
Quinidine
(Simultaneous administration with herb enhance both effects and side effects)
Saluretics
(Simultaneous administration with herb enhance both effects and side effects)

STROPHANTHUS GRATUS
Calcium Salts
(Simultaneous administration with herb enhance both effects and side effects)
Glucocorticoids
(Simultaneous administration with herb enhance both effects and side effects)
Laxatives
(Simultaneous administration with herb enhance both effects and side effects)
Quinidine
(Simultaneous administration with herb enhance both effects and side effects)
Saluretics
(Simultaneous administration with herb enhance both effects and side effects)

STROPHANTHUS KOMBÉ
(*See under* Strophanthus)

STROPHANTHUS GRATUS
(*See under* Strophanthus Gratus)

STROPHANTHUS HISPIDUS
(*See under* Kombé Seed)

SYMPATHOMIMETIC AGENTS
Digitalis
(Increases risk of cardiac arrhythmias)
Digitalis Lanata
(Risk of cardiac arrhythmias)
Indian Squill
(Can increase the risk of cardic arrhythmias when given simultaneously with this herb)
Rauwolfia
(Increases blood pressure)
Squill
(Increases risk of cardiac arrhythmias)
St. John's Wort
(St. John's Wort may have MAO inhibitor properties and caution should be used with sympathomimetic agents)

TANACETUM PARTHENIUM
(*See under* Feverfew)

THEOPHYLLINE
St. John's Wort
(The herb induces the cytochrome P450 enzyme system and will lower theophylline serum levels)

THIAZIDE DIURETICS
Aloe
(Increased potassium loss)
Buckthorn
(Increases hypokalemic effects)
Cascara Sagrada
(Increases hypokalemic effect)
Licorice
(Additive effect of hypokalemia)
Uva-Ursi
(The sodium-sparing effect of Uva-Ursi may antagonize the diuretic effect of thiazide diuretics)

THYROID PREPARATIONS
Bugleweed
(Effect not specified)

TRAZODONE HYDROCHLORIDE
Wormwood
(Wormwood preparations should not be administered with drugs known to lower the seizure threshold)

TRICYCLIC ANTIDEPRESSANTS
Belladonna
(Increases anticholinergic effect of herb)
Henbane
(Increased anticholinergic action)
Scopolia
(Increased effect when given simultaneously with herb)
Wormwood
(Wormwood preparations should not be administered with drugs known to lower the seizure threshold)

TRIGONELLA FOENUM-GRAECUM
(*See under* Fenugreek)

URGINEA INDICA
(*See under* Indian Squill)

URGINEA MARITIMA
(*See under* Squill)

URINARY TRACT ACIDIFIERS
Uva-Ursi
(Drugs or foods that acidify the urine will decrease the antibacterial effect of Uva-Ursi)

UVA-URSI
Loop Diuretics
(The sodium-sparing effect of Uva-Ursi may antagonize the diuretic effect of the loop diuretics)
Medication and Food that Increase Uric Acid Levels
(Decreases effect of herb)
Non-Steroidal Anti-Inflammatory Drugs
(Uva-Ursi may potentiate the gastrointestinal irritation caused by NSAIDs)
Thiazide Diuretics
(The sodium-sparing effect of Uva-Ursi may antagonize the diuretic effect of thiazide diuretics)
Urinary Tract Acidifiers
(Drugs or foods that acidify the urine will decrease the antibacterial effect of Uva-Ursi)

UZARA
Digoxin
(Herb contains cardiac glycosides and may have additive effect when taken with digoxin, possibly increasing digoxin toxicity)

VACCINIUM MYRTILLUS
(*See under* Bilberry)

VACCINIUM VITIS-IDAEA
(*See under* Alpine Cranberry)

VALERIAN
Alcohol
(Additive depressive effects with Valerian)
Hypnotics
(Additive effect when taken with Valerian)

VALERIANA OFFICINALIS
(*See under* Valerian)

VITEX AGNUS-CASTUS
(*See under* Chaste Tree)

WARFARIN SODIUM

Arnica
(Additive anticoagulant effect)
Bilberry
(Increases prothrombin time; caution should be observed when used concurrently)
Feverfew
(Increased antithrombotic effect)
German Chamomile
(Hydroxycoumarin component in Chamomile may elevate prothrombin times)
Papaya
(Increased INR levels)

WHITE WILLOW

Alcohol
(Enhances toxicity of salicylates)
Antiplatelet Drugs
(Additive effect with salicylates)
Barbiturates
(Enhances toxicity of salicylates)
Carbonic Anhydrase Inhibitors
(Potentiates action of salicylates)
Non-Steroidal Anti-Inflammatory Drugs
(Use with caution; effect not specified)
Salicylates
(Use with caution; effect not specified)

WILD YAM

Estrogen
(Additive effect)
Indomethacin
(Wild Yam may decrease the anti-inflammatory effect of indomethacin)

WORMWOOD

Phenothiazines
(Wormwood preparations should not be administered with drugs known to lower the seizure threshold)
Trazodone Hydrochloride
(Wormwood preparations should not be administered with drugs known to lower the seizure threshold)
Tricyclic Antidepressants
(Wormwood preparations should not be administered with drugs known to lower the seizure threshold)

XYSMALOBIUM UNDULATUM

(*See under* Uzara)

YOHIMBE BARK

Antihypertensive agents, unspecified
(May need to adjust antihypertensive medications due to hypertensive effect of Yohimbe)
Ethanol
(Increased anxiogenic effects)
Morphine Sulfate
(Potentiates effects of morphine)
Naltrexone Hydrochloride
(Potentiates Yohimbe side effects)
OTC stimulants
(Potentiates hypertensive effect)

YOHIMBINE HYDROCHLORIDE

Milk Thistle
(Silymarin antagonizes the effect of yohimbine)

Safety Guide

This guide lists botanicals in three precautionary categories:

- *Not for use during pregnancy*
- *Not for use while nursing*
- *For use only under supervision*

All common, scientific, and brand names of each potentially harmful botanical are listed alphabetically. Generally accepted common names that serve as monograph titles appear in bold type. Scientific names are shown in italic type. Brand names are followed by the supplier's name in parentheses. If an entry lists two page numbers, the first refers to a photograph of the plant or product in the Identification Guide, the second to the herbal monograph. For additional information on potential adverse effects, be sure to check the appropriate underlying monograph.

Not for use during pregnancy

Absinthe G-26, 829
Achillea millefolium G-26, 833
Adiantum capillus-veneris 491
Akebia 189
Akebia quinata 189
Alant G-10, 266
Alcohol Free Chaste Tree Berry Liquid (Nature's Answer) 176
Alcohol Free Kava Kava Liquid (Nature's Answer) 443
Alcohol Free Sage Liquid (Nature's Answer) 655
Alcohol Free Yarrow Flowers Liquid (Nature's Answer) 833
Alder Buckthorn G-12, 317
Alder Dogwood G-12, 317
Alexandrian Senna G-22, 684

ALKANET
(Alkanna tinctoria) G-3, 13

Alkanet Root G-3, 13
Alkanna tinctoria G-3, 13

ALOE
(Aloe barbadensis; Aloe capensis; Aloe vera) G-3, 16

Aloe 99 Gel (Lee) 16
Aloe barbadensis G-3, 16
Aloe capensis G-3, 16
Aloe ferox 16
Aloe vera G-3, 16
Aloe Vera Capsules (ADH, Herbal Harvest, National Vitamin, Nature's Bounty, Nature's Way) 16
Aloe Vera Concentrate 5000 Capsules (Mason Vitamins) 16
Aloe Vera Mild Stimulant Laxative Capsules (Nature's Herbs) 16
Aloe Vera Super-Strength Liquid (Pharmaceutical Labs) 16

AMARGO
(Quassia amara) G-3, 23

AMERICAN LIVERLEAF
(Hepatica nobilis) 26

American Saffron 652

AMMONIAC GUM
(Dorema ammoniacum) 29

Anchusa G-3, 13

ANGELICA
(Angelica archangelica) G-3, 32

Angelica archangelica G-3, 32
Angelica Root Liquid Fluid Extract (Nature's Answer) 32
Angel's Wort G-3, 32

ANISE
(Pimpinella anisum) G-3, 35

Apium graveolens G-8, 172
Arabian Coffee G-9, 202
Arabica Coffee G-9, 202
Aralia racemosa G-23, 711
Arberry G-25, 779
Arborvitae G-24, 759

Not for use while nursing

For use only under supervision

Manufacturers Index

This index provides you with contact information for each supplier whose products appear in the herbal monographs. The names of the products follow the company's contact information. If an entry lists two page numbers, the first refers to a photograph of the product in the Identification Guide, the second to the herbal monograph in which the product appears.

ACTION LABS, INC.
280 Adams Boulevard
Farmingdale, NY 11735

Direct Inquiries to:
(800) 932-2953
FAX: (516) 694-6493

Herbal Products Available:
Garl-Action Tablets 327
Gin-Action Tablets 346
Ginseng Power Max 4X Capsules 346
Ginseng Power Max 4X Liquid 346
Super Bilberry Plus Tablets 75
Super Ginkgo Biloba Plus Tablets 342
Super Milk Thistle Plus Tablets 516
Super Saw Palmetto Plus Tablets 664
Super St. John's Wort Plus Tablets 719
Wild Oats Liquid 551
Wild Oats Tablets 551
Yohimbe Power Max 1500 for Women Tablets 843
Yohimbe Power Max 1500 Tablets 843
Yohimbe Power Max 2000 Capsules 843
Yohimbe Power Max 2000 Liquid 843
Yohimbized 1000 Liquid 843

ADH HEALTH PRODUCTS INC.
215 North Route 303
Congers, NY 10920-1726

Direct Inquiries to:
(914) 268-0027
FAX: (914) 268-2988

Herbal Products Available:
Aloe Vera Capsules 16
Barley Grain Capsules 63
Bilberry Extract Capsules 75
Borage Oil Capsules 114
Butcher's Broom Capsules 132
Cat's Claw Capsules 160
Cayenne Peppers Capsules 165
Damiana Leaves Capsules 244
Dandelion Root Capsules 245
Devil's Claw Capsules 247
Echinacea Capsules 261
Evening Primrose Oil Capsules 298
Garlic Tablets 327
Ginkgo Biloba Capsules 342
Ginseng American Capsules 346
Ginseng Chinese Capsules 346
Goldenseal Capsules 355
Gotu Kola Capsules 359
Hawthorne Capsules 271
Sarsaparilla Capsules 661
Saw Palmetto Capsules 664
Uva Ursi Leaf Capsules 779
Valerian Root Capsules 783
White Willow Bark Capsules 807

ADVANCED NUTRITIONAL TECHNOLOGY, INC.
6988 Sierra Court
Dublin, CA 94568

Direct Inquiries to:
(800) 624-6543
(925) 828-2128
FAX: (925) 828-6848

Herbal Products Available:
Activin Capsules 362
Flaxseed Oil Capsules 313
Garlic Oil Capsules 327
Ginseng Korean Capsules 346
New Energy Capsules 313

AIM FOR HERBS
16 Kingston Street
Somerville, MA 02144

Direct Inquiries to:
(888) 752-1352
www.aimforherbs.com

Herbal Products Available:
Activated Ginkgo Tablets 342

ALVITA TEA COMPANY
600 East Quality Drive
American Fork, UT 84003-3302

Direct Inquiries to:
(800) 258-4828
FAX: (801) 763-0789
www.alvita.com

Herbal Products Available:
Alvita Astragalus Root Tea Bags 54
Caffeine-Free Ginger Root Tea Bags 339
Chinese Green Tea Tea Bags 369

AMERICAN PHARMACAL, INC.
1201 Douglas Avenue
Kansas City, KS 66103

Direct Inquiries to:
(800) 349-4923
FAX: (210) 349-9043

Herbal Products Available:
Ginseng Capsules 346

AMERICAN PHARMACEUTICAL CO.
12 Dwight Place
Fairfield, NJ 07004

Direct Inquiries to:
(973) 515-1000

FAX: (973) 515-9766

Herbal Products Available:

Garlic Tablets 327

APOTHECARY PRODUCTS
11531 Rupp Drive
Burnsville, MN 55337

Direct Inquiries to:
(800) 328-2742
FAX: (800) 328-1584

Herbal Products Available:

Alfalfa Tablets 12
Cayenne Herbal Capsules 165
Echinacea Root Herbal Capsules 261
Garlic Oil Capsules 327
Garlic Tablets 327
Ginkgo Biloba Plus Capsules ... 342
Ginseng Siberian Capsules 346
Goldenseal Root Capsules 355
Guarana Tablets 376
Papaya Digestive Enzyme Tablet 565
Red Clover Herbal Capsules 633
Sarsaparilla Root Capsules 661
Valerian Root Tablets 783
White Willow Bark Capsules ... 807

AURA CACIA
101 Arbuckle Road
Weaverville, CA 96093

Direct Inquiries to:
(800) 437-3301
FAX: (800) 717-4375
www.auracacia.com

Herbal Products Available:

Ginger Root Oil 339
Juniper Berry Oil 440
Myrrh Commiphora Oil 534
Red Thyme Oil 761
White Thyme Oil 761
Wild Chamomile Oil 331

BASIC VITAMINS
P.O. Box 412
Vandalia, OH 45377

Direct Inquiries to:
(800) 782-2742
FAX: (937) 898-0500
www.basicvitamins.com

Herbal Products Available:

Alfalfa Tablets 12
Garlic Oil Capsules 327
Garlic Tablets 327
Ginseng Capsules 346

BAYER CORP., CONSUMER CARE DIVISION
36 Columbia Road
P.O. Box 1910
Morristown, NJ 07962-1910

Direct Inquiries to:
(800) 348-2240

Herbal Products Available:

One-A-Day Cholesterol Health Tablets G-29, 327
One-A-Day Cold Season Tablets G-29, 261
One-A-Day Garlic Capsules G-29, 327
One-A-Day Memory & Concentration Tablets G-29, 342
One-A-Day Menopause Health Tablets G-29, 92
One-A-Day Prostate Health Capsules G-29, 664
One-A-Day Tension & Mood Tablets G-29, 719

BERGEN BRUNSWIG DRUG COMPANY
4000 Metropolitan Drive
Orange, CA 92868

Direct Inquiries to:
(714) 385-4000
FAX: (714) 385-8830

Herbal Products Available:

Bilberry Capsules 75
Cat's Claw Capsules 160
Cayenne Capsules 165
Echinacea Capsules 261
Evening Primrose Oil Capsules 298
Feverfew Capsules 306
Garlic Oil Capsules 327
Garlic Tablets 327
Ginger Root Capsules 339
Ginkgo Biloba Capsules 342
Ginseng Capsules 346
Ginseng Natural Tablets 346
Ginseng Root Korean White Capsules 346
Ginseng Root Siberian Capsules 346
Golden Seal Root Capsules 355
Gotu Kola Capsules 359
Grape Seed Capsules 362
Green Tea Capsules 369
Kava Kava Capsules 443
Saw Palmetto Capsules 664
St. John's Wort Capsules 719
Valerian Root Capsules 783

BIOGLAN PHARMA, INC.
900 West Valley Road
Suite 400
Wayne, PA 19087

Direct Inquiries to:
(610) 225-0200
FAX: (610) 225-0160

Herbal Products Available:

Zostrix Cream 165

BIO-TECH PHARMACAL, INC.
P.O. Box 1992
Fayetteville, AR 72702

Direct Inquiries to:
(800) 345-1199
FAX: (501) 443-5643

Herbal Products Available:

Bioflax Capsules 313
Garlic Capsules 327
Wild Yam Capsules 817

BOERICKE & TAFEL
2381 Circadian Way
Santa Rosa, CA 95407

Direct Inquiries to:
(800) 876-9505
(707) 571-8202
FAX: (707) 571-8237

Herbal Products Available:

Califlora Calendula Gel 497

BOIRON USA
6 Campus Boulevard
Newtown Square, PA 19073

Direct Inquiries to:
(800) 264-7661
FAX: (610) 325-7480

Herbal Products Available:

Calendula Gel 497
Calendula Lotion 497
Calendula Ointment 497

BOSCOGEN INC.
11 Morgan
Irvine, CA 92618

Direct Inquiries to:
(949) 380-4317
FAX: (949) 583-2016
www.boscogen.com

Herbal Products Available:

Lynae Ginse-Cool Chewable Tablets 346

BRECKENRIDGE PHARMACEUTICAL, INC.
P.O. Box 206
Boca Raton, FL 33429

Direct Inquiries to:
(800) 367-3395
(561) 367-8512
FAX: (561) 367-8107

Herbal Products Available:

St. John's Wort Capsules 719

E.T. BROWNE DRUG COMPANY
140 Sylvan Avenue
P.O. Box 1613
Englewood Cliffs, NJ 07632

Direct Inquiries to:
(201) 947-3050
FAX: (201) 947-9276

Herbal Products Available:
Palmers Aloe Vera Formula Cream 16

CARDINAL HEALTH, INC.
5555 Glendon Court
Dublin, OH 43016
Direct Inquiries to:
(614) 757-5000
Herbal Products Available:
Bilberry Capsules 75
Echinacea Capsules 261
Garlic Capsules 327
Garlic Oil Natural Capsules 327
Ginkgo Biloba Capsules 342
Ginseng Siberian Capsules 346
Saw Palmetto Capsules 664
Valerian Root Capsules 783

CELESTIAL SEASONINGS, INC.
4600 Sleepytime Drive
Boulder, CO 80301-3292
Direct Inquiries to:
(303) 530-5300
FAX: (303) 581-1294
www.celestialseasonings.com
Herbal Products Available:
Echinacea Capsules 261
Garlic Tablets 327
Ginkgo Biloba Capsules 342
Ginseng Energy Capsules 346
Green Tea Extract Capsules 369
Kava Kava Capsules 443
Panax Ginseng Capsules 346
Saw Palmetto Capsules 664
St. John's Wort Capsules 719

CONTRACT PHARMACAL CORPORATION
160 Commerce Drive
Hauppauge, NY 11788
Direct Inquiries to:
(631) 231-4610
FAX: (631) 231-4156
Herbal Products Available:
Echinacea Capsules 261
Garlic Tablets 327
Ginseng Capsules 346
St. John's Wort Tablets 719

ENZYMATIC THERAPY
825 Challenger Drive
Green Bay, WI 54311
Direct Inquiries to:
(800) 783-2286
E-mail: etmail@enzy.com
www.enzy.com
Herbal Products Available:
Hypericalm Capsules 719

FAMILY PHARMACY
P.O. Box 1027
Southeastern, PA 19398-1027
Direct Inquiries to:
(800) 333-7347
FAX: (610) 695-8604
Herbal Products Available:
Garlic Oil Capsules 327
Garlic Tablets 327
Ginseng Vitamin Capsules 346

FREEDA VITAMINS, INC.
36 E. 41st Street
New York, NY 10017
Direct Inquiries to:
(800) 777-3737
(212) 685-4980
FAX: (212) 685-7297
Herbal Products Available:
Alfalfa Concentrate Tablets 12
Cabbage Tablets 134
Garlic Tablets 327
Guar Gum Powder 376
Pacific Kelp Tablets 122
Papaya Tablets 565

FRONTIER
P.O. Box 299
Norway, IA 52318
Direct Inquiries to:
(800) 786-1388
FAX: (800) 717-4372
Herbal Products Available:
Alfalfa Leaf Capsules 12
American Ginseng Root Capsules 346
Bilberry Leaf Capsules 75
Black Cohosh Capsules 92
Black Walnut Hulls Capsules 134
Blessed Thistle Capsules 107
Burdock Root Capsules 128
Butcher's Broom Root Capsules 132
Cascara Sagrada Bark Capsules 153
Catnip Leaf Capsules 164
Cat's Claw Inner Bark Capsules 160
Cayenne 30,000 Heat Units Capsules 165
Certified Organic Nettle Leaf Capsules 729
Certified Organic Red Raspberry Leaf Capsules 630
Chamomile Flowers Capsules 331
Chickweed Herb Capsules 180
Damiana Leaf Capsules 244
Dandelion Root Capsules 245
Devil's Claw Root Tuber Capsules 247
Echinacea Angustifolia Herb Capsules 261
Echinacea purpurea Root Capsules 261
Elder Flowers Capsules 287
Eleuthero Ginseng Root Capsules 346
Eyebright Herb Capsules 300
Fenugreek Seed Capsules 304
Garlic Capsules 327
Ginger Root Capsules 339
Ginkgo Leaf Capsules 342
Goldenseal Leaf Capsules 355
Goldenseal Root Capsules 355
Gotu Kola Capsules 359
Guggul Resin Capsules 534
Hawthorne Berries Capsules 271
Horsetail Grass Capsules 409
Kava Kava Root Capsules 443
Korean Ginseng Root Capsules 346
Licorice Root Capsules 469
Marshmallow Root Capsules 505
Mullein Leaf Liquid 532
Nettle Leaf Capsules 729
Passion Flower Capsules 573
Red Clover Herb Capsules 633
Red Raspberry Leaves Capsules 630
Sarsaparilla Root Capsules 661
Saw Palmetto Berries Capsules 664
Senna Leaf Capsules 684
Skullcap Herb Capsules 678
Slippery Elm Bark Capsules 697
St. John's Wort Herb Capsules 719
Uva Ursi Leaf Capsules 779
Valerian Root Capsules 783
White Willow Bark Capsules 807
Wild Yam Root & Rhizome Extract Liquid 817
Wild Yam Root Capsules 817
Yarrow Flowers Capsules 33
Yellow Dock Root Capsules 835

FUTUREBIOTICS
145 Ricefield Lane
Hauppauge, NY 11788
Direct Inquiries to:
(800) 367-5433
www.futurebiotics.com

GLENWOOD
82 North Summit Street
Tenafly, NJ 07670

Direct Inquiries to:
(800) 664-1449
(732) 981-9780
FAX: (732) 981-9790

THE GREEN TURTLE BAY VITAMIN CO., INC.
56 High Street
P.O. Box 642
Summit, NJ 07902

Direct Inquiries to:
(800) 887-8535
(908) 277-2240
FAX: (908) 273-9116
E-mail: mail@energywave.com
www.energywave.com

HEALTH FROM THE SUN
P.O. Box 179
Newport Beach, NH 03773

Direct Inquiries to:
(800) 447-2249
FAX: (603) 763-9159
www.hfts.com

HEALTH PRODUCTS CORPORATION/ HEALTH BRAND
Health Vitamin Company, Inc.
1060 Nepperhan Avenue
Yonkers, NY 10703-1432

Direct Inquiries to:
(914) 423-2900
FAX: (914) 963-6001

HERB PHARM
P.O. Box 116
Williams, OR 97544

Direct Inquiries to:
(800) 599-2392
(541) 846-6262
FAX: (800) 545-7392
E-mail: Herbpharm@aol.com
www.herb-pharm.com

HERBAL HARVEST
90 Orville Drive
Bohemia, NY 11716

Direct Inquiries to:
(631) 567-9500
FAX: (631) 244-2136

HUMCO
7400 Alumax Drive
Texarkana, TX 75501

Direct Inquiries to:
(800) 662-3435
FAX: (903) 831-7736

IRWIN NATURALS
10549 West Jefferson Boulevard
Culver City, CA 90232

Direct Inquiries to:
(800) 841-8448
FAX: (310) 202-9454

THE KEY COMPANY
1313 W. Essex Ave.
P.O. Box 220370
St. Louis, MO 63122

Direct Inquiries to:
(800) 325-9592
(314) 965-6699
FAX: (314) 965-7629

KISS MY FACE
P.O. Box 224
Gardiner, NY 12525
Direct Inquiries to:
(800) 262-KISS
(914) 255-0884
FAX: (914) 255-4312
www.kissmyface.com
Herbal Products Available:
Natural Honey & Calendula Moisturizer for Extra Dry Skin 497

KONSYL PHARMACEUTICALS
4200 South Hulen
Fort Worth, TX 76109
Direct Inquiries to:
(800) 356-6795
(817) 763-8011
FAX: (817) 731-9389
www.konsyl.com
Herbal Products Available:
Konsyl Easy Mix 612
Konsyl for Kids 612
Konsyl Powder Sugar Free 612

LEE PHARMACEUTICALS
1434 Santa Anita Avenue
P.O. Box 3836
South El Monte, CA 91733-3312
Direct Inquiries to:
(800) 950-5337
FAX: (626) 442-6994
Herbal Products Available:
Aloe 99 Gel 16
Sundance Aloe Vera Gel 16

LICHTWER PHARMA U.S., INC.
Foster Plaza 9
750 Holiday Drive
Pittsburgh, PA 15220
Direct Inquiries to:
(412) 928-9334
FAX: (412) 928-9655
Herbal Products Available:
Ginkai Tablets G-29, 342
Ginsai Capsules 346
Kira Tablets G-29, 719
Kwai Garlic Tablets G-29, 327

MAJOR PHARMACEUTICALS
31778 Enterprise Drive
Livonia, MI 48150
Direct Inquiries to:
(800) 875-0123
FAX: (734) 762-9730
Herbal Products Available:
Alfalfa Tablets 12
Bilberry Capsules 75
Cayenne Pepper Capsules 165
Echinacea Root Capsules 261
Evening Primrose Capsules 298
Eyebright Capsules 300
Garlic Capsules 327
Garlin Tablets 327
Ginkgo Biloba Capsules 342
Ginkgo Biloba Tablets 342
Ginseng Capsules 346
Ginseng Korean Capsules 346
Ginseng Siberian Capsules 346
Golden Seal Root Capsules 355
Gotu Kola Capsules 359
Grape Seed Extract Capsules 362
Kava Kava Root Capsules 443
Kelp Tablets 122
Licorice Root Capsules 469
Milk Thistle Capsules 516
Oat Bran Tablets 551
Papaya Tablets 565
Saw Palmetto Capsules 664
Valerian Root Capsules 783

MARLEX PHARMACEUTICALS, INC.
50 McCullough Drive
Southgate Center
New Castle, DE 19720
Direct Inquiries to:
(302) 328-3355
FAX: (302) 328-6968
Herbal Products Available:
Papaya Chewable Tablets 565
Papaya Coated Tablets 565

MASON VITAMINS, INC.
5105 N.W. 159th Street
Miami Lakes, FL 33014
Direct Inquiries to:
(800) 327-6005
FAX: (800) 328-3944
www.masonvitamins.com
Herbal Products Available:
Alfalfa Fortified Tablets 12
Alfalfa Tablets 12
Aloe Vera Concentrate 5000 Capsules 16
Bilberry Capsules 75
Cat's Claw Capsules 160
Cayenne Capsules 165
Echinacea Capsules 261
Evening Primrose Oil Capsules 298
Feverfew Capsules 306
Garlic Capsules 327
Garlic Oil Capsules 327
Garlic Tablets 327
Garlic-X Tablets 327
Ginger Capsules 339
Ginger Root Capsules 339
GinkAlert Tablets 342
Ginkgo Biloba Capsules 342
Ginkgo Biloba Extract Capsules 342
Ginseng Complex Korean Capsules 346
Ginseng Korean Capsules 346
Ginseng Korean Tablets 346
Ginseng Siberian Capsules 346
Goldenseal Capsules 355
Goldenseal Root Capsules 355
Gotu Kola Capsules 359
G-Sana Capsules 346
Guarana Capsules 122
Hawthorn Berry Capsules 271
Kava Kava Capsules 443
Kelp Tablets 122
Licorice Capsules 469
Milk Thistle Capsules 516
Oat Bran Tablets 551
Papaya Enzyme with Papain Tablet 565
Saw Palmetto Capsules 664
St. John's Wort Capsules 719
Total Gar Capsules 327
Valerian Capsules 783
Valerian Root Tablets 783
Yohimbe Capsules 843
Yohimbe Super Potent Tablets 843

McKESSON DRUG COMPANY
One Post Street
San Francisco, CA 94104-5296
Direct Inquiries to:
(415) 983-8300
FAX: (415) 983-7160
Herbal Products Available:
Cayenne Capsules 165
Echinacea Capsules 261
Ginseng Capsules 346
Ginseng Concentrate Capsules 346
Golden Seal Root Capsules 355
Gotu Kola Herb Capsules 359
Valerian Root Capsules 783

McZAND HERBAL, INC.
P.O. Box 5312
Santa Monica, CA 90409
Direct Inquiries to:
(800) 800-0405
FAX: (310) 822-1050
Herbal Products Available:
Alfalfa Liquid 12
Astragalus Root Liquid 54
Black Walnut Liquid 134
Blue Cohosh Liquid 109
Cat's Claw Capsules 160

THE MEDICINE SHOPPE
1100 North Lindbergh
St. Louis, MO 63132

Direct Inquiries to:
(800) 325-1397
(314) 993-6000
FAX: (314) 872-5500

Herbal Products Available:

MERICON INDUSTRIES, INC.
8819 N. Pioneer Road
Peoria, IL 61615-1561

Direct Inquiries to:
(800) 242-6464
FAX: (309) 693-2158
E-mail: monocal@aol.com

Herbal Products Available:

NATIONAL VITAMIN COMPANY, INC.
2075 West Scranton Avenue
Porterville, CA 93257-8358

Direct Inquiries to:
(800) 538-5828
FAX: (209) 781-8878

Herbal Products Available:

NATROL
21411 Prairie Street
Chatsworth, CA 91311

Direct Inquiries to:
(800) 326-1520
www.natrol.com

Herbal Products Available:

NATURALIFE CORPORATION
10 Mountain Springs Parkway
Springville, UT 84663

Direct Inquiries to:
(800) 531-3233
FAX: (800) 489-3302

Herbal Products Available:

NATURE MADE
1150 Aviation Place
San Fernando, CA 91340

Direct Inquiries to:
(800) 276-2878
www.naturemade.com

Herbal Products Available:

NATURE'S ANSWER
320 Oser Avenue
Hauppauge, NY 11788

Direct Inquiries to:
(800) 439-2324
(516) 231-7492
FAX: (516) 951-2499
www.naturesanswer.com

Herbal Products Available:

NATURE'S BOUNTY, INC.

90 Orville Drive
Bohemia, NY 11716

Direct Inquiries to:
(631) 567-9500
FAX: (631) 244-2136

Herbal Products Available:

NATURE'S HERBS

150 Motor Parkway
Hauppauge, NY 11788

Direct Inquiries to:
(516) 467-3140
www.naturesherbs.com

Herbal Products Available:

NATURE'S RESOURCE
1150 Aviation Place
San Fernanado, CA 91340

Direct Inquiries to:
(800) 314-4372
www.naturesresource.com

Herbal Products Available:

NATURE'S WAY
10 Mountain Springs Parkway
Springville, UT 84663
Direct Inquiries to:
(800) 962-8873
FAX: (801) 489-1700
www.naturesway.com

Herbal Products Available:

NEUROVITES
P.O. Box 180
Rockaway Beach, OR 97136
Direct Inquiries to:
(503) 228-4119
FAX: (503) 228-4119

Herbal Products Available:

NOVARTIS CONSUMER HEALTH, INC.
560 Morris Avenue
Summit, NJ 07901-1312
Direct Inquiries to:
(800) 452-0051
FAX: (800) 635-2801

Herbal Products Available:

NOVOGEN, INC.
1 Landmark Square, 2nd Floor
Stamford, CT 06901-2628
Direct Inquiries to:
(888) NOVOGEN
E-mail: info@novogen.com
www.novogen.com

Herbal Products Available:

PD-RX PHARMACEUTICALS INC.
727 North Ann Arbor Avenue
Oklahoma City, OK 73127
Direct Inquiries to:
(800) 299-7379
FAX: (405) 942-5471

Herbal Products Available:

PERRIGO
117 Water Street
Allegan, MI 49010
Direct Inquiries to:
(800) 827-2296
FAX: (616) 673-9122

Herbal Products Available:

PHARMACEUTICAL LABORATORIES, INC.
1170 Corporate Drive W.
Suite 102
Arlington, TX 76006-6813
Direct Inquiries to:
(817) 633-1461
FAX: (817) 633-8146

Herbal Products Available:

PHARMANEX, INC.
625 Cochran Street
Simi Valley, CA 93065-1939
Direct Inquiries to:
(800) 999-6229
FAX: (805) 582-9301

Herbal Products Available:

PHARMATON NATURAL HEALTH PRODUCTS
900 Ridgebury Road
P.O. Box 368
Ridgefield, CT 06877
Direct Inquiries to:
(203) 798-4157
FAX: (203) 798-5771

Herbal Products Available:

PHYTOPHARMICA
825 Challenger Drive
Green Bay, WI 54311
Direct Inquiries to:
(800) 553-2370 (Doctors and Pharmacists)
(800) 644-0799 (Consumers)

Herbal Products Available:

PNC, PHARMACISTS' NUTRITION CENTER
9775 SW Commerce Circle
Suite C4
Wilsonville, OR 97070-9602
Direct Inquiries to:
(877) 376-6762
(503) 682-1415
FAX: (503) 682-0845
E-mail: pnc@nfformulas.com

Herbal Products Available:

PROCTER & GAMBLE
P.O. Box 5516
Cincinnati, OH 45201
Direct Inquiries to:
(800) 358-8707
(513) 558-4422

Herbal Products Available:

THE PURDUE FREDERICK COMPANY
100 Connecticut Avenue
Norwalk, CT 06850-3590
Direct Inquiries to:
(800) 877-5666
FAX: (800) 877-3210

Herbal Products Available:

RAINBOW LIGHT NUTRITIONAL SYSTEMS
125 McPherson Street
Santa Cruz, CA 95060
Direct Inquiries to:
(800) 635-1233
(831) 429-9089
FAX: (831) 429-0189

Herbal Products Available:

REESE PHARMACEUTICAL COMPANY
10617 Frank Ave.
P.O. Box 1957
Cleveland, OH 44106
Direct Inquiries to:
(800) 321-7178
FAX: (216) 231-6444
E-mail: reese@apk.net
www.reesechemical.com

Herbal Products Available:

REPUBLIC DRUG COMPANY, INC.
175 Great Arrow
Buffalo, NY 14207
Direct Inquiries to:
(800) 828-7444
FAX: (716) 874-6060

Herbal Products Available:

REXALL CONSUMER PRODUCTS
Div. of Rexall Sundown, Inc.
6111 Broken Sound Parkway, NW
Boca Raton, FL 33487-3693
Direct Inquiries to:
(800) 255-7399
FAX: (561) 995-6881
www.rexallsundown.com

Herbal Products Available:

Herbal Products Available:

Bilberry Tablets 75
Psyllium Husks Capsules 612

ZAYCO, INC.
4275 Executive Square
Suite 800
La Jolla, CA 92037

Direct Inquiries to:
(888) 776-6005
FAX: (760) 770-2612

Herbal Products Available:

St. John's Wort Transdermal Patch 719

ZENITH GOLDLINE PHARMACEUTICALS
4400 Biscayne Boulevard
Miami, FL 33137

Direct Inquiries to:
(800) 327-4114
FAX: (954) 575-4319

Herbal Products Available:

Bilberry Capsules 75
Echinacea Capsules 261
Garlic Tablets 327
Ginkgo Biloba Capsules 342
Ginseng Korean Capsules 346
Golden Seal Root Capsules 355
Gotu Kola Capsules 359
Saw Palmetto Capsules 664
St. John's Wort Capsules 719
Valerian Root Capsules 783

Herb Identification Guide

In this full-color photo section, you'll find hundreds of pictures of herbs and leading commercial preparations.

The first part of the section is an Herb Identification Guide with photos of over 380 common medicinal plants. Each herb is labeled with its generally accepted common name immediately above the photo, and its scientific name immediately below. The pictures are arranged alphabetically by common name.

Following these photos is a Product Identification Guide in which you'll find a representative selection of popular commercial formulations. The pictures on these pages are arranged alphabetically by manufacturer and product name.

Please note that the plants are not reproduced in actual size, and that the scale of the photos varies. For the average dimensions of the plant and its component structures, please check the Description section of the corresponding herbal monograph.

ABSCESS ROOT

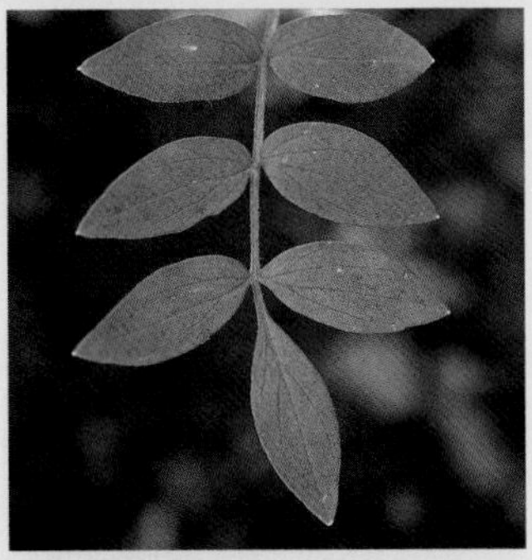

Polemonium reptans

ADONIS

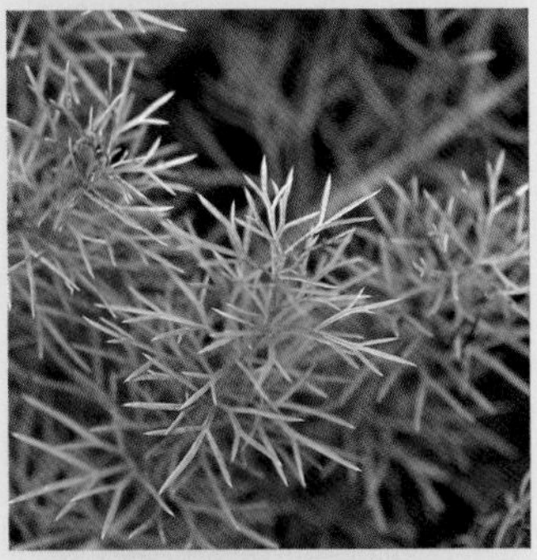

Adonis vernalis

ADRUE

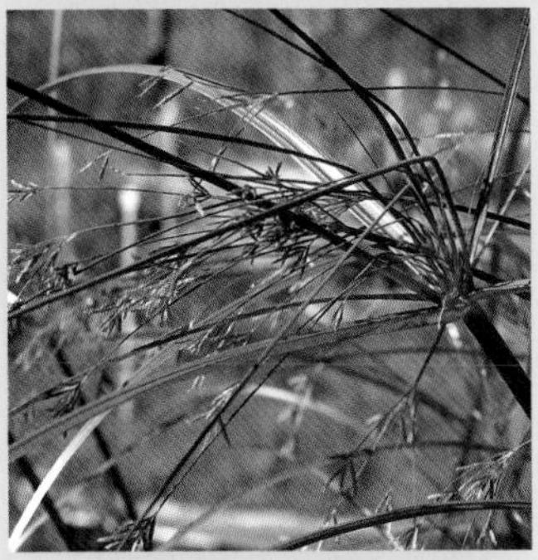

Cyperus articulatus

AGA

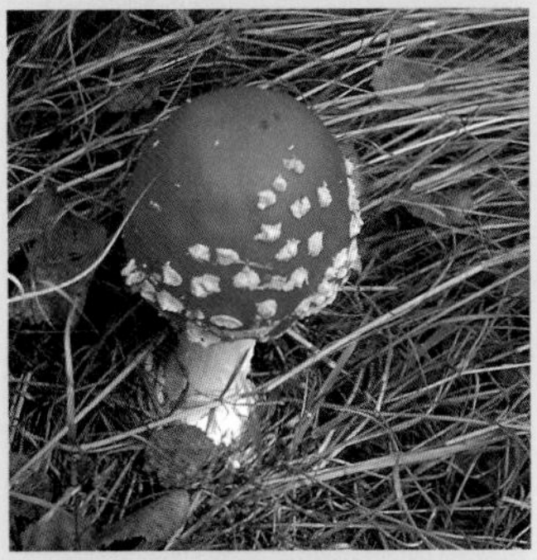

Amanita muscaria

AGRIMONY

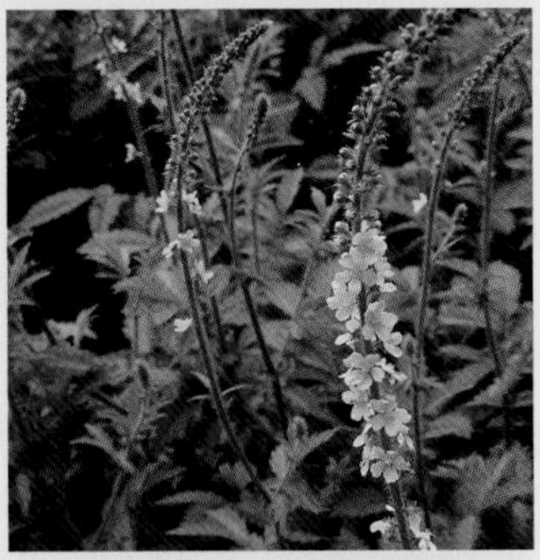

Agrimonia eupatoria

ALFALFA

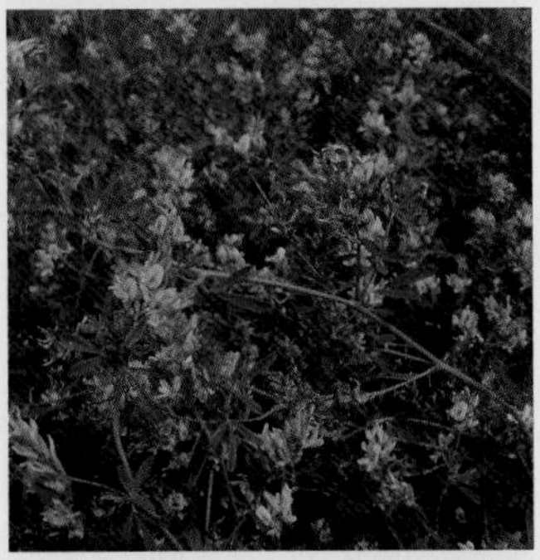

Medicago sativa

ALISMA

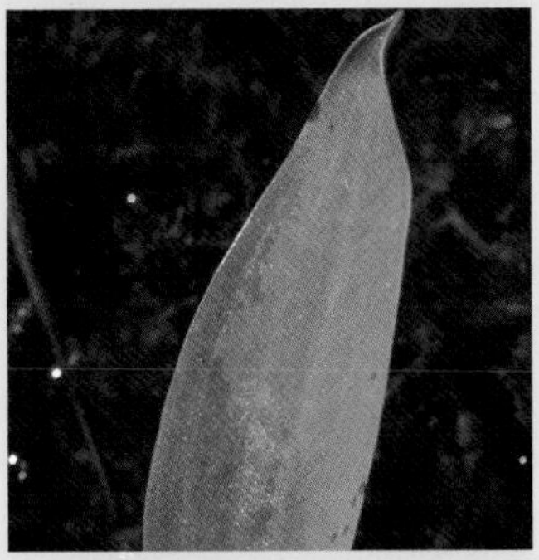

Alisma plantago-aquatica

ALKANET

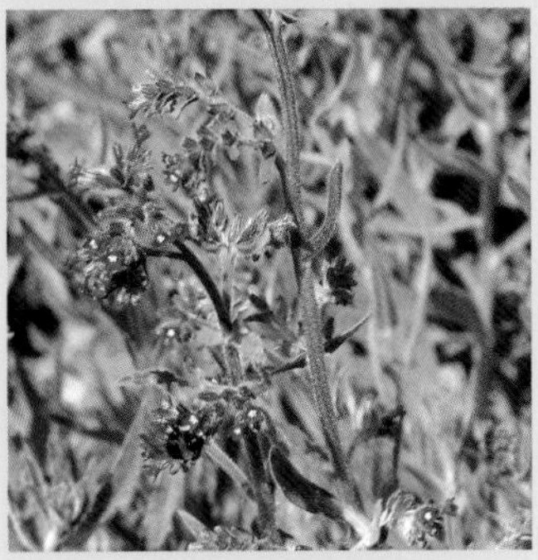

Alkanna tinctoria

ALOE

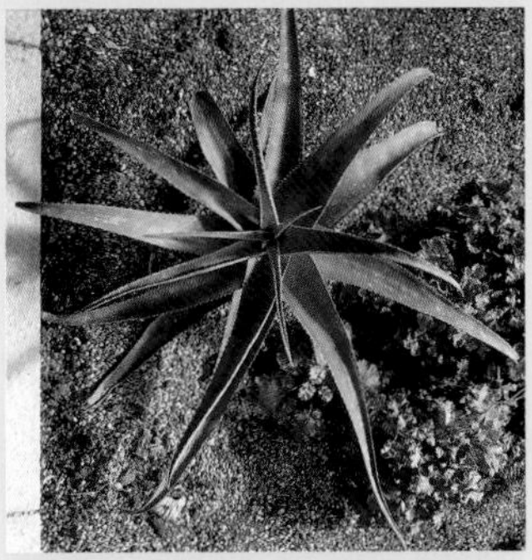

Aloe species

ALPINE CRANBERRY

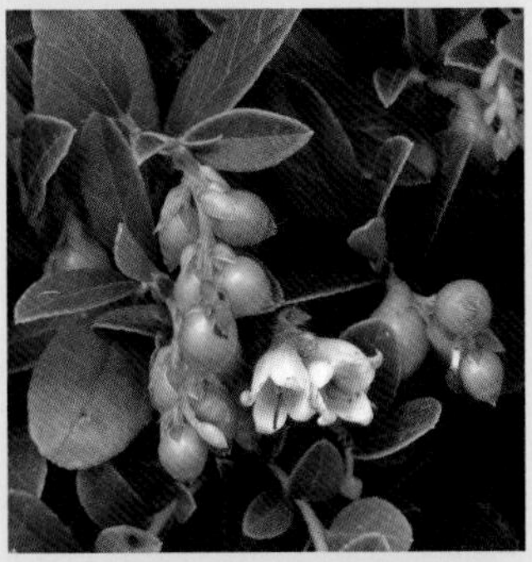

Vaccinium vitis-idaea

AMARANTH

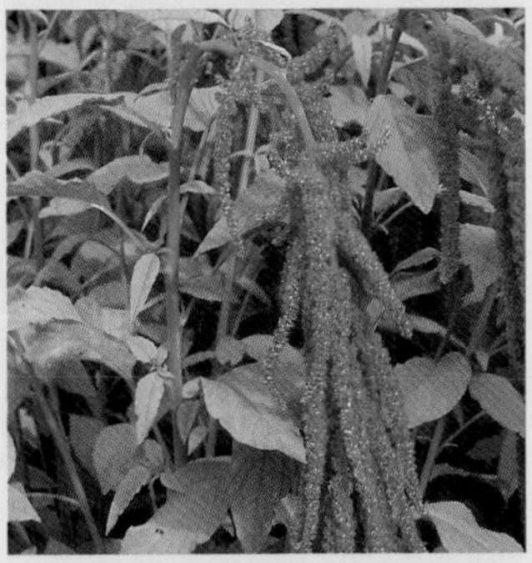

Amaranthus species

AMARGO

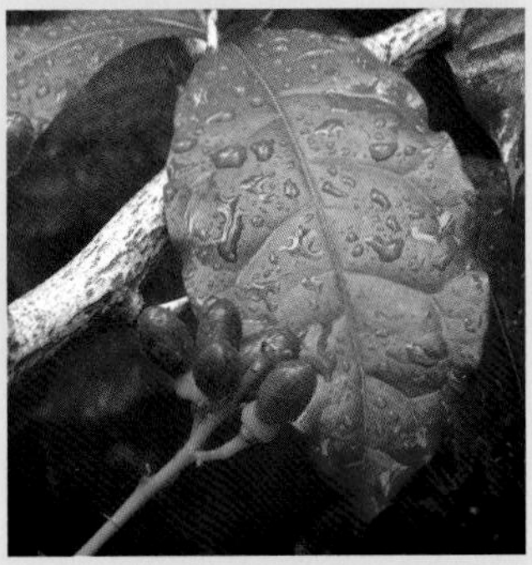

Quassia amara

AMERICAN IVY

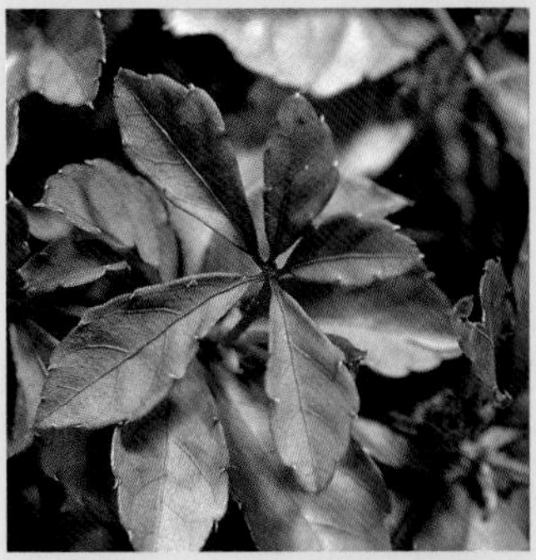

Parthenocissus quinquefolia

AMERICAN WHITE POND LILY

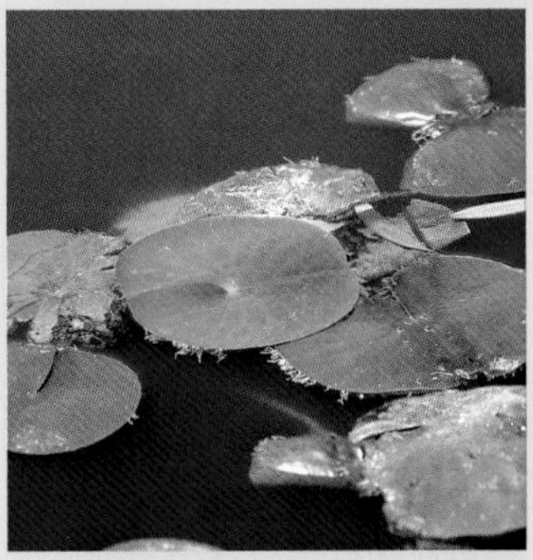

Nymphaea odorata

ANGELICA

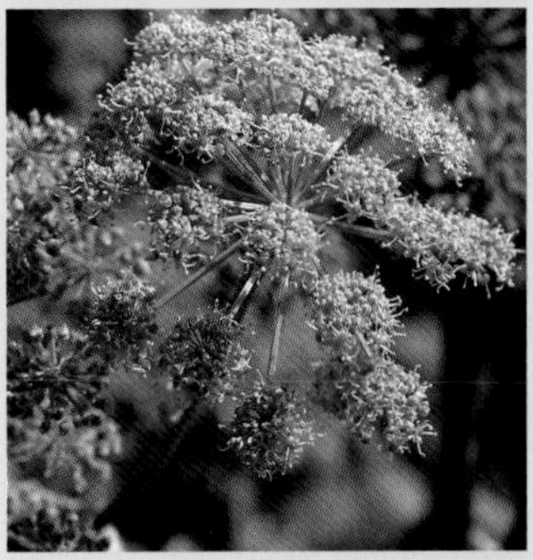

Angelica archangelica

ANISE

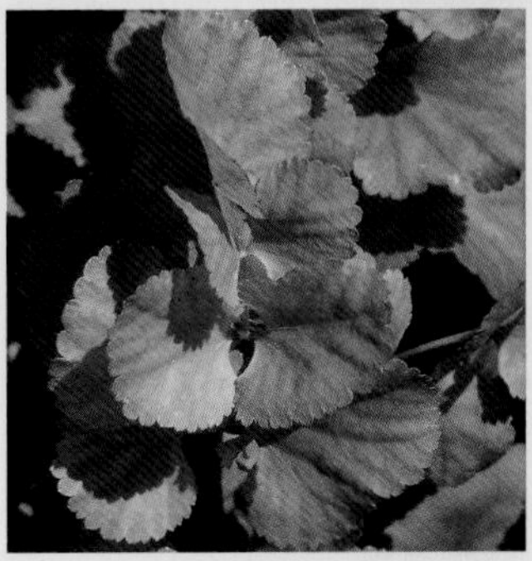

Pimpinella anisum

APPLE TREE

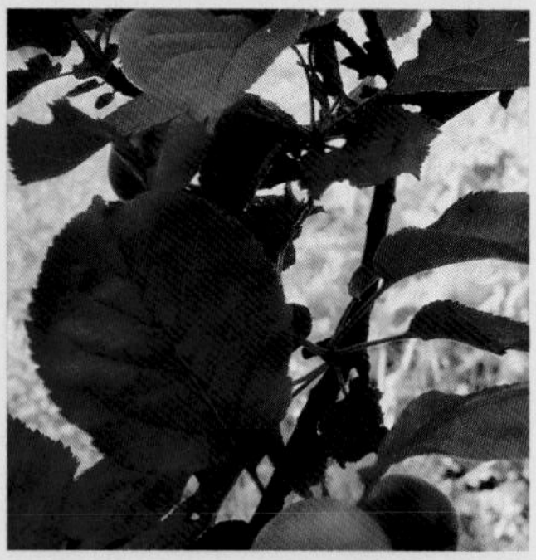

Malus domestica

ARECA NUT

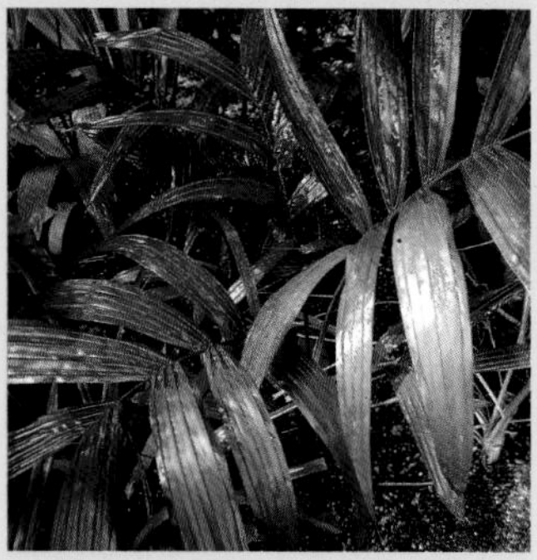

Areca catechu

ARTICHOKE

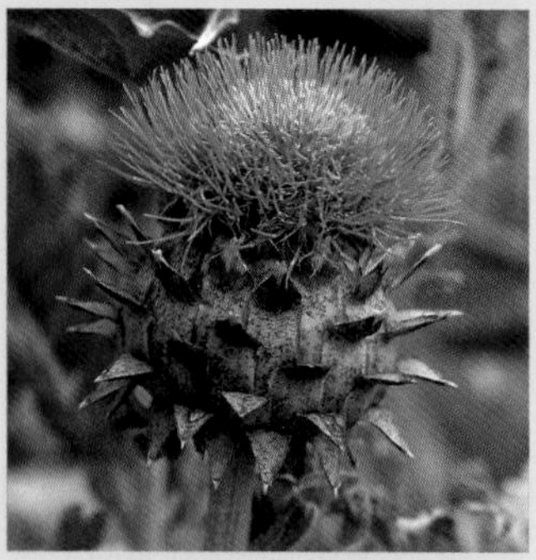

Cynara scolymus

ASH

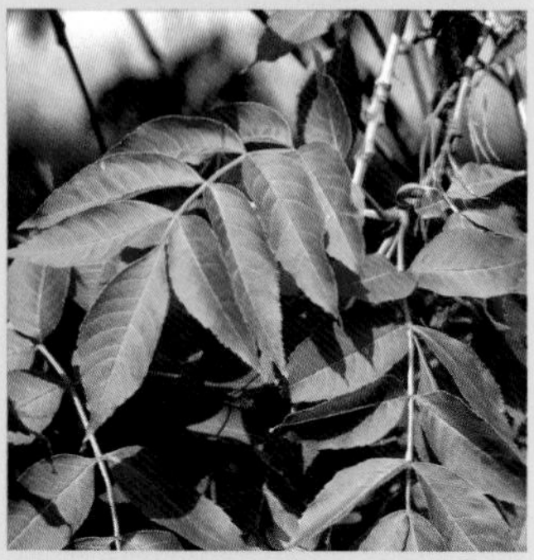

Fraxinus excelsior

ASPARAGUS

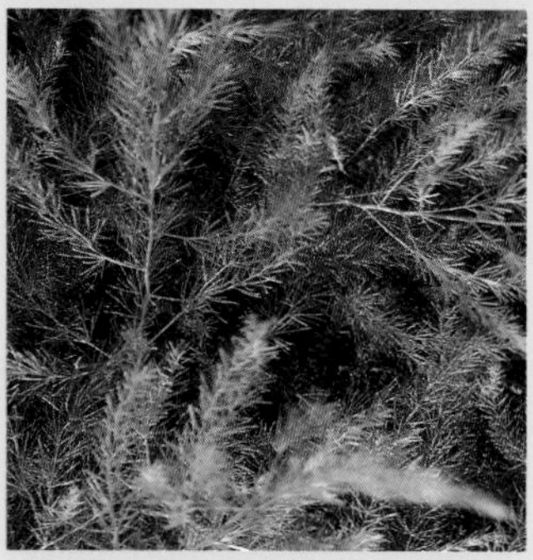

Asparagus officinalis

BALMONY

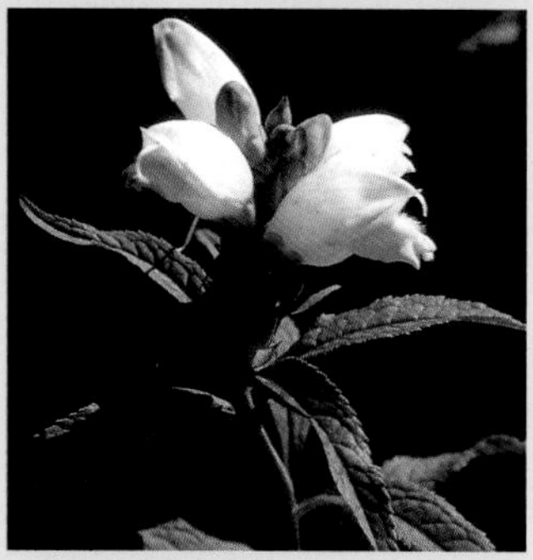

Chelone glabra

BAMBOO

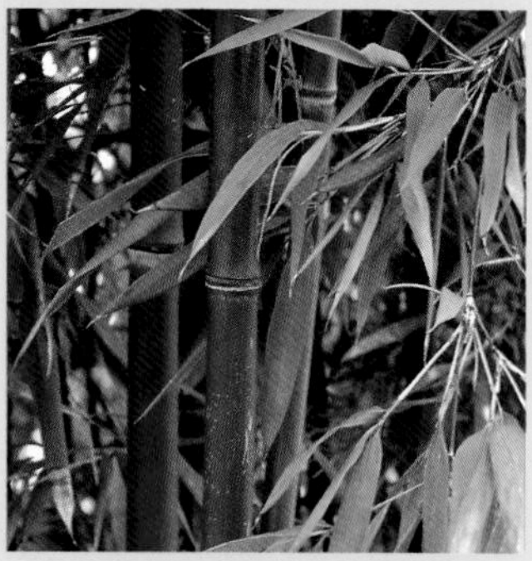

Arundinaria japonica

BARBERRY

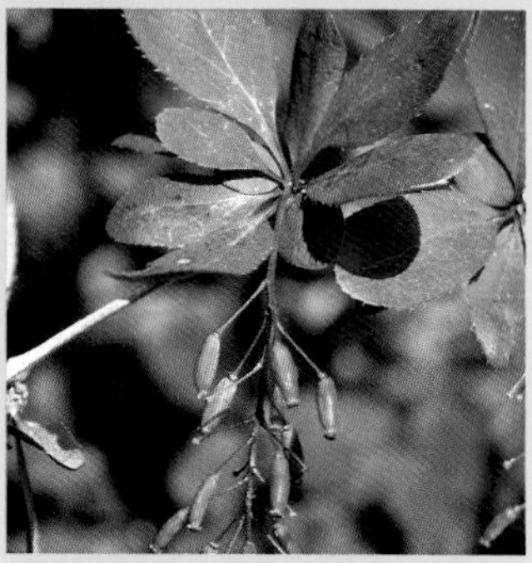

Berberis vulgaris

BARLEY

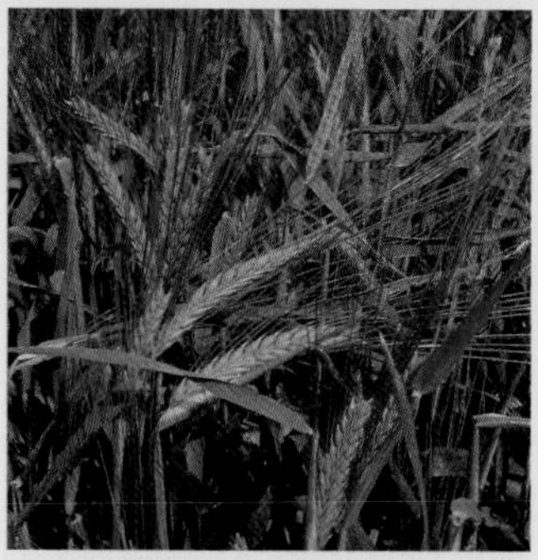

Hordeum species

BASIL

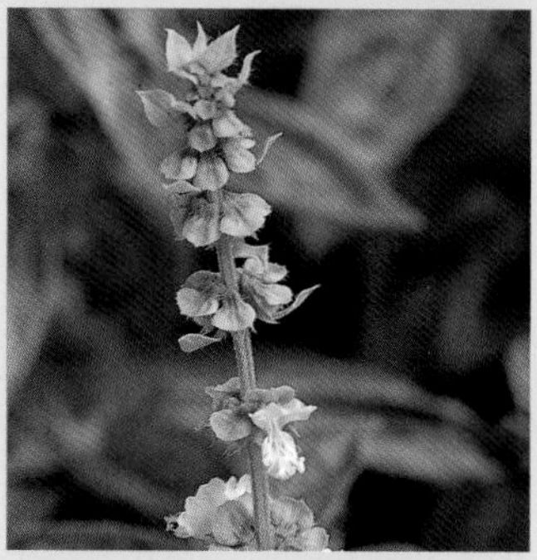

Ocimum basilicum

BEAN POD

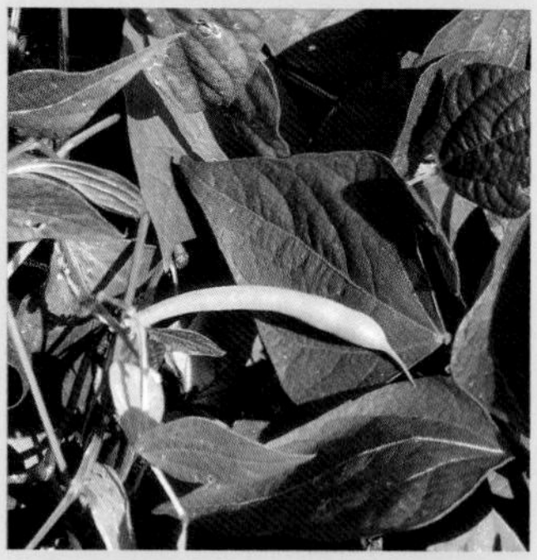

Phaseolus vulgaris

BEET

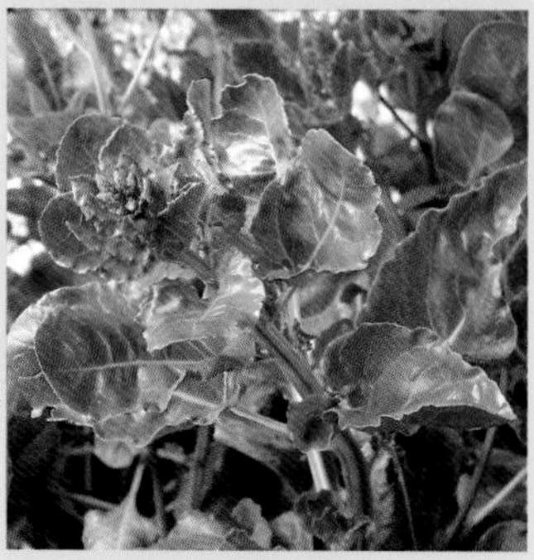

Beta vulgaris

BELLADONNA

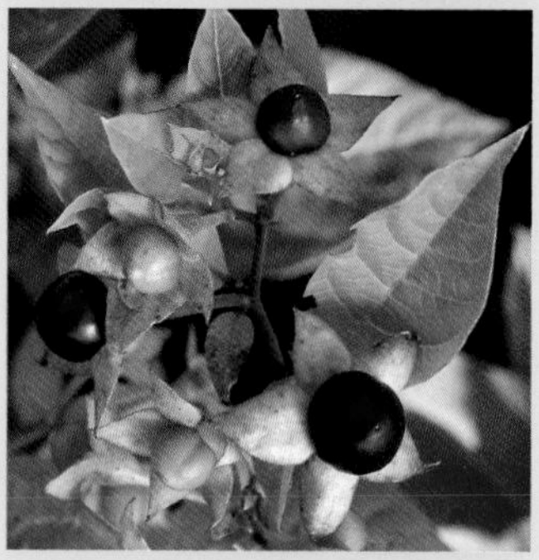

Atropa belladonna

BENNET'S ROOT

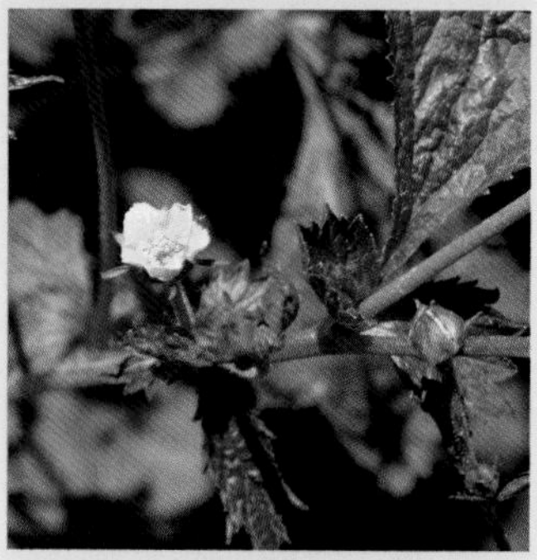

Geum urbanum

BETEL NUT

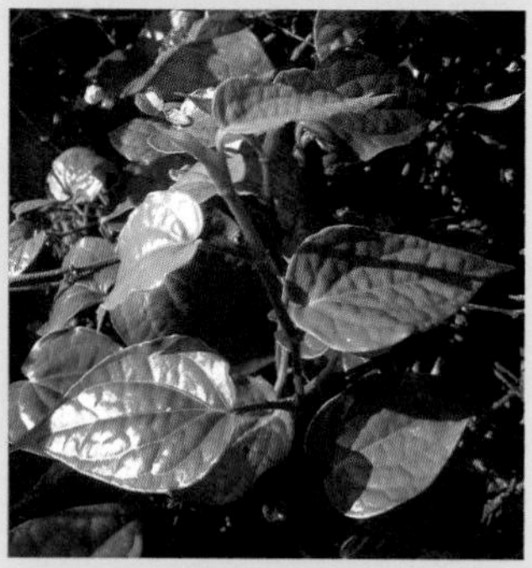

Piper betle

BETH ROOT

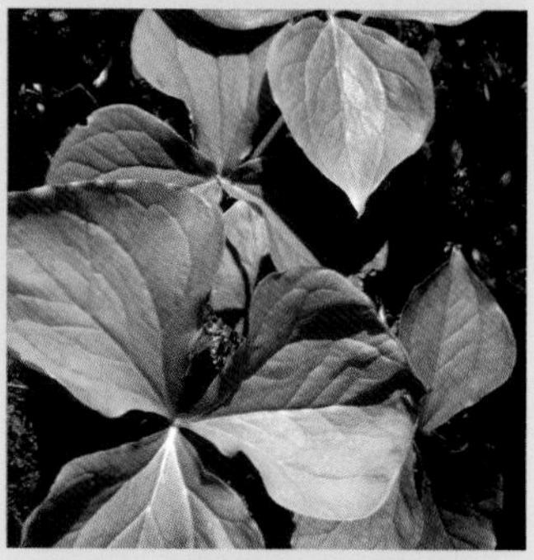

Trillium erectum

BILBERRY

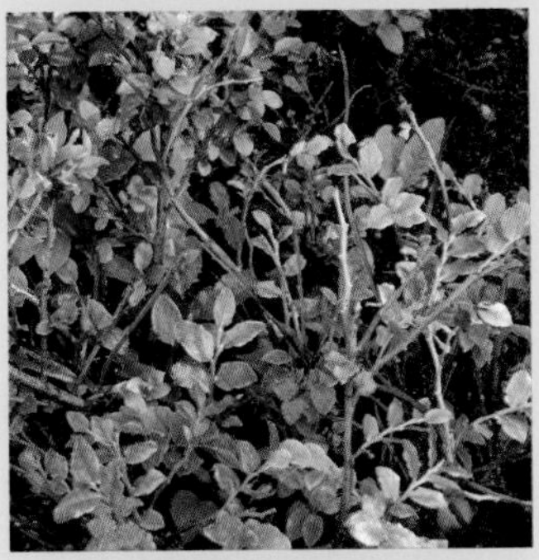

Vaccinium myrtillus

BIRCH

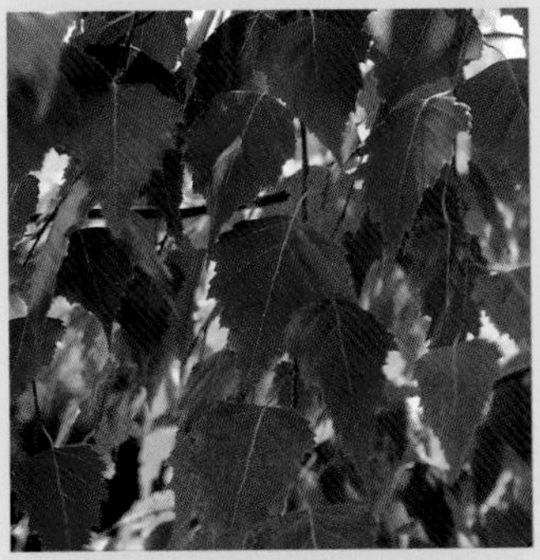

Betula species

BIRTHWORT

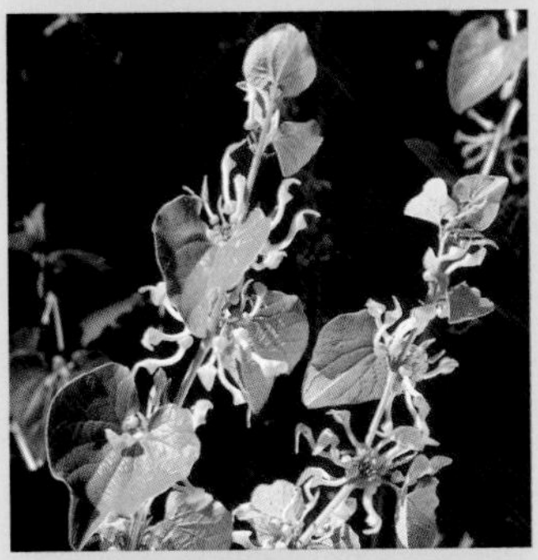

Aristolochia clematitis

BISHOP'S WEED

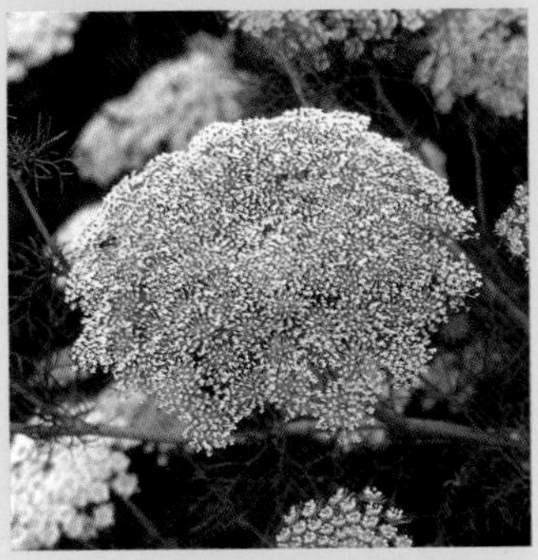

Ammi visnaga

BISTORT

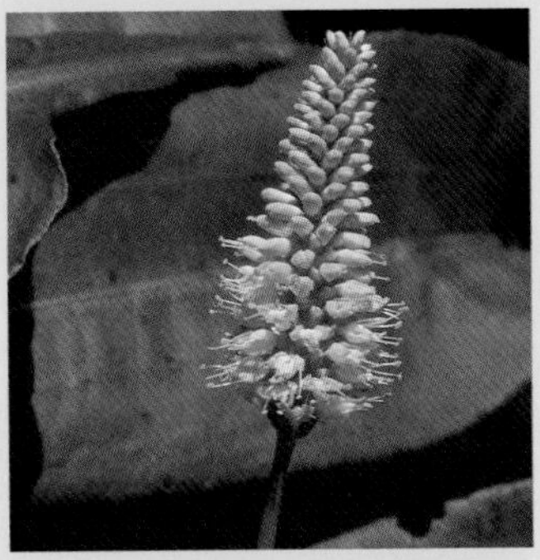

Persicaria bistorta

BITTER APPLE

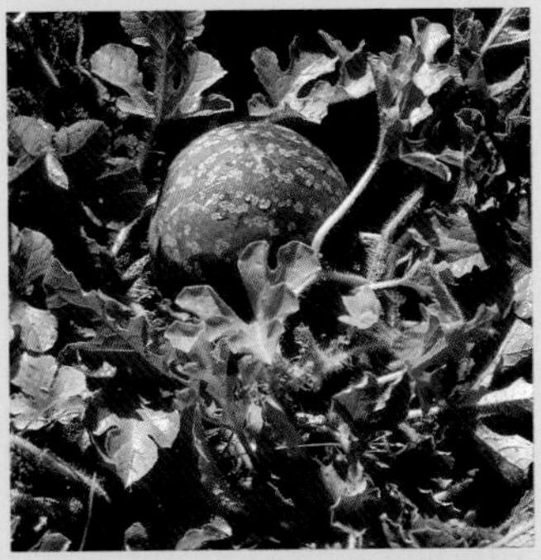

Citrullus colocynthis

BITTER ORANGE

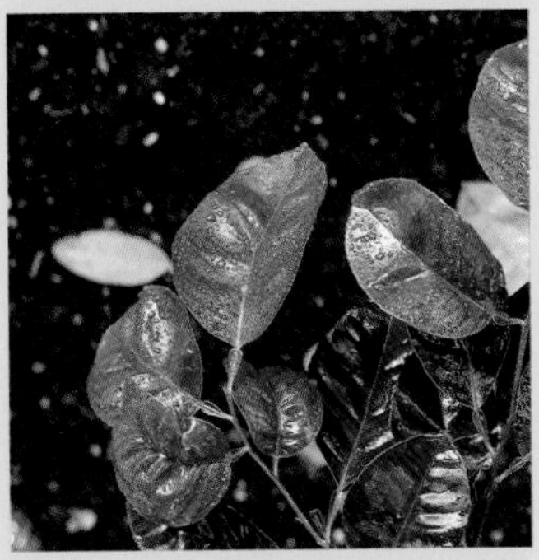

Citrus aurantium

BITTERSWEET NIGHTSHADE

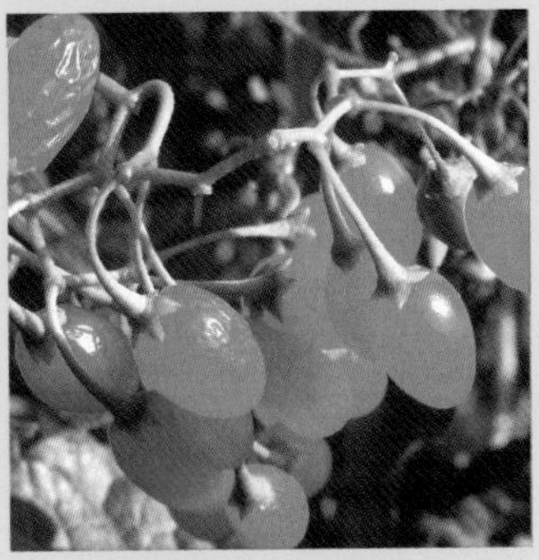

Solanum dulcamara

BLACK ALDER

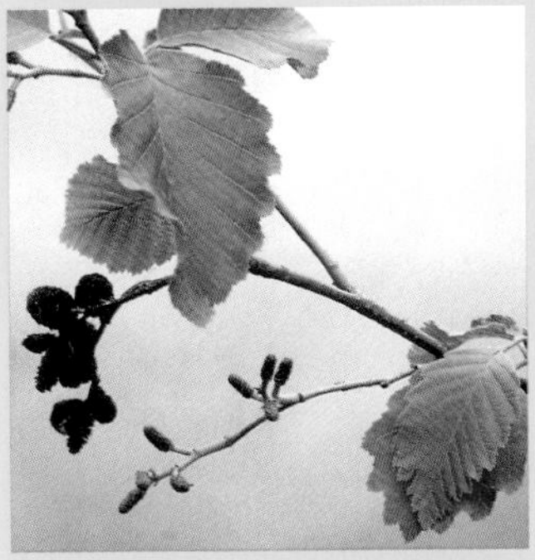

Alnus glutinosa

BLACK BRYONY

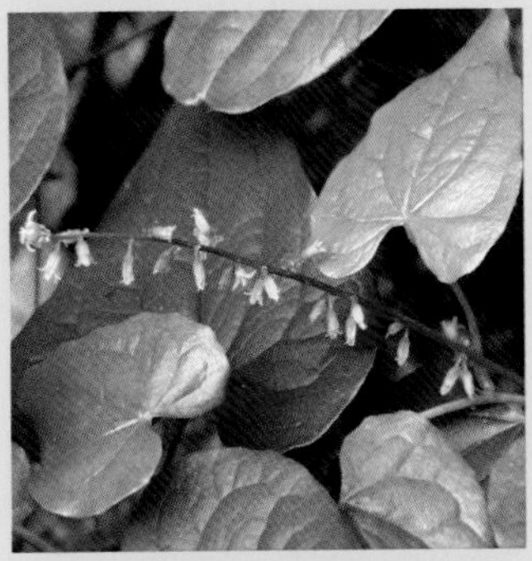

Tamus communis

BLACK COHOSH

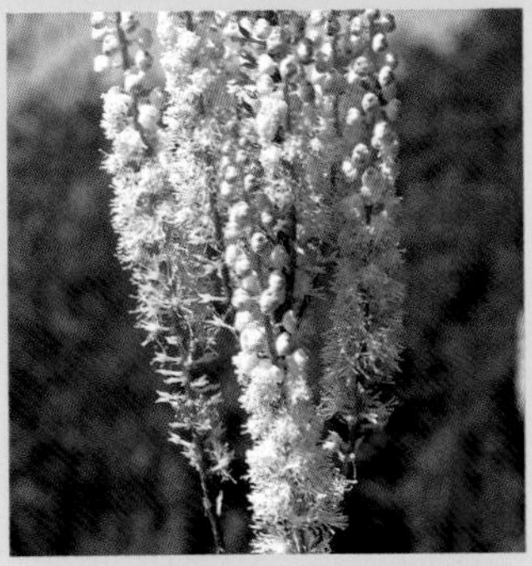

Cimicifuga racemosa

BLACK CURRANT

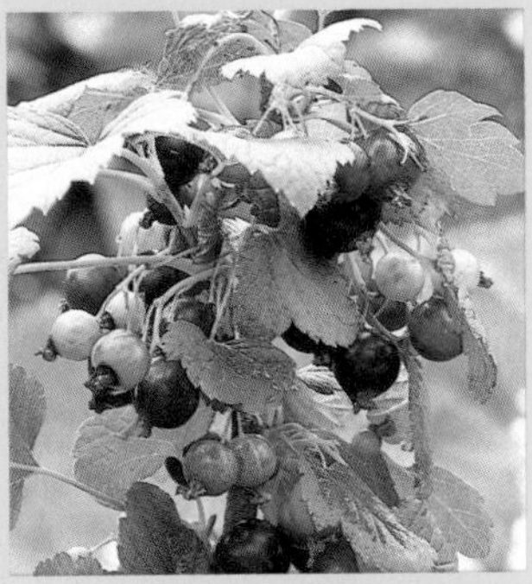

Ribes nigrum

BLACK HAW

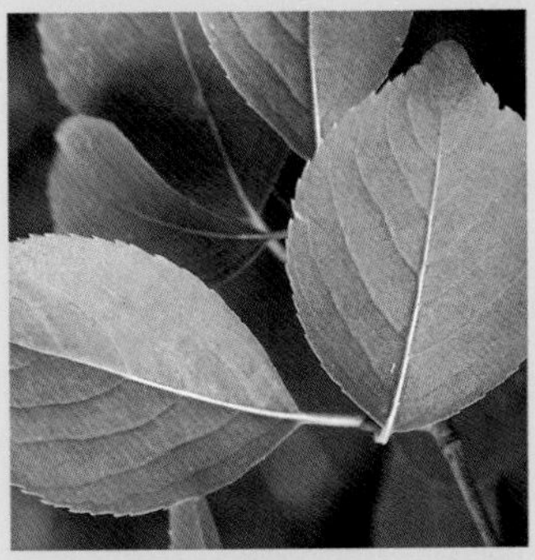

Viburnum prunifolium

BLACK HELLEBORE

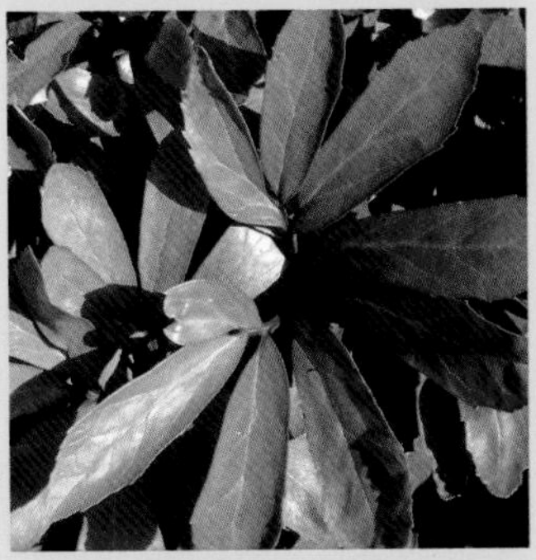

Helleborus niger

BLACK HOREHOUND

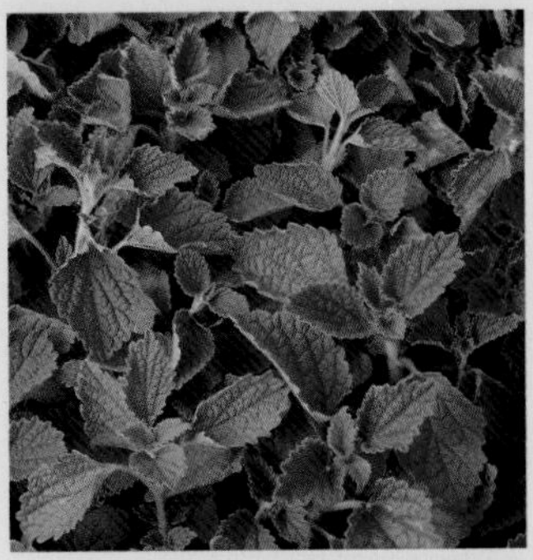

Ballota nigra

BLACK MUSTARD

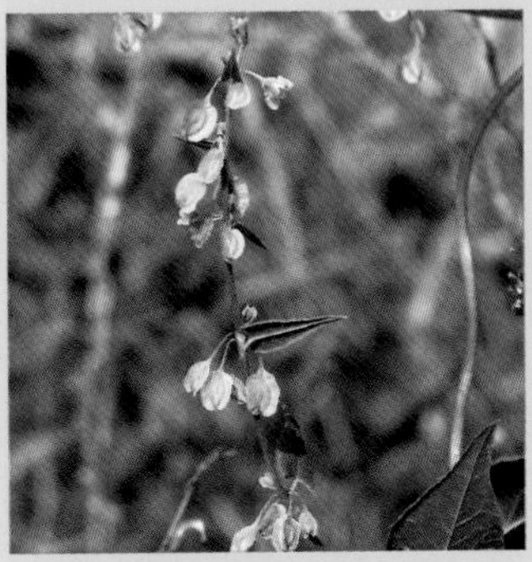

Brassica nigra

BLACK NIGHTSHADE

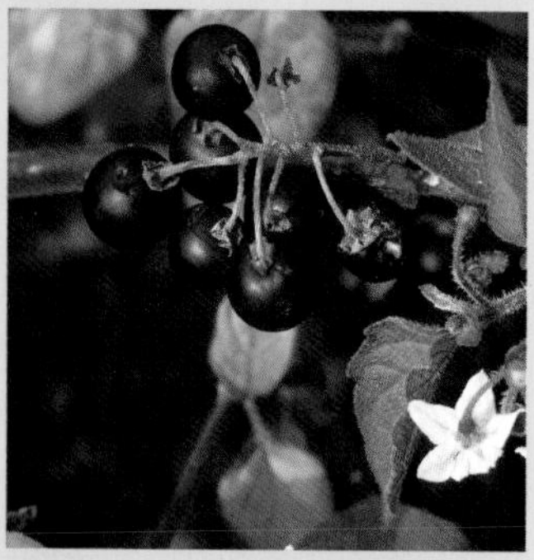

Solanum nigrum

BLACK PEPPER

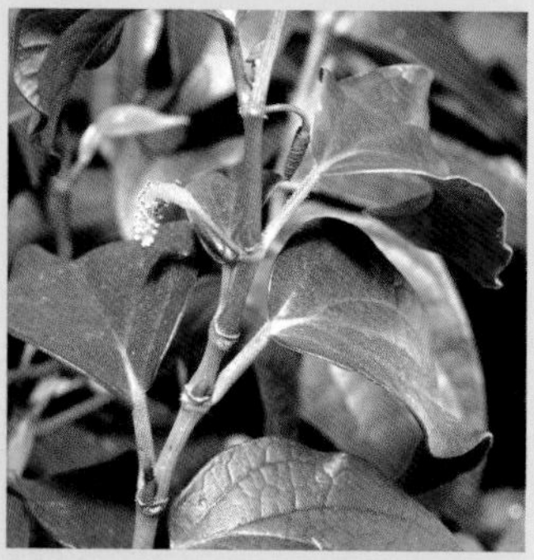

Piper nigrum

BLACKBERRY

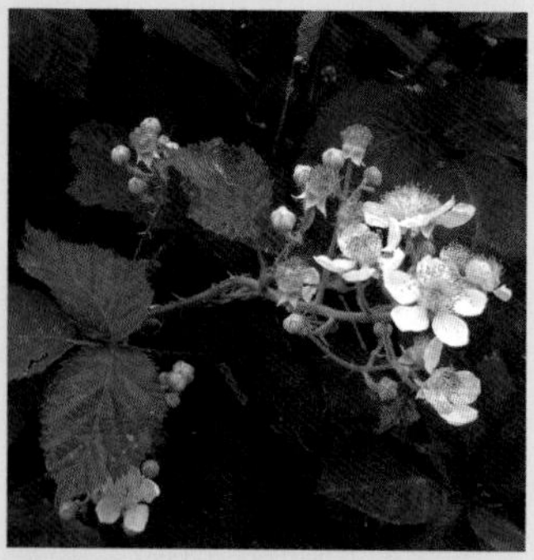

Rubus fruticosus

BLADDERWORT

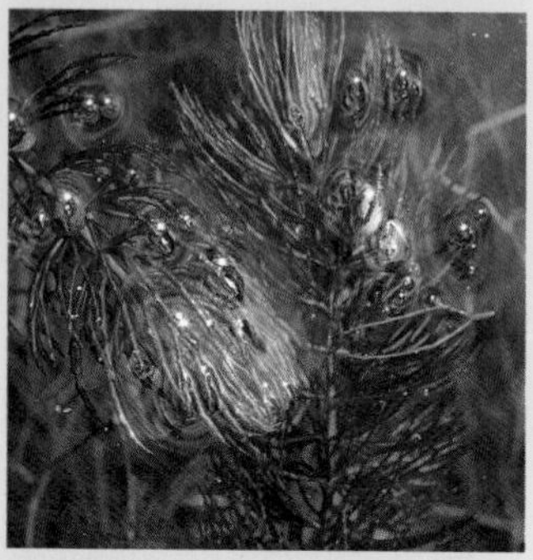

Utricularia vulgaris

BLESSED THISTLE

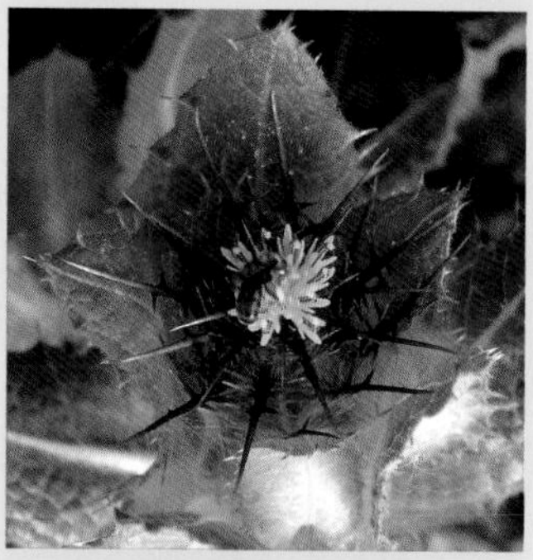

Cnicus benedictus

BOG BEAN

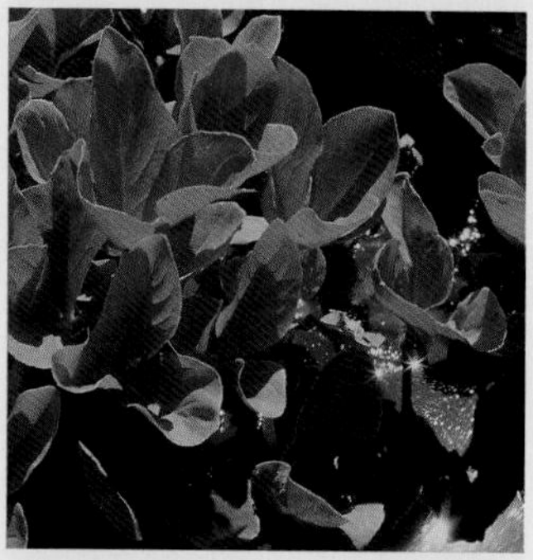

Menyanthes trifoliata

BOG BILBERRY

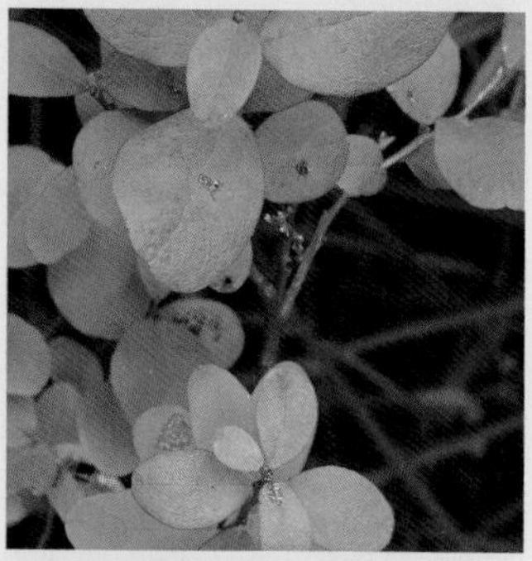

Vaccinium uliginosum

BOLDO

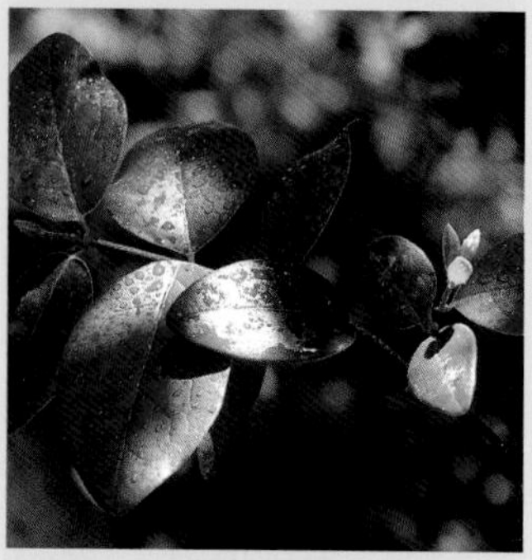

Peumus boldus

BONESET

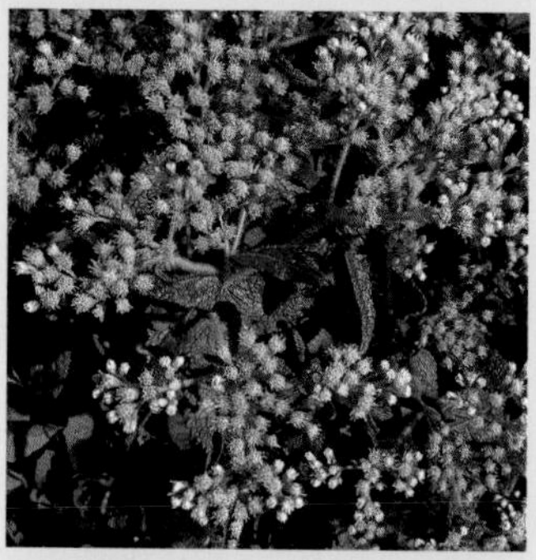

Eupatorium perfoliatum

BORAGE

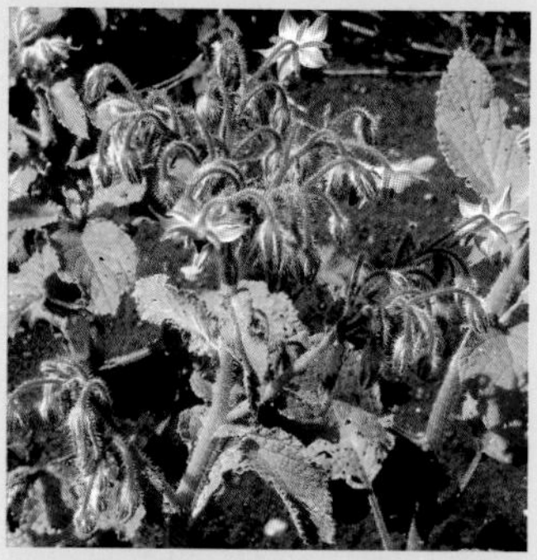

Borago officinalis

BOXWOOD

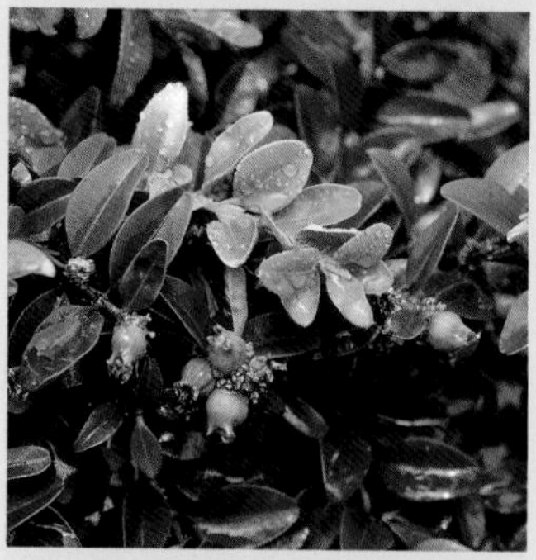

Buxus sempervirens

BROOKLIME

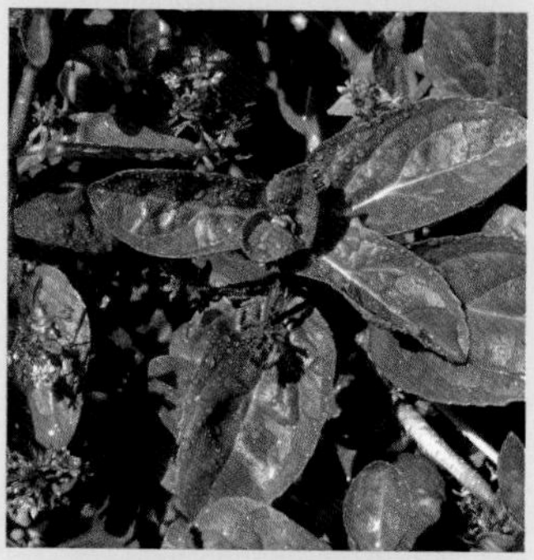

Veronica beccabunga

BUCKTHORN

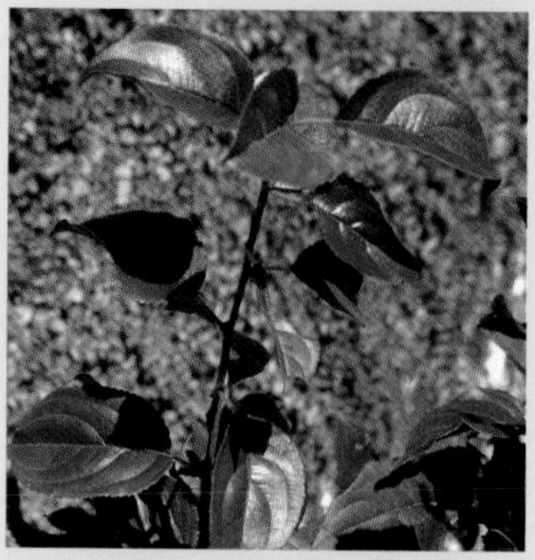

Rhamnus catharticus

BUCKWHEAT

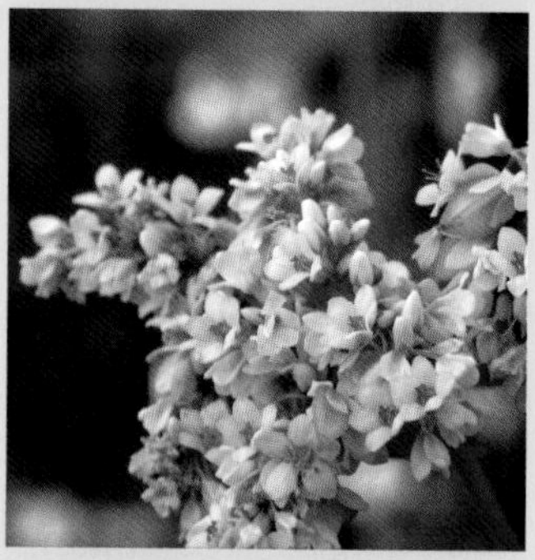

Fagopyrum esculentum

BUGLE

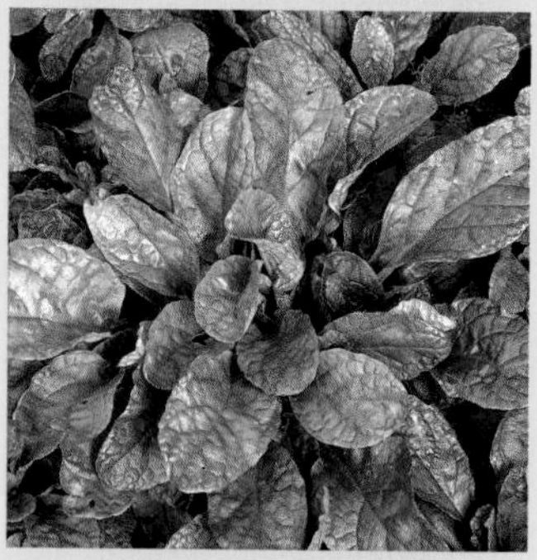

Ajuga reptans

BUGLEWEED

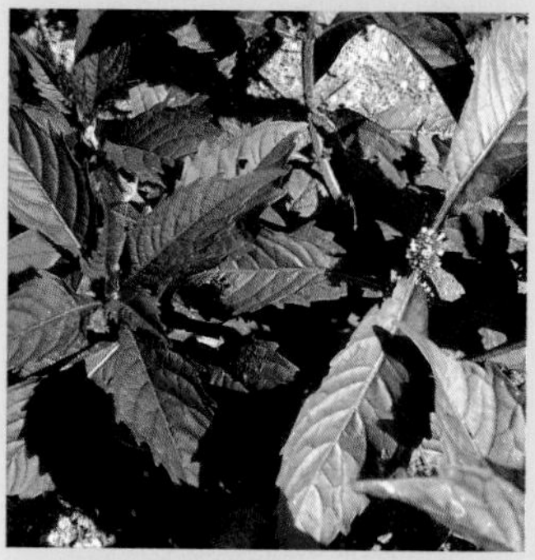

Lycopus virginicus

BURDOCK

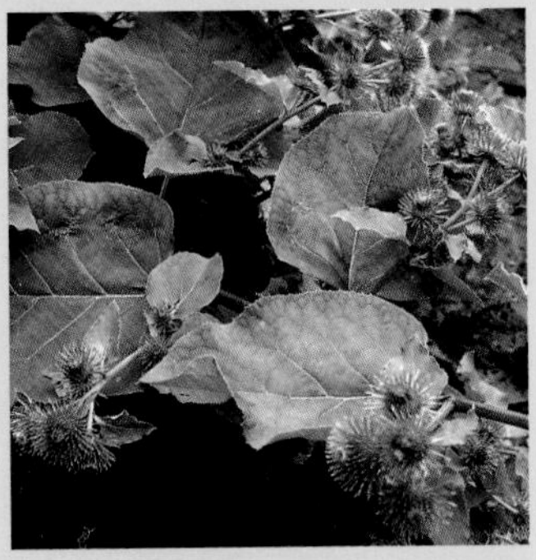

Arctium lappa

BURNING BUSH

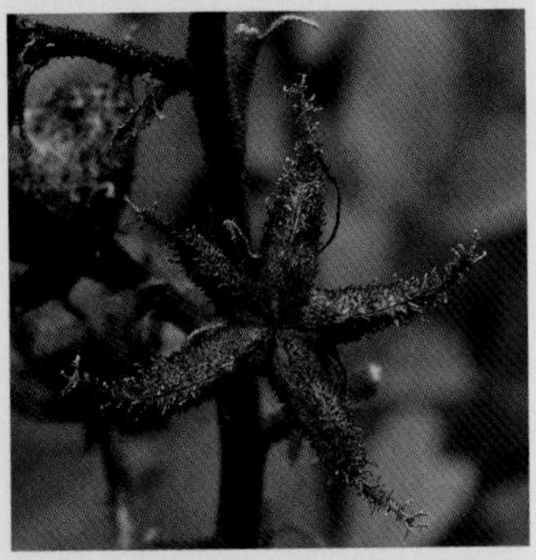

Dictamnus albus

BURR MARIGOLD

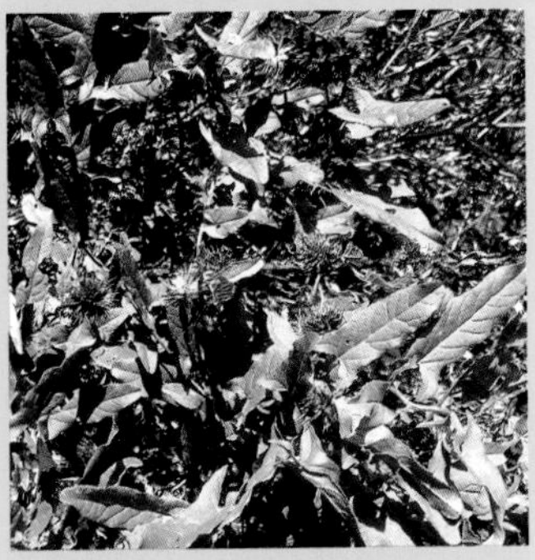

Bidens tripartita

BUTCHER'S BROOM

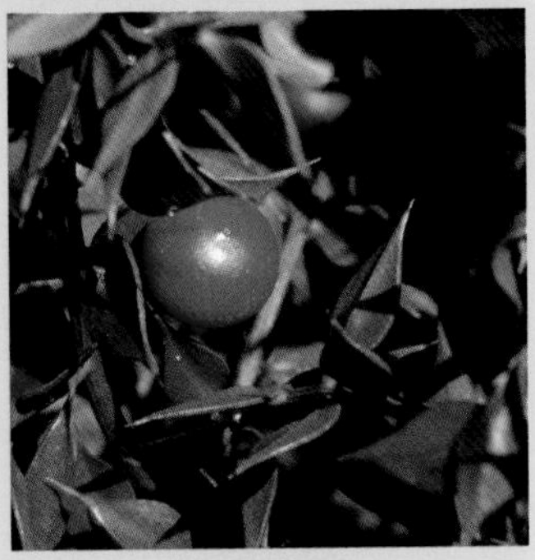

Ruscus aculeatus

CABBAGE

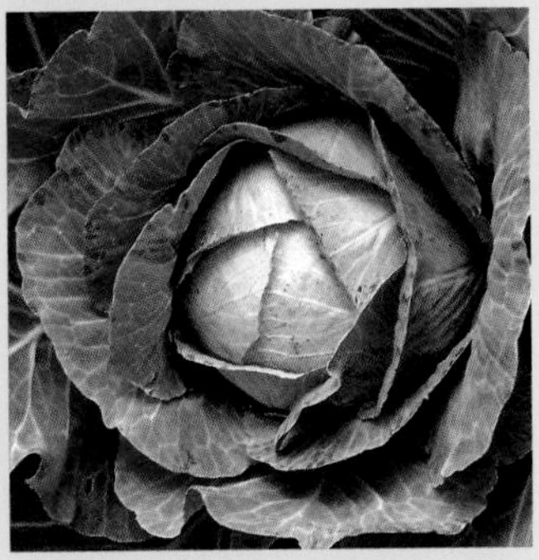

Brassica oleracea

CAJUPUT

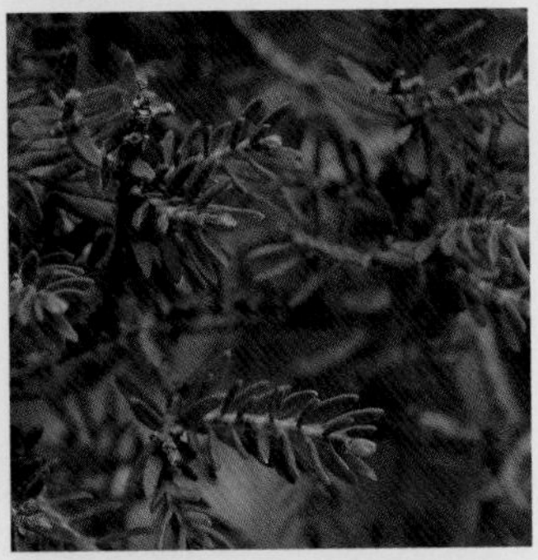

Melaleuca leucadendra

CALAMUS

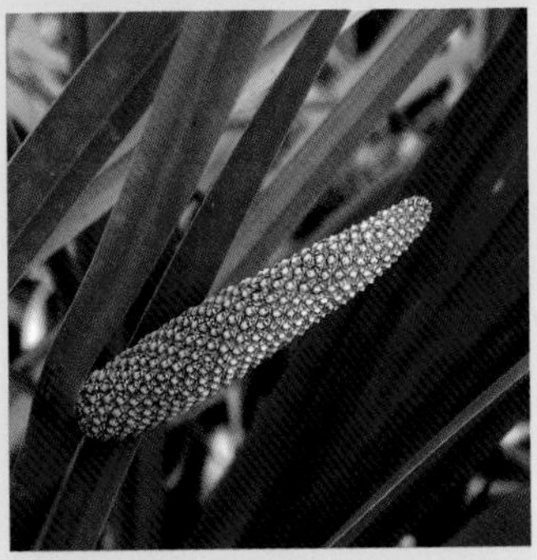

Acorus calamus

CALIFORNIA POPPY

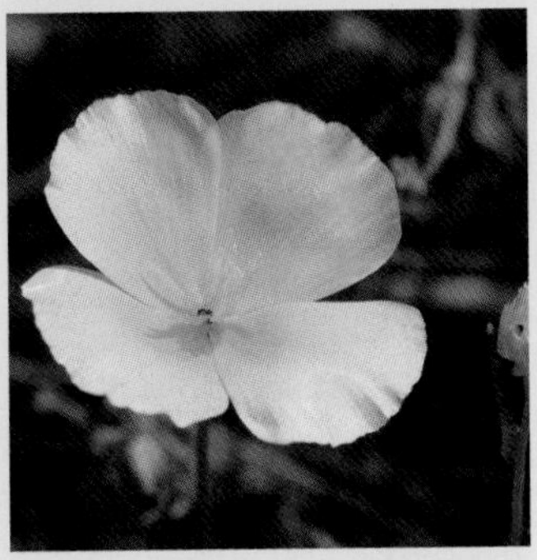

Eschscholtzia californica

CAMPHOR TREE

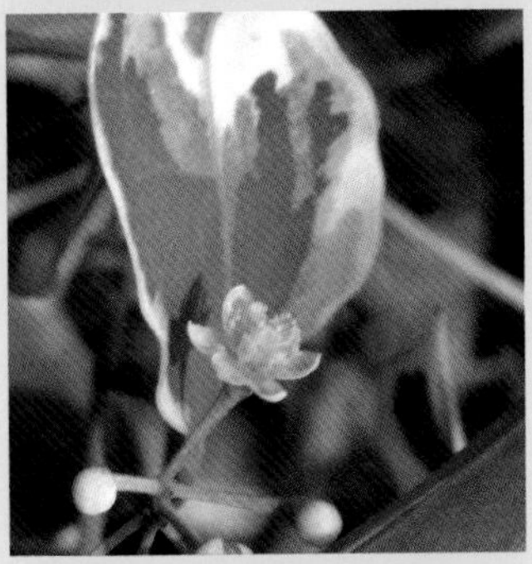

Cinnamomum camphora

CANADIAN FLEABANE

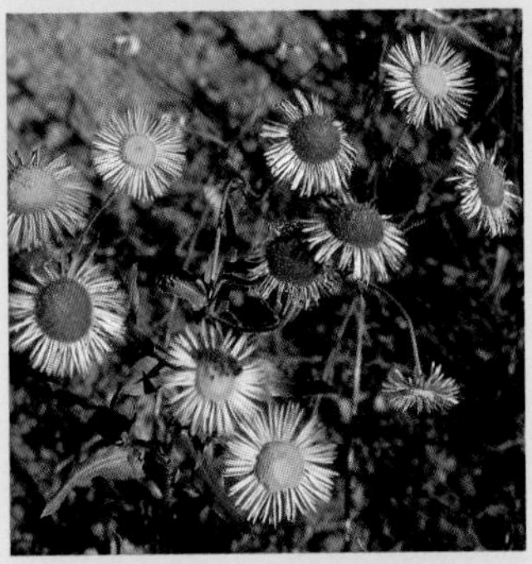

Erigeron canadensis

CARAWAY

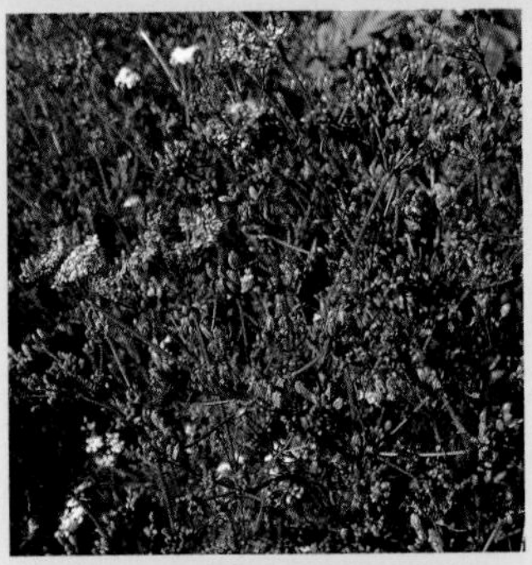

Carum carvi

CARDAMOM

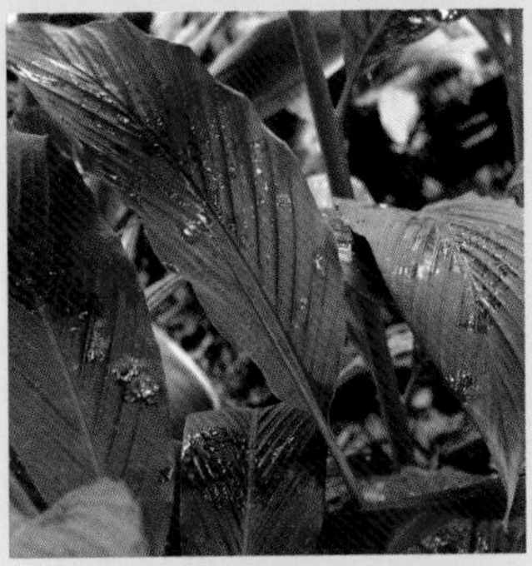

Elettaria cardamomum

CAROB

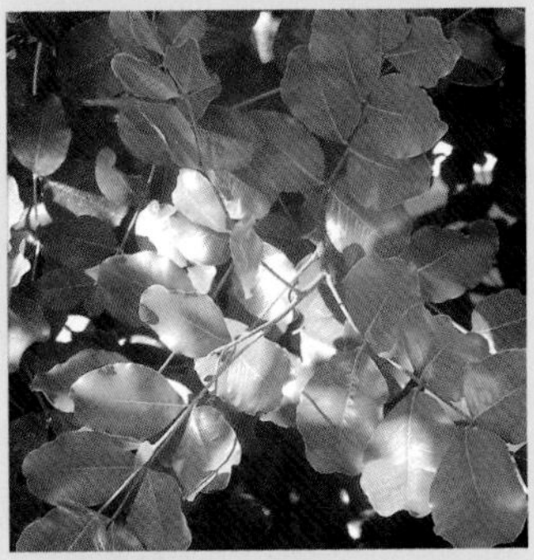

Ceratonia siliqua

CASCARA SAGRADA

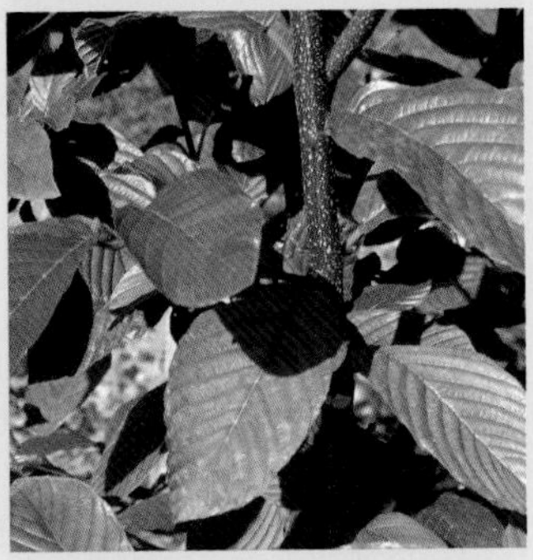

Rhamnus purshiana

CASHEW

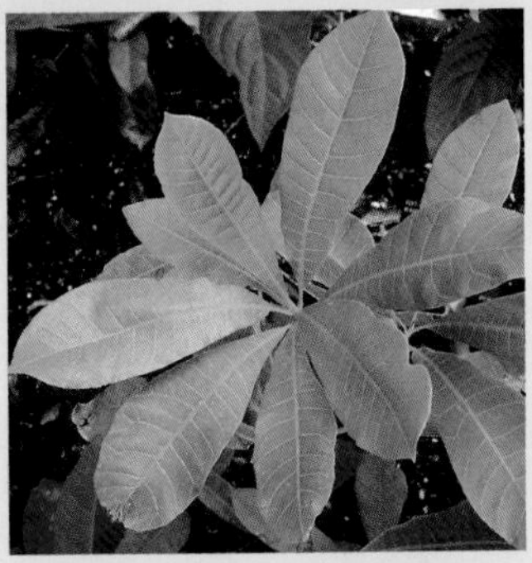

Anacardium occidentale

CASTOR OIL PLANT

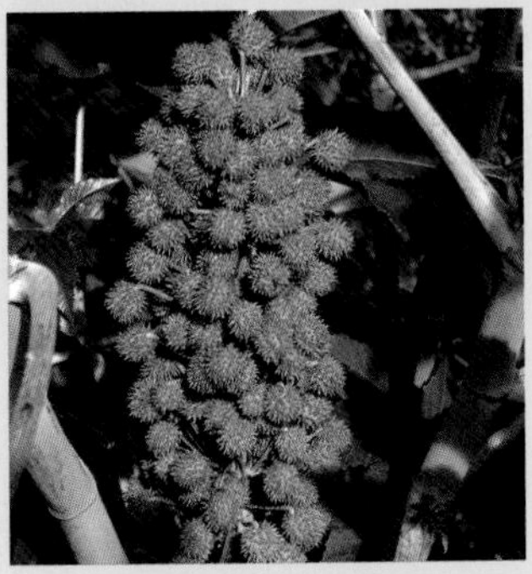

Ricinus communis

CATNIP

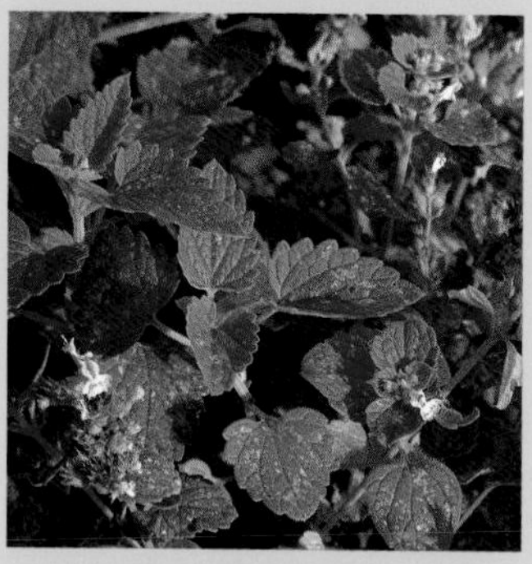

Nepeta cataria

CAT'S FOOT

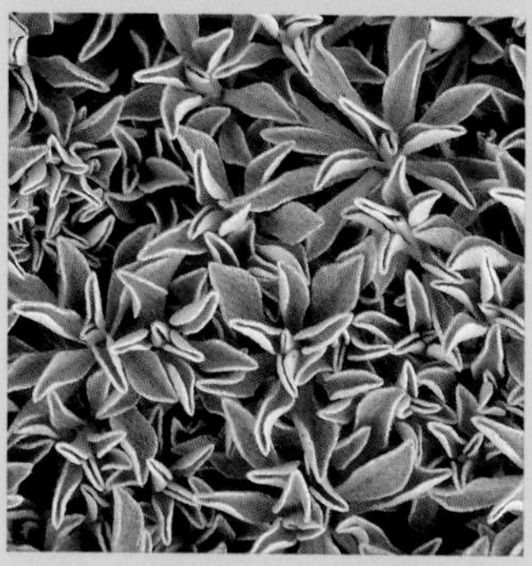

Antennaria dioica

CAYENNE

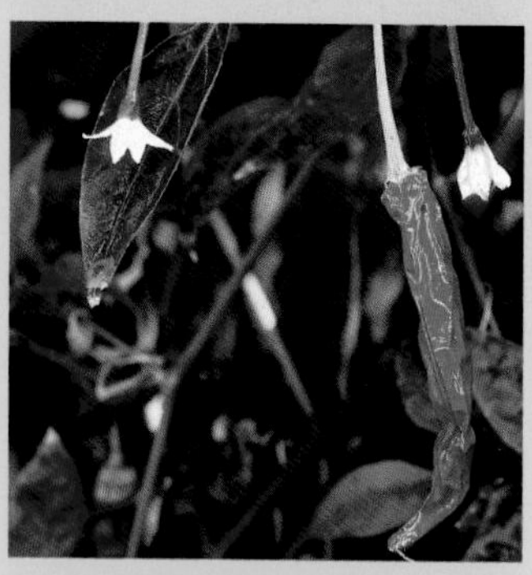

Capsicum annuum

CELANDINE

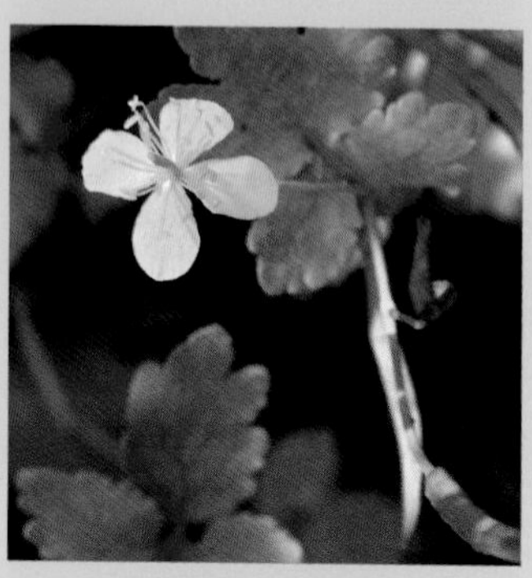

Chelidonium majus

CELERY

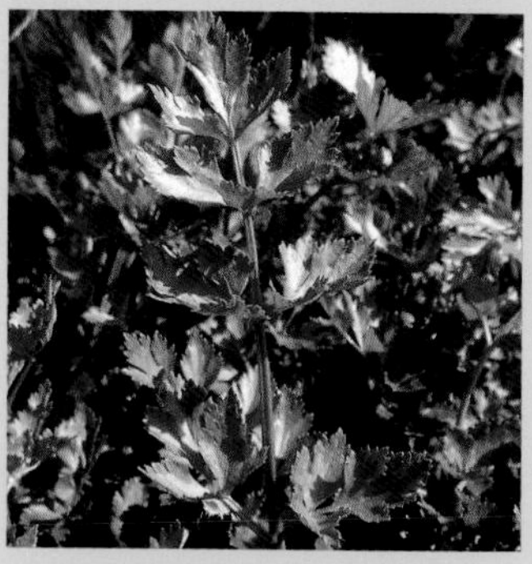

Apium graveolens

CENTAURY

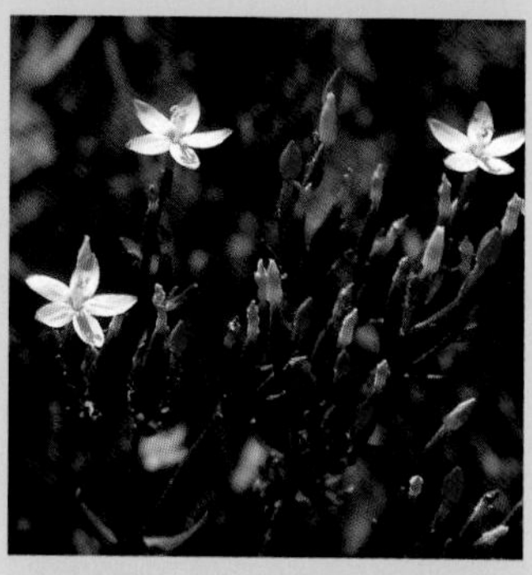

Centaurium erythraea

CHASTE TREE

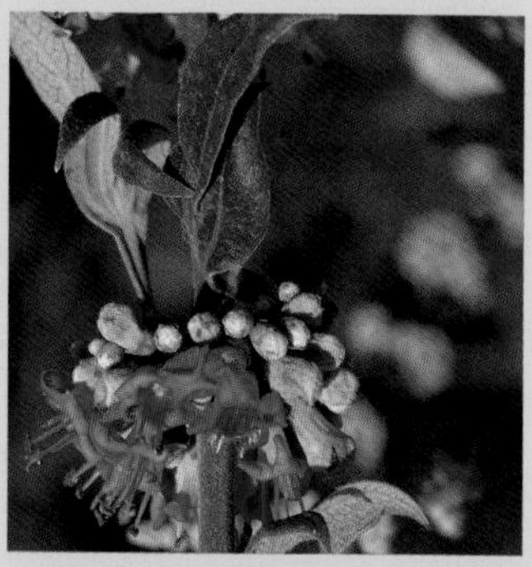

Vitex agnus-castus

CHERRY LAUREL

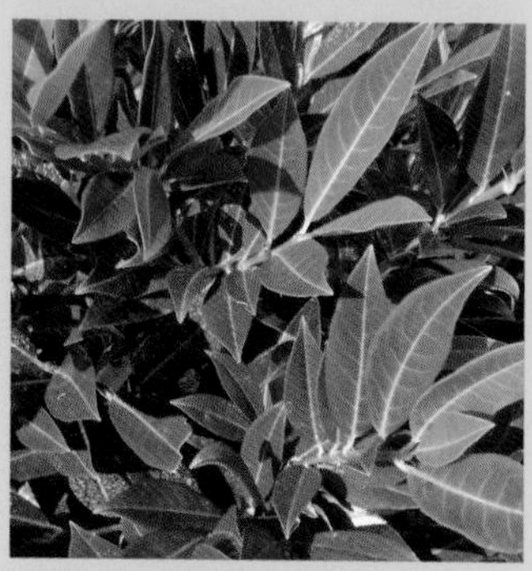

Prunus laurocerasus

CHICORY

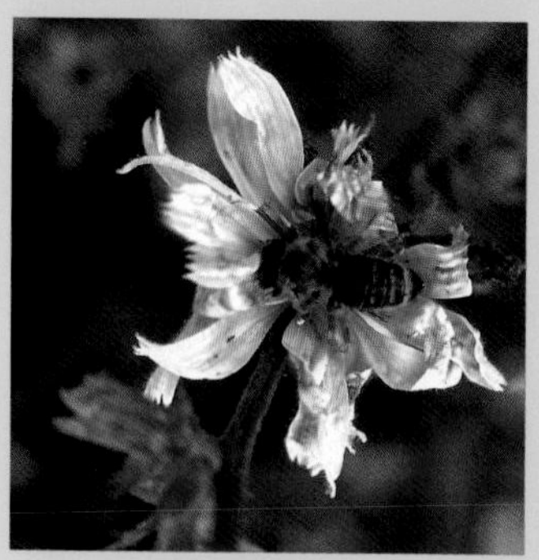

Cichorium intybus

CHINESE RHUBARB

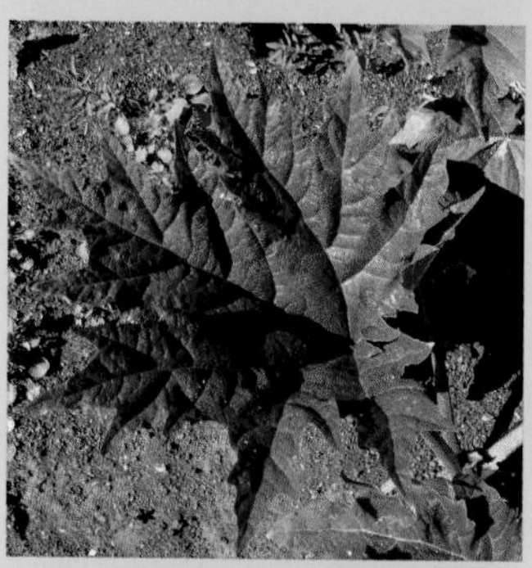

Rheum palmatum

CHIVE

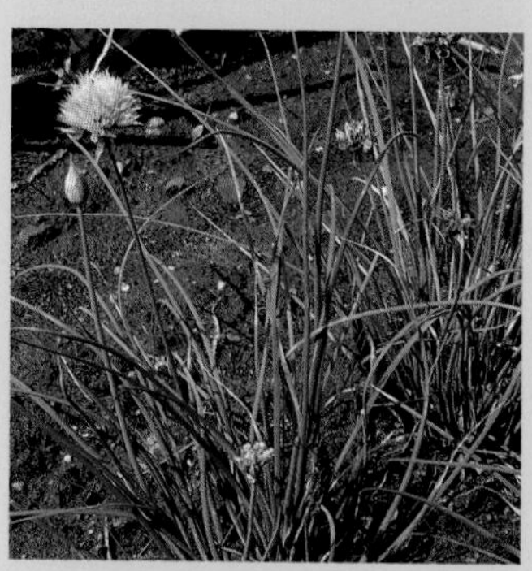

Allium schoenoprasum

CINNAMON

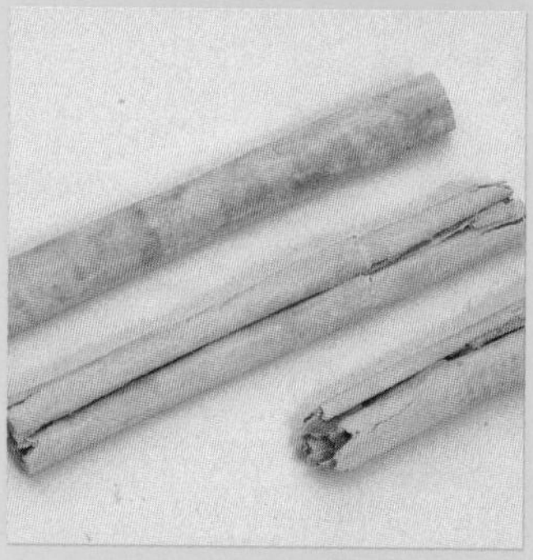

Cinnamomum verum

CINQUEFOIL

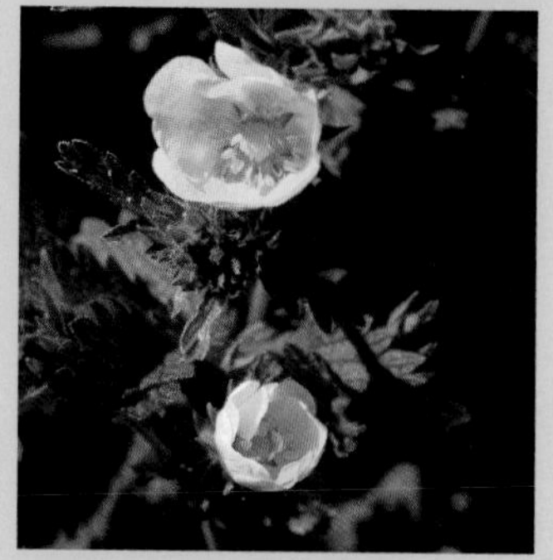

Potentilla erecta

CLEMATIS

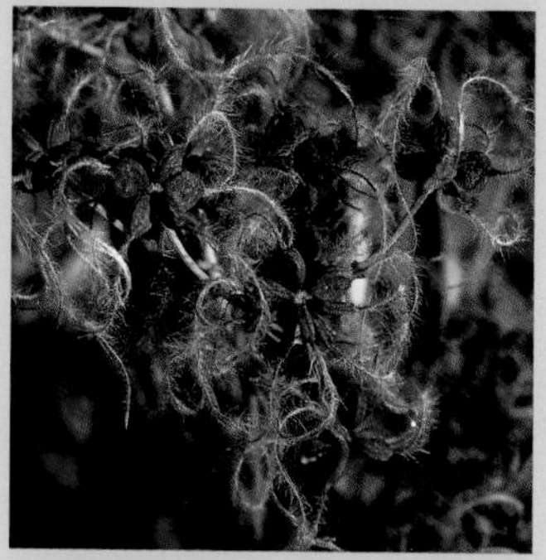

Clematis recta

CLOVE

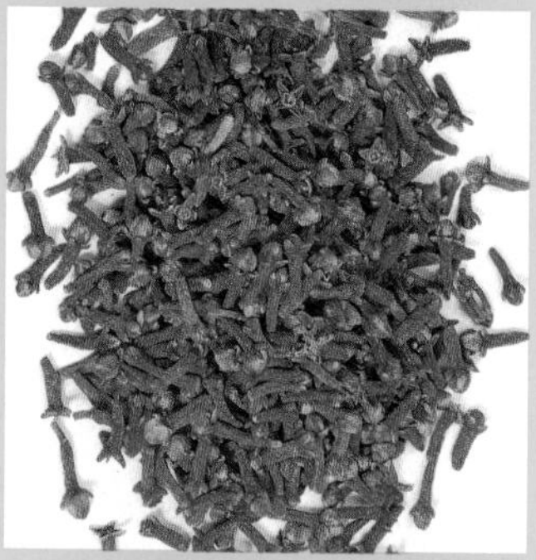

Syzygium aromaticum

COCOA

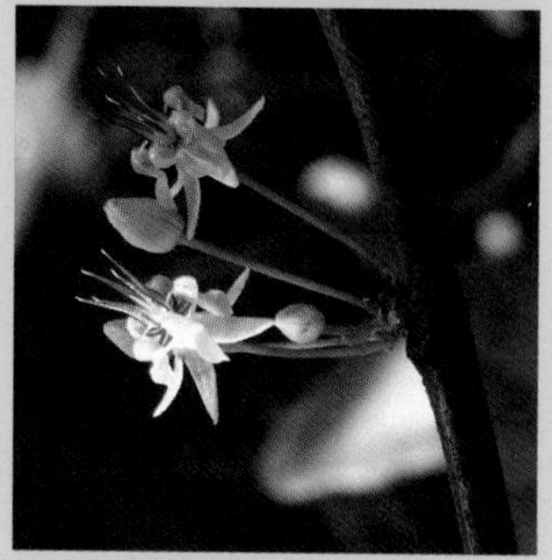

Theobroma cacao

COCONUT PALM

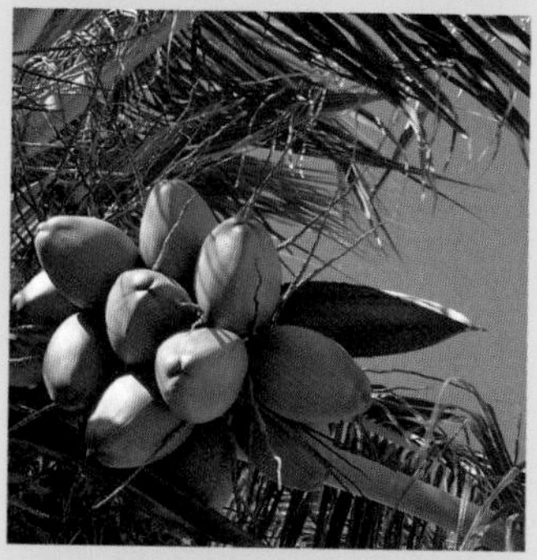

Cocos nucifera

COFFEE

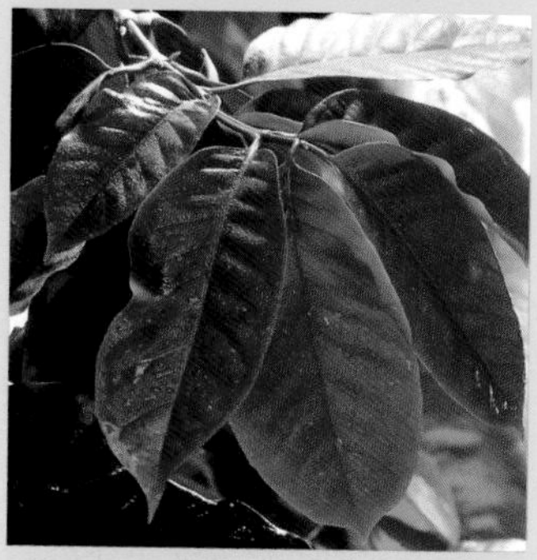

Coffea arabica

COLCHICUM

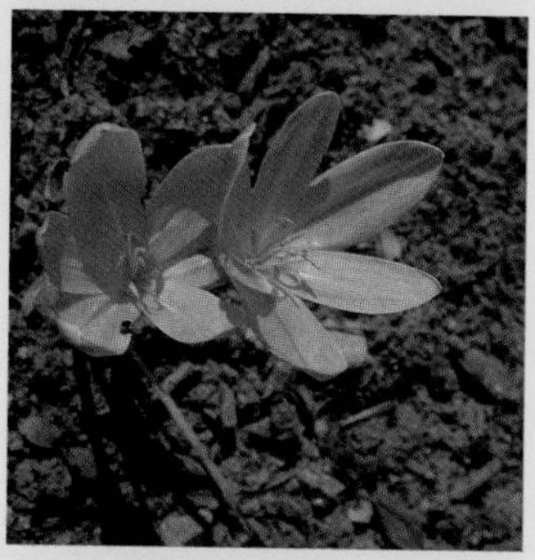

Colchicum autumnale

COLT'S FOOT

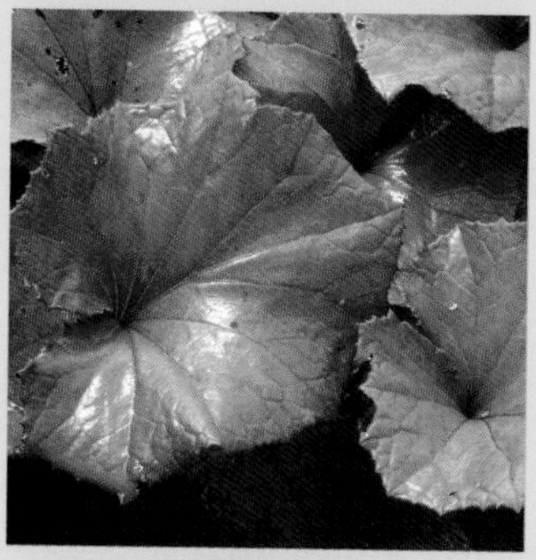

Tussilago farfara

COLUMBINE

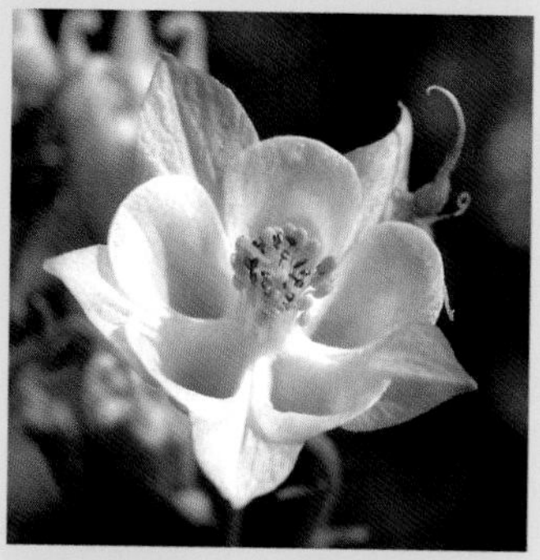

Aquilegia vulgaris

COMFREY

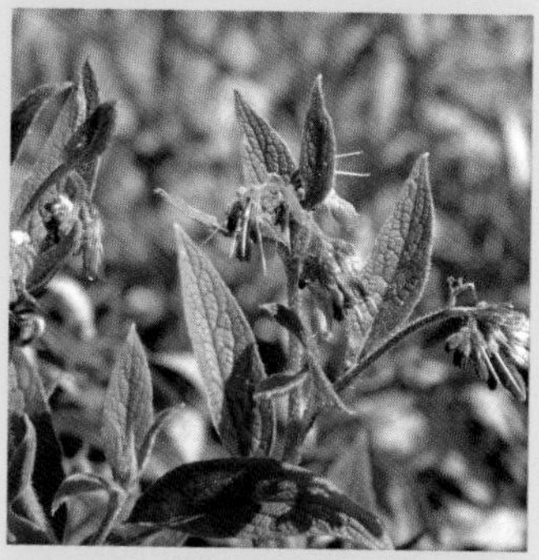

Symphytum officinale

COMMON KIDNEY VETCH

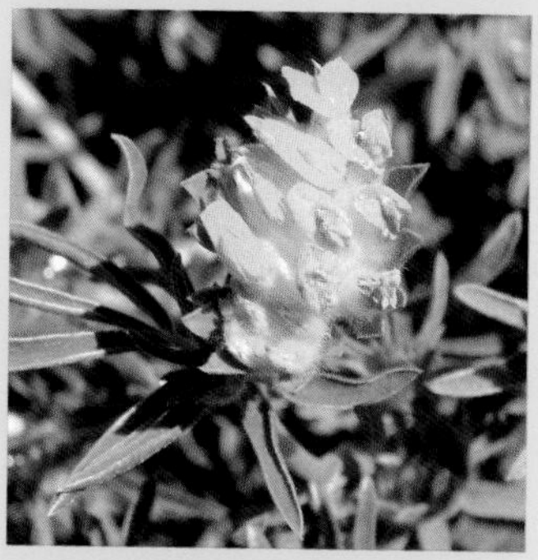

Anthyllis vulneraria

COOLWORT

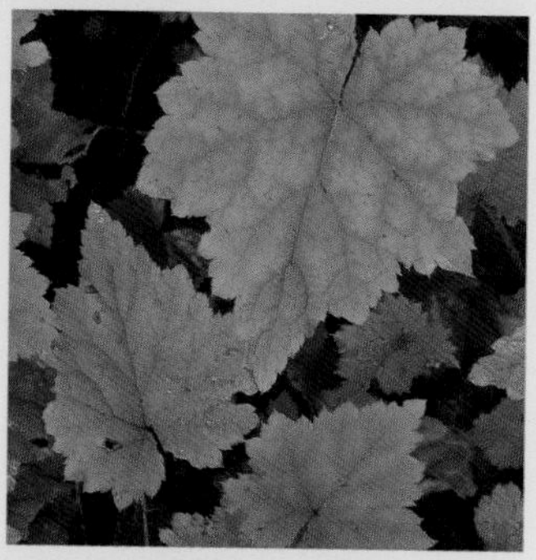

Tiarella cordifolia

CORIANDER

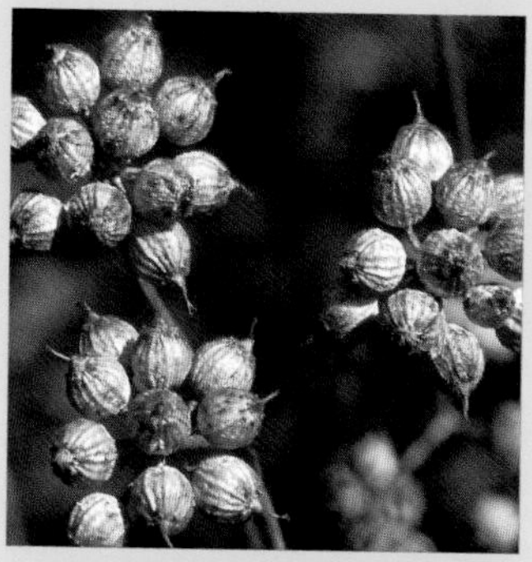

Coriandrum sativum

CORNFLOWER

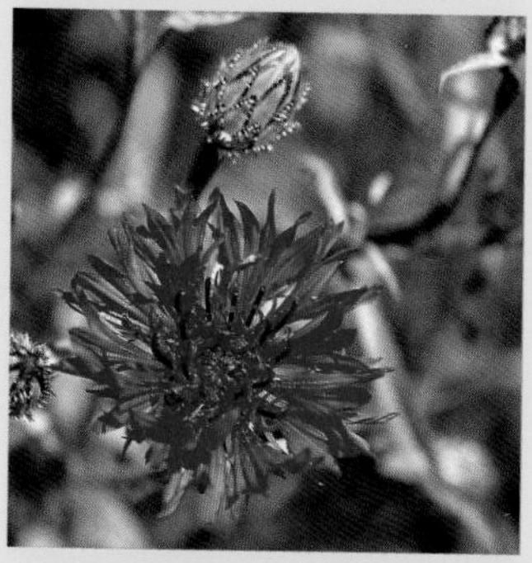

Centaurea cyanus

CUMIN

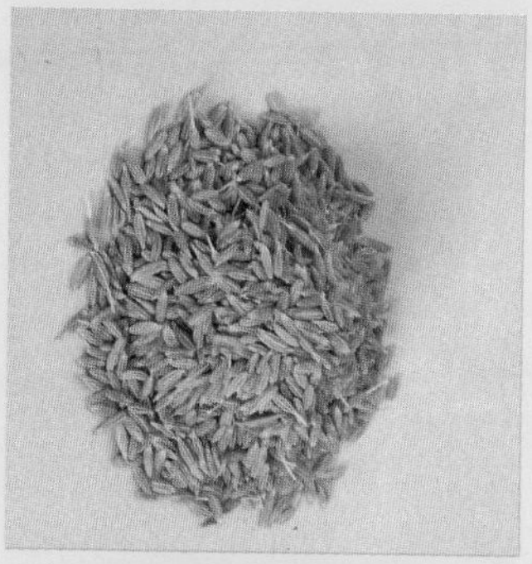

Cuminum cyminum

CUP PLANT

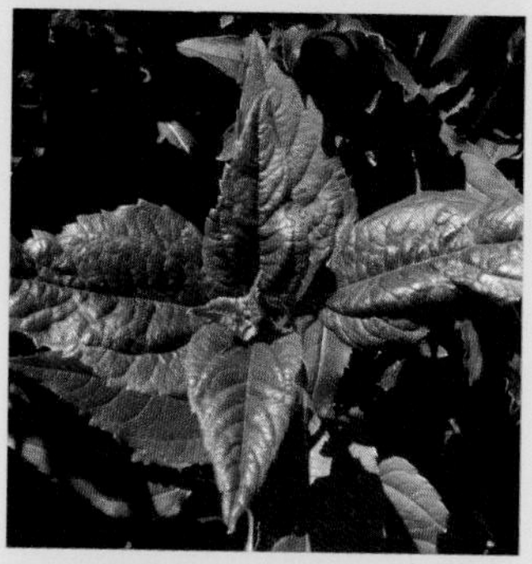

Silphium perfoliatum

CURCUMA

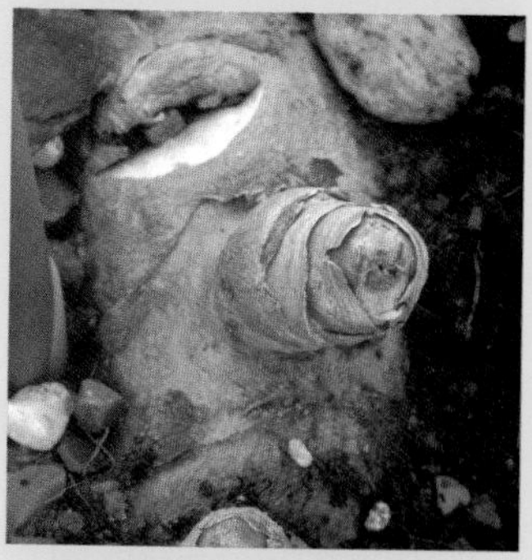

Curcuma xanthorrhizia

CYPRESS

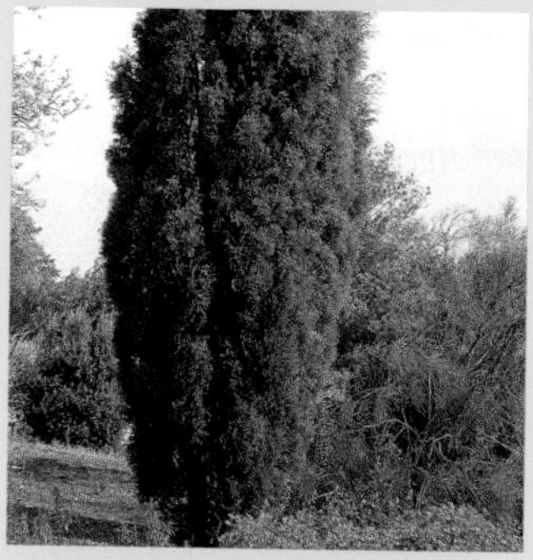

Cupressus sempervirens

CYPRESS SPURGE

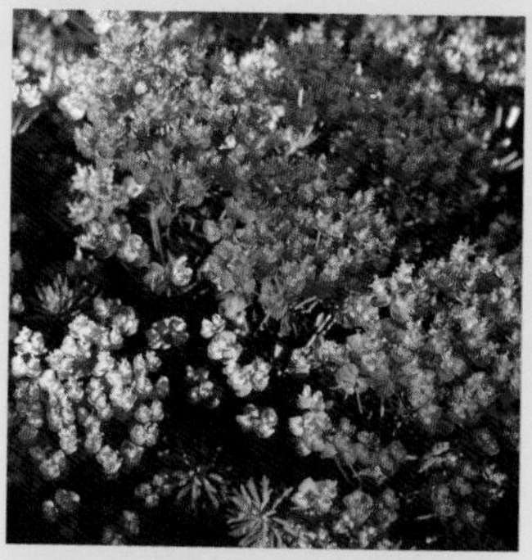

Euphorbia cyparissias

DANDELION

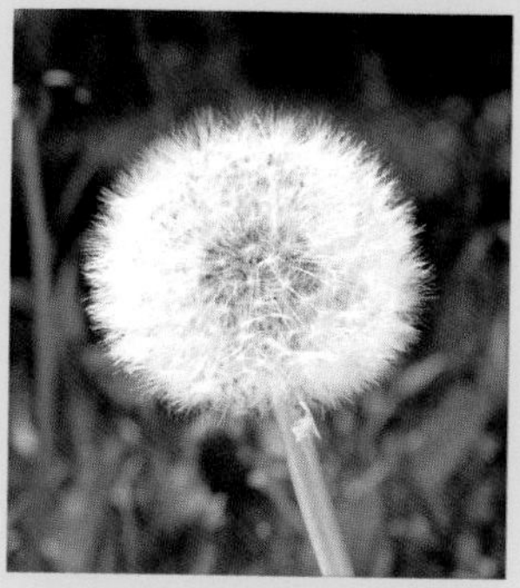

Taraxacum officinale

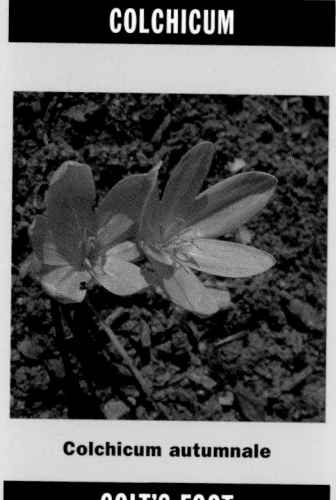

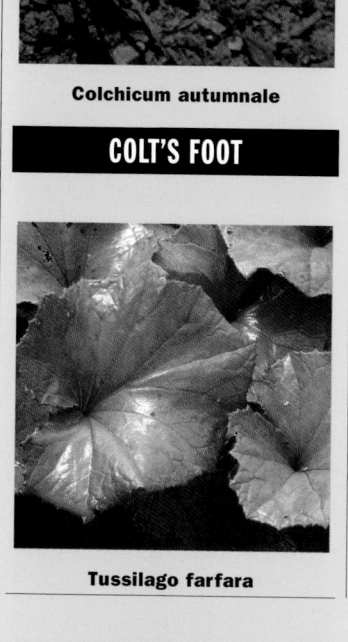

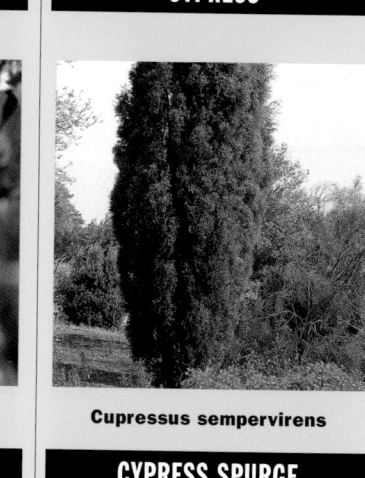

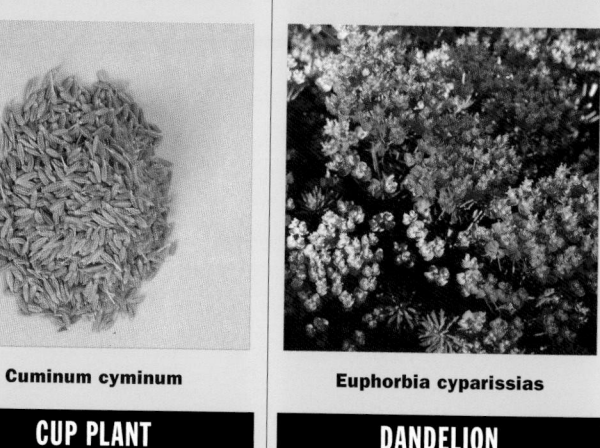

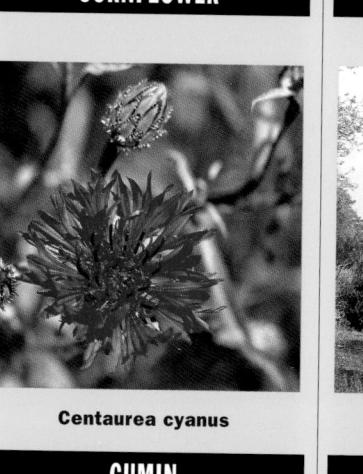

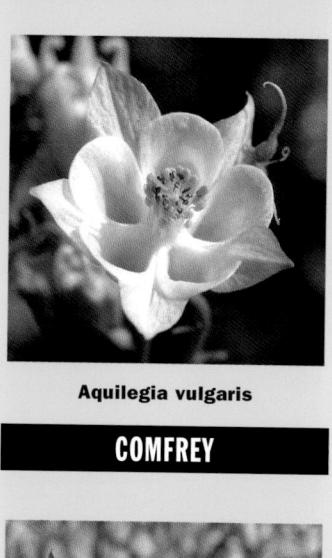

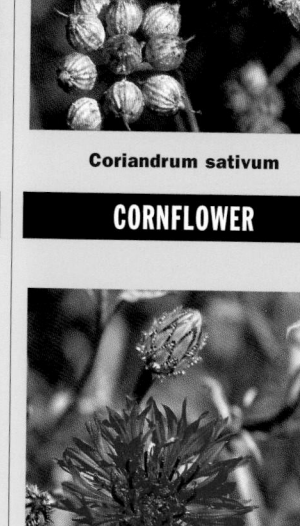

DATE PALM

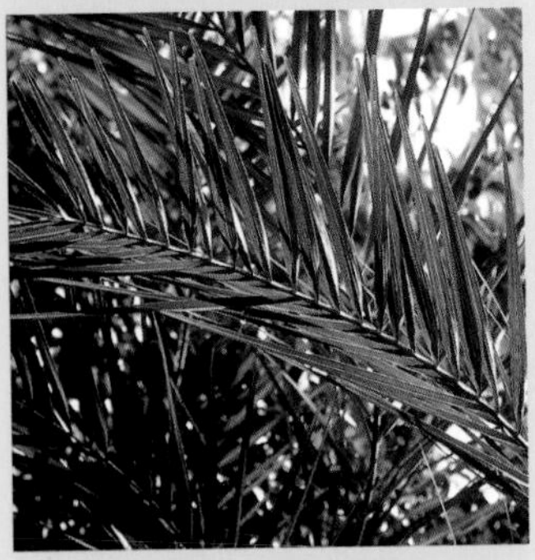

Phoenix dactylifera

DIGITALIS

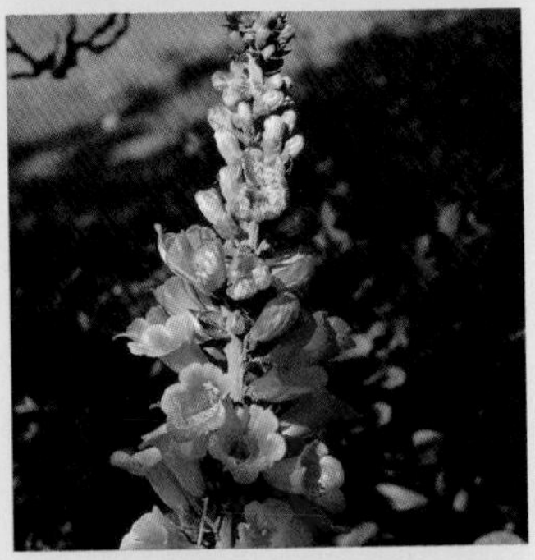

Digitalis purpurea

DILL

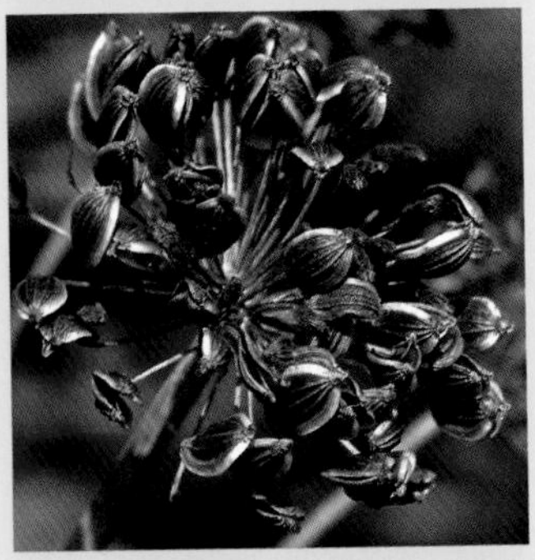

Anethum graveolens

DODDER

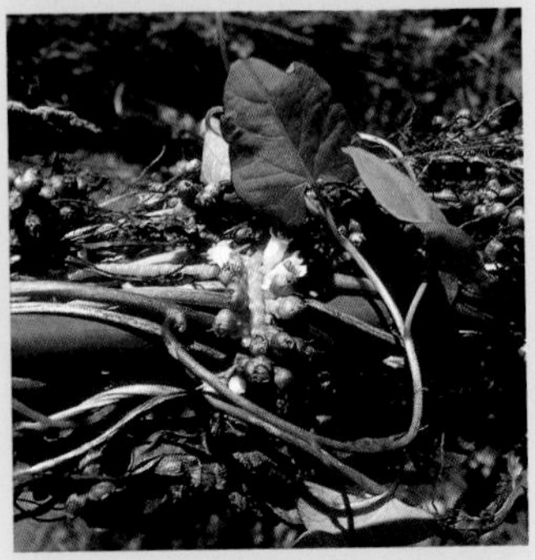

Cuscuta epithymum

DOG ROSE

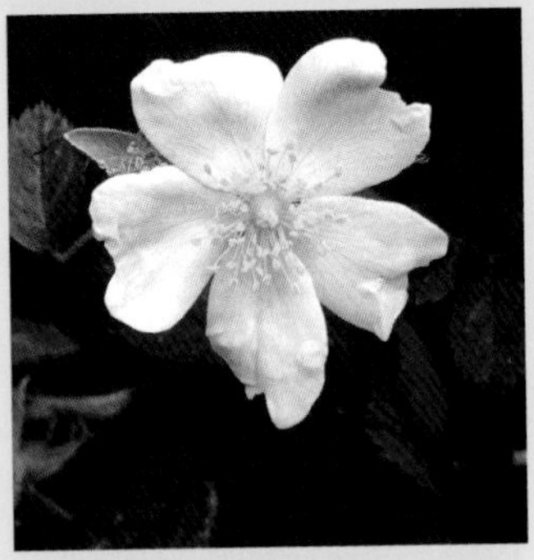

Rosa canina

DOGWOOD

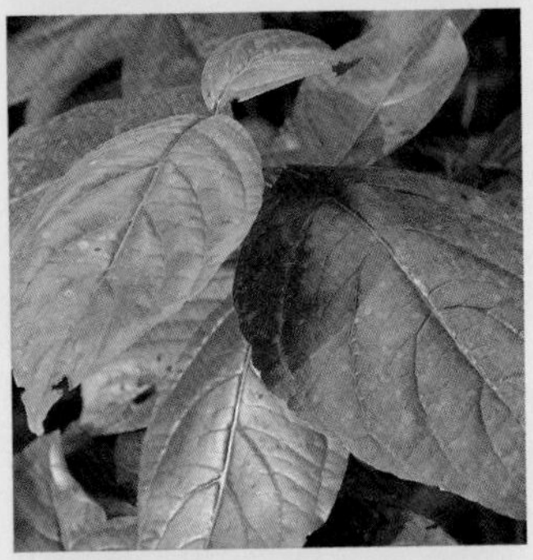

Cornus florida

DUCKWEED

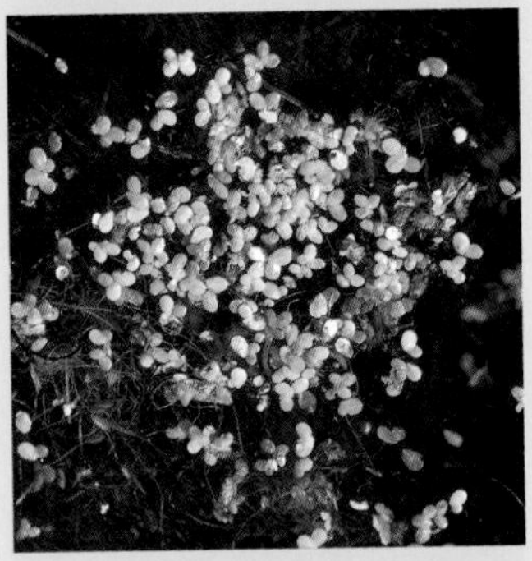

Lemna minor

DYER'S BROOM

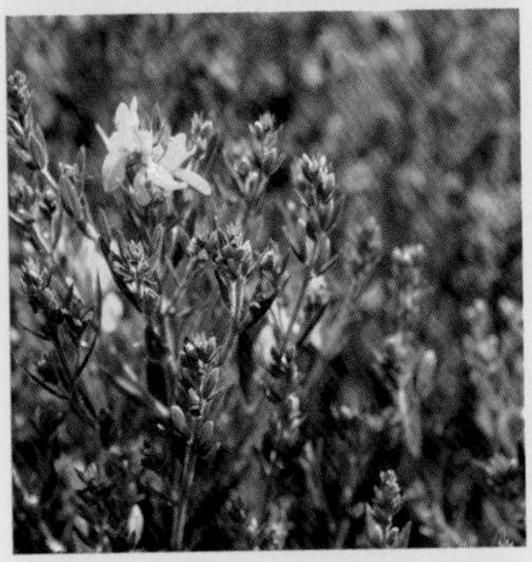

Genista tinctoria

ECHINACEA PURPUREA

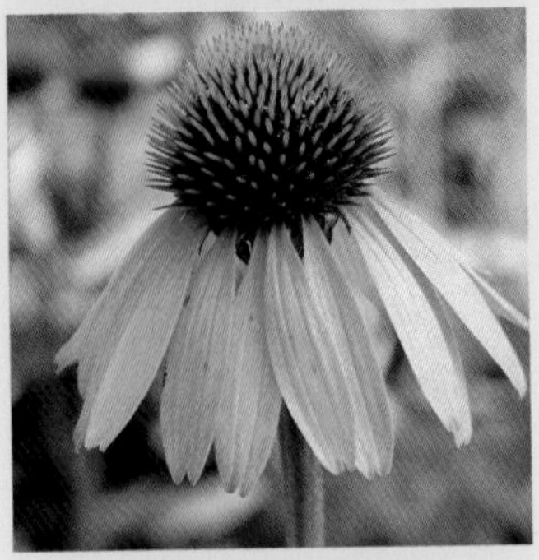

Echinacea purpurea

ELECAMPANE

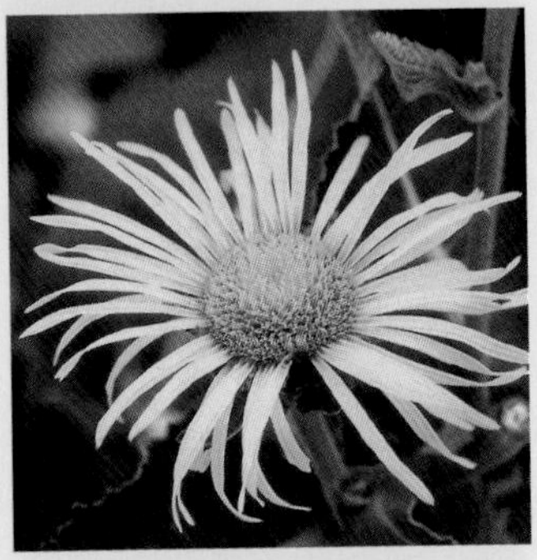

Inula helenium

ELM BARK

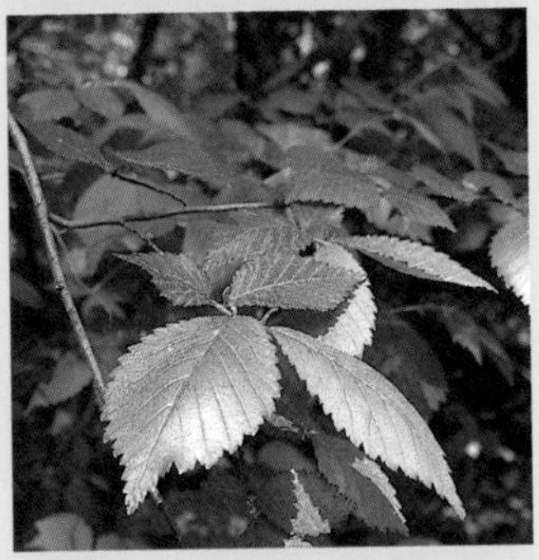

Ulmus minor

ENGLISH CHAMOMILE

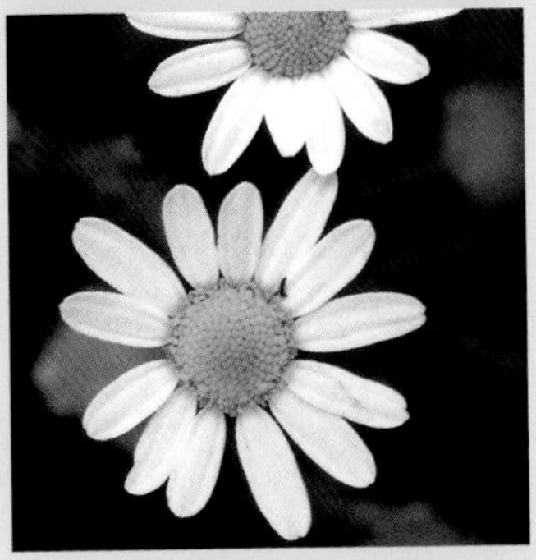

Chamaemelum nobile

ENGLISH HAWTHORN

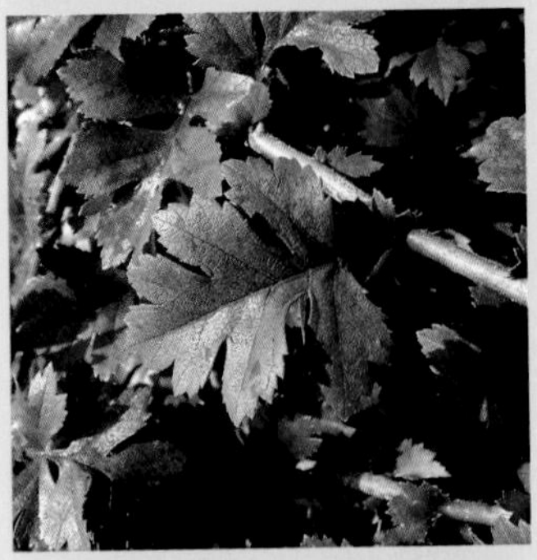

Crataegus laevigata

ENGLISH HORSEMINT

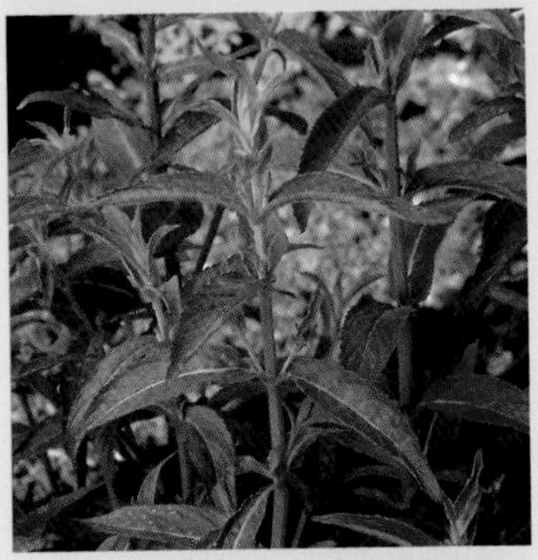

Mentha longifolia

ENGLISH IVY

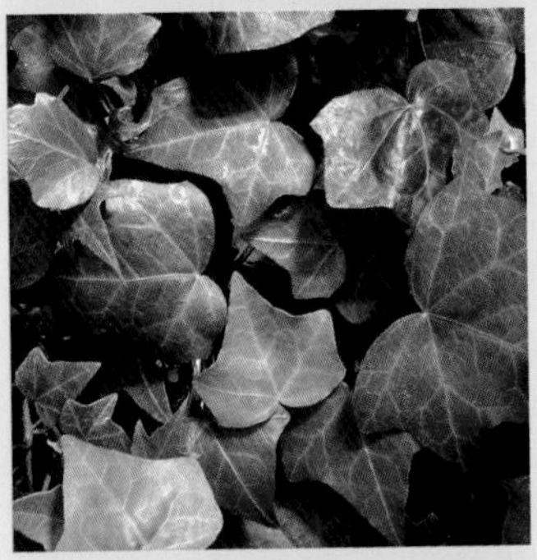

Hedera helix

ENGLISH LAVENDER

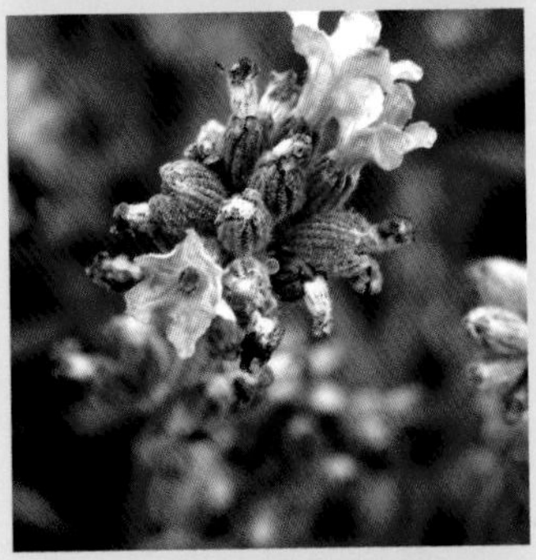

Lavandula angustifolia

ENGLISH PLANTAIN

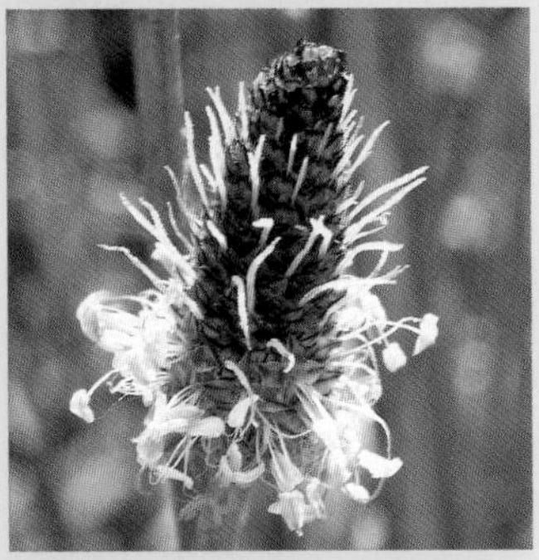

Plantago lanceolata

ERYNGO

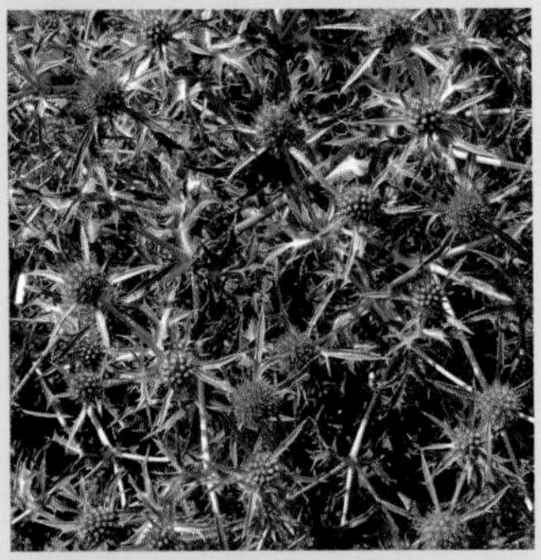

Eryngium campestre

EUCALYPTUS

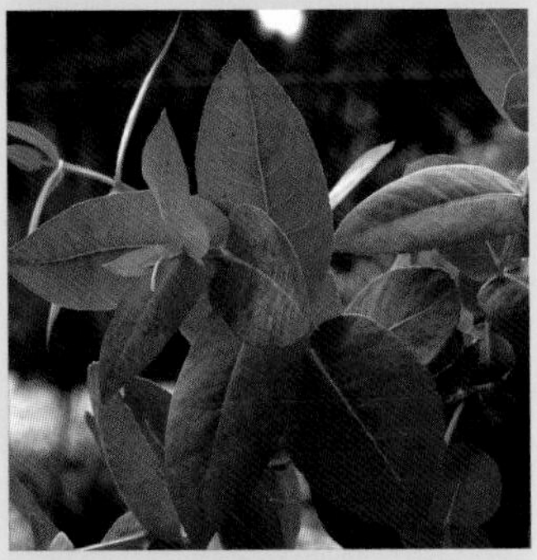

Eucalyptus globulus

EUROPEAN ELDER

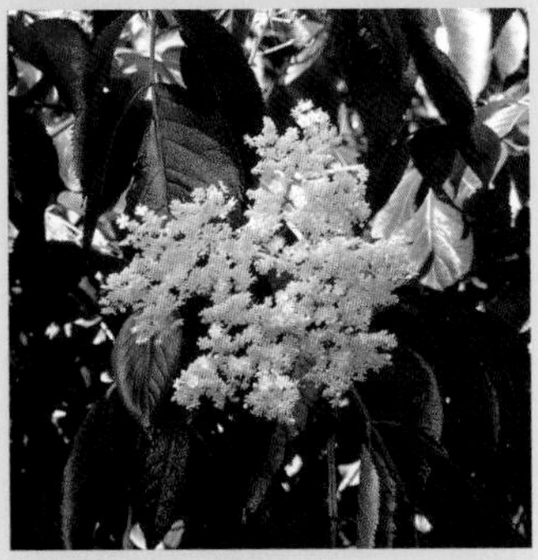

Sambucus nigra

EUROPEAN FIVE-FINGER GRASS

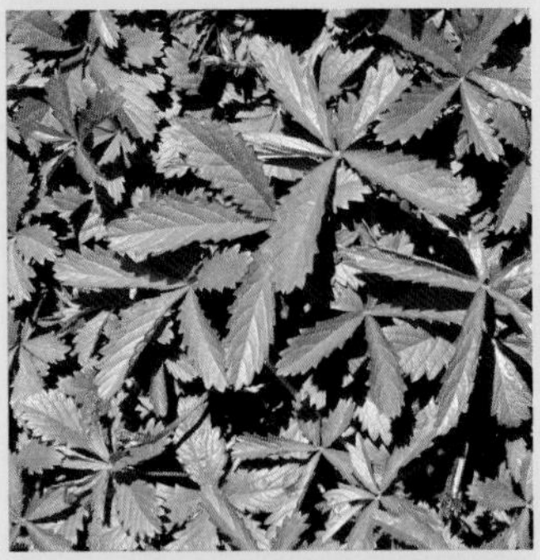

Potentilla reptans

EUROPEAN GOLDEN ROD

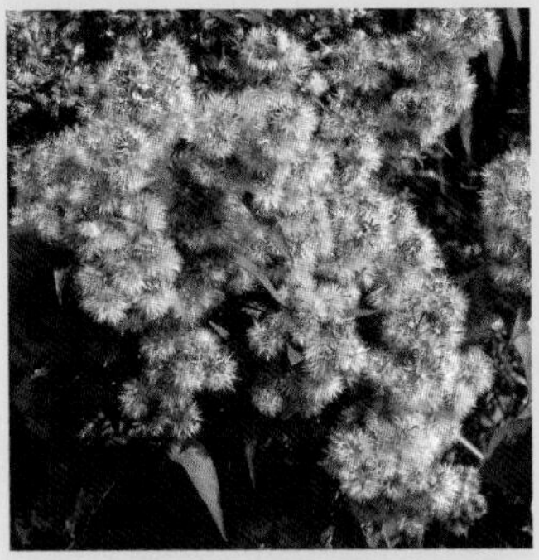

Solidago virgaurea

EUROPEAN MISTLETOE

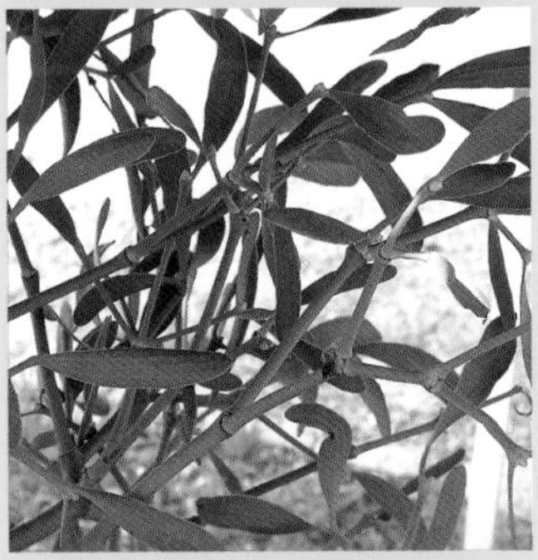

Viscum album

EUROPEAN PEONY

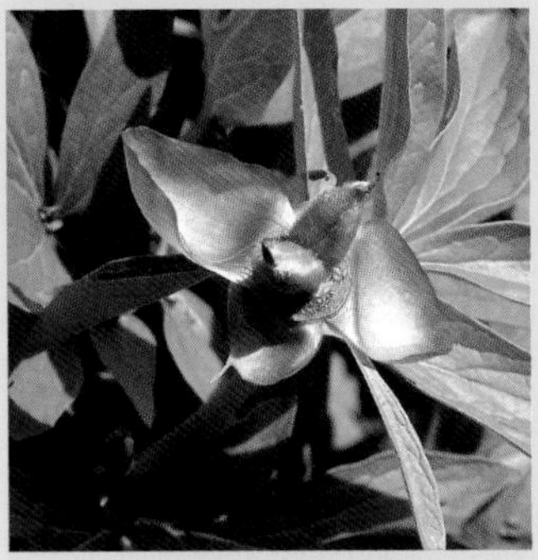

Paeonia officinalis

EUROPEAN WATER HEMLOCK

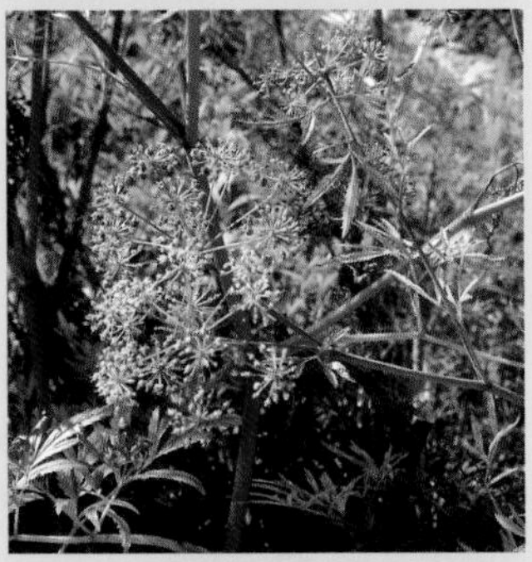

Cicuta virosa

EVENING PRIMROSE

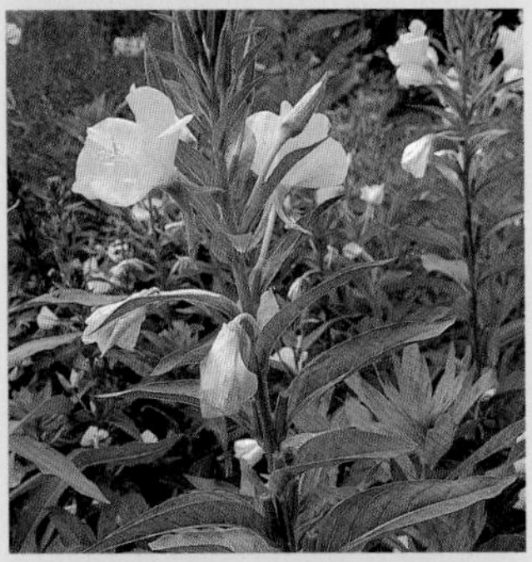

Oenothera biennis

FENNEL

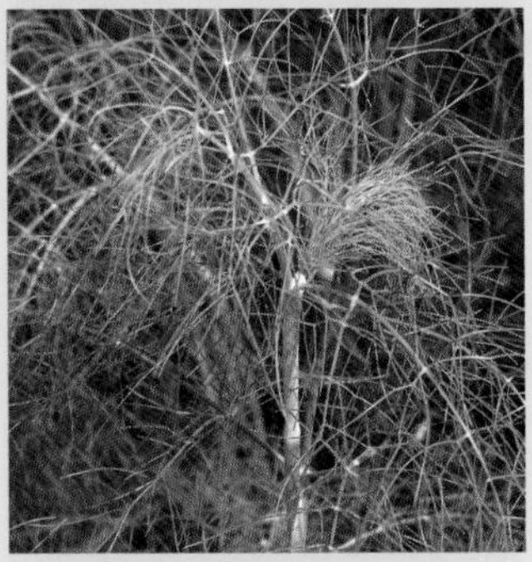

Foeniculum vulgare

FENUGREEK

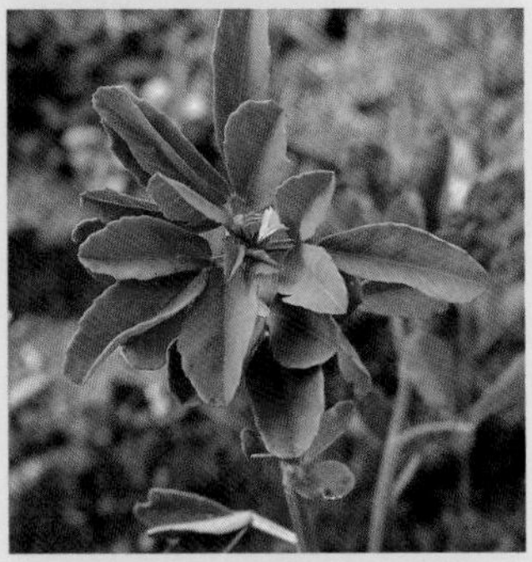

Trigonella foenum-graecum

FEVERFEW

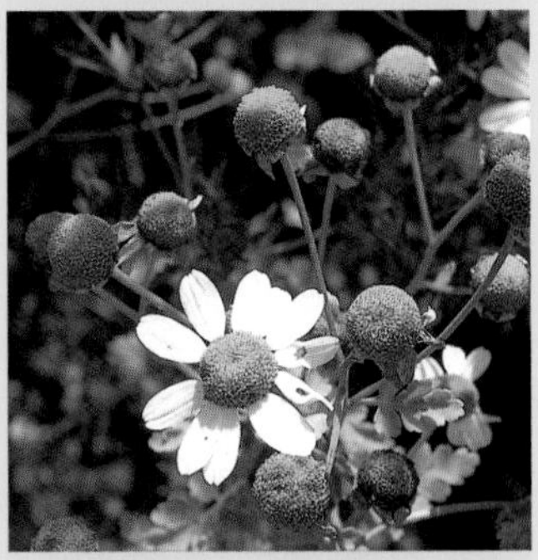

Tanacetum parthenium

FIELD SCABIOUS

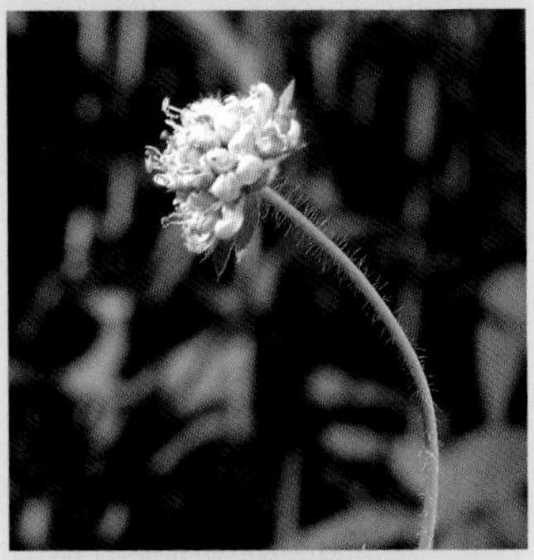

Knautia arvensis

FIGS

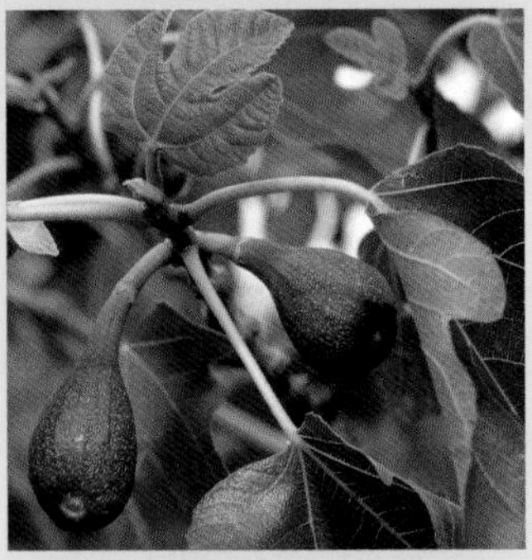

Ficus carica

FIGWORT

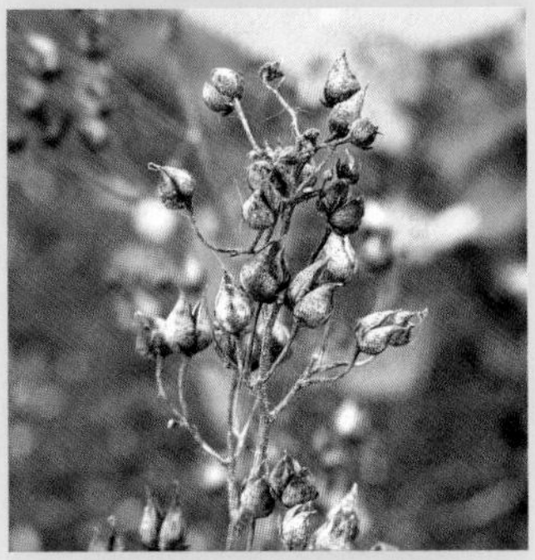

Scrophularia nodosa

FLAX

Linum usitatissimum

FOOL'S PARSLEY

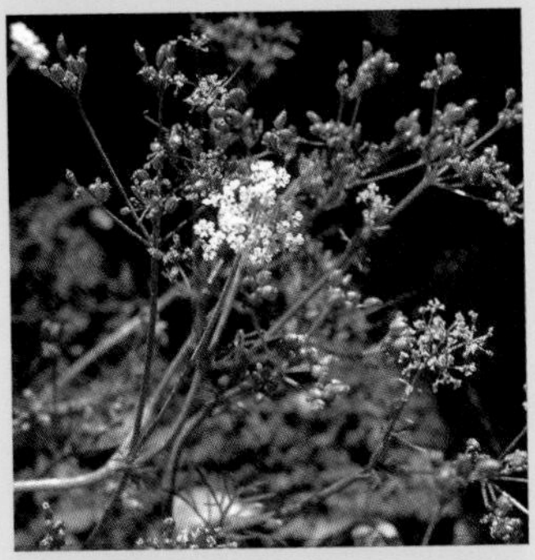

Aethusa cynapium

FORGET-ME-NOT

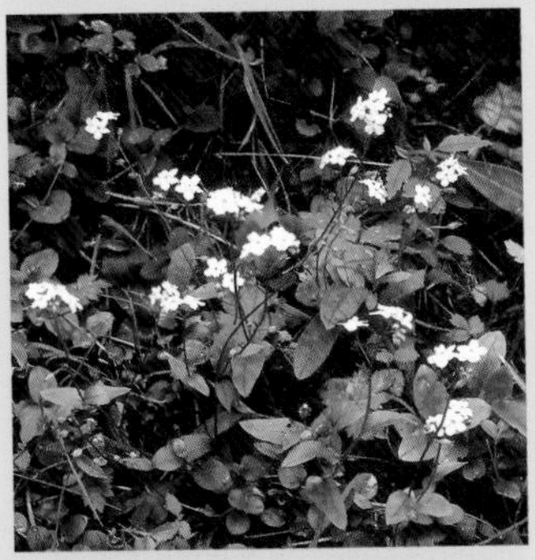

Myosotis arvensis

FRANGULA

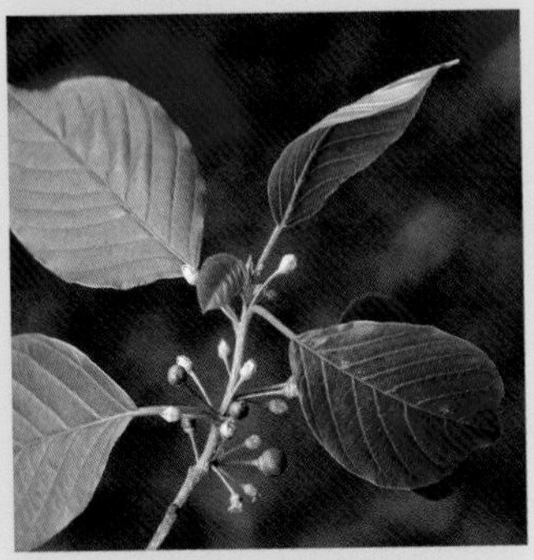

Rhamnus frangula

FRENCH TARRAGON

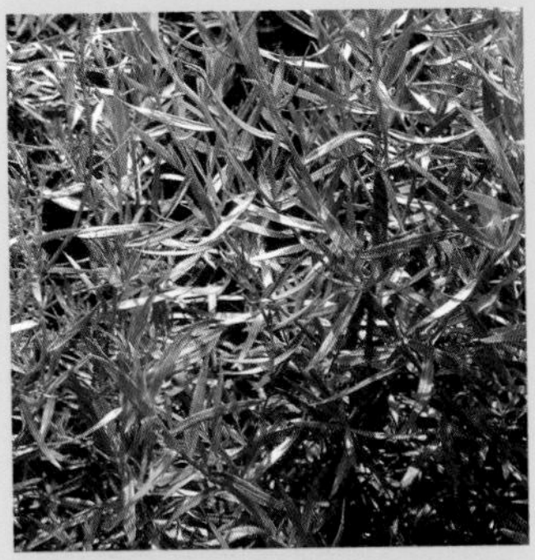

Artemisia dracunculus

FRINGETREE

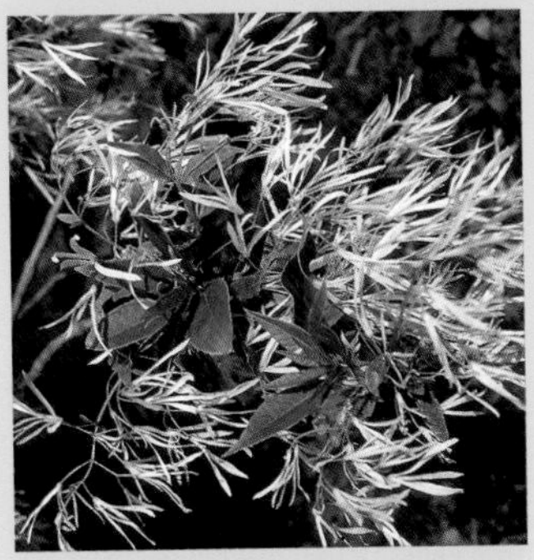

Chionanthus virginicus

FROSTWORT

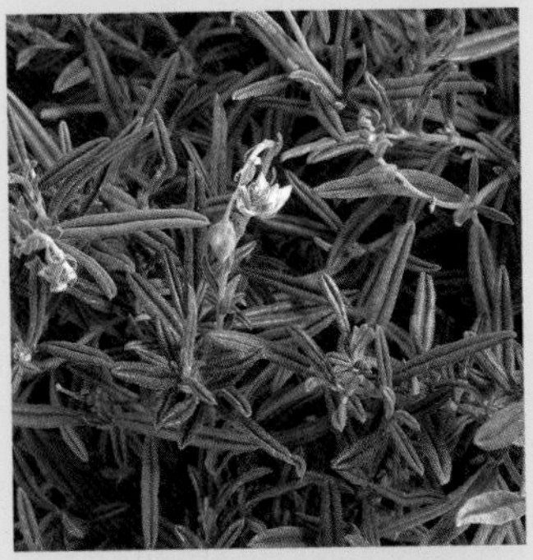

Helianthemum canadense

FUMITORY

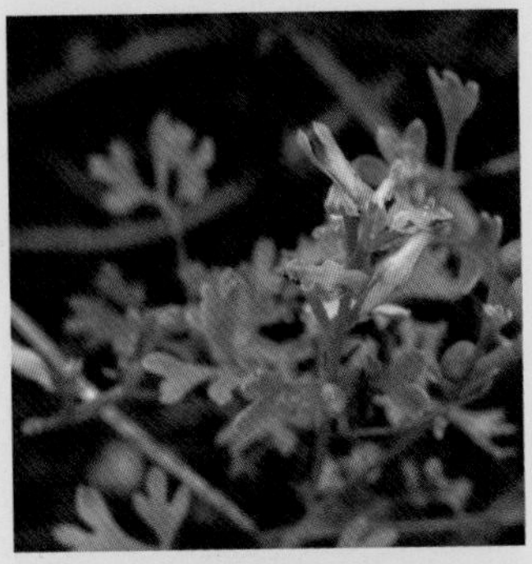

Fumaria officinalis

GAMBOGE

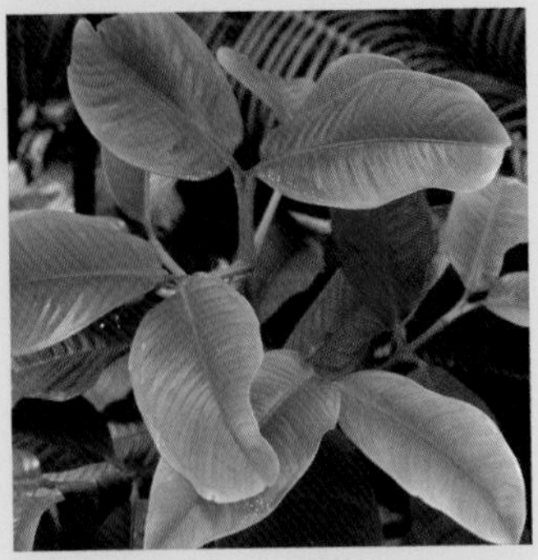

Garcinia hanburyi

GARDEN CRESS

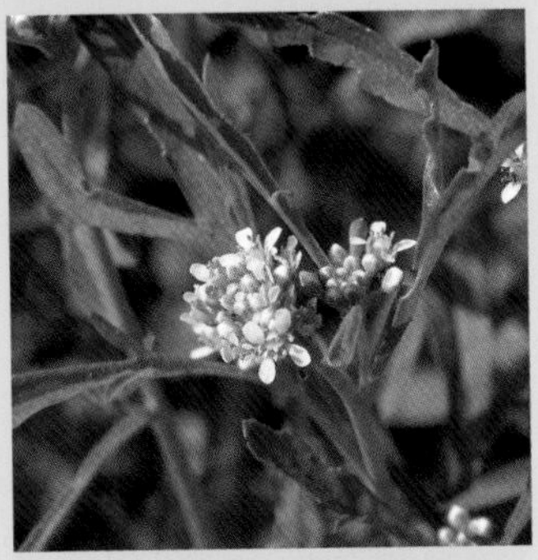

Lepidium sativum

GARLIC

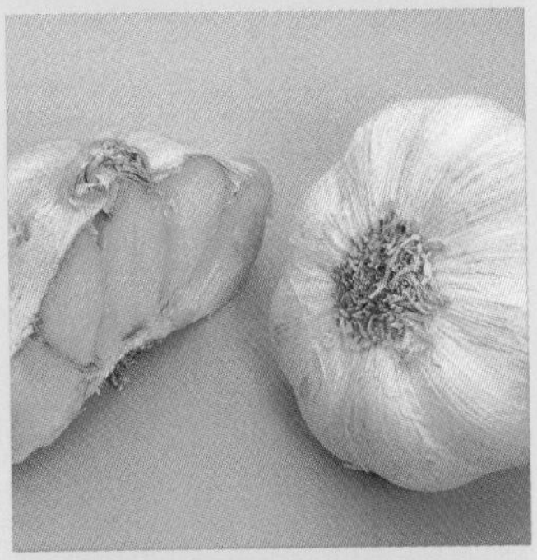

Allium sativum

GERMAN CHAMOMILE

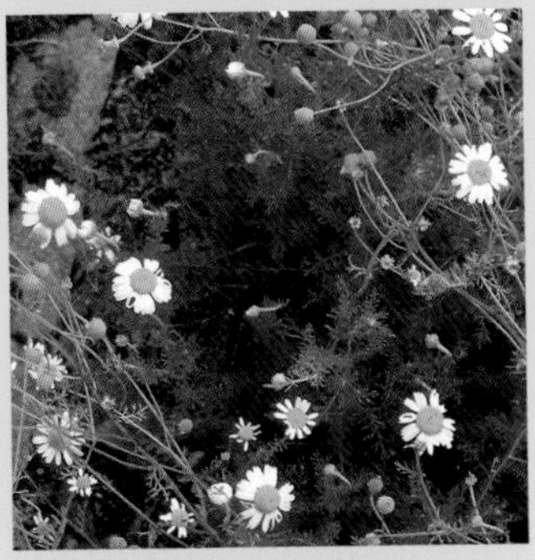

Matricaria recutita

GERMANDER

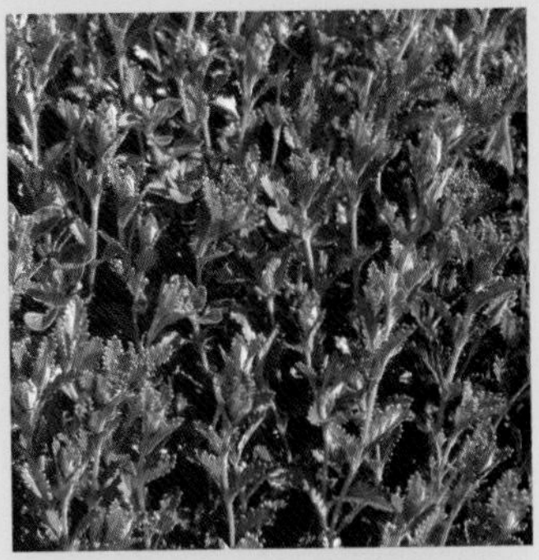

Teucrium chamaedrys

GINGER

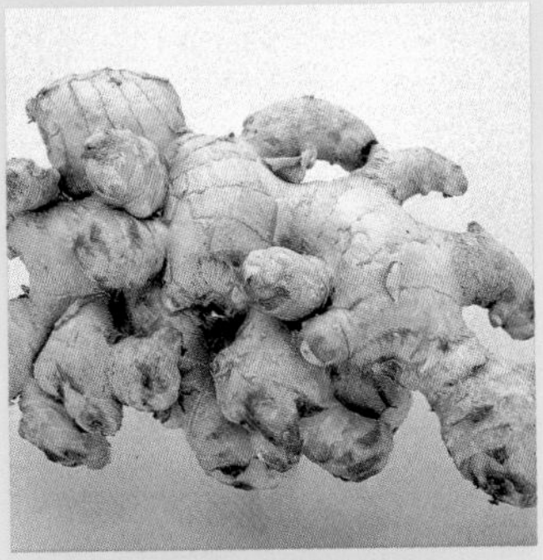

Zingiber officinale

GINKGO

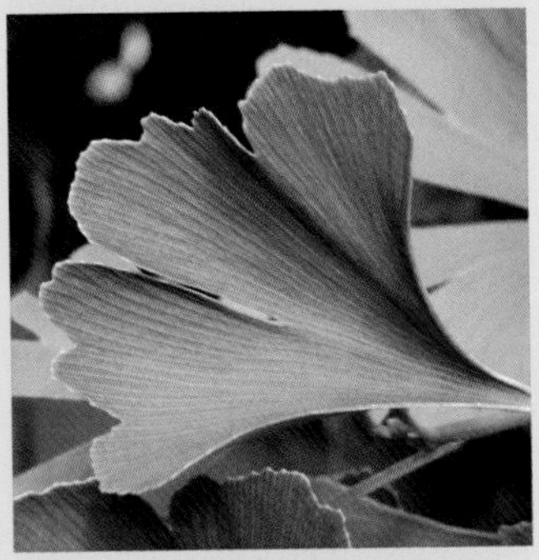

Ginkgo biloba

GLOBE FLOWER

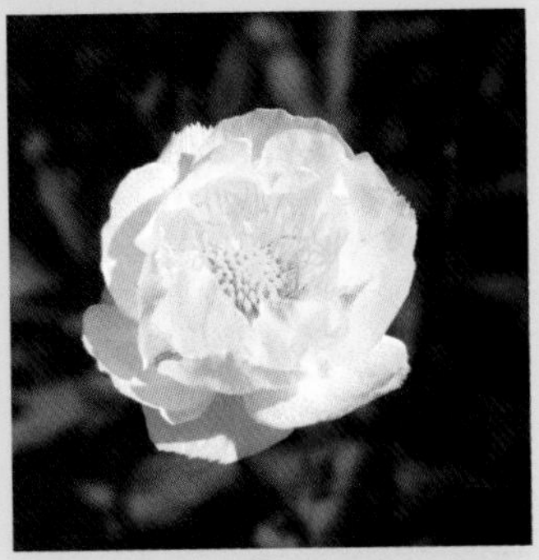

Trollius europaeus

GOAT'S RUE

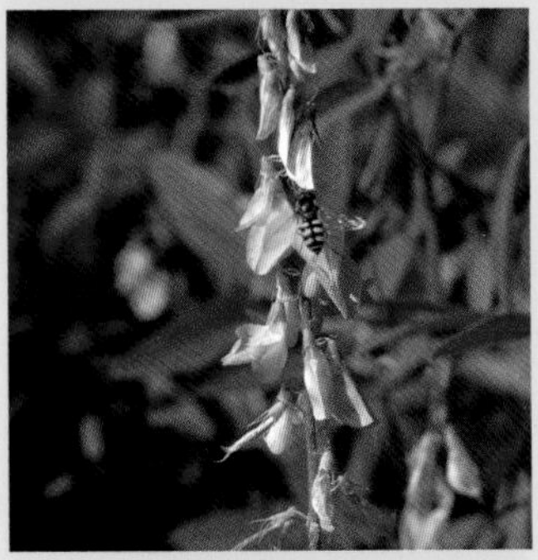

Galega officinalis

GOLDEN SHOWER TREE

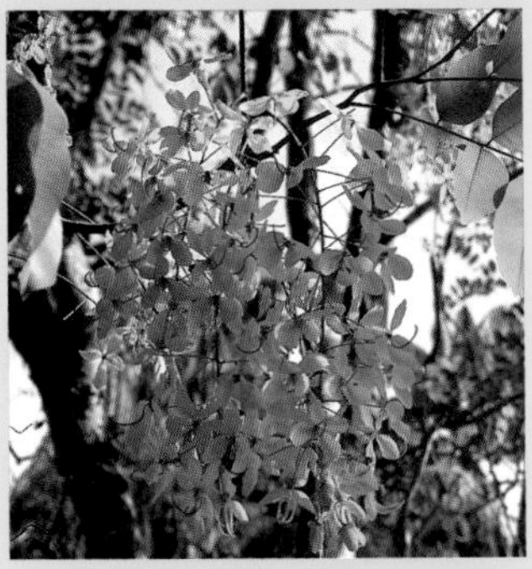

Cassia fistula

GOLDENSEAL

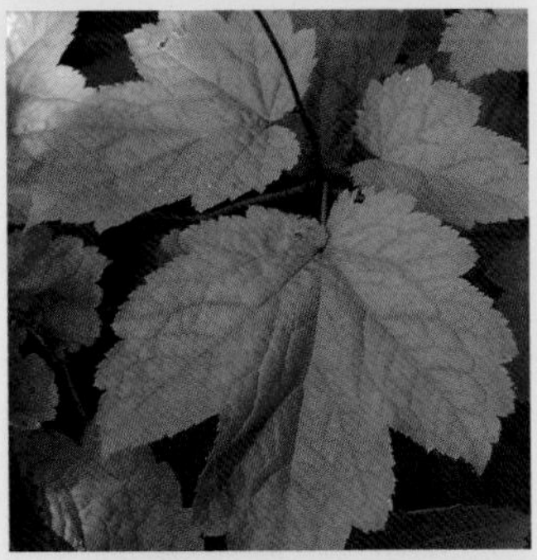

Hydrastis canadensis

GOTU KOLA

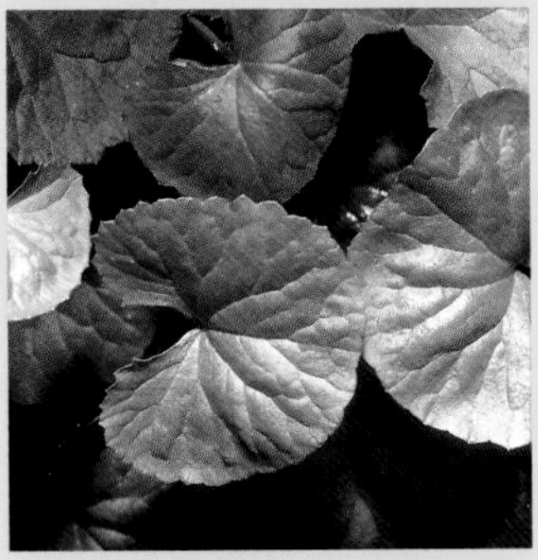

Centella asiatica

GOUTWEED

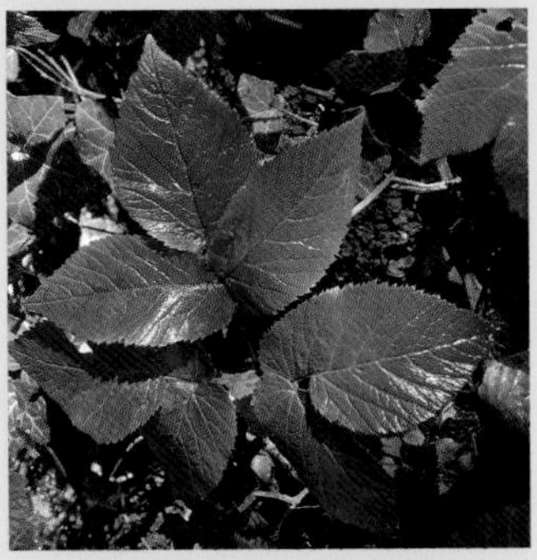

Aegopodium podagraria

GRAINS OF PARADISE

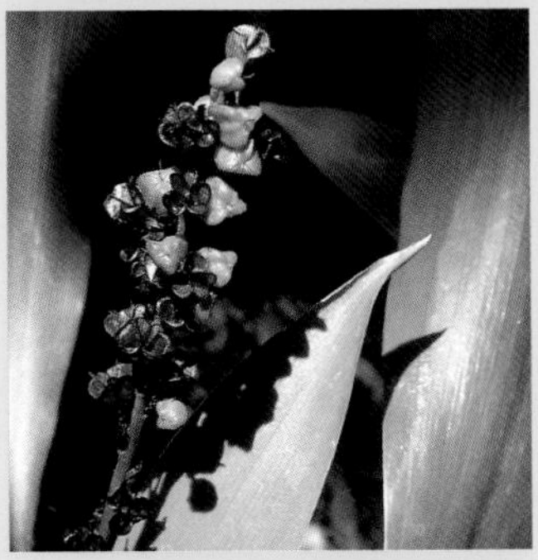

Aframomum melegueta

GRAPE

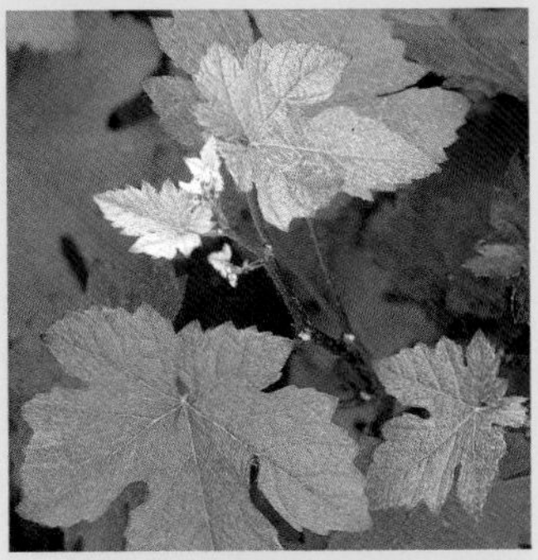

Vitis vinifera

GREAT BURNET

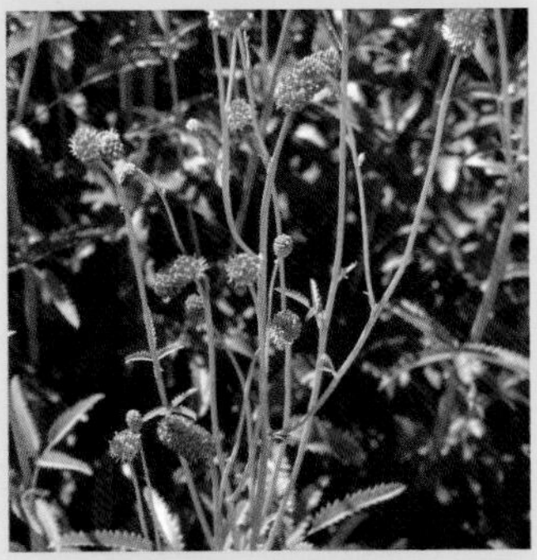

Sanguisorba officinalis

GREATER BINDWEED

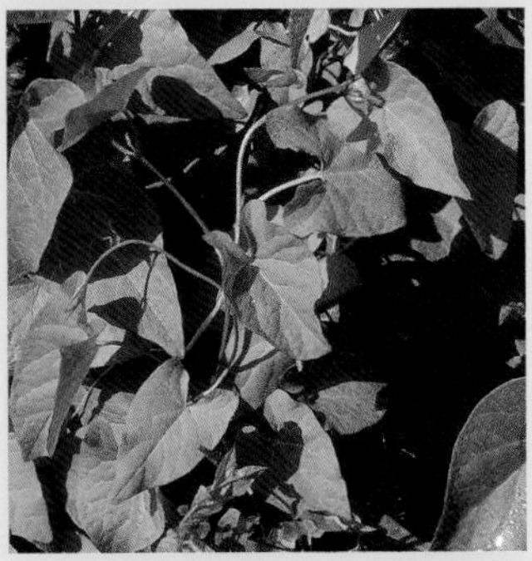

Calystegia sepium

GREEN TEA

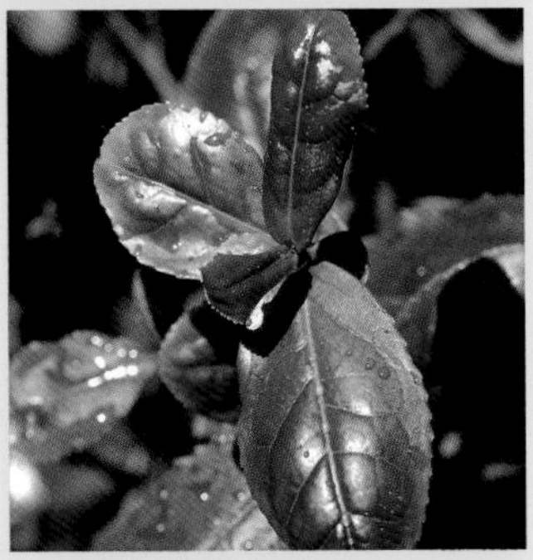

Camellia sinensis

GROUND PINE

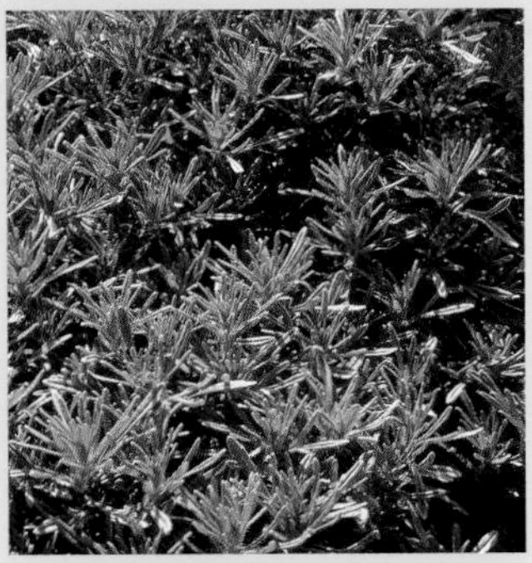

Ajuga chamaepitys

HEATHER

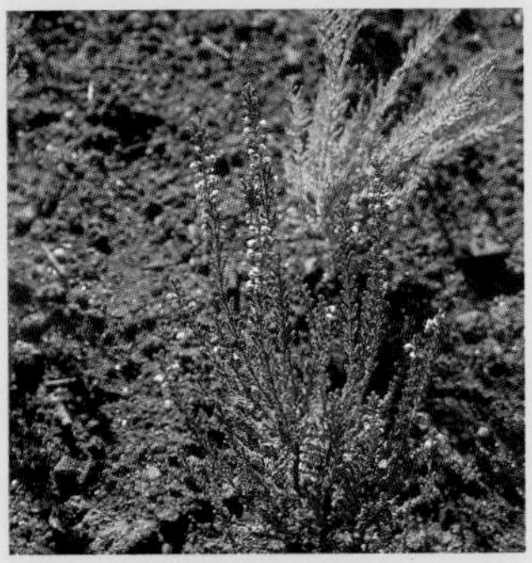

Calluna vulgaris

HEDGE-HYSSOP

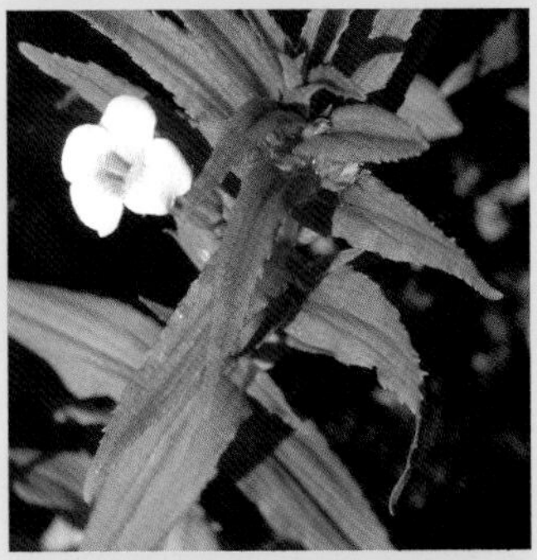

Gratiola officinalis

HEMLOCK

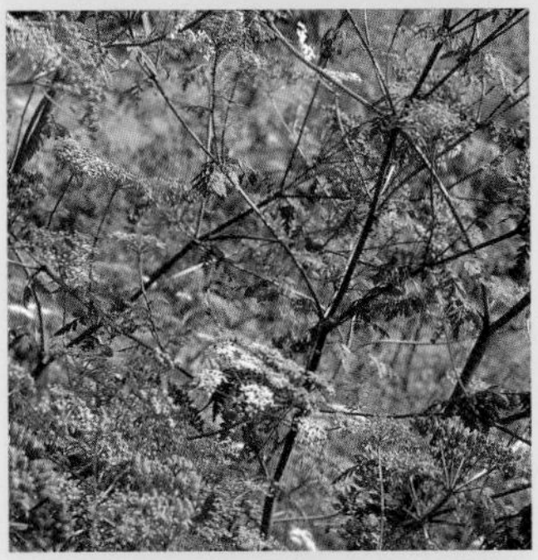

Conium maculatum

HEMP AGRIMONY

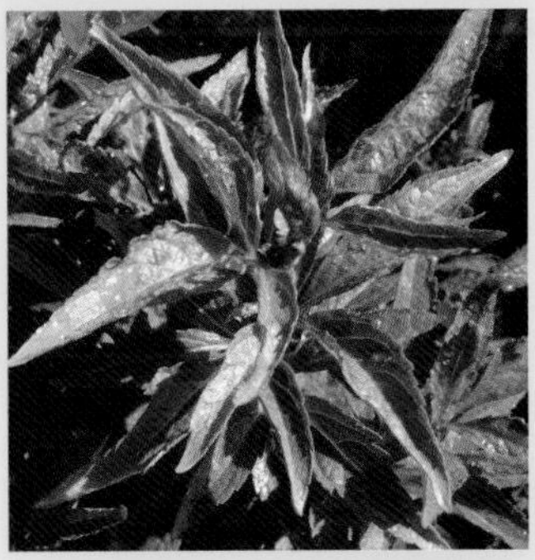

Eupatorium cannabinum

HEMPNETTLE

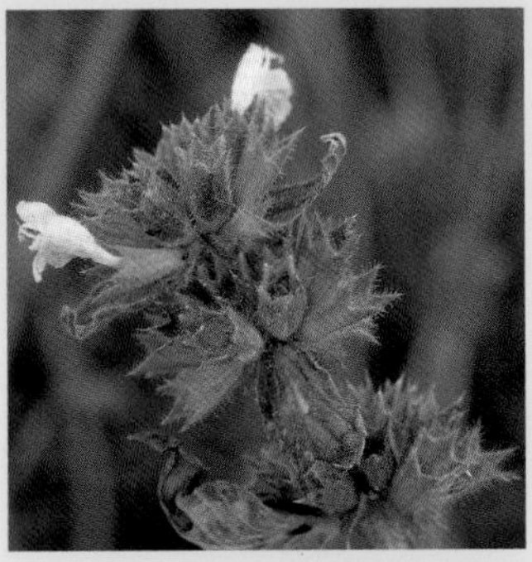

Galeopsis segetum

HENBANE

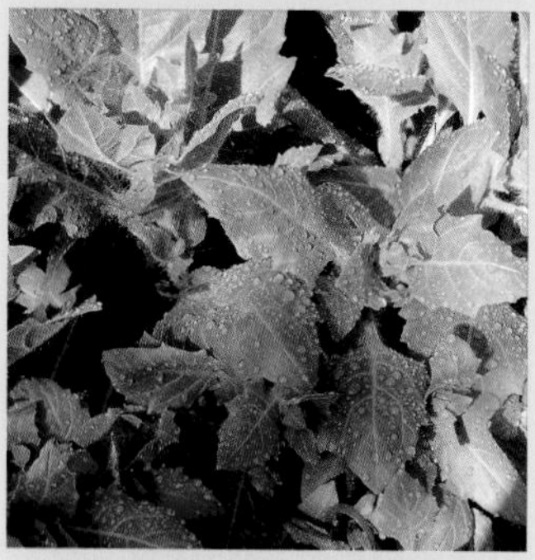

Hyoscyamus niger

HENNA

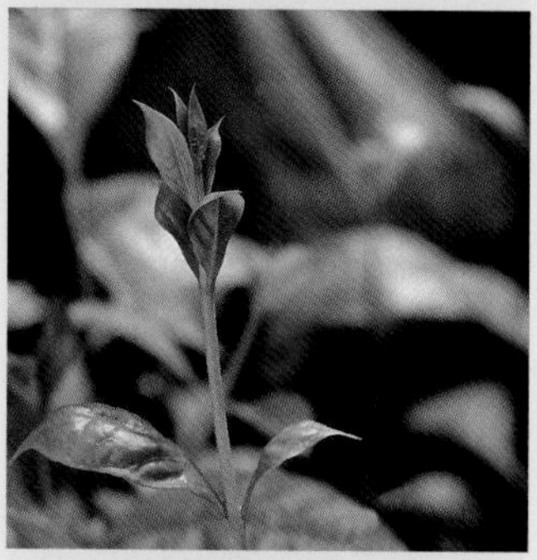

Lawsonia inermis

HERB PARIS

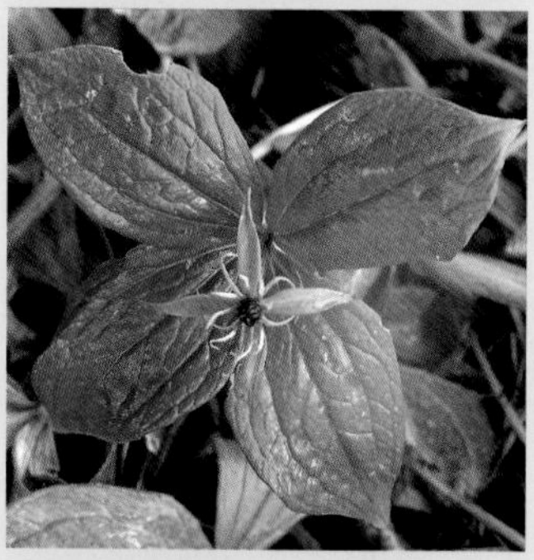

Paris quadrifolia

HERB ROBERT

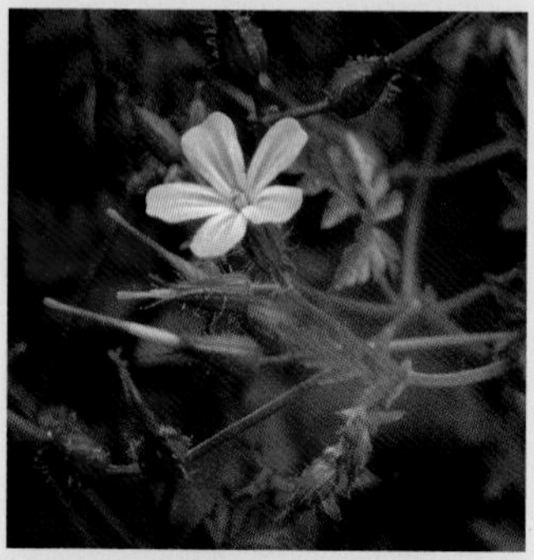

Geranium robertianum

HIBISCUS

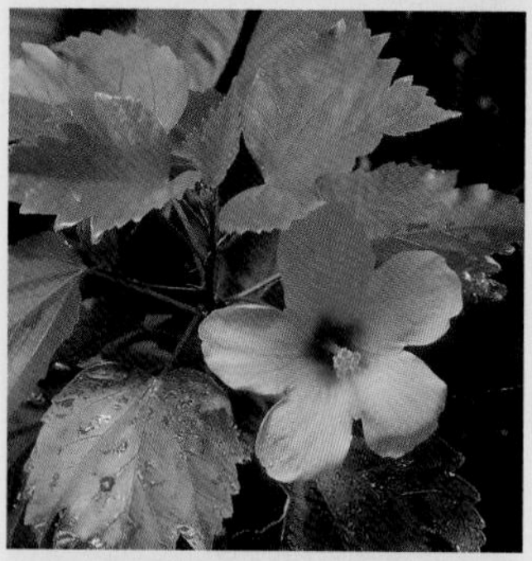

Hibiscus sabdariffa

HIGH MALLOW

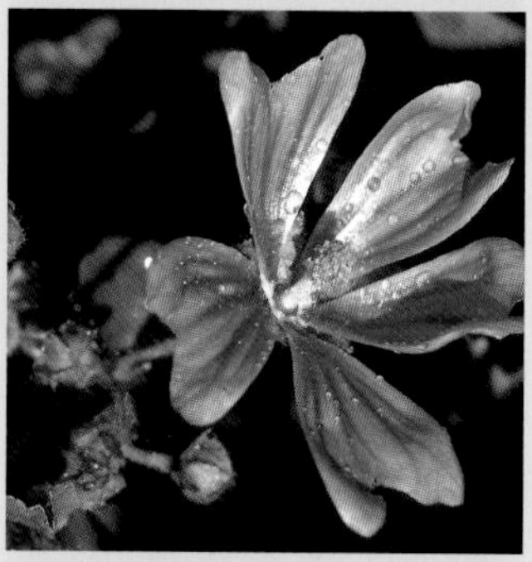

Malva sylvestris

HOGWEED

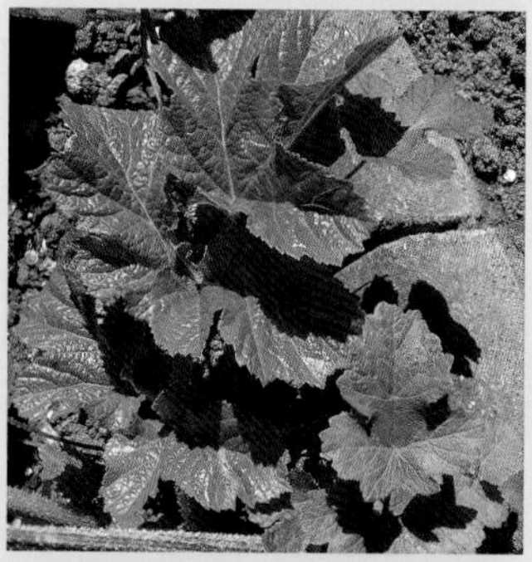

Heracleum sphondylium

HOLLY

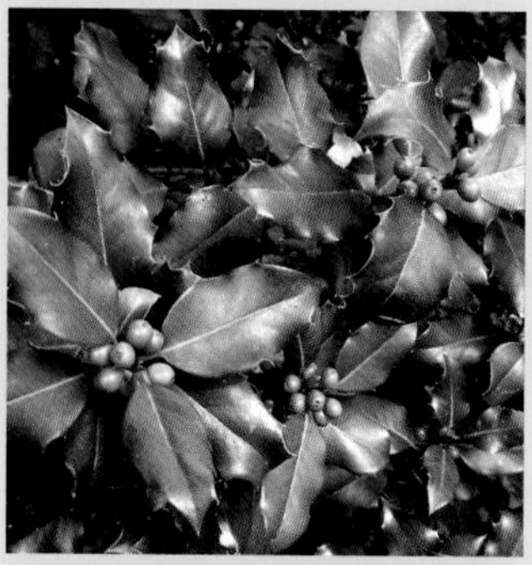

Ilex aquifolium

HOLLYHOCK

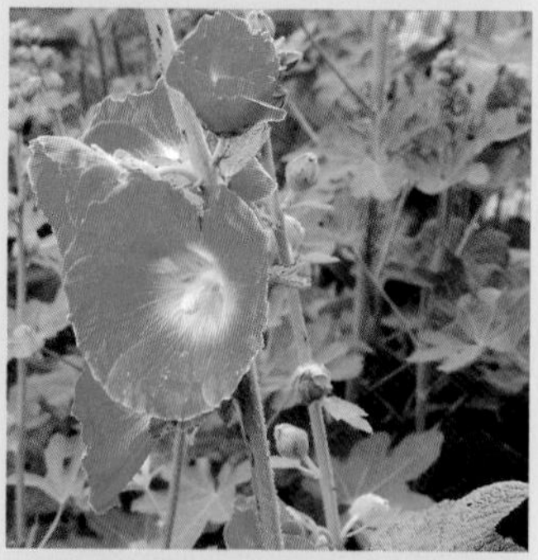

Alcea rosea

HOPS

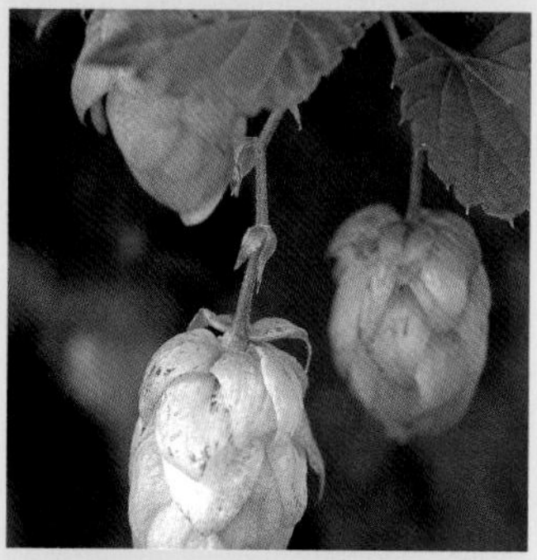

Humulus lupulus

HOREHOUND

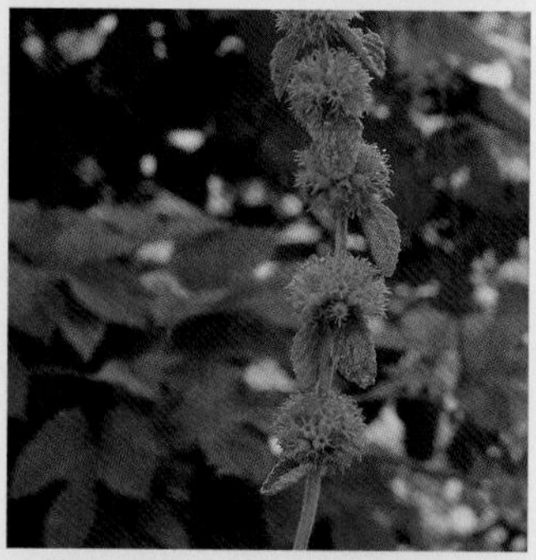

Marrubium vulgare

HORSE CHESTNUT

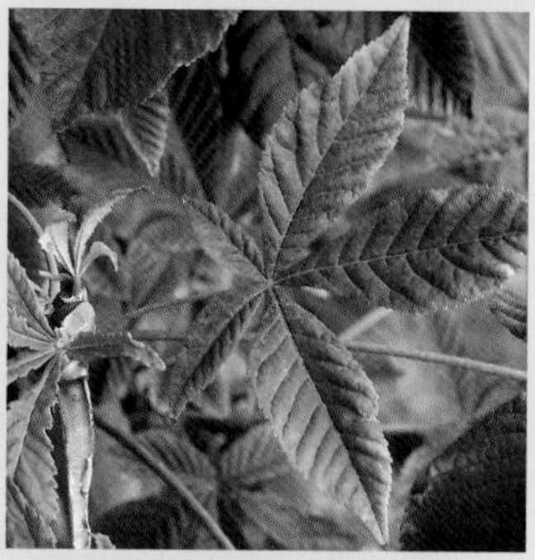

Aesculus hippocastanum

HORSERADISH

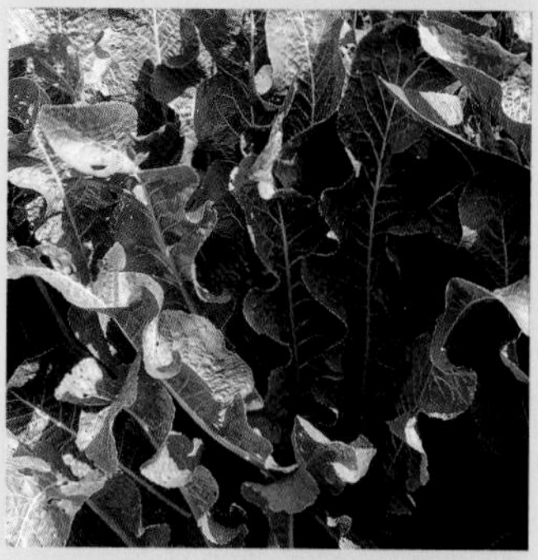

Armoracia rusticana

HORSETAIL

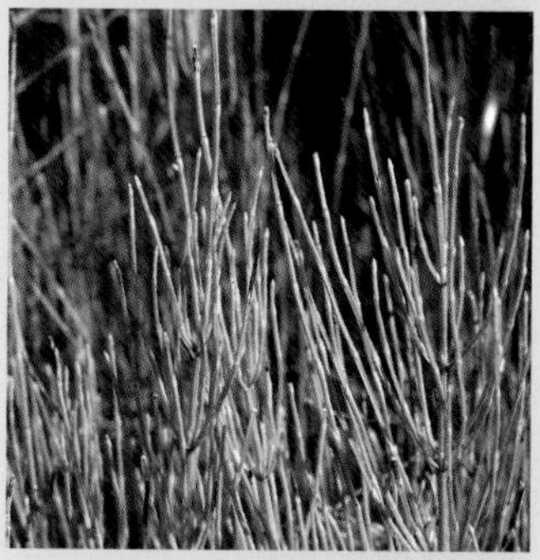

Equisetum arvense

HOUSELEEK

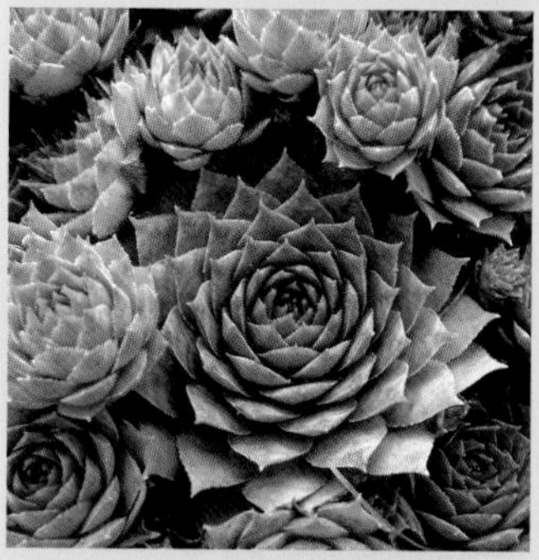

Sempervivum tectorum

HYDRANGEA

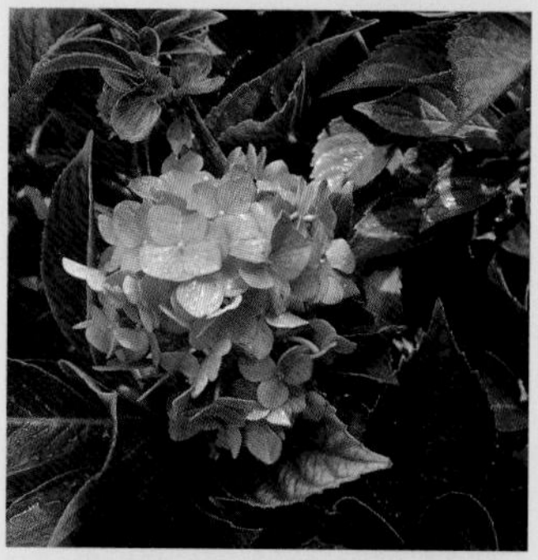

Hydrangea arborescens

HYSSOP

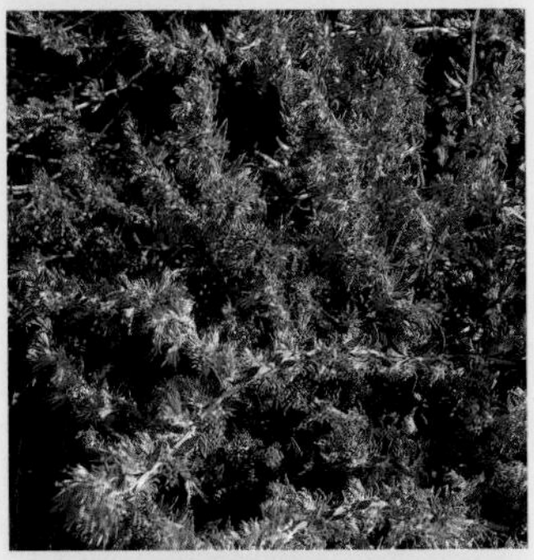

Hyssopus officinalis

JABORANDI

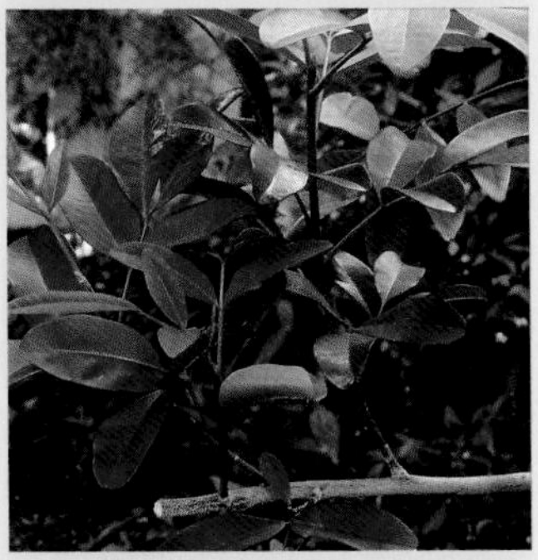

Pilocarpus microphyllus

JACOB'S LADDER

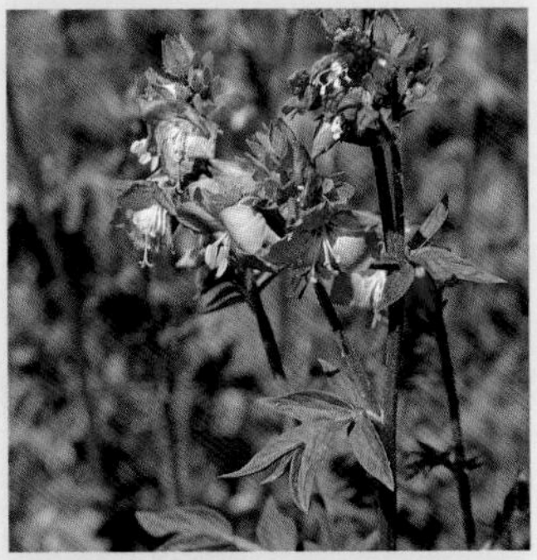

Polemonium caeruleum

JALAP

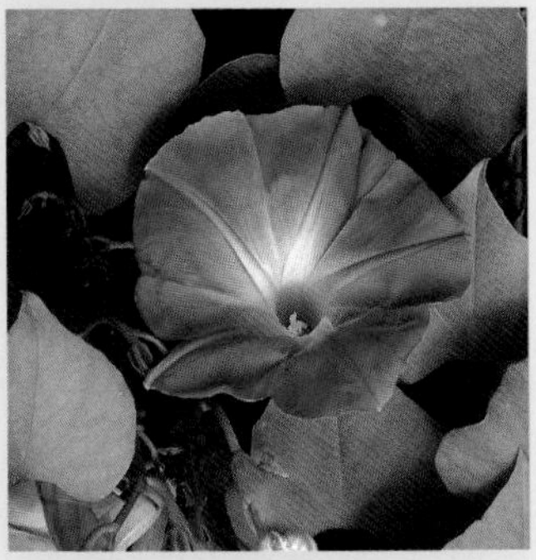

Ipomoea purga

JASMINE

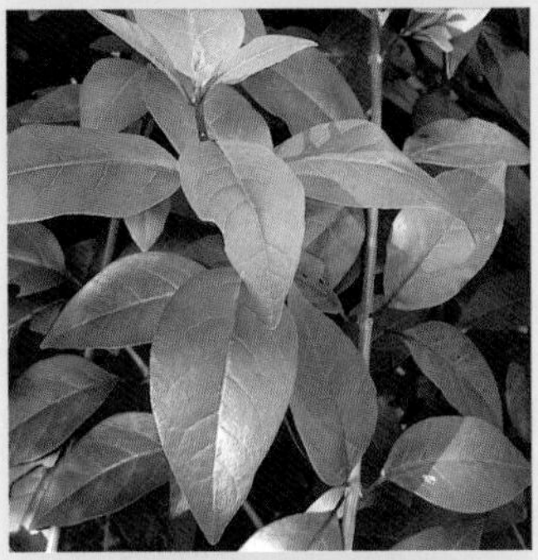

Jasminum officinale

JIMSON WEED

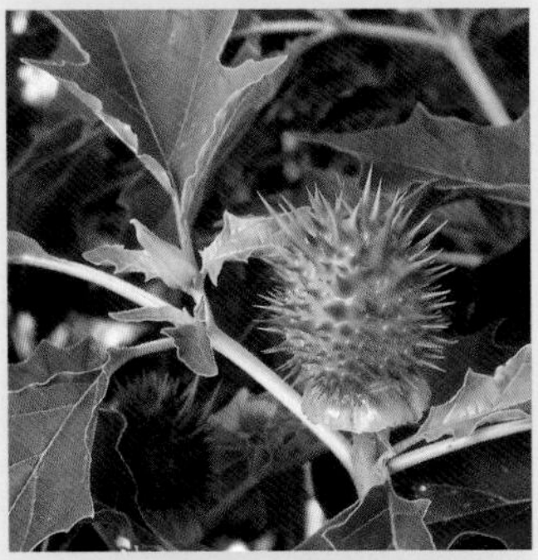

Datura stramonium

JOJOBA

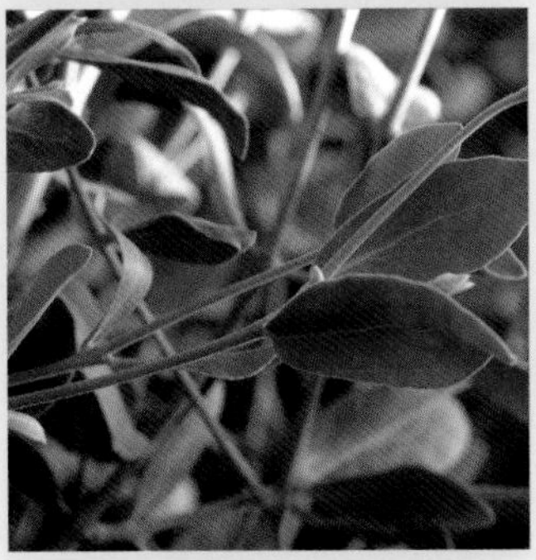

Simmondsia chinesis

JUNIPER

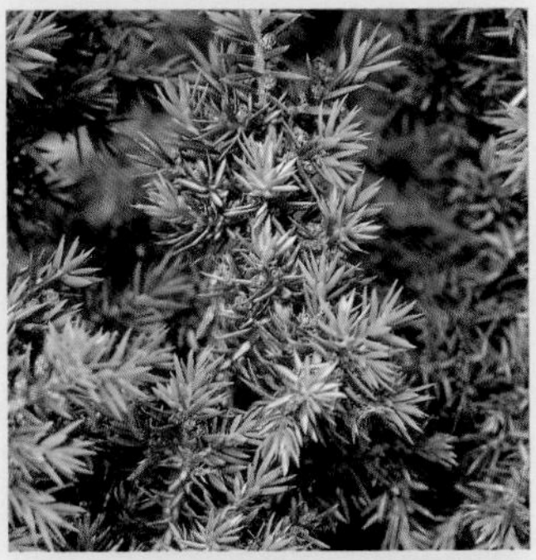

Juniperus communis

KAVA KAVA

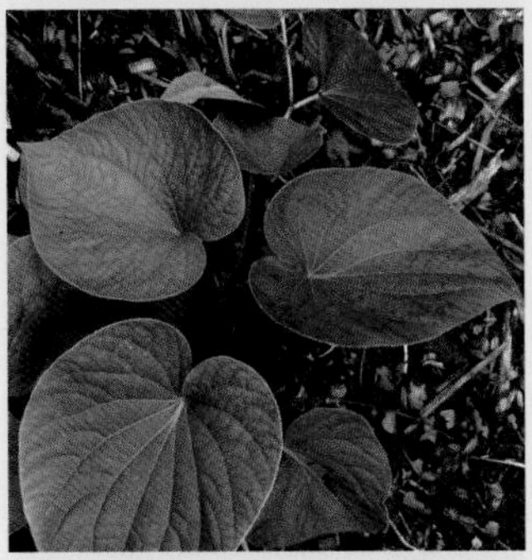

Piper methysticum

KNOTWEED

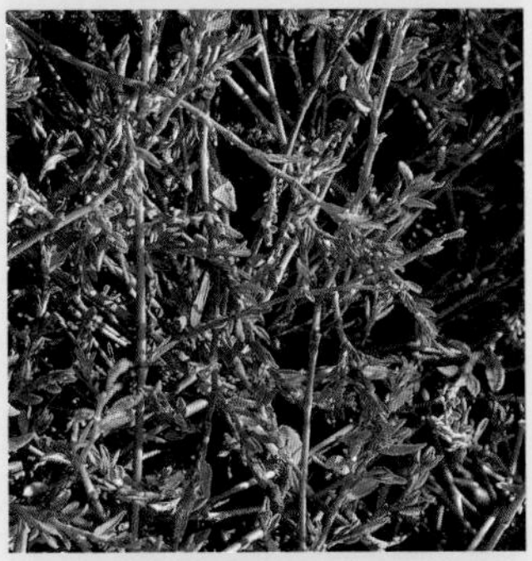

Polygonum aviculare

LADY FERN

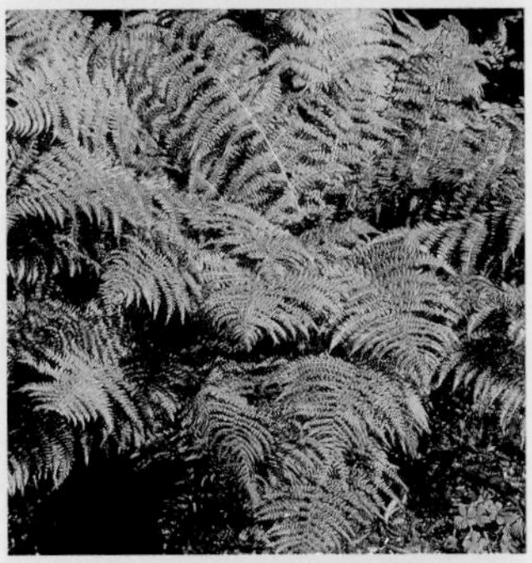

Athyrium filix-femina

LADY'S BEDSTRAW

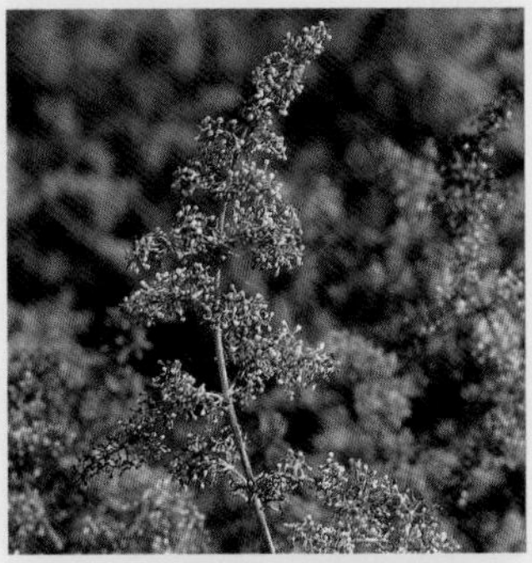

Galium verum

LADY'S MANTLE

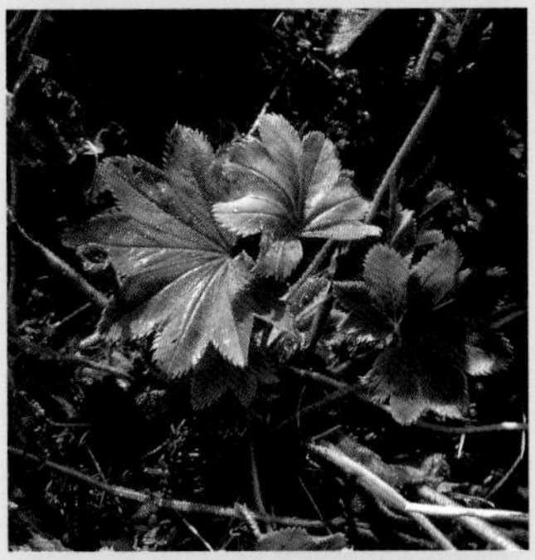

Alchemilla vulgaris

LARCH

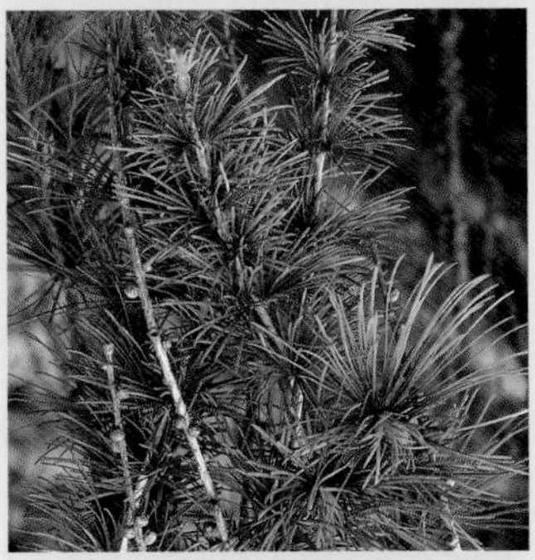

Larix decidua

LARKSPUR

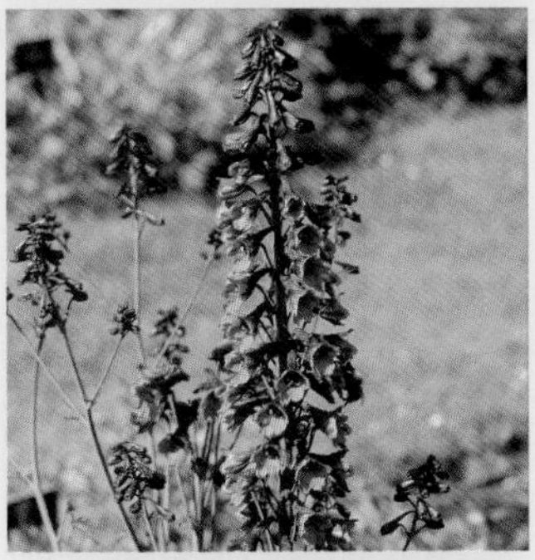

Delphinium consolida

LAUREL

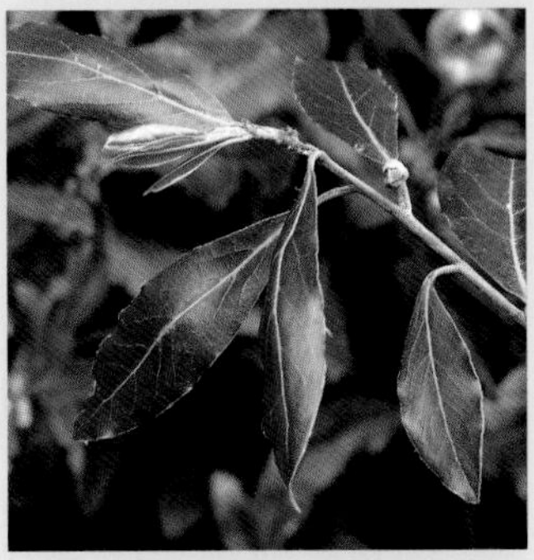

Laurus nobilis

LAVENDER COTTON

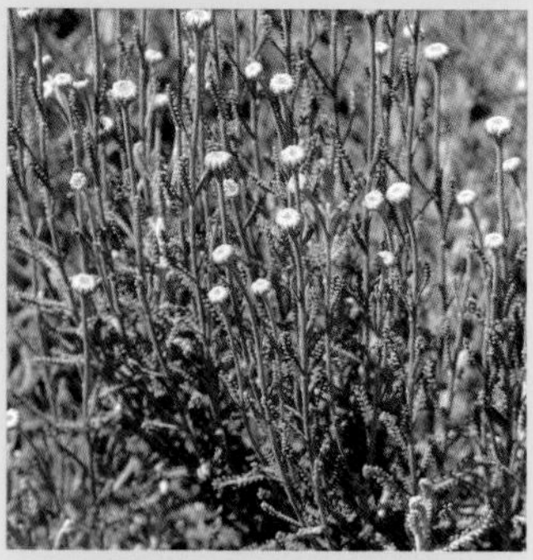

Santolina chamaecyparissias

LEMON BALM

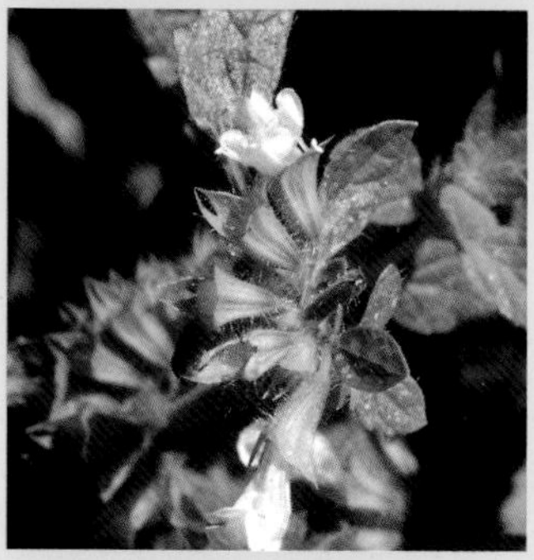

Melissa officinalis

LEMONGRASS

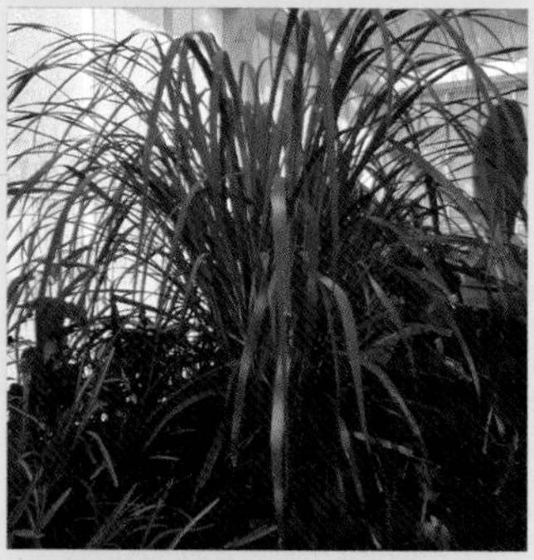

Cymbopogon citratus

LEVANT COTTON

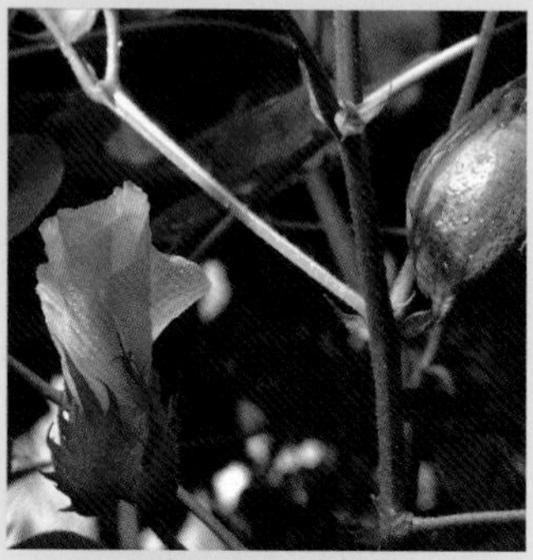

Gossypium herbaceum

LICORICE

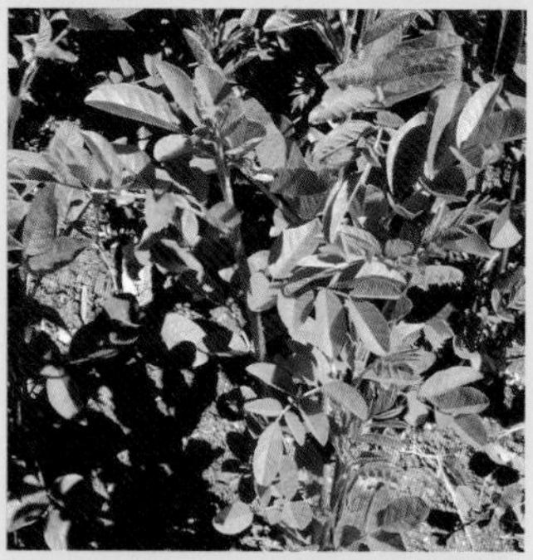

Glycyrrhiza glabra

LILY-OF-THE-VALLEY

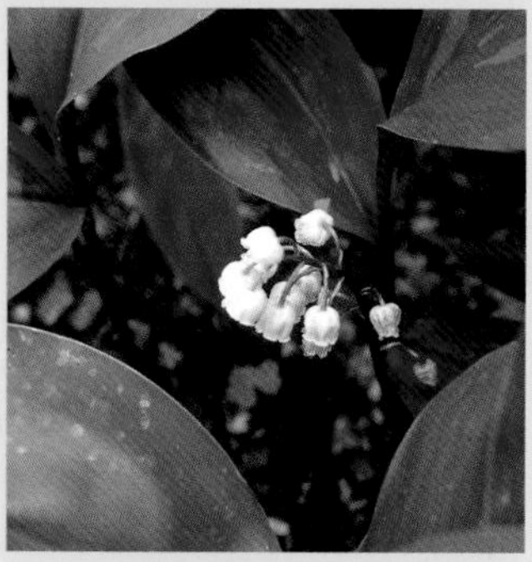

Convallaria majalis

LIME

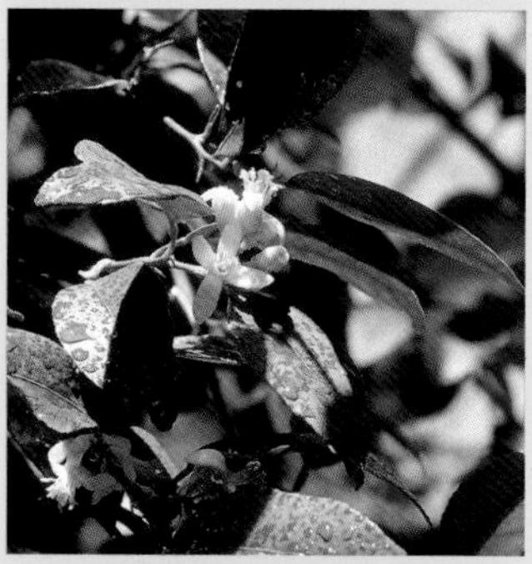

Citrus aurantifolia

LINDEN

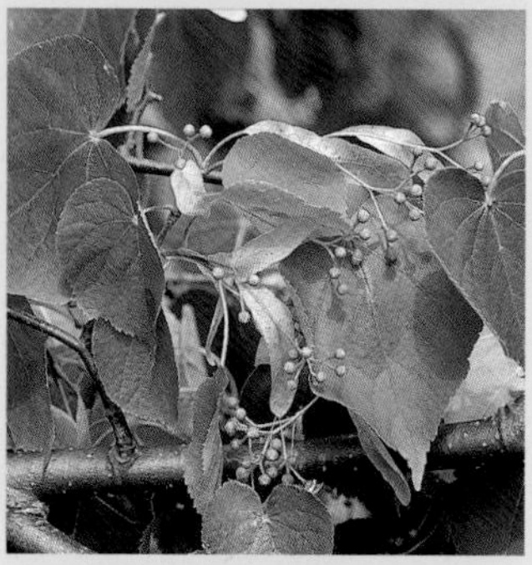

Tilia species

LOBELIA

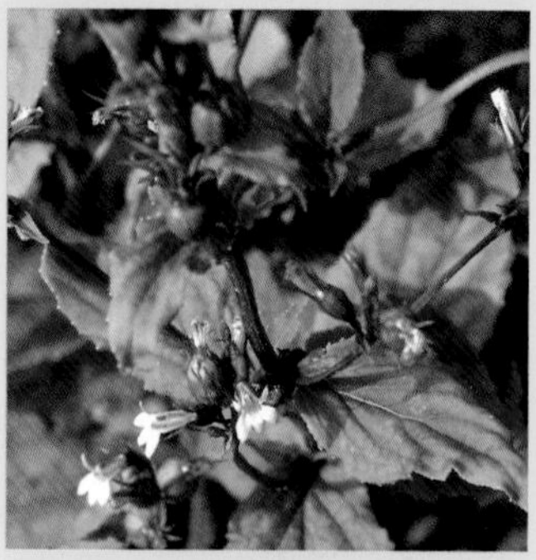

Lobelia inflata

LOOSESTRIFE

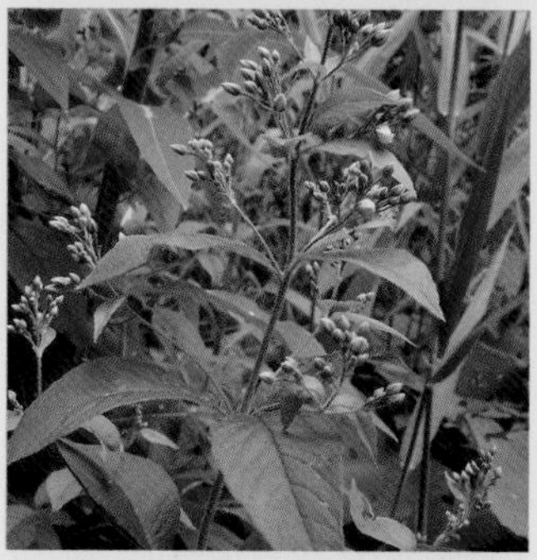

Lysimachia vulgaris

LOTUS

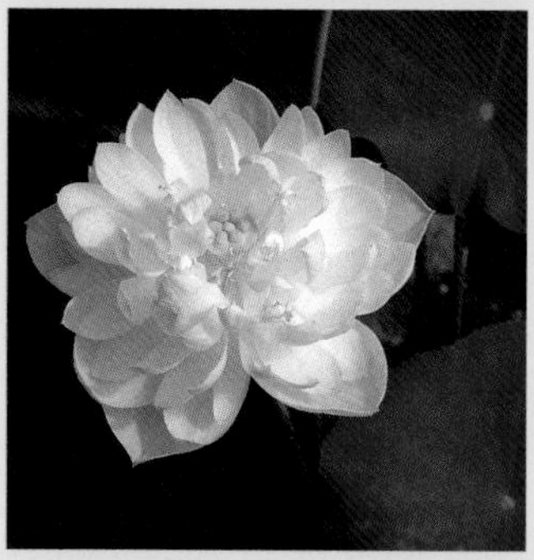

Nelumbo nucifera

LOVAGE

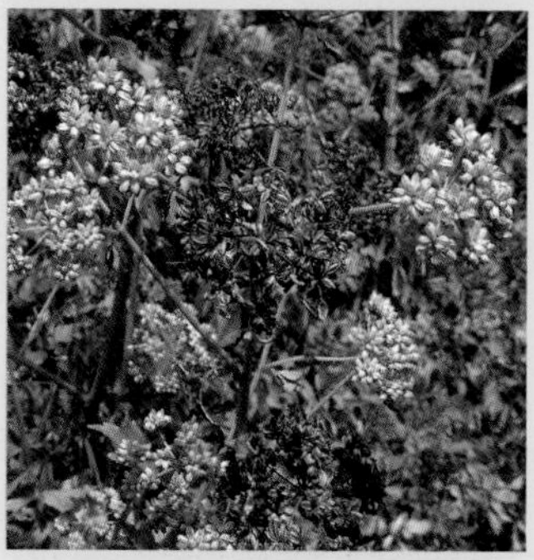

Levisticum officinale

LUFFA

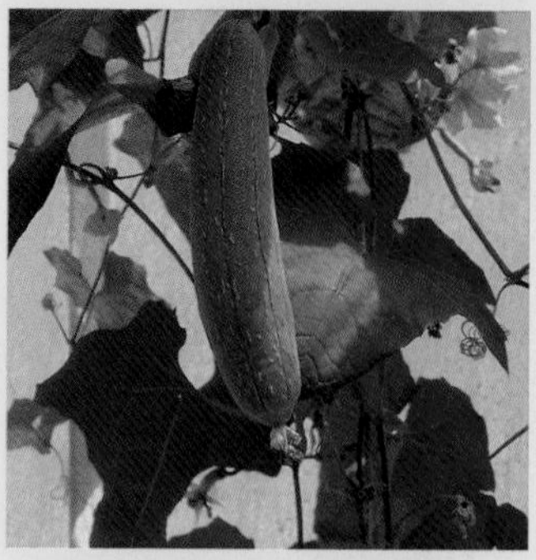

Luffa aegyptica

LUNGWORT

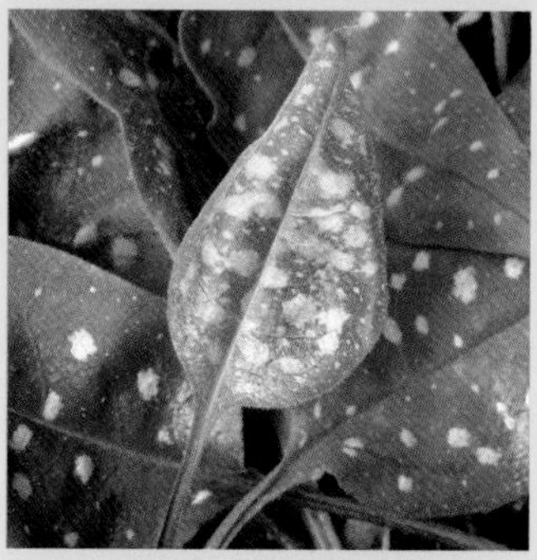

Pulmonaria officinalis

MADDER

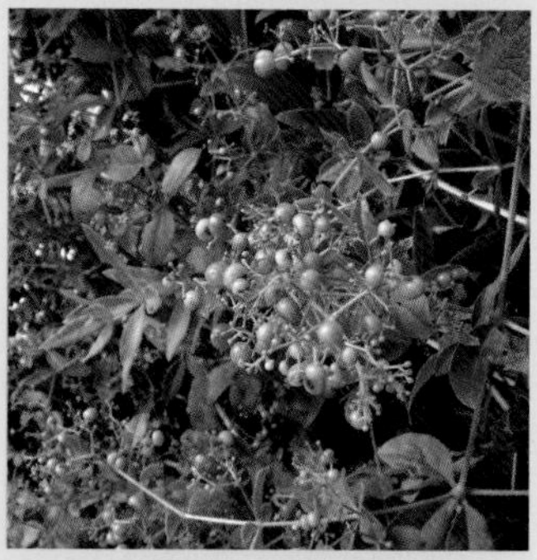

Rubia tinctorum

MA-HUANG

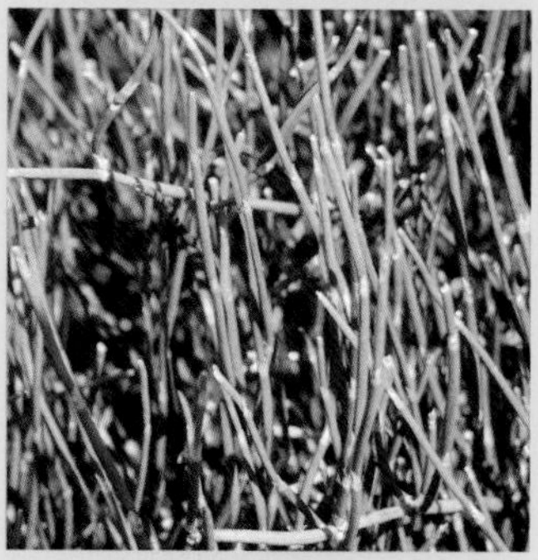

Ephedra sinica

MALABAR NUT

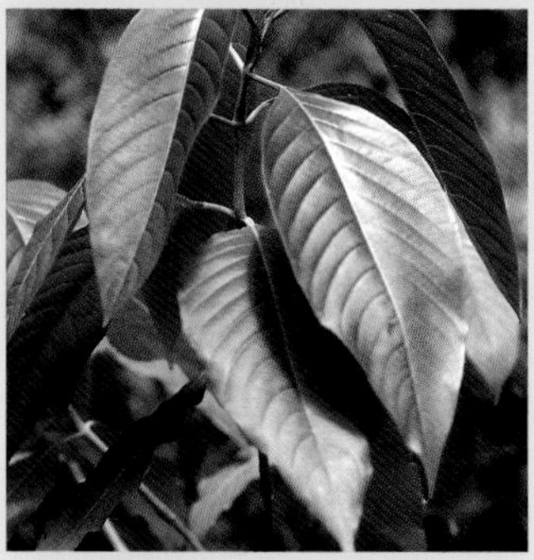

Justicia adhatoda

MALE FERN

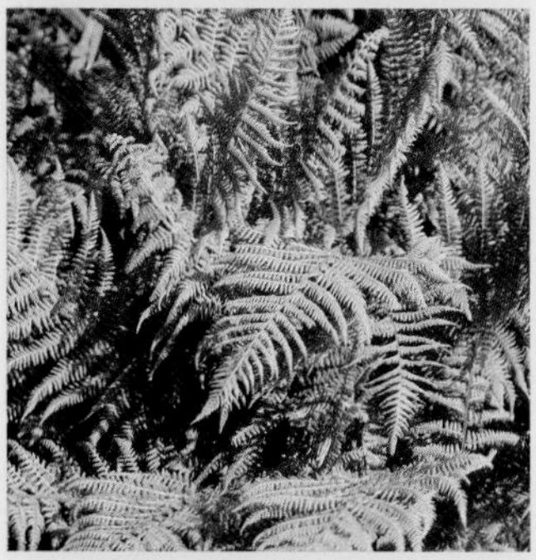

Dryopteris filix-mas

MANDRAKE

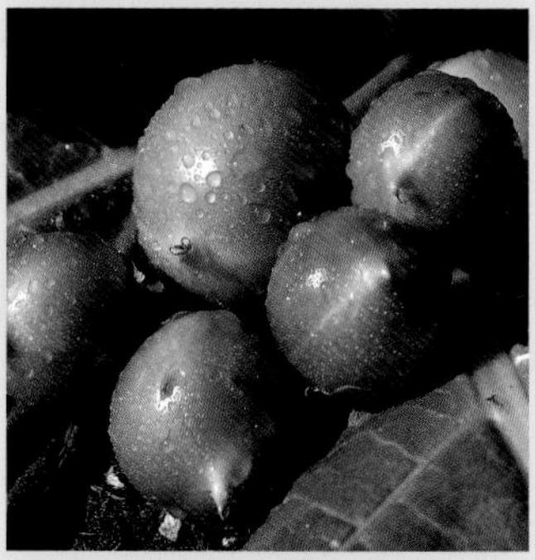

Mandragora officinarum

MANNA

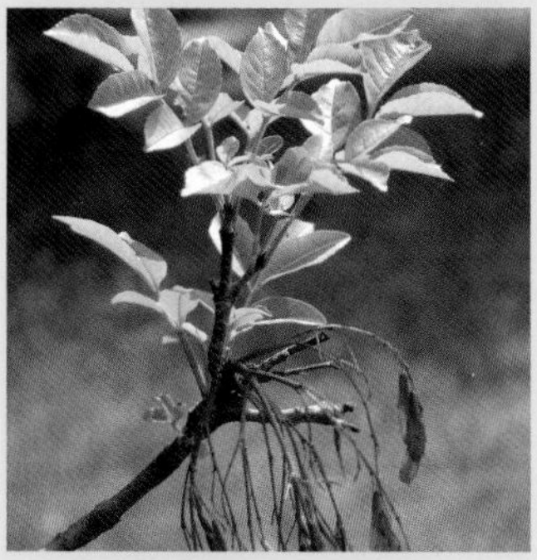

Fraxinus ornus

MARIGOLD

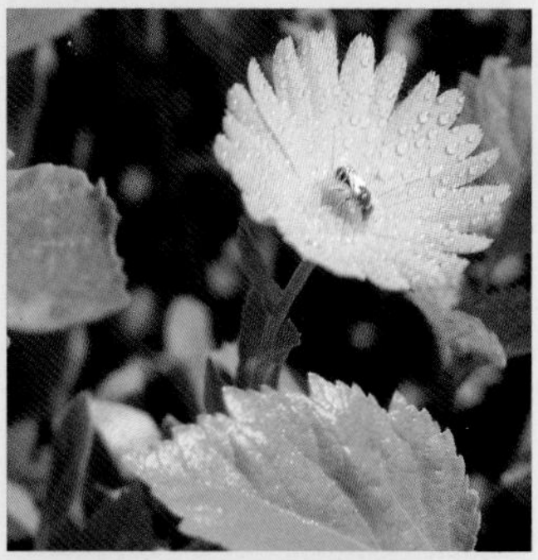

Calendula officinalis

MARIJUANA

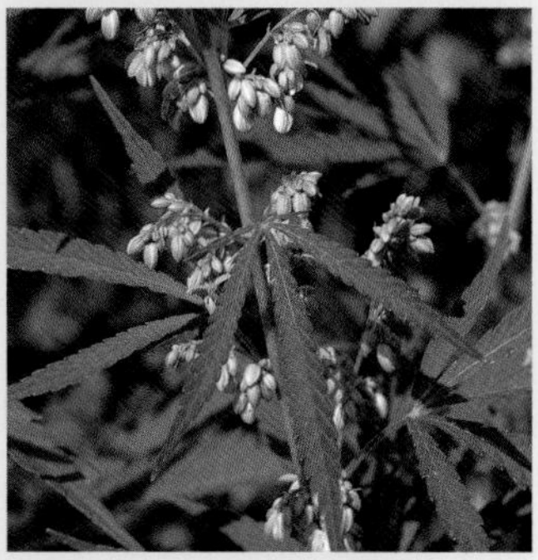

Cannabis sativa

MARSH BLAZING STAR

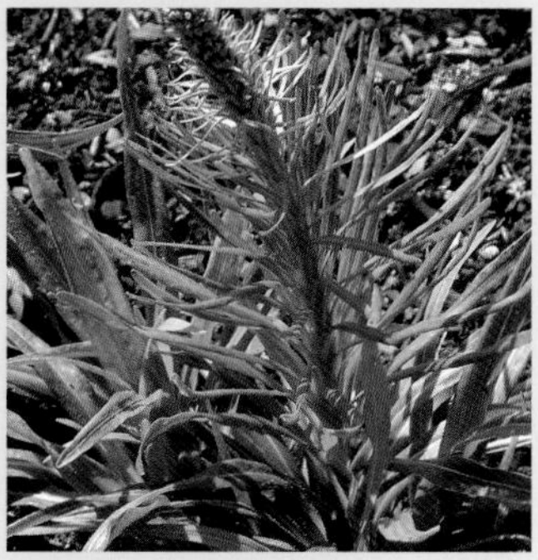

Liatris spicata

MARSH MARIGOLD

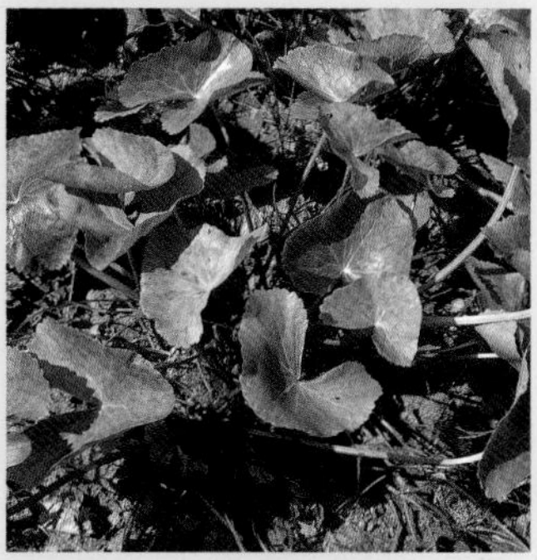

Caltha palustris

MASTIC TREE

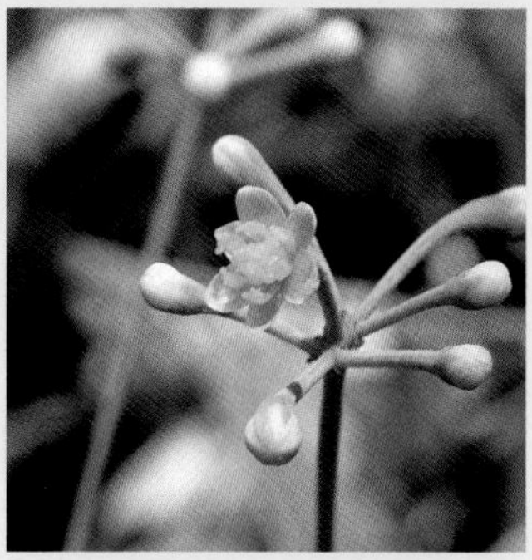

Pistacia lentiscus

MATÉ

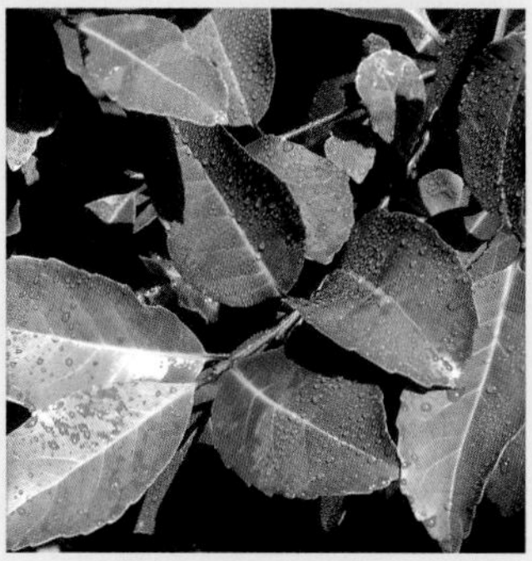

Ilex paraguariensis

MAYAPPLE

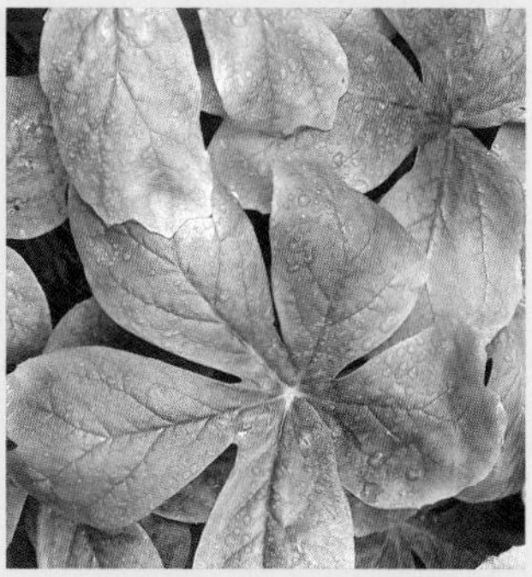

Podophylium peltatum

MEADOWSWEET

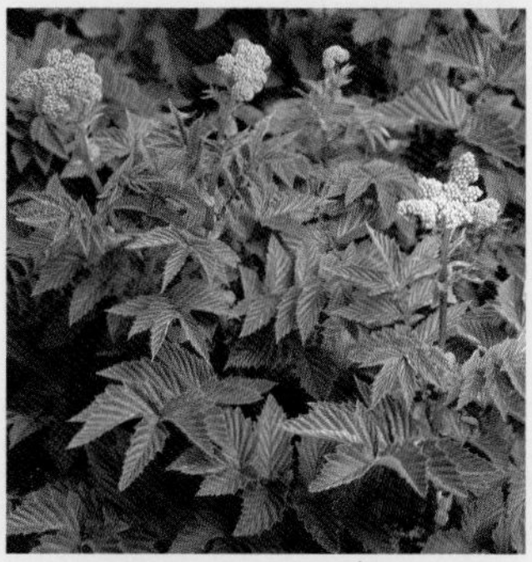

Filipendula ulmaria

MERCURY HERB

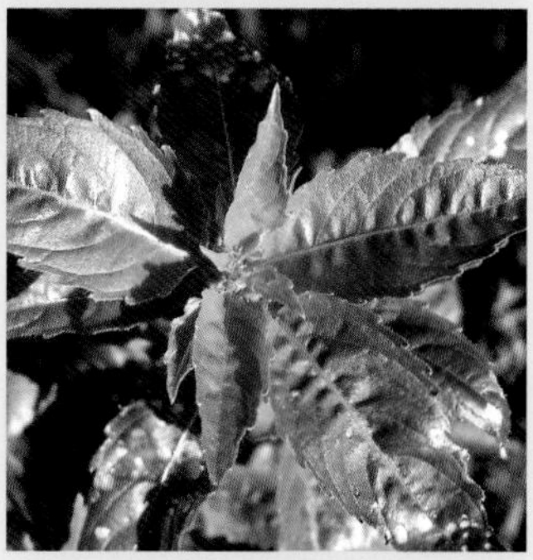

Mercurialis annua

MEZEREON

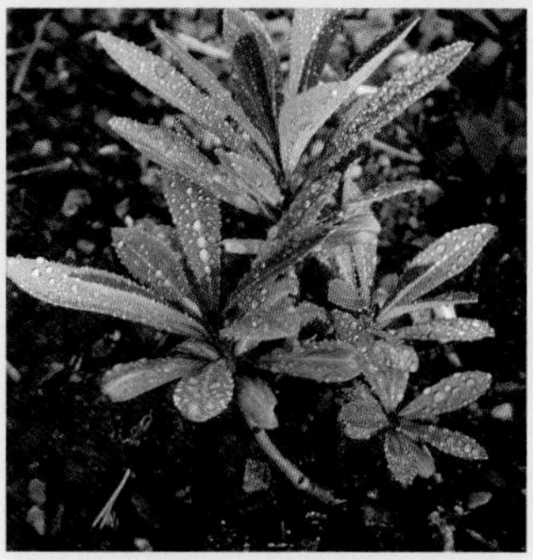

Daphne mezereum

MILK THISTLE

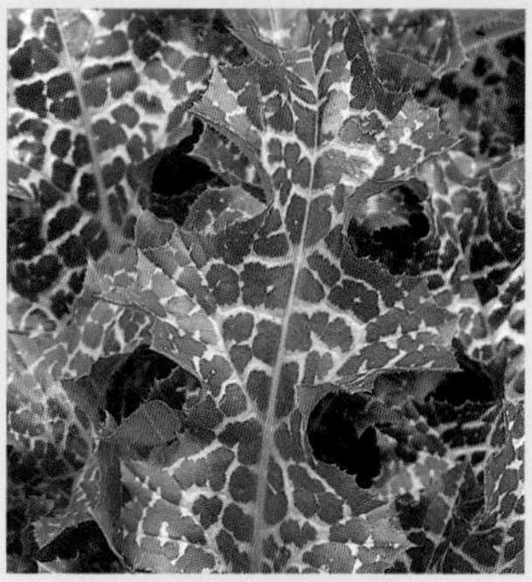

Silybum marianum

MONEYWORT

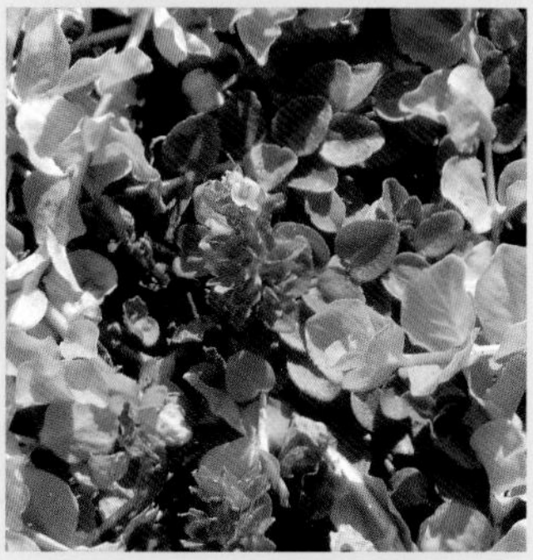

Lysimachia nummularia

MONKSHOOD

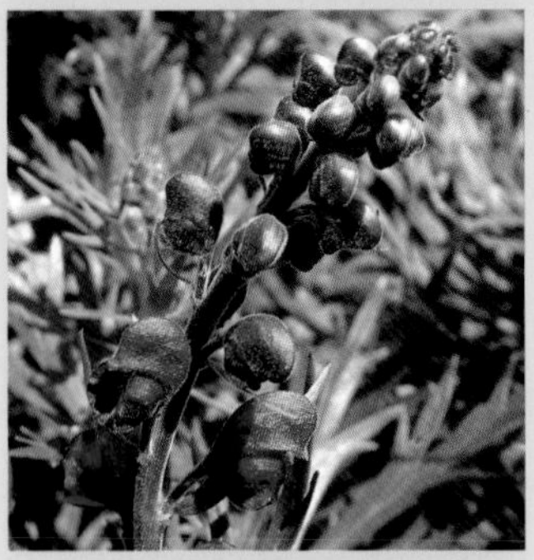

Aconitum napellus

MOTHERWORT

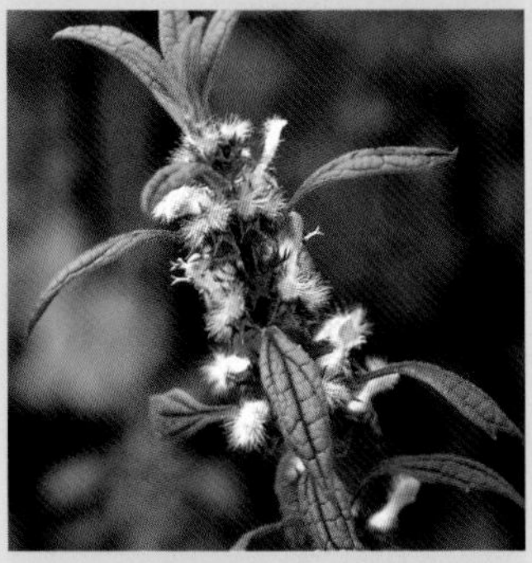

Leonurus cardiaca

MOUNTAIN ASH BERRY

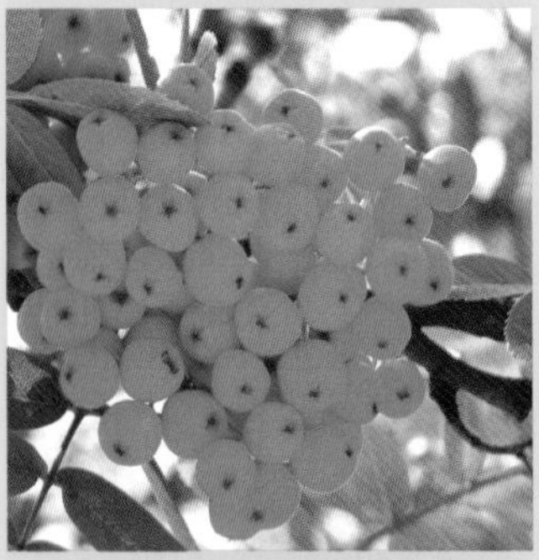

Sorbus aucuparia

MOUNTAIN GRAPE

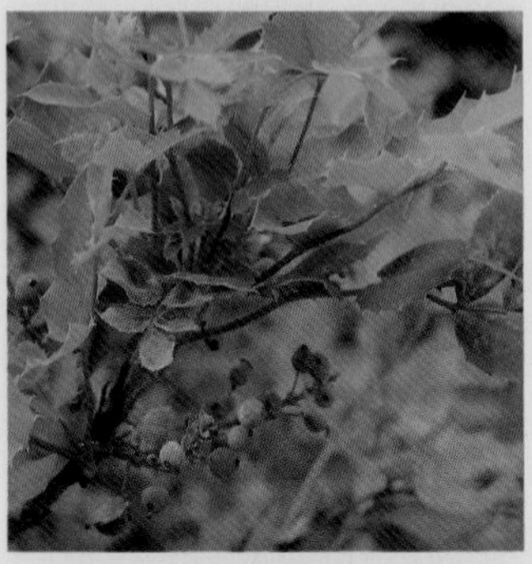

Mahonia aquifolium

MOUNTAIN LAUREL

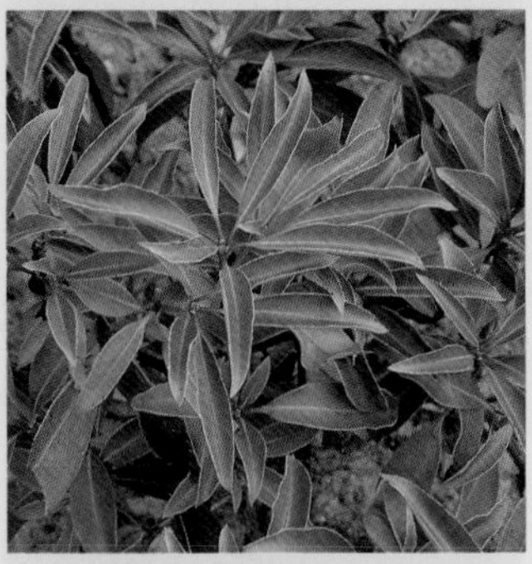

Kalmia latifolia

MUGWORT

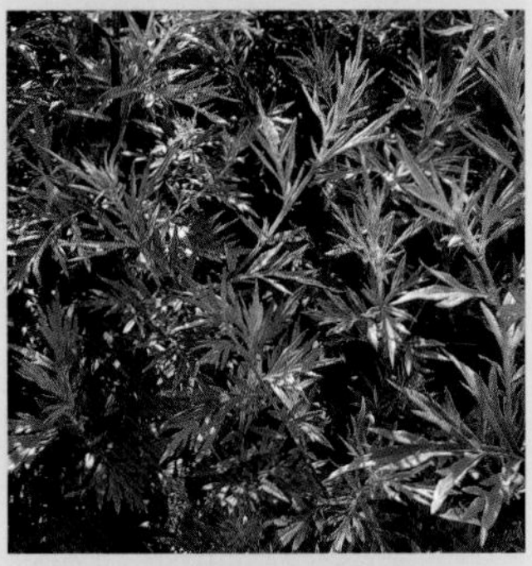

Artemisia vulgaris

MULLEIN

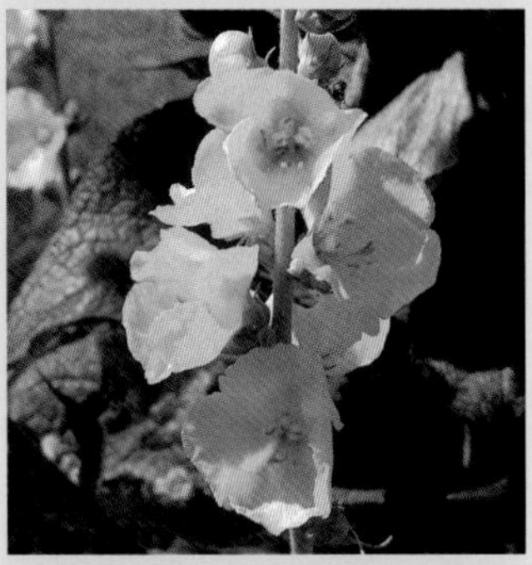

Verbascum densiflorum

MYRRH

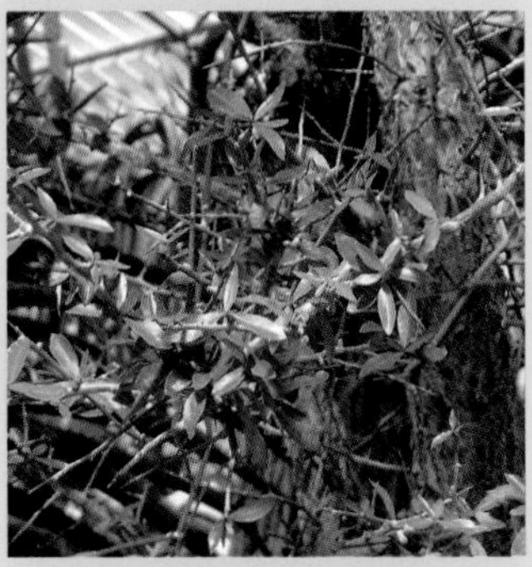

Commiphora molmol

MYRTLE

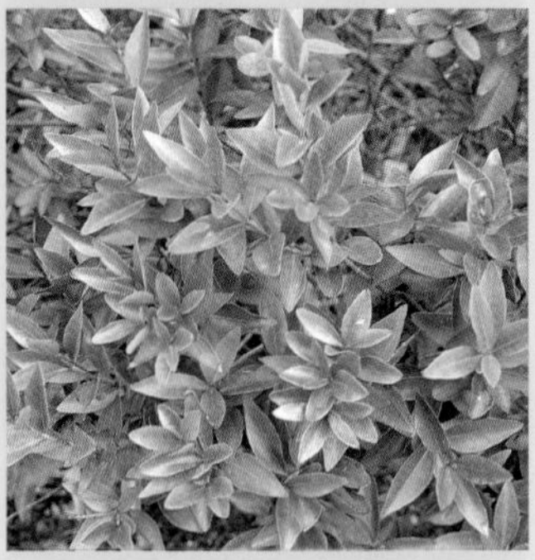

Myrtus communis

NASTURTIUM

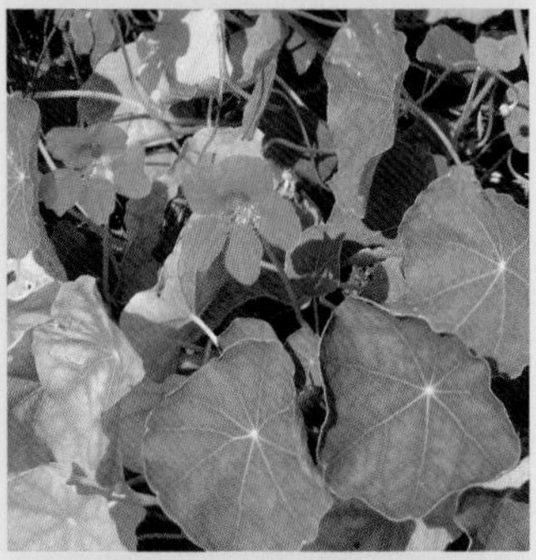

Tropaeolum majus

NEEM

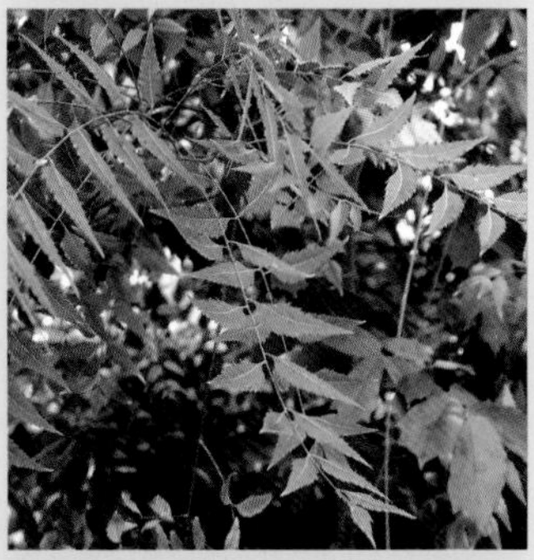

Antelaea azadirachta

NONI

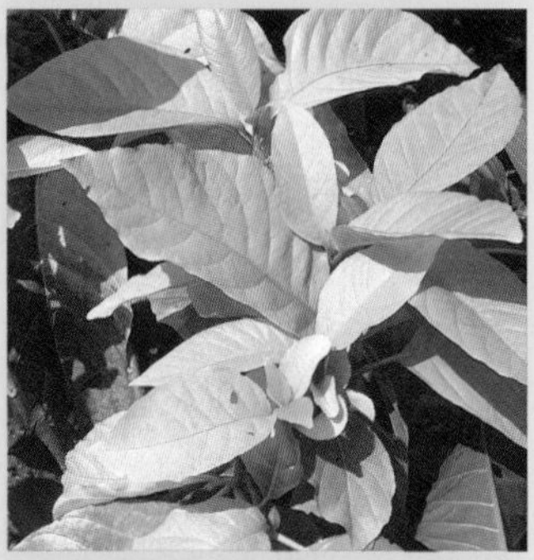

Morinda citrifolia

NUTMEG

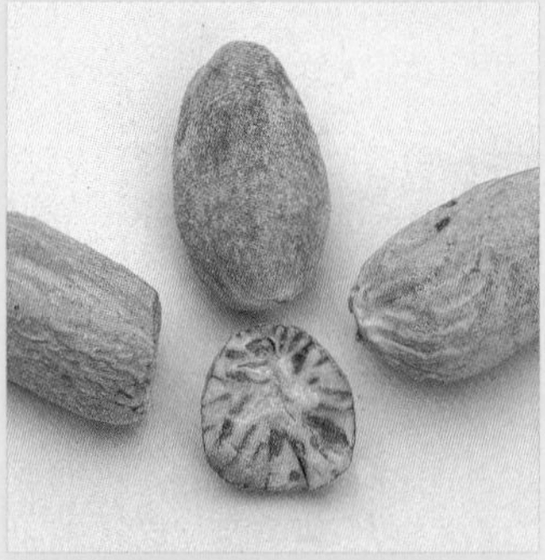

Myristica fragrans

NUX VOMICA

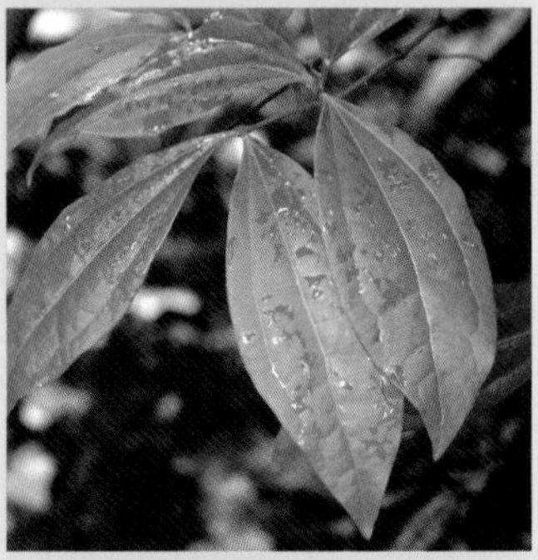

Strychnos nux vomica

OAK

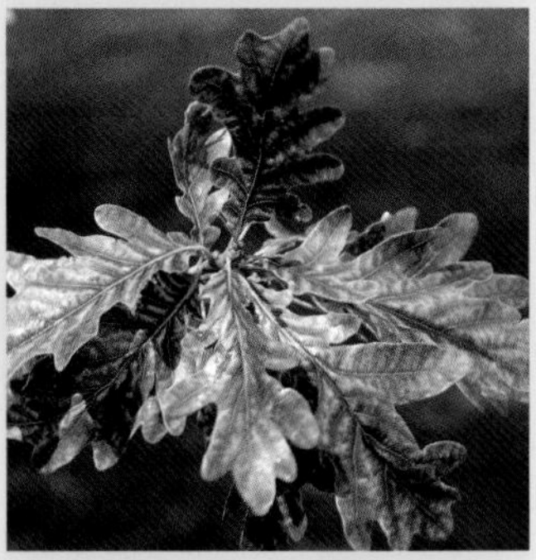

Quercus robur

OATS

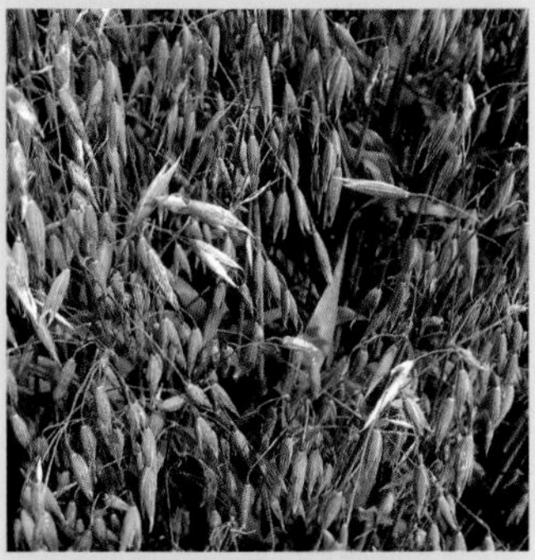

Avena sativa

OILSEED RAPE

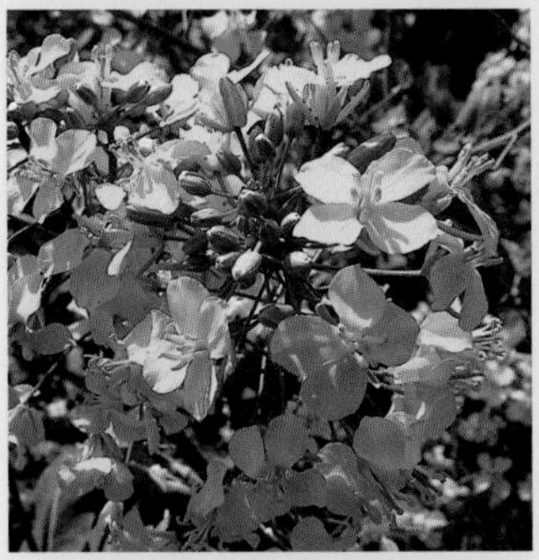

Brassica napus

OLEANDER LEAF

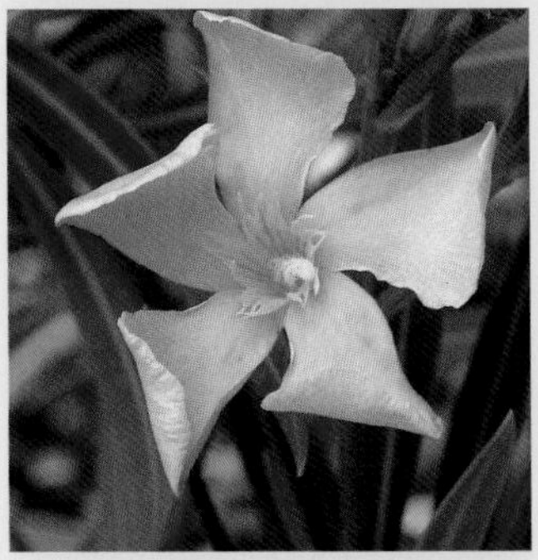

Nerium oleander

OLIVE

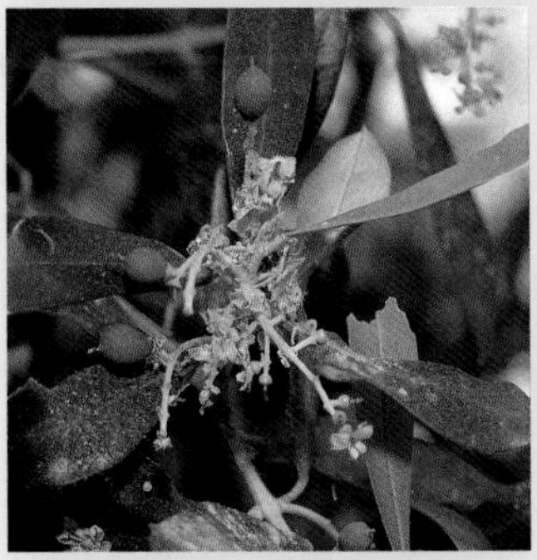

Olea europaea

ONION

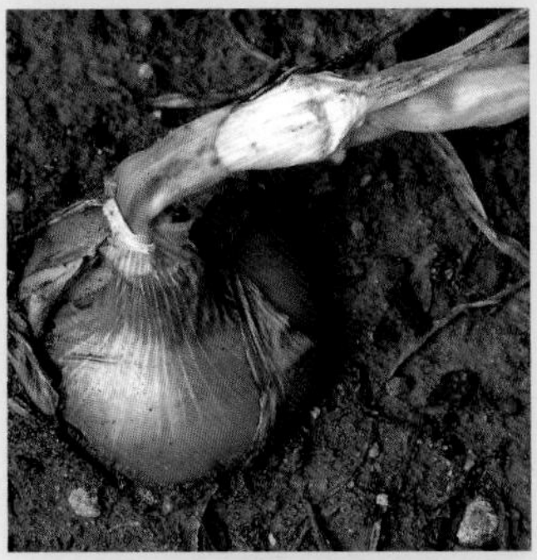

Allium cepa

OREGANO

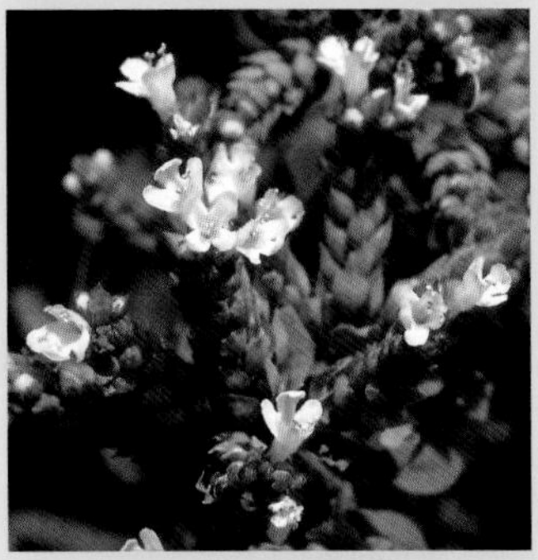

Origanum vulgare

ORRIS

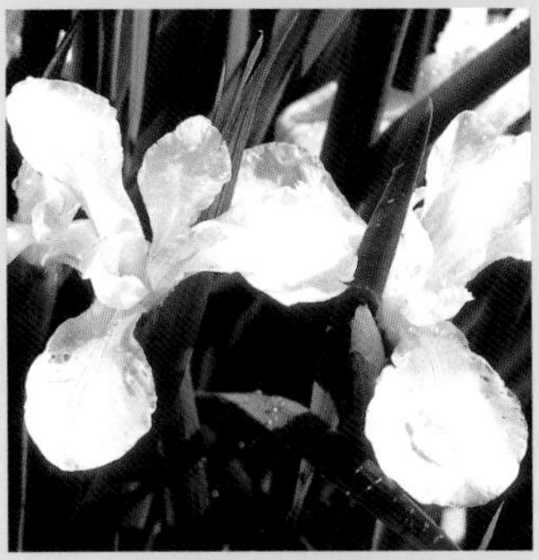

Iris species

PAPAYA

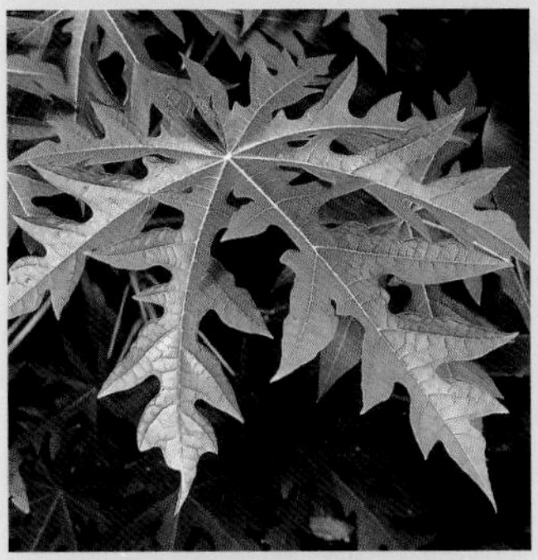

Carica papaya

PARSLEY

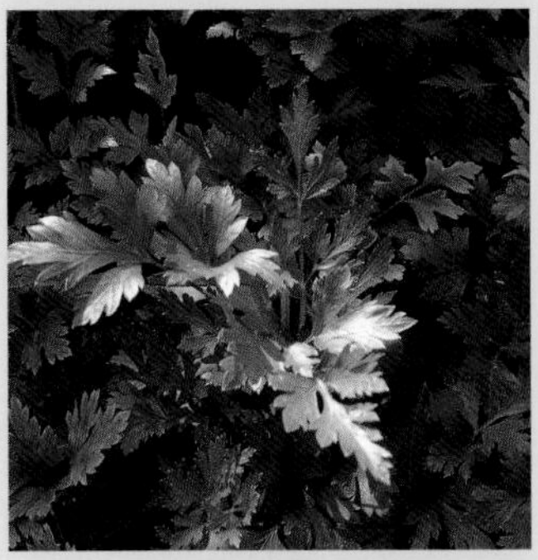

Petroselinum crispum

PARSNIP

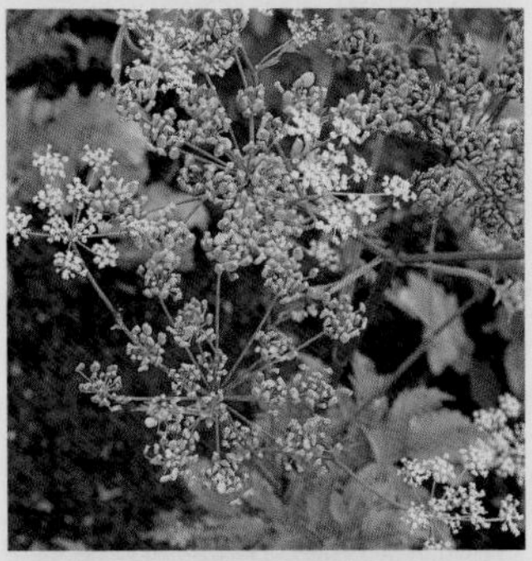

Pastinaca sativa

PASSION FLOWER

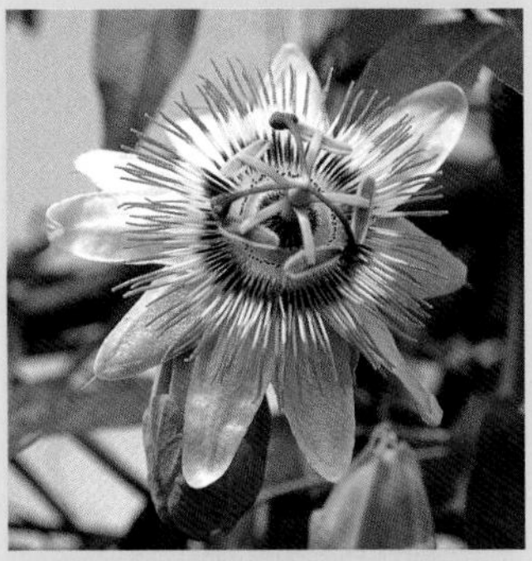

Passiflora incarnata

PATCHOULI

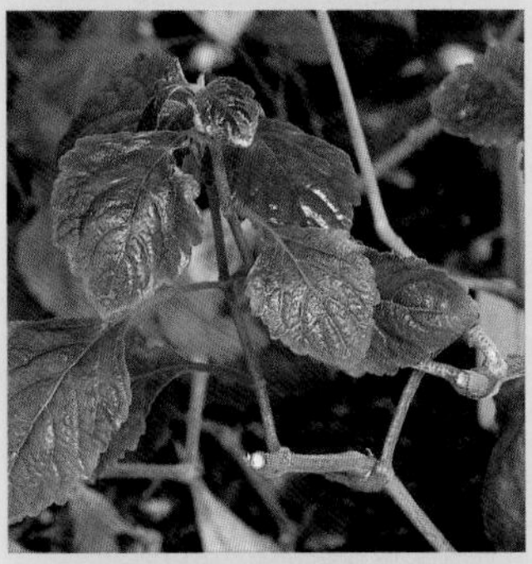

Pogostemon cablin

PEPPERMINT

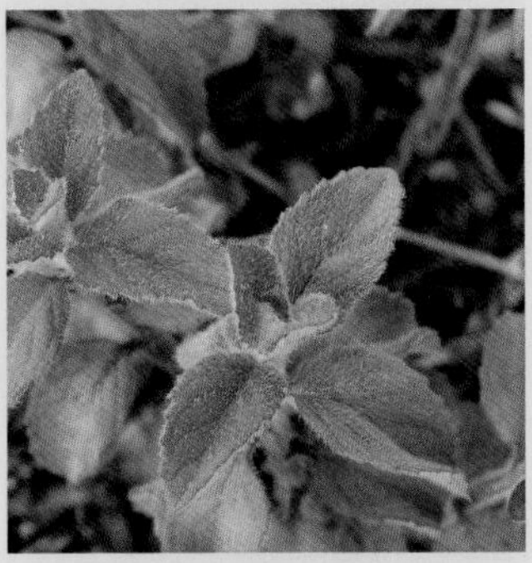

Mentha piperita

PETASITES

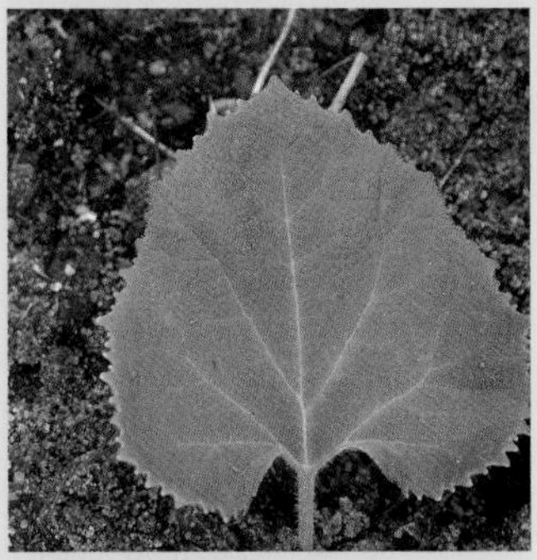

Petasites hybridus

PEYOTE

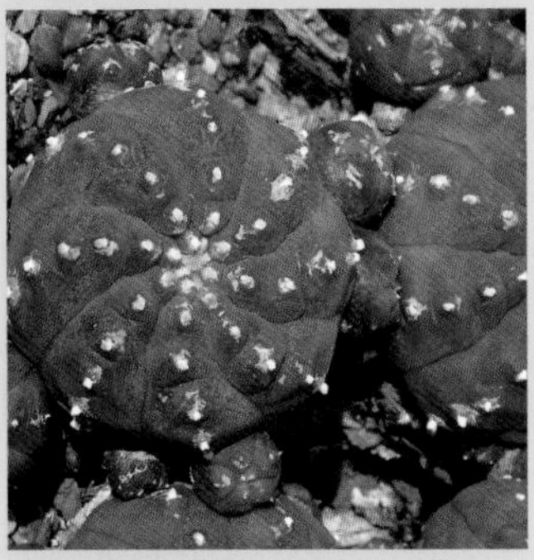

Lophophora williamsii

PIMPINELLA

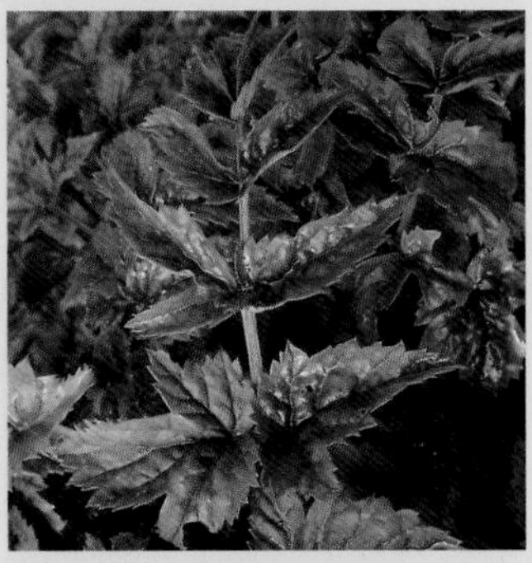

Pimpinella major

PINUS BARK

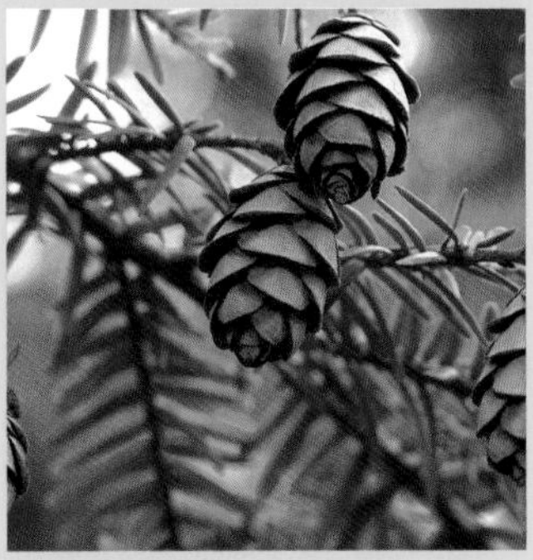

Tsuga canadensis

PITCHER PLANT

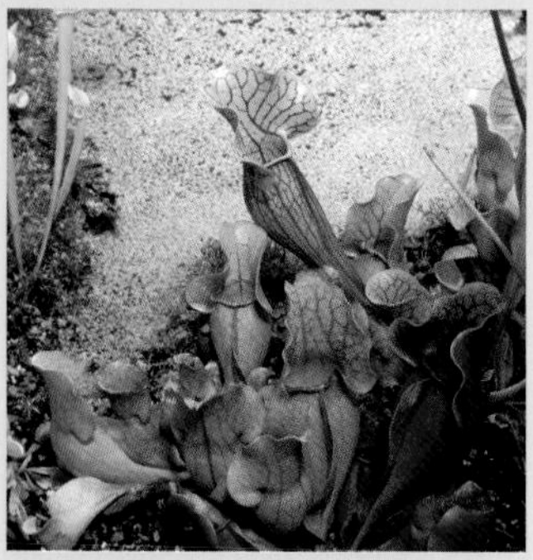

Sarracenia purpurea

PLEURISY ROOT

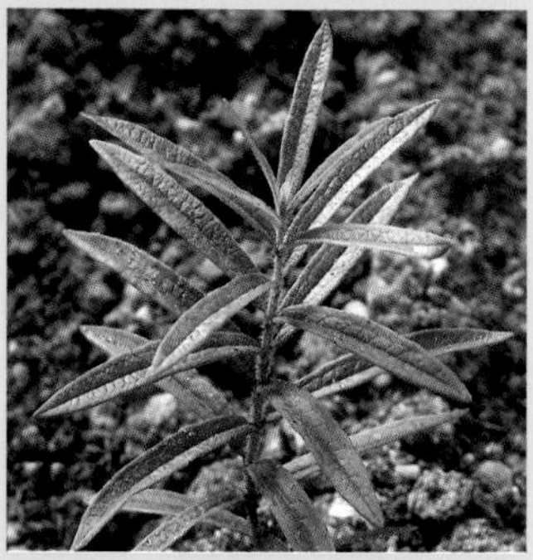

Asclepias tuberosa

POISONOUS BUTTERCUP

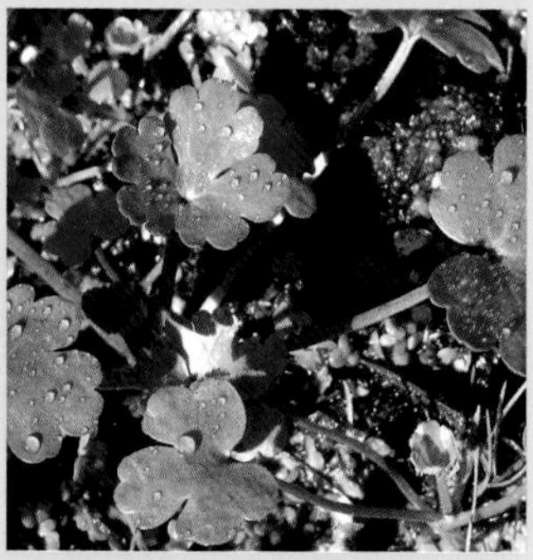

Ranunculus sceleratus

POKE

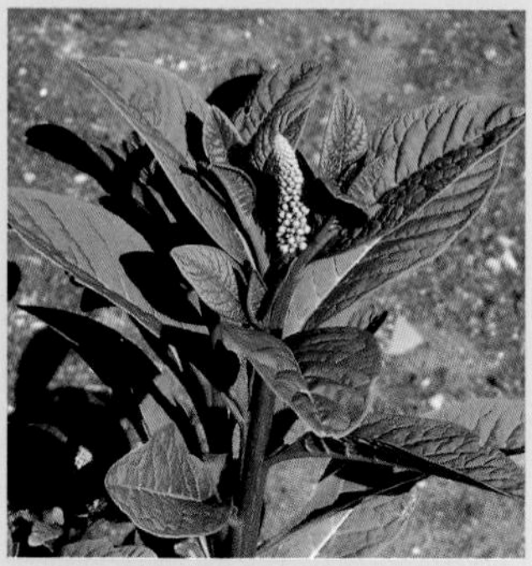

Phytolacca americana

POMEGRANATE

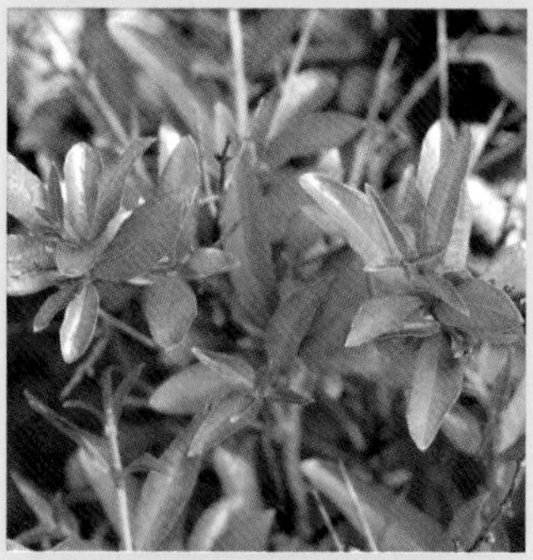

Punica granatum

POPLAR

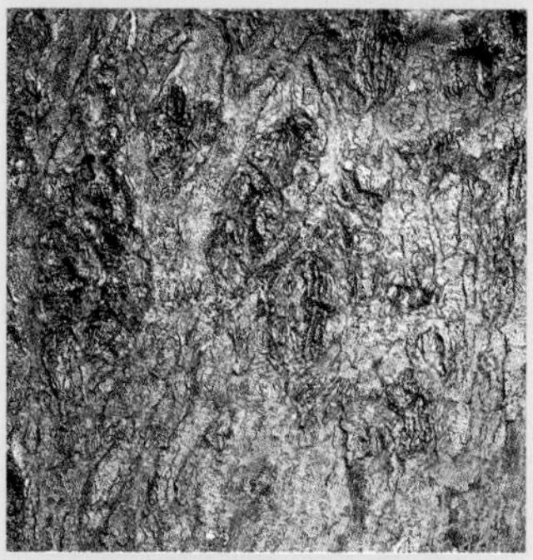

Populus species

POPPYSEED

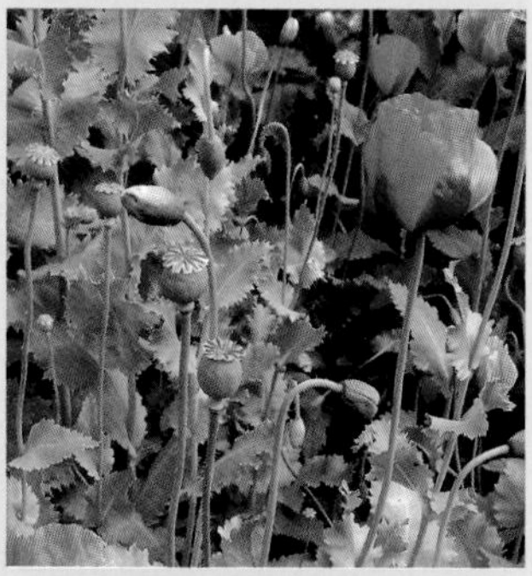

Papaver somniferum

POTENTILLA

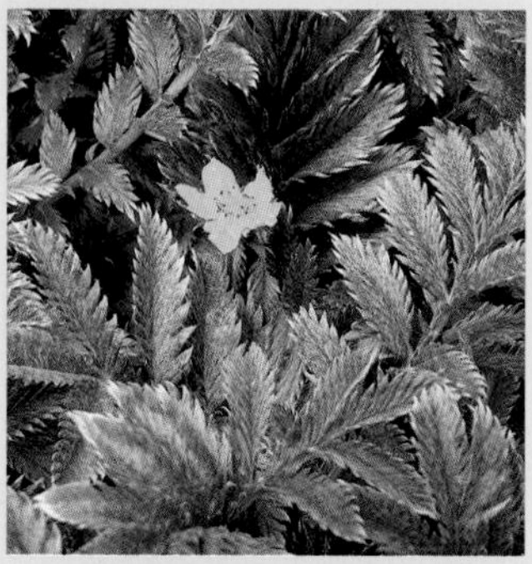

Potentilla anserina

PREMORSE

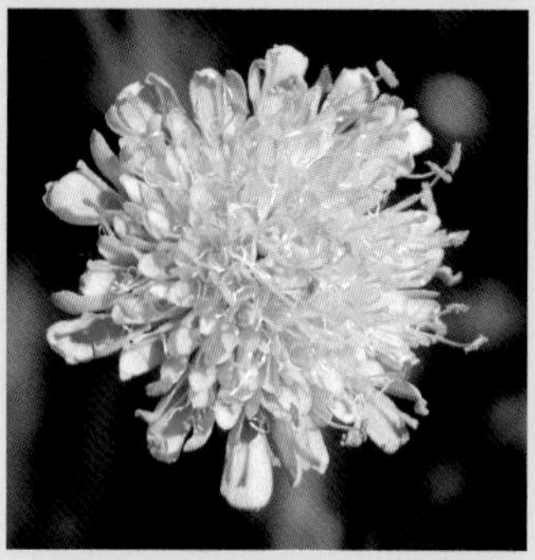

Scabiosa succisa

PSYLLIUM SEED

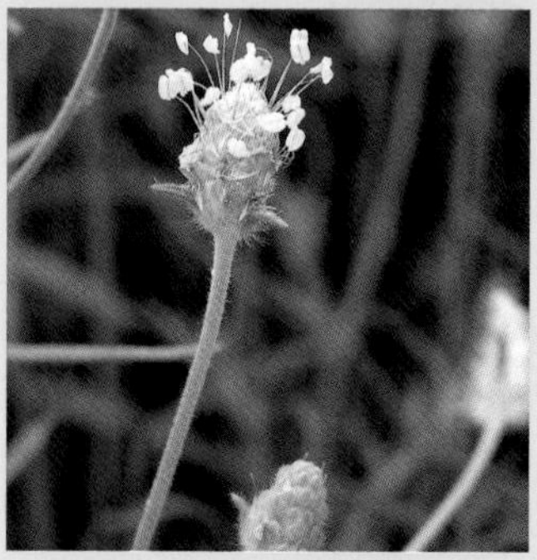

Plantago afra

PUMPKIN

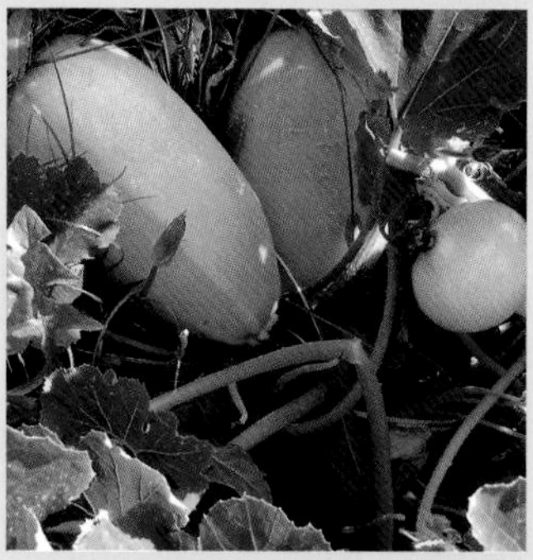

Cucurbita pepo

PURPLE LOOSESTRIFE

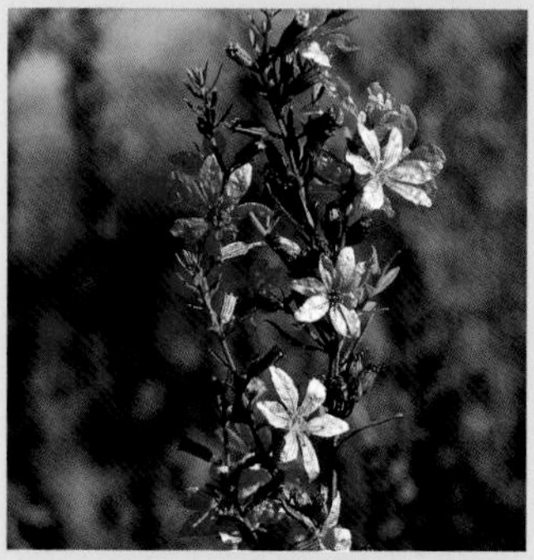

Lythrum salicaria

QUILLAJA

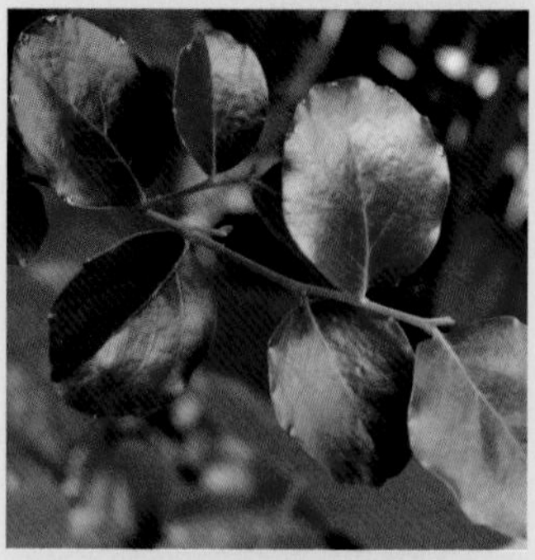

Quillaja saponaria

QUININE

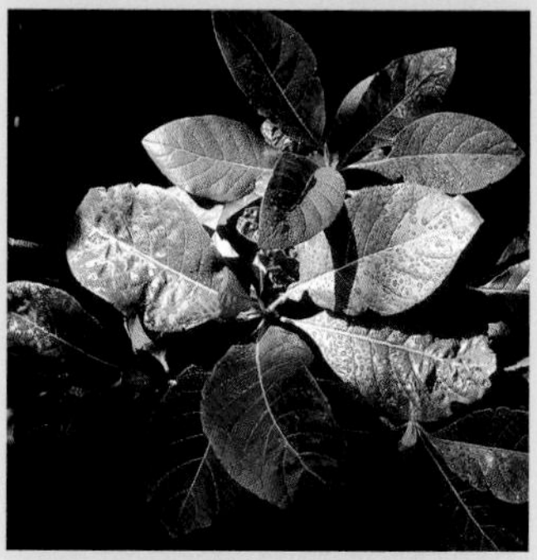

Cinchona pubescens

RADISH

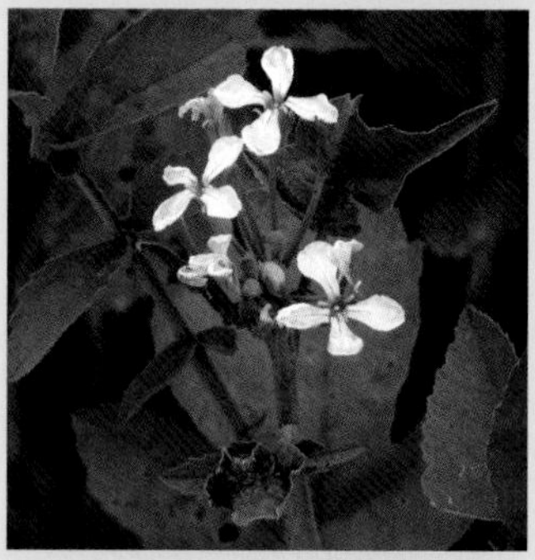

Raphanus sativus

RAGWORT

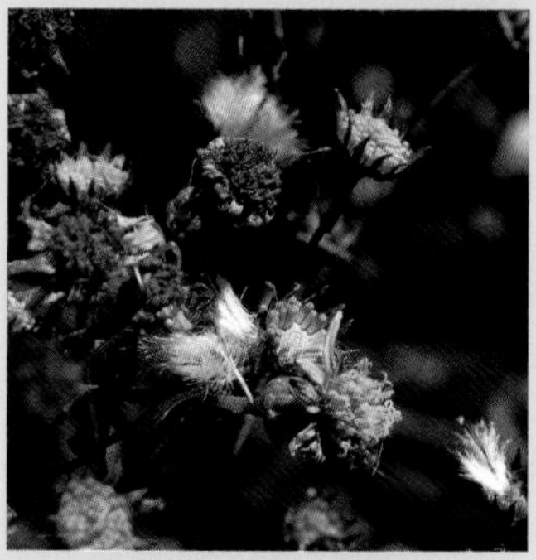

Senecio jacobaea

RASPBERRY

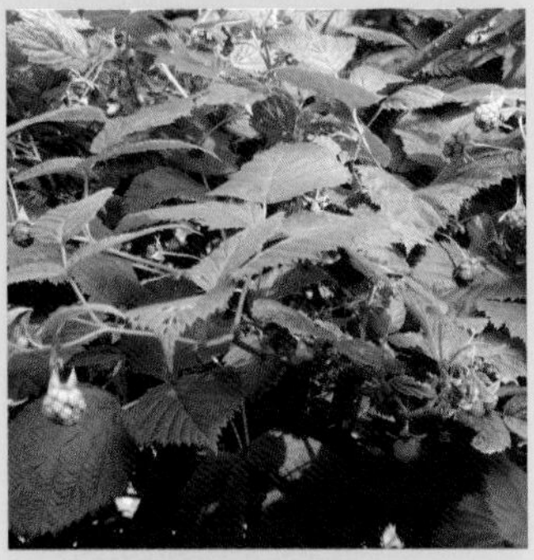

Rubus idaeus

RED-SPUR VALERIAN

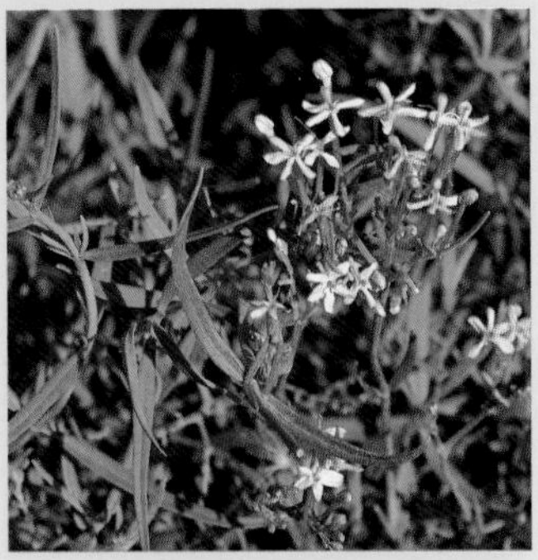

Centranthus ruber

RUE

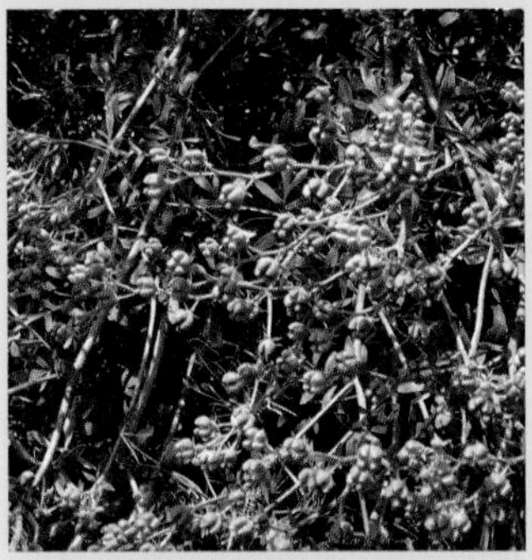

Ruta graveolens

SARSAPARILLA

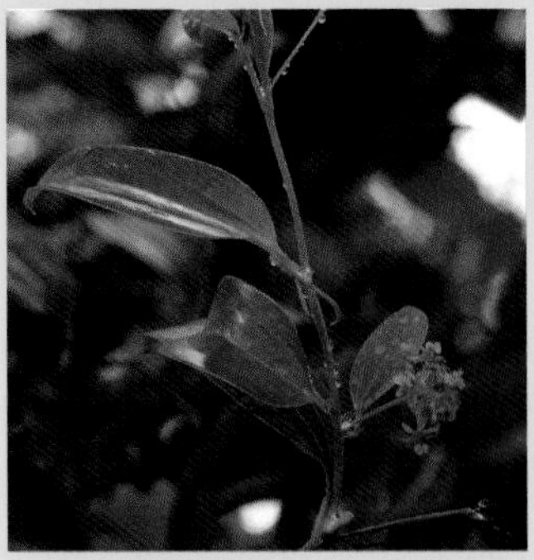

Smilax species

RED CLOVER

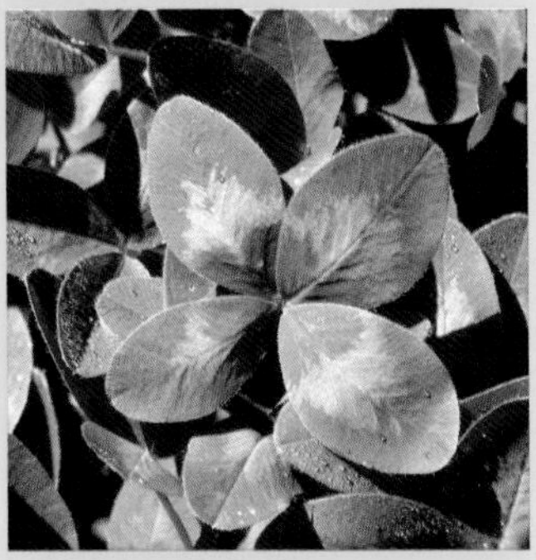

Trifolium pratense

RICE

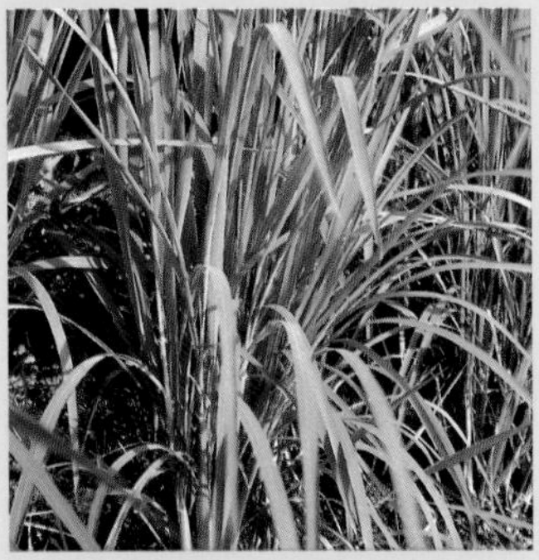

Oryza sativa

RUPTUREWORT

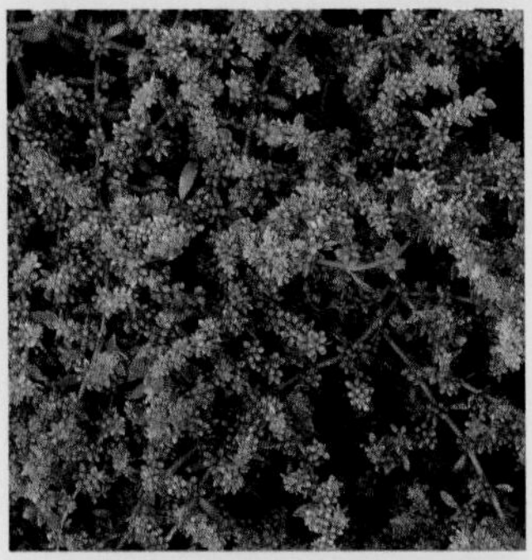

Herniaria glabra

SASSAFRAS

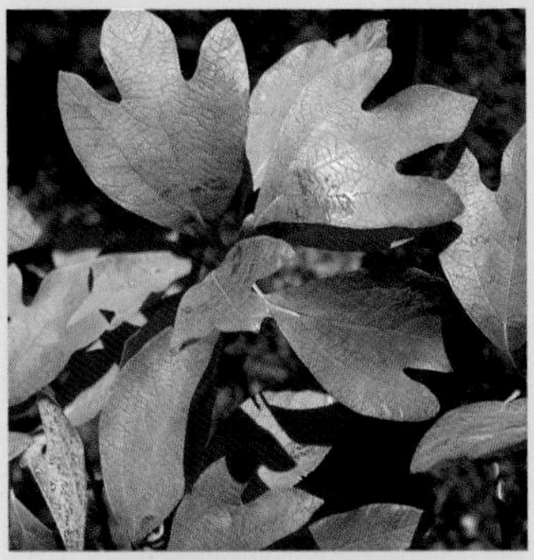

Sassafras albidum

RED CURRANT

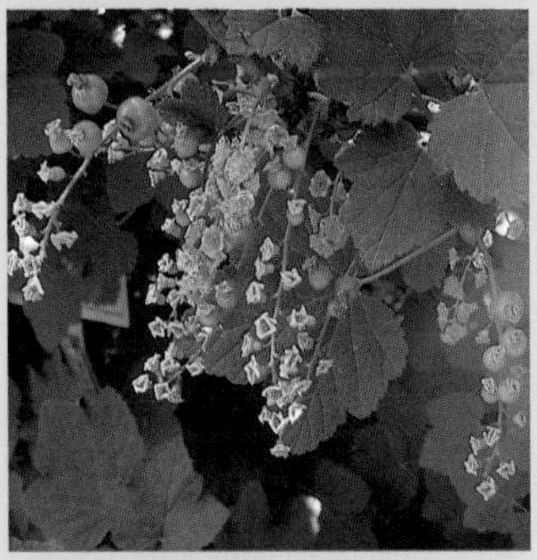

Ribes rubrum

ROSEMARY

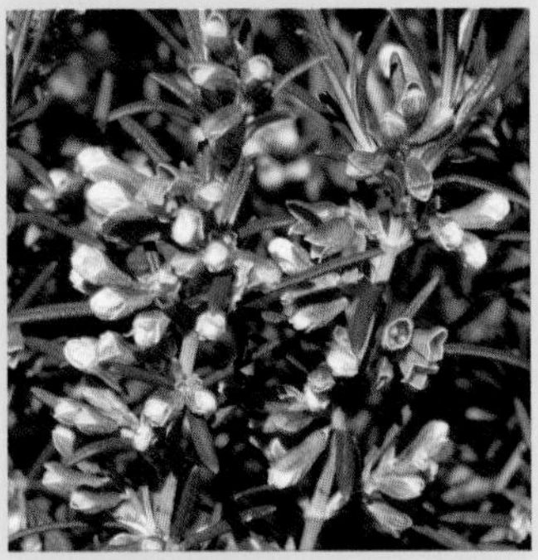

Rosmarinus officinalis

SAFFRON

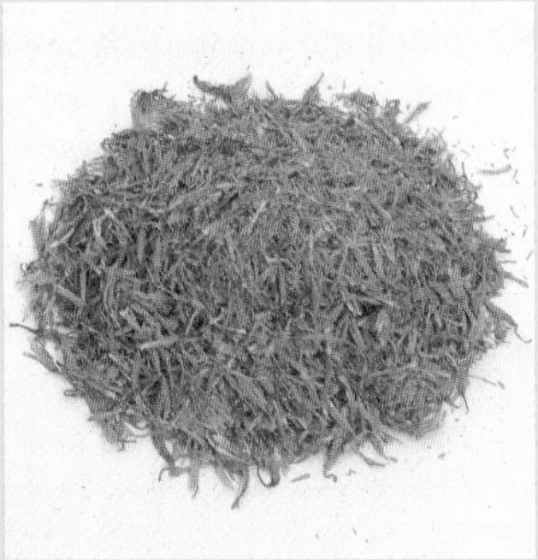

Crocus sativus

SAVIN TOPS

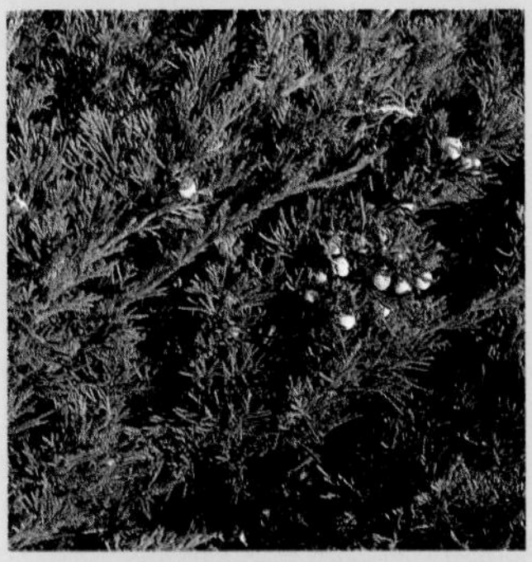

Juniperus sabina

RED MAPLE

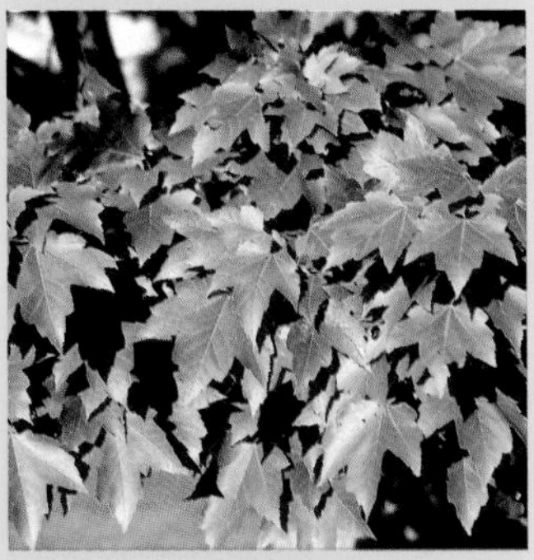

Acer rubrum

ROSINWEED

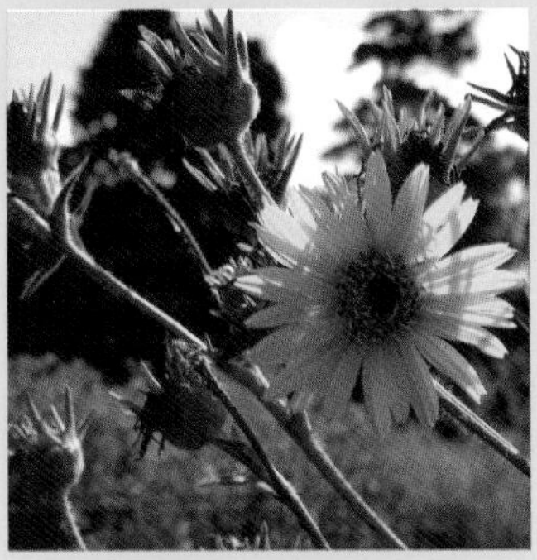

Silphium laciniatum

SAGE

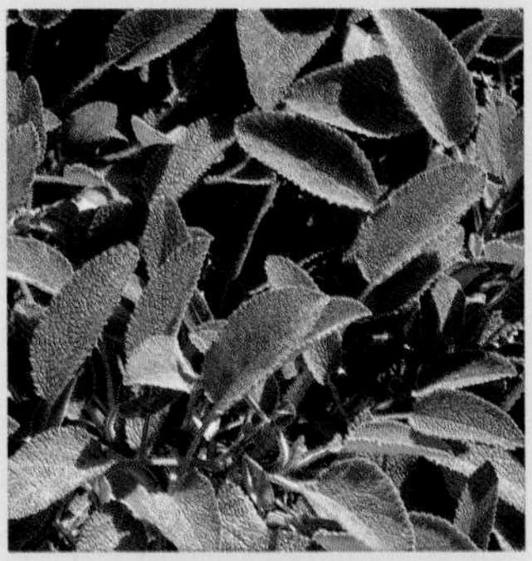

Salvia officinalis

SAW PALMETTO

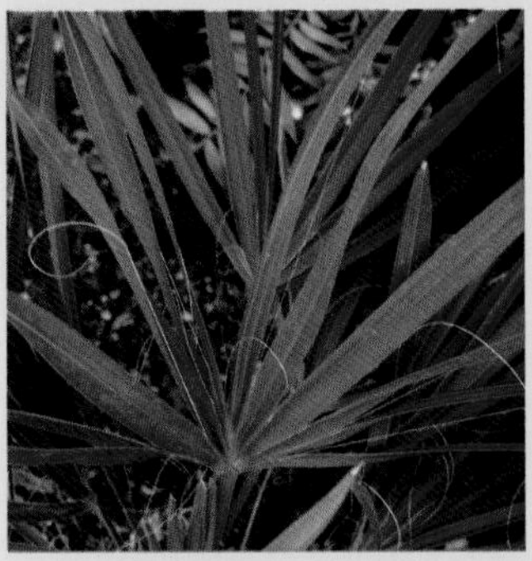

Serenoa repens

SCARLET PIMPERNEL

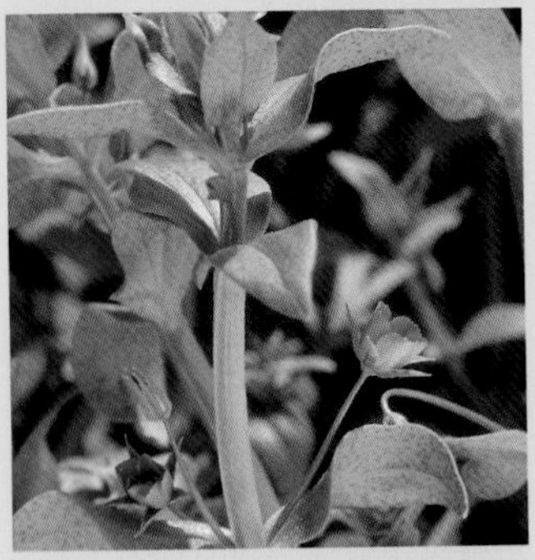

Anagallis arvensis

SCOTCH BROOM

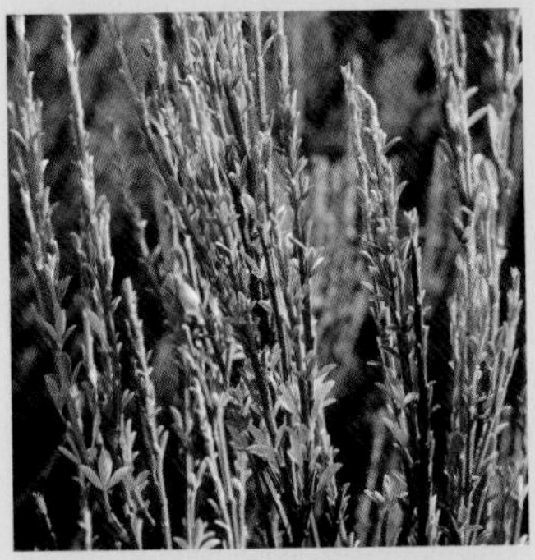

Cytisus scoparius

SCOTCH PINE

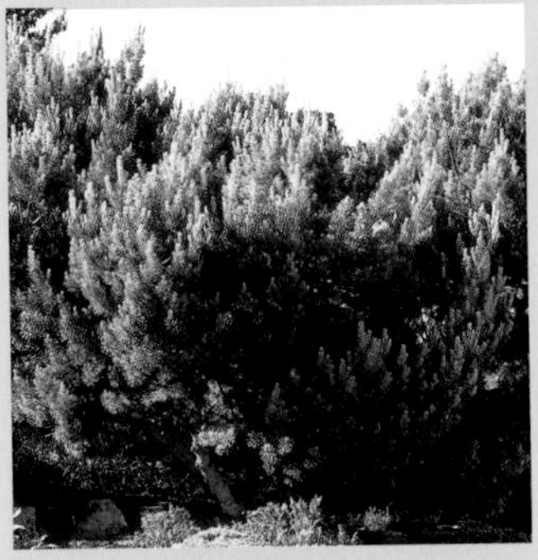

Pinus species

SCOTCH THISTLE

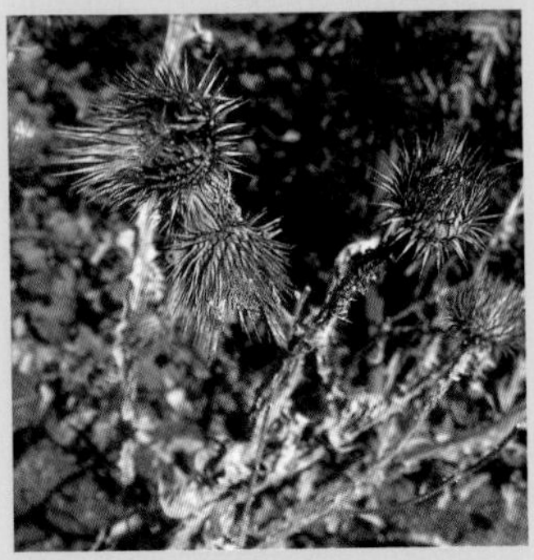

Onopordum acanthium

SCULLCAP

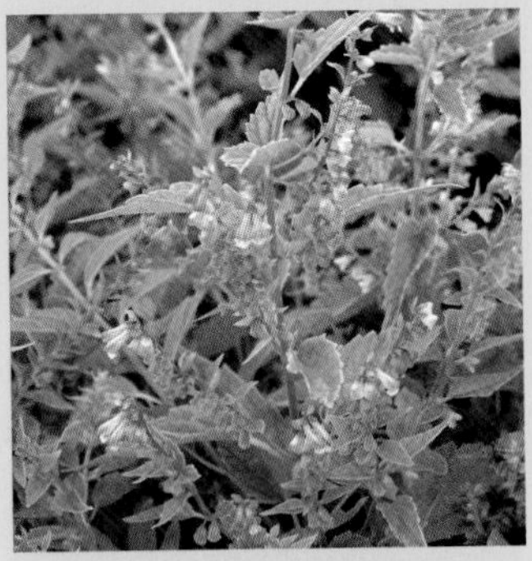

Scutellaria lateriflora

SCURVY GRASS

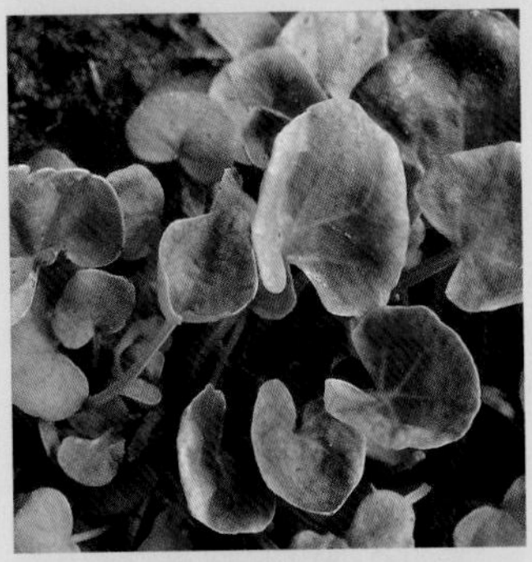

Cochlearia officinalis

SEA BUCKTHORN

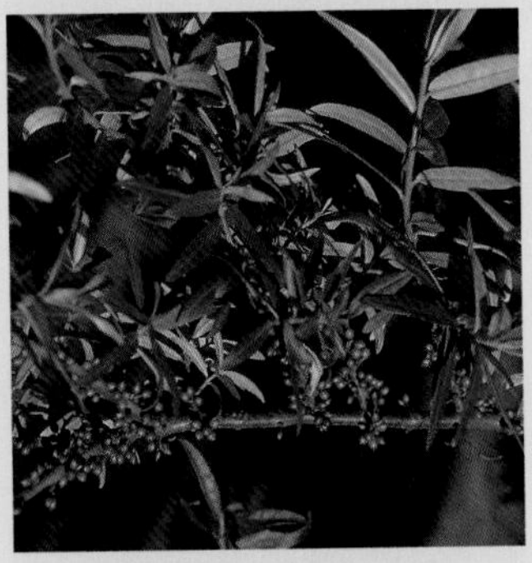

Hippophaë rhamnoides

SELF-HEAL

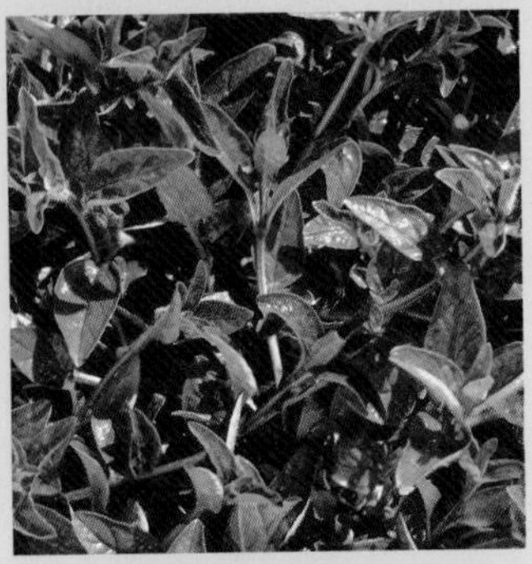

Prunella vulgaris

SENNA

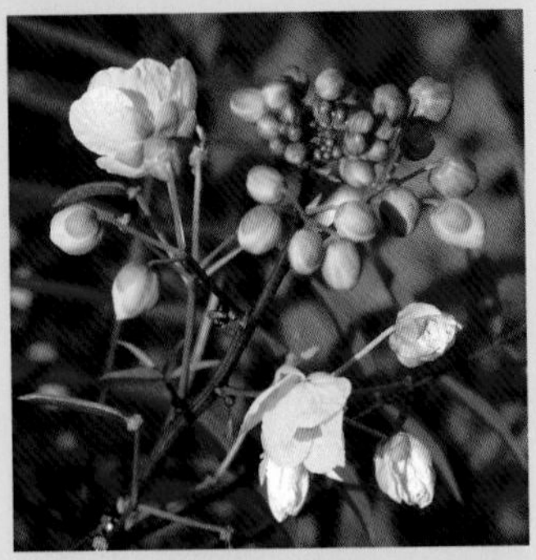

Cassia senna

SHEPHERD'S PURSE

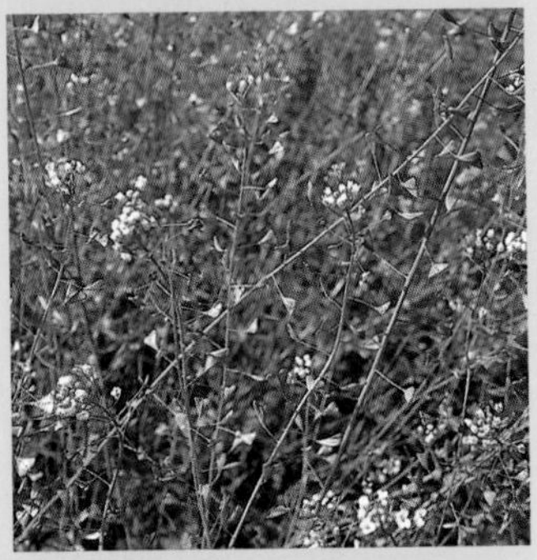

Capsella bursa-pastoris

SKIRRET

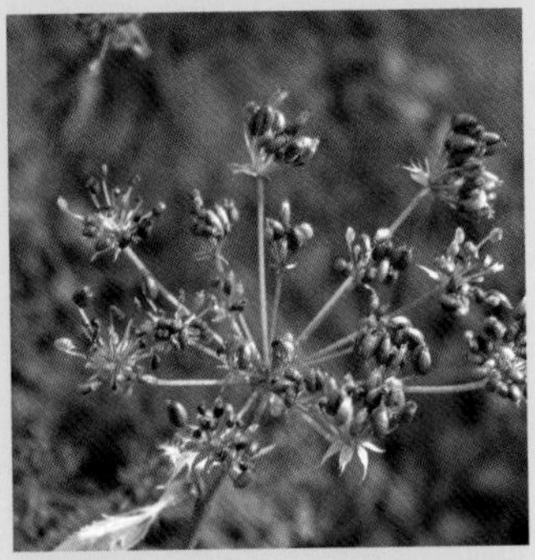

Sium sisarum

SLOE

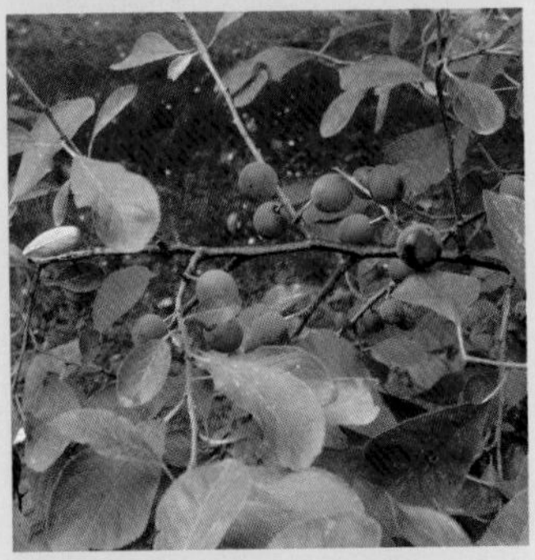

Prunus spinosa

SOAPWORT

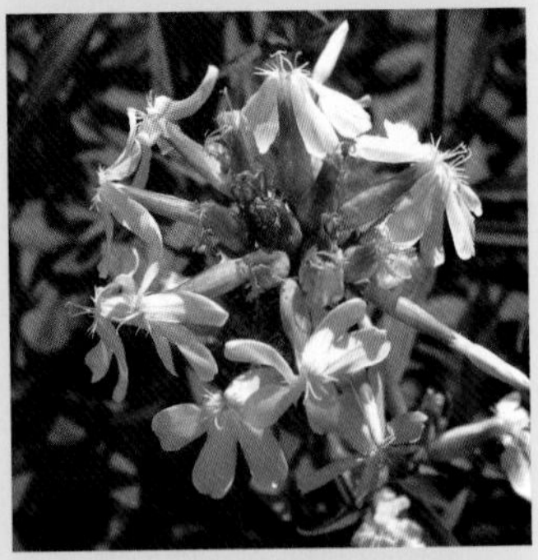

Saponaria officinalis

SOLOMON'S SEAL

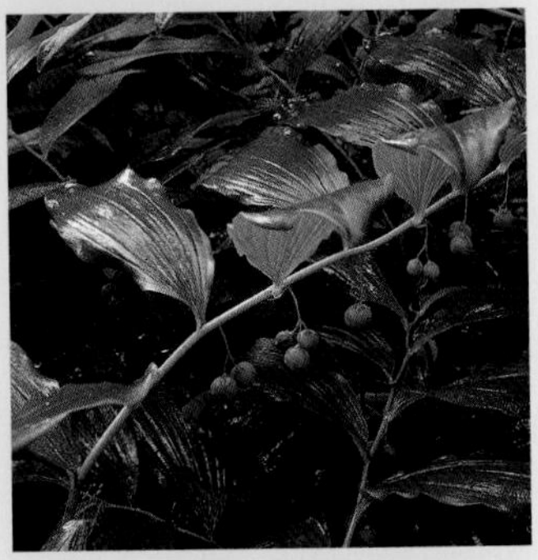

Polygonatum multiflorum

SOUTHERN BAYBERRY

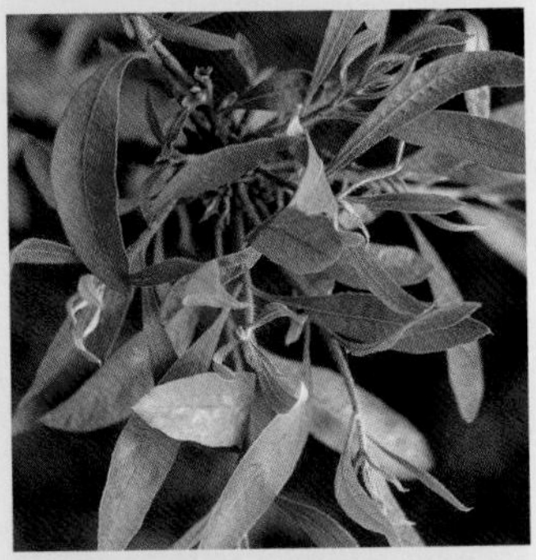

Myrica cerifera

SOYBEAN

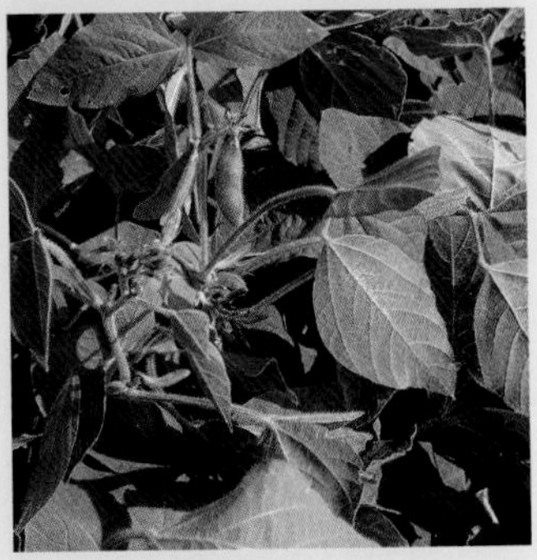

Glycine soja

SPEARMINT

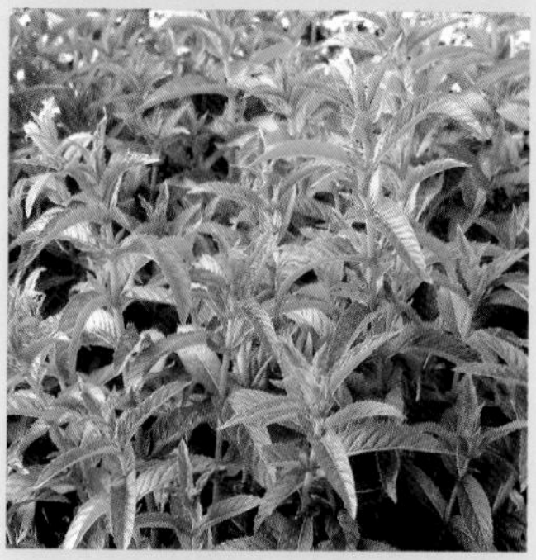

Mentha spicata

SPEEDWELL

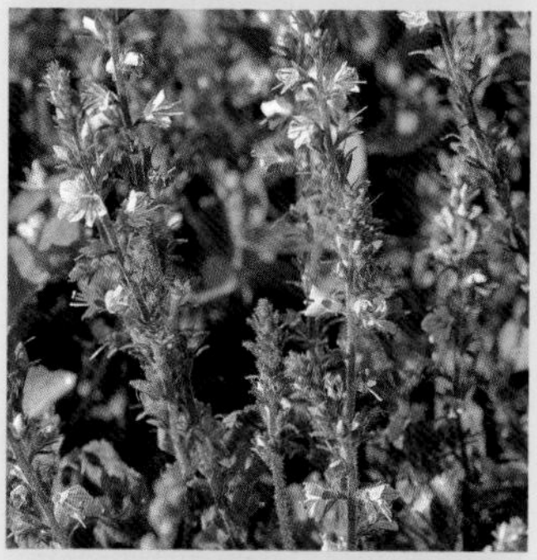

Veronica officinalis

SPIKENARD

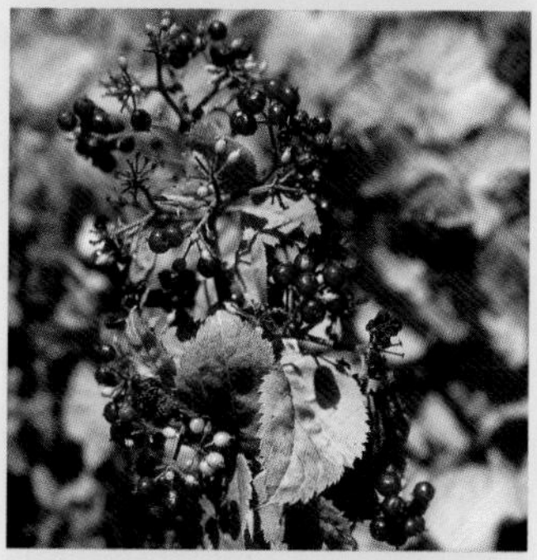

Aralia racemosa

SPINACH

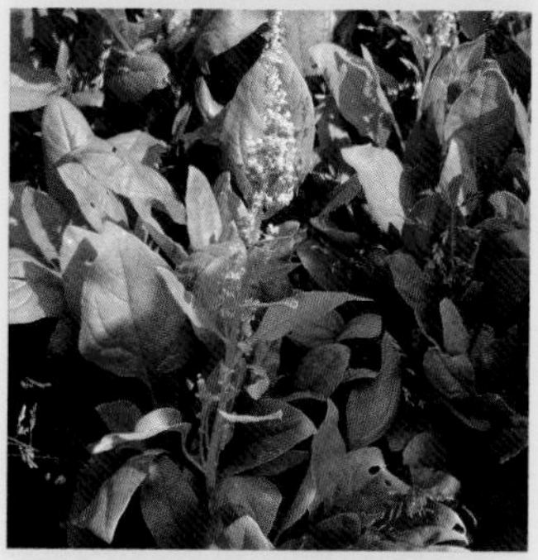

Spinacia oleracea

SPINY REST HARROW

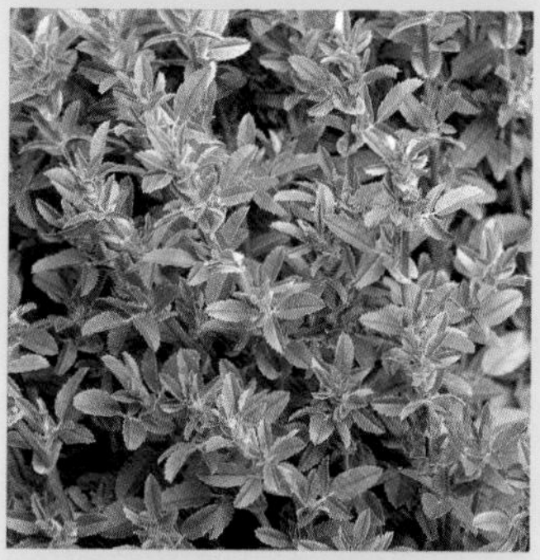

Ononis spinosa

SQUILL

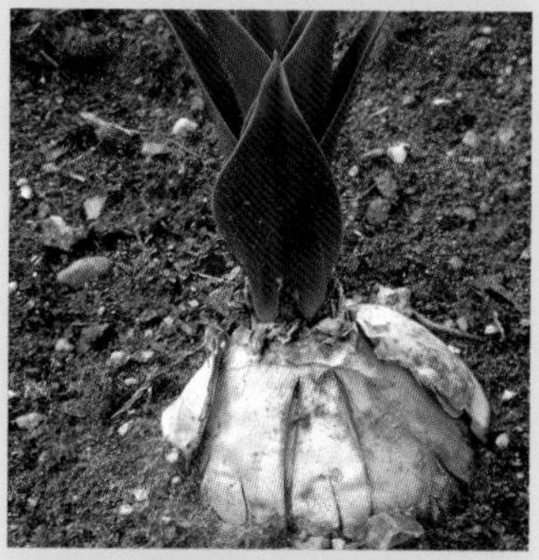

Urginea maritima

ST. JOHN'S WORT

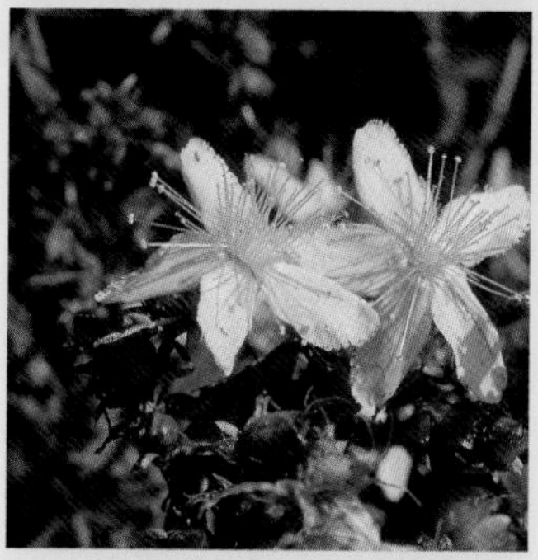

Hypericum perforatum

STAR ANISE

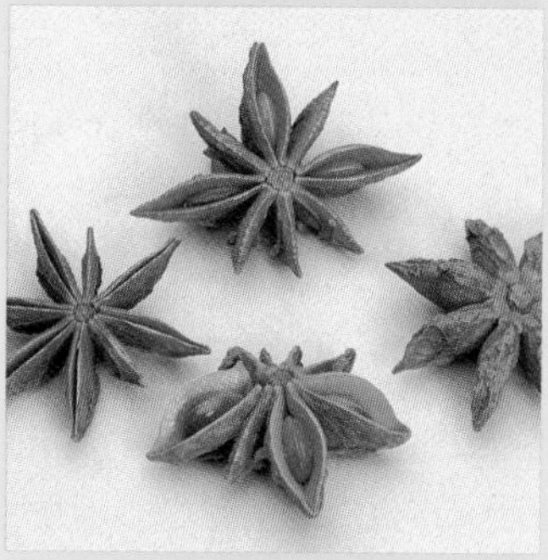

Illicium verum

STINGING NETTLE

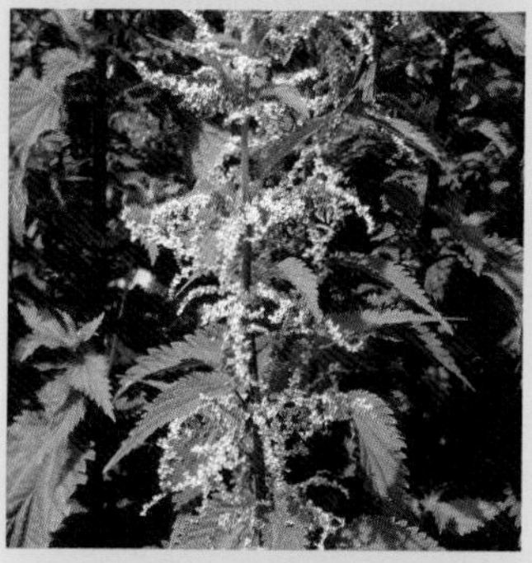

Urtica dioica

STONE ROOT

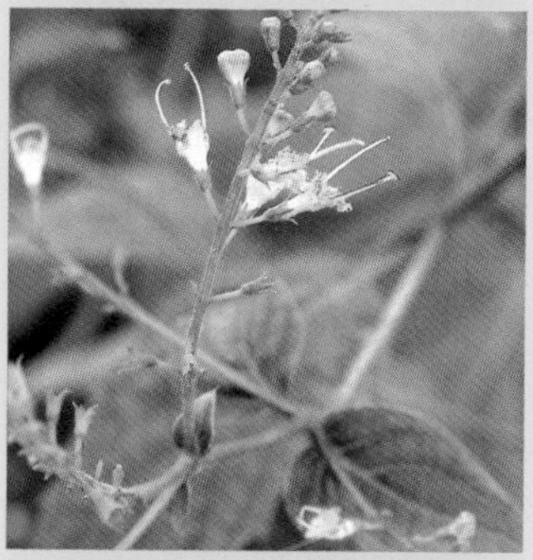

Collinsonia canadensis

STORAX

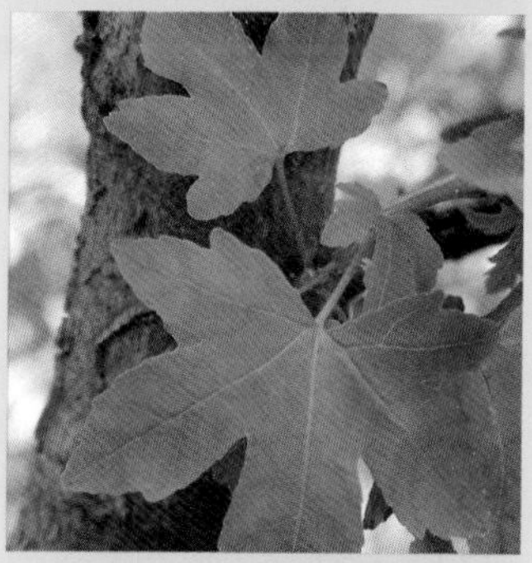

Liquidambar orientalis

STRAWBERRY

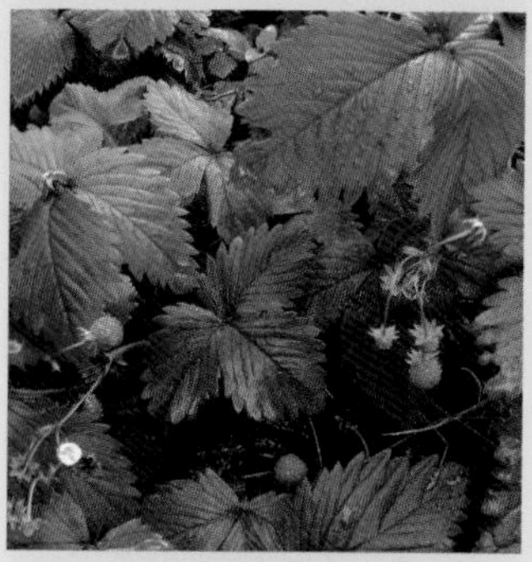

Fragaria vesca

SUMBUL

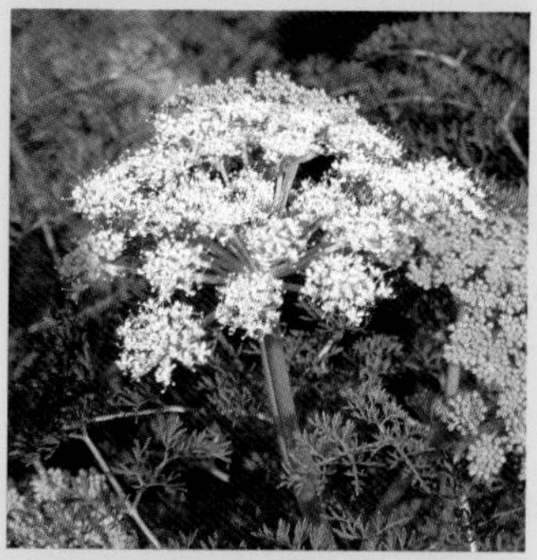

Ferula sumbul

SUMMER SAVORY

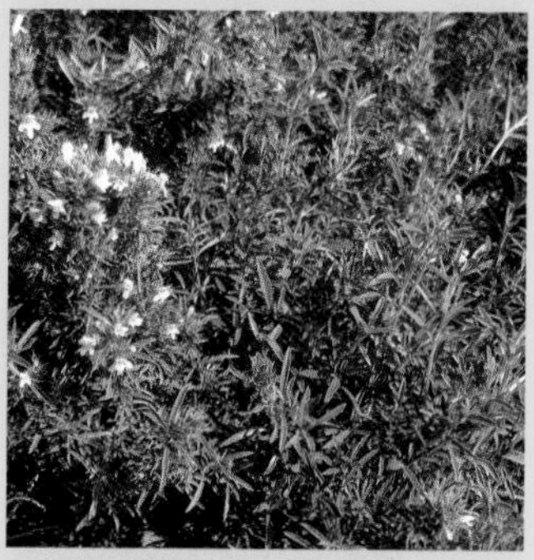

Satureja hortensis

SUNFLOWER

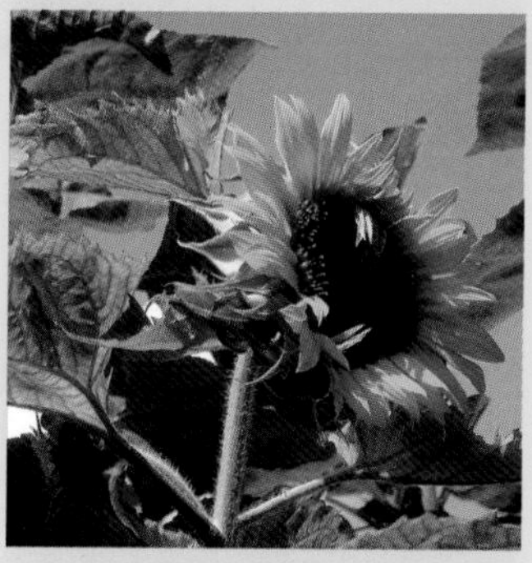

Helianthus annuus

SWAMP MILKWEED

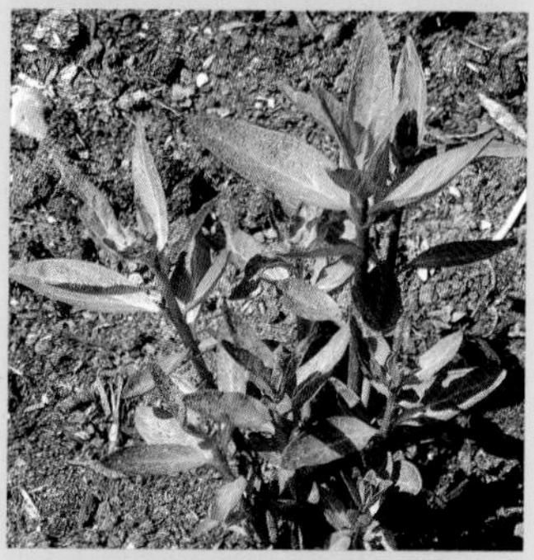

Asclepias incarnata

SWEET CICELY

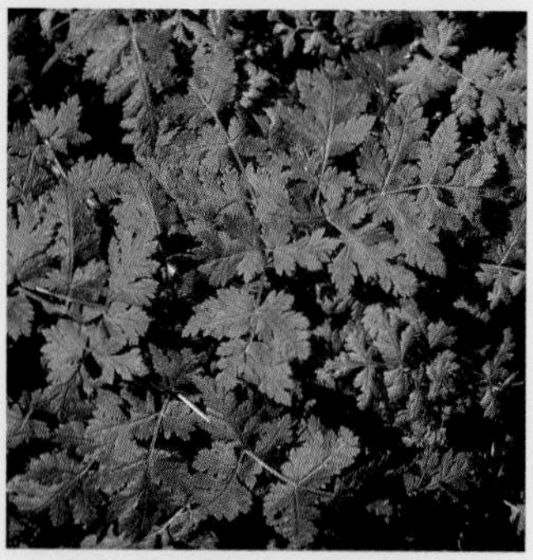

Myrrhis odorata

SWEET CLOVER

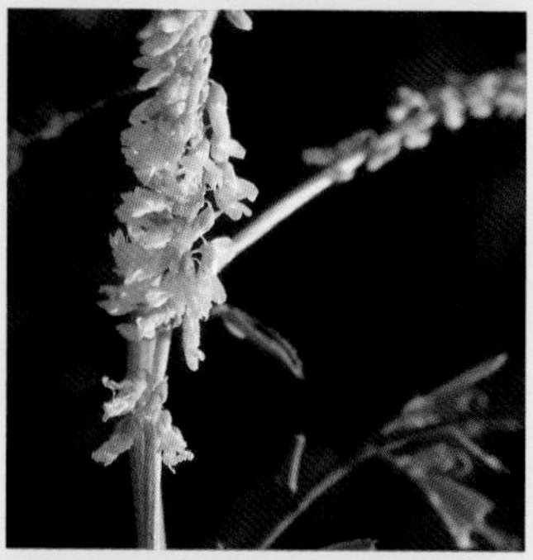

Melilotus officinalis

SWEET GALE

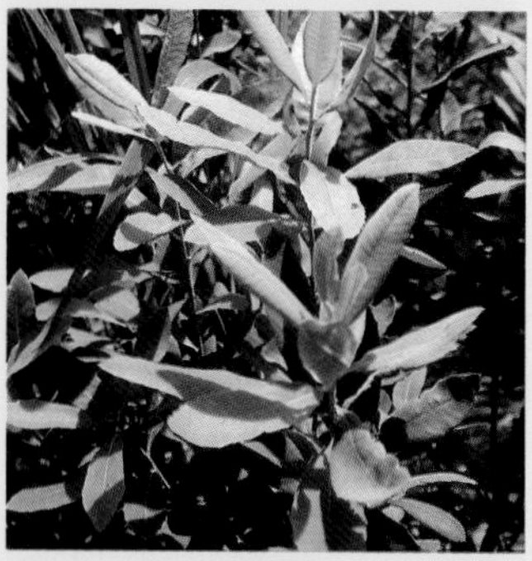

Myrica gale

SWEET MARJORAM

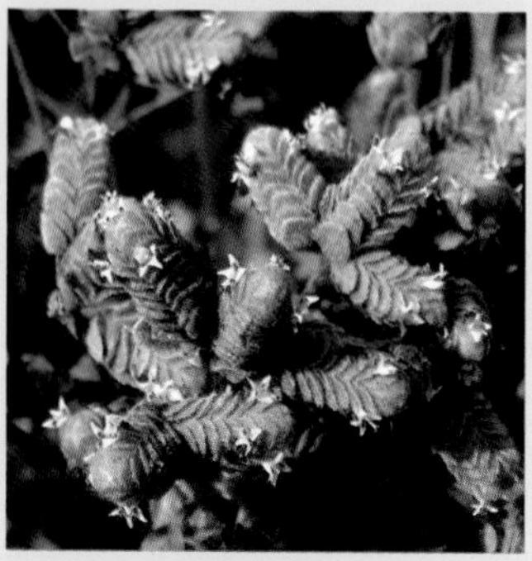

Origanum majorana

SWEET ORANGE

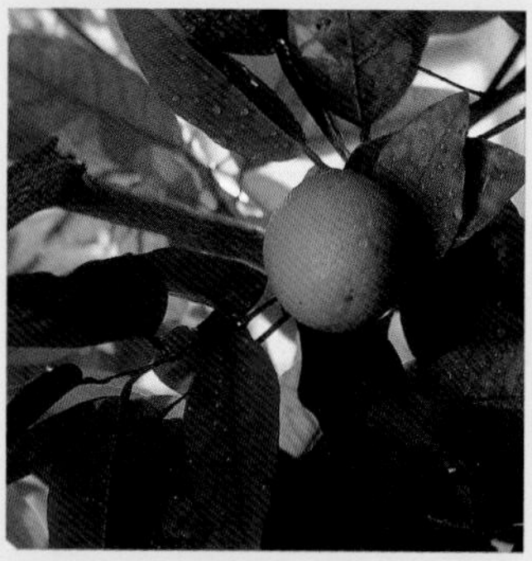

Citrus sinensis

SWEET VERNAL GRASS

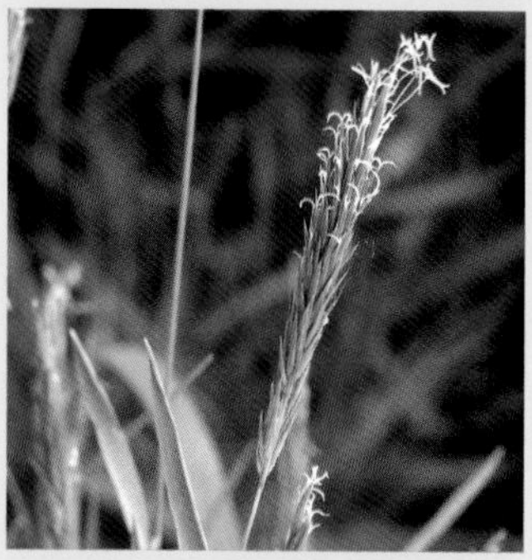

Anthoxanthum odoratum

SWEET VIOLET

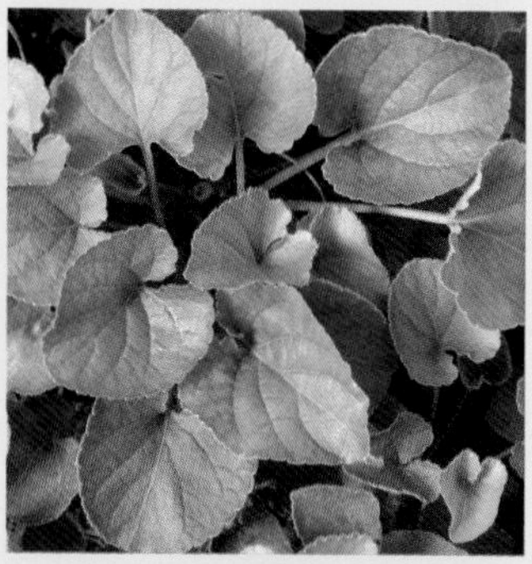

Viola odorata

SWEET WOODRUFF

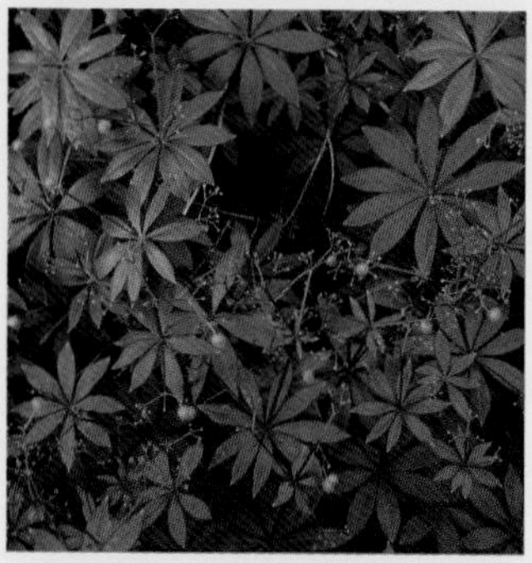

Galium odoratum

TANSY

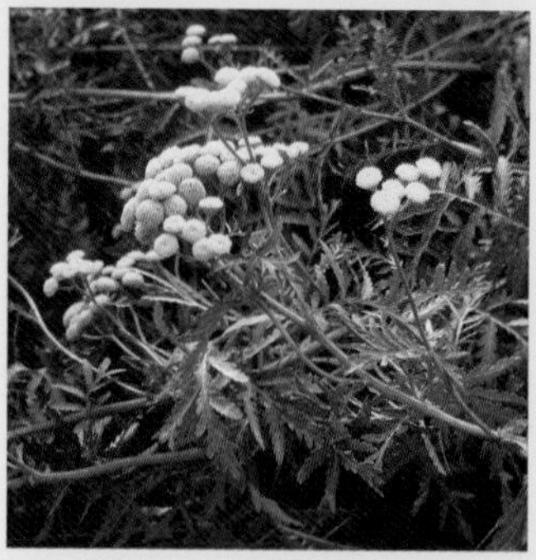

Tanacetum vulgare

TAUMELLOOLCH

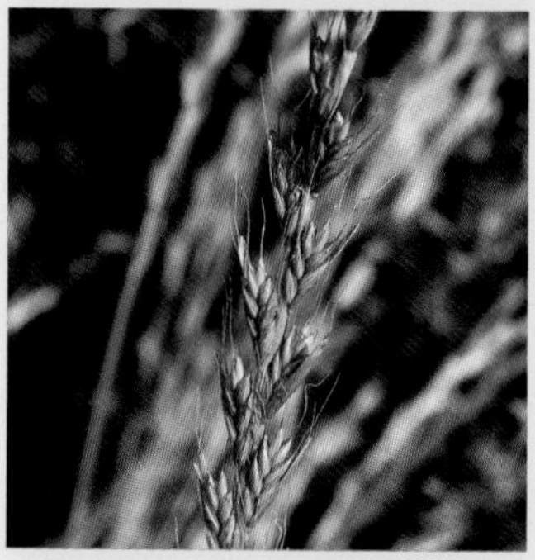

Lolium temulentum

TEAZLE

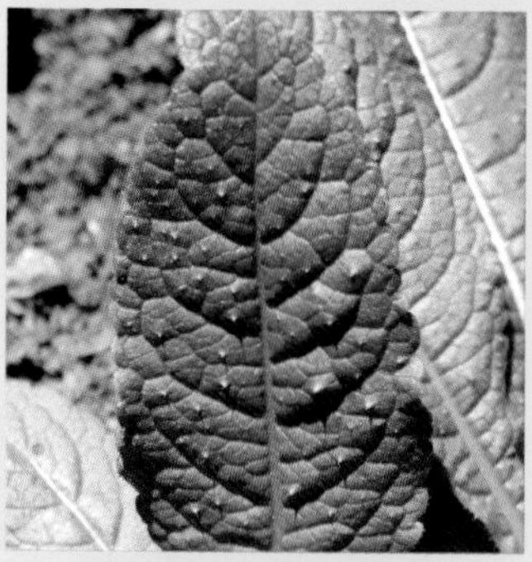

Dipsacus silvestris

THUJA

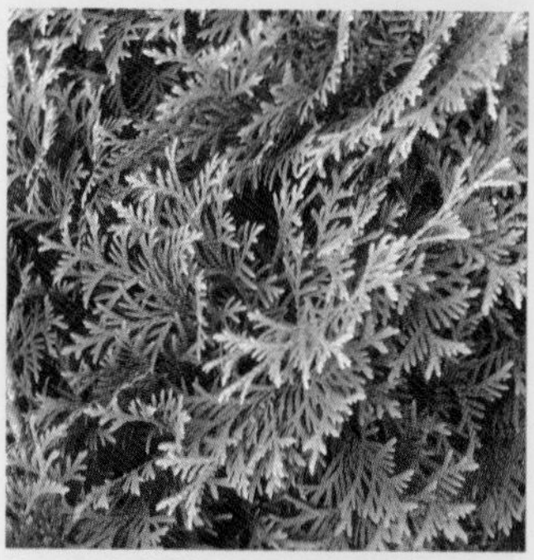

Thuja occidentalis

THYME

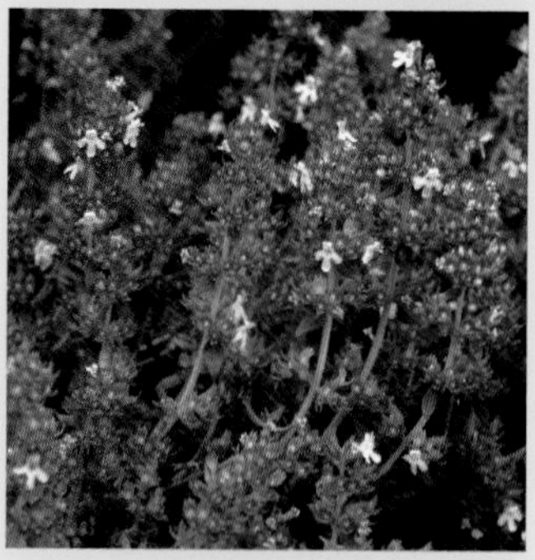

Thymus vulgaris

TOBACCO

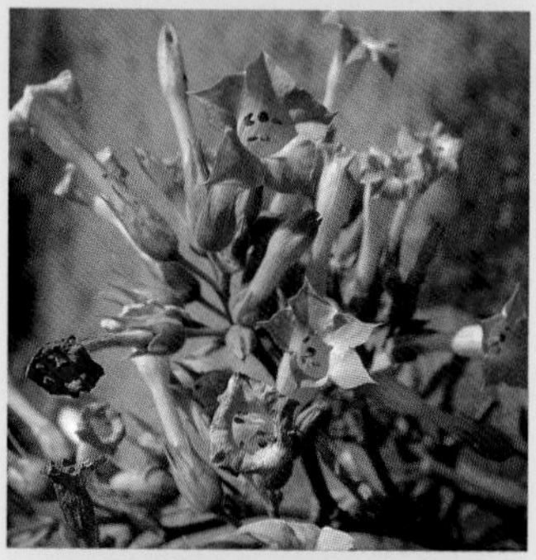

Nicotiana tabacum

TOLU BALSAM

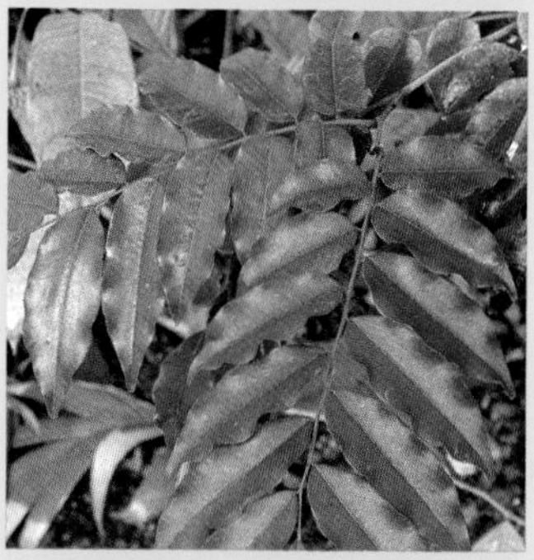

Myroxylon balsamum

TOMATO

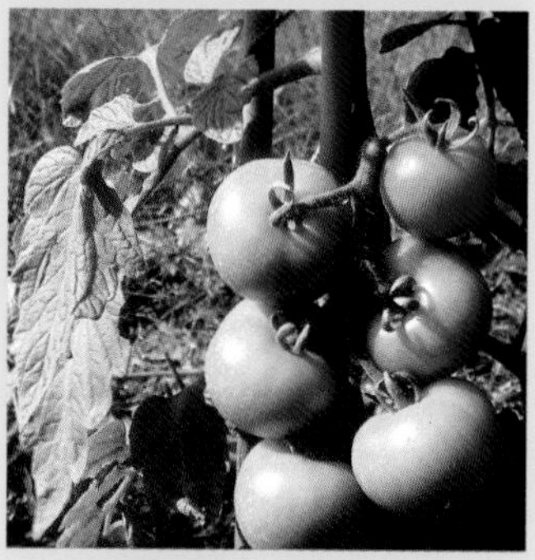

Lycopersicon esculentum

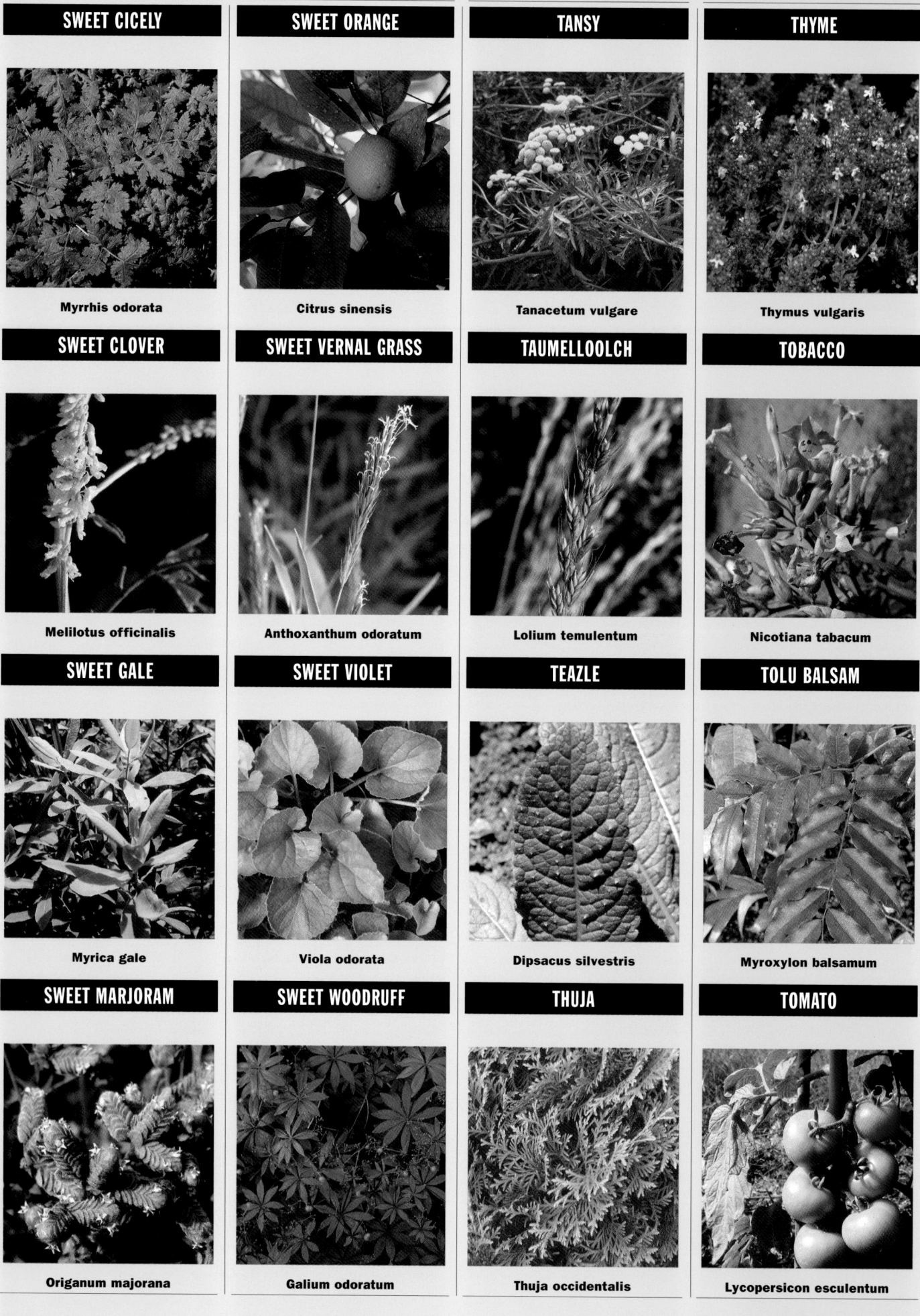

TRAVELLER'S JOY

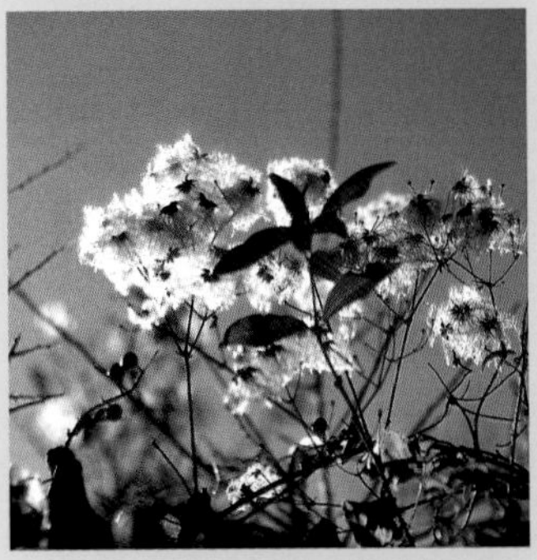

Clematis vitalba

TRITICUM

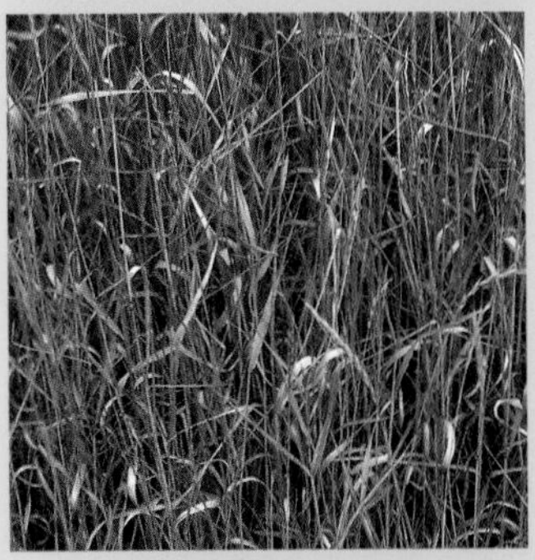

Agropyron repens

UVA-URSI

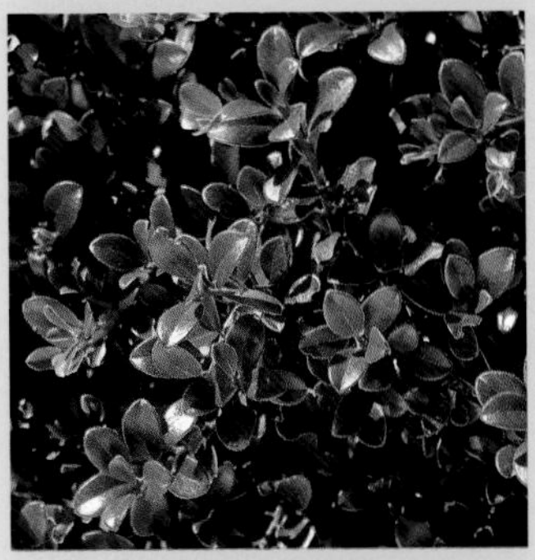

Arctostaphylos uva-ursi

VALERIAN

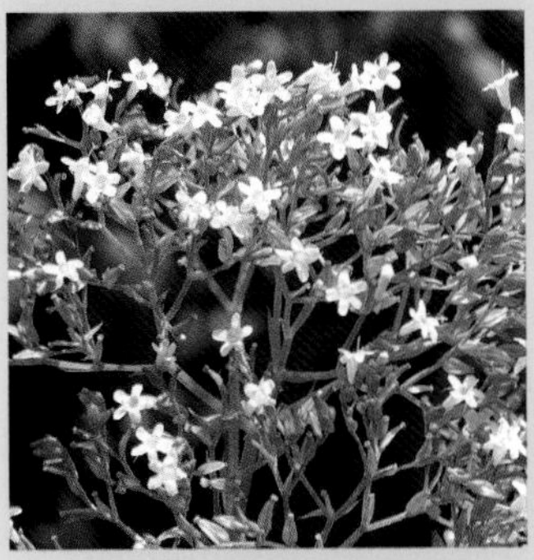

Valeriana officinalis

VERVAIN

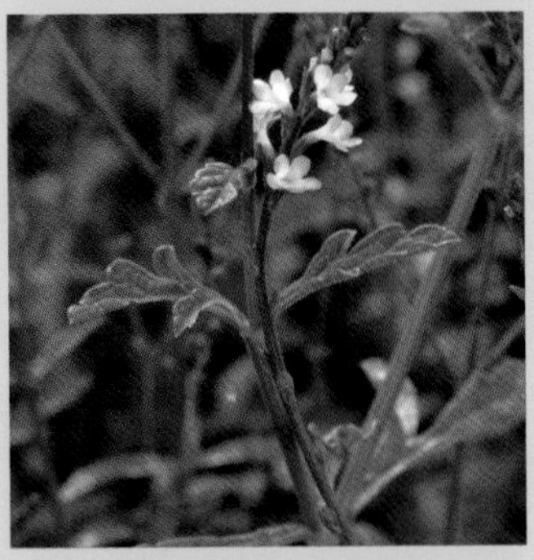

Verbena officinalis

WAHOO

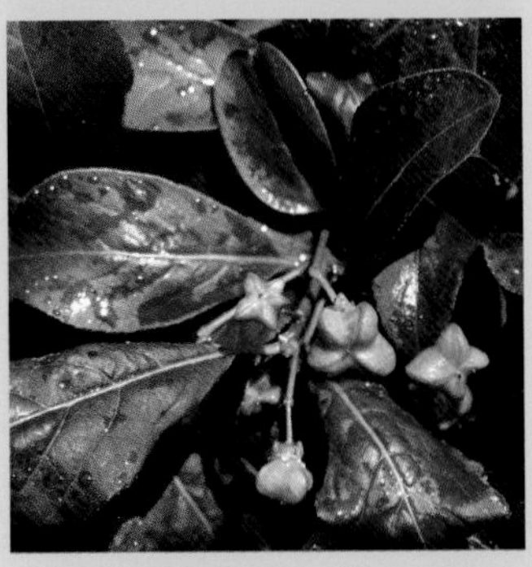

Euonymus atropurpurea

WALLFLOWER

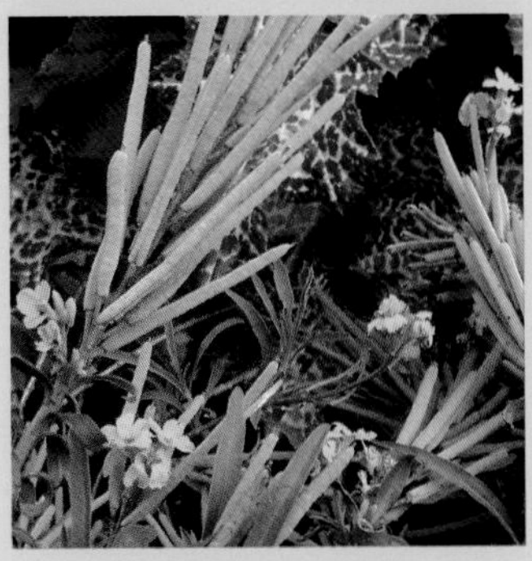

Cheiranthus cheiri

WALNUT

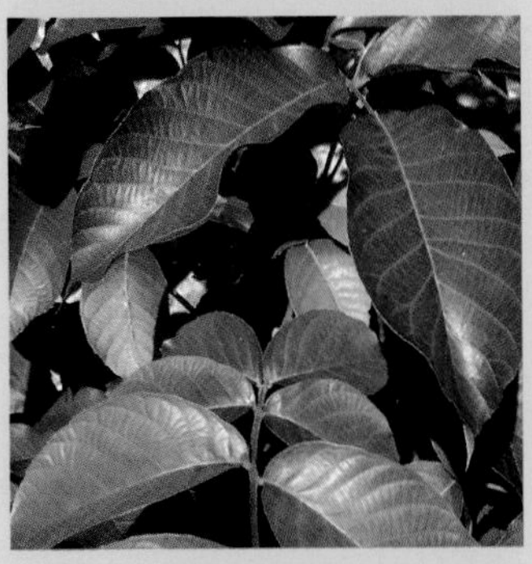

Juglans regia

WATER AVENS

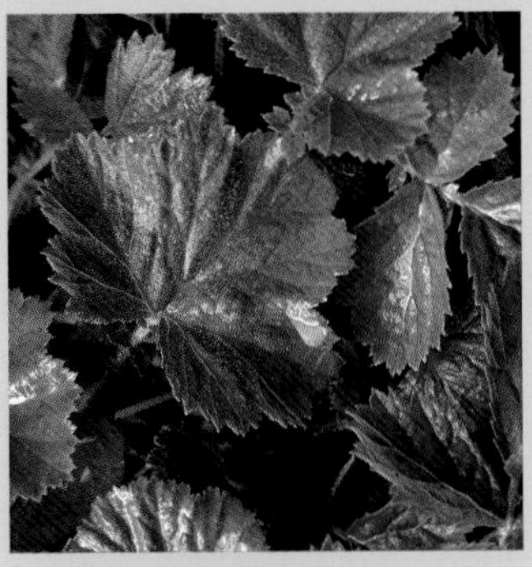

Geum rivale

WATER FENNEL

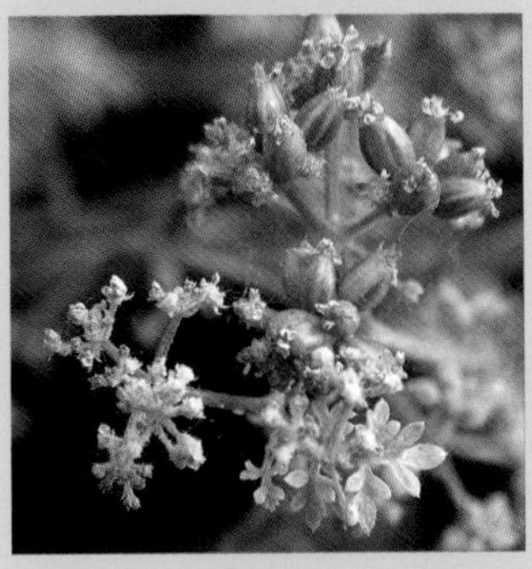

Oenanthe aquatica

WHITE BRYONY

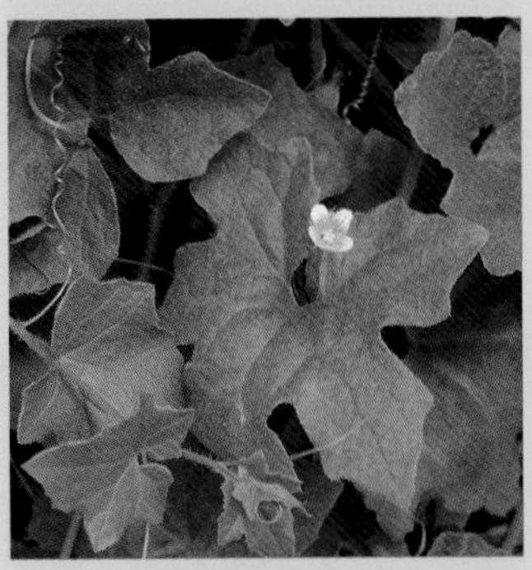

Bryonia alba

WHITE HELLEBORE

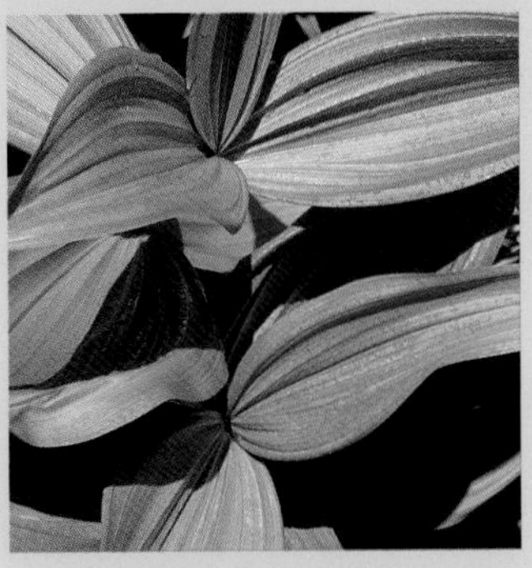

Veratrum album

WHITE MUSTARD

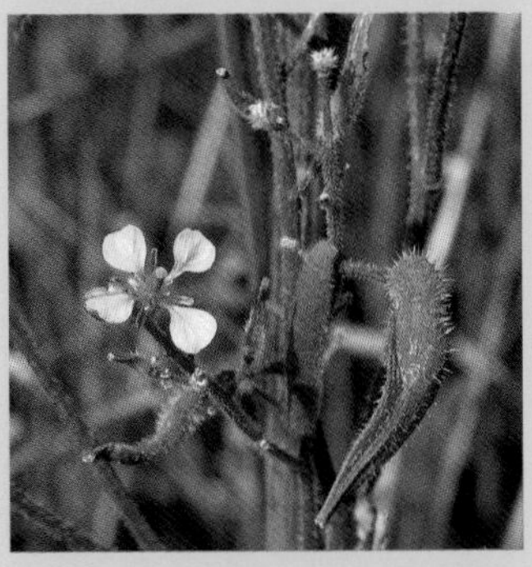

Sinapis alba

WHITE NETTLE

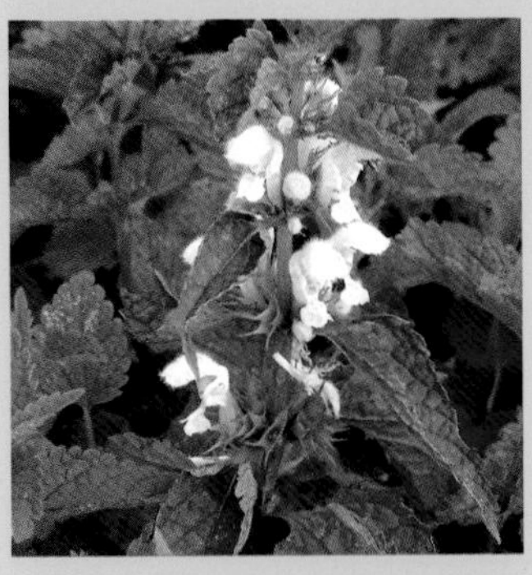

Lamium album

WHITE WILLOW

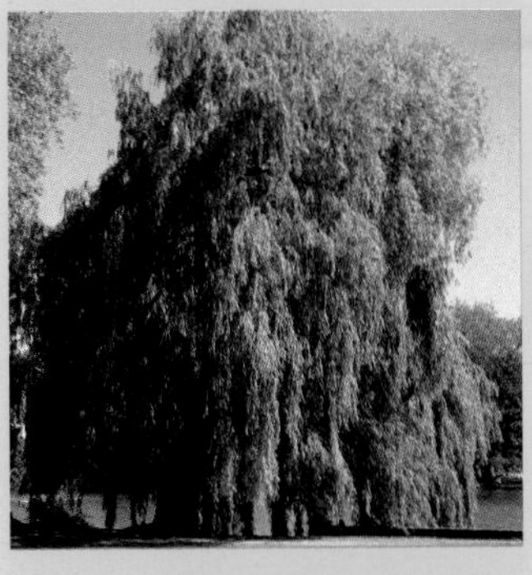

Salix species

WILD CARROT

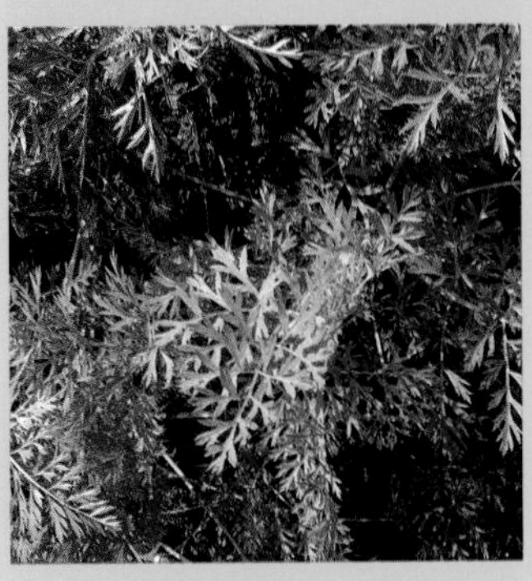

Daucus carota

WILD DAISY

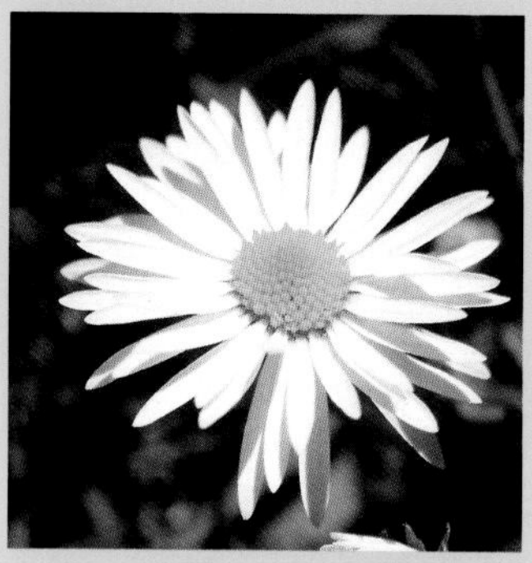

Bellis perennis

WILD INDIGO

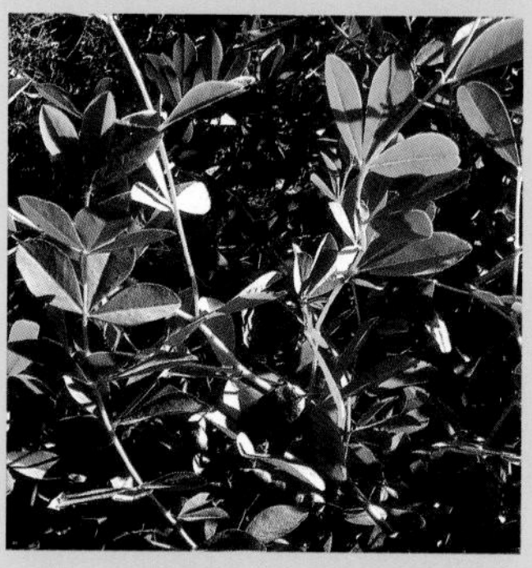

Baptisia tinctoria

WILD MINT

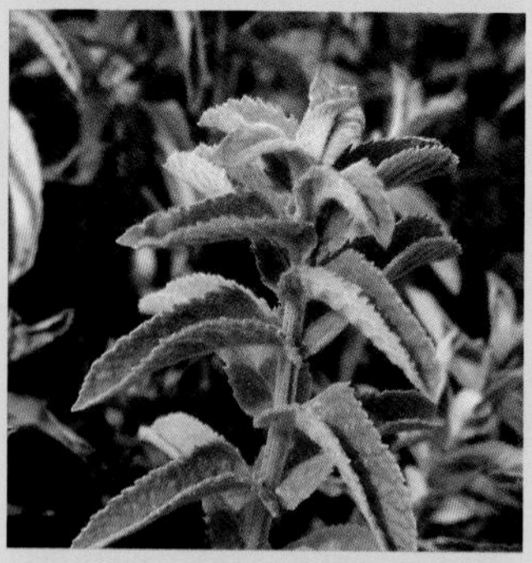

Mentha aquatica

WILD RADISH

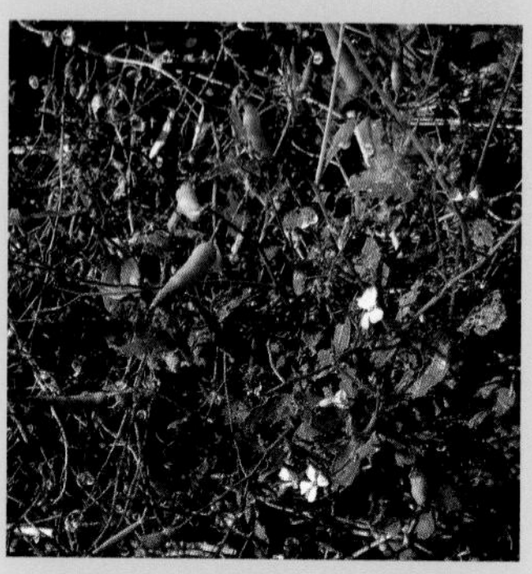

Raphanus raphanistrum

WILD THYME

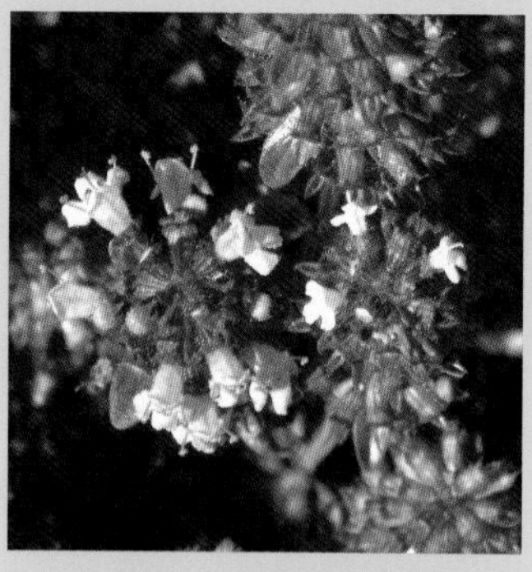

Thymus serpyllum

WILD YAM

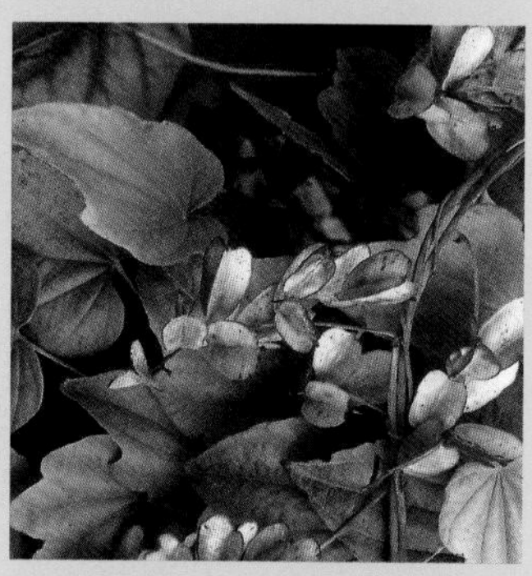

Dioscorea villosa

WILLOW HERB

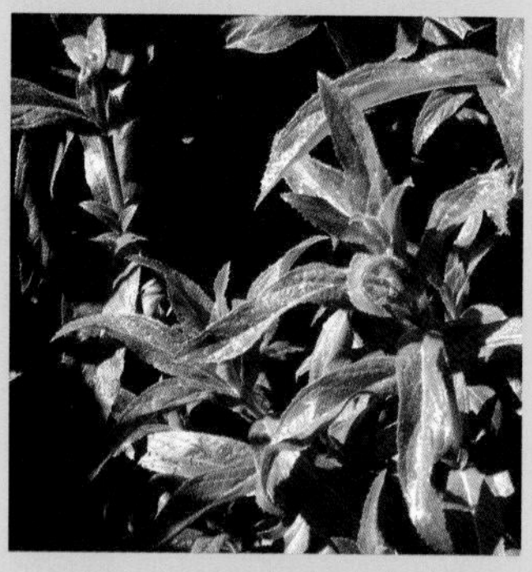

Epilobium angustifolium

WINTER CHERRY

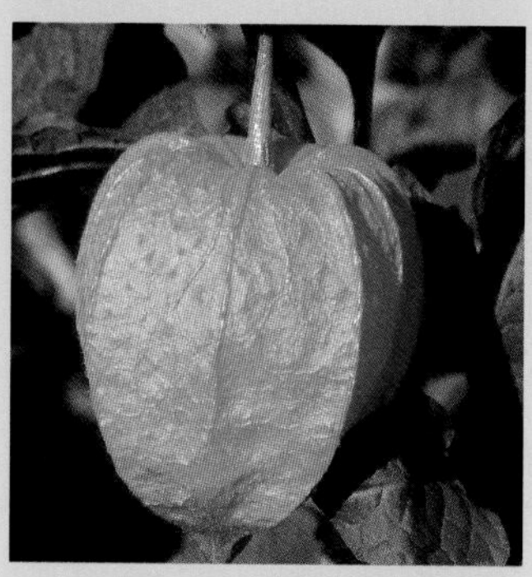

Physalis alkekengi

WITCH HAZEL

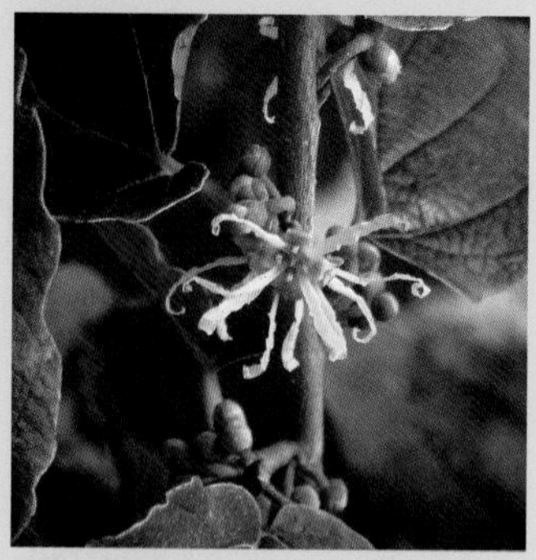

Hamamelis virginiana

WOOD BETONY

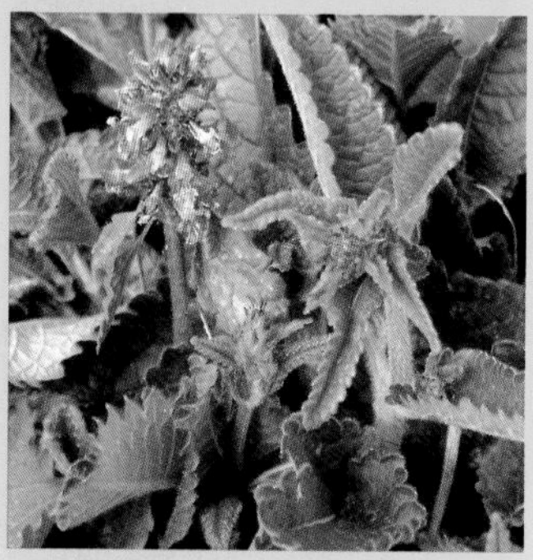

Betonica officinalis

WOOD SAGE

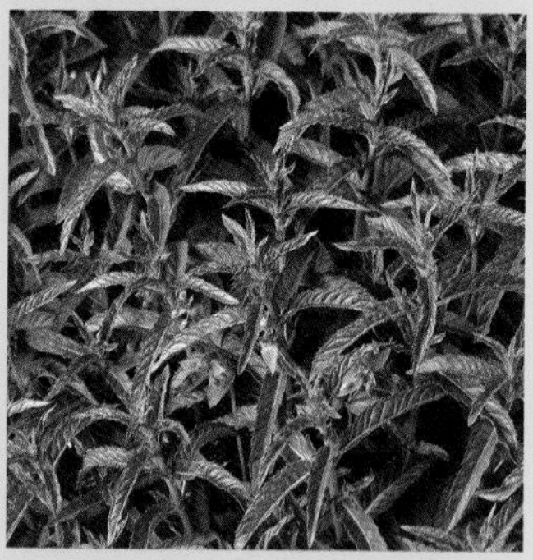

Teucrium scorodonia

WORMSEED OIL

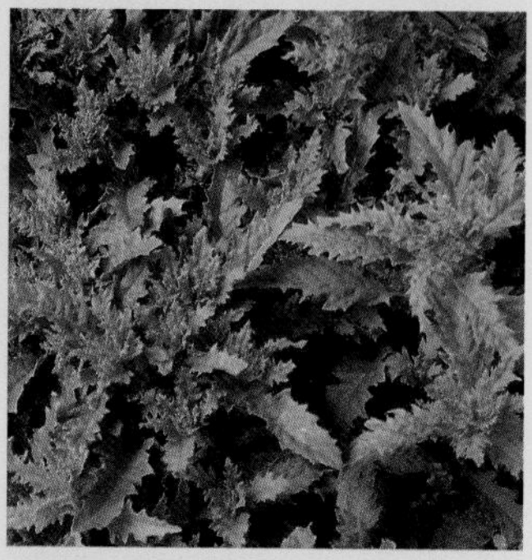

Chenopodium ambrosioides

WORMWOOD

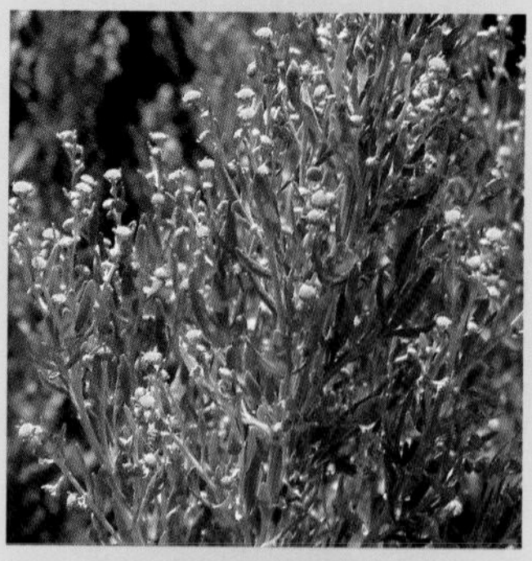

Artemisia absinthium

YARROW

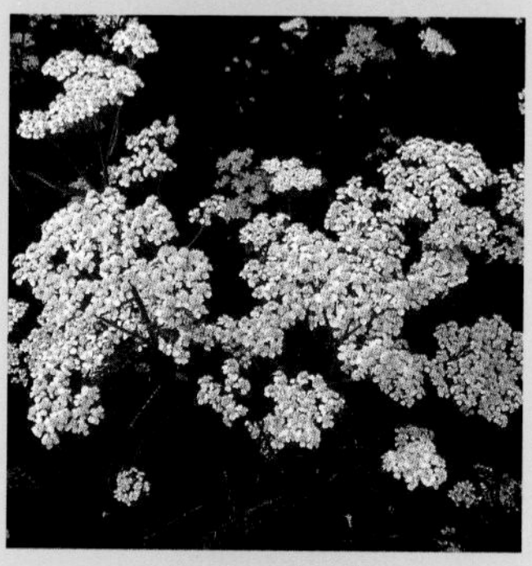

Achillea millefolium

YEW

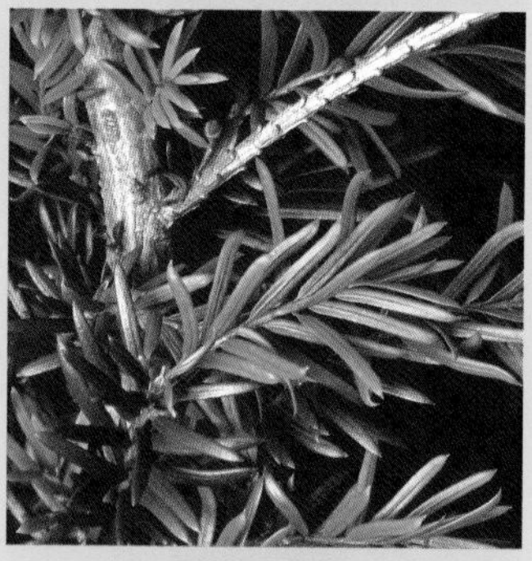

Taxus baccata

ZEDOARY

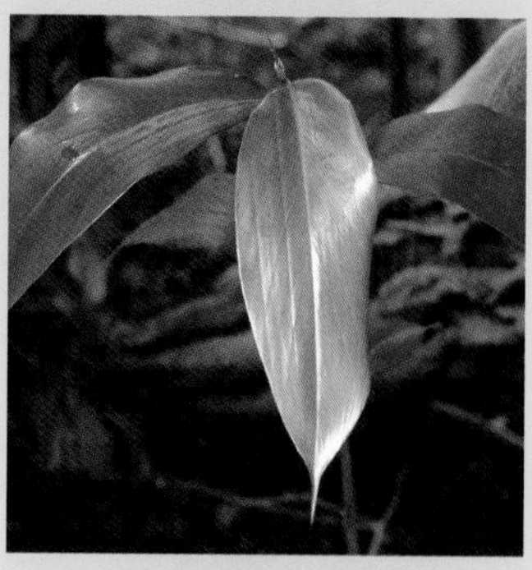

Curcuma zedoaria

Product Identification Guide

Shown here are selected herbal preparations and their packaging. The photos are arranged alphabetically by manufacturer and brand name. The company's name appears above the product; its brand name below.

BAYER CORPORATION

BAYER CORPORATION
CONSUMER CARE DIVISION

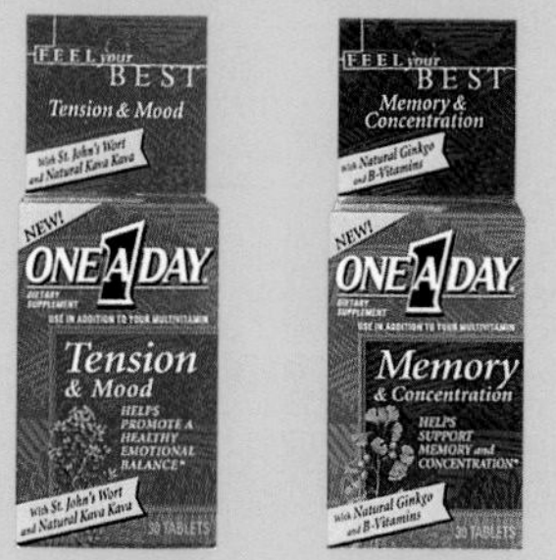

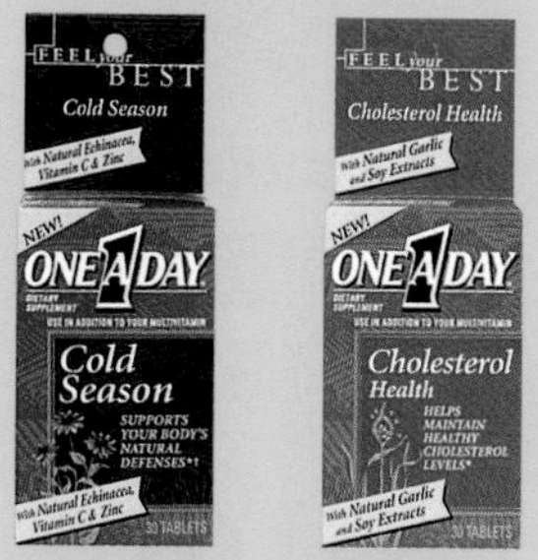

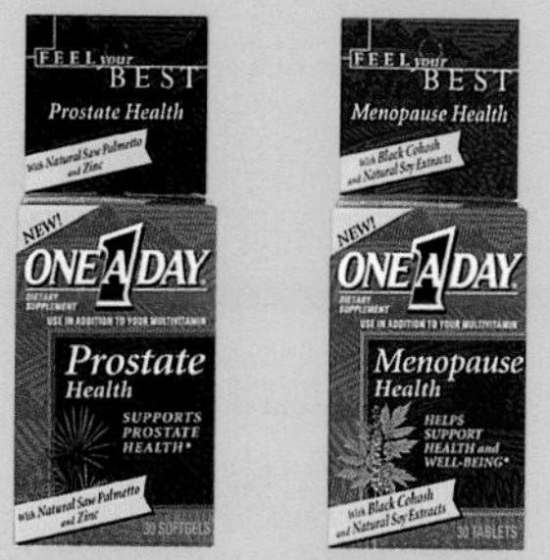

Specialized Nutritional Supplements

Tension & Mood,
Memory & Concentration,
Cold Season, Cholesterol Health,
Prostate Health, Menopause Health

One-A-Day®

BAYER CORPORATION
CONSUMER CARE DIVISION

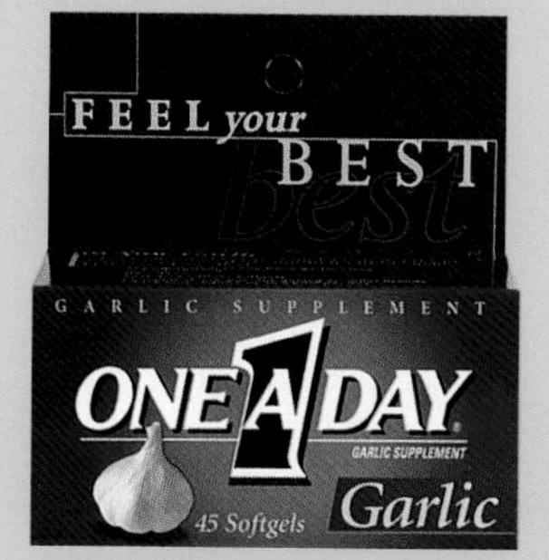

One-A-Day®
Garlic Softgels

LICHTWER PHARMA

LICHTWER PHARMA

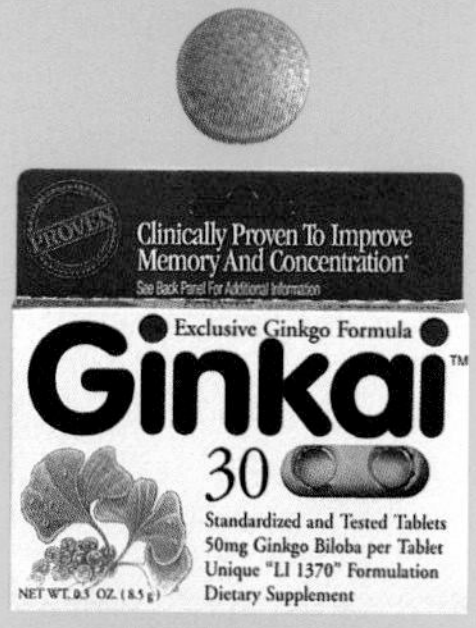

50 mg Ginkgo Biloba
Clinically Proven to Improve
Memory and Concentration

Ginkai®

LICHTWER PHARMA

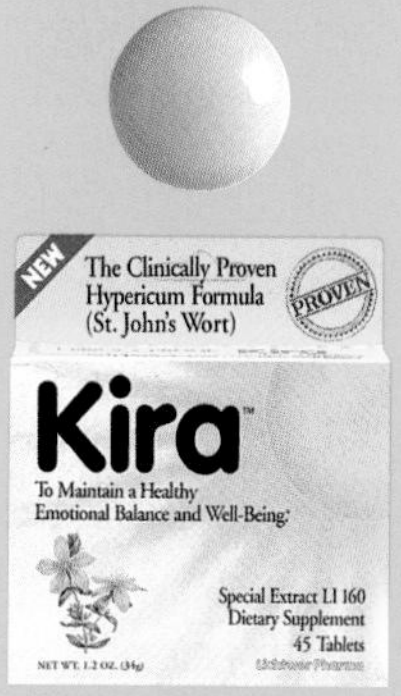

Standardized St. John's Wort Extract
To Maintain a Healthy Emotional Balance and Well-Being

Kira®

LICHTWER PHARMA

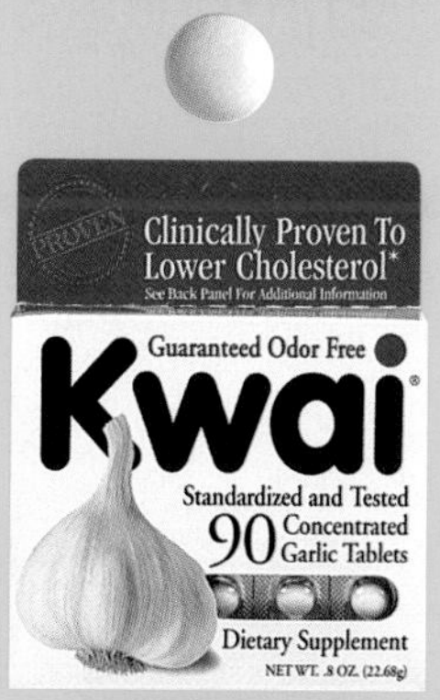

Concentrated Garlic Tablets
Clinically Proven to Lower Cholesterol

Kwai®

NATROL

NATROL

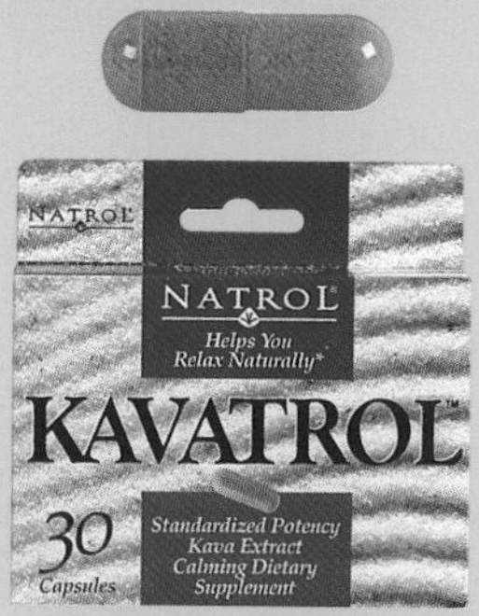

Standardized Potency Kava Extract

Kavatrol™

NOVARTIS

NOVARTIS CONSUMER HEALTH, INC.

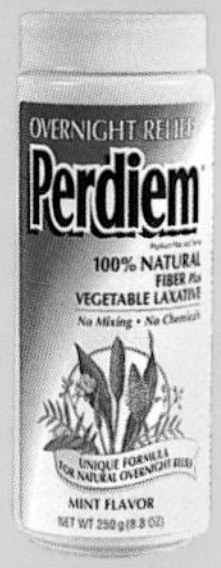

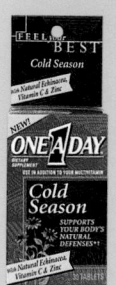

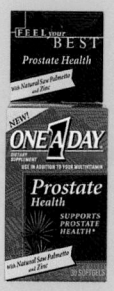

100% Natural Vegetable Laxative
250 gm and 400 gm

Perdiem®
Overnight Relief

NOVARTIS CONSUMER HEALTH, INC.

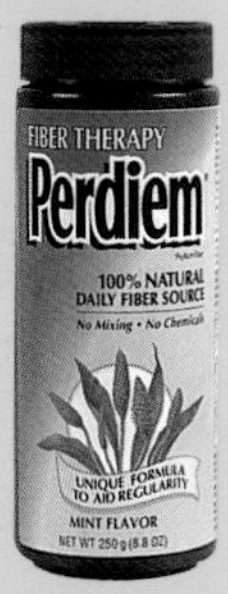

100% Natural
Daily Fiber Source
available in 250 gm

Perdiem® Fiber Therapy

NOVOGEN

NOVOGEN

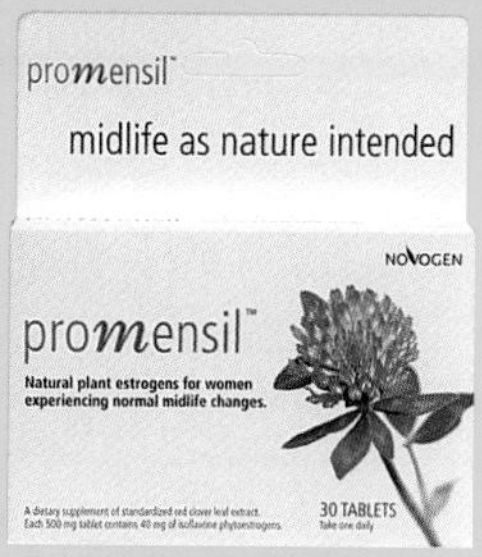

30 Tablets
Natural plant estrogens for women experiencing normal midlife changes.

Promensil™

TO DOUBLE-CHECK SAFETY:

Take a quick glance at the Safety Guide, which lists herbs to be avoided while pregnant and nursing, and those to be used only under supervision.

PHARMANEX, INC.

PHARMANEX, INC.

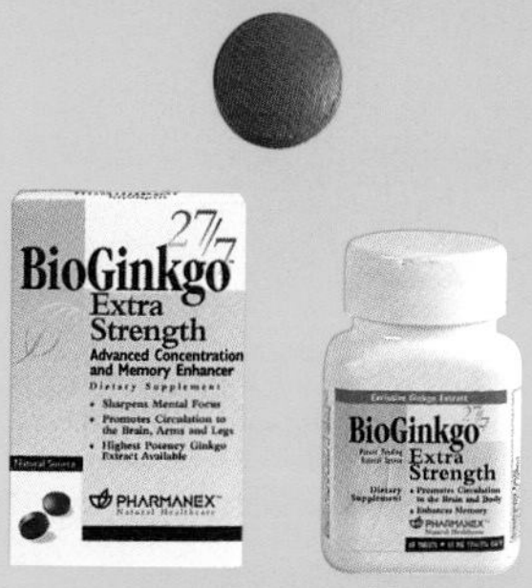

60 mg
Extra Strength Ginkgo biloba
Available in 60 ct.

BioGinkgo 27/7®

PHARMATON

PHARMATON

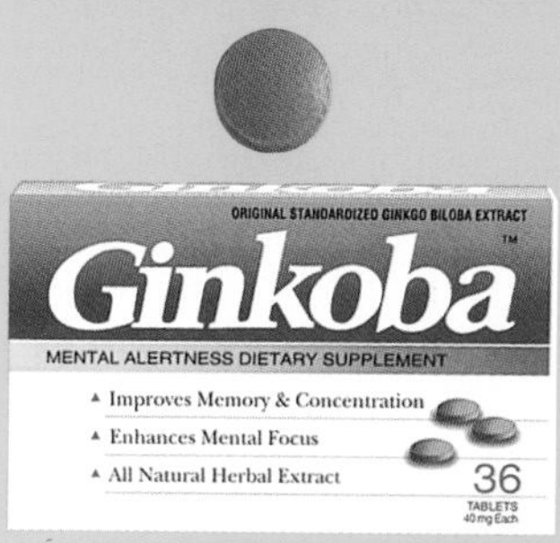

40 mg

Ginkoba™

PHARMATON

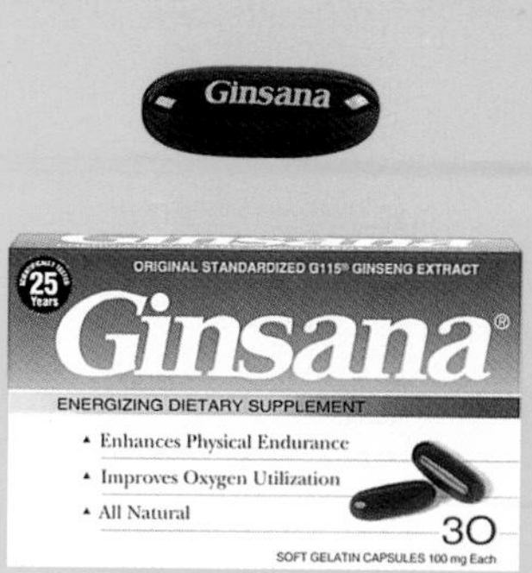

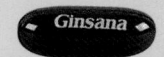

100 mg
Capsules

Ginsana®

PHARMATON

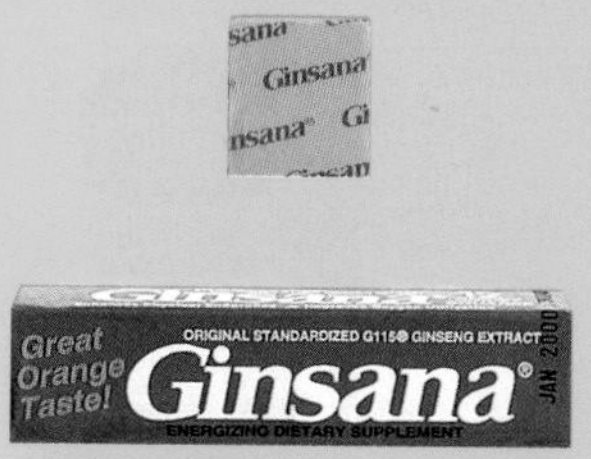

50 mg
Chewy Squares

Ginsana®

PHARMATON

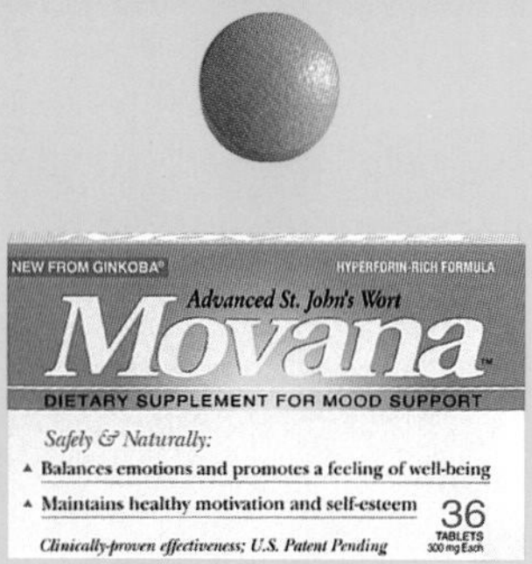

300 mg
Dietary Supplement for Mood Support

Movana™

PHARMATON

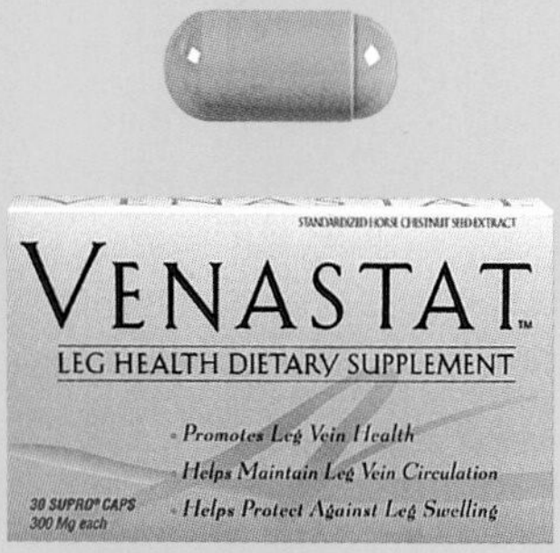

Dietary Supplement for Leg Health

Venastat™

PHYTOPHARMICA

PHYTOPHARMICA

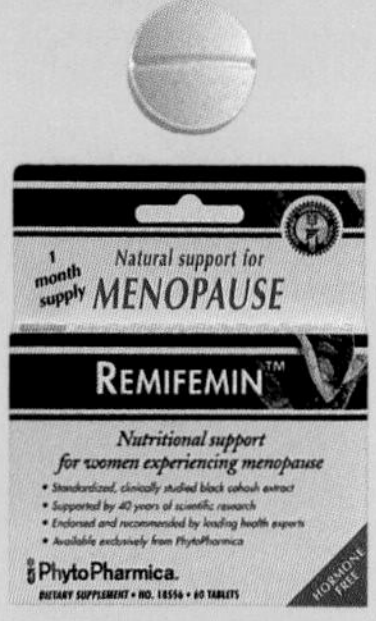

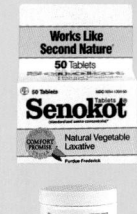

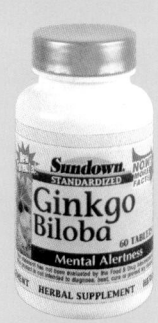

60 and 120 tablets
Natural support for menopause.
Also available in Remifemin™ Plus,
with St. John's Wort.

Remifemin™

PROCTER & GAMBLE

PROCTER & GAMBLE

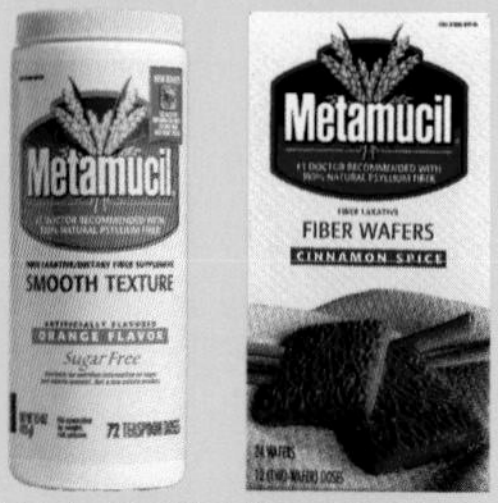

Available in 48, 72, 114 and 180 dose canisters and cartons of 30 one-dose packets.
Also available in sugar free.
Cinnamon Spice and Apple Crisp Wafers available in 12-dose cartons.

Metamucil®

PURDUE FREDERICK

THE PURDUE FREDERICK COMPANY

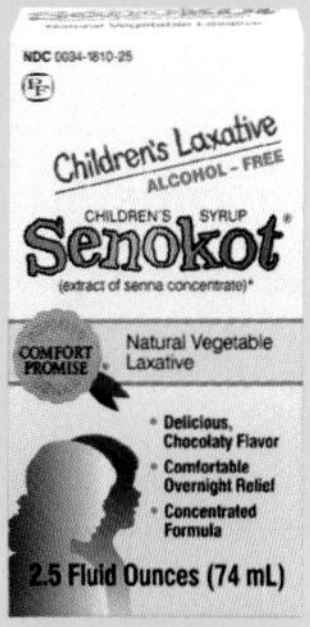

Natural Vegetable Laxative
Children's Syrup

Senokot®

THE PURDUE FREDERICK COMPANY

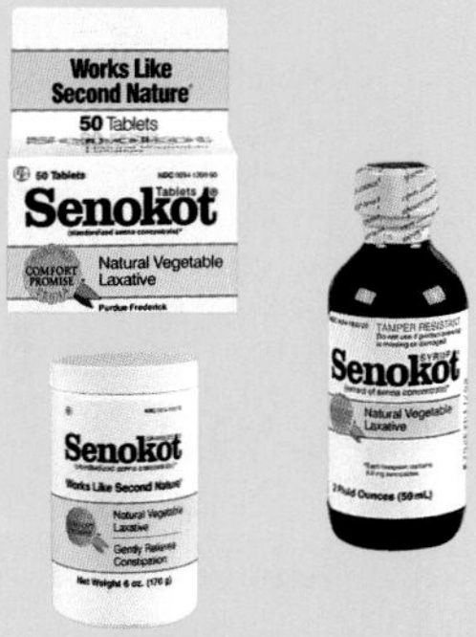

Natural Vegetable Laxative
Available in Tablets, Granules, and Syrup.

Senokot®

REXALL SUNDOWN

REXALL SUNDOWN

Ginkgo Biloba

REXALL SUNDOWN

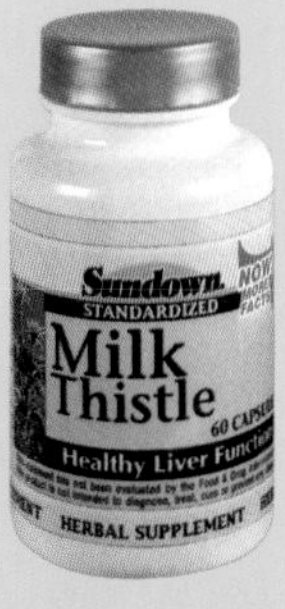

Milk Thistle

REXALL SUNDOWN

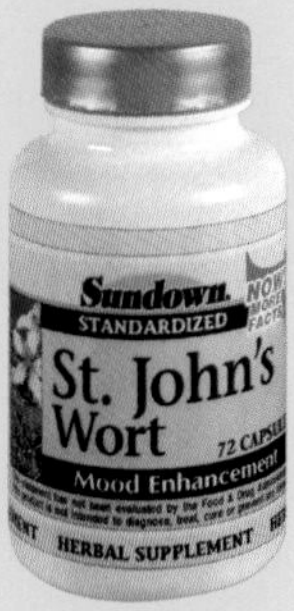

St. John's Wort

REXALL SUNDOWN

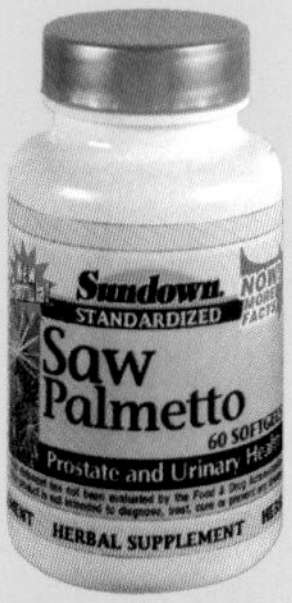

Saw Palmetto

WAKUNAGA

WAKUNAGA CONSUMER PRODUCTS

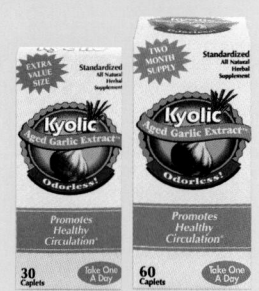

Aged Garlic Extract™

Kyolic®

WARNER-LABMERT

WARNER-LAMBERT CONSUMER HEALTHCARE

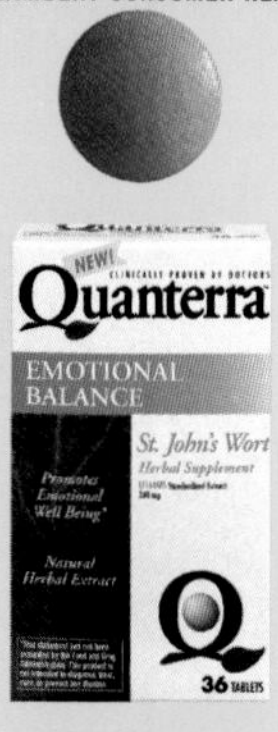

Quanterra™
Emotional Balance

WARNER-LAMBERT CONSUMER HEALTHCARE

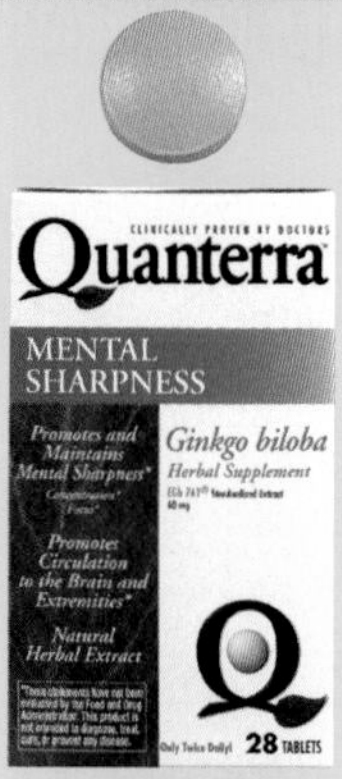

Quanterra™
Mental Sharpness

WARNER-LAMBERT CONSUMER HEALTHCARE

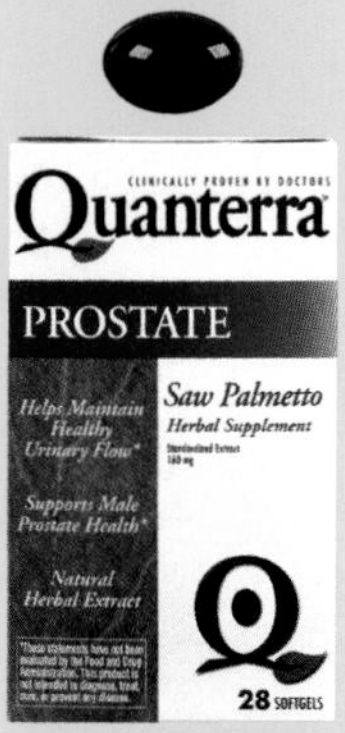

Quanterra™ Prostate

WARNER-LAMBERT CONSUMER HEALTHCARE

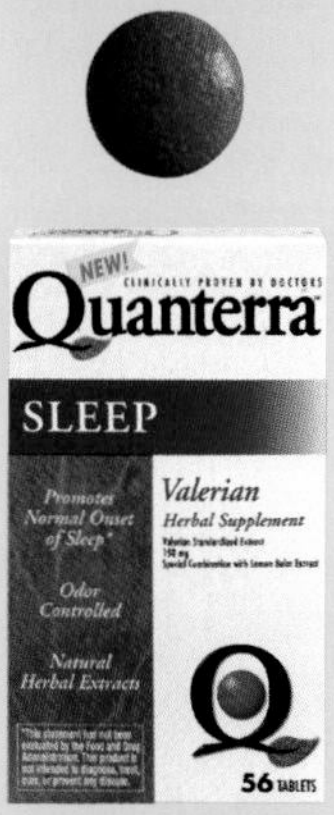

Quanterra™ Sleep

WARNER-LAMBERT CONSUMER HEALTHCARE

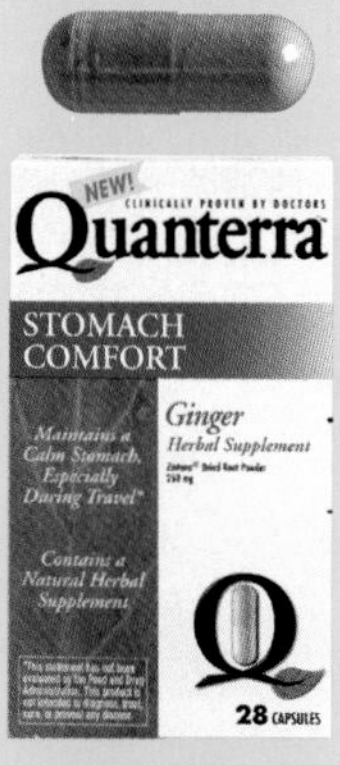

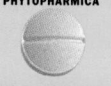

Quanterra™
Stomach Comfort

WHITEHALL-ROBINS

WHITEHALL-ROBINS

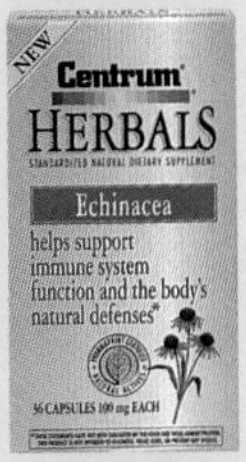

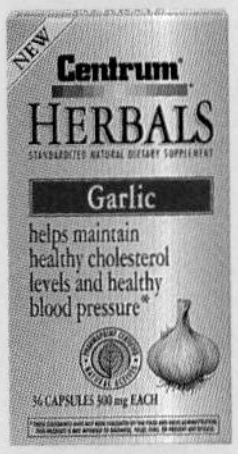

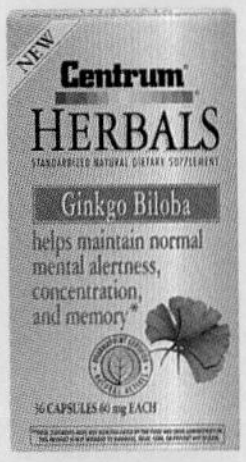

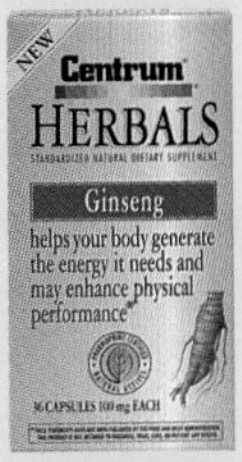

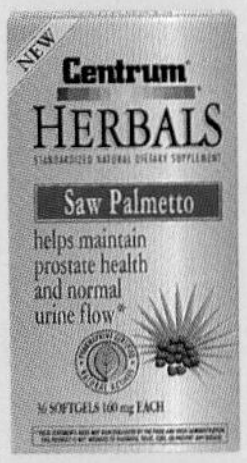

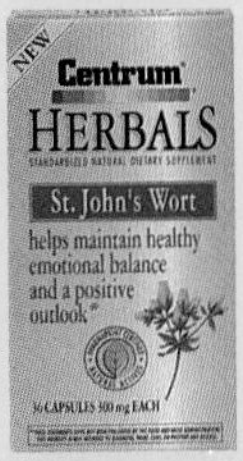

Echinacea, Garlic,
Ginkgo Biloba, Ginseng,
Saw Palmetto, St. John's Wort

Centrum® Herbals

Herbal Monographs

This section contains comprehensive profiles of some 700 medicinal herbs, including the findings of the German Regulatory Authority's herbal watchdog agency, commonly called "Commission E." This agency has conducted an intensive assessment of the peer-reviewed literature on some 300 common botanicals, weighing the quality of the clinical evidence and identifying the uses for which the herb can reasonably be considered effective. Its conclusions represent the best expert consensus on medicinal herbs currently to be found.

For those herbs not considered by Commission E, *Physicians' Desk Reference* has augmented this section with the results of an exhaustive literature review conducted by the respected PhytoPharm U.S. Institute of Phytopharmaceuticals under the direction of noted botanist, Dr. Joerg Gruenwald. These monographs, some 400 in number, provide a detailed introduction to an array of exotic botanicals that you'll be hard pressed to find in any other source.

To make the information in the monographs as useful and accessible as possible, *PDR* has echoed the structure of standard U.S. product labeling. Each monograph contains up to ten standard sections, covering considerations ranging from description to dosage. Specifically, here's what you will find:

■ **Title:** Each monograph begins with the herb's generally accepted common name, followed by its scientific name. In addition, all monographs are cross-referenced by their botanical designation.

■ **Trade Names:** Listed here are common commercial preparations of the herb.

■ **Description:** This section provides a detailed botanical overview of the herb, including information on its medicinal parts; flower and fruit; leaves, stem, and root; unique characteristics, habitat, production, related plants, and additional common names and synonyms.

■ **Actions and Pharmacology:** Here you'll find data on the active compounds or heterogeneous mixtures found in the plant, followed by a summary of the herb's clinical effects. If various parts of the plant possess different pharmacological activity, the parts are discussed individually, here and throughout the remainder of the monograph.

■ **Indications and Usage:** Information on the uses of the herb is listed under five categories, as applicable:
— Approved by Commission E
— Unproven Uses
— Chinese Medicine
— Indian Medicine
— Homeopathic

Approved uses are presented in list fashion. Other uses are described with provisos as necessary regarding route and form of administration.

■ **Contraindications:** Although most natural remedies can be used under all medical circumstances, a few pharmacologically potent herbs must be avoided in the presence of certain medical conditions. If any such contraindications exist, they are summarized here.

■ **Precautions and Adverse Reactions:** Found in this section are any cautions or special considerations regarding safe use of the herb, including any restrictions on use in pregnancy or childhood. Although most herbal remedies are notably free of known side effects, any reported in the available literature are noted here.

■ **Overdosage:** As we all know, "natural" is not synonymous with "benign," and an overdose of many "healing" herbs can have serious—even fatal—consequences. Whenever adverse effects of overdose have been found in the literature, they are reported here, along with the appropriate medical interventions to be undertaken when an overdose occurs.

■ **Dosage:** Listed here are common modes of administration, forms and strengths of available commercial preparations, methods for preparing the natural herb, and representative dosage recommendations drawn from the literature. Note, however, that dosage recommendations can be used only as a general guide. The potency of individual preparations and extracts is subject to substantial variation, so the manufacturer's directions should be consulted whenever available.

■ **Literature:** This section provides you with a unique bibliography of the technical literature. Because German researchers have been particularly active in the herbal arena, you will find an unusual number of German-language citations. However, work in the English literature is included as well.

PDR for Herbal Medicines is the product of one of the most thorough and inclusive examinations of the herbal literature ever undertaken. Nevertheless, it's important to remember that it merely summarizes and synthesizes key data from the underlying research reports, and of necessity includes neither every published report nor every recorded fact.

As in all scientific investigation, conclusions regarding the effectiveness of the herbs discussed in this compendium are based on the preponderance of current evidence and cannot be considered firm or final. The publisher does not warrant that any herb will unfailingly and uniformly exhibit the properties ascribed to it by Germany's Commission E or any other scientific authority.

In the United States, herbal products are marketed under the provisions of the Dietary Supplement and Health Education Act of 1994, which prohibits their sale for the diagnosis, treatment, cure, or prevention of any disease. Enumeration of specific commercial preparations within an herbal monograph should not be construed as a claim or warranty of their efficacy for any purpose, by either the manufacturer or the publisher. Furthermore, it should be understood that, just as omission of a product does not signify rejection, inclusion of a product does not imply endorsement, and that the publisher is not advocating the use of any product or substance described herein.

Please remember, too, that dosing of herbal preparations is highly dependent on a variety of factors, such as cultivation and harvesting conditions, the specific parts of the plant to be processed, the extraction methods employed, and the dosage form chosen by the manufacturer. Since there are no official standards governing the production of herbal medicines in the United States, and the potency and the purity of herbal products are subject to substantial variation, dosage ranges set forth in the herbal monographs must be employed only as general guidelines.

In addition, the publisher does not guarantee that every possible hazard, adverse effect, contraindication, precaution, or consequence of overdose is included in the summaries presented here. The publisher has performed no independent verification of the data reported herein, and expressly disclaims responsibility for any error, whether inherent in the underlying literature or resulting from erroneous translation, transcription, or typography.

Abelmoschus moschatus

See Muskmallow

Abies alba

See White Fir

Abrus precatorius

See Jequirity

Abscess Root

Polemonium reptans

DESCRIPTION

Medicinal Parts: The medicinal part is the dried root.

Flower and Fruit: The hanging blue flowers are in loose terminal, glandular-haired panicles.

Leaves, Stem and Root: The plant grows to about 25 cm. It has creeping roots and a thin rhizome, which produces numerous stems and numerous pale, thin, glabrous and brittle roots. The glabrous stems are heavily branched and bear alternate or opposite, pinnatifid leaves with 6 or 7 pairs of leaflets.

Habitat: The plant is found in the U.S.

Production: Abscess Root is the rhizome of Polemonium reptans.

Not to be Confused With: The plant is known as False Jacob's Ladder because it has an astringent action similar to true Jacob's Ladder.

Other Names: American Greek Valerian, Blue Bells, False Jacob's Ladder, Sweatroot

ACTIONS AND PHARMACOLOGY

COMPOUNDS

Triterpene saponins

EFFECTS

Abscess root has astringent, diaphoretic and expectorant effects.

INDICATIONS AND USAGE

Unproven Uses: The drug is used for febrile and inflammatory disorders.

PRECAUTIONS AND ADVERSE REACTIONS

No health hazards or side effects are known in conjunction with the proper administration of designated therapeutic dosages.

DOSAGE

Mode of Administration: It is ground as a drug for infusion.

LITERATURE

Hegnauer R, Chemotaxonomie der Pflanzen, Bde 1-11, Birkhäuser Verlag Basel, Boston, Berlin 1962-1997.

Acacia

Acacia arabica

DESCRIPTION

Medicinal Parts: The medicinal parts are the bark, the gum and the fruit of the plant.

Flower and Fruit: The flowers are yellow and sweetly scented. Two to 6 inflorescence peduncles with capitula-like inflorescences grow from the axils of the upper leaflets. The flowers have short calyces with numerous overlapping sepals. The completely fused petals are almost twice as large as the sepals. The fruit is a 12 to 16 cm long and 1.5 cm wide pod. The pod is straight or lightly curved, flat to convex, and pinched in to create segments. It is matte-black to dark-red. The seeds are 7 x 6 mm and the same color as the pod.

Leaves, Stem and Root: Acacia arabica is a 6 m high tree with a compact, round to flat crown. Older branches are bare, younger ones measuring 15 to 20 mm in diameter are covered in hairy down. The bark is black and fissured; the coloring in the fissure changes to red-brown. There are stipule thorns at the nodes. The leaflets of the double-pinnate leaves are in 3 to 12 pairs on the bare to downy petiole, which is covered with glands. The leaflets are oblong, blunt, and bare or thinly ciliate.

Habitat: The plant is indigenous to the Nile area, Ethiopia, East Africa, Angola, Mozambique, South Africa, Arabia, Iran, Afghanistan and India.

Production: The bark is collected from plants that are at least 7 years old and then left to mature for a year.

Not to be Confused With: The bark of the Australian species Acacia decurrens, which is commercially available under the same name.

Other Names: Acacia Bark, Babul Bark, Wattle Bark, Indian Gum, Black Wattle

ACTIONS AND PHARMACOLOGY

COMPOUNDS

Tannins

EFFECTS

The drug has an astringent effect.

INDICATIONS AND USAGE

Unproven Uses: The drug is used as a decoction for gum disease and inflammations of the mucous membrane of the mouth and throat (rarely used today).

Indian Medicine: Acacia is used as a decoction in the treatment of diarrhea and vaginal secretions, and as an enema for hemorrhoids.

PRECAUTIONS AND ADVERSE REACTIONS

Large doses taken internally can lead to indigestion and constipation.

LITERATURE

Berger F, Handbuch der Drogenkunde, W Maudrich Verlag Wien 1964.

Hänsel R, Keller K, Rimpler H, Schneider G (Hrsg.), Hagers Handbuch der Pharmazeutischen Praxis, 5. Aufl., Bde 4-6 (Drogen), Springer Verlag Berlin, Heidelberg, New York, 1992-1994.

Trease GE, Evans WC (Eds.), Pharmacognosy, 12th Ed., Bailliere Tindall 1983.

Acacia arabica

See Acacia

Acacia catechu

See Catechu

Acacia senegal

See Gum Arabic

Acalypha indica

See Indian Nettle

Acer rubrum

See Red Maple

Achillea millefolium

See Yarrow

Achillea ptarmica

See Sneezewort

Aconitum napellus

See Monkshood

Acorus calamus

See Calamus

Actaea spicata

See Baneberry

Adam's Needle

Yucca filamentosa

DESCRIPTION

Medicinal Parts: The medicinal parts are the leaves and the roots of non-flowering plants.

Flower and Fruit: The flowers are ivory-colored and located in nodding, many-blossomed terminal panicles. The perigone is simple, campanulate, tinged greenish on the outside, with 6 tepals. The flower has 6 stamens, and the stigma is 3-sectioned.

Leaves, Stem and Root: The plant is 120 to 240 cm in height. The leaves are in a basal rosette. They are sword-shaped and erect with a recurved tip. They are short-thorned, broadly grooved and covered on the margin with long, twisted, whitish or yellowish threads.

Habitat: The plant is indigenous to the southern United States and is cultivated mainly as an ornamental plant in Europe.

Production: Adam's Needle leaves are the leaves of Yucca filamentosa.

ACTIONS AND PHARMACOLOGY

COMPOUNDS

Steroid saponins (from the roots; the saponins from the leaves remain uninvestigated): protoyuccoside C, yuccoside B, yuccoside E, yuccoside C, aglycones including sarsapogenin, tigogenin

EFFECTS

No information is available.

INDICATIONS AND USAGE

Unproven Uses: The plant is used for liver and gallbladder disorders.

PRECAUTIONS AND ADVERSE REACTIONS

No health hazards or side effects are known in conjunction with the proper administration of designated therapeutic dosages. Intake can lead to stomach complaints because of the saponin content.

DOSAGE

Mode of Administration: Adam's Needle is available in ground form and in extracts.

LITERATURE

Kern W, List PH, Hörhammer L (Hrsg.), Hagers Handbuch der Pharmazeutischen Praxis, 4. Aufl., Bde. 1-8: Springer Verlag Berlin, Heidelberg, New York, 1969.

Madaus G, Lehrbuch der Biologischen Arzneimittel, Bde 1-3, Nachdruck, Georg Olms Verlag Hildesheim 1979.

Adiantum capillus-veneris

See Maidenhair

Adonis

Adonis vernalis

DESCRIPTION

Medicinal Parts: The medicinal part is derived from the aerial parts of the herb, which are collected during the flowering season and dried.

Flower and Fruit: The erect, solitary, terminal flower is 4 to 7 cm in diameter and the 5 broad-ovate, downy sepals are half as long as the petals. The 10 to 20 petals are narrow, wedge-shaped, simple or finely serrated at the tip. They are 20 to 40 mm long and lemon-yellow, splayed, glossy, reddish on the outside or greenish-tinged. There are numerous stamens and carpels. The small fruit forms a globose capitulum. The fruit is tomentose, wrinkled, laterally veined and keeled with a sideways-facing, hook-shaped beak. The fruit are arranged on the spindle-shaped, oblong receptacle.

Leaves, Stem and Root: The plant is 10 to 40 cm high with a sturdy, black-brown rhizome. The stem is erect, undivided, covered with scales at the base, vertically grooved and succulent. There are few branches. The leaves have many slits and a curved, glabrous or sparsely haired tip. The middle leaves are half-clasping.

Characteristics: Adonis is a poisonous plant.

Habitat: This Siberian/east European plant is found in the north as far as the central Urals and southwest Sweden. In central Europe, it is limited to the basins of the Weichsel and the Oder as far as the Main and Rhine.

Production: The drug is gathered in forests and should be dried quickly.

Not to be Confused With: Other Adonis species may be added to Adonidis herba.

Other Names: False Hellebore, Yellow Pheasant's Eye, Oxeye, Sweet Vernal, Pheasant's Eye, Red Morocco, Rose-a-Rubie

ACTIONS AND PHARMACOLOGY

COMPOUNDS

Cardioactive steroid gylcosides (cardenolids): including adonitoxin, k-strophanthoside, k-strophanthoside-β and cymarin

Flavonoids: including vitexin and luteolin

EFFECTS

Adonis has a positive inotropic effect. Animal tests demonstrated a tonic effect on the veins. The adonitoxin component is slightly more toxic than coumarin.

The drug is insufficiently documented.

INDICATIONS AND USAGE

Approved by Commission E:

- Arrhythmia
- Nervous heart complaints

Unproven Uses : The drug is used for mild impairment of heart functions (NYHA I and II), especially when accompanied by nervous symptoms.

In Russian folk medicine, the drug is used for dehydration, cramps, fever and menstrual disorders, but efficacy is unproven.

Homeopathic Uses: Preparations of Adonis vernalis are used for cardiac insufficiency.

CONTRAINDICATIONS

Adonis is contraindicated in conjunction with digitalis glycoside therapy and also in potassium deficiency.

PRECAUTIONS AND ADVERSE REACTIONS

General: Despite the strong efficacy of the drug's cardioactive steroid gylcosides in parenteral application, serious poisoning in the course of per oral administration is hardly to be expected due to the low resorption rate.

Drug Interactions: Enhancement of efficacy, and thus also of side effects, with simultaneous administration of quinidine, digoxin, calcium, saluretics, laxatives and extended therapy with glucocorticoids.

OVERDOSAGE

For possible symptoms of overdose and treatment of poisonings see *Digitalis folium.*

DOSAGE

Mode of Administration: Comminuted herb and preparations thereof for internal use.

Daily Dosage: The average daily dose is 0.5 gm of standardized Adonis powder. The maximum single dose is 1.0 gm; maximum daily dose is 3.0 gm.

Homeopathic Dosage: From D2: 5 to 10 drops, 1 tablet or 5 to 10 globules, 1 to 3 times daily; Injection solution: 1 ml once a week sc. From D4: Injection solution: 1 ml twice weekly sc.

Storage: Adonis herb and powder should be stored carefully. Adonis powder should be stored away from light in tightly sealed containers.

LITERATURE

Brevoort P, Der Heilpflanzenmarkt der USA - Ein Überblick. In: ZPT 18(3):155-162. 1997.

ESCOP-Monographs. In: ESCOP-Monographs Fascicule I and II. 1996.

Hiller KO, Rahlfs V, Therapeutische Äquivalenz eines hochdosierten Phytopharmakons mit Amytriptylin bei ängstlich-depressiven Versimmungen - Reanalyse einer randomisierten Studie unter besonderer Beachtung biometrischer und klinischer Aspekte. In: Forsch.

Karrer W, (1950) Helv Chim Acta 33:433.

Lee MK, et al., Antihepatotoxic activity of Icariin, a major constituent of Epimedium koreanum. In: PM 61(6):523-526. 1995.

Loew, Buch. In: Loew D, Rietbrock N: Phytopharmaka II: Forschung und klinische Anwendung, Steinkopff Verlag, Darmstadt, 1996.

Loew DA, Loew AD, Pharmakokinetik von herzglykosidhaltigen Pflanzenextrakten. In: ZPT 15(4):197-202. 1994.

Loew D, Phytotherapie bei Herzinsuffizienz. In: ZPT 18(2):92-96. 1997.

Martinez-Vazquez M, Ramirez Apan TO, Hidemi Aguilar M, Bye R, Analgesic and antipyretic activities of an aqueous extract and of the flavone Linarin of Buddleia cordata. In: PM 62:137-140. 1996.

Reinhard KH, Uncaria tomentosa (WILLD.) DC. - Cat's claw, Una de gato oder Katzenkralle Protrait einer Arzneipflanze. In: ZPT 18(2):112-121. 1997.

Sandberg F, Thorsen R, (1962) Lloydia 25(3):201.

Schulz V, Hübner WD, Ploch M, Klinische Studien mit Psycho-Phytopharmaka. In: ZPT 18(3):141-154. 1997.

Winkler C and Wichtel M, (1985) Pharm Acta Helv 60(9/10): 234.

Further information in:

Frohne D, Pfänder HJ, Giftpflanzen - Ein Handbuch für Apotheker, Toxikologen und Biologen, 4. Aufl., Wiss. Verlags-Ges Stuttgart 1997.

Hänsel R, Keller K, Rimpler H, Schneider G (Hrsg.), Hagers Handbuch der Pharmazeutischen Praxis, 5. Aufl., Bde 4-6 (Drogen), Springer Verlag Berlin, Heidelberg, New York, 1992-1994.

Lewin L, Gifte und Vergiftungen, 6. Aufl., Nachdruck, Haug Verlag, Heidelberg 1992.

Madaus G, Lehrbuch der Biologischen Arzneimittel, Bde 1-3, Nachdruck, Georg Olms Verlag Hildesheim 1979.

Roth L, Daunderer M, Kormann K, Giftpflanzen, Pflanzengifte, 4. Aufl., Ecomed Fachverlag Landsberg Lech 1993.

Schulz R, Hänsel R, Rationale Phytotherapie, Springer Verlag Heidelberg 1996.

Steinegger E, Hänsel R, Pharmakognosie, 5. Aufl., Springer Verlag Heidelberg 1992.

Teuscher E, Biogene Arzneimittel, 5. Aufl., Wiss. Verlagsges. Stuttgart 1997.

Teuscher E, Lindequist U, Biogene Gifte - Biologie, Chemie, Pharmakologie, 2. Aufl., Fischer Verlag Stuttgart 1994.

Wagner H, Wiesenauer M, Phytotherapie. Phytopharmaka und pflanzliche Homöopathika, Fischer-Verlag, Stuttgart, Jena, New York 1995.

Adonis vernalis

See Adonis

Adrue

Cyperus articulatus

DESCRIPTION

Medicinal Parts: Adrue root is used in the West Indies for its anti-emetic properties.

Flower and Fruit: The tubers are blackish and top-shaped, with bristly remains of former leaves. The plant is sometimes connected in twos or threes by narrow underground stems. The transverse section is pale, showing a central column with darker vascular bundles.

Characteristics: Adrue has an aromatic odor and a bitter taste, reminiscent of Lavender.

Habitat: Turkey, region of the river Nile, Jamaica.

Production: Adrue root is the root of Cyperus articulatus. The roots are collected in the autumn, scalded or steamed, and then dried in the sun.

Other Names: Guinea Rush

ACTIONS AND PHARMACOLOGY

COMPOUNDS

Volatile oil: containing above all sesquiterpene hydrocarbons and sesqiterpene alcohols, including cyperenone

EFFECTS

Adrue has anti-emetic, carminative and sedative properties.

INDICATIONS AND USAGE

Unproven Uses: Preparations of the root are used for digestive disorders, nausea and flatulence.

Chinese Medicine: Used for pre- and post-natal headaches, epigastric pain, vomiting with bleeding, hematuria, leucorrhea, menstrual irregularities, tension and pain in the breasts and amenorrhea.

PRECAUTIONS AND ADVERSE REACTIONS

Health risks or side effects following the proper administration of designated therapeutic dosages are not recorded.

DOSAGE

Mode of Administration: Available as a liquid extract for internal use.

Daily Dosage: 6 to 9 gm of drug

Storage: Should be stored in a cool and dry place, protected from insects.

LITERATURE

Bum EN et al., Extracts from rhizomes of Cyperus articulatus displace 3H CGP39653 and 3H glycine binding from cortical membranes and selectively inhibit NMDA receptor-mediated neurotransmission. J Ethnopharmacol, 54:103-11, 1996 Nov

Kern W, List PH, Hörhammer L (Hrsg.), Hagers Handbuch der Pharmazeutischen Praxis, 4. Aufl., Bde 1-8, Springer Verlag Berlin, Heidelberg, New York, 1969.

Mongelli E, Desmarchelier C, Coussio J, Ciccia G, Antimicrobial activity and interaction with DNA of medicinal plants from the Peruvian Amazon region. Rev Argent Microbiol, 27:199-203, 1995 Oct-Dec

Pinder AR, (1976) Tetrahedron 23:2172.

Aegle marmelos

See Bael

Aegopodium podagraria

See Goutweed

Aesculus hippocastanum

See Horse Chestnut

Aethusa cynapium

See Fool's Parsley

Aframomum melegueta

See Grains-of-Paradise

African Potato

Hypoxis rooperi

DESCRIPTION

Medicinal Parts: The medicinal part is the plant's rhizome tuber.

Flower and Fruit: Four to 10 flowers are arranged in racemes on a long peduncle; the pedicles are 1.2 to 2.5 cm long. The 6 tepals are approximately 18 mm long, elongate, free and yellow. There are 6 stamens, and the ovary is inferior, 3-chambered, top-shaped and thickly pubescent. The fruit is a densely pubescent capsule approximately 12 mm long and split in the middle. The seeds are black and warty.

Leaves, Stem and Root: The plant is a herbaceous perennial with 12 to 18 leaves that are 30 to 60 cm long, 2.4 to 4 cm wide, lanceolate, acuminate, firm with a ciliate margin and short hairs underneath. The leaves grow from a globose shoot, which has a diameter of 5 to 8 cm and is crowned with a ring of bristle-like hairs.

Habitat: Hypoxis rooperi is indigenous to South Africa.

Production: Bantu tulip is the fresh or dried rhizome tuber of Hypoxis rooperi. The plant is collected in the wild, cut and then dried in the sun.

Other Names: Bantu Tulip, Sterretjie

ACTIONS AND PHARMACOLOGY

COMPOUNDS

Lignans (3.5 to 4.5%): particularly hypoxoside (norlignan glucoside)

Steroids: sterols, including beta-sitosterol (ca. 0.2%), beta-sitosterol glucoside

Polysaccharides: starch

EFFECTS

The phytosterols, which have not as yet been more closely identified (beta-sitosterol is possibly the chief active ingredient), are said to have anti-exudative effects in animal experiments. The positive effect of the drug on benign prostate hyperplasia (reduction of the residual urine volume, increase of the uroflow, improvement of subjectively experienced complaints) is explained by the phytosterols' inhibition of local prostaglandin synthase.

INDICATIONS AND USAGE

Unproven Uses: Used internally for micturition complaints resulting from benign prostate hyperplasia, cystitis (South Africa/decoction) and lung disease (Botswana). It is used externally as a vulnerary (Africa). Efficacy for these indications has not yet been proven.

PRECAUTIONS AND ADVERSE REACTIONS

No health hazards are known in conjunction with the proper administration of designated therapeutic dosages.

DOSAGE

Mode of Administration: Whole and cut drug preparations for internal and external use.

How Supplied: Commercially produced capsules.

LITERATURE

Bräuer H, Schomann C, Tolerance of beta-sitosterin from Hypoxis rooperi in patients with limited liver function. Results of a controlled double-blind study, Fortschr Med, 96:833-4, 1978 Apr 20.

Hänsel R, Keller K, Rimpler H, Schneider G (Ed.), Hagers Handbuch der Pharmazeutischen Praxis, 5. Aufl., Bde 4 - 6 (Drogen), Springer Verlag Berlin, Heidelberg, New York, 1992-1994.

Aga

Amanita muscaria

DESCRIPTION

Medicinal Parts: The fungus is used to prepare homeopathic dilutions.

Flower and Fruit: Aga belongs to the group of lamella fungi, genus Amanita. The hymenium in the inside of the fruiting body is exposed by unfolding the cap on the underside.

Characteristics: The poisonous fungus has a basidia which is dirty white, as are the cuffs and underside of the cap. The mushroom's cap is orange at first, then strong red with a few dirty white to yellow spots.

Habitat: Aga grows in the Northern Hemisphere as far north as the tundra and thrives in sandy, acid soils.

Production: Aga is the above-ground part of Amanita muscaria.

Other Names: Fly Agaric

ACTIONS AND PHARMACOLOGY

COMPOUNDS

Ibotenic acid (0.17% to 1%)

Muscimol

Muscarine (traces)

Muscazone

Betalains (skin pigment): muscaflavin, muscaaurins and muscapurpurins

Amavandin (compound containing vanadium)

EFFECTS

The drug, containing ibotenic acid, has a psychotropic and hallucinogenic effect and is toxic in higher doses. The decarboxylation product muscimol is similar in structure to the neurotransmitter GABA and attaches itself to the latter's receptor complex as a selective and direct antagonist. The drug is initially stimulating then paralyzing in its effect.

INDICATIONS AND USAGE

Homeopathic Uses: The fungus is used to treat neuralgias, fever, anxiety, alcohol poisoning and joint pains.

PRECAUTIONS AND ADVERSE REACTIONS

The drug is highly toxic. Signs of poisoning include dizziness, vomiting, abdominal pain, movement disorders, muscle cramps and psychic stimulation, followed by deep sleep.

OVERDOSAGE

The intake of more than 10 g of the fresh mushroom can lead to coordination disorders, confusion, illusions and manic attacks. Higher dosages (over 100 g of fresh mushrooms) lead to unconsciousness, asphyxiation, coma and death.

The treatment of poisoning includes emptying the gastrointestinal tract and the use of sedatives. In case of shock, a plasma volume expander should be used. Artificial respiration should be administered for respiratory arrest.

DOSAGE

Mode of Administration: In homeopathy, dilutions of the mother tincture are used.

LITERATURE

Hastings MH, et al., Brain Res 360:248. 1985.

Hatfield GM, Brady LR, JNP 38:36, 1975.

Marmo E, Med Res Rev 8:441, 1988.

Schwarz B, Ein Männlein steht im Walde. In: PZ 139(13):1040. 1994.

Further information in:

Benjamin DR, Mushroom poisoning in infants and children: the Amanita pantherina/muscaria group. J Toxicol Clin Toxicol, 256:13-22, 1992

Bresinsky A, Bresl H, Giftpilze. Ein Handbuch für Apotheker, Ärzte und Biologen, Wiss. Verlagsges. mbH, Stuttgart 1885.

Lewin L, Gifte und Vergiftungen, 6. Aufl., Nachdruck, Haug Verlag, Heidelberg 1992.

Madaus G, Lehrbuch der Biologischen Arzneimittel, Bde 1-3, Nachdruck, Georg Olms Verlag Hildesheim 1979.

Roth L, Daunderer M, Kormann K, Giftpflanzen, Pflanzengifte, 4. Aufl., Ecomed Fachverlag Landsberg Lech 1993.

Teuscher E, Lindequist U, Biogene Gifte - Biologie, Chemie, Pharmakologie, 2. Aufl., Fischer Verlag Stuttgart 1994.

Agar

Gelidium amansii

DESCRIPTION

Medicinal Parts: The medicinal part of the plant is the seaweed's gelatinous extract known as Agar or Agar-Agar.

Flower and Fruit: This perennial seaweed grows up to 1 m long. The thallus sprouts from a permanent base every year and is heavily branched. It is cylindrical or flattened, pinnately subdivided and tough. The brownish-white, translucent thallus has prickly appendages on the branchings. The fruit is spherical.

Characteristics: Agar is colorless and tasteless. It is capable of absorbing up to 200 times its volume of water to form a jelly.

Habitat: The plant is indigenous to the Pacific coasts of Japan and China, Sri Lanka and also the South African coasts.

Production: Agar, or Agar-Agar, is the purified and bleached gel derived from algae mucilage of the Rhodophyceae Gelidium amansii (Lamour), which has been dried and cut into thread-like strips. An aqueous extract is obtained from the algae through autoclaving (pressure-cooking), using over-heated steam. It is then chilled in ice cells and cooled into ice-blocks, which are crushed and thawed. Water separates from the gel during the thawing process. The gel mass is dried using warm air.

Other Names: Agar-Agar, Japanese Isinglass

ACTIONS AND PHARMACOLOGY

COMPOUNDS

Heteropolysaccharides: made up of D-galactose- and 3,6-anhydro-L-galactose- components, partially bearing sulfate or pyruvic acid residues, low-sulfate fraction designated agarose

EFFECTS

The drug has a laxative effect due to its ability, similar to that of cellulose, to absorb and retain large quantities of water and swell in the intestine. The mucilaginous substances cause an increase in the bulk of the content of the intestine that stimulates the intestinal muscles, thereby aiding peristalsis.

INDICATIONS AND USAGE

Unproven Uses: The drug is used as a mild laxative.

PRECAUTIONS AND ADVERSE REACTIONS

No health hazards or side effects are known in conjunction with the proper administration of designated therapeutic dosages.

DOSAGE

Mode of Administration: The drug is used internally.

Daily Dosage: Laxative: Take 1 to 2 teaspoons of the powder, always with some liquid, fruit or jam before meals, 1 to 3 times daily. Never take dry!

Storage: Dried Agar can be kept tightly sealed for up to 5 years without being opened and tested.

LITERATURE

Ataki C, Chem Soc Japan 29:543. 1956.

Franz G (Hrsg.), Polysaccharide. Springer Verlag Berlin, Heidelberg, New York 1991.

Kern W, List PH, Hörhammer L (Hrsg.), Hagers Handbuch der Pharmazeutischen Praxis, 4. Aufl., Bde. 1-8, Springer Verlag Berlin, Heidelberg, New York, 1969.

Murano E et al., Pyruvate-rich agarose from the red alga Gracilaria dura. In: PM 58(Suppl. 7)

Schmid OJ, Marina (Hamburg) 1:54. 1959.

Steinegger E, Hänsel R, Pharmakognosie, 5. Aufl., Springer Verlag Heidelberg 1992.

Teuscher E, Biogene Arzneimittel, 5. Aufl., Wiss. Verlagsges. Stuttgart 1997.

Vessal M, Mehrani HA, Omrani GH, Effects of an aqueous extract of Physalis alkekengi fruit on estrus cycle, reproduction and uterine craetive kinase BB-isoenzyme in rats. In: ETH 34(1):69-78. 1991.

Agrimonia eupatoria

See Agrimony

Agrimony

Agrimonia eupatoria

DESCRIPTION

Medicinal Parts: The drug consists of the flowering plant, which is cut a few fingers width above the ground and dried.

Flower and Fruit: The flowers are yellow, arranged along small, spike-like racemes. They have an epicalyx and 5 sepals, 5 ovate petals, 5 to 20 stamens and 2 ovaries. The calyx is rough-haired with deep furrows. The fruit is obconical and thorny (burdocks).

Leaves, Stem and Root: The plant is fifty to 100 cm high, with a villous, erect stem. The leaves are alternate and irregularly pinnate. The leaflets are deeply serrate and downy beneath.

Characteristics: Agrimony has a slight pleasant fragrance and a tangy, bitter taste.

Habitat: The plant is indigenous to middle and northern Europe, temperate Asia and North America.

Production: Agrimony herb consists of the dried, above-ground parts of Agrimonia eupatoria and/or Agrimonia procera gathered just before or during flowering, as well as its preparations in effective dosage.

Other Names: Stickwort, Cocklebur, Liverwort, Common Agrimony, Philanthropos, Church Steeples, Sticklewort

ACTIONS AND PHARMACOLOGY

COMPOUNDS

Catechin tannins

EFFECTS

Agrimony is an astringent.

INDICATIONS AND USAGE

Approved by Commission E:

- Diarrhea
- Inflammation of the skin
- Inflammation of the mouth and pharynx

Unproven Uses: Agrimony is used internally for mild, nonspecific, acute diarrhea, cholestasis, inflammation of oral and pharyngeal mucosa, inflammation of kidney and bladder, diabetes and childhood bedwetting; externally for poorly healing wounds, chronic pharyngitis, psoriasis, seborrhoeic eczema as well in hip-baths for lower abdominal conditions.

Chinese Medicine: Agrimony is used as a hemostyptic. It is also used for certain forms of cancer and as an anthelmintic.

PRECAUTIONS AND ADVERSE REACTIONS

No health hazards or side effects are known in conjunction with the proper administration of designated therapeutic dosages. Because of the constituent tannins, the intake of larger quantities could lead to digestive complaints and constipation.

DOSAGE

Daily Dosage: Internally, the average daily dose is 3 to 6 gm of herb or equivalent preparations. Externally, a poultice prepared from a decoction (10%) several times a day is applied.

LITERATURE

Bilai AR, et al., A flavonol glycoside from Agrimonia eupatoria. In: PH 32:1078. 1993.

Chon SC, et al., (1987) Med Pharmacol Exp 16(5):407-413.

Drozd GA, et al., (1983) Khim Prir Soed 1:106.

Patrascu V, et al., (1984) Ser. Dermato-Venerol 29(2):153-157.

Peter-Horvath M, et al., (1964) Rev Med 10(2):190-193.

Further information in:

Kern W, List PH, Hörhammer L (Hrsg.), Hagers Handbuch der Pharmazeutischen Praxis, 4. Aufl., Bde. 1-8, Springer Verlag Berlin, Heidelberg, New York, 1969.

Madaus G, Lehrbuch der Biologischen Arzneimittel, Bde 1-3, Nachdruck, Georg Olms Verlag Hildesheim 1979.

Teuscher E, Biogene Arzneimittel, 5. Aufl., Wiss. Verlagsges. Stuttgart 1997.

Wichtl M (Hrsg.), Teedrogen, 4. Aufl., Wiss. Verlagsges. Stuttgart 1997.

Agropyron repens

See Triticum

Agrostemma githago

See Corn Cockle

Ailanthus altissima

See Tree of Heaven

Ajuga chamaepitys

See Ground Pine

Ajuga reptans

See Bugle

Akebia quinata

See Chocolate Vine (Mu-Tong)

Alcea rosea

See Hollyhock

Alchemilla vulgaris

See Lady's Mantle

Alchornea floribunda

See Iporuru

Aletris

Aletris farinosa

DESCRIPTION

Medicinal Parts: The medicinal part is the dried Aletris farinosa rhizome with roots. Fresh underground parts dug up after flowering are also used.

Flower and Fruit: The plant has numerous white, tubular-oblong, campanulate flowers. The flowers, with a few small bracts, are in terminal, spike-like racemes on stalks that reach up to 1 m. The perianth is tubular, covered in scales and shrinks when ripe. Later, the perianth springs open in a beak shape. The fruit is an ovoid capsule containing many oblong ribbed seeds.

Leaves, Stem and Root: The leaves are erect-oblong, lanceolate and 2 to 20 cm long. The rhizome is brownish-gray, flattened and has a diameter of up to 1 cm, but usually measures less. The upper part is covered in leaf bases and stem scars. The fracture is floury and white.

Characteristics: The plant has a sweet taste, becoming bitter and soapy. The odor is mild.

Habitat: The plant is found in the northeast U.S., south to Gulf of Mexico, southern Canada.

Production: Aletris root is the rhizome of Aletris farinosa. It is gathered in the wild and air-dried in the shade.

Other Names: Star Grass, Colic-Root, Starwort, Blazing Star, Ague-Root, Aloe-Root, Ague Grass, Black-Root, Bitter Grass, Crow Corn, Bettie Grass, Devil's Bit, True Unicorn Star-Grass, True Unicorn Root

ACTIONS AND PHARMACOLOGY

COMPOUNDS

Saponins

Volatile oil

Resins

Bitter principles

Starch

EFFECTS

The active agents increase motility and act as a tonic. There may be an estrogenic principle but a possible estrogenic effect has not been sufficiently researched.

INDICATIONS AND USAGE

Unproven Uses: In the U.S., the plant is used for gynecological disorders or "female complaints," in particular dysmenorrhea, amenorrhea and complaints associated with prolapses vaginae.

Preparations of Aletris are also used for loss of appetite, venous dyspepsia, flatulence and nervous digestive complaints. In Argentina, it is used to treat chronic bronchitis.

Homeopathic Uses: Prolapsed uterus, gastrointestinal complaints.

PRECAUTIONS AND ADVERSE REACTIONS

No health hazards or side effects are known in conjunction with the proper administration of designated therapeutic dosages.

DOSAGE

Mode of Administration: Available in the forms of powdered root, liquid extract and infusions for internal use.

Preparation: To prepare an infusion, 1.5 gm of the drug is added to 100 ml of water. A fluid extract (1:1) is produced with ethanol water (45%).

Daily Dosage: Approximately 6 gm. The recommended single dose is 0.3 to 0.6 gm to be taken 3 times daily. Infusion: 1.5 gm of the drug to 100 ml water. Fluid extract (1:1), produced with ethanol water (45%).

Homeopathic Dosage: 5 to 10 drops, 1 tablet or 5 to 10 globules; Injection solution: 1 ml once a week sc (HAB1).

LITERATURE

Costello CH, Lynn EV, (1950) J Am Pharm Ass 39:117.

Marker RE et al., (1940) J Chem Soc 60:2620.

Further information in:

Hänsel R, Keller K, Rimpler H, Schneider G (Hrsg.), Hagers Handbuch der Pharmazeutischen Praxis, 5. Aufl., Bde 4 - 6 (Drogen), Springer Verlag Berlin, Heidelberg, New York, 1992-1994.

Madaus G, Lehrbuch der Biologischen Arzneimittel, Bde 1-3, Nachdruck, Georg Olms Verlag Hildesheim.

Wagner H, Wiesenauer M, Phytotherapie. Phytopharmaka und pflanzliche Homeopathika, Fischer-Verlag, Stuttgart, Jena, New York.

Aletris farinosa

See Aletris

Alfalfa

Medicago sativa

TRADE NAMES

Alfalfa, Alfalfa Concentrate, Alfalfa Fortified, Alfalfa Natural, Alfalfa Organics, Alfalfa Whole Juice Concentrate Alfamin

DESCRIPTION

Medicinal Parts: The medicinal parts are the whole flowering plant or the germinating seeds.

Flower and Fruit: The clover-like flowers can be yellow to violet-blue. They are 9 to 10 mm long and appear in oblong, many-blossomed racemes. The fruit is a spiralled pod with 2 or 3 twists; the center is hollow and not thorny.

Leaves, Stem and Root: The annual, succulent plant grows from 45 to 100 cm high. The stems are erect, smooth and sharply angled. The leaves are trifoliate, petiolate, and alternate. The leaflets are thorny-tipped, dentate toward the front, obovate, and villous beneath. The stipules are ovate, lanceolate, slightly dentate and acuminate.

Characteristics: The taste is unpleasantly salty, bitter and dry.

Habitat: The plant is indigenous to the Mediterranean region and has been widely cultivated elsewhere for centuries.

Other Names: Lucerne, Purple Medick, Purple Medicle, Buffalo Herb, Purple Medic

ACTIONS AND PHARMACOLOGY

COMPOUNDS: IN THE FOLIAGE

Carotinoids: including among others, lutein

Triterpene saponins: sojasapogenols A-E aglycones medicagenic acid, hederagenin

Isoflavonoids: including among others, formononetin glycosides, genistein, daidzein

Coumestans: coumestrol, 3′-methoxy coumestrol, lucernol, sativol, trifoliol

Triterpenes: including among others, stigmasterol, spinasterol

Cyanogenic glycosides: (corresponding to less than 80 mg HCN/100 g)

COMPOUNDS: IN THE SEEDS

L-canavaine

Betaine: stachydrine, homostachydrine

Trigonelline

Fatty oil

EFFECTS

The saponin contents act on the cardiovascular, nervous, and digestive systems.

INDICATIONS AND USAGE

Unproven Uses: In folk medicine, the drug is used in the treatment of diabetes and malfunctioning of the thyroid gland.

Alfalfa has isolated use as a diuretic and aromatic.

PRECAUTIONS AND ADVERSE REACTIONS

No health hazards or side effects are known in conjunction with the proper administration of designated therapeutic dosages.

LITERATURE

Berrang B, (1974) Phytochemistry 13:2253.

Gestetner B, (1974) Phytochemistry 10:2221.

Keeler RF, (1975) Lloydia 38:56.

Larher F et al., (1983) Plant Sci Lett 29(2/3):315.

Malinow MR et al., (1977) Steroids 29:105.

Morton JF, (1975) Morris Arbor Bull 26:24.

Nowacki E et al., (1976) Biochem. Physiol Pflanz. 169:183.

Tapper BA et al., (1975) J Sci Food Agric 26:277.

Further information in:

Hegnauer R, Chemotaxonomie der Pflanzen, Bde 1-11, Birkhäuser Verlag Basel, Boston, Berlin 1962-1997.

Kern W, List PH, Hörhammer L (Hrsg.), Hagers Handbuch der Pharmazeutischen Praxis, 4. Aufl., Bde. 1-8, Springer Verlag Berlin, Heidelberg, New York, 1969.

Leung AY, Encyclopedia of Common Natural Ingredients Used in Food, Drugs and Cosmetics, John Wiley & Sons Inc., New York 1980.

Madaus G, Lehrbuch der Biologischen Arzneimittel, Bde 1-3, Nachdruck, Georg Olms Verlag Hildesheim 1979.

Teuscher E, Lindequist U, Biogene Gifte - Biologie, Chemie, Pharmakologie, 2. Aufl., Fischer Verlag Stuttgart 1994.

Wagner H, Wiesenauer M, Phytotherapie. Phytopharmaka und pflanzliche Homöopathika, Fischer-Verlag, Stuttgart, Jena, New York 1995.

Alisma plantago-aquatica

See Alisma (Ze-Xie)

Alisma (Ze-Xie)

Alisma plantago-aquatica

DESCRIPTION

Medicinal Parts: The medicinal part is the fresh rhizome.

Flower and Fruit: The peduncle is triangular. There are long-pedicled, white or reddish flowers in leafless, loose panicles. There are 3 sepals, 3 petals and 3 stamens in the flower. The fruit is small and obtuse and is formed by 15 to 30 ovaries.

Leaves, Stem and Root: The water leaves are ribbon-like. There are long-stemmed, swimming leaves. The aerial leaves are basal, long-stemmed, cordate or oblong-ovate, and spoon-like.

Characteristics: The rootstock of Alisma has a bitter taste; it is poisonous when fresh.

Habitat: The plant is distributed widely throughout Europe, northern Asia and North America.

Other Names: Mad-Dog Weed, Water Plantain, Ze-Xie

ACTIONS AND PHARMACOLOGY

COMPOUNDS

Triterpenes: including alisol-A, alisol-B, alisol-C and their monoacetates

Sesquiterpenes (guaian type): alismol, alismol oxide

Flavone sulfate

Caffeic acid derivatives: chlorogenic acid sulfate

EFFECTS

No information is available.

INDICATIONS AND USAGE

Unproven Uses: Alisma is used for diseases of the bladder and urinary tract.

Chinese Medicine: The drug is used to lower blood sugar, blood pressure and cholesterol levels; it is also used as a diuretic.

PRECAUTIONS AND ADVERSE REACTIONS

No health hazards or side effects are known in conjunction with the proper administration of designated therapeutic dosages.

DOSAGE

Mode of Administration: The drug is available as an extract for oral use. The root is also used in homeopathy.

LITERATURE

Kern W, List PH, Hörhammer L (Hrsg.), Hagers Handbuch der Pharmazeutischen Praxis, 4. Aufl., Bde 1-8, Springer Verlag Berlin, Heidelberg, New York, 1969.

Murata T et al., (1968) Tetrahedron Letteers 103:849.

Murata T et al., Chem Pharm Bull 18:1369. 1970.

Oshima Y et al., PH 22:183. 1983.

Alkanet

Alkanna tinctoria

DESCRIPTION

Medicinal Parts: The medicinal part is the root of the plant (the dried roots and rhizomes).

Flower and Fruit: The calyx is 4 to 5 mm in the flower, 5 to 6 mm in the fruit and eglandular. The corolla is blue and glabrous outside. The funnel is as long as or slightly longer than the calyx. The limb is 6 to 7 mm in diameter. There are 5 stamens, and the anthers are fused with the corolla tube. The nutlets are 2 mm in diameter, irregularly reticulate and tuberculate.

Leaves, Stem and Root: Alkanet is a short-bristled, perennial half-rosette shrub. The stems are 10 to 20 cm, procumbent or ascending and glandular. The basal leaves are 6 to 15 cm by 0.7 to 1.5 cm, linear-lanceolate; the lower ones are cauline, oblong-linear and cordate at base. The bracts are slightly longer than calyx and oblong-lanceolate. The neck of the root is covered with the remains of leaves and the stems. The root is spindle-shaped, curved, up to 25 cm long and 1.5 cm thick, with purplish root bark.

Habitat: The plant is indigenous to southeastern Europe and some parts of Turkey and Hungary. It is cultivated in other parts of Europe, Britain and northern Africa.

Production: Alkanna rhizomes are the dried roots and rhizomes of Alkanna tinctoria Tausch.

Other Names: Anchusa, Dyer's Bugloss, Spanish Bugloss, Alkanet Root, Alkanna

ACTIONS AND PHARMACOLOGY

COMPOUNDS

Naphthazarine derivatives: including the ester of the (-)-alkannin (stained red)

Pyrrolizidine alkaloids

Tannins

EFFECTS

Antimicrobial action: In the agar diffusion test, Alkanet root extracts and Alkannin esters impaired the growth of *Staphylococcus aureus* and *Staphylococcus epidermidis*, however Alkannin worked only against *Candida albicans.*

Healing action for wounds: In a double-blind study, 72 patients suffering from ulcers of the leg (Ulcus cruris) caused by varicose veins, were treated with Histoplastin Red® over a period of three years. After 5 to 6 weeks of daily administration, 80% of the patients' ulcers had healed or were considerably reduced in size.

The results are difficult to assess, as details concerning the patients, the treatment pattern and control groups are unavailable.

INDICATIONS AND USAGE

Unproven Uses: Used by the ancient Greeks to heal wounds; also for skin diseases and diarrhea.

PRECAUTIONS AND ADVERSE REACTIONS

Hepatotoxicity and carcinogenity are expected, due to the pyrrolizidine alkaloids with 1,2-unsaturated necic parent substances in its makeup. Alkanna should not be taken internally for this reason and is recommended for external use only.

DOSAGE

Mode of Administration: Seldom used as a drug. Internal administration is not recommended, due to the drugs toxic characteristics and its uncertain efficacy. Alkannin and extracts of the root are used externally in pharmacy.

Preparations: Extractum alcannae: almost black, green glistening mass (no extraction information).

Histoplastin Red® Ointment: The ointment approved in Greece, contains 76.5 gm loosely defined ethereal oily Alkanet root extract with lipophil ointment base (beeswax, mastic rubber and olive oil q.s. ad 100 gm).

Daily Dosage: Maximum 0.1 mcg pyrrolizidine alkaloids with 1.2 unsaturated necin framework and their N-oxides.

LITERATURE

Majlathova L, (1971) Nahrung 15:505.

Papageorgiou VP, (1980) Planta Med 38(3):193-203.

Papageorgiou VP, PM 31:390-394. 1977.

Papageorgiou VP, Digenis GA, PM 39:81-84. 1980.

Röder E, Pyrrolizidinhaltige Arzneipflanzen. In: DAZ 132(45):2427-2435. 1992.

Röder E, et al., PH 23:2125-2126. 1984.

Wiedenfield H et al., (1985) Arch Pharm 318(4):294.

Further information in:

Hänsel R, Keller K, Rimpler H, Schneider G (Hrsg.), Hagers Handbuch der Pharmazeutischen Praxis, 5. Aufl., Bde 4-6 (Drogen), Springer Verlag Berlin, Heidelberg, New York, 1992-1994.

Wichtl M (Hrsg.), Teedrogen, 4. Aufl., Wiss. Verlagsges. Stuttgart.

Alkanna tinctoria

See Alkanet

Allium cepa

See Onion

Allium sativum

See Garlic

Allium schoenoprasum

See Chives

Allium ursinum

See Bear's Garlic

Almond

Prunus species

DESCRIPTION

Medicinal Parts: The medicinal part is the ripe fruit.

Flower and Fruit: The flowers are very short-petioled in pairs and appear before the leaves. The petals are 19 to 20 mm long, pale pink to whitish with dark veins. The fruit is oblong-ovoid, compressed, 3.5 to 4.6 cm long by 2.5 to 3 cm wide, gray-green, velvet-downy and pubescent. The nut shell is yellow, hard, compressed, broad- and sharp-edged, punctate externally with irregular grooves, smooth and glossy inside and thick- or thin-skinned. The seed is cinnamon brown, flattened, and 2 cm long by 1.2 to 1.5 cm wide.

Leaves, Stem and Root: The plant is of medium height, seldom reaching 12 m. It is a tree or shrub with mildly red-tinged branches, thorny in its wild form but not in the cultivated form. The leaves have a 1.2 to 1.5 cm long, glandular petiole and glabrous, oblong-lanceolate-acuminate or serrate, tough, glossy, dark green blades.

Habitat: The tree is indigenous to Western Asia and is extensively cultivated in many regions.

Production: Bitter almonds are the fruits of Prunus dulcis var. amara (also of Prunus armeniaca).

Sweet almonds are the fruits of Prunus amygdalus var. dulcis.

Other Names: Greek Nuts, Jordan Almond, Bitter Almond, and Sweet Almond

ACTIONS AND PHARMACOLOGY

COMPOUNDS: BITTER ALMONDS

Cyanogenic glycosides, amygdalin, 0.2 to 8.5% (corresponding to 12 to 500 mg prussic acid per 100 gm)

Fatty oil (non-dehydrating, 38 to 60%): chief fatty acids oleic acid (77%) and linoleic acid (17 to 20%)

Mucilages (3 to 3%): arabinogalactans

Proteic substances (25 to 35%)

EFFECTS: BITTER ALMONDS

There is no reliable information available.

COMPOUNDS: SWEET ALMONDS

Fatty oil (non-dehydrating, 43 to 57%): chief fatty acids oleic acid (77%) and linoleic acid (17 to 20%)

Mucilages (3 to 4%): arabinogalactans

Proteic substances (20 to 25%)

EFFECTS: SWEET ALMONDS

Sweet Almonds have a demulcent effect.

INDICATIONS AND USAGE

BITTER ALMONDS

Unproven Uses: Bitter Almonds were used in the past as a remedy for coughs, vomiting and nausea in the form of bitter almond water.

SWEET ALMONDS

Unproven Uses: Sweet Almonds are used topically in skin care and liniments.

PRECAUTIONS AND ADVERSE REACTIONS

BITTER ALMONDS

To be used only under the supervision of an expert qualified in the appropriate use of this substance.

SWEET ALMONDS

No health hazards or side effects are known in conjunction with the proper administration of designated therapeutic topical dosages.

OVERDOSAGE

BITTER ALMONDS

10 bitter almonds are said to be fatal for a child, 60 for an adult (a fatal dosage would presumably be already reached at a lower level, given disadvantageous conditions - higher cyanide level in the almonds, intensive chewing). Recommended antidotes include injection of solutions of dicobalt-EDTA or thiosulfates or else application of methemoglobin-forming substances, such as amyl nitrite. At the same time, vomiting should be induced or the stomach emptied.

Circulation support measures and/or artificial respiration may be required.

DOSAGE

BITTER ALMONDS

Mode of Administration: The drug is obsolete and no longer used.

SWEET ALMONDS

Mode of Administration: Sweet Almonds fatty oil is used as an ointment base and in the production of natural cosmetics.

LITERATURE

BITTER ALMONDS

Fincke H, Z Untersuch Lebensm 52:423. 1926.

Le Quesne PW et al., JNP 48:496. 1985.

Opdyke DLJ, (1976) Food Cosmet Toxicol: 14.

Salvo F et al., Riv Ital Sostanze Grasse 57:24. 1980.

Saura-Calixto F et al., Fette, Seifen, Anstrichm 87:4. 1985.

Further information in:

Kern W, List PH, Hörhammer L (Hrsg.), Hagers Handbuch der Pharmazeutischen Praxis, 4. Aufl., Bde. 1-8, Springer Verlag Berlin, Heidelberg, New York, 1969.

Madaus G, Lehrbuch der Biologischen Arzneimittel, Bde 1-3, Nachdruck, Georg Olms.

Steinegger E, Hänsel R, Pharmakognosie, 5. Aufl., Springer Verlag Heidelberg 1992.

Teuscher E, Biogene Arzneimittel, 5. Aufl., Wiss. Verlagsges. Stuttgart 1997.

SWEET ALMONDS

Fincke H, Z Untersuch Lebensm 52:423. 1926.

Le Quesne PW et al., JNP 48:496. 1985.

Opdyke DLJ, (1976) Food Cosmet Toxicol: 14.

Rosenthaler L, Ber Pharm Ges 30:13. 1920.

Salvo F et al., Riv Ital Sostanze Grasse 57:24. 1980.

Saura-Calixto F et al., Fette, Seifen, Anstrichm 87:4. 1985.

Sommer W, Dissertation Albrechts-Universität Kiel. 1984.

Further information in:

Frohne D, Pfänder HJ, Giftpflanzen - Ein Handbuch für Apotheker, Toxikologen und Biologen, 4. Aufl., Wiss. Verlags-Ges Stuttgart 1997.

Kern W, List PH, Hörhammer L (Hrsg.), Hagers Handbuch der Pharmazeutischen Praxis, 4. Aufl., Bde. 1-8, Springer Verlag Berlin, Heidelberg, New York, 1969.

Lewin L, Gifte und Vergiftungen, 6. Aufl., Nachdruck, Haug Verlag, Heidelberg 1992.

Roth L, Daunderer M, Kormann K, Giftpflanzen, Pflanzengifte, 4. Aufl., Ecomed Fachverlag Landsberg Lech 1993.

Teuscher E, Lindequist U, Biogene Gifte - Biologie, Chemie, Pharmakologie, 2. Aufl., Fischer Verlag Stuttgart 1994.

Alnus glutinosa

See Black Alder

Aloe

Aloe barbadensis/capensis/vera

TRADE NAMES

Aloe Vera (available from numerous manufacturers), Herbal Sure Aloe Vera, Aloe Vera Mild Stimulant Laxative, Aloe 99 Gel, Sundance Aloe Vera Gel, Chantal Aloe Vera Cream, Palmers Aloe Vera Formula Cream, Aloe Vera Super Strength, Herbal Sure Aloe Vera

DESCRIPTION

Medicinal Parts: The medicinal part of the plant is dried juice of the leaves.

Flower and Fruit: The inflorescence is forked once or twice and is 60 to 90 cm high. The raceme is dense, cylindrical and narrows toward the top. The terminal raceme is up to 40 cm high while the lower ones are somewhat shorter. The bracts are almost white, and the flowers are yellow, orange or red, and are 3 cm long.

Leaves, Stem and Root: The lily-like succulent-leafed rosette shrub either does not have a stem or has a 25 cm stem. The stem has about 25 leaves in an upright dense rosette. The lanceolate leaf is thick and fleshy, 40 to 50 cm long and 6 to 7 cm wide at the base. The upper surface is concave, gray-green, often with a reddish tinge, which sometimes appears in patches in the young plants. The leaf margin has a pale pink edge and 2 mm long pale teeth.

Habitat: Aloe is thought to have originated in the Sudan and the Arabian Peninsula. Today the species is cultivated and found in the wild in northern Africa, the Near East, Asia, and in the southern Mediterranean region. The plant is cultivated in subtropical regions of the United States and Mexico, and on the Dutch Antilles, as well as coastal regions of Venezuela.

Production: Curacao Aloe consists of the dried latex of the leaves of Aloe barbadensis (syn. Aloe vera), as well as its preparations. Aloe is harvested from August until October. The juice is dried using various methods.

Not to be Confused With: Confusion sometimes arises with Agave americana, known as American Aloe, which is not a true Aloe.

ACTIONS AND PHARMACOLOGY

COMPOUNDS: ALOE BARBADENSIS

Anthracene derivatives: particularly anthrone-10-C-glycosyls, including aloin A, aloin B, 7-hydroxyaloins A and B, and 1,8-dihydroxy ions, including aloe-emodin, and 6'cinnamic acid esters of these compounds

2-alkylchromones: including aloe resins B, C and D

Flavonoids

COMPOUNDS: ALOE CAPENSIS

Anthracene derivatives: particularly anthrone-10-C-glycosyls, including aloin A, aloin B, 5-hydroxyaloin, and 1,8-dihydroxy anthraquinones, including aloe-emodin, and mixed anthrone-C- and O-glycosides, including aloinosides A and B

2-alkylchromones: including aloe resins A, B, C and D

Flavonoids

EFFECTS

Laxative Effects

Aloe anthranoids such as 1,8-dihydroxy-anthracene derivatives exert a laxative effect. The laxative action is due to anti-absorption osmotic properties. The compounds induce active secretion of electrolytes and water in the lumen of the bowel. Absorption of electrolytes and water from the colon is inhibited resulting in a volume increase. The volume increase of the bowel content leads to an increase in pressure and stimulates intestinal peristalsis. There is some evidence that endogenous nitric oxide modulates the diarrhea effect of aloe. Studies demonstrate a laxative effect 9 hours after ingestion (Izzo, 1999).

Antibacterial/Antiviral Effects

Aloe-emodin exerts dose-dependent growth inhibition of *H. pylori* through inhibition of arylamine N-acetyltransferase (NAT) activity (Wang, 1998). Aloe-emodin has shown antibacterial effects on four strains of methicillin-resistant *Staphylococcus aureus* (Hatano, 1999). Aloe emodin inactivates enveloped viruses and is directly viracidal to *herpes simplex virus type 1* and *type 2*, *varicella-zoster virus*, *pseudorabies virus*, and *influenza virus* (Sydiskis, 1991).

Antineoplastic Effects

Emodin suppresses tyrosine kinase activity of HER-2/neu-encoded p185neu receptor tyrosine kinase resulting in antineoplastic effects. This is beneficial in controlling HER-2/neu overexpressing cancer cells (Zhang, 1998).

Effects of topical Aloe plants

Aloe vera depresses action potential generation and conduction at neuromuscular junction processes which result in analgesic and anti-inflammatory effects (Friedman, 1999). Ultraviolet radiation (UV) suppresses delayed type hypersensitivity (DTH) by altering the function of immune cells in the skin and causing the release of immunoregulatory cytokines. Extracts of crude Aloe barbadensis gel inhibits this photosuppression by preventing suppression of DTH responses and reducing the amount of keratinocyte derived immunosuppressive cytokines (IL-2) (Byeon, 1998; Strickland, 1999). Aloe vera gel contains small molecular modulators that prevent UVB-induced immune suppression in the skin. The immunomodulators restore the UVB-induced damages on epidermal Langerham cells (Lee, 1999).

Aloe vera increases collagen content of the granulation tissue and its degree of crosslinking to contribute to wound healing (Chithra, 1998). Aloe vera acts as a modulatory system toward wounds with anti-inflammatory effects (Davis, 1991). The use of Aloe vera has been associated with a delay in wound healing compared to standard treatment (Schmidt, 1991). Aloe vera gel exerts anti-inflammatory activity through its inhibitory action on the arachidonic acid pathway via cyclooxygenase (Vazquez, 1996). Due to its anti-thromboxane effects, Aloe vera decreases the morbidity of progressive dermal ischemia in frostbite (Heggers, 1987). Aloe vera contains a carboxypeptidase that inactivates bradykinin, salicylates, and a substance that inhibits thromboxane formation (Fujita, 1976; Klein, 1988).

CLINICAL TRIALS

Psoriasis

A double-blind, placebo-controlled study was conducted to evaluate the clinical efficacy and tolerability of topical Aloe vera extract 0.5% (in hydrophilic base) in patients with psoriasis vulgaris. There were 60 patients with slight to moderate chronic plaque-type psoriasis determined by the Psoriasis Area and Severity Score (PASI). The extract was applied topically three times daily for 5 consecutive days per week with a maximum of 4 weeks active treatment. The study period was for 16 weeks with monthly check-ups for a period of 12 months. Aloe vera extract cream had a significantly higher cure rate and clearing of psoriatic plaques compared to placebo. The PASI score was also decreased in the Aloe treatment group compared to placebo. The Aloe-treatment group had no adverse drug related symptoms and the drug was well tolerated (Syed, 1996).

Radiation-Induced Skin Toxicity

A phase III, double-blind, placebo-controlled study evaluated Aloe vera gel for use as a prophylactic agent for radiation-induced skin toxicity. A total of 194 women receiving breast or chest wall irradiation were included in the study. Skin dermatitis was scored weekly during the trial by patients and by health care providers. Aloe vera gel did not protect against radiation therapy-induced dermatitis (Williams, 1996).

INDICATIONS AND USAGE

ALOE BARBADENSIS AND CAPENSIS

Approved by Commission E:

- Constipation

ALOE BARBADENSIS

Unproven Uses: The drug is used for evacuation relief in the presence of anal fissures after recto-anal operations. In European folk medicine the drug is employed for its ability to influence digestion.

Chinese Medicine: The most common use in Chinese medicine is for treatment of fungal diseases.

Indian Medicine: Uses in Indian medicine include stomach tumors, constipation, colic, skin diseases, amenorrhea, worm infestation, and infections.

ALOE CAPENSIS

Unproven Uses: Aloe capensis has been used as a stool softener in the presence of anal fissures, hemorrhoids, and after recto-anal operations. The fresh juice is used for eye inflammations and for syphillis in South Africa.

Homeopathic Uses: The herb is used for gastrointestinal disorders, hemorrhoids, and constipation.

CONTRAINDICATIONS

Aloe is contraindicated in cases of intestinal obstruction, acutely inflamed intestinal diseases (e.g., Crohn's disease, ulcerative colitis), appendicitis and abdominal pain of unknown origin.

PRECAUTIONS AND ADVERSE REACTIONS

General: If cramping of the gastrointestinal tract after single dosing occurs, the dosage should be reduced. Spasmodic gastrointestinal complaints are a side effect to the drug's purgative effect. Heart arrhythmias, nephropathies, edema and accelerated bone deterioration may occur in rare cases. Prolonged use of Aloe may lead to pigmentation in the intestinal mucosa (pseudomelanosis coli), a harmless side effect, which usually reverses upon discontinuation of the drug. Long-term use can also lead to albuminuria and hematuria.

Hypersensitivity: Hypersensitivity, manifested by generalized nummular eczematous and papular dermatitis, have been reported after long-term use of oral and topical Aloe preparations (Morrow, 1980).

Loss of Electrolytes: Long-term use can cause loss of electrolytes, in particular potassium. The loss of potassium can result in hyperaldosteronism, inhibition of intestinal motility and enhancement of the effect of cardioactive medications.

Malignancy: Prolonged use of anthracene drugs increases the relative risk of colon carcinoma (Siegers, 1993). Recent studies fail to demonstrate a connection between the administration of anthracene drugs and frequency of carcinomas in the colon (Schorkhuber, 1998). Low molecular weight compounds found in Aloe vera gel are cytotoxic (Avila, 1997). The component 1,8-dihydroxyanthraquinone inhibits the catalytic activity of topoisomerase II resulting in genotoxicity and mutagenicity (Mueller, 1999).

Tissue Damage: Chronic treatment with high doses of Aloe reduces vasoactive intestinal peptide and somatostatin levels, which may damage enteric nervous tissue (Tzavella, 1995).

Drug Interactions:

Cardiac glycosides and antiarrhythmic drug—Chronic use of Aloe can lead to potassium loss, which can increase the actions of cardiac glycosides and antiarrhythmic drugs.

Thiazide diuretics, loop diuretics, licorice and corticosteroids—There is an increase in the possibility of potassium deficiency when Aloe is used along with these agents.

Pregnancy: Aloe should not be used during pregnancy.

Pediatric Use: Aloe should not be prescribed to children under 12 years of age.

DOSAGE

Mode of Administration: Due to the side effects of the drug, it is rarely used and is not recommended. Aloe powder, aqueous- and aqueous-alcoholic extracts in powdered or liquid form are available for oral use.

How Supplied:

Capsule—250 mg, 470 mg

Cream

Gel—99%, 72%

Softgel—1000 mg

Preparation: A stabilized aloe extract is prepared with hot water. The extract will have a content of 19% to 21% aloin.

Daily Dosage: The recommended daily dosage is 20 to 30 mg hydroxyanthracene derivatives/day, calculated as anhydrous aloin. The recommended single dosage is 0.05 g aloe powder from Aloe barbadensis or 0.05 to 0.2 g aloe powder of Aloe capensis in the evening. Aloe capensis can be given as a single dose of 0.1 g in the evening.

Homeopathic Dosage: For Aloe capensis, administer 5 drops, 1 tablet, 10 globules, or parenterally 1-2 ml three times daily (HAB1).

Note: The smallest dosage needed to maintain a soft stool should be used. Stimulating laxatives must not be used over an extended period of time (1 to 2 weeks) without medical advice.

Storage: Aloe should be protected from light and moisture.

LITERATURE

Anonym, Aloe und Aloine - Aktuelles über weltweit verwendete Arzneistoffe. In: DAZ 135(39):3644-3645. 1995.

Avila H, Rivero J, Herrera F, Fraile G, Cytotoxicity of a low molecular weight fraction from Aloe vera (Aloe barbadensis Miller) gel. Toxicon 1997 Sep;35(9):1423-30.

BGA, Arzneimittelrisiken: Anthranoide. In: DAZ 132(21):1164. 1992.

Byeon SW, Pelley RP, Ullrich SE et al., Aloe barbadensis extracts reduce the production of interleukin-10 after exposure to ultraviolet radiation. J Invest Dermatol 1998 May;110(5): 811-7.

Che QM, Akao T, Hattori M, Kobashi K, Namba T, Metabolism of barbaloin by intestinal bacteria. 2. Isolation of human intestinal bacterium capable of tranforming barbaloin to Aloe-emodin anthrone. In: PM 57:15. 1991.

Chithra P, Sajithlal GB, Chandrakasan G, Influence of Aloe vera on collagen turnover in healing of dermal wounds in rats. Indian J Exp Biol 1998 Sep;36(9):896-901.

Davis RH, Parker WL, Samson RT, Murdoch DP, Isolation of a stimulatory system in an Aloe extract. J Am Podiatr Med Assoc 1991 Sep;81(9):473-8.

Friedman RN, Si K, Initial characterization of the effects of Aloe vera at a crayfish neuromuscul junction. Phytother Res 1999 Nov;13(7):580-583.

Fujita K, Ito S, Teradaira R, Beppu H, Properties of a carboxypeptidase from aloe. Biochem Pharmacol 1979 Apr 1;28(7):1261.

Hatano T, Uebayashi H, Ito H et al., Phenolic constituents of Cassia seeds and antibacterial effect of some naphthalenes and anthraquinones on methicillin-resistant Staphylococcus aureus. Chem Pharm Bull (Tokyo) 1999 Aug;47(8):1121-7.

Heggers JP, Robson MC, Manavalen K et al., Experimental and clinical observations on frostbite. Ann Emerg Med 1987 Sep;16(9):1056-62.

Hutter JA et al., Anti-inflammatory C-glucosyl chromone from Aloe barbadensis. In: JNP 59(5):541-543. 1996.

Izzo AA, Sautebin L, Borrelli F et al., The role of nitric oxide in aloe-induced diarrhoea in the rat. Eur J Pharmacol 1999 Feb 26;368(1):43-8.

Klein AD, Penneys NS, Aloe vera. J Am Acad Dermatol 1988 Apr;18(4 Pt 1):714-20.

Klimpel BE et al., Anthranoidhaltige Laxantien - ein Risiko für die Entwicklung von Tumoren der ableitenden Harnwege. In: PUZ 26(1):33, Jahrestagung der DPhG, Berlin, 1996. 1997.

Koch A, Investigations on the laxative action of aloin in the human colon. In: PM 59(7)89. 1993.

Koch A, Metabolisierung von Aloin. Korrelation zwischen In-vitro- und in-vivo-Versuchen. In: DAZ 135(13):1150-1152. 1995.

Lee CK, Han SS, Shin YK et al., Prevention of ultraviolet radiation-induced suppression of contact hypersensitivity by Aloe vera gel components. Int J Immunopharmacol 1999 May;21(5):303-10.

Morrow D, Rapaport M, Strick R. Hypersensitivity to aloe. Arch Dermatol 1980 Sep;116(9):1064-5.

Mueller S, Stopper H. Characterization of the genotoxicity of anthraquinones in mammalian cells. Biochim Biophys Acta 1999 Aug 5;1428(2-3):406-14.

Park MK et al., Neoaloesin A: A new C-glucofuranosyl chromone from Aloe barbadensis. In: PM 62(4):363-365. 1996.

Schmidt JM, Greenspoon JS, Aloe vera dermal wound gel is associated with a delay in wound healing. Obstet Gynecol 1991 Jul;78(1):115-7.

Shida T et al., (1985) Planta Med 51(3):273.

Sigers C, von Hertzberg-Lottin E, Otte M, Schneider B. Anthranoid laxative abuse—a risk for colorectal cancer? Gut 1993 Aug;34(8):1099-101.

Schorkhuber M, Richter M, Dutter A, et al. Effect of anthraquinone-laxatives on the proliferation and urokinase secretion of normal, premalignant and malignant colonic epithelial cells. Eur J Cancer 1998 Jun;34(7):1091-8.

Strickland FM, Darvill A, Albersheim P et al., Inhibition of UV-induced immune suppression and interleukin-10 production by plant oligosaccharides and polysaccharides. Photochem Photobiol 1999 Feb;69(2):141-7.

Sydiskis RJ, Owen DG, Lohr JL et al., Inactivation of enveloped viruses by anthraquinones extracted from plants. Antimicrob Agents Chemother 1991 Dec;35(12):2463-6.

Syed TA, Ahmad SA, Holt AH et al., Management of psoriasis with Aloe vera extract in a hydrophilic cream: a placebo-controlled, double-blind study. Trop Med Int Health 1996 Aug;1(4):505-9.

Tzavella K, Riepl RL, Klauser AG et al., Decreased substance P levels in rectal biopsies from patients with slow transit constipation. Eur J Gastroenterol Hepatol 1996 Dec;8(12):1207-1211.

Tzeng SH, Ko WC, Ko FN, Teng CM, Inhibition of platelet aggregation by some flavonoids. In: Thromobosis Res 64:91. 1991.

Vazquez B, Avila G, Segura D, Escalante B, Anti-inflammatory activity of extracts from Aloe vera gel. J Ethnopharmacol 1996 Dec;55(1):69-75.

Wang HH, Chung JG, Ho CC, Wu LT, Chang SH. Aloe-emodin effects on arylamine N-acetyltransferase activity in the bacterium Helicobacter pylori. Planta Med 1998 Mar;64(2):176-178.

Westendorf J, Phytotherapie: Anthranoide in Arzneipflanzen. In: DAZ 133(25):2345. 1993.

Williams MS, Burk M, Loprinzi CL et al., Phase III double-blind evaluation of an aloe vera gel as a prophylactic agent for radiation-induced skin toxicity. nt J Radiat Oncol Biol Phys 1996 Sep 1;36(2):345-9.

Yoig A, Egusa T, Arase M, Tanabe M, Tsujitt, Isolation and characterization of the glycoprotein fraction with proliferation-promotory activity on human and hamster cells in vitro. In: PM 63:18-21. 1997.

Zhang L, Tizard IR, Activation of a mouse macrophage cell line by acemannan: the major carbohydrate fraction from Aloe vera gel. Immunopharmacology 1996 Nov;35(2):119-28.

Further information in:

Hänsel R, Keller K, Rimpler H, Schneider G (Hrsg.), Hagers Handbuch der Pharmazeutischen Praxis, 5. Aufl., Bde 4-6 (Drogen), Springer Verlag Berlin, Heidelberg, New York, 1992-1994.

Hausen BM, Allergiepflanzen - Pflanzenallergene, Ecomed Fachverlag Landsberg Lech 1988.

Hoppe HA, (1975-1987) Drogenkunde, 8. Aufl., Bde 1-3, W. de Gruyter Verlag, Berlin, New York.

Lewin L, Gifte und Vergiftungen, 6. Aufl., Nachdruck, Haug Verlag, Heidelberg 1992.

Steinegger E, Hänsel R, Pharmakognosie, 5. Aufl., Springer Verlag Heidelberg 1992.

Teuscher E, Biogene Arzneimittel, 5. Aufl., Wiss. Verlagsges. Stuttgart 1997.

Wagner H, Wiesenauer M, Phytotherapie. Phytopharmaka und pflanzliche Homöopathika, Fischer-Verlag, Stuttgart, Jena, New York 1995.

Wichtl M (Hrsg.), Teedrogen, 4. Aufl., Wiss. Verlagsges. Stuttgart 1997.

Aloe barbadensis/capensis/vera

See Aloe

Aloysia triphylla

See Lemon Verbena

Alpine Cranberry

Vaccinium vitis-ideae

DESCRIPTION

Medicinal Parts: The medicinal parts are the dried leaves and the ripe dried fruit.

Flower and Fruit: The white to reddish-tinged flowers are in clusters of various sizes. The 10 stamens are pubescent at the base and the anthers are two-tipped and have no appendage. The white berries initially turn scarlet and contain numerous rust-brown seeds that are 1.5 to 2 mm long.

Leaves, Stem and Root: The plant is a low shrub up to 30 cm high with scaly underground runners. The shoots sprout from the axillary buds of the runners. The sprouts are downy when young and later become glabrous. The leaves are alternate, short-petioled, obovate and coriaceous. The upper surface is dark green and the under surface pale green and covered in glandular hairs.

Habitat: The plant is common in the Northern Hemisphere.

Production: Cranberry leaves are the foliage leaves of Vaccinium vitis-ideae. Collection takes place in uncultivated regions (Scandinavia, England). The leaves are dried in the open air.

Other Names: Cowberry, Red Bilberry, Whortleberry

ACTIONS AND PHARMACOLOGY

COMPOUNDS

Hydroquinone glycosides: arbutin (3-5%), pyroside (6'-acetyl-arbutin), hydroquinone gentiobioside, 2-O-caffeoyl arbutin

Tannins (10-20%): chiefly condensed tannins, proanthocyainidine

Flavonoids: including among others, avicularin, hyperoside, quercitrin, isoquercitrin

Triterpenes: including among others, beta-amyrin, oleanolic acid, ursolic acid

EFFECTS

The drug is antiviral and a urine disinfectant due to the tannin fraction. It also raises cyclooxigenase activity through the flavonol glycosides.

INDICATIONS AND USAGE

Unproven Uses: Alpine Cranberry is used to treat urinary tract irritation, gout, rheumatism, and calculus (stone complaints). It is also considered a substitute for Bearberry leaves.

CONTRAINDICATIONS

The drug is contraindicated in pregnancy, nursing, and in children under 12 years of age.

PRECAUTIONS AND ADVERSE REACTIONS

No health hazards are known in conjunction with the proper administration of designated therapeutic dosages. Individuals with gastric sensitivity may experience queasiness and vomiting following intake of preparations made from the drug with high tannin content. Liver damage is conceivable with administration of the drug over extended periods, particularly with children, due to the possible hepatotoxicity of the hydroquinones released.

Because the urine-disinfecting effect of the hydroquinones released in the urinary tract only occurs in an alkali environment, the simultaneous administration of medication and food that increases uric acid concentration in the bladder should be avoided.

DOSAGE

Mode of Administration: Available as whole, cut, and powdered drug.

Daily Dose: The internal dose is 2 gm as a single dose; as a decoction, the concentration is 2 gm per cup.

Storage: Store the drug in a tightly sealed container and protect it from light.

LITERATURE

Friedrich H, Naturwissenschaften 48:304. 1961.

Frohne D, Pfänder HJ, Giftpflanzen - Ein Handbuch für Apotheker, Toxikologen und Biologen, 4. Aufl., Wiss. Verlags-Ges. Stuttgart 1997.

Hänsel R, Keller K, Rimpler H, Schneider G (Hrsg.), Hagers Handbuch der Pharmazeutischen Praxis, 5. Aufl., Bde 4-6 (Drogen): Springer Verlag Berlin, Heidelberg, New York, 1992-1994.

Sticher O et al., PM 35:253. 1979.

Thieme H et al., PA 24:236. 1969.

Thieme H, Winkler HJ, PA 21:182. 1966.

Teuscher E, Biogene Arzneimittel, 5. Aufl., Wiss. Verlagsges. Stuttgart 1997.

Thompson RS et al., J Chem Soc Perkin Tarns I:1387. 1972.

Alpine Ragwort

Senecio nemorensis

DESCRIPTION

Medicinal Parts: The medicinal part is the herb.

Flower and Fruit: The composite flower heads are in a dense, usually heavily blossomed corymb. The involucre bracts are grass- or olive-green and often tinged greenish-black at the tips. The florets are yellow. The fruit is 4 mm long, long-stemmed and glabrous. During flowering, the pappus is only as long as the disc florets. By the time the fruit ripens, the pappus is 3 times as long as the fruit.

Leaves, Stem and Root: This geophytic perennial has runners that are fleshy, 20 cm long and 5 cm thick. The stem is erect, 40 to 140 cm high with rounded ribs. The stem is green or, in particularly sunny locations, reddish-brown. The stem is glabrous to sparsely pubescent or short-downy. The foliage leaves are lanceolate-ovate, oblong-elliptic to oblong-lanceolate, acute or acuminate and serrate to double-serrate-dentate. The upper cauline leaves are usually petiolate, almost glabrous above to sparsely pubescent. The lower surface of the leaf is sparsely or moderately scattered and appressed pubescent.

Habitat: The plant grows in many regions of southern and western Europe and is cultivated in some eastern European countries.

Other Names: Squaw Weed, Life Root

ACTIONS AND PHARMACOLOGY

COMPOUNDS

Pyrrolizidine alkaloids (0.01-0.1%): including among others, senecionine, fuchsisencionine, 7-angeloylretronecin, bulgarsenine, nemorensin, platyphyllin, sarracin

Sesquiterpenes of the eremophilane-type: including among others, nemosenine A-D

Flavonoids: including among others, rutin, quercitrin

Hydroxycoumarins: including among others, esculetin

Volatile oil (0.1%)

EFFECTS

The drug is hemostyptic and hypoglycemic. The pyrrolizidine alkaloids are hepatotoxic and carcinogenic.

INDICATIONS AND USAGE

Unproven Uses: Folk medicine uses of Life Root have included diabetes mellitus, hemorrhage, high blood pressure, spasms and as a uterine stimulant. The drug is also used in bleeding as a result of tooth extraction.

PRECAUTIONS AND ADVERSE REACTIONS

Life Root should not be taken internally. Hepatotoxicity and carcinogenicity are possible due to the presence of pyrrolizidine alkaloids with 1,2-unsaturated necic parent substances.

DOSAGE

Mode of Administration: Internal use is not recommended.

How Supplied: Forms of commercial pharmaceutical preparations include drops.

Preparation: To prepare a tea, pour boiling water over 1 teaspoonful (approximately 1 g) of finely cut drug, steep for 5 to 10 minutes, then strain.

Daily Dosage: A cup of the tea may be taken several times a day. (See precautions and adverse reactions).

LITERATURE

Gottlieb R et al., DAZ 130:285. 1990.

Röder E et al., PH 16:1462. 1977.

Röder E, Pyrrolizidinhaltige Arzneipflanzen. In: DAZ 132(45):2427-2435. 1992.

Wiedenfeld H et al., Arch Pharm 315:165. 1982.

Wiedenfeld H et al., Arch Pharm 318:294. 1985.

Wiedenfeld H et al., PH 18:1083. 1979.

Wiedenfeld H et al., PM 41:124. 1981.

Wiedenfeld H et al., PM 46:426. 1986.

Wiedenfeld H et al., Sci Pharm 57:97. 1989.

Further information in:

Hänsel R, Keller K, Rimpler H, Schneider G (Hrsg.), Hagers Handbuch der Pharmazeutischen Praxis, 5. Aufl., Bde 4-6

(Drogen): Springer Verlag Berlin, Heidelberg, New York, 1992-1994.

Steinegger E, Hänsel R, Pharmakognosie, 5. Aufl., Springer Verlag Heidelberg 1992.

Teuscher E, Lindequist U, Biogene Gifte - Biologie, Chemie, Pharmakologie, 2. Aufl., Fischer Verlag Stuttgart 1994.

Wagner H, Wiesenauer M, Phytotherapie. Phytopharmaka und pflanzliche Homöopathika, Fischer-Verlag, Stuttgart, Jena, New York 1995.

Wichtl M (Hrsg.), Teedrogen, 4. Aufl., Wiss. Verlagsges. Stuttgart 1997.

Alpinia officinarum

See Lesser Galangal

Alstonia constricta

See Fever Bark

Althaea officinalis

See Marshmallow

Amanita muscaria

See Aga

Amaranth

Amaranthus hypochondriacus

DESCRIPTION

Medicinal Parts: The entire plant is used medicinally

Flower and Fruit: The inflorescence is bifurcated, solitary and oblong-spicate in dense spike-like terminal clusters with very short internodes, often composed of twigs. In some species they are all in the leaf axils. The plant is monoecious, dioecious or mixed. Bracteoles are 4 to 6 mm, ovate, with a mucro that is about twice as long as the perianth. The perianth segments are narrowly ovate, usually acute and about as long as the fruit. The segments are dry-skinned, whitish- or reddish-green to red. The ovary is ovate. The fruit is one-seeded, ovate, dry-skinned, and forms a transversely dehiscing capsule. Seeds are lentil-shaped, erect, circular, smooth and usually black.

Leaves, Stem and Root: The plant is a tall, glabrous annual, occasionally perennial, and grows up to 2 m tall. It is erect, glabrous or sparsely pubescent above. The leaves are rhomboid-ovate and alternate, with occasionally undulating or ruffled margins.

Habitat: Amaranth is common in temperate and warm climates.

Production: Amaranth is the complete plant in flower of Amaranthus hypochondriacus.

Other Names: Lady Bleeding, Lovely Bleeding, Love-Lies-Bleeding, Red Cockscomb, Velvet Flower, Pilewort, Prince's Feather

ACTIONS AND PHARMACOLOGY

COMPOUNDS

Saponins

Betacyans

Protoalkaloids

EFFECTS

The drug is said to have an astringent effect (possibly due to the saponins, betacyans and protoalkaloids). There are no studies available on efficacy.

INDICATIONS AND USAGE

Unproven Uses: Amaranth has been used for diarrhea, ulcers, and inflammation of the mouth and throat.

PRECAUTIONS AND ADVERSE REACTIONS

No health hazards or side effects are known in conjunction with the proper administration of designated therapeutic dosages.

DOSAGE

Mode of Administration: Amaranth is administered orally as a liquid extract.

LITERATURE

Martindale. The Extra Pharmacopoeia, 27th Ed. Pub. The Pharmaceutical Press (1977) UK.

Amaranthus hypochondriacus

See Amaranth

Amargo

Quassia amara

DESCRIPTION

Medicinal Parts: The medicinal part is the wood of the trunk and branches.

Flower and Fruit: The flowers are small and pale yellowish green. The sepals are round to ovate, fused at the base and imbricate. There are 5 petals, 10 stamens and 5 carpels. The style is fused from bottom to top. The fruit is a pea-sized drupe, which ripens from December to January. They are black, glossy, solitary, clavate and have a thin skin.

Leaves, Stem and Root: The plant is a 15 to 30 m high tree with a diameter of 1 m. The bark is smooth and grayish. The alternate leaves are odd pinnate. The leaflets are opposite, oblong, acuminate and uneven at the base.

Habitat: The plant grows in Jamaica

Production: Quassia Wood is the wood of Quassia amara or Picrasma excelsa.

Not to be Confused With: The wood of Rhus metopium

Other Names: Bitter Wood, Jamaica Quassia, Surinam Quassia, Japanese Quassia, Bitter Ash

ACTIONS AND PHARMACOLOGY

COMPOUNDS

Triterpenes: decanor-triterpenes (picrasan derivatives, quassinoids, simaroubolides) chief components quassin (nigakilactone D, 0.1 to 0.2%), isoquassin (picrasmine), neoquassin and 18-hydroxyquassin

Indole alkaloids of:

-beta-carboline type, including 1-vinyl-4,8-dimethoxy-beta-carboline

-canthinone type, including 2-methoxy-6-one, 3-methylcanthine-5,6-dione

EFFECTS

The amaroid drug (quassinoids) stimulates secretion of gastric juices, increases appetite and aids digestion. It may also have a choleretic effect.

INDICATIONS AND USAGE

Homeopathic Uses: Quassia amara is used for gallbladder complaints, as bitter tonic, purgative and as anthelmintic (for ascarid and threadworms).

CONTRAINDICATIONS

Contraindicated in pregnancy.

PRECAUTIONS AND ADVERSE REACTIONS

General: No health hazards or side effects are known in conjunction with the proper administration of designated therapeutic dosages. Internal administration can be followed occasionally by dizziness and headache, as well as by uterine pain.

Pregnancy: Not to be used during pregnancy.

OVERDOSAGE

Overdosage could lead to mucous membrane irritation, followed by vomiting. Use over prolonged periods of time may lead to weakened vision and total blindness.

DOSAGE

Mode of Administration: Quassia Wood is used in homeopathic dilutions and in commercial pharmaceutical preparations.

Daily Dosage: 500 mg

Storage: Quassia should be protected from light and kept dry.

LITERATURE

Barbetti P et al., Quassinoids from Quassia amara. In: PH 32:1007. 1993.

Bray DH et al., (1987) Phytother Res 1 (1):22.

Geissmann T, (1964) Ann Rev Pharmacol 4:305.

Kupchan SM, Streelman DR, (1976) J Org Chem 41:3481.

Murae T et al., (1973) Tetrahedron 29:1515.

Murae T et al., (1975) Chem Pharm Bull 23 (9):2191.

Njar VCO et al., 2-Methoxycanthin-6-on: a new alkaloid from the stem wood of Quassia amara. In: PM 59(3):259. 1992.

Njar VCO et al., Antifertility activity of Quassia amara: Quassin inhibits the steroidgenesis in rat Leydig cells in vitro. In: PM 61(2):180-182. 1995.

Ohmoto T, Koike K. (1983) Chem Pharm Bull 31:3198.

Polonsky J, (1973) Fortschr. Chem Org Naturst 30. 101.

Wagner H et al., (1979) Planta Med 36:113.

Wagner H et al., (1980) Planta Med 38:204.

Further information in:

Kern W, List PH, Hörhammer L (Hrsg.), Hagers Handbuch der Pharmazeutischen Praxis, 4. Aufl., Bde 1-8, Springer Verlag Berlin, Heidelberg, New York, 1969 (unter Pirola rotundifolia).

Leung AY, Encyclopedia of Common Natural Ingredients Used in Food Drugs and Cosmetics, John Wiley & Sons Inc., New York 1980.

Lewin L, Gifte und Vergiftungen, 6. Aufl., Nachdruck, Haug Verlag, Heidelberg 1992.

Madaus G, Lehrbuch der Biologischen Arzneimittel, Bde 1-3, Nachdruck, Georg Olms Verlag Hildesheim 1979.

Roth L, Daunderer M, Kormann K, Giftpflanzen, Pflanzengifte, 4. Aufl., Ecomed Fachverlag Landsberg Lech 1993.

Schulz R, Hänsel R, Rationale Phytotherapie, Springer Verlag Heidelberg 1996.

Steinegger E, Hänsel R, Pharmakognosie, 5. Aufl., Springer Verlag Heidelberg 1992.

Teuscher E, Biogene Arzneimittel, 5. Aufl., Wiss. Verlagsges. Stuttgart 1997.

Wagner H, Wiesenauer M, Phytotherapie. Phytopharmaka und pflanzliche Homöopathika, Fischer-Verlag, Stuttgart, Jena, New York 1995.

Wichtl M (Hrsg.), Teedrogen, 4. Aufl., Wiss. Verlagsges. Stuttgart 1997.

American Adder's Tongue

Erythronium americanum

DESCRIPTION

Medicinal Parts: The medicinal parts are the leaves and tubers.

Flower and Fruit: The flowers are terminal, large, hanging, lily-like and are 2.5 cm in diameter. The bracts of the involucre are sharply revolute, bright yellow and often tinged purple and sprinkled at the base. There are 6 stamens. The fruit is a fusiform nodule about 2 cm long.

Leaves, Stem and Root: The plant grows from a small, ovate fern-colored corm to between 2 and 2.5 cm long. It is perennial with a bulbous light brown root. The stem is thin and about 25 cm high. There are only 2 leaves which are lanceolate, and pale green. They have purplish or brownish spots, are about 6 cm long by 2 to 3 cm wide, minutely wrinkled and with parallel veins. The petioles are 5 to 7.5 cm long.

Characteristics: The fresh leaves have emollient and anti-scrofulous properties when applied as a poultice.

Habitat: The plant grows in the eastern U.S. as far south as Florida and as far north and west as Ontario and Arkansas.

Production: American Adder's Tongue leaves are the fresh leaves of Erythronium americanum.

Other Names: Dog's Tooth Violet, Erythronium, Lamb's Tongue, Rattlesnake Violet, Serpent's Tongue, Snake Leaf, Yellow Snakeleaf, Yellow Snowdrop

ACTIONS AND PHARMACOLOGY

COMPOUNDS

Alpha-methylene-gamma-butyrolactones: tuliposides

EFFECTS

When used internally, the drug is emetic. Externally it is an emollient.

INDICATIONS AND USAGE

Unproven Uses: The plant is used externally for ulcers.

PRECAUTIONS AND ADVERSE REACTIONS

The plant has a strongly sensitizing effect. Reciprocal reactions occur with tulip, fritallaria, lily, alstroemeria and Bomarea species. Nothing is known regarding health hazards or side effects in connection with the administration of the drug.

DOSAGE

Mode of Administration: Fresh leaves are applied topically as a poultice or administered internally as an infusion.

LITERATURE

Cavallito CJ, Haskell TH, (1946) J Am Chem Soc 66:2332.

Hausen B, Allergiepflanzen, Pflanzenallergene, ecomed Verlagsgesellsch. mbH, Landsberg 1988.

Kern W, List PH, Hörhammer L (Hrsg.), Hagers Handbuch der Pharmazeutischen Praxis, 4. Aufl., Bde 1-8, Springer Verlag Berlin, Heidelberg, New York, 1969.

Teuscher E, Lindequist U, Biogene Gifte - Biologie, Chemie, Pharmakologie, 2. Aufl., Fischer Verlag Stuttgart 1994.

American Bittersweet

Celastrus scandens

DESCRIPTION

Medicinal Parts: The medicinal parts are the root and the bark of the plant.

Flower and Fruit: The twining shrub is up to 8 m tall. The leaves are 5 to 12.5 cm long, ovate to ovate-lanceolate and serrate. There are numerous very small greenish flowers on terminal racemes 10 cm long. The orange-yellow seed capsules are 1 cm in diameter.

Habitat: The plant is indigenous to North America.

Production: American Bittersweet root and bark are the root and bark of Celastrus scandens.

Other Names: Waxwork, False Bittersweet

ACTIONS AND PHARMACOLOGY

COMPOUNDS

Tannins

Celastrol (yellow quinoide nortriterpene)

EFFECTS

American Bittersweet has diuretic and diaphoretic effects.

INDICATIONS AND USAGE

Unproven Uses: The drug has been used for rheumatism, menstrual disorders and liver disorders, but is rarely used today.

PRECAUTIONS AND ADVERSE REACTIONS

No health hazards or side effects are known in conjunction with the proper administration of designated therapeutic dosages.

DOSAGE

No information is available.

LITERATURE

Hegnauer R, Chemotaxonomie der Pflanzen, Bde 1-11, Birkhäuser Verlag Basel, Boston, Berlin 1962-1997.

Kern W, List PH, Hörhammer L (Hrsg.), Hagers Handbuch der Pharmazeutischen Praxis, 4. Aufl., Bde. 1-8, Springer Verlag Berlin, Heidelberg, New York, 1969.

American Hellebore

Veratrum viride

DESCRIPTION

Medicinal Parts: The medicinal parts are the dried rhizome and the roots.

Flower and Fruit: The terminal inflorescence is a panicle made up of spike-like racemes. The flowers are short-pedicled and often unisexual. The perigone has 6 tepals and is almost free. The anther is reniform. The fruit is capsule-like with numerous seeds and dividing membranes. The seeds are flattened, light-brown and winged all around. The embryo is small and set in the tip of the fusiform endosperm.

Leaves, Stem and Root: The species are perennial herbs with strong leafy stems. The leaves are spiralled, broadly elliptical to linear-lanceolate, heavily ribbed and drawn together in a broad sheath. The leaves of Veratrum viride are oval to linear.

Characteristics: Characteristics of the species Veratrum viride is very similar to Veratrum album.

Habitat: The herb is indigenous to the swamps and moist ground from Canada to Georgia and westward to Minnesota.

Production: American Hellebore root is the rhizome of Veratrum viride.

Not to be Confused With: The rhizome from Symplocarpus foetidus is thicker than that of Veratrum viride and more porous.

Other Names: Bugbane, Devil's Bite, Earth Gall, Indian Poke, Itchweed, Tickleweed

ACTIONS AND PHARMACOLOGY

COMPOUNDS

Steroid alkaloids (1%): including among others, some of the solanidane-type, isorubijervine, rubijervine- C-nor-D-homo-sterane-type: including among others, protoverine, protover-atrine A and B. In contrast with Veratrum album, the less toxic alkaloids of the solanidane-type are here in the majority.

EFFECTS

The herb reduces blood pressure and slows down the pulse due to the alkaloid germitrin. When used externally, it is hyperemic, hyperalgic, and locally anaesthetic. The drug is extremely toxic.

INDICATIONS AND USAGE

Unproven Uses: The drug is obsolete due to the high risk of side effects. Historically, American Hellebore was used internally to treat pneumonia, peritonitis, epilepsy, pain, asthma, colds, cholera, croup, consumption, dyspepsia, fever, hypertension, herpes, gout, headache, inflammation, neuralgia, whooping cough, puerperal fever, scarlet fever, sciatica, rheumatism, shingles, toothache, scrofulous, tumors, and typhus. It was used externally for throat infections and tonsillitis (as a gargle solution), neuralgia, and skin irritations.

PRECAUTIONS AND ADVERSE REACTIONS

The drug is severely toxic and has numerous severe side effects, even in therapeutic dosages. It is no longer administered in allopathic medicine. The alkaloids are severely mucous membrane-irritating, and because they inhibit inactivation of the sodium ion channels after resorption, the alkaloids have a paralyzing effect on numerous excitable cells, in particular those governing cardiac activity.

OVERDOSAGE

The first symptoms of poisoning are sneezing, lacrimation, salivation, vomiting, diarrhea, burning sensation in the mouth and pharyngeal space, and inability to swallow; then, following resorption: paresthesia, vertigo, possible blindness, paralysis of the limbs; also mild convulsions, lowering of cardiac frequency, cardiac arrhythmias and hypotension. Death occurs either through systolic cardiac arrest or through asphyxiation. The alkaloids can also be absorbed through uninjured skin.

Following gastrointestinal emptying (inducement of vomiting, gastric lavage with burgundy-colored potassium permanganate solution, sodium sulphate), installation of activated charcoal and shock prophylaxis (appropriate body position, quiet, warmth), the therapy for poisoning consists of treating spasms with diazepam or certain barbiturates (i.v.), bradycardia with atropine and hypotension with peripherally active circulatory medications. Electrolyte substitution may be necessary and possible cases of acidosis should be treated with sodium bicarbonate infusions. Intubation and oxygen respiration may also be necessary.

DOSAGE

Mode of Administration: The herb can be found in whole and powdered forms.

Daily Dose: The daily dose is 100 mg.

Storage: The drug should be clearly labeled as ''poisonous'' and stored in a safe place.

LITERATURE

Brossi, B, In: Brossi A, Cordell GA (Eds), The Alkaloids. Vol. 41. Academic Press, 1250 Sixth Avenue, San Diego, CA 92101. 1992.

Frohne D, Pfänder HJ, Giftpflanzen - Ein Handbuch für Apotheker, Toxikologen und Biologen, 4. Aufl., Wiss. Verlags-Ges. Stuttgart 1997.

Kern W, List PH, Hörhammer L (Hrsg.), Hagers Handbuch der Pharmazeutischen Praxis, 4. Aufl., Bde 1-8: Springer Verlag Berlin, Heidelberg, New York, 1969.

Kupchan, S M et al., (1961) Lloydia 24(1):17.

Madaus G, Lehrbuch der Biologischen Arzneimittel, Bde 1-3, Nachdruck, Georg Olms Verlag Hildesheim 1979.

Roth L, Daunderer M, Kormann K, Giftpflanzen, Pflanzengifte, 4. Aufl., Ecomed Fachverlag Landsberg Lech 1993.

Teuscher E, Lindequist U, Biogene Gifte - Biologie, Chemie, Pharmakologie, 2. Aufl., Fischer Verlag Stuttgart 1994.

American Ivy

Parthenocissus quinquefolia

DESCRIPTION

Medicinal Parts: The medicinal parts are the bark, the branch tips, the fresh leaves, the berries and the resin.

Flower and Fruit: The inflorescences are fairly small and appear in yellowish-green racemes. They produce dark-purple, pea-sized berries; the seeds are cordate.

Leaves, Stem and Root: American Ivy is a high-climbing shrub with dark green branches, which sometimes develop adventitious roots. The flowering branches turn into regular, double-rowed creepers, which diminish toward the top. The leaves are long-petioled and divided into 5 elliptical, ovate or obovate, roughly serrate or dentate leaflets. The leaflets have broad, suddenly acuminate and usually somewhat rounded-off teeth. The upper surface is dark green, and the undersurface is whitish-green and matte.

Habitat: Parthenocissus quinquefolia originated in North America and is cultivated worldwide.

Production: American Ivy bark is the bark of the trunk and branches of Parthenocissus quinquefolia.

Other Names: American Woodbine, Creeper, False Grapes, Five Leaves, Ivy, Virginia Creeper, Wild Woodbine, Wild Woodvine, Woody Climber

ACTIONS AND PHARMACOLOGY

COMPOUNDS

Up to 2% oxalic acid is contained in the berries, however there is no information available on the constituents of the rind.

EFFECTS

The plant is diaphoretic, astringent and tonic.

INDICATIONS AND USAGE

Unproven Uses: American Ivy is used for digestive disorders.

PRECAUTIONS AND ADVERSE REACTIONS

The berries are considered poisonous, however no health hazards or side effects are known in conjunction with the proper administration of designated therapeutic dosages. Older scientific literature describes the death of a child following intake of the berries (Lewin, 1992).

DOSAGE

Mode of Administration: The drug is ground for use as an infusion.

LITERATURE

Kern W, List PH, Hörhammer L (Hrsg.), Hagers Handbuch der Pharmazeutischen Praxis, 4. Aufl., Bde 1-8, Springer Verlag Berlin, Heidelberg, New York, 1969.

Lewin L, Gifte und Vergiftungen, 6. Aufl., Nachdruck, Haug Verlag, Heidelberg 1992.

Roth L, Daunderer M, Kormann K, Giftpflanzen, Pflanzengifte, 4. Aufl., Ecomed Fachverlag Landsberg Lech 1993.

American Liverleaf

Hepatica nobilis

DESCRIPTION

Medicinal Parts: The drug is the herb, without roots, harvested at flowering season.

Flower and Fruit: The flowering stems are axillary, numerous, pubescent and erect. They are usually reddish and have 3 entire-margined, ovate, unpetiolate, calyx-like bracts, up to 1 cm long, directly under the upright flower. The 6 to 8 bracts are sky blue, paler on the outside, occasionally pink or white, narrow-ovate, entire-margined and dropping. There are no nectaries. The stamens are almost white with red connective. The stigma is head-like. The fruit is oblong with a short beak fitted into the semi-globular receptacle.

Leaves, Stem and Root: The herb is a 7 to 15 cm high, hardy perennial with a short, fibrous, dark brown rhizome. The numerous leaves are basal, long-petioled, coriaceous, green above and usually more or less violet beneath. They are cordate and 3-lobed at the base, deeply indented, broadly ovate, with blunt to acute lobes. The young leaves, including the stems, are densely covered in silky white hairs. The leaves later become glabrous and appear after flowering. Liverwort is a protected species in Germany, Austria, Switzerland, Italy, the Czech Republic, Slovakia and Hungary.

Habitat: The plant is indigenous to almost all of Europe except the Atlantic regions, Denmark and northwest Germany. It is also indigenous to Korea, Japan and temperate North America.

Production: American Liverleaf consists of the fresh or dried above-ground parts of Hepatica nobilis. The herb is harvested when in bloom and air-dried in the shade. The roots must be left in the ground because they are a protected species.

Other Names: Herb Trinity, Kidneywort, Liverleaf, Liverweed, Round-Leaved Hepatica, Trefoil

ACTIONS AND PHARMACOLOGY

COMPOUNDS

Protoanemonine-forming agents (0.07% in the freshly harvested plant, based on weight): presumably, the glycoside ranunculin changes enzymatically when the plant is cut into small pieces (and probably also during dehydration) into the pungent, volatile protoanemonine that quickly dimerizes to anemonine. Once dried, the plant is not capable of protoanemonine formation.

Flavonoids: including isoquercitrin, astragalin, querci-meritrin

Saponins

EFFECTS

The main active agents are lactone-forming glycosides, flavo-glycosides and anthocyane. The fresh plant contains protoanemonine, which causes skin irritation.

INDICATIONS AND USAGE

Unproven Uses: Preparations of American Liverleaf herb are used for liver ailments, liver diseases of all origins, jaundice, gallstones and gravel.

PRECAUTIONS AND ADVERSE REACTIONS

Health risks or side effects following the proper administration of designated therapeutic dosages are not recorded. Extended skin contact with the freshly harvested, bruised plant can lead to blister formation and cauterizations that are difficult to heal due to the resulting protoanemonine, which is severely irritating to the skin and mucous membranes. If taken internally, severe irritation to the gastrointestinal tract, combined with colic and diarrhea, as well as irritation of the urinary drainage passages, are possible.

Symptomatic treatment for external contact consists of mucilaginosa, following irrigation with diluted potassium permanganate solution. In case of internal contact, administration of activated charcoal should follow gastric lavage.

DOSAGE

Mode of Administration: The drug can be taken internally or used externally as a rinse.

Preparation: To make a rinse, a cataplasm can be made of the squeezed fresh plant; alcohol can be used if necessary. A liniment can be made with added fats, oils or alcohol.

Daily Dosage: When used internally, a single dose consists of 2 to 4 gm as an infusion, or 2 to 3 cups from a 3 to 6% infusion. The daily dosage is 4 teaspoonfuls, or 3.8 gm drug.

LITERATURE

Hänsel R, Keller K, Rimpler H, Schneider G (Hrsg.), Hagers Handbuch der Pharmazeutischen Praxis, 5. Aufl., Bde 4-6 (Drogen), Springer Verlag Berlin, Heidelberg, New York, 1992-1994.

Madaus G, Lehrbuch der Biologischen Arzneimittel, Bde 1-3, Nachdruck, Georg Olms Verlag Hildesheim 1979.

Roth L, Daunderer M, Kormann K: Giftpflanzen, Pflanzengifte, 4. Aufl., Ecomed Fachverlag Landsberg Lech 1993.

Ruijgrok HWL, PM 11:338-347. 1963.

Teuscher E, Lindequist U, Biogene Gifte - Biologie, Chemie, Pharmakologie, 2. Aufl., Fischer Verlag Stuttgart 1994.

American Pawpaw

Asimina triloba

DESCRIPTION

Medicinal Parts: The medicinal parts are the seeds, bark and leaves.

Flower and Fruit: The axillary flowers are dull purple and solitary. They are about 3.5 cm wide. The petals are round, ovate and marbled. The outer ones are almost circular and 3 to 4 times as long as the sepals. The fruit is yellowish, oblong-ovoid. The fleshy pods are about 7.5 by 2.5 cm and contain 3 flat, brown seeds. The seeds are slightly polished with darker brown lines on the surface. They are oblong-oval, with a grayish hilum at one end. The taste and smell are resinous.

Leaves, Stem and Root: The American Pawpaw grows up to 6 m in height. The young shoots and leaves are covered in rust-colored down and later become glabrous. The leaves are thin (20-25 cm long and 7 cm wide), smooth, entire, ovate and acuminate. The plant's leaves and flowers appear simultaneously.

Characteristics: The fruit has an unpleasant smell when unripe, but when it ripens after a frost, it smells, faintly of custard. This characteristic gives rise to one of its common names—Custard Apple.

Habitat: The plant is found in the west, south and central U.S., also India and parts of Asia and Africa.

Production: American Pawpaw seeds are the seeds of Asimina triloba.

Other Names: Custard Apple

ACTIONS AND PHARMACOLOGY

COMPOUNDS

Benzyl isoquinoline alkaloids: including anolobine

Polyketides: including asimicine

Fatty oil

EFFECTS

No information is available.

INDICATIONS AND USAGE

Homeopathic Uses: In homeopathy, American Pawpaw is used in the treatment of scarlet fever, fevers and vomiting, as well as for mouth and throat inflammation.

PRECAUTIONS AND ADVERSE REACTIONS

The drug has a nauseant effect. Allergic individuals may be susceptible to severe urticaria.

DOSAGE

Mode of Administration: The mother tincture is used in homeopathic dilutions.

LITERATURE

He K, Shi G, Zhao GX, Zeng L, Ye Q, Schwedler JT, Wood KV, McLaughlin JL, Three new adjacent bis-tetrahydrofuran acetogenins with four hydroxyl groups from Asimina triloba. J Nat Prod, 59:1029-34, 1996.

He K, Zhao GX, Shi G, Zeng L, Chao JF, McLaughlin JL, Additional bioactive annonaceous acetogenins from Asimina triloba (Annonaceae). Bioorg Med Chem, 5:501-6, 1997.

Kern W, List PH, Hörhammer L (Hrsg.), Hagers Handbuch der Pharmazeutischen Praxis, 4. Aufl., Bde. 1-8, Springer Verlag Berlin, Heidelberg, New York, 1969.

Lewin L, Gifte und Vergiftungen, 6. Aufl., Nachdruck, Haug Verlag, Heidelberg 1992.

Oliver-Bever B (Ed.), Medicinal Plants of Tropical West Africa, Cambridge University Press Cambridge, London 1986.

Ratnayake S, Rupprecht JK, Potter WM, McLaughlin JL, Evaluation of various parts of the paw paw tree Asimina triloba (Annonaceae) as commercial sources of the pesticidal annonaceous acetogenins. J Econ Entomol, 55:2353-6, 1992.

Woo MH, Cho KY, Zhang Y, Zeng L, Gu ZM, McLaughlin JL, Asimilobin and cis- and trans-murisolinones novel bioactive Annonaceous acetogenins from the seeds of Asimina triloba. J Nat Prod, 4:1533-42, 1995.

Zhao G, Hui Y, Rupprecht JK, McLaughlin JL, Wood KV, Additional bioactive compounds and trilobacin a novel highly cytotoxic acetogenin from the bark of Asimina triloba. J Nat Prod, 55:347-56, 1992.

Zhao GX, Chao JF, Zeng L, McLaughlin JL, (24-cis)-asimicinone and (24-trans)-asimicinone: two novel bioactive ketolactone acetogenins from Asimina triloba (Annonaceae). Nat Toxins, 4:128-34, 1996.

Zhao GX, Chao JF, Zeng L, Rieser MJ, McLaughlin JL, The absolute configuration of adjacent bis-THF acetogenins and asiminocin a novel highly potent asimicin isomer from Asimina triloba. Bioorg Med Chem, 4:25-32, 1996.

American White Pond Lily

Nymphaea odorata

DESCRIPTION

Medicinal Parts: The medicinal parts are the cut and dried rhizome, the fresh rhizome and the rhizome with the roots.

Flower and Fruit: The androgynous flowers are solitary, 7 to 15 cm across and radial-symmetrical. They grow from the rhizome and extend above the water by means of a long stem. The 4 sepals are almost free, oblong-ovate, pale green on the outside and greenish-white on the inside. The pure white 23 to 32 petals are free, elliptical-lanceolate, narrower than the sepals and arranged on the axis like a screw. The numerous carpels are sunk into the beaker-shaped axis in a ring and are partially fused with it. The fruit is a berry-like capsule, which ripens under water. The seeds are small, ovate, approximately 2.5 mm long, smooth and have an aril. The flowers open as the sun rises, close a few hours later (before the intense midday heat) and remain closed until the next morning. The size of the plant varies according to depth of water.

Leaves, Stem and Root: The fragrant water lily is an aquatic plant with a strong horizontal rhizome, which grows under water. The leaves are swimming, alternate, long-petioled and have 4 air channels in the petiole. The lamina is oval-orbicular, large (15-30 cm long) and has a wedge-shaped deep indentation at the base. It is entire-margined, coriaceous, green above and purple-brown beneath. The petiole is greenish and is usually purple-tinged. The stipules are triangular to reniform.

Characteristics: The flowers have a sweet fragrance.

Habitat: The plant is indigenous to the eastern part of North America. It is found as far south as Mexico, El Salvador and the West Indies, and has been naturalized in parts of western Europe.

Production: American White Pond Lily root is the rhizome of Nymphaea odorata and other varieties. The drug is derived from the cut and dried rhizome and, in powdered form, is yellowish to gray-brown.

Other Names: Water Cabbage, Cow Cabbage, Water Lily, Water Nymph

ACTIONS AND PHARMACOLOGY

COMPOUNDS

Tannins (gallotannins, ellagitannins)

Only a very small amount of research work has been carried out on the drug, but American White Pond Lily root is known to contain large amounts of gallic and ellagic tannins.

EFFECTS

The astringent and antiseptic effects of the American White Pond Lily can be attributed to the high tannin content. Only limited amounts of research have been carried out on the drug.

INDICATIONS AND USAGE

Unproven Uses: Chronic diarrhea is a common internal application. Externally, the plant has been used in the treatment of vaginal conditions and as a gargle in the treatment of diseases of the mouth and throat. Traditional folk medicine uses also included dysentery, gonorrhea and leukorrhea, and the leaves and roots were applied as a mash poultice for boils, tumors, scrofulous sores and inflamed skin.

Homeopathic Uses: Morning diarrhea is one use in homeopathy.

PRECAUTIONS AND ADVERSE REACTIONS

No health hazards or side effects are known in conjunction with the proper administration of designated therapeutic dosages.

OVERDOSAGE

No poisonings have yet been observed among humans but animal experiments have been performed with fatal results. Even though very high dosages were used with the animals, these results should be taken as a warning to exercise care.

DOSAGE

Mode of Administration: As a decoction or liquid extract used for washes, poultices and gargles or taken internally.

Preparation: The fluid extract is produced by percolation: 1:1 using ethanol 25%.

Daily Dosage: Internally: in a single dose of 1 to 2 g drug as an infusion; 1 to 4 ml of liquid extract.

Homeopathic Dosages: 5 drops, 1 tablet or 10 globules every 30 to 60 minutes (acute) or 1 to 3 times daily (chronic); parenterally: 1 to 2 ml sc acute, 3 times daily; chronic: once a day (HAB1).

LITERATURE

Hänsel R, Keller K, Rimpler H, Schneider G (Hrsg.), Hagers Handbuch der Pharmazeutischen Praxis, 5. Aufl., Bde 4-6 (Drogen), Springer Verlag Berlin, Heidelberg, New York, 1992-1994.

Madaus G, Lehrbuch der Biologischen Arzneimittel, Bde 1-3, Nachdruck, Georg Olms Verlag Hildesheim 1979.

Odinstsova NV, (1960) Farmakol i Toxicol 23:132.

Roth L, Daunderer M, Kormann K, Giftpflanzen, Pflanzengifte, 4. Aufl., Ecomed Fachverlag Landsberg Lech 1993.

Su KL et al., (1983) Lloydia 36:72 and 80.

Ammi visnaga

See Bishop's Weed

Ammoniac Gum

Dorema ammoniacum

DESCRIPTION

Medicinal Parts: The medicinal part of the plant is a resin exuded from the flowers and stems.

Flower and Fruit: The inflorescence is an umbel which grows from the axils of the upper leaves. Because of the very short flower stems, the individual inflorescences appear very globular. The flower structures are in fives, the flowers radial and small, the calyx teeth indistinct, the petals white with revolute tips. There are 5 stamens. The ovary is inferior, 2-chambered, densely haired, with a conical style cushion with 2 styles. The fruit is double achene.

Leaves, Stem and Root: This herbaceous perennial grows up to 2.5 m high. The leaves are arranged in spirals, with clearly developed sheaths, and the lamina is often only rudimentary. The stem is hollow, gnarled, blue-striped, and up to 5 cm thick. The taproot is tuberous.

Habitat: The plant is found growing in areas from Iran to southern Siberia.

Production: Ammoniac gum is the naturally-exuding gum resin latex of Dorema ammoniacum hardened in the air and collected in the wild.

Not to be Confused With: Confusion may occur with North African and Cyrenian ammoniac.

ACTIONS AND PHARMACOLOGY

COMPOUNDS

Resin (60 to 70%): chief component ammoresinol

Water-soluble polysaccharides (10 to 20%)

Volatile oil (0.1 to 0.3%): chief components linalool, linalyl acetate, citronellyl acetate

EFFECTS

The drug is credited with being mildly diuretic, sudorific, spasmolytic, expectorate and menstruation-promoting in its effect, although research data regarding these effects is not available.

INDICATIONS AND USAGE

Unproven Uses: Uses dating back to ancient times include ingestion for its expectorant effect in chronic bronchitis, especially in the elderly. Because of the resin's purported diuretic, antispasmodic and stimulant properties, it was often employed internally as a diaphoretic and emmenagogue as well as externally as a plaster for swellings of the joints and indolent tumors. In the late 19th century, it was used as an expectorant for chronic catarrh and externally in plasters to relieve hyperadenosis and in compresses for abscesses. More recently, internal folk medicine uses include chronic bronchitis, asthma, sciatica and joint pain as well as conditions of the liver and spleen. Among external uses are treatment of wounds and abscesses as well as lymph node swelling.

Homeopathic Uses: Homeopathic uses include bronchitis.

CONTRAINDICATIONS

The drug is contraindicated during pregnancy due to the existence of indications of a menstruation-inducing effect.

PRECAUTIONS AND ADVERSE REACTIONS

According to older sources, repeated visual disorders and glaucoma-like states appeared following ingestion of the drug, however no health hazards have been verified in conjunction with the proper administration of designated therapeutic dosages.

DOSAGE

Mode of Administration: Preparations for internal and external use

Preparation:

Ammoniacum depuratum — 1000 parts coarse ammoniac powder are heated with 1500 parts ethanol 60% in a steam bath while being constantly stirred until an emulsion is formed. It is then pressed through linen and evaporated until a few drops can be worked in the hand without becoming sticky.

Combination — Ammoniac emulsion: toluene: distilled water; 1:2:30

Daily Dosage: 0.3 to 1 g drug

Homeopathic Dosage: 5 drops, 1 tablet or 10 globules every 30 to 60 minutes (acute) and 1 to 3 times daily (chronic); parenterally: 1 to ml sc acute: 3 times daily; chronic: once a day (HAB1); special doses for children

Storage: The drug should be stored over chalk in a container that protects it from light.

LITERATURE

Blaschek W, Hänsel R, Keller K, Reichling J, Rimpler G, Schneider G (Eds) Hagers Handbuch der Pharmazeutischen Praxis. Folgeb nde 1 und 2. Drogen A-Z. Springer. Berlin, Heidelberg 1998.

Amomum aromaticum

See Nepalese Cardamom

Anacardium occidentale

See Cashew

Anacyclus pyrethrum

See Pellitory

Anagallis arvensis

See Scarlet Pimpernel

Anamirta cocculus

See Fish Berry

Ananas comosus

See Pineapple

Andira araroba

See Goa Powder

Anemarrhena asphodeloides

See Anemarrhena (Zhi-Mu)

Anemarrhena (Zhi-Mu)

Anemarrhena asphodeloides

DESCRIPTION

Medicinal Parts: The medicinal part of the plant is the rhizome.

Flower and Fruit: The inflorescence is spike-like, and the flowers are clustered and radial. The perianth structures are in sixes. The tepals are free and all the same. There are 3 stamens and a 3-carpeled, fused ovary, with 1 to 3 seeds in each chamber. The fruit is a globose capsule, which opens on 3 sides.

Leaves, Stem and Root: Anemarrhena asphodeloides is a herbaceous perennial, and extends up to 60 cm high. The leaves are grass-like and clustered at the base.

Habitat: The plant is native to northern China, Korea and Japan.

Production: Zhi-Mu is the dried rhizome of Anemarrhena asphodeloides. It is best harvested in the third year of cultivation in spring or autumn. The rhizome is then air-dried.

ACTIONS AND PHARMACOLOGY

COMPOUNDS

Steroid saponins (6%): aglycones sarsapogenin, markogenin, neogitonin, particularly sarsapogenin-3-timobioside and markogenin-3-timobioside

Water-soluble polysaccharides: anemarans A to D

Lignans: hinoki resinol, among others

Xanthones: mangiferin (1.3%)

EFFECTS

A variety of experiments have been able to demonstrate antipyretic and cortisone-like effects for the drug with its steroid saponin content. In addition, inhibitions of platelet aggregation, of Na, K-ATP-ase and of DNA-polymerase were observed. The timosaponin A-III isolated from the drug reduced the serum levels of a 1-fetoprotein in animal experiments.

INDICATIONS AND USAGE

Unproven Uses: Zhi-Mu is used for agitation (in Oriental medicine).

Chinese Medicine: In China, Zhi-Mu is used for febrile conditions and inflammation, diabetes, dry cough, ''bone fever'' and general dehydration, painful stool or strangury. It is also as a decoction for typhus, scarlet fever and tuberculosis.

PRECAUTIONS AND ADVERSE REACTIONS

No health hazards are known in conjunction with the proper administration of designated therapeutic dosages.

OVERDOSAGE

The ingestion of large dosages of the drug may lead to gastroenteritis, intestinal colic and diarrhea, due to the saponin content. The drug is not to be administered in the presence of diarrhea.

DOSAGE

Mode of Administration: Whole and cut drug preparations for internal use.

Daily Dosage: 6 to 12 gm of drug often used with other herbs in teas.

Storage: Should be stored in a dry and well-aired place.

LITERATURE

Dong JX, Han GY, A new active steroidal saponin from Anemarrhena asphodeloides. Planta Med, 57:460-2, 1991 Oct.

Dong JX, Han GY, Studies on the active constituents of Anemarrhena asphodeloides bunge. Yao Hsueh Hsueh Pao, 27:26-32, 1992.

Hänsel R, Keller K, Rimpler H, Schneider G (Ed), Hagers Handbuch der Pharmazeutischen Praxis, 5. Aufl., Bde 4 - 6 (Drogen), Springer Verlag Berlin, Heidelberg, New York, 1992-1994.

Li PM, Zhong JL, Chen RQ, Zhang XK, Ho KL, Chiu JF, Huang DP, Zhi-mu saponin inhibits alpha-fetoprotein gene expression in developing rat liver. Int J Biochem, 21:15-22, 1989.

Liu JQ, Wu DW, 32 cases of postoperative osteogenic sarcoma treated by chemotherapy combined with Chinese medicinal herbs. Planta Med, 21: 1997.

Ma B, Wang B, Dong J, Yan X, Zhang H, Tu A, New spirostanol glycosides from Anemarrhena asphodeloides. Letter Planta Med, 63:376-9, 1997 Aug.

Miura T, Kako M, Ishihara E, Usami M, Yano H, Tanigawa K, Sudo K, Seino Y, Antidiabetic effect of seishin-kanro-to in KK-Ay mice. Planta Med, 21:320-2, 1997 Aug.

Nakashima N, Kimura I, Kimura M, Matsuura H, Isolation of pseudoprototimosaponin AIII from rhizomes of Anemarrhena asphodeloides and its hypoglycemic activity in streptozotocin-induced diabetic mice. J Nat Prod, 57:Kimura I, Matsuura H.

Takahashi M, Konno C, Hikino H, Isolation and hypoglycemic activity of anemarans A, B, C and D, glycans of Anemarrhena asphodeloides rhizomes. Planta Med, 57:100-2, 1985 Apr.

Anemone nemorosa

See Wood Anemone

Anethum graveolens

See Dill

Angelica

Angelica archangelica

TRADE NAMES

Nature's Answer Angelica Root Liquid

DESCRIPTION

Medicinal Parts: The medicinal parts are the seed, whole herb and root.

Flower and Fruit: The flowers are greenish-white to yellowish and are arranged in 20 to 40 rayed compact umbels without an involucre. The tiny epicalyx has numerous sepals with minute tips. The petals have an indented, indistinguishable tip. The elliptic fruit is 7 mm long by 4 mm wide and winged. The outer fruit membrane separates from the inner one.

Leaves, Stem and Root: The plant is 50 to 250 cm tall. The rhizome is short, strong, fleshy and has long fibrous roots. The stem is erect, often as thick as an arm at the base. It is round, finely grooved, hollow and tinged reddish below. The leaves are very large, 60 to 90 cm and tri-pinnate with a hollow petiole. Leaflets are ovate and unevenly serrate. The leaf sheaths are large and swollen.

Characteristics: The plant has a strong tangy odor. The taste is sweetish to burning tangy.

Habitat: Angelica is thought by some botanists to be indigenous to Syria, Holland or Poland. Today it is found growing in the wild on the coasts of the North and Baltic Seas as far north as Lapland. It is a protected species in Iceland, and is cultivated in other regions. Other species are found in America (A. atropurpurea), in Europe (A. sylvestris) and in China/Asia (A. sinensis).

Production: Angelica seed consists of the fruit of Angelica archangelica, which is harvested from July onward. After drying in the air or in ovens, the umbels are threshed to separate the seeds. Angelica herb consists of the above-ground parts of Angelica archangelica. Angelica root is the dried root and rhizome of Angelica archangelica.

Other Names: European Angelica, Garden Angelica, Angel's Wort

ACTIONS AND PHARMACOLOGY

COMPOUNDS: ANGELICA FRUIT

Volatile oil: constituents include hexylmethyl phthalate, alpha-pinene, beta-phellandrene, borneol, camphene, beta-bisabolene, beta-caryophyllene, macrocyclic lactones (odor-determining) such as 15-oxypentadecenlactone

Furanocoumarins: including angelicin, bergaptene, imperatorin, oxypeucedanin, xantholtoxin

Fatty oil

Phytosterols: including beta-sitosterol, sigmasterol

EFFECTS: ANGELICA FRUIT

The furanocoumarins in the fruit are cytostatic and phototoxic. The spasmolytic, gastric juice-stimulating and cholagogic effect of the herb could be explained by the aromatic-amaroid structure.

COMPOUNDS: ANGELICA LEAVES

Volatile Oil (0.015 to 0.1%): chief constituents myrcene (17 to 29%), p-cymene, limonene, cis-and trans-ocimene, alpha-phellandrene, beta-phellandrene, alpha-pinene

Furanocoumarins: including angelicin, bergaptene, imperatorin, isoimperatorin, oxypeucedanin, archangelicin

EFFECTS: ANGELICA LEAVES

The essential oils and furanocoumarins from the leaves have a strong irritant effect on the skin and mucous membranes (angelica dermatitis). The spasmolytic, gastric juice-stimulating and cholagogic effect of the herb could be explained by the aromatic-amaroid structure.

COMPOUNDS: ANGELICA ROOT

Volatile oil: chief components are alpha- and beta-phellandrenes, alpha-pinenes, macrocyclic lactones, including penta- and heptadecanolide

Furanocoumarins: including bergaptene, xanthotoxin, scopoletin, umbelliferone

Caffeic acid derivatives: including chlorogenic acid

Flavonoids

EFFECTS: ANGELICA ROOT

The root acts as an antispasmodic, cholagogue and stimulatory for secretion of gastric juices.

INDICATIONS AND USAGE

ANGELICA FRUIT

Approved by Commission E:

- Fevers and colds
- Infections of the urinary tract
- Dyspeptic complaints
- Loss of appetite

Unproven Uses: Preparations of angelica seed are used internally for conditions of the kidneys and efferent urinary tract, the intestinal tract and the respiratory tract, as well as for rheumatic and neuralgic complaints. Preparations are also used as a diaphoretic and have been used in the past for malaria. Externally, an ointment from the seeds is used for body lice.

ANGELICA LEAVES

Unproven Uses: Preparations from the leaves have been used as a diuretic and diaphoretic.

ANGELICA ROOT

Approved by Commission E:

- Dyspeptic complaints
- Loss of appetite

Unproven Uses: In folk medicine, preparations of the root are used as a mild rubefacient, for coughs, bronchitis, menstruation complaints, loss of appetite, dyspeptic complaints with mild gastrointestinal cramps, liver and biliary duct conditions.

PRECAUTIONS AND ADVERSE REACTIONS

ANGELICA FRUIT AND HERB

General: No health hazards or side effects are known in conjunction with the proper administration of designated therapeutic dosages. Photodermatosis is possible following contact with the plant juice.

Pregnancy: Preparations are not to be used during pregnancy.

ANGELICA ROOT

No health hazards or side effects are known in conjunction with the proper administration of designated therapeutic dosages. The furocoumarins contained in angelica root sensitize the skin to light and can lead to inflammation of the skin in combination with UV rays. It is therefore advisable to avoid sunbathing and intensive UV radiation for the duration of treatment with Angelica or its preparations.

DOSAGE

ANGELICA ROOT

Mode of Administration: Comminuted herb and other oral galenic preparations for internal use.

How Supplied:

Fluid Extract — 1:1

Oil

Tincture — 1:5

Preparation: There is no information on preparation in the literature.

Daily Dosage: 4.5 gm of drug, 0.5 to 3.0 gm of liquid extract (1:1); 1.5 gm of tincture (1:5); 10 to 20 drops of essential oil.

LITERATURE

ANGELICA FRUIT AND HERB

Amling R, Phytotherapeutika in der Neurologie. In: ZPT 12(1):9. 1991.

Ashraf M et al., (1980) Pak J Sci Ind Res 23 (1-2):73.

Chang, EH et al., (Eds), Advances in Chinese Medicinal Materials Research, World Scientific Pub. Co. Singapore 1985.

Escher S, Keller U et al., (1979) Helv Chim Acta 62 (7):2061.

Glowniak K et al., Localisation and seasonal changes of psoralen in Angelica fruits. In: PM 62, Abstracts of the 44th Ann Congress of GA, 76. 1996.

Lemmich J et al., (1983) Phytochemistry 23 (2):553-555.

Leung AY, Encyclopedia of Common Natural Ingredients used in Food Drugs and Cosmetics, John Wiley & Sons Inc., New York, 1980.

Opdyke DLJ, (1975) Food Cosmet Toxicol: 13, Suppl 713.

Sethi OP, Shah AK, (1979) Ind J Pharm Sci 42 (6): C11.

Shimizu M, Matsuzawa T, Suzuki S, Yoshizaki M, Morita N, Evaluation of Angelicae radix (Touki) by inhibitory effect on platelet aggregation. In: Chem Pharm Bull 39:2046. 1991.

Taskinen J, (1975) Acta Chem Scan 29 (5):637 et (7) 757.

Tastrup O et al., (1983) Phytochemistry 22 (9):2035.

Zotikov YM et al., (1978) Rastit Resur 14 (4):579.

Further information in:

Kern W, List PH, Hörhammer L (Hrsg.), Hagers Handbuch der Pharmazeutischen Praxis, 4. Aufl., Bde. 1-8, Springer Verlag Berlin, Heidelberg, New York, 1969.

Madaus G, Lehrbuch der Biologischen Arzneimittel, Bde 1-3, Nachdruck, Georg Olms Verlag Hildesheim 1979.

ANGELICA ROOT

Amling R, Phytotherapeutika in der Neurologie. In: ZPT 12(1):9. 1991.

Ashraf M et al., (1980) Pak J Sci Ind Res 23 (1-2):73.

Chang, EH et al., (Eds), Advances in Chinese Medicinal Materials Research, World Scientific Pub. Co., Singapore 1985.

Chalchat JC, Garry RPh, J Essent Oil Res 5:447. 1993.

Escher S, Keller U et al., (1979) Helv Chim Acta 62 (7):2061.

Glowniak K et al., Localisation and seasonal changes of psoralen in Angelica fruits. In: PM 62, Abstracts of the 44th Ann Congress of GA, 76. 1996.

Harkar S, Razdan TK, Waight ES, Steroids, chromoines and coumarins from Angelica officinalis. In: PH 23:419-426. 1983.

Härmälä P, Kaltia S, Vuorela H, PM 58:287. 1992.

Lemmich J et al., (1983) Phytochemistry 23 (2):553-555.

Leung AY, Encyclopedia of Common Natural Ingredients used in Food Drugs and Cosmetics, John Wiley & Sons Inc., New York, 1980.

Nykanen I et al., Essent Oil Res 3:229. 1991.

Opdyke DLJ, (1975) Food Cosmet Toxicol: 13, Suppl 713.

Sethi OP, Shah AK, (1979) Ind J Pharm Sci 42 (6):C11.

Shimizu M, Matsuzawa T, Suzuki S, Yoshizaki M, Morita N, Evaluation of Angelicae radix (Touki) by inhibitory effect on platelet aggregation. In: Chem Pharm Bull 39:2046. 1991.

Sun H, Jakupovic J, PA 41:888. 1986.

Taskinen J, (1975) Acta Chem Scan 29 (5):637 et (7) 757.

Tastrup O et al., (1983) Phytochemistry 22 (9):2035.

Zotikov YM et al., (1978) Rastit Resur 14 (4):579.

Further information in:

Hausen B, Allergiepflanzen, Pflanzenallergene, ecomed Verlagsgesellsch. mbH, Landsberg 1988.

Kern W, List PH, Hörhammer L (Hrsg.), Hagers Handbuch der Pharmazeutischen Praxis, 4. Aufl., Bde. 1-8, Springer Verlag Berlin, Heidelberg, New York, 1969.

Madaus G, Lehrbuch der Biologischen Arzneimittel, Bde. 1-3, Nachdruck, Georg Olms Verlag Hildesheim 1979.

Roth L, Daunderer M, Kormann K, Giftpflanzen, Pflanzengifte, 4. Aufl., Ecomed Fachverlag Landsberg Lech 1993.

Schulz R, Hänsel R, Rationale Phytotherapie, Springer Verlag Heidelberg 1996.

Steinegger E, Hänsel R, Pharmakognosie, 5. Aufl., Springer Verlag Heidelberg 1992.

Teuscher E, Lindequist U, Biogene Gifte - Biologie, Chemie, Pharmakologie, 2. Aufl., Fischer Verlag Stuttgart 1994.

Teuscher E, Biogene Arzneimittel, 5. Aufl., Wiss. Verlagsges. Stuttgart 1997.

Wagner H, Wiesenauer M, Phytotherapie. Phytopharmaka und pflanzliche Homöopathika, Fischer-Verlag, Stuttgart, Jena, New York 1995.

Wichtl M (Hrsg.), Teedrogen, 4. Aufl., Wiss. Verlagsges. Stuttgart 1997.

Angelica archangelica

See Angelica

Angostura

Galipea officinalis

DESCRIPTION

Medicinal Parts: The medicinal part is the dried bark of the tree.

Flower and Fruit: The flowers are in terminal, peduncled and closed racemes. The fruit is a 5-valved capsule, of which 2 or 3 are often sterile. There are 2 round, black seeds in each capsule and usually only one seed is fertile.

Leaves, Stem and Root: Galipea officinalis is a small 4 to 5 m high tree, which is 7.5 to 12.5 cm in diameter and has a straight trunk and irregular branches. The bark is smooth and gray. It is slightly curved or quilled. The outer layer is sometimes soft and spongy; the inner surface is yellowish-gray. The transverse section is dark brown. The bright green leaves are smooth, glossy, alternate and petiolate. They sometimes have white spots. The 3 leaflets are oblong, pointed and 4 cm long.

Characteristics: The flowers have a strong scent, which initially resembles that of tobacco. The taste is bitter.

Habitat: Angostura is indigenous to Venezuela and tropical regions of South America.

Production: Angostura is the whole or ground bark of Galipea officinalis.

Other Names: Cusparia Bark, True Angostura

ACTIONS AND PHARMACOLOGY

COMPOUNDS

Volatile oil : chief constitents galipol, (-)- cadinene, galipene

Quinolin alkaloids: including cusparine including galipine, galipoline, quinaldine, cuspareine, galipoidine, 1-methyl-2-quinolone

Angustorine (bitter iridoid glycoside)

EFFECTS

Angostura stimulates gastric juices and acts as a tonic. In larger doses, the drug also has an emetic and strong laxative effect.

INDICATIONS AND USAGE

Unproven Uses: Folk medicine indications include diarrhea; it is also used as a febrifuge.

PRECAUTIONS AND ADVERSE REACTIONS

No health hazards or side effects are known in conjunction with the proper administration of designated therapeutic dosages. The administration of larger doses can lead to nausea and vomiting.

LITERATURE

Brieskorn CH, Beck V, (1971) Phytochemistry 10:3205.

Hoppe HA, (1975-1987) Drogenkunde, 8. Aufl., Bde 1-3, W. de Gruyter Verlag, Berlin, New York.

Kern W, List PH, Hörhammer L (Hrsg.), Hagers Handbuch der Pharmazeutischen Praxis, 4. Aufl., Bde 1-8, Springer Verlag Berlin, Heidelberg, New York, 1969.

Leung AY, Encyclopedia of Common Natural Ingredients Used in Food Drugs and Cosmetics, John Wiley & Sons Inc. New York 1980.

Madaus G, Lehrbuch der Biologischen Arzneimittel, Bde 1-3, Nachdruck, Georg Olms Verlag Hildesheim 1979.

Roth L, Daunderer M, Kormann K, Giftpflanzen, Pflanzengifte, 4. Aufl., Ecomed Fachverlag Landsberg Lech 1993.

Anise

Pimpinella anisum

DESCRIPTION

Medicinal Parts: The medicinal parts are the essential oil from the ripe fruit and the dried fruit.

Flower and Fruit: The inflorescences are medium-sized umbels with about 7 to 15 scattered pubescent rays. There is usually no involucre, but sometimes there is a single bract. There are barely any sepals. The petals are white, about 15 mm long, and have a ciliate margin. They have small bristles on the outside and a long indented tip. The fruit is downy, ovate to oblong and flattened at the sides.

Leaves, Stem and Root: The plant is an annual herb about 0.5 m high; it is downy all over. The root is thin and fusiform, and the stem is erect, round, grooved and branched above. The lower leaves are petiolate, orbicular-reniform, entire and coarsely dentate to lobed. The middle leaves are orbicular and 3-lobed, or 3-segmented with ovate or obovate segments. The upper leaves are short-petioled to sessile with narrow sheaths; they are pinnatisect with narrow tips.

Characteristics: The taste is sweet and the odor characteristic.

Habitat: The origin of the plant is unknown but it probably came from the Near East. Today, it is cultivated mainly in southern Europe, Turkey, central Asia, India, China, Japan, Central and South America.

Production: Anise consists of the dried fruits of Pimpinella anisum.

ACTIONS AND PHARMACOLOGY

COMPOUNDS

Volatile oil (2 to 6%): chief constituent trans-anethole (94%), including as well chavicol methyl ether (estragole, 2%), anis aldehyde (1.4%)

Caffeic acid derivatives: including chlorogenic acid (0.1%), other caffeoyl quinic acids

Flavonoids: including apigenin-7-O-glucoside, isoorientin, isovitexin, luteolin-7-O-glucoside

Fatty oil (30%)

Proteic substances (20%)

EFFECTS

The drug is said to have an expectorant, mildly spasmolytic and antibacterial effect based on the essential oil. The data is empirical and there are no recent studies available.

Aniseed oil (main constituent trans-anethol) has an antibacterial, antiviral, insect repellent effect and in animal experiments it has been shown to be expectorant, spasmolytic and estrogenic.

INDICATIONS AND USAGE

Approved by Commission E:

- Common cold
- Cough/bronchitis
- Fevers and colds
- Inflammation of the mouth and pharynx
- Dyspeptic complaints
- Loss of appetite

The drug is used internally for dyspeptic complaints. It is used both internally and externally for catarrhs of the respiratory tract.

Unproven Uses: In folk medicine, Anise is used internally for whooping cough, flatulence, colic-like pain, as a digestive, for menstruation disturbances, liver disease and tuberculosis.

Homeopathic Uses: Pimpinella anisum is used for shoulder pain and lumbago.

CONTRAINDICATIONS

Anise is contraindicated in patients allergic to anise and anethole.

PRECAUTIONS AND ADVERSE REACTIONS

No health hazards or side effects are known in conjunction with the proper administration of designated therapeutic dosages. Sensitization has been observed very rarely.

DOSAGE

Mode of Administration: As a comminuted drug for infusions and other galenic preparations for internal use or for inhalation. The purpose of an external application of an Anise preparation is the inhalation of essential oil.

Daily Dosage: Internal average daily dose is 3 g drug (depending on the preparation).

Tea — Drink 1 cup mornings and/or evenings (expectorant); 1 dessertspoon per day (gastrointestinal complaints); infants 1 teaspoon (added to the bottle).

Infusion — single dose: 0.5 to 1 g before meals.

External application — inhalation of the essential oil.

Homeopathic Dosage: 5 drops, 1 tablet or 10 globules every 30 to 60 minutes (acute) or 1 to 3 times daily (chronic); parenterally: 1 to 2 ml sc acute, 3 times daily; chronic: once a day (HAB1).

LITERATURE

Albert Puleo M, (1980) J Ethnopharmacol 2(4):337.

Czygan FC, Anis (Anisi fructus DAB 10) - Pimpinella anisum. In: ZPT 13(3):101. 1992.

Drinkwater NR, Miller EC, Miller JA, Pitot HC, (1976) Hepatocarcinogenicity of estragole and 1'-hydroxyestragole in the mouse and mutagenicity of 1-acetoxystragole in bacteria. J Natl Canc Inst 57:1323-1331.

Gershbein LL, (1977) Food Cosmet Toxicol 15(3):173.

Kartnig T et al., (1975) Planta Med 27:1.

Kubeczka KH et al., (1976) Z Naturforsch 31b:283.

Kubeczka KH, Formacek V, New Constituents from the Essential Oils of Pimpinella. In: Brunke EJ (Ed.) Progress in Essential Oil Research, Walter de Gruyter & Co, Berlin 1986. 1986.

Kunzemann J, Herrmann K, (1977) Z Lebensm Unters Forsch 164:194.

Mueller-Limmroth W, Froenlich HH, (1980) Fortschr Med 98 (3):95.

Nofal MA, (1981) Ain Chams Univ Fac Agric Res Bull 1602: 1-10.

Reichling J, Merkel B, Elicitor-Induced Formation of Coumarin Derivatives of Pimpinella anisum. In: PM 59(2):187. 1993.

Truhaut R, LeBourhis B, Attia M, Glomot R, Newman J, Caldwell J, (1989) Chronic toxicity/carcinogenicity study of trans-anethole in rats. Food chem Tox 27:11-20.

Further information in:

Hänsel R, Keller K, Rimpler H, Schneider G (Hrsg.), Hagers Handbuch der Pharmazeutischen Praxis, 5. Aufl., Bde 4-6 (Drogen), Springer Verlag Berlin, Heidelberg, New York, 1992-1994.

Hausen B, Allergiepflanzen, Pflanzenallergene, ecomed Verlagsgesellsch. mbH, Landsberg 1988.

Leung AY, Encyclopedia of Common Natural Ingredients Used in Food Drugs and Cosmetics, John Wiley & Sons Inc., New York, 1980.

Madaus G, Lehrbuch der Biologischen Arzneimittel, Bde 1-3, Nachdruck, Georg Olms Verlag Hildesheim 1979.

Schulz R, Hänsel R, Rationale Phytotherapie, Springer Verlag Heidelberg 1996.

Steinegger E, Hänsel R, Pharmakognosie, 5. Aufl., Springer Verlag Heidelberg 1992.

Teuscher E, Biogene Arzneimittel, 5. Aufl., Wiss. Verlagsges. Stuttgart 1997.

Wagner H, Wiesenauer M, Phytotherapie. Phytopharmaka und pflanzliche Homöopathika, Fischer-Verlag, Stuttgart, Jena, New York, 1995.

Wichtl M (Hrsg.), Teedrogen, 4. Aufl., Wiss. Verlagsges. Stuttgart 1997.

Antelaea azadirachta

See Neem

Antennaria dioica

See Cat's Foot

Anthoxanthum odoratum

See Sweet Vernal Grass

Anthyllis vulneraria

See Common Kidney Vetch

Aphanes arvensis

See Parsley Piert

Apium graveolens

See Celery

Apocynum cannabinum

See Indian Hemp

Apple Tree

Malus domestica

DESCRIPTION

Medicinal Parts: The medicinal parts are the fresh false fruit, the dried fruit peels, and the inflorescences with their leaves and solid peduncles.

Flower and Fruit: The flowers are umbelled racemes with only a few blossoms. The petals are obovate, up to 2.5 cm long, stemmed, white, pink, or pink on the outside and white on the inside. The carpels are fused with the false fruit.

Leaves, Stem and Root: The plant is a 6 to 10 m high tree or shrub. Boughs and branches are initially villous-haired, later becoming glabrous. The leaves are alternate, ovate, usually shortly acuminate and finely crenate-serrate.

Habitat: The plant is cultivated in the temperate regions of the Northern Hemisphere, and occasionally grows wild.

Production: Medicinal and pharmaceutical preparations of apples come in liquid and dried pectin forms. The source material is the apple residue with 10% to 20% pectin in the dried mass. The residue is extracted at pH 1.5 to 3 and 60° to 100° C.

ACTIONS AND PHARMACOLOGY

COMPOUNDS: IN THE FRUIT PULP

Fruit acids: the chief acid is malic acid (0.2 to 1.5%); in unripe apples quinic acid; including as well citric acid, succinic acid, lactic acid

Caffeic acid derivatives: including 5-caffeoyl quinic acid

Aromatic substances: in particular 2-trans-hexenal, 3-cis-hexenal, 2-trans-hexenol, 3-cis-hexenol, beta-damascenone, ethyl butyrate, methyl butyric acid hexylester; in some strains, 1-methoxy-4-(2-propenyl)benzole

Pectins

Tannins

Vitamins: in particular ascorbic acid (3 to 30 mg/100 gm)

COMPOUNDS: IN THE SEEDS

Cyanogenic glycoside: amygdalin (0.5 to 1.5%, corresponding to 30 to 90 mg HCN/100 gm)

Fatty oil

EFFECTS

Pectin is a swelling agent. Apple pectins have a mild binding effect.

INDICATIONS AND USAGE

Unproven Uses: Finely ground fruit or preparations that contain liquid or dry pectin are used for milder forms of dyspepsia, diarrhea and digestive complaints, especially in children.

PRECAUTIONS AND ADVERSE REACTIONS

No health hazards or side effects are known in conjunction with the proper administration of designated therapeutic dosages.

DOSAGE

Mode of Administration: The fruit is available for oral use in the grated or chopped form. The skin peel can be used in teas. Medicinal and pharmaceutical preparations of apples come in liquid and dried pectin forms.

LITERATURE

Belitz HD, Grosch W, Lehrbuch der Lebensmittelchemie, 4. Aufl., Springer Verlag Berlin, Heidelberg, New York 1992.

Hänsel R, Keller K, Rimpler H, Schneider G (Hrsg.), Hagers Handbuch der Pharmazeutischen Praxis, 5. Aufl., Bde 4-6 (Drogen), Springer Verlag Berlin, Heidelberg, New York, 1992-1994.

Kern W, List PH, Hörhammer L (Hrsg.), Hagers Handbuch der Pharmazeutischen Praxis, 4. Aufl., Bde. 1-8, Springer Verlag Berlin, Heidelberg, New York, 1969.

Madaus G, Lehrbuch der Biologischen Arzneimittel, Bde 1-3, Nachdruck, Georg Olms Verlag Hildesheim 1979.

Roth L, Daunderer M, Kormann K, Giftpflanzen, Pflanzengifte, 4. Aufl., Ecomed Fachverlag Landsberg Lech 1993.

Teuscher E, Lindequist U, Biogene Gifte - Biologie, Chemie, Pharmakologie, 2. Aufl., Fischer Verlag Stuttgart 1994.

Aquilegia vulgaris

See Columbine

Arachis hypogaea

See Peanut

Aralia racemosa

See Spikenard

Arctium lappa

See Burdock

Arctostaphylos uva-ursi

See Uva-Ursi

Areca catechu

See Areca Nut

Areca Nut

Areca catechu

DESCRIPTION

Medicinal Parts: The medicinal part of the plant is the nut.

Flower and Fruit: The plant is an erect palm growing up to 30 m high. The trunk has a girth of about 50 cm. The numerous feathery leaflets are 30 to 60 cm long, confluent and glabrous. The flowers are on branching spadix. The male flowers are numerous and above, the female solitary and below. The ovoid drupe has a fibrous layer under the yellow shell and one-seeded stone. The seeds are conical or nearly spherical and about 2.5 cm in diameter. They are very hard, and contain a deep brown testa showing fawn marbling.

Characteristics: The taste is slightly acrid and astringent, and the odor faint.

Habitat: The plant is found in the East Indies, cultivated in parts of Asia and eastern Africa.

Production: Areca or Betel Nuts are the fresh seeds of Areca catechu.

Not to be Confused With: Piper Betel, also called Betel, the leaf of which is chewed.

Other Names: Betel Nut, Pinang

ACTIONS AND PHARMACOLOGY

COMPOUNDS

Pyridine alkaloids: arecoline, guvacoline (ester alkaloids), as well as arecaidine, guvacine

Tannins: catechin type

EFFECTS

The drug acts on the parasympathetic nervous system with an effect that is more muscarinic than nicotinic. It stimulates secretion in the salivary, bronchial and intestinal glands and causes tremors and bradycardia. Chewing mouthfuls of betel leads to a saponification of the ester alkaloids and the resulting arecaidine produces euphoria. The drug also causes cramps in the muscles of intestinal parasites and stimulates the vagus nerve. Central nervous system stimulation has been observed in mice.

INDICATIONS AND USAGE

Unproven Uses: Betel Nut is no longer frequently prescribed in human medicine. However, the nuts are chewed as a recreational drug by an estimated 450 million people because of their intoxicating qualities. Fresh slices of the seed are part of the "betel titbit" used in eastern Asia. (Arecoline is converted in the central nervous system to the stimulant arecaidine through chewing.) That practice is being discouraged because of its link with some forms of oral cancer. In veterinary medicine, the drug is used as a vermifuge for tape worms in cattle and dogs, as well as for intestinal colic in horses.

Chinese Medicine: Uses in Chinese medicine include chronic hepatitis, edema, oliguria, diarrhea and digestive problems.

Indian Medicine: The juice of young seeds is used as a laxative in Indian medicine. A decoction of the root is used for cracked lips.

PRECAUTIONS AND ADVERSE REACTIONS

Due to its arecoline content, the drug appears parasympathomimetic. It leads to increased salivation, in high doses to bradycardia, tremor, reflex excitability, spasms and eventual paralysis. Long-term use of the drug as a stimulant can result in malignant tumors of the oral cavity through formation of nitrosamines. When the nuts are chewed, the mouth and lips are stained red, as are the feces.

OVERDOSAGE

The toxic dose for humans is 8 to 10 g of the drug. Atropine is given as the antidote. Chewing the "nut" leads to a saponification of the ester alkaloids. The resulting arecaidine produces euphoria.

DOSAGE

Mode of Administration: In the past, Areca Nut was used in chewing balm for gum disease and as a vermifuge. Today, it is only used as a vermifuge in veterinary medicine for house pets. Therapeutic use is insignificant.

Storage: Must be stored separately, protected from light and in well-sealed containers.

LITERATURE

Aue W, Pharm Zentralhalle 136:728. 1967.

Hirono I, J Environ Sci Health C3(2):145. 1985.

Huang JL, McLeish MJ, J Chromatogr 475:447. 1989.

Juptner H, (1968) Z Tropenmed Parasit 19:254.

Lewin L, Über Areca catechu, Chavica Betle und das Betelkauen. In: Monographie, Stuttgart, F. Enke, 1889.

Schneider E, PUZ 15:161. 1986.

Further information in:

Frohne D, Pfänder HJ, Giftpflanzen - Ein Handbuch für Apotheker, Toxikologen und Biologen, 4. Aufl., Wiss. Verlags-Ges Stuttgart 1997.

Kern W, List PH, Hörhammer L (Hrsg.), Hagers Handbuch der Pharmazeutischen Praxis, 4. Aufl., Bde. 1-8, Springer Verlag Berlin, Heidelberg, New York, 1969.

Lewin L, Gifte und Vergiftungen, 6. Aufl., Nachdruck, Haug Verlag, Heidelberg 1992.

Roth L, Daunderer M, Kormann K, Giftpflanzen, Pflanzengifte, 4. Aufl., Ecomed Fachverlag Landsberg Lech 1993.

Tang W, Eisenbrand G, Chinese Drugs of Plant Origin, Springer Verlag Heidelberg 1992.

Teuscher E, Lindequist U, Biogene Gifte - Biologie, Chemie, Pharmakologie, 2. Aufl., Fischer Verlag Stuttgart 1994.

Arenaria Rubra

Spergularia rubra

DESCRIPTION

Medicinal Parts: The medicinal part is the herb.

Flower and Fruit: The bracts of the inflorescence are almost as large as the leaves. The sepals and petals are 3 to 4 mm. The petals are usually pink, sometimes white. There are 5 to 10 stamens. The capsule is 4 to 5 mm and about equal in size to the sepals. The seeds are 0.45 to 0.55 mm, unwinged, dark brown, subtrigonal and more or less flattened.

Leaves, Stem and Root: The plant is annual to perennial with a slender to somewhat woody taproot, which is smooth and somewhat sticky. From beneath, it produces numerous, 5 to 22 cm long, diffuse, decumbent or procumbent stems. The leaves are narrow, linear and have very short, lanceolate, acute, silver, scarious stipules.

Habitat: The plant is common in Europe, Russia, Australia, North America and Asia.

Production: Arenaria Rubra is the aerial part of Spergularia rubra.

Other Names: Common Sandspurry, Sabline Rouge, Sandwort

ACTIONS AND PHARMACOLOGY

COMPOUNDS

Triterpene saponins

Resins

EFFECTS

The herb has diuretic effects.

INDICATIONS AND USAGE

Unproven Uses: Arenaria Rubra is used for conditions of the urinary tract, such as cystitis, dysuria and urinary calculus.

PRECAUTIONS AND ADVERSE REACTIONS

No health hazards or side effects are known in conjunction with the proper administration of designated therapeutic dosages.

DOSAGE

Mode of Administration: The herb is used internally as a liquid extract.

LITERATURE

Kern W, List PH, Hörhammer L (Hrsg.), Hagers Handbuch der Pharmazeutischen Praxis, 4. Aufl., Bde 1-8: Springer Verlag Berlin, Heidelberg, New York, 1969.

Arisaema atrorubens

See Jack-in-the-Pulpit

Aristolochia clematitis

See Birthwort

Arjun Tree

Terminalia arjuna

DESCRIPTION

Medicinal Parts: The medicinal parts of the tree are the bark and fruit.

Flower and Fruit: The flowers are arranged in upright, apical panicles. The upper flowers of the panicles are usually only male. The flowers are small and fused; their structures are in fours or fives. The sepals are almost glabrous; the calyx tube has 4 to 5 short, triangular lobes. The petals are inconspicuous. There are 10 stamens and inferior, single-chambered, brownish or reddish pubescent ovary. The style is long and projects above the bud. The fruit is an over 2-cm long, glabrous, ovoid 4- to 5-sided drupe with 5 thick, narrow wings.

Leaves, Stem and Root: Arjun tree grows up to 30 m high. The leaves are opposite, 12 to 30 cm long and coriaceous with approximately 6-mm long petioles, which have 2 glands at the upper end. The lamina is elongate-elliptical, blunt or with a short tip. The base is narrow or cordate and has a finely crenate margin. The trunk is grooved with a thick bark.

Habitat: India

Production: Arjun Tree bark is the dried trunk bark of Terminalia arjuna. It is collected in wild areas.

Other Names: White Murda

ACTIONS AND PHARMACOLOGY

COMPOUNDS

Tannins: gallotannins, ellagitannins

Steroids: sterols, including beta-sitosterol

Triterpenes: arjunolic acid and its glucosides, oleanolic acid

Flavonoids: including arjunolon, baicalein

EFFECTS

Clinical experiments with the bark powder have demonstrated efficacy against congestive cardiac insufficiency and hypertonia. Various extracts caused lowered blood pressure, bradycardia and positively inotropic effects in animal experiments. Spasmolytic and hemostyptic qualities have also been described. The substance is said to be sedative and potentiates the activity of barbiturates.

INDICATIONS AND USAGE

Indian Medicine: Arjun tree is used for fractures, ulcers, discharge of the urethra, leucorrhea, diabetes, anemia, cardiopathy, hyperhydrosis, asthma, bronchitis, states of exhaustion, tumors, dysentery, internal and external hemorrhaging, liver cirrhosis and high blood pressure.

PRECAUTIONS AND ADVERSE REACTIONS

No health hazards are known in conjunction with the proper administration of designated therapeutic dosages.

DOSAGE

Mode of Administration: Powdered drug and liquid preparations for internal use.

Preparation: The following basic forms are used in Indian medicine in many compound preparations.

Arjunatvagadi — An aqueous decoction.

Pardhadyaristam — An aqueous decoction with grapes and final fermentation.

Arjunaghrtam — A paste of the powdered drug with purified butter, heated and filtered.

Arjunatvak — The powdered drug.

Daily Dosage: Since the Indian medicine is dosed according to the individual patient, there is no exact information available. There was, however, one study carried out with a daily dose of 3.88 gm powdered drug.

LITERATURE

Bharani A, Ganguly A, Bhargava KD, Salutary effect of Terminalia Arjuna in patients with severe refractory heart failure. Int J Cardiol, 49:191-9, 1995 May.

Chauhan S, Agarwal S, Mathur R, Vasal assault due to Terminalia arjuna W. & A. bark in albino rats. Andrologia, 53:491-4, 1990 Sep-Oct.

Dwivedi S, Jauhari R, Beneficial effects of Terminalia arjuna in coronary artery disease. Indian Heart J, 49:507-10, 1997 Sep-Oct.

Hänsel R, Keller K, Rimpler H, Schneider G (Ed), Hagers Handbuch der Pharmazeutischen Praxis, 5. Aufl., Bde 4 - 6 (Drogen), Springer Verlag Berlin, Heidelberg, New York, 1992-1994.

Kandil FE, Nassar MI, A tannin anti-cancer promoter from Terminalia arjuna. Phytochemistry, 53:1567-8, 1998 Apr.

Kaur S, Grover IS, Kumar S, Antimutagenic potential of ellagic acid isolated from Terminalia arjuna. Indian J Exp Biol, 53:478-82, 1997 May.

Pettit GR, Hoard MS, Doubek DL, Schmidt JM, Pettit RK, Tackett LP, Chapuis JC, Antineoplastic agents 338. The cancer cell growth inhibitory. Constituents of Terminalia arjuna (Combretaceae). J Ethnopharmacol, 53:57-63, 1996 Aug.

Pettit GR, Hoard MS, Doubek DL, Schmidt JM, Pettit RK, Tackett LP, Chapuis JC, Hypocholesterolaemic effects of Terminalia arjuna tree bark. J Ethnopharmacol, 53:165-9, 1997 Feb.

Pettit GR, Hoard MS, Doubek DL, Schmidt JM, Pettit RK, Tackett LP, Chapuis JC, On the ethnomedical significance of the Arjun tree, Terminalia arjuna (Roxb.) Wight & Arnot. J Ethnopharmacol, 53:173-90, 1987 Jul.

Seth SD, Maulik M, Katiyar CK, Maulik SK, Role of Lipistat in protection against isoproterenol induced myocardial necrosis in rats: a biochemical and histopathological study. Indian J Physiol Pharmacol, 42:101-6, 1998 Jan.

Singh N, Kapur KK, Singh SP, Shanker K, Sinha JN, Kohli RP, Mechanism of cardiovascular action of Terminalia arjuna. Planta Med, 53:102-4, 1982 Jun.

Srivastava N, Prakash D, Behl HM, Biochemical contents, their variation and changes in free amino acids during seed germination in Terminalia arjuna. Int J Food Sci Nutr, 53:215-9, 1997 May.

Armoracia rusticana

See Horseradish

Arnica

Arnica montana

DESCRIPTION

Medicinal Parts: The medicinal parts of Arnica are the ethereal oil of the flowers, the dried flowers, the leaves collected before flowering and dried, the roots, and the dried rhizome and roots.

Flower and Fruit: The terminal composite flower is found in the leaf axils of the upper pair of leaves. They have a diameter of 6 to 8 cm, are usually egg yolk-yellow to orange-yellow, but occasionally light yellow. The receptacle and epicalyx are hairy. The 10 to 20 female ray flowers are lingui-form. In addition, there are about 100 disc flowers, which are tubular. The 5-ribbed fruit is black-brown and has a bristly tuft of hair.

Leaves, Stem and Root: Arnica is a herbaceous plant growing 20 to 50 cm high. The brownish rhizome is 0.5 cm thick by 10 cm long, usually unbranched, 3-sectioned and sympodial. The rhizome may also be 3-headed with many yellow-brown secondary roots. Leaves are in basal rosettes. They are in 2 to 3 crossed opposite pairs and are obovate and entire-margined with 5 protruding vertical ribs. The glandular-haired stem has 2 to 6 smaller leaves, which are ovate to lanceolate, entire-margined or somewhat dentate.

Characteristics: The flower heads are aromatic; the taste is bitter and irritating.

Habitat: Arnica is found in Europe from Scandinavia to southern Europe. It is also found in southern Russia and central Asia.

Production: Arnica flower consists of the fresh or dried inflorescence of Arnica montana or Arnica chamissonis. The flower should be dried quickly at 45° to 50°C.

Not to be Confused With: Other yellow-flowering Asteracea.

Other Names: Arnica Flowers, Arnica Root, Leopard's Bane, Mountain Tobacco, Wolfsbane

ACTIONS AND PHARMACOLOGY

COMPOUNDS

Sesquiterpene lactones of the pseudo-guaianolid-type: particularly esters of the helenalin- and 11,13-dihydrohelenalins with short-chained fatty acids such as acetic acid, isobutyric acid, 2- methyl-butyric acid, methylacrylic acid, isovaleric acid or tiglic acid

Volatile oil: with thymol, thymol esters, free fatty acids

Polyynes: including tri-dec-1-en-penta-3,5,7,9 11-in

Hydroxycumarines

Caffeic acid derivatives: including chlorogenic acid, 1,5-dicaffeoyl quinic acid

Flavonoids: numerous flavone and flavonol glycosides and their aglycones

EFFECTS

Arnica preparations have an antiphlogistic, analgesic and antiseptic effect when applied topically, due to the sesquiterpene lactone componant. The flavonoid bonds, essential oils and polyynes may also be involved. In cases of inflammation, Arnica preparations also show analgesic and antiseptic activity. The sesquiterpenes (helenalin) in the drug have an antimicrobial effect in vitro and an antiphlogistic effect in animal tests. A respiratory-analeptic, uterine tonic and cardiovascular effect (increase of contraction amplitude with simultaneous increase in frequency, i.e. positive inotropic effect) was demonstrated.

INDICATIONS AND USAGE

Approved by Commission E:

- Fever and colds
- Inflammation of the skin
- Cough/bronchitis
- Inflammation of the mouth and pharynx
- Rheumatism
- Common cold
- Blunt injuries
- Tendency to infection

Unproven Uses: External folk medicine uses include consequences of injury such as traumatic edema, hematoma, contusions, as well as rheumatic muscle and joint problems. Other applications are inflammation of the oral and throat region, furunculosis, inflammation caused by insect bites and phlebitis. In Russian folk medicine, the drug is used to treat uterine hemorrhaging. Furthermore, the drug is used for myocarditis, arteriosclerosis, angina pectoris, exhaustion, cardiac insufficiency, sprains, contusions and for hair loss due to psychological causes. While some uses are plausible, most are unproven.

PRECAUTIONS AND ADVERSE REACTIONS

General: The risks connected with the external, appropriate administration of therapeutic dosages of the drug are minimal. Frequent administration, in particular of the undiluted tincture, as well as with contacts with the plant, can nevertheless lead to sensitization.

Allergy-related skin rashes with itching, blister formation, ulcers and superficial necroses can result from repeated contact with, among other things, cosmetics containing Arnica flowers or other composites (for example tansy, chrysanthemums, sunflowers). External application of very high concentrations can also result in primary blister formation and necroses.

Drug Interactions: The coumarin componant may theoretically interact with warfarin, resulting in an additive anticoagulant effect.

OVERDOSAGE

Overdoses taken internally can lead to poisonings, characterized by severe mucous membrane irritation (vomiting, diarrhea, mucous membrane hemorrhage) and a brief stimulation of cardiac activity followed by cardiac muscle palsy. For that reason, internal administration of the drug is strongly discouraged.

DOSAGE

Mode of Administration: Arnica is used in the form of the whole herb, cut herb or herb powder for infusions, extracts, and tinctures; gel, oil and poultice for external application.

How Supplied: Commercial pharmaceutical preparations include gels, ointments, tinctures, oils and plasters.

Preparation: Arnica tincture (3x to 10x dilutions with water) is used to prepare a poultice. A tincture is prepared using 1 part Arnica flowers and 10 parts ethanol 70% v/v (according to DAB 10). Arnica oil is an extract of 1 part herb and 5 parts slightly warmed fatty oil. Ointments are made up with up to 15% Arnica oil or with 10 to 25% tinctures in a neutral ointment base. Mouthwashes are prepared as a tincture in 10x dilution.

Daily Dose: Tincture for cataplasm: tincture in 3x to 10x dilution. For mouth rinses: tincture in 10x dilution. Ointments should contain a maximum of 15% Arnica oil.

Storage: When stored, the drug should be tightly sealed and protected from light.

LITERATURE

Anonym, Arnikablüten nur äußerlich. In: DAZ 131(38):1949. 1991.

Beekman AC et al., Structure-cytotoxicity relationship of some helenanolide-type sesquiterpene lactones. In: JNP 60(3):252-257. 1997.

Brandt L, (1967) Scand J Haematol Suppl 2.

Brock FE, Arnica montana bei Venenleiden. In: ZPT 12(5):141. 1992.

Hall, IH et al., (1979) J Pharm Sci 68:537.

Halub M et al., (1975) Phytochemistry 14:1659.

Hörmann HP, Kortin HC, (1995) Allergic acute contact dermatitis due to Arnica tincture self-medication. Phytomedicine 4:315-317.

Kaziro, GSN et al., (1984) Br. J Oral Maxillofacial Surg 22:42.

Merfort I, (1984) Planta Med 50 (1):107.

Merfort I, (1985) Planta Med 51 (2):136.

Schmidt Th J et al., Sesquiterpen lactones and inositol esters from Arnica angustifolia. In: PM 61(6):544-550. 1995.

Thesen R, Phytotherapeutika - nicht immer harmlos. In: ZPT 9(49):105. 1988.

Weil D, Reuter HD, Einfluβ von Arnika-Extrakt und Helenalin auf die Funktion menschlicher Blutplättchen. In: ZPT 9(1):26. 1988.

Willuhn G et al., (1984) Planta Med 50 (1):35.

Willuhn G, Leven W, Luley C, Arnikablüten DAB 10. Untersuchung zur qualitativen und quantitativen Variabilität des Sesquiterepnelactongehaltes der offizinellen Arzneidroge. In: DAZ 134(42):4077. 1994.

Willuhn G, Leven W, Qualität von Arnikazubereitungen. In: DAZ 135(21):1939-1942. 1995.

Woerdenbag HJ et al., Cytotoxicity of flavonoids and sesquiterpene lactones from Arnica species. In: PM 59(7)81. 1993.

Further information in:

Frohne D, Pfänder HJ, Giftpflanzen - Ein Handbuch für Apotheker, Toxikologen und Biologen, 4. Aufl., Wiss. Verlags-Ges Stuttgart 1997.

Hänsel R, Keller K, Rimpler H, Schneider G (Hrsg.), Hagers Handbuch der Pharmazeutischen Praxis, 5. Aufl., Bde 4-6 (Drogen): Springer Verlag Berlin, Heidelberg, New York, 1992-1994.

Hausen B, Allergiepflanzen, Pflanzenallergene, ecomed Verlagsgesellsch. mbH, Landsberg 1988.

Leung AY, Encyclopedia of Common Natural Ingredients Used in Food Drugs and Cosmetics, John Wiley & Sons Inc., New York 1980.

Lewin L, Gifte und Vergiftungen, 6. Aufl., Nachdruck, Haug Verlag, Heidelberg 1992.

Lyss G, Schmidt TJ, Merfort I, Pahl HL, Helenalin an anti-inflammatory sesquiterpene lactone from Arnica selectively inhibits transcription factor NF-kappaB. Biol Chem, 378:951-61, 1997.

Lyss G, Schmidt TJ, Merfort I, Pahl HL, Immunologic studies of plant combination preparations. *In-vitro* and *in-vivo* studies on the stimulation of phagocytosis. Arzneimittelforschung, 378:1072-6, 1991.

Lyss G, Schmidt TJ, Merfort I, Pahl HL, Postpartum homeopathic Arnica montana: a potency-finding pilot study. Br J Clin Pract, 378:951-61, 1997.

Madaus G, Lehrbuch der Biologischen Arzneimittel, Bde 1-3, Nachdruck, Georg Olms Verlag Hildesheim 1979.

Puhlmann J, Zenk MH, Wagner H, Immunologically active polysaccharides of Arnica montana cell cultures. Phytochemistry, 111:1141-5, 1991.

Roth L, Daunderer M, Kormann K, Giftpflanzen, Pflanzengifte, 4. Aufl., Ecomed Fachverlag Landsberg Lech 1993.

Schroeder H, Loesche W, Strobach H, Leven W, Willuhn G, Till U, Schroer K, Helenalin and 11 alpha13-dihydrohelenalin two constituents from Arnica montana L. inhibit human platelet function via thiol-dependent pathways. Thromb Res, 57:839-45, 1990.

Schulz R, Hänsel R, Rationale Phytotherapie, Springer Verlag Heidelberg 1996.

Steinegger E, Hänsel R, Pharmakognosie, 5. Aufl., Springer Verlag Heidelberg 1992.

Teuscher E, Lindequist U, Biogene Gifte - Biologie, Chemie, Pharmakologie, 2. Aufl., Fischer Verlag Stuttgart 1994.

Teuscher E, Biogene Arzneimittel, 5. Aufl., Wiss. Verlagsges. Stuttgart 1997.

Tveiten D, Bruseth S, Borchgrevink CF, L hne K Effect of Arnica D 30 during hard physical exertion. A double-blind randomized trial during the Oslo Marathon 1990. Tidsskr Nor Laegeforen, 111:3630-1, Dec 10, 1991.

Wagner H, Wiesenauer M, Phytotherapie. Phytopharmaka und pflanzliche Homöopathika, Fischer-Verlag, Stuttgart, Jena, New York 1995.

Wichtl M (Hrsg.), Teedrogen, 4. Aufl., Wiss. Verlagsges. Stuttgart 1997.

Arnica montana

See Arnica

Arrach

Chenopodium vulvaria

DESCRIPTION

Medicinal Parts: The whole fresh, flowering plant has medicinal properties.

Flower and Fruit: The flowers are small, yellow-green and inconspicuous. They grow in clusters in leafless, compact spikes at the tip of the stem. The fruit is enclosed by the involucre. The seeds are black and glossy.

Leaves, Stem and Root: The plant is 15 to 40 cm high. The stems are branched from low down. The leaves are broad, rhomboid, entire-margined and petiolate. The whole plant is floury-dusty.

Characteristics: Arrach has a distinctive unpleasant smell of musty herring brine.

Habitat: Europe, northern Africa and the Caucacus

Production: Arrach is the complete flowering plant of Chenopodium vulvaria.

Other Names: Stinking Arrach, Stinking Goosefoot, Dog's Arrach, Goat's Arrach, Goosefoot, Stinking Motherwort, Netchweed, Oraches

ACTIONS AND PHARMACOLOGY

COMPOUNDS

Mono-, di- and trimethylamine : only in the fresh plant due to their volatility

Betaine

Tannins

EFFECTS

No substantiated information is available.

INDICATIONS AND USAGE

Unproven Uses: Arrach is used internally and externally to relieve cramps and as an emmenagogue.

PRECAUTIONS AND ADVERSE REACTIONS

No health hazards or side effects are known in conjunction with the proper administration of designated therapeutic dosages. The offensive smell often precludes continued use.

DOSAGE

Mode of Administration: Arrach is used externally and as an extract.

LITERATURE

Roth L, Daunderer M, Kormann K, Giftpflanzen, Pflanzengifte, 4. Aufl., Ecomed Fachverlag Landsberg Lech 1993.

Arrowroot

Maranta arundinacea

DESCRIPTION

Medicinal Parts: The medicinal parts are the starch from the rhizome tubers and the dried rhizome.

Flower and Fruit: The flowers are in pairs, 3.5 cm long and pedicled. They have 3 green, lanceolate sepals and a white, tubular-fused corolla with 1 hanging and two erect tips. The stamens are in 2 circles; the first consists of 2 petal-like staminoids, the second of 1 hood-like. There is 1 thickened stamen partly developed like a petal. The ovary is inferior and 3-sectioned. Only 1 carpel is developed. The fruit is 1-valved and has 1 seed.

Leaves, Stem and Root: The plant is a herbaceous perennial, 1 to 2 m high with thin, reed-like, branched and cane-like stems. The rhizome produces, along with the usual root, a sturdy, fusiform, swollen, up to 8 cm thick and 35 cm long tuber. The tuber is thickly covered with whitish, scaly stipules. The leaves are obovate, light green, lightly pubescent and short-petioled. They have long sheaths and up to 13 cm long and 6 cm ovate-lanceolate leaf blades.

Habitat: The plant is indigenous to Central America and is found today in all tropical regions around the world.

Production: Arrowroot is the rhizome of Maranta arundinacea. The drug itself is a white powder extracted from the rhizome. The rhizome is washed, peeled and macerated, and the starch is then extracted, using water in a process of elutriation. The resulting starch mass is purified by repeated sieving and dried in the sun.

Not to be Confused With: Cheaper starches, such as potato, maize, wheat, or rice starch. These are often used as substitutes.

Other Names: Maranta

ACTIONS AND PHARMACOLOGY

COMPOUNDS

Starch (25-27%, with respect to the fresh bulbs): as Marantae amylum, maranta starch, medicinal arrowroot

Other constituent elements are not known.

EFFECTS

Animal tests: In rats that received a Marantae-rich diet, a reduction in the increase of the cholesterin levels in the aorta and heart muscle was reported. The effect was put down to an increased elimination of bile acids.

In humans, the drug is a demulcent and soothing agent.

INDICATIONS AND USAGE

Unproven Uses: Arrowroot is used as a nutritive (nutritional food stuff) for infants and convalescents, a dietary aid in gastrointestinal disorders, and also for diarrhea, especially in pediatrics. In folk medicine, it is used in acute diarrhea.

Indian Medicine: Arrowroot is used in dysentery, diarrhea, dyspepsia, bronchitis, coughs and as a particularly nourishing food for children, the chronically ill and convalescents.

PRECAUTIONS AND ADVERSE REACTIONS

No health hazards or side effects are known in conjunction with the proper administration of designated therapeutic dosages.

DOSAGE

Mode of Administration: The powder is boiled with water.

Storage: Arrowroot should be stored in tightly sealed containers.

LITERATURE

Hänsel R, Keller K, Rimpler H, Schneider G (Hrsg.), Hagers Handbuch der Pharmazeutischen Praxis, 5. Aufl., Bde 4-6 (Drogen), Springer Verlag Berlin, Heidelberg, New York, 1992-1994.

Artemisia absinthium

See Wormwood

Artemisia cina

See Wormseed

Artemisia dracunculus

See French Tarragon

Artemisia vulgaris

See Mugwort

Artichoke

Cynara scolymus

DESCRIPTION

Medicinal Parts: The medicinal parts are the dried whole or cut basal leaves and the dried or fresh herb from the artichoke.

Flower and Fruit: Globose, thorny capitual of lingual florets grows at the end of the stem. The epicalyx is ovate to globose. The bracts are fleshy and taper into a flattened greenish or purple tip. The petals are blue, lilac or white. The fruit is a pubescent achaene 4 to 5 mm in diameter and 7 to 8 mm long. It is flecked brown and glossy.

Leaves, Stem and Root: Cynara scolymus is a perennial plant with a short rhizome and a strong, erect, glabrous stalk. The stalk is up to 2 m high, thickly covered in lanceolate, prickly pinnate to double pinnate leaves. The upper surface is bare and light green; the lower surface is gray and tomentose.

Habitat: The plant is found in the Mediterranean region, the Canary Islands and South America. It is cultivated elsewhere.

Production: Artichoke root is the dried root of Cynara scolymus. Artichoke leaf consists of the fresh or dried basal leaves of Cynara scolymus. Artichoke is cultivated and dried with extreme care.

Other Names: Garden Artichoke, Globe Artichoke

ACTIONS AND PHARMACOLOGY

COMPOUNDS: ARTICHOKE LEAF

Caffeic acid derivatives: chlorogenic acid, neochlorogenic acid, cryptochlorogenic acid, cynarin

Flavonoids (0.5%): in particular rutin

Sesquiterpene lactones (0 to 4%): cynaropicrin, dehydrocynaropicrin, grossheimin, cynaratriol

COMPOUNDS: ARTICHOKE ROOT

Caffeic acid derivatives, including chlorogenic acid sesquiterpene lactones, are not contained in the rhizome.

EFFECTS: ARTICHOKE LEAF AND ROOT

The main active principles are sesquiterpenes (amaroids), hydroxy cinnamic acid and flavonoids. The drug has a cholagogic, hepatotoxic and lipid-reducing effect. A choleretic effect has been observed in rats (effect of the cinnamic acid). The cholesterol levels were reduced in the rats; a hepatostimulating and bitter effect on the gastrointestinal tract has also been documented.

INDICATIONS AND USAGE

ARTICHOKE LEAF

Approved by Commission E:

- Liver and gallbladder complaints
- Loss of appetite

ARTICHOKE LEAF AND ROOT

Unproven Uses: Artichoke is used for dyspeptic problems and also for prophylactic treatment against the return of gallstones.

In folk medicine, Artichoke is also used for digestion complaints and as a tonic in convalescence.

CONTRAINDICATIONS

ARTICHOKE LEAF AND ROOT

Because of the stimulating effect of the drug upon the biliary tract, it should not be administered if there is a bile duct blockage. Colic can occur where the patient suffers from gallstones.

PRECAUTIONS AND ADVERSE REACTIONS

ARTICHOKE LEAF AND ROOT

Health risks or side effects following the proper administration of designated therapeutic dosages are not recorded. The plant possesses a medium potential for sensitization through skin contact. Allergic reactions occur in particular when there is frequent on-the-job contact with artichokes. There are cross-reactions with other composites (including chrysanthemes, arnica pyrethrum).

DOSAGE

ARTICHOKE LEAF

Mode of Administration: Dried, comminuted drug, pressed juice of fresh plant and other galenical preparations for internal use.

Daily Dosage: The average daily dose is 6 gm of drug; single dose is 500 mg of dry extract.

Storage: Artichoke should be protected from light and insects in well-sealed containers.

LITERATURE

Adzet T, Puigmacia M, J Chromatogr 348:447-453. 1985.

Brand N, Cynara scolymus L. - Die Artischocke. In: ZPT 11(5):169. 1990.

Fintelmann V, Antidyspetische und lipidsenkende Wirkung von Artischockenblätterextrakt. In: ZPT 17(5) Beilage ZFA. Zeitschrift für Allgem Med. 1996.

Fintelmann V, Menβen HG, Artischockenblätterextrakt Aktuelle Erkenntnis zur Wirkung als Lipidsenker und Antidyspeptikum. In: DAZ 136(17):1405-1414. 1996.

Hinou J, Harvala C, Philianos S, Polyphenolic substances of Cynara scolymus L. leaves. Ann Pharm Fr, 47:95-8, 1989

Khalkova Zh, Vangelova K, Zaikov Kh, An experimental study of the effect of an artichoke preparation on the activity of the sympathetic-adrenal system in carbon disulfide exposure. Probl Khig, 53:162-71, 1995

Kirchhoff R, Beckers CH, Kirchhoff GM, Trinczek-Gärtner H, Petrowicz O, Reimann HJ (1994) Increase in choleresis by means of artichoke extract. Phytomedicine 1:107-115.

Maros T, Seres-Sturm L, Racz G, Rettegi C, Kovacs VV, Hints M, Quantitative analysis of cynarin in the leaves of the artichoke (Cynara scolymus L.) Farm Zh, 18:56-9, 1965

Meding B, Allergic contact dermatitis from artichoke Cynara scolymus. Contact Dermatitis, 18:314, 1983 Jul

Reuter HD, Pflanzliche Gallentherapeutika (Teil I) und (Teil II). In: ZPT 16(1):13-20, 77-89. 1995.

Schilcher H, Pharmazeutische Aspekte pflanzlicher Gallentherapeutika. In: ZPT 16(4):211-222. 1995.

Schmidt M, Phytotherapie: Pflanzliche Gallenwegstherapeutika. In: DAZ 135(8):680-682. 1995.

Sokolova VE, Liubartseva LA, Vasilchenkoo EA, Effect of artichoke (Synara scolymus) on some aspects of nitrogen metabolism in animals. Farmakol Toksikol, 53:340-3, 1970 May-Jun

Wasielewski S, Artischockenblätterextrakt: Prävention der Arteriosklerose?. In: DAZ 137(24):2065-2067. 1997.

Further information in:

Adzet T, Camarasa J, Laguna JC, Hepatoprotective activity of polyphenolic compounds from Cynara scolymus against CCl4 toxicity in isolated rat hepatocytes. J Nat Prod, 50:612-7, 1987 Jul-Aug

Gebhardt R, Antioxidative and protective properties of extracts from leaves of the artichoke (Cynara scolymus L.) against hydroperoxide-induced oxidative stress in cultured rat hepatocytes. Toxicol Appl Pharmacol, 144:279-86, 1997 Jun

Hänsel R, Keller K, Rimpler H, Schneider G (Hrsg.), Hagers Handbuch der Pharmazeutischen Praxis, 5. Aufl., Bde 4-6 (Drogen), Springer Verlag Berlin, Heidelberg, New York, 1992-1994.

Hausen B, Allergiepflanzen, Pflanzenallergene, ecomed Verlagsgesellsch. mbH, Landsberg 1988.

Khalkova Zh, Vangelova K, Zaikov Kh, Inefficiency of cynarin as therapeutic regimen in familial type II hyperlipoproteinaemia. Atherosclerosis, 53:249-53, 1977 Feb

Khalkova Zh, Vangelova K, Zaikov Kh, Traditional medicine in health care. J Ethnopharmacol, 53:19-22, 1995

Maros T, Seres-Sturm L, Racz G, Rettegi C, Kovacs VV, Hints M, Effect of Cynara scolymus-extracts on the regeneration of rat liver. Arzneimittelforschung, 18:884-6, 1968 Jul

Maros T, Seres-Sturm L, Racz G, Rettegi C, Kovacs VV, Hints M, On the determination of o-dihydrophenols of caffeic acid type present in artichoke leaves (Cynara scolymus L.) Ann Pharm Fr, 18:419-27, 1965 Jun

Ruppelt BM, Pereira EF, Goncalves LC, Pereira NA, Pharmacological screening of plants recommended by folk medicine as anti-snake venom. Analgesic and anti-inflammatory activities. Mem Inst Oswaldo Cruz, 53:203-5, 1991

Schulz R, Hänsel R, Rationale Phytotherapie, Springer Verlag Heidelberg 1996.

Steinegger E, Hänsel R, Pharmakognosie, 5. Aufl., Springer Verlag Heidelberg 1992.

Teuscher E, Lindequist U, Biogene Gifte - Biologie, Chemie, Pharmakologie, 2. Aufl., Fischer Verlag Stuttgart 1994.

Teuscher E, Biogene Arzneimittel, 5. Aufl., Wiss. Verlagsges. mbH Stuttgart 1997.

Wagner H, Wiesenauer M, Phytotherapie. Phytopharmaka und pflanzliche Homöopathika, Fischer-Verlag, Stuttgart, Jena, New York 1995.

Arum

Arum maculatum

DESCRIPTION

Medicinal Parts: The medicinal part is the root of the plant.

Flower and Fruit: The flowers are pale yellowish-green. They are surrounded by a bulbous spath and therefore are not visible. A violet or brown-red spadix emerges from the bract with 2 circles of bristles underneath. Under the bristles are the male flowers, and under these are the female flowers. The spath doubles the length of the spadix. The whole structure forms a typical insect trap. The fruit is a scarlet berry.

Leaves, Stem and Root: Arum maculatum is a 30 to 60 cm spit- to arrow-shaped plant. It is long-stemmed, glossy, often brown-speckled and basal. The petiole is spread to a sheath at the base. The root-stock is tuberous, ovoid and floury-fleshy, varying in size between that of a hazelnut and a pigeon's egg.

Characteristics: Arum maculatum bears attractive scarlet berries that yield an acrid juice that is poisonous and can be fatal if ingested by small children.

Habitat: The plant is indigenous to parts of Europe, to Britain and the U.S.

Production: Arum root is the fresh rhizome of Arum maculatum collected before removing the leaves.

Other Names: Adder's Root, Bobbins, Cocky Baby, Cuckoo Pint, Cypress Powder, Dragon Root, Friar's Cowl, Gaglee, Kings and Queens, Ladysmock, Lords and Ladies, Parson and Clerk, Portland Arrowroot, Quaker, Ramp, Wake Robin

ACTIONS AND PHARMACOLOGY

COMPOUNDS

Mucilages: glucomannane

Starch

Lectins

EFFECTS

The glucomannans, bassorin and starch contained in the drug have a strong irritant and swelling effect on the mucous membranes. The diaphoretic and expectorant effect attributed to the drug may be due to the strong actions of these constituents.

INDICATIONS AND USAGE

Unproven Uses: Arum is used for colds and inflammation of the throat.

PRECAUTIONS AND ADVERSE REACTIONS

The intake of plant parts leads to severe mucous membrane irritations (swelling of the tongue, bloody vomiting, bloody diarrhea), presumably due to lesions of the membrane from the very sharp-edged oxalate needles and the introduction of impurities into the wounds. Decoctions of the roots in therapeutic dosages can be taken without risk. Caution is advised even though the level of cyanogenic glycosides is too low to be able to bring about signs of poisoning and other soluble poisonous substances have not been shown to be present.

DOSAGE

No dosage information is available.

LITERATURE

Akhtardziev K et al., (1984) Farmatsiya 34(3):1.

Koch H, Steinegger E, Components of Arum maculatum L. (woven arrowroot). In: Pharm Acta Helv 54(2):33-36. 1979.

Mladenov IV, (1982) C R Acad Bulg Sci 35(8):116.

Mladenov I, Bulanov I, Stamenova M, Ribarova F, The composition and structure of isolectins from Arum maculatum. Eksp Med Morfol, 29:36-9, 1990.

Moore THS, Vet Rec 89:569. 1971.

Nahrstedt A, Triglochinin in Arum maculatum. In: PH 14(12):1870-1871. 1975.

Poisonous Plants in Britain and Their Effects on Animals and Man, Ministry of Agriculture, Fisheries and Food, Pub; HMSO (1984) UK.

Proliac A, Chaboud A, Raynaud J, Isolement et identification de trois C- glycosylflavonews dans les tiges feuilleés d'Arum dracunculus. In: PA:47:646-647. 1992.

Further information in:

Allen AK, Purification and characterization of an N-acetyllactosamine-specific lectin from tubers of Arum maculatum. Biochim Biophys Acta, 317 (Pt 1):129-32, 1995.

Bulanov I, Mladenov I, Boianovska V, Gateva I, Stanislavov R, The effect of lectins on human spermatozoa in the capillary sperm penetration test. Eksp Med Morfol, 317 (Pt 1):42-5, 1990.

Frohne D, Pfänder HJ, Giftpflanzen - Ein Handbuch für Apotheker, Toxikologen und Biologen, 4. Aufl., Wiss. Verlags-Ges Stuttgart 1997.

Jaspersen-Schib R, Theus L, Guirguis-Oeschger M, Gossweiler B, Meier-Abt PJ, Serious plant poisonings in Switzerland 1966-1994. Case analysis from the Swiss Toxicology Information Center. Schweiz Med Wochenschr, 60:1085-98, 1996.

Lewin L, Gifte und Vergiftungen, 6. Aufl., Nachdruck, Haug Verlag, Heidelberg 1992.

Madaus G, Lehrbuch der Biologischen Arzneimittel, Bde. 1-3, Nachdruck, Georg Olms Verlag Hildesheim 1979.

Ministry of Agriculture Fisheries and Food (Ed) Poisonous Plants in Britain and Their Effects on Animals and Man, HMSO, UK 1984

Roth L, Daunderer M, Kormann K, Giftpflanzen, Pflanzengifte, 4. Aufl., Ecomed Fachverlag Landsberg Lech 1993.

Teuscher E, Lindequist U, Biogene Gifte - Biologie, Chemie, Pharmakologie, 2. Aufl., Fischer Verlag Stuttgart 1994.

Arum maculatum

See Arum

Arundinaria japonica

See Bamboo

Asa Foetida

Ferula foetida

DESCRIPTION

Medicinal Parts: The medicinal part is the oily gum-resin extracted from the plant.

Flower and Fruit: The flowers appear after 5 years in yellow umbels on a 10 cm thick naked stem. They are numerous, pale greenish-yellow to white. The fruit is ovate, flat, thin, flaky, reddish-brown with distinct oil marks.

Leaves, Stem and Root: The plant is a herbaceous monoecious perennial, 1.5 to 2 m high with a large, fleshy rhizome, which is 14 cm thick at the crown. The leaves are large, bipinnate, and radical.

Characteristics: The fruit has milky juice and a strong smell.

Habitat: Afghanistan and eastern Iran.

Production: Asa foetida is the gum resin of Ferula foetida.

Other Names: Devil's Dung, Food of the Gods, Gum Asafoetida

ACTIONS AND PHARMACOLOGY

COMPOUNDS

Volatile oil: chief constituent is sec-propenyl-isobutyl disulphide

Gum resin: consisting mainly of ferulic acid esters, farnesiferol A, B, C and bassorin-like mucilage

Sesquiterpenoide coumarins: including asafoetida

EFFECTS

Asa foetida has a mild intestinal disinfectant effect; its sedative effect is uncertain. In animal experiments it has antitumoural and mild mutagenic effect on *Salmonella typhimurium.*

INDICATIONS AND USAGE

Unproven Uses: The drug is used for chronic gastritis, dyspepsia and irritable colon.

Chinese Medicine: In China, the drug is used for infestation with intestinal parasites.

Indian Medicine: In India, Asa foetida is used to treat asthma, whooping cough, flatulence, constipation, diseases of the liver and spleen and for epilepsy.

Homeopathic Uses: Ferula foetida is used for low acid levels in the stomach, stomach pressure, flatulence and loose stools.

PRECAUTIONS AND ADVERSE REACTIONS

General: No health hazards or side effects are known in conjunction with the proper administration of designated therapeutic dosages. The intake of larger dosages can lead to swelling of the lips, digestive complaints (belching, flatulence, diarrhea), discomfort and headache. Convulsions are possible in susceptible individuals. Swelling of the genital organs has been observed following external administration on the abdomen.

Pregnancy: Not to be used during pregnancy.

DOSAGE

Mode of Administration: The drug is available as an extract.

Preparation: Gum-resin is obtained by incising the roots, which contain a fetid juice. This solidifies to a brown resin, sometimes with a pinkish tint, in sticky lumps. The final product has a pungent, acrid, persistent, alliaceous odor.

Daily Dosage: Tincture: 20 drops as a single dose.

Homeopathic Dosage: D3 and D4 dilutions.

LITERATURE

Buddrus J et al., (1985) Phytochemistry 24(4):869.

Kern W, List PH, Hörhammer L (Hrsg.), Hagers Handbuch der Pharmazeutischen Praxis, 4. Aufl., Bde 1-8, Springer Verlag Berlin, Heidelberg, New York, 1969.

Lewin L, Gifte und Vergiftungen, 6. Aufl., Nachdruck, Haug Verlag, Heidelberg 1992.

Madaus G, Lehrbuch der Biologischen Arzneimittel, Bde 1-3, Nachdruck, Georg Olms Verlag Hildesheim 1979.

Naimie H et al., (1972) Collect Czec Chem Commun 37:1166.

Rajanikanth B et al., (1984) Phytochemistry 23(4):899.

Roth L, Daunderer M, Kormann K, Giftpflanzen, Pflanzengifte, 4. Aufl., Ecomed Fachverlag Landsberg Lech 1993.

Asarum

Asarum europaeum

DESCRIPTION

Medicinal Parts: The primary medicinal part is the root of the plant. However, the leaves have been used to a lesser extent.

Flower and Fruit: The end of the stem forms a short-pedicled, slightly hanging flower. The perigone forms a campanulate tube with a 3 to 4 lobed margin. It is brownish on the outside, dark and purple on the inside. There are 2 groups of 6 stamens on the ovaries, which are fused with the tube and are flattened above. The style is thick, short and not hollow; the stigma is 6-rayed. The fruit is a many-seeded, indehiscent capsule divided into many chambers by false membranes. In each capsule there are numerous boat-shaped seeds with a spongy appendage.

Leaves, Stem and Root: Asarum europaeum is a shaggy-haired perennial growing 4 to 10 cm high. It has a thin, creeping rhizome that is branched and usually has 3 to 4 scale-like, brownish-green stipules. It has an ascending short-scaled stem, with the terminal flower at the tip. There are 2 to 4 long-petioled, almost opposite, broad, reniform leaves. They are entire-margined, coriaceous, dark-green glossy above, pale and matte beneath, deeply reticulate and evergreen.

Characteristics: The rhizome has a pepper-like smell; the leaves and flowers have an unpleasant camphor smell. Asarum europaeum is a protected species.

Habitat: The plant is indigenous to the northern parts of southern Europe, central and east-central Europe as far as the Crimea and eastward into western Siberia as well as an enclave in the Atai. Asarum is cultivated in the U.S.

Production: Asarum root is the root of Asarum europaeum, which is gathered in August and air-dried in the shade. Asarum is primarily collected in the wild, but is cultivated in the U.S.

Not to be Confused With: Can be confused with other valerian types and with Arnica montana, Genum urbanum, Valeriana officinalis and Viola ordorata. The mistaken powder can be identified by the presence of fibers, stone cells, oxalate filament agglomerations and the absence of starch.

Other Names: Asarabacca, Coltsfoot, False Coltsfoot, Fole's Foot, Hazelwort, Public House Plant, Snakeroot, Wild Ginger, Wild Nard

ACTIONS AND PHARMACOLOGY

COMPOUNDS

Volatile oil: composition depends upon breed but possible constituents include asarone trans-isoasarone, trans-isoeugenol methyl ether, trans-isoelemicin or eudesmol, possibly in addition to sesquiterpene hydrocarbons, -alcohols, -furans,-carbonyl compounds

Caffeic acid derivatives: including chlorogenic acid, isochlorogenic acid

Flavonoids

EFFECTS

Asarum acts as an expectorant, bronchial spasmolytic, superficial relaxant and local anesthetic. Studies of the plant's emetic action exist for Asari root and herb. However, self-experiment with 100 gm trans-isoasaron taken orally caused severe vomiting.

The surface-tension-reducing effect of trans-isoasaron and trans-isomethyleugenol was studied in vitro, using stalagmometry. Both substances showed a concentration-dependent surface activity, which surpassed the effect of the control substance tyloxapol in a normal treatment concentration.

In studies of Asarum's spasmolytic effect, bronchial spasms induced in a guinea pig by histamine were inhibited in vivo by trans-isoasaron, depending on the dose. The survival rate was determined subsequent to the addition of a histamine-containing aerosol 30 minutes after trans-isoasarin had been administered. The control substance here was clemizole hydrochloride, which has a similarly inhibiting effect.

The action of trans-isoasaron and of isomethyleugenol as a local anesthetic was tested on 10 volunteer subjects, in order to compare it with benzocaine (anesthetic index AI = 1). The results showed a dose-related action for both drugs, with the following anesthetic indexes of AI = 0.72 for trans-isoasarin and AI = 0.47 for trans-isomethyleugenol.

The only available studies of Asarum's antibacterial effect are those carried out on Asari root and herb. A double-blind clinical trial with a placebo as alternative was carried out on 30 patients with acute bronchitis, 30 with chronic bronchitis and an additional 30 with bronchial asthma. Eighty percent of the patients with acute bronchitis, 58% of the patients with chronic bronchitis and 68% of the patients with bronchial asthma were cured or showed improvement in both their subjective and objective states. The contrast with the placebo groups was significant. The treatment consisted of a daily dose of 3 x 2 tablets, purified dry (GB) or powdered (US) extract (30 mg phenylpropanol derivatives) taken over an average of 7 days. However, to obtain conclusive results, further trials are needed over a longer period and with more patients. The drug's efficacy was also tested in a multicentric field trial, a clinically controlled study and an open bicentric study. However, the results are only useful to a small extent, as there is an absence of details about placebo groups, trial parameters, and statistical analysis.

INDICATIONS AND USAGE

Unproven Uses: The purified dry extract of Asarum europaeum rootstock is used for inflammatory conditions of the lower respiratory system (acute and chronic bronchitis), for various causes of bronchial spasms and for bronchial asthma. Asari root and Asari root with herb are used for similar indications in folk medicine. In the past, the drugs were used as emetics. Some other uses are as antitussives (cough remedies), sneezing-powder for chronic rhinitis, for inflammation of the eye, for pneumonia, angina pectoris, migraines, liver disease and jaundice, for dehydration, as an emmenagogue (menstrual stimulant) and for artificial abortion. The dried, powdered leaves have been used as an ingredient of some snuffs, helping to expel mucus from the respiratory passages.

Homeopathic Uses: Homeopathic uses include diarrhea, irritation of mucous membranes and exhaustion.

PRECAUTIONS AND ADVERSE REACTIONS

Older scientific literature contains reports of signs of poisoning including burning of the tongue, gastroenteritis, diarrhea, erysipeloid skin rashes and hemiparesis. An extremely susceptible mouse strain developed hepatoma after exposure to asarone. Administration of the drug is not advised.

CONTRAINDICATIONS

Asarum is not to be used during pregnancy.

DOSAGE

Mode of Administration: Asarum is taken as a sneezing-powder, or orally as a purified dry extract in the form of coated tablets and pills. It is obsolete as a drug.

How Supplied: Commercial pharmaceutical preparations include coated tablets and confectionery tea mixtures.

Preparation: The air-dried rootstock is extracted with an organic solvent, which can be mixed with water. The liquid extract is separated from the solvent by means of vacuum distillation. The watery portion remaining is diluted with an equal amount of distilled water, and further extraction takes place. Then the organic liquid extract is mixed with a suitable excipient according to the desired percentage of trans-isoasaron. Afterward, the extract is dried and rubbed. Trans-isoasaron can also be produced from asarylaldehyde by means of Perkin's cinnamic synthesis. As sneezing-powder, the average content of the drug is 20%.

Daily Dosage: The average daily oral dose of the dry extract for adults and children aged 13 and over is 30 mg, which corresponds to 30 mg phenylpropane derivatives and should be spread over 2 to 3 doses per day. Children aged 2 and over can take an extract corresponding to 5 mg phenylpropanol derivatives 3 times daily. The average single dose of the drug is 0.1 gm.

Homeopathic Dosage: 5 to 10 drops, 1 tablet, 5 to 10 globules 1 to 3 times daily or 1 ml injection solution twice weekly sc; ointments 1 to 2 times daily; D1 and D2 should not be taken for longer than 1 month (HAB1).

Storage: Coated tablets and pills that contain the purified dry extract or the tincture from the rhizome can be stored for a period of 28 days in conditions of high temperature, humidity and light. Under preferred storage conditions (i.e.

brown glass, away from light), they can be stored for up to 2 years, after which period stability should be checked.

LITERATURE

Doskotch RW, Vanevenhoven PW, (1967) Lloydia 30:141.

Gracza L, (1987) Pharmazie 42 (2):141.

Gracza L, In vitro studies on the expectorant effect of the phenylpropane derivatives from hazlewort. 12. The active agents in Asarum europaeum. In: PM 42(2):155. 1981.

Gracza L, Phytobiological (phytophamacological) studies on phenylpropane derivatives from Asarum europaeum L. 10. Actice principles of Asarum europaeum L. In: Arzneim Forsch 30(5):767-771. 1980.

Gracza L, Über die Wirkstoffe von Asarum europaeum. 16. Mitt., Die lokalanästhetische Wirkung der Phenylprpanderivate. In: PM 48(3):153-157. 1983.

Mose JR, Lukas G, (1961) Arzneim Forsch 11:33.

Rosch A, (1984) Z Phytother 5(6):964.

Trennheuser L, Dissertation Saarbrücken. 1961.

Further information in:

Frohne D, Pfänder HJ, Giftpflanzen - Ein Handbuch für Apotheker, Toxikologen und Biologen, 4. Aufl., Wiss. Verlags-Ges Stuttgart 1997.

Hänsel R, Keller K, Rimpler H, Schneider G (Hrsg.), Hagers Handbuch der Pharmazeutischen Praxis, 5. Aufl., Bde. 4-6 (Drogen), Springer Verlag Berlin, Heidelberg, New York, 1992-1994.

Lewin L, Gifte und Vergiftungen, 6. Aufl., Nachdruck, Haug Verlag, Heidelberg 1992.

Madaus G, Lehrbuch der Biologischen Arzneimittel, Bde. 1-3, Nachdruck, Georg Olms Verlag Hildesheim 1979.

Roth L, Daunderer M, Kormann K, Giftpflanzen, Pflanzengifte, 4. Aufl., Ecomed Fachverlag Landsberg Lech 1993.

Teuscher E, Lindequist U, Biogene Gifte - Biologie, Chemie, Pharmakologie, 2. Aufl., Fischer Verlag Stuttgart 1994.

Asarum europaeum

See Asarum

Asclepias incarnata

See Swamp Milkweed

Asclepias tuberosa

See Pleurisy Root

Ash

Fraxinus excelsior

DESCRIPTION

Medicinal Parts: The medicinal parts are the dried leaves, the fresh bark, the branch bark, and the fresh leaves.

Flower and Fruit: The flowers are in richly blossomed panicles, the terminal ones appearing on the new flowering branches. They are usually androgynous, occasionally male, polygamous or dioecious. They have no calyx or corolla. The anthers of the male flowers are dark purple and are on short filaments. The female flowers consist of 1 inferior ovary with a 2-lobed stigma and 2 split staminoids. The fruit is a narrow lanceolate to oblong-obovate nutlet hanging on a thin stem. The fruit is 25 to 50 mm long and 7 to 10 mm wide, glossy brown, 1-seeded with a veined winged border.

Leaves, Stem and Root: The ash is an impressive 15 to 30 m tall tree with a gray-brown, smooth, later fissured and wrinkled bark and large, black-brown, pubescent buds. The leaves are entire-margined, opposite and odd pinnate. There are 9 to 15 leaflets. The leaflets are sessile, usually 5 to 11 cm long by 1 to 3 cm wide, oblong-ovate to lanceolate, long acuminate, finely and sharply serrate. They are glabrous above, rich green, loosely tomentose or almost glabrous, and greenish brown beneath.

Habitat: The plant is distributed in most parts of Europe except the northern, southern and eastern edges.

Production: Ash bark consists of the bark of young branches of Fraxinus excelsior. Ash leaf consists of the leaf of Fraxinus excelsior. The leaves are harvested in spring and air-dried.

Not to be Confused With: It may be confused with Ailanthus glandulosa.

Other Names: Bird's Tongue, European Ash, Common Ash, Weeping Ash

ACTIONS AND PHARMACOLOGY

COMPOUNDS: ASH LEAF

Flavonoids: including rutin (0.1-0.9%)

Tannins

Mucilages (10-20%)

Mannitol (16-28%)

Triterpenes, phytosterols

Iridoide monoterpenes: including syringoxide, deoxy-syringoxidin

COMPOUNDS: ASH BARK

Hydroxycoumarins: aesculin, fraxin, aesculetin, fraxetin, fraxidin, isofraxidin, fraxinol, scopoletine

Tannins

Iridoide monoterpenes: including 10-hydroxyligstroside

EFFECTS: ASH BARK

The main active principle is coumarin. Preparations of fresh ash bark showed an analgesic, anti-oxidative, and antiphlogistic action. Cyclo AMP phosphodiesterase is inhibited and an anti-oxidative (radical trapping action) effect was proven for scopoletine, isofraxin and fraxin.

INDICATIONS AND USAGE

ASH LEAF

Unproven Uses: Preparations of Ash leaf are used for arthritis, gout, bladder complaints, as well as a laxative and diuretic. In folk medicine Ash leaf is used internally for fever, rheumatism, gout, edema, stones, constipation, stomach symptoms and worm infestation; and externally for lower leg ulcers and wounds.

ASH BARK

Unproven Uses: Preparations of Ash bark are used for fever and as a tonic.

PRECAUTIONS AND ADVERSE REACTIONS

Health risks or side effects following the proper administration of designated therapeutic dosages are not recorded.

DOSAGE

Mode of Administration: Since the efficacy for the claimed applications has not been documented, therapeutic application cannot be recommended. The efficacy of Ash in fixed combinations must be verified specifically for each preparation.

Storage: Should be protected from light.

LITERATURE

Carnat A, Lamaison JL, Dubnand F, Plant Méd Phytothér 24:145-151. 1990.

Genius OB, DAZ 120:1505-1506. 1980.

Jensen SR, Nielsen BJ, PH 15:221-223. 1976.

Marekov N et al., Khim Ind 58:132-135. 1986.

Tissut M, Ravane P, PH 19:2077-2081. 1980.

Yamagami I, Suzuki Y, Koichiro I, Pharmacological studies on the components of Fraxinus japonica. In: Nippon Yakurigaku Zasshi 64(6):714-729 (jap.). 1968.

Further information in:

Hänsel R, Keller K, Rimpler H, Schneider G (Hrsg.), Hagers Handbuch der Pharmazeutischen Praxis, 5. Aufl., Bde 4-6 (Drogen), Springer Verlag Berlin, Heidelberg, New York, 1992-1994.

Madaus G, Lehrbuch der Biologischen Arzneimittel, Bde 1-3, Nachdruck, Georg Olms Verlag Hildesheim 1979.

Poisonous Plants in Britain and their Effects on Animals and Man, Ministry of Agriculture Fisheries and Food, HMSO UK 1984.

Asiatic Dogwood

Cornus officinalis

DESCRIPTION

Medicinal Parts: The medicinal part of the tree is the fruit.

Flower and Fruit: The umbels contain 20 to 30 flowers surrounded by 4 yellow-green, 6 to 8 mm long, elliptical-acuminate bracts. The flower structures are in fours and the diameter of the flower is 4 to 5 mm including the disc. The calyx is fused and has 4 tips. There are 4 free petals, 4 stamens and a 2-chambered ovary, with 1 ovule per chamber. The drupe is elongate- elliptical, approximately 15 mm long and red with an elongate, 2-chambered stone kernel.

Leaves and Branches: Cornus officinalis is shrub or tree, that grows up to 4 m high. The leaves are opposite, simple and 4 to 10 cm long. The petiole is 6 to 10 cm long. The lamina is ovate-elliptical or ovate, long acuminate, rounded at the base, yellow-brown and pubescent beneath. The branches are smooth, bluish-green and the bark peels off.

Habitat: China, Japan

Production: Cornus fruit is the dried fruit pulp of Cornus officinalis. Fruits are harvested in the late autumn or the beginning of winter. They are scalded with boiling water or gently heated. Cleaning of the raw drug follows kernel extraction and drying.

ACTIONS AND PHARMACOLOGY

COMPOUNDS

Iridoids: iridoid glycosides, including loganin, cornuside, sweroside, morronoside

Tannins: gallotannins, including cornusiens-A to -G, tellimagrandin I and II, camptothins-A and -B

Triterpenes: including oleanolic acid, ursolic acid

Anthocyans

EFFECTS

The drug has an astringent effect due to its tannin content. It has exhibited diuretic, blood pressure-lowering and leukocytopoiesis-promoting effects in clinical tests.

INDICATIONS AND USAGE

Unproven Uses: In folk medicine, the drug has been used for impotency, loss of semen, lumbago-sciatica syndrome, night sweats and vertigo.

Chinese Medicine: In China, Asiatic Dogwood is used for liver and renal disorders, tinnitus, hyperhidrosis, impotency and low back and knee pain.

PRECAUTIONS AND ADVERSE REACTIONS

No health hazards are known in conjunction with the proper administration of designated therapeutic dosages.

DOSAGE

Mode of Administration: Whole herb preparations and liquid preparations for internal use

Preparation: The fruit is boiled or steamed with wine until all the liquid has been drawn out.

Daily Dosage: 5 to 12 gm of drug.

Chinese Medicine Dosage: 3 to 9 gm of drug daily.

Storage: The herb should be protected from insects and stored in dry place.

LITERATURE

Hänsel R, Keller K, Rimpler H, Schneider G (Ed) Hagers Handbuch der Pharmazeutischen Praxis. 5. Aufl., Bde 4 - 6 (Drogen), Springer Verlag Berlin, Heidelberg, New York, 1992-1994.

Jeng H, Wu CM, Su SJ, Chang WC A substance isolated from Cornus officinalis enhances the motility of human sperm. Am J Chin Med, 25:301-6, 1997.

Jeng H, Wu CM, Su SJ, Chang WC Observations on the biological characteristics of Cornus officinalis Chung Yao Tung Pao, 25:8-11, Jul, 1985.

Asimina triloba

See American Pawpaw

Asparagus

Asparagus officinalis

DESCRIPTION

Medicinal Parts: The medicinal parts of the plant are the herb and the rhizome with roots.

Flower and Fruit: Thin pedicles measuring from 2 to 20 mm long, grow 1 to 3 flowers from the nodes. The plants are usually dioecious. The perigone of the male flowers is about 5 mm long, funnel-shaped and whitish to greenish-yellow. The perigone is longer than the cauline leaves and has oblanceolate sections that are twice as long as the perigone tube. The stamens are oblong and almost as long the filaments. The perigone of the female flowers is much smaller. The fruit is a pea-sized, brick-red round berry that is up to 8 mm thick. The seeds are black with wrinkly stripes and are 3 to 4 mm wide.

Leaves, Stem and Root: Asparagus officinalis is a perennial with a short, woody rootstock. In the wild, the plant typically reaches heights of 30 to 100 cm, but cultivated plants may grow to 150 cm. The stem is erect, glabrous and smooth, later inclined with numerous erect to leaning branches. The scale sections at the base have short spurs. The round, needle-like phylloclades are in clusters of 4 to 15 that are 5 to 25 cm long and about 0.5 cm thick. The root-stock is short and thick. It produces a few ascending shoots that are as thick as a finger, fleshy, white, and red or blue-reddish tinged. (This is the edible asparagus.) The female plants are often slimmer than the male, which are shorter and stockier.

Characteristics: The fruit is considered to be poisonous, but that has not been substantiated.

Habitat: The plant grows in central and southern Europe, the Middle East, western Siberia and northern Africa. It is cultivated in many places.

Production: Asparagus herb consists of the above-ground parts of Asparagus officinalis. Asparagus root consists of the rhizome with roots of Asparagus officinalis, which are dug up and air-dried in autumn, and also the fresh underground shoots.

Not to be Confused With: This variety is sometimes confused with other types of asparagus cultivated in the Mediterranean region.

Other Names: Sparrow Grass

ACTIONS AND PHARMACOLOGY

COMPOUNDS: ASPARAGUS HERB

Flavonoids: including rutin, hyperoside, isoquercitrin

Steroid saponins

EFFECTS: ASPARAGUS HERB

Animal experiments indicate the herb has a mild diuretic action.

COMPOUNDS: ASPARAGUS RHIZOME AND ROOT

Steroid saponins: including asparagosides A, B, D, F, G, H, I, the bitter steroid saponins, aspartic saponin I

Amino acids: among them sulphur-containing aspartic acid, the esters 3-mercapto- butyric acid, 3-methylthio-isobutyric acid, diisobutyric acid disulphide

Fructans: asparagose, asparagosine

EFFECTS: ASPARAGUS RHIZOME AND ROOT

Animal tests indicate that the root has a diuretic effect. The main active principles are flavonol glycoside and furostanol and spirostanol glycosides, mainly derivatives of sarsapogenin. The distinctive odor of the urine after an individual has eaten asparagus is said to be caused by methylmercaptan.

INDICATIONS AND USAGE

ASPARAGUS HERB

Unproven Uses: Preparations of Asparagus are used as a diuretic, although the effectiveness for the claimed application has not been sufficiently documented.

ASPARAGUS RHIZOME AND ROOT

Approved by Commission E:

- Infections of the urinary tract
- Kidney and bladder stones

Unproven Uses: Traditional uses of the root include application for non-specific inflammatory diseases of the efferent urinary tract and for prevention of kidney and bladder stones (irrigation therapy). Among other folk medicine uses are dropsy, rheumatic conditions, liver disease, bronchial asthma and gout. These applications have not been proven.

Chinese Medicine: The root is used to treat irritable cough, coughing with blood, dry mouth and throat, and constipation.

Homeopathic Uses: Uses in homeopathy include kidney stones and cardiac insufficiency.

CONTRAINDICATIONS

ASPARAGUS RHIZOME AND ROOT

Because of the irritating effect of saponin, the drug should not be administered in the presence of kidney diseases. In the case of reduced cardiac and/or kidney function, irrigation therapy should not be attempted.

PRECAUTIONS AND ADVERSE REACTIONS

ASPARAGUS HERB

No health hazards or side effects are known in conjunction with the proper administration of designated therapeutic dosages. The plant has a low sensitization potential through skin contact. The berries are considered poisonous, although there is no proof of this.

ASPARAGUS RHIZOME AND ROOT

No health hazards or side effects are known in conjunction with the proper administration of designated therapeutic dosages. When used in irrigation therapy, ensure ample fluid intake. There is a low sensitization potential, particularly among workers in canning factories who can become prone to asparagus scabies.

DOSAGE

ASPARAGUS RHIZOME AND ROOT

Mode of Administration: The cut rhizome is used for teas, as well as other galenic preparations for internal use. When used in flushing-out therapy, ensure ample fluid intake.

How Supplied: Commercial pharmaceutical preparations of Asparagus root are available in tablet form.

Daily Dosage: The daily dosage is 45 to 80 g. A typical single dose is 800 mg of the drug.

Homeopathic Dosage: 5 to 10 drops, 1 tablet or 5 to 10 globules 1 to 3 times daily, or 1 ml injection solution twice weekly sc (HAB1).

LITERATURE

ASPARAGUS HERB

Goryanu GM et al., (1976) Khim Prir Soed 3: 400 et 6: 762.

Kawano K et al., (1975) Agric Biol Chem 39: 1999.

Shiomi N et al., (1976) Agric Biol Chem 40: 567.

Tagasuki M et al., (1975) Chem Letters 1: 43.

Woeldecke M, Hermann K, (1974) Z Lebensm Forsch Unters 25: 459.

Further information in:

Frohne D, Pfänder HJ, Giftpflanzen - Ein Handbuch für Apotheker, Toxikologen und Biologen, 4. Aufl., Wiss. Verlags-Ges Stuttgart 1997.

Hänsel R, Keller K, Rimpler H, Schneider G (Hrsg.), Hagers Handbuch der Pharmazeutischen Praxis, 5. Aufl., Bde 4-6 (Drogen), Springer Verlag Berlin, Heidelberg, New York, 1992-1994.

Hausen B, Allergiepflanzen, Pflanzenallergene, ecomed Verlagsgesellsch. mbH, Landsberg 1988.

Lewin L, Gifte und Vergiftungen, 6. Aufl., Nachdruck, Haug Verlag, Heidelberg 1992.

Madaus G, Lehrbuch der Biologischen Arzneimittel, Bde 1-3, Nachdruck, Georg Olms Verlag Hildesheim 1979.

Roth L, Daunderer M, Kormann K, Giftpflanzen, Pflanzengifte, 4. Aufl., Ecomed Fachverlag Landsberg Lech 1993.

Teuscher E, Lindequist U, Biogene Gifte - Biologie, Chemie, Pharmakologie, 2. Aufl., Fischer Verlag Stuttgart 1994.

ASPARAGUS RHIZOME AND ROOT

Goryanu GM et al., (1976) Khim Prir Soed 3: 400 et 6: 762.

Kawano K et al., Agric Biol Chem (Tokyo) 41:1. 1977.

Lazurevskii GV et al., Doklady Akademii Nauk SSSR 231:1479. 1976.

Pant G et al., PH 27:3324. 1988.

Shao Y et al., Steroidal saponins from Asparagus officinalis and their cytotoxic activity. In: PM 63(3):258-262. 1997.

Shiomi N et al., (1976) Agric Biol Chem 40: 567.

Tagasuki M et al., (1975) Chem Letters 1: 43.

Woeldecke M, Hermann K, (1974) Z Lebensm Untersuch Forsch 25: 459

Further information in:

Frohne D, Pfänder HJ, Giftpflanzen - Ein Handbuch für Apotheker, Toxikologen und Biologen, 4. Aufl., Wiss. Verlags-Ges Stuttgart 1997.

Hänsel R, Keller K, Rimpler H, Schneider G (Hrsg.), Hagers Handbuch der Pharmazeutischen Praxis, 5. Aufl., Bde 4-6 (Drogen), Springer Verlag Berlin, Heidelberg, New York, 1992-1994.

Hausen B, Allergiepflanzen, Pflanzenallergene, ecomed Verlagsgesellsch. mbH, Landsberg 1988.

Leung AY, Encyclopedia of Common Natural Ingredients Used in Food Drugs and Cosmetics, John Wiley & Sons Inc., New York 1980.

Lewin L, Gifte und Vergiftungen, 6. Aufl., Nachdruck, Haug Verlag, Heidelberg 1992.

Madaus G, Lehrbuch der Biologischen Arzneimittel, Bde 1-3, Nachdruck, Georg Olms Verlag Hildesheim 1979.

Roth L, Daunderer M, Kormann K, Giftpflanzen, Pflanzengifte, 4. Aufl., Ecomed Fachverlag Landsberg Lech 1993.

Teuscher E, Lindequist U, Biogene Gifte - Biologie, Chemie, Pharmakologie, 2. Aufl., Fischer Verlag Stuttgart 1994.

Asparagus officinalis

See Asparagus

Aspidosperma quebracho-blanco

See Quebracho

Astragalus gummifer

See Tragacanth

Astragalus (Huang-Qi)

Astragalus species

TRADE NAMES

Astragalus (available from numerous manufacturers), Astragalus Root, Superior Chinese Astragalus, Astragalus Vegicaps, Astragalus Extract, Alvita Astragalus Root

DESCRIPTION

Medicinal Parts: The primary medicinal parts of the herb are the roots.

Flower and Fruit: The flower racemes are apical, and most are axillary. The inflorescenses have many small, blue, purple or blue-purple flowers. Two to three days following bloom, pods will develop in a square shape of a cross section with two chambers. There are 10 dark brown seeds in each chamber. The seeds are 6 to 13 mm long.

Leaves, Stem and Root: The plant is a perennial and has several stems 1.5 to 2.0 m in height. The stems are covered with pinnate leaves with T-shaped soft hairs. The primary root is thick, long and contains many lateral roots. There is a secondary root beginning 20 to 30 feet below the soil surface.

Characteristics: The plant is cold tolerant and also able to grow in high temperatures.

Habitat: Astragalus australis is an endemic plant of the Olympic Mountains, Washington. Other species are grown in northern and southern parts of China, Japan, and Korea.

Other Names: Beg Kei, Bei Qi, Hwanggi, Membranous Milk Vetch, Astragali, Tragacanth

ACTIONS AND PHARMACOLOGY

COMPOUNDS

Triterpene glycosides: brachyosides A, B, and C, and cyclocephaloside II, astrachrysoside A

Saponins: astragalosides I, II, and IV, isoastragaloside I, 3-0-beta-D-xylopyranosyl-cycloastragenol, cyclocanthoside E, soyasaponin I and cycloastragenol

Tragacanth (from the sap)

Sterols: daucosterol and beta-sitosterol

Fatty acids: including heptenoic acid, tetradecanoic acid, pentadecanoic acid, hexadecanoic acid, octadecenoic acid, octadecanoic acid, octadecadienoic acid, linolenic acid, eicosanoic acid, eicosenoic acid and docosanoic acid

Isoflavonoid compounds: astrasieversianin XV (II), 7,2′-dihydroxy-3′,4′-dimethoxy-isoflavane-7-O-beta-D-glucoside (III)

Amino acids: gamma-L-glutamyl-Se-methyl-seleno-L-cysteine, Se-methylseleno-L-cysteine

Polysaccharides

EFFECTS

Antiviral—Astragalus membranaceus inhibits the replication of coxsackie B-3 virus (CB3V)-RNA, a virus that causes myocarditis in animal models (Peng, 1995). The herb demonstrated significantly higher survival rates and lower abnormal action potential in animal models infected with CB3V, suggesting its possible use for prevention and treatment of acute myocarditis involving CB3V (Rui, 1994).

Antioxidant—Astragalus membranaceus inhibits lipid peroxidation in rat heart mitochondria (Hong, 1994).

Cardiovascular Effects—Astragalus membranaceus increases cardiac output in patients with angina pectoris (Lei, 1994). Astragaloside IV improves left ventricular end-diastolic volume, left ventricular end-systolic volume and slows heart rate in heart failure. The compound also alleviates chest distress and dyspnea associated with heart failure (Luo, 1995). The herb has therapeutic effects on sodium and water retention in aortocaval fistula-induced heart failure, improving cardiac and renal functions in heart failure. The mechanism is partly through correction of abnormal mRNA expressions of hypothalmic arginine vasopresin system and aquaporin-2, and amelioration of blunted renal response to atrial natriuretic peptide (Ma, 1998).

Fibrinolytic—Astragaloside IV increases the fibrinolytic potential of endothelial ells by upregulating the expression of tissue-type plasminogen activator and by downregulating the expression of plasminogen activator inhibitor type 1 (Zhang, 1997).

Gastrointestinal Effects—The herb strengthens the movement and muscle tonus in the intestine, especially the jejunum, to increase movements in the digestive tract, as evidenced by positive effects on the cycle duration of interdigestive myoelectric complex (Lei, 1994).

Hepatoprotective—An ethanol extract of the root of Astragalus membranaceus alleviated liver injury through a reduction of elevated SGPT levels and subacute toxicity. The herb also decreased loss of righting reflex and protected hepatic cells from pathological changes (Zhang, 1990).

Immuno-modulating—The herb stimulates macrophages, promotes antibody formation, and increases T lymphocyte proliferation. F3, an immuno-regulatory component of the herb reverses macrophage suppression induced by urological tumors (Rittenhouse, 1991). Astragalus membranaceus extracts enhance the antibody response to a T-dependent antigen associated with an increase of Th cell activity in normal and immunodepressed animal models (Zhao, 1990). A fractionated extract of Astragalus membranaceus potentiates lymphokine-activated killer (LAK) cell cytotoxicity generated by low-dose recombinant interleukin-2 (rIL-2). This immune response occurs through a 10-fold potentiation of rIL-2 activity manifested by tumor cell killing activity resulting from LAK cell generation (Chu, 1990).

Memory Improvement—Aqueous extracts of Astragalus demonstrated improvement of anisodine-induced impairment on memory acquisition as well as the alcohol-elicited deficit of memory retrieval (a reduction in errors and prolonged latent period) (Hong, 1994).

CLINICAL TRIALS

Immune-stimulating

The effect of pure Astragalus preparation (PAP) in treating 115 patients with leukopenia was determined after 8 weeks of therapy. Group I was treated by a concentrated PAP (10 ml, equivalent to 15 grams of Astragalus), and group II was treated with a different concentrated PAP (10 ml, equivalent to 5 grams of Astragalus). Both treatment groups received a dose of 10 ml twice daily. The effectiveness was statistically different between the groups with 82.76% and 47.37% in Group I and II, respectively. The total effective rate was 65.22%. The average WBC count of group I was significantly higher than that of group II with a significant rise of the WBC counts in both groups after treatment (Weng XS, 1995).

Cardiovascular Effects

The effect of Astragalus membranaceus on left ventricular function and oxygen free radicals was evaluated in 43 cardiac patients. All patients in the treatment group had experienced their myocardial infarction within the past 36 hours. The herb demonstrated a strengthening of left ventricular function and an effect of anti-oxygen free radicals for a cardiotonic action. The herb decreased the ratio of pre- ejection period/left ventricular ejection time, increased the superoxide dismutase activity of red blood cells and reduced lipid peroxidation content (Chen, 1995).

INDICATIONS AND USAGE

Unproven Uses: The herb has been used for respiratory infections, immune depression, cancer, heart failure, viral infections, liver disease and kidney disease. Astragalus has also been used as a diuretic.

Chinese Medicine: The herb has been used alone and in combination for liver fibrosis, acute viral myocarditis, heart failure, small cell lung cancer, amenorrhea, and antiviral.

PRECAUTIONS AND ADVERSE REACTIONS

General: Caution should be taken with patients receiving immunosuppressive therapy, such as transplant patients, or patients with autoimmune diseases. Extracts of Astragalus lusitanicus in animal models resulted in toxic excitatory cardiac effects and respiratory depression, involving skeletal muscle and neurological systems (Abdennebi, 1998).

Neurological Dysfunction: Due to the selenium content in Astragalus, toxic doses may result in neurological dysfunction leading to paralysis (Panter, 1996).

Drug Interactions:

Cyclophosphamide—Although enhancement of the antibody response through an increase of Th cell activity was seen in cyclophosphamide immunosuppressed animal models, another study demonstrated the herb does not prevent cyclophosphamide-induced myelosuppression. Astragalus membranaceus given concomitantly with cyclophosphamide showed no difference in terms of nadir count, time to nadir and time to recovery for both the ANC and the platelet counts (Khoo, 1995; Zhao, 1990).

Anticoagulants/Antiplatelets/Antithrombotic Agents—Due to the increased fibrinolysis effect of astragaloside IV, concomitant use with anticoagulants, antiplatelets or antithrombotic agents may potentiate the risk of bleeding (Zhang, 1997).

DOSAGE

How Supplied:

Capsule—200 mg, 250 mg, 400 mg, 450 mg, 470 mg, 500 mg, 520 mg

Liquid

Tea Bag

Daily Dosage: The dried root is administered as 2-6 grams daily, and the fluid extract as 4 to 12 milliliters daily (Bone, 1997). The powdered root capsule (250 mg-500 mg) has been administered as two capsules three times daily (Foster, 1998).

LITERATURE

Abdennebi EH, el Ouazzani N, Lamnaouer D., Clinical and analytical studies of sheep dosed with various preparations of Astragalus lusitanicus. Vet Hum Toxicol 1998 Dec;40(6):327-31.

Barneby, R. 1964. Atlas of North American astragalus part II. Mem. New York Bot. Gard. Vol. 13.

Bedir D; Calis I; Aquino R et al. Secondary metabolites from the roots of Astragalus trojanus. J Nat Prod 1999 Apr;62(4):563-8.

Bedir E; Calis I; Aquino R et al. Cycloartane triterpene glycosides from the roots of Astragalus brachypterus and Astragalus microcephalus. J Nat Prod 1998 Dec;61(12):1469-72.

Bone K: Clinical Applications of Ayurvedic and Chinese Herbs: Monographs for the Western Herbal Practitioner. Phytotherapy Press, Queensland, Australia 1997.

Chen LX; Liao JZ; Guo WQ. Effects of Astragalus membranaceus on left ventricular function and oxygen free radical in acute myocardial infarction patients and mechanism of its cardiotonic action. Chung Kuo Chung Hsi I Chieh Ho Tsa Chih 1995 Mar;15(3):141-3.

Chen M; Liu F. Chemical constituents of the seed oil of Astragalus complanatus R. Brown. Chung Kuo Chung Yao Tsa Chih 1990 Apr;15(4):225-6, 255.

Chu D; Sun Y; Lin J et al. F3, a fractionated extract of Astragalus membranaceus, potentiates lymphokine-activated killer cell cytotoxicity generated by low-dose recombinant interleukin-2. Chung Hsi I Chieh Ho Tsa Chih 1990 Jan;10(1):34-6, 5.

Chu DT; Lin JR; Wong W. The in vitro potentiation of LAK cell cytotoxicity in cancer and aids patients induced by F3—a fractionated extract of Astragalus membranaceus. Chung Hua Chung Liu Tsa Chih 1994 May;16(3):167-71.

Foster S. Astragalus: A superior herb. Herbs for Health 1998; Sept/Oct:40-41.

Guo XW; Zhang XX; Zhang ZM; Li FD. Characterization of astragalus sinicus rhizobia by restriction fragment length polymorphism analysis of chromosomal and nodulation genes regions. Curr Microbiol 1999 Dec;39(6):358-0364.

Hirotani M; Zhou Y; Rui H; Furuya T. Cycloartane triterpene glycosides from the hairy root cultures of Astragalus membranaceus. Phytochemistry 1994 Nov;37(5):1403-7.

Hong CY; Lo YC; Tan FC et al. Astragalus membranaceus and Polygonum multiflorum protect rat heart mitochondria against lipid peroxidation. Am J Chin Med 1994;22(1):63-70.

Hong GX; Qin WC; Huang LS. Memory-improving effect of aqueous extract of Astragalus membranaceus (Fisch.) Bge. Chung Kuo Chung Yao Tsa Chih 1994 Nov;19(11):687-8, 704.

Kaye TN. From flowering to dispersal: reproductive ecology of an endemic plant, Astragalus australis var. olympicus (Fabaceae). Am J Bot 1999 Sep;86(9):1248.

Khoo KS; Ang PT. Extract of astragalus membranaceus and ligustrum lucidum does not prevent cyclophosphamide-induced myelosuppression. Singapore Med J 1995 Aug;36(4):387-90.

Lei ZY; Qin H; Liao JZ. Action of Astragalus membranaceus on left ventricular function of angina pectoris. Chung Kuo Chung Hsi I Chieh Ho Tsa Chih 1994 Apr;14(4):199-202, 195.

Li SQ; Yuan RX; Gao H. Clinical observation on the treatment of ischemic heart disease with Astragalus membranaceus. Chung Kuo Chung Hsi I Chieh Ho Tsa Chih 1995 Feb;15(2):77-80.

Luo HM; Dai RH; Li Y. Nuclear cardiology study on effective ingredients of Astragalus membranaceus in treating heart failure. Chung Kuo Chung Hsi I Chieh Ho Tsa Chih 1995 Dec;15(12):707-9.

Ma J; Peng A; Lin S. Mechanisms of the therapeutic effect of astragalus membranaceus on sodium and water retention in experimental heart failure. Chin Med J (Engl) 1998 Jan;111(1):17-23.

Nigam SN; McConnell WB. Seleno amino compounds from Astragalus bisulcatus. Isolation and identification of gamma-L-glutamyl-Se-methyl-seleno-L-cysteine and Se-methylseleno-L-cysteine. Biochim Biophys Acta 1969 Nov 18;192(2):185-90.

Panter KE, Hartley WJ, James LF, et al. Comparative toxicity of selenium from seleno-DL-methionine, sodium selenate, and Astragalus bisulcatus in pigs. Fundam Appl Toxicol 1996 Aug;32(2):217-23.

Peng T; Yang Y; Riesemann H; Kandolf R. The inhibitory effect of astragalus membranaceus on coxsackie B-3 virus RNA replication. Chin Med Sci J 1995 Sep;10(3):146-50.

Rittenhouse JR; Lui PD; Lau BH. Chinese medicinal herbs reverse macrophage suppression induced by urological tumors. J Urol 1991 Aug;146(2):486-90.

Rui T; Yang YZ; Zhou TS. Effect of Astragalus membranaceus on electrophysiological activities of acute experimental Coxsackie B3 viral myocarditis in mice. Chung Kuo Chung Hsi I Chieh Ho Tsa Chih 1994 May;14(5):292-4, 26.

Wang HK; He K; Xu HX, et al. The structure of astrachrysosid A and the study of 2D-NMR on astrasieversianin XV and 7,2′-dihydroxy-3′,4′-dimethoxy-isoflavane-7-O- beta-D-glycoside. Yao Hsueh Hsueh Pao 1990;25(6):445-50.

Weng XS. Treatment of leucopenia with pure Astragalus preparation—an analysis of 115 leucopenic cases. Chung Kuo Chung Hsi I Chieh Ho Tsa Chih 1995 Aug;15(8):462-4.

Zhang WJ; Wojta J; Binder BR. Regulation of the fibrinolytic potential of cultured human umbilical vein endothelial cells: astragaloside IV downregulates plasminogen activator inhibitor-1 and upregulates tissue-type plasminogen activator expression. J Vasc Res 1997 Jul-Aug;34(4):273-80.

Zhang ZL; Wen QZ; Liu CX. Hepatoprotective effects of astragalus root. J Ethnopharmacol 1990 Sep;30(2):145-9.

Zhao KS; Mancini C; Doria G. Enhancement of the immune response in mice by Astragalus membranaceus extracts. Immunopharmacology 1990 Nov-Dec;20(3):225-33.

Zheng Z; Liu D; Song C et al. Studies on chemical constituents and immunological function activity of hairy root of Astragalus membranaceus. Chin J Biotechnol 1998;14(2):93-7.

Astragalus species

See Astragalus (Huang-Qi)

Athyrium filix-femina

See Lady Fern

Atractylodes japonica

See Japanese Atractylodes

Atractylodes lancea

See Southern Tsangshu (Cang-Zhu)

Atropa belladonna

See Belladonna

Avena sativa

See Oats

Averrhoa carambola

See Carambola

Avocado

Persea americana

DESCRIPTION

Medicinal Parts: The medicinal parts are the dried leaves, the fresh leaves, the whole fruit including the seed and the oil extracted from the leaves.

Flower and Fruit: The flowers are in compact or loose racemes. They are 5 to 8.2 mm long and greenish. The inner and outer perianth circles are 4 to 6 mm long and elliptical to oval-elliptical. The anthers are 3.5 mm long, and the filaments are 2.3 mm. The ovary is oval or pear-shaped and downy. It develops into a drupe, which is green and fleshy and up to 18 cm long. The drupe is smooth with thick oily flesh and a very large seed.

Leaves, Stem and Root: The avocado is a tree up to 40 m in height and with a trunk 60 cm in diameter. The leaves are 6 to 30 cm long and 3.5 to 19 cm wide. They are narrow to broadly elliptical. The leaf surface is sticky, while the lower surface is downy.

Habitat: The plant originated in central and southern South America and is cultivated in all tropical and subtropical regions today.

Production: Avocado oil comes from the fruit of Persea americana. Avocado oil is recovered from the pericarp of Persea americana and refined if necessary.

ACTIONS AND PHARMACOLOGY

COMPOUNDS

Fatty oil: chief fatty acids oleic acid, palmitic acid, linoleic acid, palmitoleic acid (tocopherols, vitamin E)

EFFECTS

Avocado oil is an emollient, which improves rough ichtyotic skin.

INDICATIONS AND USAGE

Avocado is a main ingredient in so-called natural cosmetics.

PRECAUTIONS AND ADVERSE REACTIONS

No health hazards or side effects are known in conjunction with the proper administration of designated therapeutic dosages.

DOSAGE

Mode of Administration: As an active or inactive ingredient in various preparations (bath oils, ointments, etc.).

Storage: Oils from different batches should not be mixed. The drug should be stored in a sealed container away from light and moisture.

LITERATURE

Albert K, Pharm Ztg 131:2279. 1986.

Hänsel R, Keller K, Rimpler H, Schneider G (Hrsg.), Hagers Handbuch der Pharmazeutischen Praxis, 5. Aufl., Bde 4-6 (Drogen), Springer Verlag Berlin, Heidelberg, New York, 1992-1994.

Heller H, Asche W, Seifen Oele Fette Wachse 111:164. 1985.

Teuscher E, Biogene Arzneimittel, 5. Aufl., Wiss. Verlagsges. Stuttgart 1997.

Bael

Aegle marmelos

DESCRIPTION

Medicinal Parts: The medicinal parts are the unripe fruit, the root, the leaves and the branches.

Flower and Fruit: The plant has greenish-white flowers. The yellow fruit is globular or ovoid, with a hard shell. The fruit is divided internally like an orange. The flesh is reddish, with numerous seeds covered in a layer of latex.

Characteristics: The taste is mucilaginous and slightly sour.

Habitat: This plant is native to India but has spread over wide areas of southeast Asia.

Other Names: Bel, Bengal Quince

ACTIONS AND PHARMACOLOGY

COMPOUNDS

Tannins

Saccharides

Starch

Fatty oil

Furocoumarins

Furoquinolin alkaloids

EFFECTS

Bael has a digestive and an astringent effect.

INDICATIONS AND USAGE

Indian Medicine: Bael is used, especially in Indian medicine, for constipation and diarrhea.

PRECAUTIONS AND ADVERSE REACTIONS

No health hazards or side effects are known in conjunction with the proper administration of designated therapeutic dosages.

OVERDOSAGE

Digestive complaints and constipation are possible with the intake of large quantities, due to the constituent tannins.

DOSAGE

Mode of Administration: Available as a liquid extract for internal use.

LITERATURE

Oliver-Bever B (Ed., 1986), Medicinal Plants of Tropical West Africa, Cambridge University Press UK.

Sharma BR and Sharma P, (1981) Planta Med 43:102.

Schimmer O, Furochinolinalkaloide als biologisch aktive Naturstoffe. In: ZPT 12(5):151. 1991.

Balloon-Flower (Jie-Geng)

Platycodon grandiflorum

DESCRIPTION

Medicinal Parts: The medicinal parts of the plant are the main and secondary roots.

Flower and Fruit: The flowers are at the tip of the leading shoot. The flower structures are in fives and are fused. The calyx tube is appressed to the ovary; the corolla is 5-lobed, blue, occasionally white with a diameter of approximately 5 cm. The 5 stamens are free and the ovary inferior with numerous ovules. The fruit is an obovoid, multi-chambered, dehiscent capsule. The seeds are ovoid, light to dark brown, smooth, 1.7 to 2.2 mm long, 1 to 1.2 mm wide and flattened.

Leaves, Stem and Root: The plant is a herbaceous perennial growing to 90 cm high. The leaves are almost sessile with a simple lamina, bluish-green above and gray-green beneath, irregularly crenate-serrate and entire at the base. The plant has a hardy (approximately 3 cm thick) taproot and hardy secondary roots.

Habitat: Balloon-Flower is indigenous to China, Japan, Korea and Siberia.

Production: The plant is collected in the wild and air-dried. Balloon-Flower root is the dried main and secondary root of Platycodon grandiflorum.

Other Names: Chinese Bell-Flower, Japanese Bell-Flower

ACTIONS AND PHARMACOLOGY

COMPOUNDS

Triterpene saponins (1.7%): including platycodin, platycoside C, aglycone platycodigenin, including glycosides of polygalic acid, platycogenic acids A to C

Volatile oil (0.2 to 0.3%)

Steroids: sterols, including delta7-stigmasterol, alpha-spinasterol

EFFECTS

The saponin fraction contained in the drug has inhibiting effects upon gastric secretion and exhibits both ulcer-protective and ulcer-healing effects. In addition, a mild antibacterial effect was able to be demonstrated. The plant is said to have a sedative effective on the respiratory organs and to encourage expectoration. The antitussive, anti-inflammatory and sedative effects require further clinical testing for verification.

INDICATIONS AND USAGE

Chinese Medicine: Jie-Geng is mainly used as an expectorant for bronchitis, sore throat, tonsillitis and other conditions of the respiratory tract. Efficacy as an expectorant is plausible due to the saponin content; efficacy for the other indications has not been proven.

PRECAUTIONS AND ADVERSE REACTIONS

No health hazards are known in conjunction with the proper administration of designated therapeutic dosages.

DOSAGE

Mode of Administration: Preparations of whole, cut and powdered drug are for internal use.

Preparation: Liquid extract: root powder 1:1 25% ethanol

Daily Dosage:

Powder — 6 g daily; 0.5 g as a single dose

Decoction — 1 g daily; 0.2 g as a single dose

Storage: Store tightly sealed and protected from light.

LITERATURE

Hänsel R, Keller K, Rimpler H, Schneider G (Ed), Hagers Handbuch der Pharmazeutischen Praxis, 5. Aufl., Bde 4 - 6 (Drogen), Springer Verlag Berlin, Heidelberg, New York, 1992-1994.

Kim KS, Ezaki O, Ikemoto S, Itakura H, Effects of Platycodon grandiflorum feeding on serum and liver lipid concentrations in rats with diet-induced hyperlipidemia. J Nutr Sci Vitaminol (Tokyo), 41:485-91, 1995 Aug.

Kim KS, Ezaki O, Ikemoto S, Itakura H, Effects of Platycodon grandiflorum feeding on serum and liver lipid concentrations in rats with diet-induced hyperlipidemia. Yakugaku Zasshi, 41:485-91, 1995 Aug.

Kim KS, Ezaki O, Ikemoto S, Itakura H Rat plasma corticosterone secretion-inducing activities of total saponin and prosapogenin methyl esters from the roots of Platycodon grandiflorum A.DC. Yakugaku Zasshi, 41:1191-4, 1995 Aug.

Ballota nigra

See Black Horehound

Balmony

Chelone glabra

DESCRIPTION

Medicinal Parts: The medicinal part is the fresh herb picked during the flowering season

Flower and Fruit: The inflorescence is a short terminal spike of bilabiate white, purple, cream or pink flowers. The lower lip is awned in the tube and the cordate anthers are downy. The seeds are round and bitter.

Leaves, Stem and Root: The plant is small and erect, and may reach up to 60 cm in height. It is a perennial herb with angular, smooth stems and a horizontally spreading root system. The leaves are opposite, oblong-lanceolate, on short petioles.

Characteristics: The leaves have a tea-like smell and an extremely bitter taste.

Habitat: Northeastern U.S. and Canada

Production: Balmony is the above-ground part of Chelone glabra.

Other Names: Turtlebloom, Turtle Head, Chelone, Shell-flower, Salt-Rheum Weed, Bitter Herb, Hummingbird Tree, Snakehead

ACTIONS AND PHARMACOLOGY

COMPOUNDS

Iridoide monoterpenes: catalpol

Resin: (bitter-tasting)

EFFECTS

No information available.

INDICATIONS AND USAGE

Homeopathic Uses: Chelone glabra is used in the treatment of liver disorders, digestive disorders and worm infestation.

PRECAUTIONS AND ADVERSE REACTIONS

No health hazards or side effects are known in conjunction with the proper administration of designated therapeutic dosages.

DOSAGE

Mode of Administration: The herb is available in homeopathic dilutions.

LITERATURE

Belofsky G et al., PH 28:1601. 1989.

Kern W, List PH, Hörhammer L (Hrsg.), Hagers Handbuch der Pharmazeutischen Praxis, 4. Aufl., Bde. 1-8, Springer Verlag Berlin, Heidelberg, New York, 1969.

Bamboo

Arundinaria japonica

DESCRIPTION

Medicinal Parts: The medicinal parts are the young shoots of the plant.

Flower and Fruit: Greenish-yellow, round culms exceeding 3 m in height are surrounded at the culm nodes by dry leaf sheaths, which do not fall off. The upper surface of the leaves are shiny and dark green; the underside is matte and gray-green. The leaf margins are sharply serrated.

Habitat: The plant is indigenous to the tropics, southern subtropics and Asia.

Production: Bamboo sprouts are the young shoots of Arundinaria japonica.

ACTIONS AND PHARMACOLOGY

COMPOUNDS

Soluble mono-, oligo-, and polysaccharides

Silicic acid: to some extent water-soluble

EFFECTS

No information is available.

INDICATIONS AND USAGE

Bamboo is seldom used for medicinal purposes in Western medicine.

Chinese Medicine: The drug is used for asthma, coughs and disorders of the gallbladder.

PRECAUTIONS AND ADVERSE REACTIONS

No health hazards or side effects are known in conjunction with the proper administration of designated therapeutic dosages.

DOSAGE

Mode of Administration: The juice from the young shoots is hardened as bamboo sugar and used internally.

LITERATURE

No literature is available.

Baneberry

Actaea spicata

DESCRIPTION

Medicinal Parts: The medicinal part is the root.

Flower and Fruit: The white flowers are in ovate racemes. They have 4 to 6 bracts, white stamens and 1 ovary. The fruit is a black, many-seeded berry.

Leaves, Stem and Root: The plant grows 30 to 60 cm tall. It is large, long-petioled, trifoliate and pinnate. The leaflets are pinnatisect and serrate. The stem is erect and glabrous.

Characteristics: Baneberry is poisonous, as are several other plants with similar qualities.

Habitat: The plant grows in most of Europe and in moderate and arctic regions of Asia.

Production: Baneberry or Herb Christopher root is the root of Actaea spicata.

Not to be Confused With: Helleborus niger is occasionally used as a substitute by mistake.

Other Names: Bugbane, Herb Christopher, Toadroot

ACTIONS AND PHARMACOLOGY

COMPOUNDS

Isoquinoline alkaloids: magnoflorine, corytuberine

Triterpene glycosides: including actein

Trans-aconitic acid

EFFECTS

The drug, which contains alkaloids (magnoflorine) and saponins, was shown to inhibit growth of *Mycobacterium tuberculosis*. An antirheumatic effect is being investigated.

INDICATIONS AND USAGE

Unproven Uses: Baneberry is used as an emetic and purgative.

Homeopathic Uses: The drug is used in homeopathy for rheumatic conditions, especially those of the smaller joints.

PRECAUTIONS AND ADVERSE REACTIONS

No health hazards or side effects are known in conjunction with the proper administration of designated therapeutic dosages.

DOSAGE

Mode of Administration: In homeopathy, Baneberry is available as dilutions of the mother tincture.

LITERATURE

Fardella G, Corsano St, Preliminary study on actein biosynthesis. In: Ann Chim(Rom)63:333-337. 1973.

Frohne D, Pfänder HJ, Giftpflanzen - Ein Handbuch für Apotheker, Toxikologen und Biologen, 4. Aufl., Wiss. Verlags-Ges Stuttgart 1997.

Kern W, List PH, Hörhammer L (Hrsg.), Hagers Handbuch der Pharmazeutischen Praxis, 4. Aufl., Bde. 1-8, Springer Verlag Berlin, Heidelberg, New York, 1969.

Madaus G, Lehrbuch der Biologischen Arzneimittel, Bde 1-3, Nachdruck, Georg Olms Verlag Hildesheim 1979.

Nikonow GK, Syrkina SA, Chemische Untersuchungen der aktiven Prinzipien von Actaea spicata L. In: Pharm Zentralhalle 103(8):601. 1964.

Banisteriopsis caapi

See Yage

Baptisia tinctoria

See Wild Indigo

Barberry

Berberis vulgaris

DESCRIPTION

Medicinal Parts: The medicinal part is the fruit and the root bark.

Flower and Fruit: The flowers are 5 to 7 cm long in yellow, dense, hanging clusters. The 6 sepals are yellow and the 6 petals have orange-colored honey glands at the base. The 6 stamens burst open at the side. The ovary is superior with a flat stigma. The edible fruit is a bright scarlet, oblong-cylindrical berry, 10 to 12 mm long and 6 mm thick. The exocarp is membranous-coriaceous. There are usually 2 seeds.

Leaves, Stem and Root: Barberry is a deciduous, heavily branched, thorny bush up to 2 m high. The thorny branches are angular, deeply grooved, initially brownish yellow, later more white-gray. The thorns are 1 to 2 cm long and stick out horizontally. The leaves are in bunches and are obovate to elliptoid, 2 to 4 cm long and narrow. They are dark green and reticulate, the margin is dentate.

Characteristics: The flowers have a repulsive smell; the stamens lie on the carpels at the slightest touch. The flesh of the fruit is juicy and sour.

Habitat: Europe, northern Africa, parts of America and central Asia.

Production: Barberries are the ripe fruit of Berberis vulgaris. Barberry root bark or berberis bark is the dried root bark of Berberis vulgaris. Berberis aquifolium is a closely-related American variety that is often used in commercially available Oregon Grape products.

Not to be Confused With: There is a possiblity of confusion with the fruits of other berberidis types. The commercial drug often consists of admixtures; between 15% and 50% of branch and trunk bark.

Other Names: Berberry, Pipperidge, Jaundice Berry, Sow Berry, Mountain Grape, Oregon Grape

ACTIONS AND PHARMACOLOGY

COMPOUNDS: BARBERRY FRUIT

Isoquinoline alkaloids (at the most, traces)

Anthocyans

Chlorogenic acid

Malic acid, acetic acid

EFFECTS: BARBERRY ROOT BARK

Source of vitamin C. In various metabolic processes, vitamin C increases immune system activity, stimulates iron absorption, and prevents scurvy. There is a mild diuretic effect due to the acid content.

COMPOUNDS: BARBERRY ROOT BARK

Isoquinoline alkaloids: in particular berberine, berbamine, oxyacanthin, further to include columbamine, palmatine, jatrorrhizine, magnoflorine.

EFFECTS: BARBERRY ROOT BARK

Cardiovascular effect: Fractions from the root extracts, which contain 80% berberine and other alkaloids, have been shown to reduce the blood pressure of cats for several hours. With varying doses, both positive and negative inotropic effects on the cats' hearts were recorded.

Cholagogue effect: A homeopathic mother tincture increased the bile flow in guinea pigs by an average of 20%. An extract with 80% berberine and additional alkaloids stimulated the bile excretion of rats by 72%.

Antipyretic effect: Aqueous tinctures have an anti-febrile effect on a feverish rabbit.

Antibiotic effect

Stimulation of intestinal peristalsis

INDICATIONS AND USAGE

BARBERRY FRUIT

Unproven uses: Decoction or alcoholic extract for lung, spleen and liver diseases. Jam or wine made from the fresh berries can relieve constipation and stimulate the appetite. Alcoholic extracts have been used for heartburn and stomach cramps. Extracts have also been used for susceptibility to infection, feverish colds, and diseases of the urinary tract. Used in the pharmaceutical industry as a syrup for masking flavor.

BARBERRY ROOT BARK

Unproven uses: Barberry has been used for opium or morphine withdrawal. In folk medicine, the bark is used for liver malfunctions, gallbladder disease, jaundice, splenopathy, indigestion, diarrhea, tuberculosis, piles, renal disease, urinary tract disorders, gout, rheumatism, arthritis, lumbago, malaria, and leishmaniasis.

PRECAUTIONS AND ADVERSE REACTIONS

BARBERRY FRUIT AND ROOT BARK

No health hazards or side effects are known in conjunction with the proper administration of designated therapeutic dosages.

OVERDOSAGE

BARBERRY ROOT BARK

Dosages over 4 mg will bring about light stupor, nosebleeds, vomiting, diarrhea and kidney irritation. The treatment for poisonings is to be carried out symptomatically.

DOSAGE

BARBERRY FRUIT

Mode of Administration: Barberry is used internally in tea mixtures and combination preparations.

Preparation: To prepare a tea infusion, pour approximately 150 ml of hot water into 1 to 2 teaspoons of whole or squashed Barberries and strain after 10 to 15 minutes.

BARBERRY ROOT BARK

How Supplied:

Liquid—1:1, 1:5

Tea

Preparation: A tincture 1:10 is prepared according to the German Pharmacopeia 10th ed.

To extract the pure alkaloids from berberis roots, use 0.3% sulphuric acid mixed with 10% sodium chloride. The precipitated berberine hydrochloride is washed with mildly hydrochloric water and dried. It is then dissolved in water (pH 8) and filtered. The filtrate is heated to 70° C and set to pH 2.0 using hydrochloric acid. The precipitate of pure berberine hydrochloride is then washed and dried.

Daily Dosage: The dosage of the infusion is 2 g in 250 ml water, to be sipped. The tincture dosage is 20 to 40 drops daily.

LITERATURE

Andronescu E et al., (1973) Clujul. Med 46: 627.

Chen MQ et al., (1965) Acta Pharm Sinica 12 (3): 185.

Cordell GA, Farnsworth NR, (1977) Lloydia 40: 1.

Ikram M, (1975) Planta Med 28: 253.

Lahiri SC et al., (1958) Ann Biochem Exp Med India 18: 95.

Liu CX et al., (1979) Chinese Traditional and Herbal Drugs Communications 9: 36.

Naidovich LP et al., (1976) Farmatsiya 24: 33.

Subbaiah TV, Amin AH, (1967) Nature 215: 527.

Ubebaba K et al., (1984) Jpn J Pharmacol 36 (Suppl): 352.

Willaman JJ, Hui-Li L, (1970) Lloydia 33 (3A): 1.

Further information in:

Frohne D, Pfänder HJ, Giftpflanzen - Ein Handbuch für Apotheker, Toxikologen und Biologen, 4. Aufl., Wiss. Verlags-Ges Stuttgart 1997.

Hänsel R, Keller K, Rimpler H, Schneider G (Hrsg.), Hagers Handbuch der Pharmazeutischen Praxis, 5. Aufl., Bde 4-6 (Drogen), Springer Verlag Berlin, Heidelberg, New York, 1992-1994.

Madaus G, Lehrbuch der Biologischen Arzneimittel, Bde 1-3, Nachdruck, Georg Olms Verlag Hildesheim 1979.

Roth L, Daunderer M, Kormann K, Giftpflanzen, Pflanzengifte, 4. Aufl., Ecomed Fachverlag Landsberg Lech 1993.

Teuscher E, Lindequist U, Biogene Gifte - Biologie, Chemie, Pharmakologie, 2. Aufl., Fischer Verlag Stuttgart 1994.

Wagner H, Wiesenauer M, Phytotherapie. Phytopharmaka und pflanzliche Homöopathika, Fischer-Verlag, Stuttgart, Jena, New York 1995.

Barley

Hordeum distichon

TRADE NAMES

Barley (available from numerous manufacturers and as combination product), Barley Grain

DESCRIPTION

Medicinal Parts: The medicinal part is the polished grain without the husk.

Flower and Fruit: The spike is 7 to 15 cm long. The long form is nodding and the shorter one erect and compressed at the side that does not bear spikelets. The spike spindle is tough and loosens the spikelets when ripe. The lateral spikelets are unbearded, male or sexless. The middle spikelet is seed-bearing with a beard up to 15 cm long.

Leaves, Stem and Root: The plant is an annual that grows 60 to 130 cm high. It has a long hollow stalk and lanceolate leaves. The leaflets are very wide, long and glabrous.

Habitat: Barley is cultivated worldwide.

Production: Barley seeds are the seeds of Hordeum distichon.

Other Names: Pearl Barley, Pot Barley, Scotch Barley

ACTIONS AND PHARMACOLOGY

COMPOUNDS

Polysaccharides: starch (50%), fructans

Mono- and oligosaccharides: saccharose, raffinose, glucodi-fructose, glucose, fructose

Proteins (10%): including, among others, prolamines: hordein- glutelins: hordenine (not to be confused with the amine of the same name, see below)- albumins and globulins

Prolamines: hordein

Glutelins: hordenine (not to be confused with the amine of the same name, see below)

Albumins and globulins

Fatty oil (2%): chief fatty acids linoleic and oleic acid

Vitamins: Vitamin E, nicotinic acid, pantothenic acid, vitamins B6, B2, folic acid

Hydroxycoumarins (only in the stalks): including, among others, umbelliferone, scopoletin, herniarin, aesculetin (in the sprouts)

Amines: tyramine, hordenine (dimethyltyramine), gramine also with certain strains (dimethy- laminomethylindol)

EFFECTS

Barley is soothing on the alimentary tract.

INDICATIONS AND USAGE

Unproven Uses: Barley has been used for convalescents and in the treatment of diarrhea, gastritis and inflammatory bowel conditions.

PRECAUTIONS AND ADVERSE REACTIONS

General: No health hazards or side effects are known in conjunction with the proper administration of designated therapeutic dosages.

Pregnancy: Not to be used during pregnancy.

DOSAGE

Mode of Administration: Barley is used as a malt extract, in preparations and in combinations.

How Supplied:

Capsules - 450 mg

LITERATURE

Bergantino E, Sandon'a D, Cugini D, Bassi R, The photosystem II subunit CP29 can be phosphorylated in both C3 and C4 plants as suggested by sequence analysis. Plant Mol Biol, 36:11-22, 1998 Jan

Davies TG, Theodoulou FL, Hallahan DL, Forde BG, Cloning and characterisation of a novel P-glycoprotein homologue from barley. Gene, 199:195-202, 1997 Oct 15

Dhar ML et al., (1968) Indian J Exp Biol 6:232.

Kern W, List PH, Hörhammer L (Hrsg.), Hagers Handbuch der Pharmazeutischen Praxis, 4. Aufl., Bde. 1-8, Springer Verlag Berlin, Heidelberg, New York, 1969.

Labbe M, (1936) J Canad Med Assoc 34:141.

Oliver-Bever B (Ed), Medicinal Plants of Tropical West Africa. Cambridge University Press, Cambridge, London 1986

Pajuelo P, Pajuelo E, Forde BG, Marquez AJ, Regulation of the expression of ferredoxin-glutamate synthase in barley. Planta, 203:517-25, 1997 Dec

Rudi H et al., A (His)6-tagged recombinant barley endosperm ADP-glucose pyrophosphorylase expressed in the baculovirus-insect cell system is insensitive to allosteric regulation by 3-phosphoglycerate and inorganic phosphate. FEBS Lett, 419, 1997

Schuurink RC, Shartzer SF, Fath A, Jones RL, Characterization of a calmodulin-binding transporter from the plasma membrane of barley aleurone. Proc Natl Acad Sci U S A, 95:1944-9, 1998 Feb 17

Barosma species

See Short Buchu

Basil

Ocimum basilicum

DESCRIPTION

Medicinal Parts: The medicinal parts of the plant are the fresh or dried herb as well as the oil extracted from the dried aerial parts.

Flower and Fruit: The white, labiate flowers are in 6-blossomed, pedicled, almost sessile axillary false whorls. The calyx is bilabiate, and the corolla is 4-lobed. The lower lip is simple; the 4 stamens lie on it.

Leaves, Stem and Root: The plant grows from 20 to 40 cm high. The stem is erect, branched from the base up and downy. The leaves are ovate or oblong. They are long-petioled, acuminate, irregularly dentate or entire-margined.

Characteristics: Basil has a characteristic odor and sharp taste.

Habitat: The plant probably originated in India, Afghanistan, Pakistan and northern India, and now is cultivated worldwide.

Production: Basil herb consists of the dried, above-ground parts of Ocimum basilicum. Oil of basil is the essential oil extracted from the dried aerial parts of Ocimum basilicum by steam distillation.

Other Names: St. Josephwort

ACTIONS AND PHARMACOLOGY

COMPOUNDS: BASIL HERB

Volatile oil: chief constituents are chavicol methyl ether (estragole), linalool and eugenol

Caffeic acid derivatives

Flavonoids

EFFECTS: BASIL HERB

In vitro, Basil is antimicrobial.

COMPOUNDS: BASIL OIL

Chief constituents: estragole (chavicol methyl ether), linalool, eugenol

EFFECTS: BASILOIL

In vitro, the oil demonstrates an antimicrobial effect.

INDICATIONS AND USAGE

BASIL HERB

Unproven Uses: Preparations of basil are used for supportive therapy for feelings of fullness and flatulence, for the stimulation of appetite and digestion, and as a diuretic.

Chinese Medicine: Basil herb is used for disturbances of renal function, gum ulcers and as a hemostyptic both before and after birth.

Indian Medicine: Among uses in Indian medicine are earaches, rheumatoid arthritis, anorexia, itching and skin diseases, amenorrhea and dysmenorrhea, malaria and other febrile illnesses.

BASIL OIL

Unproven Uses: Among traditional uses for the oil are wounds, rheumatic complaints, colds and chills, contusions, joint pains and depression.

PRECAUTIONS AND ADVERSE REACTIONS

BASIL HERB

General: No health hazards or side effects are known in conjunction with the proper administration of designated therapeutic dosages.

Pregnancy: The herb contains about 0.5% essential oil with up to 85% estragole. Because of the high estragole content in the essential oil, the herb should not be taken during pregnancy.

BASIL OIL

General: No health hazards or side effects are known in conjunction with the proper administration of designated therapeutic dosages. However, pending final determination of the drug's carcinogenic potential, one should completely forgo administration of the drug.

Pregnancy: Because a mutagenic effect in vitro and a carcinogenic effect in animal experiments have been demonstrated for estragole, oil of basil should not be administered during pregnancy or while nursing.

Pediatric Use: Basil oil should not be given to infants or small children.

DOSAGE

Until the final determination of the drug's carcinogenic potential, one should completely forgo its administration.

LITERATURE

Balambal R et al., (1985) J Assoc Phys (India) 33(8):507.

Czygan FCh, Balsilikum - Ocimum basilicum L. Portrait einer Arzneipflanze. In: ZPT 18(1):58-66. 1997.

Jain ML, Jain SR, (1972) Planta Med 22:66.

Lemberkovics É et al., Formation of essential oil and phenolic compounds during the vegetation period in Ocimum basilicum. In: PM 59(7)00. 1993.

Miller EC et al., (1983) Cancer Res 43:1124.

Opdyke DLJ, (1973) Food Cosmet Toxicol 11:867.

Wagner H, Nörr H, Winterhoff H, Drogen mit "Adaptogenwirkung" zur Stärkung der Widerstandskräfte. In: ZPT 13(2):42. 1992.

Further information in:

Kern W, List PH, Hörhammer L (Hrsg.), Hagers Handbuch der Pharmazeutischen Praxis, 4. Aufl., Bde. 1-8, Springer Verlag Berlin, Heidelberg, New York, 1969.

Leung AY, Encyclopedia of Common Natural Ingredients Used in Food Drugs and Cosmetics, John Wiley & Sons Inc., New York 1980.

Madaus G, Lehrbuch der Biologischen Arzneimittel, Bde 1-3, Nachdruck, Georg Olms Verlag Hildesheim 1979.

Simon JE, Chadwick AF, Craker LE (Eds.), Herbs. An Indexed Bibliography 1971-80. Archon Books, USA 1984.

Wichtl M (Hrsg.), Teedrogen, 4. Aufl., Wiss. Verlagsges. Stuttgart 1997.

Bean Pod

Phaseolus vulgaris

DESCRIPTION

Medicinal Parts: The medicinal parts are the ripe, dried pods and the beans.

Flower and Fruit: The white, pink and lilac flowers are in lightly blossomed, peduncled racemes, which are shorter than their leaves. The calyx is bilabiate. The carina, stamens and style are twisted in a spiral. The fruit is a straight, smooth, hanging pod with a number of reniform seeds.

Leaves, Stem and Root: The annual plant grows from 30 to 60 cm high. It is heavily branched but not twining. The leaves are trifoliate, the leaflets are broad ovate and acuminate. The terminal leaflet is rhomboid.

Habitat: The plant is indigenous to America and is cultivated worldwide today.

Production: The seed-free pods of Phaseolus vulgaris are collected during the harvest season.

Other Names: Common Bean, Green Bean, Kidney Bean, Navy Bean, Pinto Bean, Snap Bean, String Bean, Wax Bean

ACTIONS AND PHARMACOLOGY

COMPOUNDS

Lectins: complex termed phytomitogen (tetrameric glycoproteins)

Saponins

L-pipecolic acid

Flavonoids

EFFECTS

A weak diuretic action has been demonstrated in animal and human experiments. Chromium salts present in the Bean Pod may produce an antidiabetic effect.

INDICATIONS AND USAGE

Approved by Commission E:

- Infections of the urinary tract
- Kidney and bladder stones

Unproven Uses: Bean Pod is used as a supportive treatment for inability to urinate. In folk medicine, it is used as a diuretic and antidiabetic.

PRECAUTIONS AND ADVERSE REACTIONS

No health hazards or side effects are known in conjunction with the proper administration of designated therapeutic dosages, in the form of heated infusions.

OVERDOSAGE

Poisonings following the intake of large quantities of fresh green bean husks (or of raw green beans) are not to be entirely ruled out, due to the lectins content, which varies greatly among the individual species. Symptoms include vomiting, diarrhea and gastroenteritis. The lectins are destroyed in the process of cooking.

DOSAGE

Mode of Administration: As a comminuted herb for decoctions and other galenic preparations for internal use. The drug is a component of various kidney and bladder teas and of standardized preparations of natural diuretics and antidiabetics.

Preparation: To make an infusion, pour boiling water over 2.5 gm drug and strain after 10 to 15 minutes while still covered (1 teaspoonful = 1.5 gm drug).

Daily Dosage: The recommended daily dosage is 5 to 15 gm of herb.

LITERATURE

Kern W, List PH, Hörhammer L (Eds.), Hagers Handbuch der Pharmazeutischen Praxis, 4. Aufl., Bde. 1-8, Springer Verlag Berlin, Heidelberg, New York, 1969.

Madaus G, Lehrbuch der Biologischen Arzneimittel, Bde 1-3, Nachdruck, Georg Olms Verlag Hildesheim 1979.

Pusztai A et al., Recent advances in the study of the nutrtional toxicity of kidney bean (Phaseolus vulgaris) lectins in rat. In: Toxicon 20(1): R195. 1982.

Roth L, Daunderer M, Kormann K, Giftpflanzen, Pflanzengifte, 4. Aufl., Ecomed Fachverlag Landsberg Lech 1993.

Steinegger E, Hänsel R, Pharmakognosie, 5. Aufl., Springer Verlag Heidelberg 1992.

Teuscher E, Lindequist U, Biogene Gifte - Biologie, Chemie, Pharmakologie, 2. Aufl., Fischer Verlag Stuttgart 1994.

Wagner H, Wiesenauer M, Phytotherapie. Phytopharmaka und pflanzliche Homöopathika, Fischer-Verlag, Stuttgart, Jena, New York 1995.

Wichtl M (Ed.), Teedrogen, 4. Aufl., Wiss. Verlagsges. Stuttgart 1997.

Bear's Garlic

Allium ursinum

DESCRIPTION

Medicinal Parts: The fresh herb and fresh bulb are the medicinal parts of the plant.

Flower and Fruit: The sheath of the terminal inflorescence is made up of 3 ovate-lanceolate, acute, early-falling leaves, which are almost as long as the peduncle. The inflorescence is a loose, flat, 2.5 to 6 cm wide cyme with 6 to 20 florets. The florets are erect, outward-inclined, pointed or blunt. They are pure white and have 6 star-shaped, splayed petals. Six stamens are wedge-shaped, only fused at the base and only half as long as the involucre. One superior ovary is formed out of 3 carpels and 3 deep grooves. The 3-valved capsule contains black, angular seeds.

Leaves, Stem and Root: The plant's compact stem is upright, 10 to 50 cm high, double-edged, half-cylindrical or triangular-to-round in shape. The leaf blade is flat, narrow-elliptical-lanceolate to narrow-ovate and acute. It is 6 to 20 cm long and thin, with a base that is rounded to cordate and narrows suddenly to a 5 to 20 cm long petiole. The leaf's dark-green underside is covered with irregular horizontal veins that face upward, leaving the paler upper surface facing toward the ground. The bulb is almost cylindrical, 2 to 6 cm long, about 1 cm wide and surrounded by transparent or white skins.

Characteristics: Bear's garlic forms many onions and has a distinctive leek odor.

Habitat: Bear's Garlic is indigenous to almost all of Europe and Turkey, but not in the Hungarian plain and the evergreen Mediterranean region. It is also found in the Caucasus and Siberia as far as Kamtschatka.

Production: Bear's garlic is fresh or dried herb of Allium ursinum.

Not to be Confused With: One case was reported of confusion with colchicum leaves.

Other Names: Ramsons, Broad-Leaved Garlic

ACTIONS AND PHARMACOLOGY

COMPOUNDS

Alliins (alkylcysteine sulphoxides): in particular methyl alliin (methyl-L-(+)-cysteine sulphoxide) and allylalliin (allyl-L-(+)-cysteine sulphoxide) and presumably their gamma-glutamyl conjugates, that readily transform into the so-called alliaceous oils, for example into dimethyl-disulphide-mono-S-oxide, allicin (diallyl-disulphide-mono-S-oxide) and allyl-methyl-disulphide mono-S-oxide and the corresponding dialkyldi- or oligosulphides

EFFECTS

The diverse sulphur bonds are said to be lipid-reducing, anti-oxidative, aggregation inhibiting and ACE inhibiting.

INDICATIONS AND USAGE

Unproven Uses: The drug is used internally for gastrointestinal complaints, fermentative dyspepsia, flatulence, high blood pressure and arteriosclerosis; externally for chronic rashes.

Homeopathic Uses: Uses in homeopathy include digestive disorders.

PRECAUTIONS AND ADVERSE REACTIONS

No health hazards or side effects are known in conjunction with the proper administration of designated therapeutic dosages.

DOSAGE

Mode of Administration: The drug is used internally as well as externally.

Preparation: Extract of Bear's Garlic.

Daily Dosage: Due to low concentration of the active substance, the drug must be administered in higher doses than Allium sativum.

Homeopathic Dosage: 5 drops, 1 tablet or 10 globules every 30 to 60 minutes for acute conditions, and 1 to 3 times daily for chronic; parenterally: 1 to 2 ml daily sc (HAB1).

LITERATURE

Landshuter J et al., Comparative biochemical studies on a purified C-S-lyase preparation from wild garlic. In: PM 58(7)66. 1992.

Sendl A, Bärlauch: Alternative zu Knoblauch. In: Naturw. Rdsch 7/94. 1994.

Sendl A, Phytotherapie: Bärlauch und Knoblauch im Vergleich. In: DAZ 133(5):392. 1993.

Veit M, Bärlauch (Allium ursinum) als Ersatz für Knoblauch (Allium sativum). In: ZPT 13(6):201. 1993.

Wagner H, Ebl G, Lotter H, Guinea M, Evaluation of natural products as inhibitors of angiotensin I-converting enzyme (ACE). In: Pharm Pharmacol Letters 1(1):15-18. 1991.

Wagner H, Sendl A, Bärlauch und Knoblauch. In: DAZ 130(33):1809. 1990.

Further information in:

Hänsel R, Keller K, Rimpler H, Schneider G (Hrsg.), Hagers Handbuch der Pharmazeutischen Praxis, 5. Aufl., Bde 4-6 (Drogen), Springer Verlag Berlin, Heidelberg, New York, 1992-1994.

Madaus G, Lehrbuch der Biologischen Arzneimittel, Bde 1-3, Nachdruck, Georg Olms Verlag Hildesheim 1979.

Teuscher E, Biogene Arzneimittel, 5. Aufl., Wiss. Verlagsges. Stuttgart 1997.

Wagner H, Wiesenauer M, Phytotherapie. Phytopharmaka und pflanzliche Homöopathika, Fischer-Verlag, Stuttgart, Jena, New York 1995.

Wichtl M (Hrsg.), Teedrogen, 4. Aufl., Wiss. Verlagsges. Stuttgart 1997.

Beet

Beta vulgaris

DESCRIPTION

Medicinal Parts: The root is the medicinal part.

Flower and Fruit: The flowers bloom in clusters of 2 to 4 in panicle-like leafy inflorescences.

Leaves, Stem and Root: The beet is a 0.5 to 1.5 m perennial with a swollen, edible tuber that is red or white. The large, upright leaves have long stalks and grow in rosettes that arise basally from the top of the tuber. They are deep green and tinged with red.

Habitat: The Beet is indigenous to the coastal regions of Europe, North Africa, and Asia from Turkey to India. Red Beets, Sugar Beets and the white variety are all widely cultivated.

Other Names: Chard

ACTIONS AND PHARMACOLOGY

COMPOUNDS

Saccharose (up to 27% in the pressed sugar beet)

Other oligosaccharides: refined sugar, ketose

Polysaccharides: including galactans, arabans, pectin

Fruit acids: including L(-)-malic acid, D(+)-tartaric acid, oxaluric acid, adipic acid, citric acid, glycolic acid, glutaric acid

Amino acids: including asparagine, glutamine

Betaine (trimethylglycine)

Triterpene saponins

EFFECTS

Beet is said to have antihepatotoxic effects; in animal tests, the drug effectively keeps fat from depositing in the liver. This is probably due to the herb's concentration of betaine, which is a methyl group donor in the liver's transmethylation process.

INDICATIONS AND USAGE

Unproven Uses: Beet is used as supportive therapy in diseases of the liver and fatty liver.

Indian Medicine: The drug is used for coughs and infections.

PRECAUTIONS AND ADVERSE REACTIONS

No health hazards or side effects are known in conjunction with the proper administration of designated therapeutic dosages.

OVERDOSAGE

Taking very large quantities could lead to hypocalcemia and kidney damage because of the drug's oxaluric acid content.

DOSAGE

Mode of Administration: Beet is available as a granular powder in standardized form.

Daily Dosage: For the first 14 days, take 10 gm of drug after meals throughout the course of the day. For long-term treatment, the dose is 5 gm per day for at least 3 months.

LITERATURE

Kern W, List PH, Hörhammer L (Hrsg.), Hagers Handbuch der Pharmazeutischen Praxis, 4. Aufl., Bde 1-8, Springer Verlag Berlin, Heidelberg, New York, 1969.

Behen

Moringa oleifera

DESCRIPTION

Medicinal Parts: The medicinal parts of the plant are the leaves, bark, nuts and root, which have had numerous uses in traditional medicine.

Flower and Fruit: The inflorescence is a leaf-axillary panicle. The flowers are zygomorphic with their structures in fives and a bowel-shaped receptacle. The sepals are linear-lanceolate, irregular and revolute. The petals are spatulate, veined, irregular and white or yellow. There are 5 stamens, and a superior ovary developing from 3 fused carpels. The fruit is a hanging capsule opening on 3 sides, up to 1.2 m long and triangular with 9 ribs. The seeds are triangular, light brown to black, with 3 thin, whitish wings, approximately the size of a hazelnut.

Leaves, Stem and Root: The leaves of the tree are alternate, 30 to 60 cm long, and incompletely triple-pinnate. The leaflets are 12 to 20 mm long and elliptical. The branches are slim.

Characteristics: The flowers are extremely fragrant, and the leaves, root and fruit taste like horseradish.

Habitat: The tree is indigenous to India.

Production: Behen root is the fresh or dried root of Moringa oleifera. Behen nuts are the ripe unpeeled seeds of Moringa oleifera.

Other Names: Ben Nut Tree, Drumstick Tree, Indian Horseradish

ACTIONS AND PHARMACOLOGY

COMPOUNDS: BEHEN ROOT

Glucosinolates: 4-(alpha-L-rhamnosyloxy)benzyl glucosinolate (ca. 1%), yielding 4-(alpha-L-rhamnosyloxy)benzyl isothiocyanate following enzymatic segregation with myrosinase, glucotropaeolin (ca. 0.05%), yielding benzyl isothiocyanate

EFFECTS: BEHEN ROOT

The root is antimicrobial in effect, due to the mustard oils it contains. Applied as a cataplasm, it triggers local hyperemias due to the irritating effect of the isothiocyanates. Dried extracts of the root are abortive and contraceptive in their effect.

COMPOUNDS: BEHEN SEEDS

Glucosinolates (up to 9% in the defatted seeds): 4-(alpha-L-rhamnosyloxy)benzyl glucosinolate, yielding 4-(alpha-L-rhamnosyloxy)benzyl isothiocyanate following enzymatic segregation with myrosinase

Phenol carboxylic acids: 1-beta-D-glucosyl-2,6-dimethyl benzoate

Fatty oil (20 to 50%): chief fatty acids oleic acid (60 to 70%), palmitic acid (3 to 12%), stearic acid (3 to 12%), including as well behenic acid, eicosanoic acid, lignoceric acid

EFFECTS: BEHEN SEEDS

The seeds are antimicrobial in effect, due to the mustard oils they contain.

INDICATIONS AND USAGE

BEHEN ROOT

Unproven Uses: The root has been used internally in folk medicine for gastrointestinal complaints, epilepsy, paralyses, cardiac and blood pressure disturbances, fever (particularly intermittent), scurvy, dizziness and colds. External indications include gingivitis, worm diseases, snake bites, abscesses, inflammation, rheumatism and poorly healing wounds. Root paste has been used to treat worms, rheumatism and headaches.

Indian Medicine: Indications have included smallpox and rheumatism. Efficacy for rheumatism seems plausible because of the stimulating effect of the isothiocyanates. Efficacy for the other indications has not yet been proven.

BEHEN SEEDS

Unproven Uses: Folk medicine indications for internal use are constipation, warts and worms (Central America); for diarrhea (Chad); for splenomegaly, colic, dyspepsia, fever, inflammation of the skin, edema, diabetes, abdominal tumors, paralyses and lumbago (Saudi Arabia). The seeds are used externally for dandruff in Nigeria.

Indian Medicine: Behen seeds are used for fever and as an aphrodisiac. Efficacy for these indications has not yet been proven.

PRECAUTIONS AND ADVERSE REACTIONS

BEHEN ROOT

No health hazards are known in conjunction with the proper administration of designated therapeutic dosages. The ingestion of larger quantities can lead to nausea, dizziness and vomiting.

BEHEN SEEDS

No health hazards are known in conjunction with the proper administration of designated therapeutic dosages.

The single peroral administration of a dosage of 5 g of the drug/kg body weight to a mouse led to hyperkeratosis in the stomach and to liver cell steatosis. Administration of 22 to 50 mg/kg body weight, parenterally, of the glucosinolate mentioned above proved to be fatal for mice.

CONTRAINDICATIONS

BEHEN ROOT

Behen preparations are contraindicated during pregnancy because of their possible abortive effect.

DOSAGE

BEHEN ROOT

Mode of Administration: Preparations of the whole and powdered root are administered internally and externally.

BEHEN SEEDS

Mode of Administration: Preparations of the seed are used internally and externally.

LITERATURE

Hänsel R, Keller K, Rimpler H, Schneider G (Ed), Hagers Handbuch der Pharmazeutischen Praxis, 5. Aufl., Bde 4 - 6 (Drogen), Springer Verlag Berlin, Heidelberg, New York, 1992-1994.

Belladonna

Atropa belladonna

DESCRIPTION

Medicinal Parts: The medicinal parts are the leaves and roots.

Flower and Fruit: The flowers are solitary and hanging. The calyx is fused at the base, has 5 divisions and is spread like a star when the fruit ripens. The violet corolla is a campanulate tube, 2.5 to 3.5 cm long, dirty yellow on the inside with crimson veins. There are 5 stamens and 1 style with a 2-lobed stigma. The ovary is superior. The fruit is a cherry-sized globose berry. The fruit is initially green, then becomes black and glossy with numerous black, ovoid seeds.

Leaves, Stem and Root: Atropa belladonna is a perennial, herbacious plant 1 to 2 m high with a many-headed cylindrical rhizome. The woody stem is erect, branched, bluntly angular and hairy. The leaves are ovately pointed, entire-margined, downy and up to 15 cm long. The lower leaves are alternate. Near the inflorescence the leaves are in pairs of 1 large and 1 small.

Characteristics: Belladonna has a strong narcotic smell, a sharp and bitter taste, and is poisonous.

Habitat: The plant is found throughout western, central and southern Europe, in the Balkans, southeast Asia, Iran, northern Africa, Denmark, Sweden and Ireland. It is cultivated in other countries, particularly England, France and the U.S.

Production: Belladonna leaf consists of the dried leaves, or the dried leaves together with the flowering branch tips, of Atropa belladonna. The leaves are collected in the wild from May to July. They are dried at a temperature not exceeding 60°C. Belladonna root consists of the dried roots and rhizomes of Atropa belladonna. The roots of 2- to 4-year-old plants are dug up in mid-October to mid-November or shortly before the start of the flowering season. They are cleaned and dried at a maximum temperature of 50°C.

Not to be Confused With: Belladonna leaf should not be confused with Ailanthus altissimus, Phytolacca americana or Scopolia carniolica. Belladonna root should not be confused with Atropa acuminata. It is sometimes adulterated with Phytolacca americana and Scopolia cariolica.

Other Names: Deadly Nightshade, Devil's Cherries, Devil's Herb, Divale, Dwale, Dwayberry, Great Morel, Naughty Man's Cherries, Poison Black Cherry

ACTIONS AND PHARMACOLOGY

COMPOUNDS: BELLADONNA LEAF

Tropan alkaloids: chief alkaloid (-)-hyoscyamine, which during drying transforms to some extent into atropine, as well as apoatropine, scopolamine and tropine

Flavonoids

Hydroxycoumarins: including scopoline, scopoletine

Tannins

COMPOUNDS: BELLADONNA ROOT

Tropan alkaloids: chief alkaloid (-)-hyoscyamine, in drying transformed to some extent during dehydration into atropine as well as apoatropine, 3alpha-phenylacetoxytropane, tropine, cuskhygrine, scopolamine, pseudotropine

EFFECTS: BELLADONNA LEAF AND ROOT

The tropane alkaloids in the drug (atropine, scopolamine, tropine etc.) are responsible for the anti-cholinergic-parasympatholytic, spasmolytic, positive, dromotropic and chronotropic effect. Atropa belladonna preparations act as a parasympatholytic or anticholinergic via a competitive antagonism of the neuromuscular transmitter acetylcholine. This antagonism concerns mainly the muscarine-like effect of acetylcholine and less the nicotine-like effects on the ganglions and the neuromuscular end plate. Atropa belladonna preparations release peripheral effects targeted on the vegetative nervous system and the smooth muscle system, as well as the central nervous system. Because of the parasympatholytic properties, the drug can cause relaxation of organs with smooth muscles and relieve spastic conditions, especially in the gastrointestinal tract and bile ducts. Additionally, Belladonna use may result in muscular tremor or rigidity due to effects on the central nervous system. Atropa belladonna preparations have a positive dromotropic as well as a positive chronotropic effect on the heart. The drug has always been important in folk medicine for its hallucinogenic effect.

INDICATIONS AND USAGE

BELLADONNA LEAF

Approved by Commission E:

- Liver and gall bladder complaints

Unproven Uses: Belladonna leaf is used for spasms and colic-like pain in the gastrointestinal tract and bile ducts. External uses include gout and ulcers. In folk medicine, the drug is contained in medicinal plasters and is applied for neuro-vegetative disorders, hyperkinesis, hyperhidrosis and bronchial asthma.

Homeopathic Uses: Homeopathic uses include meningitis as well as inflammations (accompanied by fever) of the tonsils, respiratory organs, the urogenital tract, the skin, the joints and the gastrointestinal tract.

BELLADONNA ROOT
Approved by Commission E:
■ Liver and gall bladder complaints

Unproven Uses: The drug is used for arrhythmia, cardiac insufficiency NYHA I and II, nervous heart complaints, and colic-like pains in the gastrointestinal tract and bile ducts. In folk medicine, a drug from the leaves is preferred for pain in the gastrointestinal area, for asthma, bronchitis and muscular pain. (Also see Belladonna leaf.)

PRECAUTIONS AND ADVERSE REACTIONS

BELLADONNA LEAF AND ROOT
General: No health hazards are known in conjunction with the proper administration of designated therapeutic dosages. The following could occur as side effects, particularly with overdoses: erubescence, dryness of the mouth, mydriasis, and tachycardiac arrhythmias. These are early signs of atropine poisoning. Other side effects may include hypocycloses, heat accumulation through reduction of perspiration, micturation difficulties and obstipation. Because of potential ramifications, Belladonna should be used only under the supervision of an expert familiar with the appropriate use of this substance.

Pediatric Use: The fatal dose in children is considerably less than that of adults.

Drug Interactions: Tricyclic antidepressants, amantadine and quinidine will increase the anticholinergic effect.

OVERDOSAGE

BELLADONNA LEAF AND ROOT
High dosages lead to central excitation that may produce restlessness, compulsion to talk, hallucinations, delirium and manic attacks, followed by exhaustion and sleep. The fatal dose depends on the atropine content; asphyxiation can occur with 100 mg atropine, which corresponds to 5 to 50 g of Belladonna. Treatment of poisonings consists of gastric lavage, application of wet cloths to reduce body temperature (avoid antipyretics), oxygen respiration for breathing distress, intubation, parenteral physostigmine salts as an antidote, diazepam for spasm and chlorpromazine for serious excitation. (Also see side effects listed under PRECAUTIONS AND ADVERSE REACTIONS, which may be early signs of poisoning.)

DOSAGE

BELLADONNA LEAF
Mode of Administration: The comminuted drug is used for decoctions and dried extracts, and the powdered drug is used internally for galenic preparations. Due to the toxicity, the drug must be handled with care.

How Supplied: Forms of commercial pharmaceutical preparations include coated and uncoated tablets, drops, tea, juice, syrup, ampules, capsules, suppositories, plaster and ophthalmic drops.

Daily Dosage: When using Belladonna powder (belladonnae pulvis normatus-total alkaloid content 0.28% to 0.32% German pharmacopoeia 10), the average single dose is 0.05 to 0.10 g. The maximum single dose is 0.20 g, which is equivalent to 0.60 mg total alkaloids, calculated as hyoscyamine. The maximum daily dosage is 0.60 g, which is equivalent to 1.8 mg total alkaloids, calculated as hyoscyamine.

For Belladonna extract, the average single dose is 0.01 g. The maximum single dose is 0.05 g, which is equivalent to 0.73 mg total alkaloids, calculated as hyoscyamine. The maximum daily dosage is 0.150 g, which is equivalent to 2.2 mg total alkaloids, calculated as hyoscyamine.

Storage: Belladonna leaves and various leaf preparations have specific storage requirements. Store leaves and powders tightly sealed and protected from light. Extracts require protection from moisture and light as well as a temperature of approximately 30°C. Store tinctures tightly sealed without exposure to direct sunlight or extreme heat to attain a shelf life of approximately 3.5 years.

BELLADONNA ROOT
Mode of Administration: As a comminuted drug for infusions and dried extracts and as a powdered drug for other galenic preparations for internal use.

Daily Dosage: The average daily dosage is 0.3 g, which is equivalent to 1.5 mg total alkaloids, calculated as hyoscyamine. Single doses range from 0.05 g to a maximum of 0.1 g.

For Belladonna extract, the total alkaloids range from 1.3% to 1.45% (German pharmacopoeia 10). Single doses of the extract range from 0.01 g to 0.05 g. The maximum daily dosage is 0.15 g, which is equivalent to 2.2 mg total alkaloids, calculated as hyoscyamine.

For Belladonna tincture, a single dose of 0.5 to 2 ml is given 3 times daily.

Homeopathic Dosage: 5 to 10 drops, 1 tablet, 5 to 10 globules, 1 to 3 times daily or 1 ml injection solution twice weekly sc. From D3: one suppository 2 to 3 times daily; ointments 1 to 2 times daily (HAB1).

Storage: Belladonna root should be stored for a maximum of 3 years in well-sealed containers protected from light and insects.

LITERATURE

BELLADONNA LEAF AND ROOT

Fintelmann V, Phytopharmaka in der Gastroenterologie. In: ZPT 15(3):137. 1994.

Hartmann Th et al., Reinvestigation of the alkaloid composition of Atropa belladonna plants, roots cultures, and cell suspension. In: PM 53:390-395. 1986.

Phillipson JD et al., (1975) Phytochemistry 14: 999-1003.

Further information in:

Frohne D, Pfänder HJ, Giftpflanzen - Ein Handbuch für Apotheker, Toxikologen und Biologen, 4. Aufl., Wiss. Verlags-Ges Stuttgart 1997.

Hänsel R, Keller K, Rimpler H, Schneider G (Hrsg.), Hagers Handbuch der Pharmazeutischen Praxis, 5. Aufl., Bde 4-6 (Drogen), Springer Verlag Berlin, Heidelberg, New York, 1992-1994.

Leung AY, Encyclopedia of Common Natural Ingredients Used in Food Drugs and Cosmetics, John Wiley & Sons Inc., New York 1980.

Lewin L, Gifte und Vergiftungen, 6. Aufl., Nachdruck, Haug Verlag, Heidelberg 1992.

Madaus G, Lehrbuch der Biologischen Arzneimittel, Bde 1-3, Nachdruck, Georg Olms Verlag Hildesheim 1979.

Roth L, Daunderer M, Kormann K, Giftpflanzen, Pflanzengifte, 4. Aufl., Ecomed Fachverlag Landsberg Lech 1993.

Steinegger E, Hänsel R, Pharmakognosie, 5. Aufl., Springer Verlag Heidelberg 1992.

Teuscher E, Biogene Arzneimittel, 5. Aufl., Wiss. Verlagsges. Stuttgart 1997.

Teuscher E, Lindequist U, Biogene Gifte - Biologie, Chemie, Pharmakologie, 2. Aufl., Fischer Verlag Stuttgart 1994.

f Wagner H, Wiesenauer M, Phytotherapie. Phytopharmaka und pflanzliche Homöopathika, Fischer-Verlag, Stuttgart, Jena, New York 1995.

BELLADONNA ROOT

Fintelmann V, Phytopharmaka in der Gastroenterologie. In: ZPT 15(3):137. 1994.

Hartmann Th et al., Reinvestigation of the alkaloid composition of Atropa belladonna plants, roots cultures, and cell suspension. In: PM 53:390-395. 1986.

Phillipson JD et al., (1975) Phytochemistry 14: 999.

Further information in:

Frohne D, Pfänder HJ, Giftpflanzen - Ein Handbuch für Apotheker, Toxikologen und Biologen, 4. Aufl., Wiss. Verlags-Ges Stuttgart 1997.

Hänsel R, Keller K, Rimpler H, Schneider G (Hrsg.), Hagers Handbuch der Pharmazeutischen Praxis, 5. Aufl., Bde 4-6 (Drogen), Springer Verlag Berlin, Heidelberg, New York, 1992-1994.

Leung AY, Encyclopedia of Common Natural Ingredients Used in Food Drugs and Cosmetics, John Wiley & Sons Inc., New York 1980.

Lewin L, Gifte und Vergiftungen, 6. Aufl., Nachdruck, Haug Verlag, Heidelberg 1992.

Madaus G, Lehrbuch der Biologischen Arzneimittel, Bde 1-3, Nachdruck, Georg Olms Verlag Hildesheim 1979.

Roth L, Daunderer M, Kormann K, Giftpflanzen, Pflanzengifte, 4. Aufl., Ecomed Fachverlag Landsberg Lech 1993.

Steinegger E, Hänsel R, Pharmakognosie, 5. Aufl., Springer Verlag Heidelberg 1992.

Teuscher E, Lindequist U, Biogene Gifte - Biologie, Chemie, Pharmakologie, 2. Aufl., Fischer Verlag Stuttgart 1994.

Teuscher E, Biogene Arzneimittel, 5. Aufl., Wiss. Verlagsges. Stuttgart 1997.

Wagner H, Wiesenauer M, Phytotherapie. Phytopharmaka und pflanzliche Homöopathika, Fischer-Verlag, Stuttgart, Jena, New York 1995.

Bellis perennis

See Wild Daisy

Bennet's Root

Geum urbanum

DESCRIPTION

Medicinal Parts: The medicinal parts of the plant are the dried flowering herb, the dried or fresh underground parts and the roots.

Flower and Fruit: The inflorescence is a loose panicled, umbelled cyme with a few terminal and erect flowers. The pedicles are short-haired. The sepals are 3 to 8 cm long with long tips, pubescent on the outside and glabrous on the inside, except for a tomentose border. The epicalyx bracts are half as long as the sepals, pubescent on both sides and narrowly lanceolate. The yellow petals are 3 to 7 mm long, slightly stemmed, and drop easily. The style is jointed and the stigma flat. The small fruits have no stems and are pubescent.

Leaves, Stem and Root: The plant is a semi-rosette shrub with a primary root that dies off early and is replaced by adventitious roots. The rhizome is simple, thick, cylindrical and crooked. The stem is erect, soft-haired, 15 to 70 cm high; it sprouts from the basal rosette. The basal leaves are rosette-like and pinnate. The cauline leaves are trifoliate to tri-pinnate and the stipules are small, fused with the stem in the lower part, and ovate-lanceolate roughly dentate to pinnatesect.

Characteristics: The plant's root has a clove-like scent.

Habitat: Bennet's Root is found in central and southern Europe, central Asia and North America.

Production: Bennet's Root herb is the aerial part of Geum urbanum. Bennet's Root (root) is the root of Geum urbanum, which is usually harvested in May and then air-dried or dried artificially at a maximum of 35° C.

Other Names: Avens Root, Colewort, Herb Bennet, City Avens, Wild Rye, Way Bennet, Goldy Star, Geum, European Avens, Blessed Herb, Star of the Earth, Yellow Avens

ACTIONS AND PHARMACOLOGY

COMPOUNDS: BENNET'S ROOT HERB

Tannins: gallo tannins, ellagitannins, including sanguiin H-6, casuarictin, penduncalagin, potentillin, tellimagrandin I

EFFECTS: BENNET'S ROOT HERB

The drug has an astringent effect.

COMPOUNDS: BENNET'S ROOT (ROOT)

In the freshly harvested rhizome:

Tannins

Gein (eugenol-vicianose): transformed through drying or size reduction into eugenol

In the dried rhizome and the roots:

Volatile oil (traces): chief components - eugenol, additionally cis- and trans-myrtanal, cis- and trans-myrtanol

EFFECTS: BENNET'S ROOT (ROOT)

The drug has an astringent effect.

INDICATIONS AND USAGE

BENNET'S ROOT HERB

Unproven Uses: Although rarely used today, folk medicine indications have included use of the drug for digestive complaints and diarrhea, febrile illnesses, and for muscle and nerve pain. Use as a bath additive for hemorrhoids seems plausible due the astringent content.

BENNET'S ROOT (ROOT)

Unproven Uses: Internal folk medicine applications include use for digestive problems such as loss of appetite and diarrhea. The root of Bennet's Root has been used externally as a gargle for gum and mucous membrane inflammations and as a bath additive or poultice for frost bite, hemorrhoids and skin diseases. Efficacy appears plausible due to the astringent properties of the tannins.

Homeopathic Uses: Homeopathic applications include use for inflammations of the bladder and urinary tract.

PRECAUTIONS AND ADVERSE REACTIONS

Health risks or side effects following the proper administration of designated therapeutic dosages are not recorded.

DOSAGE

BENNET'S ROOT HERB

The herb is rarely used medicinally today. It is found in some pharmaceutical preparations.

BENNET'S ROOT (ROOT)

Mode of Administration: Infusions are drunk or applied as an external wash or poultice.

Preparation: To prepare an internal infusion, boil 1/2 to 1 teaspoon coarsely powdered drug in water for 10 minutes and filter. Prepare an external infusion by adding 1 teaspoon coarsely powdered drug to cold water, bringing it briefly to the boil, leaving it to steep for 10 minutes and then straining.

Daily Dosage: Infusion (internal): 1 cup lukewarm several times a day. Infusion (external): Use several times a day for washes or poultices.

Homeopathic Dosage: 5 drops, 1 tablet or 10 globules every 30 to 60 minutes (acute) or 1 to 3 times a day (chronic); parenterally: 1 to 2 ml sc acute, 3 times daily; chronic: once a day (HAB1).

LITERATURE

BENNET'S ROOT HERB

Hänsel R, Keller K, Rimpler H, Schneider G (Hrsg.), Hagers Handbuch der Pharmazeutischen Praxis, 5. Aufl., Bde 4-6 (Drogen), Springer Verlag Berlin, Heidelberg, New York, 1992-1994.

Madaus G, Lehrbuch der Biologischen Arzneimittel, Bde 1-3, Nachdruck, Georg Olms Verlag Hildesheim 1979.

Psenák M et al., (1970) Planta Med 19(2):154.

Vollmann C, Schultze W, Nelkenwurz. In: DAZ 135(14):1238-1248. 1995.

Vollmann C, Untersuchung der Nelkenwurz. In: DAZ 131(40):2081. 1991.

BENNET'S ROOT (ROOT)

Hänsel R, Keller K, Rimpler H, Schneider G (Hrsg.), Hagers Handbuch der Pharmazeutischen Praxis, 5. Aufl., Bde 4-6 (Drogen), Springer Verlag Berlin, Heidelberg, New York, 1992-1994.

Madaus G, Lehrbuch der Biologischen Arzneimittel, Bde 1-3, Nachdruck, Georg Olms Verlag Hildesheim 1979.

Psenák M et al., (1970) Planta Med 19(2):154.

Wichtl M (Hrsg.), Teedrogen, 4. Aufl., Wiss. Verlagsges. Stuttgart 1997.

Vollmann C, Schultze W, Nelkenwurz. In: DAZ 135(14):1238-1248. 1995.

Vollmann C, Untersuchung der Nelkenwurz. In: DAZ 131(40):2081. 1991.

Benzoin

Styrax benzoin

DESCRIPTION

Medicinal Parts: The medicinal part of the plant is the balsamic resin obtained from the mechanically damaged trunk.

Flower and Fruit: The flowers are in terminal or axillary panicled racemes. The flowers are fused and their structures are in fives. The calyx is campanulate, weakly 5 toothed, densely silky tomentose and red-brown on the inside. The corolla is 6 to 11 mm long with 5 tips, brown-red, silky tomentose on the outside and at the margin. There are 8 to 10 stamens fused below to a tube and a 1-chambered ovary above and 2- to 3-chambered ovary below. The fruit is nut-like, appressed pubescent with a diameter of up to 3 cm. The seeds are light brown with 6 longitudinal stripes and are up to 2 cm long.

Leaves, Stem and Root: Styrax benzoin is an evergreen tree, which grows up to 30 m high. The leaves are alternate and the petioles are rust brown-downy pubescent. They are approximately 1 cm long. The lamina is 8 to 13 cm long, 2.5 to 5 cm wide, ovate or elongate with a rounded base and irregularly curved-dentate margin. The lamina is covered with white and brown star hairs beneath. The bark is wine-red and the wood is white.

Characteristics: The flowers have a strong fragrance.

Habitat: The plant is native to western Java and Sumatra.

Production: Sumatra benzoin (Gum benzoin) is the balsamic resin from the damaged trunk of Styrax benzoin and Styrax paralleloneurum. The optimal age of trees to be harvested is 7 years. The tree is cut, causing it to exude resin to heal the cuts. The resin is then collected in a vessel and left to melt to a homogenous mass in the sun.

Other Names: Benjamin Tree

ACTIONS AND PHARMACOLOGY

COMPOUNDS

Ester mixture (70 to 80%): composed of coniferyl benzoate and cinnamyl benzoate, as well as cinnamyl cinnamoate (styracin), propyl cinnamoate

Phenylacrylic acids: cinnamic acid (10%)

Benzoic acid (to 30%)

Resins

EFFECTS

The expectorant effect with which the drug is credited could not be proven experimentally (it possibly originated in connection with an "aroma therapy," due to its vanilla content).

INDICATIONS AND USAGE

Unproven Uses: Benzoin is used for respiratory catarrh.

Chinese Medicine: In China, benzoin is used for stroke, syncopes, post partal syncope due to heavy loss of blood, and for chest and stomach pain.

PRECAUTIONS AND ADVERSE REACTIONS

No health hazards are known in conjunction with the proper administration of designated therapeutic dosages.

DOSAGE

Mode of Administration: Whole herb preparations are for internal use.

Storage: Benzoin should be tightly sealed and stored below 25°C.

LITERATURE

Bacchi EM, Sertié JA, Villa N, Katz H, delta7-stigmasteryl-3 betaD-glucoside from Styrax officinalis. Part II. Planta Med, 61:221-2, 1976 Nov.

Bacchi EM, Sertié JA, Villa N, Katz H, Preliminary investigations on the herba of Styrax officinalis. I. Planta Med, 61:290-3, 1973 Nov.

Hänsel R, Keller K, Rimpler H, Schneider G (Ed), Hagers Handbuch der Pharmazeutischen Praxis, 5. Aufl., Bde 4 - 6 (Drogen), Springer Verlag Berlin, Heidelberg, New York, 1992-1994.

James WD, White SW, Yanklowitz B, Allergic contact dermatitis to compound tincture of benzoin. J Am Acad Dermatol, 11:847-50, 1984 Nov.

Berberis vulgaris

See Barberry

Bergenia crassifolia

See Elephant-Ears

Beta vulgaris

See Beet

Betel Nut

Piper betle

DESCRIPTION

Medicinal Parts: The main medicinal parts are the dried leaves; the roots and the fruit are also used.

Flower and Fruit: The inflorescences are compact, hanging, cylindrical and 3.5 to 5 cm long spikes of yellow-green flowers. There are 2 stamens in the male flowers. The female stamens have an ovary, which is pubescent at the top and has 3 to 5 stigmas. The fruit is globular, fleshy and about 6 mm in diameter. The fruit is yellow and becomes red when ripe. The seeds are also globular.

Leaves, Stem and Root: The plant is a dioecious or monoecious woody climber that can grow to 15 m. It has numerous small and short adventitious roots. The stem is thickened at the nodes, and the younger parts are glabrous. The leaves have a 2.5 to 5 cm long petiole, are broadly cordate, 5 to 18 cm long and half as wide. The leaves are glabrous, light green and glossy on both surfaces with 5 to 7 radiating ribs.

Habitat: Piper betle is found in tropical southern Asia and has been introduced to east Africa, Madagascar and the West Indies.

Production: Betel Nut leaves are the leaves of Piper betle. When the leaves are green, they are gathered, pressed and dried.

Other Names: Betel

ACTIONS AND PHARMACOLOGY

COMPOUNDS

Volatile oil (0.8-1.8%): chief components- chavibetol (betel phenol), eugenol, additionally allylpyrocatechol (hydroxy-chavicol), allylpyrocatechol-mono and -diacetate, anethole, chavibetolacetate, chavicol, methyl eugenol, safrol

Neolignans: including crotepoxide, piperbetol, piperol, among others

EFFECTS

The essential oils are antimicrobial and immune-modulating. The Betel leaf is centrally sedating.

INDICATIONS AND USAGE

Unproven Uses: In folk medicine, Betel Nut is used for coughs, as an expectorant for stomach ailments, diphtheria and inflammation of the middle ear.

Indian Medicine: In India, Betel Nut is used to treat asthma, bronchitis, coughs, dyspepsia, rheumatism, leprosy, severe thirst, alcoholism, syncopes, toothache and impotency.

PRECAUTIONS AND ADVERSE REACTIONS

No health hazards or side effects are known in conjunction with the proper administration of designated therapeutic dosages.

DOSAGE

Mode of Administration: Today, the drug is obsolete.

LITERATURE

Das PC, Sarkar AK, (1979) Acta Physiol Pol. 30(3):389.

Rawat AKS et al., Ind Perf 31:146-149. 1987.

Sharma ML et al., Ind Perf 26:134-137. 1982.

Further information in:

Hänsel R, Keller K, Rimpler H, Schneider G (Hrsg.), Hagers Handbuch der Pharmazeutischen Praxis, 5. Aufl., Bde 4-6 (Drogen), Springer Verlag Berlin, Heidelberg, New York, 1992-1994.

Roth L, Daunderer M, Kormann K, Giftpflanzen, Pflanzengifte, 4. Aufl., Ecomed Fachverlag Landsberg Lech 1993.

Beth Root

Trillium erectum

DESCRIPTION

Medicinal Parts: The medicinal parts are the rhizome and the dried root and the leaves.

Flower and Fruit: The plant has solitary, terminal, hanging flowers. The 3 green, persistent sepals and the 3 large, white to red or yellow, wilting sepals are characteristic.

Leaves, Stem and Root: The plant is a perennial, smooth herb with an erect stem, which grows from 25 to 40 cm high. It bears 3 whorled, terminal leaves under the flower, which are broad, rhomboid and lightly curled. The rhizome is matte brown, subconical, more or less compressed, 3 to 5 cm long and 2 to 3 cm in diameter. It is often ringed with oblique lines and with numerous wrinkled root fibres on the upper surface.

Characteristics: The taste is sweetish then acrid and the odor is characteristic.

Habitat: The plant is indigenous to the central and western U.S.

Production: Beth Root Stock is the rhizome of Trillium erectum, Trillium pendulum and other varieties.

Other Names: Birthroot, Indian Shamrock, Lamb's Quarters, Wake-Robin, Indian Balm, Ground Lily, Coughroot, Jew's-Harp Plant, Milk Ipecac, Pariswort, Rattlesnake Root, Snakebite, Three-Leaved, Nightshade

ACTIONS AND PHARMACOLOGY

COMPOUNDS

Steroid saponins: including among others, trillin (disogenin monoglucoside), trillarin (disogenin diglucoside), aglycones including cryptogenin, chlorogenin, nologenin

Tannins

EFFECTS

The drug has astringent and expectorant properties. It can severely irritate the area to which it has been applied; the irritation can cause vomiting.

INDICATIONS AND USAGE

Unproven Uses: Internally, Beth Root is used internally for long and heavy menstruation and externally, it is used for varicose veins, ulcers, hematoma, and hemorrhoidal bleeding.

CONTRAINDICATIONS

The drug should not be used during pregnancy.

PRECAUTIONS AND ADVERSE REACTIONS

No health hazards or side effects are known in conjunction with the proper administration of designated therapeutic dosages. In higher dosages, the drug is said to be nauseant, and to have the effect of promoting labor and menstruation.

Pregnancy: In high dosages, the drug promotes labor; therefore, it should not be used during pregnancy.

DOSAGE

Mode of Administration: The ground drug and liquid extract are used for infusions and poultices.

Daily Dosage: The usual dose is 2 to 4 gm dissolved in liquid as an infusion.

LITERATURE

Fukuda N et al., (1981) Chem Pharm Bull 29 (2):325.

Hegnauer R, Chemotaxonomie der Pflanzen, Bde 1-11: Birkhäuser Verlag Basel, Boston, Berlin 1962-1997.

Kern W, List PH, Hörhammer L (Hrsg.), Hagers Handbuch der Pharmazeutischen Praxis, 4. Aufl., Bde. 1-8: Springer Verlag Berlin, Heidelberg, New York, 1969.

Madaus G, Lehrbuch der Biologischen Arzneimittel, Bde 1-3, Nachdruck, Georg Olms Verlag Hildesheim 1979.

Nakano K et al., (1982) J Chem Soc Chem Commun. 789.

Nakano K et al., (1982) Yakugaku Zasshi 102(11):1031.

Nakano K et al., (1983) Phytochemistry 22 (5):1249.

Roth L, Daunderer M, Kormann K, Giftpflanzen, Pflanzengifte, 4. Aufl., Ecomed Fachverlag Landsberg Lech 1993.

Wolters B, Zierpflanzen aus Nordamerika. In: DAZ 137(26):2253-2261. 1997.

Betonica officinalis

See Wood Betony

Betula species

See Birch

Bidens tripartita

See Burr Marigold

Bilberry

Vaccinium myrtillus

TRADE NAMES

Bilberry, Bilberry Extract, Bilberry Herb (available from numerous manufacturers,) Time Release Bilberry Power, Standardized Bilberry Extract, Super Bilberry Plus, Bilberry Power, Bilberry Leaf

DESCRIPTION

Medicinal Parts: The medicinal parts are the dried leaves, the ripe, dried fruit and the ripe fresh fruit.

Flower and Fruit: The flowers are axillary and solitary. They are 4 to 7 mm long, short-pedicled, greenish and tinged with pale pink. The calyx is fused to the ovary, persistent and indistinctly 5-lobed. The corolla is globular-jug-shaped and has 5 tips. There are 8 to 10 stamens, which are enclosed and shorter than the styles. They have glabrous filaments that widen toward the base and 2 horn-like yellow-brown anthers, whose spurred appendage is erect. The fruit is a globular, blue-black, frosted, many-seeded berry with purple pulp.

Leaves, Stem and Root: The plant is a deciduous, dwarf shrub with sharp-edged, green branches 15 to 50 cm high. The leaves are alternate, ovate or oblong-ovate, acuminate and finely serrate.

Habitat: The plant is common to central and northern Europe, Asia and North America.

Production: The leaves and fruit of Bilberry are collected in the wild from July to August and dried in the shade.

Not to be Confused With: Myrtilli folium should not be confused with the fruits of Vaccinium uliginosum.

Other Names: Whortleberry, Blueberry, Burren myrtle, Dyeberry, Huckleberry, Hurtleberry, Wineberry, Black Whortles, Hurts, Bleaberry, Airelle, Trackleberry

ACTIONS AND PHARMACOLOGY

COMPOUNDS: BILBERRY LEAF

Catechin tannins (1 to 7%): including oligomeric proanthocyandins

Flavonoids: including among others, avicularin, hyperoside, isoquercitrin, quercitrin, meratine, astragaline

Iridoide monoterpenes: asperuloside, monotropein

Caffeic acid derivatives: chlorogenic acid

Phenolic acids: including among others, salicylic acid, gentisic acid

Quinolizidine alkaloids: myrtine, epimyrtine (hybrids of Vaccinium myrtillus x V. vitis-idaea contain arbutin [hydroquine glucosides]).

EFFECTS: BILBERRY LEAF

The drug is astringent and useful for treating diarrhea due to the catechin tannin content. The drug is antiviral and, in animal experiments, lipid-lowering.

It is thought that the chromium content of the drug is responsible for a possible antidiabetic effect.

COMPOUNDS: BILBERRY FRUIT

Fruit acids: including among others, quinic acid (3-5%), malic acid, citric acid

Tannins (5-12%): chiefly catechin tannins, including oligomeric procyanidins

Anthocyanoides (0.1% -0.5%): chief components delphinidine-3-O-arabinoside, delphinidine-3-O-galactoside, delphinidine-3-O-glucoside, cyanidin, petunidin, peonidin, malvidin

Flavonoids: including among others, hyperoside, isoquercitrin, quercitrin, astragaline

Iridoids: including asperuloside, onotropein (only in the unripe fruits)

Caffeic acid derivatives: chlorogenic acid

Pectins

EFFECTS: BILBERRY FRUIT

The drug is an astringent and has anti-diarrheal action due to the catechin tannin content which is also responsible for the wound healing effect.

Limited data show that the bilberry anthranocyoside is anti-exudative, vessel-protective, inhibits platelet aggregation in human blood and has an anti-ulcer effect.

Several animal studies have demonstrated that anthocyanosides have a collagen stabilizing effect, and provide protection againts ischemia reperfusion injury (Bertuglia, 1995.) Increased synthesis of connective tissue is one of the contributing factors that may lead to blindness caused by diabetic retinopathy. Anthocyanides have been shown to slow the synthesis of polymeric collagen in diabetic patients (Boniface, 1996.)

CLINICAL STUDIES

One case study involving 20 patients with diabetic retinopathy that were treated with 400 mg of Bilberry extract twice daily demonstrated increased conjunctival capillary resistance in the subjects that were evaluated. The authors of the study concluded that Bilberry provides protection against hemorrhage of the retina (Sevin, 1996.)

INDICATIONS AND USAGE

BILBERRY LEAF

Unproven Uses: Bilberry has been used in Diabetes Mellitus (for prevention and treatment); complaints of the gastrointestinal tract, kidney and urinary tract, arthritis, gout and dermatitis. External uses include inflammation of the oral mucosa, eye inflammation, burns and skin diseases.

BILBERRY FRUIT

- Diarrhea
- Inflammation of the mouth and pharynx

Internally, Bilberry is used for nonspecific, acute diarrhea (particularly in light cases of enteritis). Externally the berry is used for mild inflammation of the mucous membranes of mouth and throat.

Unproven Uses: Well constructed clinical studies in humans that give conclusive support for use of Bilberry in the treatment of diabetic retinopathy or as a treatment for improving night vision are not available. There is moderate support in animal model trials that support the vasoprotective and anti-edema properties of Bilberry. The literature also demonstrates efficacy in animal models for the treatment of diabetes, hyperlipidemia and gastric ulcers. Folk medicine uses include internal use for vomiting, bleeding and hemorroids and external use for poorly healing skin ulcers and wound healing.

PRECAUTIONS AND ADVERSE REACTIONS

BILBERRY LEAF

General: No health hazards or side effects are known in conjunction with the proper administration of designated therapeutic dosages. Digestive complaints due to the high tannin content are possible.

Drug Interactions: Bilberry has a platelet aggregation inhibiting effect. There is a possiblility that the herb can interact with other platelet aggregation inhibitors such as aspirin and anticoagulants like warfarin.

BILBERRY FRUIT

No health hazards or side effects are known in conjunction with the proper administration of designated therapeutic dosages.

OVERDOSAGE

BILBERRY LEAF

The signs of poisoning observed in animal experiments (including cachexia, anemia, icterus) appeared only in conjunction with the chronic administration of high dosages and are presumably effects of the tannins.

DOSAGE

BILBERRY LEAF

Preparation: To prepare an infusion, pour boiling water over 1 g finely cut drug (1 teaspoonful = approximately 0.6g) and strain after 10 to 15 minutes. Not to be taken over a long duration.

Daily Dosage: The daily dosage of tea is 1 cup 2 to 3 times daily. For an infusion, a single dose is equal to 1 g per cup.

BILBERRY FRUIT

Mode of Administration: Tablets, capsules, macerated drug for infusions for internal use and local application.

How Supplied:

Most commercially available capsules and tablets are standardized at 25 to 36% anthocyanoside content.

Capsule — 40 mg, 60 mg, 80 mg, 125 mg, 160 mg, 310 mg, 400 mg, 500 mg, 1000 mg

Tablet — 40 mg

Preparation: To prepare an infusion, use 5 to 10 g mashed drug in cold water; bring to a simmer for 10 minutes, then strain (1 teaspoonful = 4 g drug). A 10% decoction is prepared for external use.

Daily Dose: 20 to 60 g of unprocessed fruit for internal use. Externally use a 10% infusion. For commercially available tablets and capsules that are standardized to 36% anthocyanosides, the recommended dose is 60 to 160 mg three times daily.

LITERATURE

BILBERRY LEAF

Bertuglia S, Malandrino S,Colantuoni A Effect of Vaccinium myrtillus anthocyanosides on ischaemia reperfusion injury in hamster cheek pouch microcirculation. Pharmacol Res, 84:183-7, Mar-Apr, 1995.

Bettini V et al., (1984) Fitoterapia 55(6):323.

Bettini V et al., (1985) Fitoterapia 56(1):3.

Bomser J et al., In vitro anticancer activity of fruit extracts from Vaccinium species. In: PM 62(3):212-216. 1996.

Bosio E et al., Ginkgo biloba L. and Vaccinium myrtillus L. extracts prevent photo-induced oxidation of low density lipoproteins. In: PM 62, Abstracts of the 44th Ann Congress of GA, 24. 1996.

Cignarella A, Bertozzi D, Pinna C, Puglisi L, Hypolipidemic activity of Vaccinium myrtillus leaves on an model of genetically hyperlipidemic rat. In: PM 58(Suppl. 7):A581. 1992.

Colantuoni A, Bertuglia S, Magistretti MJ, Donato L Effects of Vaccinium Myrtillus anthocyanosides on arterial vasomotion. Arzneimittelforschung, 84:905-9, Sep, 1991.

Dombrowicz E, Zadernowski R, Swiatek L Phenolic acids in leaves of Arctostaphylos uva ursi L. Vaccinium vitis idaea L. and Vaccinium myrtillus L. Pharmazie, 84:680-1, Sep, 1991.

Frohne D, Vaccinium myrtillus L.- Die Heidelbeere. In: ZPT 11(6):209-211. 1999.

Kyerematen G, Sandberg F, (1986) Acta Pharm Suec. 23:101.

Sticher O et al., (1979) Planta Med 35:253.

Further information in:

Hänsel R, Keller K, Rimpler H, Schneider G (Hrsg.), Hagers Handbuch der Pharmazeutischen Praxis, 5. Aufl., Bde 4-6 (Drogen): Springer Verlag Berlin, Heidelberg, New York, 1992-1994.

Madaus G, Lehrbuch der Biologischen Arzneimittel, Bde 1-3, Nachdruck, Georg Olms Verlag Hildesheim 1979.

Roth L, Daunderer M, Kormann K, Giftpflanzen, Pflanzengifte, 4. Aufl., Ecomed Fachverlag Landsberg Lech 1993.

Teuscher E, Biogene Arzneimittel, 5. Aufl., Wiss. Verlagsges. Stuttgart 1997.

Wichtl M (Hrsg.), Teedrogen, 4. Aufl., Wiss. Verlagsges. Stuttgart 1997.

BILBERRY FRUIT

Bertuglia S, et al. Effect of Vacciniu myrtillus anthocyanosides on ischaema reperfusion injury in hamster cheek pouch microcirculation. Pharmaol Res:31; 183-187. 1995.

Bettini V et al., (1984) Fitoterapia 55(6):323.

Bettini V et al., (1985) Fitoterapia 56(1):3.

Bomser J et al., In vitro anticancer activity of fruit extracts from Vaccinium species. In: PM 62(3):212-216. 1996.

Boniface R & Robert AM: Influence of anthocyanosides on human connective tissue metabolism. Klin Monatsbl Augenheilkd 209(6):368-372. 1996.

Bosio E et al., Ginkgo biloba L. and Vaccinium myrtillus L. extracts prevent photo-induced oxidation of low density lipoproteins. In: PM 62, Abstracts of the 44th Ann Congress of GA, 24. 1996.

Cignarella A, Bertozzi D, Pinna C, Puglisi L, Hypolipidemic activity of Vaccinium myrtillus leaves on an model of genetically hyperlipidemic rat. In: PM 58(Suppl. 7):A581. 1992.

Frohne D, Vaccinium myrtillus L.- Die Heidelbeere. In: ZPT 11(6):209-211. 1999.

Kyerematen G, Sandberg F, (1986) Acta Pharm Suec 23:101.

Sevin R, Cuendent JF. Effects d'unne association d'anthocyanosides de myrtille et de beta-carotene sur la resistance capillaire des diabetiques. Ophthalmologica: 152:109-117. 1966.

Sticher O et al., (1979) Planta Med 35:253.

Further information in:

Hänsel R, Keller K, Rimpler H, Schneider G (Hrsg.), Hagers Handbuch der Pharmazeutischen Praxis, 5. Aufl., Bde 4-6 (Drogen), Springer Verlag Berlin, Heidelberg, New York, 1992-1994.

Madaus G, Lehrbuch der Biologischen Arzneimittel, Bde 1-3, Nachdruck, Georg Olms Verlag Hildesheim 1979.

Roth L, Daunderer M, Kormann K, Giftpflanzen, Pflanzengifte, 4. Aufl., Ecomed Fachverlag Landsberg Lech 1993.

Steinegger E, Hänsel R, Pharmakognosie, 5. Aufl., Springer Verlag Heidelberg 1992.

Teuscher E, Biogene Arzneimittel, 5. Aufl., Wiss. Verlagsges. Stuttgart 1997.

Wichtl M (Hrsg.), Teedrogen, 4. Aufl., Wiss. Verlagsges. Stuttgart 1997.

Birch

Betula species

DESCRIPTION

Medicinal Parts: The medicinal parts are the bark, leaves and buds.

Flower and Fruit: The male flowers of Betula pendula are sessile and oblong-cylindrical 6 to 10 cm long. The female catkins are petioled, cylindrical and 2 to 4 cm long by 8 to 10 mm thick when fully grown. They are densely flowered, first yellow-green, later light green. The fruit scales are brownish and pubescent or glabrous. The middle lobes are small, short-triangular and shorter than the broad, always revolute side lobes. The fruit wings are half-oval and 2 to 3 times as broad as the fruit.

The male catkins of Betula pubescens are sessile and oblong-cylindrical. They are initially upright, later hanging, 2.5 to 4 cm long and 6 to 10 mm thick, greenish to light brown. The middle lobes of the fruit scales protrude clearly, are usually linguiform-elogated and generally longer than the usually sharp-cornered, clearly evolute side lobes. The fruit scales are about as broad as the fruit.

Leaves, Stem and Root: Betula pendula is a tree that grows up to 30 cm high, with a snow white bark that usually peels off in horizontal strips or changes into a black, stony, hard bark. Young branches are glabrous and thickly covered in warty resin glands. The petioled leaves are dark green above, a lighter gray-green below. They have serrate margins and particularly tightly packed veins. The lamina are about 3 to 7 cm long by 2 to 5 cm wide, rhomboid-triangular, acuminate, glabrous, densely covered in glands, and have a doubly serrate margin. They are dark green and glabrous above and a lighter green below; they are initially downy and later pubescent in the vein axils.

Habitat: Betula pendula and Betula pubescens are indigenous to Europe from the northern Mediterranean regions to Siberia and to temperate regions of Asia.

Production: Birch leaf consists of the fresh or dried leaf of Betula pendula (syn. Betula verrucosa), Betula pubescens, or of both species. The leaves are collected in the wild during the spring and dried at room temperature in the shade. Birch tar (Betulae oleum empyreumaticum retificatum) is a clear, dark brown oil obtained from Betula pendula or Betula pubescens through a distillation process.

ACTIONS AND PHARMACOLOGY

COMPOUNDS: BIRCH LEAF

Triterpene alcohol ester with saponin-like effect: betula-triterpene saponins

Flavonoids: including hyperoside, quercetin, myricetin digalactosides

Proanthocyanidins

Volatile oil: including sesquiterpene oxide

Monoterpene glucosides: including betula alboside A and B, roseoside

Caffeic acid derivatives: including chlorogenic acid

Ascorbic acid

3,4'-dihydroxy propiophenone-3-beta-D-glucoside

EFFECTS: BIRCH LEAF

Birch leaves have a mild saluretic effect and are antipyretic. In animal tests, they have been shown to increase the amount of urine.

COMPOUNDS: BIRCH TAR

Phenols (6%): including among others guaiacol, cresole, catechol, pyrogallol, 5-propyl-pyrogallol dimethyl ether and 5-methyl-pyrogallol dimethyl ether

EFFECTS: BIRCH TAR

The aliphatic and aromatic hydrocarbons in birch tar are irritating to the skin and have an antiparasitic effect. Its use for diverse skin conditions and for parasitic infestation such as scabies seems plausible.

INDICATIONS AND USAGE

BIRCH LEAVES

Approved by Commission E:

- Infections of the urinary tract
- Kidney and bladder stones
- Rheumatism

Unproven Uses: The leaves are used in flushing-out therapy for bacterial and inflammatory diseases of the urinary tract and for kidney gravel. They are also used in adjunct therapy for rheumatic ailments, for increasing amount of urine. In folk medicine, the leaves are used as a blood purifier, and for gout and rheumatism. Externally, the leaves are used for hair loss and dandruff.

BIRCH TAR

Unproven Uses: External birch tar uses include parasitic infestation of the skin with subsequent hair loss, rheumatism and gout (ointment); dry eczema and dermatoses (liquid preparations), psoriasis and other chronic skin diseases. Birch tar is a constituent of "Unguentum contra scabiem" that is used for the treatment of scabies.

CONTRAINDICATIONS

BIRCH LEAF

The drug should not be used for edema when there is reduced cardiac or kidney function.

PRECAUTIONS AND ADVERSE REACTIONS

BIRCH LEAF

No health hazards or side effects are known in conjunction with the proper administration of designated therapeutic dosages.

BIRCH TAR

No health hazards are known in conjunction with the proper administration of designated therapeutic dosages. Birch tar can cause irritations on sensitive skin. Administration of the drug is not advisable, due to the possible presence of cancerogenic hydrocarbons.

DOSAGE

BIRCH LEAF

Mode of Administration: Comminuted herb or dry extracts are used for teas; other galenic preparations and freshly pressed plant juices can also be used internally.

Preparation: Tea is prepared by pouring 150 ml hot water over 1 to 2 dessertspoons of drug and then straining the leaves out after 15 minutes.

Daily Dosage: The average daily dose is 2 to 3 g drug several times a day with a caution to ensure ample intake of fluid (minimum 2 liters per day). A fresh cup of tea is taken between meals 3 to 4 times a day

Storage: Birch leaf should be stored in sealed containers protected from light and moisture.

BIRCH TAR

Mode of Administration: Birch Tar is used in combination preparations as external ointments and liniments.

Storage: Birch tar should be stored in tightly sealed containers.

LITERATURE

BIRCH LEAF

Anonym, Phytotherapie: Pflanzliche Antirheumatika - was bringen sie. In: DAZ 136(45):4012-4015. 1996.

Bufe A, Spangfort MD, Kahlert H, Schlaak M, Becker WM, The major birch pollen allergen Bet v 1 shows ribonuclease activity. Planta, 175:413-5, 1996.

Cadot P, LeJoly M, Van Hoeyveld EM, Stevens EA, Influence of the pH of the extraction medium on the composition of birch (Betula verrucosa) pollen extracts. Allergy, 108:431-7, 1995 May.

Carnat A, Lacouture I, Fraisse D, Lamaison JL, Standardization of the birch leaf. Ann Pharm Fr, 175:231-5, 1996.

Cirla AM, Sforza N, Roffi GP, Alessandrini A, Stanizzi R, Dorigo N, Sala E, Della Torre F, Preseasonal intranasal immunotherapy in birch-alder allergic rhinitis. A double-blind study. Allergy, 175:299-305, 1996 May.

Czygan FC, Betula pendula - Die Birke. Z Phytother 10(1989): 135-139.

Davidov MI, Goriunov VG, Kubarikov PG, Phytoperfusion of the bladder after adenomectomy. Urol Nefrol (Mosk), 175:19-20, 1995 Sep-Oct.

Fountain DW, Berggren B, Nilsson S, Einarsson R, Expression of birch pollen-specific IgE-binding activity in seeds and other plant parts of birch trees (Betula verrucosa Ehrh.). Int Arch Allergy Immunol, 98:370-6, 1992.

Hasler A et al., High-performance liquid chromatographic determination of five widespread flavonoid aglycones. J. Chromatogr. 508, 1(1990): 236-40.

Hiller K, Pharmazeutische Bewertung ausgewählter Teedrogen. In: DAZ 135(16):1425-1440. 1995.

Hörhammer L, Wagner H, Luck R, Arch Pharm 290:338-341. 1957.

Karatodorof K, Kalarova R, (1977) Izn Durzh Inst Kontrol Lek Sredstva 10:103-9.

Keinanen M, Comparison of methods for extraction of flavonoids from birch leaves carried out using high-performance liquid chromatography. J. Agric. Food Chem. 41, 11(1993): 1986-90.

Kiiskinen M, Korhonen M, Kangasjaervi J, Immunological study of the HLA class II antigen associated with birch pollen allergy. Nippon Jibiinkoka Gakkai Kaiho, 35:541-50, 1992 Apr.

Lee MW et al., Phenolic compounds of the leaves of Betula. Arch. Pharmaceutical. Res. 15, 3(1992): 211-14.

Olsen OT et al., A double-blind randomized study investigating the efficacy and specificity of immunotherapy with Artemisia vulgaris or Phleum pratense/betula verrucosa. Allergol Immunopathol (Madr), 23:73-8, 1995 Mar-Apr.

Ossipov V et al., HPLC isolation and identification of flavonoids from white birch. Biochem Syst. Ecol. 23, 3(1995): 213-22.

Pietta PG et al., HPLC determination of the flavonoid glycosides from Betulae folium. Chromatographia, 28, 5-6(1989): 311-12.

Pisha E et al., Discovery of betulinic acid as a selective inhibitor of human melanoma that functions by induction of apoptosis. In: Nature Medicine 1:1046-1051. 1995.

Ramirez J, Carpizo JA, Ipsen H, Carreira J, Lombardero M, Quantification in mass units of Bet v 1 the main allergen of Betula verrucosa pollen by a monoclonal antibody based-ELISA. Clin Exp Allergy, 27:926-31, 1997 Aug.

Rickling B, Glombitza KW, Saponins in the leaves of birch? Hemolytic dammarane triterpenoids esters of Betula pendula. Planta Med 59 (1993), 77.

Schilcher H, Boesel R, Effenberger ST Segebrecht S, Neuere Untersuchungsergebnisse mit aquaretisch, antibakteriell und prostatotrop wirksamen Arzneipflanzen. In: ZPT 10(3):77. 1989.

Schilcher H, Rau H, Nachweis der aquaretischen Wirkung von Birkenblätter- und Goldrutenauszügen im Tierversuch. Urologe B 28(1988): 274-280.

Sökeland J, Phytotherapie in der Urologie. In: ZPT 10(1):8. 1989.

Spangfort MD, Ipsen H, Sparholt SH, Aasmul-Olsen S, Osmark P, Poulsen FM, Larsen M, M rtz E, Roepstorff P, Larsen JN, Characterisation of recombinant isoforms of birch pollen allergen Bet v 1. Adv Exp Med Biol, 175:251-4, 1996.

Tschesche R, Ciper F, Breitmeier E, Chem Ber 110:3111-3117. 1977.

Valenta R, Duchene M, Ebner C, Valent P, Sillaber C, Deviller P, Ferreira F, TeJkl M, Edelmann H, Kraft D, et al., Profilins constitute a novel family of functional plant pan-allergens. J Exp Med, 175:377-85, 1992 Feb 1.

Further information in:

Hänsel R, Keller K, Rimpler H, Schneider G (Hrsg.), Hagers Handbuch der Pharmazeutischen Praxis, 5. Aufl., Bde 4-6 (Drogen), Springer Verlag Berlin, Heidelberg, New York, 1992-1994.

Madaus G, Lehrbuch der Biologischen Arzneimittel, Bde 1-3, Nachdruck, Georg Olms Verlag Hildesheim 1979.

Steinegger E, Hänsel R, Pharmakognosie, 5. Aufl., Springer Verlag Heidelberg 1992.

Teuscher E, Biogene Arzneimittel, 5. Aufl., Wiss. Verlagsges. Stuttgart 1997.

Wagner H, Wiesenauer M, Phytotherapie. Phytopharmaka und pflanzliche Homöopathika, Fischer-Verlag, Stuttgart, Jena, New York 1995.

Wichtl M (Hrsg.), Teedrogen, 4. Aufl., Wiss. Verlagsges. Stuttgart 1997.

BIRCH TAR

Kreitmair H, PA 8:534-536. 1953.

Nowak GA, Am Perf Cosmet 81:37-39. 1966.

Further information in:

Hänsel R, Keller K, Rimpler H, Schneider G (Hrsg.), Hagers Handbuch der Pharmazeutischen Praxis, 5. Aufl., Bde 4-6 (Drogen), Springer Verlag Berlin, Heidelberg, New York, 1992-1994.

Leung AY, Encyclopedia of Common Natural Ingredients Used in Food Drugs and Cosmetics, John Wiley & Sons Inc., New York 1980.

Birthwort

Aristolochia clematitis

DESCRIPTION

Medicinal Parts: The medicinal parts are the aerial portion (when in blossom) and the root.

Flower and Fruit: The plant has dirty yellow flowers, usually in axillary groups of 7. The perigone forms a straight tube, which is bulbous beneath and has a linguiform, oblong-ovate, obtuse border. There are 6 stamens, the style is upward growing, and the stigma is 6-lobed. The flower briefly traps the insects that pollinate it. The fruit is a globose, pear-shaped capsule.

Leaves, Stem and Root: The plant grows to a height of 30 to 100 cm. The stem is erect, simple, grooved and glabrous. The leaves are alternate, long-petioled, cordate-reniform, yellow-green with prominent ribs.

Characteristics: The plant has a fruit-like fragrance and is poisonous.

Habitat: Indigenous to Mediterranean regions, Asia Minor and the Caucasus, but is also found in numerous other regions.

Production: Birthwort is the aerial part of Aristolochia clematitis.

ACTIONS AND PHARMACOLOGY

COMPOUNDS

Aristolochic acids (10-nitro-phenanthrene-1-acids): in particular aristolochic acids I and II

Isoquinoline alkaloids: including magnoflorin, corytuberin

Volatile oil (0.03 to 0.2%): chief constituents alpha-pinene, alpha-terpineol

EFFECTS

The aristolochic acids have a phagocytosis- and metabolism-activating effect. They are also thought to improve the production of lymphokinins. Activation of phagocytes has been demonstrated in animal tests in rabbits and guinea pigs, along with an increase in serum bactericides and stimulation of β-lysine. In addition, in animal tests, immune resistance to Herpes simplex viruses of the eye was proven. In the ring test, stimulation and formation of granulation tissue was demonstrated in rats. In mice, there was a clear increase in the survival rate in cases of general infection. No significant results were recorded in cases where infections had no or only a low leucocytic immune reaction. The drug's pure aristolochic acid acts similarly to colchicine; it is nephrotoxic, carcinogenic and mutagenic.

INDICATIONS AND USAGE

Unproven Uses: Birthwort is used to stimulate the immune system and in the treatment of allergically caused gastrointestinal and gallbladder colic. The plant is used in a wide variety of ways in the folk medicine of nearly all European countries.

Chinese Medicine: Uses in Chinese medicine include joint pain, stomachache, malaria and abscesses.

Homeopathic Uses: Homeopathic indications include gynecological disorders and climacteric symptoms, as well as the treatment of wounds and ulcers. It is also used as a treatment after major surgery and in ear-nose-throat treatments.

CONTRAINDICATIONS

Birthwort is contraindicated during pregnancy.

PRECAUTIONS AND ADVERSE REACTIONS

General: Birthwort is highly toxic. The intake of acutely toxic doses leads to vomiting, gastroenteritis, spasms, severe kidney damage and eventually to death by kidney failure. The chronic intake of low dosages among both humans and laboratory animals led to the development of tumors. Because of the genotoxic and carcinogenic effects of the aristolochic acids, the drug is not to be administered even in small dosages.

Pregnancy: Birthwort is not to be used during pregnancy.

DOSAGE

Mode of Administration: Birthwort is used as a tincture in an ethanol solution. No further information is available.

How Supplied: Birthwort is available in homeopathic dilutions of D11.

LITERATURE

Che CT et al., (1984) J Nat Prod 47(2):331.

Fanselow G, Der Einfluβ von Pflanzenextrakten (Echinacea purpurea, Aristolochia clematitis) und homöopathischen Medikamenten auf die Phagocytoseleistung humaner Granulocyten in vitro. In: Dissertation Berlin. 1981.

Henrickson CU, (1970) Z Immunitäts Forsch 5:425.

Mengs U, Klein M, Genotoxic Effects of Aristolochic Acid in the Mouse Micronucleus Test. In: PM 52(6):502. 1988.

Mix DB et al., (1982) J Nat Prod 45(6):657.

Siess M, Seybold G, Untersuchungen über die Wirkung von Pulsatilla pratensis, Cimicifuga racemosa und Aristolochia clematis auf den Östrus infantiler und kastrierter weiβer Mäuse. In: Arzneim Forsch 10:514. 1960.

Strauch R, Hiller K, (1974) Pharmazie 29(10/11):656.

Tympner KD, (1981) Z Angew Phytother 5:181.

Further information in:

Chan H, But P (Eds.), Pharmacology and Applications of Chinese Materia Medica, Vol. 1, Ed. World Scientific Singapore 1986.

Frohne D, Pfänder HJ, Giftpflanzen - Ein Handbuch für Apotheker, Toxikologen und Biologen, 4. Aufl., Wiss. Verlags-Ges Stuttgart 1997.

Kern W, List PH, Hörhammer L (Hrsg.), Hagers Handbuch der Pharmazeutischen Praxis, 4. Aufl., Bde. 1-8, Springer Verlag Berlin, Heidelberg, New York, 1969.

Lewin L, Gifte und Vergiftungen, 6. Aufl., Nachdruck, Haug Verlag, Heidelberg 1992.

Madaus G, Lehrbuch der Biologischen Arzneimittel, Bde. 1-3, Nachdruck, Georg Olms Verlag Hildesheim 1979.

Roth L, Daunderer M, Kormann K, Giftpflanzen, Pflanzengifte, 4. Aufl., Ecomed Fachverlag Landsberg Lech 1993.

Steinegger E, Hänsel R, Pharmakognosie, 5. Aufl., Springer Verlag Heidelberg 1992.

Teuscher E, Lindequist U, Biogene Gifte - Biologie, Chemie, Pharmakologie, 2. Aufl., Fischer Verlag Stuttgart 1994.

Bishop's Weed

Ammi visnaga

DESCRIPTION

Medicinal Parts: The medicinal part is the fruit.

Flower and Fruit: The rays are slender and patent in the flower, becoming erect, thickened and indurate in the fruit. The bracts are 1 to 2-pinnatisect, equaling or exceeding the rays, and the bracteoles are subulate. The pedicles are erect, stout and rigid in the fruit. The fruit is 2 to 2.5 mm long.

Leaves, Stem and Root: Bishop's Weed is a robust annual or biennial that grows up to 100 cm tall. The lower leaves are pinnate, the others are 2 to 3 pinnate. All of the leaves have narrow linear or filform lobes.

Habitat: The plant grows in the Mediterranean region, and is cultivated in the U.S., Mexico, Chile and Argentina.

Production: Bishop's Weed fruit consists of the dried, ripe fruits of Ammi visnaga.

Other Names: Khella, Khella Fruits, Greater Ammi

ACTIONS AND PHARMACOLOGY

COMPOUNDS

Furochromones: particularly khellin, visnagin, khellol and khellol glucoside

Pyranocoumarins: particularly visnadin and samidin

Flavonoids: including quercetin and isohamnetin and their 3-sulfates

Volatile oil

Fatty oil

EFFECTS

The drug intensifies coronary and myocardial circulation, acting as a mild positive ionotrope. It has an antispasmodic effect on smooth muscles.

INDICATIONS AND USAGE

Unproven Uses: Bishop's Weed has been used for angina pectoris, cardiac insufficiency, paroxysmal tachycardia, extra systoles, hypertonia, asthma, whooping cough and cramp-like complaints of the abdomen.

PRECAUTIONS AND ADVERSE REACTIONS

Infrequently, a cholestatic jaundice (reversible) is observed following administration of the drug. The drug also possesses a phototoxic effect.

OVERDOSAGE

Long-term use or overdose of the drug can lead to queasiness, dizziness, loss of appetite, headache or sleep disorders. Very high dosages, corresponding to over 100 mg khellin, may cause elevated levels (reversible) of liver enzymes in blood plasma.

DOSAGE

No information is available.

LITERATURE

Duarte J et al., Effects of visnadine on rat vascular smooth muscle. In: PM 63(3):233-236. 1997.

Greinwald R, Stobernack HP, Ammi visnaga - Das Bischhofskraut. In: ZPT 11(2):65. 1990.

Le Quesne PW et al., JNP 48:496. 1985.

Martelli P et al., J Chromatogr 301:297. 1984.

Trunzler G, Phytotherapeutische Möglichkeiten bei Herz- und arteriellen Gefäßerkrankungen. In: ZPT 10(5):147. 1989.

Further information in:

Kern W, List PH, Hörhammer L (Hrsg.), Hagers Handbuch der Pharmazeutischen Praxis, 4. Aufl., Bde. 1-8, Springer Verlag Berlin, Heidelberg, New York, 1969.

Madaus G, Lehrbuch der Biologischen Arzneimittel, Bde 1-3, Nachdruck, Georg Olms Verlag Hildesheim 1979.

Schulz R, Hänsel R, Rationale Phytotherapie, Springer Verlag Heidelberg 1996.

Steinegger E, Hänsel R, Pharmakognosie, 5. Aufl., Springer Verlag Heidelberg 1992.

Teuscher E, Biogene Arzneimittel, 5. Aufl., Wiss. Verlagsges. Stuttgart 1997.

Wagner H, Wiesenauer M: Phytotherapie. Phytopharmaka und pflanzliche Homöopathika, Fischer-Verlag, Stuttgart, Jena, New York 1995.

Wichtl M (Hrsg.), Teedrogen, 4. Aufl., Wiss. Verlagsges. Stuttgart 1997.

Bistort

Persicaria bistorta

DESCRIPTION

Medicinal Parts: The medicinal parts are the leaves and the rhizome.

Flower and Fruit: The flowering stem terminates in a compact, cylindrical, false spike of flesh-colored flowers without a terminal bud. The pedicle is winged. The flowers consist of 5 sepals, 8 stamens and an ovary with 2 to 3 styles. The flowers are in pairs, one of which is complete, the other only having a rudimentary ovary. Only the latter ripens. The complete flowers can be cross-pollinated by insects. The fruit is a three-seeded achene. The ripe seeds are small, brown and glossy.

Leaves, Stem and Root: The plant is a perennial, 30 cm to 1 m high herb on a thick, somewhat flattened and twisted S-shaped rhizome. The radical, oval leaves grow out of the rhizome to form basal rosette leaves with cordate bases, which are blue-green above and somewhat undulate.

Habitat: The plant is indigenous to Europe, North America and Asia.

Production: Bistort root and rhizome is the subterranean part of Persicaria bistorta. The root-stocks of the older plants are harvested, cleaned and freed from green parts and rootlets. The stronger parts are then cut up, and this material is dried in the sun.

Other Names: Adderwort, Dragonwort, Easter Giant, Easter Mangiant, Oderwort, Osterick, Patience Dock, Red Legs, Snakeweed, Sweet Dock

ACTIONS AND PHARMACOLOGY

COMPOUNDS

Tannins (15-36%): chiefly catechin tannins, small quantity of gallo tannins

Starch (in the root 30%)

EFFECTS

The active agents are the galenic tannin substance, starch, catechin and silicic acid. Higher concentrations of the root cause an increase in the formation of mucous. It is also an astringent.

INDICATIONS AND USAGE

Unproven Uses: The herb is used in the treatment of digestive disorders, particularly diarrhea and for internal bleeding. Externally, it is used as a gargle for mouth and throat infections and as an ointment for wounds.

Chinese Medicine: Preparations from the rhizome are used for epilepsy, fever, tetanus, carbuncles, snake and mosquito bites, scrofulous and cramps in the hands and feet.

PRECAUTIONS AND ADVERSE REACTIONS

No health hazards or side effects are known in conjunction with the proper administration of designated therapeutic dosages.

DOSAGE

Mode of Administration: Internally as a powdered drug for infusion, or externally as an extract or ointment.

Preparation:

Infusion (internal) — Macerate 50 g drug in 1 l water for 6 hours, percolate and sweeten as required (Penso, 1987).

Infusion (external) — Boil 60 g drug with 1 l water for 15 minutes, percolate and cool (Penso, 1987).

Liquid extract — drug 1:1 in 25% ethanol (BHP83).

Tincture — drug 1:5 in 25% ethanol (BHP83).

Daily Dosage:

Internal Dosage

Powder—in the form of 0.25 g gelatine capsules, 2 to 4 capsules every 3 hours.

Decoction—1 to 2 g for each decoction, 3 times a day.

Infusion—200 ml every 3 hours.

Liquid extract—1 to 2 ml 3 times daily.

Tincture—1 to 3 ml 3 times daily.

External Dosage

Decoction—poultice applied every 2 hours.

LITERATURE

Gonnet JF, (1981) Biochem Syst Ecol 9(4):299.

Kern W, List PH, Hörhammer L (Hrsg.), Hagers Handbuch der Pharmazeutischen Praxis, 4. Aufl., Bde. 1-8, Springer Verlag Berlin, Heidelberg, New York, 1969.

Penso G, Medico Farmaceutica, Milano, 1987.

Rao PRSP, Rao EV, (1977) Curr. Sci 48(18):640.

Bitter Apple

Citrullus colocynthis

DESCRIPTION

Medicinal Parts: The medicinal part of the plant is the dried pulp.

Flower and Fruit: The flowers are yellow and appear singly in the leaf axils. The fruit is about the size of an apple. It is yellow, smooth, dry and very bitter. When ripe, the fruit contains white spongy flesh within the coriaceous peel, with numerous ovate, white or brownish seeds. The seeds are 0.75 cm long and 0.5 cm wide, ovate, compressed, without an edge, oily and somewhat shiny.

Leaves, Stem and Root: Bitter Apple is an annual similar to a watermelon plant. The stems are leafy and rough-haired. The leaves are alternate on long petioles. They are triangular, divided, variously indented, obtuse and pubescent. The upper surface is delicate green, the lower surface rough and pale.

Characteristics: Bitter Apple (the drug) is highly poisonous.

Habitat: Bitter Apple is indigenous to Turkey and southern Mediterranean countries. It is also found in Sri Lanka, Egypt, Syria and the Arabian Gulf.

Production: Bitter Apples are the ripe fruits of Citrullus colocynthis that have been removed from the harder outer layer.

Other Names: Colocynth Pulp, Bitter Cucumber

ACTIONS AND PHARMACOLOGY

COMPOUNDS

Cucurbitacins: including cucurbitacin E-, J-, L-glucosides

Caffeic acid derivatives: chlorogenic acid

Fatty oil (in the seeds)

EFFECTS

Bitter Apple irritates the intestinal mucous membrane, increasing liquid production.

INDICATIONS AND USAGE

Unproven Uses: Preparations of Bitter Apple are used as a drastic purgative in fixed combinations in the treatment of acute and chronic constipation with various causes. It is also used in pregnancy and in the treatment of liver and gallbladder disorders.

Indian Medicine: Acitis and elephantiasis are among the conditions treated with Bitter Apple in Indian medicine.

PRECAUTIONS AND ADVERSE REACTIONS

The drug is severely poisonous. It has a strongly irritating (and painful) effect on mucous membranes due to its cucurbitacin glycoside content, out of which cucurbitacins are released in watery environments.

OVERDOSAGE

Vomiting, bloody diarrhea, colic, and kidney irritation follow the intake of toxic dosages (0.6 to 1 g), and then increased diuresis that progresses to anuria. Lethal dosages (starting at 2 g) lead to convulsions, paralysis and, if untreated, to death through circulatory collapse. The treatment for poisonings should proceed symptomatically following gastric lavage. Administration in allopathic dosages is no longer defensible.

LITERATURE

Habs M et al., (1984) J Cancer Res Clin Oncol 108(1):154.

Konopa J et al., In: Advances in Antimicrobial and Antineoplastic Chemotherapy, Vol. 2, Ed. M. Semonsky, Avicenna Press Prague 1972.

Lavie D et al., (1964) Phytochemistry 3:52.

Rawson MD, (1966) Lancet 1:1121.

Further information in:

Hegnauer R, Chemotaxonomie der Pflanzen, Bde 1-11, Birkhäuser Verlag Basel, Boston, Berlin 1962-1997.

Kern W, List PH, Hörhammer L (Hrsg.), Hagers Handbuch der Pharmazeutischen Praxis, 4. Aufl., Bde. 1-8, Springer Verlag Berlin, Heidelberg, New York, 1969.

Lewin L, Gifte und Vergiftungen, 6. Aufl., Nachdruck, Haug Verlag, Heidelberg 1992.

Madaus G, Lehrbuch der Biologischen Arzneimittel, Bde 1-3, Nachdruck, Georg Olms Verlag Hildesheim 1979.

Roth L, Daunderer M, Kormann K, Giftpflanzen, Pflanzengifte, 4. Aufl., Ecomed Fachverlag Landsberg Lech 1993.

Wagner H, Wiesenauer M, Phytotherapie. Phytopharmaka und pflanzliche Homöopathika, Fischer-Verlag, Stuttgart, Jena, New York 1995.

Bitter Candytuft

Iberis amara

DESCRIPTION

Medicinal Parts: The medicinal parts are the ripe seeds and the whole flowering plant.

Flower and Fruit: The stemmed flowers are arranged in racemes; there are 4 orbicular, diagonally splayed sepals approximately 2 mm long with white or reddish membranous margins and 4 obovate-elongate white petals, the outer ones approximately 6 mm, the inner ones 3 mm long. The plant has 2 short and 4 long stamens and a superior 4-carpled ovary; the carpels are fused. The fruit is a small pod, 4 to 5 mm long, almost circular with wide-winged fruit sides and a tough margin. Each of the 2 chambers has only 1 seed. The seeds are semi-ovoid, 2.5 to 3 mm long, flat and approximately 1 mm thick. They are usually narrow-winged at the margin, brown and smooth.

Leaves, Stem and Root: The plant is an herb, occasionally biennial, up to 40 cm high. The leaves are elongate-cuneiform and obtuse. The lower leaves are often spatulate and narrow toward the petiole. The upper leaves are sessile, usually with 2 to 4 blunt teeth at wide intervals and a ciliate margin. The stem is upright with splayed branches and downy-haired at the edges.

Habitat: The plant is found in most parts of western, central and southern Europe, in the Caucasus, and also in Algeria.

Production: Bitter Candytuft seeds are the ripe seeds of Iberis amara, which are collected in the wild and cultivated. Bitter Candytuft herb is the fresh, whole flowering plant of cultivated Iberis amara.

Other Names: Clown's Mustard, White Candytuft

ACTIONS AND PHARMACOLOGY

COMPOUNDS: BITTER CANDYTUFT SEEDS

Cucurbitacins (0.2 to 0.4%): particularly cucurbitacins E and I

Glucosinolates (1%): glucoiberin, glucocheiroline, glucoiberviridine

Fatty oil (12%): chief fatty acids are behenic acid (45%), oleic acid (20%), palmitic acid (10%) and linolenic acid (10%)

EFFECTS: BITTER CANDYTUFT SEEDS

The cucurbitacins contained in the seeds are toxic, cytotoxic and generally irritating to the small and large intestines. Furthermore, the seeds exhibit a mildly antimicrobial and fungistatic effect.

COMPOUNDS: BITTER CANDYTUFT HERB

Cucurbitacins: particularly cucurbitacins E and I

Flavonoids: including kempferol-3-O-arabinosido-7-O-rhamnoside, kempferol-7-O-rhamnoside, quercetin-3-O-glucosido-7-O-rhamnoside (high concentration in the flowers)

EFFECTS: BITTER CANDYTUFT HERB

The chief active ingredients of the fresh plant are cucurbitacins. A significant anti-edematous effect was exhibited in animal experiments. Its nature as a bitter substance makes its administration both as a choleretic and for stimulating the secretion of gastric juices appear plausible.

INDICATIONS AND USAGE

BITTER CANDYTUFT SEEDS

Unproven Uses: Folk medicine uses for the drug have included problems with cardiac arrhythmia and insufficiency.

Homeopathic Uses: Homeopathic uses include cardiac arrhythmia and insufficiency.

BITTER CANDYTUFT HERB

Unproven Uses: Folk medicine usage includes digestion problems.

PRECAUTIONS AND ADVERSE REACTIONS

BITTER CANDYTUFT SEEDS

The drug is toxic, due to its cucurbitacin content. Symptoms of poisoning could include vomiting, diarrhea, colic and kidney irritation. Cases of poisonings, however, have not been documented.

BITTER CANDYTUFT HERB

No risks are known in connection with the administration of homeopathic dosages of the drug. The drug is mildly toxic due to its (low) level of cucurbitacins. Symptoms of poisoning could include vomiting, diarrhea, colic and kidney irritation. Cases of poisonings have, however, never been documented.

OVERDOSAGE

BITTER CANDYTUFT SEEDS

In case vomiting has not already occurred, gastric lavage should be induced using burgundy-colored potassium permanganate solution and sodium sulfate.

Following gastrointestinal emptying and installation of activated charcoal, begin therapy for poisoning. Diazepam (i.v.) for muscle spasm may be necessary, along with electrolyte substitution and treatment for possible cases of acidosis with sodium bicarbonate infusions. In the event of shock, plasma volume expanders should be infused. Monitoring of kidney function is imperative. Intubation and oxygen respiration also may be necessary.

DOSAGE

BITTER CANDYTUFT SEEDS

How Supplied: Commercially prepared pharmaceutical compounds only.

Homeopathic Dosage: 5 drops, 1 tablet, 10 globules, every 30 to 60 minutes (acute) and 1 to 3 times daily (chronic); parenterally: 1 ml sc: 3 times daily (acute); 1 ml sc once a day (chronic) (HAB1).

BITTER CANDYTUFT HERB

How Supplied: Only available in commercial pharmaceutical compound preparations.

LITERATURE

Hänsel R, Keller K, Rimpler H, Schneider G (Ed), Hagers Handbuch der Pharmazeutischen Praxis, 5. Aufl., Bde 4 - 6 (Drogen), Springer Verlag Berlin, Heidelberg, New York, 1992-1994.

Kowalewski Z, Wierzbicka K, Flavonoid compounds in the blossoms of Iberis amara, L Planta Med, 20:328-39, 1971 Dec.

Uhlenbruck G, Dahr W, Studies on lectins with a broad agglutination spectrum. XII. N-acetyl-D-galactosamine specific lectins from the seeds of Soja hispida, Bauhinia purpurea, Iberis amara, Moluccella laevis and Vicia graminea. Vox Sang, 21:338-51, 1971 Oct.

Bitter Milkwort

Polygala amara

DESCRIPTION

Medicinal Parts: The medicinal part is the flowering plant with root.

Flower and Fruit: The blue or occasionally white or pink flowers are in many-blossomed racemes. Of the 5 sepals, the 2 lateral ones are large, petal-like, patent and 3-veined. The other 3 are smaller; the middle vein is green. The 3 petals are fused together with the stamens. These form 2 clusters in 2 green pockets on the larger, lower petal. The 2 upper petals form a kind of upper lip. The ovary is superior and bilocular with a spoon-like style. The fruit is an obcordate capsule, compressed at the sides and enclosed in the sepals.

Leaves, Stem and Root: The plant grows from 5 to 15 cm high. The stems are branched at the base, decumbent or ascending. The basal leaves form a rosette, while the cauline leaves are alternate, oblong-cuneate or obovate-lanceolate.

Habitat: The plant is indigenous to Europe.

Production: Bitter Milkwort herb, including its roots, is the complete plant of *Polygala amara*.

Other Names: European Bitter Polygala, European Senega Snakeroot, Evergreen Snakeroot, Flowering Wintergreen, Little Pollom

ACTIONS AND PHARMACOLOGY

COMPOUNDS

Saponins (1-2%)

Bitter principles: polygalin (polygamarin)

Phenol glycosides: monotropitoside (methyl salicylic acid-primveroside)

Polygalite (acerite, 1,5-anhydrosorbite)

EFFECTS

The drug is mildly expectorant.

INDICATIONS AND USAGE

Unproven Uses: Bitter Milkwort is used for conditions of the respiratory tract, cough and bronchitis.

PRECAUTIONS AND ADVERSE REACTIONS

No health hazards or side effects are known in conjunction with the proper administration of designated therapeutic dosages.

DOSAGE

Preparation: The drug is contained in tea for the treatment of bronchitis.

LITERATURE

Hegnauer R, Chemotaxonomie der Pflanzen, Bde 1-11, Birkhäuser Verlag Basel, Boston, Berlin 1962-1997.

Kern W, List PH, Hörhammer L (Hrsg.), Hagers Handbuch der Pharmazeutischen Praxis, 4. Aufl., Bde. 1-8, Springer Verlag Berlin, Heidelberg, New York, 1969.

Madaus G, Lehrbuch der Biologischen Arzneimittel, Bde 1-3, Nachdruck, Georg Olms Verlag Hildesheim 1979.

Bitter Orange

Citrus aurantium

DESCRIPTION

Medicinal Parts: The medicinal parts are the fresh and dried fruit peel, the flowers, the seeds and the extracted essential oil.

Flower and Fruit: The flowers are arranged singly or in clusters in the axils, and are very fragrant. The calyx is cup-shaped, and the 5 thick fleshy petals are an intense white and revolute. The fruit is about 7.5 cm in diameter (similar in size to a cherry), subglobose, slightly flattened at both ends, 10- to 12-locular. The peel is thick, rough and orange when ripe. The fruit pulp is acidic. The core is hollow when ripe.

Leaves, Stem and Root: Bitter Orange is an evergreen tree with a rounded crown and smooth grayish-brown bark. The branches are angular when young, becoming terete and glabrous soon after, with a few stout but flexible axillary spines. The alternate leaves are 7.5 to 10 cm, broadly elliptoid, subacute at the apex, cuneate or rounded below. The upper surface is a shiny dark green and the underside paler. Petioles are broadly winged, tapering to a wingless base.

Habitat: The plant is indigenous to tropical Asia but is widely cultivated in other regions today, such as the Mediterranean.

Production: Bitter Orange flower consists of the dried flowers of Citrus aurantium. The oil is obtained by steam distillation of the fresh, fully opened flowers. Bitter Orange peel consists of the dried outer peel of ripe fruits of Citrus aurantium separated from the white pulp layer.

Other Names: Orange, Neroli, Bigarade Orange

ACTIONS AND PHARMACOLOGY

COMPOUNDS: BITTER ORANGE FLOWER AND FLOWER OIL

Volatile oil: chief constituents linalool, linalyl acetate, alpha-pinenes, limonene, nerol

Methyl anthranilate

Limonoids: (triterpenoide bitter principles)

Flavonoids

EFFECTS: BITTER ORANGE FLOWER AND FLOWER OIL

No substantiated information available. Efficacy of the use of an extraction of the blossoms as a neurostimulant is not confirmed.

COMPOUNDS: BITTER ORANGE PEEL

Volatile oil: chief constituents (+) -limonene, nerol, geraniol, linalool, linalyl-, neryl-, geranyl- and citronellyl acetate, typical constituent methyl anthranilate

Flavonoids: among them the bitter compounds neohesperidin dyhydrochalcone and naringin as well as the lipophilic compounds sinensetin, nobiletin, tangeretin

Furocoumarins

EFFECTS: BITTER ORANGE PEEL

Bitter Orange has a mild spasmolytic effect on the gastrointestinal tract and increases gastric juice secretion.

INDICATIONS AND USAGE

BITTER ORANGE FLOWER AND FLOWER OIL

Unproven Uses: Preparations of Bitter Orange flower and flower oil are used as a preventive measure for gastric and nervous complaints, gout, sore throat, as a sedative, for nervous tension and sleeplessness. Fold medicine uses include chronic bronchitis.

Chinese Medicine: Uses in Chinese medicine include pain in the epigastrum, vomiting and anorexia.

BITTER ORANGE PEEL

Approved by Commission E:

- Loss of appetite
- Dyspeptic complaints

Unproven Uses: Folk medicine uses include loss of appetite and dyspeptic symptoms.

Chinese Medicine: Bitter Orange peel is used for coughs, colds, anorexia, to reduce apathy and for uterine and anal prolapse.

PRECAUTIONS AND ADVERSE REACTIONS

BITTER ORANGE FLOWER AND FLOWER OIL

No health hazards or side effects are known in conjunction with the proper administration of designated therapeutic dosages.

BITTER ORANGE PEEL

No health hazards or side effects are known in conjunction with the proper administration of designated therapeutic dosages. An elevation of UV-sensitivity is possible with light-skinned individuals due to the phototoxic effect of the furocoumarins. Frequent contact with the drug or with the volatile oil (such as the exposure experienced by workers in the liquor industry) can cause a sensitization that results in erythema, swelling, blisters, pustules, dermatoses leading to scab formation and pigment spots.

DOSAGE

BITTER ORANGE PEEL

Mode of Administration: Cut and coarsely powdered drug for teas, other bitter-tasting galenic preparations for oral application.

How Supplied: Commercial pharmaceutical preparations include drops, tonics and tea mixtures.

Preparation: To prepare a tea, add 1 tsp of drug to 150 ml of hot water, let stand for 10 minutes, then strain.

Daily Dosage:

Drug: 4 to 6 g

Extract: 1 to 2 g

Tea: 1 cup 1 hour before meals

Tincture (according to DAB 7): 2 to 3 g

LITERATURE

BITTER ORANGE FLOWER AND OIL

Slater CA, (1961) J Sci Agric Food 12:732.

Stanley WL, Jurd L, (1971) J Agric Food Chem 19:1106.

Tatum JH, Berry RE, (1977) Phytochemistry 16:109.

Further information in:

Kern W, List PH, Hörhammer L (Hrsg.), Hagers Handbuch der Pharmazeutischen Praxis, 4. Aufl., Bde. 1-8, Springer Verlag Berlin, Heidelberg, New York, 1969.

Leung AY, Encyclopedia of Common Natural Ingredients Used in Food Drugs and Cosmetics, John Wiley & Sons Inc., New York 1980.

Madaus G, Lehrbuch der Biologischen Arzneimittel, Bde 1-3, Nachdruck, Georg Olms Verlag Hildesheim 1979.

Roth L, Daunderer M, Kormann K, Giftpflanzen, Pflanzengifte, 4. Aufl., Ecomed Fachverlag Landsberg Lech 1993.

Tang W, Eisenbrand G, Chinese Drugs of Plant Origin, Springer Verlag Heidelberg 1992.

Wichtl M (Hrsg.), Teedrogen, 4. Aufl., Wiss. Verlagsges. Stuttgart 1997.

BITTER ORANGE PEEL

Clavarano I, Essenze Deriv. Agrum 36:5. 1966.

Horowitz RM, Gentili B, Tetrahedron 19:773. 1963.

Slater CA, (1961) J Sci Agric Food 12:732.

Stanley WL, Jurd L, (1971) J Agric Food Chem 19:1106.

Tatum JH, Berry RE, (1977) Phytochemistry 16, 109.

Further information in:

Kern W, List PH, Hörhammer L (Hrsg.), Hagers Handbuch der Pharmazeutischen Praxis, 4. Aufl., Bde. 1-8, Springer Verlag Berlin, Heidelberg, New York, 1969.

Leung AY, Encyclopedia of Common Natural Ingredients Used in Food Drugs and Cosmetics, John Wiley & Sons Inc., New York 1980.

Lewin L, Gifte und Vergiftungen, 6. Aufl., Nachdruck, Haug Verlag, Heidelberg 1992.

Madaus G, Lehrbuch der Biologischen Arzneimittel, Bde 1-3, Nachdruck, Georg Olms Verlag Hildesheim 1979.

Roth L, Daunderer M, Kormann K, Giftpflanzen, Pflanzengifte, 4. Aufl., Ecomed Fachverlag Landsberg Lech 1993.

Steinegger E, Hänsel R, Pharmakognosie, 5. Aufl., Springer Verlag Heidelberg 1992.

Tang W, Eisenbrand G, Chinese Drugs of Plant Origin, Springer Verlag Heidelberg 1992.

Teuscher E, Biogene Arzneimittel, 5. Aufl., Wiss. Verlagsges. Stuttgart 1997.

Wichtl M (Hrsg.), Teedrogen, 4. Aufl., Wiss. Verlagsges. Stuttgart 1997.

Bittersweet Nightshade

Solanum dulcamara

DESCRIPTION

Medicinal Parts: The medicinal part is the stem of the plant.

Flower and Fruit: The violet flowers are arranged in 10 to 20 blossomed, long-peduncled and hanging, panicle-like forms. The calyx is fused, 5-tipped and does not drop. The corolla has a very short tube and 5 long tips, which become revolute when mature. At the base of each tip, there are 2 green spots surrounded by white. There are 5 stamens with golden yellow anthers, which lean toward each other, and 1 superior ovary. The fruit is an oblong, scarlet and many-seeded berry.

Leaves, Stem and Root: The plant is a subshrub from 30 to 150 cm in height with a creeping, branched rhizome. The stem is twining or creeping, woody below, angular and usually glabrous. The leaves are petiolate, the upper and lower ones are usually cordate and acute. The middle leaves are usually pinnatesect with 1 pair of lateral segments and a large terminal segment.

Habitat: The plant is common in Europe, northern Africa, eastern and western Asia, and North America.

Production: Bittersweet Nightshade consists of the dried, 2- to 3-year-old stems of Solanum dulcamara harvested in spring prior to leafing, or late autumn after the leaves have dropped.

Other Names: Bittersweet, Dulcamara, Felonwort, Felonwood, Scarlet Berry, Violet Bloom, Blue Nightshade, Fever Twig, Nightshade, Woody, Staff Vine

ACTIONS AND PHARMACOLOGY

COMPOUNDS

Steroid alkaloid glycosides: (0.07 to 0.4%) the alkaloid spectrum varies widely with the variety

Tomatidenol variety—alpha-solamarine, beta-solamarine

Soladulcidine variety—soladulcidinetetraoside

Solasodine variety—solasonine, solamargine

Steroid saponins

Mixed varieties also occur.

EFFECTS

The main active principles are the steroid alkaloid glycosides whose resorption is probably promoted by the saponins. They stimulate phagocytosis, are hemolytic, cytotoxic, antiviral, anticholinergic and have local anaesthetic properties.

Solasodin has a cortisone-like effect. A desensitizing and cardiotonic effect has been observed in clinical trials with patients suffering from rheumatic polyarthritis.

Its use as an expectorant may be due to the saponin content.

INDICATIONS AND USAGE

Approved by Commission E:

- Eczema
- Furuncles
- Acne
- Warts

Unproven Uses: In folk medicine, Bittersweet Nightshade is used internally for nose bleeds, rheumatic conditions, asthma and bronchitis, and to stimulate the immune system; externally for herpes, eczema, abscesses and contusions.

Homeopathic Uses: Solanum dulcamara is used for inflammation of the respiratory and gastrointestinal tracts, the joints and skin, and for febrile infections. Efficacy has not been proven.

CONTRAINDICATIONS

Bittersweet Nightshade is contraindicated in pregnancy and nursing mothers.

PRECAUTIONS AND ADVERSE REACTIONS

Health risks or side effects following the proper administration of designated therapeutic dosages are not recorded. Toxic effects should not be seen in dosages under approximately 25 gm due to the low alkaloid content of the stem.

OVERDOSAGE

Poisonings among children are known through the unripe berries. More than 10 berries cause nausea, vomiting, dilated pupils and diarrhea. Lethal dosage is estimated to be 200 berries.

DOSAGE

Mode of Administration: Comminuted herb is used in teas and other galenic preparations for internal use. The drug is also used externally in compresses and rinses.

Preparation: A decoction is prepared by adding 1 to 2 g of drug to 250 ml water.

Daily Dosage: The average daily internal dose is 1 to 3 gm of the drug. Externally, the herb is used as infusions or decoctions that have strengths equivalent to 1 to 2 gm of the drug per 250 ml of water.

Homeopathic Dosage: 5 drops, 1 tablet or 10 globules every 30 to 60 minutes (acute) or 1 to 3 times a day (chronic); parenterally: 1 to 2 ml, sc, acute: 3 times daily; chronic: once a day (HAB1)

LITERATURE

Frohne D, (1992) Solanum dulcamara L. - Der Bittersüße Nachtschatten. Portrait einer Arzneipflanze. Z Phytother 14: 337-342.

Hölzer I, (1992) Dulcamara-Extrakt bei Neurodermitis und chronischem Ekzem. Ergebnisse einer klinischen Prüfung. Jatros Dermatologie 6: 32-36.

JNP 56(3):430-431. 1993.

Kupchan SM et al., (1965) Science 150:1827.

Rönsch H, Schreiber K, Stubbe H, Naturwissenschaften 55:182. 1968.

Willaman JJ, Hui-Li L, (1970) Lloydia 33 (3A):1.

Willuhn G, Kothe U, (1983) Arch Pharm 316(8):678-687.

Willuhn G, Phytopharmaka in der Dermatologie. In: ZPT 16(6):325-342. 1995.

Wolters B, Antibiotische Wirkung von Solanum dulcamara. In: Naturwissenschaften 51:111. 1964.

Wolters B, Der Anteil der Steroidsaponine an der antibiotischen Wirkung von Solanum dulcamara. In: PM 13:2. 1965.

Wolters B, (1965) Planta Med 13:189.

Further information in:

Frohne D, Pfänder HJ, Giftpflanzen - Ein Handbuch für Apotheker, Toxikologen und Biologen, 4. Aufl., Wiss. Verlagsges. mbH Stuttgart 1997.

Hänsel R, Keller K, Rimpler H, Schneider G (Hrsg.), Hagers Handbuch der Pharmazeutischen Praxis, 5. Aufl., Bde 4-6 (Drogen): Springer Verlag Berlin, Heidelberg, New York, 1992-1994.

Madaus G, Lehrbuch der Biologischen Arzneimittel, Bde 1-3, Nachdruck, Georg Olms Verlag Hildesheim 1979.

Roth L, Daunderer M, Kormann K, Giftpflanzen, Pflanzengifte, 4. Aufl., Ecomed Fachverlag Landsberg Lech 1993.

Schulz R, Hänsel R, Rationale Phytotherapie, Springer Verlag Heidelberg 1996.

Steinegger E, Hänsel R, Pharmakognosie, 5. Aufl., Springer Verlag Heidelberg 1992.

Teuscher E, Biogene Arzneimittel, 5. Aufl., Wiss. Verlagsges. mbH Stuttgart 1997.

Teuscher E, Lindequist U, Biogene Gifte - Biologie, Chemie, Pharmakologie, 2. Aufl., Fischer Verlag Stuttgart 1994.

Wagner H, Wiesenauer M, Phytotherapie. Phytopharmaka und pflanzliche Homöopathika, Fischer-Verlag, Stuttgart, Jena, New York 1995.

Black Alder

Alnus glutinosa

DESCRIPTION

Medicinal Parts: The medicinal parts of the plant are the bark and leaves.

Flower and Fruit: Black Alder is monoecious. Male flowers are arranged in stemmed catkins. Female flowers form ovoid fruit, which turns woody and remains on the tree the whole year.

Leaves, Stem and Root: The plants grow as a shrub or tree extending up to 25 m high. Black Alder has gray branches and orange-colored wood. The obovate leaves have double-serrate margins; the young leaves are very sticky.

Habitat: Black Alder originated in the damp regions of Europe, Asia and North America. The plant now grows in much of the Northern Hemisphere.

Production: Black (English) Alder bark is the bark and branch rind of Alnus glutinosa. It is gathered from the shrubs or trees growing wild.

Other Names: Common Alder, Owler, Tag Alder

ACTIONS AND PHARMACOLOGY

COMPOUNDS

Tannins

Flavonoids: in particular hypericin

Steroids: beta-sitosterol

Triterpenes: especially alpha-amyrenone, lupenone, taraxerol, glutenone

EFFECTS

The decoction is a tonic and has astringent and hemostatic properties, which may be due to the tannins (20%), flavone glycosides and triterpenes.

INDICATIONS AND USAGE

Unproven Uses: Black Alder is used as a decoction for gargles in the treatment of streptococcal sore throat and pharyngitis, and for intestinal bleeding. The bark is considered to be effective for intermittent fever.

PRECAUTIONS AND ADVERSE REACTIONS

No health hazards or side effects are known in conjunction with the proper administration of designated therapeutic dosages.

DOSAGE

Mode of Administration: Leaves and bark are prepared as infusions and decoctions for internal and local use. Mention is made of an ophthalmic powder.

Preparations: The bark is prepared as a decoction.

LITERATURE

Freudenberg K, Weinges K, (1967) Tetrahedron Letters 17: 19.

Hänsel R, Keller K, Rimpler H, Schneider G (Hrsg.), Hagers Handbuch der Pharmazeutischen Praxis, 5. Aufl., Bde 4-6 (Drogen), Springer Verlag Berlin, Heidelberg, New York, 1992-1994.

Hoppe, HA (1975-1987) Drogenkunde, 8. Aufl., Bde 1-3, W. de Gruyter Verlag, Berlin, New York.

Black Bryony

Tamus communis

DESCRIPTION

Medicinal Parts: The medicinal part is the root.

Flower and Fruit: The flowers are small greenish-white and in loose clusters. They consist of 6 petals and are found on various plants in fertile and infertile form. The fertile flowers develop into crimson berries.

Leaves, Stem and Root: Tamus communis is a glabrous climber. The stem dies back in winter but the root is perennial. The leaves are cordate, smooth, acute and glossy. The root is almost cylindrical with a diameter of 2 to 3 cm. The root is 6 to 8 cm long and has scattered, thin root fibers. Externally, the root is blackish-brown. Internally, it is whitish and produces a slimy paste when it is peeled.

Characteristics: The taste of the root is acrid and the odor is slightly earthy.

Habitat: The plant is indigenous to parts of Europe.

Production: Black Bryony root is the root of Tamus communis. The roots are gathered at the end of the vegetation period. They are dug up and the bark is peeled off and cut into slices or pieces. During this procedure, gloves should be worn to protect the hands, as the fresh roots cause serious reddening of the skin.

Other Names: Blackeye Root

ACTIONS AND PHARMACOLOGY

COMPOUNDS

Histamine-oxalate: in the form of skin- and mucous membrane-irritating needles

Mucilages (2.5-5%)

Volatile oil (1%)

Phenanthrene derivatives

Steroid saponins, aglycone diosgenin

EFFECTS

Black Bryony stimulates the external nerve ends. A substance similar to histamine increases blood circulation in areas of the skin to which it is applied.

INDICATIONS AND USAGE

Unproven Uses: The plant is used for agitation and redness of the skin, bruises, strains, torn muscles, gout and other rheumatic disorders. Black Bryony is also used for irritation of the intestine mucous membrane and as an emetic. It is also used as a tonic for hair loss, as it improves blood circulation to the scalp.

PRECAUTIONS AND ADVERSE REACTIONS

Skin contact with the fresh plant leads to the formation of rashes, swelling, pustules and wheals, due to the skin- and mucous membrane-irritating oxalate needles and histamine. Internal administration triggers signs of severe irritation in the mouth, pharyngeal space and gastrointestinal tract, combined with vomiting and intense diarrhea. Extracts from the plant are toxicologically harmless. Skin lesions are treated with cortisone foam and sterile coverings; tetanus prophylaxis might be required. If taken by mouth, following gastric lavage with burgundy-colored potassium permanganate solution and administration of activated charcoal, treat spasms with diazepam (i.v.) and colic with atropine. Monitoring of kidney function is essential. Intubation and oxygen respiration may also be necessary.

DOSAGE

Mode of Administration: The ground root is applied externally as a lotion.

LITERATURE

Aquino R et al., (1985) J Nat Prod 48(3):502.

Aquino R et al., (1985) J Nat Prod 48(5):811.

Barbakadze V, Usov AI, Isolation and characterisation of glucans from roots of Tamus communis L. In: PM 62, Abstracts of the 44th Ann Congress of GA, 127. 1996.

Frohne D, Pfänder HJ, Giftpflanzen - Ein Handbuch für Apotheker, Toxikologen und Biologen, 4. Aufl., Wiss. Verlags-Ges. Stuttgart 1997.

Ireland CR et al., (1981) Phytochemistry 20:1569.

Kern W, List PH, Hörhammer L (Hrsg.), Hagers Handbuch der Pharmazeutischen Praxis, 4. Aufl., Bde. 1-8: Springer Verlag Berlin, Heidelberg, New York, 1969.

Lewin L, Gifte und Vergiftungen, 6. Aufl., Nachdruck, Haug Verlag, Heidelberg 1992.

Roth L, Daunderer M, Kormann K, Giftpflanzen, Pflanzengifte, 4. Aufl., Ecomed Fachverlag Landsberg Lech 1993.

Teuscher E, Lindequist U, Biogene Gifte - Biologie, Chemie, Pharmakologie, 2. Aufl., Fischer Verlag Stuttgart 1994.

Black Catnip

Phyllanthus amarus

DESCRIPTION

Medicinal Parts: The whole, dried herb is the medicinal part.

Flower and Fruit: The flowers are axillary. The male flower has 5, 0.5 mm long, acute, pale-green sepals with a white margin. There are 3 stamens with the filaments forming a 0.2 mm high column. The female flowers have an apically thickened pedicle and 5 ovate-elongate, up to 1 mm long, yellowish-green sepals. The ovary is 0.3 mm in diameter and 3-chambered. The fruit is ochre to olive with 3 pressed lobes, 2 mm in diameter and 1 mm long.

Leaves and Stem: Black catnip is a monoecious, occasionally dioecious, upright or ascending herb, which grows up to 60 cm high, or occasionally higher. The bracts and stipules are linear-lanceolate, 1 mm long, cream with a brownish middle rib. The stem is round, greenish or reddish, glabrous and woody at the base.

Habitat: Africa, Asia and America.

Production: Black catnip herb is the aerial part of Phyllanthus amarus. The harvested herb is dried.

Not to be Confused With: May be confused with Phyllanthus urinaria, P. niruri, P. debilis and P. fraternus.

ACTIONS AND PHARMACOLOGY

COMPOUNDS

Tannins: gallotannins, including amarine, phyllanthusin D, geraniine, corilagin, elaecarpusin

Flavonoids: including rutin, quercetin-3-O-glucoside

Lignans: phyllantin (0.8%, extremely bitter), hypophyllanthin

EFFECTS

The drug, which contains tannins and lignans, is antiviral and antimicrobial in effect.

INDICATIONS AND USAGE

Unproven Uses: The herb is used for fever (Cuba, Nigeria), for malaria (Cuba, Bahamas), diarrhea, tachycardia and female sterility (Congo), constipation with spasms and colic, as a diuretic (Nigeria) and for diabetes (Dominican Republic).

Indian Medicine: Black catnip is used for stomach conditions, ascites, jaundice, diarrhea, dysentery, intermittent fever, conditions of the urogenital tract, eye disease, scabies, ulcers and wounds.

PRECAUTIONS AND ADVERSE REACTIONS

No health hazards are known in conjunction with the proper administration of designated therapeutic dosages.

DOSAGE

Mode of Administration: Whole herb preparations for internal and external use.

Preparation: Decoction: 10 plants to 1-liter water

Daily Dosage: No exact doses are known.

LITERATURE

Blaschek W, Hänsel R, Keller K, Reichling J, Rimpler G, Schneider G (Eds), Hagers Handbuch der Pharmazeutischen Praxis. Folgebände 1 und 2. Drogen A-Z. Springer. Berlin, Heidelberg 1998.

Blumberg BS, Millman I, Venkateswaran PS, Thyagarajan SP, Hepatitis B virus and hepatocellular carcinoma - treatment of HBV carriers with Phyllanthus amarus. Cancer Detect Prev, 14:195-201, 1989.

Blumberg BS, Millman I, Venkateswaran PS, Thyagarajan SP, Hepatitis B virus and primary hepatocellular carcinoma: treatment of HBV carriers with Phyllanthus amarus. Vaccine, 8 Suppl: 86-92, 1990 Mar.

Lee CD, Ott M, Thyagarajan SP, Shafritz DA, Burk RD, Gupta S, Phyllanthus amarus down-regulates hepatitis B virus mRNA transcription and replication. Eur J Clin Invest, 26:1069-76, 1996 Dec.

Leelarasamee A, Trakulsomboon S, Maunwongyathi P, Somanabandhu A, Pidetcha P, Matrakool B, Lebnak T, Ridthimat W, Chandanayingyong D, Failure of Phyllanthus amarus to eradicate hepatitis B surface antigen from symptomless carriers. Lancet, 2:1600-1, 1990 Jun 30.

Niu JZ, Wang YY, Qiao M, Gowans E, Edwards P, Thyagarajan SP, Gust I, Locarnini S, Effect of Phyllanthus amarus on duck hepatitis B virus replication in vivo. J Med Virol, 32:212-8, 1990 Dec.

Ott M, Thyagarajan SP, Gupta S, Phyllanthus amarus suppresses hepatitis B virus by interrupting interactions between HBV enhancer I and cellular transcription factors. Eur J Clin Invest, 27:908-15, 1997 Nov.

Srividya N, Periwal S, Diuretic, hypotensive and hypoglycaemic effect of Phyllanthus amarus. Indian J Exp Biol, 74:861-4, 1995 Nov.

Thamlikitkul V, Wasuwat S, Kanchanapee P, Efficacy of Phyllanthus amarus for eradication of hepatitis B virus in chronic carriers. J Med Assoc Thai, 74:381-5, 1991 Sep.

Thyagarajan SP, Jayaram S, Valliammai T, Madanagopalan N, Pal VG, Jayaraman K, Phyllanthus amarus and hepatitis B. Lancet, 2:949-50, 1990 Oct 13.

Thyagarajan SP, Subramanian S, Thirunalasundari T, Venkateswaran PS, Blumberg BS, Beneficial effects of Phyllanthus amarus for chronic hepatitis B. J Hepatol, 2:405-6, 1991 May.

Thyagarajan SP, Subramanian S, Thirunalasundari T, Venkateswaran PS, Blumberg BS, Effect of Phyllanthus amarus on chronic carriers of hepatitis B virus. Lancet, 2:764-6, 1988 Oct 1.

Thyagarajan SP, Subramanian S, Thirunalasundari T, Venkateswaran PS, Blumberg BS, In vitro effect of Phyllanthus amarus on hepatitis B virus. Indian J Med Res, 2:71-3, 1991 Mar.

Black Cohosh

Cimicifuga racemosa

TRADE NAMES

Black Cohosh (available from a number of manufacturers) and sometimes sold as Black Cohosh Root, Black Cohosh Power, Wild Countryside Black Cohosh, NuVeg Black Cohosh Root, Remifemin

DESCRIPTION

Medicinal Parts: The medicinal part is the fresh and dried root.

Flower and Fruit: The inflorescence is a long-peduncled, drooping raceme, 30 to 90 cm long with white flowers. There are 3 to 8 petals without nectaries, and the sepals enclose the flower bud.

Leaves, Stem and Root: The plant grows 1 to 1.5 m high. It is leafy, with a sturdy, blackish rhizome, which is cylindrical, tough and knotty. The straight, strong, dark brownish roots sprout from the underground rhizome and are roughly quadrangular and grooved. The transverse root section shows wedge-shaped bundles of white wood. The rhizome section shows a large black medulla surrounded by a ring of paler, woodier wedges. The leaves are double-pinnate, smooth and crenate-serrate.

Habitat: Black Cohosh is native to Canada and the U.S.; it is cultivated in Europe.

Production: The medicinally used part of the plant consists of the dried rhizome of Cimicifuga racemosa with attached roots.

Other Names: Black Snake Root, Rattleroot, Rattleweed, Squaw Root, Bugbane, Bugwort, Cimicifuga, Richweed

ACTIONS AND PHARMACOLOGY

COMPOUNDS

Triterpenes : triterpene glycoside, including actein, 27-deoxyactein, cimifugoside

Quinolizidine alkaloids: cytisine, methyl cytisine

Phenylpropane derivatives: including isoferulic acid

EFFECTS

The active ingredients in the root are the triterpine glycosides such as cimifugaside, 27-deoxyactein and the actein. The increase in luteinizing hormone (LH) that occurs as estrogen levels decrease is implicated as the cause of menopausal symptoms. Compounds of the rootstock of Cimicifuga racemosa bind to the estrogen receptor where it selectively suppresses LH secretion with no effect on FSH. The result is an estrogenic effect, which will decrease climacteric symptoms such as hot flashes, diaphoresis and psychological disturbances (Duker, 1991; Lehmann-Wilenbrock, 1988).

There have been conflicting reports stating Cimicifuga racemosa has no estrogen-like action (Einer-Jensen, 1996; Liske, 1998). The herb did not appear to have an effect on levels of LH, FSH, sex hormone-binding globulin (SHBG), prolactin and estradiol in a study that concluded the therapeutic effects seen are not attributable to estrogenic or other endocrine-system effects (Liske, 1998).

The improvement in premenstrual symptoms, dysmenorrhea and menopause may be due to the relaxing of uterine tissue (Tyler, 1997).

CLINICAL TRIALS

A placebo-control, open study was conducted to determine the effects of commercially available Cimicifuga racemosa extract (Remifemin) on LH and FSH secretion in 110 menopausal women. After 2 months of therapy with 8 mg daily of the drug, FSH levels in the Remifemin treatment group and placebo group were similar. LH secretion was significantly reduced in the Remifemin treatment group, which points to the estrogenic effect of Cimicifuga racemosa preparations (Duker, 1991).

Sixty hysterectomized patients, under 40 years of age, with at least one intact ovary were involved in a study to determine the effect of Cimicifuga racemosa extract (Remifemen 8 mg), estriol (1 mg), conjugated estrogens (1.25 mg) and an estrogen-gestagen product on menopausal symptoms. The evaluation of menopausal symptoms was determined by the Kupperman-Index. The study also included evaluation of the trophic disorders of the genitals, including FSH and LH serum concentration measurement. There was a significant decrease in menopausal symptoms determined by the Kupperman-Index in all treatment groups. There was a moderate decline in the serum gonadotropin concentration in each group, with no significant therapeutic difference between the groups. Cimicifuga racemosa was as effective as the estrogen products in decreasing menopausal symptoms in young patients who have undergone a hysterectomy (Lehmann-Willenbrock, 1988).

In an open study including 50 patients with menopausal complaints, the effect of Cimicifuga racemosa extract

(Remifemen) 40 drops twice daily was determined after a duration of 3 months. The participants had either refused hormone treatment or had conditions where hormone treatment was contraindicated. The efficacy of the herb was measured according to the Kupperman-Index, Profile of Mood States (POMS) scale and the Clinical Global Impressions (CGI) scale. A significant improvement in menopausal complaints for all testing protocols were recorded. (Vorberg, 1984).

Note: Cimicifuga racemosa should not be substituted for hormone replacement therapy with estrogen. There is no information to date that the herb contains cardioprotective effects or protective effects against osteoporosis, as those seen with estrogen therapy.

INDICATIONS AND USAGE

Approved by Commission E:

- Climacteric complaints
- Premenstrual syndrome (PMS)

Unproven Uses: In folk medicine, the plant is used for rheumatism, sore throats and bronchitis. The tincture is also used as a sedative, for choreic states (involuntary, rapid motions), fever, lumbago (pain in the lumbar region) and snakebite. The herb is also available commercially in combination with St. John's Wort for depressive moods associated with premenstrual and menopausal symptoms.

Chinese Medicine: The Chinese have used Black Cohosh for the above indications as well as for measles in the pre-exanthem stage.

CONTRAINDICATIONS

The use of Black Cohosh is contraindicated during pregnancy due to an increased risk of spontaneous abortion.

PRECAUTIONS AND ADVERSE REACTIONS

General: No health hazards or side effects are known in conjunction with the proper administration of designated therapeutic dosages, although occasional stomach complaints have been observed.

Drug Interactions: Black Cohosh can potentiate the effect of antihypertensive medications. The concomitant use of these drugs may result in hypotension (Einer-Jensen, 1996; Lehmann-Willenbrock, 1988).

OVERDOSAGE

An intake of very high dosages of the drug (5 g) or an extract (12 g) leads to vomiting, headache, dizziness, limb pains and lowered blood pressure.

DOSAGE

Mode of Administration: Galenic preparations for internal use.

How Supplied:

Capsules — 60 mg, 80 mg, 450 mg, 540 mg, 545 mg

Drops

Solutions

Tablets — 60 mg, 120 mg.

Daily Dosage: Alcoholic-aqueous extracts (ethanolic-aqueous 40-60% (V/V) or isopropanolic-aqueous 40% (V/V)) corresponding to 40 mg drug. The herb is not recommended for treatment longer than 6 months unless advised by a physician.

LITERATURE

Benoit PS et al., (1976) Lloydia 39:160.

Berger S, Junior P, Kopanski L, 27-Desoxyactein: a New Polycyclic Triterpenoid Glycoside from Actaea racemosa. In: PM 54:579-780. 1988.

Beuscher N, Cimicifuga racemosa L. - Die Traubensilberkerze. In: ZPT 16(5):301-310. 1995.

Corsano S, Panizzi L, Sull' Acteina, principio attivo della Actaea racemosa. In: Atti Acca Nazl Lincei, Rend, Classe Sci, Fis. Mat. Nat 38:600-604. 1965.

Daiber W, Klimakterische Beschwerden: ohne Hormone zum Erfolg! In: Ärztl Praxis 35:1946-1947. 1983.

Duke JA, Handbook of Medicinal Herbs. Boca Raton: CRC, 1985.

Düker EM, Kopanski L, Jarry H, Wuttke W, (1991) Effects of extracts from cimicifuga racemosa on gonadotropin release in menopausal women and ovariectomized rats. Planta Med 57:420-424.

Einer-Jensen N, Zhao J, Andersen KP, Kristoffersen K, Cimicifuga and Melbrosia lack oestrogenic effects in mice and rats. In: Maturitas 25(1995):149-153. 1996.

Földes J, Die Wirkungen eines Extraktes aus Cimicifuga racemosa. In: Ärztl Forsch 13:623-624. 1959.

Genazzani, E et al., (1962) Nature 194:544.

Gerhard I, Liske E, Wüstenberg P, Behandlung von psychovegetativen Beschwerden im Klimakterium mit Remifemin(R)plus (Poster). In: ZPT 16(5, Supplement):21, 6. Phytotherapiekongreβ in Berlin. 1995.

Görlich N, Behandlung ovarieller Störungen in der Allgemeinpraxis. In: Ärztl Praxis 14:1742-1743. 1962.

Harnischfeger G, Cillien N, Influence of Cimicifuga racemosa extract fractions on the proliferation of human carcinoma cells in vitro with regard to their estrogen receptor sensitivity. In: PM 62, Abstracts of the 44th Ann Congress of GA, 40. 1996.

Harnischfeger G, Stolze H, Bewährte Wirksubstanzen aus Naturstoffen. Traubensilberkerze. In: Notabene medici 10:446-450. 1980.

Jarry H, Gorkow Ch, Wuttke W, (1995) Treatment of Menopausal Symptoms with Extracts of Cimicifuga Racemosa,

In vivo and in vitro Evidence for Estrogenic Activity. In, Loew D, Netbrock N (Hrsg) Phytopharmaka in Forschung und klinischer Anwendung. Steinkopff Verlag, Darmstadt, S 99-112.

Jarry H, Harnischfeger G, (1985) Studies on the endocrine effects of the contents of Cimicifuga racemosa, 1. Influence on the serum concentration of pituitary hormones in ovariectomized rats. Planta Med 51:46-49.

Jarry H, Harnischfeger G, Düker E, (1985) Studies on the endocrine effects of the contents of Cimicifuga racemosa, 2. In vitro binding of compounds to extrogen receptors. Planta Med 51:316-319.

Jarry H, Isolierung pharmakogologisch aktiver Substanzen aus Cimicifuga racemosa. In: Dissertation, math.-naturwiss. 1984.

Jarry H, Ludwig L, Stephan A, Wuttke W, Erste Beweise für eine direkte Wirkung von Inhaltsstoffen von Cimicifuga racemosa auf die in-vitro- Steroidsekretion von porcinen Granulosa- und Lutealzellen (Poster). In: ZPT 16(5, Supplement):7-8, 6. Phytotherapiek.

Kesselkauf O, Über die Behandlung klimakterischer Beschwerden mit Remifemin. In: Med Monatsschr 11:87-88. 1957.

Krämer H, Geisenhofer H, Erfahrungen mit dem Cimicifuga-Präparat Remifemin. In: Therapie der Gegenwart 97:238-239. 1958.

Lauritzen C, Nichthormonale Therapie klimakterischer Beschwerden. In: Gynäkol Praxis 14:43-56. 1990.

Lehmann-Willenbrock E, Riedel HH, Clinical and endocrinologic studies of the treatment of ovarian insufficiency manifestations following hysterectomy with intact adnexa. Zentralbl Gynakol 1988.110(10):611-8.

Liske E, Therapeutic efficacy and safety of Cimicifuga racemosa for gynecologic disorders. Adv Ther 1998 Jan-Feb;15(1):45-53.

Liske E, Wustenberg P, Therapy of climacteric complaints with Cimicifuga racemosa: herbal medicine with clinically proven evidence. Menapause. 1998 5:250.

Neβelhut T, Schellhase C, Dietrich R, Kuhn W, Untersuchungen zur proliferativen Potenz von Phytopharmaka mit östrogenähnlicher Wirkung bei Mammakarzinomzellen. In: Arch Gynecol Obstetrics 254:817-818. 1993.

Pethö A, Umstellung einer Hormonbehandlung auf ein pflanzliches Gynäkologikum möglich? In: Ärztl Praxis 47:1551-1553. 1987.

Radics L et al., (1975) Tetrahedron Letters 48:4287.

Shibata M et al., (1980) Yakugaku Zasshi 100:1143.

Shibata M, (1977) J Chem Soc Jpn 97:911.

Stoll W, (1987) Phytotherapeutikum beeinfluβ atrophisches Vaginalepithel, Doppelblindversuch Cimicifuga vs. Östrogenpräparat. Therapeutikon 1:23-32.

Stolze H, Der andere Weg klimakterische Beschwerden zu behandeln. In: Gyne 1:14-16. 1982.

Suntry L, (1984) Pat. JP 84/20298 Japan.

Tyler VE, The bright side of black cohosh. Prevention Magazine, April 1997.

Vorberg G, Treatment of menopausal symptoms. ZFA 1984;60:626-629.

Warnecke G, (1985) Beeinflussung klimakterischer Beschwerden durch ein Phytotherapeutikum. Erfolgreiche Therapie mit Cimicifuga- Monoextrakt. Med Welt 36:871-874.

Winterhoff H, (1993) Arzneipflanzen mit endokriner Wirksamkeit. Z Phytother 14:83-94.

Further information in:

Chan EH et al., (Eds), Advances in Chinese Medicinal Materials Research, World Scientific Pub. Co. Singapore 1985.

Kern W, List PH, Hörhammer L (Hrsg.), Hagers Handbuch der Pharmazeutischen Praxis, 4. Aufl., Bde. 1-8, Springer Verlag Berlin, Heidelberg, New York, 1969.

Leung AY, Encyclopedia of Common Natural Ingredients Used in Food Drugs and Cosmetics, John Wiley & Sons Inc., New York 1980.

Lewin L, Gifte und Vergiftungen, 6. Aufl., Nachdruck, Haug Verlag, Heidelberg 1992.

Madaus G, Lehrbuch der Biologischen Arzneimittel, Bde 1-3, Nachdruck, Georg Olms Verlag Hildesheim 1979.

Roth L, Daunderer M, Kormann K, Giftpflanzen, Pflanzengifte, 4. Aufl., Ecomed Fachverlag Landsberg Lech 1993.

Schulz R, Hänsel R, Rationale Phytotherapie, Springer Verlag Heidelberg 1996.

Steinegger E, Hänsel R, Pharmakognosie, 5. Aufl., Springer Verlag Heidelberg 1992.

Teuscher E, Biogene Arzneimittel, 5. Aufl., Wiss. Verlagsges. mbH Stuttgart 1997.

Wagner H, Wiesenauer M, Phytotherapie. Phytopharmaka und pflanzliche Homöopathika, Fischer-Verlag, Stuttgart, Jena, New York 1995.

Black Currant

Ribes nigrum

TRADE NAMES

Bio-EFA Black Currant, Black Currant, Black Currant Oil, Black Currant Seed Oil

DESCRIPTION

Medicinal Parts: The medicinal parts are the leaves collected after the flowering season and dried, the fresh ripe fruit with the tops and stems and the fresh leaves collected in summer.

Flower and Fruit: The flowers form richly blossomed racemes. Each is in the axil of a pubescent bract, which is shorter than the petiole. The petiole is pinnate has 2 small bracteoles. The sepals are together with the 5 small stamens on the campanulate flower axis within which the single-valved ovary and the divided style is sunk. The hanging flowers are self-pollinating. The multi-seeded, black, glandular punctuate berries develop from the ovary.

Leaves, Stem and Root: The plant is a sturdy perennial bush up to 2 m high. The branches are pale, hard and initially pubescent. The leaves are alternate, petiolate, becoming quickly glabrous on the upper surface and have numerous yellow resin glands on the undersurface. The 3- to 5-lobed leaf blade has a cordate base and doubly dentate margin.

Habitat: The plant is indigenous to Eurasian forests as far as the Himalayas, Canada and Australia and is cultivated in many regions.

Production: Black currant leaves are the leaves of Ribes nigrum collected during or shortly after the flowering season. Leaves are harvested from cultivated crops during or shortly after flowering. They are air-dried in the shade or carefully at a maximum temperature of 60° C.

Black currant fruits are the ripe fruits, with stalks attached, of Ribes nigrum. Fruits are harvested when fully ripe, and utilized immediately or deep frozen.

Other Names: Quinsy Berries, Squinancy Berries

ACTIONS AND PHARMACOLOGY

COMPOUNDS: BLACK CURRANT LEAVES

Flavonoids: including astragalin, isoquercitrin, rutin

Oligomeric proanthocyanidins

Ascorbic acid (vitamin C, 0.1 to 0.27% of fresh weight)

Volatile oil (traces)

EFFECTS: BLACK CURRANT LEAVES

A salidiuretic effect is attributed to the drug through a 'diuretic factor' that is not closely defined. In animal experiments, a hypotensive, anti-exudative and prostaglandin-release inhibiting effect has been proven.

COMPOUNDS: BLACK CURRANT FRUITS

Ascorbic acid (vitamin C, 0.1 to 0.3%)

Anthocyans: chiefly cyanidin-3-O-rutinoside and delphinidin-3-O-rutinoside

Phenol caroboxylic acid derivatives: caffeoyl-, p-cumaroyl- and feruloyl-quinic acids; p-cumaroyl and feruloyl glucoses

Flavonoids: chief components isoquercitrin, myricetin glucoside, rutin

Fruit acids (3.5%): malic acid, citric acid, isocitric acid

Invert sugar

Pectins

COMPOUNDS: BLACK CURRANT SEEDS

Fatty oil (30%) with high gamma linolenic acid content

Monosaccharides: invert sugar

EFFECTS: BLACK CURRANT FRUIT AND SEEDS

The extract of the drug that contains anthocyane has a hypotensive and spasmolytic effect in animal experiments. In addition, an antimicrobial and xanthine-oxidase and lipoperoxidase inhibiting effect has been proven.

INDICATIONS AND USAGE

BLACK CURRANT LEAVES

Unproven Uses: Black Currant leaves are used internally to increase micurition. In folk medicine they are used internally for arthritis, gout and rheumatism, diarrhea, colic, jaundice and liver ailments, painful micturition, urinary stones, convulsive coughs and whooping cough. Black Currant is used externally for treatment of wounds and insect bites.

BLACK CURRANT FRUITS

Unproven Uses: In folk medicine Black Currant fruit is used internally to relieve colds, hoarseness and coughs, diarrhea and stomachache. It is also used as a source of vitamin C. Preparations are used on mucous membranes as a gargle for hoarseness, strep throat and other inflammations of the oral cavity.

Black currant dried berries are used for bladder complaints, venous insufficiency, hemorrhoids, bruising and petechiae

CONTRAINDICATIONS

BLACK CURRANT LEAVES

Contraindicated in edema resulting from reduced cardiac and renal activity.

PRECAUTIONS AND ADVERSE REACTIONS

BLACK CURRANT LEAVES AND FRUITS

No health hazards or side effects are known in conjunction with the proper administration of designated therapeutic dosages.

DOSAGE

BLACK CURRANT LEAVES

Mode of Administration: Black currant leaves are available as whole, crude and powder drug for internal use.

Preparation: To prepare a tea, add 1 to 2 heaped teaspoons (2 to 4 gm) Black currant leaves to boiling water (150 ml), and strain after 10 minutes.

Daily Dosage:

Tea — 1 cup to be drunk several times a day.

Poultice — freshly rubbed Black Currant leaves or leaves soaked in warm water are dried and used as a compress. Place dried drug on wounds and fresh rubbed leaves on insect bites.

Storage: Should be protected from light and moisture

BLACK CURRANT FRUITS

Mode of Administration: Black Currant fruit is available as whole drug for internal use.

Daily Dosage:

Syrup — 5 to 10 ml, by the tablespoon, taken several times daily, or eaten as jelly or sweets.

Gargle — with the juice and equal parts of warm water.

LITERATURE

BLACK CURRANT LEAVES

Kyerematen G, Sandberg F, (1986) Acta Pharm Suecica 23:101.

Lietti A et al., (1976) Arzneim Forsch 26(5):829.

Senchute GV, Boruch IF, (1976) Rastit Resur 12(1):113.

Further information in:

Hänsel R, Keller K, Rimpler H, Schneider G (Hrsg.), Hagers Handbuch der Pharmazeutischen Praxis, 5. Aufl., Bde 4-6 (Drogen): Springer Verlag Berlin, Heidelberg, New York, 1992-1994.

Wichtl M (Hrsg.), Teedrogen, 4. Aufl., Wiss. Verlagsges. Stuttgart 1997.

BLACK CURRANT FRUITS

Kyerematen G, Sandberg F, (1986) Acta Pharm Suecica 23:101.

Lietti A et al., (1976) Arzneim Forsch 26(5):829.

Senchute GV, Boruch IF, (1976) Rastit Resur 12(1):113.

Further information in:

Hänsel R, Keller K, Rimpler H, Schneider G (Hrsg.), Hagers Handbuch der Pharmazeutischen Praxis, 5. Aufl., Bde 4-6 (Drogen): Springer Verlag Berlin, Heidelberg, New York, 1992-1994.

Black Haw

Viburnum prunifolium

DESCRIPTION

Medicinal Parts: The medicinal part is the bark of the trunk and the root.

Flower and Fruit: The flowers of the Viburnum species are white and in richly blossomed, flat, apical cymes. The central florets are campanulate and fertile; the lateral ones are much larger, rotate and infertile. The calyx margin is small and 5-tipped. The corolla of the fertile florets is campanulate and 5-petalled. There are 5 stamens, a semi-inferior ovary and 3 sessile stigmas. The fruit of the Black Haw is a shiny, black, juicy berry. The fruit of Viburnum opulus is red.

Leaves, Stem and Root: Black Haw is a deciduous tree 5 m tall. It has gray-brown bark and green, grooved branches. The leaves are opposite, petiolate, 3 to 5 lobed, roughly dentate, green on both surfaces and softly pubescent beneath.

Habitat: The plant is indigenous to the eastern and central U.S.

Production: Black Haw bark is the bark of the trunk and branches of Viburnum prunifolium.

Other Names: Stagbush, American Sloe, European Cranberry, Cramp Bark, Guelder Rose, Snowball Tree, King's Crown, High Cranberry, Red Elder, Rose Elder, Water Elder, May Rose, Whitsun Rose, Dog Rowan Tree, Whitsun Bosses, Silver Bells, Wild Guelder Rose

ACTIONS AND PHARMACOLOGY

COMPOUNDS

Flavonoids: amentoflavon (a biflavone)

Triterpenes: including among others oleanolic acid, ursolic acid as well as their acetates

Hydroxycoumarins: scopoletin, aesculetin, scoplin

Caffeic acid derivatives: chlorogenic acid, isochlorogenic acid

Phenol carboxylic acids: salicylic acid, salicin

Tannins (2%)

Arbutin (traces)

EFFECTS

The drug has a spasmolytic and, to date, an undefined effect on the uterus.

INDICATIONS AND USAGE

Unproven Uses: Black Haw is used for complaints of dysmenorrhea.

PRECAUTIONS AND ADVERSE REACTIONS

No health hazards or side effects are known in conjunction with the proper administration of designated therapeutic dosages.

DOSAGE

Mode of Administration: An extract is used as a constituent of a tea mixture made from Black Haw bark, Camomile flowers, and Peppermint leaves.

LITERATURE

Handjieva N et al., PH 27:3175. 1988.

Hörhammer L, Wagner H, Reinhardt H, Chemistry, pharmacology, and pharmaceutics of the components of Viburnum prunifolium and V. opulus. In: Botan Mag (Tokyo) 79(Oct./Nov.): 510-525. 1966.

Jarboe CH et al., (1967) J Med Chem 10: 448.

Jarboe CH et al., (1969) J Org Chem 34: 4202.

Jensen SR et al., PH 24:487. 1985.

Further information in:

Fenaroli's Handbook of Flavor Ingredients, Vol. 1, 2nd Ed., CRC Press 1975.

Kern W, List PH, Hörhammer L (Hrsg.), Hagers Handbuch der Pharmazeutischen Praxis, 4. Aufl., Bde. 1-8: Springer Verlag Berlin, Heidelberg, New York, 1969.

Roth L, Daunderer M, Kormann K, Giftpflanzen, Pflanzengifte, 4. Aufl., Ecomed Fachverlag Landsberg Lech 1993.

Wichtl M (Hrsg.), Teedrogen, 4. Aufl., Wiss. Verlagsges. Stuttgart 1997.

Black Hellebore

Helleborus niger

DESCRIPTION

Medicinal Parts: The medicinal parts of the plant are the dried rhizome with or without roots and the fresh underground parts.

Flower and Fruit: The flower is white with a greenish margin, reddish on the outside. It is hanging and splayed. There are 5 broadly ovate, campanualate bracts with red-brown borders, which tend toward each other. The petals are altered to nectaries. There are numerous yellow stamens. The fruit is a pod-like, many-seeded follicle with a curved beak and horizontal stripes. The seeds are matte black, ovate and have a long swelling on them.

Leaves, Stem and Root: The plant is a perennial subshrub up to 50 cm high. The stem is erect, glabrous, branched, woody at the base and almost leafless. The basal leaves are long-petioled, thickish, coriaceous, glabrous, dark green above with a lighter underside.

Characteristics: The plant is poisonous; rhizome is black-brown.

Habitat: The plant is indigenous to the forests of southern and central Europe.

Production: Black Hellebore root is the root of Helleborus niger.

Not to be Confused With: Helleborus foetidus, Helleborus niger and Helleborus viridis are different plants with different active compounds. They may be confused with the subterranean parts of Trollius eurpaeus, Aconitum napellus, Astrantia major, Actaea spicata and Adonis vernalis.

Other Names: Christe Herbe, Christmas Rose, Melampode

ACTIONS AND PHARMACOLOGY

COMPOUNDS: HELLEBORUS FOETIDUS

Steroid saponins: mixture known as helleborin

COMPOUNDS: HELLEBORUS NIGER

Steroid saponins: mixture known as helleborin

Cardioactive steroid glycosides (bufadienolide): including hellebrin, deglucohellebrin (only traces)

Alkaloids: celliamine, sprintillamine

COMPOUNDS: HELLEBORUS VIRIDIS

Steroid saponins: mixture known as helleborin

Cardioactive steroid glycosides (bufadienolide): including hellebrin, deglucohellebrin

Alkaloids: celliamine, sprintillamine, sprintillin

EFFECTS: ALL SPECIES

The plant is said to have a typical saponin effect (irritates mucous membranes) and is in general extremely toxic.

Note that other varieties of Helleborus also contain hellebrin with a digitalis-like effect.

INDICATIONS AND USAGE

Unproven Uses: In folk medicine, Black Hellebore is used as a laxative, for nausea, worm infestation, to regulate menstruation and as an abortifacient, as well as for acute nephritis. Also used in the treatment of head colds.

Homeopathic Uses: Used to treat acute diarrhea, encephalitis, cephalitis, kidney inflammation and states of confusion.

PRECAUTIONS AND ADVERSE REACTIONS

General: The mucous membrane-irritating saponin effect of the drug is the chief focus in cases of poisoning. Symptoms include scratchy feeling in mouth and throat, salivation, nausea, vomiting, diarrhea, dizziness, shortness of breath, possible spasm and asphyxiation. Disorders of cardiac function (cardiac arrhythmias are to be expected with large intakes of the rhizome of Helleborus viridis). Poisonings are recorded among the animals that feed on the plant. Following stomach and intestinal emptying (gastric lavage, sodium sulfate) and the administration of activated charcoal, therapy for poisonings consists of diazepam for spasm and electrolyte replenishment and sodium bicarbonate infusions for any acidosis that may arise. Intubation and oxygen respiration may also be necessary.

Pregnancy: In folk medicine, Black Hellebore is used as an abortifacient.

DOSAGE

Mode of Administration: Black Hellebore is obsolete and dangerous as a drug in allopathic doses.

Daily Dosage: The average dose is 0.05 gm; the maximum single dose is 0.2 gm; the largest daily dose is 1.0 gm. A powder with a medium content of 10% is used for head colds.

Homeopathic Dosage: 5 drops, 1 tablet or 10 globules every 30 to 60 minutes (acute) or 1 to 3 times daily (chronic); parenterally: 1 to 2 ml sc acute, 3 times daily; chronic: once a day (HAB34).

LITERATURE

Frohne D, Pfänder HJ, Giftpflanzen - Ein Handbuch für Apotheker, Toxikologen und Biologen, 4. Aufl., Wiss. Verlagsges. mbH Stuttgart 1997.

Glombitza KW et al., Do roots of Helleborus niger contain cardioactive substances. In: PM 55:107. 1989.

Hänsel R, Keller K, Rimpler H, Schneider G (Hrsg.), Hagers Handbuch der Pharmazeutischen Praxis, 5. Aufl., Bde 4-6 (Drogen), Springer Verlag Berlin, Heidelberg, New York, 1992-1994.

Lewin L, Gifte und Vergiftungen, 6. Aufl., Nachdruck, Haug Verlag, Heidelberg 1992.

Madaus G, Lehrbuch der Biologischen Arzneimittel, Bde 1-3, Nachdruck, Georg Olms Verlag Hildesheim 1979.

Petricic J et al., Acta Pharm Jugosl 27:127. 1977.

Petricic J, Acta Pharm Jugosl 24:179. 1974.

Poisonous Plants in Britain and their effects on Animals and Man, Ministry of Agriculture Fisheries and Food, Pub; HMSO, UK 1984.

Roth L, Daunderer M, Kormann K, Giftpflanzen, Pflanzengifte, 4. Aufl., Ecomed Fachverlag Landsberg Lech 1993.

Teuscher E, Lindequist U, Biogene Gifte - Biologie, Chemie, Pharmakologie, 2. Aufl., Fischer Verlag Stuttgart 1994.

Wißner W, Kating H, Botanische und phytochemische Untersuchung an europäischen und kleinasiatischen Arten der Gattung Helleborus. In: PM 26:128-143, 228-249, 364-374. 1974.

Black Horehound

Ballota nigra

DESCRIPTION

Medicinal Parts: The aerial parts of the plant are used medicinally.

Flower and Fruit: The clearly stemmed flowers are 1 to 1.5 cm long. They are arranged in 4 to 10 fairly loose and often short-stemmed cymes in the axils of the cauline leaves. The bracteoles are arrow-shaped and soft. They are half as long as the funnel-shaped calyx, which is downy to silky-shaggy haired. The calyx has 5 awned tips. The corolla is usually reddish-lilac, occasionally white. It contains a straight tube that grows out of the calyx tube and has a ring of hairs at the base. It has an elliptoid, slightly domed upper lip, which is slightly compressed from the outside. There is an equally long, downward hanging, white-marked lower lip, and an obovate, often edged or weakly dentate middle lip. The stamens are slightly hairy at the base and have small, distinctly spreading pollen sacks. The plant produces a hard fruit. The nuts are ovoid, 12 mm long and quite smooth.

Leaves, Stem and Root: Horehound is a perennial 0.30 to 1 m high shrub with a short creeping rhizome and upright, sturdy, angular, branched stems. The whole plant is pubescent and fresh green. In the autumn, the plant is often tinged brown-violet. The opposite leaves have a 0.5 to 1 cm long petiole. The lower leaves are larger and have an ovate to almost round, 2 cm long by 1.5 to 3.5 cm wide leaf blade. They are weakly cordate, blunt or wedge-shaped at the base and finely crenate to roughly and unevenly serrate. Both sides are pubescent, the upper surface often becoming glabrous and somewhat glossy.

Characteristics: The whole plant has an unpleasant smell of essential oil.

Habitat: The plant is considered to be a weed in western, central and northern Europe, but was intentionally introduced to the U.S.

Production: Black Horehound is the aerial part of Ballota nigra, gathered when in bloom. It is collected in the wild or from cultivated plants propagated by sowing seeds or planting cuttings at the end of winter. The harvest is in July and August. There are no special conditions for drying.

Not to be Confused With: The drug can be confused with Folia melissae. Adulterations with hybrids of Marubium vulgare have been found on the market.

Other Names: Black (Stinking) Horehound

ACTIONS AND PHARMACOLOGY

COMPOUNDS

Diterpenes, marrubiin: 7-acetoxymarrubiin, ballotinon, ballotenol, ballonigrin (to some extent bitter principles)

Volatile oil (traces, unpleasant smell)

Caffeic and ferulic acid derivatives: including chlorogenic acid

Tannins

EFFECTS

Horehound acts as a stimulant, antiemetic and antispasmodic; however, the mode of action has not been satisfactorily explained. According to older literature, a drop in arterial blood pressure and bradycardia occurred in a dog when it was injected intravenously with an infusion (2.5g infusion per kg body weight). When a decoction of the fresh plant was administered intravenously, the volume of gall secretions tripled within 30 minutes.

INDICATIONS AND USAGE

Unproven Uses: Internally, Horehound is used as a sedative in cases of hysteria and hypochondria, as a spasmolytic for stomach cramps and complaints, for whooping cough and to increase bile flow. Horehound is also used to treat nervous, upset stomach, nausea and vomiting. In France, it is traditionally used in the symptomatic treatment of nervous disorders in adults and children, especially for mild sleep disorders and for the symptomatic treatment of coughs. Furthermore, Horehound enemas and suppositories are used against worm infestation. Externally, Horehound is used for gout. The drug's efficacy has not been adequately proven.

PRECAUTIONS AND ADVERSE REACTIONS

No health hazards or side effects are known in conjunction with the proper administration of designated therapeutic dosages.

DOSAGE

Mode of Administration: The drug is used internally in the form of liquid extracts and tinctures. It is also used externally.

Preparation: Liquid extract: 1:1 in 25% ethanol. Tincture: 1:10 with 45% ethanol. Alcohol tincture from the fresh plant with 90% alcohol.

Daily Dose: Single dose of the drug is 2 to 4 g (as an infusion); Liquid extract: 1 to 3 ml; Tincture: 1 to 2 ml.

LITERATURE

Balansard J, Compt Rend Soc Biol 115:1295-1297. 1933.

Kooiman P, (1972) Acta Bot Nederl 21 (4): 417.

Savona G et al., (1976) J Chem Soc (P) 1: 1607-1609.

Savona G et al., (1977) J Chem Soc (P) 1: 322-324 et 497-499.

Savona G et al., La chimica e lĺndustria 58:378. 1976.

Seidel V et al., Phenylpropanoid glycosides from Ballota nigra. In: PM 62(2):186-187. 1997.

Further information in:

Hänsel R, Keller K, Rimpler H, Schneider G (Hrsg.), Hagers Handbuch der Pharmazeutischen Praxis, 5. Aufl., Bde 4-6 (Drogen), Springer Verlag Berlin, Heidelberg, New York, 1992-1994.

Black Mulberry

Morus nigra

DESCRIPTION

Medicinal Parts: The medicinal parts are the ripe berries and the root bark.

Flower and Fruit: The plant is monoecious or dioecious. The greenish flowers are in catkin-like inflorescences. The male flowers are ovate to cylindrical; the female flowers ovate or globular. The flowers have a 4-bract involucre, which enlarges and becomes fleshy in the female flowers. The female flowers have 2 stigmas, the male flowers have 4 stamens. All of the fruit from the catkins develops into blackberry-like false berries, which are really a series of fleshy drupes that are edible and pleasant-tasting.

Leaves, Stem and Root: The tree grows from 6 to 12 m high. The bark is gray-brown. The leaves are alternate with flat-grooved, somewhat hairy petioles. They are cordate or ovate, sessile, unevenly lobed, and serrate with short rough hairs on the upper surface.

Habitat: The plant is cultivated worldwide in temperate regions.

Other Names: Purple Mulberry, White Mulberry

ACTIONS AND PHARMACOLOGY

COMPOUNDS: IN THE FRUIT

Fruit acids (1.9%): including malic acid, citric acid

Saccharose (10%)

Pectins

Ascorbic acid (0.17%)

Flavonoids: including, among others rutin

COMPOUNDS: IN THE LEAVES

Flavonoids: including among others rutin (2-6%)

The constituents of the rhizome rind are not known.

EFFECTS

The active agents are sugar, acids, pectin and rutin, but there is no information available regarding their effects.

INDICATIONS AND USAGE

Unproven Uses: The drug is used as a mild laxative and in the treatment of inflammations of the mucous membranes of the respiratory system.

PRECAUTIONS AND ADVERSE REACTIONS

No health hazards or side effects are known in conjunction with the proper administration of designated therapeutic dosages.

DOSAGE

Mode of Administration: The drug is used internally as a comminuted drug, juice or syrup.

Daily Dosage: The average daily dose is 2 to 4 ml of syrup.

LITERATURE

Deshpande VH, (1968) Tetrahedron Lett 1715.

Kern W, List PH, Hörhammer L (Hrsg.), Hagers Handbuch der Pharmazeutischen Praxis, 4. Aufl., Bde 1-8, Springer Verlag Berlin, Heidelberg, New York, 1969.

Kimura Y et al., (1986) J Nat Prod 94(4):639.

Madaus G, Lehrbuch der Biologischen Arzneimittel, Bde 1-3, Nachdruck, Georg Olms Verlag Hildesheim 1979.

Nomura T et al., (1983) Planta Med 47:151.

Oliver-Bever B (Ed.), Medicinal Plants of Tropical West Africa, Cambridge University Press, Cambridge 1986.

Black Mustard

Brassica nigra

DESCRIPTION

Medicinal Parts: The medicinal parts are the seeds from which oil is extracted.

Flower and Fruit: The inflorescences are terminal or axillary and compressed into a semi-sphere. The flowers have 4 free sepals, 4 free petals, 6 stamens and 1 ovary. The sepals are 3.5 to 4.5 mm long and appear linear because of slits on the edge. They are yellowish-green, usually glabrous, upright and slightly splayed. The yellow petals are twice as long as the calyx, obovate, rounded at the tip and narrowed to a stem at the base. The ovary is on the receptacle. The style is thin and has a semi-globose, cushion-like stigma. The fruit is an erect pod, which is linear and rounded or angular with a thin dividing wall. It is 10 to 25 mm long and pressed onto the stem. The seed is globose, brown, matte and punctate.

Leaves, Stem and Root: Black Mustard is an annual that grows up to 1 m tall and is slim-branched with thin fusiform roots. The stem grows up to 1 m. It is almost round and bristly-haired at the base, with a bluish bloom toward the top. The stem is glabrous with upright branches almost in bushels. The leaves are petiolate, up to 12 cm long and 5 cm wide. The lower leaves are grass-green and covered in 1 mm long bristles. They are pinnatifid and densely dentate, with 2 to 4 obtuse lobes on each side and a large end section. The upper stem and branch leaves are smaller, usually glabrous and blue-green, ovate or lanceolate and slightly dentate.

Habitat: Black Mustard grows in temperate regions worldwide.

Production: Mustard seeds are the seeds of Brassica nigra.

ACTIONS AND PHARMACOLOGY

COMPOUNDS

Glucosinolates: chiefly sinigrin (allylglucosinolates, 1-5%); grinding the seeds into powder and then rubbing with warm water (not with hot water because enzymes would be destroyed), as well as chewing, releases the volatile mustard oil allylisothiocyanate

Fatty oil (30-35%)

Proteins (40%)

Phenyl propane derivatives: including sinapine (choline ester of sinapic acid, 1%)

EFFECTS

The hyperemic effect is the main effect and is employed for various indications where increased blood flow is desired. The drug contains glucosinolates whose main constituent, sinigrin, is converted through enzymatic hydrolysis to allyl mustard oil. This causes a stabbing pain and an intense reddening of the skin. Upon contact with the skin, Allylsen oil causes the severity of the inflammation to increase, potentially to the extent were blisters and necrosis may occur.

INDICATIONS AND USAGE

Unproven Uses: External uses include bronchial pneumonia, sinusitis, pleurisy, lumbago and sciatica for which a mustard poultice is applied, sometimes to achieve an antirheumatic effect (mustard spirit 2%). Foot baths and full baths are used to prompt increased circulation (headaches and mild glaucoma) or to stimulate the cardiopulmonary system (frost bite and vascular disease).

Homeopathic Uses: Uses in homeopathy include irritation of the upper respiratory tract and the gastrointestinal tract.

CONTRAINDICATIONS

Use of Black Mustard is contraindicated in individuals with gastrointestinal ulcers or inflammatory kidney diseases.

PRECAUTIONS AND ADVERSE REACTIONS

General: No health hazards or side effects are known in conjunction with the proper administration of designated therapeutic dosages. Gastrointestinal complaints (and, rarely, kidney irritation) could occur following internal administration, due to the mucus-membrane-irritating effect of the mustard oil. The drug possesses minimal potential for sensitization; contact allergies have been observed. The draining effect associated with the drug's administration makes it inadvisable in the presence of varicosis and venous disorder.

Sneezing, coughing and possible asthmatic attacks can result from breathing the allylisothiocyanate that arises with the preparation and application of mustard poultices. Eyes should be protected when preparing or using the poultices because the vapors can cause eye irritation. Long-term external application or too-intensive reactions upon the skin can lead to injury such as blister formation, suppurating ulcerations and necroses. Mustard poultices are to be removed after no more than 30 minutes.

Drug Interactions: Avoid concomitant use of preparations containing ammonia, because ammonia with mustard oil forms inactive thiosinamine.

Pediatric Use: Black Mustard should not be administered to children under 6 years of age.

OVERDOSAGE

Internal overdosage can lead to vomiting, stomach pain and diarrhea. In severe cases, these can be accompanied by somnolence, cardiac weakness, breathing difficulties and even to death through coma. Following installation of activated charcoal and shock prophylaxis (suitable body position, quiet, warmth), the therapy for poisonings consists of administering mucilaginosa for the protection of mucus membranes and generous amounts of fluids. Possible cases of acidosis should be treated with sodium bicarbonate infusions. In case of shock, plasma volume expanders should be infused. Cardiac massage, intubation and oxygen respiration may also be necessary.

DOSAGE

Mode of Administration: Used externally as a mustard plaster, foot bath or full bath. On rare occasions, Black Mustard is used as a constituent in antirheumatic preparations and cardiac ointments.

How Supplied: Allyl mustard oil: 1 to 3% solution, ointments, emulsions and other rubs (including a rheumatism liniment) are available from commercial sources.

Preparation: To prepare a mustard poultice, mix approximately 100 g mustard flour with lukewarm water and pack in linen. Use on the chest should not exceed 10 minutes (with a maximum of 3 to 5 minutes for children). Limit use on the face to 3 to 4 minutes and take care to avoid the eye area. When mustard paper is used, it is immersed in warm water and then placed on the painful area of skin.

To prepare a full mustard bath, mix 100 to 200 g mustard flour with cold water and press through a cloth into the warm bath. A mustard footbath should be prepared in a bucket or other container that allows the warm water to extend up the leg to the desired position. Add 1 to 3 dessertspoons of mustard flour and stir.

Daily Dosage: The poultice is placed on the chest for about 10 minutes (with a maximum of 3 to 5 minutes for children). Foot bath use should be limited to 10 minutes.

Homeopathic Dosage: 5 drops, 1 tablet, 10 globules every 30 to 60 minutes (acute) or 1 to 3 times daily (chronic); parenterally: 1 to 2 ml sc; acute: 3 times daily; chronic once a day (HAB34).

Storage: The stored drug should be protected from light.

LITERATURE

Halva S et al., Agric Sci Finl 58:157. 1986.

Hänsel R, Keller K, Rimpler H, Schneider G (Hrsg.), Hagers Handbuch der Pharmazeutischen Praxis, 5. Aufl., Bde 4-6 (Drogen): Springer Verlag Berlin, Heidelberg, New York, 1992-1994.

Hill CB et al., J Am Soc Hort Sci 112(2):309. 1987.

Leung AY, Encyclopedia of Common Natural Ingredients Used in Food Drugs, Cosmetics, John Wiley & Sons Inc., New York 1980.

Madaus G, Lehrbuch der Biologischen Arzneimittel, Bde 1-3, Nachdruck, Georg Olms Verlag Hildesheim 1979.

Roth L, Daunderer M, Kormann K, Giftpflanzen, Pflanzengifte, 4. Aufl., Ecomed Fachverlag Landsberg Lech 1993.

Steinegger E, Hänsel R, Pharmakognosie, 5. Aufl., Springer Verlag Heidelberg 1992.

Teuscher E, Lindequist U, Biogene Gifte - Biologie, Chemie, Pharmakologie, 2. Aufl., Fischer Verlag Stuttgart 1994.

Teuscher E, Biogene Arzneimittel, 5. Aufl., Wiss. Verlagsges. Stuttgart 1997.

Wichtl M (Hrsg.), Teedrogen, 4. Aufl., Wiss. Verlagsges. Stuttgart 1997.

Black Nightshade

Solanum nigrum

DESCRIPTION

Medicinal Parts: The medicinal parts are the dried herb collected during the flowering season, the whole fresh plant collected during the flowering season and the whole fresh plant with berries.

Flower and Fruit: The small white flowers are in 6- to 10-blossomed, umbel-like, nodding, axillary inflorescences. The calyx is 5-tipped and does not drop. The corolla is 5-tipped with a short tube. There are 5 stamens with clavate anthers inclining toward each other. The corolla is rotate and has 1 superior ovary. The fruit is a pea-sized black, occasionally green or yellow, berry.

Leaves, Stem and Root: Solanum nigrum is an annual plant 10 to 50 cm in height. The stem is erect, leafy and angular with outward-inclined branches. The leaves are fleshy, petiolate, rhomboid or ovate. They narrow to a cuneate base, which is crenate-dentate and glabrous or sparsely pubescent.

Characteristics: The plant has a musk-like odor when wilting and is poisonous.

Habitat: The plant is found worldwide.

Production: Black Nightshade is the herb of Solanum nigrum picked in uncultivated regions (the wild) and dried in the open air.

Not to be Confused With: Black Nightshade was often called Petty (a corruption of ''petit'') Morel, to distinguish it from the Deadly Nightshade, or Great Morel, as it is also poisonous but apparently less so.

Other Names: Garden Nightshade, Petty Morel, Poisonberry

ACTIONS AND PHARMACOLOGY

COMPOUNDS

Steroid alkaloid glycosides: in the foliage and in unripe fruits (0-2.0%). Ripe fruits are, as a rule, free of alkaloids.

Chief alkaloids: solasonine, solamargine, β-solamargine

Steroid saponins: with tigogenin as an aglycone

EFFECTS

According to folk medicine, the herb should work as an antispasmodic, pain reliever, sedative and narcotic; however, there are no studies available. In animal experiments, the steroid alkaloid glycosides have a local anesthetic effect, increase sleep duration and significantly inhibit the occurrence of acetlysalicylic acid-induced stomach ulcers. The effect is attributed to the inhibition of pepsin and hydrochloric acid secretion.

INDICATIONS AND USAGE

Unproven Uses: Internally, Black Nightshade is used for gastric irritation, cramps and whooping cough. Externally, the herb is used for psoriasis, hemorrhoids, abscesses, eczema and bruising.

Chinese Medicine: Black Nightshade is used for furuncles, carbuncles, abscesses, erysipelas, sprains, strains, contusions, chronic bronchitis and acute hepatitis.

Indian Medicine: Black Nightshade is used for rheumatic pain, coughs, asthma, bronchitis, wounds, swellings, ulcers, flatulence, dyspeptic complaints, vomiting, dysuria, earache, hiccups, eye disease, leprosy and skin diseases.

Homeopathic Uses: Black Nightshade is used for cerebral and meningeal irritation.

PRECAUTIONS AND ADVERSE REACTIONS

No health hazards or side effects are known in conjunction with the proper administration of designated therapeutic dosages.

OVERDOSAGE

Overdoses resulting from the intake of large quantities of fresh foliage with high alkaloid content could lead to gastrointestinal signs of irritation, characterized by queasiness, vomiting, headache and, in rare cases, mydriasis.

DOSAGE

Mode of Administration: The herb is available as a ground drug, tincture and liquid extract for internal and external use.

Preparation: To prepare a rinse or moist compress, add a handful of drug to 1 liter of water and boil for 10 minutes. A tincture is prepared in a ratio of 1:1 with 95% ethanol.

Daily Dosage: Externally, use as a compress or rinse. Internally, the dose is 10 drops of liquid extract 2 to 3 times daily, or 5 to 10 gm of tincture daily.

Homeopathic Dosage: 5 drops, 1 tablet or 10 globules every 30 to 60 minutes (acute) or 1 to 3 times daily (chronic); parenterally: 1 to 2 ml sc; acute, 3 times daily; chronic: once a day (HAB34)

LITERATURE

Frohne D, Pfänder HJ, Giftpflanzen - Ein Handbuch für Apotheker, Toxikologen und Biologen, 4. Aufl., Wiss. Verlags-Ges. Stuttgart 1997.

Hänsel R, Keller K, Rimpler H, Schneider G (Hrsg.), Hagers Handbuch der Pharmazeutischen Praxis, 5. Aufl., Bde 4-6 (Drogen): Springer Verlag Berlin, Heidelberg, New York, 1992-1994.

Johnson R, Lee JS, Ryan CA, Regulation of expression of a wound-inducible tomato inhibitor I gene in transgenic nightshade plants. Plant Mol Biol, 45:349-56, 1990 Mar.

Lewin L, Gifte und Vergiftungen, 6. Aufl., Nachdruck, Haug Verlag, Heidelberg 1992.

Madaus G, Lehrbuch der Biologischen Arzneimittel, Bde 1-3, Nachdruck, Georg Olms Verlag Hildesheim 1979.

Moundipa PF, Domngang FM, Effect of the leafy vegetable Solanum nigrum on the activities of some liver drug-metabolizing enzymes after aflatoxin B1 treatment in female rats. Br J Nutr, 45:81-91, 1991 Jan.

Ridout CL et al., PA 44:732. 1989.

Roth L, Daunderer M, Kormann K, Giftpflanzen, Pflanzengifte, 4. Aufl., Ecomed Fachverlag Landsberg Lech 1993.

Schreiber K, Kulturpflanze 11:451-501. 1963.

Sultana S, Perwaiz S, Iqbal M, Athar M, Crude extracts of hepatoprotective plants Solanum nigrum and Cichorium intybus inhibit free radical-mediated DNA damage. J Ethnopharmacol, 45:189-92, 1995 Mar.

Teuscher E, Biogene Arzneimittel, 5. Aufl., Wiss. Verlagsges. Stuttgart 1997.

Black Pepper

Piper nigrum

DESCRIPTION

Medicinal Parts: The medicinal parts are the berries, which have been freed from the pericarp, and the dried berry-like fruit, which has been collected before ripening.

Flower and Fruit: The inflorescences are pendulous, axillary spikes 5 to 15 cm long containing over 100 inconspicuous white florets. The florets have 1 large ovary with 3 stigmas, 2 stamens and a reduced perianth. Red berry-like drupes form the 30 to 50 flowers, which are fertilized.

Leaves, Stem and Root: The plant is actually a liane, which in cultivation is trained on posts or wire. It can grow to over 6 m. The stem is strong and woody, and the leaves are cordate, glossy and pale green. The leaves are 5 to 10 cm wide, 8 to 18 cm long and are on 5 cm long petioles.

Habitat: The plant grows wild in southern India and is cultivated in tropical Asia and the Caribbean.

Production: Black Peppers are the dried fruits of Piper nigrum, harvested before ripening. The whole ears are plucked and separated from the spindles that have been dried, or the fruit is first brushed from the spindles and then dried. Once the shell has been removed, the green stone-fruit is sun-dried or roasted, after which it blackens.

Not to be Confused With: Foreign fruits of the Piperacae family. It is most frequently confused with peppershells, pepper spindles or stiles, i.e. by-products of the extraction of white pepper from black pepper.

Other Names: Piper, Pepper Bark

ACTIONS AND PHARMACOLOGY

COMPOUNDS

Volatile oil (1.2-2.6%): chief components- sabinene (15-25%), limonene (15-20%), caryophyllene (10-15%), beta-pinene (10-12%), alpha-pinene (8-12%), delta3-carene (5%)

Acid amides (pungent substances): chief components- piperine, additionally including among others piperylin, piperolein A and B, cumaperine

3,4-dihydroxy phenyl ethanol glycosides (substratum for the enzymatic black colouring of the fresh fruits)

Polysaccharides (45%)

Fatty oil (10%)

EFFECTS

The drug stimulates the thermal receptors and increases secretion of saliva and gastric mucous. It has an antimicrobial effect. It influences liver and metabolic functions, and has an insecticidal effect.

INDICATIONS AND USAGE

Unproven Uses: Folk medicine uses include stomach disorders and digestion problems, neuralgia and scabies.

Chinese Medicine: Black Pepper is used for vomiting, diarrhea and gastric symptoms in China.

Indian Medicine: Indian uses include arthritis, asthma, fever, coughs, catarrh, dysentery, dyspepsia, flatulence, hemorrhoids, hiccoughs, urethral discharge and skin damage.

Homeopathic Uses: Piper nigrum is used for irritation of the mucous membranes and galactorrhea.

PRECAUTIONS AND ADVERSE REACTIONS

No health hazards or side effects are known in conjunction with the proper administration of designated therapeutic dosages.

DOSAGE

Mode of Administration: Black Pepper is used internally for stomach disorders and externally as an irritant ointment for neuralgia and scabies.

Daily Dosage: Single doses range from 0.3 to 0.6 gm. The daily dosage is 1.5 gm.

Homeopathic Dosage: 5 to 10 drops, 1 tablet or 5 to 10 globules 1 to 3 times a day or from D4: 1 ml injection solution sc twice weekly (HAB1).

LITERATURE

Atal CK et al., (1975) Lloydia 38:256.

Freist W, Der scharfe Geschmack des Pfeffers - Ein altes Rätsel, nur teilweise gelöst. In: Chemie i.u. Zeit 23(3):135-142. 1991.

Kapil A, Piperine. A Potent Inhibitor of Leishmania donovani Promastigotes in vitro. In: PM 59(5):474. 1993.

Koul IB, Kapil A, Evaluation of the Liver Protective Potential of Piperine, an Active Principle of Black and Long Peppers. In: PM 59(5):413. 1993.

Raina ML et al., (1976) Planta Med 30:198.

Richard ML et al., (1976) J Food Sci 36:584.

Schröder, Buch. In: Schröder R: Kaffee, Tee und Kardamom, Ulmer-Verlag, Stuttgart. 1991.

Traxter JT, (1971) J Agric Food Chem 19:1135.

Further information in:

Fenaroli's Handbook of Flavor Ingredients, Vol. 1. 2nd Ed. Pub. CRC Press Boca Raton 1975.

Hänsel R, Keller K, Rimpler H, Schneider G (Hrsg.), Hagers Handbuch der Pharmazeutischen Praxis, 5. Aufl., Bde 4-6 (Drogen), Springer Verlag Berlin, Heidelberg, New York, 1992-1994.

Leung AY, Encyclopedia of Common Natural Ingredients Used in Food Drugs and Cosmetics, John Wiley & Sons Inc., New York 1980.

Steinegger E, Hänsel R, Pharmakognosie, 5. Aufl., Springer Verlag Heidelberg 1992.

Teuscher E, Biogene Arzneimittel, 5. Aufl., Wiss. Verlagsges. Stuttgart 1997.

Black Root

Leptandra virginica

DESCRIPTION

Medicinal Parts: The medicinal part is the dried rhizome with the roots. The roots have a very different action according to whether they are used fresh or dry. The dried root is milder.

Flower and Fruit: The stems end in terminal, 15 to 25 cm long spikes of white flowers.

Leaves, Stem and Root: The plant is a perennial herb, which grows to about 120 cm high. The rhizome is horizontal, cylindrical, branched and dark red to dark purple-brown on the outside. The simple, erect stems grow in intervals of 1.2 to 3.2 cm from the rhizome. They are smooth and finely downy. The leaves are whorled (4 to 7 in one whorl), lanceolate, on short petioles, pointed and finely serrate.

Habitat: Indigenous to the eastern U.S. but grows elsewhere.

Production: Black Root and its rhizome are the complete underground parts of Leptandra virginica.

Other Names: Bowman's Root, Physic Root, Hini, Oxadoddy, Tall Speedwell, Tall Veronica, Whorlywort, Culveris Root

ACTIONS AND PHARMACOLOGY

COMPOUNDS

Volatile oil: composition unknown

Cinnamic acid derivatives: including among others 4-methoxycinnamic acid, 3,4-dimethoxycinnamic acid and their esters

Tannins

The constituents of the drug have not been fully investigated.

EFFECTS

The drug has diaphoretic, carminative and cathartic effects. It is also a cholagogue and a laxative.

INDICATIONS AND USAGE

Unproven Uses: Black Root is used for chronic constipation and liver and gallbladder disorders. It is also used as an emetic.

Homeopathic Uses: The drug is used for diarrhea and inflammation of the liver and gallbladder.

PRECAUTIONS AND ADVERSE REACTIONS

No health hazards are known in conjunction with the proper administration of designated therapeutic dosages. The emetic and laxative effects of the drug are used therapeutically.

DOSAGE

Homeopathic Dosage: 5 drops, 1 tablet or 10 globules every 30 to 60 minutes (acute) or 1 to 3 times daily (chronic); parenterally: 1 to 2 ml sc, acute: 3 times daily; chronic: once a day (HAB1).

LITERATURE

Hänsel R, Keller K, Rimpler H, Schneider G (Hrsg.), Hagers Handbuch der Pharmazeutischen Praxis, 5. Aufl., Bde 4-6 (Drogen), Springer Verlag Berlin, Heidelberg, New York, 1992-1994 (unter Veronica virginica).

Lewin L, Gifte und Vergiftungen, 6. Aufl., Nachdruck, Haug Verlag, Heidelberg 1992.

Madaus G, Lehrbuch der Biologischen Arzneimittel, Bde 1-3, Nachdruck, Georg Olms Verlag Hildesheim 1979.

Wagner H, Wiesenauer M, Phytotherapie. Phytopharmaka und pflanzliche Homöopathika, Fischer-Verlag, Stuttgart, Jena, New York 1995.

Blackberry

Rubus fruticosus

DESCRIPTION

Medicinal Parts: The medicinal parts are the leaves, roots and berries.

Flower and Fruit: The white or sometimes pale pink flowers are in cymes. The calyx is 5-sepaled, the corolla is 5-petalled. There are numerous stamens and ovaries. The small fruit forms a black or reddish-black aggregate fruit, the blackberry.

Leaves, Stem and Root: The plant is a fast-growing, thorny bush up to 2 m high. The generally blunt stems are densely covered in tough thorns that creep or curve backward. The leaves are usually 5-paired pinnate, glabrous above, and gray to white tomentose beneath.

Habitat: The plant is indigenous to Europe and has naturalized in America and Australia.

Production: Blackberry root consists of the underground parts of Rubus fruticosus as well as its preparations. Blackberry leaf consists of the dried, fermented or unfermented leaf, gathered during the flowering period, of Rubus fruticosus as well as its preparations.

Other Names: Blackberry, American, Dewberry, Bramble, Goutberry, High Blackberry, Thimbleberry

ACTIONS AND PHARMACOLOGY

COMPOUNDS: BLACKBERRY ROOT

Saponins

Tannins

EFFECTS: BLACKBERRY ROOT

There is no reliable information available.

COMPOUNDS: BLACKBERRY LEAF

Fruit acids: including citric acid, isocitric acid

Flavonoids

Tannins (8 to 14%): gallo tannins, dimeric ellagitannins

EFFECTS: BLACKBERRY LEAF

Blackberry leaf has astringent and antidiarrheal effects due to the high tannin content.

INDICATIONS AND USAGE

BLACKBERRY ROOT

Unproven Uses: Blackberry root is used in folk medicine as a prophylaxis for dropsy. It is also used in gastrointestinal conditions.

BLACKBERRY LEAF

Approved by Commission E:

- Diarrhea
- Inflammation of the mouth and pharynx

Blackberry leaf is used for non-specific, acute diarrhea and mild inflammation of the mucosa of the oral cavity and throat.

PRECAUTIONS AND ADVERSE REACTIONS

BLACKBERRY ROOT AND LEAF

No health hazards or side effects are known in conjunction with the proper administration of designated therapeutic dosages.

DOSAGE

BLACKBERRY ROOT

No information is available

BLACKBERRY LEAF

Mode of Administration: Balckberry leaf is available as crude drug for infusions and other preparations for internal use, as well as for mouthwashes. The drug is a component of various tea mixtures.

Daily Dosage: 2 to 5 gm drug. To prepare a tea, scald 1.5 gm drug, steep for 10 to 15 minutes, strain (1 teaspoon equivalent to approximately 0.6 gm drug).

LITERATURE

BLACKBERRY LEAF

Henning W, (1981) Lebensm Unters Forsch 173:180.

Gupta RK et al., J Chem Soc Perkin I:2525. 1982.

Mukherjee M et al., PH 23:2881. 1984.

Wollmann Ch et al., PA 19:456. 1964.

Further information in:

Kern W, List PH, Hörhammer L (Hrsg.), Hagers Handbuch der Pharmazeutischen Praxis, 4. Aufl., Bde. 1-8: Springer Verlag Berlin, Heidelberg, New York, 1969.

Leung AY, Encyclopedia of Common Natural Ingredients Used in Food, Drugs, Cosmetics, John Wiley & Sons Inc., New York 1980.

Madaus G, Lehrbuch der Biologischen Arzneimittel, Bde 1-3, Nachdruck, Georg Olms Verlag Hildesheim 1979.

Wichtl M (Hrsg.), Teedrogen, 4. Aufl., Wiss. Verlagsges. Stuttgart 1997.

BLACKBERRY ROOT

Henning W, (1981) Lebensm Unters Forsch 173:180.

Further information in:

Kern W, List PH, Hörhammer L (Hrsg.), Hagers Handbuch der Pharmazeutischen Praxis, 4. Aufl., Bde. 1-8: Springer Verlag Berlin, Heidelberg, New York, 1969.

Leung AY, Encyclopedia of Common Natural Ingredients Used in Food, Drugs, Cosmetics, John Wiley & Sons Inc., New York 1980.

Bladderwort

Utricularia vulgaris

DESCRIPTION

Medicinal Parts: The medicinal part is the whole plant.

Flower and Fruit: The vertical peduncle is 10 to 35 cm high and bears 4 to 15 flowers in a loose raceme. The petioles are short and campanulate, 13 to 20 mm long with a bilabiate margin.

Leaves, Stem and Root: Utricularia vulgaris is a water plant, which appears at flowering time. The water shoot is 60 cm long with double-rowed leaves facing all directions. The water leaves are 1 to 8 cm long and have 2 to 3 large lobes. Each lobe is pinnatifid and ends in numerous tips. There are 8 to 209 tubes per leaf.

Habitat: Europe

Production: Bladderwort is the whole plant of Utricularia vulgaris.

ACTIONS AND PHARMACOLOGY

COMPOUNDS

Iridoids: including globularin, scutellarioside II

Phenylpropane derivatives: 1-p-cumaroyl-glucoside

EFFECTS

The plant has diuretic, antispasmodic and anti-inflammatory effects.

INDICATIONS AND USAGE

The drug was formerly used internally in the treatment of urinary tract disorders and externally for burns. The active substances in Bladderwort increase gallbladder secretions; consequently, the drug is used to treat skin and mucous membrane inflammation.

PRECAUTIONS AND ADVERSE REACTIONS

No health hazards or side effects are known in conjunction with the proper administration of designated therapeutic dosages.

DOSAGE

Mode of Administration: The drug is obsolete in many parts of Germany. Bladderwort is used internally and externally in other parts of the world.

Preparation: To prepare a diuretic infusion for internal use, add 2 gm of drug per 100 ml of water. To prepare an anti-inflammatory infusion for external use, add 6 gm of drug per 100 ml of water.

Daily Dosage: Internally, as a diuretic infusion, drink two small cups daily. Externally, the anti-inflammatory infusion is used in mouthwashes, cleansers, cosmetics and face packs.

LITERATURE

Baumgartner DL, Laboratory evaluation of the bladderwort plant, Utricularia vulgaris (Lentibulariaceae), as a predator of late instar Culex pipiens and assessment of its biocontrol potential. J Am Mosq Control Assoc, 23:504-7, 1987 Sep.

Hegnauer R, Chemotaxonomie der Pflanzen, Bde 1-11: Birkhäuser Verlag Basel, Boston, Berlin 1962-1997.

Bladderwrack

Fucus vesiculosus

TRADE NAMES

Bladderwrack (available from numerous manufacturers and as combination product)

DESCRIPTION

Medicinal Parts: The medicinal parts are the dried thallus and the fresh thallus of Bladderwrack.

Flower and Fruit: Some thallus ends look grainy and it is here that the reproductive organs are found. The fructifications consisting of 3 cm long ovoid receptacles are found in the tips of these thalli. They are either cordate or ovately flattened with grainy bladders.

Leaves, Stem and Root: The plant is often over 1 m long, olive green when fresh and black brown when dry. The stem of the thallus is flat, repeatedly bifurcated and has a midrib along the whole length. Beside this midrib there are often scattered pores and numerous air-filled bladders.

Habitat: The plant is found on the North Sea coast, the western Baltic coast, and on the Atlantic and Pacific coasts.

Production: Bladderwrack consists of the dried thallus of Fucus vesiculosus, of Ascophyllum nodosum, or of both species, as well as their preparations. The algae are harvested when the tide is out, then washed in fresh water and dried at 60° C.

Other Names: Seawrack, Kelpware, Black-Tang, Bladder Fucus, Cutweed, Fucus, Quercus marina, Kelp-Ware, Rockwrack

ACTIONS AND PHARMACOLOGY

COMPOUNDS

Inorganic iodine salts

Organically-bound iodine: in particular in proteins and lipids, also present as diiodothyrosine

Polysaccharides: including alginic acid, fucane, fucoidine (strongly sulfated)

Polyphenold: Phlorotannins

EFFECTS

The drug is antimicrobial, has a hypoglycemic effect in animal experiments and leads in vitro to hemaglutination of human erythrocytes because of the polyphenolic substances.

Its use in the treatment of thyroid conditions associated with hypethyrosis has merit because of the high iodine content. There is information on its apparent usefulness in weight reduction, which must be strongly criticized for the reasons given above.

INDICATIONS AND USAGE

Unproven Uses: Preparations of Bladderwrack are used internally for diseases of the thyroid, obesity, overweight, arteriosclerosis and digestive disorders and externally for sprains.

Homeopathic Uses: In Homeopathy Fucus vesiculosus is used for obesity and goitre.

PRECAUTIONS AND ADVERSE REACTIONS

General: Dosages above 150 gm iodide/day carry with them the danger of induction or worsening of a hyperthyroidism. For that reason, the drug should no longer be administered due to its variable iodide content (0.03 - 1%). Allergic reactions have been known to occur.

Pregnancy: Not to be used during pregnancy.

Drug Interactions: Bladderwrack has a hypoglycemic effect. Theoretically, there may be an interaction with other anti-hyperglycemic medications. Monitor patients carefully if they are concurrently using glucose lowering agents.

DOSAGE

Mode of Administration: Bladderwrack is available as drops and fluid extract for internal use.

How Supplied: Fluid Extract: 1:1

Daily Dosage:
Infusion — single dose: 5 to 10 gm drug 3 times daily.

Extract — single dose: 4 to 8 ml 3 times daily.

Homeopathic Dosage: 5 drops, 1 tablet or 10 globules every 30 to 60 minutes (acute) and 1 to 3 times daily (chronic); parenterally: 1 to 2 ml sc acute: 3 times daily; chronic: once a day (HAB34).

Maximum daily intake of iodine is limited to 120 µg.

Storage: Should be protected from light.

LITERATURE

Béress A, Wassermann O, Bruhn T, Béress L, A new procedure for the isolation of anti-HIV compounds (polysaccharides and polyphenols) from the marine alga Fucus vesiculosus. In: JNP 56(4):478-488. 1993.

Criado MT et al., (1983) IRC Med Sci 11(3):286.

Curro F et al., (1976) Arch Med Interna 28(1):19.

Frohne D, Phytotherapeutika und Schilddrüse. In: Intern Praxis 32(1)158. 1992.

Glombitza KW et al., (1977) Planta Med 32(1):33.

Glombitza KW, Lentz G (1981) Tetrahedron 37(22):3861.

Phillips DJH (1979) Environ Pollut 18(1):31.

Quang-Liem P, Laur MH (1974) Biochimie 56(6/7):925.

Quang-Liem P, Laur MH (1976) Biochimie 58(11/12):1367.

Stahl E et al., DAZ 115:1893. 1975.

Further information in:

Hänsel R, Keller K, Rimpler H, Schneider G (Hrsg.), Hagers Handbuch der Pharmazeutischen Praxis, 5. Aufl., Bde 4-6 (Drogen), Springer Verlag Berlin, Heidelberg, New York, 1992-1994.

Madaus G, Lehrbuch der Biologischen Arzneimittel, Bde 1-3, Nachdruck, Georg Olms Verlag Hildesheim 1979.

Steinegger E, Hänsel R, Pharmakognosie, 5. Aufl., Springer Verlag Heidelberg 1992.

Teuscher E, Biogene Arzneimittel, 5. Aufl., Wiss. Verlagsges. mbH Stuttgart 1997.

Wichtl M (Hrsg.), Teedrogen, 4. Aufl., Wiss. Verlagsges. Stuttgart 1997.

Blessed Thistle

Cnicus benedictus

TRADE NAMES

Blessed Thistle is available from a number of manufacturers.

DESCRIPTION

Medicinal Parts: The dried leaves and upper stems, including the inflorescence, and the flowering parts of the plant.

Flower and Fruit: The blossom is a pale yellow composite, its solitary flower sessile on the tips of the twigs. The florets are tubular. The few lateral florets are sterile, have 3-part borders and are smaller than the numerous androgynous florets. The epicalyx is ovate. The inner bracts end in a long, rigid and pinnatifid thorn. The outer bracts terminate in a simple thorn. They are broad, leafy and connected with the cordate-oblong leaflets of the epicalyx by numerous web-like hairs. The fruit has a tuft of hair.

Leaves, Stem and Root: The thistle grows to 30 to 50 cm high. The stems are heavily branched, thistle-like, villous and glutinous pubescent. The leaves are oblong, emarginate to pinnatifid, thorny-dentate, and roughly reticulate.

Characteristics: The plant has a strong and bitter taste.

Habitat: The thistle comes from southern Europe but is cultivated in other regions of the continent.

Production: Blessed Thistle herb consists of the dried leaves and upper stems, including inflorescence, of Cnicus benedictus.

Other Names: St. Benedicts Thistle, Cardin, Holy Thistle, Spotted Thistle

ACTIONS AND PHARMACOLOGY

COMPOUNDS

Sesquiterpene lactone-bitter principles: chief components cnicin, additionally, salonitenolide, artemisiifolin

Lignans (also bitter): trachelogenin, arctigenin, nor-tracheloside

Volatile oil: components including n-nonane, n-undecane, n-tridecane, dodeca-1,11-dien-3,5,7,9-tetrain (polyyne), p-cymene, fenchon, citral, cinnamaldehyde

Triterpenes: alpha-amyrin, multiflorenol

Flavonoides: including apigenin-7-O-glucoside, luteolin, astragalin

EFFECTS

The main constituent is the amaroid cnicin, which is antimicrobial, cytotoxic and antitumoural. The amaroids stimulate the secretion of saliva and gastric juices. In animal tests an anti-edemic effect was demonstrated.

INDICATIONS AND USAGE

Approved by Commission E:

- Dyspeptic complaints
- Loss of appetite

Unproven Uses: St. Benedict Thistle is used as a cholagogue. Internal folk medicine applications include loss of appetite, anorexia, fever and colds, and as a diuretic. External application for wounds and ulcers is noted.

CONTRAINDICATIONS

St. Benedict Thistle is not to be used during pregnancy.

PRECAUTIONS AND ADVERSE REACTIONS

Health risks or side effects following the proper administration of designated therapeutic dosages are not recorded. The drug exhibits a strong potential for sensitization (cross-reactions with mugwort and cornflower, among others); however, allergic reactions have been seen only rarely.

DOSAGE

Mode of Administration: Comminuted drug and dried extracts for infusions or other bitter-tasting galenic preparations for internal use.

How Supplied:

Capsules — 340 mg, 360 mg

Extract — 1:1

Tablets

Preparation: Infusions are prepared by pouring boiling water over 1.5 to 2 gm of drug, allowing to set, then straining after 10 to 20 minutes.

Daily Dosage: Four to 6 gm of drug. The dosage for the aromatic bitter is 1 cup 1/2 hour before meals. One cup of tea is taken 3 times a day.

LITERATURE

Banhaelen M, Vanhaelen-Fastre R, (1975) Phytochemistry 14: 2709.

Farnsworth NR et al., (1975) J Pharm Sci 64(4):535.

Harnischfeger G, Stolze H, notabene medici 11:652. 1981.

Urzúa A, Acuna P, (1983) Fitoterapia 4:175

Vanhaelen-Fastre R, PM 24:165. 1973.

Vanhaelen-Fastre R, Vanhaelen M, (1976) Planta Med 29:179.

Further information in:

Fenaroli's Handbook of Flavor Ingredients, Vol. 1, 2nd Ed., CRC Press 1975.

Hausen B, Allergiepflanzen, Pflanzenallergene, ecomed Verlagsgesellsch. mbH, Landsberg 1988.

Kern W, List PH, Hörhammer L (Hrsg.), Hagers Handbuch der Pharmazeutischen Praxis, 4. Aufl., Bde. 1-8, Springer Verlag Berlin, Heidelberg, New York, 1969.

Madaus G, Lehrbuch der Biologischen Arzneimittel, Bde 1-3, Nachdruck, Georg Olms Verlag Hildesheim 1979.

Roth L, Daunderer M, Kormann K, Giftpflanzen, Pflanzengifte, 4. Aufl., Ecomed Fachverlag Landsberg Lech 1993.

Steinegger E, Hänsel R, Pharmakognosie, 5. Aufl., Springer Verlag Heidelberg 1992.

Teuscher E, Biogene Arzneimittel, 5. Aufl., Wiss. Verlagsges. mbH Stuttgart 1997.

Wagner H, Wiesenauer M, Phytotherapie. Phytopharmaka und pflanzliche Homöopathika, Fischer-Verlag, Stuttgart, Jena, New York 1995.

Wichtl M (Hrsg.), Teedrogen, 4. Aufl., Wiss. Verlagsges. Stuttgart 1997.

Bloodroot

Sanguinaria canadensis

DESCRIPTION

Medicinal Parts: The medicinal parts are roots and the whole plant.

Flower and Fruit: The plant bears a white flower with 8 to 12 petals on a 15 cm long scape. It is wax-like and has golden stamens. The seed is an oblong, narrow capsule approximately 2.5 cm long.

Leaves, Stem and Root: The perennial plant grows to about 15 cm high. The rhizome is thick, round, fleshy and slightly curved at the end. It is 2.5 to 10 cm long and has orange-red rootlets. The 1 basal palmately-lobed leaf appears when the flower dies. The down-covered, grayish green leaf is clasping, 15 to 25 cm long and has 5 to 9 lobes. Protruding ribs are recognizable on the under surface.

Habitat: The plant is indigenous to the northeastern U.S.

Production: Canadian Bloodroot is the root-stock (rhizome) of Sanguinaria canadensis.

Other Names: Indian Paint, Tetterwort, Red Root, Paucon, Coon Root, Snakebite, Sweet Slumber, Indian Plant, Pauson, Sanguinaria

ACTIONS AND PHARMACOLOGY

COMPOUNDS

Isoquinoline alkaloids of the benzophenanthridine type (4-7%): chief alkaloid sanguinarine, further including among others, chelerythrine, oxysanguinarine; protoberberine-type: berberine, coptisine; protopine-type: protopine, alpha- and beta-allocryptopine

Resins

Starch

EFFECTS

The alkaloid sanguinarin is antimicrobial and anti-inflammatory. Its use as an antiplaque agent and for gingivitis is plausible and has been documented in diverse studies. The alkaloids initially act as a narcotic, causing severe cramping that is followed by a local paralysis of sensitive nerve endings.

INDICATIONS AND USAGE

The drug was formerly used as an expectorant, as an active antiplaque agent, and as a mouthwash.

CONTRAINDICATIONS

Bloodroot is not to be used during pregnancy.

PRECAUTIONS AND ADVERSE REACTIONS

No health hazards or side effects are known in conjunction with the proper administration of designated therapeutic dosages.

OVERDOSAGE

The drug has an emetic effect in dosages above 0.03 g, and was previously used therapeutically. Higher dosages of the drug severely irritate the mucus membranes. Overdoses can cause vomiting, diarrhea, intestinal colic, and possible collapse.

DOSAGE

Mode of Administration: The drug is obsolete in most countries. Bloodroot is still used in homeopathic preparations, as an ingredient in some pharmaceutical preparations, and as a component of toothpaste and mouthwashes.

LITERATURE

Anonym, Medizinische Mundpflege mit Sanguinaria-Extrakt. In: DAZ 131(16):XLII. 1991.

Collins KR, Pat. EP 25649 (1981) Europe.

Elliott JQ, Pat. US 4515779 (1985) USA.

Ladanyi P, Pat. CH 638973 (1983) Switzerland.

Maiti M et al., Febs Lett 142:280.

Further information in:

Frohne D, Pfänder HJ, Giftpflanzen - Ein Handbuch für Apotheker, Toxikologen und Biologen, 4. Aufl., Wiss. Verlags-Ges. Stuttgart 1997.

Kern W, List PH, Hörhammer L (Hrsg.), Hagers Handbuch der Pharmazeutischen Praxis, 4. Aufl., Bde 1-8: Springer Verlag Berlin, Heidelberg, New York, 1969.

Lewin L, Gifte und Vergiftungen, 6. Aufl., Nachdruck, Haug Verlag, Heidelberg 1992.

Madaus G, Lehrbuch der Biologischen Arzneimittel, Bde 1-3, Nachdruck, Georg Olms Verlag Hildesheim 1979.

Roth L, Daunderer M, Kormann K, Giftpflanzen, Pflanzengifte, 4. Aufl., Ecomed Fachverlag Landsberg Lech 1993.

Wagner H, Wiesenauer M, Phytotherapie. Phytopharmaka und pflanzliche Homöopathika, Fischer-Verlag, Stuttgart, Jena, New York 1995.

Blue Cohosh

Caulophyllum thalictroides

TRADE NAMES

Blue Cohosh Root Liquid (available from numerous manufacturers and as a combination product)

DESCRIPTION

Medicinal Parts: Medicinal parts are the dried rhizome and roots and preparations of the fresh roots.

Flower and Fruit: The inflorescence on the terminal leaf is panicled, 3 to 6 cm long and surrounded by a leaf-like bract. The flowers are yellowish-green to purple and are 1 cm in diameter. The 6 sepals are arranged in 2 rows. The 6 petals are markedly reduced, inconspicuous and gland-like. The 6 stamens are as long as the petals. The ovary opens before it is ripe and contains 2 dark blue 5 to 8 mm long, roundish seeds on solid stems. These resemble drupes because of the fleshy seed-shell.

Leaves, Stem and Root: The plant is a leafy, 30 to 70 cm high erect perennial with a brownish-gray, branched rhizome. The leaves are inserted in the middle of the shoot with a large, almost sessile leaf, which is tri-pinnate and resembles 3 foliage leaves. The leaflets are stemmed, obovate, finely divided into 3 lobes, and wedge-shaped at the base.

Characteristics: Taste is sweetish, then bitter; almost odorless.

Habitat: The plant is found in the damp woods of the eastern part of North America.

Production: Blue Cohosh is the dried root and root-stock of Caulophyllum thalictroides. It is collected in the wild.

Other Names: Papoose Root, Squawroot, Blueberry Root, Beechdrops, Blue Ginseng, Yellow Ginseng

ACTIONS AND PHARMACOLOGY

COMPOUNDS

Quinolizidine alkaloids: main alkaloids (-)-anagyrines, (-)-N-methyl-cytisines, and (-)-baptifoline

Isoquinoline alkaloids: magnoflorine

Triterpene saponins: caulophyllosaponin

Caulosapogenin

EFFECTS

An unspecified glycoside, which has been localized from the drug and then injected into the ears of rabbits, causes a strong local irritation. Applying a solution into the rabbit's eyes leads to inflammation. Glycoside is supposed to have an oxytoxic effect.

The weak estrogenic, spasmolytic effect is probably caused by, as yet unknown constituents; the ensuing nicotine effect is possibly caused by N-methylcytisine.

INDICATIONS AND USAGE

Unproven Uses: Internally it has been used for amenorrhoea, dysmenorrhoea, threatened miscarriage, contraction-like spasms, rheumatic symptoms, and in particular conditions resulting from uterus atonia.

Indian Medicine: In India, the drug is known as a treatment for gynecological disorders. In English and American medicine, the drug has been used since the beginning of the 20th century for worm infestation, dehydration, menstrual ailments, cramps, and mainly to stimulate contractions and act as an antispasmodic during labor.

Homeopathic Uses: Uses include for problems of menstruation and labor, as well as rheumatism of the fingers and toes.

PRECAUTIONS AND ADVERSE REACTIONS

General: No health hazards or side effects are known in conjunction with the proper administration of designated therapeutic dosages.

Pregnancy: The drug should not be taken during the first three months of pregnancy due to its estrogenic effect and possible teratogenic action of the anagyrines.

DOSAGE

Mode of Administration: The drug is used internally as a decoction or a liquid extract.

How Supplied:
Liquid — 1:1

Preparation: Infusion (no specifications); liquid extract 1:1 in ethanol 70% (V/V)

Daily Dosage: The average single dose is 0.3 to 1 gm of drug; 0.5 to 1 ml of liquid extract.

Homeopathic Dosage: 5 drops, 1 tablet, 10 globules 30 to 60 minutes (acute) or 1 to 3 times a day (chronic); parenterally: 1 to 2 ml 3 times a day sc (HAB34).

LITERATURE

Benoit PS et al., (1976) Lloydia 39:160.

Di Carlo FI et al., (1964) J Reticuloendothelial Soc 1:224.

Flom MS et al., (1967) J Pharm Sci 56:1515-1517.

Strigina LI et al., (1975) Phytochemistry 15:1583.

Strigina LI et al., (1976) Khim Prir Soedin 5:619.

Further information in:

Hänsel R, Keller K, Rimpler H, Schneider G (Hrsg.), Hagers Handbuch der Pharmazeutischen Praxis, 5. Aufl., Bde 4-6 (Drogen), Springer Verlag Berlin, Heidelberg, New York, 1992-1994.

Hegnauer R, Chemotaxonomie der Pflanzen, Bde 1-11, Birkhäuser Verlag Basel, Boston, Berlin 1962-1997.

Madaus G, Lehrbuch der Biologischen Arzneimittel, Bde 1-3, Nachdruck, Georg Olms Verlag Hildesheim 1979.

Roth L, Daunderer M, Kormann K, Giftpflanzen, Pflanzengifte, 4. Aufl., Ecomed Fachverlag Landsberg Lech 1993.

Bog Bean

Menyanthes trifoliata

DESCRIPTION

Medicinal Parts: The medicinal part of the plant is the dried herb.

Flower and Fruit: The flowers are white or reddish-white, medium-sized and have many blossomed racemes on long, leafless peduncles. There are 5 sepals. The corolla is fused with 5 tips and is pubescent inside. There are 5 reddish stamens and 1 superior ovary. The fruit is an ovate capsule.

Leaves, Stem and Root: Menyanthes trifoliata is a perennial green, glabrous aquatic plant that grows from 15 to 30 cm high. The herb has a small, finger-thick creeping rhizome. The decumbent stem varies in length according to conditions. Leaf sheaths surround the stem. The leaves are on long, fleshy, grooved petioles. They are trifoliate, 5 cm long and 2.5 cm wide, and have obovate leaflets.

Characteristics: The herb has a strong bitter taste.

Habitat: The plant is indigenous to Europe, Asia and America.

Production: Bog Bean leaf consists of the leaf of Menyanthes trifoliata.

Other Names: Buck Bean, Bog Myrtle, Brook Bean, Marsh Clover, Moonflower, Trefoil, Water Shamrock

ACTIONS AND PHARMACOLOGY

COMPOUNDS

Iridoide monoterpenes (bitter principles): chief components 7', 8'-dihydrofoliamenthin, additionally including among others sweroside, loganin, menthiafolin, foliomenthin

Monoterpene alkaloids: including gentianin E

Flavonoids: including among others rutin, hyperoside, trifolin

Hydroxycoumarins: scopoletin

Caffeic acid derivatives

Pyrridine alkaloids: including gentianine, gentianidine

Triterpene glycosides: lupeol, beta-amyrenol, betulin, betulinic acid, alpha-spinasterol, stigmast-7-enol

EFFECTS

The drug stimulates saliva and gastric juice secretion. An antimicrobial effect has been demonstrated in vitro.

INDICATIONS AND USAGE

- Dyspeptic complaints
- Loss of appetite

Because it is a bitter and promotes gastric secretion, the drug is used for loss of appetite and peptic discomfort.

Unproven Uses: Folk medicine uses, particularly in European countries, include diseases of the digestive system and fevers.

Chinese Medicine: Insomnia, weak stomach and intestines, spleen disorders, intermittent fever, headache, breathing difficulties, amenorrhea, ear ache, jaundice, edema, gout, scabies and furuncles are among the applications in Chinese medicine.

CONTRAINDICATIONS

Use of the drug is contraindicated for patients with diarrhea, dysentery or colitis.

PRECAUTIONS AND ADVERSE REACTIONS

No health hazards or side effects are known in conjunction with the proper administration of designated therapeutic dosages.

OVERDOSAGE

Symptoms of overdose include vomiting and diarrhea.

DOSAGE

Mode of Administration: Comminuted herb for teas and other bitter-tasting preparations for internal use.

Preparation: Pour boiling water over 0.5 to 1 g of the finely cut drug (1 teaspoonful = 0.9 g) or place the drug in cold water and bring rapidly to a boil. Allow either preparation to steep for 5 to 10 minutes, then strain.

How Supplied: The drug is a component of standardized preparations of various tonics.

Daily Dosage: The average daily dose is 1.5 to 3 g of the drug. The dosage for the infusion is 1/2 cup, unsweetened, before each meal.

LITERATURE

Battersby AR et al., (1967) J Chem Soc Chem Commun. 1277.

Ciaceri G, (1972) Fitoterapia 43:134.

Janeczko Z et al., A triterpenoid glycoside from Menyanthes trifoliata. In: PH 29(12):3885-3887. 1990.

Junior P, Weitere Untersuchungen zur Verteilung und Straktur der Bitterstoffe von Menyanthes trifoliata. In: PM 32(12): 112. 1989.

Phillipson JD, Anderson LA, (1984) Pharm J 233:80 et 111.

Swaitek L et al., (1986) Planta Med 6:60P.

Tumón H et al., The effect of Menyanthes trifolita L. on acute renal failure might due to PAF-inhibition. In: Phytomedicine 1:39-45. 1994.

Further information in:

Fenaroli's Handbook of Flavor Ingredients, Vol. 1., 2nd Ed., CRC Press Boca Raton 1975.

Kern W, List PH, Hörhammer L (Hrsg.), Hagers Handbuch der Pharmazeutischen Praxis, 4. Aufl., Bde. 1-8, Springer Verlag Berlin, Heidelberg, New York, 1969.

Madaus G, Lehrbuch der Biologischen Arzneimittel, Bde 1-3, Nachdruck, Georg Olms Verlag Hildesheim 1979.

Roth L, Daunderer M, Kormann K, Giftpflanzen, Pflanzengifte, 4. Aufl., Ecomed Fachverlag Landsberg Lech 1993.

Steinegger E, Hänsel R, Pharmakognosie, 5. Aufl., Springer Verlag Heidelberg 1992.

Teuscher E, Biogene Arzneimittel, 5. Aufl., Wiss. Verlagsges. Stuttgart 1997.

Wichtl M (Hrsg.), Teedrogen, 4. Aufl., Wiss. Verlagsges. Stuttgart 1997.

Bog Bilberry

Vaccinium uliginosum

DESCRIPTION

Medicinal Parts: The medicinal part is the dried ripe fruit.

Flower and Fruit: The flowers are arranged in axils of small leaves at the end of short lateral branches. They are hanging and white or reddish in color. The pedicle is encircled at the base with a light brown bud husk. The calyx is fused with the ovary. The fruit is a round or pear-shaped, blue-frosted, 7 to 10 cm long, multi-seeded berry. The light brown seeds are sickle-shaped with sharp ends, and have a punctate-reticulate skin.

Leaves, Stem and Root: The plant is an angular shrub up to 80 cm high with round, gray-brown, glabrous branches and a creeping rhizome. The leaves are deciduous, obovate or oblong, entire, tough and short-petioled. The undersurface has a protruding, reticulate vein system and is blue-green. The upper surface of the leaves is light matte-green to almost white.

Habitat: The plant is common throughout the Northern Hemisphere.

Production: Bog Bilberries and leaves are the ripe fruit and leaves of Vaccinium uliginosum. The collection or picking occurs in uncultivated regions. The drug is either air-dried in the shade or dried artificially.

Not to be Confused With: The Bog Bilberry has smaller flowers and berries than the common Bilberry (Vaccinium myrtillus; see separate entry).

ACTIONS AND PHARMACOLOGY

COMPOUNDS: IN THE LEAVES

Tannins: catechin tannins

Triterpenes: alpha-amyrin, friedelin, ursolic acid

Sterols: beta-sitosterol, beta-sitosterol-3-O-beta-glucoside

Flavonoids: including hyperoside

COMPOUNDS: IN THE FRUITS

Anthocyans: including chief components: malvidin-3-O-glucoside, delphinidine-3-O-glucoside, delphinidine-3-O-arabinoside

Organic acids: including benzoic acid

Flavonoids: including hyperoside, myricetin, myricetin-5'-methyl ether

EFFECTS

No information is available.

INDICATIONS AND USAGE

Unproven Uses: Bog Bilberry is used for gastric and intestinal catarrh, diarrhea and bladder complaints.

PRECAUTIONS AND ADVERSE REACTIONS

No health hazards or side effects are known in conjunction with the proper administration of designated therapeutic dosages.

OVERDOSAGE

Signs of poisoning following consumption of large quantities of the fruits have occurred very rarely. Signs include queasiness, vomiting, states of intoxication, feelings of weakness and visual disorders. Presumably, these poisonings can be traced back to the plant being infested with the lower fungus *Sclerotinia megalospora.*

DOSAGE

Mode of Administration: The drug is used internally as a liquid extract (tea).

Preparation: To prepare a tea, pour 250 ml of cold water over 2 heaping teaspoons of drug; steep for 10 to 12 hours and strain.

Daily Dosage: Drink 1 cup of the prepared tea, unsweetened, once or twice a day.

LITERATURE

Frohne D, Pfänder HJ, Giftpflanzen - Ein Handbuch für Apotheker, Toxikologen und Biologen, 4. Aufl., Wiss. Verlags-Ges. Stuttgart 1997.

Hänsel R, Keller K, Rimpler H, Schneider G (Hrsg.), Hagers Handbuch der Pharmazeutischen Praxis, 5. Aufl., Bde 4-6 (Drogen): Springer Verlag Berlin, Heidelberg, New York, 1992-1994.

Lewin L, Gifte und Vergiftungen, 6. Aufl., Nachdruck, Haug Verlag, Heidelberg 1992.

Roth L, Daunderer M, Kormann K, Giftpflanzen, Pflanzengifte, 4. Aufl., Ecomed Fachverlag Landsberg Lech 1993.

Teuscher E, Lindequist U, Giftstoffe mikrobieller Endo- und Epiphyten. Gefahren für Mensch und Tier. In: DAZ 132(42):2231. 1992.

Boldo

Peumus boldo

DESCRIPTION

Medicinal Parts: The medicinal parts are the leaves.

Flower and Fruit: The inflorescences are racemes of whitish or pinkish campanulate flowers. The berries are small, yellowish-green and edible.

Leaves, Stem and Root: The plant is a strongly aromatic, heavily branched evergreen shrub 5 to 6 m tall. The leaves are sessile, opposite, oval, about 5 cm long with an entire and slightly revolute margin. They are rather thick and coriaceous with a protruding midrib and a row of small glands on the upper surface. Both surfaces are slightly pubescent.

Characteristics: Boldo has a bitter, aromatic odor and a camphoraceous, lemony taste.

Habitat: The plant is indigenous to Chile and Peru. It is naturalized in mountainous Mediterranean regions and on the western coast of the U.S.

Production: Boldo leaf consists of the dried leaves of Peumus boldus.

Other Names: Boldu, Boldus

ACTIONS AND PHARMACOLOGY

COMPOUNDS

Isoquinoline alkaloids of the aporphine type (0.25-0.5%): main alkaloid boldine (0.1%)

Volatile oil (2-3%): chief components are p-cymene, cineol, ascaridiole

Flavonoids: including rhamnetin-3-O-arabinoside-3'-O-rhamnoside (peumoside), isorhamnetin-3-O-glucoside-7-O-rhamnoside (boldoside), isorhamnetin dirhamnoside (fragroside)

EFFECTS

Boldo has been shown to be antispasmodic, choleretic and to increase gastric secretions.

INDICATIONS AND USAGE

Approved by Commission E:

■ Dyspeptic complaints

CONTRAINDICATIONS

Boldo is contraindicated in patients with bile duct obstruction and those with severe liver diseases. Patients who have gallstones should consult a physician before using the drug.

PRECAUTIONS AND ADVERSE REACTIONS

No health hazards or side effects are known in conjunction with the proper administration of designated therapeutic dosages. The volatile oil should not be used, because it contains up to 40% of the toxin ascaridole.

OVERDOSAGE

Signs of paralysis are reported to appear following intake of very high dosages. A case is described in the older scientific literature in which depression, color hallucinations, sound hallucinations and partial motor aphasia occurred following the consumption of boldine over a period of months.

DOSAGE

Mode of Administration: Comminuted herb for infusions and other, virtually ascaridol-free preparations for internal application. Because of the ascaridol content, essential oil and distillates of Boldo leaf should not be used.

Daily Dosage: The average daily dosage is 4.5 gm

LITERATURE

Betts TJ, J Chromatogr 511:373. 1990.

Bombardelli E et al., (1976) Fitoterapia 47:3.

Kern W, List PH, Hörhammer L (Eds.), Hagers Handbuch der Pharmazeutischen Praxis, 4. Aufl., Bde. 1-8, Springer Verlag Berlin, Heidelberg, New York, 1969.

Kreitmar H, (1952) Pharmazie 7:507.

Leung AY, Encyclopedia of Common Natural Ingredients Used in Food Drugs and Cosmetics, John Wiley & Sons Inc., New York 1980.

Madaus G, Lehrbuch der Biologischen Arzneimittel, Bde 1-3, Nachdruck, Georg Olms Verlag Hildesheim 1979.

Reuter HD, Pflanzliche Gallentherapeutika (Teil I) und (Teil II). In: ZPT 16(1):13-20 u. 77-89. 1995.

Roth L, Daunderer M, Kormann K, Giftpflanzen, Pflanzengifte, 4. Aufl., Ecomed Fachverlag Landsberg Lech 1993.

Schulz R, Hänsel R, Rationale Phytotherapie, Springer Verlag Heidelberg 1996.

Steinegger E, Hänsel R, Pharmakognosie, 5. Aufl., Springer Verlag Heidelberg 1992.

Teuscher E, Biogene Arzneimittel, 5. Aufl., Wiss. Verlagsges. Stuttgart 1997.

Urzúa A, Acuna P, (1983) Fitoterapia 4:175.

Wichtl M (Eds.), Teedrogen, 4. Aufl., Wiss. Verlagsges. Stuttgart 1997.

Wolters B, Arzneipflanzen und Volksmedizin Chiles. In: DAZ 134(39):3693. 1994.

Boneset

Eupatorium perfoliatum

DESCRIPTION

Medicinal Parts: The medicinal part is the herb after flowering.

Flower and Fruit: There are numerous flower heads in terminal, large and slightly convex cymose-paniculate inflorescences. They consist of 10 to 12 white, inconspicuous florets with bristly pappus whose hairs are arranged in a single row. The fruit is a tufted achene.

Leaves, Stem and Root: Eupatorium perfoliatum is a perennial herb with a horizontal hairy rootstock. The stems are rough-haired and grow to about 1.5 m. The leaves are opposite, 10 to 15 cm long, lanceolate, crenate, tapering to narrow point and fused at the base. They have shiny yellow points due to the resin glands, which are visible on the undersurface.

Characteristics: The taste is astringent and persistently bitter.

Habitat: The herb is indigenous to the eastern U.S.

Production: Boneset is the complete aerial part of Eupatorium perfoliatum.

Other Names: Agueweed, Crosswort, Feverwort, Indian Sage, Sweating Plant, Teasel, Thoroughwort, Vegetable Antimony

ACTIONS AND PHARMACOLOGY

COMPOUNDS

Flavonoids: including eupatorin, astragalin, rutin, hyperoside

Sesquiterpene lactones: including eupafolin, euperfolitin, eufoliatin, eufoliatorin, euperfolide

Immunostimulating polysaccharides (heteroxylans)

EFFECTS

The herb acts as an antiphlogistic, a diaphoretic and a bitter, in addition to stimulating the body's immune system. In a comparative study of the homeopathic preparation Eupatorium D2 with aspirin in the treatment of feverish catarrh, a similar positive tendency was observed. In vitro, the phagocytic action of granulocytes was increased.

INDICATIONS AND USAGE

Unproven Uses: On rare occasions, Boneset is used in folk medicine.

Homeopathic Uses: Boneset is used as a treatment for flu and febrile diseases.

PRECAUTIONS AND ADVERSE REACTIONS

Health risks or side effects following the proper administration of designated therapeutic dosages are not recorded. Sensitization after skin contact with the plant is possible. Older scientific literature (Lewin) calls attention to the fact that the drug can lead to enhanced outbreaks of sweat and diarrhea in therapeutic use.

DOSAGE

Mode of Administration: Boneset is used in homeopathic preparations and dilutions.

LITERATURE

Antibiotika und Immunabwehr. In: Symbiose 4(2):20. 1992.

Benoit PS et al., (1976) Lloydia 39:160.

Bohlmann F et al., (1977) Phytochemistry 16:1973.

Elsässer-Beile U, Willenbacher W, Bartsch HH, Gallati H, Schulte Mönting J, Kleist von S et al., Cytokine production in leukocyte cultures during therapy with echinacea extract. In: J Clin Lab Analysis 10(6):441-445. 1996.

Herz W et al., (1977) J Org Chem 42(13):2264.

Vollmar A et al., (1986) Phytochemistry 25:377.

Wagner H (1972) Phytochemistry 11:1504.

Röder E, Pyrrolizidinhaltige Arzneipflanzen. In: DAZ 132(45):2427-2435. 1992.

Woerdenbag HJ, Eupatorium perfoliatum L.- der ''durchwachsene'' Wasserhanf. In: ZPT 13(4):134-139. 1992.

Further information in:

Chan, EH et al., (Eds), Advances in Chinese Medicinal Materials Research, World Scientific Pub. Co. Singapore 1985.

Kern W, List PH, Hörhammer L (Hrsg.), Hagers Handbuch der Pharmazeutischen Praxis, 4. Aufl., Bde. 1-8, Springer Verlag Berlin, Heidelberg, New York, 1969.

Leung AY, Encyclopedia of Common Natural Ingredients Used in Food, Drugs and Cosmetics, John Wiley & Sons Inc., New York 1980.

Lewin L, Gifte und Vergiftungen, 6. Aufl., Nachdruck, Haug Verlag, Heidelberg 1992.

Madaus G, Lehrbuch der Biologischen Arzneimittel, Bde 1-3, Nachdruck, Georg Olms Verlag Hildesheim 1979.

Roth L, Daunderer M, Kormann K, Giftpflanzen, Pflanzengifte, 4. Aufl., Ecomed Fachverlag Landsberg Lech 1993.

Wagner H, Wiesenauer M, Phytotherapie. Phytopharmaka und pflanzliche Homöopathika, Fischer-Verlag, Stuttgart, Jena, New York 1995.

Borage

Borago officinalis

TRADE NAMES

Borage Oil capsules are available from numerous manufacturers.

DESCRIPTION

Medicinal Parts: The medicinal parts are the dried Borage flowers and the dried or fresh foliage, stems and leaves.

Flower and Fruit: The flowers are in separate, terminal, erect, leafy racemes. The calyx is divided almost to the base into 5 rough-haired tips. The 1.5 to 2.5 cm wide corolla is usually sky blue (occasionally white) and has a short tube. The scales of the tube are white. The 5 stamens have a broadened filament and a violet, spur-like appendage. The anthers are black-violet. The style is thread-like with a head-like stigma. The ovary is divided into 4 valves. The small nut is elongate-ovate, about 7 to 10 mm long, light brown, keeled, ribbed, warty and rough.

Leaves, Stem and Root: Borage is an annual, succulent, bristly-haired herb, 15 to 60 cm high. The erect, vertically grooved stems are covered in rough, whitish hairs. The leaves are alternate, clasping, solitary, entire-margined and hairy. They are also folded, curved in at the margins, green on top and whitish on the underside. The leaves are 3 to 10 cm long and elliptoid to ovate.

Characteristics: Borage has a taste similar to cucumber.

Habitat: Borage originated in the Mediterranean region, but is now found all over Europe and the U.S.

Production: Borage oil is the fatty oil of the seeds of Borago officinalis. Borage leaves are the dried leaves and inflorescence of Borago officinalis. The herb most often grows wild, but is cultivated on a small scale in Yugoslavia, Rumania, Bulgaria and Turkey. Borage is harvested during the flowering period. Due to the plant's very high water content, it should be artificially dried at 40°C.

Not to be Confused With: The herb can be confused with Echium vulgare.

Other Names: Burrage, Bugloss, Burage

ACTIONS AND PHARMACOLOGY

COMPOUNDS: BORAGE OIL

Fatty oil: chief fatty acid is gamma-linolenic acid (17-25%), linoleic acid

EFFECTS: BORAGE OIL

The drug acts as an astringent and as a sequestering agent.

COMPOUNDS: BORAGE LEAF

Pyrrolizidine alkaloids: supinin, lycopsamin, 7-acetyl-lycopsamin, intermedin, 7-acetyl- intermedine, amabiline, thesinine

Silicic acid (to some extent water-soluble)

Mucilages

Tannins

EFFECTS: BORAGE LEAF

The tannins in Borage leaves have an astringent effect and the mucins a sequestering effect.

INDICATIONS AND USAGE

BORAGE OIL

Unproven Uses: The oil is used for neurodermatitis and as a food supplement.

BORAGE LEAF

Unproven Uses: In folk medicine, Borage is used as a sequestering and mucilaginous agent for coughs and throat illnesses and as a bronchial treatment. It is also used as an anti-inflammatory agent for kidney and bladder disorders, as an astringent and to treat rheumatism. Preparations using Borage are also used for blood purification and dehydration; the prevention of chest and peritoneal inflammation and rheumatism of the joints; as a pain-relieving, cardiotonic, sedative, sudorific; as a performance-enhancing agent; and for phlebitis and menopausal complaints.

PRECAUTIONS AND ADVERSE REACTIONS

BORAGE OIL

No health hazards or side effects are known in conjunction with the proper administration of designated therapeutic dosages.

BORAGE LEAF

Even though the hepatotoxic and hepatocarcinogenic pyrrolizidine alkaloid content is small, the drug should not be administered. External use may present less of a potential for problems.

DOSAGE

BORAGE OIL

Mode of Administration: In capsules, sometimes in combination with vitamins.

How Supplied:

Capsules — 500mg, 1000 mg

BORAGE LEAF

Storage: The drug should be protected from light and moisture.

LITERATURE

BORAGE OIL

Fell KR, Peck JM, (1968) Planta Med 4: 411.

Hänsel R, Keller K, Rimpler H, Schneider G (Hrsg.), Hagers Handbuch der Pharmazeutischen Praxis, 5. Aufl., Bde 4-6 (Drogen), Springer Verlag Berlin, Heidelberg, New York, 1992-1994.

Ippen H, Gamma-Linolensäure besser aus Nachtkerzen- oder aus Borretschöl? In: ZPT 16(3):167-170. 1995.

Luthy J et al., (1984) Pharm Acta Helv 59 (9/10): 242.

BORAGE LEAF

Dodson CD, Stermitz FR, JNP 49(4):727-728. 1986.

Frohne D, Pfänder HJ, Giftpflanzen - Ein Handbuch für Apotheker, Toxikologen und Biologen, 4. Aufl., Wiss. Verlags-Ges Stuttgart 1997.

Hänsel R, Keller K, Rimpler H, Schneider G (Hrsg.), Hagers Handbuch der Pharmazeutischen Praxis, 5. Aufl., Bde 4-6 (Drogen), Springer Verlag Berlin, Heidelberg, New York, 1992-1994.

Larson KM, Stermitz FR, JNP 47(4):747-748. 1984.

Röder E, Pyrrolizidinhaltige Arzneipflanzen. In: DAZ 132(45):2427-2435. 1992.

Teuscher E, Lindequist U, Biogene Gifte - Biologie, Chemie, Pharmakologie, 2. Aufl., Fischer Verlag Stuttgart 1994.

Borago officinalis

See Borage

Boswellia carteri

See Frankincense

Boxwood

Buxus sempervirens

DESCRIPTION

Medicinal Parts: The medicinal parts are the dried Boxwood tree leaves and the woody aerial parts of the plant.

Flower and Fruit: Clusters of axillary yellow flowers open in early spring. The male flowers are evenly shaped and have 4 tepals, 4 stamens and a small rudimentary ovary. The female flowers have 4 to 8 tepals, 3 fused carpels with 3 free, short, thick styles. The fruit is a capsule with oblong, 5 to 6 mm long seeds.

Leaves, Stem and Root: Boxwood is an evergreen monoecious shrub or tree growing to a height of 6 m with variable forms and leaf shapes. The green branches are initially pubescent, later glabrous, olive green, angular and densely covered with ovate leaves, which are usually opposite. The upper surface of the leaves is smooth, coriaceous, dark green and very glossy. The lower surface is lighter in shade, and the lamina margin is smooth.

Characteristics: The leaves have a nauseous taste.

Habitat: The plant is found mainly in southern and central Europe with a clear division into east and west regions, i.e., northwest Spain and southern France in the west and the Balkans to northern Greece and Asia Minor in the east. It is otherwise extensively cultivated.

Production: Boxwood leaves are the leaves of Buxus sempervirens. They are collected from the wild.

Other Names: Dudgeon, Bush Tree

ACTIONS AND PHARMACOLOGY

COMPOUNDS

Steroid alkaloids: including cyclobuxine-D, cyclobuxine-B, cycloprotobuxine-A, cycloprotobu

EFFECTS

The cycloprotobuxine in the drug was shown to have a cytotoxic effect in vitro as well as an inhibitory effect on the growth of *mycobacterium tuberculosis.*

In animal tests, an inhibition of motility, including tetanus, spinal paralysis and respiratory paralysis, was demonstrated.

A hypotensive effect has been described.

INDICATIONS AND USAGE

Unproven Uses: In folk medicine preparations were used internally for rheumatism and constipation (decoction), as a diaphoretic (aqueous extract), for malaria (tincture) and pneumonia (ethanol extract), and externally for rashes, hair loss, gout and rheumatic complaints (ointment)

Homeopathic Uses: Buxus sempervirens is used for greasy scalp with dandruff and for hair loss.

PRECAUTIONS AND ADVERSE REACTIONS

No health hazards or side effects are known in conjunction with the proper administration of designated therapeutic dosages. Contact dermatitis, in particular through contact with the freshly harvested plant, is possible.

OVERDOSAGE

The intake of toxic dosages of the drug leads to vomiting, diarrhea, severe clonic spasms, eventually to signs of paralysis and ultimately to fatal asphyxiation. The fatal dosage in dogs is 0.1 gm of the alkaloid mixture/kg body weight (approximately 5 to 10 gm of the drug/kg body weight). The treatment for poisonings proceeds through suppression of the spasms with diazepam or barbiturates (no more than absolutely necessary) followed by gastric lavage and possible oxygen respiration. Phenothiazines and analeptics are not to be administered.

DOSAGE

Mode of Administration: Boxwood is obsolete as a drug.

Homeopathic Dosage: 5 to 10 drops, 1 tablet or 5 to 10 globules, 1 to 3 times daily or 1 ml injection solution sc twice weekly. (HAB34)

LITERATURE

Atta-ur-Rahman et al., Alkaloids from Buxus species. In: PH 31(8):2933-2935. 1992.

Atta-ur-Rahman et al., New alkaloids from Buxus sempervirens. In: JNP 52:1319-1322. 1989.

Atta-ur-Rahman et al., Steroidal alkaloids from leaves of Buxus sempervirens. In: PH 30(4):1295-1298. 1991.

Frohne D, Pfänder HJ, Giftpflanzen - Ein Handbuch für Apotheker, Toxikologen und Biologen, 4. Aufl., Wiss. Verlags-Ges Stuttgart 1997.

Hänsel R, Keller K, Rimpler H, Schneider G (Hrsg.), Hagers Handbuch der Pharmazeutischen Praxis, 5. Aufl., Bde 4-6 (Drogen), Springer Verlag Berlin, Heidelberg, New York, 1992-1994.

Khodshaev BU et al., (1984) Khim Prir Soedin 6:802.

Lewin L, Gifte und Vergiftungen, 6. Aufl., Nachdruck, Haug Verlag, Heidelberg 1992.

Roth L, Daunderer M, Kormann K, Giftpflanzen, Pflanzengifte, 4. Aufl., Ecomed Fachverlag Landsberg Lech 1993.

Teuscher E, Lindequist U, Biogene Gifte - Biologie, Chemie, Pharmakologie, 2. Aufl., Fischer Verlag Stuttgart 1994.

Willaman JJ, Hui-Li L, (1970) Lloydia 33(3A):1.

Brassica napus

See Oilseed Rape

Brassica nigra

See Black Mustard

Brassica oleracea

See Cabbage

Brassica rapa

See Wild Turnip

Brazilian Pepper Tree

Schinus terebinthifolius

DESCRIPTION

Medicinal Parts: Medicinal properties have been attributed to the bark, leaves, fruit and seeds.

Flower and Fruit: The flowers are in panicles up to 15 cm long. The flowers are small, ivory white to greenish, and the structures are in five. The calyx is 5-tipped. There are 5 petals, 10 stamens and a superior ovary developing from a single carpel and a style in 3 sections. The fruit is a bright pink to red, glossy, single-drupe with a diameter of approximately 5 mm, a thin pergament-like exocarp, an oleo-resin-rich mesocarp and a hard endocarp.

Leaves, Stem and Root: The leaves are alternate, up to 40 cm long, odd pinnate, with 7 to 13 leaflets up to 8 cm long, 1 to 2 cm wide, sessile, elongate, glossy, finely serrate or jagged-edged. The branches do not hang down.

Characteristics: The fruit is aromatic and sweetish.

Habitat: Indigenous to Central America and South America.

Production: Brazilian peppers (Pink peppers) are the ripe unpeeled seeds of Schinus terebinthifolius Raddi, which are harvested in winter (May to August) and then air- or freeze-dried.

Other Names: Christmas-Berry Tree, Florida Holly

ACTIONS AND PHARMACOLOGY

COMPOUNDS

Volatile oil (2.0 to 10.0%): chief components including limonene, alpha-phellandrene, beta-phellandrene, alpha-pinene, beta-pinene, including as well p-cymol, sabinene, terpinolene, in some chemical varieties up to 50% delta3-carene

Alkyl phenols (0.1%): cardanols, cardols, 2-methyl cardolenes

Fatty oil (in the seeds 20 to 60%)

Flavonoids: including biflavonoids, for example amentoflavone

Triterpenes: masticadienonic acid, 3-epimasticadienonic acid

EFFECTS

The ''antibiotic activity'' with which the drug is credited has not yet been proven. Its use on wounds and inflammatory alterations of the skin appears plausible, due to the antimicrobial, astringent and anti-inflammatory characteristics of the gallic acid it contains.

INDICATIONS AND USAGE

Unproven Uses: Internal folk medicine uses have included treatment of tumors and as a diuretic. In Brazil, a liquid extract and tincture are prepared from the bark and used internally as a stimulant, tonic and astringent, and externally for rheumatism, gout and syphilis. The leaf and fruit have been added to baths for wounds and ulcers. (Hager, 1949.) The effect seems plausible due to the gallic acid content but has not yet been sufficiently clinically proven.

PRECAUTIONS AND ADVERSE REACTIONS

No health hazards are known in conjunction with the proper administration of designated therapeutic dosages, although there is some danger of sensitization (alkyl phenols). Sensitizations occur particularly frequently in North America. Stomach upset and vomiting have been observed following the ingestion of a number of the fruits.

CONTRAINDICATIONS

Should not be administered to individuals with a pre-existing sensitivity to alkyl phenols.

DOSAGE

Mode of Administration: Whole drug, tincture and extract for internal and external use.

Daily Dosage: There is no information in the literature.

Storage: Store tightly sealed and protected from light in a cool, dry place.

LITERATURE

Hänsel R, Keller K, Rimpler H, Schneider G (Ed), Hagers Handbuch der Pharmazeutischen Praxis, 5. Aufl., Bde 4 - 6 (Drogen), Springer Verlag Berlin, Heidelberg, New York, 1992-1994.

Hayashi T, Nagayama K, Arisawa M, Shimizu M, Suzuki S, Yoshizaki M, Morita N, Ferro E, Basualdo I, Berganza LH, Pentagalloylglucose, a xanthine oxidase inhibitor from a Paraguayan crude drug, Molle-i (Schinus terebinthifolius). J Nat Prod, 39:210-1, 1989 Jan-Feb.

Jain MK, Yu BZ, Rogers JM, Smith AE, Boger ET, Ostrander RL, Rheingold AL, Specific competitive inhibitor of secreted phospholipase A2 from berries of Schinus terebinthifolius. Phytochemistry, 39:537-47, 1995 Jun.

Ramos Ruiz A, De la Torre RA, Alonso N, Villaescusa A, Betancourt J, Vizoso A, Screening of medicinal plants for induction of somatic segregation activity in Aspergillus nidulans. J Ethnopharmacol, 39:123-7, 1996 Jul 5.

Brewer's Yeast

Saccharomyces cerevisiae

DESCRIPTION

Medicinal Parts: The medicinal part is the mature, debittered, bottom-fermented Brewer's Yeast.

Flower and Fruit: The cells may be single, in pairs, in chains or aggregate. On a suitable solid fertile base the individual cell colonies have smooth margins, are slightly convex to flat and are whitish to cream-yellow. Older individual colonies are slightly raised, smooth or slightly lobed (sometimes in sections), or folded, and are yellowish to light brown. The vegetative reproduction is via multilateral budding. Ascospores are produced from the vegetative cells. There are normally 1 to 4, occasionally more, round, smooth-walled ascospores per ascus.

Characteristics: Brewer's Yeast is found extensively in the wild, and it lives as a saprophytic parasite or symbiotically.

Habitat: Brewer's Yeast is grown worldwide.

Production: Medicinal yeast consists of fresh or dried cells of *Saccharomyces cerevisiae* and/or of *Candida utilis.*

ACTIONS AND PHARMACOLOGY

COMPOUNDS

Vitamins of the B group (per 100 gm): thiamin 8-15 mg, riboflavin 4-8 mg, nicotinic acid amide 45-90 mg, pantothenic acid 7-25 mg, pyridoxine 4-10 mg, biotin 20 µg, folic acid 1-5 mg, vitamin B-12 20 µg

Polysaccharides: mannans, glucans

Proteins

Amines

Sterols: ergosterol, zymosterol

EFFECTS

The yeast is antibacterial and stimulates phagocytosis.

INDICATIONS AND USAGE

Approved by Commission E:

- Dyspeptic complaints
- Eczema, furuncles, acne
- Loss of appetite

Unproven Uses: Brewer's Yeast is used for constipation and itching skin diseases.

PRECAUTIONS AND ADVERSE REACTIONS

General: Health risks or side effects following the proper administration of designated therapeutic dosages are not recorded. The intake of large quantities can cause gas. Allergic intolerance reactions are possible (itching, urticaria, exanthema, Quinck's disease). Migraine headaches can be triggered in susceptible patients.

Drug Interactions: The simultaneous intake of monoamine oxidase inhibitors can cause an increase in blood pressure.

DOSAGE

Mode of Administration: Medicinal yeast and galenic preparations are available for internal use. Pharmaceutical forms include tablets and compound preparations.

Daily Dosage: The average daily dosage is 6 gm.

Storage: Store in air-tight containers protected from light.

LITERATURE

Aflmann C, Mikroorganismen:Biotherapeutika bei Infektionskrankheiten. In: DAZ 136(46):4136-4137. 1996.

Anonym, Hefepräparate haben sich bewährt. In: PTA 5(9):433. 1991.

Böckeler W, Thomas G, (1989): In-vitro-Studien zur destabilisierenden Wirkung lyophilisierter Saccharomyces cerevisiae Hansen CBS 5926-Zellen auf Enterobakterien. Läßt sich diese Eigenschaft biochemisch erklären? In, Müller J, Ottenjann R, Seifert J (Hrsg), Ökosystem Darm, Springer Verlag, S 142-153.

Czerucka D, Roux 1, Rampal P, (1994) Saccharomyces boulardii inhibits sectretagogue-mediated adenosin-cyclic monophosphate induction in intestinal cells. Gastroenterology 106:65-72.

Ewe K, (1983) Obstipation - Pathophysiologie, Klinik, Therapie. Int Welt 6:286-292.

Gedek B, Hagenhoff G, (1989) Orale Verabreichung von lebensfähigen Zellen des Hefestammes Saccharomyces cerevisiae

Hansen CBS 5926 und deren Schicksal während der Magen-Darm-Passage. Therapiewoche 38 (Sonderheft): 33-40.

Höchter W, Chase D, Hagenhoff G, (1990) Saccharomyces boulardii bei akuter Erwachsenediarrhoe. Münch Med Wschr 132: 188-192.

Hojgaard L, Arffmann S, Jorgeasen M, Krag E, (1981) Tea consumption, a cause of constipation. Br Med J 282: 864.

Jahn HU, Zeitz M, (1991) Immunmodulatorische Wirkung von Saccharomyces boulardii beim Menschen. In: Seifert J, Ottenjann R, Zeitz M, Bockemühl J (Hrsg) Ökosystem Darm III. Springer-Verlag, S 159-164.

Kollaritsch HH, Tobüren D, Scheiner O, Wiedermann G, (1988) Prophylaxe der Reisediarrhoe. Münch Med Wschr 130: 671-673.

Massot J, Desconclois M, Astoin J, (1982) Protection par Saccharomyces boulardii de la diarrhée Escherichia coli du souriceau. Ann Pharm Fr 40: 445-449.

Plein K, Hotz J, (1993) Therapeutic effect of Saccaromyces boulardii on mild residual symptoms in a stable phase of Crohn's disease with special respect to chronic diarrhea - a pilot study. Z Gastroenterol 31: 129-134.

Schmidt CH, (1977) Unspezifische Steigerung der Phagozytoseaktivitäten von Peritoneal-makrophagen nach oraler Gabe verschiedener Hefepräparationen. Dissertation Freie Universität Berlin.

Sinai Y, Kaplan A, Hai Y et al., (1974) Enhancement of resistance to infectious disease by oral administration of Brewer's Yeast. Infection Immunol 9: 781-787

Surawicz Ch, Elmer GW, Speelman P, McFarland LV, Chinn J, van Belle G, (1989) Die Prophylaxe Antibiotika-assoziierter Diarrhöen mit Saccharomyces boulardii. Eine prospektive Studie. Gastroenterol 96: 981-988.

Tempé JD, Steidel AL, Blehaut H, Hasselmann M, Lutun PH, Maurier F, (1983) Prévention par Saccharomyces boulardii des diarrhées de l'alimentation entérale débit continu. La Semaine des Paris 59: 1409-1412.

Weber R, Regio Seminar Pharma: Reisemedizinische Beratung. In: DAZ 135(25):2352-2354. 1995.

Further information in:

Hänsel R, Keller K, Rimpler H, Schneider G (Hrsg.), Hagers Handbuch der Pharmazeutischen Praxis, 5. Aufl., Bde 4-6 (Drogen), Springer Verlag Berlin, Heidelberg, New York, 1992-1994 (unter Saccharomyces).

Schulz R, Hänsel R, Rationale Phytotherapie, Springer Verlag Heidelberg 1996.

Teuscher E, Biogene Arzneimittel, 5. Aufl., Wiss. Verlagsges. mbH Stuttgart 1997.

Wagner H, Wiesenauer M, Phytotherapie. Phytopharmaka und pflanzliche Homöopathika, Fischer-Verlag, Stuttgart, Jena, New York 1995.

British Elecampane (Xuan-Fu-Hua)

Inula britannica

DESCRIPTION

Medicinal Parts: The medicinal part is the flower.

Flower and Fruit: The semi-globose composite flowers are surrounded by bracts; they have a diameter of 2.5 to 5 cm, are single or in umbelliferous racemes with bracts arranged in a number of rows. The lingual florets are yellow and up to 1 mm wide, the tubular florets are 5-tipped, androgenous and numerous. The anther has an appendage tail. The fruit is a cylindrical, long-ribbed, 1.3 mm long achene. The pappus is single-rowed, approximately 5 mm long and consists of fine, rough bristles.

Leaves, Stem and Root: This herbaceous perennial grows up to 60 cm high. The leaves are alternate and simple. The lower leaves narrow into the short petiole, entire or dentate. The upper leaves are sessile and rounded at the base, lanceolate, sparsely pubescent above, and are covered below in dense silky hairs or almost glabrous. The stem is upright, round, weakly ribbed, silky-haired to almost glabrous. The root is creeping.

Habitat: The plant is indigenous to Asia and Europe.

Production: Elecampane flowers are the inflorescences of Inula britannica and Inula japonica, dried in the sun or shade after harvesting.

Not to be Confused With: Arnicae flos

Other Names: Alant-Okleuveasis

ACTIONS AND PHARMACOLOGY

COMPOUNDS

Sesquiterpenes: sesquiterpene lactones, particularly gaillardin but also including britanin

Flavonoids: including isoquercitrin

Caffeic acid derivatives: including chlorogenic acid

EFFECTS

It has been reported that a watery extract of the sesquiterpene-containing drug inhibits in vitro cAMP-phosphodiesterase up to 60%, and prevents the infection of human embryo muscle cells with the herpes simplex virus II. The drug is also assumed to possess potential for sensitization, due to the sesquiterpene lactones with exocyclic methylene groups it contains. The secretolytic and emetic effect with which the drug is credited has not been documented. The flower of the East Asian species is used as a depurative.

INDICATIONS AND USAGE

Unproven Uses: Indications in folk medicine include feelings of fullness in the chest and diaphragm area, vomiting, coughs and symptoms of the efferent urinary tract.

PRECAUTIONS AND ADVERSE REACTIONS

No health hazards are known in conjunction with the proper administration of designated therapeutic dosages.

DOSAGE

Mode of Administration: Whole and powdered drug.

Preparation: The drug is roasted with a honey solution until it is no longer sticky. A decoction is prepared by boiling 3 to 9 g drug in a sealed sachet.

Storage: Store in a dry place.

LITERATURE

Hänsel R, Keller K, Rimpler H, Schneider G (Ed), Hagers Handbuch der Pharmazeutischen Praxis, 5. Aufl., Bde 4 - 6 (Drogen), Springer Verlag Berlin, Heidelberg, New York, 1992-1994.

Iijima K, Kiyohara H, Tanaka M, Matsumoto T, Cyong JC, Yamada H Preventive effect of taraxasteryl acetate from Inula britannica subsp. japonica on experimental hepatitis in vivo. Planta Med, 61:50-3, 1995 Feb.

Broad Bean

Vicia faba

DESCRIPTION

Medicinal Parts: The medicinal part is the fresh flower.

Flower and Fruit: The white or bluish short-pedicled flowers have black spots on the standard. They are arranged in groups of 2 to 4 in the upper leaf axils. The calyx tips are uneven, with the upper ones shorter than the lower. The pod is leathery and velvety on the flat surface. The seeds are large, flat, ovate or oblong, and brown.

Leaves, Stem and Root: The plant is 60 to 125 cm high. The stem is erect and has no climbers. The leaves are pinnate and the leaflets elliptical, fleshy, blue-green and terminate acutely. The stipules are ovate and semi-saggitate.

Habitat: The plant is indigenous to the temperate regions of the world.

Production: Broad Beans are the seeds of Vicia faba.

ACTIONS AND PHARMACOLOGY

COMPOUNDS

Pyrimidine derivatives: vicine (vicioside, 0.4-0.8%), convicine (0.1-0.6%)

Lectins: The isolectins mixture is referred to as favine

L-3,4-dihydroxyphenylalanine (L-DOPA, up to 8%)

Starch

Proteins (26%)

Tannins (2%)

EFFECTS

No information is available.

INDICATIONS AND USAGE

Unproven Uses: Formerly, Broad Bean flowers were used in the treatment of coughs and kidney and genital complaints. Externally, they are used as a poultice for skin inflammation, warts and burns.

Homeopathic Uses: An essence of the fresh plant after flowering is used in homeopathy.

PRECAUTIONS AND ADVERSE REACTIONS

No health hazards or side effects are known in conjunction with the proper administration of designated therapeutic dosages. Following division of the glycosides in the intestine resorption and oxidation through dehydration of SH-groups in the erythrocyte membrane, the pyrimidine derivatives can, in high dosages, lead to hemolysis.

OVERDOSAGE

The intake of large quantities of raw or only briefly cooked seeds can lead to queasiness, vomiting, diarrhea and feelings of vertigo. In severe cases, overdosage may lead to acute hemolytic anemia with fever, icterus, hemoglobinuria, oliguria and anuria, particularly among individuals with genetically caused glucose-6-phosphate-dehydrogenase deficiency (inadequate protection of the erythrocytes by glutathione), which is also known as favism. Favism is treated by transfusion of washed erythrocytes and administration of prednisone. Elevations in blood pressure are also possible due to the L-DOPA content of the seeds.

DOSAGE

Mode of Administration: Broad Bean preparations are now obsolete.

LITERATURE

Chevion M, Maer J, Glaser G, Naturally occuring food toxicant: favism-producing agents. In: CRC Handbook of Naturally Occuring Food Toxicants, CRC Press, Boca Raton, Florida. 1983.

Kern W, List PH, Hörhammer L (Hrsg.), Hagers Handbuch der Pharmazeutischen Praxis, 4. Aufl., Bde. 1-8: Springer Verlag Berlin, Heidelberg, New York, 1969.

Teuscher E, Lindequist U, Biogene Gifte - Biologie, Chemie, Pharmakologie, 2. Aufl., Fischer Verlag Stuttgart 1994.

Vered Y et al., The influence of Vicia faca (Broad bean) seedlings on urinary sodium excretion. In: PM 63(3):237-240. 1997.

Brooklime

Veronica beccabunga

DESCRIPTION

Medicinal Parts: The medicinal parts are the fresh flowering plant freed from the root, the fresh aerial parts collected during the flowering season and the whole plant.

Flower and Fruit: The flowers are in loose, axillary, diagonal clusters. The accompanying leaves are linear, as long as or shorter than the flowers. The peduncles and pedicles are glabrous. The calyx is dorsiventral and divided into 4. The sepals are lanceolate to spatulate and acuminate; the front ones are larger than the back ones. The corolla is rotate with a very short tube, 4 to 9 mm wide and azure blue. The ovary is green and the stigma capitual-like. The fruit is a cordate, almost globular, narrow-winged capsule. The seeds are 0.6 mm long and 0.45 mm wide. They are yellow, oval and flatly convex with a fairly smooth back.

Leaves, Stem and Root: The plant is a perennial with a creeping rhizome. The stem is ascending, up to 50 cm high, round and filled with latex. The leaves are petiolate, ovate or broad elliptical, obtuse, narrowly serrate, glabrous and glossy.

Habitat: The plant is indigenous to almost all of Europe, western and northern Asia and northern Africa, and is naturalized in eastern North America.

Production: Brooklime is the aerial part of Veronica beccabunga. The collection or picking occurs in uncultivated regions in Europe, west and north Asia, North Africa and North America.

Other Names: Beccabunga, Mouth-Smart, Neckweed, Speedwell, Water Purslane, Water Pimpernel

ACTIONS AND PHARMACOLOGY

COMPOUNDS

Iridoide monoterpenes: aucubin (0.8%)

Flavonoids: including among others scutellarin glycosides

The drug has not been extensively investigated.

EFFECTS

Brooklime has a diuretic effect.

INDICATIONS AND USAGE

Unproven Uses: Brooklime is used to lessen the elimination of urine. It is also used for constipation, liver complaints, dysentery and lung conditions. The drug has also been reported to be effective against bleeding of the gums.

PRECAUTIONS AND ADVERSE REACTIONS

No health hazards or side effects are known in conjunction with the proper administration of designated therapeutic dosages.

LITERATURE

Hänsel R, Keller K, Rimpler H, Schneider G (Hrsg.), Hagers Handbuch der Pharmazeutischen Praxis, 5. Aufl., Bde 4-6 (Drogen): Springer Verlag Berlin, Heidelberg, New York, 1992-1994.

Inouye H et al., (1974) Planta Med 25:285.

Kato Y, (1946) Folia Pharmacol Jap 42:37 (via CA 47: 1843).

Swiatek L et al., Acta Pol Pharm 25:597. 1968.

Broom Corn

Sorghum vulgare

DESCRIPTION

Medicinal Parts: The medicinal parts are the seeds.

Flower and Fruit: The flowers and inflorescences are large spadix-like and solitary. They may also be in pairs and terminal on long, stiff, indistinct panicles. The panicles may be bushy-branched or occasionally tangled-branched. The individual spikelets are usually ovate to round, and the spelts are usually broad-lanceolate. The spelts become hard, shiny and dentated at the tip. The seeds are small, round and white.

Leaves, Stem and Root: The plant is reed-like and similar to maize but is not as tall.

Habitat: The plant is common in Spain, Italy and southern Europe. It is widely cultivated in the U.S.

Production: Broom Corn seeds are the seeds of Sorghum vulgare.

Other Names: Darri, Durri, Guinea Corn, Sorghum

ACTIONS AND PHARMACOLOGY

COMPOUNDS

Cyanogenic glycosides: dhurrin (in the fruits, in contrast with the foliage [250-700 mg/100 gm] only in very low concentrations: 0.005-5 mg/100 gm)

Starch (70%)

Proteins (10%)

Fatty oil (3%)

Vitamins of the B group: thiamin (B1), riboflavine (B2)

EFFECTS

Broom Corn is a demulcent that is soothing to the alimentary tract.

INDICATIONS AND USAGE

Unproven Uses: Preparations of the seeds are used for digestive disorders, but it is mainly used as a cereal grain.

PRECAUTIONS AND ADVERSE REACTIONS

No health hazards or side effects are known in conjunction with the proper administration of designated therapeutic dosages.

DOSAGE

Mode of Administration: Broom Corn can be administered as an infusion, but is mostly used as a cereal grain.

LITERATURE

Erb N et al. PM 41:84. 1981.

Kern W, List PH, Hörhammer L (Hrsg.), Hagers Handbuch der Pharmazeutischen Praxis, 4. Aufl., Bde. 1-8: Springer Verlag Berlin, Heidelberg, New York, 1969.

Seigler D, Cyanogene Glykoside (Vortragsref.). In: DAZ 132(25):1365. 1992.

Teuscher E, Lindequist U, Biogene Gifte - Biologie, Chemie, Pharmakologie, 2. Aufl., Fischer Verlag Stuttgart 1994.

Brown Kelp

Macrocystis pyrifera

DESCRIPTION

Medicinal Parts: The medicinal part is the thallus.

Flower and Fruit: This brown algae grows up to 100 m long. Generations switch between sporophyte and gametophyte. The haploid male or female gametophytes are tiny plantlets. The 50 to 100 m long sporophyte is made up of root-like rhizoids, a rope-like cauloid, and phylloids that are leaf-like, coriaceous-thick sections with a large elongate to pear-shaped air-bladder at the base. The rhizoids form a conical adhesive disc of up to 1 m in diameter. The phylloids grow up to 1 m long, are attached to the cauloid-like leaflets and are covered with sporangia.

Habitat: Found along the west coast of United States (primarily California) and along the coast of Chile.

Production: Brown algae thallus is the dried thallus, usually only the phylloid, of Macrocystis pyrifera. (Macrocystis integrifolia may be added.) The algae are harvested using vessels called mowing ships.

Other Names: Giant Kelp, Long-Bladder Kelp, Sea Kelp

ACTIONS AND PHARMACOLOGY

COMPOUNDS

Alginic acid (15 to 20%)

Polysaccharides: fucoidan, laminaran

Iodine (0.1 to 0.5%): to some extent organically bound

Proteins

Cyclitols: laminitol (4-C-methyl-meso-inositol)

Sugar alcohols: mannitol

EFFECTS

Brown algae thallus serves chiefly as a source of iodine. The drug has also been demonstrated to have an influence on the immune system, as well as antiviral qualities. In a study with 400 women, the daily intake of 5.5 g of macrocystis powder over a period of 6 to 8 weeks led to an elevation of hemoglobin levels of 86% over normal values. Although licensed as a substance to aid weight loss, no adequate experimental data are available to support that effect.

INDICATIONS AND USAGE

Unproven Uses: Folk medicine uses include weight reduction. The drug is used as a commercial pharmaceutical preparation in the U.S. for anemia in pregnancy. In Japan the drug is used for hypertension.

PRECAUTIONS AND ADVERSE REACTIONS

No health hazards are known in conjunction with the proper administration of designated therapeutic dosages.

CONTRAINDICATIONS

Brown Kelp should not be used by individuals with a familial disposition to thyroid illness or hyperthyroidism.

OVERDOSAGE

Long-term administration of daily dosages that exceed 150 micrograms iodine carry with them the danger of worsening an existing hyperthyroidism. Quantities over 300 micrograms iodine per day can precipitate hyperthyroidism.

DOSAGE

Mode of Administration: Brown Kelp preparations are available for internal use.

Storage: Store in tightly sealed container.

LITERATURE

Hänsel R, Keller K, Rimpler H, Schneider G (Ed), Hagers Handbuch der Pharmazeutischen Praxis, 5. Aufl., Bde 4 - 6 (Drogen), Springer Verlag Berlin, Heidelberg, New York, 1992-1994.

Zeller SG, Gray GR, Analysis of Macrocystis pyrifera and Pseudomonas aeruginosa alginic acids by the reductive-cleavage method. Carbohydr Res, 226:313-26, 1992 Mar 30.

Brunfelsia hopeana

See Manaca

Bryonia alba

See White Bryony

Bryonia cretica

See Red Bryony

Buckthorn

Rhamnus catharticus

DESCRIPTION

Medicinal Parts: The medicinal parts are the whole, ripe, dried fruit and the fresh ripe fruit.

Flower and Fruit: The small, dioecious, greenish-yellow flowers are in axillary cymes. The calyx is fused, has 4 segments and droops. The petals are small and are on the edge of the calyx tube, which has short stamens. The ovary is 4-valved with a style that is divided in 4. The fruit is a pea-sized, black berry-like drupe. The seeds are 5 mm long and triangular with a narrow split, which separates slightly at the end and is surrounded by a cartiliginous margin.

Leaves, Stem and Root: The plant occurs in a variety of forms, usually as a bush that is up to 3 m in height, but occasionally as a tree with a bent trunk that grows up to 8 m. The boughs are usually stiffly spread; the branches are more or less clearly opposite, glossy, glabrous or occasionally pubescent and end in a thorn. The leaves are clustered on the older branches, opposite on the younger ones. They are ovate or elliptical, finely serrate with 2 to 3 lateral ribs curved towards the midrib.

Characteristics: The flowers are fragrant, the heartwood is orange-red.

Habitat: The plant is common all over Europe, Western Asia and North Africa.

Production: Buckthorn, consists of the dried ripe berries of Rhamni catharticus and its preparations. Buckthorn is harvested in uncultivated regions in autumn and dried.

Not to be Confused With: May be confused with the fruit of Frangula alnus.

Other Names: Hartsthorn, Common Buckthorn, Purging Buckthorn, Waythorn, Highwaythorn, Ramsthorn

ACTIONS AND PHARMACOLOGY

COMPOUNDS

Anthracene derivatives (2 to 7%): anthranoids, chief components glucofrangulin A, diacetylglucofrangulin, frangulin A

Flavonoids (1 to 2%): including catharticin (rhamnocitrin-3-O-rhamnoside), xanthorhamnine (rhamnetin-3-O-rhamnoside)

Tannins (3 to 4%): oligomeric proanthocyanidins

EFFECTS

The drug has a laxative effect because of the anthranoid content. Anthranoids have an anti-absorptive hydrogogic effect resulting in a more liquid stool and an increase in volume of the content of the intestine.

INDICATIONS AND USAGE

Approved by Commission E:

- Constipation

Buckthorn is used internally for constipation and for bowel movement relief in cases of anal fissures and hemorrhoids. It is used after recto-anal surgery and in preparation for diagnostic intervention in the gastrointestinal tract and to achieve softer stool.

Unproven Uses: In folk medicine it is used as a diuretic (in 'blood-purifying' remedies).

Homeopathic Uses: Rhamnus catharticus is used for poor digestion.

CONTRAINDICATIONS

Contraindicated in intestinal obstruction, acute inflammatory intestinal diseases, appendicitis and abdominal pain of unknown origin. Use during pregnancy or while nursing only after consulting a physician. The drug is not to be administered to children under 12 years of age.

PRECAUTIONS AND ADVERSE REACTIONS

General: Spasmodic gastrointestinal complaints could occur as a side effect to the drug's purgative effect. Long-term use leads to loss of electrolytes, especially potassium ions. This may lead to hyperaldosteronism, inhibition of intestinal motility and enhancement of the effect of cardioactive steroids, which in rare cases may result in cardiac arrhythmias. Nephropathies, edema and accelerated bone deterioration may be the result of long term use.

Drug-Interactions: Resorption of other medications could be reduced due to the laxative effect. In the case of chronic use/overuse, a potassium deficiency leads to an increase in the effect of cardiac glycosides as well as effecting heartbeat-regulating drugs.

Pregnancy: Not to be used during pregnancy.

OVERDOSAGE

The intake of large quantities of the fresh berries could lead to European cholera or kidney irritation. The question of the increase in probability of developing colonic carcinomas following long-term administration of anthracene drugs has not yet been fully clarified. Recent studies show no connection between the administration of anthracene drugs and the frequency of carcinoma of the colon.

DOSAGE

Mode of Administration: Buckthorn is available in solid pharmaceutical forms and in commercial compounded preparations for oral intake. It is also available parenterally for homeopathic use.

Preparation: To prepare a tea, pour boiling water over 4 gm cut drug and strain after 10 to 15 minutes or put the drug in cold water, bring to boil, boil for 2 to 3 minutes and strain while still warm. (1 teaspoon corresponds to approximately 3.8 gm drug).

Daily Dosage: 2 to 5 gm drug corresponding to 20 to 30 mg hydroxyanthracene derivative per day calculated as glucofrangulin A

Tea — 1 cup mornings and evenings.

The individual dose is the minimum dose required to produce a soft stool. Administration should be limited to a few days.

Homeopathic Dosage: from D3: 5 drops, 1 tablet or 10 globules every 30 to 60 minutes (acute) or 1 to 3 times daily (chronic); parenterally: 1 to 2 ml sc acute: 3 times daily; chronic: once a day (HAB1)

Storage: Buckthorn should be protected from light.

LITERATURE

Anonym, Abwehr von Arzneimittelrisiken, Stufe II. In: DAZ 136(38):3253-2354. 1996.

Anonym, Anwendungseinschränkungen für Anthranoid-haltige Abführmittel angeordnet. In: PUZ 25(6):341-342. 1996.

BGA, Arzneimittelrisiken: Anthranoide. In: DAZ 132(21):1164. 1992.

Belkin M et al., (1952) J Nat Cancer Inst 13:742.

Coskun M, Int J Pharmacogn 30:151. 1992.

Demirezer LÖ, Glucofrangulinanthrone A/B, deren Oxidationsformen und davon abgeleitete Zuckerester aus Rhamnus-Arten. In: Dissertation Universität Frankfurt/Main. 1991.

Klimpel BE et al., Anthranoidhaltige Laxantien - ein Risiko für die Entwicklung von Tumoren der ableitenden Harnwege. In: PUZ 26(1):33, Jahrestagung der DPhG, Berlin, 1996. 1997.

Rauwald HW Just, J-D, (1981) Planta Med 42:244.

Thesen R, Phytotherapeutika - nicht immer harmlos. In: ZPT 9(49):105. 1988.

Further information in:

Frohne D, Pfänder HJ, Giftpflanzen - Ein Handbuch für Apotheker, Toxikologen und Biologen, 4. Aufl., Wiss. Verlags-Ges. Stuttgart 1997.

Hänsel R, Keller K, Rimpler H, Schneider G (Hrsg.), Hagers Handbuch der Pharmazeutischen Praxis, 5. Aufl., Bde 4-6 (Drogen): Springer Verlag Berlin, Heidelberg, New York, 1992-1994.

Lewin L, Gifte und Vergiftungen, 6. Aufl., Nachdruck, Haug Verlag, Heidelberg 1992.

Madaus G, Lehrbuch der Biologischen Arzneimittel, Bde 1-3, Nachdruck, Georg Olms Verlag Hildesheim 1979.

Roth L, Daunderer M, Kormann K, Giftpflanzen, Pflanzengifte, 4. Aufl., Ecomed Fachverlag Landsberg Lech 1993.

Steinegger E, Hänsel R, Pharmakognosie, 5. Aufl., Springer Verlag Heidelberg 1992.

Thomson RH, Naturally Occuring Quinones, 2nd Ed., Academic Press New York 1971.

Teuscher E, Lindequist U, Biogene Gifte - Biologie, Chemie, Pharmakologie, 2. Aufl., Fischer Verlag Stuttgart 1994.

Teuscher E, Biogene Arzneimittel, 5. Aufl., Wiss. Verlagsges. Stuttgart 1997.

Wichtl M (Hrsg.), Teedrogen, 4. Aufl., Wiss. Verlagsges. Stuttgart 1997.

Buckwheat

Fagopyrum esculentum

DESCRIPTION

Medicinal Parts: The medicinal parts are the fresh aerial parts, and the leaves and flowers collected during the flowering season and later dried.

Flower and Fruit: Short, compact, long-peduncled thryses form in the leaf axils and at the end of the branches. The involucre is 3 to 4 mm long. It has 5 bracts, is pink or white and usually green at the base. The floret has 8 stamens with golden yellow nectaries at the base. The fruit is a sharply triangular achaene.

Leaves, Stem and Root: Buckwheat is an annual 15 to 60 cm high plant with an erect, usually red stem covered in alternating, sagittate and sessile leaves. The lobes are obtuse or rounded with sweeping borders. The lower leaves are petioled, the upper ones less so. The root is fusiform. Tatar Buckwheat (Fagopyrum tataricum), which is used in the pharmaceutical industry, is easily distinguishable from Fagopyrum esculentum by its green flowers, usually green stems, and curved, dentated and squat achaenes.

Habitat: The plant is indigenous to central Asia and is cultivated in Europe.

Production: Buckwheat herb consists of the flower and leaves of Fagopyrum esculentum, which are harvested during flowering season and dried. The harvest takes place 50 to 60 days after sowing and before the fruit forms. There is a slight loss of rutin if it is quickly dried (20 to 40 minutes) at high temperatures (105° to 135° C).

ACTIONS AND PHARMACOLOGY

COMPOUNDS

Flavonoids: rutin (up to 8% in the leaves), quercitrin, hyperoside

Anthracene derivatives (naphthadianthrones, chiefly in the blossoms): fagopyrine (0.01%), protofagopyrine

EFFECTS

Buckwheat increases the venous tone (antiedematic, capillary sealing), which can be attributed to the rutin in the herb.

INDICATIONS AND USAGE

Unproven Uses: In folk medicine, the drug is used as a venous and capillary tonic and as a prophylaxis to prevent general hardening of the arteries. The drug alleviates venous stasis and varicose veins.

Homeopathic Uses: Buckwheat is used to treat skin and liver diseases with itching and headache.

PRECAUTIONS AND ADVERSE REACTIONS

Health risks or side effects following the proper administration of designated therapeutic dosages are not recorded.

OVERDOSAGE

The intake of large quantities of the Buckwheat plant leads to phototoxicoses in animals due to the photosensitizing effect of the naphthadianthrones. There are no dangers for humans in the application of therapeutic dosages.

DOSAGE

Mode of Administration: Buckwheat is taken orally as tablets and in teas.

Preparation: Follow package instructions for making Buckwheat tea.

Homeopathic Dosage: 5 drops, 1 tablet or 10 globules every 30 to 60 minutes (acute) or 1 to 3 times daily (chronic); from D6: parenterally: 1 to 2 ml sc, acute, 3 times daily; chronic: once a day (HAB1).

LITERATURE

Adamek B, Drozdzik M, Samochowiec L, Wojcicki J, Clinical effect of buckwheat herb, Ruscus extract and troxerutin on retinopathy and lipids in diabetic patients. In: Phytotherapy Res 10(8):659-662. 1996.

Anonym, Nicht-Brotgetreidearten: Alternative Körner unter der Lupe. In: DAZ 136(38):3229-2330. 1996.

Bässler R, PA 12:758-772 et 834-841. 1985.

Couch JF, Naghski J, Krewson CF, Science 103:197-198. 1974.

Gaidies I, Buchweizen, eine Venenhilfe. In: PTA 6(7):439. 1992.

Hagels H et al., Two anthraquinones and a bianthraquinone from Fagopyrum tataricum. In: PM 62, Abstracts of the 44th Ann Congress of GA, 125. 1996.

Ihme N et al., Leg oedema protection from a buckwheat herb tea in patients with chronic venous insufficiency: A single centre, randomised, double blind, placebo controlled clinical trial. In: European J Clin Pharmacol 50(6)443-447. 1996.

Koscielny J, Radtke H, Hoffmann KH, Jung F, Müller A, Grützner KI, Kiesewetter H, Fagorutin-Tee bei chronisch venöser Insuffizienz (CVI). In: ZPT 17(3):145-159. 1996.

Samel D, de Witte P, Fagopyrins from Fagopyrum esculentum and their PTK inhibitory activity. In: PM 61(Abstracts of 43rd Ann Congr):67. 1995.

Further information in:

Hänsel R, Keller K, Rimpler H, Schneider G (Hrsg.), Hagers Handbuch der Pharmazeutischen Praxis, 5. Aufl., Bde 4-6 (Drogen): Springer Verlag Berlin, Heidelberg, New York, 1992-1994.

Lewin L, Gifte und Vergiftungen, 6. Aufl., Nachdruck, Haug Verlag, Heidelberg 1992. (unter Buchweizen).

Roth L, Daunderer M, Kormann K, Giftpflanzen, Pflanzengifte, 4. Aufl., Ecomed Fachverlag Landsberg Lech 1993.

Teuscher E, Lindequist U, Biogene Gifte - Biologie, Chemie, Pharmakologie, 2. Aufl., Fischer Verlag Stuttgart 1994.

Wagner H, Wiesenauer M, Phytotherapie. Phytopharmaka und pflanzliche Homöopathika, Fischer-Verlag, Stuttgart, Jena, New York 1995.

Bugle

Ajuga reptans

DESCRIPTION

Medicinal Parts: The medicinal parts are the aerial parts collected during the flowering season and dried.

Flower and Fruit: The flowers are 1 to 1.5 cm long. The flowers are in spikes. They are located in the axils of undivided bracts at the end of the stem. The 5-tipped, hairy çalyx is short-stemmed, erect, labiate and campanulate. The tips are triangular and about as long as the tube. The corolla is bright violet-blue, pink or white. It is downy-haired on the outside with a long straight tube, which has a circle of hairs under the stamen. There are 4 stamens with yellow anthers. The 4 mericarps are 2 mm long and finely reticulate.

Leaves, Stem and Root: Ajuga reptans is a shrub, up to 30 cm high with overground rooting runners sprouting from the rosette-like basal leaves. The flower stem is quadrangular, villous above and glabrous below. The rest of the plant is glabrous. The basal leaves are large, long-petioled, spatulate and dentate. The cauline leaves are crossed opposite, short-petioled, small and oval. The lowest or at least the third-lowest stem is flower-bearing. There are some upper false whorls, which are compressed into a false spike.

Habitat: The plant is found in Europe, Britain, and parts of Asia and northern Africa.

Production: The aerial parts of Ajuga reptans are picked when in bloom and dried. Gathered in uncultivated areas (the wild).

Other Names: Bugula, Middle Comfrey, Middle Confound, Sicklewort, Carpenter's Herb

ACTIONS AND PHARMACOLOGY

COMPOUNDS

Iridoid glycosides and ajugols

Phytoecdysone: ajugalactone

Diterpene bitter principles

Caffeic acid derivatives: including rosemary acid

EFFECTS

There is no information available.

INDICATIONS AND USAGE

Unproven Uses: Internally, Bugle is used as an astringent for inflammation of the mouth and larynx. It is also used for gallbladder and stomach disorders. Externally, the plant is used for the treatment of wounds.

PRECAUTIONS AND ADVERSE REACTIONS

No health hazards or side effects are known in conjunction with the proper administration of designated therapeutic dosages.

DOSAGE

Mode of Administration: Bugle is used topically, in alcoholic extracts, as a water infusion and in teas.

LITERATURE

Breschi M, Martinotti E, Catalano S, Flamini G, Morelli I, Pagni A, Vasoconstrictor activity of 8-O-Acetylharpagide from Ajuga reptans. In: JNP 55: 1145-1148. 1992.

Camps F, et al., (1985) An Quim 81C(1):74-75.

Camps F, et al., (1981) Rev Latinoamj Quim 12:81-88. 1981.

Camps F, Coll J, (1993) Insect allochemicals from Ajuga plants. In: PH 32:1361.

Hänsel R, Keller K, Rimpler H, Schneider G (Hrsg.), Hagers Handbuch der Pharmazeutischen Praxis, 5. Aufl., Bde 4-6 (Drogen), Springer Verlag Berlin, Heidelberg, New York, 1992-1994.

Komissarenko NF, et al., (1976) Khim Prir Soedin 11:109-110. 1976.

Kooiman P, (1972) Acta Bot Nederl. 21(4):417.

Ruhdorfer J, Rimpler H, (1981) Z Naturforsch 36c:697-707. 1981.

Bugleweed

Lycopus virginicus

DESCRIPTION

Medicinal Parts: The medicinal part is the fresh or dried herb collected during the flowering season.

Flower and Fruit: The flowers are small, almost radial in dense axillary whorls. The calyx is campanulate with a glabrous tube and 4 or 5 regular, usually erect, tips. The corolla is whitish with the tube only partly showing and a few uneven lobes. The epicalyx and calyx sepals are shorter than in the European variety. There are only 2 fertile stamens with initially parallel, later spreading pollen sacs. The upper stamens are reduced to staminoids or completely disappear. The fruit is a flattened, rectangular, stunted, and smooth nutlet.

Leaves, Stem and Root: The plant is a herbaceous perennial with runners. The quadrangular, 60 cm high smooth stems grow from the perennial creeping root. The stems bear pairs of opposite, short-petioled leaves. The upper ones are dentate and pointed; the lower ones wedge-shaped to entire-margined. They are glabrous and glandular-punctate on the lower surface.

Habitat: The plant grows in North America. Lycopus europaeus, Gypsywort, is a close European relative.

Production: Bugleweed consists of the fresh or dried, aboveground parts of Lycopus europaeus and/or Lycopus virginicus, as well as preparations collected in the wild and air-dried.

Other Names: Sweet Bugle, Water Bugle, Virginia Water Horehound, Gypsywort

ACTIONS AND PHARMACOLOGY

COMPOUNDS

Caffeic acid derivatives: rosmaric acid, lithospermic acid and their oligomerics created through oxidation

Flavonoids: including acacetine-, apigenein-, luteolin glycosides, among them cosmosiin, genkwanin, pilloin, apigenin-, acacetine- and luteolin-7-O-glucuronides.

Diterpenes: tetrahydroxy-delta8(9)-pimaric acid methyl ester

Volatile oil (0.1%)

EFFECTS

Bugleweed has antigonadotropic and antithyrotropic effects. It inhibits the peripheral de-iodination of T4. The phenolic constituents of the drug have an atigonadotropic effect. They cause a lowering of the prolactin level and have a depressant effect on the thyroid as a result of an inhibition of iodine transport and the release of preformed thyroid hormone.

INDICATIONS AND USAGE

Approved by Commission E:

- Nervousness and insomnia
- Premenstrual syndrome (PMS)

Unproven Uses: Bugleweed is used for mild thyroid hyperfunction associated with disturbances of the autonomic nervous system. It is also used for tension and pain in the breast (mastodynia). In folk medicine, it is used for functional and organic cardiac conditions, liver and kidney disease.

Homeopathic Uses: Lycopus virginicus is used to treat hyperthyroidism in homeopathic preparations.

CONTRAINDICATIONS

The drug is contraindicated in hypofunction of the thyroid and thyroid gland enlargement without function disturbance. There should not be any simultaneous administration of thyroid hormone preparations.

PRECAUTIONS AND ADVERSE REACTIONS

General: No health hazards or side effects are known in conjunction with the proper administration of designated therapeutic dosages.

Drug Interactions: No simultaneous administration of thyroid preparations. Administration of Lycopus preparations disturbs the administration of diagnostic procedures with radioactive isotopes.

OVERDOSAGE

Enlargement of the thyroid gland is possible only through administration of the drug in very high dosage. Sudden discontinuation of Lycopus preparation can lead to a rebound phenomenon with increased TSH secretion and prolactin secretion, as well as an increase of the hyperthyroid symptom complex and mastodynia.

DOSAGE

Mode of Administration: Comminuted herb, freshly pressed juice and other galenic preparations for internal use.

Daily Dosage: The average daily dose is 1 to 2 gm of the drug for teas, and water-ethanol extracts containing the equivalent of 20 mg of the drug.

Each patient has his own individual optimal level of thyroid hormone. Only rough estimations of dosage are possible for thyroid disorders, in which age and weight must be considered.

Homeopathic Dosage: 5 drops, 1 tablet or 10 globules every 30 to 60 minutes (acute) or 1 to 3 times daily (chronic); parenterally: 1 to 2 ml sc acute, 3 times daily; chronic: once a day (HAB1)

LITERATURE

Auf'mkolk M, (1985) Endocrinology 116(5):1687.

Bucar R et al., Flavonoid glycosides from Lycopus europaeus. In: PM 61(5):489. 1995.

Frömbling-Borges A, (1987) Intrathyreoidale Wirkung von Lycopus europaeus, Pflanzensäuren, Tyrosinen, Thyroninen und Lithiumchlorid. Darstellung einer Schilddrüsensekretions-blockade. Inauguraldissertation. Westfälische Wilhelms-Universität Münster.

Frömbling-Borges A, Intrathyreoidale Wirkung von Lycopus europaeus, Pflanzensäuren, Kaliumjodid und Lithiumchlorid. In: ZPT 10(1):1. 1990.

Gumbinger HG et al., (1981) Contraception 23(6):661.

Hegnauer R, Kooiman P, (1978) Planta Med 33(1):13.

Jeremic D et al., (1985) Tetrahedron 41(2):357.

John M, Gumbinger HG, Winterhoff H, The oxidation of caffeic acid derivatives as model reaction for the formation of potent gonadotropin inhibitors in plant extracts. In: PM 59(3):195. 1993.

Jung F, Kiesewetter H, Mrowietz C, Pindur G, Heiden M, Miyashita C, Wenzel E, Akutwirkungen eines zusammen-gesetzten Knoblauchpräparates auf die Fließfähigkeit des Blutes. In: ZPT 10(3):87. 1989.

Kartnig T, Lycopus europaeus L. - Wolfsfuß oder Wolfstrapp. In: ZPT 10(1):31. 1989.

Kern W, List PH, Hörhammer L (Hrsg.), Hagers Handbuch der Pharmazeutischen Praxis, 4. Aufl., Bde. 1-8, Springer Verlag Berlin, Heidelberg, New York, 1969.

Schulz R, Hänsel R, Rationale Phytotherapie, Springer Verlag Heidelberg 1996.

Kooiman P, (1972) Acta Bot Neerl 21(4)417.

Sourgens H et al., (1982) Planta Med 45:78.

Teuscher E, Biogene Arzneimittel, 5. Aufl., Wiss. Verlagsges. Stuttgart 1997.

Wagner H, Wiesenauer M, Phytotherapie. Phytopharmaka und pflanzliche Homöopathika, Fischer-Verlag, Stuttgart, Jena, New York 1995.

Bulbous Buttercup

Ranunculus bulbosus

DESCRIPTION

Medicinal Parts: The medicinal parts are the latex and the fresh flowering herb with root.

Flower and Fruit: The large golden yellow flowers consist of 5 sepals hanging down, 5 petals on grooved stems and numerous stamens and ovaries. The small fruit has a short curved beak.

Leaves, Stem and Root: The plant grows from 10 to 30 cm high and has a tuber on the underground part of the stem. The basal leaves are long-petioled, trifoliate with orbicular and pinnasect leaflets. The middle one has a longer petiole and is sheath-like at the base. The stems are branched and tuberously thickened at the base. The plant is appressed pubescent above and patently pubescent below.

Habitat: The plant grows in the northern parts of Europe and in the northeastern U.S.

Production: Bulbous Buttercup is the whole plant in flower of Ranunculus bulbosus with root.

Other Names: Crowfoot, Cuckoo Buds, Frogwort, King's Cup, Meadowbloom, Pilewort, St. Anthony's Turnip, Frogsfoot, Goldcup

ACTIONS AND PHARMACOLOGY

COMPOUNDS

The glycoside ranunculin: changes enzymatically when the plant is cut into small pieces, and probably also when it is dried, into the pungent, volatile protoanemonine that quickly dimerizes to non-mucous-membrane irritating anemonine. When dried, the plant is not capable of protoanemonine formation.

EFFECTS

The active agents cause signs of toxic irritation; the drug is also said to cause symptoms of drowsiness and tiredness.

INDICATIONS AND USAGE

Homeopathic Uses: The herb is used for skin diseases, rheumatism, gout, neuralgia, influenza and meningitis.

CONTRAINDICATIONS

The administration of the drug during pregnancy is absolutely contraindicated.

PRECAUTIONS AND ADVERSE REACTIONS

General: No health hazards or side effects are known in conjunction with the proper administration of designated therapeutic dosages of the dehydrated drug.

Extended skin contact with the freshly harvested, bruised plant can lead to blister formation and cauterizations that are difficult to heal due to the resulting protoanemonine, which is severely irritating to skin and mucous membranes. If taken internally, severe irritation to the gastrointestinal tract, combined with colic and diarrhea, as well as irritation of the urinary drainage passages, are possible. Symptomatic treatment for external contact should consist of mucilage, after irrigation with diluted potassium permanganate solution; in case of internal contact, activated charcoal should follow gastric lavage.

Pregnancy: The administration of the drug during pregnancy is absolutely contraindicated.

OVERDOSAGE

Death by asphyxiation following the intake of large quantities of protoanemonine-forming plants has been observed in animal experiments.

DOSAGE

Mode of Administration: The herb is used as an extract in homeopathic dilutions.

LITERATURE

Bonora A et al., PH 26:2277. 1987.

Frohne D, Pfänder HJ, Giftpflanzen - Ein Handbuch für Apotheker, Toxikologen und Biologen, 4. Aufl., Wiss. Verlags-Ges. Stuttgart 1997.

Kern W, List PH, Hörhammer L (Hrsg.), Hagers Handbuch der Pharmazeutischen Praxis, 4. Aufl., Bde. 1-8: Springer Verlag Berlin, Heidelberg, New York, 1969.

Madaus G, Lehrbuch der Biologischen Arzneimittel, Bde 1-3, Nachdruck, Georg Olms Verlag Hildesheim 1979.

Roth L, Daunderer M, Kormann K, Giftpflanzen, Pflanzengifte, 4. Aufl., Ecomed Fachverlag Landsberg Lech 1993.

Ruijgrok HWL, PM 11:338-347. 1963.

Teuscher E, Lindequist U, Biogene Gifte - Biologie, Chemie, Pharmakologie, 2. Aufl., Fischer Verlag Stuttgart 1994.

Bupleurum chinense

See Chinese Thoroughwax (Chai-Hu)

Burdock

Arctium lappa

TRADE NAMES

Burdock Root (available from numerous manufacturers).

DESCRIPTION

Medicinal Parts: The medicinal parts of the plant are the ripe seed and the fresh or dried roots.

Flower and Fruit: The crimson flowers grow in long-peduncled, loose cymes. The heads are fairly large, globose and almost glabrous. All flowers are funnel-shaped and androgynous. The bracts are green and coriaceous with a barb-shaped inward-curving tip. The fruit is compressed and has a bristly tuft, which falls off easily. The fruits separate from their stems on ripening.

Leaves, Stem and Root: The plant grows to a height of 80 to 150 cm. The stem is erect, rigid, grooved, branched and downy to wooly. The leaves are alternate, petiolate, broad to ovate-cordate. They are blunt and slightly wooly to hairy on the underside. The lowest leaves are very large and have a latex-filled stem.

Habitat: Burdock grows in Europe, northern Asia and North America.

Production: Burdock root consists of the fresh or dried underground parts of Arctium lappa, Arctium minus and/or Arctium tomentosum. Roots are gathered in the autumn of the plant's first year or the early part of the second year.

Other Names: Bardana, Beggar's Buttons, Burr Seed, Clot-Bur, Cockle Buttons, Cocklebur, Fox's Clote, Great Burr, Happy Major, Hardock, Hareburr, Lappa, Love Leaves, Personata, Philanthropium, Thorny Burr

ACTIONS AND PHARMACOLOGY

COMPOUNDS

Volatile oil (small amounts) of very complex make-up: including, among others, phenylacetaldehyde, benzaldehyde, 2-alkyl-3-methoxy-pyrazines

Lignans: neoarchtiin A

Sesquiterpene lactones

Polyynes: chief components are trideca-1, 11-dien-3, 5,7,9-tetrain, as well as sulfur derivatives

Caffeic acid derivatives: including chlorogenic acid, isochlorogenic acid

Polysaccharides: insulin (fructose), mucilage's (xyloglucans, acidic xylans)

Triterpenes: including alpha-amyrin, omega-taraxasterol, present to some extent as acetic acid ester

Phytosterols: beta-sitosterol, stigmasterol, campesterol and their esters

Tannins

EFFECTS

In vitro, the drug shows mild antimicrobial activity. No other information is available.

INDICATIONS AND USAGE

Unproven Uses: Preparations of Burdock Root are used for ailments and complaints of the gastrointestinal tract, as a diaphoretic and diuretic, and for blood purifying. Externally, they are used for ichthyosis, psoriasis and seborrhea of the scalp. The claimed efficacies have not been documented.

Chinese Medicine: Burdock is used to treat carbuncles, ulcers and erythema of the skin as well as sore throats. Efficacy has not been proven.

PRECAUTIONS AND ADVERSE REACTIONS

No health hazards or side effects are known in conjunction with the proper administration of designated therapeutic dosages. There is a slight potential for sensitization via skin contact with the drug.

DOSAGE

Mode of Administration: Administered as a drug and, for external use, in the form of burdock oil (extract with fat oil).

How Supplied:

Capsules — 460 mg and 475 mg

Fluid Extract — 1:1

LITERATURE

Bryson PD et al., (1978) J Am Med Ass 239 (20):2157.

Dombradi G, (1970) Chemotherapy 15:250.

Ichihara A et al., (1968) Tetrahedron 44:3961.

Ichihara A et al., (1978) Tetrahedron Letters 33:305.

Morita K et al., (1984) Mutat Res 129(1):25.

Naya K et al., (1972) Chem Letters 3:235.

Schulte K et al., (1967) Arzneim Forsch 17:829.

Takeda H, Kiriyami S, (1979) J Nutr 109(3):388.

Tsujita J et al., (1979) Nutr Rep Int 20(5):635.

Yamada Y et al., (1975) Phytochemistry 14:582.

Yamanouchi S et al., (1976) Yakugaku Zasshi 96(12):1492.

Further information in:

Hausen B, Allergiepflanzen, Pflanzenallergene, ecomed Verlagsgesellsch. mbH, Landsberg 1988.

Kern W, List PH, Hörhammer L (Hrsg.), Hagers Handbuch der Pharmazeutischen Praxis, 4. Aufl., Bde. 1-8, Springer Verlag Berlin, Heidelberg, New York, 1969.

Leung AY, Encyclopedia of Common Natural Ingredients Used in Food Drugs and Cosmetics, John Wiley & Sons Inc., New York, 1980.

Madaus G, Lehrbuch der Biologischen Arzneimittel, Bde 1-3, Nachdruck, Georg Olms Verlag Hildesheim 1979.

Schulte KE et al Arzneim Forsch 17 (1967), 825.

Wichtl M (Hrsg.), Teedrogen, 4. Aufl., Wiss. Verlagsges. Stuttgart 1997.

Burning Bush

Dictamnus albus

DESCRIPTION

Medicinal Parts: The medicinal parts are the dried and occasionally the fresh leaves, the fresh or dried root, and the fresh or dried root rind.

Flower and Fruit: The flowers are terminal racemes and pink with dark veins. They are large and irregular, with 5 sepals and 5 petals. There are 2 bracteoles that are slightly zygomorphous. The 10 stamens are long, threadlike and bent forward. The ovaries have 5 carpels fused at the base on a short gynophore. The fruit is a capsule that bursts open into mericarps ejecting the seeds.

Leaves, Stem and Root: The plant is a 0.5 to 1.5 m high perennial. Numerous erect, unbranched and sticky-glandular-haired shoots grow from the root. The leaves are alternate, odd, 7 to 11 pinnate and transparently punctuated with oil glands.

Characteristics: The plant has a strong lemon or cinnamon fragrance. The oil is easily inflammable.

Habitat: The plant is indigenous to central Europe and parts of Asia, and is cultivated in the northern U.S.

Not to be Confused With: Burning Bush herb can be confused with that of the herb Dictamni cretici. Previous sources cite a confusion between Burning Bush root and Carophyllaceen root.

Other Names: Fraxinella, Dittany, Gas Plant, Diptam

ACTIONS AND PHARMACOLOGY

COMPOUNDS: BURNING BUSH ROOT

Volatile oil: chief components are the fraxinellone derivatives, thymol methylether, beta-pinene, pregeijerene, geijerene

Furoquinoline alkaloids: including skimmianine, gamma-fagarine, dictamnine

Limonoids: including limonin, obacunone, dictamdiol, limonin diosphenol

EFFECTS: BURNING BUSH ROOT

In vitro, a mutagenic effect on *Salmonella typhimurum* and a phototoxic effect on bacteria and yeasts have been observed.

In animal tests, a contraceptive effect was observed through the inhibition of implantation, as well as a slight increase in hair growth of shaved mice after the application of an alcoholic extract.

COMPOUNDS: BURNING BUSH HERB

Volatile oil: chief components (according to breed) anethole (+) estragole, anethole (+) myrcene, limonene, 1,8-cineol, p-cymene (+) estragole

Furoquinoline alkaloids: including skimmianine, gamma-fagarine, dictamnine

Furocoumarins: including psoralen, xanthotoxin, auraptene, bergaptenE

Limonoids: including limonin, obacunone, obacunone acid

Flavonoids: including rutin, diosmin, isoquercitrin

EFFECTS: BURNING BUSH HERB

See Burning Bush root.

A 40% reduction in egg laying by *Clonorchis sinensis* (Chinese liver fluke) was observed when infected rabbits were given an evaporated extract of the drug.

INDICATIONS AND USAGE

BURNING BUSH ROOT

Unproven Uses: Infusion of the root is used to treat stomach disorders, cramps and worm infestation, and to promote menstruation.

In Greece, it is used as a tonic and a stimulant.

Chinese Medicine: Burning Bush root is used for jaundice, inflammation of the skin, rheumatic ailments, fever, hemorrhage of the womb, thread fungus, as a sedative, tonic and for nervous crying in children. It is also found in decoctions for the external treatment of eczema, impetigo and scabies.

Indian Medicine: Burning Bush root is used for amenorrhea and the regulation of labor.

BURNING BUSH HERB

Unproven Uses: In the Middle Ages, the drug was used as a cure or remedy for wounds, to promote menstruation and to aid the expulsion of afterbirth. It served as a urinary aid and was used in the treatment of epilepsy, in combination with mistletoe and peony.

At the end of the 19th century, the drug was applied as an ointment for rheumatism. The infusion is used as a remedy for worm infestation, to treat stomach disorders and cramps and to promote menstruation. In Greece, it is used as a tonic and stimulant.

PRECAUTIONS AND ADVERSE REACTIONS

BURNING BUSH ROOT AND HERB

Health risks or side effects following the proper administration of designated therapeutic dosages are not recorded. The plant can trigger phototoxicoses through skin contact. The furoquinoline derivatives have a mutagenic effect in the Ames test.

DOSAGE

BURNING BUSH ROOT

Mode of Administration: Mostly obsolete as a drug. It is occasionally used in tea mixtures.

Preparation: To prepare a tea infusion, add 1 teaspoon of drug to 2 glasses of hot water.

Daily Dosage: Drink the tea preparation throughout the day.

BURNING BUSH HERB

Mode of Administration: Mostly obsolete as a drug. The herb is sometimes used internally as an infusion.

Preparation: An infusion is prepared by adding 20 gm of dried herb to 1 liter of water; or 1 gm fresh or 2 gm dried herb to 1 cup of water.

Daily Dosage: Drink one cup of the infusion 2 to 3 times daily after meals.

LITERATURE

Kanamori H, Sakamoto I, Mizuta M, Chem Pharm Bull 34:1826. 1986.

Reisch J, PM 15:320. 1967.

Renner W, PA 12:763-776. 1962.

Renner W, PA 17:763. 1962.

Szenedrei K, Novak I, Varga E, Buzas G, PA 23:76-77. 1968.

Further information in:

Hänsel R, Keller K, Rimpler H, Schneider G (Hrsg.), Hagers Handbuch der Pharmazeutischen Praxis, 5. Aufl., Bde 4-6 (Drogen), Springer Verlag Berlin, Heidelberg, New York, 1992-1994.

Hausen B, Allergiepflanzen, Pflanzenallergene, ecomed Verlagsgesellsch. mbH, Landsberg 1988.

Madaus G, Lehrbuch der Biologischen Arzneimittel, Bde 1-3, Nachdruck, Georg Olms Verlag Hildesheim 1979.

Roth L, Daunderer M, Kormann K, Giftpflanzen, Pflanzengifte, 4. Aufl., Ecomed Fachverlag Landsberg Lech 1993.

Teuscher E, Lindequist U, Biogene Gifte - Biologie, Chemie, Pharmakologie, 2. Aufl. Fischer Verlag Stuttgart 1994.

Burr Marigold

Bidens tripartita

DESCRIPTION

Medicinal Parts: The whole Burr Marigold plant is used medicinally.

Flower and Fruit: The flower heads are solitary, erect or inclined, 15 to 25 mm long and wide, generally with no lingual blossoms. There are two rows of bracts. The inner row is ovate and brownish-yellow; the outer is oblong and green. The petals are brownish-yellow. The fruit is glabrous, distinctly compressed, brownish-green, with thorny edges and 2 to 4 awns.

Leaves, Stem and Root: Bidens tripartita is an erect annual growing 15 to 100 cm high with a fibrous fusiform root. The stem is erect, heavily branched, glabrous or somewhat downy ,and often brownish-red. The leaves are dark green, opposite and narrow to a short, winged petiole. The leaves are usually 3 to 5 lobed, ovate-rhomboid to lanceolate with pointed, roughly dentate tips and straight or narrowly curved teeth.

Habitat: The plant is found in damp regions throughout Europe.

Production: Burr Marigold is the aerial part of Bidens tripartita.

Other Names: Water Agrimony

ACTIONS AND PHARMACOLOGY

COMPOUNDS

Flavonoids: including isookanin-7-O-glucoside and tridecane derivatives such as trideca-1,12-dien-3,5,7,9-tetrain

Hydroxycoumarins: including umbelliferone, scopoletin

Polyynes (tridecane derivatives): including trideca-1,12-dien-3,5,7,9-tetrain

Water-soluble polysaccharides

Bitter principles

Tannins

Volatile oil: including eugenol, ocimene, cosmene

EFFECTS

Astringent, diaphoretic and diuretic effects are attributed to the plant, but remain unproven. In a study that has not been described in detail, a choleretic effect caused by the flavones and flavonoids was proven.

INDICATIONS AND USAGE

Unproven Uses: Folk medicine uses include gout, hematuria, loss of hair, scurvy and toothache. The roots were used for scorpion bites. It was used for other indications when a diuretic, diaphoretic or astringent effect was desired.

PRECAUTIONS AND ADVERSE REACTIONS

No health hazards or side effects are known in conjunction with the proper administration of designated therapeutic dosages.

DOSAGE

No information is available.

LITERATURE

Bauer R, Neues von "immunmodulierenden Drogen" und "Drogen mit antiallergischer und antiinflammatorischer Wirkung". In: ZPT 14(1):23-24. 1993.

Ben'ko GN, (1983) Rastit Resur 19 (4),516.

Morozova SS et al., (1981) Rastit Resur 17 (1),101.

Further information in:

Alvarez L, Marquina S, Villarreal ML, Alonso D, Aranda E, Delgado G, Anti-inflammatory activity of Taiwan folk medicine "ham-hong-chho" in rats. Am J Chin Med, 62:273-8, 1995.

Alvarez L, Marquina S, Villarreal ML, Alonso D, Aranda E, Delgado G, Bioactive polyacetylenes from Bidens pilosa. Planta Med, 62:355-7, 1996.

Alvarez L, Marquina S, Villarreal ML, Alonso D, Aranda E, Delgado G, Constituents and biological activity of Bidens pilosa L. grown in Egypt. Acta Pharm Hung, 62:317-23, 1991.

Brandao MG et al., Antimalarial activity of extracts and fractions from Bidens pilosa and other Bidens species (Asteraceae) correlated with the presence of acetylene and flavonoid compounds. J Ethnopharmacol, 57:131-8, 1997.

de Tommasi N, Pizza C, Aquino R, Cumanda J, Mahmood N, Flavonol and chalcone ester glycosides from Bidens leucantha. J Nat Prod, 60:270-3, 1997 Mar

Geissberger P, Sequin U, Constituents of Bidens pilosa L.: do the components found so far explain the use of this plant in traditional medicine? Acta Trop, 57:251-61, 1991.

Jaeger AK, Hutchings A, van Staden J, Screening of Zulu medicinal plants for prostaglandin-synthesis inhibitors. J Ethnopharmacol, 52:95-100, 1996.

Kern W, List PH, Hörhammer L (Hrsg.), Hagers Handbuch der Pharmazeutischen Praxis, 4. Aufl., Bde. 1-8, Springer Verlag Berlin, Heidelberg, New York, 1969.

Martin Calero M et al., Healing process induced by a flavonic fraction of Bidens aurea on chronic gastric lesion in rat. Role of angiogenesis and neutrophil inhibition. Z Naturforsch C , 51:570-7, 1996.

Morozova SS et al Rastit Resur 17 (1981), 101 Further information in: Kern, W.; List, P.H.; Hörhammer, L. (Ed.): Hagers Handbuch der Pharmazeutischen Praxis. 4. Aufl., Bde. 1-8, Springer Verlag Berlin, Heidelberg, New York 1969.

Butcher's Broom

Ruscus aculeatus

TRADE NAMES

Butcher's Broom (available from numerous manufactures), Butcher's Broom Root, Curcu Capsules

DESCRIPTION

Medicinal Parts: The medicinal parts are the herb and the rhizome.

Flower and Fruit: The small greenish white flowers are solitary or in a few clusters and grow from the middle of the leaves. They are dioecious. The corolla is deeply divided into 6 segments. In one variety the stamens are fused at the base. In fertile varieties the style is surrounded by a honey gland. The fertile flowers develop into cherry-sized, scarlet berries, which ripen in September and remain on the tree all winter.

Leaves, Stem and Root: The plant is a perennial evergreen subshrub that grows 20 to 80 cm high. The stems are erect, woody and heavily branched. The leaves are small, brown-membranous, triangular to lanceolate, and scale-like. The phylloclades (short shoots spread like leaves) are oblong, stiff, double-rowed, up to 2.5 cm long and terminate in a sharp tip.

Habitat: The plant is indigenous to almost all of Europe, western Asia and North Africa.

Production: Butcher's Broom consists of the dried rhizome and root of Ruscus aculeatus.

Other Names: Kneeholm, Pettigree, Sweet Broom, Knee Holly, Jew's Myrtle

ACTIONS AND PHARMACOLOGY

COMPOUNDS

Steroid saponins (4-6%): chief components, ruscine, ruscoside, aglycones neoruscogenin, ruscogenin

Benzofuranes: euparone, ruscodibenzofurane

EFFECTS

In animal tests, there was an increase in venous tone and an electrolyte-like reaction on the cell wall of capillaries. Butcher's Broom is antiphlogistic and diuretic.

INDICATIONS AND USAGE

Approved by Commission E:

- Hemorrhoids
- Venous conditions

The herb is used as supportive therapy for discomfort of chronic venous insufficiency, such as pain and heaviness, as well as cramps in the legs, itching, and swelling. Butcher's Broom also is used as therapy for hemorrhoid complaints, such as itching and burning.

PRECAUTIONS AND ADVERSE REACTIONS

No health hazards or side effects are known in conjunction with the proper administration of designated therapeutic dosages. Stomach complaints and queasiness can occur in rare cases.

DOSAGE

Mode of Administration: Extracts and their preparations for internal use.

How Supplied:
Capsules — 75 mg, 370 mg, 470 mg, 475 mg

Daily Dosage: Raw extract, equivalent to 7 to 11 mg total ruscogenin (determined as the sum of neoruscogenin and ruscogenin obtained after fermentation or acid hydrolysis).

LITERATURE

Adamek B, Drozdzik M, Samochowiec L, Wojcicki J, Clinical effect of buckwheat herb, Ruscus extract and troxerutin on retinopathy and lipids in diabetic patients. In: Phytotherapy Res 10(8):659-662. 1996.

Bombardelli E et al., (1972) Fitoterapia 43:3.

Dunaouau CH et al., Triterpenes and sterols from Ruscus aculeatus. In: PM 62(2):189-190. 1997.

Rauwald HW, Janβen B, Desglucoruscin and Desglucoruscosid als Leitstoffe des Ruscus-aculeatus-Wurzelstock. Analytische Kennzeichnung mittel HPLC und DC. In: PZW 133(1):61-68. 1988.

Schiebel-Schlosser G, Stechender Mäusedorn, eine Venenhilfe. In: PTA 8(7):586. 1994.

Vanhoutte PM (1986) in: Advances in Medicinal Phytochemistry, Ed. D Barton, WD Ollis, Pub. John Wiley 1986.

Further information in:

Kern W, List PH, Hörhammer L (Hrsg.), Hagers Handbuch der Pharmazeutischen Praxis, 4. Aufl., Bde. 1-8: Springer Verlag Berlin, Heidelberg, New York, 1969.

Steinegger E, Hänsel R, Pharmakognosie, 5. Aufl., Springer Verlag Heidelberg 1992.

Teuscher E, Biogene Arzneimittel, 5. Aufl., Wiss. Verlagsges. Stuttgart 1997.

Wagner H, Wiesenauer M, Phytotherapie. Phytopharmaka und pflanzliche Homöopathika, Fischer-Verlag, Stuttgart, Jena, New York 1995.

Wichtl M (Hrsg.), Teedrogen, 4. Aufl., Wiss. Verlagsges. Stuttgart 1997.

Buttercup

Ranunculus acris

DESCRIPTION

Medicinal Parts: The medicinal part is the herb.

Flower and Fruit: The golden-yellow, medium-sized flowers are on long, round pedicles. The 5 sepals and 5 petals are close. There are numerous stamens and ovaries. The broad obovate petals are very glossy and have a broad scale on the surface. The small fruit is in an almost globular capitulum.

Leaves, Stem and Root: The leafy plant grows from 30 to 80 cm. The erect stem has few branches. The petioles and pedicles are appressed and downy. The basal leaves are long-petioled and palmate with rhomboid tips, which are divided into 2 or 3. The similar cauline leaves are shorter-petioled.

Characteristics: The fresh herb is spicy and poisonous; once dried, it is no longer poisonous.

Habitat: The plant is indigenous to northern Europe.

Production: Buttercup is the fresh herb Ranunculus acris.

Other Names: Acrid Crowfoot, Batchelor's Buttons, Blisterweed, Burrwort, Globe Amaranth, Gold Cup, Meadowbloom, Yellows, Yellowweed

ACTIONS AND PHARMACOLOGY

COMPOUNDS

Glycoside ranunculin: as protoanemonine-forming agent in the freshly harvested plant (0.36-2.66% of the fresh weight) that changes enzymatically when the plant is cut into small pieces, and probably also while it is drying, into the pungent, volatile protoanemonine that quickly dimerizes to non-mucous-membrane-irritating anemonine. Once dried, the plant may not be capable of protoanemonine formation.

Saponins

EFFECTS

The active agents are ranunculin, protoanemonin and anemonin. On contact with the skin, the juice of the plant causes redness, swelling and blisters. If taken internally, it can lead to burning in the mouth, vomiting, stomachache and pains in the liver.

INDICATIONS AND USAGE

Unproven Uses: Buttercup is used for blisters, bronchitis, chronic skin complaints, neuralgia and rheumatism.

PRECAUTIONS AND ADVERSE REACTIONS

No health hazards or side effects are known in conjunction with the proper administration of designated therapeutic dosages of the dehydrated drug. Extended skin contact with the freshly harvested, bruised plant can lead to blister formation and cauterizations that are difficult to heal due to the resulting protoanemonine, which is severely irritating to skin and mucous membranes. If taken internally, severe irritation to the gastrointestinal tract, combined with colic and diarrhea, as well as irritation of the urinary drainage passages, may occur.

Symptomatic treatment for external contact should consist of mucilaginosa, after irrigation with diluted potassium permanganate solution. In case of internal contact, administration of activated charcoal should follow gastric lavage.

OVERDOSAGE

Death by asphyxiation following the intake of large quantities of protoanemonine-forming plants has been observed in animal experiments.

DOSAGE

Mode of Administration: Buttercup is available as a ground dried herb and as an extract.

LITERATURE

Bonora A et al., PH 26:2277. 1987.

Frohne D, Pfänder HJ: Giftpflanzen - Ein Handbuch für Apotheker, Toxikologen und Biologen, 4. Aufl., Wiss. Verlags-Ges. Stuttgart 1997

Hegnauer R, Chemotaxonomie der Pflanzen, Bde 1-11: Birkhäuser Verlag Basel, Boston, Berlin 1962-1997.

Kern W, List PH, Hörhammer L (Hrsg.), Hagers Handbuch der Pharmazeutischen Praxis, 4. Aufl., Bde. 1-8: Springer Verlag Berlin, Heidelberg, New York, 1969.

Roth L, Daunderer M, Kormann K, Giftpflanzen, Pflanzengifte, 4. Aufl., Ecomed Fachverlag Landsberg Lech 1993.

Ruijgrok HWL, PM 11:338-347. 1963.

Teuscher E, Lindequist U: Biogene Gifte - Biologie, Chemie, Pharmakologie, 2. Aufl., Fischer Verlag Stuttgart 1994.

Butternut

Juglans cinerea

TRADE NAMES

Black Walnut (Juglans nigra), Black Walnut Hulls, Alcohol Free Black Walnut Green Hulls

DESCRIPTION

Medicinal Parts: The medicinal parts are the bark of the tree and root.

Flower and Fruit: The tree has male catkins and female flowers. The male catkins are 5 to 8 cm long. The fruit is 4 to 6.5 cm and ovoid-oblong. The fruit is pubescent, viscid and strong smelling. The hard nut is ovoid-oblong with 4 prominent and 4 less prominent sharp ridges and many broken grooves between them.

Leaves, Stem and Root: Butternut tree grows up to 30 m tall. The bark is gray and deeply fissured. The leaf scars have a prominent pubescent band on their upper edge. The 6 to 12 cm long leaflets are oblong-lanceolate, acuminate and appressed-serrate. They are finely pubescent above, glandular and pubescent beneath.

Habitat: Butternut is indigenous to the forests of the U.S.

Production: Butternut bark is the inner rind of Juglans cinerea.

Other Names: White Walnut, Oil Nut, Lemon Walnut, and Black Walnut

ACTIONS AND PHARMACOLOGY

COMPOUNDS

Fatty oil

Tannins

Juglone

Juglandis folium

EFFECTS

Vermifuge, laxative, tonic.

INDICATIONS AND USAGE

Unproven Uses: Preparations of the bark are used for disorders of the gallbladder, for hemorrhoids and in the treatment of skin diseases. Juglone has antimicrobial, antineoplastic and antiparasitic properties as well as being a gentle laxative.

PRECAUTIONS AND ADVERSE REACTIONS

No health hazards or side effects are known in conjunction with the proper administration of designated therapeutic dosages.

DOSAGE

Mode of Administration: Available preparations include liquid and dry extracts that are used internally and externally.

How Supplied:

Capsules — 95 mg, 500 mg, 3.5 gm

Fluid Extract - 1:1

LITERATURE

Hegnauer R, Chemotaxonomie der Pflanzen, Bde 1-11, Birkhäuser Verlag Basel, Boston, Berlin 1962-1997.

Kern W, List PH, Hörhammer L (Hrsg.), Hagers Handbuch der Pharmazeutischen Praxis, 4. Aufl., Bde. 1-8, Springer Verlag Berlin, Heidelberg, New York, 1969.

Madaus G, Lehrbuch der Biologischen Arzneimittel, Bde 1-3, Nachdruck, Georg Olms Verlag Hildesheim 1979.

Buxus sempervirens

See Boxwood

Cabbage

Brassica oleracea

TRADE NAMES

Cabbage Tables (available from various manufacturers)

DESCRIPTION

Medicinal Parts: The medicinal parts of the plant are the fresh cabbage head and juice derived from the fresh leaves.

Flower and Fruit: The inflorescences have long-pedicled flowers. The flowers are large and have 4 erect, narrowly elliptoid sepals 6 to 12 mm long. The 4 petals are about twice as long as the calyx and are sulphur yellow. The margin broadens at the tip and narrows at the base to an equally long wedge-shaped funicle stem. The stamens are erect and close to the ovary. The central honey gland is almost erect. The fruit is oblong, pod-like, almost cylindrical and has a domed lid. The dividing wall of the fruit is thin as well as pitted and folded between the dark brown seeds, which have a diameter of 1.5 to 4 mm.

Leaves, Stem and Root: The plant can be annual, biennial or perennial. It is about 2 m high and has thin roots. The stem is woody from the first year and is covered in leaf nodes. It has a bluish bloom and is branched toward the top. The leaves are fleshy, blue-green and glabrous. The lower leaves are petiolate, lyre-shaped, pinnatifid or simple. The upper leaves are oblong to linear-oblong, usually entire-margined and narrowed to rounded at the base and sessile.

Habitat: Wild Cabbage was originally found in the Mediterranean region. Today it grows wild as far north as southern England and Helgoland, and cultivated varieties are found in temperate and damp climates worldwide.

Production: White cabbage juice is the juice of Brassica oleracea.

Other Names: Colewort

ACTIONS AND PHARMACOLOGY

COMPOUNDS

Mustard oils (breakdown products of the glucosinolates accompanying cell destruction): allyl mustard oil, methyl sulfinyl alkyl isothiocyanates, methyl sulfonyl alkyl isothiocyanates

3-hydroxy-methyl-indole

5-vinyl-oxazolidine-2-thion (goitrin)

Rhodanides

Alkyl nitriles

Amino acids: including S-methyl cysteine sulphoxide, S-methyl methionine sulphoxide and, when extracted from red cabbage, also anthocyans, including cyanidine-5-0-glucoside-3-0-sophoroside

EFFECTS

Cabbage protects the mucous membrane of the stomach from gastric hydrochloric acid. The gastroprotective effect of the juice is attributed to the regenerative ability of the mucous membrane that is caused by an anti-ulcer factor (vitamin U).

INDICATIONS AND USAGE

Unproven Uses: Folk medicine uses include drinking the juice for Roemheld syndrome, gastritis, gastric and duodenal ulcers, gastralgia and subacidity.

Homeopathic Uses: Preparations of the flowering herb are used for hypothyroidism.

Indian Medicine: Cabbage leaves are used for disorders of the thyroid, gastrointestinal tract, itching and cough, as well as for asthma, gout and hemorrhoids.

PRECAUTIONS AND ADVERSE REACTIONS

No health hazards or side effects are known in conjunction with the proper administration of designated therapeutic dosages.

DOSAGE

Mode of Administration: The drug is available as a standard preparation or prepared from chopped and pressed Cabbage for internal use. Also available in homeopathic preparations.

How Supplied:
Tablet — 500 mg

Preparation: White cabbage (Brassica Oleracea Var. Capitata) extract is prepared by processing leaves by mashing or using a centrifuge. The resulting mass is pressed through a linen cloth.

Daily Dosage: To augment a bland diet take 1 liter of juice daily for at least 3 weeks but not more than 6 weeks as a dietary additive.

For gastralgia and subacidity, the dose is 1 teaspoonful to be taken before meals, 3 times daily.

Homeopathic Dosage: 5 drops, 1 tablet, 10 globules every 30 to 60 minutes (acute) or 1 to 3 times daily (chronic); parenterally: 1 to 2 ml sc; acute: 3 times daily; chronic: once a day (HAB34).

Storage: The fresh juice will keep for approximately 24 hours if kept cool.

LITERATURE

Josefsson E, PH 6:1617-1627. 1967.

Kaoulla N et al., PH 19:1053-1056. 1980.

Larson KM, Stermitz FR, JNP 47(4):747-748. 1984.

Petroski RJ, Tookey HL, PH21:1903-1905. 1982.

Slominski BA, Campbell LD, J Agric Food Chem 37:1297-1302. 1989.

Further information in:

Hänsel R, Keller K, Rimpler H, Schneider G (Hrsg.), Hagers Handbuch der Pharmazeutischen Praxis, 5. Aufl., Bde 4-6

(Drogen), Springer Verlag Berlin, Heidelberg, New York, 1992-1994.

Kern W, List PH, Hörhammer L (Hrsg.), Hagers Handbuch der Pharmazeutischen Praxis, 4. Aufl., Bde. 1-8, Springer Verlag Berlin, Heidelberg, New York, 1969.

Teuscher E, Lindequist U, Biogene Gifte - Biologie, Chemie, Pharmakologie, 2. Aufl., Fischer Verlag Stuttgart 1994.

Caesalpinia bonducella

See Divi-Divi

Cajuput

Melaleuca leucadendra

DESCRIPTION

Medicinal Parts: The medicinal part is the oil distilled from the fresh leaves and twigs.

Flower and Fruit: The tree has racemes of small, sessile, creamy white flowers on long terminal spikes up to 15 cm long, which themselves terminate in a tuft of leaves. The flowers have numerous stamens extending to 15 mm.

Leaves, Stem and Root: Melaleuca leucadendra is a large tree up to 40 m tall with a flexible trunk and irregular pendulous branches. The tree is covered in a pale, lamellate bark, which is soft and spongy and occasionally peels off its layers. The leaves are alternate, entire-margined, oblong-lanceolate, tapering, ash-colored and on short petioles.

Characteristic: It has an odor reminiscent of camphor and eucalyptus.

Habitat: The plant is indigenous to Southeast Asia and the tropical regions of Australia. It is cultivated elsewhere.

Production: Cajuput oil consists of the essential oil of Melaleuca leucadendra. It is extracted from the fresh leaves and twig tips of a number of varieties collected from the wild or from cultivation, followed by air-drying and aqueous steam distillation.

Other Names: White Tea Tree, Swamp Tea Tree, Paperbark Tree, White Wood

ACTIONS AND PHARMACOLOGY

COMPOUNDS

Chief constituents: cineol, (+)-alpha-terpineol, (-)-alpha-terpineol, (+)-alpha-terpineol valerate, (-)- alpha-terpineol valerate, furthermore alpha-pinenes and bicyclic sesquiterpenes, non-rectified oils also contain 3,5-dimethyl-4, 6-di-O-methyl-phloroacetophenone

EFFECTS

In vitro, the drug has an antimicrobial and a rubefacient effect.

INDICATIONS AND USAGE

Approved by Commission E:

- Rheumatism
- Neurogenic pain
- Temporary relief of muscular pain
- Tendency to infection
- Wounds and burns

Unproven Uses: The drug is used for painful muscles and joints in rheumatic disorders, sciatica, lumbago, slipped disk and low back pain. Cajuput is also used for muscular tension and pain following sports injuries such as sprains, bruising, and pulled muscles or ligaments.

CONTRAINDICATIONS

No internal administration of the drug should take place in the presence of inflammatory illnesses of the gastrointestinal area or of the biliary ducts, nor in the presence of severe liver diseases. Preparations containing the oil should not be applied to the faces of infants or small children (glottal spasm or bronchial spasm or even asthma-like attacks or respiratory failure might occur).

PRECAUTIONS AND ADVERSE REACTIONS

General: No health hazards or side effects are known in conjunction with the proper administration of designated therapeutic dosages; however, contact dermatitis is possible.

Pediatric Use: The drug should not be applied to the facial area, in particular not around the nose, of infants and small children (glottal spasms could occur).

OVERDOSAGE

Overdoses of cajuput oil (more than 10 gm) could lead to life-threatening poisonings, due to the high cineole content. Symptoms include including loss of blood pressure, circulatory disorders, collapse and respiratory failure. Vomiting is not to be induced in the case of poisoning, because of the danger of aspiration. Following administration of activated charcoal, the therapy for poisonings consists of treating spasms with diazepam (i.v.), treating colic with atropine, electrolyte substitution and treating possible cases of acidosis with sodium bicarbonate infusions. Intubation and oxygen respiration may also be necessary.

DOSAGE

Mode of Administration: Cajuput oil is used only for external purposes.

LITERATURE

Fenaroli's Handbook of Flavor Ingredients, Vol. 1. 2nd Ed., CRC Press 1975.

Kern W, List PH, Hörhammer L (Hrsg.), Hagers Handbuch der Pharmazeutischen Praxis, 4. Aufl., Bde 1-8, Springer Verlag Berlin, Heidelberg, New York, 1969.

Leung AY, Encyclopedia of Common Natural Ingredients Used in Food Drugs and Cosmetics, John Wiley & Sons Inc., New York 1980.

Lowry JB, (1973) Nature 241:61.

Opdyke DLJ, (1976) Food Cosmet Toxicol:14.

Steinegger E, Hänsel R, Pharmakognosie, 5. Aufl., Springer Verlag Heidelberg 1992.

Teuscher E, Biogene Arzneimittel, 5. Aufl., Wiss. Verlagsges. Stuttgart 1997.

Calabar Bean

Physostigma venenosum

DESCRIPTION

Medicinal Parts: The medicinal parts are the seeds.

Flower and Fruit: The inflorescences are pendulous racemes of bean-like flowers. The fruit is a dark brown pod up to 15 cm long containing two or three dark brown or blackish kidney-shaped seeds that are about 2.5 cm long. They are rounded at the ends, uneven and somewhat polished with the hilum extending along the whole convex side. The cotyledons are whitish.

Leaves, Stem and Root: The plant is a large, perennial, twining, woody climber with large, pinnate, trifoliate leaves.

Habitat: The plant is indigenous to western Africa and is cultivated in India and parts of South America.

Production: The Calabar Bean is the seed of Physostigma venenosum.

Other Names: Chop Nut, Ordeal Bean

ACTIONS AND PHARMACOLOGY

COMPOUNDS

Indole alkaloide (0.3 - 0.5%): main alkaloid physostigmine, secondary alkaloids include physovenine, geneserine, eseramine

Starch (up to 50%)

Proteic substances

Fatty oil

EFFECTS

The main alkaloid, physostigmine, is miotic, spasmogenic, negatively chronotropic and curare-antagonistic. It causes an increase in tone in the parasympathetic system and the striated muscles. In particular, it causes the pupils to contract, thus reducing intraocular pressure. It is a glandular stimulant and increases peristalsis of the gastrointestinal tract. It reduces heart rate and is a curare antidote.

INDICATIONS AND USAGE

Unproven Uses: The drug is frequently used in the treatment of glaucoma. It is also a poison antidote. Its use in the treatment of Alzheimer's disease to reduce memory loss and confusion is being investigated.

PRECAUTIONS AND ADVERSE REACTIONS

The drug is only used in the extraction of physostigmine. Symptoms of poisoning include: diarrhea, dizziness, nausea, salivation, stupor, sweats and vomiting.

OVERDOSAGE

Lethal doses can cause muscle twitching, spasms, tachycardia and cyanosis through asphyxiation. Following gastric lavage, poisonings are treated with atropine; in the case of spasms, diazepam is also used. Forced diuresis can be useful. The lethal dose for an adult is 6 to 10 mg of physostigmine (corresponding to approximately 2 to 3 Calabar Beans). Poisonings are possible through inappropriate administration of physostigmine eye drops, due to drainage into the mouth or nose.

DOSAGE

Mode of Administration: As an eye medication, in drops and ointments. It is used as an antidote in the form of an injection solution. For gastrointestinal use, it has been replaced by synthetic prostigmine.

Daily Dosage: Apply 1 to 2 eye drops 3 times daily to the conjunctival sac.

LITERATURE

Die G, 125 Jahre Physostigmin. In: ZPT 11(2):7. 1990.

Morbus A, Was gibt es Neues aus der Forschung? In: DAZ 133(23):2090. 1993.

Kern W, List PH, Hörhammer L (Eds.), Hagers Handbuch der Pharmazeutischen Praxis, 4. Aufl., Bde. 1-8, Springer Verlag Berlin, Heidelberg, New York, 1969.

Madaus G, Lehrbuch der Biologischen Arzneimittel, Bde 1-3, Nachdruck, Georg Olms Verlag Hildesheim 1979.

Roth L, Daunderer M, Kormann K, Giftpflanzen, Pflanzengifte, 4. Aufl., Ecomed Fachverlag Landsberg Lech 1993.

Steinegger E, Hänsel R, Pharmakognosie, 5. Aufl., Springer Verlag Heidelberg 1992.

Teuscher E, Lindequist U, Biogene Gifte - Biologie, Chemie, Pharmakologie, 2. Aufl., Fischer Verlag Stuttgart 1994.

Teuscher E, Biogene Arzneimittel, 5. Aufl., Wiss. Verlagsges. Stuttgart 1997.

Calamint

Calamintha nepeta

DESCRIPTION

Medicinal Parts: The medicinal parts are the dried foliage, stems, leaves and flowers.

Flower and Fruit: The medium-sized to large flowers are 5 to 20 blossomed cymes. The pedicle is 0 to 22 mm long and the tubular calyx is 3 to 7 mm by 1 to 1.5 mm in size and slightly downy to very downy on the inside. The upper tips are 0.5 to 1.5 mm and the lower ones are 1 to 2 mm, downy. They occasionally have long, ciliate hairs. The corolla is white to lilac and purple.

Leaves, Stem and Root: Calamint is a perennial, 30 to 80 cm high, slightly to densely downy shrub. The leaves are oval, obtuse, almost entire-margined or lightly to deeply crenate-serrate, with 9 teeth on each side.

Habitat: Britain, Europe, northern Africa

Production: Calamint is the above-ground part of Calamintha nepeta. It is collected in the wild.

Other Names: Basil Thyme, Mountain Mint, Mountain Balm, Mill Mountain

ACTIONS AND PHARMACOLOGY

COMPOUNDS

Volatile oil (0.35%: including pulegone, menthone, menthol and its ester, β-bisobolen, cineol, thymol

Triterpenes: including calaminthadiol, ursolic acid

EFFECTS

The drug is a diaphoretic and expectorant.

INDICATIONS AND USAGE

Unproven Uses: Calamint has been used for febrile colds and respiratory diseases. The drug is also used in folk medicine for hiccups, tinnitus, as a diuretic and for stomach complaints.

PRECAUTIONS AND ADVERSE REACTIONS

No health hazards or side effects are known in conjunction with the proper administration of designated therapeutic dosages.

DOSAGE

No information is available.

LITERATURE

de Pooter HL, Goetghebeur P. Schamp P, PH 26(12):3355-3356. 1987.

Hänsel R, Keller K, Rimpler H, Schneider G (Hrsg.), Hagers Handbuch der Pharmazeutischen Praxis, 5. Aufl., Bde 4-6 (Drogen), Springer Verlag Berlin, Heidelberg, New York, 1992-1994.

Kokkalo E, Stefanaou E, Flavour Fragrance J 5(1):23-26. 1990.

Calamintha nepeta

See Calamint

Calamus

Acorus calamus

DESCRIPTION

Medicinal Parts: The medicinal part is the rhizome after the removal of all other material.

Flower and Fruit: Green flowers, like small dice, form a tightly packed, slim, conical spadix. The plant is non-fruit-bearing and propagates from the rhizome.

Leaves, Stem and Root: The plant grows from 60 to 100 cm tall. The stem is triangular and sprouts from a horizontal, round root-stock, which has the thickness of a thumb. The upper shoot forms a grooved flower sheath. The leaves are oblong, sword-shaped and arranged in two rows. The leaves have no stems.

Characteristics: The rhizome has an intensely aromatic fragrance and a tangy, pungent and bitter taste. The leaves often undulate on the margins.

Habitat: Today Calamus is found all over the world. It probably originated in India and North America.

Production: Calamus root-stock is the dried, coarsely ground and mostly peeled, root-stock of Acorus calamus. Calamus oil is extracted from the same plant.

Other Names: Sweet Flag, Sweet Sedge, Grass Myrtle, Myrtle Flag, Sweet Grass, Sweet Myrtle, Sweet Rush, Sweet Root, Sweet Cane, Gladdon, Myrtle Sedge, Cinnamon Sedge

ACTIONS AND PHARMACOLOGY

COMPOUNDS

Volatile oil: chief constituents are heavily dependent upon the chemical strain (di-, tri-, tetraploid); beta-asarone (cis-isoasarone), alpha- and gamma-asarone, beta- gurjuns, acorone (bitter), ZZ-Deca-4,7-dienal (odor-determining)

EFFECTS

Calamus is an aromatic, bitter stomachic, which stimulates appetite and digestion. It has spasmolytic, carminative and sedative effects, in addition to being externally hyperemic.

INDICATIONS AND USAGE

Unproven Uses: The drug is used in the form of teas, for dyspeptic disorders, gastritis and ulcers. It is used externally for rheumatism, gum disease and tonsillitis.

Indian Medicine: Calamus is used for dyspeptic complaints, worms, pain syndrome and toothache.

Chinese Medicine: Acorus calamus stimulates peptic juices for disorders of the gastrointestinal tract. It is used externally for fungal infections.

PRECAUTIONS AND ADVERSE REACTIONS

No health hazards or side effects are known in conjunction with the proper administration of designated therapeutic dosages. Long-term use of this drug should be avoided. Malignant tumors appeared in rats that received Indian Calmus oils over an extended period (tetraploid strain, over 80% β-asarone in volatile oil).

DOSAGE

Mode of Administration: Calamus preparations are for internal and external use. Preparations are used as a bitter, stomachic, carminative, digestant, sedative, rubefacient, balneotherapeutic and corrigent. Calamus is available in tea mixtures, as an oil or extract and as a bath oil.

Preparation: Steep with hot water to make a tea. For use in a bath, add 250 to 500 gm of the drug to the bath water.

Storage: Store for a maximum of 18 months. If in powder form, however, do not keep for more than 24 hours.

LITERATURE

Iguchi M et al., (1973) Tetrahedron Letters 29:2759.

Keller K et al., (1985) Planta Med 51(1):6.

Keller K, Stahl E, Composition of the essential oil from beta-asarone free calamus. In: PM 47(2):71. 1983.

Keller K, Stahl E, Kalmus: Inhalsstoffe und β-Asarongehalt bei verschiedenen Herkünften. In: DAZ 122(48):2463-2466. 1982.

Mazza G, Gas chromatographic and mass spectrometric studies of the constituents of the rhizome of calamus. In: J Chromatogr 328:179-206. 1985.

Rohr M, Naegeli P, (1979) Phytochemistry 18(2):279 and 328.

Saxena DB, Phenyl indane from Acorus calamus. In: PH 25(2):553. 1986.

Schneider K, Jurenitsch J, Kalmus als Arzneidroge: Nutzen oder Risiko. In: Pharmazie 47(2):79-85. 1992.

Stahl E, Keller K, Classification of typical commercial Calamus drugs. In: PM 43(2):128-140. 1981.

Taylor JM et al., Toxicity of oil of calamus (Jammu variety). In: Toxicol Appl Pharmacol 10:405 (Abstract). 1967.

Further information in:

Chan, EH et al. (Eds.), Advances in Chinese Medicinal Materials Research, World Scientific Pub. Co. Singapore 1985.

Kern W, List PH, Hörhammer L (Hrsg.), Hagers Handbuch der Pharmazeutischen Praxis, 4. Aufl., Bde 1-8, Springer Verlag Berlin, Heidelberg, New York, 1969.

Leung AY, Encyclopedia of Common Natural Ingredients Used in Food, Drugs and Cosmetics, John Wiley & Sons Inc., New York 1980.

Madaus G, Lehrbuch der Biologischen Arzneimittel, Bde 1-3, Nachdruck, Georg Olms Verlag Hildesheim 1979.

Roth L, Daunderer M, Kormann K, Giftpflanzen, Pflanzengifte, 4. Aufl., Ecomed Fachverlag Landsberg Lech 1993.

Steinegger E, Hänsel R, Pharmakognosie, 5. Aufl., Springer Verlag Heidelberg 1992.

Teuscher E, Biogene Arzneimittel, 5. Aufl., Wiss. Verlagsges. Stuttgart 1997.

Teuscher E, Lindequist U, Biogene Gifte - Biologie, Chemie, Pharmakologie, 2. Aufl., Fischer Verlag Stuttgart 1994.

Wagner H, Wiesenauer M, Phytotherapie. Phytopharmaka und pflanzliche Homöopathika, Fischer-Verlag, Stuttgart, Jena, New York 1995.

Wichtl M (Hrsg.), Teedrogen, 4. Aufl., Wiss. Verlagsges. Stuttgart. 1997.

Calendula officinalis

See Marigold

California Peppertree

Schinus molle

DESCRIPTION

Medicinal Parts: Medicinal properties have been attributed to the plant's leaves, bark, fruit and gum resin.

Flower and Fruit: The flowers are in apical, heavily branched, hanging, 5 to 30 cm long panicles. The flowers are small, yellowish-white, and their structures are in fives. The calyx is 5-tipped. The flower has 5 petals, 10 stamens and a superior ovary that develops from a carpel. The style is divided into 3. The fruit is a coral red, single-seeded drupe with a diameter of approximately 7 mm, a thin pergament-like exocarp, an oleo-resin-rich mesocarp and a hard endocarp.

Leaves, Stem and Root: The tree is an evergreen, up to 15 m high. The leaves are alternate, up to 25 cm long and odd pinnate. There are 17 to 35 leaflets, 1.6 to 6 cm long, 2 to 8 mm wide, sessile, linear-lanceolate, punctate with oil glands and dentate. The branches hang down.

Characteristics: The leaves give off a pepper-like smell when rubbed; the fruit is aromatic and somewhat sweet.

Habitat: The tree is indigenous to Central America and South America.

Production: California Peppertree (or Peruvian Peppertree) leaves are the leaflets of Schinus molle. California Peppertree fruits are ripe unpeeled drupes of Schinus mollek, which are air- or freeze-dried.

Not to be Confused With: Other Schinus species.

Other Names: Australian Pepper Tree, Brazilian Pepper Tree, False Pepper, Peruvian Mastix Tree, Peruvian Peppertree, Weeping Pepper Tree

ACTIONS AND PHARMACOLOGY

COMPOUNDS: CALIFORNIA PEPPERTREE LEAVES

Volatile oil (0.2 to 1.0%): chief components including alpha-phellandrene, beta-phellandrene, limonene, including as well T-cadinol, elemol, germacrene D, gamma-eudesmol

Flavonoids: including kaempferol, myricetin, quercetin

Resins

Mucilages

EFFECTS: CALIFORNIA PEPPERTREE LEAVES

The leaves contain unknown bitter substances and tannins, which make administration for inflammatory alterations of the skin and oral mucous membranes plausible.

COMPOUNDS: CALIFORNIA PEPPERTREE FRUIT

Volatile oil (2.0 to 5.0%): chief components including alpha-phellandrene, beta-phellandrene, limonene, alpha-pinene, beta-pinene, including as well camphene, carvacrol, p-cymol, 4-ethyl phenol

Triterpenes: including 3-epiisomasticadienolalic acid, 3-epimasticadienolic acid, isomasticadienonic acid, masticadienonic acid

Fatty oil (in the seeds 6 to 14%)

Resins (with long-chained fatty acids, C22 to C28)

EFFECTS: CALIFORNIA PEPPERTREE FRUIT

The fruit resin is purgative in effect. The essential oil is fungicidal and is said to be excreted primarily through the lungs and the kidneys. No experimental data are available for the traditional areas of administration.

INDICATIONS AND USAGE

CALIFORNIA PEPPERTREE LEAVES

Unproven Uses: Internal uses in folk medicine include infections of the pharynx, respiratory tract conditions, rheumatism (decoction), for leucorrhea, suppuration of the mucous membranes and hypertension (infusion), for swellings, loss of teeth, conjunctivitis (leaf juice), and as a diuretic. External indications are considered to include uterus prolapse, eye inflammations, joint pains, colds (used as healing baths), as a vulnerary and for rheumatism.

CALIFORNIA PEPPERTREE FRUIT

Unproven Uses: Used internally as a stomachic, tonic, for nausea, vomiting, anuria, gastric complaints, loss of appetite, conditions of the respiratory tract, blennorrhagia, for muscular pain and as a diuretic. Preparations from the fruit are used externally for rheumatism.

PRECAUTIONS AND ADVERSE REACTIONS

CALIFORNIA PEPPERTREE LEAVES AND FRUIT

No health hazards are known in conjunction with the proper administration of designated therapeutic dosages.

DOSAGE

CALIFORNIA PEPPERTREE LEAVES

Preparation: To prepare an infusion, use 30 g drug to 500 ml water.

Daily Dosage: For inflammation of the mucous membranes, gargle with infusion 3 times daily. For wound cleansing, wash wounds with infusion.

CALIFORNIA PEPPERTREE FRUIT

Mode of Administration: Whole and cut drug are used in preparations for internal and external use.

Daily Dosage: No information is given in the literature.

Storage: Tightly sealed, cool, dry and protected from light.

LITERATURE

Dikshit A, Naqvi AA, Husain A, Schinus molle: a new source of natural fungitoxicant. Appl Environ Microbiol, 38:1085-8, 1986 May.

Hänsel R, Keller K, Rimpler H, Schneider G (Ed), Hagers Handbuch der Pharmazeutischen Praxis, 5. Aufl., Bde 4 - 6 (Drogen), Springer Verlag Berlin, Heidelberg, New York, 1992-1994.

Vargas Correa JB, Sβnchez Sol s L, Farfβn Ale JA, Noguchi H, Moguel Ba~nos MT, Vargas de la Pe~na MI, Allergological study of pollen of mango (Magnifera indica) and cross reactivity with pollen of piru (Schinus molle). Rev Alerg, 38:134-8, 1991 Sep-Oct.

California Poppy

Eschscholtzia californica

DESCRIPTION

Medicinal Parts: The medicinal parts of Eschscholtzia californica are the aerial parts collected during the flowering season and dried.

Flower and Fruit: The bright yellow-to-orange flowers are solitary, axillary and long-pedicled. They are 2.5 to 4 cm in diameter with a cup-shaped receptacle. The sepals are fused. Four crenate petals, orange-red at the base, form an open dish. The stigma is thread-like. There are numerous yellow stamens. The fruit is an oblong, 4 to 6 cm pod-like exploding capsule, which spreads small globular seeds.

Leaves, Stem and Root: Eschscholtzia californica is a bluish-green annual or perennial that grows 30 to 60 cm high. The leaves are sparse. The strongly pinnatifid leaves have linear sections and taper to a thin tip.

Habitat: The plant grows in California and is cultivated in central Europe and southern France.

Production: The Californian Poppy herb consists of the aerial parts of Eschscholtzia californica. It is collected in uncultivated regions.

ACTIONS AND PHARMACOLOGY

COMPOUNDS

Isoquinoline alkaloids: The main alkaloid is californidine. Included are others, such as eschscholzine (escholzine), protopine, alpha-allocryptopine, beta-allocryptopine.

Cyanogenic glycosides (in the freshly-harvested plant)

EFFECTS

The main active principle californidine has sleep-inducing, sedative, anxiolytic and spasmolytic effects. In mice, a hot water extract had a significant sleep-inducing effect. In other animal experiments an anxiolytic and spasmolytic effect was proven.

INDICATIONS AND USAGE

Unproven Uses: Preparations of the drug are used for insomnia, aches, nervous agitation, enuresis nocturna in children, diseases of the bladder and liver, reactive agitative and masked depressions, melancholia, neurasthenia, neuropathy, organic neuroses, vegetative-dystonic disorders, mood swings, weather sensitivity, vasomotor dysfunctions, vegetative-endocrine syndrome, constitutional weakness of the nervous system and vasomotor cephalgia. The tea is used as a sedative.

Homeopathic Uses: Eschscholtzia californica is used to treat insomnia.

PRECAUTIONS AND ADVERSE REACTIONS

General: Health risks or side effects following the proper administration of designated therapeutic dosages are not recorded.

Pregnancy: Not to be used during pregnancy.

DOSAGE

Mode of Administration: The drug is rarely prescribed, yet is a component of some standardized preparations in combination with plant sedatives. Medical or clinical documentation and other experimental material about phytotherapeutic application of the Californian Poppy herb are unavailable. As the efficacy of the claimed uses has not been documented, a therapeutic application cannot be justified.

Preparation: The tea is prepared using 2 gm herb per 150 ml water. The liquid extract (Extractum Eschscholziae) should be prepared according to the German Pharmacopoeia (DAB)10.

Daily Dosage: The tea is taken as a drink. The average single dose for the liquid extract is 1 to 2 ml.

Homeopathic Dosage: from D2: 5 drops, 1 tablet or 10 globules every 30 to 60 minutes (acute) or 1 to 3 times daily (chronic); from D4: parenterally: 1 to 2 ml sc acute: 3 times daily; chronic: once a day (PF X).

LITERATURE

Hänsel R, Keller K, Rimpler H, Schneider G (Hrsg.), Hagers Handbuch der Pharmazeutischen Praxis, 5. Aufl., Bde 4-6 (Drogen), Springer Verlag Berlin, Heidelberg, New York, 1992-1994.

Jain L et al., Alkaloids of Eschscholtzia californica. In: PM 62(2):188. 1997.

Lewin L, Gifte und Vergiftungen, 6. Aufl., Nachdruck, Haug Verlag, Heidelberg 1992.

Roth L, Daunderer M, Kormann K, Giftpflanzen, Pflanzengifte, 4. Aufl., Ecomed Fachverlag Landsberg Lech 1993.

Sturm S, Stuppner H, Mulinacci N, Vincieri F, Capillary zone electrophoretic analysis of the main alkaloids from Eschscholtzia californica. In: PM 59(7)25. 1993.

Teuscher E, Lindequist U, Biogene Gifte - Biologie, Chemie, Pharmakologie, 2. Aufl., Fischer Verlag Stuttgart 1994.

Weischer ML, Okpanyi SN, Pharmakologie eines pflanzlichen Schlafmittels. In: ZPT 15(5):257-262. 1994.

Calluna vulgaris

See Heather

Calotropis

Calotropis procera

DESCRIPTION

Medicinal Parts: The medicinal parts are the dried root and root bark. The bark with its outer cork layer removed is known as Mudar, and is used medicinally.

Flower and Fruit: The fragrant flowers are 2.5 cm in diameter and form umbel-like flower clusters. The erect petals are whitish and have purple spots on the upper half. The bracts of the corolla are smooth or downy with a divided tip. The ovate follicles are 7.5 to 10 cm long by 5 to 7.5 cm wide. The seeds have a tuft of silky hair.

Leaves, Stem and Root: This upright herbacious perennial normally grows to a height of 1.8 to 2.4 m. The leaves are short-petioled, 6 to 15 cm long by 4.5 to 8 cm wide, oblong-elliptoid to broadly ovate. The bark appears in irregular short pieces, slightly quilled or curved and about 0.3 - 0.5 cm thick. The external portion is grayish-yellow, soft and spongy. The internal portion is yellowish-white. The fracture is short.

Characteristics: The taste is acrid and bitter.

Habitat: Indigenous to parts of Asia, India, Africa, Pakistan and on the Sunda Islands

Production: Calotropis bark is the dried root bark of Calotropis procera.

Other Names: Mudar Bark, Mudar Yercum

ACTIONS AND PHARMACOLOGY

COMPOUNDS

Cardioactive steroids (cardenolids): including calotropin, calactin, uscharidin

EFFECTS

The cardenolid glycocides calotropine shows an anti-tumor effect in vitro on human epidermoid carcinoma cells of the rhinopharynx. It is also works as an expectorant and a diuretic.

INDICATIONS AND USAGE

Unproven Uses: The powdered root bark is used to treat dysentery. It has a similar effect to that of the ipecacuanha root. In Indian and African folk medicine, the bark is used to treat epilepsy, hysteria, cramps, cancer, warts, leprosy, elephantitis, worms, fever, gout and snake bites. In particular, the milky juice is used against boils, ulcers, swellings and rheumatism. In Africa, it is used to treat toothache, syphilis, digestive disorders and diarrhea.

Indian Medicine: The smoke (fumes) from the bark is used for coughs and asthma and as a sudorific.

Homeopathic Uses: Calotropis procera is used for obesity.

PRECAUTIONS AND ADVERSE REACTIONS

No health hazards or side effects are known in conjunction with the proper administration of designated therapeutic dosages.

OVERDOSAGE

The drug is highly toxic. Higher dosages cause vomiting, diarrhea, bradycardia and convulsions. Very high dosages may cause death. Following gastric lavage, treatment for poisonings should proceed symptomatically (for further measures, see Digitalis).

DOSAGE

Mode of Administration: Calotropis is used in a ground form, as a powder, as smoke (fume) and also topically.

Daily Dosage: As an expectorant and diaphoretic 200 mg to 600 mg; as an emetic 2 gm to 4 gm.

Homeopathic Dosage: from D4: 5 to 10 drops, 1 tablet, 5 to 10 globules 1 to 3 times daily; from D6: 1 ml injection solution sc twice weekly (HAB1).

LITERATURE

Hänsel R, Keller K, Rimpler H, Schneider G (Hrsg.), Hagers Handbuch der Pharmazeutischen Praxis, 5. Aufl., Bde 4-6 (Drogen), Springer Verlag Berlin, Heidelberg, New York, 1992-1994.

Seiber JN et al., (1982) Phytochemistry 21(9):2343.

Willaman JJ, Hui-Li L, (1970) Lloydia 33(3A):1.

Calotropis gigantea

See Giant Milkweed

Calotropis procera

See Calotropis

Caltha palustris

See Marsh Marigold

Calystegia sepium

See Greater Bindweed

Camellia sinensis

See Green Tea

Camphor Tree

Cinnamomum camphora

DESCRIPTION

Medicinal Parts: The medicinal part is camphor oil extracted from the tree.

Flower and Fruit: The flowers are small, white and sessile on 1 to 1.5 mm long pedicles. The petals are pubescent on the inside. The flowers are caespitose, on long axillary petioles. The 1.5 mm stamens form 3 circles and are pubescent with broad, sessile-cordate glands. The fruit is a purple-black, 1-seeded, 10 to 12 mm oval drupe.

Leaves, Stem and Root: The plant is an evergreen tree growing up to 50 m tall and 5 m in diameter. The trunk is erect at the lower part and knottily branched above. The leaves are alternate on long petioles, oval-lanceolate, acuminate, grooved and glossy. They are light yellowish-green above and paler beneath; they grow to 5 to 11 cm long by 5 cm across.

Habitat: Camphor trees are indigenous to Vietnam and an area extending from southern China to southern Japan.

Production: Purified camphor is obtained from the chipped wood of the Cinnamomum camphora tree using steam distillation followed by sublimation to yield the oil.

Other Names: Gum Camphor, Laurel Camphor, Cemphire

ACTIONS AND PHARMACOLOGY

COMPOUNDS

Camphora is a single substance: D(+) -camphor ((1R,4R)-1,7,7-trimethyl-bicyclo[2.2.1]heptan-2-on), extracted from the volatile oil of the trunk of the camphor tree, Cinnamomum camphora. L(-)-camphor also occurs in nature. Synthetic camphor is DL-camphor.

EFFECTS

Used externally, camphor acts as a bronchial secretolytic and hyperemic. Internally, the effect is that of a respiratory analeptic and bronchospasmolytic. It should be noted that the effect only sets in at dosages considered toxic. An antibacterial effect has been noted in vitro, with cineol the main active principle.

INDICATIONS AND USAGE

Approved by Commission E:

- Arrhythmia
- Cough/bronchitis
- Hypotension
- Nervous heart complaints
- Rheumatism

Unproven Uses: External uses in folk medicine include muscular rheumatism and cardiac symptoms. Among internal uses are hypotonic circulatory regulation disorders and digestive complaints. Inflammation of respiratory-tract mucous membranes is treated with both internal and external applications.

Indian Medicine: Uses include muscle pain, cardiac insufficiency and asthma.

CONTRAINDICATIONS

Camphor should not be used during pregnancy.

PRECAUTIONS AND ADVERSE REACTIONS

General: Local administration can lead to skin irritation, as well as to resorbent and/or airborne poisonings. Contact eczema occasionally appears following the application of oily salves containing camphor. The drug is sometimes used as a hashish substitute because 6 to 10 g leads to intoxication.

Pediatric Use: Camphor salves should not be administered to infants.

OVERDOSAGE

Symptoms of poisonings that have been seen, particularly in children, include intoxicated states, delirium, spasms and respiratory control disturbances. Treatment proceeds symptomatically. Less than 1 g can be a lethal dosage for young children. For adults, the lethal dosage is considered to be approximately 20 g. However, toxicity in adults has been noted after use of as little as 2 g.

DOSAGE

Mode of Administration: As a liquid (camphor spirit) for topical application or inhalation, and also semi-solid ointments and liniments. Internally, in liquid or solid preparations.

How Supplied: Commercial pharmaceutical preparations include creams, ointments, balms and gels.

Daily Dosage: Internal average daily dosage: 2 to 4 g drug; 0.05 to 0.2 g essential oil. For external use, camphor spirit (DAB10) 9.5 to 10.5% camphor to be rubbed in several times a day. Depending on prescribed application, concentrations generally are not higher than 25% for adults and no higher than 5% for small children.

Storage: Camphor should be stored in containers filled so there is no empty air space left and also should be protected from light.

LITERATURE

Bean NE, Camphora -curriculum vitae of a perverse terpene. In: Chem in Brain 8(9):386. 1972.

Burrow A, Eccles R, Jones AS, (1983) The effects of camphor, eucalyptus and menthol vapor on nasal resistance to airflow and nasal sensation. Acta Otolaryng (Stockholm) 96:157-161.

Stone JE, Blundell MJ, (1951) Anal Chem 23:771.

Takaoka D et al., (1975) Nippon Kagaku Kaishi 12:2192.

Further information in:

Bruchhausen F von, Ebel S, Frahm AW, Hackenthal E (Hrsg.), Hagers Handbuch der Pharmazeutischen Praxis, 5. Aufl., Bde 7-9 (Stoffe), Springer Verlag Berlin, Heidelberg, New York, 1993.

Lewin L, Gifte und Vergiftungen, 6. Aufl., Nachdruck, Haug Verlag, Heidelberg 1992.

Madaus G, Lehrbuch der Biologischen Arzneimittel, Bde 1-3, Nachdruck, Georg Olms Verlag Hildesheim 1979.

Roth L, Daunderer M, Kormann K, Giftpflanzen, Pflanzengifte, 4. Aufl., Ecomed Fachverlag Landsberg Lech 1993.

Steinegger E, Hänsel R, Pharmakognosie, 5. Aufl., Springer Verlag Heidelberg 1992.

Teuscher E, Lindequist U, Biogene Gifte - Biologie, Chemie, Pharmakologie, 2. Aufl., Fischer Verlag Stuttgart 1994.

Teuscher E, Biogene Arzneimittel, 5. Aufl., Wiss. Verlagsges. Stuttgart 1997.

Wagner H, Wiesenauer M, Phytotherapie. Phytopharmaka und pflanzliche Homöopathika, Fischer-Verlag, Stuttgart, Jena, New York 1995.

Canadian Fleabane

Erigeron canadensis

DESCRIPTION

Medicinal Parts: The medicinal parts are the dried aerial parts of the plant and the fresh aerial parts of the flowering plant.

Flower and Fruit: Canadian Fleabane has very small yellowish-white composite flowers in long, terminal, branched panicle-like inflorescences. The involucre is in a number of rows. The composite head has numerous florets. The ray florets are linguiform, female, white or reddish. The disc florets are tubular and androgynous. The stamens are fused. The fruit is an achaene, 1.2 to 1.5 mm long, brownish and has short appressed hair.

Leaves, Stem and Root: Erigeron canadensis is an annual or biennial 30 to 100 cm high. The root is thin and fusiform, the stem erect, roundish, slightly ribbed, greenish with paler ribs and is covered in scattered patent hairs. It is branched from the peduncle. The leaves are alternate, pointed, ciliate, narrowly lanceolate and up to 10 cm wide and tapering to the petiole.

Habitat: The plant is indigenous to America but is found globally today.

Production: Canadian Fleabane is the flowering plant and seeds (without the root) of Erigeron canadensis. The plant is collected in the wild in high summer, then hung in bundles to dry.

Other Names: Coltstail, Flea Wort, Horseweed, Prideweed

ACTIONS AND PHARMACOLOGY

COMPOUNDS

Volatile oil: including (++)-limonene, alpha-cis-bergamots, beta-trans-farnesene, beta-pinenes, myrcene, cis, cis-matricariamethyl ester (polyyne)

Tannins

EFFECTS

The drug is reported to have anti-edema and antiphlogistic effects.

INDICATIONS AND USAGE

Unproven Uses: The drug is used for diarrhea, dysentery, as an antithelmintic, a mild hemostyptic, for uterine bleeding, gout, rheumatic symptoms, dropsy, tumors, and bronchitis. In African folk medicine, it is used in the treatment of granuloma annulare, sore throats, urinary tract infections and for medicinal baths.

Homeopathic Uses: Erigeron canadensis is used for bleeding of the bladder, hemorrhoids, menorrhagia and metrorrhagia, gastritis, hepatitis and cholecystitis

PRECAUTIONS AND ADVERSE REACTIONS

Health risks or side effects following the proper administration of designated therapeutic dosages are not recorded.

DOSAGE

Mode of Administration: The drug is used topically and in alcoholic extracts.

Daily Dosage: Tea: 3 cups daily after meals; Liquid extract: approximately 2 teaspoons.

Homeopathic Dosage: 5 drops, 1 tablet or 10 globules every 30 to 60 minutes (acute) or 1 to 3 times daily (chronic); parenterally: 1 to 2 ml 3 times daily sc (HAB1).

LITERATURE

Grancia D et al., (1985) Ceskoslov Farm 34(6):209.

Hänsel R, Keller K, Rimpler H, Schneider G (Hrsg.), Hagers Handbuch der Pharmazeutischen Praxis, 5. Aufl., Bde 4-6 (Drogen), Springer Verlag Berlin, Heidelberg, New York, 1992-1994 (unter Conyza).

Lasser B et al., (1983) Naturwissenschaften 70:95.

Madaus G, Lehrbuch der Biologischen Arzneimittel, Bde 1-3, Nachdruck, Georg Olms Verlag Hildesheim 1979.

Wagner H, Wiesenauer M, Phytotherapie. Phytopharmaka und pflanzliche Homöopathika, Fischer-Verlag, Stuttgart, Jena, New York 1995.

Canadian Golden Rod

Solidago canadensis

DESCRIPTION

Medicinal Parts: The medicinal parts are the dried aerial parts collected during the flowering season, the fresh inflorescences and the flowering twigs.

Flower and Fruit: The yellow composite flowers are in erect racemes facing all directions and are simple or compound. They are medium-sized. The involucral bracts are imbricate and arranged in numerous rows. The ray florets are narrow, lingual and female. The disc florets are funnel-shaped, 5-tipped and androgynous. The fruit is an achene, which is cylindrical with numerous ribs. It is brown, sparsely pubescent and 3.5 to 4.5 mm long with a tuft of hair.

Leaves, Stem and Root: The plant is a perennial that ranges in size from a few centimeters to over 1 m. The rhizome is cylindrical, noded, diagonally ascending and short. The stem is erect, cane-like, angularly grooved above, usually red-tinged beneath, and glabrous to loosely appressed pubescent higher up. The basal leaves are long-petioled, elliptical, acuminate and narrowing to the winged stem. The lower ones are serrate and the upper ones entire-margined.

Habitat: The plant is indigenous to Europe, Asia and North America.

Production: Golden Rod is the aerial part of Solidago virgaurea. It occurs in the wild in Hungary, former Yugoslavia, Bulgaria and Poland. Golden Rod herb consists of the above-ground parts of Solidago serotina (synonym S. gigantea). Solidago canadensis and its hybrids are gathered during the flowering season and carefully dried.

Not to be Confused With: Despite qualitative and quantitative differences in their effects, drugs containing Solidago gigantea or Solidago canadensis are exchanged with Solidago virgaurea on the market; confusions with Senecio species are also conceivable.

Other Names: Aaron's Rod, Woundwort

ACTIONS AND PHARMACOLOGY

COMPOUNDS: CANADIAN GOLDEN ROD

Triterpene saponins: bisdemosides of the bayogenin, bearing acylglycosidically-bound arabino residue

Polysaccharides (water-soluble): beta-1,2-fructans, acidic polysaccharides

Volatile oil (0.6%): chief components curlone, germacrene D, alpha-pinene, beta-sesquiphellandrene, limonene

Diterpenes of the trans-clerodane and ladanum types

Carotenoids (as blossom pigments)

Flavonoids (2.4%): rutin (1.4%), including as well hyperoside, quercitrin, astragalin

Caffeic acid derivatives: including chlorogenic acid

COMPOUNDS: CANADIAN GOLDEN ROD (GIGANTEA VARIETY)

Triterpene saponins (9%): bisdesmoside of the bayogenins: GS1-GS4

Volatile oil (0.5%): chief components gamma-cadinene-diterpenes of the cis-clerodane-type, including among others 6-deoxysolidagolactone IV-18,19-olide

Carotenoids (as blossom pigments)

Flavonoids (3.8%): quercitrin (1.3%), further including among others hyperoside, rutin, isoquercitrin

Caffeic acid derivatives: including among others chlorogenic acid

EFFECTS: CANADIAN GOLDEN ROD

Canadian Golden Rod is diuretic, weakly spasmolytic and, because of the saponin componant, antiphlogistic.

INDICATIONS AND USAGE

Approved by Commission E:

- Infections of the urinary tract
- Kidney and bladder stones

Unproven Uses: The herb is used as a flushing-out therapy for inflammatory diseases of the lower urinary tract.

CONTRAINDICATIONS

Irrigation therapy is contraindicated in cases of edema resulting from reduced cardiac and/or kidney function.

PRECAUTIONS AND ADVERSE REACTIONS

No health hazards or side effects are known in conjunction with the proper administration of designated therapeutic dosages. The drug possesses a weak potential for sensitization. Care must be taken in patients with chronic renal diseases, and the drug should be used in this patient population only under the supervision of a doctor.

DOSAGE

SOLIDAGINIS VIRGAUREAE HERBA

Mode of Administration: As chopped drug by itself or in combination preparations.

Daily Dosage: The daily dosage is 6 to 12 gm of comminuted drug prepared as an infusion. Fluid intake of at least 2 liters daily is recommended.

Storage: The drug must be protected from light and moisture.

LITERATURE

Bader G et al., (1987) Pharmazie 42(2):140.

Goswami A et al., (1984) Phytochemistry 23(4):837.

Metzer J et al., (1984) Pharmazie 39(12):869.

Lassere B et al., (1983) Naturwissenschaft 70:95.

Reznicek G et al., PM 55:623. 1989.

Reznicek G et al., Tetrahedron Lett 30:4097. 1989.

Reznicek G, Freiler M, Schader M, Schmidt U, Determination of the content and the composition of the main saponins from Solidago gigantea AIT. Using high-perfomance liquid chromatography. In: J Chromatogr A 755(1):133-37. 1996.

Tiansheng L et al., Polyacetylenes and diterpenes from Solida canadensis. In: PH 32:1483. 1993.

Weyerstahl P, Marshall H, Christiansen C, Kalemba D, Góra J, Constituents of the essential oil of Solidago canadensis (''Goldenrod'') from Poland. In: PM 59(3):281. 1993.

Further information in:

Hänsel R, Keller K, Rimpler H, Schneider G (Hrsg.), Hagers Handbuch der Pharmazeutischen Praxis, 5. Aufl., Bde 4-6 (Drogen): Springer Verlag Berlin, Heidelberg, New York, 1992-1994.

Hausen B, Allergiepflanzen, Pflanzenallergene, ecomed Verlagsgesellsch. mbH, Landsberg 1988.

Madaus G, Lehrbuch der Biologischen Arzneimittel, Bde 1-3, Nachdruck, Georg Olms Verlag Hildesheim 1979.

Roth L, Daunderer M, Kormann K, Giftpflanzen, Pflanzengifte, 4. Aufl., Ecomed Fachverlag Landsberg Lech 1993.

Steinegger E, Hänsel R, Pharmakognosie, 5. Aufl., Springer Verlag Heidelberg 1992.

Teuscher E, Biogene Arzneimittel, 5. Aufl., Wiss. Verlagsges. Stuttgart 1997.

Wagner H, Wiesenauer M, Phytotherapie. Phytopharmaka und pflanzliche Homöopathika, Fischer-Verlag, Stuttgart, Jena, New York 1995.

Wichtl M (Hrsg.), Teedrogen, 4. Aufl., Wiss. Verlagsges. Stuttgart 1997.

Canarium species

See Chinese Olive

Cane-Reed

Costus specious

DESCRIPTION

Medicinal Parts: The medicinal part of the plant is the rhizome.

Flower and Fruit: The inflorescence is ovoid, apical and 4 to 7 cm long. The zygomorphic flowers are each supported by one narrow, ovate, acuminate, coriaceous, thickly haired, red to red-brown bract. There is a bracteole, which is approximately 2 cm long, violet to brown-red and sparsely pubescent. The calyx is approximately 2.5 cm long, green to red-brown and tubular. The 3 petals are approximately 6 cm long, white to pale pink and silky haired. The corolla tube is approximately 1.5 cm long. The lobes are elliptical to ovate and 6 to 7 cm long. The lobes are white to pale pink, with a yellow lip in the center made up of 5 stamens. When spread out, the lobe is broad obviate and crenate. There is 1 fertile stamen, which is white to yellowish and up to 5 cm long. The style is thread-like and the ovary 3-chambered and inferior. The fruit is a light red, loculicidal capsule. The seeds are black, 2 to 4 mm wide, with a narrow, fleshy aril.

Leaves, Stem and Root: Costus specious is a herbaceous perennial, upright, up to 3 m high. The leaves have tubular sheaths, which are 0.7 to 1.2 cm in diameter and a pubescent to glabrous. The ligula is 1 to 2 mm long; the leaves are 12 to 25 cm long, 3 to 6 cm wide, narrow elliptical, thorny-tipped, glabrous above and downy-haired beneath. The stem is upright. The rhizome is up to 50-cm long, 3 cm thick and rich in starch.

Habitat: India

Production: Kust or costus root is the dried rhizome of Costus speciosus.

Not to be Confused With: Confusion may occur with Saussurea lappa and Canella winterana. The drug itself is used to adulterate Gloroisa superba.

ACTIONS AND PHARMACOLOGY

COMPOUNDS

Steroid saponins (1 to 4%): chief components dioscin and gracillin, aglycones diosgenin, tigogenin

Steroids: sterols, including beta-sitosterol, beta-sitosterol glucoside

Curcuminoids (3 %): including curcumin

EFFECTS

The saponin fraction of the drug exhibits estrogenic, antiexudative, spasmolytic, choleretic and anesthesia-prolonging effects.

INDICATIONS AND USAGE
Indian Medicine: for febrile conditions, coughs, skin conditions, retention of the placenta, post-partum bleeding, threatening abortion, insufficient uterine contractility and snake bites.

PRECAUTIONS AND ADVERSE REACTIONS
No health hazards are known in conjunction with the proper administration of designated therapeutic dosages. It is conceivable that gastric complaints and nausea might be experienced, as well as kidney irritation, due to the high level of saponin content.

OVERDOSAGE
Overdose could lead to European cholera, increased diuresis and shock.

DOSAGE
Mode of Administration: Whole herb preparations, cut and powdered drug for internal use.

LITERATURE
Hänsel R, Keller K, Rimpler H, Schneider G (Ed) Hagers Handbuch der Pharmazeutischen Praxis. 5. Aufl., Bde 4 - 6 (Drogen), Springer Verlag Berlin, Heidelberg, New York, 1992-1994

Canella
Canella winterana

DESCRIPTION
Medicinal Parts: The medicinal part is the bark of the tree.

Flower and Fruit: The flowers are small and seldom open. They are violet and fused in clusters to the tips of the branches. The involucre is sometimes fused at the base. The stamens are fused to form a pollen tube. The fruit is an elongate berry with 4 reniform seeds. The fruit changes color from green to blue and then to a shiny black.

Leaves, Stem and Root: Canella winterana is a tree that grows up to 15 m and is only branched at the top. The bark is whitish-yellowish on the outside and chalk-like on the inside. The leaves are alternate, oblong, thick, and are a dark, intense laurel-green shade.

Habitat: The tree is indigenous to the Caribbean and Florida.

Not to be Confused With: It is often sold as the rarer Cortex winteranus.

Other Names: Canella alba, White Cinnamon, White Wood, Wild Cinnamon

ACTIONS AND PHARMACOLOGY
COMPOUNDS

Volatile oil (1%): chief components eugenol, cineol, pinene, caryophyllene, myristicin

Resins (8%)

Sesquiterpenes: including muzigadial, warburganal (pungent-tasting dialdehydes)

Mannitol (6-8%)

Starch (12%)

EFFECTS

Canella has a stimulant and tonic effect. The sesquiterpenes contained in the bark have antimycotic and molluscacidal effects.

INDICATIONS AND USAGE
Unproven Uses: In Central and South America, Canella is used internally to treat upset stomach, fever and conditions of the mouth and throat; it is used externally for rheumatism. In the West Indies, it is used to treat scurvy and as a spice.

PRECAUTIONS AND ADVERSE REACTIONS
No health hazards or side effects are known in conjunction with the proper administration of designated therapeutic dosages.

DOSAGE
Mode of Administration: Canella is available in whole, cut and powdered forms.

LITERATURE
El Feraly M et al., (1980) J Nat Prod 43:407.

Kern W, List PH, Hörhammer L (Hrsg.), Hagers Handbuch der Pharmazeutischen Praxis, 4. Aufl., Bde 1-8, Springer Verlag Berlin, Heidelberg, New York, 1969.

Morton JF, An Atlas of Medicinal Plants of Middle America, Charles C. Thomas USA 1981.

Canella winterana
See Canella

Cannabis sativa
See Marijuana

Capsella bursa-pastoris
See Shepherd's Purse

Capsicum species

See Cayenne

Carambola

Averrhoa carambola

DESCRIPTION

Medicinal Parts: The medicinal part is the fruit.

Flower and Fruit: Cymose inflorescences grow from the trunk. The flowers are radial, and their structures are arranged in fives. The petals are free; there are 10 stamens and a 5-chambered ovary. The fruit is a berry, approximately 10 cm long. The berry is acuminate, 5-sided and star-shaped in cross-section. It is translucently amber-yellow.

Leaves, Stem and Root: Averrhoa carambola is a tree, that grows up to 5 m high. The leaves are alternate, odd pinnate and 10 to 12 cm long.

Habitat: India

Production: The fruit of the Carambola tree is the ripe fruit of Averrhoa carambola.

ACTIONS AND PHARMACOLOGY

COMPOUNDS

Oxalic acid (0.3% of fresh weight)

Vitamin C (0.05% of fresh weight)

Monosaccharides/polysaccharides

Carotinoids

EFFECTS

No definitive data available.

INDICATIONS AND USAGE

Indian Medicine: Carambola is used for diarrhea, vomiting, severe thirst, hemorrhoids, intermittent fever, scabies and liver pain.

PRECAUTIONS AND ADVERSE REACTIONS

There is no evidence of any health risks connected with limited consumption of the fruit or the preserves made from them. Nevertheless, due to the high oxalate content, which corresponds approximately to that of rhubarb stalks, the ingestion of large amounts over extended periods should be avoided.

DOSAGE

No information is available.

LITERATURE

Neto MM, Robl F, Netto JC, Depressant action of averrhoa carambola. Med J Malaysia, 13:279-80, 1980 Mar.

Neto MM, Robl F, Netto JC, Intoxication by star fruit (Averrhoa carambola) in six dialysis patients? (Preliminary report) news. Nephrol Dial Transplant, 13:570-2, 1998 Mar.

Caraway

Carum carvi

DESCRIPTION

Medicinal Parts: The medicinal part is the fruit and the oil obtained from the squashed fruit when ripe.

Flower and Fruit: The main trunk and the side branches each terminate in a compound flowering umbel of 8 to 16 umbel rays. The epicalyx and calyx are almost non-existent. The florets are white or reddish and very small. The fruit is a schizocarp that is glabrous, oblong and elliptoid. It consists of 2 mericarps that are 3 to 6 mm long, sickle-shaped, brownish with 5 lighter, angular main ribs (caraway seeds).

Leaves, Stem and Root: Carum carvi is usually a biennial, 30 to 100 cm high plant with a fleshy, fusiform tap root. The stem is erect, angular, grooved, filled with latex, glabrous and branched from the ground up. The rosette leaves and the cauline leaves are glabrous and in part tri-pinnate. The lower pinna are typically crossed.

Characteristics: The plant has a caraway taste and an aromatic smell.

Habitat: Caraway is found in Europe, Siberia, the Caucasus, the Near East, the Himalayas, Mongolia and Morocco. Found wild in North America after being introduced.

Production: Caraway oil consists of the essential oil extracted from the ripe fruits of Carum carvi. Caraway is harvested when completely ripe and threshed 3 weeks later. The oil is recovered from the crushed seeds by a process of aqueous steam distillation.

Not to be Confused With: Carvon is occasionally added in synthetic form.

ACTIONS AND PHARMACOLOGY

COMPOUNDS

In the berries: volatile oil, fatty oil, polysaccharides, proteins, furocoumarins (traces)

In volatile oil: in particular D-(+)-carvone and D-(+)-limonene

EFFECTS

In animal tests the drug had a spasmolytic effect. The antimicrobial effect has been demonstrated against *bacillus, pseudomonas*, and *candida*; *dermatomyces* are also inhibited. The choleretic effect has been described in a study which is not accessible.

INDICATIONS AND USAGE

Approved by Commission E:

- Dyspeptic complaints

Unproven Uses: Caraway is used for gastrointestinal cramps, flatulence and feelings of fullness, as well as nervous cardiac-gastric complaints.

In folk medicine, Caraway is used to improve lactation in nursing mothers, as an emmenagogue and to settle the stomach. The essential oil is used as constituent in mouthwashes and bath additives.

PRECAUTIONS AND ADVERSE REACTIONS

No health hazards or side effects are known in conjunction with the proper administration of designated therapeutic dosages.

OVERDOSAGE

An intake of larger dosages of the volatile oil (see for example in caraway liquor) for extended periods can lead to kidney and liver damage.

DOSAGE

Mode of Administration: Preparations from the essential oil are for internal use. The comminuted fresh drug is used for infusions and other galenic preparations.

How Supplied: Powder, capsules, film tablets, coated tablets, drops and tea.

Preparation: An infusion is prepared by pressing 1 to 2 teaspoonfuls of seeds before using and pouring 150 ml of hot water over it, draining after 10 to 15 minutes.

Daily Dosage: The average single dose of oil is 2 to 3 drops on sugar; caraway, 1 to 5 gm. The average daily dose of oil is 3 to 6 drops; caraway, 1.5 to 6 gm.

Storage: Protect from light and moisture in glass or metal containers.

LITERATURE

Debelmas AM, Rochat J, (1967) Plant Med Phytother 1:23.

Harries N et al., (1978) J Clin Pharm 2:171.

Hopf H, Kandler O, (1977) Phytochemistry 16:1715.

Koedam A, Scheffer JJC, Barheim Svendsen A, Z Lebensm Unters Forsch 168:106-111. 1979.

Salveson A et al., Sci Pharm 46(2):93-100. 1978.

Further information in:

Chan, EH et al. (Eds), Advances in Chinese Medicinal Materials Research, World Scientific Pub. Co. Singapore 1985.

Hänsel R, Keller K, Rimpler H, Schneider G (Hrsg.), Hagers Handbuch der Pharmazeutischen Praxis, 5. Aufl., Bde 4-6 (Drogen), Springer Verlag Berlin, Heidelberg, New York, 1992-1994.

Leung AY, Encyclopedia of Common Natural Ingredients Used in Food Drugs and Cosmetics, John Wiley & Sons Inc., New York 1980.

Madaus G, Lehrbuch der Biologischen Arzneimittel, Bde 1-3, Nachdruck, Georg Olms Verlag Hildesheim 1979.

Schulz R, Hänsel R, Rationale Phytotherapie, Springer Verlag Heidelberg 1996.

Simon JE, Chadwick AF, Craker LE (Eds.), Herbs. An Indexed Bibliography 1971-80. Archon Books, USA 1984.

Steinegger E, Hänsel R, Pharmakognosie, 5. Aufl., Springer Verlag Heidelberg 1992.

Teuscher E, Biogene Arzneimittel, 5. Aufl., Wiss. Verlagsges. mbH Stuttgart 1997.

Wichtl M (Hrsg.), Teedrogen, 4. Aufl., Wiss. Verlagsges. Stuttgart 1997.

Cardamom

Elettaria cardamomum

DESCRIPTION

Medicinal Parts: The medicinal parts are the oil extracted from the seeds and fruit plus seeds harvested shortly after ripening.

Flower and Fruit: The flowering shoots grow on the stem very close to the ground. The panicle branches can grow up to 8 cm. The flowers are alternate and covered by sheath-like bracts before opening. The calyx is slightly wider above, finely striped, obtusely 3-tipped and does not droop. The corolla is greenish white. The lobes are rounded, somewhat curly, white with a yellowish border with blue veins and lines in the center. The only fertile stamen is set into the edge of the petals. The sterile stamens are arranged beside the styles on the receptacle. The pollen is globular and prickly. The ovary is inferior, oblong, obovate with 3 valves, each with 12 horizontal ovules. The fruit is 6 to 18 mm long, 6 to 10 mm thick, short-stemmed, ovate or elliptical to oblong. The seeds are light brown, gray or dark red brownish. They are very roughly wrinkled, 4 to 5 mm long, irregular edged and the whole seed is surrounded by an almost colorless seed coat. Mysore and Malabar cardamoms are usually blanched pale and have a smooth surface. They are sold commercially less often than the Green Aleppy or Ceylon varieties.

Leaves, Stem and Root: Elettaria cardamomum is a perennial with a thick, tuberous rhizome and numerous long roots. There are up to 30 erect, glabrous, green stems that are 2 to 3 m high. The leaves are in 2 rows with a leaf membrane at the end of a soft-haired sheath. The leaf surface is lanceolate, clearly acuminate and up to 60 cm long. The leaves are entire-margined, downy above, silky-haired beneath and punctuated by numerous small oil cells. The seeds are about 4 mm diameter and dark-reddish-brown.

Characteristics: Cardamom has an aromatic and pleasant odor. The taste is aromatic and pungent.

Habitat: The plant is indigenous in southern India and Sri Lanka and is cultivated in tropical regions in southeast Asia and Guatamala.

Production: Cardamom consists of the dried, almost ripe, greenish to yellow-gray fruit of Elettaria cardamomum. Medicinal use is limited to the seed, which is removed from its fruit capsule. The main harvest is in October and November of the third year after planting. The fruit is then dried either in the sun or in so-called 'curing houses' and then sorted according to size, form, color etc.

ACTIONS AND PHARMACOLOGY

COMPOUNDS

Volatile oil: composition varies according to the specific strain, chief components cineol, alpha-terpinyl acetate, linalyl acetate

Fatty oil

Starch

EFFECTS

The drug is a cholagogue and has virustatic properties. The essential oil (monoterpene) of the drug is antibacterial and antimycotic. In animal experiments the essential oil caused an increase in the secretion of bile and a reduction of gastric juice production.

INDICATIONS AND USAGE

Approved by Commission E:

- Common cold
- Cough/bronchitis
- Fevers and colds
- Inflammation of the mouth and pharynx
- Liver and gallbladder complaints
- Loss of appetite
- Tendency to infection

Unproven Uses: Cardamom is also used for dyspepsia. In folk medicine it is used for digestive complaints, vomiting and diarrhea, morning sickness and loss of appetite as well as Roemheld syndrome.

Chinese Medicine: Cardamom is used for stomachache, nausea, vomiting and flatulence.

Indian Medicine: In Indian medicine, Cardamom is used for disorders of the efferent urinary tract.

PRECAUTIONS AND ADVERSE REACTIONS

No health hazards or side effects are known in conjunction with the proper administration of designated therapeutic dosages. The drug can trigger gallstone colic, due to its motility-enhancing effect.

DOSAGE

Mode of Administration: Ground seeds, as well as galenic preparations for internal use.

Daily Dosage: The average daily dosage is 1.5 gm of drug. When using a tincture, the dosage range is 1 to 2 gm.

Storage: Cardamom should be stored in a cool, dry place protected from light in tightly sealed containers. The powder can be stored for a maximum of 24 hours. Loose seeds without the testa cannot be stored.

LITERATURE

Fenaroli's Handbook of Flavor Ingredients, Vol. 1, 2nd Ed., CRC Press 1975.

Hänsel R, Keller K, Rimpler H, Schneider G (Hrsg.), Hagers Handbuch der Pharmazeutischen Praxis, 5. Aufl., Bde 4-6 (Drogen), Springer Verlag Berlin, Heidelberg, New York, 1992-1994.

Haginiwa H et al., (1963) Yakagaku Zasshi 83:623.

Leung AY, Encyclopedia of Common Natural Ingredients Used in Food, Drugs and Cosmetics, John Wiley & Sons Inc., New York 1980.

Lewis YS, Nambuduri ES, Philip T, Perfum Essent Oli Res 57:623-628. 1966.

Teuscher E, Biogene Arzneimittel, 5. Aufl., Wiss. Verlagsges. mbH Stuttgart 1997.

Wagner H, Wiesenauer M, Phytotherapie. Phytopharmaka und pflanzliche Homöopathika, Fischer-Verlag, Stuttgart, Jena, New York 1995.

Carex arenaria

See German Sarsaparilla

Carica papaya

See Papaya

Carlina acaulis

See Carline Thistle

Carline Thistle

Carlina acaulis

DESCRIPTION

Medicinal Parts: The medicinal part is the root.

Flower and Fruit: The flowers are made up of individual heads that are 7 to 13 cm in diameter. The disc florets are androgynous, pink to violet, and have a 5-tipped radial corolla. The outer bracts are thorny. The middle bracts consist of glossy white, acuminate, 3 to 4 cm long leaves. The stamens have bristly-tipped appendages. The styles are cylindrical with short stigma lobes. The fruit is 5 mm long, obclavate to cylindrical, and bluntly angular with bifurcated hairs at the tip.

Leaves, Stem and Root: Carlina acaulis is a 30 cm high thistle-like, leafy plant with milky latex. The stem is compressed and under 5 cm long. The whorled to alternate leaves are flat or slightly frilled and a little tough, 10 to 20 cm long, pinnatifid to pinnatisect with broad, thorny tips. The rhizome is finger thick and has 1 or more heads.

Habitat: The plant extends from Spain, Italy and the Balkans across central Europe to central Russia.

Production: Carline Thistle (Dwarf Thistle) is the root of Carlina acaulis collected in autumn and dried. It is collected in the wild.

Not to be Confused With: Sometimes Carline Thistle is adulterated by addition of other Carlina species.

Other Names: Stemless Carlina Root, Dwarf Carline, Ground Thistle, Southernwood Root

ACTIONS AND PHARMACOLOGY

COMPOUNDS

Volatile oil: chief components carlina oxide

Inulin (18 to 20%) (fructosan)

Tannins

EFFECTS

There is no valid data on the mode of action. The essential oil hinders the growth of *Staphylococcus aureus* up to a dilution of 1:2 X 105. Carline Thistle has mild diuretic, spasmolytic and diaphoretic effects.

INDICATIONS AND USAGE

Unproven Uses: The drug is used internally for cholecystopathy, digestive insufficiency and for spasms in the alimentary canal. In Spain, it is used to treat colds and illnesses accompanied by fever.

Externally, it is used as a wash for dermatosis, and to rinse wounds and ulcers; as a mouthwash to alleviate symptoms associated with cancer of the tongue.

PRECAUTIONS AND ADVERSE REACTIONS

No health hazards or side effects are known in conjunction with the proper administration of designated therapeutic dosages.

DOSAGE

Mode of Administration: Carline Thistle is used both internally and externally.

Daily Dosage: Common preparations and doses are:

Decoction: Boil 3 gm of drug in 150 ml of water for 5 minutes, drink 3 cups daily.

Infusion: 2 teaspoons of the drug to be boiled in 1 cup of water for 10 minutes, leave to draw for half an hour, take 3 to 4 cups daily between mealtimes.

Tincture: 20 gm of chopped drug, left to draw for 10 days in 80 gm of ethanol 60%, use 40 to 50 drops, 4 to 5 times daily.

Wine: Add 50 gm of the drug to 1 L of white wine, leave to draw for a minimum of 12 days, then strain; drink one full small glass before mealtimes.

Externally it is used as a decoction; 30 gm of the drug added to 1 L of water.

Storage: Should be stored in tightly sealed containers.

LITERATURE

Hänsel R, Keller K, Rimpler H, Schneider G (Hrsg.), Hagers Handbuch der Pharmazeutischen Praxis, 5. Aufl., Bde 4-6 (Drogen), Springer Verlag Berlin, Heidelberg, New York, 1992-1994.

Schilcher H, Hagels H, Carlinae radix. Verfälschung, Verwechslung oder Ersatzdroge. In: DAZ 130(40):2186. 1990.

Wichtl M (Hrsg.), Teedrogen, 4. Aufl., Wiss. Verlagsges. Stuttgart 1997.

Carob

Ceratonia siliqua

DESCRIPTION

Medicinal Parts: The medicinal parts are the fruit and the bark.

Flower and Fruit: The inflorescence is erect and lateral in old wood. It is often bushy, clustered or catkin-like, and unisexual with erect receptacles. There is no corolla. The male flowers have 5 long filaments with long slits and opening pollen tubes. The female flowers have short-stemmed ovaries. The pods are 10 to 20 cm by 2 cm, tough leathery, brown-violet, flat and often rounded to a horn shape. There are numerous, lumpy and glossy brown seeds.

Leaves, Stem and Root: This walnut-like tree is usually under 6 m high, broad-crowned, sparsely branched and with cracked gray-brown bark. There are 2 to 4 paired pinnate leaves. The leaflets are obovate, 4 to 5 cm long, curved, glabrous, glossy dark green above and red-brown beneath.

Habitat: Indigenous to southeastern Europe and west Asia, otherwise cultivated.

Production: Carob seed flour is the ground endosperm of the seeds of Ceratonia siliqua.

Not to be Confused With: Carob Tree, Jacaranda procera or Jacaranda caroba.

Other Names: St. John's Bread, Locust Bean, Locust Pods, Sugar Pods

ACTIONS AND PHARMACOLOGY

COMPOUNDS

Mucilages: chiefly made up of galactomannanes

Proteic substances

Flavonoids: including isoschaftoside, neoschaftoside, schaftoside

EFFECTS

In various test series and studies, the effect of carob gum on the serum glucose level, the secretion and activity of digestive enzymes, the secretion of gastrointestinal hormones as well as on the serum lipid level was proven. The hypoglycaemic and hypolipidaemic effect is attributed to an increase in viscosity of the gastrointestinal content.

Effects on nitrogen balance, efficacy in infantile diarrhea, as well as an anti-exudative, anticoagulant and antiviral effects have been demonstrated.

INDICATIONS AND USAGE

Unproven Uses: Carob is used in dietary agents for acute nutritional disorders, diarrheal disorders, dyspepsia, enterocolitis, celiac disease and sprue. It is also used for habitual vomiting in babies, acetonemic vomiting, rumination, retching cough and vomiting.

Carob seed flour is used in the production of glutin-free starch bread, which is used for vomiting during pregnancy, celiac disease and obesity.

PRECAUTIONS AND ADVERSE REACTIONS

No health hazards or side effects are known in conjunction with the proper administration of designated therapeutic dosages.

DOSAGE

Mode of Administration: It is obsolete as a drug but is included in thickening powders and as a baking aid for glutin-free starch bread.

Preparation: As a baking aid or thickening agent, dissolve in cold liquid, boil for 1 to 2 minutes, cool and mix into the prepared baby food.

Daily Dosage: For a 3 to 10% arabon preparation, add 20 to 30 mg of drug to water, tea or milk, to be drunk during the course of the day. As a baking agent in glutin-free bread for babies, add 1/4 to 1/2 gm of drug (max. 2 gm) to 100 ml liquid; adults 1% to 3% additive to low-calorie starters and desserts.

LITERATURE

Kern W, List PH, Hörhammer L (Hrsg.), Hagers Handbuch der Pharmazeutischen Praxis, 4. Aufl., Bde 1-8, Springer Verlag Berlin, Heidelberg, New York, 1969.

Leung AY, Encyclopedia of Common Natural Ingredients Used in Food Drugs and Cosmetics, John Wiley & Sons Inc., New York 1980.

McLeary BV, Biomass A Cellulose and Hemicellulose 160:523. 1988.

Steinegger E, Hänsel R, Pharmakognosie, 5. Aufl., Springer Verlag Heidelberg 1992.

Tang W, Eisenbrand G, Chinese Drugs of Plant Origin, Springer Verlag Heidelberg 1992.

Teuscher E, Biogene Arzneimittel, 5. Aufl., Wiss. Verlagsges. mbH Stuttgart 1997.

Carrageen

Chondrus crispus

DESCRIPTION

Medicinal Parts: The medicinal part of carrageen, the Irish seaweed, is the thallus that has been freed from the adhesive disc then dried and bleached in the sun.

Flower and Fruit: Gamatangia: The spematangia are colorless and are at the end of the younger thallus lobes. The spermatia are 7.5 to 10 μm long and 4 to 5 μm wide; the carposporangia are 20 to 20 μm long and 14 to 25 μm wide and have no outer threads. The tetrasporangia, along with the cruciform arranged tatra spores, are in the medulla of the short side branches.

Thallus: Chondrus crispus is a perennial red algae that grows in waters up to 25 m deep. The thallus is usually yellow-green to purplish-brown when fresh, white to yellow and translucent after drying. Thallus fronds, are 10 to 30 cm long on an adhesive disc, arising from a subcylindrical stem. They then become flattened, curled and sometimes bifid. The segments are linear and usually 3 to 8 mm wide. The margin is linguiform, later repeatedly dividing into bifid thallus lobes. The thallus is cartilaginous and double-layered. The internal tissue is made up of reticulately linked cells. The bark layer is at right angles to the thallus. The bifurcated cell strings are like strings of pearls that are spread radially.

Habitat: Carrageen is found from the coast of Iceland to the Baltic, from northern Russia to the south of Spain, Morocco and the Cape Verde Islands, and also in parts of North America and some Japanese coastal regions.

Production: Carrageen is the dried and bleached thalli of Chondrus crispus as well as other varieties of Gigartina species. After being cleaned, the algae are left to bleach in the sun, then dried.

Not to be Confused With: Confusion can arise with related species of Gigartina stellata and Gigartina pistillata.

Other Names: Irish Moss, Chondrus, Carrahan, Carrageennan

ACTIONS AND PHARMACOLOGY

COMPOUNDS

Carrageenans: (carrageenine): in particular kappa-, iota- and lambda-carrageenan (muciform galactane sulphates)

Proteins

Mineral salts: including iodides and bromides

EFFECTS

The drug contains hydrocolloids of the carrageenan type. Carrageen is considered a mucilage because it hinders the effect of peptides in digestive enzymes. It also acts as an expectorant and secretory agent. In animal experiments the drug was not absorbed. There are no studies available on absorption in humans. The drug's purported demulcent and antitussive effects have not been confirmed.

INDICATIONS AND USAGE

Unproven Uses: Folk medicine internal uses of Carrageen include as roughage for constipation and as a mucilage for diarrhea, as well as for peptic ulcers. Sometimes a decoction is used for coughs, bronchitis and tuberculosis.

PRECAUTIONS AND ADVERSE REACTIONS

No health hazards or side effects are known in conjunction with the proper administration of designated therapeutic dosages. Intracutaneous injections of solutions, however, can trigger local inflammations.

DOSAGE

Mode of Administration: Seldom used as a drug, but is included in compound preparations as syrup and granules.

Preparation: Irish moss extract is prepared using a diluted, almost boiling alkali solution. Filtration and vacuum inspissation follow prior to extensive dehydration. A decoction is prepared by combining 1.5 g drug with 1 cup water.

Storage: The drug should be stored in tightly sealed containers.

LITERATURE

Chapman B, Chapman VJ, Chapman DJ, Seaweeds and their uses. Chapmann and Hall, London, New York 1980.

Stancioff DJ, Renn DW, (1975) A C S Symp Ser. 15:282.

Thomson AW, Horne CHW, (1976) Brit J Exp Pathol 57:455.

Further information in:

Hänsel R, Keller K, Rimpler H, Schneider G (Hrsg.), Hagers Handbuch der Pharmazeutischen Praxis, 5. Aufl., Bde 4-6 (Drogen), Springer Verlag Berlin, Heidelberg, New York, 1992-1994.

Steinegger E, Hänsel R, Pharmakognosie, 5. Aufl., Springer Verlag Heidelberg 1992.

Teuscher E, Biogene Arzneimittel, 5. Aufl., Wiss. Verlagsges. mbH Stuttgart 1997.

Carthamus tinctorius

See Safflower

Carum carvi

See Caraway

Cascara Sagrada

Rhamnus purshiana

TRADE NAMES

Cascara Sagrada (available from numerous manufacturers), Cascara Sagrada Bark Mild Stimulant Laxative, Cascara Sagrada Natural Laxative, Cascara Sagrada Bark

DESCRIPTION

Medicinal Parts: The medicinal part is the dried bark.

Flower and Fruit: The flowers are in axillary richly blossomed racemes. The receptacles are green and the sepals are larger than the petals. Both receptacles and sepals are white. The ovary is longer than the style and is trilocular. The fruit is dark purple and top-shaped. The seeds are ovate, black, glossy, domed on the outside and have a distinct line on the inside.

Leaves, Stem and Root: The plant is either a bush or a 6 to 18 m tall tree with branches which are gray tomentose when young. The leaves are oblong-ovate, rounded at the base or sometimes narrowing at the petiole. On the longer shoots they are up to 17 cm long and 7.5 cm wide with an 8 to 18 mm long petiole. The margins are finely dentate and the young leaves are tomentose, later becoming dark-green but not coriaceous even in autumn.

Habitat: The plant is indigenous to the western part of North America and is cultivated on the Pacific coast of the U.S., Canada and in eastern Africa.

Production: Cascara sagrada bark consists of the dried bark of Rhamnus purshiana.

Not to be Confused With: The bark of other Rhamnus species.

Other Names: Purshiana Bark, Sagrada Bark, Sacred Bark, Bitter Bark, Yellow Bark, Dogwood Bark, California Buckthorn, Chittem Bark, Cascara Buckthorn

ACTIONS AND PHARMACOLOGY

COMPOUNDS

Anthracene derivatives (8-10%): anthranoids, chief components cascarosides A and B (stereoisomeric aloin-8-glucosides), C and D (stereoisomeric 11-deoxy-aloin-8-glucosides), E and F (C-glucosyl-emodin-anthron-8-glucosides), further including aloin, 11-deoxyaloin

EFFECTS

Laxative Effects

The anthranoid compounds of Cascara are carried unabsorbed to the large intestine where the active aglycon is released by bacterial hydrolysis of the sugar. The intestinal bacterial flora reduces anthraquinone aglycons to the active components of 1,8-dihydroxy-anthracene derivatives, which have the laxative effect (de Witte & Lemli, 1990).

The anthranoids are anti-absorptive, hydrogogic and inhibit the absorption of electrolytes and water from the colon. The laxative effect is caused by an increase in the volume of the intestinal contents with the resulting increase in pressure and stimulation of intestinal peristalsis. In addition, stimulation of the active chloride secretion into the intestine by nitric-oxide-donating compounds or nitric oxide itself increases water and electrolyte content (Izzo, 1998). Aloin and other anthranoid derivatives stimulate prostaglandin production in isolated segments of intestinal tissue, thus contributing to the cathartic action (Cohen, 1982; Capasso, 1983).

CLINICAL TRIALS

Bowel Preparation

The effectiveness and acceptability of three bowel-cleansing regimens was determined in 271 patients for colonoscopy. Senna laxative (X-prep), combined with a saline enema, a polyethylene glycol electrolyte lavage solution (Golytely 4 liters) or combined regimen of Cascara-Salax laxative (PicoSalax) and 1.51 Golytely was administered. No clinically important differences were found between the three bowel preparation regimens (Borkje, 1991).

A prospective, randomized clinical trial was conducted to determine the side effects, patient acceptance, residual liquid and stool during colonoscopy and also quality of examination of three colon cleansing methods. Three hundred ambulatory patients were randomly assigned to one of the following three groups for colon preparation: Group 1, (4 liters of Golytely), group 2, (2 liters of Golytely combined with Cascara-Salax), and group 3, (X-Prep (a Senna preparation) combined with an enema). X-Prep caused significantly more abdominal cramps than Group 1 or Group 2. Vomiting was most frequent with Group 1, and the patients preferred X-Prep to 4 liters of Golytely. The cleanest colon was obtained with 4 liters of Golytely; 2 liters of Golytely with Cascara-Salax was least effective. The quality of the examination was equal in groups 1 and 3, which were both significantly better than group 2 (Hangartner, 1989).

INDICATIONS AND USAGE

Approved by Commission E:

■ Constipation

Cascara Segrada is used for constipation, relief of defecation with anal fissures, hemorrhoids, and as a recto-anal post-operative treatment. The herb is also used in preparation of diagnostic procedures of the gastrointestinal tract and to obtain a soft stool.

Unproven Uses: In Folk medicine, Cascara is used as a tonic and for cleaning wounds.

Homeopathic Uses: The herb is used for rheumatism and as a digestive aid.

CONTRAINDICATIONS

The drug is contraindicated in intestinal obstruction, acute inflammatory intestinal disease (colitis, Crohn's disease, irritable bowel), appendicitis and abdominal pain of unknown origin. Cascara drug is not to be administered to children under 12 years of age.

PRECAUTIONS AND ADVERSE REACTIONS

General: Spasmodic gastrointestinal complaints can occur as a side effect to the drug's purgative effect. In rare cases, prolonged use may lead to heart arrhythmias, nephropathies, edema and accelerated bone deterioration. Intake of the fresh rind could lead to European cholera, intestinal colic, bloody diarrhea and kidney irritation.

Electrolyte Abnormalies: Long-term use leads to loss of electrolytes, in particular potassium ions. Hyperaldosteronism, albuminuria, hematuria, inhibition of intestinal motility, and muscle weakness may occur. Enhancement of cardioactive steroids and antiarrythics may also occur as a consequense of hypokalemia.

Carcinogenesis: The probability of carcinomas in the colon following long-term administration of anthracene drugs has not yet been fully clarified. Cascara glycoside may act as weak promoters in colon carcinogenesis in animal models (Mereto, 1996). One study determined aloin-enriched diets did not promote incidence and growth of adenomas, carcinomas or significant hepatotoxicity after 20 weeks (Siegers, 1993a). Anthranoid laxative abuse is a relative risk factor for colorectal cancer (Siegerss, 1993b).

Drug Interactions:

Thiazide Diuretics/Corticoadrenal Steroids/Liquorice Root — These drugs may potentiate potassium deficiency when used concomitantly with Cascara.

Antiarrythmics — Loss of potassium associated with prolonged use of Cascara may potentiate arrhythmias when given concomitantly with antiarrhythmic medications.

Digitalis Glycosides — With prolonged use or abuse of Cascara, loss of potassium may potentiate digitalis toxicity.

Indomethacin (NSAIDS) — Indomethacin given concomitantly with anthracene derivatives had a decrease in therapeutic effect due to the inhibition of prostaglandin E2 (SEE EFFECTS) (Cohen, 1982; Capasso, 1983).

Pregnancy: Use during pregnancy or while nursing only after consulting a physician.

Nursing Mothers: Cascara has been identified by the American Academy of Pediatrics as compatible with breastfeeding (Hagemann, 1998).

Pediatric Use: The drug is not to be administered to children under 12 years of age.

DOSAGE

Mode of Administration: Liquid or solid forms of medication are exclusively for oral use. The drug is used as comminuted drug, powder or dry extracts for infusions, decoction, and as a cold maceration or elixir.

How Supplied:

Capsule — 425 mg, 440 mg, 450 mg, 850 mg

Preparation: To prepare an infusion, add 2 gm finely cut drug to boiling water and strain after 10 minutes. (1 teaspoonful = 2.5 gm drug)

Daily Dosage: Administer 20 to 30 mg hydroxyanthracene derivatives daily, calculated as cascaroside A.

Tea: Take 1 fresh cup mornings and evenings.

Homeopathic Dosage: from D3: 5 drops, 1 tablet or 10 globules every 30 to 60 minutes (acute) or 1 to 3 times daily (chronic); parenterally: 1 to 2 ml sc acute: 3 times daily; chronic: once a day (HAB34)

Note: The individually correct dosage is the smallest dosage necessary to maintain a soft stool. Stimulating laxatives must not be used over a period of more than 1 to 2 weeks without medical advice.

LITERATURE

Anonym, Abwehr von Arzneimittelrisiken, Stufe II. In: DAZ 136(38):3253-2354. 1996.

Anonym, Anwendungseinschränkungen für Anthranoid-haltige Abführmittel angeordnet. In: PUZ 25(6):341-342. 1996.

Borkje B; Pedersen R; Lund GM et al. Effectiveness and acceptability of three bowel cleansing regimens. Scand J Gastroenterol 1991 Feb;26(2):162-6.

BGA, Arzneimittelrisiken: Anthranoide. In: DAZ 132(21):1164. 1992.

Capasso F; Mascolo N; Autore G; Duraccio MR. Effect of indomethacin on aloin and 1,8 dioxianthraquinone-induced production of prostaglandins in rat isolated colon. Prostaglandins 1983 Oct;26(4):557-62.

Cohen MM. The effect of cathartics on prostaglandin synthesis by rat gastrointestinal tract. Prostaglandins Leukot Med 1982 Apr;8(4):389-97.

de Witte P, Cuveele J, Lemli J, Bicascarosides in fluid extracts of Cascara. In: PM 57:440. 1991.

de Witte P; Lemli L. The metabolism of anthranoid laxatives. Hepatogastroenterology 1990 Dec;37(6):601-5.

Evans FJ et al., (1975) J Pharm Pharmacol 27:91P.

Fairbairn JW et al., (1977) J Pharm Sci 66:1300.

Fairbairn JW, Simic S, (1964) J Pharm Pharmacol 16:450.

Griffini A et al., Isolation and characterisation of pure Cascarosides A, B, C, and D. In: PM 58(Suppl.7):A593. 1992.

Hagemann TM. Gastrointestinal medications and breastfeeding. J Hum Lact 1998 Sep;14(3):259-62.

Hangartner PJ; Munch R; Meier J et al. Comparison of three colon cleansing methods: evaluation of a randomized clinical trial with 300 ambulatory patients. Endoscopy 1989 Nov;21(6):272-5.

Helmholz H, Ruge A, Piasecki A, Schröder S, Westendorf J, Genotoxizität der Faulbaumrinde. In: PZ 138(43):3478. 1993.

Izzo AA; Mascolo N; Capasso F. Nitric oxide as a modulator of intestinal water and electrolyte transport. Dig Dis Sci 1998 Aug;43(8):1605-20.

Klimpel BE et al., Anthranoidhaltige Laxantien - ein Risiko für die Entwicklung von Tumoren der ableitenden Harnwege. In: PUZ 26(1):33, Jahrestagung der DPhG, Berlin, 1996. 1997.

Manitto P et al., Studies on cascara, part 2. Structure of cascarosides E and F. In: JNP 58(3):419-423. 1995.

Mereto E; Ghia M; Brambilla G. Evaluation of the potential carcinogenic activity of Senna and Cascara glycosides for the rat colon. Cancer Lett 1996 Mar 19;101(1):79-83.

Siegers CP; Siemers J; Baretton G. Sennosides and aloin do not promote dimethylhydrazine-induced colorectal tumors in mice. Pharmacology 1993a Oct;47 Suppl 1:205-8.

Siegers CP; von Hertzberg-Lottin E; Otte M; Schneider B. Anthranoid laxative abuse—a risk for colorectal cancer? Gut 1993b Aug;34(8):1099-101.

Thesen R, Phytotherapeutika - nicht immer harmlos. In: ZPT 9(49):105. 1988.

Further information in:

Hänsel R, Keller K, Rimpler H, Schneider G (Hrsg.), Hagers Handbuch der Pharmazeutischen Praxis, 5. Aufl., Bde 4-6 (Drogen): Springer Verlag Berlin, Heidelberg, New York, 1992-1994.

Leung AY, Encyclopedia of Common Natural Ingredients Used in Food, Drugs, Cosmetics, John Wiley & Sons Inc., New York 1980.

Lewin L, Gifte und Vergiftungen, 6. Aufl., Nachdruck, Haug Verlag, Heidelberg 1992.

Madaus G, Lehrbuch der Biologischen Arzneimittel, Bde 1-3, Nachdruck, Georg Olms Verlag Hildesheim 1979.

Roth L, Daunderer M, Kormann K, Giftpflanzen, Pflanzengifte, 4. Aufl., Ecomed Fachverlag Landsberg Lech 1993.

Steinegger E, Hänsel R, Pharmakognosie, 5. Aufl., Springer Verlag Heidelberg 1992.

Teuscher E, Lindequist U, Biogene Gifte - Biologie, Chemie, Pharmakologie, 2. Aufl., Fischer Verlag Stuttgart 1994.

Teuscher E, Biogene Arzneimittel, 5. Aufl., Wiss. Verlagsges. Stuttgart 1997.

Wichtl M (Hrsg.), Teedrogen, 4. Aufl., Wiss. Verlagsges. Stuttgart 1997.

Cascarilla

Croton eluteria

DESCRIPTION

Medicinal Parts: The medicinal part is the dried bark.

Flower and Fruit: The flowers are small, with white petals and a pleasant fragrance.

Leaves, Stem and Root: The plant is a small tree that rarely grows to more than 6 m. It has small, opposite, ovate-lanceolate leaves about 5 cm long. Scales beneath densely cover the leaves, giving them a silver-bronze appearance. Above, the scales are scattered and white. The bark occurs in short quilled pieces, usually with a chalky, more or less cracked, white surface, with black dots due to the fruit of lichens. The transverse fracture is reddish-brown.

Characteristics: The taste is aromatic and bitter.

Habitat: Indigenous to the West Indies, also grown in tropical areas of America.

Production: Cascarilla bark is the bark of Croton eluteria.

Other Names: Sweet Wood Bark, Sweet Bark, Bahama Cascarilla

ACTIONS AND PHARMACOLOGY

COMPOUNDS

Volatile oil (1.5 to 3%): chief components are p-cymene, limonene, alpha-thujone, pinenes, linalool, myrcene, terpeni-nol-4

Diterpene bitter principles: including Cascarillin A (15%)

Resins (25%)

EFFECTS

Cascarilla is a stimulant and a tonic.

INDICATIONS AND USAGE

Unproven Uses: Cascarilla is used for digestive disorders, diarrhea and vomiting.

PRECAUTIONS AND ADVERSE REACTIONS

Health risks or side effects following the proper administration of designated therapeutic dosages are not recorded.

DOSAGE

Mode of Administration: Available as a powder, liquid extract or tincture.

LITERATURE

Fenaroli's Handbook of Flavor Ingredients, Vol. 1, 2nd Ed., CRC Press 1975.

Hegnauer R, Chemotaxonomie der Pflanzen, Bde 1-11, Birkhäuser Verlag Basel, Boston, Berlin 1962-1997.

Kern W, List PH, Hörhammer L (Hrsg.), Hagers Handbuch der Pharmazeutischen Praxis, 4. Aufl., Bde 1-8, Springer Verlag Berlin, Heidelberg, New York, 1969.

Leung AY, Encyclopedia of Common Natural Ingredients Used in Food Drugs and Cosmetics, John Wiley & Sons Inc., New York 1980.

Mc Echean CE et al., J Chem Soc 166B:633. 1966.

Steinegger E, Hänsel R, Pharmakognosie, 5. Aufl., Springer Verlag Heidelberg 1992.

Cashew

Anacardium occidentale

DESCRIPTION

Medicinal Parts: The medicinal parts are the finely chopped bark, the cashew nut, the fresh leaves and extracted cashew oil.

Flower and Fruit: Flowers are in terminal, cyme-like, 10 to 20 cm long panicles and are polygamous. The pedicles are 2 to 3 mm long. The calyx is deeply divided into five sepals, which are lanceolate, erect, imbricate, glabrous inside and covered on the outside with short, thick, gray hairs. The corolla is 5-petaled. The petals are lineal-lanceolate, 7 to 8 mm long by 1 mm wide, acute, soft and gray-haired on the outside. The petals are glabrous and yellow with a red stripe on the inside that curls outward in the later stages. Seven to 10 stamens are fused at the base, but only one 8 to 9 mm long stamen is fertile; the sterile ones are shorter. Anthers are yellowish-white, oblong-ovate and burst open along a vertical slit. The gynoecium is obovate, 2 mm long, one-valved and elongates to a 4 mm long wedge-shaped style with a spot-like stigma. The flowers are followed by a fleshy, edible receptacle, which partly encloses the fruit. The fruit is reniform, with a smooth, pale grayish-brown drupe, about 2 to 3 cm long and 1 cm thick.

Leaves, Stem and Root: The Cashew is a broad evergreen tree from 6 to 10 m high with smooth glabrous branches, densely leafed toward the tops. It has short-petioled leaves that are alternate, coriaceous and entire-margined. The leaf blade is obovate, 12 to 14 cm by 6 to 8 cm with a prominent midrib and 10 to 14 veins that are almost parallel.

Habitat: The plant grows in the Caribbean and Central and South America; it is cultivated everywhere in the tropics, especially in Africa and India.

Production: Fruit of the Cashew tree is harvested with the stem removed.

Other Names: East Indian Almond

ACTIONS AND PHARMACOLOGY

COMPOUNDS: IN THE SEED CASE

Alkyl phenoles

Anacardic acid

Cardol

Methyl cardol

COMPOUNDS: IN THE SEEDS

Fatty oil

Chief fatty acids: oleic acid and linolenic acid

Proteins

Starch

EFFECTS

It has been demonstrated in vitro that the dried extract prepared with ethanol is effective against the gram-positive bacteria *Bacillus subtilis* and *Staphylococcus aureus.* It also acts as an astringent and cauterizing agent due to the phenolic skin stimulant (anacardic acid) found mostly in the skin of the fruit, but also in the fruit itself.

INDICATIONS AND USAGE

Unproven Uses: Cashew is used for gastrointestinal ailments in Brazil and Nigeria. Cashew shell oil and cashew fruit are used as skin stimulants and cauterizing agents for ulcers, warts and corns. In Brazil and Nigeria, the bark is used to make an astringent decoction to treat toothache and inflammation of the gums. External uses in Haiti include amenorrhea, and internally cashew is used for dysentery. Young leaves are used in the Philippines in the treatment of diarrhea, dysentery and hemorrhoids; older leaves are used as hot poultices for burns and skin disorders. Efficacy for these indications has not been documented.

Indian Medicine: Cashew bark is used for fevers, as a laxative and anthelmintic, and to treat diabetes insipidus. One particular form is used to treat snake bites. Cashew shell oil is used as a runefacient and skin stimulant in the treatment of leprosy, elephantitis, psoriasis and ring worm, in addition to warts and corns.

Homeopathic Uses: Cashew is used to treat severely itching rashes with blistering and also facial erysipelas.

PRECAUTIONS AND ADVERSE REACTIONS

The alkyl phenoles contained in the seed case of the nut are strong skin irritants. Contact between the seed case and skin can lead to erythemas with nodule and blister formation. Frequent contact can lead to rimose exanthemas. The roasted seeds eaten as cashew nuts are free of alkyl phenoles, as is the plant stalk.

DOSAGE

Mode of Administration: Available preparations include acajou oil, cashew oil, oleum anacardiae and fatty oil extracted from the seeds.

Preparation: Preparations are often compounds, particularly in homeopathy.

Homeopathic Dosage: Daily dosage is 5 drops, 1 tablet, 10 globules, every 30 to 60 minutes for acute conditions; or one of those options 1 to 3 times daily for chronic conditions. Parenterally: 1 to 2 ml 3 times daily; Ointments, rinses and poultices: 1 dessertspoon : 1/4L water 1 to 2 times daily (HAB34).

LITERATURE

Banerjee S, Rao AR, Promoting action of cashew nut shell oil in DMBA-initiated mouse skin tumour model system. Cancer Lett, 47:149-52, 1992 Feb 29.

Barroso MAT, Hort Sciences: 8:99. 1973.

Behl, Buch. In: Behl PN, Captain RM, Bedi BMS, Gupta S: Skin Irritant and Sensitizing plants found in India, PN Behl, India. 1967.

Kubo I, et al., Tyrosinase inhibitors from Anacardium occidentale. In: JNP 57(4):545. 1994.

Laurens A, Paris RR, (1976) Plant Med Phytother 11:16.

Nagaraja KV, Plant Foods Hum Nutr 37:307-311. 1987.

Nagaraja KV, Qual Plat - Plant Foods Hum Nutr 37:69-75. 1987.

Neuwinger HD, Arzneipflanzen Schwarzafrikas. In: DAZ 134(6):453. 1994.

Ogunlana EO, Ramstad E, (1975) Planta Med 27:354.

Paul VJ, Yeddanapalli LM, J Am Chem Soc 78:5675-5678. 1956.

Samant SK, Rege DV, Lebensm-Wiss Technol 22:164-168. 1989.

Smit HF, Woerdenbag HJ, Singh RH, Meulenbeld GJ, Labadie RP, Zwaving JH, Ayurvedic herbal drugs with possible cytostatic activity. J Ethnopharmacol, 47:75-84, 1995 Jul 7.

Sullivan JT, et al., (1982) Planta Med 44:175.

Tyman JHP, Anal Chem 48:30-34. 1976.

Tyman JHP, Kiong LS, Lipids 13:525-532. 1978.

Further information in:

Franca F, Lago EL, Marsden PD, Plants used in the treatment of leishmanial ulcers due to Leishmania (Viannia) braziliensis in an endemic area of Bahia Brazil. Rev Soc Bras Med Trop, 47:229-32, 1996 May-Jun.

George J, Kuttan R, Mutagenic carcinogenic and cocarcinogenic activity of cashewnut shell liquid. Cancer Lett, 47:11-6, 1997 Jan 15.

Gil RR, Lin LZ, Cordell GA, Kumar MR, Ramesh M, Reddy BM, Mohan GK, Narasimha AV, Rao A, Anacardoside from the seeds of Semecarpus anacardium. Phytochemistry, 58:405-7, 1995 May.

Hausen B, Allergiepflanzen, Pflanzenallergene, ecomed Verlagsgesellsch. mbH, Landsberg 1988.

Hänsel R, Keller K, Rimpler H, Schneider G (Hrsg.), Hagers Handbuch der Pharmazeutischen Praxis, 5. Aufl., Bde 4-6 (Drogen), Springer Verlag Berlin, Heidelberg, New York, 1992-1994.

Jurberg P, et al., Effect of Niclosamide (Bayluscide WP 70) Anacardium occidentale hexane extract and Euphorbia splendens latex on behavior of Biomphalaria glabrata (Say 1818) under laboratory conditions. Mem Inst Oswaldo Cruz, 58:191-4, 1995 Mar-Apr.

Kubo I, et al., Tyrosinase inhibitors from Anacardium occidentale. J Nat Prod 57 (1994), 545.

Laurens A, Paris RR, Plant Med Phytother 11 (1976), 16.

Lewin L, Gifte und Vergiftungen, 6. Aufl., Nachdruck, Haug Verlag, Heidelberg 1992.

Madaus G, Lehrbuch der Biologischen Arzneimittel, Bde 1-3, Nachdruck, Georg Olms Verlag Hildesheim 1979.

Mendes NM, de Oliveira AB, Guimaraes JE, Pereira JP, Katz N, Molluscacide activity of a mixture of 6-n-alkyl salicylic acids (anacardic acid) and 2 of its complexes with copper (II) and lead (II). Rev Soc Bras Med Trop, 47:217-24, 1990 Oct-Dec.

Oliver-Bever B (Ed.), Medicinal Plants of Tropical West Africa, Cambridge University Press Cambridge, London 1986.

Roth L, Daunderer M, Kormann K, Giftpflanzen, Pflanzengifte, 4. Aufl., Ecomed Fachverlag Landsberg Lech 1993.

Smit HF, Woerdenbag HJ, Singh RH, Meulenbeld GJ, Labadie RP, Zwaving JH, Ayurvedic herbal drugs with possible cytostatic activity. J Ethnopharmacol, 47:75-84, 1995 Jul 7.

Vijayalakshmi T, Muthulakshmi V, Sachdanandam P, Salubrious effect of Semecarpus anacardium against lipid peroxidative changes in adjuvant arthritis studied in rats. Mol Cell Biochem, 36:65-9, 1997 Oct.

Vijayalakshmi T, Muthulakshmi V, Sachdanandam P, Semecarpus anacardium-induced facial oedema. Br J Dermatol, 58:338-9, 1996 Aug.

Cassia fistula

See Golden Shower Tree

Cassia species

See Senna

Castanea sativa

See Spanish Chestnut

Castor Oil Plant

Ricinus communis

DESCRIPTION

Medicinal Parts: The medicinal parts are the oil extracted from the seeds, the fat extracted from the oil, the ripe seeds and the dried seeds.

Flower and Fruit: The inflorescences are terminal and almost panicled and 15 to 50 cm long. The pedicled female flowers are in the upper section and the male flowers are clustered in the lower section of the inflorescence. The male ones have a 3 to 5 part perianth with numerous, heavily branched stamens which bear up to 1,000 separate bursting anthers. The female perianth is divided in 5. The ovary is trilocular. The style has 3 red, doubly split stigma branches.

The fruit capsule is soft prickly or smooth and grooved, 1 to 2.5 cm in diameter. The capsule bursts open when ripe flinging out the large brightly speckled seeds.

Leaves, Stem and Root: Ricinus communis is an annual plant in Central Europe, a bi- or -triennial shrub in Southern Europe and a perennial tree in the tropics. There is a taproot and lateral roots near the surface. The stem is erect and hollow. As it grows older, the stem becomes green or brownish-red. The leaves are petioled, greenish or reddish, often frosted blue, and arranged in a spiral. The leaf blade is peltate, 10 to 60 cm long and wide. The blade is usually divided into palmate, ovate-oblong or lanceolate lobes. The ribs are palmate and the margins are irregularly serrate.

Habitat: The plant is cultivated widely today in the tropics and subtropics and in temperate latitudes where maize thrives.

Production: Castor Oil is fatty oil obtained from the seeds of Ricinus communis. It is obtained by mechanical harvesting followed by sorting. Fruits that open by bursting when ripen, must be harvested before ripening and then threshed.

Not to be Confused With: May be confused with the poisonous seeds of other Euphorbiaceae.

Other Names: Castor Bean, Mexico Seed, Castor Oil Plant, Castor Oil Bush, Palma Christi

ACTIONS AND PHARMACOLOGY

COMPOUNDS

CASTOR OIL SEEDS

Fatty oil (42 to 55%, see below for constituents)

Proteic substances (20 to 25%)

Lectins (0.1 to 0.7%): including ricin D (RCA-60, severely toxic), RCA-120 (less toxic)

Pyrridine alkaloids: ricinine (up to 0.3%)

Triglycerides: chief fatty acids ricinoleic acid (12-hydroxy-oleic acid, 85 to 90%)

Tocopherols (vitamin E)

EFFECTS

The laxative principle of Castor Oil is the ricinolic acid. Ricinolic acid is anti-absorptive and secretogogic. In animal experiments, stimulation of PgE2 synthesis in the small intestine was proven. The possible reason for effectiveness of ricini semen is the antimicrobial activity of the seeds (ricin is highly toxic).

INDICATIONS AND USAGE

Unproven Uses: Castor Oil is used internally in folk medicine for acute constipation, intestinal inflammation, for removal of worms, and as a form of birth control. The oil is used externally for inflammatory skin disorders, furuncles, carbuncles, abscesses, inflammation of the middle ear and headaches (poultice.)

Chinese Medicine: In China, Castor Oil is used to treat sore throat, facial paralysis, dry stool, furuncles, ulcers and festering inflammation of the skin.

Indian Medicine: In India, the drug is used for dyspeptic complaints and joint pains.

Homeopathic Uses: Ricinus communis is used to treat diarrhea.

CONTRAINDICATIONS

Castor Oil is contraindicated in intestinal obstruction, acute inflammatory intestinal diseases, appendicitis, abdominal pain of unknown origin, during pregnancy and while nursing. The drug is not to be administered to children under 12 years of age.

PRECAUTIONS AND ADVERSE REACTIONS

General: No health hazards or side effects are known in conjunction with the proper administration of designated therapeutic dosages of Castor Oil. Allergic skin rashes have been observed in rare cases.

Pregnancy: Not to be used during pregnancy.

OVERDOSAGE

Overdosage can lead to gastric irritation with nausea, vomiting, colic and severe diarrhea. Long-term use leads to loss of electrolytes, especially potassium ions. This effect may lead to hyperaldosteronism, inhibition of intestinal motility and enhancement of the effect of cardioactive steroids.

Castor beans are severely poisonous due to the toxic lectin content. The ricinus lectins disturb the function of ribosomes and thereby prevent protein synthesis. 12 castor beans are believed to be fatal for an adult. Symptoms include severe gastroenteritis with bloody vomiting and bloody diarrhea, kidney inflammation, loss of fluid and electrolytes and ultimately circulatory collapse. Death is usually the result of hypovolemic shock.

Following gastrointestinal emptying (inducement of vomiting, gastric lavage with burgundy-colored potassium permanganate solution, sodium sulfate) and installation of medicinal charcoal, the therapy for castor bean poisoning includes treating spasms with diazepam (i.v.), generous supplies of fluids, electrolyte substitution and treating possible cases of acidosis with sodium bicarbonate infusions. In case of shock, plasma volume expanders should be infused. Monitoring of kidney function and blood coagulation is essential. Papain activated with H2-S has been attempted as an antidote.

DOSAGE

Mode of Administration: Castor Oil is available as whole drug, in solid, semi-solid and in compounded pharmaceutical preparations for internal and external use.

Preparation: Industrial production using specific procedures.

Daily Dosage:
Internally — for acute constipation or as a laxative against worms, at least 5 (x2 g) or 10 (x1 g) capsules must be taken; Caster Oil is also available in compound preparations.

Externally — a paste made of ground seeds is applied to the affected skin areas twice daily. A course of treatment takes up to 15 days.

Homeopathic Dosage: 5 drops, 1 tablet or 10 globules every 30 to 60 minutes (acute) or 1 to 3 times daily (chronic); parenterally: 1 to 2 ml sc acute: 3 times daily; chronic: once a day (HAB34)

LITERATURE

Anonym, Pharmaceutical Care: ''Den Mißbrauch von Laxanzien vermeiden helfen''. In: DAZ 135(20):1867-1868. 1995.

BGA, Abwehr von Arzneimittelrisiken:Poly-(oxyethylen)-35-Rizinusöl. In: DAZ 132(33):1733. 1992.

Macfarlane N, Trop Sc 17:217-228. 1975.

Scarpa A, Guerci A, Various uses of the castor oil plant (Ricinus communis L.), a review. In: ETH 5(2):117. 1982.
Further information in:

Frohne D, Pfänder HJ: Giftpflanzen - Ein Handbuch für Apotheker, Toxikologen und Biologen, 4. Aufl., Wiss. Verlags-Ges. Stuttgart 1997.

Hänsel R, Keller K, Rimpler H, Schneider G (Hrsg.), Hagers Handbuch der Pharmazeutischen Praxis, 5. Aufl., Bde 4-6 (Drogen): Springer Verlag Berlin, Heidelberg, New York, 1992-1994.

Leung AY, Encyclopedia of Common Natural Ingredients Used in Food, Drugs, Cosmetics, John Wiley & Sons Inc., New York 1980.

Lewin L, Gifte und Vergiftungen, 6. Aufl., Nachdruck, Haug Verlag, Heidelberg 1992.

Madaus G, Lehrbuch der Biologischen Arzneimittel, Bde 1-3, Nachdruck, Georg Olms Verlag Hildesheim 1979.

Roth L, Daunderer M, Kormann K: Giftpflanzen, Pflanzengifte, 4. Aufl., Ecomed Fachverlag Landsberg Lech 1993.

Schulz R, Hänsel R, Rationale Phytotherapie, Springer Verlag Heidelberg 1996.

Steinegger E, Hänsel R, Pharmakognosie, 5. Aufl., Springer Verlag Heidelberg 1992.

Teuscher E, Lindequist U, Biogene Gifte - Biologie, Chemie, Pharmakologie, 2. Aufl., Fischer Verlag Stuttgart 1994.

Teuscher E, Biogene Arzneimittel, 5. Aufl., Wiss. Verlagsges. Stuttgart 1997.

Wagner H, Wiesenauer M, Phytotherapie. Phytopharmaka und pflanzliche Homöopathika, Fischer-Verlag, Stuttgart, Jena, New York 1995.

Cat's Claw

Uncaria tomentosa

TRADE NAMES

Cat's Claw (available from numerous manufacturers), Cat's Claw Power, Cat's Claw Inner Bark, Cat's Claw Bark

DESCRIPTION

Medicinal Parts: The medicinal part is the root bark

Flower and Fruit: The flowers are bisexual and sessil. The calyx is tubular 1 to 2 mm in length and 1 mm in diameter. The corolla is 7-12 mm long, 4 mm in diameter and contains 5 roundish lobes. The stamens are in fives and fused. The anthers are 1 mm in length; the stigma eliptical. The ovary is inferior. The fruits are elliptical, 6-8 mm in length and 4-6 mm wide.

Leaves, Stem and Root: Uncaria tomentosa is a large woody vine that sometimes reaches heights of 100 feet. The bark has longitudinal fissures and range from yellow to yellow-green in color. The leaves are simple, opposite, elliptic or ovate. They range in size from 7 to 18 cm in length and from 4 to 13 cm wide. The margins of the leaf are entire, with a roundish base.The spines are woody and occur in pairs. They are curved like a cat's and thorn-like.

Characteristics: The sap of Uncaria tomentosa is watery and has an astringent taste.

Habitat: Cat's Claw is indigenous to the rainforest areas of Central and South America

Production: Cat's Claw is harvested in the wild.

Not to be Confused With: There are several plants with the common name of Una de Gato. Confusion can occur with Anadenanthera flava, Bauhinia aculeata, Berberis goudotii, Celtis uguanae, Doxantha ungis catti, Mimosa albida, Pisonia aculeata, Rubus urticaefolius, the various Smilax species and Zanthoxylum panamensis (Obregon, 1995).

Other Names: Una de Gato, Paraguaya, Garbato, Tambor hausca, Toron

ACTIONS AND PHARMACOLOGY

COMPOUNDS

Alkaloids: including 5-alpha-carboxystrictosidine, isopteropodine, mitraphylline, isomitraphyllin, isorynchophylline, rynchophyllin

Triterpenes

Organic acids: oleanolic acid, ursolic acid

Glycosides: quinovic acid glycosides

Procyanidins: (-)-epicatechin, cinchonain 1 a, cinchonain 1b

Sterols: beta-sitosterol (60%), stigmasterol, capesterol

EFFECTS

Anti-inflammatory/Immunostimulating Effects — The sterol componants of Cat's Claw have been found to have anti-inflammatory activity (Senatore, 1989). Carrageenan-induced rat paw edema was shown to respond to per oral doses of various extracts of Cat's Claw dried root bark (Aquino, 1991). The beta-sitosterol fraction, which accounts for 60% of the total steroid content in the herb is thought to be responsible for most of the anti-inflammatory effect (Senatore, 1989). Uncaria tomentosa extract has been found to stimulate interleukin-1 and interleukin-6 production by alveolar macrophages (Lemaire, 1999).

Effects on Platelet Aggregation — Rhynchophylline, an alkaloid present in Cat's Claw, has been found to inhibit venous and cerebral thrombosis in rabbits. It has also demonstrated platelet aggregation inhibition (Chen, 1992).

Effects on Serotonin and Dopamine — In one study, rhynchophylline increased the serotonin levels in the hypothalamus and cortex of rat brain and reduced the dopamine levels in the cortex, amygdala, and spinal cord. Rhynchophylline increased the release of endogenous dopamine from 4 brain regions. The release of serotonin was increased in 2 brain regions (Shi, 1993).

Hirsutine, an alkaloid present in Uncaria tomentosa has a potent ganglion blocking effect. Hirsutine was found to block nicotine induced dopamine release in rat pheochromocytoma cells. Hirsutine was found to be equipotent to hexamethonium in blocking the inward current activated by nicotine (Nakazawa, 1991).

Antihypertensive Effects — Hirsutine has antihypertensive effects. This effect can partly be explained by the ability of hirsutine to reduce intracellular calcium levels by inhibiting calcium release from the calcium store and increasing calcium uptake into the calcium store. Hirsutine was also found to exhibit calcium channel blocking activity by inhibiting the calcium influx through voltage dependent calcium channels in the rat aorta (Horie, 1992).

Contraceptive Effect — There is only anecdotal evidence of the use of Cat's Claw in the prevention of pregnancy. In Peru, it has been used for this purpose for years in some rainforest tribes, but the amount of drug used would be considered very high. A decoction prepared from 11 to 13 pounds of the root is reduced to about 1 cup and taken at the time of menstruation. It is claimed that sterility can be maintained for 3 to 4 years after one dose (Cabieses, 1994).

Effects on Cancer — Aqueous extracts of Uncaria tomentosa suppressed cell growth through induction of apoptosis in two different human leukemic cell lines. Apoptosis was demonstrated by the fact that both DNA single and double strand breaks increased within 24 hours of treatment with the Uncaria tomentosa extract (Sheng, 1998).

INDICATIONS AND USAGE

Unproven Uses: The effects that have some scientific evidence of efficacy include antiviral, immunostimulating, and anti-inflammatory properties.

Cat's Claw has been used in folk medicine for rheumatic complaints, diarrhea, gastritis, treatment of wounds, as an adjunct to cancer treatment, asthma, menstrual irregularity and as a contraceptive.

CONTRAINDICATIONS

Cat's Claw is contraindicated in pregnancy and in nursing mothers.

PRECAUTIONS AND ADVERSE REACTIONS

General: Serum estradiol and progesterone levels may be reduced after long-term Cat's Claw use. In one study, long term use (8 weeks) of Uncaria tomentosa resulted in a precipitous drop in both estradiol and progesterone serum levels (Rodriguez, 1998).

Uncaria tomentosa prevented estrogen from binding to estrogen receptors on breast cancer cells (Salazar & Jayme, 1988).

There is one report of acute renal failure associated with Cat's Claw ingestion in a patient with systemic lupus erythematosus. Though the patient was taking several other medications at the time, Cat's Claw was the only agent that was discontinued. Urinalysis results gradually returned to baseline following discontinuation of the herb (Hilepo, 1997).

DOSAGE

Mode of Administration: Cat's Claw is available in a powder form, capsules and liquid for internal administration.

Preparation: To prepare a decoction, add 30 g of powder to 800 ml water; allow to simmer on the stove for 45 minutes or until there is about 500 ml liquid remaining. Allow to cool, then strain and refrigerate (Schauss, 1998).

How Supplied:
Capsule — 250 mg, 350 mg, 400 mg, 440 mg, 500 mg, 505 mg, 540 mg

Liquid — 4:1

Daily Dosage: The daily dosage is 250 to 1000 mg daily. The total alkaloid equivalent should be 10 to 30 mg. Decoction dosage is 60 ml once daily in the morning on an empty stomach (Schauss, 1998).

Storage: Cat's Claw should be stored at room temperature away from heat, moisture and direct light.

LITERATURE

Aquino R, De Feo V, De Simone F et al: Plant metabolites: new compounds and anti-inflammatory activity of Uncaria tomentosa. J Nat Prod 54(2):453-459. 1991.

Chen C, et al., Inhibitory effect of rhynchophylline on platelet aggregation and thrombosis. In: Chung Kuo Yao Li Hsueh Pao, 13(2);126-30, Mar, 1992.

Cabieses, Fernando, The saga of the Cat's Claw, In: Via Lactera Editores: Lima, Peru, 1994.

Hilepo JN, Bellucci AG & Mossey RT: Acute renal failure caused by "cat's claw" herbal remedy in a patient with systemic lupus erythematosus (letter). Nephron 77(3):361-369. 1997.

Horie S, et al., Effects of hirsutine, an antihypertensive indole alkaloid from Uncaria rhynchophylla, on intracellular calcium in rat thoracic aorta. In: Life Sci, 50(7):491-8, 1992.

Lemaire I, Assinewe V, Cano P et al: Stimulation of interleukin-1 and -6 production in alveolar macrophages by the neotropical liana, Uncaria tomentosa (una de gato). J Ethnopharmacol 64(2):109-115. 1999.

Nakazawa K, et al., Inhibition of ion channels by hirsutine in rat pheochromocytoma cells. In: Jpn J Pharmacol, 57(4):507-15, Dec, 1991.

Obregon LE: Identificacion correcta de "una de gato" (genero Uncaria). Natura Medicatrix 40(summer):28-30. 1995.

Rodriguez H, Massey PJ, Rodriguez K et al: Inhibition of steroid hormone production by a nutrition supplement "una de gato" or "cat's claw." Biol Reprod 58(1):208. 1998.

Salazar EL & Jayme V: Depletion of specific binding sites for estrogen receptor by Uncaria tomentosa. Proc Western Pharmacol Soc 41:123-124. 1998.

Schauss AG: Cat's Claw (Uncaria tomentosa). Nat Med J 1998; 1(2):16-19.

Senatore A, Cataldo A, Iaccarino FP et al: Ricerche fitochimiche e biologiche sull? Uncaria tomentosa (Italian). Boll Soc Ital Biol Sper 65:517-520. 1989.

Sheng Y, Pero RW, Amiri A et al: Induction of apoptosis and inhibition of proliferation in human tumor cells treated with extracts of Uncaria tomentosa. Anticancer Res 18(5A):3363-3368. 1998.

Shi J, et al., Effects of rhynchophylline on motor activity of mice and serotonin and dopamine in rat brain. In: Chung Kuo Yao Li Hsueh Pao, 14(2):114-117, Mar, 1993.

Cat's Foot

Antennaria dioica

DESCRIPTION

Medicinal Parts: The medicinal part is the flower.

Flower and Fruit: The plant has bright red and white, dioecious composite flowers. They are very small and are in terminal cymes. The female flowers are bright red with thread-like, cylindrical corolla. The male flowers are white with a funnel-shaped corolla. The bracts of the male are white, the female, pink. The fruit has a tuft of hair.

Leaves, Stem and Root: The plant is 7 to 20 cm tall, with leafy rooting runners. The stem is erect with basal leaves that are spatulate, green above, gray beneath, cauline, linear and erect.

Habitat: Cat's Foot is found in Europe, Asia and America as far north as the Arctic.

Production: Cat's Foot flower consists of the fresh or dried flowers of Antennaria dioica.

Not to be Confused With: Occasional confusion occurs with the flower heads of Helichrysum stoechas or Helichrysum angustifolium.

Other Names: Mountain Everlasting, Life Everlasting, Cudweed

ACTIONS AND PHARMACOLOGY

COMPOUNDS

Anthracene derivatives

Flavonoids: including luteolin and its glucosides

Bitter substances

Mucilages

Saponins

Tannins

EFFECTS

In animal tests, a mild spasmolytic and choleric effect has been reported.

INDICATIONS AND USAGE

Unproven Uses: In folk medicine, preparations of Cat's Foot flower are used as a diuretic, for diarrhea, and to treat respiratory and intestinal diseases.

PRECAUTIONS AND ADVERSE REACTIONS

No health hazards or side effects are known in conjunction with the proper administration of designated therapeutic dosages.

DOSAGE

Mode of Administration: Since the efficacy for the claimed uses is not documented, a therapeutic application cannot be recommended.

Preparation: To prepare an infusion, pour boiling water over 1 gm finely cut drug, then strain after 5 to 10 minutes.

LITERATURE

Delaveau P, et al., (1980) Planta Med 40:49.

Didry N, et al., (1982) Ann Pharm Fr 40 (1):75.

Kern W, List PH, Hörhammer L (Hrsg.), Hagers Handbuch der Pharmazeutischen Praxis, 4. Aufl., Bde. 1-8, Springer Verlag Berlin, Heidelberg, New York, 1969.

Swiatek L, et al., (1982) Planta Med 30:153, 12P.

Catechu

Acacia catechu

DESCRIPTION

Medicinal Parts: Black catechu is extracted from the heartwood in a process of distillation and is used in a variety of preparations.

Flower and Fruit: The flowers grow in closely sitting spikes from the leaf axils. The calyx is about 1 to 2 mm and covered in gray hairs. The corolla is yellow. The pod is about 10 to 15 cm long, dark brown and veined with 6 to 8 seeds.

Leaves, Stem and Root: Acacia catechu is a medium-sized tree with brown bark and downy-haired branches. The leaf stems of the double-pinnate leaves are about 15 cm long and have glands at the base and between the upper 5 to 7 cm long fronds. The leaflets are sessile, close, pale green and smaller than 1 cm. There are a few short thorns in pairs.

Habitat: The plant is indigenous to India and Burma.

Production: The heartwood is ground and boiled in water for 12 hours. The wood residue is removed and the extract steamed to the consistency of a syrup. The syrup is stirred and cooled in molds. The dried mass is broken up into irregular pieces.

Not to be Confused With: Haematoxylon campechium and the seeds of Areca catechu, tar products and admixtures of earth, alumen, iron carbonate and sand.

Other Names: Cutch

ACTIONS AND PHARMACOLOGY

COMPOUNDS

Catechins (2-12%): (+)- and (-)-catechin, (+)- and (-)-epicatechin

Catechin tannins (20-60%)

EFFECTS

Catechu is an astringent and antiseptic.

INDICATIONS AND USAGE

Unproven Uses: Internally, Catechu is used for chronic catarrh of the mucous membranes, dysentery and bleeding. Externally, Catechu is a constituent of tooth tinctures, mouth washes and gargles. It is used externally in hemostatic powders, dressing solutions and injection solutions. It is also used for colitis mucosa, gingivitis, stomatitis and pharyngitis.

Indian Medicine: Catechu is a constituent of preparations for mouth ulcers, throat infections and toothache.

Chinese Medicine: The drug is used for poorly healing ulcers, weeping skin diseases, oral ulcers with bleeding and traumatic injuries.

PRECAUTIONS AND ADVERSE REACTIONS

No health hazards or side effects are known in conjunction with the proper administration of designated therapeutic dosages.

DOSAGE

Mode of Administration: Catechu tincture can be painted on mucous membranes or used for mouth washes.

Preparation: Catechu tincture.

Daily Dosage: The average daily dose of the drug is 0.3 to 2 gm to be taken orally, 3 times daily; single dose is 0.5 gm.

Twenty drops of Catechu tincture is added to a glass of lukewarm water for use as a mouthwash, or the tincture may be applied with a brush in undiluted form to affected mucous membranes.

LITERATURE

Sham JSK et al., (1984) Planta Med 2:177.

Further information in:

Hänsel R, Keller K, Rimpler H, Schneider G (Hrsg.), Hagers Handbuch der Pharmazeutischen Praxis, 5. Aufl., Bde 4-6 (Drogen), Springer Verlag Berlin, Heidelberg, New York, 1992-1994.

Leung AY, Encyclopedia of Common Natural Ingredients Used in Food, Drugs and Cosmetics, John Wiley & Sons Inc., New York 1980.

Catha edulis

See Khat

Catnip

Nepeta cataria

TRADE NAMES

Catnip is available from numerous manufacturers, sometimes as Catnip Leaf, Catnip Herb or Catnip Herb Liquid.

DESCRIPTION

Medicinal Parts: The medicinal parts are the aerial parts of the plant.

Flower and Fruit: The inflorescence is spike-like and the lower verticillasters distant from each other. The small individual flowers are on short pedicles. The bracts are 1.5 to 3 mm and linear-awl-shaped. The sepals are 5 to 6.5 mm long and ovate. The tips are 1.5 to 2.5 mm long, linear-lanceolate and patent. The corolla is 7 to 10 mm long, slightly longer than the calyx and white with small purple spots.

Leaves, Stem and Root: The root of the plant is perennial. The stems are up to 1 m high, angular, erect and branched. They are leafy and gray-pubescent to tomentose, which gives the entire plant a whitish-gray appearance. The leaves are 2 to 8 cm, ovate, cordate at the base, crenate or serrate and gray-tomentose beneath. The petiole is 0.5 to 4 cm in length.

Characteristics: The plant has a characteristic aromatic scent, reminiscent of Mint and Pennyroyal.

Habitat: Catnip is indigenous to Europe and naturalized in the U.S.

Production: Catnip is the aerial part of Nepeta cataria. The harvesting of uncultivated plants takes place during the flowering season. The drug is manually cut during dry and sunny weather. The woodless parts of the plant are sorted out and the usable material is then left to dry in the shade.

Other Names: Catnep, Catrup, Catmint, Catswort, Field Balm

ACTIONS AND PHARMACOLOGY

COMPOUNDS

Volatile oil (0.2-0.7%): chief components are nepetalactone (share 80-95%), additionally including among others epi-nepetalactone, caryophyllene, camphor, thymol, carvacrol, pulegone

EFFECTS

Active agents are bitter and tannin substances, as well as essential oil. Catnip is considered to have antipyretic, refrigerant, antispasmodic, sedative and diaphoretic effects. The tea has a diuretic effect and increases gallbladder activity.

INDICATIONS AND USAGE

Unproven Uses: Folk medicine uses include treatment of colds, colic and fevers. It is also used for nervous disorders and migraine, since preparations from the mint have a calming effect. It is also used in the treatment of gynecological disorders. Nepeta cataria has a long tradition in England and France as a kitchen and medicinal herb and was used occasionally as a stimulating drink until the introduction of black tea.

CONTRAINDICATIONS

Catnip is not to be taken during pregnancy.

PRECAUTIONS AND ADVERSE REACTIONS

No health hazards or side effects are known in conjunction with the proper administration of designated therapeutic dosages.

DOSAGE

Mode of Administration: Orally in ground and dried forms. Flowers are usually ingested in tea form, because the important constituent elements are to some extent volatile.

How Supplied:

Capsules — 380 mg

Fluid extract — 1:1

Liquid — 1:01

Preparation: To prepare an infusion (tea), add 10 dessert-spoonfuls per liter of water, leave this to steep for 10 minutes, then strain.

Daily Dosage: 2 to 3 cups of the tea daily.

LITERATURE

Harvey JW et al., (1978) Lloydia 41:367.

Hatch RC, (1972) Amer J Vet Res 33:143.

Margolis JS, In: Complete Book of Recreational Drugs, Cliff House Books USA 1978.

Roitman JN, (1981) Lancet I:944.

Sakan T et al., (1967) Tetrahedron 23:4635.

Sastry SD et al., (1972) Phytochemistry 11:453.

Sherry CJ et al., (1981) Quart J Crude Drug Res 19(1):31.

Tagawa M, Murai F, (1983) Planta Med 47:109.

Young LA et al., In: Recreational Drugs, Berkeley Publishing Co. USA 1977.

Further information in:

Clark IM, Forde BG, Hallahan DL, Spatially distinct expression of two new cytochrome P450s in leaves of Nepeta racemosa: identification of a trichome-specific isoform. Plant Mol Biol, 33:875-85. Mar 1997.

Hallahan DL et al., Purification and characterization of an acyclic monoterpene primary alcohol:NADP+ oxidoreductase from catmint (Nepeta racemosa). Arch Biochem Biophys, 33:105-12. Apr 1, 1995.

Hegnauer R, Chemotaxonomie der Pflanzen, Bde 1-11, Birkhäuser Verlag Basel, Boston, Berlin 1962-1997.

Kern W, List PH, Hörhammer L (Hrsg.), Hagers Handbuch der Pharmazeutischen Praxis, 4. Aufl., Bde. 1-8, Springer Verlag Berlin, Heidelberg, New York, 1969.

Massoco CO, Silva MR, Gorniak SL, Spinosa MS, Bernardi MM Behavioral effects of acute and long-term administration of catnip (Nepeta cataria) in mice. Vet Hum Toxicol, 33:530-3. Dec 1995.

Osterhoudt KC, Lee SK, Callahan JM, Henretig FM, Catnip and the alteration of human consciousness. Vet Hum Toxicol, 33:373-5. Dec 1997.

Simon E, Chadwick AF, Craker LE (Eds.), Herbs. An Indexed Bibliography 1971-80 Archon Books USA 1984.

Steinegger E, Hänsel R, Pharmakognosie, 5. Aufl., Springer Verlag Heidelberg 1992.

Teuscher E, Lindequist U, Biogene Gifte - Biologie, Chemie, Pharmakologie, 2. Aufl., Fischer Verlag Stuttgart 1994.

Caulophyllum thalictroides

See Blue Cohosh

Cayenne

Capsicum species

TRADE NAMES

Cayenne (available from numerous manafacturers), Cayenne Herbal, Cayenne Peppers, Cayenne 30,000 Heat Units, Premium Cayenne, Cayenne Power Herb, Cayenne 40,000 BTU, Natural Herbal Cayenne, Zostrix

DESCRIPTION

Medicinal Parts: The fresh or dried fruits of different Capsicum species are used medicinally.

Flower and Fruit: The flowers are usually solitary, but may occasionally be in pairs or in threes. They are hanging and long-pedicled. The calyx is semi-globose to campanulate and has 5 to 7 tips. The corolla is wheel-shaped with a short tube, varying in color from white to yellow, occasionally from purple to violet with whitish-green or violet markings. There are 5 to 6 stamens with violet anthers and 5 small papillous staminoids. The ovary is superior. The dividing walls are partially underdeveloped. The seed carriers at the top are attached to the walls and fused to a column below. The berry is 1.5 to 5 cm long and up to 9 cm thick; it varies in form. The calyx remains. The wall of the fruit is tough and leathery and may be red, yellow-green or brownish. The seeds are numerous, light, yellowish-white, flat, disc, circular or kidney-shaped and thickened at the margins. The surface is pitted.

Leaves, Stem and Root: Capsicum annum is an annual (perennial in the tropics) 20 to 100 cm high plant with an erect stem, which is somewhat woody and angular. It is sparsely branched higher up. The leaves are usually solitary, long-petioled, oval, lanceolate to ovate, obtusely accuminate, wedge-shaped at the base, entire-margined or slightly curved and glabrous.

Habitat: The herb is indigenous to Mexico and Central America and is cultivated today in warmer regions of the globe.

Production: Paprika consists of the dried ripe fruit of Capsicum anuum or Capsicum fructescens. The fruit is harvested when completely ripe and dried at a maximum temperature of 35° C.

Not to be Confused With: Other varieties of Capsicum anuum.

Other Names: Capsicum, Grains of Paradise, African Pepper, Bird Pepper, Chili Pepper, Sweet Pepper, Hungarian Pepper, Red Pepper, Goat's Pod, Zanzibar Pepper, Paprika, Tabasco Pepper, chilies, Chili

ACTIONS AND PHARMACOLOGY

COMPOUNDS

Capsaicinoids (amides of the vanillyl amine with C8 - C13-fatty acids): chief components capsaicin (32-38%), dihydrocapsaicin (18-52%)

Carotinoids (0.3-0.8%): in particular capsanthin (dark red), alpha-carotin, violaxanthine, free or as fatty acid esters

Flavonoids: including apiin, luteolin-7-O-glucoside

Steroid saponins: mixture referred to as capsicidine, in the seeds

Volatile oil (0.1%): 2-methoxy-3-isobutyl pyrazine and N-(13-methyl tetradecyl)acetamide (capsiamide)

EFFECTS

Pain Modulation

The most important active ingredient in the herb is the capsaicin, which exerts hyperemic effects. Cutaneous nociceptors are also known as peripheral sensory neurons of primary sensory neurons activated by noxious stimuli (Biro, 1997; Nakamura, 1999). Peripheral fibers produce a local response consisting of edema, redness and vasodilation, while afferent fibers relay nocioceptive information to the central nervous system resulting in the perception of pain and burning. Long-term desensitization of the fibers occurs after repeated exposure to capsaicin, and results in a subsequent loss of pain sensation (Appendino, 1997).

Capsaicin binds to the C-type vanilloid receptor (VR1) and opens a cationic channel allowing the influx of calcium. The calcium influx is an excitatory response, which initiates release of neuropeptides (substance P). The neuropeptides are responsible for chemogenic pain, thermoregulation and neurogenic inflammation. By blocking the calcium channel, there will be a depletion of substance P in the sensory nerves and loss of pain (Appendino, 1997; Biro, 1997; Jung, 1999).

Antimicrobial

Capsaicin and dihydrocapsaicin have antimicrobial effects against *Bacillus cereus, Bacillus subtilis, Clostridium sporogenes, Clostridium tetani*, and *Streptococcus pyogenes* (Cichewicz, 1996). Capsaicin has shown bactericidal activity against *H. pylori* and therefore, could have a protective effect against *H. pylori*-associated gastroduodenal disease (Jones, 1997). A recent study using capsaicin from jalapeno peppers did not support the role for jalapenos in the treatment of *H. pylori* infection (Graham, 1999).

Antineoplastic

Capsaicin, once thought to be carcinogenic, has been shown to not cause any significant increase in papilloma formation, abnormal hyperplasia or inflammatory lesions. The drug does not induce the epidermal ornithine decarboxylase activity, suggesting that it lacks tumor-promotional activity (Park, 1997; Park, 1998). Chemoprotective effects of capsaicin and dihydrocapsaicin include the inhibition of microsomal monooxygenases involved in carcinogen activation (Surh, 1995).

Detoxification/Gastroprotective/Thrombolytic Effects

Capsaicin and dihydrocapsaicin have detoxification activity with pharmacologically active substances by interacting irreversibly with hepatic drug metabolizing enzymes (Surh, 1995). Capsaicin has a gastroprotective effect against gastric mucosal injury caused by aspirin (Yeoh, 1995). Capsicum has been found to induce increased fibrinolytic activity and simultaneously cause hypocoagulability of blood (Visudhiphan, 1982).

Many documented trials are based on observations of various extracts of the drug. The initial local effect is pain, then warmth, then hypersensitivity; reversible or irreversible peripheral nerve damage is possible.

CLINICAL TRIALS

Pain Modulation

The efficacy of topical capsaicin was determined in 22 patients with chronic severe painful diabetic neuropathy over an 8-week study period. The randomized, placebo-controlled study demonstrated a significant improvement with capsaicin 0.75% applied 4 times daily for the overall clinical improvement of pain status, as measured by physician's global evaluation and by a categorical pain severity scale. The capsaicin treatment group had a 16% decrease in mean pain intensity by a visual analogue scale (VAS) versus 4.1% decrease with the placebo group. The capsaicin treatment group had a 44.6% decrease in mean pain relief on VAS versus 23.2% decrease with the placebo group. Approximately 50% of subjects reported improved pain control or were cured in a follow-up, open-label study, and 25% were unchanged or worse (Tandan, 1992).

Gastroprotective Effects

The efficacy of capsaicin as a gastroprotective agent was determined in 18 healthy volunteers with normal index endoscopies. The volunteers underwent two studies four weeks apart to evaluate the effect of capsaicin against aspirin-induced gastric mucosal injury. Each volunteer took 20 g chili orally with 200 ml water in one study and 200 ml water in another study. After 30 minutes, each case was followed with 600 mg aspirin with 200 ml water. Endoscopy was repeated 6 hours later, and the gastroduodenal mucosal damage was assessed by a previously validated scoring system. The median gastric injury score in the chili group was significantly less, demonstrating a gastroprotective effect of chili in human subjects (Yeoh, 1995).

INDICATIONS AND USAGE

Approved by Commission E:

- Muscular tensions
- Rheumatism

Unproven Uses: Cayenne is used for painful muscle spasms in areas of shoulder, arm and spine. In folk medicine the herb is used for frostbite, chronic lumbago and as a gargle for hoarseness, sore throats and infected throats. The drug is also used internally for gastrointestinal disorders, seasickness and as prophylactic therapy for arteriosclerosis, stroke and heart disease.

The herb is used in cream form for circulation and as a female orgasm stimulant. Use should be limited to 2 days, and should only be used again after 2 weeks. Longer usage can cause festering dermatitis, blistering and ulceration (See PRECAUTIONS).

Indian Medicine: Cayenne is used for gout, arthritis, sciatica, coughs and hoarseness. It has been used for lowering the temperature in malaria, yellow fever, scarlet fever and typhus. It is used for cholera, edema and anorexia nervosa. It is used in compound preparations for loss of appetite, dyspepsia and diarrhea (tablets 1:1:1; Cayenne pepper, rhubarb and ginger root) and for alcoholism as an infusion (Cayenne pepper with sugar and cinnamon) to reduce the desire for alcohol.

Homeopathic Uses: The herb is used for inflammation of the efferent urinary tract, the alimentary canal, the mouth and throat, and middle ear infection.

PRECAUTIONS AND ADVERSE REACTIONS

General: There has not yet been a final determination of possible health hazards or side effects in conjunction with the proper administration of designated therapeutic dosages. Internal administration may increase gastrointestinal peristalsis resulting in diarrhea, intestinal and gallstone colics. Besides the intended stimulating effect, external applications can lead to blister and ulcer formation. Investigations into mutagenicity, teratogenicity and carcinogenicity yielded contradictory results. **Warning: Use should be limited to 2 days and should only be used again after 2 weeks. Keep away from the eyes!**

Hematologic Effects: Capsicum has been found to induce increased fibrinolytic activity and simultaneously cause hypocoagulability of blood (Visudhiphan, 1982).

Hypersensitivity: Anaphylaxis and rhinoconjunctivitis symptoms have been associated with the herb due to its antigenic components (Jensen-Jarolim, 1998; Vega de la Osada, 1998). Contact dermatitis has been reported from the direct handling of chili peppers containing capsaicin (Williams, 1995). A hypersensitivity reaction known as plasma cell gingivitis may occur with the herb, and may cause severe gingival inflammation, discomfort and bleeding (Serio, 1991). One study suggest the allergy is rarely an autonomous sensitization, but rather a consequence of pollen allergy on the basis of immunologic cross-reactivity (Ebner, 1998).

Respiratory Effects: Alveobronchiolitis and fibrotic changes have occurred as a result of a respirable paprika dust preparation used after a single intratracheal dose (Tatrai, 1992). Chronic exposure to chili peppers has been associated with an increase in cough (Blanc, 1991).

Drug Interactions: Aspirin and salicylic acid compounds-The bioavailabilities of aspirin (acetylsalicylic acid) and of salicylic acid were reduced when given concomitantly with Capsicum annuum extract, containing 100 mg of capsaicin per gram as a result of the gastrointestinal effects of capsaicin (Cruz, 1999).

OVERDOSAGE

Toxic dosages lead to life-threatening hypothemias by affecting the thermoreceptors. High doses of the drug (or the herb) administered over extended periods can cause chronic gastritis, kidney damage, liver damage and neurotoxic effects. The treatment for poisonings proceeds symptomatically.

DOSAGE

Mode of Administration: Preparations of Cayenne are exclusively for external indications in antirheumatic ointments and plasters.

How Supplied:
Capsules—400 mg, 445 mg, 450 mg, 455 mg, 500 mg

Cream—0.25% capsaicin, 0.75% capsaicin

Preparation: A liquid extract is prepared by percolating 100 gm drug with 60 gm ethanol. Other formulations include: Capsicum-oleoresin with 90% ethanol and a tincture with 90% ethanol.

Daily Dosage: External daily dose: 10 gm drug; Tincture: (1:10); Semi-solid preparations: maximum 50 mg capsaicin in 100 gm neutral base. The cream is applied to the affected area not more than 3 or 4 times daily (Zostrix Package Insert, 1998).

Internal application: Decoction: 1/2 liter water with 5 gm powdered drug, 3 gm powdered cascarilla bark and 5 gm powdered rhubarb root; 2 cups per day.

Homeopathic Dosage: 5 drops, 1 tablet or 10 globules every 30 to 60 minutes (acute) or 1 to 3 times a day (chronic); ointment: once or twice daily (HAB1)

Storage: Should be well sealed and protected from light.

LITERATURE

Anonym, Behandlung chronischer Schmerzen: Capsaicin - Lichtblick für Schmerzpatienten. In: DAZ 137(13):1027-1028. 1997.

Anonym, Phytotherapie:Pflanzliche Antirheumatika - was bringen sie? In: DAZ 136(45):4012-4015. 1996.

Bascom R, Kageysobotka A, Prous D, Effect of intranasal capsaicin on symptoms and mediator release. In: J Pharmacol Exp Ther 259(3):1323. 1991.

Biro T, Acs G, Acs P et al., Receptor advances in understanding of vanilloid receptors: a therapeutic target for treatment of pain and inflammation in skin. J Invest Dermatol 1997; 2:56-60.

Blanc P, Liu D, Juarez C, Boushey HA, Cough in hot pepper workers. Chest 1991 Jan;99(1):27-32.

Camara B, Moneger R, (1978) Phytochemistry 17:91.

Cichewicz RH, Thorpe PA, The antimicrobial properties of chile peppers (Capsicum species) and their uses in Mayan medicine. J Ethnopharmacol 1996; 52:61-70.

Cruz L, Castaneda-Hernandez G, Navarrete A et al., Ingestion of chili pepper (Capsicum annuum) reduces salicylate bioavailability after oral aspirin administration in the rat. Can J Physiol Pharmacol 1999 Jun;77(6):441-6.

Ebner C, Jensen-Jarolim E, Leitner A, Breiteneder H, Characterization of allergens in plant-derived spices: Apiaceae spices, pepper (Piperaceae), and paprika (bell peppers, Solanaceae). Allergy 1998;53(46 Suppl):52-4.

Fusco BM, Fiore G, Gallo F et al., 'Capsaicin-sensitive' sensory neurons in cluster headache: pathophysiological aspects and therapeutic indication. Headache 1994 Mar;34(3):132-7.

Gal IE, (1967) Pharmazie 22:120.

Graham DY, Anderson SY, Lang T et al., Garlic or jalapeno peppers for treatment of Helicobacter pylori infection. Am J Gastroenterol 1999 May;94(5):1200-2.

Jensen-Jarolim E, Santner B, Leitner A et al., Bell peppers (Capsicum annuum) express allergens (profilin, pathogenesis-related protein P23 and Bet v 1) depending on the horticultural strain. Int Arch Allergy Immunol 1998 Jun;116(2):103-9.

Jung J, Hwang S, Kwak J et al., Capsaicin binds to the intracellular domain of the capsaicin-activated ion channel. J Neurosci 1999 Jan 15;19(2):529-38.

Kohane D, Kuang Y, Lu N et al., Vanilloid receptor agonists potentiate the in vivo local anesthetic activity of percutaneously injected site 1 sodium channel blockers. Anesthesiology 1999 Feb;90(2):524-34.

Kreymeier J, Rheumatherapie mit Phytopharmaka. In: DAZ 137(8):611-613. 1997.

Masada Y et al., (1971) J Food Sci 36:858.

Monsereenusorn Y et al., (1982) Crit Rev Toxicol 10:321.

Nakamura A, Shiomi H, Recent advances in neuropharmacology of cutaneous nociceptors. Jpn J Pharmacol 1999 Apr;79(4):427-31.

Park KK, Surh YJ, Effects of capsaicin on chemically induced two-stage mouse skin carcinogenesis. Cancer Lett 1997 Mar 19;114(1-2):183-4.

Park K, Chun K, Yook, Surh Y, Lack of tumor promoting activity of capsaicin, a principal pungent ingredient of red pepper, in mouse skin carcinogenesis. Anticancer Res 1998 Nov-Dec;18(6A):4201-5.

Surh YJ & Lee SS, Capsaicin, a double-edged sword: toxicity, metabolism and chemopreventive potential. Life Sci 1995; 56:1845-1855.

Surh YJ, Lee RC, Park KK, Mayne ST et al., Chemoprotective effects of capsaicin and diallyl sulfide against mutagenesis or tumorigenesis by vinyl carbamate and N-nitrosodimethylamine. Carcinogenesis 1995 Oct;16(10):2467-71.

Surh YJ, Ahn SH, Kim KC et al., Metabolism of capsaicinoids: evidence for aliphatic hydroxylation and its pharmacological implications. Life Sci 1995 Mar 10;56(16):PL305-11.

Surh YJ & Lee SS, Capsaicin in hot chili pepper: carcinogen, co-carcinogen or anticarcinogen? Fd Chem Toxic 1996; 34:313-316.

Vega de la Osada F, Esteve Drauel P, Alonso Lebrero E, et al., Sensitization to paprika: anaphylaxis after intake and rhinoconjunctivitis after contact through airways. Med Clin (Barc) 1998 Sep 12;111(7):263-6.

Williams S, Clark R, Dunford J, Contact dermatitis associated with capsaicin: Hunan hand syndrome. Ann Emerg Med 1995 May;25(5):713-5.

Yeoh KG, Kang JY, Yap I et al., Chili protects against aspirin-induced gastroduodenal mucosal injury in humans. Dig Dis Sci 1995 Mar;40(3):580-3.

FURTHER INFORMATION IN:

Hänsel R, Keller K, Rimpler H, Schneider G (Hrsg.), Hagers Handbuch der Pharmazeutischen Praxis, 5. Aufl., Bde 4-6 (Drogen): Springer Verlag Berlin, Heidelberg, New York, 1992-1994.

Leung AY, Encyclopedia of Common Natural Ingredients Used in Food Drugs and Cosmetics, John Wiley & Sons Inc., New York 1980.

Lewin L, Gifte und Vergiftungen, 6. Aufl., Nachdruck, Haug Verlag, Heidelberg 1992.

Madaus G, Lehrbuch der Biologischen Arzneimittel, Bde 1-3, Nachdruck, Georg Olms Verlag Hildesheim 1979.

Roth L, Daunderer M, Kormann K, Giftpflanzen, Pflanzengifte, 4. Aufl., Ecomed Fachverlag Landsberg Lech 1993.

Steinegger E, Hänsel R, Pharmakognosie, 5. Aufl., Springer Verlag Heidelberg 1992.

Tandan R, Lewis G, Krusinski P et al., Topical capsaicin in painful diabetic neuropathy. Controlled study with long-term follow-up. Diabetes Care 1992 Oct;15(10):1434.

Teuscher E, Lindequist U, Biogene Gifte - Biologie, Chemie, Pharmakologie, 2. Aufl., Fischer Verlag Stuttgart 1994.

Teuscher E, Biogene Arzneimittel, 5. Aufl., Wiss. Verlagsges. mbH Stuttgart 1997.

Wagner H, Wiesenauer M, Phytotherapie. Phytopharmaka und pflanzliche Homöopathika, Fischer-Verlag, Stuttgart, Jena, New York 1995.

Wichtl M (Hrsg.), Teedrogen, 4. Aufl., Wiss. Verlagsges. Stuttgart 1997.

Ceanothus americanus

See New Jersey Tea

Cedar

Cedrus libani

DESCRIPTION

Medicinal Parts: The medicinal parts are the leaves, the wood and the oil.

Flower and Fruit: The male cones are 3 to 5 cm; the female cones are 7 to 12 cm and almost cylindrical-truncate or umbilicate at the apex.

Leaves, Stem and Root: The cedar is a majestic tree that grows up to 40 m in height with a rigid leading shoot and a flat crown. The young branches are glabrous. The needle-like leaves are dark green and 20 to 30 mm long.

Habitat: The Lebanon Cedar is indigenous to the Lebanese mountains and the southwest of Turkey, Cyprus, the Atlas Mountains and the Himalayas. The tree is also found in Asia and Africa.

Production: Cedar oil is the essential oil extracted from the leaves and wood of Cedrus libani.

ACTIONS AND PHARMACOLOGY

COMPOUNDS

When extracted from Cedrus libani (true cedarwood oil): borneol

When extracted from Cedrus atlantica (atlas cedarwood oil): cadinene, alpha- and gamma-atlantone

When extracted from Cedrus deodora (Himalayan cedarwood oil): alpha- and gamma-atlantone, p-methyl-delta-3-tetrahydroacetophenone, (+)-longiborneol, himachalol, all-ohimachalol

EFFECTS

Cedar has an expectorant effect.

INDICATIONS AND USAGE

Unproven Uses: Cedar wood oil is used for catarrhal conditions of the respiratory tract.

PRECAUTIONS AND ADVERSE REACTIONS

No health hazards or side effects are known in conjunction with the proper administration of designated therapeutic dosages.

DOSAGE

Mode of Administration: Externally, the drug is used as a rub (Bormelin balm). It is also used internally as an inhalation.

LITERATURE

Kern W, List PH, Hörhammer L (Hrsg.), Hagers Handbuch der Pharmazeutischen Praxis, 4. Aufl., Bde. 1-8, Springer Verlag Berlin, Heidelberg, New York, 1969.

Cedrus libani

See Cedar

Celandine

Chelidonium majus

DESCRIPTION

Medicinal Parts: The medicinal parts are the aerial parts that have been collected during the flowering season and dried. The root, which has been collected in late autumn and dried, and the fresh rhizome are also used medicinally.

Flower and Fruit: The plant has yellow flowers arranged in umbels. There are 2 sepals, 4 petals, numerous yellow stamens and 1 ovary. The fruit is pod-like and many-seeded. The seeds are black-brown and glossy.

Leaves, Stem and Root: Celandine is a 30 to 120 cm high plant with an erect stem. The stem has irregularly bifurcated, thickened nodes. The leaves are alternate and indent-pinnatifid. The upper leaves are pinnatisect, dull green above, sea-green beneath. The plant contains a dark-yellow latex.

Characteristics: Celandine has a hot and bitter taste. The latex has a narcotic fragrance.

Habitat: Celandine is found throughout Europe and the temperate and subarctic regions of Asia.

Production: Celandine herb consists of the dried, above ground parts of Chelidonium majus gathered during flowering season. The herb is collected in the wild during the flowering season and dried at high temperatures.

Greater Celandine root is the root, harvested between August and October, of Chelidonium majus. The herb is gathered in uncultivated regions and harvested commercially.

Other Names: Tetterwort

ACTIONS AND PHARMACOLOGY

COMPOUNDS: CELANDINE HERB

Isoquinoline alkaloids of the protoberberine type: including coptisine (main alkaloid), berberine

Isoquinoline alkaloids of the benzophenanthridine type: including chelidonine, sanguinarine, chelerythrine

Isoquinoline alkaloids of the protopine type: including protopin, cryptopine

Caffeic acid derivatives: including 2-(-)-coffeoyl-D-glyceric acid, coffeoyl-L-malic acid

EFFECTS: CELANDINE HERB
Celandine has mild analgesic, cholagogic, antimicrobial, oncostatic and central-sedative effects. It also acts as a spasmolytic on smooth muscles. In animal tests, Celandine is a cytostatic. It also has a nonspecific immune-stimulating effect.

Note: The blood pressure-lowering effects and the therapeutic efficacy for mild forms of hypertonia (borderline hypertonia) need further investigation.

COMPOUNDS: CELANDINE ROOT
Isoquinoline alkaloids of the protoberberine type: including coptisine (main alkaloid), berberine

Isoquinoline alkaloids of the benzophenanthridine type: including chelidonine, sanguinarine, chelerythrin

Isoquinoline alkaloids of the protopine-type: including protopin, cryptopine

Caffeic acid derivatives: including 2-(-)-coffeoyl-D-glyceric acid, coffeoyl-L-malic acid

EFFECTS: CELANDINE ROOT
Only clinical studies and experiments on the fresh plants are available. However, previous studies have shown that the extract, with an alkaloid content of 80%, should have similar effects to those of the fresh leaves. These effects include immobilization in mice, when it was applied subcutaneously and orally. On rabbit intestines it caused limpness; and in higher doses, tone reduction. When applied to the rabbit uterus, it caused contraction of the smooth muscle. Positive inotropic effects were observed in isolated cat and frog hearts; in a canine heart-lung preparation it stimulated the heart, raised blood pressure and widened the arteries.

Experimental data are unavailable, therefore the results must be considered unofficial.

An oncostatic effect was observed through the cytotoxic results of Eagle's 9 KB carcinoma of the naso-pharynx in cell cultures.

INDICATIONS AND USAGE

CELANDINE HERB
Approved by Commission E:

■ Liver and gallbladder complaints

Unproven Uses: Celandine is used for spasmodic pain of the bile ducts and the gastrointestinal tract. In folk medicine, it was used for skin conditions such as blister rashes, scabies and warts. It is said to be effective in the treatment of cholecystitis, chloelithiasis, catarrhal jaundice, gastroenteritis, and diffuse latent liver and gall bladder complaints. It has also been used for intestinal polyps and breast lumps. Other uses include angina pectoris, cramps, asthma, arteriosclerosis, high blood pressure, stomach cancer, gout, edema and hepatitis.

Chinese Medicine: Celandine is used for inflammation of the rim of the eyelid, febrile and ulcerating dermatitis, warts, edema, ascites, jaundice and stomach carcinomas

CELANDINE ROOT
Unproven Uses: In folk medicine, the fresh roots are chewed to alleviate toothache, and a powder derived from the roots is applied to ease tooth extraction.

Chinese Medicine: Preparations are used for irregular menstruation.

Homeopathic Uses: Chelidonium majus is used for inflammation, stones and chronic disorders of the hepatobiliary system, rheumatism and inflammation of the lungs and pleura.

PRECAUTIONS AND ADVERSE REACTIONS

CELANDINE HERB
General: No health hazards or side effects are known in conjunction with the proper administration of designated therapeutic dosages. Older scientific literature credits the plant with toxicity (burning in the mouth, nausea, vomiting, bloody diarrhea, hematuria, stupor), but recent studies offer no clear proof of this; animal experiments yielded no results.

No symptoms of inflammation were observed in the eyes of rabbits following introduction of the chyle. Nevertheless, contact between it and the eyes should be avoided.

Pregnancy: Not to be used during pregnancy.

CELANDINE ROOT
No health hazards or side effects are known in conjunction with the proper administration of designated therapeutic dosages. Older scientific literature credits the plant with toxicity (burning in the mouth, nausea, vomiting, bloody diarrhea, hematuria, stupor), but recent studies offer no clear proof of this. Animal experiments yielded no examples of toxicity.

DOSAGE

CELANDINE HERB
Mode of Administration: Comminuted and powdered drug for infusions and decoctions; dried extracts for liquid and solid medicinal forms for internal use.

Preparations:
Fluid extract — 1:1 in 25% ethanol.

Tincture — 1:10 in 45% ethanol (BHP83).

Tea — allow 1½ dessertspoonfuls to draw in boiling water for 10 minutes.

Infusion — 15 gm dried herb to 1 liter of water, leave to draw for 15 minutes.

Daily Dosage: The average daily dose is 2 to 4 gm of drug in liquid or solid extracts, equivalent to 12 to 30 mg total alkaloids calculated as chelidonine; fluid extract, 1 to 2 ml three times daily; decoction, 3 cups daily; infusion, 3 cups between meals.

Storage: Celandine herb should be protected carefully from light.

CELANDINE ROOT

Mode of Administration: Most standardized and compound preparations contain the extract of Celandine herb; various homeopathic preparations also contain dilutions of the fresh herb Greater Celandine.

Daily Dosage: The standard dose is 0.5 gm of drug.

Homeopathic Dosage: 5 drops, 1 tablet, 10 globules every 30 to 60 minutes (acute) or 1 to 3 times daily (chronic); parenterally: 1 to 2 ml sc acute: 3 times daily; chronic: once daily (HAB1).

Storage: Preparations must be stored carefully.

LITERATURE

CELANDINE HERB

Äberlein H et al., Chelidonium majus L, Components with in vitro affinity for GABA A receptor: Positive cooperation of alkaloids. In: PM 62(3):227-231. 1996.

Anonym, Brennpunkt ZNS. In: DAZ 137(25):2166-2167. 1997.

Arnason JT, Gurein B, Kraml MM, Mehta B, Rehmond JC, Scaiano JC, Phototoxic and photochemical properties of sanguinarin. In: Photochemistry and Photobiology 55(1):35. 1992.

Baumann J, (1975) Über die Wirkung von Chelidonium, Curcuma, Absinth und Carduus marianus auf die Galle- und Pankreassekretion bei Hepatopathien. Med Mschr 29:173.

Boegge SC et al., Reduction of ACh-induced contraction of rat isolated ileum by Coptisin, Caffeoylmalic acid, Chelidonium majus, and Corydalis lutea extracts. In: PM 62(2):173-174. 1997.

Diener H, Schöllkraut. In: PTA 8(2):145. 1994.

Dostál J et al., Structure of chelerythrine base. In: JNP 58(5):723-729. 1995.

Fulde G, Wichtl M, Analytik von Schöllkraut, Hauptalkaloid Coptisin. In: DAZ 134(12):1031. 1994.

Hahn R, Nahrstedt A, Hydroxycinnamic acid derivatives, caffeoylmalic and new caffeoylaldonic acid esters, from Chelidonium majus. In: PM 59(1):71. 1993.

Hamacher H, Haben Phytopharmaka eine Zukunft? In: DAZ 131(42):2155. 1991.

Kim DJ, Ahn B, Han BS, Tsuda H, Potential preventive effects of Chelidonium majus L (Papaveraceae) herb extract on glandular stomach tumor development in rats treated with N-methyl-N'-nitro-N nitrosoguanidine (MNNG) and hypertonic sodium chloride. In: Can.

Mitra S et al., Effect of Chelidonium majus L. on experimetal hepatic tissue injury. In: Phytother Res 10(4):354-356. 1996.

Reuter HD, Pflanzliche Gallentherapeutika (Teil I) und (Teil II). In: ZPT 16(1):13-20 u. 77-89. 1995.

Schilcher H, Pharmazeutische Aspekte pflanzlicher Gallentherapeutika. In: ZPT 16(4):211-222. 1995.

Schmidt M, Phytotherapie: Pflanzliche Gallenwegstherapeutika. In: DAZ 135(8):680-682. 1995.

Táborská E et al., The alkaloids of Chelidonium majus L. and their variability. In: PM 62, Abstracts of the 44th Ann Congress of GA, 145. 1996.

Vahlensiek U et al., The effect of Chelidonium majus herb extract on the choleresis in the isolated perfused rat liver. In: PH 61(3):267-270. 1995.

Vavreckova C, Gawlik I, Müller K, Benzophenanthridine alkaloids of Chelidonium majus: I. Inhibition of 5- and 12-lipoxygenase by a non-redox mechanism. In: PM 62(5):397-401. 1996.

Willaman JJ and Hui-Li L, (1970) Lloydia 33 (3A):1.

Further information in:

Chan, EH et al., (Eds), Advances in Chinese Medicinal Materials Research, World Scientific Pub. Co. Singapore 1985.

Frohne D, Pfänder HJ, Giftpflanzen - Ein Handbuch für Apotheker, Toxikologen und Biologen, 4. Aufl., Wiss. Verlagsges. mbH Stuttgart 1997.

Hänsel R, Keller K, Rimpler H, Schneider G (Hrsg.), Hagers Handbuch der Pharmazeutischen Praxis, 5. Aufl., Bde 4-6 (Drogen): Springer Verlag Berlin, Heidelberg, New York, 1992-1994.

Lewin L, Gifte und Vergiftungen, 6. Aufl., Nachdruck, Haug Verlag, Heidelberg 1992.

Madaus G, Lehrbuch der Biologischen Arzneimittel, Bde 1-3, Nachdruck, Georg Olms Verlag Hildesheim 1979.

Roth L, Daunderer M, Kormann K, Giftpflanzen, Pflanzengifte, 4. Aufl., Ecomed Fachverlag Landsberg Lech 1993.

Schulz R, Hänsel R, Rationale Phytotherapie, Springer Verlag Heidelberg 1996.

Steinegger E, Hänsel R, Pharmakognosie, 5. Aufl., Springer Verlag Heidelberg 1992.

Teuscher E, Lindequist U, Biogene Gifte - Biologie, Chemie, Pharmakologie, 2. Aufl., Fischer Verlag Stuttgart 1994.

Teuscher E, Biogene Arzneimittel, 5. Aufl., Wiss. Verlagsges. mbH Stuttgart 1997.

Wagner H, Wiesenauer M, Phytotherapie. Phytopharmaka und pflanzliche Homöopathika, Fischer-Verlag, Stuttgart, Jena, New York 1995.

Wichtl M (Hrsg.), Teedrogen, 4. Aufl., Wiss. Verlagsges. Stuttgart 1997.

CELANDINE ROOT

Hänsel R, Keller K, Rimpler H, Schneider G (Hrsg.), Hagers Handbuch der Pharmazeutischen Praxis, 5. Aufl., Bde 4-6 (Drogen): Springer Verlag Berlin, Heidelberg, New York, 1992-1994.

Literatur zu den Wirkungen der Inhaltsstoffe vgl. Chelidonii herba.

Celastrus scandens

See American Bittersweet

Celery

Apium graveolens

TRADE NAMES

Celery Seed, Celery Seed-Power, Celery Liquid

DESCRIPTION

Medicinal Parts: The medicinal parts are the root, above-ground foliage and stems, the fruit (seeds) of the plant and the oil extracted from the seeds.

Flower and Fruit: The umbels are greenish-white, small, 6 to 12 rayed, star-shaped and splayed. Some umbels are top-heavy, short petioled or sessile, and some are terminal and more or less long-petioled with no involucre. Petals are usually 0.5 mm, white or greenish to yellowish, cordate at the base and have indented tips. The fruit is almost spherical and somewhat compressed at the side. The 5 mm mericarps are rounded in section. They are 5-cornered with 5 equal, weakly protruding, bow-shaped main ribs. The edge of the ribs form the edge of the mericarps. The fruit axis is bristly and slightly crenate at the tip.

Leaves, Stem and Root: The glabrous plant is a biennial and reaches a height of 30 to 100 cm. The root of the wild variety is fusiform, about 5 to 7 mm thick, branched and becomes woody in the second year. The root of the cultivated variety is fleshy, roundly tuberous and reaches a diameter of over 15 cm. The stem is erect, with edged grooves, often hollow and branched. The leaves are glossy and rich green. The basal and lower cauline leaves are more or less long-petioled and pinnatifid. The upper cauline leaves are sometimes opposite. They are on short white-membrane-edged sheaths and are almost sessile and tri-pinnate. The lower leaves are roundish, almost blunt at the base with broad, lozenge-shaped, indented-serrate, blunt and short-thorned tips. The upper cauline leaves are wedge-shaped and acuminate, also 3-lobed or pinnate or lanceolate and entire-margined.

Characteristics: The plant has a strong odor.

Habitat: Celery is found in Europe from England and Lapland to southern Russia. The plant also grows in western Asia as far as eastern India; in northern and southern Africa and South America; and is cultivated and grows wild in North America, Mexico and Argentina.

Production: Celery seed consists of the fruit of Apium graveolons; celery herb consists of the fresh or dried above-ground parts of the plant; and celery root is the plant's fresh or dried underground parts.

Other Names: Smallage

ACTIONS AND PHARMACOLOGY

COMPOUNDS: CELERY SEED (FRUIT)

Volatile oil: chief constituents ((+) - limonene, beta-selinene, phthalides among them 3-butyliden phthalide, 3-butyl phthalide, 3-isovaleryliden-3a, 4-dihydrophthalid, 3-isobutyliden phthalide, sedanoid, neocnidilid)

Flavonoids: graveobioside A and B, apiin, isoquercitrin

Furocoumarins: including bergapten, isoimperatorin, isopimpinellin

Fatty oil

EFFECTS: CELERY FRUIT

In animal tests, a sedative and anticonvulsive effect was demonstrated, a diuretic effect could not be proven. The essential oil contained in the drug had a mildly inhibiting effect on bacteria and fungi.

COMPOUNDS: CELERY HERB

Volatile oil): including (+)-limonene, myrcene, beta-selinene, alpha-terpineol, carveol, dihydrocarvone, geranyl acetate, phthalides (including 3-butyliden phthalid, 3-butyl phthalid, 3-isobutyliden dihydrophthalid)

Flavonoids: including apiin, luteolin-7-O-apiosyl glucoside, chrysoeriol glucoside

Furocoumarins: including bergaptene, xanthotoxin, isopimpinellin

Caffeic acid derivatives: including chlorogenic acid

EFFECTS: CELERY HERB

In animal tests, a sedative and anticonvulsive effect was demonstrated, a diuretic effect could not be proven. The essential oil contained in the drug had a mildly inhibiting effect on bacteria and fungi.

COMPOUNDS: CELERY ROOT

Volatile oil: chief constituents (+)-limonene, beta-pinene, p-cymene, cis-, 3-methyl-4-ethyl-hexane), phthalides (including 3-butyliden phthalid, 3-butyl phthalid, ligustilid, neocnidilid)

Flavonoids: including apiin, luteolin-7-O-apiosyl glucoside

Furocoumarins: including bergaptene

Polyyne: including falcarinol, falcarindiol

EFFECTS: CELERY ROOT

In animal tests, a sedative and anticonvulsive effect was demonstrated; a diuretic effect could not be proven. The essential oil contained in the drug had a mildly inhibiting effect on bacteria and fungi.

INDICATIONS AND USAGE

CELERY FRUIT, HERB AND ROOT

Unproven Uses: Folk medicine use of celery and preparations of celery are used as a diuretic, for regulating the bowels, for glandular stimulation, rheumatic complaints, gout, gall and kidney stones. Other traditional uses include as a prophylactic for nervous agitation, for loss of appetite and exhaustion. Celery is also used as a cough treatment and as a helminthic.

Homeopathic Uses: Celery preparations are used in homeopathy for ailments of the ovaries and rheumatism.

CONTRAINDICATIONS

CELERY SEED (FRUIT)

The drug should not be used during pregnancy. Also, because of the kidney-irritating effect of the volatile oil, the drug should not be administered to individuals with kidney infections.

PRECAUTIONS AND ADVERSE REACTIONS

CELERY FRUIT, HERB AND ROOT:

No health hazards or side effects are known in conjunction with the proper administration of designated therapeutic dosages. Nevertheless, because of the kidney-irritating effect of the volatile oil, the drug should not be administered in the presence of kidney infections. Latent yeast infections of the plant could cause the furanocoumarin content of the fresh root to rise to 200 times its original level under storage conditions. For this reason, the relatively large amounts of furanocoumarins frequently to be found in stored celeriac bulbs, or in incorrectly dehydrated drug samples, could lead to phototoxicoses.

DOSAGE

CELERY SEED (FRUIT)

Mode of Administration: Whole and powdered drug, liquid extract, and as a component in a variety of tea mixtures.

How Supplied:

Capsules — 450 and 505 mg

Fluid Extract — 1:1

Preparation: To prepare a liquid extract, percolate 1 kg of seed in a specula process to 1 liter of fluid extract. The essential oil is removed after filtration with paper soaked in alcohol.

For an infusion, pour boiling water on 1 g of the squeezed drug and strain after 5 to 10 minutes.

Decoctions are prepared in a 1:5 ratio.

Daily Dosage: The daily dosage of the seeds is 1.2 to 4 g and as an infusion, 1 g drug.

Homeopathic Dosage: 5 to 10 drops, 1 tablet or 5 to 10 globules 1 to 3 times daily or 1 ml injection solution twice weekly sc (HAB34).

Storage: Celery seed should be kept tightly sealed, away from light and moisture.

CELERY HERB

Mode of Administration: Whole and cut drug as well as a variety of tea mixtures.

Preparation: Celery is contained in a variety of tea mixtures (kidney and bladder teas).

Daily Dosage: Pressed juice of the fresh plant: 23 g (15 ml) 3 times daily.

Homeopathic Dosage: 5 to 10 drops, 1 tablet or 5 to 10 globules 1 to 3 times daily or 1 ml injection solution twice weekly sc (HAB34).

Storage: The herb should be kept sealed, away from light and moisture.

CELERY ROOT

Mode of Administration: The drug is available in a few combination preparations for internal use.

Preparation: A cough mixture is prepared by boiling the root juice with sugar.

Dosage: Pressed juice of the fresh plant: 23 g (15 ml) 3 times daily.

Homeopathic Dosage: 5 to 10 drops, 1 tablet or 5 to 10 globules 1 to 3 times daily or 1 ml injection solution twice weekly sc (HAB1).

Storage: Celery root should be kept sealed, away from light and moisture.

LITERATURE

Beier RS, Oertli EH, Psoralen and other phytoalexins in celery. In: PH 22(11):2595. 1983.

Bjeldanes LF, Kim I, (1977) J Org Chem 42:2333.

Fehr D, (1979) Pharmazie 29(5):349 et 34 (10):658.

Garg SK et al., (1979) Phytochemistry 18:1580 et 1764.

Garg SK et al., (1980) Planta Med 38:363.

Gijbels MJM et al., Phthalides in roots of Apium graveolens, A. graveolens var. rapeceum, Bifora testiculata and Petroselinum crispum var. tuberosum. In: Fitoterapia 56:17. 1985.

Harborne JB, in "The Biology and Chemistry of the Umbelliferae," Ed. V. N. Heywood. Pub. Academic Press, London 1971.

Lewis DA et al., (1985) Int J Crude Drug Res 28 (1):27.

Mac Leod G, Ames JM, Volatile components of celery and celeriac. In: PH 28(7):1817-1824. 1989.

Nigg HN, Strandberg JO, Beier RC, Petersen HD, Harrison JM, Furanocoumarins in Florida celery varieties increased by fungicide treatment. In: J Agricult Food Chem 45(4):1430-1436. 1997.

Tsi D et al., Effects of aqueous celery (Apium graveolens) extract on lipid parameters of rats fed a high fat diet. In: PM 61(1):18-21. 1995.

Uhlig, JW, Chang A, Jen JJ, Effect of phthalides on celery flavor. In: J Food Sci 52(3):658-660. 1987.

Yu RS, You SQ, (1984) Acta Pharm Sinica 19 (8):566.

Further information in:

Frohne D, Pfänder HJ, Giftpflanzen - Ein Handbuch für Apotheker, Toxikologen und Biologen, 4. Aufl., Wiss. Verlags-Ges Stuttgart 1997.

Hänsel R, Keller K, Rimpler H, Schneider G (Hrsg.), Hagers Handbuch der Pharmazeutischen Praxis, 5. Aufl., Bde 4-6 (Drogen), Springer Verlag Berlin, Heidelberg, New York, 1992-1994.

Hausen B, Allergiepflanzen, Pflanzenallergene, ecomed Verlagsgesellsch. mbH, Landsberg 1988.

Leung AY, Encyclopedia of Common Natural Ingredients Used in Food Drugs and Cosmetics, John Wiley & Sons Inc., New York 1980.

Madaus G, Lehrbuch der Biologischen Arzneimittel, Bde 1-3, Nachdruck, Georg Olms Verlag Hildesheim 1979.

Teuscher E, Lindequist U, Biogene Gifte - Biologie, Chemie, Pharmakologie, 2. Aufl., Fischer Verlag Stuttgart 1994.

Wagner H, Wiesenauer M, Phytotherapie. Phytopharmaka und pflanzliche Homöopathika, Fischer-Verlag, Stuttgart, Jena, New York 1995.

Wichtl M (Hrsg.), Teedrogen, 4. Aufl., Wiss. Verlagsges. Stuttgart 1997.

Centaurea cyanus

See Cornflower

Centaurium erythraea

See Centaury

Centaury

Centaurium erythraea

DESCRIPTION

Medicinal Parts: The medicinal parts are the dried, aerial parts of the flowering plant.

Flower and Fruit: The different-sized flowers form a dense or loose cyme. They are purple to pink-red, seldom white. The calyx tube is pentangular with awl-shaped tips. There are 5 petals fused into a tube, 5 stamens mostly fused to the corolla and 1 superior, narrowly linear ovary. The stigma is 2-lobed. The fruit is a large, yellow, many-seeded capsule.

Leaves, Stem and Root: The plant is an annual that grows to between 5 and 30 cm high. The stem is erect, quadrangular and unbranched. The cauline leaves are crossed opposite, fleshy, oblong-ovate to lanceolate, and sessile. The basal leaves are rosette-like, obovate and narrowed to a petiole.

Characteristics: Centaury has a very bitter taste.

Habitat: The plant is found in the Mediterranean region and as far as Britain and Scandinavia. It is cultivated in the U.S.

Production: Centaury consists of the dried aerial parts, in flower, of Centaurium erythraea. The plant is harvested during the flowering season and dried quickly to retain the flower color.

Not to be Confused With: Other Centaurium varieties.

Other Names: Feverwort, Centaury Gentian, Filwort, Centory, Christ's Ladder, Bitter Herb, Bitterbloom, Bitter Clover, Eyebright, Rose Pink, Wild Succory, Canchalagua

ACTIONS AND PHARMACOLOGY

COMPOUNDS

Iridoide bitter principles (monoterpenes): in particular swertiamarin, including among others gentiopicrin, sweroside

Pyrridine alkaloids: gentianine, gentianidine

Xanthones: including methyl bellidifoline

EFFECTS

Centaury increases gastric secretion and salivation because of the typical bitter reaction, also antiphlogistic and antipyretic effects have been studied in various animal experiments. The effect for loss of appetite, stomach complaints and dyspepsia can also be attributed to the amaroids.

INDICATIONS AND USAGE

Approved by Commission E:

- Dyspeptic complaints
- Loss of appetite

Unproven Uses: The drug is used for loss of appetite, dyspepsia and poor gastric secretion. In folk medicine, it is used for fever, worm infestation and as a hypotensive. It is also used for diabetes in Mallorca, and for expelling kidney stones in Egypt. Externally, it is used in the treatment of wounds.

CONTRAINDICATIONS

Because of its secretion-activating effect, the drug should not be administered in the presence of stomach or intestinal ulcers.

PRECAUTIONS AND ADVERSE REACTIONS

No health hazards or side effects are known in conjunction with the proper administration of designated therapeutic dosages.

DOSAGE

Mode of Administration: Comminuted herb for infusions and other bitter-tasting preparations for internal use.

Preparation: Tea: Brew 2 to 3 gm drug with 150 ml boiling water and strain after 15 minutes; Centaurium Extract: extract of 1 part drug to 10 parts water and 1 part 98% ethanol steamed till thickened (EB6).

Liquid extract: 1:1 25% ethanol (V/V) (BHP83).

Daily Dosage: The average daily dose is 6 gm of drug or 1 to 2 gm of extract; single dose is 1 gm.

The powdered drug is taken 3 times daily on a wafer with honey; the infusion is taken 1/2 hour before meals.

The daily dose of extractum Centaurii fluidum is 2 to 5 ml.

Storage: Keep protected from light and moisture in sealed containers.

LITERATURE

Bishay DW et al., (1978) Planta Med 33:422.

D'Agostino M et al., (1985) Boll Soc Ital Biol Sper 61 (2):165.

Do T et al., PM 53:580. 1987.

Lacroix R et al., (1973) Tunisie Med 51:327.

Neshta NM et al., (1983) Khim Prir Soed 1:106.

Schimmer O, Mauthner H, Centaurium erythraea RAFN. Tausendgüldenkraut. In: ZPT 15(5):299-304. 1994.

Schimmer O, Mauthner H, Polymethoxylated xanthones from the herb of Centaurium erythraea with strong antimutagenic properties in Salmonella typhimurium. In: PM 62(6):561-564. 1996.

van der Sluis WG, Plant Syst Evol 149:253-286. 1985.

van der Sluis WG et al., (1980) Planta Med 39:268.

van der Sluis WG, PM 41:221-231. 1981.

Further information in:

Hänsel R, Keller K, Rimpler H, Schneider G (Hrsg.), Hagers Handbuch der Pharmazeutischen Praxis, 5. Aufl., Bde 4-6 (Drogen), Springer Verlag Berlin, Heidelberg, New York, 1992-1994.

Leung AY, Encyclopedia of Common Natural Ingredients Used in Food Drugs and Cosmetics, John Wiley & Sons Inc., New York 1980.

Madaus G, Lehrbuch der Biologischen Arzneimittel, Bde 1-3, Nachdruck, Georg Olms Verlag Hildesheim 1979.

Schulz R, Hänsel R, Rationale Phytotherapie, Springer Verlag Heidelberg 1996.

Steinegger E, Hänsel R, Pharmakognosie, 5. Aufl., Springer Verlag Heidelberg 1992.

Teuscher E, Biogene Arzneimittel, 5. Aufl., Wiss. Verlagsges. mbH Stuttgart 1997.

Wagner H, Wiesenauer M, Phytotherapie. Phytopharmaka und pflanzliche Homöopathika, Fischer-Verlag, Stuttgart, Jena, New York 1995.

Wichtl M (Hrsg.), Teedrogen, 4. Aufl., Wiss. Verlagsges. Stuttgart 1997.

Centella asiatica

See Gotu Kola

Centranthus ruber

See Red-Spur Valerian

Cephaelis ipecacuanha

See Ipecac

Ceratonia siliqua

See Carob

Cetraria islandica

See Iceland Moss

Chamaemelum nobile

See English Chamomile

Chaste Tree

Vitex agnus-castus

TRADE NAMES

Chasteberry Power, Vitex, Alcohol-Free Chaste Tree Berry

DESCRIPTION

Medicinal Parts: The medicinal parts are the ripe dried fruit and the dried leaves.

Flower and Fruit: The 8 to 10 cm, blue, occasionally pink flowers form terminal, branched, spike-like inflorescences. The calyx and epicalyx of the bilabiate corolla are pubescent. The fruit is a globular to oblong, 3 to 4 mm, reddish black, 4-seeded drupe. It is surrounded up to two-thirds in cup-like fashion by the calyx. The exocarp has short-stemmed, glandular hairs.

Leaves, Stem and Root: The plant is a 1 to 6 m high bush or tree with quadrangular, gray, tomentose, young branches. The leaves are deciduous, crossed-opposite, long-petioled and palmate. They have 5 to 7 entire-margined, up to 10 cm long, lanceolate leaflets. The under surface of the leaf is white and tomentose.

Habitat: The plant is indigenous to the Mediterranean region as far as western Asia.

Production: Chaste Tree fruits consist of the ripe, dried fruits of Vitex agnus-castus.

ACTIONS AND PHARMACOLOGY

COMPOUNDS

Iridoid glycosides: agnoside, aucubin

Flavonoids: including casticin, 3,6,7,4′-tetramethylether, 6-hydroxy-kempferol-3,6,7,4′-tetramethylether, 6-hydroxy-kempferol-3,6,7-trimethylether (penduletin), quercetagenin-3,6,7-trimethylether (chrysosplenol D)

Volatile oil (0.8-1.6%): including among others, 1,8-cineole, lime, alpha-pinene, beta-pinene, as well as bornyl acetate, camphor, p-cymol, sabinene

Fatty oils

EFFECTS

The drug is dopaminergic and FSH-suppressive; it also inhibits lactation (main active principles aucubin and agnoside). In addition, the drug represses the release of prolactin and improves the symptoms of PMS.

In older animal experiments, the drug was tested on the ovaries and resulted in a reduction of cystic and bleeding follicles. In other animal experiments, an inhibition of lactation and a normalization of stress-induced hyperprolactin anemia was observed. In clinical studies, the positive effect on symptoms resulting from hyperprolactin anemia was proven.

A dopaminergic effect via bonding on D2-receptors was also shown.

INDICATIONS AND USAGE

Approved by Commission E:

- Premenstrual syndrome (PMS)
- Menopausal complaints

Unproven Uses: Chaste Tree preparations are used to treat irregularities of the menstrual cycle, premenstrual complaints, menstrual disturbances caused by corpus luteum insufficiency, insufficient milk production and mastodynia. It is also used to control libido, increase milk flow, reduce flatulence, suppress appetite, and induce sleep. Additional uses include the treatment of impotency, spermatorrhea, prostatitis, swelling of the testes, sexual neurasthenia, sterility, amenorrhea, uterine pain, and swelling of the ovaries. Chaste Tree is also used to induce menstruation.

Homeopathic Uses: Chaste Tree is used for male sexual disturbances, disturbances of milk flow, and nervous depression.

CONTRAINDICATIONS

The drug is contraindicated in pregnancy and in nursing mothers.

PRECAUTIONS AND ADVERSE REACTIONS

General: Occasionally, the administration of the drug leads to the formation of rashes.

Drug Interactions: Because of the dopaminergic effect of the drug, a reciprocal weakening of the effect can occur in case of ingestion of dopamine-receptor antagonists.

Pregnancy: The drug should not be administered during pregnancy

Nursing Mothers: The drug should not be used by breast-feeding mothers.

DOSAGE

Mode of Administration: Whole and powdered drug available as capsules, drops, film tablets, and compound preparations.

How Supplied:

Capsules — 40 mg, 100 mg

Liquid Extract — 1:1

Preparation: For the dried extract, preparations of 100 gm contain 0.2 gm dried extract in a ratio of 1:5, in either ethanol or water.

Daily Dosage: The daily dosage of aqueous-alcoholic extracts is 30 to 40 mg of the drug.

Homeopathic Dosage: 5 to 10 drops, 1 tablet or 5 to 10 globules, 1 to 3 times a day; parenterally: 1 ml injection solution sc twice weekly (HAB1).

LITERATURE

Becker H, Hemmung der Prolaktinsekretion. In: T W Gynäkologie 6:2-10. 1991.

Böhnert KJ, Hahn G, Erfahrungsheilkunde 39:494-502c. 1990.

Dittmann FW, Böhnert KJ, Peeters M, Albrecht M, Lamertz M, Schmidt U, Prämenstruelles Syndrom. Behandlung mit einem Phytopharmakon. In: TW Gynäkologie 5:60-68. 1992.

Feldmann HU, Albrecht M, Lamertz M, Böhnert KJ, Therapie bei Gelbkörperschwäche bzw. prämenstruellem Syndrom mit Vitex-agnus-castus-Tinktur. In: Gyne 11:421-425. 1990.

Jarry H, Leonhardt S, Gorkow C, Wuttke W, (1994) In vitro prolactin but not LH and FSH release is inhibited by compounds in extracts of Agnus castus, direct evidence for a dopaminergic principle by the dopamine receptor assay. Exp Clin Endocrinol 102:448-454.

Jarry H, Leonhardt S, Wuttke W, Behr B, Gorkow C, (1991) Agnus castus als dopaminerges Wirkprinzip in Mastodynon N. Z Phytother 12:77-82.

Kustrac D et al., The composition of the essential oil of Vitex agnus-castus. In: PM 58(7):A681. 1992.

Lehmann-Willenbrock E, Riedel HH, (1988) Klinische und endokrinologische Untersuchungen zur Therapie ovarieller Ausfallserscheinungen nach Hysterektromie unter Belassung der Adnexe. Zent Gynäkol 110:611-618.

Loew D, Gorkow C, Schrödter A, Reitbrock S, Merz PG, Schnieders M, Sieder C, Zur dosisabhängigen Verträglichkeit eines Agnus-castus-Spezialextraktes. In: ZPT 17(4):237-243. 1996.

Merz PG, Schrödter A, Rietbrock S, Gorkow Ch, Loew D, (1995) Prolaktinsekretion und Verträglichkeit unter der Behandlung mit einem Agnus-castus-Spezialextrakt (B1095E1). Erste Ergebnisse zum Einfluβ auf die Prolaktinsekretion. In, Loew D, Rietbrock N (Hrsg) Phytopharmaka in Forschung und klinischer Anwendung. Steinkopff Verlag, Darmstadt, S. 93-97.

Propping D, Böhnert KJ, Peeters M, Albrecht M, Lamertz M, Vitex agnus-castus. Behandlung gynäkologischer Krankheitsbilder. In: Therapeutikon 5:581-585. 1991.

Reuter HD, Böhnert KJ, Schmidt U, (1995) Die Therapie des prämenstruellen Syndroms mit Vitex agnus castus. Kontrollierte Doppelblindstudie gegen Pyridoxin. Z Phytother Abstractband, S.7.

Reuter HD, Böhnert KJ, Schmidt U, Die Therapie des prämenstruellen Syndroms mit Vitex agnus castus. Kontrollierte Doppelblindstudie gegen Pyridoxin.. In: ZPT, Abstract-Band, S.7. 1995.

Röder D, Therapie von Zyklusstörungen mit Vitex agnus-castus. In: ZPT 15(3):155-159. 1994.

Wichtl M, Phytopharmaka: Agnus castus - ein Dopamin-Agonist? In: DAZ 132(8):360. 1992.

Winterhoff H, (1993) Arzneipflanzen mit endokriner Wirksamkeit. Z Phytother 14:83-94.

Winterhoff H, Gorkow C, Behr B, Die Hemmung der Laktation bei Ratten als indirekter Beweis für die Senkung von Prolaktin durch Agnus castus. In: ZPT 12(6):175-179. 1991.

Wuttke W, Gorkow Ch, Jarry J, (1995) Dopaminergic Compounds in Vitex Agnus Castus. In, Loew D, Rietbrock N (Hrsg) Phytopharmaka in Forschung und klinischer Anwendung. Steinkopff Verlag, Darmstadt, S. 81-91.

Further information in:

Hänsel R, Keller K, Rimpler H, Schneider G (Hrsg.), Hagers Handbuch der Pharmazeutischen Praxis, 5. Aufl., Bde 4-6 (Drogen): Springer Verlag Berlin, Heidelberg, New York, 1992-1994.

Lewin L, Gifte und Vergiftungen, 6. Aufl., Nachdruck, Haug Verlag, Heidelberg 1992.

Madaus G, Lehrbuch der Biologischen Arzneimittel, Bde 1-3, Nachdruck, Georg Olms Verlag Hildesheim 1979.

Schulz R, Hänsel R, Rationale Phytotherapie, Springer Verlag Heidelberg 1996.

Steinegger E, Hänsel R, Pharmakognosie, 5. Aufl., Springer Verlag Heidelberg 1992.

Teuscher E, Biogene Arzneimittel, 5. Aufl., Wiss. Verlagsges. Stuttgart 1997.

Wagner H, Wiesenauer M, Phytotherapie. Phytopharmaka und pflanzliche Homöopathika, Fischer-Verlag, Stuttgart, Jena, New York 1995.

Chaulmoogra

Hydnocarpus species

DESCRIPTION

Medicinal Parts: Chaulmoogra is found in all of the named species. The expressed oil is known as Gynocardia oil in Britain and Oleum Chaulmoograe in the U.S.

Flower and Fruit: The grayish seeds are about 2 to 3 cm long and 1.5 cm in diameter. They are irregularly angular with rounded ends. The kernel is oily and encloses two thin, heart-shaped, three-veined cotyledons and a straight radical.

Characteristics: The taste is acrid and the odor disagreeable.

Habitat: Malaysia, Indian subcontinent.

Production: Chaulmoogra seeds are the seeds of various Hydnocarpus varieties. Chaulmoogra oil is the fatty oil extracted from the seeds.

Other Names: Hydnocarpus

ACTIONS AND PHARMACOLOGY

COMPOUNDS: CHAULMOOGRA SEEDS

Fatty oil (30-40%, bitter-type consistency)

Proteins (25%)

Cyanogenic glycosides

Flavolignans

EFFECTS: CHAULMOOGRA SEEDS

The chaulmoogric acid in the drug is antimicrobial. The drug has sedative, febrifuge and dermatic effects. The flavonol lignans hydnocarpin, hydnowightin and neohydnocarpin isolated from the seeds are lipid lowering, anti-inflammatory and antitumoral in animal experiments.

COMPOUNDS: CHAULMOOGRA OIL

Triglycerides: chief fatty acids D-hydnocarpic acid, D-chaulmoogric acid, D-gorli acid (cyclopentene fatty acids)

EFFECTS: CHAULMOOGRA OIL

The chaulmoogric acid in the drug is antimicrobial.

INDICATIONS AND USAGE

Unproven Uses: Externally, preparations of Hydnocarpus are used in the treatment of various skin conditions such as psoriasis and eczema. It is also used as an injection in the treatment of leprosy.

Chinese Medicine: In China, Chaulmoogra is used for leprosy, scabies and furuncles.

Indian Medicine: Uses include leprosy, skin diseases, itching, leocodermia, eczema, flatulence and diabetes.

PRECAUTIONS AND ADVERSE REACTIONS

Coughing, dyspnea, laryngospasms, kidney damage, visual disorders, head and muscle pain, and central paralyses are side effects following intake of the oil. It is severely irritating in local application.

OVERDOSAGE

Following stomach and intestinal emptying (inducement of vomiting, gastric lavage with burgundy-colored potassium permanganate solution, sodium sulfate), the treatment for poisonings consists of the instillation of activated charcoal and shock prophylaxis (quiet, warmth), and of electrolyte substitution and the countering of any acidosis imbalance that may appear through sodium bicarbonate infusions. In the event of shock, plasma volume expanders should be infused. Monitoring of kidney function is necessary. Intubation and oxygen respiration may also be required.

The seeds are severely poisonous due to their cynagenic glycoside content. Injections of solutions of Dicobalt-EDTA or of thiosulfates, or administration of methemoglobin-forming agents, such as amyl nitrite, are recommended as antidotes. The triggering of vomiting and gastric lavage should be carried out in a parallel fashion. Circulatory support measures and artificial respiration may be required.

DOSAGE

Mode of Administration: The seeds and oil in various preparations, as powder, oil, emulsion and ointments.

LITERATURE

Kern W, List PH, Hörhammer L (Hrsg.), Hagers Handbuch der Pharmazeutischen Praxis, 4. Aufl., Bde 1-8, Springer Verlag Berlin, Heidelberg, New York, 1969.

Lefort D et al., (1969) Planta Med 17:261.

Madaus G, Lehrbuch der Biologischen Arzneimittel, Bde 1-3, Nachdruck, Georg Olms Verlag Hildesheim 1979.

Roth L, Daunderer M, Kormann K, Giftpflanzen, Pflanzengifte, 4. Aufl., Ecomed Fachverlag Landsberg Lech 1993.

Sleumer, (1947) Pharm Ztg 83:165.

Teuscher E, Biogene Arzneimittel, 5. Aufl., Wiss. Verlagsges. Stuttgart 1997.

Cheiranthus cheiri

See Wallflower

Cheken

Eugenia chequen

DESCRIPTION

Medicinal Parts: The medicinal parts are the dried leaves.

Flower and Fruit: The flowers are usually solitary, occasionally in threes. The receptacle is top-shaped and pubescent. There are 4 pubescent or ciliate sepals. The petals are white, oval and 5 to 8 mm long. The stamens are numerous but small. The ovary is glabrous. The fruit is a red or black-violet, glabrous, globular berry, 6 to 8 mm in diameter. It has 2 to 3 seeds which are dark, lentil-shaped and are about 4 mm in diameter.

Leaves, Stem and Root: The plant is an evergreen tree, which grows up to 15 m high and sometimes looks like a shrub. The leaves are coriaceous, ovate, about 1 to 1.5 cm long, 0.5 to 1 cm wide, entire-margined, very shortly petioled with numerous minute, round, translucent oil-cells.

Characteristics: The leaves have a bitter taste that is astringent and aromatic, reminiscent of bay leaves. The odor is slight and they contain an essential oil.

Habitat: Eugenia chequen grows in Chile.

Production: Cheken leaves are the leaves of Eugenia chequen.

Other Names: Arryan, Myrtus Chekan

ACTIONS AND PHARMACOLOGY

COMPOUNDS

Bitter substances

Volatile oil: including alpha-pinene, 1,8-cineol

EFFECTS

The ethanol extract inhibits xanthinoxydasis. The essential oil has a similar effect on germinating salad seeds such as auxin. An antibacterial and antimycotic effect has also been demonstrated. In the agar diffusion test, the leaf oil was effective against *Pseudomonas acruginsosa*, *Trichophyton mentagrophytes* and *Asperigillus niger.* It also affects fat metabolism: the oil is used against hyperlipoprotinemia. It is used as a tonic, a diuretic and an expectorant.

INDICATIONS AND USAGE

Unproven Uses: In South American folk medicine, a decoction of the leaves is used in the treatment of diarrhea, fever, gout, as a tonic, diuretic, an antihypertensive, and as a digestive aid.

PRECAUTIONS AND ADVERSE REACTIONS

Health risks or side effects following the proper administration of designated therapeutic dosages are not recorded.

DOSAGE

Mode of Administration: As a decoction and as a liquid extract.

Chelidonium majus

See Celandine

Chelone glabra

See Balmony

Chenopodium ambrosioides

See Wormseed Oil

Chenopodium vulvaria

See Arrach

Cherry Laurel

Prunus laurocerasus

DESCRIPTION

Medicinal Parts: The medicinal parts are the dried leaves.

Flower and Fruit: The flowers are erect and in slender racemes 10 to 12 cm long with 3 mm pedicles. The petals are obovate, 3 mm long and white. The fruit is black and globular-ovoid. The smooth kernel within the fruit is ovoid and acute, with a long black weal.

Leaves, Stem and Root: The plant is an evergreen shrub or tree, completely glabrous, and grows up to 6 m high. The bud scales drop early. The petioles are 1 cm long and glandless. The leaf blades are obovate-lanceolate and 8 to 15 cm long. They are curved, entire or with a finely serrate margin, coriaceous and bright green. The upper surface of the leaves is glossy. The lower surface has 1 to 4 protruding nectaries in the axils of the ribs.

Characteristics: Poisonous. The fruit is similar to black cherries, and smells of hydrocyanic acid.

Habitat: The plant is indigenous to parts of Asia and is cultivated in many temperate areas.

Production: Cherry Laurel leaves are the leaves of Prunus laurocerasus.

Not to be Confused With: Other forms of *Prunus* species.

Other Names: Cherry-Bay

ACTIONS AND PHARMACOLOGY

COMPOUNDS

Cyanogenic glycosides: prunasin (corresponding to 0.5-2.5%, 50-210 mg HCN/100 gm)

EFFECTS

The drug acts as a tonic for the stomach, an anti-irritant and a sedative.

INDICATIONS AND USAGE

Unproven Uses: Cherry Laurel is used to treat coughs and the common cold.

Homeopathic Uses: Cherry Laurel is used for dry coughs, whooping cough, cyanosis and spasms.

PRECAUTIONS AND ADVERSE REACTIONS

No health hazards or side effects are known in conjunction with the proper administration of designated therapeutic dosages.

OVERDOSAGE

Overdoses of Cherry Laurel water prepared from the drug can lead to fatal poisonings. Ingestion of the leathery leaves and the seeds is improbable; the fruit pulp is low in cyanogenic glycosides (yielding 5-20 mg HCN/100 gm). The recommended antidotes include the injection of solutions of Dicobalt-EDTA or thiosulfates, or the administration of methemoglobin-forming agents, e.g., amyl nitrite, 4-dimethyl aminophenol. The inducement of vomiting or gastric lavage should be done in parallel fashion. Circulatory support and artificial respiration may also be required.

DOSAGE

Mode of Administration: The drug is available as a watery extract, an aromatic, a breathing stimulant and an antispasmodic.

LITERATURE

Frohne D, Pfänder HJ, Giftpflanzen - Ein Handbuch für Apotheker, Toxikologen und Biologen, 4. Aufl., Wiss. Verlags-Ges. Stuttgart 1997.

Kern W, List PH, Hörhammer L (Hrsg.), Hagers Handbuch der Pharmazeutischen Praxis, 4. Aufl., Bde. 1-8, Springer Verlag Berlin, Heidelberg, New York, 1969.

Leung AY, Encyclopedia of Common Natural Ingredients Used in Food Drugs and Cosmetics, John Wiley & Sons Inc., New York 1980.

Madaus G, Lehrbuch der Biologischen Arzneimittel, Bde 1-3, Nachdruck, Georg Olms Verlag Hildesheim 1979.

Roth L, Daunderer M, Kormann K, Giftpflanzen, Pflanzengifte, 4. Aufl., Ecomed Fachverlag Landsberg Lech 1993.

Sommer W, Dissertation Universität Kiel. 1984.

Steinegger E, Hänsel R, Pharmakognosie, 5. Aufl., Springer Verlag Heidelberg 1992.

Teuscher E, Lindequist U, Biogene Gifte - Biologie, Chemie, Pharmakologie, 2. Aufl., Fischer Verlag Stuttgart 1994.

Teuscher E, Biogene Arzneimittel, 5. Aufl., Wiss. Verlagsges. Stuttgart 1997.

Wagner H, Wiesenauer M, Phytotherapie. Phytopharmaka und pflanzliche Homöopathika, Fischer-Verlag, Stuttgart, Jena, New York 1995.

Chickweed

Stellaria media

TRADE NAMES

Chickweed Herbs, Wild Countryside Chickweed

DESCRIPTION

Medicinal Parts: The medicinal part is the fresh flowering or dried herb.

Flower and Fruit: The solitary white flowers are located in the leaf or branch axils. They open at 9 am and, in good weather, remain open for 12 hours. The 5 double petals are shorter than the oblong-lanceolate sepals. There are 2 to 5 stamens and 3 stigma. The fruit is globular or ovate and covered in teeth. It opens when ripe and the seeds are shaken out through the movement of the plant.

Leaves, Stem and Root: The plant is 5 to 30 cm high. The stem is decumbent and weak, heavily branched and often grows to an impressive length. It creeps along the ground, is fleshy, pale green, and slightly thickened at the nodes. The leaves are opposite and orbicular-ovate. The lower ones are long-petioled and the upper ones are sessile. They are 1.25 cm long and 0.70 cm wide and sit in pairs on the stem.

Characteristics: The stem is pubescent on one side.

Habitat: The plant is found worldwide as a weed.

Production: Chickweed is the fresh herb in flower of Stellaria media.

Other Names: Adder's Mouth, Passerina, Satin Flower, Starweed, Starwort, Stitchwort, Tongue-Grass, Winterweed

ACTIONS AND PHARMACOLOGY

COMPOUNDS

Flavonoids: including, among others, rutin

Ascorbic acid (vitamin C, 0.1-0.15%)

Alkaloids

INDICATIONS AND USAGE

Unproven Uses: Internally, Chickweed is used for rheumatism, gout, stiffness of the joints, tuberculosis, and diseases of the blood. Externally, it is used for poorly healing wounds, hemorrhoids, inflammation of the eyes, eczema and other diverse skin diseases.

PRECAUTIONS AND ADVERSE REACTIONS

No health hazards or side effects are known in conjunction with the proper administration of designated therapeutic dosages.

DOSAGE

Mode of Administration: The herb is used as a tea or in the form of juice for poultices, and in baths for medicinal purposes.

LITERATURE

Tsotsoriya G et al., (1977) Kromatogr Met Farm 172 (via CA 90:51421).

Further information in:

Kern W, List PH, Hörhammer L (Hrsg.), Hagers Handbuch der Pharmazeutischen Praxis, 4. Aufl., Bde 1-8: Springer Verlag Berlin, Heidelberg, New York, 1969.

Madaus G, Lehrbuch der Biologischen Arzneimittel, Bde 1-3, Nachdruck, Georg Olms Verlag Hildesheim 1979.

Watt JM, Breyer-Brandwijk MG, The Medicinal, Poisonous Plants of Southern, Eastern Africa, 2nd Ed, Livingstone 1962.

Chicory

Cichorium intybus

DESCRIPTION

Medicinal Parts: The medicinal parts of the plant are the dried leaves and roots, which are collected in autumn; the whole plant collected and dried in the flowering season; and the fresh plant and root.

Flower and Fruit: Size: The numerous flower heads are 3 to 4 cm in diameter and are terminal or axillary, solitary or in groups, sessile or short-pedicled. The epicalyx bracts are bristly ciliate, often glandular-haired. The inner bracts are oblong-lanceolate and erect, the outer ones ovate, splayed and half as long as the inner ones. The androgynous lingual florets are usually light blue, but occasionally white or pink. The fruit is an achaene 2 to 3 mm in length. It has no hair tuft and is ovate and straw yellow to blackish.

Leaves, Stem and Root: The plant can grow to a height of 2 m and has a hardy, 10 to 30 cm long, thick root. The stem is rigidly erect, sparsely branched above and often bristly. The leaves are 10 to 30 cm long and 1 to 5 cm wide. They are obovate, oblong, shaped like a cross-cut saw or slit, with numerous stiff hairs beneath. The lowest leaves in a basal rosette are petiolate. The upper ones as well as those near the inflorescences are alternate, oblong to lanceolate, crenate-dentate and sessile.

Characteristics: Chicory has a bitter taste.

Habitat: The plant is found in Europe, the Middle East as far as Iran, north and south Africa, all of America, Australia and New Zealand.

Production: Chicory consists of the dried leaves and underground parts of Cichorium intybus, which are collected in autumn in the wild and air-dried.

Other Names: Succory, Hendibeh

ACTIONS AND PHARMACOLOGY

COMPOUNDS

Sesquiterpenes: sesquiterpene lactones, especially lactucin, lactucopicrin, 8-desoxy lactucin, guaianolid glycosides, including chicoroisides B and C, sonchuside C

Caffeic acid derivatives: chiroric acid, chlorogenic acid, isochlorogenic acid, dicaffeoyl tartaric acid

Hydroxycoumarins: including umbelliferone

Flavonoids: including hyperoside

Polyynes

EFFECTS

An anti-exudative, choleretic, negatively chronotropic and negatively inotropic effect has been described due to the plant's sesquiterpene lactones, cinnamic acid derivatives and flavonoids. Animal studies have noted a distinct reduction of pulse rate and contractility; a mildly cholagogic effect; and lowered cholesterin level in rats' livers and plasma. Application for dyspeptic complaints seems plausible because of the amaroid (guaianolide) content.

INDICATIONS AND USAGE

Approved by Commission E:

- Loss of appetite
- Dyspeptic complaints

Unproven Uses: In Folk medicine, the herb is used externally for liver complaints and as a gargle. Among internal uses are sore throat, hemorrhoids, tuberculosis, abdominal cramps, melancholy, deafness and rashes. The juice of the chicory plant is also used as a laxative for children.

Indian Medicine: Medicinal uses include headaches, dyspeptic symptoms, skin allergies, vomiting and diarrhea.

PRECAUTIONS AND ADVERSE REACTIONS

No health hazards or side effects are known in conjunction with the proper administration of designated therapeutic dosages. There is a slight potential for sensitization via skin contact with the drug.

DOSAGE

Mode of Administration: Comminuted drug for infusions as well as other bitter-tasting preparations for internal use.

How Supplied: Commercial pharmaceutical preparations include drops and compound preparations.

Preparation: Prepare an infusion by scalding 2 to 4 g drug with boiling water, allowing it to stand for 10 minutes, then straining. A tea is prepared by brewing 2 to 4 g of the whole herb with 150 to 250 ml boiling water and then straining it after 10 minutes.

Daily Dosage: 3 to 5 g comminuted drug. Single dose: 2 to 4 g whole herb for an infusion.

LITERATURE

Anonym, Abwehr von Arzneimittelrisiken, Stufe II. In: DAZ 136(38):3253-2354. 1996.

BGA, Arzneimittelrisiken: Anthranoide. In: DAZ 132(21):1164. 1992.

Balbaa S et al., (1973) Planta Med 24:133.

Benoit PS et al., (1976) Lloydia 39:160.

Kawabata S, Deki M, (1977) Kanzei Chuo Bunsek 17:63.

Müller K, Wiegrebe W, Psoriasis und Antipsoriatika. In: DAZ 137(22):1893-1902. 1997.

Noldenn U, Dissertation Universität Bonn. 1989.

Proliac A, Blanc M, (1976) Helv Chem Acta 58:2503.

Wagner, H, In 'The Biology and Chemistry of the Compositae,'' Eds V. N. Heywood et al. Academic Press, London 1977.

Further information in:

Hänsel R, Keller K, Rimpler H, Schneider G (Hrsg.), Hagers Handbuch der Pharmazeutischen Praxis, 5. Aufl., Bde 4-6 (Drogen), Springer Verlag Berlin, Heidelberg, New York, 1992-1994.

Hausen B, Allergiepflanzen, Pflanzenallergene, ecomed Verlagsgesellsch. mbH, Landsberg 1988.

Madaus G, Lehrbuch der Biologischen Arzneimittel, Bde 1-3, Nachdruck, Georg Olms Verlag Hildesheim 1979.

Chimaphila umbellata

See Pipsissewa

Chinese Cinnamon

Cinnamomum aromaticum

DESCRIPTION

Medicinal Parts: The medicinal parts are the flowers collected and dried after they have finished blossoming, and the whole or partly peeled, dried bark of thin and young branches, as well the oil extracted from them.

Flower and Fruit: The flowers are small on short, slender, silky pedicles. They are arranged in threes in cymous panicles in the leaf axils and in larger panicles at the end of the branches. The perianth is slightly silky, about 3 mm long, with oblong-lanceolate petals. The fruit is a juicy, pea-sized, elliptoid, smooth drupe.

Leaves, Stem and Root: This evergreen tree grows up to 7 m tall with aromatic bark and angular branches. The bark is brown, in quilled pieces, sometimes with the remains of the outer layer present. The 7.5 to 10 cm long leaves are oblanceolate and pubescent on 6 to 8 cm long petioles, more or less tapered toward the base. They are coriaceous, alternate and brown underneath.

Habitat: Indigenous and cultivated in southern China, Vietnam, Laos and Burma.

Production: Chinese Cinnamon consists of the completely or partly peeled, dried stem bark from the aboveground or thin-branched axis of Cinnamomum aromaticum. The drug, from branches 2 to 3 cm thick, is peeled with horn knives, freed from cork and outer rind, and dried in the sun for 24 hours.

Not to be Confused With: Chinese Cinnamon should not be confused with waste products from the production process or other barks and materials, nor with the skins of horse chestnut seeds.

Other Names: Cassia, False Cinnamon, Bastard Cinnamon, Cassia Lignea, Cassia Bark, Cassia aromaticum, Canton Cassia

ACTIONS AND PHARMACOLOGY

COMPOUNDS

Volatile oil: chief components are cinnamaldehyde, weiterhin cinnamylacetate, cinnamyl alcohol, o-methoxycinnamaldehyde, cinnamic acid, coumarin

Diterpenes: cinnzeylanoles, cinncassioles A to E

Tannins: catechin tannins

Oligomere proanthocyanidins

Mucilages

EFFECTS

The essential oil and its main constituent cinnamaldehyde are antibacterial, fungistatic, improve immune resistance in animal tests (inhibiting allergic reactions Type I and II), promote motility, inhibit ulcers and act on the digestive tract (tannin content).

INDICATIONS AND USAGE

Approved by Commission E:

- Loss of appetite
- Dyspeptic complaints

Unproven Uses: Folk medicine uses include symptomatic treatment of gastrointestinal disorders (mild, colicky upsets of the gastrointestinal tract, bloating, flatulence and diarrhea), as well as for temporary states of exhaustion and to increase weight. Efficacy has been sufficiently proven for gastric complaints and it is plausible for diarrhea, but the evidence is not sufficient for the other indications.

Chinese Medicine: Among uses in Chinese medicine are impotence, diarrhea, enuresis, rheumatic conditions, testicle hernia, menopause syndrome, amenorrhea, abortion and to stabilize immunity.

Indian Medicine: Digestive complaints, vomiting and diarrhea are the most common uses in Indian medicine.

CONTRAINDICATIONS

Use of medicinal preparations of Chinese Cinnamon is contraindicated during pregnancy.

PRECAUTIONS AND ADVERSE REACTIONS

General: No health hazards or side effects are known in conjunction with the proper administration of designated therapeutic dosages. The drug possesses a medium potential for sensitization, primarily due to the cinnamaldehyde.

Pregnancy: The drug is not to be administered in time of pregnancy.

DOSAGE

Mode of Administration: Comminuted bark for infusions, essential oil, as well as other galenic preparations for internal use.

Preparation: To prepare a tincture of Chinese Cinnamon, moisten 200 parts cinnamon bark evenly with ethanol and percolate to produce 1000 parts tincture.

Daily Dosage: 2 to 4 g drug; 0.05 to 0.2 g essential oil. The average single dose is 1 g.

Storage: Chinese Cinnamon should be stored in a cool, dry environment in tightly sealed containers.

LITERATURE

Hikino H, Economic and Medicinal Plant Research, Vol I., Academic Press UK 1985.

Lockwood GB, Die Hauptbestandteile des ätherischen Öls von Cinnamomum cassia BLUME. In: PM 36(4):380-381. 1979.

Nagai H et al., (1982) Jpn J Pharmacol 32(5):813.

Nohara T et al., (1982) Phytochemistry 21(8):2130.

Nohara T et al., (1985) Phytochemistry 24(8):1849.

Nohara T et al., Cinncassiol E, a diterpene from the bark of Cinnamomum cassia. In: PH 24:1849. 1985.

Nohara T et al., PH 21:2130-2132. 1982.

Otsuka H et al., (1982) Yakugaku Zasshi 102:162.

Sagara K et al., J Chromatogr 409:365-370. 1987.

Senayake UM et al., (1978) J Agric Food Chem 20:822.

Structure of potent antiulcerogenic compounds from Cinnamomum cassia, Tetrahedron 44:4703. 1988.

Further information in:

Chan, EH et al., (Eds), Advances in Chinese Medicinal Materials Research, World Scientific Pub. Co. Singapore 1985.

Hänsel R, Keller K, Rimpler H, Schneider G (Hrsg.), Hagers Handbuch der Pharmazeutischen Praxis, 5. Aufl., Bde 4-6 (Drogen), Springer Verlag Berlin, Heidelberg, New York, 1992-1994.

Tang W, Eisenbrand G, Chinese Drugs of Plant Origin, Springer Verlag Heidelberg 1992.

Chinese Motherwort

Leonurus japonicus

DESCRIPTION

Medicinal Parts: The fruit is said to have medicinal properties.

Flower and Fruit: The inflorescence is long with whorls of a few flowers at some distance from each other. The bracts are short and usually have a thorn-like awn. The flowers are sessile and dorsiventral. The calyx is narrow clavate, approximately 8 mm long, short-haired. The calyx teeth are upright, the lower 2 are longer than the 3 upper ones. The corolla is bilabiate, made up of 5 fused petals, approximately 10 mm long, lilac to pink. The upper lip has a purple middle lobe and the lower lip is divided into 3. There are 2 long and 2 short stamens. The ovary is superior, 2-carpled and 4-chambered. The fruit breaks up into 4 black, 3-edged, approximately 2 mm long, 1-seeded mericarps.

Leaves, Stem and Root: This herbaceous perennial grows to a height of up to 1 m. The leaves are petiolate, 5 to 10 cm long, ovate to cordate, narrowing cuneiformly at the base. The lower leaves are palmately divided to the middle; the sections are pinnatifid with linear-acuminate lobes. The upper leaves are decussate opposite, simple, lanceolate, entire and pubescent on both surfaces. The stem is gray-green, upright, branched and square; the surface is grooved, and the ribs are pubescent.

Habitat: Leonurus japonicus is found in China, North and South Korea, and Japan.

Production: Chinese Motherwort fruit is the dried fruit of Leonurus japonicus.

ACTIONS AND PHARMACOLOGY

COMPOUNDS

Diterpenes: including leonurine

Fatty oil: chief fatty acids oleic acid and linolenic acid

EFFECTS

When taken internally, the alkaloid-containing drug (chief active ingredient leonurine) is said to have a contracting effect upon the uterus and to have generally anti-inflammatory effects upon various organ systems.

Topical application is said to reduce edema connected with injuries.

Watery drug extracts reduce blood pressure in animal experiments.

INDICATIONS AND USAGE

Chinese Medicine: Chinese Motherwort is used internally for inflammation of the kidney, the throat and the retina; for disturbances of menstruation, and in obstetrics for lochiastase. Externally, the fruit is used for swelling of the tissue after trauma.

Homeopathic Uses: The drug is used as a cardiac tonic, for nervous cardiac disturbances, anxiety states and nervous breathlessness.

PRECAUTIONS AND ADVERSE REACTIONS

No health hazards are known in conjunction with the proper administration of designated therapeutic dosages.

OVERDOSAGE

Feelings of weakness, outbreaks of sweating, enhanced sensitivity to pain and feelings of closeness in the chest can all follow intake of higher dosages of the drug (starting at 30 g).

CONTRAINDICATIONS

Not to be used during pregnancy.

DOSAGE

Mode of Administration: Whole and powdered drug. Preparations are administered internally and externally

Preparation: Infusion: 4 to 10 g drug

Daily Dosage: Not specified in the literature

LITERATURE

Hänsel R, Keller K, Rimpler H, Schneider G (Ed), Hagers Handbuch der Pharmazeutischen Praxis, 5. Aufl., Bde 4 - 6 (Drogen), Springer Verlag Berlin, Heidelberg, New York, 1992-1994.

Chinese Olive

Canarium species

DESCRIPTION

Medicinal Parts: The medicinal part of the plant is the resin.

Flower and Fruit: The flowers are arranged in helicoid or scorpiod cymes; the structures are in threes. The 3 petals are thick and often coriaceous; the 3 sepals are usually fused into a cup- or jug-shaped calyx. There are 6 stamens, and the ovary is 3-chambered with an ovule in each chamber; the stigma is 3-lobed. The fruit is an ovoid drupe with a thin, resin-rich mesocarp.

Leaves, Stem and Root: The tree is monoclinous or diclinous, reaching heights up to 15 m. The leaves are odd pinnate. The leaflets are short-petiolate and very irregular. The stipules are round or slit.

Habitat: The tree is indigenous to the Spice Islands, Philippines, China, Melanesia, and Moluccas.

Production: Elemi is the oleoresin (soft) exuding from fresh cuts made in Canarium luzonicum and the residual resin (hard) left to dry on the tree. The soft elemi is obtained by cutting split secretion channels and, after knocking off the hard elemi, collecting the resin which dries on that tree.

Other Names: Elemi

ACTIONS AND PHARMACOLOGY

COMPOUNDS

Triterpenes (70 to 80%): particularly alpha- and beta-amyrin, including alpha-, beta-, gamma-, delta-elemic acid, brein, maniladiol

Volatile oil (20 to 30%): chief component limonene (25%), also including alpha-phellandrene, elemol, eudesmol, carvacrol, methyl eugenol

EFFECTS

The resin is credited with promoting the healing of wounds. An immunostimulating effect was demonstrated in animal experiments. Topical administration causes skin irritation.

INDICATIONS AND USAGE

Unproven Uses: The resin is used in folk medicine as an expectorant for coughs as well as for gastric complaints, ulcers and rheumatism (plaster).

PRECAUTIONS AND ADVERSE REACTIONS

No health hazards are known in conjunction with the proper administration of designated therapeutic dosages. According to older sources, stomach complaints, kidney irritation and hemorrhagic erosions have been observed following administration of the essential oil. Topical application causes skin irritation.

DOSAGE

Mode of Administration: Preparations of the resin are used topically.

Preparation: Elemi resin is prepared by melting the resin at low heat and putting it through a filter. This cleaning process results in a somewhat darker elemi. Plasters are prepared using 25% drug in ointment.

Storage: Store in well-sealed tins protected from light.

LITERATURE

Blaschek W, Hänsel R, Keller K, Reichling J, Rimpler G, Schneider G (Eds), Hagers Handbuch der Pharmazeutischen Praxis. Folgebände 1 und 2. Drogen A-Z. Springer. Berlin, Heidelberg 1998.

Chinese Rhubarb (Da-Huang)

Rheum palmatum

DESCRIPTION

Medicinal Parts: The medicinal parts are the dried underground parts, and most of the root bark in the dried form.

Flower and Fruit: The inflorescence is an erect panicle foliated to the tip. The flowers have narrow, red, pink or whitish yellow tepals. The tepals are curved and located far back in the mature flowers to facilitate wind pollination. The fruit is red-brown to brown, and oval. The fruit is angular, about 10.2 mm to 7.8 mm wide and usually has scarious wings. The nutlet is 6 to 10 mm long and 7 mm in diameter.

Leaves, Stem and Root: The plant is a large, sturdy herbaceous perennial. The stem grows to over 1.5 m high. The leaves are orbicular-cordate, palmate lobed, somewhat rough on the upper surface and 3 to 5 ribbed. The lobes are oblong-ovate to lanceolate, dentate or pinnatisect. The root system consists of a tuber, which after a number of years measures 10 to 15 cm in diameter and has arm-thick lateral roots.

Habitat: The plant is indigenous to the western and northwestern provinces of China and is cultivated in many regions around the world. The main producers are China and Russia.

Production: Chinese Rhubarb consists of the dried underground parts of Rheum palmatum, Rheum officinale or of both species. Stem parts, roots and most of the bark are removed from the rhizomes.

Not to be Confused With: Other Rheum species such as Rheum rhaponticum or Rheum rhabarbarum. Garden Rhubarb is Rheum ponticum.

Other Names: Rhubarb

ACTIONS AND PHARMACOLOGY

COMPOUNDS

Anthracene derivatives (3-12%): chief components 1- or 8-O-β-glucosides of the aglycones rheumemodin, aloe-emodin, rhein, chrysophanol, physcion (together 60-80%), 8,8′-diglucosides of dianthrones (10-25%), including among others, sennosides A and B

Tannins: gallo tannins, including among others galloyl glucose, galloyl saccharose, lindleyine, isolindleyine

Flavonoids (2-3%)

Naphthohydroquinone glycosides

EFFECTS

Main active principles: hydroxyanthracene derivatives, tannins and a small proportion of flavonoids

The laxative effect is due to the hydrogogic and antiabsorptive properties of the anthranoids. This effect causes an increase in the volume of the intestinal contents resulting in pressure and stimulation of intestinal peristalsis.

INDICATIONS AND USAGE

Approved by Commission E:

- Constipation

Unproven Uses: Rhubarb is used as an appetite stimulant and for digestion problems, gastrointestinal catarrh and painful teething (children). External uses include burn treatment and skin conditions.

Chinese Medicine: In China, Rhubarb is used for delirium, tenesmus, edema, amenorrhea and abdominal pain. Efficacy for digestion problems is plausible because of the tannin content but not without risk because of the anthranoids (toxicity); efficacy for the other indications has not been proven.

Homeopathic Uses: Homeopathic uses include diarrhea and teething.

CONTRAINDICATIONS

Chinese Rhubarb is contraindicated in cases of intestinal obstruction, acute inflammatory intestinal disease, appendicitis and abdominal pain of unknown origin.

PRECAUTIONS AND ADVERSE REACTIONS

General: Spasmodic gastrointestinal complaints can occur as a side effect to the drug's purgative effect. Long-term use leads to losses of electrolytes, in particular potassium ions. The loss of electrolytes may lead to hyperaldosteronism, inhibition of intestinal motility and enhancement of the effect of cardioactive steroids. Long term use may lead to heart arrhythmias, nephropathies, edema and accelerated bone deterioration.

The increased incidence of carcinoma of the colon following long-term administration of anthracene drugs has not yet been fully clarified. Recent studies show no association between the administration of anthracene drugs and the frequency of carcinoma of the colon.

Stimulating laxatives must not be used over an extended period (1 to 2 weeks) without medical advice.

Drug Interactions: Potassium deficiency can cause an increase in the effect of cardiac glycosides.

Pregnancy: Use during pregnancy or while nursing only after consulting a physician.

Pediatric Use: The drug is not to be administered to children under 12 years of age.

DOSAGE

Mode of Administration: Liquid or solid forms of medication are exclusively for oral use. The drug is available as comminuted drug, powder or dry extracts for teas, decoctions, cold macerations or elixirs. Extracts of the drug are often constituents of laxatives, cholagogics and gastrointestinal remedies, and are found in "slimming cures," "springtime tonics" and "blood purifying" teas.

Preparation: To prepare an infusion to be used as a laxative, use 1.0-2.0 gm coarse powdered drug; for a stomachic, 0.1 to 0.2 gm powdered drug stirred with sufficient liquid (may be flavored with cinnamon, ginger, or peppermint oil) or scald and strain after 5 minutes. (1 teaspoonful = approximately 2.5 gm drug)

Daily Dosage: As a laxative, the dose is 1.0 to 2.0 gm of drug prepared according to instructions above. As an astringent and stomachic, the dose is 0.1-0.2 gm.

1.2 to 4.8 gm drug corresponds to 30 to 120 mg hydroxyanthracene derivatives/day, calculated as rhein.

Tea — 1 cup mornings and/or evenings

Extract — Single dose: 0.3 to 1 gm

Laxatives should be used for the shortest possible time (maximum 1 to 2 weeks)

Homeopathic Dosage: 5 drops, 1 tablet or 10 globules every 30 to 60 minutes (acute) or 1 to 3 times daily (chronic); parenterally: 1 to 2 ml sc acute: 3 times daily; chronic: once a day (HAB1).

LITERATURE

Anonym, Abwehr von Arzneimittelrisiken, Stufe II. In: DAZ 136(38):3253-2354. 1996.

Anonym, Anwendungseinschränkungen für Anthranoid-haltige Abführmittel angeordnet. In: PUZ 25(6):341-342. 1996.

BGA, Arzneimittelrisiken: Anthranoide. In: DAZ 132(21):1164. 1992.

Fairbairn JW, (1976) Pharmacol 14(Suppl 1):48.

Foust B, In: Foust MC. Rhubarb: The Wondrous Drug. Princeton University Press, Princeton, NJ 1992.

Friedrich H, Höhle J, (1966) Arch Pharm 299:857.

Iida K et al., Potent inhibitors of tyrosinase activity and melanin biosynthesis from Rheum officinale. In: PM 61(5):425-428. 1995.

Kashiwada Y et al., (1984) Chem Pharm Bull 32(9):3461.

Klimpel BE et al., Anthranoidhaltige Laxantien - ein Risiko für die Entwicklung von Tumoren der ableitenden Harnwege. In: PUZ 26(1):33, Jahrestagung der DPhG, Berlin, 1996. 1997.

Nonaka G et al., (1977) Chem Pharm Bull 25:2300.

Oshio H et al., (1974) Chem Pharm Bull 22:823.

Sanches EF, Feritas TV, Ferreiraalves DL, Velarde DT, Diniz MR, Cordeiro MN, Agostinicotta G, Biological activities of venoms from south American snakes. In: Toxicon 30(1):95. 1992.

Tsuboi et al., (1977) Chem Pharm Bull 25:2708.

Van Os FHL, (1976) Pharmacol 14(Suppl 1):7.

Zwaving JH, (1972) Planta Med 21:254.

Zwaving JH, (1974) Pharm Weekbl 109:1169.

Further information in:

Chan EH et al., (Eds.), Advances in Chinese Medicinal Materials Research, World Scientific Pub. Co. Singapore 1985.

Hänsel R, Keller K, Rimpler H, Schneider G (Hrsg.), Hagers Handbuch der Pharmazeutischen Praxis, 5. Aufl., Bde 4-6 (Drogen): Springer Verlag Berlin, Heidelberg, New York, 1992-1994.

Leung AY, Encyclopedia of Common Natural Ingredients Used in Food Drugs, Cosmetics, John Wiley & Sons Inc., New York 1980.

Lewin L, Gifte und Vergiftungen, 6. Aufl., Nachdruck, Haug Verlag, Heidelberg 1992.

Madaus G, Lehrbuch der Biologischen Arzneimittel, Bde 1-3, Nachdruck, Georg Olms Verlag Hildesheim 1979.

Roth L, Daunderer M, Kormann K, Giftpflanzen, Pflanzengifte, 4. Aufl., Ecomed Fachverlag Landsberg Lech 1993.

Schulz R, Hänsel R, Rationale Phytotherapie, Springer Verlag Heidelberg 1996.

Steinegger E, Hänsel R, Pharmakognosie, 5. Aufl., Springer Verlag Heidelberg 1992.

Tang W, Eisenbrand G, Chinese Drugs of Plant Origin, Springer Verlag Heidelberg 1992.

Teuscher E, Lindequist U, Biogene Gifte - Biologie, Chemie, Pharmakologie, 2. Aufl., Fischer Verlag Stuttgart 1994.

Teuscher E, Biogene Arzneimittel, 5. Aufl., Wiss. Verlagsges. Stuttgart 1997.

Wichtl M (Hrsg.), Teedrogen, 4. Aufl., Wiss. Verlagsges. Stuttgart 1997.

Chinese Thoroughwax (Chai-Hu)

Bupleurum chinense

DESCRIPTION

Medicinal Parts: The medicinal part of the plant is the root.

Flower and Fruit: The inflorescence is a compound umbel. The flower structures are arranged in fives. The flowers are radial and small; the petals are yellowish, almost orbicular; the calyx teeth are insignificant. The ovary is inferior and 2-chambered. The fruit is a double achaene.

Leaves, Stem and Root: Thoroughwax is an upright herbaceous perennial, which grows about 30 to 70 cm high. The leaves are alternate, arranged in spirals, simple and entire. The stem is hollow, gnarled and branched.

Habitat: China, Japan and central Europe

Production: Bupleuri roots are the dried roots of Bupleurum chinense. They are collected in the wild.

Not to be Confused With: May be confused with Bupleurum longiradiatum.

Other Names: Chai Hu

ACTIONS AND PHARMACOLOGY

COMPOUNDS

Triterpene saponins (saikosides,1.2 to 4.9%, content declining with the diameter of the root): saikosaponins a, b1, b2, c and d, aglycones are the so-called saikogenins

Steroids: sterols, including alpha-spinasterol, stigmasterol

Polyynes: saikodiine A, B and C

EFFECTS

The drug is not usually used alone, but rather used in various drug mixtures.

The saiko saponins or saikogenins that the drug contains have exhibited antipyretic, edema-protective and anti-inflammatory effects in animal experiments. At the same time, an inducement of the depletion of corticosterone and a liver-protective effect could be demonstrated, as could a sedative and an analgesic effect. The drug is also credited with antitussive, anti-ulcerogenic and blood-pressure lowering characteristics.

INDICATIONS AND USAGE

Unproven Uses: Chinese Thoroughwax is used for inflammatory conditions (oriental regions).

Chinese Medicine: Preparations are used for shivering and fever, jaundice, chest pain, bitter taste in the mouth, nausea, vomiting, malaria and deafness.

PRECAUTIONS AND ADVERSE REACTIONS

General: No health hazards are known in conjunction with the proper administration of designated therapeutic dosages.

Pregnancy: The drug is not to be administered during pregnancy.

OVERDOSAGE

The ingestion of larger dosages of the drug may lead to gastroenteritis, intestinal colic and diarrhea, due to the saponin content.

DOSAGE

Mode of Administration: Whole drug and cut drug preparations for internal and external use.

Preparation: The drug is usually only used in Chinese and Japanese medicine in compounded preparations.

Storage: Should be well sealed (to protect against insects), and air dried.

LITERATURE

Hänsel R, Keller K, Rimpler H, Schneider G (Ed), Hagers Handbuch der Pharmazeutischen Praxis, 5. Aufl., Bde 4 - 6 (Drogen), Springer Verlag Berlin, Heidelberg, New York, 1992-1994.

Jin RL, Shi L, Kuang Y, Comparative studies on the roots of wild and cultured Bupleurum chinense. DC Chung Yao Tung Pao, 20:11-3, 61, 1988 Apr.

Ohtsu S, Izumi S, Iwanaga S, Ohno N, Yadomae T, Analysis of mitogenic substances in Bupleurum chinense by ESR spectroscopy. Biol Pharm Bull, 20:97-100, 1997 Jan.

Zhang J, Comparison on saikosaponin levels in the root of Bupleurum chinense of various sizes. Chung Yao Tung Pao, 20:13-4, 1985 Apr.

Chionanthus virginicus

See Fringetree

Chiretta

Swertia chirata

DESCRIPTION

Medicinal Parts: The medicinal part is the herb, which is cut and dried when the seed is ripe.

Flower and Fruit: The numerous flowers are small and form a yellow panicle. The fruit is a single-valved capsule, which tastes very bitter and is odorless.

Leaves, Stem and Root: The plant is an annual and grows up to 90 cm high. The branching stem is brown or purplish, 2 to

4 mm thick, cylindrical below and becoming quadrangular toward the top. The leaves are smooth, opposite, lanceolate or ovate and entire-margined with 3 to 7 longitudinal ribs.

Habitat: The plant is indigenous to northern India and Nepal.

Production: Chiretta is the aerial part of Swertia chirata.

Other Names: Chirata, Chirayta, Indian Balmony, Indian Gentian

ACTIONS AND PHARMACOLOGY

COMPOUNDS

Iridoide monoterpenes as bitter substances (1.3%): chief components swertiamarin (0.4%), sweroside (0.2%), including as well gentiopicrin, amarogentin, amaroswerin

Xanthone derivatives: including mangiferin (0.12%), swerchirin (methyl bellidifoline), swertianin, 7-O-methyl swertianin, chiratol, swertiapunicoside, chiratanin

EFFECTS

Chiretta stimulates the secretion of gastric juices. In animal experiments, an anticholinergic (due to swertiamarin), antiphlogistic, hypoglycemic (due to xanthone derivatives), and centrally suppressing effect has been described.

INDICATIONS AND USAGE

Unproven Uses: Chiretta is used for dyspeptic disorders, loss of appetite, problems with the production of gastric juices and disorders of the digestive system.

CONTRAINDICATIONS

The drug should not be used in patients who have gastric or duodenal ulcers due to the drug's stimulation of gastric juice secretion.

PRECAUTIONS AND ADVERSE REACTIONS

No health hazards or side effects are known in conjunction with the proper administration of designated therapeutic dosages.

DOSAGE

Mode of Administration: The drug is a constituent part of various preparations, especially drops.

Daily Dosage: The daily dosage is 15 to 20 drops, 3 times daily before meals. For nervous disorders, 10 to 15 drops are taken daily between meals.

LITERATURE

Dalal SR et al. (1953) J Ind Chem Soc 30: 455.

Ghosal S et al. (1973) J Pharm Sci 62: 926.

Goyal H et al. (1981) J Res Ayur Siddha 2 (3): 286.

Hikano H et al. (1984) Shoyakugku Zasshi 38: 359.

Komatsu M et al. (1971) Jpn Kokai 71 (27): 558.

Ray S et al. Amarogentin, a naturally occuring secoiridoid glycoside and a newly recognized inhibitor of topoisomerase I from Leishmania donovani. In: JNP 59(1):27-29. 1996.

Sharma PV (1982) Indian J Pharm Sci 44 (2): 36.

Further information in:

Kern W, List PH, Hörhammer L (Hrsg.), Hagers Handbuch der Pharmazeutischen Praxis, 4. Aufl., Bde. 1-8: Springer Verlag Berlin, Heidelberg, New York, 1969.

Leung AY, Encyclopedia of Common Natural Ingredients Used in Food Drugs, Cosmetics, John Wiley & Sons Inc., New York 1980.

Steinegger E, Hänsel R, Pharmakognosie, 5. Aufl., Springer Verlag Heidelberg 1992.

Chives

Allium schoenoprasum

DESCRIPTION

Medicinal Parts: The medicinal parts are the fresh or dried aerial parts of the plant.

Flower and Fruit: The cyme has numerous florets. The sheath of the inflorescence has 2 or 3 flaps. The flap is broad-ovate and shorter than the inflorescence; it is white or reddish. The florets are dense and globose with no bulbils. The petals of the perianth are lanceolate-ovate and acute or pointed. They are 7 to 11 mm long, bluish or white to yellowish, and have a dark middle stripe. The stamens are shorter than the perianth. They are awl-shaped and fused with each other and the perianth petals at the base. The perianth surrounds the capsule like a balloon.

Leaves, Stem and Root: Allium schoenoprasum is a perennial, 15 to 30 cm high plant. The base is branched with numerous erect, closely packed leaves. Thin sheaths form incomplete, oblong bulbs. The bulb skin is thin, white and splitting when mature. The stem is round, usually smooth and leafy from the lower third. The compact leaves are completely hollow, round, somewhat elastic, and gray or gray-green.

Habitat: Chives grow wild in the temperate regions of Europe and North America and are cultivated in Europe, Turkistan, North America and from Siberia to Japan.

Production: Chives are the complete aerial parts of Allium schoenoprasum, which are harvested before flowering.

Other Names: Cive Garlic, Civet, Chive

ACTIONS AND PHARMACOLOGY

COMPOUNDS

Alliins (alkyl cysteine sulfoxides): in particular, methyl alliin (S-methyl-L-(+)-cysteine sulfoxide) and pentyl alliin (S-pentyl-L-(+)-cysteine sulfoxide), as well as their gamma-glutamyl conjugates; in the course of cutting up the fresh foliage, the alliins undergo a transformation (which is triggered by fermentation) into the so-called alliaceous oils, e.g., dimethyl-disulfide-mono-S-oxide

EFFECTS

The volatile and non-volatile sulphur bonds are said to be anthelmintic. However, efficacy has not been documented in scientific studies.

INDICATIONS AND USAGE

Unproven Uses: The drug is used to expel worms and intestinal parasites.

PRECAUTIONS AND ADVERSE REACTIONS

No health hazards or side effects are known in conjunction with the proper administration of designated therapeutic dosages. The intake of large quantities can lead to stomach irritation.

DOSAGE

Mode of Administration: Chives are used fresh or dried, as a cut drug.

LITERATURE

Kameoka H, Hashimoto S, Two sulfur containing constituents from Allium schoenoprasum. In: PH 22:294-295. 1983.

Hänsel R, Keller K, Rimpler H, Schneider G (Hrsg.), Hagers Handbuch der Pharmazeutischen Praxis, 5. Aufl., Bde 4-6 (Drogen): Springer Verlag Berlin, Heidelberg, New York, 1992-1994.

Hashimoto S et al., Food Sci 48:1858. 1983.

Chocolate Vine (Mu-Tong)

Akebia quinata

DESCRIPTION

Medicinal Parts: The dried stems and fruits of the Akebia quinata are frequently used in medicine.

Flower and Fruit: The inflorescence is racemose, hanging, 5 to 9 cm long, with 1 to 3 female flowers. The pedicle is 3 to 5 cm long. There are 3 to 4 violet to pink-violet sepals up to 1.5 cm long and 5 to 7 apocarpic, blue-violet carpels. There are 4 to 15 male flowers with 3 violet to lilac sepals and 6 to 7 violet to black stamens. The fruit is an elongate pome, 6 to 9 cm long, dark violet when ripe with white spots and a coriaceous cupule. The seeds are numerous, red-brown to black, ovoid, approximately 6 mm long and embedded in jelly-like tissue.

Leaves, Stem and Root: Akebia quinata is a climbing shrub that grows up to 10 m high. The shrub is deciduous, diclinous and monoecious. The leaves are alternate and arranged in fives. The petiole and the stems of the leaflets are approximately 2 cm long. The leaflets are up to 2.5 cm long, rounded at the base and entire. The trunk is silvery or gray, with cork warts.

Characteristics: The fruit is edible.

Habitat: Japan, China, Korea

Production: Chocolate vine is the dried stem of Akebia quinata.

Other Names: Five-Leaflet Akebia, Mu Tong

ACTIONS AND PHARMACOLOGY

COMPOUNDS

Triterpene saponins: akebosides, aglycones oleanolic acid and hederagenin

Steroids: sterols, including beta-sitosterol, beta-sitosterol glucoside, betulin

Monosaccharides/oligosaccharides: saccharose

Cyclitols: meso-inositol

EFFECTS

Animal experiments have demonstrated an anti-edemic effect attributed to the saponin mixture contained in the drug. In addition, diuretic, uricosuric, centrally depressant, antipyretic, mild analgesic and motility-inhibiting (intestinal) effects have been reported, although no results of controlled clinical studies have as yet been published.

INDICATIONS AND USAGE

Unproven Uses: Preparations of the plant have been used for acute urinary tract infections and ascites.

Chinese Medicine: Mu Tong is used for laryngitis and dry coughs, urinary stones, disturbances of bladder function, galacturia, convulsions, anemia and hematuria.

PRECAUTIONS AND ADVERSE REACTIONS

No health hazards are known in conjunction with the proper administration of designated therapeutic dosages. The ingestion of larger dosages of the drug may lead to gastroenteritis, intestinal colic and diarrhea, due to the saponin content. The drug is not to be administered during pregnancy.

DOSAGE

Mode of Administration: Liquid preparations for internal use.

Daily Dosage: 3 to 9 gm in the form of a decoction.

LITERATURE

Hänsel R, Keller K, Rimpler H, Schneider G (Ed), Hagers Handbuch der Pharmazeutischen Praxis, 5. Aufl., Bde 4 - 6 (Drogen), Springer Verlag Berlin, Heidelberg, New York, 1992-1994.

Yang DJ, The study of the constituents of Clematis and Akebia spp. II. On the saponins isolated from the stem of Akebia quinata Decne. (1) (author's transl) Yakugaku Zasshi, 9:194-8, 1974 Feb.

Yang DJ, Tinnitus treated with combined traditional Chinese medicine and Western medicine. Chung Hsi I Chieh Ho Tsa Chih, 9:270-1, 259-60, 1989 May.

Chondrodendron tomentosum

See Pareira

Chondrus crispus

See Carrageen

Chrysanthemum cinerariifolium

See Pyrethrum

Chrysanthemum leucanthemum

See Ox-Eye Daisy

Cichorium intybus

See Chicory

Cicuta virosa

See European Water Hemlock

Cimicifuga racemosa

See Black Cohosh

Cinchona pubescens

See Quinine

Cinnamomum aromaticum

See Chinese Cinnamon

Cinnamomum camphora

See Camphor Tree

Cinnamomum verum

See Cinnamon

Cinnamon

Cinnamomum verum

TRADE NAMES

Cinnamon bark liquid extract is available from several manufacturers.

DESCRIPTION

Medicinal Parts: The medicinal parts are the cinnamon oil extracted from the bark, the cinnamon bark of younger branches and the cinnamon leaf oil.

Flower and Fruit: The flowers are whitish-green, inconspicuous and have an unpleasant smell. They are about 0.5 cm long; arranged in loose, axillary or terminal panicles; and covered in silky hairs. The fruit is berry-like, ovoid-oblong, short-thorned and half-enclosed by the attached epicalyx.

Leaves, Stem and Root: The plant is a heavily foliated evergreen tree 6.5 to 12 m tall with a pale brown bark in thin quills, several rolled inside one another. The branches are cylindrical with a gray-brown bark. The tough leaves, which are opposite and splayed horizontally to leaning, are initially red then turn green. They are about 12 cm by 5 cm, roundish-ovate or ovate-lanceolate to oblong, more or less acuminate and entire-margined. The leaves smell like cloves.

Habitat: Cinnamon is indigenous to Sri Lanka and southwest India.

Production: Cinnamon consists of the dried tree bark, separated from the cork and outer rind, of young shoots growing on the branches of Cinnamomum verum. The tree is widely cultivated, and the harvested bark is dried in the shade.

Not to be Confused With: Confusion can arise with other powdered cinnamon varieties.

Other Names: Ceylon Cinnamon

ACTIONS AND PHARMACOLOGY

COMPOUNDS

Volatile oil: chief components - cinnamaldehyde, weiterhin eugenol, cinnamylacetate, cinnamyl alcohol, o-methoxycinnamaldehyde, cinnamic acid

Diterpenes: cinnzeylanol, cinnzeylanin

Oligomeric proanthocyanidins

Mucilages

EFFECTS

The cinnmaldehyde in the cinnamon bark's essential oil is antibacterial, fungistatic and promotes motility. It has a mildly positive estrogen effect on the genital system of animals in tests, although the constituent responsible is unidentified. Cinnamon increases gastric secretions slightly and is an insecticide due to the diterpenes cinnzeylanin and cinnceylanol.

INDICATIONS AND USAGE

Approved by Commission E:

- Loss of appetite
- Dyspeptic complaints

Unproven Uses: In addition, folk medicine internal uses include infantile diarrhea, chills, influenza and worm infestation. Cinnamon is used externally for cleaning wounds.

Indian Medicine: Uses in Indian medicine include toothache, nausea and vomiting, and halitosis.

CONTRAINDICATIONS

Use of the drug is contraindicated during pregnancy.

PRECAUTIONS AND ADVERSE REACTIONS

General: No health hazards or side effects are known in conjunction with the proper administration of designated therapeutic dosages. The drug possesses a medium potential for sensitization because of the cinnamaldehyde content.

Pregnancy: The drug is not to be administered to pregnant women.

DOSAGE

Mode of Administration: Comminuted drug for infusions; essential oil, as well as other galenic preparations for internal use. Bath additives, drops and compound preparations for external use.

How Supplied:

Extract — 1:1

Preparation: To prepare a tea, pour hot water over 0.5 to 1 g cinnamon bark and strain after 10 minutes. A tincture is made from a maceration of 20 parts cinnamon bark + 100 parts 70% ethanol V/V (ÖAB90).

Daily Dosage: 2 to 4 g drug; 0.05 to 0.2 g essential oil. One cup of tea/infusion is taken 2 to3 times daily at mealtimes. Liquid extract is taken 3 times in 1.5 to 1 ml doses. Two to 4 ml of tincture are taken 3 times daily. The standard single dose is 0.5 to 1 g of the drug.

Storage: Protect from light and moisture in non-synthetic containers.

LITERATURE

Buchalter L, (1971) J Pharm Sci 60: 144.

Isogai A et al., (1977) Agric Biol Chem 41: 1779.

Kato Y, (1975) Koryo 113: 17, et 24.

Kaul R, Pflanzliche Procyanidine. Vorkommen, Klassifikation und pharmakologische Wirkungen. In: PUZ 25(4):175-185. 1996.

Schneider E, Cinnamomum verum - Der Zimt. In: ZPT 9(6):193. 1988.

Schröder, Buch. In: Schröder R: Kaffee, Tee und Kardamom, Ulmer-Verlag, Stuttgart. 1991.

Further information in:

Hänsel R, Keller K, Rimpler H, Schneider G (Hrsg.): Hagers Handbuch der Pharmazeutischen Praxis, 5. Aufl., Bde 4-6 (Drogen), Springer Verlag Berlin, Heidelberg, New York, 1992-1994.

Leung AY, Encyclopedia of Common Natural Ingredients Used in Food Drugs and Cosmetics, John Wiley & Sons Inc., New York 1980.

Madaus G, Lehrbuch der Biologischen Arzneimittel, Bde 1-3, Nachdruck, Georg Olms Verlag Hildesheim 1979.

Roth L, Daunderer M, Kormann K, Giftpflanzen, Pflanzengifte, 4. Aufl., Ecomed Fachverlag Landsberg Lech 1993.

Steinegger E, Hänsel R, Pharmakognosie, 5. Aufl., Springer Verlag Heidelberg 1992.

Teuscher E, Biogene Arzneimittel, 5. Aufl., Wiss. Verlagsges. mbH Stuttgart 1997.

Wichtl M (Hrsg.), Teedrogen, 4. Aufl., Wiss. Verlagsges. Stuttgart 1997.

Cinquefoil

Potentilla erecta

DESCRIPTION

Medicinal Parts: The medicinal parts are the rhizome freed from the roots, the fresh underground parts collected in the spring, the dried rhizome and the rhizome gathered in the spring.

Flower and Fruit: The small, yellow, long-pedicled flowers grow opposite the leaves or at branching points on the stem. The 4 sepals have a 4-bract epicalyx. There are 4 free petals, which are obcordate and somewhat darker at the base. There are usually 16 stamens and numerous ovaries with thread-like styles. The receptacle is domed. The fruit is nut-like, hard, 1 seeded, ovate, grooved and occasionally smooth.

Leaves, Stem and Root: The plant is about 30 cm high and a rhizomatus herbacious perennial. The rhizome is 1 to 3 cm thick, irregular, gnarled to cylindrical, woody, dark-brown outside and blood red inside. The stem is erect or decumbent, never rooting, branching. The trifoliate rosette-like basal leaves wilt early and are gone before flowering. The cauline leaves are sessile, trifoliate and appear to be in fives because of 2 stipules

Characteristics: The plant is odorless and has an astringent taste.

Habitat: The plant is found as far north as Northern Scandinavia and as far south as Northwest Africa, Italy, Central Spain and the Balkans.

Production: Cinquefoil rhizome consists of the dried rhizome, freed from the roots, of Potentilla erecta (syn: Potentilla tormentilla N.) and its preparations. After harvesting the rhizome is air-dried.

Not to be Confused With: May be confused with Radix bistortae and the rhizomes of Geum species.

Other Names: Cinquefoil, Septfoil, Thormantle, Biscuits, Bloodroot, Earthbank, Ewe Daisy, Flesh and Blood, Shepherd's Knapperty, Shepherd's Knot, English Sarsaparilla

ACTIONS AND PHARMACOLOGY

COMPOUNDS

Catechins: including (-)-gallocatechin gallate, (-)-epigallocatechin gallate, dimerics and trimerics of the catechin derivatives

Catechin tannins (15 to 20%), transformed under storage conditions into non-water soluble tanner's reds (phlobaphenes)

Flavonoids: including kaempferol

Gallo tannins (3.5%), including agrimonine, pedunculagin, levigatines B and F proanthocyanidins

Tannins (17 to 22%)

Triterpenes: including tormentoside, ursolic acid, e-epi-pomolic acid

EFFECTS

The drug is astringent, antimicrobial and molluscidal because of the tannin complex (gallic tannins and ellagic tannins). In animal experiments an antihypertensive, anti-allergic, immune-stimulating, antiviral and interferon-inducing effect has been demonstrated.

INDICATIONS AND USAGE

Approved by Commission E:

- Diarrhea
- Inflammation of the mouth and pharynx

Tormentil is used internally to treat non-specific acute diarrhea. The drug is used externally for gingivitis, stomatitis and pressure caused by prosthetic devices.

Unproven Uses: In folk medicine, the drug is used internally for acute and subacute gastroenteritis and diarrhea and externally for poorly healing wounds, frostbite, burns and hemorrhoids.

PRECAUTIONS

No health hazards are known in conjunction with the proper administration of designated therapeutic dosages. There are reports in the literature of gastric complaints or vomiting following intake of the drug or its extracts.

DOSAGE

Mode of Administration: Tormentil is available in solid, liquid and compounded preparations for internal and external use.

Preparation: To prepare a tea, 2 to 3 gm finely cut or coarsely powdered drug is added to cold water, and rapidly brought to a boil, steep for some time and then strain. A cold water decoction may be used to avoid loss of tannin strength that occurs during the boiling process (1 teaspoon is equivalent to approximately 4 gm drug).

To prepare a tincture, 1 part cut rhizome is percolated with 5 parts 70% ethanol (V/V) (DAB10)

Daily Dosage: 4 to 6 gm drug

Tincture (1:10): 10 to 20 drops to one glass of water as a rinse several times a day

Tea: 1 cup to be taken 3 to 4 times a day (acts as an anti-diarrheal agent.)

Wine decoction: For diarrhea soak 2 to 4 gm powdered drug with red wine)

Storage: The herb should be protected from light.

LITERATURE

Bilia AR, Ctalano S, Fontana C, Morelli I, Palme E, A new saponin from Potentilla tormentilla. In: PM 58(7)23. 1992.

Geiger C et al., Ellagitannins from Alchemilla xanthochlora and Potentilla erecta. In: PM 60(4):384. 1994.

Glasl H, DAZ 123:1979. 1983.

Lund K, Rimpler H, (1985) Dtsch Apoth Ztg 125(3):105.

Lund K, Rimpler H, (1985) Tormentillwurzel. Dtsch Apoth Z 125:105-107.

Lund K, Tormentillwurzelstock, Phytochemische Untersuchungen des Rhizoms von Potentilla erecta (L.) RÄUSCHEL. In: Dissertation Universität Freiburg. 1986.

Scholz E, Rimpler H, Österr Apoth Ztg 48:138. 1994.

Vennat B et al., J Pharm Belg 47:485. 1992.

Further information in:

Hänsel R, Keller K, Rimpler H, Schneider G (Hrsg.), Hagers Handbuch der Pharmazeutischen Praxis, 5. Aufl., Bde 4-6 (Drogen): Springer Verlag Berlin, Heidelberg, New York, 1992-1994.

Madaus G, Lehrbuch der Biologischen Arzneimittel, Bde 1-3, Nachdruck, Georg Olms Verlag Hildesheim 1979.

Schulz R, Hänsel R, Rationale Phytotherapie, Springer Verlag Heidelberg 1996.

Steinegger E, Hänsel R, Pharmakognosie, 5. Aufl., Springer Verlag Heidelberg 1992.

Teuscher E, Biogene Arzneimittel, 5. Aufl., Wiss. Verlagsges. Stuttgart 1997.

Wichtl M (Hrsg.), Teedrogen, 4. Aufl., Wiss. Verlagsges. Stuttgart 1997.

Citrullus colocynthis

See Bitter Apple

Citrus aurantifolia

See Lime

Citrus aurantium

See Bitter Orange

Citrus limon

See Lemon

Citrus sinensis

See Sweet Orange

Cladonia pyxidata

See Cupmoss

Claviceps purpurea

See Ergot

Cleavers

Galium aparine

DESCRIPTION

Medicinal Parts: The medicinal parts are the aerial parts collected during the flowering season and dried, as well as the fresh, flowering herb and the fresh or dried whole plant.

Flower and Fruit: There are a few small white or greenish flowers in axillary, peduncled cymes. The corolla is about 1.5 to 1.7 mm long and has a pointed tip. The pedicles do not turn back before the fruit ripens. The 4 to 7 mm long mericarps are covered in barbed bristles.

Leaves, Stem and Root : The plant is 60 to 150 cm high. The stem is decumbent or climbing, sharply quadrangular even to the point of being winged and branched. There are long cauline leaves. The margins and midrib of the leaves are thorny. The foliage leaves are arranged in false whorls of 6 or 8. They are lanceolate from a wedge-shaped base, 30 to 60 mm long and 3 to 8 mm wide, obtuse and thorny tipped.

Habitat: A common wild plant throughout Europe, in Asia from Siberia to the Himalayas, and in North and South America.

Production: Cleavers is the flowering herb of the aerial part of Galium aparine, which is gathered and then dried.

Other Names: Clivers, Goosegrass, Barweed, Hedgeheriff, Hayriffe, Eriffe, Grip Grass, Hayruff, Catchweed, Scratweed, Mutton Chops, Robin-Run-in-the-Grass, Love-Man, Goosebill, Everlasting Friendship, Bedstraw, Coachweed,

Cleaverwort, Goose Grass, Gosling Weed, Hedge-Burs, Stick-a-Back, Sweethearts

ACTIONS AND PHARMACOLOGY

COMPOUNDS

Iridoide monoterpenes: asperuloside

Benzyl isoquinoline alkaloids: including protopine

Beta-carbolin alkaloids: harmine

Quinazoline alkaloids: 1-hydroxydesoxypeganin, 8-hydroxy-2,3-dehydrodesoxypeganin

Flavonoids

EFFECTS

No information is available.

INDICATIONS AND USAGE

The drug is used internally as well as externally for ulcers, festering glands, lumps in the breast and skin rashes. It is also used for lithuresis and calculosis and as a diuretic for dropsy, bladder catarrh and retention of urine (ischuria).

Efficacy has not been proven.

PRECAUTIONS AND ADVERSE REACTIONS

Health risks or side effects following the proper administration of designated therapeutic dosages are not recorded.

DOSAGE

Mode of Administration: Used topically in alcoholic extracts. Internally as a tea and juice.

Daily Dosage: As a tea, add 4 teaspoonfuls (3.3 to 4.4 gm) of the drug to 2 glasses of hot water. Drink in sips during the course of the day.

LITERATURE

Berkowitz, WF et al., (1982) J Org Chem 47:824.

Bhan MK et al., (1976) Ind J Chem 14:475.

Buckova et al., (1970) Acta Fac Pharm Univ Comeniana 19:7.

Burnett AR, Thomsom RH, (1968) J Clin Soc (6):854.

Corrigan D et al., (1978) Phytochemistry 17:1131.

Hänsel R, Keller K, Rimpler H, Schneider G (Hrsg.), Hagers Handbuch der Pharmazeutischen Praxis, 5. Aufl., Bde 4-6 (Drogen), Springer Verlag Berlin, Heidelberg, New York, 1992-1994.

Hegnauer R, Chemotaxonomie der Pflanzen, Bde 1-11, Birkhäuser Verlag Basel, Boston, Berlin 1962-1997.

Inouye H et al., (1974) Planta Med 25:285.

Madaus G, Lehrbuch der Biologischen Arzneimittel, Bde 1-3, Nachdruck, Georg Olms Verlag Hildesheim 1979.

Clematis

Clematis recta

DESCRIPTION

Medicinal Parts: The medicinal part is the fresh, flowering plant.

Flower and Fruit: The flowers are in many blossomed terminal cymes. The individual blossoms are white and similar to Clematis vitalba, except that the bracts are only downy on the edges. The nutlet is glabrous, with a thickened edge and a long tail.

Leaves, Stem and Root: The plant grows to about 50 to 125 cm high. The stem is non-climbing, erect, leafy and glabrous. The leaves are pinnatifid. The leaflets are smaller than those of Clematis vitalba.

Characteristics: The plant is poisonous.

Habitat: The plant grows in Europe.

Production: Clematis herb is the whole fresh flowering plant of Clematis recta. The herb is gathered when the plant is in full flower. It is turned regularly while being dried in the shade.

Other Names: Upright Virgin's Bower

ACTIONS AND PHARMACOLOGY

COMPOUNDS

Protoanemonine-forming agents in the freshly harvested plant: presumably, the glycoside ranunculin changes enzymatically when the plant is cut into small pieces (and probably also when it is dried) into the pungent, volatile protoanemonine that quickly dimerises to anemonine. Once dried, the plant may not be capable of protoanemonine formation.

Saponins

EFFECTS

The fresh plant induces blistering on the skin and mucous membranes and is a fungicide. Sun plants are more effective than shade plants.

INDICATIONS AND USAGE

Unproven Uses: Clematis was formerly used as a remedy for venereal diseases (syphilis), chronic skin conditions, gout, rheumatism and bone disorders, as well as a diuretic. In the pharmaceutical industry, it is used for rheumatic pains, headaches and varicose veins. In folk medicine, it is used for blisters and as a poultice for festering wounds and ulcers.

Homeopathic Uses: Clematis is used in homeopathic dilutions for ulcers and poor wound healing.

PRECAUTIONS AND ADVERSE REACTIONS

No health hazards or side effects are known in conjunction with the proper administration of designated therapeutic dosages of the dehydrated drug. Extended skin contact with the freshly harvested, bruised plant can lead to blister formation and cauterizations that heal poorly, due to the released protoanemonine, which is severely irritating to the skin and mucous membranes. If taken internally, severe irritation to the gastrointestinal tract, combined with colic and diarrhea, as well as irritation of the urinary drainage passages, are possible.

Symptomatic treatment for external contact consists of mucilaginosa, after irrigation with diluted potassium permanganate solution. In case of internal contact, administration of activated charcoal should follow gastric lavage.

OVERDOSAGE

Death by asphyxiation following the intake of large quantities of protoanemonine-forming plants has been observed in animal experiments. The risk associated with use of this plant is less than that of many other Ranunculaceae (e.g., Anemones nemorosae) due to the relatively low levels of protoanemonine-forming agents.

DOSAGE

Mode of Administration: The drug is seldom used today. It is available in the form of decoctions, which are used for poultices, as well as extracts and drops.

Homeopathic Dosage: Clematis is used in homeopathic dilutions D3 and D4.

Storage: The herb should be stored in tightly sealed containers.

LITERATURE

Bonora A et al., PH 26:2277. 1987.

Kizu H, Shimana H, Tomimori T, Studies on the constituents of Clematis species. VI. The constituents of Clematis stans Sieb. et Zucc. Chem Pharm Bull (Tokyo), 43:2187-94, 1995 Dec.

Ruijgrok HWL, PM 11:338-347. 1963.

Shropshire CM, Stauber E, Arai M, Evaluation of selected plants for acute toxicosis in budgerigars. J Am Vet Med Assoc, 200:936-9, 1992 Apr 1.

Southwell IA et al., Protoanemonin in australian Clematis. In: PH 33:1099. 1993.

Further information in:

Kern W, List PH, Hörhammer L (Hrsg.), Hagers Handbuch der Pharmazeutischen Praxis, 4. Aufl., Bde. 1-8, Springer Verlag Berlin, Heidelberg, New York, 1969.

Lewin L, Gifte und Vergiftungen, 6. Aufl., Nachdruck, Haug Verlag, Heidelberg 1992.

Madaus G, Lehrbuch der Biologischen Arzneimittel, Bde 1-3, Nachdruck, Georg Olms Verlag Hildesheim 1979.

Roth L, Daunderer M, Kormann K, Giftpflanzen, Pflanzengifte, 4. Aufl., Ecomed Fachverlag Landsberg Lech 1993.

Teuscher E, Lindequist U, Biogene Gifte - Biologie, Chemie, Pharmakologie, 2. Aufl., Fischer Verlag Stuttgart 1994.

Wagner H, Wiesenauer M, Phytotherapie. Phytopharmaka und pflanzliche Homöopathika, Fischer-Verlag, Stuttgart, Jena, New York 1995.

Clematis recta

See Clematis

Clematis vitalba

See Traveller's Joy

Clove

Syzygium aromaticum

DESCRIPTION

Medicinal Parts: The medicinal parts are the oil extracted from the whole or macerated flower buds, the pedicles and leaves, the dried flower buds and the not quite ripe fruit.

Flower and Fruit: The flowers are in triply-triple-branched cymes. They are short-pedicled, whitish-pink, approximately 6 mm wide and have 2 scale-like bracteoles. The calyx tube is 1 to 1.5 cm long and cylindrical. The 4 sepals are fleshy and there are 4 petals. The fruit is 2 to 2.5 cm long, 1.3 to 1.5 cm wide and is crowned by 4 curved sepals. The fruit is 1-seeded.

Leaves, Stem and Root: The plant is a 20 m high, pyramid-shaped evergreen tree. The diameter of the trunk is 40 cm. The branches are almost round. The leaves are 9 to 12 cm long and 3.5 cm wide. They are coriaceous, elliptical to lanceolate, short, obtusely tipped and narrowing in a cuneate form to the petiole, which is 2.5 cm long. There is 1 main rib and more than 20 lateral ones.

Characteristics: The taste and odor are characteristic.

Habitat: The plant is indigenous to the Molucca Islands and is cultivated there and in Tanzania, Madagascar, Brazil and other tropical regions.

Production: Cloves consist of the hand-picked and dried flower buds of Syzygium aromaticum (syn. Jambosa caryophyllus, Eugenia caryophyllata).

ACTIONS AND PHARMACOLOGY

COMPOUNDS

Volatile oil (15-21%): chief components eugenol (70-90%), eugenyl acetate (aceteugenol, up to 17%), beta-caryophyllene (5-12%)

Flavonoids: including astragalin, isoquercitrin, hyperoside, quercetin-3,4′-di-O-glycoside

Tannins (10%): ellagitannins, including eugenin

Triterpenes: oleanolic acid (1%), crataegolic acid (maslic acid, 0.15%)

Steroids: sterols, including beta-sitosterol

EFFECTS

Clove is antiseptic, antibacterial, antifungal, antiviral, spasmolytic and a local anaesthetic.

INDICATIONS AND USAGE

Approved by Commission E:

- Dental analgesic
- Inflammation of the mouth and pharynx

Unproven Uses: Clove oil is used internally for stomach ulcers and externally for colds and headaches. It is also used externally as a local analgesic and dental antiseptic.

Indian Medicine: The drug is used for halitosis, toothache, eye disease, flatulence, colic, gastropathy, and anorexia.

PRECAUTIONS AND ADVERSE REACTIONS

No health hazards or side effects are known in conjunction with the proper administration of designated therapeutic dosages. Allergic reactions to eugenol occur rarely. In concentrated form, oil of clove may be irritating to mucosa.

DOSAGE

Mode of Administration: As a powdered, ground, or whole herb for the recovery of the essential oil, and other galenic preparations for topical use.

Daily Dosage: Aqueous solutions corresponding to 1 to 5% essential oil are used externally for mouthwashes. In dentistry, the undiluted essential oil is used.

Storage: Do not store the drug in plastic containers, and protect it from light.

LITERATURE

Cai L, Wu ChD, Compounds from Syzygium aromaticum possesing growth inihibitory activity against oral pathogens. In: JNP 59(10):987-990. 1996.

Debelmas AM, Rochat J, (1967) Plant Med Phytother 1:23.

Deiniger R, Gewürznelken (Syzygium aromaticum) und Nelkenöl - aktuelle Phytopharmaka. In: ZPT 12(6):205. 1992.

Kato Y, (1975) Koryo 113:17 and 24.

Narayanan CS, Matthew AG (1985) Ind Perf 29(1/2):15.

Tanaka T, Orii Y, Nonaka GI, Nishioka I, Kouno I, Syziginins A and B, two ellegitannins from Syzygium aromaticum. In: PH 43(6)1345-1348. 1996.

Willuhn G, Pflanzliche Dermatika. Eine kritische Übersicht.. In: DAZ 132(37):1873. 1992.

Further information in:

Hänsel R, Keller K, Rimpler H, Schneider G (Hrsg.), Hagers Handbuch der Pharmazeutischen Praxis, 5. Aufl., Bde 4-6 (Drogen), Springer Verlag Berlin, Heidelberg, New York, 1992-1994.

Leung AY, Encyclopedia of Common Natural Ingredients Used in Food Drugs and Cosmetics, John Wiley & Sons Inc., New York 1980.

Steinegger E, Hänsel R, Pharmakognosie, 5. Aufl., Springer Verlag Heidelberg 1992.

Teuscher E, Biogene Arzneimittel, 5. Aufl., Wiss. Verlagsges. mbH Stuttgart 1997.

Wagner H, Wiesenauer M, Phytotherapie. Phytopharmaka und pflanzliche Homöopathika, Fischer-Verlag, Stuttgart, Jena, New York 1995.

Wichtl M (Hrsg.), Teedrogen, 4. Aufl., Wiss. Verlagsges. Stuttgart 1997.

Club Moss

Lycopodium clavatum

DESCRIPTION

Medicinal Parts: The medicinal parts are the spores and the fresh plant.

Flower and Fruit: Sulfur yellow, minute spores, carried in large numbers in 2 to 3 cylindrical yellow-green cones, develop in August at the ends of leafy, 15 cm high stalks extending from aerial branches.

Leaves, Stem and Root: The plant has a 1 m long, procumbent stem with only a few roots. It is covered with yellowish-green leaves, densely arranged in spirals, which are entire-margined, linear, smooth and end in a long, white, upwardly bent hair tip. There are numerous erect, circular, 5 cm high branches on the mainstem.

Habitat: The plant is found worldwide, but it originated in China and Eastern Europe.

Production: Club Moss is the aerial part Lycopodium clavatum. It is collected in the uncultivated regions and air-dried or dried artificially at a maximum of 40° C.

Other Names: Stags Horn, Witch Meal, Wolfs Claw, Vegetable Sulfur

ACTIONS AND PHARMACOLOGY

COMPOUNDS

Alkaloids (0.2%): including among others those of the lycopodine- and lycodan-types (derived from piperidine alkaloids), chief alkaloids lycopodine and dihydrolycopodine, in traces also nicotine.

Triterpenes: including alpha-onocerin, lycoclavatol, lycoclavanol, serratendiol (demonstrated in plants of Japanese origin)

Steroids: including beta-sitosterol, campesterol and stigmasterol

Flavonoids: including among others chrysoeriol, luteolin

EFFECTS

Club Moss has a diuretic effect.

INDICATIONS AND USAGE

Unproven Uses: In folk medicine, it is used internally for bladder and kidney complaints, also for pharyngeal catarrh and tonsillitis, menstruation complaints, rheumatism and impotence; externally for wounds, itching and suppurating eczema of the skin.

Homeopathic Uses: Herb and spores are used in liver and gallbladder complaints, general blood poisoning, inflammation of the respiratory tract, disorders of the intestinal tract, varicose veins, metabolic diseases, chronic and acute skin conditions, inflammation of the female genital organs and menstruation complaints, as well as behavioral and mood disturbances.

PRECAUTIONS AND ADVERSE REACTIONS

No health hazards or side effects are known in conjunction with the proper administration of designated therapeutic dosages. Irritations should be expected with extended used of the drug.

OVERDOSAGE

Despite the toxicity of the alkaloids, no poisonings have been recorded.

DOSAGE

Mode of Administration: In folk medicine, chopped drug is used in teas.

Daily Dosage: Single dose: 1.5 gm drug. Tea: 1 cup to be taken 2 to 3 times daily.

Homeopathic Dosage: 5 drops, 1 tablet or 10 globules every 30 to 60 minutes (acute) or 1 to 3 times daily (chronic); parenterally; 1 to 2 ml sc acute, 3 times daily; chronic: once a day (HAB1)

LITERATURE

Blumenkopf TA, Heathcock CH, The Alkaloids, Vol. 5, Ed. SW Pelletier, John Wiley 1985.

Kern W, List PH, Hörhammer L (Hrsg.), Hagers Handbuch der Pharmazeutischen Praxis, 4. Aufl., Bde. 1-8, Springer Verlag Berlin, Heidelberg, New York, 1969.

Leete E, The Alkaloids, Vol. 1, Ed. SW Pelletier, John Wiley 1983.

Madaus G, Lehrbuch der Biologischen Arzneimittel, Bde 1-3, Nachdruck, Georg Olms Verlag Hildesheim 1979.

Wichtl M (Hrsg.), Teedrogen, 4. Aufl., Wiss. Verlagsges. Stuttgart 1997.

Cnicus benedictus

See Blessed Thistle

Coca

Erythroxylum coca

DESCRIPTION

Medicinal Parts: The medicinal parts are the leaves of the coca bush.

Flower and Fruit: The flowers are small and greenish white. They are in axillary clusters. The fruit is a red almost 1 cm long drupe with 1 seed.

Leaves, Stem and Root: Erythroxylum coca is a small shrub-like tree up to 5 m tall. The leaves are brownish-green, oval, thin but tough, up to 5 cm long and 2.5 cm wide with two lines on the surface parallel to the midrib. The margins are entire, the apex rounded. There are 2 faint projecting lines on the upper surface parallel to the midrib which stiffen the leaf. There are small stipules in the leaf axils, which later become brown and hard.

Habitat: The plant is indigenous to the Andes region of South America; it is cultivated in Indonesia, India and Sri Lanka.

Production: Coca leaves are the dried leaves of Erythroxylum coca.

Other Names: Bolivian Coca, Cocaine, Cuca, Peruvian Coca

ACTIONS AND PHARMACOLOGY

COMPOUNDS

Tropane alkaloids: main alkaloid (-)-cocaine, including, among others, cis-cinnamoyl cocaine, trans-cinnamoyl cocaine, also including alpha-truxillin, beta-truxillin, benzoylecgonin

EFFECTS

The leaves act as a local anesthetic and stimulate the central nervous system. In high doses, the drug causes paralysis of motor neuron fibers.

INDICATIONS AND USAGE

Unproven Uses: The plant is used in the manufacture of the local anesthetic cocaine hydrochloride. It is a model for synthetic local anesthetics. Cocaine is still occasionally used in ophthalmology.

PRECAUTIONS AND ADVERSE REACTIONS

General: Chewing an excessively large quantity of the leaves can cause psychic disturbances and hallucinations. Chronic use can lead to poor nutritional states and disinterest in work, due to the suppression of feelings of hunger and the resulting reduction in food intake. The enhanced vulnerability to illness and the reduced life expectancy are also conditioned by the immunosuppressive effect of the drug. Beyond that, the drug is probably carcinogenic in effect, embryotoxic and sensitizing. The observed dependence on the drug (cocoaism) is mainly psychically conditioned, although withdrawal symptoms are also known (need for sleep, bulimia, anxiety, irritability, tremor). For the toxicology of cocaine, consult publications (Lewin, Teuscher).

Pregnancy: Cocaine passes into the embryo or fetus and is embryotoxic.

Nursing Mothers: Cocaine passes into the mother's milk.

DOSAGE

Mode of Administration: Use of Erythroxylum coca is obsolete except for use in 2% eyedrops.

LITERATURE

Aynilian G et al., (1974) J Pharm Sci 63:1938.

Brustschmerzen und Atherosklerose durch Cocain. In: DAZ 130(49):2723. 1990.

Chen GJ, Pillai R, Erickson JR, Martinez F, Estrada ALÖ, Watso RR, Cocaine immunotoxicity - abnormal cytokine production in hispanic drug users. In: Toxicol Lett 59(1-3):81. 1991.

Evans WC, ETH 3:265. 1981.

Grieb G, Miβbildungen: Schädigt Cocain menschliche Spermien? In: DAZ 132(12):578. 1992.

Homstedt B et al., (1977) Phytochemistry 16:1753.

Moore JM et al., 1-Hydroxytropacocaine: an abundant alkaloid of Erythroxylum novogranatense var. novogranatense and var. truxillense. In: PH 36(2):357. 1994.

Novak M, Salemink C, (1987) Planta Med 53(1):113.

Novak M, Salemink CA, Khan I, ETH 10:261. 1984.

Sukrasno N, Yeoman MM, Phenylpropanoid metabolism during growth and development of Capsicum frutescens fruits. In: PH 32:839. 1993.

Tuerner CE, Ma C, Elsohly MA, ETH 3:293. 1981.

Wiggins RC, Pharmacokinetics of Cocaine in pregnancy and effects on fetal maturation. In: Clinical Pharmacokinetics 22(2):85. 1992.

Further information in:

Hänsel R, Keller K, Rimpler H, Schneider G (Hrsg.), Hagers Handbuch der Pharmazeutischen Praxis, 5. Aufl., Bde 4-6 (Drogen), Springer Verlag Berlin, Heidelberg, New York, 1992-1994.

Leung AY, Encyclopedia of Common Natural Ingredients Used in Food, Drugs and Cosmetics, John Wiley & Sons Inc., New York 1980.

Lewin L, Gifte und Vergiftungen, 6. Aufl., Nachdruck, Haug Verlag, Heidelberg 1992.

Roth L, Daunderer M, Kormann K, Giftpflanzen, Pflanzengifte, 4. Aufl., Ecomed Fachverlag Landsberg Lech 1993.

Steinegger E, Hänsel R, Pharmakognosie, 5. Aufl., Springer Verlag Heidelberg 1992.

Teuscher E, Lindequist U, Biogene Gifte - Biologie, Chemie, Pharmakologie, 2. Aufl., Fischer Verlag Stuttgart 1994.

Teuscher E, Biogene Arzneimittel, 5. Aufl., Wiss. Verlagsges. mbH Stuttgart 1997.

Cochlearia officinalis

See Scurvy Grass

Cochlospermum gossypium

See Cotton Tree

Cocillana Tree

Guraea rusbyi

DESCRIPTION

Medicinal Parts: The medicinal part of the plant is the bark.

Flower and Fruit: The flowers are radial, and their structures are in fives. They are white to yellowish and inconspicuous. The ovary is superior.

Leaves, Stem and Root: The plant grows as a tree, rising up to 5 m high. The leaves are large and pinnatifid.

Habitat: Guraea rusbyi is indigenous to Cuba, Brazil and Bolivia.

Production: Cocillana bark is the bark of the trunk of Guarea rusbyi, which is collected in the wild.

ACTIONS AND PHARMACOLOGY

COMPOUNDS

Volatile oil

Steroids: sterols, including beta-sitosterol

Tannin

Alkaloids

EFFECTS

The drug is said to be expectorate, emetic and laxative in effect. In higher dosages, it is said to be menstruation-inducing. The emetic effect is credited to the alkaloid fraction, which has not been more precisely defined. Experimental data have not been made available. The bark of the tree induces vomiting and can frequently bring on a feeling of weakness and nausea. But it can also provide a stimulatory expectorant and has been used successfully in the treatment of bronchitis and respiratory illnesses.

INDICATIONS AND USAGE

Unproven Uses: Uses in folk medicine have included treatment of chronic bronchitis and coughs and also as an emetic.

PRECAUTIONS AND ADVERSE REACTIONS

No health hazards are known in conjunction with the proper administration of designated therapeutic dosages. The drug is said to induce vomiting and diarrhea in high dosages.

CONTRAINDICATION

Because it is said to induce menstruation, it should not be administered to anyone who is pregnant.

DOSAGE

Mode of Administration: Whole, cut and powdered drug preparations for internal use.

Preparation: Tinctures are prepared using drug 1:10 60% ethanol (V/V) (BHP83). Liquid extracts contain drug 1:1 60% ethanol (V/V) (BHP83).

Daily Dosage:

Decoction — from 0.5 to 1 g drug, 3 times daily

Liquid extract — 0.5 to 1 ml, 3 times daily

Tincture — 5 to 10 ml, 3 times daily

Syrup — 2 to 4 ml, 3 times daily

Dose for children — 1/4 to 1/3 of the above doses.

LITERATURE

Blaschek W, Hänsel R, Keller K, Reichling J, Rimpler G, Schneider G (Eds), Hagers Handbuch der Pharmazeutischen Praxis. Folgebände 1 und 2. Drogen A-Z. Springer. Berlin, Heidelberg 1998.

Cocoa

Theobroma cacao

DESCRIPTION

Medicinal Parts: The medicinal parts are the seed skins that remain after making cocoa and cocoa butter; the seeds which have been partly freed from their skins and lightly roasted; and the raw, dried, unroasted seeds.

Flower and Fruit: The inflorescences are on the main trunk and thicker branches on a so-called ''flower cup.'' The cyme-like branchlets are short, noded and persistent. There are 5 sepals, which are narrow. The petals are cap-shaped and stemmed with flag-like laminas. The stamen tube, with 5 fertile stamens and 5 awl-shaped staminoids, is short. The fruit is a 15 to 25 cm long and 10 cm thick, large berry. It is oblong or obovate, thick-skinned, yellow or reddish, grooved and sometimes bumpy and cucumber-like. The 20 to 50 seeds are arranged in rows and embedded in a pink, fruity, sweetish-sour pulp. They are pressed flat, almond-shaped, reddish-brown and without endosperm.

Leaves, Stem and Root: The plant is a 4 to 6 m, occasionally up to 13 m, tall tree with an irregular knotty trunk and a broad crown. The young branches are rounded. The leaves are coriaceous or paper-like, alternate and in 2 rows on the branches. The petiole is downy, cushioned, and 1.5 to 2 cm long. The lamina is oval or elliptical, slightly asymmetrical, rounded at the base with a conspicuous tip. The upper surface is green and pale when dry. The lower surface is paler green, glabrous or has a few, tiny, simple, branched and scattered hairs.

Habitat: The plant is cultivated globally in tropical regions.

Production: Cocoa seeds consist of the seeds of Theobroma cacao, which have been removed from their shells, fermented and lightly roasted. Cocoa consists of the testae of Theobroma cacao. Cocoa butter is the hard fat obtained from the ripe cocoa seeds of Theobroma cacao. After removal of the germ-roots and the shell from the seeds, the seeds are removed from the shell and crushed. The cocoa fat is squeezed out at a temperature of 70° C to 80° C and allowed to cool.

Other Names: Cacao, Chocolate Tree

ACTIONS AND PHARMACOLOGY

COMPOUNDS: COCOA SEED

Purine alkaloids (3 to 4%): main alkaloid theobromine (2.8 to 3.5%), with a lesser amount of caffeine (0.1 to 0.4%)

Fat (50%): chief fatty acids oleic acid (33 to 39%), stearic acid (30 to 37%), palmitic acid (24 to 31%)

Proteic substances (10 to 16%)

Starch (5 to 9%)

Monosaccharides/oligosaccharides (2 to 4%): saccharose, glucose, fructose

Biogenic amines: including phenyl ethyl amine, tyramine, tryptamine, serotonin

Isoquinoline alkaloids: salsolinol

Catechin tannins (10%): including oligomeric proanthocyanidins (8%)

Oxalates (0.6 to 1%)

EFFECTS: COCOA SEED

Cocoa seeds can cause constipation because of the tannin content. The drug contains methylxanthines, mainly theobromin, which have a diuretic, broncholytic, and vasodilatory effect. They also stimulate cardiac muscle performance and act as a muscle relaxant.

COMPOUNDS: COCOA SEED COAT

Purine alkaloids: main alkaloid theobromine (0.4-1.2%) with less caffeine (0.02%)

Fat (5%)

Biogenic amine: including phenyl ethyl amine, tyramine, tryptamine, serotonin

Catechin tannins: among them, proanthocyanidins

EFFECTS: COCOA SEED COAT

Cocoa can cause constipation. Cocoa contains methylxanthines, which have a diuretic, bronchyolitic, and vasodilatory effect. They also improve cardiac muscle performance and act as a muscle relaxant.

COMPOUNDS: COCOA BUTTER

Triglycerides (melting temperature 31 to 35°C): chief fatty acids oleic acid (33 to 39%), stearic acid (30 to 37%), palmitic acid (24 to 31%)

Free fatty acids

Steroids: sterols, including beta-sitosterol

Purine alkaloids (0.001 to 0.1%)

EFFECTS: COCOA BUTTER

The main constituents are triglycerides. High doses of cocoa butter, in contrast to similar saturated fatty acids, do not cause an increase of serum cholesterol and the LDL fraction.

INDICATIONS AND USAGE

COCOA SEED

Unproven Uses: In folk medicine, Cocoa seeds are used for infectious intestinal disease, diarrhea and as a secretolytic. It is also used to regulate the thyroid and as a mild stimulant (in compound drinks containing caffeine.)

COCOA SEED COAT

Preparations of cocoa seed coat are used for liver, bladder, and kidney ailments, diabetes, as a tonic and general remedy and as an astringent for diarrhea.

COCOA BUTTER

Cocoa Butter is used by the pharmaceutical and cosmetic industries as an inactive ingredient in dermatologic preparations.

PRECAUTIONS AND ADVERSE REACTIONS

COCOA SEED

General: No health hazards or side effects are known in conjunction with either the proper administration of designated therapeutic dosages or the consumption of normal amounts of chocolate products. Large dosages lead to constipation due to the tannin content. Cocoa and cocoa products can cause allergic reactions. The amines can trigger migraine attacks.

Pediatric Use: Large quantities of chocolate products can lead to overexcitability, racing pulse and sleep disorders in children because of the caffeine content, which can be as high as 0.2% in milk chocolate and 0.4% in bitter chocolate.

COCOA SEED COAT

No health hazards or side effects are known in conjunction with the proper administration of designated therapeutic dosages. Cocoa and cocoa products can cause allergic reactions. Large dosages lead to constipation due to the tannin content. The amines can trigger migraine attacks.

COCOA BUTTER

No health hazards or side effects are known in conjunction with the proper administration of designated therapeutic dosages.

DOSAGE

COCOA BUTTER

Mode of Administration: Cocoa Butter is used as a pharmaceutical base for suppositories and vaginal globules. It is an additive for ointments and cosmetic preparations, such as skin creams and lip balms.

Storage: Store in a cool, dark place.

LITERATURE

Hänsel R, Keller K, Rimpler H, Schneider G (Hrsg.), Hagers Handbuch der Pharmazeutischen Praxis, 5. Aufl., Bde 4-6 (Drogen): Springer Verlag Berlin, Heidelberg, New York, 1992-1994.

Leung AY, Encyclopedia of Common Natural Ingredients Used in Food Drugs and Cosmetics, John Wiley & Sons Inc., New York 1980.

Lewin L, Gifte und Vergiftungen, 6. Aufl., Nachdruck, Haug Verlag, Heidelberg 1992.

Naturw R, 49:481. 1996.

Roth L, Daunderer M, Kormann K, Giftpflanzen, Pflanzengifte, 4. Aufl., Ecomed Fachverlag Landsberg Lech 1993.

Schröder B, In: Schröder R, Kaffee, Tee und Kardamom, Ulmer-Verlag, Stuttgart. 1991.

Teuscher E, Biogene Arzneimittel, 5. Aufl., Wiss. Verlagsges. Stuttgart 1997.

Teuscher E, Lindequist U, Biogene Gifte - Biologie, Chemie, Pharmakologie, 2. Aufl., Fischer Verlag Stuttgart 1994.

Coconut Palm

Cocos nucifera

DESCRIPTION

Medicinal Parts: The medicinal part of the plant is the fruit.

Flower and Fruit: The flowers are arranged in up to 1.5 m long, spindle-shaped, branching axillary inflorescences, which are surrounded by a woody spathe. On each of the 20 to 40 lateral branches of the inflorescence there is only one, 3 to 3.5 cm large, yellowish-green-white female flower. There are 200 to 300 male flowers at the apex of the single branches with their structures arranged in threes. The flowers are up to 1.5 cm wide and yellowish; the ovary is 3-carpeled and fused. The drupe is up to 30 cm long and weighs 1.5 to 2.5 kg. The exocarp is smooth and impervious to water. The mesocarp is fibrous (certain floating ability, coconut fiber) and the endocarp woody and hard. The stone kernel is incorrectly called a nut. The inconspicuous embryo is embedded in the fat rich endosperm (copra). Inside the unripe fruit there is approximately 500 ml of clear, sweet-tasting liquid (coconut milk), which reduces when the fruit ripens. At the side stem insert there are 3 shoot holes, only one of which is covered with a membrane. These allow the embryo to penetrate the surrounding fiber layer.

Leaves, Stem and Root: Coconut Palm is diclinous and monoecious. The tree grows up to 30 to 35 m high. The frond is up to 5 m long, 1 to 1.7 m wide (up to 15 kg in weight) and clasps the trunk with a wide petiole. The bark is thick and the surface is shaggy with remains of the leaf bases of fallen leaves. The trunk is divided into nodes and internodes. Adventitious roots arise from the base of the trunk.

Characteristics: One palm tree produces up to 70 ripe fruit per year.

Habitat: The native country of this species is disputed, but is believed to be the Pacific regions.

Production: Coconut oil is the fat extracted from the dried solid part of the endosperm of Cocos nucifera through cold pressing. Completely ripe fruit is harvested, followed by manual or mechanical opening of the kernel and then followed by the extraction of the endosperm (known as copra). It is dried in the sun, over a fire or in special drying houses. The pressed oil is refined and cleaned.

ACTIONS AND PHARMACOLOGY

COMPOUNDS

Fatty oil: chief fatty acids lauric acid (45 to 50%), myristic acid (13 to 20%), palmitic acid (7 to 10%), caprylic acid (5 to 10%), including as well stearic acid, linoleic acid, caproic acid.

Free fatty acids (3 to 5%)

Delta-lactones of 5-hydroxy-fatty acids: particularly delta-octalactone (as aroma compounds)

EFFECTS

Coconut oil is characterized by having a large quantity of short-chained fatty acids and a rather small amount of unsaturated fatty acids. It is chiefly used as a dietetic. An immunomodulating effect was observed in animal experiments, as was an inhibiting effect upon the growth of carcinoma cells of the colon in vitro.

INDICATIONS AND USAGE

Unproven Uses: The oil of Coconut Palm has been used for poorly healing wounds and skin infections (Africa). Internally it is used for colds and inflammation of the throat (with salt; Central America) and for tooth decay (southeast Asia).

Indian Medicine: Coconut Palm oil is used for dysuria, coughs, bronchitis and to stop hair from turning gray.

PRECAUTIONS AND ADVERSE REACTIONS

No health hazards are known in conjunction with the use of the drug as a food or as a pharmaceutical vehicle or raw substance (including its use in the extraction of short- and medium-chained fatty acids and in the manufacture of soaps and solubilizing agents).

DOSAGE

Mode of Administration: Preparations are intended for internal and external use.

Storage: Protect from light in tightly sealed containers at a maximum temperature of 25° C.

LITERATURE

Blaschek W, Hänsel R, Keller K, Reichling J, Rimpler G, Schneider G (Eds), Hagers Handbuch der Pharmazeutischen Praxis. Folgebände 1 und 2. Drogen A-Z. Springer. Berlin, Heidelberg 1998.

Eghafona NO, Immune responses following cocktails of inactivated measles vaccine and Arachis hypogaea L. (groundnut) or Cocos nucifera L. (coconut) oils adjuvant. Vaccine, 84:1703-6, 1996 Dec.

Jaggi KS, Arora N, Niphadkar PV, Gangal SV, Immunochemical characterization of cocos nucifera pollen. J Allergy Clin Immunol, 84:378-85, 1989 Sep.

Karmakar PR, Chatterjee BP, Cocos nucifera pollen inducing allergy: sensitivity test and immunological study. Indian J Exp Biol, 84:489-96, 1995 Jul.

Nalini N, Sabitha K, Chitra S, Viswanathan P, Menon VP, Antifungal activity of the alcoholic extract of coconut shell - Cocos nucifera Linn. J Ethnopharmacol, 84:291-3, 1980 Sep.

Nalini N, Sabitha K, Chitra S, Viswanathan P, Menon VP, Histopathological and lipid changes in experimental colon cancer: effect of coconut kernel (Cocos nucifera Linn.) and (Capsicum annum Linn.) red chilli powder. Indian J Exp Biol, 84:964-71, 1997 Sep.

Cocos nucifera

See Coconut Palm

Coffea arabica

See Coffee

Coffee

Coffea arabica

DESCRIPTION

Medicinal Parts: The medicinal part of the plant is the seed in various forms and stages.

Flower and Fruit: The inflorescences are axillary dense clusters with 10 to 20 flowers. The sessile or very short pedicled partial inflorescences bear dense, overlapping apical leaves. The calyx is 2.5 to 3 mm long with a blunt 5-tipped border. The corolla is white and fragrant. The stamens come from the mouth of the tube and are exserted. The ripe fruit is ellipsoid, 12 to 18 mm long by 12 to 15 mm wide with a 3 to 6 mm long stem. It is initially green, later yellow and dark red when ripe. The exocarp is tough and the mesocarp fleshy and slightly sweet. The endocarp is hard. The seeds are flat-convex with a groove on the flat adaxial side. They are 8 to 12 mm long, 5 to 8 mm wide and 3 to 5 mm thick. When fresh, the seeds are gray-green. They turn brown after roasting.

Leaves, Stem and Root: Coffea arabica is an evergreen shrub or small tree up to 8 m high with many basal branches. The young branches are glabrous and flattened, and the nodes produce many shoots. The bark of the fruiting branches is ashy-white. The leaves are 6 to 20 cm long, 2.5 to 6 cm wide and live for 2 to 3 years. They are glabrous, slightly coriaceous, dark green, glossy and elliptoid-lanceolate, with a distinct leaf tip. The border is occasionally extensively ribbed.

Habitat: Coffee's area of origin is disputed, but it is now cultivated in many tropical regions of the world, including Brazil, Mexico, Columbia and Ethiopia.

Production: Coffee charcoal is produced by roasting the outer seed parts of the green, dried fruit of Coffea arabica (and other Coffea species) until almost black, then grinding the carbonized product.

Coffee beans are the seeds of Coffea arabica, which are ripe for harvest nine months after flowering. Thereafter, they are processed using one of two methods. In the dry method, the beans are dried for 3 to 4 weeks in the sun, or mechanically with air-stream dryers. In the wet method, the beans are placed in a water-filled tank, where only the ripe ones sink to the bottom. The ripe fruit is then mechanically crushed and subsequently fermented. Fermentation lasts for approximately 48 hours (for arabica varieties). Afterward, the coffee is dried mechanically or in the sun.

Not to be Confused With: Coffee beans are not easily confused with other drugs. However, ground and roasted coffee may contain coffee substitutes such as chicory, dandelion root, figs, sugar beet root, lupin seeds, rye kernels and barleycorn.

Other Names: Arabica Coffee, Arabian Coffee, Caffea

ACTIONS AND PHARMACOLOGY

COMPOUNDS: COFFEE CHARCOAL

Purine alkaloids: main alkaloid caffeine

Trigonelline

Carbonization products of hemicelluloses

EFFECTS: COFFEE CHARCOAL

Coffee charcoal contains purine alkaloids, with caffeine as the man constituent, and is absorbent and astringent.

COMPOUNDS: COFFEE BEANS (SEEDS)

Purine alkaloids: main alkaloid caffeine (0.6 - 2.2%), with it theobromine, theophylline

Caffeic and ferulic acid ester of quinic acid: in particular chlorogenic acid

Trigonelline

Norditerpene glycoside ester: atractylosides

Diterpenes: including the diterpene alcohol fatty acid esters kahweol and cafestol

In roasted coffee beans: numerous aromatic substances yielded from carbohydrates, proteins, fats and aromatic acids through pyrolysis

EFFECTS: COFFEE BEANS

Most of the indicated effects of coffee are due to the presence of caffeine. The primary effects of caffeine can be summarized as follows: Caffeine has a positive inotropic effect. In higher concentrations, it has a positive chronotropic effect on the heart and CNS. It causes a relaxation of the smooth muscles of blood vessels (except for cerebral blood vessels) and the bronchial tubes. Moreover, caffeine works as a short-lived diuretic and produces an increase of gastric secretions and the release of catecholamines.

Caffeine works competitively to block adenosinal receptors that lie on cell surfaces in the brain, fat tissue, liver, kidneys, heart and erythrocytes.

Heart, circulation, vessels: People who normally do not drink coffee react 1 hour after an intake of 250 gm, with an increase of 10 mm Hg in their systolic blood pressure. Habitual coffee drinkers are tolerant in this regard.

Blood: After 9 weeks of an average daily intake of 5.6 cups of coffee (steeped for 10 min.), the overall and LDL cholesterol increases significantly. The use of coffee filters can reduce this by up to 80%.

Digestive tract: Oral intake of 200 mg of chlorogene acid doubles gastric secretion, as does caffeine alone.

Miscellaneous: In animal studies, a diet consisting of 20% green coffee impedes the growth of DMBA-induced tumors in hamsters by 90%.

Outcome of the stimulating effects of caffeine commence a few minutes subsequent to taking the drug. The maximum plasma concentration of caffeine is reached between 15 and 45 minutes later. The plasma half-life amounts to 4 to 6 hours.

Coffee extracts made from roasted and unroasted seeds are used analogously with other drugs containing caffeine for physical and mental fatigue. The drink can also be used therapeutically in cases of hypotonia, as an analeptic agent, in the treatment of influenza (flu) and migraine and as an additive to analgesia.

INDICATIONS AND USAGE

COFFEE CHARCOAL

Approved by Commission E:

- Diarrhea
- Inflammation of the mouth and pharynx

Unproven Uses: Coffee is used for nonspecific, acute diarrhea, and local therapy of mild inflammation of the oral and pharyngeal mucosa. In folk medicine coffee is also used for festering wounds.

COFFEE BEANS (SEEDS)

Unproven Uses: Coffee is used to treat hypotonia and as a constituent of analgesics. In folk medicine coffee is also used to increase performance capability as well as for anemia, hepatitis and edema.

Homeopathic Uses: Uses in homeopathy include insomnia and neuralgias.

Indian Medicine: Unripe seeds are used in Indian medicine for migraine and fever; ripe seeds for diarrhea; and strong coffee to treat opium and alcohol intoxication.

PRECAUTIONS AND ADVERSE REACTIONS

COFFEE CHARCOAL

General: Health risks or side effects following the proper administration of designated therapeutic dosages are not recorded.

Drug Interactions: The drug can hinder the resorption of other medicines.

COFFEE BEANS

General: Health risks following the proper administration of designated therapeutic dosages are not recorded. Quantities corresponding to as much as 500 mg caffeine daily (5 cups of coffee) spread out over the day are toxicologically harmless for healthy adults accustomed to drinking coffee. Caution is advised for persons with sensitive cardiovascular systems, kidney diseases, hyperfunction of the thyroid gland, higher disposition to convulsions and certain psychic disorders (for example, panic anxiety states). Side effects of coffee intake, mainly caused by its chlorogenic acid content, can include hyperacidity, stomach irritation, diarrhea and reduced appetite. Non-specific symptoms such as restlessness, irritability, sleeplessness, palpitations, dizziness, vomiting, diarrhea, loss of appetite and headache appear with the long-term intake of dosages exceeding 1.5 g caffeine per day. Caffeine can lead to psychic as well as physical dependency (caffeinism). Symptoms of withdrawal can include headache and sleeping disorders.

Pregnancy: Pregnant women should avoid caffeine, under no circumstances exceeding a dosage of 300 mg per day (3 cups of coffee spread out over the day).

Nursing Mothers: Infants nursing from mothers who take drinks containing caffeine may suffer from sleeping disorders.

OVERDOSAGE

Dosages exceeding 1.5 g caffeine per day can lead to stiffness, arrhythmic spasms of different muscle groups, opisthotonus and arrhythmic tachycardia. Fatal poisonings with the drug are not conceivable. The lethal dosage (LD50) for an adult is approximately 150 to 200 mg caffeine per kg body weight (for which 50 kg body weight = 7.5 g = 75 cups of coffee), although there are cases of survival also with 106 g caffeine. The death of a child following the intake of 5.3 g of caffeine has been reported. The first signs of poisonings are vomiting and abdominal spasms. The therapy for caffeine poisoning should begin with the inducement of vomiting or gastric lavage. Afterward, activated charcoal and sorbitol should be given to retard resorption. Spasms are to be treated with diazepam.

DOSAGE

COFFEE CHARCOAL

Mode of Administration: Powdered coffee charcoal and its preparations intended for internal consumption or local application.

Daily Dosage: The average daily dose for internal use is 9 g of ground drug. The average single dose is 3 g of powder.

Storage: Coffee charcoal should be stored in well-sealed containers.

COFFEE BEANS

Mode of Administration: The ground beans are used in different types of infusion, i.e. cooked coffee (filter, espresso etc.). Caffeine is used in various combinations and preparations for numerous therapeutic uses. Commercial pharmaceutical preparations include tablets, coated tablets, compresses and diverse compound preparations.

Preparation: The dried seeds are roasted until they procure a deep brown color and a characteristic aroma. This process is usually carried out in the country of consumption. During roasting, the beans float for 1.5 to 3 minutes in hot gas at 220°C to 270°C.

Daily Dosage: 15 g drug

Homeopathic Dosage: 5 drops, 1 tablet or 10 globules every 30 to 60 minutes (acute) and 1 to 3 times daily (chronic); parenterally: 1 to 2 ml sc acute, 3 times daily; chronic: once a day (HAB1)

Storage: The beans should be stored in sealed containers away from light and moisture.

LITERATURE

COFFEE CHARCOAL

Kuhn A, Schäfer G, (Kaffeekohle). In: Dtsch Med Wochenschr 23:922-923. 1939.

Further information in:

Hänsel R, Keller K, Rimpler H, Schneider G (Hrsg.), Hagers Handbuch der Pharmazeutischen Praxis, 5. Aufl., Bde 4-6 (Drogen): Springer Verlag Berlin, Heidelberg, New York, 1992-1994.

COFFEE BEANS

Anonym, Wieviel Coffein ist in welchem Produkt? In: PTA 5(1):40. 1991.

Bättig K, Kaffee in wissenschaftlicher Sicht. In: ZPT 9(3):95. 1988.

Bornkessel B, Sind Kaffeetrinker stärker gefährdet? In: DAZ 131(5):189. 1991.

Butz S, Nurses'-Health-Studie: Kaffe - kein Risikofaktor für koronare Herzkrankheit? In: DAZ 136(19):1680-1582. 1996.

Coffein: Entzugssyndrom bei Kaffeetrinkern. In: DAZ 133(6):441. 1993.

Dieudonne S, Forero ME, Llano I, Lipid analysis of Coffea arabica Linn. beans and their possible hypercholesterolemic effects. Int J Food Sci Nutr, 159:135-9, 1997 Mar.

Ferré, Buch. In: Ferré F. Kaffee-Eine Kulturgeschichte. 1992.

Garattini, Buch. In: Caffeine, Coffee, and Health. Garattini S. Monographs of the Mario Negri Institute for Pharmacological Research, Milan. Raven Press, New York. 1993.

Martin E, Cholesterolspiegel erhöhender Faktor in Kaffeelipiden. In: DAZ 130(42):2376. 1990.

Mensink RP, Lebbink WJ, Lobbezoo IE, Weusten-Van der Wouw MP, Zock PL, Katan MB, Diterpene composition of oils from Arabica and Robusta coffee beans and their effects on serum lipids in man. J Intern Med, 237:543-50, 1995 Jun.

Phillips R, Smith D, Characterization of coffea canephora alpha-D-galactosidase blood group B activity. Artif Cells Blood Substit Immobil Biotechnol, 103:489-502, 1996 Sep.

Ponepal V, Spielberger U, Riedel-Caspari G, Schmidt FW, Use of a Coffea arabica tosta extract for the prevention and therapy of polyfactorial infectious diseases in newborn calves. DTW Dtsch Tierarztl Wochenschr, 103:390-4, 1996 Oct.

Ratnayake WM, Pelletier G, Hollywood R, Malcolm S, Stavric B, Investigation of the effect of coffee lipids on serum cholesterol in hamsters. Food Chem Toxicol, 33:195-201, 1995 Mar.

Schröder, Buch. In: Schröder R: Kaffee, Tee und Kardamom, Ulmer-Verlag, Stuttgart. 1991.

Schröder-Rosenstock K, Kaffeegenuβ - ein medizinisches Problem. In: DAZ 130(35):1919. 1990.

Silnermann K et al., (Entzugssymptome nach regelmäβigem Kaffeegenuβ). In: New Engl J Med 327:1109. 1992.

Further information in:

Hänsel R, Keller K, Rimpler H, Schneider G (Hrsg.), Hagers Handbuch der Pharmazeutischen Praxis, 5. Aufl., Bde 4-6 (Drogen): Springer Verlag Berlin, Heidelberg, New York, 1992-1994.

Leung AY, Encyclopedia of Common Natural Ingredients Used in Food Drugs and Cosmetics, John Wiley & Sons Inc., New York 1980.

Lewin L, Gifte und Vergiftungen, 6. Aufl., Nachdruck, Haug Verlag, Heidelberg 1992.

Madaus G, Lehrbuch der Biologischen Arzneimittel, Bde 1-3, Nachdruck, Georg Olms Verlag Hildesheim 1979.

Roth L, Daunderer M, Kormann K, Giftpflanzen, Pflanzengifte, 4. Aufl., Ecomed Fachverlag Landsberg Lech 1993.

Teuscher E, Lindequist U, Biogene Gifte - Biologie, Chemie, Pharmakologie, 2. Aufl., Fischer Verlag Stuttgart 1994.

Teuscher E, Biogene Arzneimittel, 5. Aufl., Wiss. Verlagsges. mbH Stuttgart 1997.

Cola

Cola acuminata

DESCRIPTION

Medicinal Parts: The seeds are the medicinal parts of the plant.

Flower and Fruit: The male flowers with a diameter of 1.5 cm or the androgynous flowers with a diameter of 2.5 cm are axillary or on branches in cymes of few flowers. The 5 part chalice-shaped perigone is white to yellow and marked with red on the inside. The star-shaped fruits have 5 coriaceous, thick, dark brown, unkeeled follicles arranged at right angles to the stem. The fruits grow up to 20 cm long and 5 cm wide. There are up to 14 ovate or square seeds of about 2.5 cm diameter in 2 rows with a white fleshy seed shell. The seed kernel is usually reddish or red, occasionally white.

Leaves, Stem and Root: The plant is an evergreen tree 15 to 20 m tall. The trunk is branched down as far as the base. The bark is dark green, rough and breaks off in pieces as it ages. Branches have leaves only at their ends. The tough coriaceous leaves are 15 to 18 cm long and 10 cm wide, elliptoid to ovate, and end in a curled and spiraled tip. Both sides are dark green and glossy.

Habitat: The plant is indigenous to Togo, Sierra Leone and Angola. It is found today in all tropical regions and cultivated widely.

Production: The ripe fruit is harvested and the seeds are removed and dried. Cola nut is the endosperm freed from the testa of various Cola species, particularly Cola nitida.

Not to be Confused With: Other varieties of Cola, such as Male kola which contains no caffeine.

Other Names: Kola Tree, Guru Nut, Cola Nut, Cola Seeds, Bissy Nut

ACTIONS AND PHARMACOLOGY

COMPOUNDS

Purine alkaloids: main alkaloid caffeine (0.6 - 3.7%), additionally theobromine, theophylline

(+)-catechin, (-)-epicatechin

Catechin tannins

Oligomeric proanthocyanidins

Starch

EFFECTS

Cola's purine (caffeine) content makes it a strong CNS stimulant. In humans it acts as a respiratory analeptic, lipolytic, mildly positively chronotropic and mild diuretic. In addition, it stimulates gastric acid and increases motility of the gastrointestinal tract. In animal tests, Cola is also analeptic, lipolytic, stimulates production of gastric acid and increases gastric motility.

INDICATIONS AND USAGE

Approved by Commission E:

- Lack of stamina

Unproven Uses: Cola is used internally to decrease mental and physical fatigue. In folk medicine it is chewed to treat diarrhea, suppress hunger, thirst, morning sickness and migraine. It is also used to promote digestion. It is ground and made into poultices for wounds and inflammations. Cola is also an indigenous cult drug.

CONTRAINDICATIONS

Use of Cola is contraindicated during pregnancy. The drug should not be administered in the presence of stomach or duodenal ulcers, due to the drug's stimulation of gastric juice secretion.

PRECAUTIONS AND ADVERSE REACTIONS

Health risks following the proper administration of designated therapeutic dosages have not been recorded. Side effects that may occur include difficulty falling asleep, hyperexcitability, nervous states of restlessness and stomach complaints. Signs of poisoning following the intake of Cola drinks (20 to 60 mg caffeine per glass) or medications or stimulants containing Cola extracts are not expected. Small children should avoid the intake of large quantities of Cola drinks.

DOSAGE

Mode of Administration: Powdered drug and other galenic preparations for internal use.

How Supplied: Capsules, tablets, tonics.

Preparation: Dry extract: from the percolation 1:1 with 45% ethanol; fluid extract: percolation with 70% ethanol (V/V); Cola tincture: 1:5 with 70% ethanol; Cola wine: 50 parts fluid Cola extract with 850 parts Xeres wine and 100 parts sugar syrup.

Daily Dosage: 2 to 6 g of Cola nut drug, usually taken 1 to 3 g, 3 times daily; 0.25 to 0.75 g of Cola extract; 2.5 to 7.5 g of Cola liquid extract; 10 to 30 g of Cola tincture; 60 to 180 g of Cola wine.

Storage: Cola should be protected from light in sealed containers.

LITERATURE

Hänsel R, Keller K, Rimpler H, Schneider G (Hrsg.), Hagers Handbuch der Pharmazeutischen Praxis, 5. Aufl., Bde 4-6 (Drogen): Springer Verlag Berlin, Heidelberg, New York, 1992-1994.

Leung AY, Encyclopedia of Common Natural Ingredients Used in Food Drugs and Cosmetics, John Wiley & Sons Inc., New York 1980.

Lewin L, Gifte und Vergiftungen, 6. Aufl., Nachdruck, Haug Verlag, Heidelberg 1992.

Madaus G, Lehrbuch der Biologischen Arzneimittel, Bde 1-3, Nachdruck, Georg Olms Verlag Hildesheim 1979.

Morton, JF, An Atlas of Medicinal Plants of Middle America, Charles C. Thomas USA 1981.

Oliver-Bever B (Ed.), Medicinal Plants of Tropical West Africa, Cambridge University Press Cambridge, London 1986.

Roth L, Daunderer M, Kormann K, Giftpflanzen, Pflanzengifte, 4. Aufl., Ecomed Fachverlag Landsberg Lech 1993.

Steinegger E, Hänsel R: Pharmakognosie, 5. Aufl., Springer Verlag Heidelberg 1992.

Teuscher E, Lindequist U, Biogene Gifte - Biologie, Chemie, Pharmakologie, 2. Aufl., Fischer Verlag Stuttgart 1994.

Teuscher E, Biogene Arzneimittel, 5. Aufl., Wiss. Verlagsges. mbH Stuttgart 1997.

Cola acuminata

See Cola

Colchicum

Colchicum autumnale

DESCRIPTION

Medicinal Parts: The fresh flowers and the dried ripe seeds, collected in early summer and then sliced, as well as the tubers (fresh and dried) are the medicinal parts of the plant.

Flower and Fruit: The 5 to 20 cm flowers usually bloom in autumn. They are a bright lilac-pink, and solitary or in pairs from the corm. The 6 bracts of the involucre are fused into a long, narrow tube. The flower has 6 stamens and 3 thread-like styles. The ovaries are on the side of the corm. The 3-valved capsule is initially green, later becoming brown and wrinkled, and contains black seeds with sticky appendages.

Leaves, Stem and Root: Colchicum can grow to 40 cm in height. The 3 to 4 broadly lanceolate leaves are tulip-like; leaves appear together with the fruit in spring. They are 8 to 25 cm long, 2 to 4 cm wide and overlap at the base to form a tube.

Characteristics: All parts of the plant are very poisonous and have a disgustingly bitter and scratchy taste.

Not to be Confused With: The tubers are sometimes confused with cooking onions.

Habitat: Colchicum autumnale is primarily a central European plant found in northern Ireland, England, northern Germany, southern Poland, the Ukraine, Bulgaria, Turkey, Albania and northern Spain. It also grows in central Asia.

Production: Colchicum seeds are the dried seeds of Colchicum autumnale harvested in the wild in June or July and air-dried. Colchicum bulbs are the cut and dried tubers of the plant harvested in early summer. After the surrounding leaves have been removed, the tubers are cut into slices and dried at temperatures of 60°C or lower. Colchicum flowers are collected from the wild in late summer and autumn and then air-dried.

Other Names: Meadow Saffron, Meadow Saffran, Autumn Crocus, Naked Ladies, Upstart

ACTIONS AND PHARMACOLOGY

COMPOUNDS: COLCHICUM BULB

Tropolone alkaloids: colchicine, colchicoside and N-deacetyl-N-formyl-colchicine; companion alkaloids include demecolcine

Starch

COMPOUNDS: COLCHICUM SEEDS

Trupolone alkaloids: colchicine and colchicoside

Fatty oil

COMPOUNDS: COLCHICUM FLOWERS

Tropolone alkaloids: colchicine and N-deacetyl-N-formyl-colchicine, additional alkaloids including demecolcine

EFFECTS: COLCHICUM BULBS, SEEDS AND FLOWERS

Colchicum inhibits mitosis through the inhibition of motility, particularly of the phagocytosing lymphocytes. This is of therapeutic use for blocking the immigration and the autolysis of phagocytes in inflammatory processes and thereby producing an antiphlogistic effect.

INDICATIONS AND USAGE

COLCHICUM BULBS, SEEDS AND FLOWERS

Approved by Commission E:

- Gout
- Mediterranean fever

Unproven Uses: Due to the plant's toxicity, internal application is seldom used with the exception of acute attacks of gout and familial Mediterranean fever. Efficacy for these uses appears plausible. The drug was previously used for skin tumors, condyloma, psoriasis, necrotic vasculitis, tendovaginitis, inflammation of the gastrointestinal tract, morbus Behect, liver cirrhosis, acute and chronic leukemia; also for lice, asthma, dropsy and rheumatism.

Homeopathic Uses: In addition to acute and chronic gout, Colchici is also used for inflammation of the kidney and gastrointestinal tract, bodily secretions, tendovaginitis and acute joint rheumatism. Efficacy has not been proven.

PRECAUTIONS AND ADVERSE REACTIONS

General: The drugs are severely poisonous. Signs of poisoning, including stomachaches, diarrhea, nausea, vomiting and, less frequently, stomach and intestinal hemorrhages, can occur even with the administration of therapeutic dosages.

Kidney and liver damage, hair loss, peripheral nerve inflammation, myopathia and bone marrow damage with their resulting symptoms (leukopenia, thrombocytopenia, megaloblastic anemia, and, more rarely, aplastic anemia) have been observed following long-term administration.

Pregnancy: Colchicum is not to be used during pregnancy because of possible teratogenic damage. This also has been noted following intake of the drug by the father before conception.

OVERDOSAGE

Three to 6 hours following intake of acutely toxic dosages, burning of the mouth, difficulty swallowing and thirst appear. After 12 to 14 hours, the following appear: nausea, severe stomach pains, vomiting, diarrhea, bladder spasms, hematuria, falling blood pressure and spasms, and later, progressive paralysis. Death follows through exhaustion, asphyxiation or circulatory collapse. The fatal dosage for an adult is 5 g of the seeds, 1 to 1.5 g for a child. The fatal dosage of an intake of colchicine lies between 7 mg and 200 mg.

The treatment for poisonings, following gastric lavage and the administration of a saline purgative (such as sodium sulfate), proceeds symptomatically (diazepam for convulsion, atropine for intestinal spasm) and includes possible intubation and oxygen respiration.

DOSAGE

COLCHICUM BULBS, SEEDS AND FLOWERS

Mode of Administration: Comminuted drug, freshly pressed juice and other galenic preparations taken orally.

How Supplied: Ampules, tablets.

Daily Dosage: For an acute attack of gout, an initial oral dose corresponding to 1 mg colchicine, followed by 0.5 to 1.5 mg every 1 to 2 hours until pain subsides. Total daily dosage must not exceed 8 mg of colchicine. For prophylactic and therapeutic purposes, the dosage should correspond to 0.5 to 1.5 mg of colchicine.

Storage: All forms of the drug should be stored in containers that protect them from light and dampness. In addition, the seeds should be stored over lime.

LITERATURE

Fell KR, Ramsden D, (1967) Lloydia 30:123.

Gasisc O, Potesilova H, Santavy F, PM 30:75-81. 1976.

Gröbner W, Wlater-Sack I, Gicht und ihre medikamentöse Therapie. In: DAZ 131(35):1789. 1991.

Heide L, Traditionelle Arzneipflanzen in der Gesundsheitsversorgung der Dritten Welt. Möglichkeiten und Grenzen. In: DAZ 133(23):2067. 1993.

Potesilova H, Coll Czech Chem Comm 32:141-157. 1967.

Santavy F, Reichstein T, Helv Chim Acta 33:1606-1627. 1950.

Santavy F, Talas M, Coll Czech Chem Comm 19:141-152. 1954.

Santavy F et al., PM 43:153-160. 1981.

Santavy F et al., Coll Czech Chem Comm 48:2989-2993. 1983.

Santavy F, (1957) Pharm Zentralhalle 96:307.

Ulrichová J et al., Biochemical evaluation of colchicine and related analogs. In: PM 59(29):144. 1993.

Further information in:

Frohne D, Pfänder HJ, Giftpflanzen - Ein Handbuch für Apotheker, Toxikologen und Biologen, 4. Aufl., Wiss. Verlagsges. mbH Stuttgart 1997.

Hänsel R, Keller K, Rimpler H, Schneider G (Hrsg.), Hagers Handbuch der Pharmazeutischen Praxis, 5. Aufl., Bde 4-6 (Drogen), Springer Verlag Berlin, Heidelberg, New York, 1992-1994.

Lewin L, Gifte und Vergiftungen, 6. Aufl., Nachdruck, Haug Verlag, Heidelberg 1992.

Madaus G, Lehrbuch der Biologischen Arzneimittel, Bde 1-3, Nachdruck, Georg Olms Verlag Hildesheim 1979.

Roth L, Daunderer M, Kormann K, Giftpflanzen, Pflanzengifte, 4. Aufl., Ecomed Fachverlag Landsberg Lech 1993.

Steinegger E, Hänsel R, Pharmakognosie, 5. Aufl., Springer Verlag Heidelberg 1992.

Teuscher E, Lindequist U, Biogene Gifte - Biologie, Chemie, Pharmakologie, 2. Aufl., Fischer Verlag Stuttgart 1994.

Teuscher E, Biogene Arzneimittel, 5. Aufl., Wiss. Verlagsges. mbH Stuttgart 1997.

Colchicum autumnale

See Colchicum

Collinsonia canadensis

See Stone Root

Colombo

Jateorhiza palmata

DESCRIPTION

Medicinal Parts: The medicinal parts of the plant are the roots cut in slices when fresh and then dried.

Flower and Fruit: The plant is dioecious. The male inflorescences are 40 cm long and have green sepals, which are 2.7 to 3.2 mm long and 1.2 to 1.6 mm wide. The stamens are free and are fused at the base with the involuted margins of the petals. The female inflorescence is 8 to 10 cm long and has a 1 to 1.5 mm rust-red, pubescent ovary. The fruit is a 2 to 2.5 cm long and 1.5 to 2 cm wide globose drupe containing a moon-shaped stone.

Leaves, Stem and Root: The plant is a woody, branched liane, which can climb to tree height. The liane is initially downy, then bristly to villous. The leaves are opposite and have an 18 to 25 cm long petiole. The leaf blades are 15 to 35 cm long and 18 to 40 cm wide. They are bristly haired on both surfaces, broadly rounded, deeply cordate at the base and usually have 5 broad-ovate lobes. The root has a diameter of 3 to 8 cm. It is greenish-black. The root has a floury consistency, an indented center and a thick bark. The transverse section is yellowish, with vascular bundles in radiating lines.

Characteristics: The taste is mucilaginous and very bitter, the odor is slight.

Habitat: Indigenous to Mozambique, east Africa and Madagascar. It is cultivated elsewhere.

Production: Colombo root is the root of Jateorhiza palmata, which has been sliced horizontally and dried. The tuber roots, stemming from the rhizome, are dug up in March, washed and thinly sliced, and then dried quickly in the shade to avoid decomposition.

Other Names: Calumba

ACTIONS AND PHARMACOLOGY

COMPOUNDS

Isoquinoline alkaloids: main alkaloid palmatine, additionally jatrorrhizines (jateorhizine), columbamine, and bisjatrorrhizines

Diterpene bitter principles: including palmarin, chasmanthin and their glucosides (palmatoside A and B), columbin, jateorin and their glucosides (palmatoside D and E)

EFFECTS

The drug is no longer used as a bitter (amarum). The alkaloids have a narcotic effect. They act similarly to morphine, increasing resting muscle tone in the smooth muscle of the intestinal tract. Colombo alkaloids are said to act as a CNS paralyzing agent in frogs, and palmatin has the same effect on mammals. No further information is available.

INDICATIONS AND USAGE

Unproven Uses: In folk medicine it is used for digestive disorders accompanied by diarrhea, dyspeptic disorders, chronic diarrhea in patients with lung disease, subacidic gastritis and chronic entercolitis.

The drug is used in some European countries as an antidiarrheal agent because of its morphine-like side effects.

PRECAUTIONS AND ADVERSE REACTIONS

Health risks or side effects following the proper administration of designated therapeutic dosages are not recorded. Higher dosages of the drug may trigger vomiting and pains in the epigastrium.

OVERDOSAGE

According to older sources, very high dosages can also lead to signs of paralysis and unconsciousness (Lewin).

DOSAGE

Mode of Administration: Due to its morphine-type action, its use as an antidiarrheal agent is limited. Otherwise, the chopped root is used (no preparations known).

Preparation: Colombo liquid extract is prepared with diluted ethanol, according to the German pharmacopoeia. Colombo wine is prepared using 100 parts coarsely powdered drug and 1000 parts xeres wine. The extract is pressed out after 8 days and filtered.

Daily Dosage: The dose of the decoction is 1 dessertspoonful every 2 hours. The liquid extract standard single dose is 20 drops. Tincture of Colombo standard single dose is 2.5 gm. Colombo wine standard single dose is 5 gm.

Storage: Colombo must be kept dry at all times.

LITERATURE

Chan, EH et al. (Eds), Advances in Chinese Medicinal Materials Research, World Scientific Pub. Co. Singapore 1985.

Fenaroli's Handbook of Flavor Ingredients, Vol. 1, 2nd Ed., CRC Press 1975.

Hänsel R, Keller K, Rimpler H, Schneider G (Hrsg.), Hagers Handbuch der Pharmazeutischen Praxis, 5. Aufl., Bde 4-6 (Drogen), Springer Verlag Berlin, Heidelberg, New York, 1992-1994.

Lewin L, Gifte und Vergiftungen, 6. Aufl., Nachdruck, Haug Verlag, Heidelberg 1992.

Overton KH, Wier NG, Wylie A, J Chem Soc 1482-1490. 1966.

Steinegger E, Hänsel R, Pharmakognosie, 5. Aufl., Springer Verlag Heidelberg 1992.

Colt's Foot

Tussilago farfara

DESCRIPTION

Medicinal Parts: The medicinal parts are the dried inflorescences, the dried leaves and the fresh leaves.

Flower and Fruit: The yellow compound flowers are in small, solitary capitula at the end of the scapes. The lateral florets are lingual, narrow and female. The disc florets are tubular-campanulate, 5-petalled and male. The involucral bracts are almost as long, linear-lanceolate and have a scarious margin. The fruit is 3 to 11 mm long, cylindrical, brown, glabrous and stemmed. The pappus is in a number of rows and consists of long, glossy white hairs, which are much longer than the fruit.

Leaves, Stem and Root: The plant is a perennial, 10 to 30 cm high. It has a broadly branched, underground shoot and root system with a thin round, scaly base. There is also an up to 1.8 m long, far-reaching, creeping shoot. The flower stem is a scaly, round, tomentose scape covered with lanceolate, reddish scales, which is 30 cm long when the fruit ripens. The leaves, which appear after flowering, are basal, coriaceous, cordate-round, angular, irregularly dentate, long-petioled and tomentose beneath. The leaves can reach a diameter of up to 30 cm.

Characteristics: The taste and texture is slimy-sweet and the leaves have a honey-like smell when they are rubbed.

Habitat: The plant grows wild in most of Europe, central, western and northern Asia. It has spread to the mountains of northern Africa and has been introduced into North America.

Production: Colt's Foot flower consists of the fresh or dried flowers of Tussilago farfara. Colt's Foot herb consists of the fresh or dried, above-ground parts of Tussilago farfara. Colt's Foot root consists of the fresh or dried, below-ground parts of Tussilago farfara.

Not to be Confused With: The leaves of various Petasites species, but petasine and flavonoids can be identified using thin layer chromatography.

Other Names: British Tobacco, Bullsfoot, Butterbur, Coughwort, Flower Velure, Foal's-Foot, Horse-Foot, Horsehoof, Hallfoot, Ass's Foot, Foalswort, Fieldhove, Donnhove

ACTIONS AND PHARMACOLOGY

COMPOUNDS: COLT'S FOOT FLOWER

Mucilages (7%): acidic polysaccharides

Tannins

Triterpenes: including beta-amyrin, arnidiol, faradiol

Steroids: including beta-sitosterol

Pyrrolizidine alkaloids (traces, not in plants from all places of origin): tussilagine, isotussilagine, senkirkine, senecionine

Flavonoids

COMPOUNDS: COLT'S FOOT HERB

Mucilages (8%): acidic polysaccharides

Tannins (5%)

Triterpenes: including alpha-amyrin, beta-amyrin

Steroids: including beta-sitosterol, campesterol

Pyrrolizidine alkaloids (not in plants from all places of origin): senkirkine (0.01%), senecionine, tussilagine, isotussilagine

Flavonoids

COMPOUNDS: COLT'S FOOT ROOT

The roots have not been fully investigated. Only the presence of triterpenes and sterols has been established.

EFFECTS: COLT'S FOOT FLOWER, HERB, AND ROOT

The mucin contained in the drug has a sequestering effect and envelopes the mucous membrane with a layer that protects the throat from chemical and physical irritation and thereby reduces cough irritation. The pyrrolizidine alkaloids are antibacterial, carcinogenic, and hepatotoxic.

COMPOUNDS: COLT'S FOOT LEAF

Mucilages (8%): acidic polysaccharides

Tannins (5%)

Pyrrolizidine alkaloids (traces, not from all sources): tussilagine, isotussilagine, senkirkine 0.01%), senecionin

Steroids: including beta-sitosterol, campesterol

Triterpenes: including alpha- and beta-amyrin

Flavonoids

EFFECTS: COLT'S FOOT LEAF

The pyrrolizidine alkaloids are antibacterial, carcinogenic, and hepatotoxic. The mucin polysaccharides cause a demulcent, sequestering, and anti-inflammatory effect. In animal experiments there was evidence of a stimulating effect on the ciliated epithelium.

INDICATIONS AND USAGE

COLT'S FOOT FLOWER, HERB, AND ROOT

Unproven Uses: When added to Colt's Foot leaf, the flower, herb, and root are used to treat rheumatism.

COLT'S FOOT LEAF

Approved by Commission E:

- Cough
- Bronchitis
- Inflammation of the mouth and pharynx

Unproven Uses: Colt's Foot leaf is used for inflammation of the oral and pharyngeal mucosa. In addition, cigarettes made of the leaves are used to help cure smoking addiction.

CONTRAINDICATIONS

COLT'S FOOT FLOWER, HERB, ROOT, AND LEAF

Administration during pregnancy and while nursing is contraindicated.

PRECAUTIONS AND ADVERSE REACTIONS

COLT'S FOOT FLOWER, HERB, AND ROOT

Because of the possible hepatotoxic and carcinogenic pyrrolizidine alkaloid content, the administration of the blossoms should be avoided.

COLT'S FOOT LEAF

Colt's Foot leaves may no longer be brought into circulation in Austria. In Germany, dosages cannot exceed an intake of 10 mcg pyrrolizidine alkaloids with 1.2-unsaturated necic parent substances in the form of tea mixtures, and an intake of 1 mcg in the form of extracts.

Because even traces of the alkaloids present some danger, one should forgo any administration of the drug.

DOSAGE

COLT'S FOOT FLOWER, HERB, AND ROOT

Mode of Administration: The drug is used internally through the use of tea and standardized remedies.

Preparation: To prepare a tea, add 1.5 to 2.5 gm cut drug to boiling water, then strain after 5 to 10 minutes.

Storage: Protect the drug from light and store it tightly sealed.

COLT'S FOOT LEAF

Mode of Administration: Whole, cut, and powdered drug used in teas, infusions, extracts, and tinctures.

Preparation: To make an infusion, pour hot water over 1.5 to 2.5 gm of drug and allow to draw for 10 minutes. Other preparations are made as follows: liquid extract: 1:1 with 20% ethanol; extract: 1.1 with 25% ethanol; tincture: 1:5 with 45% ethanol.

Daily Dosage: The total daily dose is 4.5 to 6 gm of drug. The maximum daily dosage must not be more than 1 mcg of total pyrrolizidine alkaloids with 1.2 unsaturated necine structure.

The tea is given several times a day. The dosage for the extract is 2 ml 3 times daily; for the tincture, it is 8 ml 3 times daily.

Storage: Protect the drug from light and store it tightly sealed.

LITERATURE

COLT'S FOOT FLOWER, HERB, AND ROOT

Delaveau P et al., (1980) Planta Med 40:49.

Didry N et al., (1982) Ann Pharm Franc 40(1):75.

Engalycheva EI et al., (1982) Farmatsiya 31(2):37.

Franz G, PM 17:217. 1969.

Hiller K, Pharmazeutische Bewertung ausgewählter Teedrogen. In: DAZ 135(16):1425-1440. 1995.

Hirono I et al., (1976) Gann 67(1):125.

Hirono I et al., (1979) J Natl Canc Inst 63(2):469.

Ihrig M, Pyrrolizidinalkaloidhaltige Drogen im Handverkauf? In: PZ 137(40):3128. 1992.

Kraus C et al., (1985) Planta Med 51(2):89.

Miething H, Steinbach RA, Ermittlung der Freisetzungsraten des Pyrrolizidinalkaloids Senkirkin in Huflattich-Teegetränken. In: PZW 135(4):153. 1990.

Paßreiter CM, Co-occurence of 2-pyrrolidineacetic acid with four isomeric tussilaginic acids in Arnica species and Tussilago farfara. In: PM 58(7)94. 1992.

Röder E et al., (1981) Plant Med 43:99.

Röder E, Pyrrolizidinhaltige Arzneipflanzen. In: DAZ 132(45):2427-2435. 1992.

Wagner H, In: Economic and Medicinal Plant Research, Vol. 1, Academic Press, UK 1985.

Wunderer H, Zentral und peripher wirksame Antitussiva: eine kritische Übersicht. In: PZ 142(11):847-852. 1997.

Further information in:

Frohne D, Pfänder HJ, Giftpflanzen - Ein Handbuch für Apotheker, Toxikologen und Biologen, 4. Aufl., Wiss. Verlagsges. mbH Stuttgart 1997.

Hänsel R, Keller K, Rimpler H, Schneider G (Hrsg.), Hagers Handbuch der Pharmazeutischen Praxis, 5. Aufl., Bde 4-6 (Drogen): Springer Verlag Berlin, Heidelberg, New York, 1992-1994.

Madaus G, Lehrbuch der Biologischen Arzneimittel, Bde 1-3, Nachdruck, Georg Olms Verlag Hildesheim 1979.

Roth L, Daunderer M, Kormann K, Giftpflanzen, Pflanzengifte, 4. Aufl., Ecomed Fachverlag Landsberg Lech 1993.

Steinegger E, Hänsel R, Pharmakognosie, 5. Aufl., Springer Verlag Heidelberg 1992.

Teuscher E, Lindequist U, Biogene Gifte - Biologie, Chemie, Pharmakologie, 2. Aufl., Fischer Verlag Stuttgart 1994.

Teuscher E, Biogene Arzneimittel, 5. Aufl., Wiss. Verlagsges. mbH Stuttgart 1997.

Wichtl M (Hrsg.), Teedrogen, 4. Aufl., Wiss. Verlagsges. Stuttgart 1997.

COLT'S FOOT LEAF

Delaveau P et al., (1980) Planta Med 40:49.

Didry N et al., (1982) Ann Pharm Franc 40(1):75.

Engalycheva EI et al., (1982) Farmatsiya 31(2):37.

Franz G, PM 17:217. 1969.

Hiller K, Pharmazeutische Bewertung ausgewählter Teedrogen. In: DAZ 135(16):1425-1440. 1995.

Hirono I et al., (1976) Gann 67(1):125.

Hirono I et al., (1979) J Natl Canc Inst 63(2):469.

Ihrig M, Pyrrolizidinalkaloidhaltige Drogen im Handverkauf? In: PZ 137(40):3128. 1992.

Kraus C et al., (1985) Planta Med 51(2):89.

Miething H, Steinbach RA, Ermittlung der Freisetzungsraten des Pyrrolizidinalkaloids Senkirkin in Huflattich-Teegetränken. In: PZW 135(4):153. 1990.

Paβreiter CM, Co-occurence of 2-pyrrolidineacetic acid with four isomeric tussilaginic acids in Arnica species and Tussilago farfara. In: PM 58(7)94. 1992.

Röder E et al., (1981) Plant Med 43:99.

Röder E, Pyrrolizidinhaltige Arzneipflanzen. In: DAZ 132(45):2427-2435. 1992.

Wagner H, In: Economic and Medicinal Plant Research, Vol. 1, Academic Press, UK 1985.

Wunderer H, Zentral und peripher wirksame Antitussiva: eine kritische Übersicht. In: PZ 142(11):847-852. 1997.

Further information in:

Frohne D, Pfänder HJ, Giftpflanzen - Ein Handbuch für Apotheker, Toxikologen und Biologen, 4. Aufl., Wiss. Verlagsges. mbH Stuttgart 1997.

Hänsel R, Keller K, Rimpler H, Schneider G (Hrsg.), Hagers Handbuch der Pharmazeutischen Praxis, 5. Aufl., Bde 4-6 (Drogen): Springer Verlag Berlin, Heidelberg, New York, 1992-1994.

Madaus G, Lehrbuch der Biologischen Arzneimittel, Bde 1-3, Nachdruck, Georg Olms Verlag Hildesheim 1979.

Roth L, Daunderer M, Kormann K, Giftpflanzen, Pflanzengifte, 4. Aufl., Ecomed Fachverlag Landsberg Lech 1993.

Steinegger E, Hänsel R, Pharmakognosie, 5. Aufl., Springer Verlag Heidelberg 1992.

Teuscher E, Lindequist U, Biogene Gifte - Biologie, Chemie, Pharmakologie, 2. Aufl., Fischer Verlag Stuttgart 1994.

Teuscher E, Biogene Arzneimittel, 5. Aufl., Wiss. Verlagsges. mbH Stuttgart 1997.

Wichtl M (Hrsg.), Teedrogen, 4. Aufl., Wiss. Verlagsges. Stuttgart 1997.

Columbine

Aquilegia vulgaris

DESCRIPTION

Medicinal Parts: The medicinal parts are the stems and leaves, the aerial parts gathered and dried in flowering season, and the seeds and preparations of the whole plant also gathered in flowering season.

Flower and Fruit: The long-stemmed flowers are terminal, hanging, and either dark blue, dark violet, pink or white. The 5 sepals spread like petals. They are broadly ovate, and end in a blunt, green tip. The 5 petals are hood-shaped with long, inwardly hooked spurs. There are numerous stamens and usually 5 ovaries. The follicle is oblong, erect and glandular-downy. The seeds are glossy black, oval, 2.2 to 2.5 cm long by 1.5 cm wide. They are thick, blunt-tipped and anatropous. The raphe forms a distinct line on the side of the plant.

Leaves, Stem and Root: The 30- to 60-cm high plant has a many-headed, light brown and branched rhizome. The stems are erect and usually branched. They are glabrous or soft-haired. The basal leaves are long-petioled and trifoliate. The leaflets are wedge-shaped to ovoid, blunt, irregularly crenate to serrate, and bluntly lobed. The underside of the leaves are usually light green and pubescent. The cauline leaves are smaller than the basal leaves and simpler. The highest leaves are usually made up of a few elongate-ovate, entire-margined lobes.

Habitat: Columbine is indigenous to central and southern Europe and is also found in the eastern U.S. and Asia.

Production: Columbine herb is the complete aerial part of Aquilegia vulgaris harvested while in flower and dried.

Other Names: Culverwort, Capon's Feather, Culver Key

ACTIONS AND PHARMACOLOGY

COMPOUNDS

Cyanogenic glycosides: trigloquinine, dhurrin (presumably only traces)

EFFECTS

It is not known which constituents are responsible for the herb's effects. The cyanogenic glycoside trigloquinine could possibly be of toxicological interest but is probably only present in traces.

INDICATIONS AND USAGE

Unproven Uses: Columbine is used internally for scurvy and jaundice; the herb is also used to treat states of agitation due to its supposedly tranquilizing effect.

Homeopathic Uses: The herb is used to treat menopausal vomiting and dysmenorrhea in young women. It is also used to treat the sensation of a lump in the throat (globus hystericus) and nervous shaking.

PRECAUTIONS AND ADVERSE REACTIONS

No health hazards or side effects are known in conjunction with the proper administration of designated therapeutic dosages.

OVERDOSAGE

Poisonings from the leaves because of the cyanogenic glycoside content have not been observed. The amount of hydrocyanic acid that is released from the leaves is apparently too small to cause toxicity.

DOSAGE

Mode of Administration: Columbine is available in tablets and capsules for internal use.

Homeopathic Dosage: 5 to 10 drops, 1 tablet or 5 to 10 globules 1 to 3 times a day or 1 ml injection solution sc twice a week (HAB1).

LITERATURE

Bonora A et al., PH 26:2277. 1987.

Fat LTS, Proc Kon Nederl Akad Wetensch Ser C82:197. 1979.

Hänsel R, Keller K, Rimpler H, Schneider G (Hrsg.), Hagers Handbuch der Pharmazeutischen Praxis, 5. Aufl., Bde 4-6 (Drogen). Springer Verlag Berlin, Heidelberg, New York, 1992-1994.

Madaus G, Lehrbuch der Biologischen Arzneimittel, Bde 1-3, Nachdruck, Georg Olms Verlag Hildesheim 1979.

Roth L, Daunderer M, Kormann K, Giftpflanzen, Pflanzengifte, 4. Aufl., Ecomed Fachverlag Landsberg Lech 1993.

Combretum micranthum

See Opium Antidote

Comfrey

Symphytum officinale

TRADE NAMES

Comfrey (available from numerous manufacturers)

DESCRIPTION

Medicinal Parts: The medicinal parts are the fresh root and the leaves.

Flower and Fruit: The flowers are dull purple or violet. They are arranged in crowded, apical, 2-rayed hanging cymes. The calyx is fused and has 5 tips. The corolla is also fused and is cylindrical-campanulate with a pentangular tube and 5-tipped border. The tips are revolute and there are 5 awl-shaped scales in the mouth of the tube. The scales close together in a clavate form and have a glandular tipped margin. There are 5 stamens and 1 style. The ovary is 4-valved. The fruit consists of 4 smooth, glossy nutlets.

Leaves, Stem and Root: The plant grows from 30 to 120 cm in height. The root is fusiform, branched, black on the outside and white on the inside. The stem is erect and stiff-haired. The leaves are wrinkly and roughly pubescent; the lower ones and the basal ones are ovate-lanceolate and pulled together in the petiole; the upper ones are lanceolate and broad.

Characteristics: The root is slimy and horn-like when dried.

Habitat: The plant is indigenous to Europe and temperate Asia and is naturalized in the U.S.

Production: Comfrey herb consists of the fresh or dried above-ground parts of Symphytum officinale. Comfrey leaf consists of the fresh or dried leaf of Symphytum officinale. Comfrey root consists of the fresh or dried root section of Symphytum officinale.

Other Names: Ass Ear, Black Root, Blackwort, Boneset, Bruisewort, Consound, Gum Plant, Healing Herb, Knitback, Knitbone, Salsify, Slippery Root, Wallwort, Consolida, Boneset

ACTIONS AND PHARMACOLOGY

COMPOUNDS

Allantoin

Mucilages (Fructans)

Triterpene saponins: including symphytoxide A

Tannins

Silicic acid: to some extent water-soluble

Pyrrolizidine alkaloids (0.03% in the leaves): including echinatine, lycopsamine, 7-acetyl lycoposamine, echimidine, lasiocarpine, symphytine, intermedine, symveridine.

EFFECTS

Anti-inflammatory Effect—Comfrey suppresses leukocyte infiltration during the inflammation process (Shipochliev, 1981).

Demultant Effect—The mucilages act as demultants for a soothing and irritation reduction effect.

Hypotensive Effect—Symphytoxide A, a triterpene saponin, exhibited hypotensive activity in anesthetized rats (Ahmad, 1993).

Tissue/Nerve Stimulation—Allantoin, a component in Comfrey, stimulates tissue repair and wound healing through cell proliferation (Rieth, 1968). Allantoin has also had significant effect on cellular multiplication in degenerating and regenerating peripheral nerves (Loots, 1979).

CLINICAL TRIALS

The anti-inflammatory effects of Comfrey were studied in musculoskeletal disorders. Forty-one patients with musculoskeletal rheumatism were treated with either a pyrrolizidine alkaloid-free ointment or placebo for 4 weeks. The patient illnesses consisted of epicondylitis, tendovaginitis, and periarthritis. Efficacy was determined by evaluation of different pain parameters (tenderness on pressure, pain at rest, pain on exercise). There was significant improvement with the ointment compared to placebo at weeks 1, 2, and 4 in patients with epicondylitis. There was improvement with tendovaginitis at week 1 and 2, but not at week 4 with the ointment compared to placebo. There was no improvement in the peri-arthritis patients in either of the two treatment groups (Petersen, 1993).

INDICATIONS AND USAGE

Approved by Commission E:

- Blunt injuries

Externally, Comfrey is used for bruises, sprains and promotion of bone healing.

Unproven Uses: The root has been used externally as a mouthwash and gargle for gum disease, pharyngitis, and strep throat. Internally, the root has been used for gastritis and gastrointestinal ulcers. In Folk medicine, the root of the plant has been used for rheumatism, pleuritis, and as an antidiarrheal agent.

CONTRAINDICATIONS

Comfrey is contraindicated in pregnancy and in nursing mothers.

PRECAUTIONS AND ADVERSE REACTIONS

Hepatotoxicity: Internal administration of the drug, due to the presence of pyrrolizidine alkaloids, has resulted in hepatocyte membrane injury with hemorrhagic necrosis and loss of microvilli (Yeong, 1993). Hepatic veno-occlusive disease and severe portal hypertension has been associated with Comfrey ingestion, and in one case report, death resulted by liver failure (Ridker, 1989; Yeong, 1990).

Carcinogenic/Mutagenic Effects: Mutagenic effects are associated with aqueous extracts of the alkaloid fractions (Furmanowa, 1983). Hepatocelluar adenomas have been reported in animal models receiving diets containing Comfrey roots and leaves (Hirono, 1978). Comfrey also has chromosome-damaging effects in human lymphocytes (Behninger, 1989).

Gastrointestinal/Kidney/Pancreas Effects: Comfrey, through the pyrrolizidine alkaloids, has been shown to produce lesions in the gastrointestinal tract, pancreas, and renal glomeruli in animal models (Winship, 1991).

Respiratory Effects: Pulmonary endothelial hyperplasia from the pyrrolizidine alkaloids has been seen in animal models (Miskely, 1992).

Use in Pregnancy: The drug is contraindicated during pregnancy.

Use in Nursing Mothers: Use of the drug while nursing is contraindicated.

DOSAGE

Mode of Administration: The crushed root, extracts, and pressed juice of the fresh plant are used as semi-solid preparations and poultices for external use. The drug is a component of standardized preparations of analgesics, antirheumatic agents, antiphlogistics, antitussives, and expectorants.

How Supplied:

Cream—1.25 oz., 2 oz.

Preparation: To make an infusion, pour boiling water over 5 to 10 gm comminuted or powdered drug, steep 10 to 15 minutes, then strain (1 teaspoonful = 4 gm drug). For external application, a decoction of 1:10 is used, or the fresh roots are mashed.

Daily Dosage:

External Use—The daily dosage should not exceed 1 mcg of pyrrolizidine alkaloids for external preparations calculated with 5 to 7% drug, maximum 1 ppm/gm for commercial pharmaceutical preparations. The drug should be used for a maximum of 4 weeks.

Tea—When using the infusion, take 1 cup 2 to 3 times daily, but not for a long duration (SEE PRECAUTIONS).

LITERATURE

Ahmad VU; Noorwala M; Mohammad FV et al. Symphytoxide A, a triterpenoid saponin from the roots of Symphytum officinale. Phytochemistry 1993 Mar;32(4):1003-6.

Behninger C; Abel G; Roder E et al. Studies on the effect of an alkaloid extract of Symphytum officinale on human lymphocyte cultures. Planta Med 1989 Dec;55(6):518-22.

Bhandari P, Gray AI (1985) J Pharm Pharmacol 37:50P.

Branchlij et al., (1982) Experientia 38:1085.

Culvenor CJJ et al., (1980) Experientia 36:377.

Franz G, (1969) Planta Med 17:217.

Furmanowa M, Guzewska J, Beldowska B. Mutagenic effects of aqueous extracts of Symphytum officinale L. and of its alkaloid fractions. J Appl Toxicol 1983 Jun;3(3):127-30.

Furuya T, Araki K, (1968) Chem Pharm Bull 16:2512.

Garrett BJ; Cheeke PR; Miranda CL et al. Consumption of poisonous plants (Senecio jacobaea, Symphytum officinale, Pteridium aquilinum, Hypericum perforatum) by rats: chronic toxicity, mineral metabolism, and hepatic drug-metabolizing enzymes. Toxicol Lett 1982 Feb;10(2-3):183-8.

Gracza L et al., (1985) Arch Pharm 312(12):1090.

Gray AI et al., (1983) J Pharm Pharmacol 35:13P.

Hirono I, Mori H, Haga M. carcinogenic activity of Syphytum officinale. J Natl Cancer Inst 1978 Sep; 61(3):865-9.

Ihrig M, Pyrrolizidinalkaloidhaltige Drogen im Handverkauf? In: PZ137(40):3128. 1992.

Kozhina IS et al., (1970) Rastit Resur 6:345.

Loots JM; Loots GP; Joubert WS. The effect of allantoin on cellular multiplication in degenerating and regenerating nerves. S Afr Med J 1979 Jan 13;55(2):53-6.

Mascolo N et al., (1987) Phytother Res 1(1):28.

Miskelly FG & Goodyer LI: Hepatic and pulmonary complications of herbal medicines. Postgrad J 1992; 68:935-936.

Mohammad FV et al., Bisdesmosidic triterpenoidal saponins from the roots of Symphytum officinale. In: PM 61(1):94. 1995.

Mütterlein R, Arnold CG, Untersuchungen zum Pyrrolizidingehalt und Pyrrolizidinalkaloidmuster in Symphytum officinale L. In: PZ-W 138(5/6):119. 1993.

Noorwala M et al., A bisdesmosidic triterpene glycoside from roots of Symphytum officinale. In: PH 36(2):439. 1994.

Petersen G et al., Anti-inflammatory activity of a pyrrolizidine alkaloid-free extract of roots of Symphytum officinale. In: PM 59(7)A703. 1993.

Rieth H. Stimulation of tissue reparation with allantoin as adjuvant of the antifungal treatment. Mykosen 1968 Jan 1;11(1):93-4.

Ridker PN; McDermont WV. Hepatotoxicity due to comfrey herb tea. Am J Med 1989 Dec;87(6):701.

Röder E, Pyrrolizidinhaltige Arzneipflanzen. In: DAZ 132(45):2427-2435. 1992.

Shipochliev T; Dimitrov A; Aleksandrova E. Anti-inflammatory action of a group of plant extracts. Vet Med Nauki 1981;18(6):87-94.

Schoental R et al., (1970) Cancer Res 30:2127.

Stamford IF, Tavares IA, (1983) J Pharm Pharmacol 35:816.

Taylor A, Taylor NC, (1963) Proc Soc Exp Biol Med 114:772.

Weston CFM et al., (1987) Brit Med J 295:183.

White RD et al., (1983) Toxicol Letters 15:25.

Winship KA: Toxicity of comfrey. Adverse Drug React Toxicol Rev 1991; 10:47-59.

Yeong ML, Wakefield SJ, Ford HC. Hepatocyte membrane injury and bleb formation following low dose comfrey toxicity in rats. Int J Exp Pathol 1993 Apr;74(2):211-7.

Yeong ML, Swinburn B, Kennedy M, Nicholson G. Hepatic veno-occlusive disease associated with comfrey ingestion. J Gastroenterol Hepatol 1990 Mar-Apr;5(2):211-4.

Further information in:

Frohne D, Pfänder HJ: Giftpflanzen - Ein Handbuch für Apotheker, Toxikologen und Biologen, 4. Aufl., Wiss. Verlags-Ges. Stuttgart 1997.

Kern W, List PH, Hörhammer L (Hrsg.): Hagers Handbuch der Pharmazeutischen Praxis, 4. Aufl., Bde 1-8: Springer Verlag Berlin, Heidelberg, New York, 1969.

Leung AY, Encyclopedia of Common Natural Ingredients Used in Food Drugs, Cosmetics, John Wiley & Sons Inc., New York, 1980.

Madaus G, Lehrbuch der Biologischen Arzneimittel, Bde 1-3, Nachdruck, Georg Olms Verlag Hildesheim 1979.

Roth L, Daunderer M, Kormann K, Giftpflanzen, Pflanzengifte, 4. Aufl., Ecomed Fachverlag Landsberg Lech 1993.

Schulz R, Hänsel R, Rationale Phytotherapie, Springer Verlag Heidelberg 1996.

Steinegger E, Hänsel R, Pharmakognosie, 5. Aufl., Springer Verlag Heidelberg 1992.

Teuscher E, Lindequist U, Biogene Gifte - Biologie, Chemie, Pharmakologie, 2. Aufl., Fischer Verlag Stuttgart 1994.

Wagner H, Wiesenauer M: Phytotherapie. Phytopharmaka und pflanzliche Homöopathika, Fischer-Verlag, Stuttgart, Jena, New York, 1995.

Wichtl M (Hrsg.), Teedrogen, 4. Aufl., Wiss. Verlagsges. Stuttgart 1997.

Commiphora molmol

See Myrrh

Common Kidney Vetch

Anthyllis vulneraria

DESCRIPTION

Medicinal Parts: The medicinal part of the plant is the flower.

Flower and Fruit: The many-floreted capitula are in the upper bract axils. The papilonaceous flowers are almost sessile and have an upright corolla up to 20 mm long. The calyx is membranous and up to 17 mm long. It is tubular-bottle-shaped and shaggy to felt-haired. The color is yellow to white at the bottom, turning violet toward the top. The petals are whitish-yellow to yellow or occasionally crimson. They have a free standard, slightly shorter wings, and an acute, often red, carina. Ten stamens are fused into a tube. The ovaries are stemmed with a thickened style and rounded stigma. The pod-fruit is enclosed in the dried calyx. It is ovate, reticulate, dark brown, single-seeded, and does not spring open. The seed is ovate, smooth, shiny and checkered yellow-green.

Leaves, Stem and Root: Anthyllis vulneraria is a 15 to 30 cm high half-rosette shrub with a sturdy tap-root and a short, entire or often branched rhizome. The stem is upright, unbranched or branched, and tomentose. The leaves are variously pinnate, depending on where they are on the stem. All leaves are entire-margined, glabrous or slightly pubescent above, and thickly tomentose beneath. The stipules are small and generally connected to a clasping sheath.

Characteristics: Kidney Vetch has a weak aromatic odor and dry taste.

Habitat: The plant is found all across Europe to the Caucasus and the Middle East. It is found in the south to the Sahara and Ethiopia.

Production: Kidney Vetch are the flowers of Anthyllis vulneraria without their stems.Woundwort is collected in the wild and then dried quickly in the shade.

Other Names: Ladies' Fingers, Lamb's Toes, Kidney Vetch, Staunchwort, Woundwort

ACTIONS AND PHARMACOLOGY

COMPOUNDS

Tannins

Saponins

Flavonoids

Isoflavonoids

Lectins

EFFECTS

Antiviral activity was demonstrated with an ethanol extract of the plant. The flavonols quercetin and rhamnetin have a mutagenic effect. The herb's use in the treatment of ulcers and wounds may be due to the tannins (probably of the catechin type).

INDICATIONS AND USAGE

Unproven Uses: Kidney Vetch tea is used in the treatment of ulcers and wounds both internally and externally. The drug is also used in a tea for coughs that also contains ribwort, as an ingredient of blood-purifying teas, and for exposure and vomiting. It is used internally for diseases of the mouth and throat.

PRECAUTIONS AND ADVERSE REACTIONS

No health hazards or side effects are known in conjunction with the proper administration of designated therapeutic dosages.

DOSAGE

Mode of Administration: Preparations are available for internal uses, often as teas, and external uses including poultices, washes and rinses.

Preparation: To prepare tea, use 1 dessertspoonful of the flowers per 250 ml of water.

LITERATURE

Czeczot H, Tudek B, Kusztelak J, Szymczyk T, Dobrowolska B, Glinkowska G, Malinowski J, Strzelecka H, Isolation and studies of the mutagenic activity in the Ames test of flavonoids naturally occurring in medical herbs. Mutat Res, 240:209-16, 1990 Mar.

Sile A, Vanaga A, Nauka-Prakt Farm: 82-85. 1974.

Vetter J, Seregelyes-Csomos A, Magy Allatory Lapja 43(8):479-482. 1988.

Further information in:

Hänsel R, Keller K, Rimpler H, Schneider G (Hrsg.), Hagers Handbuch der Pharmazeutischen Praxis, 5. Aufl., Bde 4-6 (Drogen), Springer Verlag Berlin, Heidelberg, New York, 1992-1994.

Common Stonecrop

Sedum acre

DESCRIPTION

Medicinal Parts: The medicinal parts are the fresh or dried aerial parts collected during the flowering season.

Flower and Fruit: The flowers are leafy, twining cymes on short pedicles. There are 5 ovate sepals and 5 golden yellow petals that are 7 to 9 mm long, lanceolate and twice as long as the calyx. The fruit is a follicle, which splits after flowering to form a 5-rayed star, which is 3 to 5 mm long and has numerous seeds.

Leaves, Stem and Root: The perennial plant grows 2 to 15 cm high. It has many heavily branched shoots, which often creep underground and form grass. The leaves are thick, fleshy, almost round, acute, appressed and knobby-domed.

They are rounded at the base and have no spur-like appendage.

Characteristics: The texture is slimy and the taste hot and pepper-like.

Habitat: Common Stonecap is common to all of Europe, western Siberia, the Caucasus region and North America.

Production: The flowering parts of Sedum acre are picked while in bloom and then dried, either in the sun or, preferably, with the use of artificial heat.

Other Names: Wallpepper, Golden Moss, Wall Ginger, Bird Bread, Prick Madam, Gold Chain, Creeping Tom, Mousetail, Jach-of-the-Buttery

ACTIONS AND PHARMACOLOGY

COMPOUNDS

Piperidine alkaloids (0.3%): chief alkaloids are sedinine, sedinon

Flavonoids: including among others, glycosides of isorhamnetin, quercetin, limnocitrin

Tannins (10%)

Hydroquinone glycosides: Arbutin

Mucilages (30%)

EFFECTS

In animal experiments, the drug displayed both motility-inhibiting and motility-stimulating effects. The alkaloids and tannins may make use of the drug in the treatment of wounds plausible, but no reliable documentation is available.

INDICATIONS AND USAGE

Unproven Uses: The drug is used internally for coughs (Spain) and high blood pressure (central Europe), edema and febrile conditions. Externally, it is used for wounds and ulcers resulting from burns, hemorrhoids, warts, eczema, and oral ulcers.

Homeopathic Uses: In homeopathy, Common Stonecap is used for hemorrhoidal pain and anal fissures.

CONTRAINDICATIONS

The drug should not be administered in the presence of inflammatory diseases of the gastrointestinal tract or of the urinary drainage passages.

PRECAUTIONS AND ADVERSE REACTIONS

No health hazards or side effects are known in conjunction with the proper administration of designated therapeutic dosages.

OVERDOSAGE

Dosages consisting of over 10 g of the juice or 1 to 3.5 g of the dried foliage of the fresh plant result in queasiness, vomiting and diarrhea. However, cases of poisoning have not been recorded in recent times.

DOSAGE

Mode of Administration: Decoctions or syrups for internal use; poultice of fresh leaves for external use.

Preparation: A decoction is prepared using 1 teaspoonful of the drug in 1 cup of water. Prepare a syrup by mixing 100 g of plant juice with 180 g of sugar.

Daily Dosage: The average daily dose of the drug as a decoction is 3 g (approximately 2 teaspoonfuls). Average syrup dosage is 1 dessertspoonful every 3 hours. In external application as a poultice, the fresh plants are crushed and placed on the wart or skin area exhibiting eczema.

Homeopathic Dosage: 5 drops, 1 tablet or 10 globules every 30 to 60 minutes (acute) or 1 to 3 times daily (chronic); parenterally: 1 to 2 ml sc acute: 3 times daily; chronic: once a day (HAB34).

LITERATURE

Francis LPS, Francis GW, PM 32:268-274. 1977.

Halin F et al., Tetrahedron 41:2891. 1985.

Hootele C et al., Tetrahedron 41:5563. 1985.

Niklon B et al., Acta Pharm Jugosl 40:555. 1980.

Van der Wal R et al., PM 43:97. 1981.

Further information in:

Frohne D, Pfänder HJ, Giftpflanzen - Ein Handbuch für Apotheker, Toxikologen und Biologen, 4. Aufl., Wiss. Verlags-Ges. Stuttgart 1997.

Hänsel R, Keller K, Rimpler H, Schneider G (Hrsg.), Hagers Handbuch der Pharmazeutischen Praxis, 5. Aufl., Bde 4-6 (Drogen): Springer Verlag Berlin, Heidelberg, New York, 1992-1994.

Lewin L, Gifte und Vergiftungen, 6. Aufl., Nachdruck, Haug Verlag, Heidelberg 1992.

Madaus G, Lehrbuch der Biologischen Arzneimittel, Bde 1-3, Nachdruck, Georg Olms Verlag Hildesheim 1979.

Roth L, Daunderer M, Kormann K, Giftpflanzen, Pflanzengifte, 4. Aufl., Ecomed Fachverlag Landsberg Lech 1993.

Teuscher E, Lindequist U, Biogene Gifte - Biologie, Chemie, Pharmakologie, 2. Aufl., Fischer Verlag Stuttgart 1994.

Condurango

Marsdenia condurango

DESCRIPTION

Medicinal Parts: The medicinal part is the dried bark of the branches and trunks.

Flower and Fruit: The flowers are in umbel-like inflorescence. The calyx and the campanulate to funnel-shaped corolla have 5 sepals and petals. Pollination is only possible by insects. The fruit is a follicle containing the seeds, with a tuft of hair.

Leaves, Stem and Root: The plant is a climbing shrub with pubescent shoots. The trunk can have a diameter of 10 cm. The transverse section shows granular, yellowish-white, scattered, fine and silky fibers. The outer surface is brownish-gray, often warty, with patches of lichen. The tough, ovate, 8 to 11 cm long and 5 to 8 cm wide leaves are very pubescent. They are crossed opposite.

Characteristics: The taste is bitter and acrid. The odor is faintly aromatic.

Habitat: The plant grows on the western slopes of the Andes in Ecuador, Peru and Columbia.

Production: Condurango bark consists of the dried bark of branches and trunk of Marsdenia condurango.

Not to be Confused With: Asclepias umbellata or Elcomarrhiza amylacea

Other Names: Eagle Vine

ACTIONS AND PHARMACOLOGY

COMPOUNDS

Pregnane- and pregn-5-ene glycosides (mixture known as condurangin): including condurango glycosides A, A0, A1, B0, C, C1, D0, E0, E2

Caffeic acid derivatives: including chlorogenic acid, neochlorogenic acid

Flavonoids: including trifoliin, hyperoside, quercitrin, rutin, and saponarin

EFFECTS

The drug contains bitter condurango glycosides (condurangin). As with other amaroid drugs, a reflexive increase of saliva and gastric juice secretion is to be expected. The drug stimulates the secretion of saliva and gastric juices. It has an antitumoral effect in animals.

INDICATIONS AND USAGE

Approved by Commission E:

- Dyspeptic complaints
- Loss of appetite

Unproven Uses: Condurango is used for loss of appetite. In folk medicine, it is used for atonia of the stomach, painful nutritional disorders, for stomach cancer to alleviate nausea, as an appetite stimulant and to increase tolerance of food.

Homeopathic Uses: Condurango is used for cracked skin, constriction of the alimentary canal, and for ulceration of the lips and anus.

PRECAUTIONS AND ADVERSE REACTIONS

Health risks or side effects following the proper administration of designated therapeutic dosages are not recorded.

DOSAGE

Mode of Administration: Comminuted drug for infusions and other bitter-tasting preparations for internal use.

Preparation: An infusion is prepared by adding 1.5 gm comminuted drug to cold water and bringing to a boil; strain when cold. The drug is also added to wine; 50 to 100 gm of the drug per liter.

Daily Dosage: The average daily dose of aqueous extract is 0.2 to 0.5 gm; tincture, 2 to 5 gm; liquid extract, 2 to 4 gm; bark, 2 to 4 gm; Infusion and wine: 1 cup or 1 liquor glass 30 minutes before meals.

Homeopathic Dosage: 5 drops, 1 tablet or 10 globules every 30 to 60 minutes (acute) or 1 to 3 times daily (chronic); parenterally: 1 to 2 ml sc acute, 3 times daily; chronic: once a day. Apply ointment 1 to 2 times a day (acute and chronic) (HAB1).

Storage: Condurango should be kept tightly sealed and protected from light.

LITERATURE

Berger S et al., Arch Pharm 320:924. 1987.

Berger S et al., PH 27:1451. 1988.

Hayashi K et al., (1980) Chem Pharm Bull 28:1954.

Hayashi K et al., (1981) Chem Pharm Bull 29:2725.

Steinegger E, Koch H, Pharm Acta Helv 56:244 et 57:211. 1982.

Takase M et al., (1982) Chem Pharm Bull 30:2429.

Tschesche R, Kohl H, Tetrahedron 24:4359. 1968.

Further information in:

Hänsel R, Keller K, Rimpler H, Schneider G (Hrsg.), Hagers Handbuch der Pharmazeutischen Praxis, 5. Aufl., Bde 4-6 (Drogen): Springer Verlag Berlin, Heidelberg, New York, 1992-1994.

Madaus G, Lehrbuch der Biologischen Arzneimittel, Bde 1-3, Nachdruck, Georg Olms Verlag Hildesheim 1979.

Steinegger E, Hänsel R, Pharmakognosie, 5. Aufl., Springer Verlag Heidelberg 1992.

Teuscher E, Biogene Arzneimittel, 5. Aufl., Wiss. Verlagsges. mbH Stuttgart 1997.

Wichtl M (Hrsg.), Teedrogen, 4. Aufl., Wiss. Verlagsges. Stuttgart 1997.

Congorosa

Maytenus ilicifolia

DESCRIPTION

Medicinal Parts: The medicinal part of the plant is the dried leaf.

Flower and Fruit: The flowers are in clusters in the leaf axils; the bracts have a reddish border. The flowers are radial; their structures are in fives. The calyx is reddish and 5-tipped. The petals are free, oval to elliptical and yellow. The male flowers have 5 stamens approximately 2 mm long with their ovary covered by a disc. The female flowers have 1 mm long stamens and a 2-carpeled, fused ovary on a thick fleshy disc. The fruit is a reddish, 2-chambered capsule. The seeds are reddish with a thin aril.

Leaves, Stem and Root: Congorosa grows as a dioecious evergreen shrub or tree, reaching up to 5 m high. The leaves are alternate, 2 to 15 cm long and 1 to 7 cm wide. They are elliptical to lanceolate, coriaceous and covered on both sides with 4 to 7 prickly teeth. Sometimes the leaves are completely entire, with very narrow, dropping stipules.

Habitat: The plant is indigenous to South America.

Production: Congorosa leaves (Argentinean name) are the dried leaves of Maytenus ilicifolia.

Not to be Confused With: Congorosa is sometimes confused with (and adulterated with) Yerba Mate.

ACTIONS AND PHARMACOLOGY

COMPOUNDS

Macrocyclic alkaloids (0.00005%): maytansinoides, including maytansine, maytanprine, maytanbutine

EFFECTS

The quinoid triterpene maytenin contained in the drug exhibits antimicrobial and tumor-inhibiting properties, particularly in topical administration for the treatment of basal cell carcinomas. Maytansine exhibits significant cytotoxic and antitumoral efficacy (similar to that of vinca alkaloids). Additionally, an ulcer-preventing effect has been demonstrated in both animal and human studies.

INDICATIONS AND USAGE

Unproven Uses: Congorosa is used mainly in South American folk medicine. In Brazil, external uses focus primarily on skin conditions such as eczema and skin ulcers. Internal uses include skin cancer, gastrointestinal complaints, gastrointestinal ulcers, hyperacidity, flatulence, gastralgia, dyspepsia, pain, states of exhaustion and anemia.

In Argentina, Congorosa is used for asthma, alcoholism and as a vulnerary. Other varieties are also used for inflammatory swelling and eye conditions.

PRECAUTIONS

No health hazards are known in conjunction with the proper administration of designated therapeutic dosages. Animal experiments revealed embryotoxic and teratogenic effects of maytansines (no detailed description of dosage or experimental procedure available). Should not be used during pregnancy.

CONTRAINDICATIONS

Congorosa preparations are contraindicated during pregnancy.

DOSAGE

Mode of Administration: Preparations are available for internal and external use.

How Supplied: Capsules

Daily Dosage:

Infusion/decoction (2 to 5%) — 100 to 400 ml internally. Externally as required.

Powder — 5 to 20 g

Liquid extract — 5 to 20 ml

Extract — 1 to 4 g

Tincture — 25 to 100 ml

Elixir/wine/syrup — 50 to 100 ml

LITERATURE

Hänsel R, Keller K, Rimpler H, Schneider G (Ed), Hagers Handbuch der Pharmazeutischen Praxis, 5. Aufl., Bde 4 - 6 (Drogen), Springer Verlag Berlin, Heidelberg, New York, 1992-1994.

Lima OG de, Coelho JS, Weigert E, Albuquerque IL d', Lima D de A, Moraes e Souza MA, Antimicrobial substances from higher plants. XXXVI. On the presence of maytenin and pristimerine in the cortical part of the roots of Maytenus ilicifolia from the South of Brazil. Rev Inst Antibiot (Recife), 11:35-8, 1971 Jun.

Conium maculatum

See Hemlock

Contrayerva

Dorstenia contrayerva

DESCRIPTION

Medicinal Parts: The medicinal parts are the roots of a number of species.

Flower and Fruit: The plant has long-pedicled, greenish flowers.

Leaves, Stem and Root: The plant is a perennial, growing to a height of up to 30 cm. It is stemless with palmate leaves. The rhizome is about 2 to 4 cm long and 1 cm thick. It is reddish-brown on the outside, paler on the inside and rough with leaf scars. The rhizome is nearly cylindrical and tapers suddenly at the end into a tail-like root with numerous curled, wiry rootlets.

Characteristics: The taste is slightly aromatic, then acrid.

Habitat: Contrayerva is found in Mexico, Peru and the West Indies.

Production: Contrayerva root is the rhizome of Dorstenia contrayerva and related varieties.

ACTIONS AND PHARMACOLOGY

COMPOUNDS

Cardioactive steroids (cardenolides): syriogenin

Furocoumarins

Volatile oil

EFFECTS

Diaphoretic and stimulant.

INDICATIONS AND USAGE

Unproven Uses: Preparations of the root are used as a stimulant and to treat low stamina. It has also been used as an antidote for snakebite (uncertain mechanism).

PRECAUTIONS AND ADVERSE REACTIONS

Health risks or side effects following the proper administration of designated therapeutic dosages are not recorded. The plant can trigger phototoxicoses through skin contact.

DOSAGE

Mode of Administration: Ground root as an infusion.

LITERATURE

Casagrande C et al., Tetrahedron 30:3587. 1974.

Hegnauer R, Chemotaxonomie der Pflanzen, Bde 1-11, Birkhäuser Verlag Basel, Boston, Berlin 1962-1997.

Kanamori H, Sakamoto I, Mizuta M, Chem Pharm Bull 34:1826. 1986.

Renner W, PA 17:763. 1962.

Reisch J, PM 15:320. 1967.

Szenedrei K, Novak I, Varga E, Buzas G, PA 23:76-77. 1968.

Renner W, PA 12:763-776. 1962.

Lewin L, Gifte und Vergiftungen, 6. Aufl., Nachdruck, Haug Verlag, Heidelberg 1992.

Convallaria majalis

See Lily-of-the-Valley

Coolwort

Tiarella cordifolia

DESCRIPTION

Medicinal Parts: The medicinal part is the herb.

Flower and Fruit: The plant has inconspicuous white flowers in racemes. The buds are pink-tinged. The few seeds are somewhat clavate. They have a light acrid taste and are odorless.

Leaves, Stem and Root: The plant is a 15 to 20 cm high herbaceous perennial, which produces runners. The simple leaves are usually slightly 5-lobed and cordate. The basal leaves are often deep red-orange. The cauline leaves have deep red spots and veins, although the latter are often lacking.

Habitat: The plant is indigenous to North America from Virginia to Canada.

Production: Coolwort is the aerial part of Tiarella cordifolia.

Other Names: Foam Flower, Mitrewort

ACTIONS AND PHARMACOLOGY

COMPOUNDS

The effective agents of the plant are unknown.

EFFECTS

The herb is a diuretic and a tonic.

INDICATIONS AND USAGE

Unproven Uses: Coolwort is used for conditions of the urinary tract and digestive disorders.

PRECAUTIONS AND ADVERSE REACTIONS

No health hazards or side effects are known in conjunction with the proper administration of designated therapeutic dosages.

DOSAGE

Mode of Administration: The drug is ground for infusions.

LITERATURE

No literature is available.

Copaiba Balsam

Copaifera langsdorffi

DESCRIPTION

Medicinal Parts: The medicinal parts are the resin oil (containing resin and essential oil) tapped from drillings in the trunk.

Flower and Fruit: The flowers are small and yellow.

Leaves, Stem and Root: Copaifera langsdorffi is an evergreen tree up to 18 m high with compound leaves.

Characteristics: The resin oil consists of resin and essential oil. The resin oil (oleoresin) ranges in viscosity from very liquid to a resin-like substance, and in color from a pale yellow to a red or fluorescent tint. The taste is unpleasant and there is a characteristic smell. A single tree can yield up to 40 liters.

Habitat: Copaiba Balsam is indigenous to tropical regions of South America and South Africa.

Production: Copaiba Balsam is extracted from Copaifera reticulata and other varieties from cavities drilled into the tree trunk.

Other Names: Copaiva

ACTIONS AND PHARMACOLOGY

COMPOUNDS

Volatile oil: chief constituent alpha- and beta-caryophyllene, beta-bisabolene, L-cadinene, -)-alpha-copaene

Resins: in particular, diterpenoid oleoresins including eperu-8(20)-en-15,18-dicarboxylic acid, (-)-16beta-kaurane-19-carboxylic acid, copaiferic acid, (+)-hardwickiic acid, copalic acid

EFFECTS

Possible bacteriostatic effect on the urinary tract. The sesquiterpenes give the drug an antimicrobial effect.

INDICATIONS AND USAGE

Unproven Uses: The obsolete drug is still used in some homeopathic preparations. Folk medicine employed Copaiba Balsam as a stimulant, laxative and diuretic for conditions such as infections of the urinary tract, chronic inflammation of the mucous membranes of the lungs, kidney stones and gonorrhea.

PRECAUTIONS AND ADVERSE REACTIONS

The drug is irritating to the mucous membranes and toxic in large amounts. Stomach pains appear after the intake of 5 g of the drug. Repeated doses bring about summer cholera, shivers, tremor, pains in the groin and insomnia. Skin contact can lead to contact dermatitis such as erythema, papular or vesicular rash, urticaria and petechias. Occasionally, the rashes leave brown spots after healing.

LITERATURE

Delle Monache G et al., (1971) Tetrahedron Letters 8:659.

Ferrari M et al., (1971) Phytochemistry 10:905.

Further information in:

Fenaroli's Handbook of Flavor Ingredients, Vol. 1. 2nd Ed. CRC Press 1975.

Kern W, List PH, Hörhammer L (Hrsg.), Hagers Handbuch der Pharmazeutischen Praxis, 4. Aufl., Bde. 1-8, Springer Verlag Berlin, Heidelberg, New York, 1969.

Leung AY, Encyclopedia of Common Natural Ingredients Used in Food Drugs and Cosmetics, John Wiley & Sons Inc., New York 1980.

Lewin L, Gifte und Vergiftungen, 6. Aufl., Nachdruck, Haug Verlag, Heidelberg 1992.

Madaus G, Lehrbuch der Biologischen Arzneimittel, Bde 1-3, Nachdruck, Georg Olms Verlag Hildesheim 1979.

Roth L, Daunderer M, Kormann K, Giftpflanzen, Pflanzengifte, 4. Aufl., Ecomed Fachverlag Landsberg Lech 1993.

Steinegger E, Hänsel R, Pharmakognosie, 5. Aufl., Springer Verlag Heidelberg 1992.

Copaifera langsdorffi

See Copaiba Balsam

Coptis trifolia

See Goldthread

Coral Root

Corallorhiza odontorhiza

DESCRIPTION

Medicinal Parts: The medicinal parts are the roots of the parasite.

Flower and Fruit: The plant has 10 to 20 flowers in terminal panicles. The flower heads are hood-like, reddish or purplish on the outside, paler and flecked with purple lines on the inside. One petal forms a lip with purple spots and a purple rim. The fruit is a large, bent-back, ribbed, long capsule.

Leaves, Stem and Root: Coral Root is a perennial found growing around the roots of trees in woodlands. The rhizome is small, brown, coral-like, about 2 to 3 cm long and 2 mm in thickness, with minute warts and transverse scars. The fracture is short and horny.

Characteristics: The taste is sweetish, then bitter. The odor is strong and peculiar when fresh.

Habitat: The parasite is indigenous to the U.S.

Production: Coral Root is the rhizome of Corallorhiza odontorhiza.

Other Names: Crawley Root, Scaly Dragon's Claw, Chicken Toe, Crawley, Fever Root, Turkey Claw

ACTIONS AND PHARMACOLOGY

COMPOUNDS

Unknown

EFFECTS

Coral Root has diaphoretic, febrifuge and sedative effects.

INDICATIONS AND USAGE

Unproven Uses: Coral Root is used for colds. It is very efficient at inducing perspiration. Its scarcity prevents its wider use.

PRECAUTIONS AND ADVERSE REACTIONS

Health risks or side effects following the proper administration of designated therapeutic dosages are not recorded.

DOSAGE

Mode of Administration: Internally as a liquid extract.

LITERATURE

No references are available

Corallorhiza odontorhiza

See Coral Root

Coriander

Coriandrum sativum

DESCRIPTION

Medicinal Parts: The medicinal parts are the coriander oil and dried ripe fruit.

Flower and Fruit: The flowers are white, compact, 3 to 5 blossomed umbels with no involucre. The floret has a 3-bract epicalyx. The border of the calyx has 5 tips. The corolla of the androgynous lateral florets is splayed. The fruit is globular and has a diameter of 3 cm, is straw yellow to brownish, and drops without dividing.

Leaves, Stem and Root: Coriandrum sativum is a 20 to 70 cm high plant with a bug-like smell. The root is thinly fusiform. The stem is erect, round, glabrous and branched above. The leaves are light green, entire below and double-pinnate above.

Characteristics: The fresh herb and unripe fruit have a bug-like smell. Ripe fruit has a pleasant, tangy smell and taste.

Habitat: The herb is found in the Mediterranean region, central and eastern Europe, eastern Asia, and North and South America.

Production: Coriander consists of the ripe, dried, spherical fruit of Coriandrum sativum and its varieties vulgare A. and microcarpum. The fruit is threshed when it is rust red and is dried in lofts.

Not to be Confused With: Grains and legumes.

ACTIONS AND PHARMACOLOGY

COMPOUNDS

Volatile oil (0.4 to 1.7%): chief components D-(+)-linalool (coriandrol, share 60 to 75%), including in addition borneol, p-cymene, camphor, geraniol, limonene, alpha-pinene; the unusual, bug-like smell is caused by the trans-tridec-2-enale content

Fatty oil (13 to 21%): chief fatty acids petroselic acid, oleic acid, linolenic acid

Hydroxycoumarins: including umbelliferone, scopoletin

EFFECTS

The essential oil of coriander stimulates the secretion of gastric juices and is a carminative and spasmolytic; in vitro it has antibacterial and antifungal effects.

INDICATIONS AND USAGE

Approved by Commission E:

- Dyspeptic complaints
- Loss of appetite

Unproven Uses: Coriander is used for dyspeptic complaints, loss of appetite and complaints of the upper abdomen.

In folk medicine, Coriander is also used for digestive and gastric complaints; in other cultures for coughs, chest pains, bladder complaints, leprosy rash, fever, dysentery, externally for headaches, oral and pharyngeal disorders, halitosis, post-partum complications; the folk indications have not been proven.

Chinese Medicine: Coriander is used in China for loss of appetite, the pre-eruptive phase of chickenpox and measles, hemorrhoids and rectal prolapse.

Indian Medicine: In India, Coriander is used to treat nose bleeds, coughs, hemorrhoids, scrofulous, painful micturation, edema, bladder complaints, vomiting, amoebic dysentery and dizziness.

PRECAUTIONS AND ADVERSE REACTIONS

Health risks or side effects following the proper administration of designated therapeutic dosages are not recorded. The drug possesses a weak potential for sensitization.

DOSAGE

Mode of Administration: Crushed and powdered drug, as well as other galenic preparations for internal indication.

Preparations: Coriander extract 1:2 is prepared by percolating 1 weight part of the drug with 45% ethanol so that 2 weights tincture is produced. The infusion is prepared by pouring 150 ml of boiling water over 2 tsp. of crushed drug and straining after 15 minutes.

Daily Dosage: The average daily dose is 3.0 gm of drug. The single dose is 1 gm.

Infusion — 1 fresh cup between meals.

Tincture — 10 to 20 drops after meals.

Storage: The non-comminuted drug is stored at a maximum temperature of 25°C, protected from light in well-sealed containers.

LITERATURE

Calcandi V, Ciropol-Calcandi I, Georgescu E, PA 16(6):331-334. 1961.

Diedreichsen A et al., Chemotypes of Coriandrum sativum L. in the Gatersleben Genebank. In: PM 62, Abstracts of the 44th Ann Congress of GA, 82. 1996.

Formacék, Buch. In: Formacék, V, Kubeczka KH: Essential Oils Analysis by Capillary Gas Chromatography and Carbon-13-NMR Spectroscopy, John Wiley & Sons, Chicester, New York, Brisbane, Toronto, Singapore 1982.

Gijbels MJM et al., (1982) Fitoterapia 53(1/2):17.

Ram AS, Devi HM, (1983) Indian J Bot 6(1):21.

Schratz E, Quadry SMJS, PM 14(3):310-325. 1966.

Further information in:

Fenaroli's Handbook of Flavor Ingredients, Vol. 1, 2nd Ed., CRC Press 1975.

Hänsel R, Keller K, Rimpler H, Schneider G (Ed), Hagers Handbuch der Pharmazeutischen Praxis. 5. Aufl., Bde 4 - 6 (Drogen), Springer Verlag Berlin, Heidelberg, New York, 1992-1994

Leung AY, Encyclopedia of Common Natural Ingredients Used in Food, Drugs and Cosmetics. John Wiley & Sons Inc. New York 1980.

Mascolo N et al., Phytother Res 1 (1987), 28.

Simon JE, Chadwick AF, Craker LE (Eds.), Herbs. An Indexed Bibliography 1971-80. Archon Books, USA 1984.

Steinegger E, Hänsel R, Pharmakognosie, 5. Aufl., Springer Verlag Heidelberg 1992.

Teuscher E, Biogene Arzneimittel, 5. Aufl., Wiss. Verlagsges. mbH Stuttgart 1997.

Wichtl M (Hrsg.), Teedrogen, 4. Aufl., Wiss. Verlagsges. Stuttgart 1997.

Coriandrum sativum

See Coriander

Corn Cockle

Agrostemma githago

DESCRIPTION

Medicinal Parts: The medicinal part of the herb is the seed.

Flower and Fruit: The flowers are apical or arranged in twos or threes like a curled cyme; the 5 sepals of the calyx have 2 to 4 cm long tips that project above the corolla; the flower tube is 14 to 18 mm. The 5 petals are 30 to 35 mm long, dark purple and occasionally whitish. There are 5 styles and 10 stamens. The ovary is superior, undivided and has a central placenta. The fruit capsule is 15 to 18 mm long with numerous 2.5 to 3.5 mm long, warty seeds.

Leaves, Stem and Root: Agrostemma githago is an annual herb that grows upright, up to 100 cm high. The leaves are opposite, linear-lanceolate, acuminate and up to 10 mm wide. The stem is upright, usually unbranched, shaggy-gray-pubescent. The primary root is spindle-shaped and heavily branched.

Habitat: Europe and Asia

Production: Corn cockle seed is the dried seed of Agrostemma githago.

Other Names: Cockle

ACTIONS AND PHARMACOLOGY

COMPOUNDS

Triterpene saponins: chief component is githagoside (0.04%, gypsogenine tetraglycoside), additional components are gypsogenin and quillaic acid gylcosides

Fatty oil: 6%

Steroids: sterols, including alpha-spinasterol

Unusual amino acids: orcyl alanine (0.4%)

EFFECTS

The drug exhibits an antimycotic effect. Cornflower seeds are toxic in higher dosages.

INDICATIONS AND USAGE

Unproven Uses: Folk medicine uses include gastritis, coughs, skin impurities, edema and worm purging.

Homeopathic Uses: Dilutions are used for gastritis.

PRECAUTIONS AND ADVERSE REACTIONS

No health hazards are known in conjunction with the proper administration of designated homeopathic dosages of the drug.

OVERDOSAGE

2 to 3 gm of the seeds are considered harmless to humans; poisonous levels are reached between 3 and 5 gm, due to the toxic triterpene saponin content. Dosages over 5 gm are considered lethal. Signs of poisoning include local irritation of mucous membranes (sneezing, lacrimation, conjunctivitis, salivation, nausea, vomiting, colic, diarrhea). The ingestion of toxic levels leads to headache, dizziness, restlessness, circulatory disorders, deliria and possible spasms. Death occurs through asphyxiation. Long-term ingestion of acute non-toxic dosages can cause chronic signs of poisoning. The toxins are not affected by baking or cooking.

Following gastrointestinal emptying (inducement of vomiting, gastric lavage, sodium sulfate) and the instillation of activated charcoal, the treatment for poisoning includes diazepam or barbital (i.v.) for spasms. In the event of shock, plasma volume expanders should be infused. Monitoring of kidney function is necessary. Intubation and oxygen respiration may also be required.

DOSAGE

Mode of Administration: Whole herb preparations for internal, external and parenteral uses.

Homeopathic Dosage: Parenterally: Can be given 1 ml sc., 3 times daily for acute use; and once a day for chronic use but only from D2 (HAB34). Orally: 5 drops, 1 tablet, 10 globules, every 30 to 60 minutes for acute use; and 1 to 3 times daily for chronic use.

LITERATURE

Hänsel R, Keller K, Rimpler H, Schneider G (Ed), Hagers Handbuch der Pharmazeutischen Praxis, 5. Aufl., Bde 4 - 6 (Drogen), Springer Verlag Berlin, Heidelberg, New York, 1992-1994.

Kende H, Shen TC, Nitrate reductase in Agrostemma githago. Comparison of the inductive effects of nitrate and cytokinin. Biochim Biophys Acta, 216:118-25, 1972 Nov 24.

Siepmann C, Bader G, Hiller K, Wray V, Domke T, Nimtz M, New saponins from the seeds of Agrostemma githago var. githago. Planta Med, 216:159-64, 1998 Mar.

Smith RA, Miller RE, Lang DG, Presumptive intoxication of cattle by corn cockle, Agrostemma githago (L) Scop. Vet Hum Toxicol, 216:250, 1997 Aug.

Stirpe F, Gasperi-Campani A, Barbieri L, Falasca A, Abbondanza A, Stevens WA, Ribosome-inactivating proteins from the seeds of Saponaria officinalis L. (soapwort), of Agrostemma githago L. (corn cockle) and of Asparagus officinalis L. (asparagus), and from the latex of Hura crepitans L. (sandbox tree). Biochem J, 216:617-25, 1983 D.

Corn Poppy

Papaver rhoeas

DESCRIPTION

Medicinal Parts: The medicinal parts of the plant are the flowers and seeds.

Flower and Fruit: The flowers are solitary, terminal or axillary, and have a diameter of 10 cm. The pedicles are bristly, irregularly curved and usually axillary. The two sepals are green, bristly and fall off. The 4 petals are orbicular, usually scarlet or crimson (though occasionally white or violet) with a round, shiny, often white-bordered deep-black mark at the base. The fruit capsule is broad-elliptical, dark brown and reticulate-pitted.

Leaves, Stem and Root: Poppy is an annual, occasionally biennial, multiple-stemmed plant 25 to 90 cm high. The stems are erect to semi-erect, simple or branched with stiff, protruding hairs. They have basal rosette lanceolate leaves and deeply indented cauline leaves. The foliage leaves are oblong-lanceolate, pinnatifid to pinnatisect and very bristly.

Habitat: The plant is indigenous to Europe, northern Africa and temperate regions in Asia, and has been introduced in North and South America.

Production: Corn Poppy flower consists of the dried petals of Papaver rhoeas as well as its preparations.

Not to be Confused With: Confusion can occur with Papaver dibium and Papaver argemone.

Other Names: Copperose, Corn Rose, Cup-Puppy, Headache, Headwark, Red Poppy

ACTIONS AND PHARMACOLOGY

COMPOUNDS

Isoquinoline alkaloids (0.1%): chief alkaloids rhoeadine, isorhoeadine, rhoeagenine, coptisine, isocorydine, stylopine

Anthocyans: including among others mecocyanin (cyanidin-3-isosophoroside), cyanin

Mucilages

EFFECTS

No information is available other than that the drug, which contains alkaloids (not opium alkaloids), is said to be convulsive.

INDICATIONS AND USAGE

Unproven Uses: Corn Poppy flower is used for diseases and disorders of the respiratory tract, for disturbed sleep, as a sedative and for the relief of pain. In folk medicine, it is used to make a cough syrup for children, as a tea for insomnia, for pain relief and as a sedative.

Homeopathic Uses: Homeopathy uses Corn Poppy flower for states of agitation and excitation and also for spasms of the hollow organs.

PRECAUTIONS AND ADVERSE REACTIONS

No health hazards or side effects are known in conjunction with the proper administration of designated therapeutic dosages. The drug itself is non-toxic due to the low level of alkaloid content, but reports exist in the scientific literature of children being poisoned by intake of the fresh foliage (with blossoms). Poisoning symptoms include vomiting and stomach pain.

DOSAGE

Mode of Administration: As a component of "metabolic" teas.

Preparation: To prepare a tea, use 1 g of the flowers to 1 cup hot water. To make an infusion, scald 2 teaspoonfuls drug, steep for 10 minutes and strain (1 teaspoonful is equal to approximately 8 g drug). A poultice is prepared using 1 to 2 teaspoonfuls of tincture to 250 ml of water. (Prepare tincture in accordance with HAB1 guidelines.)

Daily Dosage: As an expectorant for inflammation of the bronchial mucous membranes, drink 1 cup infusion 2 to 3 times a day. The infusion may be sweetened with honey.

Homeopathic Dosage: Full bath: 2/3 dessertspoon tincture in a bath (correspondingly less for partial baths).

Storage: Corn Poppy flower should be thoroughly dried before storing in a tightly sealed container that protects it from light.

LITERATURE

El-Masry S et al., (1981) Planta Med 41:61.

Fairbairn JW, Williamson EM, (1978) Phytochemistry 17:2087.

Frohne D, Pfänder HJ, Giftpflanzen - Ein Handbuch für Apotheker, Toxikologen und Biologen, 4. Aufl., Wiss. Verlags-Ges. Stuttgart 1997.

Gasic O et al., Hem Pregl 33:23. 1992.

Kalaw Y, Sariyar S, PM 55:488. 1989.

Kern W, List PH, Hörhammer L (Hrsg.), Hagers Handbuch der Pharmazeutischen Praxis, 4. Aufl., Bde 1-8: Springer Verlag Berlin, Heidelberg, New York, 1969.

Lewin L, Gifte und Vergiftungen, 6. Aufl., Nachdruck, Haug Verlag, Heidelberg 1992.

Roth L, Daunderer M, Kormann K, Giftpflanzen, Pflanzengifte, 4. Aufl., Ecomed Fachverlag Landsberg Lech 1993.

Teuscher E, Lindequist U, Biogene Gifte - Biologie, Chemie, Pharmakologie, 2. Aufl., Fischer Verlag Stuttgart 1994.

Wichtl M (Hrsg.), Teedrogen, 4. Aufl., Wiss. Verlagsges. Stuttgart 1997.

Willaman JJ, Hui-Li L, (1970) Lloydia 33 (3A): 1.

Corn Silk

Zea mays

DESCRIPTION

Medicinal Parts: The medicinal part is the seed.

Flower and Fruit: The plant is monoecious. The male flowers form terminal racemes of spikes with 2-flowered husks. The female flowers are axillary. The spikes are at varying distances from the ground and are enclosed in a number of thin leaves, the sheath-like maize husk. The spikes consist of a cylindrical substance, the cob, on which the seeds are arranged in 8 rows of 40 or more. Single whitish-green threads of a silky appearance grow from the eyes of the seeds and hang outside the husk, where they catch the pollen. The Maize seeds are usually yellow but can be darker to almost black.

Leaves, Stem and Root: The plant is 1 to 3 m high and sturdy with a solid stem covered in alternate, over 4 cm wide, linear leaves.

Habitat: The plant is indigenous to America and is cultivated all over the world as green fodder or as a cereal crop.

Production: Corn Silk flowers are the styles and stigmas of Zea mays. The styles of the female flowers, as they begin to grow out of the pillow-lace, are gathered for medicinal or therapeutic purposes. They are removed by hand and dried in the shade.

Other Names: Indian Corn, Maize, Stigmata maydis

ACTIONS AND PHARMACOLOGY

COMPOUNDS

Volatile oil (0.2%): including among others carvacrol, alpha-terpineol, menthol, thymol

Flavonoids: including among others maysin, maysin-3'-ethyl ether

Bitter substances

Saponins (2-3%)

Tannins: the main one is probably proanthocyanidins

Sterols: including among others beta-sitosterol, ergosterol

Alkaloids (0.05%)

6-methoxybenzoxazolinone

Fatty oil (2%)

EFFECTS

The active agents are saponin, essential oil and tannin. Maize stimulates the cardiac muscles, increases blood pressure, acts as a diuretic and sedates the digestive tract.

INDICATIONS AND USAGE

Unproven Uses: Maize is used for disorders of the urinary tract.

Chinese Medicine: Maize is used in the treatment of liver disorders.

PRECAUTIONS AND ADVERSE REACTIONS

No health hazards or side effects are known in conjunction with the proper administration of designated therapeutic dosages.

DOSAGE

Mode of Administration: Liquid extract, in medicinal preparations and combinations.

Preparation: Prepare an infusion using 2 teaspoons of drug per cup of water. A tincture is prepared by adding 20 gm of drug to 100 ml of 20% alcohol (leave to stand for 5 days).

Daily Dosage: Drink 1 cup of infusion every other day. Take 2 to 3 teaspoons of tincture per day.

LITERATURE

Chan H, But P, Pharmacology, Applications of Chinese Materia Medica, Vol 1, World Scientific Singapore 1986.

Hahn SJ, (1973) K'at'ollick Taehak Uihak Nonmun J 25:127 (via [5]).

Hegnauer R, Chemotaxonomie der Pflanzen, Bde 1-11: Birkhäuser Verlag Basel, Boston, Berlin 1962-1997.

Kern W, List PH, Hörhammer L (Hrsg.), Hagers Handbuch der Pharmazeutischen Praxis, 4. Aufl., Bde 1-8: Springer Verlag Berlin, Heidelberg, New York, 1969.

Leung AY, Encyclopedia of Common Natural Ingredients Used in Food Drugs, Cosmetics, John Wiley & Sons Inc., New York 1980.

Madaus G, Lehrbuch der Biologischen Arzneimittel, Bde 1-3, Nachdruck, Georg Olms Verlag Hildesheim 1979.

Paris F, Schauenberg P, Guide des Plantes Medicinales, Delachaux et Niestle Switzerland 1969.

Cornflower

Centaurea cyanus

DESCRIPTION

Medicinal Parts: The medicinal parts are the fast-growing ray flowers and the dried ray florets, which have been separated from the receptacle and epicalyx, and to a lesser extent the tubular florets, which have usually been separated from the ovaries.

Flower and Fruit: The 3 cm wide flowers are solitary and terminal. The tubular flowers are blue, the cultivated ones are usually all purple-violet, pale pink or white. The lateral florets are larger, in rays and funnel-shaped. The oblong gray fruit is an achaene with the remains of a tuft of hair.

Leaves, Stem and Root: Growing 20 to 70 cm high, the annual or biennial plant contains fusiform, pale tap roots. It has a rosette of basal leaves and an erect, branched, spider-web-pubescent angular stem, covered in alternate, faintly linear-lanceolate leaves. The basal leaves are lyre-shaped, pinnatafid and long-petioled. The upper leaves are non-compound.

Habitat: The plant is probably indigenous to the Middle East, but is cultivated worldwide because of grain production.

Production: Cornflower consists of the quickly dried flowers of Centaurea cyanus. The plant is harvested during the flowering season from June to August.

Other Names: Centaurea, Bachelor's Buttons, Bluebonnet, Bluebottle, Blue Centaury, Cyani, Bluebow, Hurtsickle, Blue Cap, Cyani-flowers

ACTIONS AND PHARMACOLOGY

COMPOUNDS

Anthocyans: chief components succinylcyanin (centaurocyanin, cyanidine-3-O-(6-O-succinyl-beta-D-glucosyl)-5-O-beta-D-glucoside)

Flavonoids

Bitter principles (structure unknown)

EFFECTS

The drug has an antibacterial effect in vitro (centaurocyanin), but only for the aerial parts of the plant without the flowers.

INDICATIONS AND USAGE

Unproven Uses: Cornflowers and their preparations are used internally for fever, constipation, leucorrhea, menstrual disorders and vaginal candida, and as a laxative, tonic and bitter. The flowers are also used as a diuretic and an expectorant, or as a stimulant for liver and gall bladder function. Externally, Cornflowers are used in preparation of eye washes for eye inflammation and conjunctivitis, and for eczema of the scalp.

PRECAUTIONS AND ADVERSE REACTIONS

Health risks or side effects following the proper administration of designated therapeutic dosages are not recorded. The drug possesses a weak sensitization potential.

DOSAGE

Mode of Administration: Cornflower is rarely used today. Occasionally, it is used as an inactive ingredient in tea mixtures.

Preparation: The infusion is prepared by adding 1 gm of drug per cup.

Dosage: The tea should be drunk several times daily.

Storage: Store carefully and protect from light.

LITERATURE

Bandyukova V, Khalmatov K, (1967) Khim Prir Soedin 3:57.

Hänsel R, Keller K, Rimpler H, Schneider G (Hrsg.), Hagers Handbuch der Pharmazeutischen Praxis, 5. Aufl., Bde 4-6 (Drogen), Springer Verlag Berlin, Heidelberg, New York, 1992-1994.

Kakegawa K et al., PH 26:2261-2263. 1987.

Suljok G, László-Bencsik A, PH 24:1121-1122. 1985.

Takeda K et al., PH 27:1228-1229. 1988.

Cornus florida

See Dogwood

Cornus officinalis

See Asiatic Dogwood

Corydalis cava

See Corydalis (Yan-Hu-Suo)

Corydalis (Yan-Hu-Suo)

Corydalis cava

DESCRIPTION

Medicinal Parts: The medicinal parts are the tubers collected and dried when the plant is dormant. The fresh tuber collected just before flowering is also used.

Flower and Fruit: Flowers first appear in the fourth or fifth year. There are 4 to 5 racemes of 6 to 12 blooms, which are symmetrically 2-sided. There are 2 entire-margined bracts under the racemes. The flowers are dull red or yellowish-white, seldom lilac, brown-red or dark blue. The sepals are very small. The upper petal is drawn out into a downward curved spur; the front end is curved upward like a lip. The inner petals form a hood-like protective cover for the 6 stamens fused into 2 bundles. There is one ovary. The fruit is a pale green pod 20 to 25 cm long. The seeds are 3 mm wide, black, round, smooth and glossy.

Leaves, Stem and Root: The plant is perennial and grows to about 15 to 30 cm. A number of erect stems grows from the tuberous rhizome, which quickly becomes hollow. The stems bear the racemes and the 2 leaves. The 2 leaves under the racemes are long-petioled, double trifoliate, sea green above, and whitish green beneath.

Characteristics: The flowers have a slight fragrance of resin.

Habitat: The plant is indigenous to southern and central Europe.

Production: Corydalis tubers are the rhizomes of Corydalis cava. The tubers are dug up in autumn or in spring, once the ground has thawed. They are thoroughly cleaned, the roots and greenery are removed, and the remainder is sliced. The material is dried in a well-aired place, turned regularly and kept in temperatures not exceeding 40°C.

Other Names: Early Fumitory, Turkey Corn, Squirrel Corn, Yan-Hu-Suo

ACTIONS AND PHARMACOLOGY

COMPOUNDS

Isoquinoline alkaloids: very complex, breed-specific mixture of approximately 40 alkaloids, including (+)-bulbocapnine and (+)-corytuberin (aporphine-type) as well as (-)-corydaline (berberine-type)

EFFECTS

The full extract has a mildly sedative, sleep-inducing, spasmolytic, tranquilizing and hallucinogenic effect. It suppresses the CNS, reduces blood pressure and impedes movement of the small intestine.

INDICATIONS AND USAGE

Unproven Uses: Formerly, Corydalis was used for hyperkinetic conditions. Today, it is occasionally used for treat melancholia, pathological neuroses and mild forms of depression, as well as for severe nerve damage, trembling limbs and emotional disturbances.

Folk medicine: Corydalis was used in the past for worm infestation, menstruation disorders, Ménier's disease and

Parkinson's. Externally, the plant was used for poorly healing wounds and ulcers.

Homeopathic Uses: Used for inflammations of the respiratory tract and the eyes, rheumatism, hyperorexia, diarrhea and furunculosis.

PRECAUTIONS AND ADVERSE REACTIONS

Health risks or side effects following the proper administration of designated therapeutic dosages are not recorded. Poisonings among humans have not yet been observed.

OVERDOSAGE

Clonic spasms with musculature tremor occur with overdosages.

DOSAGE

Mode of Administration: The drug is available as a full extract in ready-made preparations.

Daily Dosage: Externally: as a compress, 3 to 5 gm of drug to 1/8 Liter of water.

Homeopathic Dosage: Oral: 5 drops, 1 tablet or 10 globules every 30 to 60 minutes (acute) or 1 to 3 times daily (chronic); parenterally: 1 to 2 ml sc acute: 3 times daily; chronic: once a day; eye drops 1 to 3 times daily; liquid dilutions D2 to D6: 20 to 60 drops; D12 to D30: 15 to 45 drops (HAB1).

LITERATURE

Frohne D, Pfänder HJ, Giftpflanzen - Ein Handbuch für Apotheker, Toxikologen und Biologen, 4. Aufl., Wiss. Verlagsges. mbH Stuttgart 1997.

Hänsel R, Keller K, Rimpler H, Schneider G (Hrsg.), Hagers Handbuch der Pharmazeutischen Praxis, 5. Aufl., Bde 4-6 (Drogen), Springer Verlag Berlin, Heidelberg, New York, 1992-1994.

Lewin L, Gifte und Vergiftungen, 6. Aufl., Nachdruck, Haug Verlag, Heidelberg 1992.

Madaus G, Lehrbuch der Biologischen Arzneimittel, Bde 1-3, Nachdruck, Georg Olms Verlag Hildesheim 1979.

Roth L, Daunderer M, Kormann K, Giftpflanzen, Pflanzengifte, 4. Aufl., Ecomed Fachverlag Landsberg Lech 1993.

Santavy F, in Manske RHF (Ed.), The Alkaloids, Vol XII, Academic Press New York, p. 333-354. 1970.

Slavík J, Slavíkova L, Collect Czech Chem Commun 44:2261-2273. 1979.

Steinegger E, Hänsel R, Pharmakognosie, 5. Aufl., Springer Verlag Heidelberg 1992.

Teuscher E, Lindequist U, Biogene Gifte - Biologie, Chemie, Pharmakologie, 2. Aufl., Fischer Verlag Stuttgart 1994.

Corynanthe pachyceras

See Hwema Bark

Costus

Saussurea costus

DESCRIPTION

Medicinal Parts: The medicinal part of the plant is the root.

Flower and Fruit: The flowers are in tough, orbicular, axillary or apical capitula with a diameter of 2.5 to 3.8 cm surrounded by an involucre. The epicalyx sepals are in a number of rows, ovate to lanceolate, acuminate, stiff and revolute. The tubular florets are dark blue to black-violet. The fruit is an achene up to 8 mm long with a brownish, feather-like pappus that is up to 1.7 cm long.

Leaves, Stem and Root: Saussurea costus is a herbaceous upright perennial growing to a height of up to 2 m. The leaves are alternate, the lamina simple, irregular dentate, basal, 0.5 to 1.2 m long and triangular. The petiole is lobed-winged. The cauline leaves are smaller, petiolate or sessile with 2 clasping lobes at the base. The plant has a strong, hard root up to 6 cm thick.

Habitat: The plant is indigenous to India and China.

Production: Indian Costus roots are the dried roots of Saussurea costus, which are harvested in September and October when the concentration of essential oils is highest.

Not to be Confused With: Because of the similarity in name, confusion sometimes occurs with Costus speciosus. The plant is also confused with Inula racemosa. In the past, confusion existed with many plants such as Byronia or Galanga, which went under the name of Kostus. However, differentiation has been established.

ACTIONS AND PHARMACOLOGY

COMPOUNDS

Volatile oil (1 to 6%): chief components dehydrocostus lactone (35%) and costunolid (15%), including as well alpha-, beta- and gamma-costol, elemol, cyclocostunolide; aroma bearers include acetic acid, 4-ethyl octanoic acid, heptanoic acid, 3-methyl butyric acid, 7-octenoic acid, isopropyliden pentanoic acid

Resins (6%)

Polysaccharides: inulin (18%)

Lignans: including olivil-4″-O-beta-D-glucoside

Sesquiterpenes: saussureamines A to E

Steroids: sterols, including beta-sitosterol, stigmasterol

EFFECTS

The drug contains large quantities of essential oil with the sesquiterpene lactones, costunolid and dehydrocostus lactone. Various drug extracts exhibit antimicrobial and fungistatic efficacy, and have an influence over liver metabolism and liver sugar levels. The saussure amines it contains inhibit the formation of stress-related stomach ulcers. A bronchospasmolytic effect has also been described. A dry extract of the drug administered in 500 mg dosages p.o. 3 times daily over a 3-month period led to a statistically significant reduction of angina pectoris attacks among patients with coronary heart disease.

INDICATIONS AND USAGE

Indian Medicine: The root has been used in India since ancient times as a universal antidote and as a contraceptive (Tschirch manual). It was also used medicinally as an aromatic and stimulant (according to Hoppe's work on drugs - 1958).

Chinese Medicine: Internal uses include gastric complaints, flatulence, coughs, cholera, loss of appetite and asthma. Externally, it has been used for poorly healing wounds and skin conditions. Efficacy for these indications has not yet been proven.

PRECAUTIONS AND ADVERSE REACTIONS

No health hazards are known in conjunction with the proper administration of designated therapeutic dosages. It is conceivable that the plant could cause allergic reactions due to its sesquiterpene lactone content, but no cases of this have as yet been documented.

DOSAGE

Mode of Administration: Whole and powdered drug preparations for internal and external use.

LITERATURE

Cheminat A, Stampf JL, Benezra C, Farrall MJ, Fr chet JM, Allergic contact dermatitis to costus: removal of haptens with polymers. Acta Derm Venereol, 61:525-9, 1981.

Hänsel R, Keller K, Rimpler H, Schneider G (Ed), Hagers Handbuch der Pharmazeutischen Praxis, 5. Aufl., Bde 4 - 6 (Drogen), Springer Verlag Berlin, Heidelberg, New York, 1992-1994.

Costus specious

See Cane-Reed

Cotton

Gossypium hirsutum

DESCRIPTION

Medicinal Parts: The medicinal parts are the seeds.

Flower and Fruit: Single axillary, radial flowers are structured in fives. The calyx is approximately 4.5 cm long, fused, divided into 5 and surrounded by 3 large, deeply dentate, epicalyx sepals. The 5 petals are 5 to 7 cm long, free, white to cream-yellow. The stamens are numerous, and the filaments are fused into a tube. The ovary is superior, and the carpels are fused. There is 1 style, with 3 to 5 stigmas that project through the stamen tube. The fruit is a walnut-sized capsule that opens on 3 to 5 sides and has 8 to 10 reniform, 3 to 5 mm thick, black seeds. These are covered in single-celled hair up to 46 mm long.

Leaves, Stem and Root: This evergreen shrub grows up to 2 m high and is typically cultivated as an annual. The leaves are alternate, long-petiolate, 3- to 7-lobed, with serrate margins, a rounded base and stipules that drop.

Habitat: The plant is indigenous to the U.S., China, Commonwealth of Independent States, India, Pakistan and Egypt.

Production: Cotton seeds are the ripe seeds of Gossypium hirsutum, Gossypium oleum and Gossypium herbaceum, as well as other cultivated Gossypium species. Cotton seed oil is the refined, fatty oil from the seeds. The oil is extracted using solvents or pressing followed by refinement with a yield of approximately 19%. Gossypium semen is derived from the industrial extraction of cottonseed oil.

Not to be Confused With: Mistaken identity can occur with sesame and kapok oil, which are sometimes used to adulterate Cotton oil preparations.

Other Names: American Cotton Plant, Cotton Seed

ACTIONS AND PHARMACOLOGY

COMPOUNDS: COTTON OIL

Fatty oil: chief fatty acids include linoleic acid (55%), palmitic acid (22%), oleic acid (15%), myristic acid (5%), as well as stearic acid, eicosanoic acid, di- cyclopropene-fatty acids malvalic acid and sterculiac acid

Lignans: gossypol (traces)

Steroids: sterols, particularly beta-sitosterol, as well as campesterol, stigmasterol, delta7-stigmasterol, 24-methyl cycloartenol

Tocopherols (vitamin E): including 0.04% alpha-tocopherol, 0.04% gamma-tocopherol

EFFECTS: COTTON OIL

The oil contains large amounts of unsaturated fatty acids and is chiefly used as a dietetic.

COMPOUNDS: COTTON SEED

Fatty oil (20 to 30%): chief fatty acids include linoleic acid (55%), palmitic acid (22%), oleic acid (15%), myristic acid (5%), as well as stearic acid, eicosanoic acid, the cyclopropene-fatty acids malvalic acid and sterculic acid

Protein (20 to 25%)

Lignans: (+)-gossypol and (-)-gossypol (0.1 to 6.0%, yellow to red in color); there are also cultivated forms that are low in gossypol (gossypol content < 0.01%)

Flavonoids

Monosaccharides/oligosaccharides (7%): saccharose, raffinose, stachyose, glucose, fructose

EFFECTS: COTTON SEED

The pigment substance gossypol contained in the seeds inhibits enzymes of the energy metabolism, decouples the respiratory chain from the oxidative phosphorylation, reduces the cellular ATP concentration, lessens membrane potentials and inhibits the acrosomal sperm proteinase acrosine (anti-fertility effect). A cytostatic effect has been demonstrated.

INDICATIONS AND USAGE

COTTON OIL

Unproven Uses: Folk medicine indications for Gossypii oleum have included hypercholesteremia and vitamin E deficiency. It is also used when a non-nitrogenous or parenteral nourishment is required.

INDICATIONS AND USAGE

COTTON SEED

Indian Medicine: Among indications in Indian medicine are headache, coughs, dysentery, constipation, gonorrhea, chronic cystitis, fever, poor lactation, epilepsy and snake bites. Reference is also made to use as an abortifacient and aphrodisiac. Efficacy for these indications has not yet been proven.

PRECAUTIONS AND ADVERSE REACTIONS

COTTON OIL

No health hazards are known in conjunction with the proper administration of designated therapeutic dosages. Animal experiments over a period of several weeks involving the administration of cyclopropene-fatty acids led to elevated cholesterol and triglyceride blood levels in rabbits and to a delayed sexual development in young female rats.

COTTON SEED

The drug is toxic, due to its gossypol content. Chronic ingestion of Cotton seed will lead to fertility disorders in men. After feeding sheep and cattle a total of 2 to 3 kg of Cotton seed press cakes over a period of 3 to 4 weeks, gastroenteritis, kidney damage with hematuria and icterus were observed. Death occurred 24 to 48 hours after first appearance of symptoms. Eye damage (Cotton seed blindness) was also noted.

DOSAGE

COTTON OIL

Preparation: Emulsion 10 to 15%: sterilization is carried out at 150° C for 1 hour.

Daily Dosage: Emulsion 40%: 60 ml p.o. in a single dose.

LITERATURE

Hänsel R, Keller K, Rimpler H, Schneider G (Ed.), Hagers Handbuch der Pharmazeutischen Praxis, 5. Aufl., Bde 4 - 6 (Drogen), Springer Verlag Berlin, Heidelberg, New York, 1992-1994.

Cotton Tree

Cochlospermum gossypium

DESCRIPTION

Medicinal Parts: The medicinal parts of the plant is the root, which yields a laxative, and the hard exudate of the aromatic bark.

Flower and Fruit: The flowers are in apical, sparsely flowered panicles. Flowers are 11 to 15 cm in diameter with 4 to 5 free silky-haired sepals, 4 to 5 gold-yellow petals and numerous stamens. The superior ovary has 5 carpels with many ovules attached to the walls. The fruit is an oval, dark-brown, hanging capsule 5 to 10 cm long, 4 cm thick and loculicidal. The seeds are reniform, approximately 7 mm long, 5 mm wide and villous.

Leaves, Stem and Root: Cochlospermum gossypium grows as a tree, rising up to 10 m high. The leaves are 10 to 20 cm wide and palmate-lobed. The 3 to 5 lobes are acuminate, or digitate; the petioles are 6 to 17 cm long. The young branches are velvet-haired and tinged reddish, the older ones are glabrous and ash gray.

Habitat: The tree is indigenous to India, Southeast Asia, Kenya and Mauritius.

Production: Cotton Tree gum is made up of the irregularly formed, leathery clumps of the exudate from the bark of Cochlospermum gossypium.

Other Names: Cotton Shell

ACTIONS AND PHARMACOLOGY

COMPOUNDS

Water-soluble polysaccharides: partially-acetylated, acidic heteroglycans

EFFECTS

The drug (acetylized acid polysaccharide) is laxative in effect.

INDICATIONS AND USAGE

Unproven Uses: The drug is used in folk medicine for constipation and sluggishness of the bowels.

Indian Medicine: Uses include coughs, diarrhea, dysentery, pharyngitis and venereal disease.

PRECAUTIONS AND ADVERSE REACTIONS

No health hazards are known in conjunction with the proper administration of designated therapeutic dosages, nor with the drug's use as a pharmaceutical vehicle.

DOSAGE

Preparation: There is no information in the literature.

Daily Dose: A single dose of 3 g drug with plenty of liquid

LITERATURE

Blaschek W, Hänsel R, Keller K, Reichling J, Rimpler G, Schneider G (Eds), Hagers Handbuch der Pharmazeutischen Praxis. Folgeb nde 1 und 2. Drogen A-Z. Springer. Berlin, Heidelberg 1998.

Cowhage

Mucuna pruriens

DESCRIPTION

Medicinal Parts: The medicinal parts of the plant are the hairs on the pod and the seeds.

Flower and Fruit: The flowers grow in racemes in twos and threes. They are large and white, with a bluish-purple papilionaceous corolla. The pod is pubescent, thick and leathery and averages about 10 cm in length. Pods have the shape of the sound opening in a violin. They are dark brown, covered with 0.25 cm long stiff hairs and contain 4 to 6 seeds. The seeds are made up of conical, sharply acuminate cells less than 1 mm in diameter and barbed at the apex. They are extremely irritating to the skin and must be handled with caution.

Leaves, Stem and Root: The plant is a climbing legume with long, thin branches and opposite, lanceolate leaves 15 to 30 cm in length. The petioles are pubescent.

Habitat: The plant is indigenous to tropical regions, especially India and the West Indies.

Production: Cowhage bean pods are the bean pods of Mucuna pruriens. The drug is derived from the hair of the pods.

Other Names: Cowitch, Couhage, Kiwach

ACTIONS AND PHARMACOLOGY

COMPOUNDS

Serotonin: 5-methyl-N,N-dimethyl-tryptamine

EFFECTS

Externally, Cowhage is a cutaneous stimulant and rubefacient. Internally, the drug has an anthelmintic effect. Carminative, hypotensive, hypoglycemic and cholesterol-reducing effects have also been described.

Experiments carried out on frogs demonstrated that prurieninin slowed down the heart rate, lowered blood pressure and stimulated intestinal peristalisis. The reduction in blood pressure was caused by the release of histamines; the spasmolysis of smooth muscle by indole bases.

INDICATIONS AND USAGE

Unproven Uses: The drug is used externally for rheumatic disorders and muscular pain, and internally for the treatment of worm infestation.

Indian Medicine: Uses in Indian medicine include gonorrhea, sterility and general debility.

PRECAUTIONS AND ADVERSE REACTIONS

Once in contact with the skin, the stinging hairs lead to extremely aggressive itching and burning, accompanied by long-lasting inflammation, caused by the injection-like introduction of serotonin and proteins (mucunain, proteolytic enzyme). The intake of the hairs for the purpose of fighting intestinal worms should be avoided. Internal administration of the drug in the form of extracts may be harmless due to the difficulty involved in resorbing the active ingredients.

DOSAGE

Mode of Administration: The drug is used internally in extract form and powder form.

LITERATURE

Bell EA, Jansen DH, (1971) Nature 229:136.

Ghosal S et al., (1971) Planta Med 24:434.

Hegnauer R, Chemotaxonomie der Pflanzen, Bde 1-11, Birkhäuser Verlag Basel, Boston, Berlin 1962-1997.

Infante ME, Perez AM, Simao MR, Manda F, Baquete EF, Fernandes AM, Cliff JL, Outbreak of acute toxic psychosis attributed to Mucuna pruriens. Lancet, 29:1129. Nov 3, 1990.

Kern W, List PH, Hörhammer L (Hrsg.), Hagers Handbuch der Pharmazeutischen Praxis, 4. Aufl., Bde. 1-8, Springer Verlag Berlin, Heidelberg, New York, 1969.

Madaus G, Lehrbuch der Biologischen Arzneimittel, Bde 1-3, Nachdruck, Georg Olms Verlag Hildesheim 1979.

Manyam BV, Paralysis agitans and levodopa in 'Ayurveda : ancient Indian medical treatise. Mov Disord, 29:47-8. 1990.

Morton JF, An Atlas of Medicinal Plants of Middle America, Charles C Thomas USA 1981.

Revilleza MJ, Mendoza EM, Raymundo LC, Oligosaccharides in several Philippine indigenous food legumes: determination localization and removal. Plant Foods Hum Nutr, 29:83-93. Jan, 1990.

Roth L, Daunderer M, Kormann K, Giftpflanzen, Pflanzengifte, 4. Aufl., Ecomed Fachverlag Landsberg Lech 1993.

Steinegger E, Hänsel R, Pharmakognosie, 5. Aufl., Springer Verlag Heidelberg 1992.

Teuscher E, Lindequist U, Biogene Gifte - Biologie, Chemie, Pharmakologie, 2. Aufl., Fischer Verlag Stuttgart 1994.

Teuscher E, Biogene Arzneimittel, 5. Aufl., Wiss. Verlagsges. Stuttgart 1997.

Woerdenbag HJ, Pras N, Frijlink HW, Lerk CF, Malingre TM, Antidiabetic evaluation of Mucuna pruriens Linn seeds. JPMA J Pak Med Assoc, 29:147-50. Jul, 1990.

Cowslip

Primula veris

DESCRIPTION

Medicinal Parts: The medicinal parts are the roots and flowers.

Flower and Fruit: The flowers are in richly blossomed umbels with a short peduncle. The flowers are turned to one side and grow in clusters (up to 25) from the center of the leaf rosette. The calyx is cylindrical and appressed with a green margin. The remaining part of the calyx is yellow and it is 12 to 15 cm long. The corolla is odorless, usually sulfur yellow and has a tube with 5 triangular, orange spots. The fruit is an oval capsule with 1.5 to 2.5 mm-long brown, warty seeds.

Leaves, Stem and Root: This 10 cm high plant is a herbaceous perennial with a short sturdy rhizome. The green plant parts are covered in 2 mm long segmented hairs. The leaves are revolute in the bud. They are wrinkled, ovate or ovate-oblong and are rounded at the base. They narrow quickly to the winged stems. During the flowering season they are irregularly dentate with blunt teeth. They are 3 to 6 cm long during the flowering season, but grow larger later. The upper side of the leaf is glabrous.

Habitat: The plant is indigenous to all of Central Europe as far as the Southern European mountains. There are many subspecies.

Production: Cowslip flower consists of the dried, whole flowers with calyx of Primula veris and/or Primula elatior as well as their preparations. Cowslip root consists of the dried rhizome with roots of Primula veris and/or Primula elatior as well as their preparations. Cowslip root is harvested at best in the third year of growth.

Other Names: Oxlip, True Cowslip, Peagles, English Cowslip, Butter Rose, Herb Peter Paigle, Key Flower, Key of Heaven, Fairy Caps, Petty Mulleins, Buckles, Crewel, Palsywort, Plumrocks, Mayflower, Password, Primrose, Arthritica, Our Lady's Keys

ACTIONS AND PHARMACOLOGY

COMPOUNDS: COWSLIP FLOWER

Flavonoids (3%): including rutin, kaempferol-3-O-rutinoside, isorhamnetin-3-O-glucoside; isorhamnetin rhamnosyl robinoside, isorhamnetin robinoside, isorhamnetin rutinoside, kaempferol robinoside, limocitrin-3-O-glucoside, quercetin gentiobioside, quercetin-3-O-glucoside, quercetin robinoside

Primine

Triterpene saponins

EFFECTS: COWSLIP FLOWER

The drug has an expectorant effect, which is due to the flavonoid and saponin content. An increase of the volume of bronchial secretion has been demonstrated in animal experiments.

COMPOUNDS: COWSLIP ROOT

Phenol glycosides (0.2 to 2.3%, high values in the Spring): primulaverin (3%, 2-hydroxy-5-methoxy- benzoic acid methyl ester-O-xyloglucoside) changing over during dehydration into the characteristic-smelling 5-methoxy-methyl salicylate

Triterpene saponins (5 to 10%): chief components primulic acid A (chief aglycone protoprimulagenin)

EFFECTS: COWSLIP ROOT

The saponin content gives the drug expectorant and diuretic effects. Recent studies on these effects are not available. The mode of action is postulated to be due to vagal stimulation.

INDICATIONS AND USAGE

COWSLIP FLOWER

Approved by Commission E:

■ Cough/Bronchitis

Unproven Uses: Cowslip flower is used internally for catarrh of the respiratory tract. In folk medicine it is used for insomnia, anxiety states, as a cardiac tonic for feelings of dizziness and cardiac insufficiency. It is also used as a nerve tonic for shaking limbs, headaches and neuralgia.

Homeopathic Uses: Primula veris is used to treat headaches and skin rashes

COWSLIP ROOT

Approved by Commission E:

■ Cough/Bronchitis

Unproven Uses: Cowslip root is used internally for catarrh of the respiratory tract. In folk medicine it is used internally for whooping cough, asthma, gout, rheumatic arthritis, bladder and kidney disease, migraine, dizziness, stomach cramps, scurvy and neuralgia. Externally it is used for headaches and skin impurities.

CONTRAINDICATIONS

COWSLIP FLOWER

Contraindicated in known allergies to Cowslip.

PRECAUTIONS AND ADVERSE REACTIONS

COWSLIP FLOWER

No health hazards or side effects are known in conjunction with the proper administration of designated therapeutic dosages. The epigeal organs of the Primula species possess a very high potential for sensitization due to the primine content. In the cases of Primula veris and P. elatior, the primine content is quite low, but sensitizations are nevertheless possible.

COWSLIP ROOT

No health hazards or side effects are known in conjunction with the proper administration of designated therapeutic dosages.

OVERDOSAGE

COWSLIP FLOWER

Overdose could lead to gastric complaints and nausea.

COWSLIP ROOT

Overdose could lead to queasiness, nausea, gastric complaints and diarrhea.

DOSAGE

COWSLIP FLOWER

Mode of Administration: Cowslip preparations are available as solid and liquid pharmaceutical forms for oral intake and also available parenterally for homeopathic use.

Preparations: Tea: boiling water is poured over 2 to 4 gm drug and strained after 10 minutes (1 teaspoon corresponds to approximately 1.3 gm drug).

Liquid extract — drug 1:1 with 25% ethanol (V/V) (BHP83)

Daily Dosage: The average daily dose is 3 gm of drug. The single dose is 1 gm of drug.

Tea — 1 cup several times a day. As a bronchial tea, several cups a day, possibly sweetened with honey

Liquid extract — 1 to 2 ml 3 times a day

Homeopathic Dosage: 5 drops, 1 tablet or 10 globules every 30 to 60 minutes (acute) or 1 to 3 times daily (chronic); parenterally: 1 to 2 ml sc acute: 3 times daily; chronic: once a day (HAB34); different doses for children.

Storage: Should be protected from light and moisture.

COWSLIP ROOT

Preparations: Tea: 0.2 to 0.5 gm finely cut drug are added to cold water and brought to the boil, left to draw for 5 minutes and strained (1 teaspoon corresponds to approximately 3.5 gm drug).

Extract: Percolation with 50 parts water and 50 parts ethanol, then filtration and vacuum drying. The residue is dissolved in 60 parts ethanol and 40 parts water and neutralized with ammonia. It is then cooled for 24 hours and filtered again. It is finally dehydrated to produce a dry extract under low pressure. (ÖAB90)

Liquid extract: the Primula extract is dissolved in a mixture of ethanol (30 parts), glycerol 85% (20 parts) and water (20 parts) and filtered when cool. (ÖAB90)

Tincture: 20 parts root and 100 parts diluted ethanol are processed to a tincture in accordance with the ÖAB VII maceration procedure.

Syrup: 1.5 parts Cowslip are dissolved in 20 parts water while being heated. It is then mixed with 10 parts 85% glycerol and 68.5 parts simple syrup. (ÖAB90)

Daily Dosage: The average daily dose is 1 gm of drug. The single dose is 0.5 gm of drug.

Tincture: The daily dose is 7.5 gm.

Extract: The single dose is 0.1 to 0.2 gm.

Liquid extract: The single dose is 0.5 gm.

Tea: as an expectorant, 1 cup every 2 to 3 hours, sweetened with honey

Storage: Cowslip should be protected from light.

LITERATURE

COWSLIP FLOWER

Büechi S, Antivirale Saponine, pharmakologische und klinische Untersuchungen. In: DAZ 136(2):89-98. 1996.

Busse WW et al., (1984) J All Clin Immunol. 73:801.

Çalis I, Yürüker A, Rüegger H, Wright AD, Sticher O, Triterpene saponins from Primula veris ssp. macrocalyx and Primula elatiro ssp. meyeri. In: JNP 55:1299-1306. 1992.

Grecu VL, Cucu V, (1975) Planta Med 25:247.

Karl C et al., (1981) Planta Med 41:96.

Middleton E, Drzewiecki G, (1984) Biochem. Pharmacol. 33:3333.

Thieme H, Winkler HJ, (1971) Pharmazie 7:434.

Further information in:

Hänsel R, Keller K, Rimpler H, Schneider G (Hrsg.), Hagers Handbuch der Pharmazeutischen Praxis, 5. Aufl., Bde 4-6 (Drogen), Springer Verlag Berlin, Heidelberg, New York, 1992-1994.

Madaus G, Lehrbuch der Biologischen Arzneimittel, Bde 1-3, Nachdruck, Georg Olms Verlag Hildesheim 1979.

Steinegger E, Hänsel R, Pharmakognosie, 5. Aufl., Springer Verlag Heidelberg 1992.

Teuscher E, Lindequist U, Biogene Gifte - Biologie, Chemie, Pharmakologie, 2. Aufl., Fischer Verlag Stuttgart 1994.

Teuscher E, Biogene Arzneimittel, 5. Aufl., Wiss. Verlagsges. Stuttgart 1997.

Wichtl M (Hrsg.), Teedrogen, 4. Aufl., Wiss. Verlagsges. Stuttgart 1997.

COWSLIP ROOT

Büechi S, Antivirale Saponine, pharmakologische und klinische Untersuchungen. In: DAZ 136(2):89-98. 1996.

Busse WW et al., (1984) J All Clin Immunol. 73:801.

Çalis I, Yürüker A, Rüegger H, Wright AD, Sticher O, Triterpene saponins from Primula veris ssp. macrocalyx and Primula elatiro ssp. meyeri. In: JNP 55:1299-1306. 1992.

Grecu VL, Cucu V, (1975) Planta Med 25:247.

Karl C et al., (1981) Planta Med 41:96.

Middleton E, Drzewiecki G, (1984) Biochem. Pharmacol. 33:3333.

Thieme H, Winkler HJ, (1971) Pharmazie 7:434.

Wagner H et al., Radix-Primulae-Extrakte. HPLC-Analyse. In: DAZ 126:1489-1493. 1986.

Further information in:

Hänsel R, Keller K, Rimpler H, Schneider G (Hrsg.), Hagers Handbuch der Pharmazeutischen Praxis, 5. Aufl., Bde 4-6 (Drogen), Springer Verlag Berlin, Heidelberg, New York, 1992-1994.

Madaus G, Lehrbuch der Biologischen Arzneimittel, Bde 1-3, Nachdruck, Georg Olms Verlag Hildesheim 1979.

Steinegger E, Hänsel R, Pharmakognosie, 5. Aufl., Springer Verlag Heidelberg 1992.

Teuscher E, Biogene Arzneimittel, 5. Aufl., Wiss. Verlagsges. Stuttgart 1997.

Wichtl M (Hrsg.), Teedrogen, 4. Aufl., Wiss. Verlagsges. Stuttgart 1997.

Cranesbill

Geranium maculatum

DESCRIPTION

Medicinal Parts: The medicinal parts are the plant's dried rhizome and the leaves.

Flower and Fruit: The inflorescence is a terminal, cymose umbel. The flowers are radial with the structures arranged in fives with a 2.5 to 4 cm diameter. There are 5 free, pubescent sepals, 5 free purple petals and 10 stamens. The ovary is formed from 5 carpels, which are fused to the sides of the central column with their long awns. The fruit is a schizocarp, which breaks up into 5 mericarps with beak-like extensions and 1 seed each.

Leaves, Stem and Root: The herbaceous perennial grows upright, rising to 60 cm high. The leaves are opposite, in fives with cuneiform lobes and whitish-green spots when older. Leaves growing from the rhizome are large with long, pubescent petioles; those growing from the trunk have short petioles; stipules are present. The stem is upright, green, pubescent and dichotomously branched. The rhizome is thick, cylindrical and branched.

Habitat: The plant is found throughout Europe, but also in North America from Newfoundland to Manitoba and as far south as Georgia and Missouri. It grows in shady and moist ground in mixed and deciduous forests.

Production: American Cranesbill herb is the dried aerial herb of Geranium maculatum harvested during the flowering season. American Cranesbill root is the dried rhizome of Geranium maculatum, which is collected in late summer and autumn.

Other Names: Alumroot, Crowfoot, Geranium, Spotted Cranesbill, Spotted Geranium, Storksbill, Wild Cranesbill

ACTIONS AND PHARMACOLOGY

COMPOUNDS: CRANESBILL HERB

Tannins (30%): gallotannins

COMPOUNDS: CRANESBILL ROOT

Tannins (10 to 28%): gallotannins

EFFECTS

The tannins give the drug astringent, hemostyptic and tonic properties.

INDICATIONS AND USAGE

Unproven Uses: Folk medicine indications have included hemorrhoids, duodenal ulcers, diarrhea, metrorrhagia, heavy menstruation and dysmenorrhea. Efficacy for these internal use indications has not yet been proven.

Homeopathic Uses: The drug is used for stomach ulcers and bleeding of the mucous membranes, but efficacy for these indications has not yet been proven.

PRECAUTIONS AND ADVERSE REACTIONS

No health hazards are known in conjunction with the proper administration of designated therapeutic dosages. Because of its high tannin content, the intake of preparations of the drug could lead to digestive disorders. Individuals with sensitive stomachs could experience nausea and vomiting.

DOSAGE

CRANESBILL HERB

Daily Dosage: Powder/Infusion: 1 to 2 g, 3 times daily.

Homeopathic Dosage: Literature notes the drug's importance as a homeopathic medicine, but does not state dosage.

CRANESBILL ROOT

Preparation: Liquid extract - drug 1:1 45% ethanol (V/V) percolated (BHP83).

Daily Dosage:

Decoction — 1 to 2 g drug, 3 times daily

Liquid extract — 1 to 2 ml, 3 times daily

Tincture — 2 to 4 ml, 3 times daily.

Homeopathic Dosage: 5 to 10 drops, 1 tablet or 5 to 10 globules, 1 to 3 times daily, or 1 ml injection solution sc twice weekly (HAB34).

LITERATURE

Hänsel R, Keller K, Rimpler H, Schneider G (Ed.), Hagers Handbuch der harmazeutischen Praxis, 5. Aufl., Bde 4 - 6 (Drogen), Springer Verlag Berlin, Heidelberg, New York, 1992-1994.

Crataegus laevigata

See English Hawthorn

Crithmum maritimum

See Samphire

Crocus sativus

See Saffron

Croton eluteria

See Cascarilla

Croton Seeds

Croton tiglium

DESCRIPTION

Medicinal Parts: The seeds are the medicinal parts. The oil is extracted from the seeds and is toxic; 1 ml can be fatal.

Flower and Fruit: Croton tiglium is a shrub or tree that grows up to 6 m. The leaves are alternate, smooth, ovate or acuminate. They are dark green above and paler beneath, with an unpleasant smell. There are inconspicuous flowers in terminal racemes. The seeds have a brown, mottled appearance. The outer layer of the seed is easily removed, leaving a hard, black coat.

Characteristics: Croton Seed oil is yellowish or reddish-brown and rather viscid, with an unpleasant odor. It is toxic and should be handled with extreme care.

Habitat: The tree is found throughout Asia and China.

Production: Croton oil is extracted from the seeds of Croton tiglium.

Other Names: Tiglium, Tiglium Seeds

ACTIONS AND PHARMACOLOGY

COMPOUNDS

Diterpenes: phorbol ester, including 12-O-tridecane olyphorbol-13-acetate (TPA, myristoylphoarbolacetate, MPA)

Fatty oil

EFFECTS

Croton Seed oil is a laxative, skin-irritant, co-carcinogenic, nephrotoxic. It is a drastic irritant. TPA is a carcinogen, affecting prostaglandin metabolism.

INDICATIONS AND USAGE

Unproven Uses: At present, it is used only in Chinese medicine and in very small doses as a remedy for gall bladder colic, obstruction of the bowels and malaria. The drug is obsolete in Europe.

Chinese Medicine: In China, Croton Seed oil is used for edema, furuncles, constipation, chest and stomach pain, worm infestation and sore throat.

Indian Medicine: Indian uses include constipation, abdominal disorders, worm infestation, convulsions and attacks of dizziness.

PRECAUTIONS AND ADVERSE REACTIONS

The phorbol esters of the oils are severe co-carcinogenics. Therapeutic uses as well as skin or mucous membrane contacts with the drug are to be strictly avoided. The drug possesses acute toxicity. When applied to the skin, it brings about itching, burning and after a time, blisters. If taken internally, it leads to burning in the mouth, vomiting, dizziness, stupor, painful bowel movements and ultimately to collapse.

OVERDOSAGE

One to 2 drops are already acutely toxic; the lethal dosage is put at 20 drops. After stomach and intestinal emptying, treatment of poisonings can only proceed symptomatically.

DOSAGE

Mode of Administration: Croton Seed oil is obsolete as drug.

LITERATURE

Berenblum I, Shubik P, (1947) Brit J Cancer 1:379.

Evans FJ (Ed.), Naturally Occurring Phorbol Esters, CRC Press 1986.

Evans FJ, Taylor SE, (1983) Prog Chem Org Nat Prod 44:1.

Hecker E, (1968) Cancer Res 28:2338.

McEchean CE et al., J Chem Soc 166B:633. 1966.

Nishizuka Y, (1984) Nature 308:693.

Further information in:

Chan, EH et al., (Eds): Advances in Chinese Medicinal Materials Research, World Scientific Pub. Co. Singapore 1985.

Kern W, List PH, Hörhammer L (Hrsg.), Hagers Handbuch der Pharmazeutischen Praxis, 4. Aufl., Bde 1-8, Springer Verlag Berlin, Heidelberg, New York, 1969.

Lewin L, Gifte und Vergiftungen, 6. Aufl., Nachdruck, Haug Verlag, Heidelberg 1992.

Madaus G, Lehrbuch der Biologischen Arzneimittel, Bde 1-3, Nachdruck, Georg Olms Verlag Hildesheim 1979.

Roth L, Daunderer M, Kormann K, Giftpflanzen, Pflanzengifte, 4. Aufl., Ecomed Fachverlag Landsberg Lech 1993.

Steinegger E, Hänsel R, Pharmakognosie, 5. Aufl., Springer Verlag Heidelberg 1992.

Teuscher E, Lindequist U, Biogene Gifte - Biologie, Chemie, Pharmakologie, 2. Aufl., Fischer Verlag Stuttgart 1994.

Wagner H, Wiesenauer M, Phytotherapie. Phytopharmaka und pflanzliche Homöopathika, Fischer-Verlag, Stuttgart, Jena, New York 1995.

Croton tiglium

See Croton Seeds

Cubeb

Piper cubeba

DESCRIPTION

Medicinal Parts: The medicinal parts are the dried, not fully ripe fruit.

Flower and Fruit: The male flowering spikes are about 4 cm long and have 2 or 3 stamens. The female spikes are made up of about 50 individual flowers, which mostly consist of the oblong ovary of 4 fused carpels with 4 sessile stigmas. The infructescence is 4 to 5 cm long. When ripe, the base of the ovary grows into a stem-like, cylindrical lower part. The upper portion of the fruit is globular and holds the seed, which contains a tiny embryo in a small cavity at the apex.

Leaves, Stem and Root: The plant is a 5 to 15 m high dioecious climbing shrub. The branches are initially pubescent, later glabrous. The leaves are glabrous, entire-margined, coriaceous, ovate to oblong-elliptical and up to 15 cm long and 6 cm wide.

Characteristics: The odor is warm and reminiscent of turpentine.

Habitat: The plant is indigenous to Indonesia and is cultivated in Sri Lanka, India and Malaysia.

Production: Cubebs are the fruit of Piper cubeba. The fruit is harvested when still green and dried in the sun.

Other Names: Java Pepper, Tailed Cubebs, Tailed Pepper

ACTIONS AND PHARMACOLOGY

COMPOUNDS

Volatile oil (10 to 20%): chief constituents alpha- and beta-cubebenes (11%), copaene (10%), cubebol (10%), delta-cadinene (9%), humulenes

Lignans: chief components (-)-cubebin, additionally (-)-cubebinin, dihydroclusin, (-)-dihydrocubebin, hinokinin

Resins

Fatty oil (12%)

EFFECTS

The sesquiterpene-rich essential oil is said to be expectorant in chronic bronchitis. The resinous acids in the drug are said to have an antiseptic and astringent effect on the urinary tract. There is no information on the mode of action.

INDICATIONS AND USAGE

Unproven Uses: Folk medicine uses include treatment for urinary tract diseases, flatulence and stomach complaints, headaches (dizziness), chronic bronchitis, to increase libido and for poor memory.

Homeopathic Uses: Piper cubeba is used for inflammation of the mucous membrane of the urogenital tract.

PRECAUTIONS AND ADVERSE REACTIONS

Health risks or side effects following the proper administration of designated therapeutic dosages are not recorded.

OVERDOSAGE

High dosages (over 8 gm) cause irritation of the urinary passages, kidney and bladder pains, albuminuria and urination problems. Beyond this, vomiting, diarrhea, cardiac pain and skin rashes can occur. After stomach and intestinal emptying, treatment of poisonings should proceed symptomatically.

DOSAGE

Mode of Administration: Cubeb is contained in medicinal preparations, such as bath additives.

Daily Dosage:

Powder — 2 to 4 g daily for internal administration

Extract (1:1) — daily dose: 2 to 4 ml

Tincture (1:5) — daily dose: 2 to 4 ml

Homeopathic Dosage: 5 to 10 drops, 1 tablet or 5 to 10 globules 1 to 3 times a day or 1 ml injection solution sc twice weekly (HAB1); children's dosage does not equal adult dose.

LITERATURE

Batterbee, J E et al., (1969) J Chem Soc (c), 2470.

Ikeda RM, (1962) J Food Sci 27:455.

Koul SK et al., Phenylpropanoids and (-)-ledol from Piper species. In: PH 32:478. 1993.

Lawrence BM, Perfum Flavor 5:28. 1980.

Ohta Y et al., (1966) Tetrahedron Letters 52:6365.

Opdyke DLJ, (1976) Food Cosmet Toxicol 14.

Prabhu BR, Mulchandani, NB, (1985) Phytochemistry 24 (2), 329.

Further information in:

Hänsel R, Keller K, Rimpler H, Schneider G (Hrsg.), Hagers Handbuch der Pharmazeutischen Praxis, 5. Aufl., Bde 4-6 (Drogen), Springer Verlag Berlin, Heidelberg, New York, 1992-1994.

Leung AY, Encyclopedia of Common Natural Ingredients Used in Food Drugs and Cosmetics, John Wiley & Sons Inc., New York 1980.

Lewin L, Gifte und Vergiftungen, 6. Aufl., Nachdruck, Haug Verlag, Heidelberg 1992.

Madaus G, Lehrbuch der Biologischen Arzneimittel, Bde 1-3, Nachdruck, Georg Olms Verlag Hildesheim 1979.

Roth L, Daunderer M, Kormann K, Giftpflanzen, Pflanzengifte, 4. Aufl., Ecomed Fachverlag Landsberg Lech 1993.

Cucurbita pepo

See Pumpkin

Cudweed

Gnaphalium uliginosum

DESCRIPTION

Medicinal Parts: The aerial parts are the medicinal parts of the plant.

Flower and Fruit: The composite flower heads are 3 to 4 mm by 5 mm, sessile and in terminal racemes of 3 to 10. They are shorter than the leaves growing from the leaf axil. The involucral bracts are oblong to linear and brownish. There are 50 to 150 female florets, 5 to 8 hermaphrodite florets. The achaene is 0.5 mm oblong-cylindrical. The pappus is 1.5 mm.

Leaves, Stem and Root: The stems are 5 to 20 cm high and branched. The leaves are 10 to 50 mm by 2 to 5 mm, linear-lanceolate to oblong-obovate. They are downy and greenish above; whitish and even more downy beneath.

Habitat: The plant is native to many parts of Europe, the Caucasus and west Asia. It has been introduced into America.

Production: Cudweed is the aerial part of Gnaphalium uliginosum.

Other Names: Cotton Weed, Dysentery Weed, Everlasting, Mouse Ear, Wartwort, Cotton Dawes

ACTIONS AND PHARMACOLOGY

COMPOUNDS

Volatile oil

Tannins

The constituents of the drug have not been extensively investigated.

EFFECTS

Cudweed is an astringent and a stomachic. According to unconfirmed sources, the drug also has antidepressive, aphrodisiac and hypotensive effects.

INDICATIONS AND USAGE

Unproven Uses: The drug is used as a gargle and rinse in the treatment of diseases of the mouth and throat.

PRECAUTIONS AND ADVERSE REACTIONS

Health risks or side effects following the proper administration of designated therapeutic dosages are not recorded.

DOSAGE

Mode of Administration: Liquid extract used as a gargle and rinse.

LITERATURE

Kern W, List PH, Hörhammer L (Hrsg.), Hagers Handbuch der Pharmazeutischen Praxis, 4. Aufl., Bde. 1-8, Springer Verlag Berlin, Heidelberg, New York, 1969.

Cumin

Cuminum cyminum

DESCRIPTION

Medicinal Parts: The medicinal parts are the Cumin oil extracted from the ripe fruit and the ripe, dried fruit.

Flower and Fruit: The flowers are in umbels radiating in groups of 3 to 5. The petals are white or red, oblong and deeply bordered with a long indented tip. The involucral bracts are long and simple. The style is short and turned outward at the end. The ovary is inferior and 3-locular. The fruit is a schizocarp, about 6 mm long and 1.5 mm wide and crowned with awl-shaped calyx tips. The mericarp is almost round in transverse section, with 5 thread-like, bristly main ribs and bristly secondary ribs.

Leaves, Stem and Root: The plant is a delicate, glabrous annual 10 to 50 cm high. The stem is bifurcated at the base and glabrous. The leaves are glabrous and finely pinnatifid with oblong-linear tips, of which the lower are mostly doubly trifoliate.

Habitat: The plant is indigenous to Turkestan (Hager) or northern Egypt (Grieve), but is cultivated today in the whole of the Mediterranean region as well as in Iran, Pakistan, India, China, the U.S. and South America.

Production: Cumin is the dried ripe fruit of Cuminum cyminum.

Not to be Confused With: Certain Indian products, such as Carum carvi and the fruit of the earth chestnut, Bunium bulbocastanium can be mistaken for or confused with Cumin. Synthetic coloring is frequently added to Turkish products.

ACTIONS AND PHARMACOLOGY

COMPOUNDS

Volatile oil (2 to 5%): chief components cuminaldehyde, gamma-terpenes, beta-pinenes, p-cymene, 1,3-p-menthandial

Fatty oil (10 to 15%): chief fatty acids petroselic acid, palmitic acid

Proteic substances (15 to 20%)

EFFECTS

Antimicrobial: The drug contains fatty oil (mainly petroselic acid and oil acid) and has an antimicrobial effect. A powder suspension of the drug has diverse inhibitory effects; it stunts mycelium growth, toxin production or afla-toxin production in *Aspergillus ochraceus*, *C. versicolor*, and *C. flavus*.

Influence on blood-clotting: A dried Cumin ether extract inhibits (in vitro) arachidon acid-induced plate aggregation in platelet-rich human plasma.

Mutagenic effect: In comparison to *Salmonella thyphimurum* TA 100, a mutagenic effect of the polar fractions of chloroform extract and methanol extract of Cumin did appear.

Influence of pharmacological metabolism: An injection of a dried ether extract prolonged the phenobarbituate hypnosis of female albino mice, up to 120%; a higher dose shortened it to 83%.

Estrogenic effect: An acetone extract of cumin, administered to female albino rats (ovariectomised, ovaries have been removed) led, depending on the dosage, to an increase in the weight of the uterus, an increase in the amount of protein in the endometrium and an increase of alkali phosphates.

Other effects (for which there are no experimental results) include the following: obstructive influence on fertility, galactogen, antispasmodic, diuretic and aphrodisiac.

Cumin also has carminative, stimulant and analgesic effects.

INDICATIONS AND USAGE

Unproven Uses: In folk medicine, Cumin is used as a carminative for stomach disorders, diarrhea and colic, particularly in veterinary medicine.

In America, Africa and India the drug is used as an abortive and as an emmenagogue.

In Indonesia, Cumin is used in cases of bloody diarrhea and headache (paste is applied to the forehead). It is also taken orally for rheumatic ailments.

Indian Medicine: In India, Cumin is used as an abortifacient, for kidney and bladder stones, chronic diarrhea, leprosy and eye disease.

PRECAUTIONS AND ADVERSE REACTIONS

Health risks or side effects following the proper administration of designated therapeutic dosages are not recorded.

DOSAGE

Mode of Administration: Cumin is used both internally and externally in ground form and as a pressed oil.

Daily Dosage: The average single dose is 300 to 600 mg of drug (equivalent to 5 - 10 fruits).

LITERATURE

Hänsel R, Keller K, Rimpler H, Schneider G (Hrsg.), Hagers Handbuch der Pharmazeutischen Praxis, 5. Aufl., Bde 4-6 (Drogen): Springer Verlag Berlin, Heidelberg, New York, 1992-1994.

Harborne JB, Williams CE, (1972) Phytochemistry 11:1741.

Leung AY, Encyclopedia of Common Natural Ingredients Used in Food Drugs and Cosmetics, John Wiley & Sons Inc., New York 1980.

Tassan CG, Russel GF, J Food Sci 40:1185-1188. 1975.

Varo PT, Heinz DE, (1970) J Agric Food Chem 18:234 et 239.

Cuminum cyminum

See Cumin

Cup Plant

Silphium perfoliatum

DESCRIPTION

Medicinal Parts: The medicinal part is the root.

Flower and Fruit: The flowers are 5 to 8 cm wide, long-pedicled and clustered. The sepals are overlapping, and the petals are egg-yolk yellow. The disc-like flowers are androgynous with long thread-like styles. The lateral flowers are female and lingual. The double-winged fruit is compressed and has a pappus of lateral awns.

Leaves, Stem and Root: The perennial plant is a 1.25 to 2.5 m high plant with a branched rhizome. The erect, angular, smooth stem is branched higher up and foliated up to the tip. The leaves are opposite, rough, ovate, acuminate, crenate, dark green above and blue-green beneath. The lower leaves are up to 30 cm long, and the upper ones are oblong-ovate, sessile and fused at the base to a cup form.

Habitat: The plant is indigenous to the western U.S., Oregon and Texas.

Other Names: Ragged Cup, Indian Gum, Prairie Dock, Pilot Plant, Polar Plant, Rosinweed, Turpentine Weed

ACTIONS AND PHARMACOLOGY

COMPOUNDS

Triterpene saponins

Sesquiterpenes: including among others silphinene, silphiperfolen, 8-hydroxy-presilphiperfolane

EFFECTS

The drug is a tonic and has a diaphoretic effect.

INDICATIONS AND USAGE

Unproven Uses: Cup Plant has been used for digestive disorders.

PRECAUTIONS AND ADVERSE REACTIONS

No health hazards or side effects are known in conjunction with the proper administration of designated therapeutic dosages.

DOSAGE

Mode of Administration: Cup Root is not used in modern medicine.

LITERATURE

Davidyants ES et al., (1984) Khim Prir Soedin. 5:666.

Hegnauer R, Chemotaxonomie der Pflanzen, Bde 1-11: Birkhäuser Verlag Basel, Boston, Berlin 1962-1997.

Cupmoss

Cladonia pyxidata

DESCRIPTION

Medicinal Parts: The wineglass-shaped scyphi of Cladonia pyxidata are used medicinally.

Flower and Fruit: Cupmoss is a lichen, not a moss as the name suggests. The scyphi are grayish-white, about 2.5 cm long, wineglass-shaped, with hollow stems and terminal cups.

Characteristics: The taste is mucilaginous and slightly sweet. There is no odor.

Habitat: The plant is indigenous to North America and is also common in other areas including Great Britain.

Other Names: Chin Cups

ACTIONS AND PHARMACOLOGY

COMPOUNDS

Lichen acids: including fumaroprotocetraric acid, barbatic acid, psoromic acid

Mucilages

EFFECTS

Cupmoss has the effect of an expectorant and antitussive.

INDICATIONS AND USAGE

Unproven Uses: Cupmoss is used for coughs, bronchitis, and also in the treatment of whooping cough.

PRECAUTIONS AND ADVERSE REACTIONS

Health risks or side effects following the proper administration of designated therapeutic dosages are not recorded.

DOSAGE

Mode of Administration: Cupmoss is used internally as an infusion with honey.

LITERATURE

Hoppe HA, (1975-1987): Drogenkunde, 8. Aufl., Bde 1-3, W. de Gruyter Verlag, Berlin, New York.

Kern W, List PH, Hörhammer L (Hrsg.), Hagers Handbuch der Pharmazeutischen Praxis, 4. Aufl., Bde 1-8, Springer Verlag Berlin, Heidelberg, New York, 1969.

Cupressus sempervirens

See Cypress

Curcuma

Curcuma xanthorrhizia

DESCRIPTION

Medicinal Parts: The medicinal parts are the dried, tuberous rhizomes cut into slices.

Flower and Fruit: The inflorescence is large; it is purple or crimson. The corolla has a red margin. Otherwise it is very similar to Curcuma domestica.

Leaves, Stem and Root: The plant is a perennial, 1.75 m high and leafy. The leaves are in long thin sheaths on the rhizome. The leaf blades are broadly lanceolate or oblong and have a narrow, purple mark on the midrib. The main rhizome is thickened like a tuber, ovate, the size of a fist with numerous roots and thin lateral rhizomes. The roots terminate partially in ovate tubers.

Habitat: Curcuma is indigenous to the forests of Indonesia and the Malaysian peninsula. It is cultivated mainly on Java, in Malaysia, Thailand and the Philippines.

Production: Japanese turmeric consists of the sliced, dried, tuberous rhizomes of Curcuma xanthorrhiza. Curcuma is cultivated and harvested in the second year of growth. After the rhizome has been washed, the main thick root is isolated, cut and dried at a temperature of 50°C.

Not to be Confused With: The rhizome of Curcuma domestica.

Other Names: Tewon Lawa, Temu Lawak

ACTIONS AND PHARMACOLOGY

COMPOUNDS

Volatile oil (3 to 12%): chief components ar-curcumene (alpha-curcumene), xanthorrhizol, beta-curcumene, germacrene, furanodien, furanodienone

Curcuminoids (0.8 to 2%): including curcumin, demethoxycurcumin

Non-phenolic diarylheptanoids: alnustone

Starch (30-40%)

EFFECTS

Curcuma acts in a manner similar to turmeric root but is mainly choleretic and antitumoral (animal testing).

INDICATIONS AND USAGE

Approved by Commission E:

- Liver and gallbladder complaints
- Loss of appetite

Unproven Uses: Curcuma is used for dyspepsia, particularly feelings of fullness after meals and meteorism.

In Indonesia it has long been used for liver and gallbladder complaints.

PRECAUTIONS AND ADVERSE REACTIONS

Health risks or side effects following the proper administration of designated therapeutic dosages are not recorded. Stomach complaints can occur following extended use or in the case of overdose. Because of the stimulating effect of the drug on the biliary tract, it should not be administered if there is a bile duct blockage. Colic can occur when the patient suffers from gallstones.

DOSAGE

Mode of Administration: Comminuted drug for infusions and other galenic forms for internal use.

Preparation: The infusion is prepared by pouring 1 cup of boiling water over 1/2 tsp. of drug and straining after 10 minutes.

Daily Dosage: The average daily dose is 2 gm of drug; infusion: 2 to 3 times daily between meals.

Storage: It should be protected from light.

LITERATURE

Anonym, Brennpunkt ZNS. In: DAZ 137(25):2166-2167. 1997.

Baumann J, (1975) Über die Wirkung von Chelidonium, Curcuma, Absinth und Carduus marianus auf die Galle- und Pankreassekretion bei Hepatopathien. MedMschr 29:173.

Claeson P et al., Non-phenolic linear diarylheptanoids from Curcuma xanthorrhiza: a novel type of topical anti-inflammatory agents: Structure-activity relationship. In: PM 62(3):236-240. 1996.

Guttenberg A, (1926) Das Cholagogum Curcumen. Klein Wschr 5:1998-1999.

Maiwald L, Schwantes PA, (1991) Curcuma xanthorrhiza Roxb., eine Heilpflanze tritt aus dem Schattendasein. Z Phytother 12:35-445.

Reuter HD, Pflanzliche Gallentherapeutika (Teil I) und (Teil II). In: ZPT 16(1):13-20 u. 77-89. 1995.

Sabieraj J, Wirkung von Curcuma xanthorrhiza. In: DAZ 131(13):609. 1991.

Schilcher H, Pharmazeutische Aspekte pflanzlicher Gallentherapeutika. In: ZPT 16(4):211-222. 1995.

Schmidt M, Phytotherapie: Pflanzliche Gallenwegstherapeutika. In: DAZ 135(8):680-682. 1995.

Veit M, Beeinflussung der Leukotrien-Biosynthese durch Curcumin. In: ZPT 14(1):46. 1993.

Further information in:

Hänsel R, Keller K, Rimpler H, Schneider G (Hrsg.), Hagers Handbuch der Pharmazeutischen Praxis, 5. Aufl., Bde 4-6 (Drogen), Springer Verlag Berlin, Heidelberg, New York, 1992-1994.

Madaus G, Lehrbuch der Biologischen Arzneimittel, Bde 1-3, Nachdruck, Georg Olms Verlag Hildesheim 1979.

Steinegger E, Hänsel R, Pharmakognosie, 5. Aufl., Springer Verlag Heidelberg 1992.

Tang W, Eisenbrand G, Chinese Drugs of Plant Origin, Springer Verlag Heidelberg 1992.

Teuscher E, Biogene Arzneimittel, 5. Aufl., Wiss. Verlagsges. mbH Stuttgart 1997.

Wichtl M (Hrsg.), Teedrogen, 4. Aufl., Wiss. Verlagsges. Stuttgart 1997.

Curcuma domestica

See Turmeric

Curcuma xanthorrhizia

See Curcuma

Curcuma zedoaria

See Zedoary

Cuscuta epithymum

See Dodder

Cyamopsis tetragonoloba

See Guar Gum

Cyclamen

Cyclamen europaeum

DESCRIPTION

Medicinal Parts: The medicinal part is the dried rhizome with the roots.

Flower and Fruit: The flowers are pinkish-red, solitary and nodding on erect stems. The 5 sepals are ovate, pointed and dentate. The corolla is a short campanulate tube with 5 revolute tips; it is darker at the base. There are 5 stamens and 1 ovary. The fruit is a capsule, which opens on 5 sides.

Leaves, Stem and Root: The plant grows from about 5 to 10 cm. The rhizome is a disc-like tuber. The leaves are long-petioled, orbicular or cordate, crenate, glabrous, with a white edge above and red beneath. The petioles and pedicles are roughly glandular.

Characteristics: The flowers are fragrant and poisonous.

Habitat: The plant is found in the Alps and the alpine regions of southern Europe.

Other Names: Groundbread, Sowbread, Swinebread, Ivy-Leafed Cyclamen

ACTIONS AND PHARMACOLOGY

COMPOUNDS

Triterpene saponins: including cyclamine, deglucocyclamine I, deglucocyclamine II

EFFECTS

No information is available.

INDICATIONS AND USAGE

Unproven Uses: The drug is used to treat menstrual complaints, emotional disorders/nervous states and digestive problems.

Homeopathic Uses: Cyclamen is used for migraine and its accompanying autonomic symptoms, and for the treatment of premenstrual syndrome.

PRECAUTIONS AND ADVERSE REACTIONS

The intake of even small dosages (0.3 gm) can lead to nausea, vomiting, diarrhea and stomach pain.

OVERDOSAGE

High dosages can cause spasm and asphyxiation. Following gastric lavage and the administration of activated charcoal, the treatment for poisoning should proceed symptomatically (e.g., treatment of convulsions with diazepam, treatment of colic with atropine).

DOSAGE

Mode of Administration: Cyclamen is used in homeopathic treatments. It is also used topically and in alcoholic extracts.

LITERATURE

Braccini I, Herve du Penhoat C, Michon V, Goldberg R, Clochard M, Jarvis MC, Huang ZH, Gage DA, Structural analysis of cyclamen seed xyloglucan oligosaccharides using cellulase digestion and spectroscopic methods. Carbohydr Res, 276:167-81, 1995 Oct 16.

Calis I, Satana ME, Ÿçker A, Kelican P, Demirdamar R, Alacam R, Tanker N, Ruegger H, Sticher O, Triterpene saponins from Cyclamen mirabile and their biological activities. J Nat Prod, 60:315-8, 1997 Mar.

Calis I, Ÿçker A, Tanker N, Wright AD, Sticher O, Triterpene saponins from Cyclamen coum var. coum. Planta Med, 276:166-70, 1997 Apr.

Jaspersen-Schib R, Theus L, Guirguis-Oeschger M, Gossweiler B, Meier-Abt PJ, Serious plant poisonings in Switzerland 1966-1994. Case analysis from the Swiss Toxicology Information Center. Schweiz Med Wochenschr, 60:1085-98, 1996 Jun 22.

Tschesche R, Mercker HJ, Wulff G, Liebig Ann Chem 721:194. 1969.

Tschesche R, Striegler H, Fehlhaber HW, Liebig Ann Chem 691:165. 1966.

Further information in:

Frohne D, Pfänder HJ: Giftpflanzen - Ein Handbuch für Apotheker, Toxikologen und Biologen, 4. Aufl., Wiss. Verlagsges. mbH Stuttgart 1997.

Kern W, List PH, Hörhammer L (Hrsg.), Hagers Handbuch der Pharmazeutischen Praxis, 4. Aufl., Bde 1-8, Springer Verlag Berlin, Heidelberg, New York, 1969.

Lewin L, Gifte und Vergiftungen, 6. Aufl., Nachdruck, Haug Verlag, Heidelberg 1992.

Madaus G, Lehrbuch der Biologischen Arzneimittel, Bde 1-3, Nachdruck, Georg Olms Verlag Hildesheim 1979.

Roth L, Daunderer M, Kormann K, Giftpflanzen, Pflanzengifte, 4. Aufl., Ecomed Fachverlag Landsberg Lech 1993.

Steinegger E, Hänsel R, Pharmakognosie, 5. Aufl., Springer Verlag Heidelberg 1992.

Teuscher E, Lindequist U, Biogene Gifte - Biologie, Chemie, Pharmakologie, 2. Aufl., Fischer Verlag Stuttgart 1994.

Wagner H, Wiesenauer M, Phytotherapie. Phytopharmaka und pflanzliche Homöopathika, Fischer-Verlag, Stuttgart, Jena, New York 1995.

Cyclamen europaeum

See Cyclamen

Cydonia oblongata

See Quince

Cymbopogon citratus

See Lemongrass

Cynanchum vincetoxicum

See German Ipecac

Cynara scolymus

See Artichoke

Cynoglossum officinale

See Hound's Tongue

Cyperus articulatus

See Adrue

Cypress

Cupressus sempervirens

DESCRIPTION

Medicinal Parts: The medicinal parts are the cones, branches and oil.

Leaves, Stem and Root: Cupressus sempervirens is a tree that grows up to 30 m tall. The leaves are 0.5 to 1 mm, dark green and obtuse. The male cones are 4 to 8 mm, the female are 25 to 40 mm. They are elliptical-oblong (rarely globose), green when young and shining yellowish-gray when ripe, with 8 to 14 short and obtusely spiked scales. There are 8 to 20 seeds on each scale.

Habitat: The plant is indigenous to Turkey and is cultivated throughout the Mediterranean region.

ACTIONS AND PHARMACOLOGY

COMPOUNDS

Chief components: alpha-pinene, D-camphene, D-silvestrene, p-cymene, L-cadinene, cedrol, terpinenol-4, terpineol, acetyl- and isovalerianyl esters of monoterpene alcohols

EFFECTS

Cypress acts as an expectorant.

INDICATIONS AND USAGE

Unproven Uses: The drug is used externally for head colds, coughs and bronchitis.

PRECAUTIONS AND ADVERSE REACTIONS

Health risks or side effects following the proper administration of designated therapeutic dosages are not recorded. Kidney irritation is likely with intake of larger dosages.

DOSAGE

Mode of Administration: Occasionally, Cypress is used externally as an ointment.

LITERATURE

Kern W, List PH, Hörhammer L (Hrsg.), Hagers Handbuch der Pharmazeutischen Praxis, 4. Aufl., Bde 1-8, Springer Verlag Berlin, Heidelberg, New York, 1969.

Cypress Spurge

Euphorbia cyparissias

DESCRIPTION

Medicinal Parts: The medicinal part of the plant is the flowering plant with the root.

Flower and Fruit: The flowers are in terminal cymes. They are yellow-green but usually red after flowering. What appear to be flowers are in fact inflorescences. In the jug-shaped invulucres there is 1 hanging pistil with a 3 valved ovary and 3 styles each with 2 stigmas and numerous stamens. Four half-moon-shaped nectaries are at the edge. The fruit is covered in small papilla.

Leaves, Stem and Root: The plant is about 15 to 30 cm high. The stem is erect, unbranched, and glabrous. The leaves are alternate, sessile, linear, entire-margined and very narrow on the non-flowering branches.

Characteristics: The entire plant contains white latex, which is poisonous.

Habitat: Indigenous to Europe and Mediterranean.

Production: Cypress Spurge herb and root is the whole plant in flower and root of Euphorbia cyparissias.

ACTIONS AND PHARMACOLOGY

COMPOUNDS

Diterpenes: ingenan-di- and triester, for example 13-hydroxy-ingenol-3-(2,3-dimethylbutyryl)-13- dodecanoate, 13-hydroxy-ingenol-5-(2,3-dimethylbutyryl)-13-dodecanoate, 13-hydroxy-ingenol-3-(2,3-dimethylbutyryl)-13-decanoate

Triterpenes

EFFECTS

The diterpene esters in the drug are severely toxic, a strong irritant, drastically purgative and encourage growth of tumors.

In animal tests and in vitro there are indications of a cytotoxic, non-specific immune-stimulating, antiphlogistic and strongly laxative effect.

INDICATIONS AND USAGE

Unproven Uses: In folk medicine Cypress Spurge is used internally for constipation, toothache and as a diuretic (macerate). It is used externally for warts and corns (ointment).

Homeopathic Uses: Euphorbia cyparissias is used for diseases of the respiratory organs, diarrhea, and skin diseases.

PRECAUTIONS AND ADVERSE REACTIONS

The Ingenan esters are severely inflammatory in their effect and cocarcinogenic. Administration of the drug should be avoided because of the cocarcinogenic effect.

A particular danger exists with the chyle of the freshly harvested plant, but the ingenan ester retains its efficacy even after drying, which means that the drug also is acutely toxic. If it gets on the skin, the chyle causes reddening, itching, burning and blisters.

In the eye, the chyle leads to swelling of the lids, conjunctival inflammation and corneal defects. If taken internally, the chyle in the drug causes burning in the mouth and vomiting. Very high dosages cause pupil enlargement, dizziness, stupor, painful bowel movements, cardiac rhythm disorders and ultimately collapse. Skin contact with the chyle requires thorough cleaning. Contact with the eye requires thorough rinsing with water. Following stomach and intestinal emptying, the treatment of poisonings is carried out symptomatically.

DOSAGE

Mode of Administration: Cypress Spurge is used only in homeopathic dilutions.

Daily Dosage: Macerate/decoction: 0.5 to 1 gm daily

Homeopathic Dosage: from D4: 5 drops, 1 tablet or 10 globules every 30 to 60 minutes (acute) or 1 to 3 times daily (chronic); From D6 parenterally: 1 to 2 ml sc acute: 3 times daily; chronic: once a day. Children should be given a weaker dose (HAB1)

LITERATURE

Frohne D, Pfänder HJ, Giftpflanzen - Ein Handbuch für Apotheker, Toxikologen und Biologen, 4. Aufl., Wiss. Verlagsges. mbH Stuttgart 1997.

Kern W, List PH, Hörhammer L (Hrsg.), Hagers Handbuch der Pharmazeutischen Praxis, 4. Aufl., Bde. 1-8, Springer Verlag Berlin, Heidelberg, New York, 1969.

Lewin L, Gifte und Vergiftungen, 6. Aufl., Nachdruck, Haug Verlag, Heidelberg 1992.

Madaus G, Lehrbuch der Biologischen Arzneimittel, Bde 1-3, Nachdruck, Georg Olms Verlag Hildesheim 1979.

Öksüz S et al., Biological active compounds. In: PM 60(6):594-596. 1994.

Ott HH, Hecker E, Experientia 37:88. 1981.

Roth L, Daunderer M, Kormann K, Giftpflanzen, Pflanzengifte, 4. Aufl., Ecomed Fachverlag Landsberg Lech 1993.

Teuscher E, Lindequist U, Biogene Gifte - Biologie, Chemie, Pharmakologie, 2. Aufl., Fischer Verlag Stuttgart 1994.

Cypripedium calceolus

See Nerve Root

Cytisus laburnum

See Laburnum

Cytisus scoparius

See Scotch Broom

Daemonorops draco

See Dragon's Blood (Xue-Jie)

Daffodil

Narcissus pseudonarcissus

DESCRIPTION

Medicinal Parts: The medicinal parts are the bulb, the leaves and the flowers, or the whole flowering plant without the roots.

Flower and Fruit: The flowers are solitary and bending on compressed 2-edged pedicles. They are pale yellow. At the base of the flower there is a dry, membranous sheath that is split higher at the side. The perigone is 6-tipped and splayed like a plate. The secondary corolla is egg-yolk yellow and cylindrical, with an undulating, folded, unevenly crenate margin. The stamens are fused to the tube. The ovary is inferior, the style is thread-like and the stigma obtuse.

Leaves, Stem and Root: The plant grows from 15 to 30 cm high. The leaves are basal, sprouting from an ovate, brown bulb. They are erect, linear, flatly grooved, and have 2 grooves rather than a keel.

Characteristics: Daffodil has a weak unpleasant odor and is poisonous.

Habitat: The plant is found all over Europe and is cultivated elsewhere.

Production: Daffodil is the flowering plant Narcissus pseudonarcissus without the root.

Other Names: Lent Lily

ACTIONS AND PHARMACOLOGY

COMPOUNDS

Amaryllidacae alkaloids (0.08-0.15% in the bulb, with considerably less in the foliage): including, among others, hemanthamine, galanthine, galanthamine, pluviine, masonine, homolycorine

Chelidonic acid

EFFECTS

No information is available.

INDICATIONS AND USAGE

Unproven Uses: Daffodil is used for irritation of the mucous membranes, such as bronchial catarrh, whooping cough, colds and asthma.

PRECAUTIONS AND ADVERSE REACTIONS

No health hazards or side effects are known in conjunction with the proper administration of designated therapeutic dosages. The plant possesses a weak potential for sensitization, a condition called "daffodil itch."

OVERDOSAGE

Overdosage or accidental intake of the bulbs (e.g., confusing them with cooking onions) can lead to poisoning. Symptoms include vomiting, salivation, diarrhea and central nervous disorders following resorption.

DOSAGE

Mode of Administration: Daffodil is available ground and as an extract. It is also found in homeopathic remedies.

LITERATURE

Furusawa E, Suzuki N, Ramanathan S, Furusawa S, Cutting W, Effect of long-term administration of Narcissus alkaloid on Rauscher leukemia and combinations with standard drugs. In: Proc Soc Exp Biol Med 140:1034-1040. 1972.

Moraes-Cerdeira RM et al., Alkaloid content of different bulb parts of Narcissus cv. Ice follies. In: PM 63(1):93-94. 1997.

Suzuki N, Tania S, Furusawa S, Furusawa E, Therapeutic activity of narcissus alkaloids on Rauscher leukemia: Antiviral affect in vitro and rational drug combination in vivo. In: Proc Soc Expl Biol Med 145:771-777. 1974.

Tojo E, (+)-Narcidine, a new alkaloid from Narcissus pseudonarcissus. In: JNP 54: 1387. 1991.

Further information in:

Frohne D, Pfänder HJ, Giftpflanzen - Ein Handbuch für Apotheker, Toxikologen und Biologen, 4. Aufl., Wiss. Verlags-Ges. Stuttgart 1997.

Hausen B, Allergiepflanzen, Pflanzenallergene, ecomed Verlagsgesellsch. mbH, Landsberg 1988.

Kern W, List PH, Hörhammer L (Hrsg.): Hagers Handbuch der Pharmazeutischen Praxis, 4. Aufl., Bde. 1-8, Springer Verlag Berlin, Heidelberg, New York, 1969.

Lewin L, Gifte und Vergiftungen, 6. Aufl., Nachdruck, Haug Verlag, Heidelberg 1992.

Madaus G, Lehrbuch der Biologischen Arzneimittel, Bde 1-3, Nachdruck, Georg Olms Verlag Hildesheim 1979.

Roth L, Daunderer M, Kormann K, Giftpflanzen, Pflanzengifte, 4. Aufl., Ecomed Fachverlag Landsberg Lech 1993.

Teuscher E, Lindequist U, Biogene Gifte - Biologie, Chemie, Pharmakologie, 2. Aufl., Fischer Verlag Stuttgart 1994.

Damiana

Turnera diffusa

TRADE NAMES

Damiana Leaves (from various manufacturers), Wild Countryside Damiana Leaves

DESCRIPTION

Medicinal Parts: The medicinal parts are the leaves harvested during the flowering season.

Flower and Fruit: The flowers are yellow, solitary and axillary. The fruit is a small, globular, many-seeded capsule, which breaks up into 3 parts. It is aromatic and resinous.

Leaves, Stem and Root: The plant is a small shrub that grows up to 60 cm high. The leaves are 1 to 2.5 cm long and up to 6 mm wide. They are smooth and pale green on the upper surface and glabrous with a few scattered hairs on the ribs underneath. The leaves are ovate-lanceolate, short-petioled and have 2 glands at the base. They have a few serrate teeth and recurved margins.

Habitat: The plant is found mainly in the region of the Gulf of Mexico, the Caribbean and southern Africa.

Production: Damiana leaf consists of the leaf of Turnera diffusa and its variations. Damiana herb consists of the herb of Turnera diffusa and its variations.

ACTIONS AND PHARMACOLOGY

COMPOUNDS

Volatile oil (0.5-0.9%): chief components 1,8-cineole, alpha- and beta-pinene, p-cymene, as well as thymol, alpha-copene, gamma-cadinene, calamene

Tannins (4%)

Resins (7%)

Hydroquinone glycosides: arbutin (0.2-0.7%)

Cyanogenic glycosides: tetraphylline B (barterin)

EFFECTS

No information is available.

INDICATIONS AND USAGE

Unproven Uses: Damiana preparations are used as an aphrodisiac and for prophylaxis and treatment of sexual disorders.

PRECAUTIONS AND ADVERSE REACTIONS

No health hazards or side effects are known in conjunction with the proper administration of designated therapeutic dosages.

DOSAGE

How Supplied:

Capsules — 380 mg, 384 mg, 395 mg, 450 mg

Fluid Extract — 1:1

LITERATURE

Auterhoff H, Häufel HP, (1968) Arch Pharm 301:537.

Dominguez XA, Hinojosa M, (1976) Planta Med 30:68.

Hegnauer R, Chemotaxonomie der Pflanzen, Bde 1-11: Birkhäuser Verlag Basel, Boston, Berlin 1962-1997.

Hoppe HA, (1975-1987) Drogenkunde, 8. Aufl., Bde 1-3: W de Gruyter Verlag, Berlin, New York.

Jin J, (1966) Lloydia 29(3):250.

Kern W, List PH, Hörhammer L (Hrsg.), Hagers Handbuch der Pharmazeutischen Praxis, 4. Aufl., Bde 1-8: Springer Verlag Berlin, Heidelberg, New York, 1969.

Madaus G, Lehrbuch der Biologischen Arzneimittel, Bde 1-3, Nachdruck, Georg Olms Verlag Hildesheim 1979.

Steinegger E, Hänsel R, Pharmakognosie, 5. Aufl., Springer Verlag Heidelberg 1992.

Wagner H, Wiesenauer M, Phytotherapie. Phytopharmaka und pflanzliche Homöopathika, Fischer-Verlag, Stuttgart, Jena, New York 1995.

Dandelion

Taraxacum officinale

TRADE NAMES

Dandelion Root (available from various manufacturers) Alcohol-Free Dandelion, Wild Countryside Dandelion Root

DESCRIPTION

Medicinal Parts: The medicinal parts are the dried leaves harvested before the flowering season, the dried root collected in autumn, the dried aerial parts with the rhizome harvested before the flowering season and the whole fresh plant.

Flower and Fruit: The flower is a golden yellow composite flower. The composite head is solitary and has a diameter of 3 to 5 cm. All the florets are lingual and androgynous. The epicalyx is oblong-campanulate. The tepals are arranged in 3 imbricate rows, 2 of which are turned back. The inner one is long acuminate with a white margin and erect. The receptacle has no bracts. The fruit is small, long-beaked, light gray-brown, ribbed and has a parachute-like tuft of hair.

Leaves, Stem and Root: The plant is perennial, hardy and is found in a number of forms. It grows to about 30 cm tall and has a short rhizome. The rhizome turns into a many-headed, 20 to 50 cm long and 2 cm thick taproot. The hollow stem is erect or ascending. The basal leaves are glabrous or villous, usually deeply notched, lanceolate and lobed like a saw. They narrow to a red-violet tinged petiole and end in a large deltoid tip.

Characteristics: The flower opens in the morning and closes in the evening remaining closed all night and in dull weather. The plant parts contain bitter latex.

Habitat: Dandelion grows in most temperate regions of Europe and Asia.

Production: Dandelion root with herb consists of the entire Taraxacum officinale plant gathered while flowering. It is air dried.

Not to be Confused With: Cichorium intybus and the leaves of various Leontodon species.

Other Names: Blowball, Cankerwort, Lion's Tooth, Priest's Crown, Swine Snout, Wild Endive

ACTIONS AND PHARMACOLOGY

COMPOUNDS

Sesquiterpene lactones (bitter substances): including, among others, taraxinacetyl-1′-O-glucosides, 11,13-dihydrotaraxinacetyl-1′-O-glucosides, taraxacolide-1′-O-glucosides, 4alpha,15,11beta,13-tetrahydroridentin B

Triterpenes and sterols: beta-sitosterol, beta-sitosterol-glucosides, taraxasterol, psi-taraxasterol, taraxerol, taraxol

Flavonoids: including among others, apigenin-7-O-glucosides, luteolin-7-O-glucosides

Mucilages

Inulin (2-40%, high values in autumn)

EFFECTS

The amaroids in Dandelion are cholagogic and secretolytic in the upper intestinal tract. The saluretic effect demonstrated in animal experiments requires further investigation.

INDICATIONS AND USAGE

Approved by Commission E:

- Dyspeptic complaints
- Infections of the urinary tract
- Liver and gallbladder complaints
- Loss of appetite

Unproven Uses: Dandelion is used internally for disturbances in bile flow, inflammatory conditions of the efferent urinary tract, and dyspepsia. It is also used for liver and gallbladder disorders, hemorrhoids, congestion in the portal system, gout, rheumatic disorders, eczema, and other skin disorders. The drug has a diuretic effect and is used for kidney and bladder complaints and kidney stone formation. A diabetic infusion is made from the roots and leaves.

Chinese Medicine: The drug is used for acute mastitis, urinary disorders, and agalactia.

Indian Medicine: The drug is used for chronic ulcers, tuberculosis, flatulence, colic, kidney disease, gout, jaundice, and biliary stones.

CONTRAINDICATIONS

Contraindications include closure of the biliary ducts, gallbladder empyema, and ileus. Consultation with a doctor is necessary in the presence of biliary ailments.

PRECAUTIONS AND ADVERSE REACTIONS

No health hazards are known in conjunction with the proper administration of designated therapeutic dosages. Superacid gastric complaints are possible due to the drug's secretion-stimulating effect. The drug possesses weak potential for sensitization reactions.

DOSAGE

Mode of Administration: Whole, cut, and powdered drug is available in the form of drops, tinctures, juice, and in compound preparations.

How Supplied:

Capsules—425 mg, 475 mg, 515 mg, 520 mg,

Liquid—1:1

Preparation: To make a tea, use 1 to 2 teaspoonfuls finely cut drug with 150 ml rapidly boiled water; strain after 15 minutes and drink warm.

To make a decoction, use 3 to 4 gm cut and powdered drug per cup of water. To make an infusion, use 3 to 4 gm cut drug per 1 cup of water.

For an extract, mix 1 part coarsely powdered Dandelion root with 8 parts of water and 1 part spirit of wine.

Daily Dosage: When using a tincture, the recommended dosage is 10 to 15 drops 3 times daily. A cup of the freshly made tea can be taken mornings and evenings.

Storage: The drug should be protected from light and moisture.

LITERATURE

Baba K et al., (1981) Yakugaku Zasshi 101(6):538.

Böhm K, (1959) Untersuchungen über choleretische Wirkungen einiger Arzneipflanzen. Arzneim Forsch Drug Res 9:376.

Budzianowski J, Coumarins, caffeoyltartaric acids and their artifactual estres from Taraxacum officinale. In: PM 63(3):288. 1997.

Czygan FC, Taraxacum officinale WIGGERS - Der Löwenzahn. In: ZPT 11(3):99. 1990.

Hänsel R et al., (1980) Phytochemistry 19:857.

Kotobuki Seiyaku KK, (1981) Pat. JP 81/10117 Japan.

Mascolo N et al., (1987) Phytother Res 1(1):28.

Rauwald HW, Huang DT, (1985) Phytochemistry 24(7):1557.

Further information in:

Hänsel R, Keller K, Rimpler H, Schneider G (Hrsg.), Hagers Handbuch der Pharmazeutischen Praxis, 5. Aufl., Bde 4-6 (Drogen): Springer Verlag Berlin, Heidelberg, New York, 1992-1994.

Hausen B, Allergiepflanzen, Pflanzenallergene, ecomed Verlagsgesellsch. mbH, Landsberg 1988.

Leung AY, Encyclopedia of Common Natural Ingredients Used in Food, Drugs, Cosmetics, John Wiley & Sons Inc., New York 1980.

Madaus G, Lehrbuch der Biologischen Arzneimittel, Bde 1-3, Nachdruck, Georg Olms Verlag Hildesheim 1979.

Roth L, Daunderer M, Kormann K, Giftpflanzen, Pflanzengifte, 4. Aufl., Ecomed Fachverlag Landsberg Lech 1993.

Steinegger E, Hänsel R, Pharmakognosie, 5. Aufl., Springer Verlag Heidelberg 1992.

Teuscher E, Lindequist U, Biogene Gifte - Biologie, Chemie, Pharmakologie, 2. Aufl., Fischer Verlag Stuttgart 1994.

Teuscher E, Biogene Arzneimittel, 5. Aufl., Wiss. Verlagsges. Stuttgart 1997.

Wagner H, Wiesenauer M, Phytotherapie. Phytopharmaka und pflanzliche Homöopathika, Fischer-Verlag, Stuttgart, Jena, New York 1995.

Wichtl M (Hrsg.), Teedrogen, 4. Aufl., Wiss. Verlagsges. Stuttgart 1997.

Daphne mezereum

See Mezereon

Date Palm

Phoenix dactylifera

DESCRIPTION

Medicinal Parts: The medicinal part is the fruit.

Flower and Fruit: The flowers are androgynous and are in branched, cob-like inflorescences. The 3 carpels form 1 ovary. The fruit is a 1-seeded berry about 5 cm long (the date with the characteristic seed).

Leaves, Stem and Root: The Date Palm is a woody plant growing primarily in girth. The leaves form a large long-petioled tuft at the top of the trunk. The lamina are frond-like pinnatifid.

Habitat: Date Palm is found from India to northern Africa.

Production: Dates are the fruits of Phoenix dactylifera.

ACTIONS AND PHARMACOLOGY

COMPOUNDS: IN THE FRUIT PULP

Sugar (50%): saccharose, inverted sugar

Leucoanthocyanidine

Piperidine derivatives: pipecolic acid, 5-hydroxy-pipecolic acid, baikiaine

COMPOUNDS: IN THE SEEDS

Fatty oil (10%)

EFFECTS

No information is available.

INDICATIONS AND USAGE

Indian Medicine: Date Palm is used for bronchitis, clouding of the cornea, headaches, inflamed wounds, kidney disease and gastric complaints.

PRECAUTIONS AND ADVERSE REACTIONS

No health hazards or side effects are known in conjunction with the proper administration of designated therapeutic dosages.

DOSAGE

Preparation: Honey made from dates is produced in Algeria using juice-rich dates, which are dried in the sun; the leftover liquid results in date honey. Date honey is used to treat chest complaints.

LITERATURE

Kern W, List PH, Hörhammer L (Hrsg.), Hagers Handbuch der Pharmazeutischen Praxis, 4. Aufl., Bde 1-8, Springer Verlag Berlin, Heidelberg, New York, 1969.

Wylegalla R, Biblische Botanik: Pflanzen und Früchte aus dem gelobten Land. In: DAZ 137(11):867-869. 1997.

Datura stramonium

See Jimson Weed

Daucus carota

See Wild Carrot

Delphinium consolida

See Larkspur

Delphinium staphisagria

See Stavesacre

Devil's Claw

Harpagophytum procumbens

TRADE NAMES

Devil's Claw (available from a number of manufacturers), Devil's Claw Secondary Root, Devil's Claw Root Tuber

DESCRIPTION

Medicinal Parts: The medicinal parts are the dried tubular secondary roots and the thick lateral tubers.

Flower and Fruit: The flowers grow on short pedicles in the leaf axils and are solitary, large and foxglove-like. The petals are pale-pink to crimson. The seed capsules are bivalvular, compressed at the sides and ovate. The capsules are 7 to 20 cm long, 6 cm in diameter, and very woody with longitudinally striped rind. They have a double row of elastic, arm-like, branched appendages with an anchor-like hook. The capsules contain about 50 dark oblong seeds with a rough surface.

Leaves, Stem and Root: The plant is perennial and leafy. It has a branched root system and branched, prostrate shoots 1 to 1.5 m long. The leaves are petiolate and lobed, and may be opposite or alternate. The aerial parts of the plant die back in the dry season. The tuber (storage) roots are formed from the main and lateral roots. The main roots have obtuse, quadrangular, upright collar-like sections, 10 to 20 cm long and 30 to 60 cm thick, which are covered in a fissured cork layer. The nodes of the lateral roots are up to 60 mm thick and 20 cm long, and are light-brown to red-brown on the outside. The roots extend out to an area of about 150 cm around the plant and grow down to a depth of 30 to 60 cm.

Characteristics: The dried, pulverized secondary tubers and roots are yellowish-gray to bright pink and horn-like in their hardness. They have a bitter taste.

Habitat: The plant originated in South Africa and Namibia, and has spread throughout the Savannas and the Kalahari.

Production: Devil's Claw root consists of the dried lateral roots and secondary tubers of Harpagophytum procumbens. The lateral roots are cut into slices or pieces, or pulverized immediately after digging because they harden and become very difficult to cut once dry.

Other Names: Grapple Plant, Wood Spider

ACTIONS AND PHARMACOLOGY

COMPOUNDS

Liridoide monoterpenes: including harpagoside (extremely bitter), harpagide, procumbide

Phenylethanol derivatives: including acteoside (verbascoside); isoacteoside

Oligosaccharides: stachyose

Harpagoquinones (traces)

EFFECTS

Devil's Claw stimulates gastric juice secretion and is choleretic. Anti-inflammatory, analgesic (and thus anti-arthritic) effect has been shown in animal experiments.

INDICATIONS AND USAGE

Approved by Commission E:

- Dyspeptic complaints
- Loss of appetite
- Rheumatism

Unproven Uses: In folk medicine, Devil's Claw is used as an ointment for skin injuries and disorders. The dried root is used for pain relief; pregnancy discomforts; arthritis; allergies; metabolic disorders; and kidney, bladder, liver and gallbladder disorders. In South Africa it is used for fevers and digestive disorders. Devil's Claw is also used for supportive therapy of degenerative disorders of the CNS system.

Homeopathic Uses: Chronic rheumatism is the primary use for Devil's Claw in homeopathy.

CONTRAINDICATIONS

The drug should not be used in the presence of stomach or duodenal ulcers, due to the drug's stimulation of gastric juice secretion.

PRECAUTIONS AND ADVERSE REACTIONS

Health risks or side effects following the proper administration of designated therapeutic dosages are not recorded. The drug has a sensitizing effect.

DOSAGE

Mode of Administration: As comminuted drug for infusions and other preparations for internal use, as an ointment for external use.

How Supplied:

Capsules — 405 mg, 480 mg, 510 mg, 520 mg

Tablets

Preparation: To make an infusion, use 1 teaspoonful (equivalent to 4.5 g) comminuted drug with 300 ml boiling water. Steep for 8 hours and strain.

Daily Dosage: For loss of appetite, the recommended dosage is 1.5 g of drug; otherwise 4.5 g of drug is used. The infusion can be taken 3 times a day.

Homeopathic Dosage: 5 to 10 drops, 1 tablet or 5 to 10 globules 1 to 3 times a day, or from D3 1 ml injection solution sc twice weekly (HAB1). The ointment is applied 1 to 3 times a day. For external use, 1 dessertspoon of the tincture should be diluted with 250 ml and used for washes or poultices.

Storage: Store Devil's Claw in a container that protects it from light and moisture.

LITERATURE

Abramowitz M, (1979) Med Letters 21:30.

Amling R, Phytotherapeutika in der Neurologie. In: ZPT 12(1):9. 1991.

Anonym, Phytotherapie:Pflanzliche Antirheumatika - was bringen sie? In: DAZ 136(45):4012-4015. 1996.

Baghdikian B et al., An analyticyl study, anti-inflammatory and analgesic effects of Harpagophytum procumbens and Harpagophytum zeyheri. In: PM 63(2):171-176. 1997.

Carle R, Pflanzliche Antiphlogistika und Spasmolytika. In: ZPT 9(3):67. 1988.

Circosta C et al., (1984) J Ethnopharmacol 11:259.

Eichler O, Koch C, (1970) Arzneim Forsch 20(1):107.

Erdos A et al., (1978) Planta Med 34:97.

Haag-Berrurier, M et al., (1978) Plant Med Phytother 12(3):197.

Kreymeier J, Rheumatherapie mit Phytopharmaka. In: DAZ 137(8):611-613. 1997.

Lichti H, Von Wartburg A, (1964) Tetrahedron Letters 15:835.

Sticher O, (1977) Dtsch Apoth Ztg 32:1279.

Tunmann P, Stierstorfer N, Tetrahedron Letters 15:1697.

Wenzel P, Wegener T, (1995) Teufelskralle. Ein pflanzliches Antirheumatikum. Dtsch Apoth Ztg 135(13):1131-1144.

Wolf E, Teufelskralle hat Entzündungen im Griff. In: PZ 142(14):1122. 1997.

Further information in:

Hänsel R, Keller K, Rimpler H, Schneider G (Hrsg.), Hagers Handbuch der Pharmazeutischen Praxis, 5. Aufl., Bde 4-6 (Drogen), Springer Verlag Berlin, Heidelberg, New York, 1992-1994.

Schulz R, Hänsel R, Rationale Phytotherapie, Springer Verlag Heidelberg 1996.

Steinegger E, Hänsel R, Pharmakognosie, 5. Aufl., Springer Verlag Heidelberg 1992.

Teuscher E, Biogene Arzneimittel, 5. Aufl., Wiss. Verlagsges. mbH Stuttgart 1997.

Wagner H, Wiesenauer M, Phytotherapie. Phytopharmaka und pflanzliche Homöopathika, Fischer-Verlag, Stuttgart, Jena, New York 1995.

Wichtl M (Hrsg.), Teedrogen, 4. Aufl., Wiss. Verlagsges. Stuttgart 1997.

Dicentra cucullaria

See Turkey Corn

Dictamnus albus

See Burning Bush

Digitalis

Digitalis purpurea

DESCRIPTION

Medicinal Parts: The medicinal parts are the dried leaves (in powder form), the ripe dried seeds, the fresh leaves of the 1-year-old plant or the leaves of the 2-year-old plant collected at the beginning of flowering. In the past, the drug of Digitalis purpurae was the raw material employed in isolating the cardiac glycosides. Today, Digitalis lantana is used.

Flower and Fruit: The flowers are carmine red with white-edged spots on the inside. The flowers appear in long hanging racemes. They have 5 free, short-tipped sepals. The corolla is about 4 cm long, campanulate, bilabiate with an obtuse upper lip and an ovate tip on the lower lip. The flower is glabrous on the outside and has a white awn on the inside. There are 2 long and 2 short stamens, and 1 superior ovary. The fruit is a 2-valved, ovate, glandular, villous capsule.

Leaves, Stem and Root: The plant is a biennial with a branched tap root. In the first year it develops a leaf rosette. In the second it produces a 2 m high, erect, unbranched, gray, tomentose stem. The leaves are alternate, ovate, tapering upward and petiolate. Almost all leaves are crenate; only the highest ones are entire-margined.

Characteristics: The plant is very poisonous; it tastes hot-bitter with a slightly unpleasant odor.

Habitat: Digitalis is indigenous to Europe. It was introduced to the east and the American continent.

Production: Digitalis leaves are the leaves of Digitalis purpurea or of Digitalis lanata. Digitalis lanata corresponds to Digitalis purpurea but has a milder effect. The rose leaves are harvested during the first period of vegetation in early autumn. The drying period is decisive for the content of cardenolide glycosides. The temperature for drying is 30° C to 50° C.

Not to be Confused With: Confusion seldom occurs due to cultivation under controlled conditions.

Other Names: Foxglove, Dead Men's Bells, Dog's Finger, Fairy Fingers, Fairy Gloves, Finger Flower, Folks' Glove, Lion's Mouth, Ladies' Glove, Witches' Gloves, Gloves of Our Lady, Fairy Caps, Fairy Thimbles, Virgin's Glove

ACTIONS AND PHARMACOLOGY

COMPOUNDS

Cardioactive steroid glycosides (cardenolides 0.5 to 1.5%): including ones of the -

- *A-sequence (aglycone digitoxigenin):* purpurea glycoside A (primary glycoside), digitoxin (secondary glycoside)

- *B-sequence (aglycone gitoxigenin):* purpurea glycoside B (primary glycoside), gitoxin (secondary glycoside), Digitalinum verum

- *E-sequence (aglycone gitaloxigenin):* glucoverodoxin, glucogitaloxin, gitaloxin

Pregnane glycosides: including digipurpurin, diginin, digitalonin

Steroid saponin: including desgalactotigonin, digitonine, purpureagitoside

Anthracene derivatives: anthraquinones

EFFECTS

The drug contains cardioactive cardenolide glycosides that are positively inotropic, negatively chronotropic and improve the contraction power of cardiac muscle.

INDICATIONS AND USAGE

Unproven Uses: In folk medicine, the drug's use originated in Ireland, then came to Scotland and England and finally to central Europe. It was used to treat ulcers in the lower abdomen, boils, headaches, abscesses and paralysis. Externally, the drug was used for the granulation of poorly healing wounds and to cure ulcers. Furthermore, the drug was used for cardiac insufficiency, especially high blood pressure.

Use of the raw product has become obsolete because the effect is not reproducible. The use of pure glycosides is recommended instead. Digitoxin is available in mono preparations (extract) and is used as an isolated pure substance.

Homeopathic Uses: Digitalis purpurea is used for cardiac insufficiency and migraine.

PRECAUTIONS AND ADVERSE REACTIONS

General: Because of the narrow therapeutic range of digitalis glycosides, a certain percentage of patients may experience side effects immediately upon administration of therapeutic dosages: hypertonia in gastrointestinal area, loss of appetite, vomiting, diarrhea and headache.

Drug Interactions: The simultaneous administration of arrhythmogenic substances (sympathomimetics, methylxanthines, phosphodiesterase inhibitors, quinidine) increases the risks of cardiac arrhythmias.

OVERDOSAGE

With overdosage, in addition to the already-mentioned symptoms, the following can also occur:

Heart: cardiac rhythm disorders, all the way up to life-threatening ventricular tachycardia, atrial tachycardia with atrioventricular block

Central nervous system: stupor, visual disorders, depression, confused states, hallucinations, psychoses

Lethal dosages lead to heart failure or asphyxiation. Administration over extended periods leads in rare cases to gynecomastia. Because of the difficulties in standardizing the drug, the administration of pure glycosides is to be preferred (digitoxin).

The first measures to be taken in case of poisoning are gastric lavage and activated charcoal instillation. All other measures proceed according to the symptoms. For loss of potassium, careful replenishment is necessary. For ectopic irritation build-up in the ventricle, administration of phenytoin as an antiarrhythmatic is recommended. Lidocaine should be used in cases of ventricular extrasystole, and for partial atrioventricular block, atropine is recommended. The prophylactic installation of a pacemaker is often necessary. For elimination of the glycosides hemoperfusion is possible, the administration of cholestyramine for interrrupting the enterohepatic circulation and/or the application of digitoxin antibodies (antigen-binding fragments, digitalis antidote {Boehringer Mannheim}, is very likely only fully effective with digitoxin poisoning).

The drugs and pure glycosides should be administered in the following situations (among others): atrioventricular block of the 2nd and 3rd degree, hypercalcaemia, hypocalcaemia, hypertrophic cardiomyopathy, carotid sinus syndrome, ventricular tachycardia, thoracic aortic aneurysm, WPW-syndrome.

DOSAGE

Mode of Administration: Today, the drug is obsolete. Due to the lack of reproductivity of content, the use of appropriate pure glycosides is advisable. Digitoxin is contained in mono preparations (extract) and used as an isolated pure substance.

Preparation: Tincture: shaken for 1 day in 25% ethanol at a ratio of 1:10.

The manufacture of the digoxin and digitoxin is a complicated process that involves fermentation, extraction and evaporation.

Storage: Store carefully away from sources of light.

LITERATURE

Brisse B, Anwendung pflanzlicher Wirkstoffe bei kardialen Erkrankungen. In: ZPT 10(4):107. 1989.

Buschauer A, Entwicklung neuer positiv inotroper Arzneistoffe: Suche nach einm ''Digitalisersatz''. In: PZW 134(1)3. 1989.

Cohn JN, (1974) J Am Med Ass 229: 1911.

Höltje HD, Molecular Modelling von Digitaloiden. In: PZ 137(37):2812. 1992.

Ikeda Y et al., Quantitative HPLC analysis of cardiac glycosides in Digitalis purpurea. In: JNP 58(6):897-901. 1995.

Lichius JJ, Weber R, Kirschke M, Liedtke S, Brieger D, Neues vom Fingerhut und seinen Kaffeesäureestern. In: DAZ 135(40):3794-3800. 1995.

Lustenberger, B, In: Lustenberger J (Basler Dissertationen zur Geschichte der Pharmazie und Naturwissenschaften, Bd. 4), Der Weg zur Etablierung der Reinglykoside in der Digitalistherapie. Juris Druck - Verlag Dietikon. 1993.

Rall B, Herzinsuffizienz: Was bringt die Digitalis-Therapie? In: DAZ 137(3):126-27. 1997.

Thomas R et al., (1974) J Pharm Sci 63:1649.

Tschesche R, Brügmann G, Tetrahedron 20:1469-1475. 1964.

Voigt G, Hiller K, Sci Pharm 55:201-207. 1987.

Wichtl M, Bühl W, Huesmann G, DAZ 127:2391-2400. 1987.

Further information in:

Frohne D, Pfänder HJ, Giftpflanzen - Ein Handbuch für Apotheker, Toxikologen und Biologen, 4. Aufl., Wiss. Verlagsges. mbH Stuttgart 1997.

Hänsel R, Keller K, Rimpler H, Schneider G (Hrsg.), Hagers Handbuch der Pharmazeutischen Praxis, 5. Aufl., Bde 4-6 (Drogen), Springer Verlag Berlin, Heidelberg, New York, 1992-1994.

Lewin L, Gifte und Vergiftungen, 6. Aufl., Nachdruck, Haug Verlag, Heidelberg 1992.

Madaus G, Lehrbuch der Biologischen Arzneimittel, Bde 1-3, Nachdruck, Georg Olms Verlag Hildesheim 1979.

Roth L, Daunderer M, Kormann K, Giftpflanzen, Pflanzengifte, 4. Aufl., Ecomed Fachverlag Landsberg Lech 1993.

Steinegger E, Hänsel R, Pharmakognosie, 5. Aufl., Springer Verlag Heidelberg 1992.

Teuscher E, Lindequist U, Biogene Gifte - Biologie, Chemie, Pharmakologie, 2. Aufl., Fischer Verlag Stuttgart 1994.

Teuscher E, Biogene Arzneimittel, 5. Aufl., Wiss. Verlagsges. mbH Stuttgart 1997.

Wagner H, Wiesenauer M, Phytotherapie. Phytopharmaka und pflanzliche Homöopathika, Fischer-Verlag, Stuttgart, Jena, New York 1995.

Digitalis Lanata

Digitalis lanata

DESCRIPTION

Medicinal Parts: The leaves are the medicinal part of the plant.

Flower and Fruit: The inflorescence is long and densely flowered, with racemes facing all directions. The bracts are glandular-haired with ciliate edges. The flower structures are in fives. The sepals are fused, the calyx tubular. The petals are fused to a campanulate corolla, which is glandular-haired on, the outside, white with yellow-brown spots, 18 to 25 mm long and unevenly bilabiate. The upper lip has 4 points, and is flat and hem-like. The lower lip is almost as long as the corolla tube and is turned away from it. There are 4 stamens, often stretching out of the corolla tube. The ovaries are superior, 2-chambered, clavate, glandular-haired, gradually merging into the stigmas. The fruit is a 10 mm long septicidal, brittle capsule. The seeds are approximately 1.5 mm long and red-brown.

Leaves, Stem and Root: Digitalis lanata is a herbaceous biennial or perennial, upright, up to 1.2 m high. The leaves are sessile, simple, narrow-lanceolate, 15 to 35 cm long, entire and ciliate in the upper area of the shoot axis. The stem is upright, usually green, grooved-edged, usually glabrous below and long woolly-haired in the upper half. The plant has a primary root with no shoot-bearing roots.

Habitat: The plant's habitat extends from Greece and the Balkans across the northern coast of the Black Sea to the Caucasus and the Caspian Sea.

Production: Woolly foxglove leaves are the dried leaves of Digitalis lanata. Annual cultivation begins with sowing in April; harvesting is between September and November. The roughly cut leaves are dried for 10 to 12 hours at 50° C.

ACTIONS AND PHARMACOLOGY

COMPOUNDS

Cardioactive steroid glycosides (cardenolides) (0.5 to 1.5%) of the following series, including:

A-series (aglycone digitoxigenin): including lanatoside A (0.05 to 0.25%) glucodigifucoside (0.01 to 0.15%), glucoevatromonoside (0.02 to 0.05%), digitoxin, alpha- and beta-acetyldigoxin

B-series (aglycone gitoxigenin): lanatoside B (0.01 to 0.15%), glucogitoroside (0.02 to 0.12%), Digitalinum verum (0.02 to 0.12%), gitoxin, alpha- and beta-acetylgitoxin

C-series (aglycone digoxigenin): lanatoside C (0.08 to 0.24%), desacetyl lanatoside C, digoxin

D-series (aglycone diginatigenin): lanatoside D, diginatin, diginatigenin gitaloside

E-series (aglycone gitaloxigenin): lanatoside E, glucoveredoxin (0.01 to 0.14%), glucoverodoxin (0.02 to 0.12%), gitaloxin

Pregnane derivatives: including digifolein, glucodigifolein, diginin, digipronin, lanafolein, gitonine

Steroid saponins: including lanagitosides I and II, tigonin, desglucolanatigonin, aglycones including tigogenin, digalogenin, digitogenin, gitogenin

EFFECTS

The cardioactive cardenolide glycosides contained in the drug are positively inotropic and negatively chronotropic. Digitalis lanata is known to be highly resorbent when administered orally. It produces rapid results and wide-ranging effects; has strong diuretic properties; is quickly abating; and demonstrates good tolerability. Digitalis lanata has three times the physiological effect of Digitalis purpurea and is preferred for its fast-acting effect. Despite these qualities, the drug is now obsolete and has been replaced by pure cardenolide glycosides.

INDICATIONS AND USAGE

Because of the unsatisfactory reproducibility during production, this drug is obsolete today; the pure cardenolide glycosides are used. The simultaneous administration of arrhythmogenic substances (sympathomimetics, methyl xanthines, phosphodiestrase inhibitors, quinidine) increases the risk of cardiac arrhythmias.

PRECAUTIONS AND ADVERSE REACTIONS

General: Because of the difficulties involved in standardizing the drug, the administration of pure glycosides is to be preferred (digitoxin, digoxin, alpha-acetyldigoxin, beta-acetyldigoxin, lanatoside C, deslanoside). Patients receiving no more than therapeutic dosages might experience the following side effects: hypertonias in gastrointestinal area, loss of appetite, vomiting, diarrhea and headache.

Drug Interactions: Neither the drug nor pure glycosides should be administered in the presence of first- and second-degree AV-Block, hypercalcemia, hypokaliemia, hypertrophic cardiomyopathy, carotid sinus syndrome, ventricle tachycardia, thoracic aortic aneurysm or WPW syndrome.

OVERDOSAGE

With overdosage, in addition to the symptoms above, the following can also occur:

Heart: Cardiac rhythm disorders as serious as life-threatening ventricular tachycardias and atrial tachycardias with atrioventricular block.

Central nervous system: Dizziness, vision disorders, depressions, states of confusion, hallucinations, psychoses.

Lethal dosages (for humans, 2 to 3 g of the drug) initially lead to signs of nausea, vomiting and diarrhea caused by irritation of the gastrointestinal tract. Slowed pulse, extrasystoles and conduction disturbances result from resorption. These are followed by ventricular fibrillation and later death from cardiac arrest.

The first-aid measures to be taken with poisonings are gastric lavage and instillation of medicinal charcoal. All other measures proceed according to the symptoms: careful potassium substitution for potassium; phenytoin as an antiarrhythmic for ectopic stimulation formation in the ventricle; lidocaine for ventricular extrasystole; atropine for partial atrioventricular block.

The prophylactic insertion of a cardiac pacemaker is recommended. Hemoperfusion for the elimination of the glycosides and cholestyramine administration for the interruption of the enterohepatic circulation are possible.

DOSAGE

Mode of Administration: The drug is not used today. The following preparation and supply information is for historical reference.

How Supplied: Whole and powdered drug.

Preparation: Tincture; powder: ethanol 25%; 1:10; succussed for 24 hours.

Storage: Store securely and protect from light.

LITERATURE

Hänsel R, Keller K, Rimpler H, Schneider G (Ed.), Hagers Handbuch der Pharmazeutischen Praxis. 5. Aufl., Bde 4 - 6 (Drogen), Springer Verlag Berlin, Heidelberg, New York, 1992-1994.

Kallfelz HC, Reinhardt D, Treatment of heart insufficiency in infancy and childhood with a combined drug made of digitalis lanata glycosides, Ther Ggw, 110:357-8 passim, 1971 Mar.

Pitra J, Horβk P, Cardiac glycosides. XII. Digoxin, the fermented drug of undulating foxglove (Digitalis lanata EHRH) Cesk Farm, 21:142-4, 1972 May.

Schneider KW, Gattenlöhner W, Different changes of central hemodynamic: due to Digitalis purpura and ianata preparations, Verh Dtsch Ges Inn Med, 77:980-2, 1971.

Digitalis lanata

See Digitalis Lanata

Digitalis purpurea

See Digitalis

Dill

Anethum graveolens

DESCRIPTION

Medicinal Parts: The medicinal part is the seed, the fresh or dried leaves and the upper stem.

Flower and Fruit: The yellow flowers are in large, 20 to 50 rayed umbels. There is no involucre or calyx. The petals have an inward-curving point, which is not indented. The fruit is flattened and oval with a rib on the back, which is sharp-edged. Ribs that appear on the edge have a winged edge.

Leaves, Stem and Root: The plant is 40 to 120 cm tall. The stem is erect, round, smooth, dark-green and white-striped. The stem is branched above, with a bluish bloom. The leaves are double and more pinnate, feathery, white-tipped leaflets with a deep groove on the upper surface. The leaf sheath is oblong with a thick-skinned edge.

Characteristics: Dill has an aromatic scent.

Habitat: The plant is indigenous to the Mediterranean region, southern Russia, and cultivated throughout Europe as well as North and South America.

Production: Dill herb consists of the fresh or dried leaf and upper stem of Anethum graveolens. Dill seed consists of the dried fruit of Anethum graveolens.

Other Names: Dilly

ACTIONS AND PHARMACOLOGY

COMPOUNDS: DILL HERB

Volatile oil (0.5 to 1.5%): chief constituents are carvone, dill apiole, (+) limonene

Phthalides

EFFECTS: DILL HERB

No information is available.

COMPOUNDS: DILL FRUIT

Volatile oil (2.5 to 4.0%): chief constituents are carvone (approximately 50%), dill apiole, (+) — limonene

Phtalides

Fatty oil

Furanocoumarins: including bergaptene

Hydroxycoumarins: including umbelliferone

EFFECTS: DILL FRUIT

The fruit of the Dill plant has an antispasmodic effect on the smooth muscles of the gastrointestinal tract, and a bacteriostatic effect.

INDICATIONS AND USAGE

DILL HERB

Unproven Uses: Dill herb is used for prevention and treatment of diseases and disorders of the gastrointestinal tract, kidney and urinary tract, for sleep disorders and for spasms.

DILL FRUIT

Approved by Commission E:

- Dyspeptic Complaints

Indian Medicine: Dill is used for halitosis, worm infestation, complaints of the repiratory tract and syphilis.

PRECAUTIONS AND ADVERSE REACTIONS

DILL HERB

No health hazards or side effects are known in conjunction with the proper administration of designated therapeutic dosages.

DILL FRUIT

No health hazards or side effects are known in conjunction with the proper administration of designated therapeutic dosages. Photodermatosis is possible after contact with the juice of the freshly harvested plant.

DOSAGE

DILL FRUIT

Mode of Administration: Whole seeds and crushed fruits are used to make teas and other galenic preparations for internal application.

Daily Dosage: The average daily dosage of the seeds is 3 gm; essential oil daily dose is 0.1 to 0.3 gm.

LITERATURE

DILL HERB

Badoc A, Contribution à l'étude du genre Anethum. In: Mémoire Diplome supérieur Rech Biol et Physiol, Univ Sci Techn Lille Flandres Artois No. 122, Dec. 1986.

Debelmas AM, Rochat J, (1967) Plant Med Phytother 1:23.

Dranik LI, (1970) Khim Prir Soed 6:268.

Gijbels MJ et al., (1983) Sci Pharm 51:414.

Harborne JB, (1969) Phytochemistry 8:1729.

Kosawa M et al., (1976) Chem Pharm Bull 24:220.

Poggendorf A, Göckeritz D, Pohloudek-Fabini R, Der Gehalt an ätherischem Öl in Anethum graveolens. In: PA 32(10):607. 1977.

Varo PT, Heinz DE, (1970) J Agric Food Chem 18:234 et 239.

Further information in:

Kern W, List PH, Hörhammer L (Hrsg.), Hagers Handbuch der Pharmazeutischen Praxis, 4. Aufl., Bde. 1-8, Springer Verlag Berlin, Heidelberg, New York, 1969.

Madaus G, Lehrbuch der Biologischen Arzneimittel, Bde 1-3, Nachdruck, Georg Olms Verlag Hildesheim 1979.

DILL FRUIT

Badoc A, Contribution à l'étude du genre Anethum. In: Mémoire Diplome supérieur Rech Biol et Physiol, Univ Sci Techn Lille Flandres Artois No. 122, Dec. 1986.

Debelmas AM, Rochat J, (1967) Plant Med Phytother 1:23.

Dranik LI, (1970) Khim Prir Soed 6:268.

Gijbels MJ et al., (1983) Sci Pharm 51:414.

Harborne JB, (1969) Phytochemistry 8:1729.

Kosawa M et al., (1976) Chem Pharm Bull 24:220.

Poggendorf A, Göckeritz D, Pohloudek-Fabini R, Der Gehalt an ätherischem Öl in Anethum graveolens. In: PA 32(10):607. 1977.

Varo PT, Heinz DE, (1970) J Agric Food Chem 18:234 et 239.

Further information in:

Kern W, List PH, Hörhammer L (Hrsg.), Hagers Handbuch der Pharmazeutischen Praxis, 4. Aufl., Bde. 1-8, Springer Verlag Berlin, Heidelberg, New York, 1969.

Madaus G, Lehrbuch der Biologischen Arzneimittel, Bde 1-3, Nachdruck, Georg Olms Verlag Hildesheim 1979.

Dionaea muscipula

See Venus Flytrap

Dioscorea villosa

See Wild Yam

Dipsacus silvestris

See Teazle

Dipteryx odorata

See Tonka Beans

Divi-Divi

Caesalpinia bonducella

DESCRIPTION

Medicinal Parts: The medicinal part of the plant is seed.

Flower and Fruit: The flowers are dorsiventrally zygomorphous and arranged in dense clusters. The sepals are free or fused at their base, or fused to the base of the petals and stamens to form the corolla. The petals are separate from each other but have an ascending bud covering. There are twice as many stamens as petals, usually 10. The ovary always has only 1 carpel. The fruit is indehiscent or a legume with yellow nuts.

Leaves, Stem and Root: Divi-Divi is a tree or shrub that grows to a height of 9 m, with alternate entire-margined or double-pinnate thorny leaves.

Habitat: Sri Lanka, Brazil, South America

Production: Nikkar nuts are the seeds of Caesalpinia bonducella.

Other Names: Nikkar Nuts, Nichol Seeds, Gray Nicker

ACTIONS AND PHARMACOLOGY

COMPOUNDS

Fatty oil (20 to 25%, bonduc nut oil): chief fatty acids are linoleic acid, oleic acid, palmitic acid, stearic acid

Proteins

Starch

Diterpenes: including, among others, alpha-, beta-, gamma-, eta-caesalpine

Saponins

EFFECTS

Divi-Divi is a febrifuge and tonic.

INDICATIONS AND USAGE

Indian Medicine: The roasted seeds are used in febrile illnesses and in the treatment of diabetes.

PRECAUTIONS AND ADVERSE REACTIONS

No health hazards or side effects are known in conjunction with the proper administration of designated therapeutic dosages.

DOSAGE

Mode of Administration: Seeds are ground and roasted for internal use.

LITERATURE

Balmain et al., Tetrahedron 1967:5027. 1967.

Hoppe HA, (1975-1987) Drogenkunde, 8. Aufl., Bde 1-3, W. de Gruyter Verlag, Berlin, New York.

Kern W, List PH, Hörhammer L (Hrsg.), Hagers Handbuch der Pharmazeutischen Praxis, 4. Aufl., Bde 1-8, Springer Verlag Berlin, Heidelberg, New York, 1969.

Dodder

Cuscuta epithymum

DESCRIPTION

Medicinal Parts: The medicinal parts are the aerial parts of the plant.

Flower and Fruit: The flowers are reddish, wax or flesh-colored. They are arranged in small clusters. The calyx is divided into 5 and the corolla is fused to a 4 to 5 tipped tube with fringed scales inside. There are 5 stamens and 1 ovary.

Leaves, Stem and Root: The plant is a leafless parasite up to 150 cm high. The stem is yellow or reddish, thread-like, branched, with sucking roots, and climbing.

Habitat: The plant grows in Europe, Asia and South Africa.

Production: Dodder is the whole plant of Cuscuta epithymum.

Other Names: Lesser Dodder, Dodder of Thyme, Devil's Guts, Beggarweed, Hellweed, Strangle Tare, Scaldweed

ACTIONS AND PHARMACOLOGY

COMPOUNDS

Saponins

Tannins

A purgative principle

The drug has been subjected to very little investigation.

EFFECTS

Dodder has hepatic and laxative effects.

INDICATIONS AND USAGE

Unproven Uses: Dodder is used for disorders of the urinary tract, spleen and liver.

PRECAUTIONS AND ADVERSE REACTIONS

Health risks or side effects following the proper administration of designated therapeutic dosages are not recorded. It is conceivable that the drug triggers intestinal colic in cases of overdosage.

LITERATURE

Kern W, List PH, Hörhammer L (Hrsg.), Hagers Handbuch der Pharmazeutischen Praxis, 4. Aufl., Bde. 1-8, Springer Verlag Berlin, Heidelberg, New York, 1969.

Pagnani F, Ciarallo G, (1974) Boll Chim Farm 113(1):30.

Dog Rose

Rosa canina

DESCRIPTION

Medicinal Parts: The medicinal parts are the petals, the Rose hips with and without seeds and the seeds.

Flower and Fruit: The pink flowers are usually solitary or in clusters of 2 or 3. The receptacle deepens to form a cup whose upper edge the 5 pinnatifid sepals and 5 petals and numerous stamens sit. There are long white silky hairs in the receptacles and numerous ovaries. The ovaries grow into stiff-haired nuts surrounded by the receptacle and become the scarlet 'rosehip'.

Leaves, Stem and Root: The plant is an approximately 1 to 3 m high shrub with hanging branches and erect root shoots that are covered in tough, sickle-shaped prickles that are appressed below. The leaves are pinnatifid with 5 to 7 leaflets. They are markedly petiolate, obovate, smooth-margined, glabrous, glossy and dark green above, lighter and simple-serrate beneath.

Characteristics: The sepals revolute at the end of the flowering period and drop when the fruit ripens.

Habitat: Rosa canina grows in Europe and North Africa and is extensively cultivated.

Production: Dog Rose fruit consist of the ripe, dried fruit (nutlet) of various species of the genus Rosa particularly Rosa moschata. The fruits are secondary products of Dog Rose shells. Dog Rose shells consist of the ripe, fresh or dried, opened seed receptacle, whole or cut and freed from hairs, of Rosa canina, Rosa pendulina, Rosa rugosa, Rosa moschata and other Rosa species. The ripe receptacles are harvested by hand and dried in the air, sun or in drying plants at a maximum temperature of 80° C. The dry Dog Roses are broken up and the fruit and skins are separated by sieving.

Other Names: Brier Hip, Hip, Rose Hip, Sweet Briar, Brier Rose, Eglantine Gall, Hogseed, Dog-Berry, Sweet Brier, Wild Brier, Witches' Brier

ACTIONS AND PHARMACOLOGY

COMPOUNDS: DOG ROSE FRUITS

Fatty oil (8 to 10%)

Tocopherol (vitamin E)

Volatile oil (0.3%)

Proteic substances

EFFECTS: DOG ROSE FRUITS

The pectin and fruit acid content are responsible for the diuretic and laxative effect.

COMPOUNDS: DOG ROSE SHELLS

Carotinoids

Flavonoids

Fruit acids: malic acid, citric acid

Monosaccharides/oligosaccharides (12 to 15%): invert sugar, saccharose

Pectins

Tannins

Vitamins: ascorbic acid (vitamin C, 0.2 to 2.4%)

EFFECTS: DOG ROSE SHELLS

The drug is a vitamin C supplement

INDICATIONS AND USAGE

DOG ROSE FRUITS

Unproven Uses: Dog Rose fruits are used in folk medicine for disorders of the efferent urinary tract and the kidneys, kidney stones, rheumatic conditions such as rheumatism, and gout, colds, scurvy and febrile conditions.

DOG ROSE SHELLS

Unproven Uses: Dog Rose shells are used in folk medicine for colds and 'flu,' intestinal conditions, digestive complaints, vitamin C deficiency, gallstones, subacidic-stomach, infectious diseases, conditions of the efferent urinary tract, edema, rheumatism and gout, bleeding and leucorrhea.

PRECAUTIONS AND ADVERSE REACTIONS

DOG ROSE FRUITS AND SHELLS

No health hazards or side effects are known in conjunction with the proper administration of designated therapeutic dosages.

DOSAGE

DOG ROSE FRUITS

Mode of Administration: Dog Rose fruits are available as whole and powdered drug.

Daily Dosage: The single dose is 2 gm drug.

Storage: Dog Rose should be stored in a dry and dark place.

DOG ROSE SHELLS

Mode of Administration: Dog Rose shells are available as whole, crude and powdered drug.

Daily Dosage: Tea: 2 to 5 gm drug added to 1 cup and steeped for 10 to 15 minutes

Storage: Should be stored in dark place.

LITERATURE

DOG ROSE SHELLS

Czygan FC, Rosa canina L. - Die Hunds- oder Heckenrose. In: ZPT 10(5):162. 1989.

Jaretzky R, Pharm Zentralh 82:229. 1941.

Kurucu S, Coskun M, Kartal M, High pressure liquid chromatographic determination of ascorbic acid in the fruits of some Rosa species growing in Turkey. In: PM 58(7)75. 1992.

Luckner M, Beβler O, PA 21:197. 1966.

Further information in:

Kern W, List PH, Hörhammer L (Hrsg.), Hagers Handbuch der Pharmazeutischen Praxis, 4. Aufl., Bde. 1-8: Springer Verlag Berlin, Heidelberg, New York, 1969.

Leung AY, Encyclopedia of Common Natural Ingredients Used in Food, Drugs, Cosmetics, John Wiley & Sons Inc., New York 1980.

Madaus G, Lehrbuch der Biologischen Arzneimittel, Bde 1-3, Nachdruck, Georg Olms Verlag Hildesheim 1979.

Steinegger E, Hänsel R, Pharmakognosie, 5. Aufl., Springer Verlag Heidelberg 1992.

Teuscher E, Biogene Arzneimittel, 5. Aufl., Wiss. Verlagsges. Stuttgart 1997.

Wagner H, Wiesenauer M, Phytotherapie. Phytopharmaka und pflanzliche Homöopathika, Fischer-Verlag, Stuttgart, Jena, New York 1995.

Wichtl M (Hrsg.), Teedrogen, 4. Aufl., Wiss. Verlagsges. Stuttgart 1997.

DOG ROSE FRUITS

Czygan FC, Rosa canina L. - Die Hunds- oder Heckenrose. In: ZPT 10(5):162. 1989.

Jaretzky R, Pharm Zentralh 82:229. 1941.

Luckner M, Beβler O, PA 21:197. 1966.

Further information in:

Kern W, List PH, Hörhammer L (Hrsg.), Hagers Handbuch der Pharmazeutischen Praxis, 4. Aufl., Bde. 1-8: Springer Verlag Berlin, Heidelberg, New York, 1969.

Leung AY, Encyclopedia of Common Natural Ingredients Used in Food, Drugs, Cosmetics, John Wiley & Sons Inc., New York 1980.

Dogwood

Cornus florida

DESCRIPTION

Medicinal Parts: The medicinal part is the dried bark. Fresh bark is also used occasionally.

Flower and Fruit: The flowers are sessile, small, greenish, and in clusters of 12 to 20 at the splayed end of a tough, 3 cm long stem. The bracts are white or pale reddish, ovate to long and are longer than the inflorescence. The petals are about 4 mm long. The fruit is a scarlet berry.

Leaves, Stem and Root: The plant is a deciduous shrub or a 4 to 9 m high tree, which is heavily branched and has a dark gray, thick and rough bark. The branches are smooth and covered in leaf scars. The leaves are 7 to 10 cm long, opposite, petiolate, entire, ovate acuminate at both ends, and somewhat rough. The upper surface is dark green. In autumn the upper surface is bright red to violet. The underside is always whitish-green. The leaves are slightly pubescent when young.

Habitat: Cornus florida is indigenous to eastern and southern North America; other varieties are found in Europe.

Production: American Boxwood bark and root-bark are the dried and occasionally fresh bark and root-bark of Cornus florida. It is collected in the wild.

Other Names: Dog-Tree, Box Tree, Boxwood, Budwood, False Box, Cornelian Tree, Cornel, Bitter Redberry, Green Ozier, Swamp Dogwood, Silky Cornel, Osier, Rose Willow

ACTIONS AND PHARMACOLOGY

COMPOUNDS

Steroid saponins: including sarsapogenin-O-beta-D-galactoside, sarsapogenin-O-beta-D-xylosyl-(1(2)-beta-D-galactoside

Iridoide monoterpenes: cornin (verbenalin)

Tannins

EFFECTS

Effect on mollusks: The drug destroys the biomphalaria glabratus snails (carrier of bilharziose).

Cardiac effect: Heart activity, at different levels up to the cessation of heartbeat, is examined depending on the concentration of the methanol extract.

Antiplasmodic effect: Induced malaria on chicks and Peking ducks was treated for 5 days with a water-insoluble fraction. As a result, antiplasmodic activity toward *P. cathemerium* could be observed, similar to that deployed by quinine and sulfadiazine. To date, the results cannot be sufficiently assessed.

The bark works as a tonic, an astringent and a stimulant.

INDICATIONS AND USAGE

Unproven Uses: In North America, the dried bark was used in folk medicine for strength, to stimulate appetite, for fever and for chronic diarrhea. It is used externally as an astringent for wounds and boils. Formerly, it was in use as a replacement for quinine. It is still used for headaches and fatigue.

Homeopathic Uses: Uses include for poor digestion and chronic attacks of fever.

PRECAUTIONS AND ADVERSE REACTIONS

Health risks or side effects following the proper administration of designated therapeutic dosages are not recorded.

DOSAGE

Mode of Administration: Formerly the drug was used internally as a tincture as an alternative to quinine and externally as a liquid extract.

Homeopathic Dosage: Oral: 5 drops, 1 tablet or 10 globules every 30 to 60 minutes (acute) or 1 to 3 times a day (chronic); parenterally: 1 to 2 ml sc acute, 3 times daily; chronic: once a day (HAB34).

Preparation: Decoction or infusion (no specifications).

LITERATURE

Caetano-Anolles G, Trigiano RN, Windham MT, Sequence signatures from DNA amplification fingerprints reveal fine population structure of the dogwood pathogen Discula destructiva. FEMS Microbiol Lett, 145:377-83, 1996 Dec 15

Jacobs, B, In: Jacobs ML, Burlage HM: Index of Plants of North Carolina with Reputed Medicinal Uses, USA. 1958.

Jensen SR, Kjaer A, Nielsen BJ, Biochem Syst Ecol 3:75-78. 1975.

Hänsel R, Keller K, Rimpler H, Schneider G (Hrsg.), Hagers Handbuch der Pharmazeutischen Praxis, 5. Aufl., Bde 4-6 (Drogen), Springer Verlag Berlin, Heidelberg, New York, 1992-1994.

Hostettmann K, Hostettmann-Kaldas M, Nakanishi K, Helv Chim Acta 61:1990. 1978.

Dorema ammoniacum

See Ammoniac Gum

Dorstenia contrayerva

See Contrayerva

Dragon's Blood (Xue-Jie)

Daemonorops draco

DESCRIPTION

Medicinal Parts: The medicinal part is the red resin from the fruit, which is extracted from both Daemonorops draco and Daemonorops propinquis.

Flower and Fruit: The flowers are arranged along the branch. The fruit is a cherry-sized berry ending in a point. When the fruit are ripe, they are covered in a reddish, resinous substance, which is separated in various ways.

Leaves, Stem and Root: Dragon's Blood is a tree with long, thin, flexible stems, which are inclined to climb when they are older. The leaves have thorny petioles, which grow into long appendages. The bark is covered in hundreds of flattened thorns.

Habitat: Malaysia, Indonesia.

Production: Dragon's Blood resin is the resin of Daemonorops draco.

Other Names: Dracorubin, Sanguis Draconis, Draconis Resina, Xue-Jie

ACTIONS AND PHARMACOLOGY

COMPOUNDS

Ester resins (dracoresin): benzoyl ester of dracoresinotannol

Dracoresen

Flavane quinones: including dracorubin (dracocarmin), dracorhodin, both colored an intense red

EFFECTS

Dragon's Blood has an astringent effect.

INDICATIONS AND USAGE

Unproven Uses: The resin is used for diarrhea, digestive disorders and as a coloring agent.

PRECAUTIONS AND ADVERSE REACTIONS

Health risks or side effects following the proper administration of designated therapeutic dosages are not recorded.

DOSAGE

Mode of Administration: The resin is used in a powder form.

LITERATURE

Hegnauer R, Chemotaxonomie der Pflanzen, Bde 1-11, Birkhäuser Verlag Basel, Boston, Berlin 1962-1997.

Kern W, List PH, Hörhammer L (Hrsg.), Hagers Handbuch der Pharmazeutischen Praxis, 4. Aufl., Bde 1-8, Springer Verlag Berlin, Heidelberg, New York, 1969.

Merlini L, Gasini G, J Chem Soc Perkin I 1976:1570. 1976.

Rao SR et al., JNP 45:646. 1982.

Drimys winteri

See Winter's Bark

Drosera ramentacea

See Sundew

Dryas octopetala

See Mountain Avens

Dryopteris filix-mas

See Male Fern

Duckweed

Lemna minor

DESCRIPTION

Medicinal Parts: The medicinal part is the whole fresh plant.

Flower and Fruit: The plant flowers infrequently. The tiny inconspicuous flowers have 2 unevenly sized stamens and 1 pistil. A delicate membranous bract surrounds 3 flowers, which are located on the edge of the stem. The fruit is tubular with 1 ovule. The seeds have longitudinal ribs.

Leaves, Stem and Root: Lemna minor is a water plant with leaf-like organs that are 2 to 6 mm long. They are flat, have 3 to 5 ribs, and are sometimes pigmented with red. Two to six leaf-like shoots stick together, and each bears a root with a rounded root cover.

Characteristics: The plant has leaf-like shoots with 1 root per leaf.

Habitat: The plant is found worldwide in cooler, oceanic climates. The plant is not found in east Asia and South Africa.

Production: Duckweed is the fresh plant Lemna minor.

ACTIONS AND PHARMACOLOGY

COMPOUNDS

Flavonoids: in particular C-glucosyl-flavone, including among others orientin, isoorientin, vitexin, isovitexin, lutonarin, vicenin-1; also O-glycosides, including among others apigenin-7-O-glucoside, luteolin-7-O-glycoside

Cyclopentane fatty acids, with structure resembling prostaglandin

Polysaccharides: apiogalacturonans

Cardiac steroids (cardenolides)

EFFECTS

No information is available.

INDICATIONS AND USAGE

Unproven Uses: Duckweed is used internally for inflammation of the upper respiratory tract and externally for gout and rheumatism.

Chinese Medicine: Duckweed is used for measles, edema, joint pain, dysuria, acne, erysipelas and epilepsy.

Homeopathic Uses: Duckweed is used for chronic colds.

PRECAUTIONS AND ADVERSE REACTIONS

No health hazards or side effects are known in conjunction with the proper administration of designated therapeutic dosages.

DOSAGE

Mode of Administration: The plant is available as fresh or ground herb and as an extract.

Homeopathic Dosage: 5 drops, 1 tablet or 10 globules every 30 to 60 minutes (acute) or 1 to 3 times daily (chronic); parenterally: 1 to 2 ml s.c., acute: 3 times daily; chronic: once a day (HAB1).

LITERATURE

Hänsel R, Keller K, Rimpler H, Schneider G (Hrsg.), Hagers Handbuch der Pharmazeutischen Praxis, 5. Aufl., Bde 4-6 (Drogen), Springer Verlag Berlin, Heidelberg, New York, 1992-1994.

Madaus G. Lehrbuch der Biologischen Arzneimittel, Bde 1-3, Nachdruck, Georg Olms Verlag Hildesheim 1979.

Dusty Miller

Senecio bicolor

DESCRIPTION

Medicinal Parts: The medicinal parts are the fresh plant harvested before flowering, the herb of the flowering plant, and the whole fresh, flowering plant.

Flower and Fruit: The plant has numerous yellow capitula, 12 to 15 cm in diameter, on short peduncles. The calyx only has a few sepals. There are 10 to 12 lingual florets. The fruit is striped.

Leaves, Stem and Root: Senecio cineraria is a semi-shrub that grows up to 80 cm high. The stem is erect, heavily branched at the base, and sometimes snow-white tomentose. The leaves are densely pubescent beneath and more or less cobwebbed on the upper surface. They may have sparse greenish hairs. The lower leaves are oval to lanceolate, pinnatifid, and the outer lobes are usually longer than they are wide.

Habitat: The plant is indigenous to the Mediterranean region, naturalized in North America and cultivated as an ornamental plant in many countries.

Production: Cineraria juice is the juice of the whole Senecio cinerarian plant.

Other Names: Cineraria Maritima

ACTIONS AND PHARMACOLOGY

COMPOUNDS

Pyrrolizidine alkaloids (0.9% in the blossoming foliage): including, among others, jaconine, jacobine, otosenine, retrorsine, senecionine, seneciphylline

Polyynes

EFFECTS

The active agents are the alkaloids jacobin, senecionin, and otosenin These pyrrolizidine alkaloids are hepatotoxic and carcinogenic.

INDICATIONS AND USAGE

Unproven Uses: Though no longer recommended, the plant previously was administered for ailments of the eye, as an emmenagogic, and in cataplasms and oral rinses.

Homeopathic Uses: In homeopathy, the juice is used to treat eye-sight problems (for the treatment of spots before the eyes), migraine, and as an emmenagogue.

PRECAUTIONS AND ADVERSE REACTIONS

Dusty Miller should not be taken internally (except in homeopathic dosages) because of the potential hepatotoxicity and carcinogenicity of the pyrrolizidine alkaloids and the 1,2-unsaturated necic parent substances.

DOSAGE

Mode of Administration: The use of the sterilized juice is no longer recommended for internal use, nor is any other preparation of Dusty Miller.

LITERATURE

Adams R et al., J Am Chem Soc 71:1953-1956. 1941.

Barger G et al., J Chem Soc:584. 1937.

Habib AM, PM 26:279. 1974.

Klasek A et al., Coll Czech Chem Comm 40:2524. 1975.

Nachmann RJ, PH 22:780-782. 1983.

Resch JF et al., PM 47:255. 1983.

Röder E, DAZ 132:2427. 1992.

Willaman JJ, Hui-Li L, (1970) Lloydia 33(3A):1.

Further information in:

Hänsel R, Keller K, Rimpler H, Schneider G (Hrsg.), Hagers Handbuch der Pharmazeutischen Praxis, 5. Aufl., Bde 4-6 (Drogen): Springer Verlag Berlin, Heidelberg, New York, 1992-1994 (unter Senecio bicolor).

Madaus G, Lehrbuch der Biologischen Arzneimittel, Bde 1-3, Nachdruck, Georg Olms Verlag Hildesheim 1979 (unter Cineraria maritima).

Teuscher E, Lindequist U, Biogene Gifte - Biologie, Chemie, Pharmakologie, 2. Aufl., Fischer Verlag Stuttgart 1994 (unter Senecio bicolor).

Dwarf Elder

Sambucus ebulus

DESCRIPTION

Medicinal Parts: The medicinal parts are the dried leaves, the ripe, dried or fresh fruit and the dried roots.

Flowers and Fruit: The reddish-white flowers are in a terminal, umbrella-like, richly blossomed, paniculate cyme with 3 main branches. The calyx margin is 5-tipped. The corolla has fused petals and is rotate with 5 acuminate tips. The 5 stamens have dark red anthers and an inferior, 3-valved ovary with 3 stigmas. The fruit is a black, globular, berry-like drupe with at least 3 to 4 ovate seeds. When ripe, the fruit stems are erect and violet or crimson.

Leaves, Stem and Root: Dwarf Elder is a perennial, herb-like plant 0.5 to 2 m high with a sturdy, finger-thick, branched rhizome that creeps deeply and horizontally. The stems are leafy, erect, sturdy and branched above. They die off in autumn. The leaves are crossed opposite, odd-pinate with 3 to 4 pairs of ovate-lanceolate leaflets and 2 large, ovate-lanceolate, and serrate stipules.

Characteristics: The fragrance is similar to that of sunflowers or almond.

Habitat: The plant is found from southern Sweden throughout central and southern Europe, in northern Africa, in western Asia as far as Iran, and in North America.

Production: Dwarf Elder root is the root of Sambucus ebulus, which is collected in the spring or late autumn and then air-dried.

Other Names: Danewort, Walewort, Blood Elder, Blood Hilder

ACTIONS AND PHARMACOLOGY

COMPOUNDS

Iridoides: ebuloside, 6′-0-apiosyl-ebuloside, 7,7-0-dihydroebuloside, secoebuloside, isoswer-oside

Nauseant, purgative resins with unresolved structure

EFFECTS

The drug is said to be a mild diuretic.

INDICATIONS AND USAGE

Unproven Uses: Dwarf Elder is used in folk medicine as an ingredient in different teas prepared to assist in weight reduction and alleviate rheumatism. The drug also is used for constipation and as an emetic and to treat edema and kidney disease.

PRECAUTIONS AND ADVERSE REACTIONS

Health risks or side effects following the proper administration of designated therapeutic dosages are not recorded.

OVERDOSAGE

According to older scientific reports, large quantities of all parts of the plant, (in particular the raw berries) leads to vomiting, bloody diarrhea, cyanosis, dizziness, headache, and unconsciousness. Cases of death are also mentioned.

DOSAGE

Mode of Administration: Dwarf Elder is obsolete as a drug in most countries. It is found in some tea mixtures, but is not used in medicinal preparations.

LITERATURE

Gross GA, Phytochemische Untersuchungen von Inhaltsstoffen der Zwergholunderwurzel, Dissertation Zürich. 1985.

Frohne D, Pfänder HJ, Giftpflanzen - Ein Handbuch für Apotheker, Toxikologen und Biologen, 4. Aufl., Wiss. Verlagsges. mbH Stuttgart 1997.

Hänsel R, Keller K, Rimpler H, Schneider G (Hrsg.), Hagers Handbuch der Pharmazeutischen Praxis, 5. Aufl., Bde 4-6 (Drogen): Springer Verlag Berlin, Heidelberg, New York, 1992-1994.

Lewin L, Gifte und Vergiftungen, 6. Aufl., Nachdruck, Haug Verlag, Heidelberg 1992.

Madaus G, Lehrbuch der Biologischen Arzneimittel, Bde 1-3, Nachdruck, Georg Olms Verlag Hildesheim 1979.

Petkov V, Markovska V, (1981) Plant Med Phytother 15(3):172.

Roth L, Daunderer M, Kormann K, Giftpflanzen, Pflanzengifte, 4. Aufl., Ecomed Fachverlag Landsberg Lech 1993.

Dyer's Broom

Genista tinctoria

DESCRIPTION

Medicinal Parts: The entire plant has medicinal applications.

Flower and Fruit: The flowers are in short, terminal racemes. They are golden yellow and bean-shaped, 1.5 to 2 cm long and are on pedicles, which are shorter than the calyx. The petal stems of the 4 lower petals are initially straight, but in moments of tension, when for instance, they are touched by an insect, they curl down suddenly and the flower opens. The fruit is a smooth pod 2.5 to 3.5 cm long. It is brown, compressed at the sides, and contains 5 to 10 seeds.

Leaves, Stem and Root: The plant is a 30 to 60 cm high, always thornless subshrub with a creeping, woody rhizome. The florescent green stems are smooth and produce fairly rigid, smooth or pubescent forked branches, which sprout lanceolate leaves. The leaves are alternate, glabrous, entire-margined, 1.25 to 2.5 cm long, nearly sessile, and with a ciliate margin. The stipules are linear-awl-shaped.

Habitat: Dyer's Broom is indigenous to the Mediterranean region, the Canary Islands, Europe and western Asia, and cultivated elsewhere, including the eastern U.S.

Production: Dyer's Broom leaves are the green leaves of Genista tinctoria.

Other Names: Dyer's Weed, Dyer's Greenwood, Dyer's Whin, Furze, Green Broom, Greenweed, Wood Waxen

ACTIONS AND PHARMACOLOGY

COMPOUNDS

Quinolizidine alkaloids: main alkaloids — cytisine, methylcytisine, anagyrine, as well as isosparteine, lupanine, tinctorin

Flavonoids: in particular luteolin glycosides

Isoflavonoids: genistein, genistin

Lectins

EFFECTS

The drug acts as a purifier, cathartic, diuretic, purgative and emetic. It increases heart rate, strengthens the walls of blood vessels, stimulates kidney blood circulation and affects metabolism.

INDICATIONS AND USAGE

Unproven Uses: Formerly, the drug was used as a purgative and to remove bladder stones, as well as for digestive disorders and gout. Once an infusion has been taken, breathing deepens and pain in the lumbar and pelvic region is alleviated.

PRECAUTIONS AND ADVERSE REACTIONS

General: Health risks or side effects following the proper administration of designated therapeutic dosages are not recorded. Overdosage can lead to diarrhea and to symptoms of a cystine poisoning. Anagyrine has exhibited teratogenic effect in animal experiments.

Pregnancy: Not to be used during pregnancy.

DOSAGE

Mode of Administration: The drug is used internally as an infusion.

Preparations: To prepare an infusion, use 1 teaspoonful of the ground drug per cup of water.

Daily Dosage: Drink 1 to 2 cups of infusion daily.

LITERATURE

Atkinson JE et al., (1969) Tetrahedron 25:1507.

Bricout J, (1974) Phytochemistry 13:2819.

Harborne JB, (1969) Phytochemistry 8:1449.

Hrochova V, Sitaniova H, Farm Obz 51:131. 1982.

Inouye H et al., (1968) Tetrahedron Letters 4429.

Inouye H et al., (1970) Chem Pharm Bull 18:1856.

Lewis JR, Gupta P, (1971) J Chem Soc Chem Comm 4:629.

Rulko F, (1976) Pr Nauk Akad. Med Wroclawin 8:3.

Sadritdinov F, (1971) Farmakol Alkaloidov Serdechnykh Glikozidov 146.

Swietek L, Dombrowicz E, (1984) Farm Pol 40(12):729.

Ulubelen A et al., (1971) Lloydia 34(2):258.

Further information in:

Chan, EH et al. (Eds), Advances in Chinese Medicinal Materials Research, World Scientific Pub. Co. Singapore 1985.

Kern W, List PH, Hörhammer L (Hrsg.), Hagers Handbuch der Pharmazeutischen Praxis, 4. Aufl., Bde. 1-8, Springer Verlag Berlin, Heidelberg, New York, 1969.

Leung AY, Encyclopedia of Common Natural Ingredients Used in Food Drugs and Cosmetics, John Wiley & Sons Inc., New York 1980.

Lewin L, Gifte und Vergiftungen, 6. Aufl., Nachdruck, Haug Verlag, Heidelberg 1992.

Madaus G, Lehrbuch der Biologischen Arzneimittel, Bde 1-3, Nachdruck, Georg Olms Verlag Hildesheim 1979.

Roth L, Daunderer M, Kormann K, Giftpflanzen, Pflanzengifte, 4. Aufl., Ecomed Fachverlag Landsberg Lech 1993.

Teuscher E, Lindequist U, Biogene Gifte - Biologie, Chemie, Pharmakologie, 2. Aufl., Fischer Verlag Stuttgart 1994.

Wichtl M (Hrsg.), Teedrogen, 4. Aufl., Wiss. Verlagsges. Stuttgart 1997.

Echinacea

Echinaceae species

TRADE NAMES

Echinacea (available from numerous manafacturers), Echinacea Root, Echinacea Standardized, Echinacea Root Herbal, Echinacea angustifolia Herb, Echinacea purpurea Root

DESCRIPTION

Medicinal Parts: The medicinal parts are, depending on varieties, the roots, leaves or the whole plant in various stages of development.

Flower and Fruit: The flower-heads are large and solitary on terminal peduncles with spreading ray florets. The bracts are in a number of rows. The bracts are leafy, rigid, thorny tipped, and longer than the conical erect disc florets. The reddish or occasionally white florets are conspicuous. The ligual florets are usually sterile and 3 cm long. The pappus is small or absent.

Leaves, Stem and Root: Echinacea is usually a perennial herb and grows up to 45 cm. in height. The leaves are large, solitary, opposite or alternate and are smooth-margined. They are 7 to 20 cm long and have a rough surface. The leaves are entire-margined and are on slender petioles. A transverse section of the rhizome shows a thin bark and a yellowish, porous wood, which is flecked with black.

Characteristics: The taste is slightly sweet then bitter leaving a tingling sensation on the tongue. The odor is faintly aromatic.

Habitat: Echinacea purpurea and Echinaceae pallida grow in the middle or eastern U.S. and is cultivated in Europe.

Production: Echinacea purpurea herb consists of the fresh, above-ground parts, harvested at flowering time. The root consists of the fresh or dried underground part, gathered in autumn. Echinacea pallida herb consists of the fresh or dried above-ground parts, collected at the time of flowering. Echinacea angustifolia herb and root consist of the fresh or dried roots, or above-ground parts collected at the time of flowering.

Not to be Confused With: The herbs and roots of Echinacea purpurea, Echinacea angustifolia and Echinacea pallida have different medicinal properties. Some Echinacea species may be confused with or adulterated with Parthenium integrifoium.

Other Names: Black Sampson, Niggerhead, Rudbeckia, Sampson Root, Purple Coneflower, Hedgehog, Red Sunflower

ACTIONS AND PHARMACOLOGY

COMPOUNDS: ECHINACEA PURPUREA HERB

Water-soluble immunostimulating polysaccharides (4-O-methylglucuronylarabinoxylans, acidic arabinorhamno-galactans)

Volatile oil (under 0.08-0.32%): components including germacrene alcohol, borneol, bornylacetate, pentadeca-8-en-2-on, germacrene D, caryophyllene, caryophyllene epoxide

Flavonoids: ferulic acid derivatives including cichoriic acid, cichoriic acid methyl ester, 2-O- caffeoyl-3-O-feruloyl-tartaric acid, 2,3-O-diferuloyl tartaric acid 2-O-caffeoyl tartaric acid

Alkamides: including undeca-2E,4Z-dien-8,10-diin acid- and dodeca-2E,4E-8Z,10E/Z- tetraen acid isobutylamide

Polyenes: trideca-1,11-dien-3,5,7,9,-tetraine, trideca-1-en-3,5,7,9,11-pentaine, trideca-8,10,12-trien-2,4,6-triine, pontica epoxide

COMPOUNDS: ECHINACEA PURPUREA ROOT

Water-soluble immunostimulating polysaccharides

Water-soluble immunostimulating glycoproteins

Volatile oil (0.2%): components including caryophyllene, humules, caryophyllene epoxide, dodeca-2,4-dien-1-yl-isovalerate, germacrene D, palmitic acid, linolenic acid

Caffeic and ferulic acid derivatives (0.6-2.1%): including cichoriic acid, cichoriic acid methyl ester, 2-O- caffeoyl tartaric acid

Alkamides (0.01-0.04%): including undeca-2E,4Z-dien-8,10-diinacetyl- and dodeca-2E,4E-8Z,10E/Z-tetracetyliso-butylamide

Polyynes (0.01mg/%): including trideca-1-en-3,5,7,9,11-pentain, trideca-1,11-dien-3,5,7,9,-tetraine, trideca-8,10,12-trien-2,4,6-triine, pontica epoxide

Effective pyrrolizidine alkaloids: tussilagine, isotussilagine

COMPOUNDS: ECHINACEA PALLIDA HERB

Volatile oil (0.1%)- including 1,8-pentadecadien

Flavonoids: in particular rutin

Caffeic acid derivatives: Cichoriic acid, chlorogenic acid, isochlorogenic acid, verbascoside

Alkamides: including dodeca-2E,4E-8Z,10E-tetracetyliso-butylamide

COMPOUNDS: ECHINACEA PALLIDA ROOT

Water-soluble immunstimulating polysaccharides (arabino-rhamnogalactans)

Volatile oil (0.2 - 2%): chief components include pentadeca-8Z-en-2-on, pentadeca-1,8Z-dien, 1-pentadecan

Caffeic acid derivatives: echinacoside

Alkamides: including isomeric dodeca-2E,4E-8Z,10E/Z-tetraenic acid-isobutylamide

Polyynes: including trideca-1-en-3,5,7,9,11-pentain, pontica epoxide

COMPOUNDS: ECHINACEA ANGUSTIFOLIA HERB

Volatile oil (under 0.1%): typical components consist of epishyobunol, beta-farnesene, alpha- and beta-pinenes, myrcene, carvomenthene, caryophyllene

Flavonoids

Caffeic acid derivatives: cichoriic acid, chlorogenic acid, isochlorogenic acid, verbascoside, echinacoside

Alkamides: including dodeca-2E,4E-8Z,10E-tetracetyl-isobutylamide

Polyynes: including trideca-1-en-3,5,7,9,11-pentaine, pontica epoxide

COMPOUNDS: ECHINACEA ANGUSTIFOLIA ROOT

Volatile oil (under 1%): components include dodeca-2,4-dien-1-ylisovalerate, as well as palmitic acid, linolenic acid

Flavonoids

Caffeic acid derivatives (0.3 to 1.3%): echinacoside, cynarin

Alkamides (0.01%): including dodeca-2E,4E-8Z,10E/Z- tetracetyl isobutylamide

Polyynes: including trideca-1-en-3,5,7,9,11-pentaine, pontica epoxide, in dehydrated roots only traces

EFFECTS: ALL VARIETIES

General

Echinacea activity is directed towards the nonspecific cellular immune system. The herb exerts anti-inflammatory, immunostimulating, bactericidal, and wound healing actions, depending on the type of plant species. The main active principles of the immunostimulating, antibacterial and virostatic drug are the alkamides, glycoproteins, caffeic acid derivatives (cichoriic acid and echinosides) and polysaccarides.

Immunostimulating

Ethanolic root extracts of the Echinacea purpurea, Echinacea pallida and Echinacea angustifolia were shown to cause a 23% increase of the phagocytosis rate in granulocyte smears *in vitro* (Jurcic, 1989; Melchart 1995). Confirmed by the carbon clearance test and granulocyte tests, the ethanolic root extracts significantly enhance phagocytosis (Bauer, 1988). The ethanolic extracts of aerial parts of Echinacea angustifolia and Echinacea purpurea exert immunostimulatory effects also through metabolic and bactericidal activities of peritoneal macrophages. The ethanolic extracts of both Echinacea plants also increase the total weight of the spleen (Bukovsky, 1993).

Anti-Inflammatory

Polyunsaturated alkamides in Echinacea angustifolia exert anti-inflammatory effects through inhibition of cyclooxygenase and 5-lipoxygenase (Muller-Jakic, 1994). The polysaccharide fraction of Echinacea angustifolia exerts anti-inflammatory effects (Tubaro, 1987), and the polysaccharide from Echinacea purpurea induces an acute phase reaction. The acute phase reaction occurs with enhancing the spontaneous motility of PMN and increasing the ability of these cells to kill bacteria such as staphylococci. (Roesler, 1991).

Cytokine Stimulation

Arabinogalactan, a highly purified polysaccharide from plant cell cultures of Echinacea purpurea, is effective in activating macrophage cytotoxicity actions against tumor cells and microorganisms (Leishmania enriettii). This polysaccharide induces macrophages to produce tumor necrosis factor (TNF-alpha), interleukin-1 (IL-1), interleukin-6 (IL-6), interleukin-10 (IL-10) and interferon-beta. The component also induces a slight increase in T-cell proliferation (Burger, 1997; Luettig, 1989; Roesler, 1991). Extracts of Echinacea purpurea stimulate cell-mediated immunity through the production of lymphokines by lymphocytes (Coeugniet, 1987). Echinacea purpurea herb has shown some short-term viral resistance against influenza, herpes, and vesicular stomatitis viruses, which has been credited to an interferon-like effect (Wacker, 1978).

Collagen Protectant

The caffeic acid derivatives exert a protective effect on the free-radical-induced degradation of Type III collagen. Collagen degradation was inhibited the greatest by echinacoside and chicoriic acid, then cynarine and chlorogenic acid. The collagen protection from free radical damage is through a scavenging effect on reactive oxygen species and/or C-, N-, S-centered secondary radicals. These activities may be useful for the treatment/protection of photodamage of the skin by UVA/UVB radiation, in which oxidative stress plays a critical role (Facino, 1995).

CLINICAL TRIALS

A randomized, placebo-controlled, double-blind trial evaluated the effect of a fluid extract of Echinacea purpurea on the incidence and severity of colds and respiratory infections. There were 109 patients with a history of more than 3 colds or respiratory infections in the previous year included in the study. The fluid extract, given 4 mL twice daily for 8 weeks, did not significantly decrease the incidence, duration or severity of colds and respiratory infections compared to placebo (Grimm, 1999).

The efficacy and safety of Echinaforce® (Echinacea purpurea preparation from 95% herb and 5% root), Echinacea concentrate (same preparation at 7 times higher concentration), and special Echinacea purpurea root preparation were evaluated in the treatment of the common cold. There were 559 volunteers with a common cold included in the study. The participants received 2 tablets 3 times daily. The primary endpoint was the relative reduction of the complaint index, which is a group of 12 symptoms that occur during common cold. Echinaforce® and its concentrated preparation were significantly more effective than the special extract or placebo treatment group. All treatments were well tolerated with the frequency of adverse events not significantly higher than in the placebo group (Brinkeborn, 1999).

The safety and efficacy of Echinacea angustifolia and Echinacea purpurea ethanolic root extracts for the prevention of upper respiratory tract infections (URTI) was determined in a double-blind, placebo-controlled study. The time until the first URTI (time and event) and adverse effects were evaluated in 302 patients. The root extract dosages were 50 drops twice daily for 12 weeks from Monday to Friday. The time until occurrence of a URTI was 66 days in the Echinacea angustifolia group, 69 days in the Echinacae purpura group and 65 days in the placebo group. Though the results do not prove efficacy of prophylaxis, the authors conclude that Echinacea may reduce the risk of developing a URTI by 10 to 20% (Melchart, 1998).

A randomized, placebo-controlled, double-blind study was conducted to determine the effect of an extract of Echinaceae pallidae root with influenza infections of the upper respiratory tract. A dose of 900 mg daily was evaluated for the relief of symptoms, including shortening of the illness period and curing cough and hoarseness. The length of the illness period was reduced significantly with the extract from 13 to 9 days compared with placebo. The strongest effects on the clinical symptoms were achieved after 8-10 days (Brauning, 1993).

INDICATIONS AND USAGE

ECHINACEA PURPUREA HERB

Approved by Commission E:

- Common cold
- Cough/bronchitis
- Fevers and colds
- Infections of the urinary tract
- Inflammation of the mouth and pharynx
- Tendency to infection
- Wounds and burns

Echinacea purpurea herb is used internally as supportive therapy for colds and chronic infections of the respiratory tract and lower urinary tract. It can also be applied locally to poorly healing superficial wounds.

ECHINACEA PURPUREA ROOT

Unproven Uses: Echinacea purpurea root is used for acute and chronic respiratory tract infections (of viral and bacterial origin); increased susceptibility to infection due to temporarily lowered resistance, treatment of leukopenia following radio and cytostatic therapy and in support of anti-infectious chemotherapy.

ECHINACEA PALLIDA ROOT

Approved by Commission E:

- Fevers and colds

Echinacea pallida root is used as a supportive therapy for influenza-like infections.

ECHINACEA ANGUSTIFOLIA HERB AND ROOT

Unproven Uses: In folk medicine, native Americans use the drug externally for burns, swelling of the lymph nodes, and insect bites. The drug is used internally for pain associated with headaches and stomach aches, measles, coughs and gonorrhea. The drug has also been used for rattlesnake bites. Today the drug is used for prophylaxis and treatment of 'flu' infections, sepsis, and mild to moderate cold infections. Externally, the drug is used for treatment of poorly healing wounds and inflammatory conditions such as abscesses and leg ulcers.

CONTRAINDICATIONS

ALL VARIETIES AND FORMS

Because of a possible activation of autoimmune aggressions and other overreactive immune responses, the drug should not be administered in the presence of multiple sclerosis, leukosis, collagen disease, AIDS or tuberculosis. Parenteral administration should not be used in patients with tendencies to allergies, especially allergies to members of the composite family (Asteraceae). Echinacea should not be used during pregnancy.

PRECAUTIONS AND ADVERSE REACTIONS

ALL VARIETIES AND FORMS

General: When used parenterally, dose-dependent short-term fever reactions, nausea and vomiting can occur. Caution should be exercised if the drug is administered parenterally to people with diabetes. Hypersensitivity reactions with anaphylaxis have been reported (Mullins, 1998). Rashes, itching, occasional swelling of the face, breathing difficulties, dizziness and a drop in blood pressure have been observed after administration of preparations containing Echinacea.

Fertility: High concentrations of Echinacea had adverse effects on oocytes in animal models (Ondrizek, 1999).

Pregnancy: Parenteral administration should be avoided during pregnancy.

Drug Interactions: The immune-stimulating effect of echinacea may interfere with drugs that have immunosuppressant effects. Interaction may occur when using cyclosporine or other anti-rejection drugs. Echinacea may also interfere with the cancer chemotherapeutic effect of corticosteroids.

DOSAGE

ECHINACEA PURPUREA HERB

Mode of Administration: Pressed juice and galenic preparations for internal and external use.

Preparation: The pressed juice is prepared in a concentration of 2.5:1 and is stabilized with 22% alcohol. Other complicated methods of preparation are known.

Daily Dosage: When used internally, the recommended dosage is 6 to 9 ml of the expressed juice. The recommended dosage for parenteral administration should be individualized, depending on the seriousness of the condition as well as the specific nature of the respective preparation. Parenteral application requires a gradation of dosage, especially for children. The manufacturer is required to show this information for the respective preparation. When used externally, semi-solid preparations containing at least 15% pressed juice are used for a maximum of 8 weeks.

ECHINACEA PURPUREA ROOT

Mode of Administration: Comminuted drug for decoctions and galenic preparations.

Daily Dosage: When using the tincture, 30 to 60 drops should be taken three times a day.

Storage: Echinacea should be protected from light sources, and, if possible be uncomminuted.

ECHINACEA PALLIDA HERB AND ROOT

Mode of Administration: As a liquid preparation for oral use.

Preparation: A 1:5 tincture is made using 50% (V/V) ethanol and native dried extract (50% ethanol in a 7 to 11:1 proportion)

Daily Dosage: The daily dose is 900 mg of drug. The drug should be used for a maximum of 8 weeks.

Storage: Protect from light sources. If possible, store uncomminuted.

ECHINACEA ANGUSTIFOLIA HERB AND ROOT

Mode of Administration: Since the efficacy in the claimed areas of application has not been documented, therapeutic application cannot be recommended. Because of the risks, the use of parenteral preparations is not justified.

How Supplied:

Capsule — 100mg, 125mg, 250mg, 380mg 390mg, 400mg, 430mg, 450mg, 500mg

Liquid — 120mg/5mL

Preparation: The root tea is prepared using 1/2 teaspoonful of comminuted drug with boiling water. Strain after 10 minutes.

Daily Dosage: For colds, drink 1 cup freshly made tea several times daily.

Storage: Protect from light sources. If possible, store uncomminuted.

LITERATURE

Bauer R, Arzneipflanzenporträt: Echinacea- welche Inhaltsstoffe wirken immunmodulierend? In: DAZ 132(23):1233. 1992.

Bauer R, Echinacea. In: PM 59(6):94. 1992.

Bauer R, Jurcic K, Puhlmann J, Wagner H, Immunologische in vivo- und in vitro Untersuchnugnen mit Echinacea-Extrakten. In: Arzneim Forsch 38:276-281. 1988.

Bauer R, Neues von ''immunmodulierenden Drogen'' und ''Drogen mit antiallergischer und antiinflammatorischer Wirkung''. In: ZPT 14(1):23-24. 1993.

Bauer R, Remiger P, Jurcic K, Wagner H, Beeinflussung der Phagozytoseaktivität durch Echinacea-Extrakte. In: ZPT 10:43-48. 1989.

Bauer R, Remiger P, Wagner H, Echinacea-Vergleichende DC- und HPLC-Analyse der Herba-Drogen von Echinacea purpurea, Echinacea pallida und Echinacea angustifolia. In: DAZ 128:174-180. 1988.

Bauer R, Wagner H, Echinacea - Der Sonnenhut - Stand der Forschung. In: ZPT 9(8):151. 1988.

Bauer R, Wagner H, Echinacea-Drogen - Who is who? In: ZPT 9(6):191. 1988.

Bauer R, Wagner H, Echinacea. Wissenschaftliche Verlagsgesellschaft mbH Stuttgart 1990.

Bauer, R et al., (1985) Helv Chim Acta 68:2355.

Bauer, R et al., (1987) Phytochemistry 26(4):1198.

Becker H, (1982) Dtsch Apoth Ztg 122(45):2320.

Beuscher N, Scheit KH, Bodinet C, Egert D, Modulation der körpereigenen Immunabwehr durch polymere Substanzen aus Baptisia tinctoria und Echinacea purpurea. In: Immunotherapeutic prospects of infectious diseases, Hrsg. Masihi KN, Lange W. Springer, Heidel.

Beuscher N, Über die medikamentöse Beeinflussung zellulärer Resistenzmechanismen im Tierversuch. Aktivierung von Peritonealmakrophagen der Maus durch pflanzliche Reizkörper. In: Arzneim Forsch 32(I):134-138. 1977.

Bodinet C, Beuscher N, Antiviral and immunological activity of glykoproteins from the root of Echinacea purpurea. In: PM, Abstracts of the 39th Annual Congress of Medicinal Plant Research. 1991.

Bohlmann F, Hoffman H, (1983) Phytochemistry 22(5):1173.

Bräunig B, Dorn M, Knick E, Echinaceae purpureae radix: zur Stärkung der körpereigenen Abwehr bei grippalem Infekten. In: ZPT 13(1):7. 1992.

Brinkeborn R, Shah D, Degenring F. Echinaforce and other Echinacea fresh plant preparations in the treatment of the common cold. A randomized, placebo controlled, double-blind clinical trial. Phytomedicine. 1999 Mar;6(1):1-6.

Bukovsky M, Kostalova D, Magnusova R et al: Testing for immunomodulating effects of ethanol-water extracts of the above-ground parts of the plants echinaceae Moench and Rudbeckia L. Cesk Farm 1993a;42:228-231.

Burger RA; Torres AR; Warren RP et al. Echinacea-induced cytokine production by human macrophages. Int J Immunopharmacol 1997 Jul;19(7):371-9.

Büsing KH, Hyaluronidasehemmung durch Echinacin. In: Arzneim Forsch 2:467-469. 1952.

Cheminat A, Zawatzky R, Becker H, Brouillard R, Caffeoylconjugates from Echinacea Species: Structure and biological activity. In: PH 27(9):2787-2794. 1988.

Coeugniet EG & Elek E. Immunomodulation with Viscum album and echinacea purpurea extracts. Onkologie 1987; 10(suppl 3):27-33.

Die Chemie der Pflanze (Standard, Wirksamkeit). In: Symbiose 4(3):11. 1992.

Dorn M, (1989) Milderung grippaler Effekte durch ein pflanzliches Immunstimulans. Natur- und Ganzheitsmedizin 2:314-319.

Facino RM; Carini M; Aldini G et al. Echinacoside and caffeoyl conjugates protect collagen from free radical-induced degradation: a potential use of Echinacea extracts in the prevention of skin photodamage. Planta Med 1995 Dec;61(6):510-4.

Forth H, Beuscher N, Beeinflussung der Häufigkeit banaler Erkältungsinfekte durch Esberitox. In: Z Allgemeinmed 57:2272-2275. 1981.

Grimm W, Muller H. A randomized controlled trial of the effect of fluid extract of Echinacea purpurea on the incidence and severity of colds and respiratory infections. Am J Med 1999 Fec;106(2):138-43.

Harnischfeger G, Stolze H, (1980) Notabene Medici 10:484.

Jacobson M, (1967) J Org Chem 32:1646.

Jurcic K, Melchart D, Holzmann M, Martin P, Bauer R, Doenecke A, Wagner H, Zwei Probandenstudien zur Stimulierung der Granulozytenphagozytose durch Echinacea-Extrakt-haltige Präparate. In: ZPT 10(2):67-70. 1989.

Kinkel HJ, Plate M, Tüllner HU, Objektivierbare Wirkung von Echinacin-Salbe auf die Wundheilung. In: Med Klinik 79:580-583. 1984.

Luettig B; Steinmuller C; Gifford GE et al. Macrophage activation by the polysaccharide arabinogalactan isolated from plant cell cultures of Echinacea purpurea. J Natl Cancer Inst 1989 May 3;81(9):669-75.

May G, Willuhn G, (1978) Arzneim Forsch 28:1.

Melchart D, Linde K, Worku F, Bauer R, Wagner H, (1994) Immunomodulation with Echinacea - a systematic review of controlled clinical trials. Phytomedicine 1:245-254.

Melchart D; Walther E; Linde K et al. Echinacea root extracts for the prevention of upper respiratory tract infections:a double-blind, placebo-controlled randomized trial. Arch Fam Med 1998 Nov-Dec;7(6):541-5.

Mose JR, (1983) Med Welt 34:51.

Muller-Jakic B; Breu W; Probstle A et al. In vitro inhibition of cyclooxygenase and 5-lipoxygenase by alkamides from Echinacea and Achillea species. Planta Med 1994 Feb;60(1):37-40.

Mullins RJ. Echinacea-associated anaphylaxis. Med J Aust 1998 Feb 16;168(4):170-1.

Ondrizek RR, Chan PJ, Patton WC, King A. An alternative medicine study of herbal effects on the penetration of zona-free hamster oocytes and the integrity of sperm deoxyribonucleic acid. Fertil Steril 1999 Mar;71(3):517-22.

Parnham MJ, Benefit-risk assessment of the squeezed sap of the purple coneflower (Echinacea purpurea) for long-term oral immunostimulation. In: Phytomedicine 3(1):95-102. 1996.

Proksch A, (1982) Über ein immunstimulierendes Wirkprinzip aus Echinacea purpurea. Dissertation, Ludwig-Maximilians-Universität, München.

Roesler J, Emmendorffer A, Steinmuller C et al. Application of purified polysaccharides from cell cultures of the plant echinacea purpurea to test subjects mediates activation of the phagocyte system. Int J Immunopharmacol 1991; 13:931-941.

Samochowie CE et al., (1979) Wiad Parazyt. 25(1) 77.

Schoneberger D. Einfluβ der immunstimulierenden Wirkung von Preβsaft aus herba Echinaceae purpureae auf Verlauf und Schweregrad von Erkältungskrankheiten. Forum Immunologie 1992;8:18-22.

Schulte KE et al., (1967) Arzneim Forsch 17:825.

Schulte KE, Rücker G, Perlick J, Das Vorkommen von Polyacetylen-Verbindungen in Echinacea purpurea MOENCH und Echinacea angustifolia DC. In: Arzneim-Forsch 17:825-829. 1967.

Schumacher A, Echinacea angustifolia und die spezifische und unspezifische zelluläre Immunantwort der Maus. In: Dissertation Heidelberg. 1989.

Stimpel M et al., (1984) Infect Immunol 46(3):845.

Stimpel M, Proksch A, Wagner H et al., (1984) Macrophage activation and induction of macrophage cytotoxicity by purified polysaccaride fractions from the plant Echinacea purpurea. Infect Immunity 46:845-849.

Stimpel M, Proksch A, Wagner H, Lohmann-Matthes ML, Macrophage activation and induction of macrophage cytotoxicity by purified polysccharide fraction from plant Echinacea purpurea. In: Infect Immun 46:845-849. 1984.

Tubaro A, Tragni E, Del Negro P et al: Anti-inflammatory activity of a polysaccharidic fraction of echinacea angustifolia. J Pharm Pharmacol 1987; 39:576-569.

Vergin H, Wolter R, Untersuchungen zur Phagozytose-Aktivität der isoliert perfundierten Rattenleber mit Echinacea purpurea-haltigen Präparaten. In: Natura med 1/2:27-29. 1988.

Vömel Th, (1985) Arzneim Forsch 35II(9):1437.

Von Röder E et al., (1984) Dtsch Apoth Ztg 124(45):2316.

Wacker A, Hilbig W, (1978) Planta Med 33:89.

Wacker A, Hilbig W, Virushemmung mit Echinacea purpurea. In: PM 33:89-102. 1978.

Wagner H et al., (1984) Arzneim Forsch 34:659.

Wagner H, Stuppner H, Puhlmann J, Brümmer B, Deppe K, Zenk MH, Gewinnung von immunologisch aktiven Polysacchariden aus Echinacea-Drogen und - Gewebekulturen. In: ZPT 10(2):35. 1989.

Further information in:

Hänsel R, Keller K, Rimpler H, Schneider G (Hrsg.), Hagers Handbuch der Pharmazeutischen Praxis, 5. Aufl., Bde 4-6 (Drogen), Springer Verlag Berlin, Heidelberg, New York, 1992-1994.

Schulz R, Hänsel R, Rationale Phytotherapie, Springer Verlag Heidelberg 1996.

Steinegger E, Hänsel R, Pharmakognosie, 5. Aufl., Springer Verlag Heidelberg 1992.

Teuscher E, Lindequist U, Biogene Gifte - Biologie, Chemie, Pharmakologie, 2. Aufl., Fischer Verlag Stuttgart 1994.

Teuscher E, Biogene Arzneimittel, 5. Aufl., Wiss. Verlagsges. mbH Stuttgart 1997.

Wagner H, Wiesenauer M, Phytotherapie. Phytopharmaka und pflanzliche Homöopathika, Fischer-Verlag, Stuttgart, Jena, New York 1995.

Wichtl M (Hrsg.), Teedrogen, 4. Aufl., Wiss. Verlagsges. Stuttgart 1997.

Echinaceae species

See Echinacea

Elecampane

Inula helenium

DESCRIPTION

Medicinal Parts: The medicinal part is the dried or fresh rhizome.

Flower and Fruit: The inflorescences are yellow composite flowers in loose, terminal, panicled cymes. They are 7 to 8 cm in diameter. The involucre is imbricate and cup-shaped. The inner bracts are dry at the tip and splayed, the outer ones are like leaves and ovate. The female lateral florets are narrowly linguiform. The androgynous disc florets are tubular. The receptacle is flat, slightly pitted and glabrous. The flowers are a bright yellow. The achaenes are cylindrical, 4 to 5 mm long, brown, glabrous and have 4 tips. The pappus is 8 to 10 mm long and consists of brownish, fine, rough, brittle bristles.

Leaves, Stem and Root: The plant is perennial and 80 to 180 cm high. The rhizome is short with compact branches. It is tuberous and has sturdy, 1 cm thick and 50 cm long roots. The stem is erect, branched above and villous. The leaves are large, tomentose beneath and irregularly dentate. The cauline leaves are cordate-acute. The basal leaves are oblong and petiolate.

Characteristics: The rhizome has a strong odor, the taste is pungent, bitter and tangy.

Habitat: Indigenous to Europe and temperate Asia, introduced to the U.S. and China.

Production: Elecampane root is the root of Inula helenium. It is harvested in autumn. The roots are then cut and hung up to dry or dried artificially at 50° C.

Other Names: Alant, Elfdock, Elfwort, Horse-Elder, Horse-heal, Scabwort, Wild Sunflower, Yellow Starwort, Velvet Dock

ACTIONS AND PHARMACOLOGY

COMPOUNDS

Volatile oil: chief components alantolactone, isoalantolactone, 11,13- dihydroisoalantolactone, 11,13- dihydroalantolactone (the mixture of alantolactone derivatives is also known as helenalin or elecampane camphor)

Polyynes

Polysaccharides: above all inulin (fructosan)

EFFECTS

The main active principles are alantolacton, isoalantolacton and other sesquiterpenlactones. Compounds of this kind have an antiphlogostic and antibiotic effect. Antifungal activity has also been demonstrated.

The antimicrobial and anthelmintic effect results from the sesquiterpene lactones. Alantolactone and isoalantolactone are antitumoral, and helenin shortens clotting time. Alantolactone and helenin lead to complete paralysis of the spontaneous contraction of the intestine in animal studies.

The plant has mild antiseptic and expectorant effect due to the essential oil, which contains sesquiterpene.

INDICATIONS AND USAGE

Unproven Uses: Preparations of the rhizome are used to treat bronchitis, whooping cough and bronchial catarrh. In folk medicine, Elecampane is used as a stomachic, diuretic, carminative and cholagogue, as well as for menstrual complaints.

Homeopathic Uses: Inula helenium preparations are used for stomach ulcers and chronic cough.

PRECAUTIONS AND ADVERSE REACTIONS

General: The drug is severely irritating to mucous membranes and strongly sensitizing.

Pregnancy: Not to be used during pregnancy.

OVERDOSAGE

Larger administrations of the drug lead to vomiting, diarrhea, spasms and signs of paralysis. Following gastric lavage, intestinal emptying (sodium sulfate) and the administration of activated charcoal powder, poisoning is treated with the antimetic trifluopromazine.

DOSAGE

Mode of Administration: The comminuted drug is used in tea mixtures. The extract is used as a constituent in numerous pharmaceutical preparations, including gastrointestinal remedies, alterants, gout remedies, diuretics and in numerous expectorants.

Preparation: To prepare an infusion, boiling water is poured over 1 gm of ground drug and left to draw for 10 to 15 minutes, after which time it is strained through a tea strainer (1 teaspoonful corresponds to about 4 gm drug).

Daily Dosage: Average single dose 1 gm.

Tea—1 cup is drunk 3 to 4 times daily as an expectorant; may be sweetened with honey.

Helenium Extract—The single dose is 0.5 gm.

Homeopathic Dosage: 5 drops, 1 tablet or 10 globules every 30 to 60 minutes (acute) or 1 to 3 times daily (chronic); parenterally: 1 to 2 ml sc acute, 3 times daily; chronic once a day (HAB34).

Storage: Store in a cool place, protected from light, not in plastic containers.

LITERATURE

Kerimov SS, Chishov OS, (1974) Khim Prir Soed 10:254.

Khvorost PP, Komissarenko NF, (1976) Khim Prir Soed 6:820.

Kiesewetter R, Müller M, (1958) Pharmazie 13:777.

Lauro L, Rolih C, Observations and research on an extract of Inula viscosa Ait. Boll Soc Ital Biol Sper, 66:829-34, 1990 Sep

Pazzaglia M, Venturo N, Borda G, Tosti A, Contact dermatitis due to a massage liniment containing Inula helenium extract. Contact Dermatitis, 61:267, 1995 Oct

Rosik GH et al., Khim Farm Zh 21:632-634. 1987.

Tripathi YB, Chaturvedi P, Assessment of endocrine response of Inula racemosa in relation to glucose homeostasis in rats. Indian J Exp Biol, 61:686-9, 1995 Sep

Vishnakova SA et al., (1977) Rastit Resur 13:428.

Zinchenko V et al., Rastit Res 19:544-548. 1983.

Further information in:

Alonso Blasi N, Fraginals R, Lepoittevin JP, Benezra C, A murine in vitro model of allergic contact dermatitis to sesquiterpene alpha-methylene-gamma-butyrolactones. Arch Dermatol Res, 284:297-302, 1992

Fokina GI, Frolova TV, Roikhel VM, Pogodina VV, Experimental phytotherapy of tick-borne encephalitis. Vopr Virusol, 36:18-21, 1991 Jan-Feb.

Hänsel R, Keller K, Rimpler H, Schneider G (Hrsg.), Hagers Handbuch der Pharmazeutischen Praxis, 5. Aufl., Bde 4-6 (Drogen), Springer Verlag Berlin, Heidelberg, New York, 1992-1994.

Hausen B, Allergiepflanzen, Pflanzenallergene, ecomed Verlagsgesellsch. mbH, Landsberg 1988.

Iijima K, Kiyohara H, Tanaka M, Matsumoto T, Cyong JC, Yamada H, Preventive effect of taraxasteryl acetate from Inula britannica subsp. Japonica on experimental hepatitis in vivo. Planta Med, 61:50-3, 1995 Feb.

Jiang B, Liao X, Jia X, Ye X, Ding J, Yu X, Wu Y, Studies and comparisons on chemical components of essential oils from Clematis hexapetala Pall. and Inula nervosa Wall. Chung Kuo Chung Yao Tsa Chih, 15:488-90 512, 1990 Aug.

Leung AY, Encyclopedia of Common Natural Ingredients Used in Food Drugs and Cosmetics, John Wiley & Sons Inc., New York 1980.

Madaus G, Lehrbuch der Biologischen Arzneimittel, Bde 1-3, Nachdruck, Georg Olms Verlag Hildesheim 1979.

Roth L, Daunderer M, Kormann K, Giftpflanzen, Pflanzengifte, 4. Aufl., Ecomed Fachverlag Landsberg Lech 1993.

Tang W, Eisenbrand G, Chinese Drugs of Plant Origin, Springer Verlag Heidelberg 1992.

Teuscher E, Lindequist U, Biogene Gifte - Biologie, Chemie, Pharmakologie, 2. Aufl., Fischer Verlag Stuttgart 1994.

Wagner H, Wiesenauer M, Phytotherapie. Phytopharmaka und pflanzliche Homöopathika, Fischer-Verlag, Stuttgart, Jena, New York 1995.

Wang Q, Zhou BN, Zhang RW, Lin YY, Lin LZ, Gil RR, Cordell GA, Cytotoxicity and NMR spectral assignments of ergolide and bigelovin. Planta Med, 62:166-8, 1996 Apr

Wichtl M (Hrsg.), Teedrogen, 4. Aufl., Wiss. Verlagsges. Stuttgart 1997.

Elephant-Ears

Bergenia crassifolia

DESCRIPTION

Medicinal Parts: Whole plant has medicinal properties.

Flower and Fruit: The flowers are arranged in curled cymes. Their structures are arranged in fives and they are radial with the 2 to 3 ovaries joined only at the base. The petals are red or pink-violet and up to 1.5 cm long. The ovary is superior, and the fruit has numerous seeds. The seeds are brown to brown-black, edged, up to 2 mm long and 0.5 mm thick.

Leaves, Stem and Root: Bergenia crassifolia is a herbaceous perennial that grows up to 50 cm high. The leaves are basal, oval, up to 20 cm long, over 10 cm wide, orbicular, fleshy, glabrous, with indented glands and slightly dentate. The rhizome is up to 3 cm thick, above ground and covered with the sheaths of the previous year's leaves.

Habitat: Russia, Mongolia

Production: Bergeniae rhizoma are the dried rhizomes of Bergenia crassifolia. They are collected in the wild and air-dried for 2 weeks.

Other Names: Leather Bergenia, Siberian Tea

ACTIONS AND PHARMACOLOGY

COMPOUNDS

Hydroquinone glycosides: arbutin (1.8 to 2.3%)

Phenol carboxylic acids: bergenin (6.7 to 10.1%, lactones)

Tannins (28%)

EFFECTS

The watery extracts of the drug have astringent, bacteriostatic, local hemostyptic and antiphlogistic effects, due to the tannin content and that of other phenolic constituents. The arbutin they contain exhibits urine-disinfecting effect (comparable to Uva ursi). A shortening of blood coagulation time could be demonstrated in animal experiments.

INDICATIONS AND USAGE

Unproven Uses: Elephant-Ears have been used for fever, tuberculosis, pneumonia, diarrhea, intestinal disease and rheumatism. The drug is also used for skin leishmaniosis and as a hemostyptic.

CONTRAINDICATIONS

Preparations are contraindicated in pregnancy, breast-feeding and children under 12 years of age.

PRECAUTIONS AND ADVERSE REACTIONS

No health hazards are known in conjunction with the proper administration of designated therapeutic dosages. Because of its high tannin content, the intake of preparations of the drug could lead to digestive disorders; individuals with sensitive stomachs may experience nausea and vomiting.

OVERDOSAGE

Overdose could lead to inflammatory irritation of the mucous membranes of the bladder and urinary tract, accompanied by urgency and blood in the urine. Long-term administration of the drug could lead to liver damage, due to the possible hepatotoxicity of the hydroquinone released, particularly among children.

DOSAGE

Mode of Administration: Whole drug preparations for internal and external use.

LITERATURE

Hänsel R, Keller K, Rimpler H, Schneider G (Ed), Hagers Handbuch der Pharmazeutischen Praxis, 5. Aufl., Bde 4 - 6 (Drogen), Springer Verlag Berlin, Heidelberg, New York, 1992-1994.

Kindl H, Conversion of (4-3H)L-phenylalanine into (4-3H)pyrocatechol and (3-3H)hydroquinone in leaves of Bergenia crassifolia. Hoppe Seylers Z Physiol Chem, 350:1289-90, 1969 Oct.

Elettaria cardamomum

See Cardamom

Eleutherococcus senticosus

See Siberian Ginseng

Elm Bark

Ulmus minor

DESCRIPTION

Medicinal Parts: The medicinal part is the inner bark of the young branches.

Flower and Fruit: The reddish brown flowers appear before the leaves. They are androgynous, short-pedicled and in globular clusters. The perigone is campanulate-top-shaped and greenish with a purple margin. There are 3 to 4 stamens with dark violet anthers. The tree is wind pollinated. The fruit is a broad-winged, almost circular, oval or elliptical and glabrous achaene. The reddish nutlet reaches to the front margin of the notch.

Leaves, Stem and Root: Ulmus minor is a 40 m high tree with black-brown, finely fissured bark. The branches, which develop long grooves, have alternate, petiolate, 6 to 10 cm long leaves with 8 to 12 lateral ribs. The leaves are ovate. The lamina is irregular and the margin double-serrate. The petioles are 8 to 15 mm longer than the buds, which develop in spring on short branches and form into clusters before flowering.

Habitat: The plant is indigenous to Europe as far as the Mediterranean.

Production: Smooth-leaved Elm bark is the bark of Ulmus minor. The bark is gathered for therapeutic or medicinal purposes. It is manually cut in circles and the bark is removed from the young (new) twigs (the diameter of the twig should not be more than 1 cm). The long grain and the upper layer of the bark must be removed, then the bark is dried.

ACTIONS AND PHARMACOLOGY

COMPOUNDS

Mucilage: yielding mainly D-galactose, L-rhamnose, D-galacturonic acid after hydrolysis

Tannins (3%)

Caffeic acid derivatives: chlorogenic acid

Sterols: including, among others, beta-sitosterol, stigmasterol

EFFECTS

The drug has diuretic and astringent properties.

INDICATIONS AND USAGE

Unproven Uses: Internally, the drug is used for digestive disorders and severe cases of diarrhea. Externally, it is used to treat open wounds.

PRECAUTIONS AND ADVERSE REACTIONS

No health hazards or side effects are known in conjunction with the proper administration of designated therapeutic dosages.

DOSAGE

Mode of Administration: Elm bark is used both internally and externally in various preparations.

Preparation: The ground bark is used for infusions. A decoction from the bark can be prepared using 2 teaspoons of the drug per cup of water. Externally, a 20% decoction is used, which is diluted 1:1 with water, for the treatment of festering and open wounds.

Daily Dose: The dosage of the decoction prepared from the bark is 1 cup 2 to 3 times daily. In powder form, a dose of 2 to 5 gm may be taken daily.

LITERATURE

Hänsel R, Keller K, Rimpler H, Schneider G (Hrsg.), Hagers Handbuch der Pharmazeutischen Praxis, 5. Aufl., Bde 4-6 (Drogen): Springer Verlag Berlin, Heidelberg, New York, 1992-1994.

Madaus G, Lehrbuch der Biologischen Arzneimittel, Bde 1-3, Nachdruck, Georg Olms Verlag Hildesheim 1979.

English Adder's Tongue

Ophioglossum vulgatum

DESCRIPTION

Medicinal Parts: The medicinal parts of the plant are the root and leaves.

Flower and Fruit: The plant's 12 to 40 ripe yellow sporangia on either side of the middle panicle form an acuminate spike. The tip contains no sporangia.

Leaves, Stem and Root: This fern grows from 8 to 25 cm high. The stems, covered in the remains of leaves, grow singly from the underground roots. The stems consist of a few sturdy, yellow fibers and are round, hollow and succulent. Each bears a smooth, oblong-oval, acuminate, entire frond.

Characteristics: Though a member of the Fern family, the appearance of English Adder's Tongue is not at all typically fern-like.

Habitat: The plant is indigenous to Britain.

Production: English Adder's Tongue is the aerial part of Ophioglossum vulgatum.

Not To Be Confused With: English Adder's Tongue is not related to American Adder's Tongue (Erythronium americanum).

Other Names: Serpent's Tongue, Christ's Spear

ACTIONS AND PHARMACOLOGY

COMPOUNDS

Flavonoids: including among others quercetin-3-methyl ether-7-diglucoside-4′ glucoside

The constituents of the drug have not been thoroughly investigated.

EFFECTS

See Erythronium americanum.

INDICATIONS AND USAGE

See Erythronium americanum.

PRECAUTIONS AND ADVERSE REACTIONS

No health hazards or side effects are known in conjunction with the proper administration of designated therapeutic dosages.

DOSAGE

Mode of Administration: See Erythronium americanum.

LITERATURE

Hegnauer R, Chemotaxonomie der Pflanzen, Bde 1-11, Birkhäuser Verlag Basel, Boston, Berlin 1962-1997.

English Chamomile

Chamaemelum nobile

DESCRIPTION

Medicinal Parts: The medicinal parts are the English Chamomile oil extracted from the fresh or dried filled or unfilled flower heads and the dried aerial plant parts; the dried flower heads of the cultivated, filled varieties; and the fresh aerial parts of the flowering plant.

Flower and Fruit: The stems end in 12 to 18 fruit-bearing, white florets, which are about 2 to 2.5 cm wide. The epicalyx is semi-globose. The bracts are in a number of rows and are lanceolate to spatulate with a broad membranous border. The receptacle is clavate, filled with latex, and covered at the edge with slit bracts. The linguiform florets are female and silver-white. The tubular florets are androgynous and yellow. The corolla of every floret has a short appendage at the base, which surrounds the tip of the fruit. The achaenes are 2 mm long, light brown and almost triangular with vertical ribs. The achaenes are smooth and have no pappus.

Leaves, Stem and Root: The 15 to 30 cm high plant has a deeply buried rhizome. The rhizome sprouts numerous, ascending, occasionally upright, simple or branched, rounded, vertically grooved, pubescent stems. The stems are covered in alternating, heavily segmented, gray-green to rich-green leaves that are 2 to 4 cm long.

Habitat: The plant is indigenous to southern and western Europe and northern Africa, and is cultivated all over Europe. The main exporters are Belgium, France, Great Britain and Italy, as well as Poland, the Czech and Slovakian Republics, North America and Argentina.

Production: English Chamomile consists of the dried flowers of the cultivated double flowered variety of Chamaemelum nobile. The plant is harvested in June and July, then dried at temperatures of 35°C.

Other Names: Ground Apple, Whig Plant, Roman Chamomile

ACTIONS AND PHARMACOLOGY

COMPOUNDS

Volatile oil: chief components include ester of angelic- or tiglic acid with isobutanol, isoamyl alcohol or 3-methyl-pentan-1-ol, to some extent present as hydroperoxides

Sesquiterpene lactones: in particular nobilin, besides 3-epinobilin, 1,10-epoxynobilin, 3-dehydronobilin that is present to some extent as hydroperoxides, including 1-beta-hydroperoxy-isonobilin and 4-alpha-hydroperoxy-manolide

Flavonoids: including anthemoside, cosmosioside, luteolin-7-0-glucoside

Caffeic and ferulic acid ester

Polynes: Including cis- and trans-dehydromatricaria ester

EFFECTS

In contrast to true chamomile, few studies are available. The essential oil is active against gram-positive bacteria and dermatomyces. The drug is also cytostatic and acts on the CNS, causing a reduction of aggressive behavior in animal tests. Efficacy in dyspepsia (including flatulence) may be due to the amaroids.

INDICATIONS AND USAGE

Unproven Uses: In folk medicine, the French use English Chamomile mainly for feelings of fullness, bloating and mild spasmodic gastrointestinal disturbances and sluggishness of the bowels. It is also used for menstrual complaints, nervousness, hysteria and general debility. It is used topically for inflammation of the mouth and throat, rhinitis, toothache, earache, headache and influenza. The oil is used in mouthwashes.

Homeopathic Uses: The drug is used in homeopathy to treat nervous gastrointestinal disorders, but efficacy has not been proven.

CONTRAINDICATIONS

Use of the drug is contraindicated during pregnancy.

PRECAUTIONS AND ADVERSE REACTIONS

General: No health hazards or side effects are known in conjunction with the proper administration of designated therapeutic dosages. The drug possesses a small potential for sensitization.

Pregnancy: The drug is not to be used during pregnancy.

DOSAGE

Mode of Administration: Since the efficacy for the claimed uses is not documented and there is a certain risk involved, a therapeutic application cannot be recommended. English Chamomile is used in folk medicine as a fluid extract, tincture, elixir, wine, syrup, ointment and powder.

Preparation: To prepare a decoction, add 3 g drug to 100 ml water. An infusion is prepared using 7 to 8 capitula per cup. A liquid rub is prepared using 1 dsp diluted in 250 ml water.

Daily Dosage: The average single dose of the drug is 1.5 g at the main meals. The average daily dose of an infusion is 50 ml to 200 ml. When used as a bath additive, add 50 g to 10 liters of water. Liquid rubs are applied as poultices or washes 2 to 3 times daily.

Homeopathic Dosage: 5 drops, 1 tablet or 10 globules every 30 to 60 minutes for acute conditions. For chronic conditions: 1 to 3 times daily; Parenterally: 1 to 2 ml sc acute 3 times daily; Chronic: once a day (HAB1)

Storage: Store in well-sealed glass or metal containers protected from moisture.

LITERATURE

Damiani P et al., (1983) Fitoterapia 54:213.

Herisset A et al., (1971) Plant Med Phytother 5(3):234.

Herisset A et al., (1974) Plant Med Phytother 8(4):306 and 287.

Holub M, Samek Z, (1977) Collect Czech Chem Commun 42: 1053.

Isaac O, Chamaemelum nobile (L.) Allioni - Römische Kamille. In: ZPT 14(4):212. 1993.

Further information in:

Hänsel R, Keller K, Rimpler H, Schneider G (Hrsg.), Hagers Handbuch der Pharmazeutischen Praxis, 5. Aufl., Bde 4-6 (Drogen), Springer Verlag Berlin, Heidelberg, New York, 1992-1994.

Hausen B, Allergiepflanzen, Pflanzenallergene, ecomed Verlagsgesellsch. mbH, Landsberg 1988.

Leung AY, Encyclopedia of Common Natural Ingredients Used in Food Drugs and Cosmetics, John Wiley & Sons Inc., New York 1980.

Steinegger E, Hänsel R, Pharmakognosie, 5. Aufl., Springer Verlag Heidelberg 1992.

Teuscher E, Biogene Arzneimittel, 5. Aufl., Wiss. Verlagsges. mbH Stuttgart 1997.

Wichtl M (Hrsg.), Teedrogen, 4. Aufl., Wiss. Verlagsges. Stuttgart 1997.

English Hawthorn

Crataegus laevigata

TRADE NAMES

Hawthorn, Hawthorn Extract (available from numerous manufacturers and as a combination product), Hawthorne Berries, Hawthorn Flowers, Leaves & Berries, Standardized Hawthorn Extract, Hawthorn Extract, Hawthorn Power, Time Release Hawthorn Power, HeartCare

DESCRIPTION

Medicinal Parts: The medicinal parts are generally white thorn flowers, leaves, fruit, and various mixtures of different plant parts.

Flowers and Fruit: The white flowers are in richly-blossomed cymes. The sepals are usually short, more or less triangular, entire-margined or, particularly the American variety, fairly long with glandular tips. The petals are usually separate, orbicular, crenate, white or occasionally red. There are 10 to 20 stamens and 1 to 5 carpels, which are more or less fused to the receptacle. There are 2 ovules, the upper one is sterile and covers the lower fertile one like a cap. There is 1 seed in each chamber. The false fruit is ovoid or globose and crowned by the remains of the sepals. It is red, black, or yellow and mealy.

Leaves, Stem and Root: Hawthorn is a bulky shrub or small tree, 1.5 to 4 m high with hard wood and usually thorny branches. The leaves have many forms. They are shallow, 3 to 5 lobed, with the lobes pointed forward. The leaves are unevenly serrate, obovate, yellowish-green, and glossy.

Characteristics: The flowers have an unpleasant smell and a slightly bitter taste; the fruit has a sour taste.

Habitat: The plant is indigenous to northern temperate zones of Europe, Asia, and North America.

Production: Hawthorn consists of the leaves and flowers of Crataegus laevigata and occasionally other species. The medicinal parts of the Hawthorn plant are collected in the wild and dried at room temperature.

Not to be Confused With: Hawthorn is sometimes mistaken for the flowers, leaves, and fruit of Robinia pseudoacacia, Sorbus aucuparia or Prunus spinosa.

Other Names: Haw, May, Whitethorn, Hawthorn

ACTIONS AND PHARMACOLOGY

COMPOUNDS

Flavonoides (1.8%): O-glycosides, including hyperoside (0.28%), rutin (0.17%)

6-C- and 8-C-glycosyl compounds, including vitexin (0.02%), vicenin-1, orientin

6-C- and 8-C-glycosyl compounds, linked O-glycosidically as well as with other monosaccharides, including vitexin-2''-O-alpha-L-rhamnoside (0.53%), vitexin-2''-O-alpha-L-rhamnoside-4'''-acetate

Oligomeric proanthocyanidins (2.4%)

Biogenic amines, including tyramine

Triterpenes (0.6%): including oleanolic acid, ursolic acid, 2-alpha-hydroxy oleanolic acid (crataegolic acid)

EFFECTS

The active principles are procyanidins and flavonoids. They cause an increase in coronary blood flow due to dilatory effects resulting in an improvement of myocardial blood flow. The drug is positively inotropic and positively chronotropic. The cardiotropic effect of Crataegus is said to be caused by the increased membrane permeability for calcium as well as the inhibition of phosphodiesterase with an increase of intracellular cylco-AMP concentrations. Increased coronary and myocardial circulatory perfusion and reduction in peripheral vascular resistance were observed. High doses may cause sedation. This effect has been attributed to the oligomeric procyanidins (Anonym, 1994).

Crataegus extract has been found to prolong the refractory period and increase the action potential duration in guinea pig papillary muscle. One study demonstrated that a Crataegus extract blocked the repolarizing potassium currents in ventricular myocytes of guinea pigs. This effect is similar to that of class III antiarrhythmic drugs and may explain the antiarrhythmic effect of Hawthorn (Muller, 1999).

INDICATIONS AND USAGE

Approved by Commission E:

■ Decrease in cardiac output (Stage II NYHA)

Hawthorn is used for senile heart, chronic cor pulmonale, and mild forms of bradycardial arrhythmias.

Unproven Uses: In folk medicine, Hawthorn is also used as a cardiotonic, for hypertension, ischemia of the heart, arrhythmia and as a sedative. Hawthorn has a high flavonoid content and is used to prevent collagen destruction in joints and decrease inflammation and decrease the fragility of capillaries. Hawthorn has shown some effectiveness in lowering cholesterol levels in at least one study. Several extracts from different componants of the plant have demonstrated antioxidant effects.

Chinese Medicine: In China, Hawthorn is used to reduce food stagnancy and blood stasis (Chen, 1995).

Homeopathic Uses: Therapeutic dilutions are used for cardiac insufficiency, senile cardiac insufficiency, dysrrhythmia, and angina pectoris.

CLINICAL STUDIES

Cardiac Effects

Several studies that have used animal models demonstrate the cardiac effects of Hawthorn. The influence of the main flavonoids from Hawthorn on coronary flow, heart rate, left ventricular pressure and the velocity of contraction and relaxation was investigated on isolated guinea pig hearts maintained at a constant perfusion pressure was the focus of one study. The study recorded an increase in coronary flow of 186% for one of the main glycosides, luteolin-7-glucoside; 66% for the hyperoside component and 66% for the rutin flavonoid. Coronary relaxation velocity increased by 104% in the luteolin-7-glucoside arm, 62% for hyperoside and 73% for rutin. Positive inotropic and chronotropic effects were noted for all of the above extracts as well. The beta adrenergic effects of the flavonoids were prevented by the addition of propranolol. The authors postulate that the mechanism of action for the cardiac effects of Hawthorne is due to the inhibition of the 3', 5'-cyclic adenosine monophosphate phosphodiesterase enzyme (Schussler, 1995). It should be noted that in a more recent study, the positive inotropic effect of Hawthorn was not attributed to phosphodiesterase inhibition or to a beta-sympathomimetic effect (Muller, 1999).

Another small, placebo controlled, randomized double-blind study was performed to test the efficacy of a special extract (WS 1442) of Hawthorn in a group of 30 patients with stage II NYHA cardiac insufficiency. Treatment duration was 8 weeks. Primary parameters were alteration in the pressure-x-rate product (PRP) under standardized loading on a bicycle ergometer, and the score of a subjective questionnaire on improvement of complaints. Secondary target parameters included exercise tolerance and the change in heart rate and arterial blood pressure. A statistically significant improvement in both primary and secondary parameters were noted in the WS 1442 group over that of the placebo group (Leuchtgens, 1993).

CONTRAINDICATIONS

Hawthorn is contraindicated in children under 12 years of age. Use of Hawthorn during the first trimester of pregnancy is contraindicated.

PRECAUTIONS AND ADVERSE REACTIONS

General: It is recommended that Hawthorn supplements be prescribed and monitored by a physician. During treatment with Hawthorn, the clinician should monitor heart rate and blood pressure on a regular basis.

Higher doses can produce hypotension, cardiac arrhythmia, and sedation. Less serious adverse effects include dizziness and tremor.

Accidental corneal scratches caused by thorns of hawthorn bushes have resulted in blindness in 88 out of 132 reported cases in Ireland (Duke, 1985).

Drug Interactions Hawthorn may potentiate the effects of cardiac glycosides. If Hawthorn therapy is initiated in patients taking digoxin, digitoxin or g-strophanthin, the dosage of standard cardiac glycosides should be adjusted downward.

Hawthorn may cause a hypertensive effect when used in combination with beta-blockers (Murray & Pizzorno, 1996).

Because Hawthorn has an action similar to Class III antiarrhythmics, use with other antiarrhythmics should be discouraged.

Hawthorn has been found to inhibit the inward flow of potassium channels resulting in an increased action potential in cardiac ventricular cells. Drugs that act in a similar manner such as cisapride are likely to interact with Hawthorn and should therefore not be taken in conjunction with Hawthorn.

Pregnancy: Hawthorn is contraindicated during the first trimester of pregnancy.

Nursing Mothers: There are no warnings in the literature regarding use of Hawthorn in nursing mothers.

Pediatrics: Hawthorn is not recommended for children under the age of 12 years.

OVERDOSAGE

The LD50 via intraperitoneal injection in the mouse model has been reported at a single dose of 1,170 mg/kg and 750 mg/kg in the rat. In both species, signs of overdose included sedation, dyspnea, tremor and piloerection (Schlegelilch & Heywood, 1994). The same authors reported that an oral dose if 3,000 mg/kg in mice and rats was well tolerated with no negative clinical signs or death reported in the animal models.

DOSAGE

Mode of Administration: The dried and comminuted drug for decoctions as well as liquid or dry extracts for oral intake.

How Supplied:

Capsules — 80 mg, 100 mg, 300 mg, 450 mg, 455 mg, 480 mg, 500 mg, 510 mg, 565 mg

Liquid — 250 mg/ml

Tablets — 80 mg

Daily Dosage: The average daily dose is 5 gm of drug or 160 to 900 mg extract administered in divided doses, 3 times daily, (ethanol 45% V/V or methanol 70% V/V) standardized on procyanidin or flavonoids; single dose: 1 gm of drug several times daily. The duration of treatment is minimum 6 weeks.

Homeopathic Dosage: 5 to 10 drops, 1 tablet or 5 to 10 globules 1 to 3 times a day or 1 ml injection solution sc twice a week; ointment 1 to 2 times a day (HAB1)

Storage: Hawthorn should be protected from light and moisture in well-sealed containers at temperatures below 25° C.

LITERATURE

Ammon HPT, Händel M, (1981) Crataegus, Toxikologie und Pharmakologie. Teil 1, Toxizität. Planta Med 43:105-120.

Ammon HPT, Handel M, (1981) Planta Med 43:105, 209 et 313.

Anonym, 5. Kongreβ für Phytotherapie: Phytoforschung intensiviert. In: DAZ 133(48):4593. 1993.

Anonym, Behandlung der leichten Herzinsuffiziens: Weiβdornextrakt und ACE-Hemmer im Vergleich. In: DAZ 134(39):3749. 1994.

Anonym, Phytopharmaka für ältere Menschen: Ginkgo, Kava, Hypericum und Crataegus. In: DAZ 135(5):400-402. 1995.

Anonym, Weiβdorn bei Herzinsuffiziens und Angina pectoris. In: Symbiose 4(3):16. 1992.

Bahorun T, Gressier B, Trotin F, Brunet C, Dine Th, Luyckx M, Vasseur J, Cazin M, Cazin JC, Pinkas M, Oxygen species scavenging activity of phenolic activities, fresh plant organs and pharmaceutical preparations. In: Arzneim Forsch 46(11):1086-1089. 1996.

Bahorun T, Trotin F, Pommery J, Vasseur J, Pinkas M, Antioxydant activities of Crataegus monogyna extracts. In: PM 60(4):323-328. 1994.

Beretz A et al., (1980) Planta Med 39(3):241.

Chen JD, WU YZ, Tao ZL et al: Hawthorn (shan zha) drink and its lowering effect on blood lipid levels in humans and rats. World Rev Nutr Diet 77:147-154. 1995.

Ciplea AG, Richter KD, (1988) The protective effect of Allium sativum and Crataegus on isoprenaline-induced tissue necroses in rats. Arzneim Forsch/Drug Res 38:1588-1592.

Czygan FC, Crataegus-Arten- Weiβdorn, Portrait einer Arzneipflanze. In: ZPT 15(2):117. 1994.

Dingermann T, Phytopharmaka im Alter: Crataegus, Ginkgo, Hypericum und Kava-Kava. In: PZ 140(23):2017-2024. 1995.

Duke JA: Handbook of Medicinal Herbs, 2nd ed. CRC Press, Inc, Boca Raton, FL, pp 146-147. 1985.

Eichstädt H, Bäder M, Danne O, Kaiser W, Stein U, Felix R, (1989) Crataegus-Extrakt hilft dem Patienten mit NYHA II-Herzinsuffizien Therapiewoche 39: 3288-3296.

Ficarra P et al., (1984) Farm Ed Prat 39(10)342.

Ficarra P et al., (1984) Farm Ed Prat 39(5)148.

Fischer K, Jung F, Koscielny J, Kiesewetter H, (1994) Crataegus-Extrakt vs. Methyldigoxin. Einfluβ auf Rheologie und Mikrozirkulation bei 12 gesunden Probanden. Münch Med Wschr 136 (Suppl 1), 35-38.

Förster A, Förster K, Bühring M, Wolfstädter HD, (1994) Crataegus bei mäβig reduzierter linksventrikulärer Auswurffraktion. Ergospirometrische Verlaufsuntersuchung bei 72. Patienten in doppelblindem Vergleich mit Plazebo. Münch Med Wschr 136 (Suppl 1), 21-26

Iwamoto M et al., (1981) Planta Med 42(1):1

Joseph G, Zhao Y, Klaus W (1995) Pharmakologisches Wirkprofil von Crataegus-Extrakt im Vergleich zu Epinephrin, Amrinon, Milrinon und Digoxin am isoliert perfundierten Meerschweinchenherzen. Arzneim Forsch/Drug Res 45: 1261-1265

Kaul R, Pflanzliche Procyanidine. Vorkommen, Klassifikation und pharmakologische Wirkungen. In: PUZ 25(4):175-185. 1996.

Klensch O, Nagell A, Die Darreichungsform Tee am Beispiel Weiβdornblätter mit Blüten. In: DAZ 134(32):3005. 1994.

Krzeminski T, Chatterjee SS, (1993) Ischemia and early reperfusion induced arrhythmias, beneficial effects of an extract of Crataegus oxyacantha L. Pharm Pharmacol Lett 3:45-48.

Kurcok A, (1992) Ischemia- and reperfusion-induced cardiac injury; effects of two flavonoids containing plant extracts possessing radical scavenging properties. Naunyn-Schmiedebergs's Arch Pharmacol 345 (Suppl RB 81) Abstr 322.

Kurzmann M, Schimmer O, Weiβdorn - Flavonoidmuster und DC-Identitätsprüfung. In: DAZ 136(33):2759-2764. 1996.

Leuchtgens H, Cratagus Special Extract WS 1442 in NYHA II heart failure. A placebo controlled randomized double-blind study. In: Fortschr Med 20;111(20021: 352-4 Jul 20,1993.

Loew D, (1994) Crataegus-Spezialextrakte bei Herzinsuffizien. Kassenarzt 15:43-52.

Loew D, Phytotherapie bei Herzinsuffizienz. In: ZPT 18(2):92-96. 1997.

Meier B, Neue Erkenntnisse zur Analytik und Wirksamkeit von Weiβdorn. In: DAZ 136(44):3877-3879. 1996.

Murray M & Pizzorno J: A Textbook of Natural Medicine, 2nd ed. Batyr University Publications, Seattle, WA, USA, ppV Cratag-1-4. 1996.

Muller A, Linke W, Klaus W: Crataegus extract blocks potassium currents in guinea pig ventricular cardiac myocytes. In: Planta Med 65(4): 335-9 May, 1999.

Pöpping S, Rose H, Ionescu I, Fischer Y, Kammermeier H, (1995) Effect of a Hawthorn Extract on Contraction and Energy Turnover of Isolated Rat Cordiomyocytes. Arzneim Forsch/Drug Res 45:1157-1161.

Rehwald A et al., HPLC analysis of the flavonoids of Crataegi folium cum flore. In: PM 59(7)28. 1993.

Reuter HD, Crataegus als pflanzliches Kardiakum. In: ZPT 15(2):73. 1994.

Rewerski W et al., (1971) Arzneim Forsch 21:886.

Schlegelmilch R, Heywood R, (1994) Toxicity of Crataegus (Hawthorn) Extract (WS 1442). J Am Coll Toxicol 13:103-111.

Schmidt U, Kuhn U, Ploch M, Hübner WD, (1994) Wirksamkeit des Extraktes LI 132 (600 mg/Tag) bei 8wöchiger Therapie. Plazebokontrollierte Doppelblindstudie mit Weiβdorn an 78 herzinsuffizienten Patienten im Stadium II nach NYHA. Münch Med Wschr 136(Suppl 1):13-20.

Schüssler M et al., Effect of flavonoids from Crataegus species in Langendorf perfused isolated guinea pig heart. In: PM 58(7)46. 1992.

Schuessler M et al., Cardiac effects of flavonoids from Crataegus species. In: PM 59(7)88. 1993.

Schussler M, Holzl J, Fricke U, Myocardial effects of flavonoids from Crataegus species. In: Arzneimittelforschung 45(8): 842-5, Aug, 1995.

Siegel G, Casper U, (1995) Crataegi folium cum flore. In, Loew D, Rietbrock N (Hrsg) Phytopharmaka in Forschung und klinischer Anwendung. Steinkopff Verlag, Darmstadt, S. 1-14.

Siegel G, Casper U, Walter H, Hetzer R, (1994) Weiβdorn-Extrakt LI 132. Dosis- Wirkungs-Studie zum Membranpotential und Tonus menschlicher Koronararterien und des Hundepapillarmuskels. Münch med Wschr 136(Suppl 1):45-56.

Sprecher E, Pflanzliche Geriatrika. In: ZPT 9(2):40. 1988.

Sticher O, Rehwald A, Meier B, (1994) Kriterien der pharmazeutischen Qualität von Crataegus-Extrakten. Münch Med Wschr 136(Suppl 1):69-73.

Tauchert M, Loew D, (1995) Crataegi folium cum flore bei HerzinsuffizienZ In, Loew D, Rietbrock N (Hrsg) Phytopharmaka in Forschung und klinischer Anwendung. Steinkopff Verlag, Darmstadt, S. 137-144.

Tauchert M, Ploch M, Hübner WD, (1994) Wirksamkeit des Weiβdorn-Extraktes LI 132 im Vergleich mit Captopril. Multizentrische Doppelblindstudie bei 132 Patienten mit Herzinsuffizienz im Stadium II nach NYHA. Münch Med Wschr 136(Suppl 1):27-34.

Tauchert M, Siegel G, Schulz V, (1994) Weiβdorn-Extrakt als pflanzliches Cardiacum (Vorwort). Neubewertung der therapeutischen Wirksamkeit. Münch Med Wschr 136(Suppl 1):3-5.

Trunzler G, Phytotherapeutische Möglichkeiten bei Herz- und arteriellen Gefäβerkrankungen. In: ZPT 10(5):147. 1989.

Wagner H, Grevel J, (1982) Planta Med 45:98.

Wichtl M, Pflanzliche Geriatrika. In: DAZ 132(30):1576. 1992.

Further information in:

Hänsel R, Keller K, Rimpler H, Schneider G (Hrsg.), Hagers Handbuch der Pharmazeutischen Praxis, 5. Aufl., Bde 4-6 (Drogen), Springer Verlag Berlin, Heidelberg, New York, 1992-1994.

Madaus G, Lehrbuch der Biologischen Arzneimittel, Bde 1-3, Nachdruck, Georg Olms Verlag Hildesheim 1979.

Schulz R, Hänsel R, Rationale Phytotherapie, Springer Verlag Heidelberg 1996.

Steinegger E, Hänsel R, Pharmakognosie, 5. Aufl., Springer Verlag Heidelberg 1992.

Teuscher E, Biogene Arzneimittel, 5. Aufl., Wiss. Verlagsges. mbH Stuttgart 1997.

Wagner H, Wiesenauer M, Phytotherapie. Phytopharmaka und pflanzliche Homöopathika, Fischer-Verlag, Stuttgart, Jena, New York 1995.

Wichtl M (Hrsg.), Teedrogen, 4. Aufl., Wiss. Verlagsges. Stuttgart 1997.

English Horsemint

Mentha longifolia

DESCRIPTION

Medicinal Parts: The medicinal part is the dried herb.

Flower and Fruit: The flowers are sometimes interrupted lower down by 1 cm thick, gray to white, downy, panicled, false spikes. The false spikes are arranged with linear, villous bracts, which are longer than the flowers. The calyx is fluffy and woolly pubescent with awl-shaped tips. The corolla is lilac to flesh-colored. The fruit is a finely speckled nutlet.

Leaves, Stem and Root: The plant is a perennial. It has a sturdy rhizome with underground runners. The shoots are densely covered in 1- or more-celled tomentose hairs with few glands and a mild odor. The stem is erect, simple or branched, up to 1 m high, tough and obtusely angular. The leaves are sessile, oblong-ovate to lanceolate, usually acuminate, with 6 to 12 pairs of curved pinnate veins. The underside of the leaves are gray to white tomentose.

Production: English Horsemint is the aerial part of Mentha longifolia, the dried herb.

Habitat: The plant is common in all of Europe to southern Sweden.

ACTIONS AND PHARMACOLOGY

COMPOUNDS

Volatile oil: chief components piperitone (share 60-80%), furthermore beta- caryophyllene (5-15%), germacren D (5-15%), 1,8-cineole (2-7%), limonene (1-8%), with other chemotypes chief components D-carvone, piperitone, isomenthone + menthofurane, menthone, piperitol, menthol or linalool

Flavonoids: including among others diosmin, hesperidin, quercitrin, thymonin, apigenine-7-glucuronide

EFFECTS

English Horsemint has carminative and stimulant effects.

INDICATIONS AND USAGE

Unproven Uses: The drug is used for digestive disorders, particularly for flatulence. Historically, it has been used for all kinds of pain, headaches in particular.

PRECAUTIONS AND ADVERSE REACTIONS

No health hazards or side effects are known in conjunction with the proper administration of designated therapeutic dosages.

DOSAGE

Mode of Administration: The ground drug is used internally as an infusion; it is used externally as a bath additive.

LITERATURE

Hänsel R, Keller K, Rimpler H, Schneider G (Hrsg.), Hagers Handbuch der Pharmazeutischen Praxis, 5. Aufl., Bde 4-6 (Drogen), Springer Verlag Berlin, Heidelberg, New York, 1992-1994.

English Ivy

Hedera helix

DESCRIPTION

Medicinal Parts: The medicinal parts are the leaves and berries.

Flower and Fruit: The inflorescences are greenish-yellow umbels, which form dense, semi-globular clusters. The calyx tips are short, almost triangular, tomentose and drooping. The 5 petals are oblong and slightly involute. There are 5 stamens and 1 inferior ovary with 5 valves. The style is fused into a column. The fruit is a globular, usually 5-valved berry, which becomes black and ripens in spring. It contains 3 to 5 reniform, triangular, acute seeds, which are reddish-violet when young, later dark brown, and finally black.

Leaves, Stem and Root: The plant is an evergreen perennial, which creeps or, by means of adventitious roots, climbs to a length of 3 to 15 m. The stem is branched, the leaves are alternate, petioled, glabrous, glossy, coriaceous. Younger leaves are 5-lobed; the leaves of older flowering plants are ovate-rhomboid.

Characteristics: The berries and leaves have a bitter taste.

Habitat: English Ivy is indigenous to the temperate regions of Europe, and also north and central Asia. It is cultivated in the U.S.

Production: English Ivy leaf consists of the dried leaves of Hedera helix.

Other Names: Gum Ivy, True Ivy, Woodbind

ACTIONS AND PHARMACOLOGY

COMPOUNDS

Triterpene saponins: aglycone hederagenin, oleanolic acid, bayogenin, chief components hederosaponin C (hederacoside C, slightly transforming into alpha-hederin, aglycone hederagenin), additionally hederosaponin B (hederacoside B)

Volatile oils: including some with methylethylketone, methylisobutylketone

Polyynes: including falcarinol, 11,12-didehydrofalcarinol

Steroids: sterols, including beta-sitosterol, campesterol

Flavonoids: including rutin

EFFECTS

English Ivy is an expectorant and antispasmodic. In animal experiments, the drug is anti-exudative and cytotoxic. Hedera saponin C exhibits an antiviral, antibacterial, antimycotic, anthelmintic and mollusicidal, as well as an antiflagellate, effect. The fresh leaves are an irritant to the skin and mucosa and can have an allergenic effect.

INDICATIONS AND USAGE

Approved by Commission E:

- Cough
- Bronchitis

English Ivy is a respiratory catarrh used for the symptomatic treatment of chronic inflammatory bronchial conditions.

Unproven Uses: In folk medicine, English Ivy is used internally for liver, spleen and gallbladder disorders and for gout, rheumatism and scrofulosis. Externally, it is used for burn wounds, calluses, cellulitis, inflammations, neuralgia, parasitic disorders, ulcers, rheumatic complaints and phlebitis.

Homeopathic Uses: English Ivy is administered in homeopathy for rachitic states.

PRECAUTIONS AND ADVERSE REACTIONS

Health risks or side effects following the proper administration of designated therapeutic dosages are not recorded. The drug has a medium potential for sensitization through skin contact.

DOSAGE

Mode of Administration: English Ivy is available as comminuted drug and other galenic preparations for internal external use.

How Supplied: Forms of commercial pharmaceutical preparations include drops, suppositories and tablets.

Preparation: Prepare a tea by adding 1 heaped teaspoonful of drug to 1/4 liter of hot water and steeping the mixture for 10 minutes. A poultice is prepared by mixing fresh Ivy leaves 1:3 with linseed meal. To make an infusion, add 1 heaping teaspoonful of drug to one-quarter cup boiling water and steep for 10 minutes.

Daily Dosage: Tea and other infusions can be taken internally 3 times daily. The average daily dose is 0.3 to 0.8 g of drug. Fresh leaves may be laid upon festering wounds and burns; a decoction of fresh leaves (200 gm/liter water) may be used externally for rheumatism. The daily dose of a tincture is 40 to 50 drops; single dose: 5 to 10 drops.

Homeopathic Dosage: 5 drops, 1 tablet or 10 globules every 30 to 60 minutes (acute) or 1 to 3 times daily (chronic); parenterally: 1 to 2 ml sc acute, 3 times daily; chronic: once a day (HAB1).

LITERATURE

Balansard G et al., (1980) Planta Med 39:234.

Czygan FC, Hedera helix L. - Der Efeu. In: ZPT 11(4):133. 1990.

Elias R et al., JNP 54:98-103. 1991.

Gladtke E, Zur Wirksamkeit eines Efeublätterpräparates (Prospan). In: Intern Praxis 32(1)187. 1992.

Hansen L, Boll PM, (1986) Phytochemistry 25(2):285.

Julien J et al., (1985) Planta Med (3):205.

Mahran GH et al., (1975) Planta Med 29:127.

Trute A, Gross J, Mutschler E, Nahrstedt A, In vitro antispasmodic compounds of the dry extract obtained from Hedera helix. In: PM 63(2):125-129. 1997.

Trute A, Nahrstedt A, Identification and quantitative analysis of phenolic dry extracts of Hedera helix. In: PM 63(2):177-179. 1997.

Tschesche R, Schmidt R, Wulff G, Z Naturforsch 20B:708-709. 1965.

Wulff G, DAZ 108:797-807. 1968.

Further information in:

Frohne D, Pfänder HJ, Giftpflanzen - Ein Handbuch für Apotheker, Toxikologen und Biologen, 4. Aufl., Wiss. Verlagsges. mbH Stuttgart 1997.

Hänsel R, Keller K, Rimpler H, Schneider G (Hrsg.), Hagers Handbuch der Pharmazeutischen Praxis, 5. Aufl., Bde 4-6 (Drogen), Springer Verlag Berlin, Heidelberg, New York, 1992-1994.

Hausen B, Allergiepflanzen, Pflanzenallergene, ecomed Verlagsgesellsch. mbH, Landsberg 1988.

Lewin L, Gifte und Vergiftungen, 6. Aufl., Nachdruck, Haug Verlag, Heidelberg 1992.

Madaus G, Lehrbuch der Biologischen Arzneimittel, Bde 1-3, Nachdruck, Georg Olms Verlag Hildesheim 1979.

Roth L, Daunderer M, Kormann K, Giftpflanzen, Pflanzengifte, 4. Aufl., Ecomed Fachverlag Landsberg Lech 1993.

Schulz R, Hänsel R, Rationale Phytotherapie, Springer Verlag Heidelberg 1996.

Steinegger E, Hänsel R, Pharmakognosie, 5. Aufl., Springer Verlag Heidelberg 1992.

Teuscher E, Biogene Arzneimittel, 5. Aufl., Wiss. Verlagsges. mbH Stuttgart 1997.

Teuscher E, Lindequist U, Biogene Gifte - Biologie, Chemie, Pharmakologie, 2. Aufl., Fischer Verlag Stuttgart 1994.

Wagner H, Wiesenauer M, Phytotherapie. Phytopharmaka und pflanzliche Homöopathika, Fischer-Verlag, Stuttgart, Jena, New York 1995.

Wichtl M (Hrsg.), Teedrogen, 4. Aufl., Wiss. Verlagsges. Stuttgart 1997.

English Lavender

Lavandula angustifolia

DESCRIPTION

Medicinal Parts: The medicinal parts are the essential oil extracted from the fresh flowers and/or the inflorescences, the flowers collected just before opening and dried, the fresh flowers and the dried flowers.

Flower and Fruit: The flowers are in false whorls of 6 to 10 blossoms forming interrupted terminal spikes. The pedicles are 10 to 15 cm long downy stems. The bracts are 5 mm long, ovate to broadly triangular, often brown and brown-violet or violet-tinged. The tubular calyx has 5 uneven tips, it is amethyst-colored, tomentose and after flowering it is closed by a lidlike appendage of its upper tip. The corolla is longer with a cylindrically fused base, the lips are flat, and the upper lip is larger with 2 lobes. The lower lip is 3-lobed with even tips. The stamens are enclosed in the tube. The ovary consists of 4 carpels and has a nectary below it. The fruit is a glossy brown nutlet.

Leaves, Stem and Root: English Lavender is a 60 cm high subshrub and is heavily branched with leafy, erect, rod-like, gray-green, young branches. The leaves are sessile, oblong-lanceolate, entire-margined, involute, gray, later green with glandular spots beneath.

Characteristics: The flowers have a fresh aromatic fragrance.

Habitat: The plant is indigenous to the Mediterranean region but is common in most of southern Europe and is cultivated extensively.

Production: English Lavender flower consists of the dried flower of Lavandula angustifolia, gathered shortly before fully unfolding, as well as its preparations. Flowering shoots are harvested when the middle section of the spike is flowering; it is cut 10 cm beneath the insertion of the spike. The most valuable part is the receptacle.

Not to be Confused With: Other varieties of lavender such as Lavendula intermedia (Lavendin) and Lavendula latifolia. The varieties are often mixed commercially. When the drug material has a high proportion of stem and leaf material, it is considered less valuable.

Other Names: French Lavender, Garden Lavender, Lavender

ACTIONS AND PHARMACOLOGY

COMPOUNDS

Volatile oil (1-3%): chief components (-)-linalool (making up 20-50%) and linalyl acetate (30-40%), furthermore, including among others, cis-ocimene, terpinene-4-ol, beta-caryophyllene, lavandulyl acetate

Hydroxycoumarins: including among others, umbelliferone, herniarin

Tannins (13%)

Caffeic acid derivatives: including among others, rosmaric acid

EFFECTS

The drug contains essential oil. The main active constituents are linalyl acetate and linalool.

In a 1936 study, a choleretic and cholagogic effect was described. In addition, an antimicrobial effect has been demonstrated in vitro. In animal experiments a neurodepressive effect was demonstrated (shortening of the falling-asleep period and lengthening of sleep duration) and a reduction of motor activity.

In humans, after inhalation of the drug, an effect on the limbic cortex (similar to nitrazepam) was demonstrated.

INDICATIONS AND USAGE

Approved by Commission E:

- Loss of appetite
- Nervousness and insomnia
- Circulatory disorders
- Dyspeptic compaints

Internally, English Lavender is used for mood disturbances such as restlessness or insomnia, functional abdominal complaints (nervous stomach irritations, Roehmheld syndrome, meteorism, nervous intestinal discomfort).

Externally, English Lavender is used in balneotherapy for treatment of functional circulatory disorders.

Unproven Uses: In folk medicine, English Lavender is used for migraine, cramps and bronchial asthma. Externally, it is used for rheumatic conditions (the drug as an extract in liniments), as a sedative in cases of tension, exhaustion; also for poorly healing wounds (lavender baths) and for sleep as aroma therapy (herb pillow).

PRECAUTIONS AND ADVERSE REACTIONS

No health hazards or side effects are known in conjunction with the proper administration of designated therapeutic dosages. The volatile oil possesses a weak potential for sensitization.

DOSAGE

Mode of Administration: The whole drug is used for infusions, as an extract and as a bath additive. Combinations with other sedative and/or carminative herbs may be beneficial.

Preparation: An infusion is prepared by adding 5 to 10 ml of drug per cup of hot water (150 ml), draw for 10 minutes, and strain. For external use as bath additive, 100 g of drug is scalded or boiled with 2 liters of water and added to the bath.

Daily Dosage: A tea prepared as indicated above can be administered 1 cup three times daily. One to 4 drops of Lavender oil may be placed on a sugar cube.

LITERATURE

Atanassova-Shopova S, Roussinow KS, (1970) On certain central neurotropic effects of lavender essential oil. Bull Inst Physiol 8:69-76.

Buchbauer G, Jirovet L, Jäger W, Dietrich H, Plank C, Karamat E, (1991) Aromatherapy: Evidence for Sedative Effects of the Essential Oil of Lavender after Inhalation. Z Naturforsch 46c:1067-1072.

Guillemain J, Rousseau A, Delaveau P, (1989) Effets neurodépresseurs de l'huile essentielle de Lavandula angustifolia Mill. Ann Pharmaceutiques Francaises 47:337-343.

Herisset A et al., (1971) Plant Med Phytother 5:305.

Ianova LG et al., (1977) Khim Prir Soedin 1:111.

Kaiser R, Lamparsky D, (1977) Tetrahedron Lett 7:665.

Meyer A, Der Duft des Monats: Lavendel. In: DAZ 133(40):3667. 1993.

Mukherjee BD, Trenkle RW, (1973) J Agric Food Chem 21:298.

Schilcher H, Pflanzliche Psychopharmaka. Eine neue Klassifizierung nach Indikationsgruppen. In: DAZ 135(20):1811-1822. 1995.

Schulz V, Hübner WD, Ploch M, Klinische Studien mit Psycho-Phytopharmaka. In: ZPT 18(3):141-154. 1997.

Ter Heide R et al., (1970) J Chromatography 50:127.

Timiner R et al., (1975) J Agric Food Chem 23:53.

Further information in:

Hänsel R, Keller K, Rimpler H, Schneider G (Hrsg.), Hagers Handbuch der Pharmazeutischen Praxis, 5. Aufl., Bde 4-6 (Drogen): Springer Verlag Berlin, Heidelberg, New York, 1992-1994.

Hausen B, Allergiepflanzen, Pflanzenallergene, ecomed Verlagsgesellsch. mbH, Landsberg 1988.

Madaus G, Lehrbuch der Biologischen Arzneimittel, Bde 1-3, Nachdruck, Georg Olms Verlag Hildesheim 1979.

Roth L, Daunderer M, Kormann K, Giftpflanzen, Pflanzengifte, 4. Aufl., Ecomed Fachverlag Landsberg Lech 1993.

Schulz R, Hänsel R, Rationale Phytotherapie, Springer Verlag Heidelberg 1996.

Steinegger E, Hänsel R, Pharmakognosie, 5. Aufl., Springer Verlag Heidelberg 1992.

Teuscher E, Biogene Arzneimittel, 5. Aufl., Wiss. Verlagsges. Stuttgart 1997.

Wagner H, Wiesenauer M, Phytotherapie. Phytopharmaka und pflanzliche Homöopathika, Fischer-Verlag, Stuttgart, Jena, New York 1995.

Wichtl M (Hrsg.), Teedrogen, 4. Aufl., Wiss. Verlagsges. Stuttgart 1997.

English Plantain

Plantago lanceolata

DESCRIPTION

Medicinal Parts: The medicinal parts are the dried leaves, the dried herb and the fresh plant.

Flower and Fruit: The globular or shortly cylindrical spikes are on erect or ascending, 5-grooved, appressed pubescent peduncles. The flowers are small, almost colorless behind scarious, narrow-acuminate bracts. The scarious calyx is deeply divided into 4 parts and has a cylindrical tube and a margin with 4 ovate tips. There are 4 long stamens with yellowish-white filaments and anthers and 1 superior ovary. The fruit is a bivalvular, 3 to 4 mm long capsule. The seeds are oblong, 2 mm long and blackish.

Leaves, Stem and Root: The plant is perennial and grows from 5 to 50 cm high. It has a very fibrous root. All the leaves are in basal rosettes and are lanceolate or linear-lanceolate, deeply 3 to 5 ribbed, entire-margined or short-dentate.

Habitat: The plant is widespread in the cool temperate regions of the world.

Production: English Plantain herb consists of the fresh or dried above-ground parts of Plantago lanceolata, harvested at flowering season (May to September) and dried quickly at 40 to 50° C.

Not to be Confused With: the similar Digitalis-lanata leaves.

Other Names: Buckhorn, Chimney-Sweeps, Headsman, Narrow-Leaved Plantain, Ribgrass, Ribwort, Ripplegrass, Soldier's Herb

ACTIONS AND PHARMACOLOGY

COMPOUNDS

Iridoide monoterpenes (2-3%): chief components are aucubin (rhinantin) and catalpol as well as asperuloside

Mucilages (2-6%): glucomannans, arabinogalactane, rhamnogalacturonane

Flavonoids: including among other chief components apigenine-6,8-diglucoside, luteolin-7-glucuronide

Caffeic acid esters: chlorogenic acid, neochlorogenic acid, acteoside (verbascoside)

Tannins

Hydroxycoumarins: aesculetin

Saponins (traces)

Silicic acid

EFFECTS

Liquid extract and the pressed juice of fresh Plantain herb have a proven bactericidal effect. The aucubigenin (hydrolised acubin) and an antimicrobial saponin are believed to be responsible for the antibacterial effect. In addition, acceleration of blood clotting has been demonstrated and a possible epithelization effect has been mentioned.

INDICATIONS AND USAGE

Approved by Commission E:

- Common cold
- Cough/bronchitis
- Fevers and colds
- Inflammation of the mouth and pharynx
- Inflammation of the skin

Unproven Uses: In folk medicine, the pressed juice of English Plantain is used internally for conditions of the respiratory tract, cystitis, enuresis, liver disease, stomach cramps, diarrhea and as a diuretic.

Externally the plant is used for wounds, furuncles, conjunctivitis and as a hemostyptic.

PRECAUTIONS AND ADVERSE REACTIONS

No health hazards or side effects are known in conjunction with the proper administration of designated therapeutic dosages.

DOSAGE

Mode of Administration: As a comminuted herb and other galenic preparations for internal and external use. It is available as macerations, liquid extracts, lozenges, syrup and pressed juice of the fresh plant. The drug is available in many standardized preparations of antitussives and expectorants.

Preparation: To make an infusion, pour boiling water over 2 to 4 gm cut drug (or put in cold water brought to a boil) and strain after 10 minutes (1 teaspoonful = approximately 0.7 gm drug).

Daily Dosage: The average daily dose is 3 to 6 gm of herb.

Tea—1 cup of freshly made tea to be drunk several times a day.

LITERATURE

Bräutigam M, Franz G, Schleimpolysaccharide aus Spitzwegerichblättern. In: DAZ 125:58. 1985.

Davini E, The quantitative isolation and antimicrobial activity of aglycone of aucubin. In: PH 25:2420. 1986.

Elich J, Die antibakterielle Aktivität einiger einheimischer Plantago-Arten. In: Disseration Universität Berlin. 1962.

Koedam A, Plantago - history and use. In: Pharm Weekbl 112(10):246-252. 1977.

Murai M et al., Phenylethanoids in the herb of Planatago lanceolata and inhibitory effects on arachidonic acid-induced mouse ear edema. In: PM 61(5):479-480. 1995.

Wunderer H, Zentral und peripher wirksame Antitussiva: eine kritische Übersicht. In: PZ 142(11):847-852. 1997.

Further information in:

Hänsel R, Keller K, Rimpler H, Schneider G (Hrsg.), Hagers Handbuch der Pharmazeutischen Praxis, 5. Aufl., Bde 4-6 (Drogen), Springer Verlag Berlin, Heidelberg, New York, 1992-1994.

Madaus G, Lehrbuch der Biologischen Arzneimittel, Bde. 1-3, Nachdruck, Georg Olms Verlag Hildesheim 1979.

Schulz R, Hänsel R, Rationale Phytotherapie, Springer Verlag Heidelberg 1996.

Steinegger E, Hänsel R, Pharmakognosie, 5. Aufl., Springer Verlag Heidelberg 1992.

Teuscher E, Biogene Arzneimittel, 5. Aufl., Wiss. Verlagsges. Stuttgart 1997.

Wagner H, Wiesenauer M, Phytotherapie. Phytopharmaka und pflanzliche Homöopathika, Fischer-Verlag, Stuttgart, Jena, New York 1995.

Wichtl M (Hrsg.), Teedrogen, 4. Aufl., Wiss. Verlagsges. Stuttgart 1997.

Ephedra sinica

See Ma-Huang

Epigae repens

See Trailing Arbutus

Epilobium species

See Willow Herb

Equisetum arvense

See Horsetail

Ergot

Claviceps purpurea

DESCRIPTION

Medicinal Parts: The medicinal part of the fungus is the sclerotium, which grows on rye plants and is later dried.

Flower and Fruit: Ergot is a permanent form of a fungus that is a parasite on ripening rye, wheat and other grasses. It is black, hard and much larger than the grains of rye. The cycle of the fungus begins with the infection of the ovary by an ascospore. The spore, usually deposited by a visiting insect, germinates on the stigma, and the hyphae grows down into the ovary where it appropriates food destined for the grain. When the ovary has been completely destroyed, the mycelium grows. Horizontal walls are formed and fat vacuoles become visible. The hyphae of the skin layer store purple pigment 3 weeks after the infection a long, curved, black sclerotium develops. It reaches a length of up to 8 cm and bears minute condia, which are made up of the remains of the ovary and the style embedded into the loose mycelium. The sclerotium usually falls to the ground before harvest and survives the winter. In the spring, 1 to 3 cm long red-stemmed, capitula-like, pink fruiting bodies grow out of it, which in turn produce 50 to 70 μm long thread-like ascospores.

Habitat: Claviceps purpurea grows as a parasite on rye (occasionally on other grasses), and is found in all areas of the world where rye is cultivated.

Production: Ergot consists of the sclerotium of Claviceps purpurea, a parasitic fungus harvested after it has grown on cultivated rye.

Other Names: Cockspur Rye, Hornseed, Mother of Rye, Smut Rye, Spurred Rye

ACTIONS AND PHARMACOLOGY

COMPOUNDS

Indole alkaloids (ergot alkaloids, varying by variety of ergot)

Chief alkaloid of the lysergic acid amide type: ergometrine (ergobasine)

Chief alkaloid of the lysergic acid ergopeptine type: ergotamine, ergovaline, ergosine, ergocristine, ergocornine, alpha- and beta-ergocryptine, further alkaloids of the clavine type: including among others agroclavine, elymoclavine, festuclavine

Peptide alkaloids (ergopeptine group): especially ergotamine, as well as ergovaline, ergosine, ergocristine, ergocornine, alpha- and beta-ergocryptine

Xanthone derivatives (ergochromes): including, among others, secalonic acid A to C, ergoflavin

Anthracene derivatives: including, among others, clavorubine, endocrocine

Amines: including, among others, trimethylamine, methylamine

Fatty oil

EFFECTS

The drug contains ergoline alkaloids of which only ergometrin and ergopeptine have a therapeutic and toxic effect. The action of ergot is traceable to its stimulation of the smooth musculature. However, therapeutic use cannot be recommended because of the risks involved.

INDICATIONS AND USAGE

Unproven Uses: Although the risk involved is too high to recommend therapeutic use, ergot and ergot preparations were previously used in gynecology and obstetrics. Uses included hemorrhages, climacteric hemorrhages, menorrhagia and metrorrhagia, before and after miscarriage, for removal of the placenta and shortening of the afterbirth period, for atonia of the uterus and also for migraine.

Homeopathic Uses: Uses in homeopathy include uterine and muscle spasm, convulsions, paralysis, circulatory problems accompanying arterial disease and a tendency to bleed. Efficacy has not been proven.

CONTRAINDICATIONS

Ergot is now contraindicated for all therapeutic use, but especially in the presence of peripheral blood flow disorders such as Raynaud's disease, Thrombangitis obliterans, severe arteriosclerotic vascular changes, liver function disorders, severe coronary insufficiency, kidney damage, pregnancy, nursing, infectious diseases, sepsis, hypertonia and severe hypotonia.

PRECAUTIONS AND ADVERSE REACTIONS

No health hazards are known in conjunction with the proper administration of designated therapeutic dosages, but therapeutic use is not recommended because of the many side effects. Among side effects that may occur are queasiness, vomiting, feeling of weakness in the legs, muscle pain, numbness in the fingers, angina complaints, tachycardia or bradycardia, localized edema and itching.

OVERDOSAGE

Overdosage or long-term administration can lead to thrombosis, damage to the vessels of the retina (combined with optic atrophy) gangrene of the extremities, hemiplagia and convulsions.

Symptoms of acute poisonings include queasiness, vomiting, diarrhea, thirst, skin coolness, itching of the skin, rapid and weak pulse, paresthesia, numbness of the extremities, confusion or unconsciousness.

Chronic poisonings appear as:

Ergotismus gangrenosus: characterized by painful arterial blood flow disorders of the extremities with dry gangrene, angina complaints, field of vision losses, aphasias.

Ergotismus convulsivus: characterized by muscle twitching, later clonic spasm and ultimately tonic spasms, hemiplagia, loss of consciousness and death.

Drug overdose is managed by gastrointestinal emptying through inducement of vomiting and gastric lavage with burgundy-colored potassium permanganate solution, sodium sulfate. That is followed by installation of activated charcoal and shock prophylaxis (quiet and warmth). The therapy for poisonings consists of treating angiospasms with Nitrolingual-spray and vascular massage, sedatives for spasm (diazepam or chloral hydrate), administration of blocking agents, electrolyte substitution and treating possible cases of acidosis with sodium bicarbonate infusions. Intubation and oxygen respiration may also be necessary.

DOSAGE

Homeopathic Dosage: 5 drops, 1 tablet, 10 globules every 30 to 60 minutes (acute) or 1 to 3 times a day (chronic); parenterally: 1 to 2 ml sc: acute: 3 times daily; chronic: once a day (HAB1).

Storage: Ergot must be stored in tightly sealed containers and kept in a cool place, protected from light. The powdered form should not be stored.

LITERATURE

Anon., Ergotamin. Deutsche Apotheker Ztg 134 (1994), 1887

Anon., Hepetitis C - Hohes Riskiko für Medizinberufe. In: PUZ 25(6):344. 1996.

Anon., Parkinson-Krankheit: Mehe Lebensqualität bei Kombination von L-DOPA mit Dopaminagonisten. In: PUZ 24(2):101. 1995. Anon

Anon. Vom Ergolin-Pharmakophor zu selektiven Arzneistoffen. Deutsche Apotheker Ztg 132 (1992), 1235

Crespi-Perellino N et al., JNP 50:1065-1074. 1987.

Ergotamin. In: DAZ 134(20):1887. 1994.

Flieger M et al., JNP 47:970-976. 1984.

Frohne D, Pfänder HJ: Giftpflanzen - Ein Handbuch für Apotheker, Toxikologen und Biologen, 4. Aufl., Wiss. Verlags-Ges. Stuttgart 1997.

Hänsel R, Keller K, Rimpler H, Schneider G (Hrsg.), Hagers Handbuch der Pharmazeutischen Praxis, 5. Aufl., Bde 4-6 (Drogen): Springer Verlag Berlin, Heidelberg, New York, 1992-1994.

Kobel H, Sanglier JJ, Biotechnology 4:569-609. 1986.

Lewin L, Gifte und Vergiftungen, 6. Aufl., Nachdruck, Haug Verlag, Heidelberg 1992.

Madaus G, Lehrbuch der Biologischen Arzneimittel, Bde 1-3, Nachdruck, Georg Olms Verlag Hildesheim 1979.

Marshall M, Wüstenberg P, Klinik und Therapie der chronischen venösen Insuffizienz. In: Klinik und Therapie der chronischen venösen Insuffizienz, Braun Fachverlage, Karlsruhe 1994. 1994.

Milhahn HC et al., Contributions to the dissociation between antineoplastic and mutagenic activities of the ergot minor alkaloid festucalavine by substitution at C-2. In: PM 59(7):A&83. 1993.

Militz M, Antoniusfeuer, Mutterkron und Isenheimer Altar. In: PZ 141(9):720-721. 1996.

Neurotransmitter: Serotoninagonisten und -antagonisten in der Pharmakotherapie. In: DAZ 133(51/52):4895. 1993.

Perellino NC, et al., Identification of ergobine, a new natural peptide ergot alkaloid. In: JNP 56(4):489-493. 1993.

Pertz H, Naturally occuring clavines: Antagonism/partial agonism at 5-HT2alpha receptors and antogonism at alpha1-adrenoceptors in blood vessel. In: PM 62(5)387-392. 1996.

Roth L, Daunderer M, Kormann K: Giftpflanzen, Pflanzengifte, 4. Aufl., Ecomed Fachverlag Landsberg Lech 1993.

Schlenger R, 50 Jahre LSD. In: DAZ 133(32):2903. 1993.

Schmidt M, LSD, Psilocybe, Ololiuqui. In: PTA 8(3):186. 1994.

Seeger R, Neumann HG, D-(+)-Lysergsäurediethylamid (LSD). In: DAZ 132(42):2244. 1992.

Seiffer B, Therapie der Akromegalie. In: Med Mo Pharm 15(5):159. 1992.

Stadler PA, PM 46:131-144. 1982.

Steinegger E, Hänsel R, Pharmakognosie, 5. Aufl., Springer Verlag Heidelberg 1992.

Teuscher E, Lindequist U, Biogene Gifte - Biologie, Chemie, Pharmakologie, 2. Aufl., Fischer Verlag Stuttgart 1994.

Teuscher E, Biogene Arzneimittel, 5. Aufl., Wiss. Verlagsges. Stuttgart 1997.

Vom Ergolin-Pharmakophor zu selektiven Arzneistoffen. In: DAZ 132(23):1235. 1992.

Wagner H, Wiesenauer M, Phytotherapie. Phytopharmaka und pflanzliche Homöopathika, Fischer-Verlag, Stuttgart, Jena, New York 1995.

Wang BH, Polya GM, The fungal teratogen secalonic acid D is an inhibitor of protein kinase C and of cyclic AMP-dependent protein kinase. In: PM 62(2):111-114. 1997.

Wenzlaff H, Dihydroergotamin. In: DAZ 136(26):2179-2181. 1996.

Erigeron canadensis

See Canadian Fleabane

Eriodictyon californicum

See Yerba Santa

Eryngium campestre

See Eryngo

Eryngo

Eryngium campestre

DESCRIPTION

Medicinal Parts: The medicinal parts are the dried leaves, dried flowers and dried roots.

Flower and Fruit: The plant bears small terminal cymes on oval to globular capitula on sweeping inflorescences. The linear-lanceolate to awl-shaped bracts terminate in sharp thorns. The sepals are lanceolate, terminate in thorny tips and are twice as long as the white or gray-green petals. The fruit is compressed obovate with lanceolate, pointed scales.

Leaves, Stem and Root: The plant is 15 to 60 cm high, perennial, with a whitish or yellow-green color. The bifurcated stem is erect, thick, grooved and spare. The stem forms a round bush with the branches. The leaves are tough, short-petioled or sessile. The upper leaves are clasping, double pinnatesect and thorny dentate. The root is cylindrical, thick, brown and woody.

Characteristics: The root is spicy.

Habitat: The plant grows in most parts of Europe and northern Africa and has been introduced into North America.

Production: Eryngo root is the root of Eryngium campestre, which is gathered and dried in the spring and autumn. It is gathered in uncultivated regions. The roots are halved and air-dried. Eryngo herb is the dried leaves and blossoms of Eryngium campestre.

Other Names: Eringo, Sea Holly, Sea Holme, Sea Hulver

ACTIONS AND PHARMACOLOGY

COMPOUNDS: ERYNGO ROOT

Triterpene saponins

Furanocoumarins

Pyranocoumarins: including egelinol and its angeloyl-, senecionyl- or benzyl-esters agasyllin, grandivetin and egelinol benzoate

Monoterpene glycosides of the cyclohexenol type: including 3-(beta-D-glucosyloxymethyl)-2,4,4-trimethyl-2,5-cyclohexadien-1-one

Caffeic acid ester: chlorogenic acid, rosmarinic acid

Oligosaccharides: 1-kestose

EFFECTS: ERYNGO ROOT
The root is said to be mildly expectorant and spasmolytic; however, there is no scientific evidence to support this.

COMPOUNDS: ERYNGO HERB
Triterpene saponins

Caffeic acid ester: chlorogenic acid, rosmarinic acid

Flavonoids

EFFECTS: ERYNGO HERB
The herb is said to be a mild diuretic and an expectorant; however, there is no scientific evidence to support this.

INDICATIONS AND USAGE

ERYNGO ROOT
Unproven Uses: The root is used in the treatment of bladder and kidney stones, renal colic, kidney and urinary tract inflammation, urinary retention and edema. It is also used for coughs, bronchitis, skin disorders and respiratory disorders.

ERYNGO HERB
Unproven Uses: The herb is used in the treatment of urinary tract infections and as an adjuvant to treat inflammation of the efferent urinary tract, prostatitis and bronchial catarrh.

PRECAUTIONS AND ADVERSE REACTIONS

ERYNGO ROOT AND HERB
Health risks or side effects following the proper administration of designated therapeutic dosages are not recorded.

DOSAGE

ERYNGO ROOT
Mode of Administration: The comminuted root is contained in tea mixtures, extracts, decoctions, liquids and tinctures.

Preparation: To make a tea, use 1 level teaspoonful of the ground root per cup of boiling water (30 to 40 gm per liter boiling water). Allow to draw until cold. To make a decoction, boil 4 teaspoonfuls of the ground root in 1 liter of water for 10 minutes and allow to draw for 15 minutes. The tincture is prepared by soaking 20 gm ground drug in 80 gm of 60% alcohol for 10 days.

Daily Dosage: The daily dosage is 3 to 4 cups of the tea; 2 to 3 cups of the decoction; 50 to 60 drops of the tincture in 3 or 4 divided doses; or 2 to 3 gm of the liquid extract.

ERYNGO HERB
Mode of Administration: The herb is administered as an extract and in homeopathic dilutions (from E. yuccifolium).

LITERATURE

Bhargava SK, Dixit VP, (1985) Plant Med Phytother 19(1):29.

Erdelmeier CAJ, Sticher O, (1985) Planta Med 51(5):407.

Gracza L et al., (1985) Arch Pharm 312(12):1090.

Hänsel R, Keller K, Rimpler H, Schneider G (Hrsg.), Hagers Handbuch der Pharmazeutischen Praxis, 5. Aufl., Bde 4-6 (Drogen), Springer Verlag Berlin, Heidelberg, New York, 1992-1994.

Hiller K, In "The Biology and Chemistry of the Umbelliferae". Ed. V. N. Heywood, Academic Press London 1971.

Hiller K, Linzer B, PA 22:321. 1967.

Kartnig T, Wolf J, Flavonoide aus den oberirdischen Teilen von Eryngium campestre. In: PM 59(3):285. 1993.

Lisciani R et al., (1984) J Ethnopharmacol 12(39):263.

Madaus G, Lehrbuch der Biologischen Arzneimittel, Bde 1-3, Nachdruck, Georg Olms Verlag Hildesheim 1979.

Steinegger E, Hänsel R, Pharmakognosie, 5. Aufl., Springer Verlag Heidelberg 1992.

Erysimum diffusum

See Gray Wallflower

Erythronium americanum

See American Adder's Tongue

Erythroxylum coca

See Coca

Eschscholtzia californica

See California Poppy

Eucalyptus

Eucalyptus globulus

DESCRIPTION

Medicinal Parts: The medicinal parts are the oil extracted from the fresh leaves and branch tips as well as the dried leaves.

Flower and Fruit: The flowers are solitary on short pedicles. They have a somewhat pointed, but low operculum stretching over the surface of the stamens. There are no sepals but there are numerous long stamens turned inward, which open along the whole length in 2 splits. The fruit is 10 to 15 by 15 to 30 mm and is a depressed-globose, somewhat tapering toward the base, with 4 main ribs.

Leaves, Stem and Root: Eucalyptus is a deciduous tree up to 40 m tall with silver-gray bark, which has scattered warts. The trunk is twisted. The juvenile leaves are 7 to 16 by 4 to 9 cm, ovate to broadly lanceolate, cordate, very glaucus. The mature leaves are 10 to 13 by 3 to 4 cm, lanceolate to falcate-lanceolate, acuminate, asymmetrical rounded and glossy green.

Habitat: Eucalyptus is indigenous to Australia and Tasmania. It is cultivated today in some subtropical regions of southern Europe, Africa, Asia and America.

Production: Eucalyptus oil consists of the volatile oil from various cineol-rich species of Eucalyptus, such as Eucalyptus globulus, Eucalyptus fructicetorum (syn. Eucalyptus polybractea) and/or Eucalyptus smithii. The oil is obtained by steam distillation, followed by rectification of the fresh leaves and branch tops. Eucalyptus leaf consists of the dried, mature leaves from older trees of Eucalyptus globulus. To harvest eucalyptus, the trees are cut down; drying takes place in the shade.

Not To Be Confused With: Camphor oil and by-products of turpentine manufacture; the oil is also blended with other expensive oils, such as rosemary and thyme. The properties of Eucalyptus leaves vary from species to species.

Other Names: Blue Gum, Fever Tree, Gum Tree, Red Gum, Stringy Bark Tree

ACTIONS AND PHARMACOLOGY

COMPOUNDS: EUCALYPTUS OIL

Chief constituent of the rectified volatile oil: 1,8-cineol (over 80%), furthermore p-cymene, alpha-pinenes, limonene, geraniol, camphene

EFFECTS: EUCALYPTUS OIL

Some of the subsequent properties mentioned refer to isolated cineole. As the standardized commodity, the drug contains 80 to 90% cineole.

In vitro, eucalyptus oil has an antibacterial and fungicidal effect. The drug inhibits prostaglandin biosynthesis and has a mild hyperemic, expectorant and secretolytic motor effect when used topically. In animal experiments eucalyptus was demonstrably cough relieving and displayed a surfactant effect. In vitro, the oil was enzyme inducing and improved pulmonary compliance. It is secretolytic, expectorant, mildly antispasmodic, and a mild local hyperemic.

COMPOUNDS: EUCALYPTUS LEAF

Volatile oil: chief constituent 1,8-cineol (45-75%), in additions myrtenol, alpha-pinenes, beta-pinenes, pinocarvon, gamma-terpenes, aliphatic aldehydes (butyr-, capron-, valerenaldehyde)

Euglobale: macrocarpale (with acylphloroglucinol-monoterpene or else sesquiterpene- parent substances)

Flavonoids: rutin, hyperoside, quercitrin

EFFECTS: EUCALYPTUS LEAF

The drug has been shown to be secretolytic, expectorant, weakly antispasmodic, deodorizing, cooling and diuretic. In animal experiments the blood-sugar level of uninfluenced plasma insulin was reduced. The euglobulin is said to have an anti-inflammatory and antiproliferative effect in animal experiments and inhibits in vitro TPA-induced EBV-EA activity.

INDICATIONS AND USAGE

EUCALYPTUS OIL

Approved by Commission E:

- Cough/bronchitis
- Rheumatism

Eucalyptus oil is used internally and externally for catarrh of the respiratory tract and externally for rheumatic complaints.

Unproven Uses: In folk medicine, the oil is used for asthma, coughs, diseases of the frontal sinuses, fever, flu, gastric complaints, hoarseness, incipient scarlet fever and measles, worm infestation and as an intestinal antiseptic.

EUCALYPTUS LEAF

Approved by Commission E:

- Cough/bronchitis

Eucalyptus leaf is used internally as a catarrh of the respiratory tract.

Unproven Uses: In folk medicine, it is used internally for the treatment of bladder diseases, asthma, fever, flu, whooping cough, liver and gallbladder complaints, loss of appetite and diabetes. It is used externally for wounds, acne, poorly healing ulcers, stomatitis, bleeding gums, pain and rheumatism, neuralgia, gonorrhea and as a gastrointestinal remedy.

PRECAUTIONS AND ADVERSE REACTIONS

EUCALYPTUS OIL

General: The administration of the drug leads in rare cases to nausea, vomiting and diarrhea. It should not be taken internally with inflammation of the gastrointestinal area and the biliary ducts or with severe illnesses of the liver.

Pediatric Use: Infants and small children should not have preparations containing the oil applied to their faces as this practice can lead to glottal or bronchial spasms, asthma-like attacks or even death by asphyxiation.

EUCALYPTUS LEAF

General: The administration of the drug leads in rare cases to nausea, vomiting and diarrhea. It should not be taken internally with inflammation of the gastrointestinal area and the biliary ducts or with severe illnesses of the liver. Poisonings occur with the volatile oil but are not likely with administration of the leaf drug.

Pediatric Use: Infants and small children should not have preparations containing the oil applied to their faces as this practice can lead to glottal or bronchial spasms, asthma-like attacks or even death by asphyxiation.

OVERDOSAGE

EUCALYPTUS OIL

Overdoses can lead to life-threatening poisonings. Severe poisonings are possible for children after a few drops; poisonings have been known in adults with 4 to 5 ml. Symptoms include drop in blood pressure, circulatory disorders, collapse and asphyxiation. Because of the danger of aspiration, vomiting should not be induced. Following the administration of activated charcoal, therapy consists of diazepam for spasms, atropine for colic, electrolyte replenishment and sodium bicarbonate infusions for any acidosis that may arise. Intubation and oxygen respiration may also be necessary.

DOSAGE

EUCALYPTUS OIL

Mode of Administration: Essential oil and other galenic preparations are available for internal and external application.

Preparation: 1,8-cineole is recovered through a renewed fractional distillation of the oil.

Daily Dosage: For internal use, the average daily dose is 0.3 to 0.6 gm eucalyptus oil.

Inhalation: 2 to 3 drops in boiling water, inhale the steam (single dose: 0.2 gm corresponding to 10 drops). Oil: 3 to 6 drops added in 150 ml water, to be taken several times a day.

When used externally, the concentration is 5 to 20% essential oil, in oil and semi-solid preparations and 5 to 10% essential oil, in aqueous-alcoholic preparations. If the essential oil is used, several drops may be rubbed into the skin.

Storage: Eucalyptus must be kept in appropriate, tightly sealed containers protected from light; different consignments must be stored separately.

EUCALYPTUS LEAF

Mode of Administration: Eucalyptus leaf is administered as the comminuted leaf for infusions and other galenic preparations for internal and external application. The drug may also be administered by inhalation.

Preparations:

Eucalyptus tincture — 1:5 70% ethanol (V/V)

Eucalyptus liquid extract — 60% 1:1

Eucalyptus syrup — pour 1500 ml on 100 gm cut drug and leave to draw for 6 hours and strain. 180 gm sugar is added to 100 ml infusion, brought to a simmer and filtered.

Tea — pour boiling water over 1.5 to 2 gm of the finely cut drug, cover and leave to draw for 5 to 10 minutes, strain.

Daily Dosage: The average daily dose is 4 to 6 gm of drug, divided up every 3 to 4 hours. Single dose: 1.5 gm several times a day

The average dose for the tincture is 3 to 4 gm.

Eucalyptus tea — 1 cup up to 3 times a day.

Eucalyptus syrup — 2 to 5 dessertspoons daily.

Eucalyptus powder — daily dose 4 to 16 gm; divided over 3 to 4 hours.

Storage: Eucalyptus must be kept in appropriate, tightly-sealed, non-synthetic containers; different consignments must be stored separately.

LITERATURE

EUCALYPTUS OIL

Anonym, Phytotherapie:Pflanzliche Antirheumatika - was bringen sie? In: DAZ 136(45):4012-4015. 1996.

Boland B, In: Eucalyptus leaf oils. Boland DJ, Brophy JJ, House APN (Eds.). Inkata Press, Melbourne, XII + 252 pp. 1992.

Boland DJ, Brophy JJ, House APN, Eucalyptus leave oils. In: Inkata Press Melbourne. 1991.

Boukef K et al., (1976) Plant Med Phytother 10:24, 30:119.

Burrow A, Eccles R, Jones AS, (1983) The effects of camphor, eucalyptus and menthol vapor on nasal resistance to airflow and nasal sensation. Acta Otolaryng (Stockholm) 96:157-161.

Fox N, (1977) Effect of Camphor, Eucalyptol and Menthol on the vascular state of the mucos membrane. Arch Otolaryngol 6: 112-122.

Göbel H, Schmidt G, (1995a) Effekt von Pfefferminz- und Eukalyptusölpräparationen in experimentellen Kopfschmerzmodellen. Z Phytother 16:23-33.

Göbel H, Schmidt G, Dworschak M, Stolze H, Heuss D, (1995) Essential plant oils and headache mechanisms. Phytomedicine 2: 93-102.

Göbel H, Schmidt G, Dworschak M, Stolze H, Heuss D, (1995) Essential plant oils and headache mechanisms. Phytomedicine 2: 93-103.

Göbel H, Schmidt G, Soyka D, (1994) Effect of peppermint and eucalyptus oil preparations on neurophysiological and experimental algesimetric headache parameters. Cephalalgia 14: 228-234.

Göbel H, Stolze H, Dworschak M, Heinze A, (1995) Oleum menthae piperitae, Wirkmechanismen und klinische Effektivität bei Kopfschmerz vom Spannungstyp. In: Loew D, Rietbrock N (Hrsg) Phytopharmaka in Forschung und klinischer Anwendung. Steinkopff Verlag, Darmstadt, S. 177-184.

Gräfe AK, Besonderheiten der Arzneimitteltherapie im Säuglings- und Kindesalter. In: PZ 140(30):2659-2667. 1995.

Ikeda RM et al., (1962) J Food Sci 27:455.

Linsenmann P, Hermat H, Swoboda M, (1989) Therapeutischer Wert ätherischer Öle bei chronisch-abstruktiver Bronchitis. Atemw Lungenkrankh 15:152-156.

Linsenmann P, Swoboda M, (1986) Therapeutische Wirksamkeit ätherischer Öle bei chronisch-obstruktiver Bronchitis. Therapiewoche 36:1161-1166.

Osawa K et al., Macrocarpals H, I, and J from the leaves of Eucalyptus globulus. In: JNP 59(9):824-827. 1996.

Patel S, Wiggins J, (1980) Eucalyptus oil poisoning. Arch Dis Childh 55:405-406.

Römmelt H, Schnizer W, Swoboda M, Senn E, (1988) Pharmakokinetik ätherischer Öle nach Inhalation mit einer terpenhaltigen Salbe. Z Phytother 9:14-16.

Zänker KS, Blümel G, (1983) Terpene-induced lowering of surface tension in vitro. In: A rationale for surfactant substitution. Resp Exp Med 182:33-38.

Zänker KS, Blümel G, Probst J, Reiterer W, (1984) Theoretical and experimental evidence for the action of terpens as modulators in lung function. Prog Resp Res 18:302-304.

Further information in:

Fenaroli's Handbook of Flavor Ingredients, Vol. 1, 2nd Ed., CRC Press 1975.

Frohne D, Pfänder HJ, Giftpflanzen - Ein Handbuch für Apotheker, Toxikologen und Biologen, 4. Aufl., Wiss. Verlagsges. mbH Stuttgart 1997.

Hänsel R, Keller K, Rimpler H, Schneider G (Hrsg.), Hagers Handbuch der Pharmazeutischen Praxis, 5. Aufl., Bde 4-6 (Drogen), Springer Verlag Berlin, Heidelberg, New York, 1992-1994.

Leung AY, Encyclopedia of Common Natural Ingredients Used in Food, Drugs and Cosmetics, John Wiley & Sons Inc., New York 1980.

Lewin L, Gifte und Vergiftungen, 6. Aufl., Nachdruck, Haug Verlag, Heidelberg 1992.

Madaus G, Lehrbuch der Biologischen Arzneimittel, Bde 1-3, Nachdruck, Georg Olms Verlag Hildesheim 1979.

Roth L, Daunderer M, Kormann K, Giftpflanzen, Pflanzengifte, 4. Aufl., Ecomed Fachverlag Landsberg Lech 1993.

Schulz R, Hänsel R, Rationale Phytotherapie, Springer Verlag Heidelberg 1996.

Steinegger E, Hänsel R, Pharmakognosie, 5. Aufl., Springer Verlag Heidelberg 1992.

Teuscher E, Biogene Arzneimittel, 5. Aufl., Wiss. Verlagsges. mbH Stuttgart 1997.

Wagner H, Wiesenauer M, Phytotherapie. Phytopharmaka und pflanzliche Homöopathika, Fischer-Verlag, Stuttgart, Jena, New York 1995.

Wichtl M (Hrsg.), Teedrogen, 4. Aufl., Wiss. Verlagsges. Stuttgart 1997.

EUCALYPTUS LEAF

Anonym, Phytotherapie:Pflanzliche Antirheumatika - was bringen sie? In: DAZ 136(45):4012-4015. 1996.

Boland B, In: Eucalyptus leaf oils. Boland DJ, Brophy JJ, House APN (Eds.). Inkata Press, Melbourne, XII + 252 pp. 1992.

Boland DJ, Brophy JJ, House APN, Eucalyptus leave oils. In: Inkata Press Melbourne. 1991.

Boukef K et al., (1976) Plant Med Phytother 10:24, 30:119.

Burrow A, Eccles R, Jones AS, (1983) The effects of camphor, eucalyptus and menthol vapor on nasal resistance to airflow and nasal sensation. Acta Otolaryng (Stockholm) 96:157-161.

Fox N, (1977) Effect of Camphor, Eucalyptol and Menthol on the vascular state of the mucous membrane. Arch Otolaryngol 6: 112-122.

Göbel H, Schmidt G, (1995a) Effekt von Pfefferminz- und Eukalyptusölpräparationen in experimentellen Kopfschmerzmodellen. Z Phytother 16:23-33.

Göbel H, Schmidt G, Dworschak M, Stolze H, Heuss D, (1995) Essential plant oils and headache mechanisms. Phytomedicine 2:93-102.

Göbel H, Schmidt G, Dworschak M, Stolze H, Heuss D, (1995) Essential plant oils and headache mechanisms. Phytomedicine 2:93-103.

Göbel H, Schmidt G, Soyka D, (1994) Effect of peppermint and eucalyptus oil preparations on neurophysiological and experimental algesimetric headache parameters. Cephalalgia 14: 228-234.

Göbel H, Stolze H, Dworschak M, Heinze A, (1995) Oleum menthae piperitae, Wirkmechanismen und klinische Effektivität bei Kopfschmerz vom Spannungstyp. In: Loew D, Rietbrock N (Hrsg) Phytopharmaka in Forschung und klinischer Anwendung. Steinkopff Verlag, Darmstadt, S. 177-184.

Gräfe AK, Besonderheiten der Arzneimitteltherapie im Säuglings- und Kindesalter. In: PZ 140(30):2659-2667. 1995.

Ikeda RM et al., (1962) J Food Sci 27:455.

Linsenmann P, Hermat H, Swoboda M, (1989) Therapeutischer Wert ätherischer Öle bei chronisch-abstruktiver Bronchitis. Atemw Lungenkrankh 15:152-156.

Linsenmann P, Swoboda M, (1986) Therapeutische Wirksamkeit ätherischer Öle bei chronisch-obstruktiver Bronchitis. Therapiewoche 36:1161-1166.

Osawa K et al., Macrocarpals H, I, and J from the leaves of Eucalyptus globulus. In: JNP 59(9):824-827. 1996.

Patel S, Wiggins J, (1980) Eucalyptus oil poisoning. Arch Dis Childh 55:405-406.

Römmelt H, Schnizer W, Swoboda M, Senn E, (1988) Pharmakokinetik ätherischer Öle nach Inhalation mit einer terpenhaltigen Salbe. Z Phytother 9:14-16.

Zänker KS, Blümel G, (1983) Terpene-induced lowering of surface tension in vitro. In: A rationale for surfactant substitution. Resp Exp Med 182:33-38.

Zänker KS, Blümel G, Probst J, Reiterer W, (1984) Theoretical and experimental evidence for the action of terpens as modulators in lung function. Prog Resp Res 18:302-304.

Further information in:

Fenaroli's Handbook of Flavor Ingredients, Vol. 1, 2nd Ed., CRC Press 1975.

Frohne D, Pfänder HJ, Giftpflanzen - Ein Handbuch für Apotheker, Toxikologen und Biologen, 4. Aufl., Wiss. Verlagsges. mbH Stuttgart 1997.

Hänsel R, Keller K, Rimpler H, Schneider G (Hrsg.), Hagers Handbuch der Pharmazeutischen Praxis, 5. Aufl., Bde 4-6 (Drogen), Springer Verlag Berlin, Heidelberg, New York, 1992-1994.

Leung AY, Encyclopedia of Common Natural Ingredients Used in Food, Drugs and Cosmetics, John Wiley & Sons Inc., New York 1980.

Lewin L, Gifte und Vergiftungen, 6. Aufl., Nachdruck, Haug Verlag, Heidelberg 1992.

Madaus G, Lehrbuch der Biologischen Arzneimittel, Bde 1-3, Nachdruck, Georg Olms Verlag Hildesheim 1979.

Roth L, Daunderer M, Kormann K, Giftpflanzen, Pflanzengifte, 4. Aufl., Ecomed Fachverlag Landsberg Lech 1993.

Schulz R, Hänsel R, Rationale Phytotherapie, Springer Verlag Heidelberg 1996.

Steinegger E, Hänsel R, Pharmakognosie, 5. Aufl., Springer Verlag Heidelberg 1992.

Teuscher E, Biogene Arzneimittel, 5. Aufl., Wiss. Verlagsges. mbH Stuttgart 1997.

Wagner H, Wiesenauer M, Phytotherapie. Phytopharmaka und pflanzliche Homöopathika, Fischer-Verlag, Stuttgart, Jena, New York 1995.

Wichtl M (Hrsg.), Teedrogen, 4. Aufl., Wiss. Verlagsges. Stuttgart 1997.

Eucalyptus globulus

See Eucalyptus

Eugenia chequen

See Cheken

Eugenia uniflora

See Surinam Cherry

Euonymus species

See Wahoo

Eupatorium cannabinum

See Hemp Agrimony

Eupatorium perfoliatum

See Boneset

Euphorbia cyparissias

See Cypress Spurge

Euphorbia resinifera

See Spurge

Euphrasia officinalis

See Eyebright

European Elder

Sambucus nigra

DESCRIPTION

Medicinal Parts: The medicinal parts are the bark peeled from the branches in spring and freed from the cork, the air-dried flowers, the fresh and dried leaves, the fresh and dried ripe fruit, the dried roots, and the fresh leaves and inflorescences in equal parts.

Flower and Fruit: The strongly perfumed, yellowish-white flowers are in large, flat, apical, richly and densely blossomed erect cymes with 5 main branches. The edge of the calyx is small and 5-tipped. The corolla is rotate, deep, and has 5 petals. There are 5 stamens and 1 inferior ovary. The fruit is a black-violet, berry-like drupe with blood-red juice. The seeds are brownish, ovate, and domed on the outside.

Leaves, Stem and Root: The plant is a shallow-rooted, up to 7 m high tree or bush with spreading branches containing dry white latex. The bark of the trunk is light brown to gray, and fissured. The bark on the young branches is green and covered with gray lenticles. The leaves are odd 3 to 7 pinnate. They are matte green above and light blue-green beneath. The leaflets are ovate or oblong acuminate, and densely serrate.

Characteristics: The flowers have a strong, somewhat numbing perfume.

Habitat: European Elder is indigenous to almost all of Europe.

Production: Elder flowers consist of the inflorescence of Sambucus nigra, which are collected in the wild, sifted and dried.

Not to be Confused With: Confusion sometimes arises with the flowers of Sambucus ebulus.

Other Names: Black Elder, Black-Berried Alder, Boor Tree, Elder, Bountry, Ellanwood, Ellhorn

ACTIONS AND PHARMACOLOGY

COMPOUNDS

Flavonoids (up to 3%): chief components are rutin, isoquercitrin, quercitrin, hyperoside, astragalin, nicotoflorin

Volatile oil (0.03-0.14%): higher share (65%) of free fatty acids, including among others palmitic acid (share 38%)

Caffeic acid derivatives (3%): chlorogenic acids

EFFECTS

Animal tests have shown that Alder increases bronchial secretion. A diaphoretic effect is apparent, but the mechanism is unknown.

INDICATIONS AND USAGE

Approved by Commission E:

- Cough/bronchitis
- Fevers and colds

The drug is used for colds and coughs. It is a sweat-producing remedy for the treatment of feverish colds.

Unproven Uses: In folk medicine, Elder flowers are used internally as a sudorific tea and for colds and other feverish conditions. Elder is also used as an infusion, as a gargle/mouthwash and for respiratory disorders such as coughs, head colds, laryngitis, flu, and shortness of breath. Elder is used occasionally by nursing mothers to increase lactation. Externally, herbal pillows are used for swelling and inflammation.

Homeopathic Uses: Among uses in homeopathy is inflammation of the respiratory tract.

PRECAUTIONS AND ADVERSE REACTIONS

No health hazards or side effects are known in conjunction with the proper administration of designated therapeutic dosages.

DOSAGE

Mode of Administration: Whole herb and other galenic preparations for infusions.

Preparation: To prepare an infusion, brew 2 teaspoonfuls (3 to 4 g) of elder flowers in 150 ml of boiling water and strain after 5 minutes.

Daily Dosage: The average daily dose of the drug is 10 to 15 gm. The infusion (tea) should be freshly prepared and drunk in doses of 1 to 2 cups several times—especially in the afternoon and evening.

Homeopathic Dosage: For adults, 5 drops, 1 tablet or 10 globules every 30 to 60 minutes (acute) or 1 to 3 times daily (chronic); parenterally: 1 to 2 ml sc acute: 3 times daily; chronic once a day (HAB1). Adjust dosages for children.

Storage: Elder should be stored where it is protected from light and moisture.

LITERATURE

Bauer R et al., (1985) Helv Chim Acta 68:2355.

Czygan FC, Holunder wird wieder gesellschaftsfähig. In: ZPT 15(2): 111. 1994.

Eberhardt R, Pfannhauser W, Z Lebensm Unters Forsch 181:97. 1985.

Inoue T, Sato K, (1975) Phytochemistry 14:1871.

Lawrie W et al., (1964) Phytochemistry 3:267.

Mascolo N et al., (1987) Phytother Res 1(1):28.

Paulo E, (1976) Folia Biol 24(2):213.

Petitjean-Freytet C et al., J Pharm Belg 46:241. 1991.

Richter W, Willuhn G, DAZ 114:947. 1974.

Willuhn G, Richter W, PM 31:328. 1977.

Further information in:

Hänsel R, Keller K, Rimpler H, Schneider G (Hrsg.), Hagers Handbuch der Pharmazeutischen Praxis, 5. Aufl., Bde 4-6 (Drogen): Springer Verlag Berlin, Heidelberg, New York, 1992-1994.

Leung AY, Encyclopedia of Common Natural Ingredients Used in Food, Drugs, Cosmetics, John Wiley & Sons Inc., New York 1980.

Madaus G, Lehrbuch der Biologischen Arzneimittel, Bde 1-3, Nachdruck, Georg Olms Verlag Hildesheim 1979.

Schulz R, Hänsel R, Rationale Phytotherapie, Springer Verlag Heidelberg 1996.

Steinegger E, Hänsel R, Pharmakognosie, 5. Aufl., Springer Verlag Heidelberg 1992.

Teuscher E, Biogene Arzneimittel, 5. Aufl., Wiss. Verlagsges. Stuttgart 1997.

Wagner H, Wiesenauer M, Phytotherapie. Phytopharmaka und pflanzliche Homöopathika, Fischer-Verlag, Stuttgart, Jena, New York 1995.

Wichtl M (Hrsg.), Teedrogen, 4. Aufl., Wiss. Verlagsges. Stuttgart 1997.

European Five-Finger Grass

Potentilla reptans

DESCRIPTION

Medicinal Parts: The medicinal parts are the fresh flowering plant and the roots.

Flower and Fruit: The flowers are solitary or in pairs on long thin pedicles opposite the leaves. The calyx has 5 segments and is 10 to 25 mm across. The golden yellow petals are obcordate and up to twice as long as the calyx. A ring-like swelling at the base of the stamens exudes a kind of honey. The small fruit is oblong-ovate and wrinkled.

Leaves, Stem and Root: The plant is a herbaceous perennial with a thin, divided rhizome and rosettes of basal leaves. The basal leaves produce 30 cm to 100 cm-long flowering stems from their axils, which are rooted at the nodes. The stems are pubescent or almost glabrous, have no glands and are often tinged red. The cauline leaves are long-petioled and 5 to 7 digitate. The basal stipules are fused to the petiole. The leaflets are obovate, 10 to 70 mm long, dentate to serrate and pubescent or almost glabrous.

Habitat: Europe. The plant is common in Europe, Western Asia, North America, Ethiopia and the Near East. Potentilla canadensis is indigenous to Canada and the U.S. and is very similar.

Production: European Five-Finger Grass and root is the complete plant of Potentilla reptans.

The drug is a mixture of green and brown in color and has no particular smell or taste. The roots are dug up in September/October and then dried in a sunny, airy place.

Other Names: Cinquefoil, Five Fingers, Five-Finger Blossom, Sunkfield, Synkfoyle

ACTIONS AND PHARMACOLOGY

COMPOUNDS

Tannins (6 to 12%)

Flavonoids: including quercetin-3,7-diglucuronide

EFFECTS

The drug is astringent and has wound healing effect due to the tannin content.

INDICATIONS AND USAGE

Unproven Uses: European Five-Finger Grass is used internally for diarrhea and fever; externally for inflammation of the mucous membranes of mouth and gums, toothache, and heartburn.

PRECAUTIONS AND ADVERSE REACTIONS

No health hazards or side effects are known in conjunction with the proper administration of designated therapeutic dosages. There have been complaints of gastrointestinal upset in conjunction with the drugs use reported in the literature.

DOSAGE

Mode of Administration: Available as crude drug and as an infusion for internal and external use.

Preparation: A decoction for internal use is prepared by adding 3 gm of drug per 100 ml of water. A decoction using 6 gm of drug per 100 ml of water is used for external application and mouth rinses.

Daily Dosage: Internally, 2 to 3 cups of a decoction prepared according to the formula above are administered daily. Externally, a decoction using the formula above is administered as a gargle, mouthwash or rinse. Moist compresses may be applied to affected areas of the skin.

LITERATURE

Hänsel R, Keller K, Rimpler H, Schneider G (Hrsg.), Hagers Handbuch der Pharmazeutischen Praxis, 5. Aufl., Bde 4-6 (Drogen), Springer Verlag Berlin, Heidelberg, New York, 1992-1994.

European Golden Rod

Solidago virgaurea

DESCRIPTION

Medicinal Parts: The medicinal parts are the dried aerial parts collected during the flowering season, the fresh inflorescences and the flowering twigs.

Flower and Fruit: The yellow composite flowers are in erect racemes facing all directions and are simple or compound. They are medium-sized. The involucral bracts are imbricate and arranged in numerous rows. The ray florets are narrow, lingual and female. The disc florets are funnel-shaped, 5-tipped and androgynous. The fruit is a cylindrical achene with numerous ribs. It is brown, sparsely pubescent and 3.5 to 4.5 mm long with a tuft of hair.

Leaves, Stem and Root: The plant is a perennial that ranges in size from a few centimeters to over 1 m. The rhizome is cylindrical, noded, diagonally ascending and short. The stem is erect, cane-like, angularly grooved above, usually red-tinged beneath, and glabrous to loosely appressed pubescent higher up. The basal leaves are long-petioled, elliptical, acuminate and narrowing to the winged stem. The lower ones are serrate and the upper ones entire-margined.

Habitat: The plant is indigenous to Europe, Asia and North America.

Production: Golden Rod is the aerial part of Solidago virgaurea. It occurs in the wild in Hungary, former Yugoslavia, Bulgaria and Poland

Not to be Confused With: Despite qualitative and quantitative differences in their effects, drugs containing Solidago gigantea or Solidago canadensis are exchanged with Solidago virgaurea on the market; confusions with Senecio species are also conceivable.

Other Names: Aaron's Rod, Woundwort, Goldenrod

ACTIONS AND PHARMACOLOGY

COMPOUNDS

Triterpene saponins (0.2 to 0.3%):

In the European form—3,28-bisdemosidic ester saponins, including acyl-virgaurea saponins 1, 2 and 3; the acid components are acetic acid and beta-hydroxy butyric acid; aglycone is polygalic acid.

In the Asian form—bi- or tridemosidic solidago saponins I to XXIX, acyl-virgaurea saponin 1, acylvirgaurea saponin 2, bellis saponin BA2

Volatile oil (0.4 to 0.5%, in the stored drug less than 0.2%): chief components

In the European form—alpha-pinene, beta-pinene, limonene, delta-elemene, gamma-cadinene, beta-phellandrene, myrcene

In the Asian form—limonene, germacrene-D, germacrene-B and beta-caryophyllene

Polysaccharides (water-soluble, 6 to 8%)

Diterpenes: cis-clerodane-derivatives, presumably only in the Asian variety

Carotinoids (as blossom pigments)

Flavonoids (1.1 to 2%): chief component rutin (0.8 %), including as well hyperoside, isoquercitrin, avicularin, quercetin-3-O-beta-D-robinoside, astragalin, nicotiflorin, kaempferol-3-O-beta-D-galactoside, kaempferol- 3-O-alpha-arabinoside, kaempferol-3-O-beta-D-robinobioside, isorhamnetin-3-O-beta-D-galactoside, isorhamnetin-3-O-beta-D-glucoside, isorhamnetin-3-O-beta-D-rutinoside, rhamnetin-3-O-glucorahamnoside

Phenol glucosides (hydroxy benzylbenzoyte diglucosides, 0.2 to 1.0%): leicarposide (0.2 to 1%), virgaureoside A (0.01 to 0.14%), benzyl-2,6-dimethoxy-benzoate

Caffeic acid derivatives (0.2 to 0.4%): including chlorogenic acid, neochlorogenic acid, 3,5-dicaffeoyl quinic acid

Phenol carboxylic acids: salicylic acid (0.1%), as well as vanillic acid, protocatechuic acid, ferulic acid, caffeic acid, sinapineic acid—free, estered or glycosylated

Polyynes (in the roots): 2,8-cis-trans-matricaria ester, 2,8-cis-cis-matricaria ester, cis-lachnophyllum ester, matricaric acid lactone, lachnophyllum lactone

EFFECTS

The drug has a diuretic effect due to the leiocarposide and the phenol glycosides. Golden Rod also inhibits the formation of urinary calculi. Leiocarposide displays an analgesic effect. The saponin is antimicrobial, weakly spasmolytic and anti-exudative.

INDICATIONS AND USAGE

Approved by Commission E:

- Infections of the urinary tract
- Kidney and bladder stones

Unproven Uses: In folk medicine, Golden Rod is used internally for rheumatism, gout, diabetes, hemorrhoids, prostatic hypertrophy, nervous bronchial asthma, internal bleeding, enlargement of the liver, acute exacerbation of pulmonary tuberculosis; externally for inflammations of the mouth and throat as well as festering wounds

Homeopathic Uses: Solidago virgaurea is used for renal insufficiency and liver disorders.

CONTRAINDICATIONS

Irrigation therapy is contraindicated in cases of edema resulting from reduced cardiac and/or kidney function.

PRECAUTIONS AND ADVERSE REACTIONS

No health hazards or side effects are known in conjunction with the proper administration of designated therapeutic dosages. The drug possesses a weak potential for sensitization. Care must be taken in patients with chronic renal diseases, and the drug should be used in this patient population only under physician supervision.

DOSAGE

Mode of Administration: As chopped drug by itself or in combination preparations.

Preparation: To make an infusion, 1 to 2 teaspoonfuls (3 to 5 gm) of drug is scalded with simmering water (150 ml) and strained after 15 minutes.

Daily Dosage: The daily dosage is 6 to 12 gm of comminuted drug prepared as an infusion. The infusion dosage is one cupful, 2 to 4 times daily between meals. The recommended dosage for the liquid extract is 0.5 to 2 ml liquid extract (1:1) in 25% ethanol 2 to 3 times daily. A dosage of 0.5 to 1 ml tincture (1:5) in 45% ethanol, 2 to 3 times daily is commonly used. Ample fluid intake should be ensured. In folk medicine, 0.5 to 2 gm drug as an infusion is taken 3 times daily.

Homeopathic Dosage: 5 drops, 1 tablet or 10 globules every 30 to 60 minutes (acute) or 1 to 3 times daily (chronic); parenterally: 1 to 2 ml sc, acute: 3 times daily; chronic: once a day (HAB1)

Storage: The drug must be protected from light and moisture.

LITERATURE

Bader G et al., (1987) Pharmazie 42(2):140.

Bader G, Plohmann B, Franz G, Hiller K, Saponins from Solidago virgaurea L. - Possible agent for therapy of cancer? In: PM 62, Abstracts of the 44th Ann Congress of GA, 21. 1996.

Bader G, Wray V, Hiller K, The main saponins from the aerial parts and the roots of Solidago virgaurea subsp. virgaurea. In: PM 61(2);158-161. 1995.

Goswami A et al., (1984) Phytochemistry 23(4):837.

Hiller K, Pharmazeutische Bewertung ausgewählter Teedrogen. In: DAZ 135(16):1425-1440. 1995.

Hiller K, Bader G, Goldruten-Kraut Portrait einer Arzneipflanze. In: ZPT 17(2):123-130. 1996.

Inose Y, Miyase T, Ueno A, Studies on the constituents of Solidago virga-aurea L. 1. Structural elucidation of saponins in the herb. In: Chem Pharm Bull 39: 2037. 1991.

Kalemba D, Phenolic acids in four Solidago species. In: PA 47:471-472. 1992.

Lassere B et al., (1983) Naturwissenschaft 70:95.

Metzer J et al., (1984) Pharmazie 39(12):869.

Schilcher H, Boesel R, Effenberger ST Segebrecht S, Neuere Untersuchungsergebnisse mit aquaretisch, antibakteriell und prostatotrop wirksamen Arzneipflanzen. In: ZPT 10(3):77. 1989.

Sökeland J, Phytotherapie in der Urologie. In: ZPT 10(1):8. 1989.

Vonkruedener S et al., Effects of extracts from Populus tremula L., Solidago virgaurea L. and Fraxinus excelsior L. on various myeloperoxidase systems. In: Arzneim Forsch 46(8):809-814. 1996.

Further information in:

Hänsel R, Keller K, Rimpler H, Schneider G (Hrsg.), Hagers Handbuch der Pharmazeutischen Praxis, 5. Aufl., Bde 4-6 (Drogen): Springer Verlag Berlin, Heidelberg, New York, 1992-1994.

Hausen B, Allergiepflanzen, Pflanzenallergene, ecomed Verlagsgesellsch. mbH, Landsberg 1988.

Madaus G, Lehrbuch der Biologischen Arzneimittel, Bde 1-3, Nachdruck, Georg Olms Verlag Hildesheim 1979.

Roth L, Daunderer M, Kormann K, Giftpflanzen, Pflanzengifte, 4. Aufl., Ecomed Fachverlag Landsberg Lech 1993.

Steinegger E, Hänsel R, Pharmakognosie, 5. Aufl., Springer Verlag Heidelberg 1992.

Teuscher E, Biogene Arzneimittel, 5. Aufl., Wiss. Verlagsges. Stuttgart 1997.

Wagner H, Wiesenauer M, Phytotherapie. Phytopharmaka und pflanzliche Homöopathika, Fischer-Verlag, Stuttgart, Jena, New York 1995.

Wichtl M (Hrsg.), Teedrogen, 4. Aufl., Wiss. Verlagsges. Stuttgart 1997,

European Mistletoe

Viscum album

DESCRIPTION

Medicinal Parts: The medicinal parts are the leaves and twigs collected before the berries form, the fresh herbs of certain host plants, the fresh leafy twigs with fruit collected in the autumn, the whole fresh plant collected from apple trees, the leaves and the berries.

Flower and Fruit: The flower is yellowish-green, dioecious and appears in insignificant, small, 3 to 5 flowered clusters. The perigone of the male flower is 4 tipped. The stamens are fused with the tips. The female flower is smaller and has 4 tepals with a thick stigma sitting on the short style. The fruit is a glossy, white, globular, pea-sized berry with thick sticky flesh. When ripe, it is white to yellowish or orange and has 1 to 2 oval or angular seeds.

Leaves, Stem and Root: The plant is a semi-parasitic, almost round bush growing on deciduous trees, which are 30 to 80 cm in diameter. The round branches are repeatedly bifurcated and thickened to knots at the joints and are the same yellowish-green as the leaves. The leaves are alternate, sessile, lanceolate or lanceolate-spatulate, coriaceous and evergreen.

Habitat: European Mistletoe is found mostly in Europe and as far as Iran. It is not found in America or Australia. It is cultivated in central Europe and China.

Production: European Mistletoe berries are the fresh or dried fruit of Viscum album. Mistletoe stem is the fresh or dried stem of Viscum album. Mistletoe herb consists of fresh or dried younger branches with flowers and fruits of Viscum album. The drug is collected in the wild during the spring and is air-dried or put in driers at a maximum temperature of 40° C.

Other Names: Mistletoe, Mystyldene, All-Heal, Birdlime, Devil's Fuge

ACTIONS AND PHARMACOLOGY

COMPOUNDS: EUROPEAN MISTLETOE FRUIT

Mucilage (2%, referred to as Viscin): The mock berries of the Mistletoe have not been fully investigated. Presumably, they lack the toxic lectins and viscotoxins.

EFFECTS: EUROPEAN MISTLETOE FRUIT

No information is available.

COMPOUNDS: EUROPEAN MISTLETOE STEM

The Mistletoe stems contain the same constituents as the Mistletoe foliage (*Visci albi herba*), but because of the high percentage of support elements lacking any effective ingredients, these constituents exist only in very low concentrations.

EFFECTS: EUROPEAN MISTLETOE STEM

No information is available.

COMPOUNDS: EUROPEAN MISTLETOE HERB

Lectins (glycoproteins with 11% carbohydrate): Mistletoe lectin I (ML I, VAA 1, viscumin), mistletoe lectin II (ML II), mistletoe lectin III (ML III, VAA II), the lectin fractions named are isolectin mixtures

Polypeptides (built up out of 46 amino acids, 0.05-0.1%): viscotoxins A2, A3, B, Ps 1-

Mucilages (known as viscin, 4-5%): including among others galacturonans, arabino galactans

Sugar alcohols: including among others mannitol, quebrachitol, pinitol, viscumitol

Flavonoids: including glycosides of quercetin, quercetin methyl ethers, isorhamnetin, sakuranetin and homoeriodictyol; in the subspecies V. album ssp. platyspermum: homoeriodictyol-7-O-glucoside, isorhamnetin-3-O-rutinoside, isorhamnetin-3-[apiosyl (1->6)]-glucosyl-7-O-rhamnoside, 5,7-dimethoxyflavanone-4'-O-glucoside, 3',5,7-trimethoxyflavanone-4'-O-glucoside

Phenyl alyl alcohols: including among others syringin (syrigenin-4'-O-glucosides), coniferyl-4'-[apiosyl (1-2')] glucoside

Lignans: including among others syringaresinol and its glycosides

Triterpenes: including among others alpha-amyrin (alpha-viscol), beta-amyrin acetate, betulic acid, oleanolic acid, ursolic acid

EFFECTS: EUROPEAN MISTLETOE HERB

The Mistletoe lectins in the drug are hypotensive, cytotoxic and immune-stimulating. It causes significant improvement of the symptoms of chronic joint conditions, and a significant lengthening of survival times of cancer patients as well an improvement of quality of life.

INDICATIONS AND USAGE

EUROPEAN MISTLETOE FRUIT

Unproven Uses: The fruit acts on circulation by regulating blood pressure. It is also an expectorant and a tonic. In addition, the fruit is used to treat internal bleeding, epilepsy, arteriosclerosis, cramps, gout, hysteria and major blood loss.

EUROPEAN MISTLETOE STEM

Unproven Uses: The stem of European Mistletoe is used for its calming effect; in the treatment of mental and physical exhaustion; and as a tranquilizer against nervous conditions such as agitation, anxiety and increased excitability.

EUROPEAN MISTLETOE HERB

Approved by Commission E:

- Rheumatism
- Tumor therapy (adjuvant)

Unproven Uses: For treating degenerative inflammation of the joints and as palliative therapy for malignant tumors through nonspecific stimulation. Other uses include long-term therapy for cases of mild high blood pressure and as an arteriosclerosis prophylactic.

European Mistletoe tea may be used for high blood pressure, epilepsy, whooping cough, asthma, vertiginous attack, amenorrhea, diarrhea, chorea, nervous tachycardia, hysteria and nervousness.

Chinese Medicine: The drug is used for joint pain, tendon and muscle pain, lumbago, back pain, vaginal bleeding during pregnancy and agalactia.

Homeopathic Uses: The drug is used for dizziness, high and low blood pressure, cardiac arrhythmia and joint degeneration.

CONTRAINDICATIONS

EUROPEAN MISTLETOE HERB

Contraindications for parenteral administration of the herb include protein oversensitivity, chronic-progressive infections, e.g., tuberculosis, and conditions of high fever.

PRECAUTIONS AND ADVERSE REACTIONS

EUROPEAN MISTLETOE FRUIT

No health hazards or side effects are known in conjunction with the proper administration of designated therapeutic dosages. The berries are said to have emetic and evacuant effects and to have caused the death of children. However, unambiguous proof for these effects does not exist.

EUROPEAN MISTLETOE STEM

No health hazards or side effects are known in conjunction with the proper administration of designated therapeutic dosages.

EUROPEAN MISTLETOE HERB

No health hazards are known in conjunction with the proper administration of designated therapeutic dosages. The drug is non-toxic with peroral administration. Local reactions can occur with parenteral administration of European Mistletoe extracts such as wheal formation, possibly also necrosis, chills, fever, headache, anginal complaints, orthostatic circulatory disorders and allergic reactions.

The wheal formation and the elevation of body temperature are considered signs of immune system stimulation and therefore as positive therapeutic effects.

DOSAGE

EUROPEAN MISTLETOE HERB

Mode of Administration: Whole, cut and powdered herb are available in the forms of juice, coated tablets, drops, oil preparations, ampules and compound preparations.

Preparation: A medicinal tea is prepared using 2.5 gm (1 teaspoonful) finely cut drug with 1 cup cold water, steeped for 12 hours at room temperature, then strained. European Mistletoe wine is prepared by adding 40 gm drug to 1 liter wine; the preparation is ready for use after 3 days.

A liquid extract is made in the ratio of 1:1 with diluted ethanol; a tincture is made in the ratio of 1:5 with 45% ethanol.

Daily Dosage: The recommended daily dose is 10 gm drug. The dosage of medicinal tea is 1 to 2 cups daily. European Mistletoe wine dosage is 3 to 4 glasses daily, liquid extract dosage is 1 to 3 ml 3 times daily, and the tincture dosage is 0.5 ml 3 times daily.

The dosage for the treatment of hypertonia and as an arteriosclerotic prophylactic is 2 to 6 gm of European Mistletoe powder 3 times daily by mouth.

Storage: European Mistletoe must be stored away from the light over an appropriate drying agent.

LITERATURE

EUROPEAN MISTLETOE FRUIT

Frohne D, Pfänder HJ, Giftpflanzen - Ein Handbuch für Apotheker, Toxikologen und Biologen, 4. Aufl., Wiss. Verlags-Ges. Stuttgart 1997.

Hänsel R, Keller K, Rimpler H, Schneider G (Hrsg.), Hagers Handbuch der Pharmazeutischen Praxis, 5. Aufl., Bde 4-6 (Drogen): Springer Verlag Berlin, Heidelberg, New York, 1992-1994.

Teuscher E, Lindequist U, Biogene Gifte - Biologie, Chemie, Pharmakologie, 2. Aufl., Fischer Verlag Stuttgart 1994.

EUROPEAN MISTLETOE HERB AND STEM

Anonym, Allergie auf Mistelextrakt. In: ZPT 13(3):96. 1992.

Anonym, Die Mistel. In: DAZ 136(48):4330-4332. 1996.

Anonym, Integrative Konzepte in der Onkologie: Misteltherapie (S. 19). In: NGM Suppl. 1/94:1-36. 1994.

Anonym, Misteltherapie aus schulmedizinischer Sicht. In: DAZ 131(37):1894. 1991.

Anonym, Optimale Misteldosierung. In: PZ 140(35):3082. 1995.

Anonym, Phytotherapie: Einsatz von Mistelextrakten in der Tumortherapie. In: DAZ 135(1):73. 1995.

Anonym, Sind Mistelpräparate mehr als nur Adjuvanzien in der onkologischen Therapie? In: ZPT 15(6):353-355. 1994.

Becker H, Exner J, (1980) Z Pflanzenphysiol. 97

Berg P, Stein G, Ein Inhaltsstoff allein genügt nicht, s. auch folgenden Artikel. In: ZPT 16(5):282. 1995.

Beuth HJ, Mistel: "In der Onkologie nur Präparate einsetzen, die auf Mistellektin standardisiert sind!" In: ZPT 16(1):40-41. 1995.

Beuth J, Ko HL, Gabius HJ, Burrichter H, Oette K, Pulverer G, (1992) Behavior of lymphocyte subsets, expression of activation markers in response to immunotherapy with galactoside-specific lectin from Mistletoe in breast cancer. Clin Invest 70:658-661

Beuth J, Ko HL, Pulverer G, Angewandte Lektinologie. In: DAZ 134(25):2331. 1994.

Beuth J, Lenartz D, Uhlenbruck G, Lektionoptimierter Mistelextrakt. In: ZPT 18(2):85-91. 1997.

Bloksma N et al., (1982) Planta Med 46:221.

Dumont S et al., Lectins from Mistletoe (Viscum album L.) induce the production of cytokines by cultured human monocytes. In: PM 61(Abstracts of 43rd Ann Congr):57. 1995.

Franz G, Phytotherapie in der Tumorbehandlung. In: DAZ 130(26):1443. 1990.

Franz H, (1985) Pharmazie 40(2):97.

Franz H et al., (1981) Biochem J 195:481.

Gabius HJ, Gabius S, Die Misteltherapie auf dem naturwissenschaftlichen Prüfstand. In: PZ 139(22):1745. 1994.

Hamacher H, Mistel (Viscum album L.) - Forschung und therapeutische Anwendung. In: ZPT 18(1):34-35. 1997.

Gabius HJ, Gabius S, Joshi SS, Koch B, Schroeder M, Manzke WM, Westerhausen M, (1994) From ill-defined extracts to the immunomodulatoty lectin: Will there be a reason for oncological application of Mistletoe? Planta Med 60:2-7.

Gabius HJ, Gabius S, Münchner-Phytotherapietagung 1992. Neues über die Misteltherapie. In: ZPT 14(1):17. 1993.

Gabius HJ, Mythos Mistel: Anspruch und Wirklichkeit. In: PZ 140(12):1029-1030. 1995.

Hajto T, Hostanka K, Frei K, Rordorf Chr, Gabins H-J, (1990a) Increased secretion of tumor necrosis factor interleukin 1: und interleukin 6 by Heiman mononuclear cells exposed to galactoside - specific lectin from clinically applied Mistletoe extract. Canc Res 50:3322.

Hajto T, Hostanka K, Gabius HI, (1989) Modulatory potency of the galactoside-specific lectin from Mistletoe extract (Iscador), the host defense system in vivo in rabbits, patients. Canc Res 49:4803.

Hajto T, Hostanka K, Gabius HI, (1990) Zytokine als Lectin-induzierte Mediatoren in der Misteltherapie. Therapeutikon 4:136-145.

Hamacher H, Mistel (Viscum album L.) - Forschung und therapeutische Anwendung. In: ZPT 18(1):34-35. 1997.

Hamacher H, Scheer R, Anthroposophie/Phytotherapie: Mistel-Forschung und therapeutische Anwendung. In: DAZ 136(34):2904-2905. 1996.

Hassauer W et al., (1979) Onkologie 2(1):28.

Hauser SP, (1993) Mistel - Wunderkraut oder Medikament? Therapiewoche 43(3):76-81.

Keine H, (1989) Klinische Studien zur Misteltherapie karzinomatöser Erkrankungen. Eine Übersicht. Therapeutikon 3:347-353.

Kleijnen J, Knopschild P, (1994) Mistletoe treatment for cancer. Review of controlled trials in humans. Phytomedicine 1:255-260.

Kwaja TA et al., (1980) Experientia 36:599.

Loew, B, In: Loew D, Rietbrock N: Phytopharmaka II: Forschung und klinische Anwendung, Steinkopff Verlag, Darmstadt, 1996.

Luther P et al., (1980) Int J Biochem 11:429.

Müller J, (1962) Ger Offen DE 1:130:112.

Olsnes S et al., (1982) J Biol Chem 257:1371.

Rentea R et al., (1981) Lab Invest. 44(1):43.

Saenz MT, Ahumada MC, Garcia MD, Extracts from Viscum and Crataegus are cytotoxic against larynx cancer cells. In: Z Naturforsch C 52(1-2):42-44. 1997.

Salzer G, Havelec L, (1978) Onkologie 1(6):264.

Salzer G, Müller H, (1978) Prax Klein Pneumol 32(11):721.

Samuellson G et al., (1981) Acta Pharm Sueca 18:179.

Schmidt S, Unkonventionelle Heilverfahren in der Tumortherapie. In: ZPT 17(2):115-117. 1996.

Schwarz T et al., Stimulation by a stable, standardised Mistletoe preparation of cytokine production in an in vitro human skin bioassay. In: PM 62, Abstracts of the 44th Ann Congress of GA, 1996.

Stirpe F et al., (1982) J Biol Chem 257(22):13271.

Timoshenko AV et al., Influence of the galactoside-specific lectin from Viscum album and its subunits on cell aggregation and selected intracellular parameters of rat thymocytes. In: PM 61(2):130-133. 1995.

Uhlenbrock S, Weihnachten, Miraculix und die Anthroposophie. In: PZ 140(51/52):4602-4603. 1995.

Wagner H et al., (1986) Planta Med (2):102.

Wagner H, Die Mistel in der Tumortherapie. In: DAZ 132(20):1087/1088. 1992.

Wagner H, Jordan E, (1986) Structure, properties of polysaccarides from Viscum album (L). Oncology (Suppl 1):8-15.

Wagner H, Pflanzliche Immunstimulanzien. In: DAZ 131(4):117. 1991.

Wasielewski S, Krebserkrankungen: Streit um alternative Heilverfahren in der Onkologie. In: DAZ 135(24):2234-2235. 1995.

Woynarvski JM et al., (1980) Hoppe-Seylers Z Physiol Chem 361(10):1525 et 1535.

Further information in:

Frohne D, Pfänder HJ, Giftpflanzen - Ein Handbuch für Apotheker, Toxikologen und Biologen, 4. Aufl., Wiss. Verlags-Ges. Stuttgart 1997.

Hänsel R, Keller K, Rimpler H, Schneider G (Hrsg.), Hagers Handbuch der Pharmazeutischen Praxis, 5. Aufl., Bde 4-6 (Drogen): Springer Verlag Berlin, Heidelberg, New York, 1992-1994.

Madaus G, Lehrbuch der Biologischen Arzneimittel, Bde 1-3, Nachdruck, Georg Olms Verlag Hildesheim 1979.

Roth L, Daunderer M, Kormann K, Giftpflanzen, Pflanzengifte, 4. Aufl., Ecomed Fachverlag Landsberg Lech 1993.

Schulz R, Hänsel R, Rationale Phytotherapie, Springer Verlag Heidelberg 1996.

Steinegger E, Hänsel R, Pharmakognosie, 5. Aufl., Springer Verlag Heidelberg 1992.

Teuscher E, Lindequist U, Biogene Gifte - Biologie, Chemie, Pharmakologie, 2. Aufl., Fischer Verlag Stuttgart 1994.

Teuscher E, Biogene Arzneimittel, 5. Aufl., Wiss. Verlagsges. Stuttgart 1997.

Wagner H, Wiesenauer M, Phytotherapie. Phytopharmaka und pflanzliche Homöopathika, Fischer-Verlag, Stuttgart, Jena, New York 1995.

Wichtl M (Hrsg.), Teedrogen, 4. Aufl., Wiss. Verlagsges. Stuttgart 1997.

European Peony

Paeonia officinalis

DESCRIPTION

Medicinal Parts: The medicinal parts are the dried ripe seeds, the fresh underground parts harvested in spring and the fresh root.

Flower and Fruit: The large flowers are solitary at the ends of the stems. The calyx consists of 5 green, partly corolla-like sepals. The wild species has 5 to 8 ovate, red petals that are 4 to 5 cm long; the cultivated forms have many more. The stamens are light-red with long yellow anthers. The 2 or 3 ovaries have red stigmas and develop into tomentose follicles containing numerous, dark, glossy, pea-sized seeds.

Leaves, Stem and Root: In its winter state, the plant has a turnip-like rhizome and close, gnarled root fibers that are brown on the outside and white inside. The stem is leafy, erect, lightly branched and glabrous, with a stalk about 50 cm high. The leaves are alternate, more or less petiolate with a dark green glossy upper surface and a light green finely pubescent undersurface.

Habitat: The plant is indigenous to the mountains of southern Europe from Portugal to Albania and Hungary, as far as Asia Minor. It is widely cultivated as a garden plant.

Production: European Peony flower consists of the petals of Paeonia officinalis and/or Paeonia mascula. European Peony root consists of the dried secondary roots of Paeonia officinalis and/or Paeonia mascula. The cultivated Peony roots are dug up in spring, cleaned and dried in the sun or artificially. The flowers are harvested in dry weather shortly after the end of flowering and dried quickly in the shade or in moderate sunshine.

Other Names: Peony, Piney

ACTIONS AND PHARMACOLOGY

COMPOUNDS: EUROPEAN PEONY FLOWERS

Anthocyans: in particular paeonin (paeonidin-3,5-diglucoside)

Tannins (pentagalloyl glucose)

Flavonoids: in particular kaempferol glycosides

EFFECTS: EUROPEAN PEONY FLOWERS

The plant contains anthocyanin glycosides and tannins (main active principle: paeonidin-3, 5-diglucoside). Animal tests have demonstrated strong uterine contraction, tone reduction in the gastrointestinal tract and a drop in blood pressure. Anticonvulsive and analgesic effects could not be demonstrated, although hypertonia has been reported in animal tests.

COMPOUNDS: EUROPEAN PEONY ROOT

Monoterpenes: monoterpene ester glucosides of the pinane-type: chief component paeoniflorine (1.5 to 3.5%)

EFFECTS: EUROPEAN PEONY ROOT

The plant contains anthocyanin glycosides and tannins (main active principle: paeonidin-3, 5-diglucoside). Animal tests have demonstrated strong uterine contraction, tone reduction in the gastrointestinal tract and a drop in blood pressure. Anticonvulsive and analgesic effects could not be demonstrated.

INDICATIONS AND USAGE

EUROPEAN PEONY ROOT

Unproven Uses: In folk medicine, European Peony root is used for neurasthenia and neurasthenia syndrome, neuralgia, migraines and allergic disorders such as excitability, epilepsy and whooping cough.

Homeopathic Uses: Among uses in homeopathy are hemorrhoids and other anal conditions.

EUROPEAN PEONY FLOWERS

Unproven Uses: The flowers were formerly used as a folk medicine remedy for epilepsy, as an emetic, emmenagogue and abortifacient, for diseases of the skin and mucous membranes, fissures, anal fissures associated with hemorrhoids, gout, rheumatoid arthritis and ailments of the respiratory tract.

Homeopathic Uses: Homeopathic uses include hemorrhoids and other anal conditions.

PRECAUTIONS AND ADVERSE REACTIONS

No health hazards are known in conjunction with the proper administration of designated therapeutic dosages. Side effects that may occur, particularly in cases of overdosages, include gastroenteritis with vomiting, colic and diarrhea. Because efficacy has not been documented, therapeutic use cannot be recommended.

DOSAGE

EUROPEAN PEONY FLOWERS

Mode of Administration: Therapeutic use cannot be recommended because efficacy has not been proven.

How Supplied: Forms of commercial pharmaceutical preparations include drops and compound preparations.

Preparation: To make an infusion, use 1 g Tree Peony flowers per cup water.

Daily Dosage: Drink one cup of infusion per day.

Homeopathic Dosage: 5 drops, 1 tablet or 10 globules every 30 to 60 minutes (acute) or 1 to 3 times daily (chronic). Parenterally: 1 to 2 ml sc acute, 3 times daily; chronic: once a day (HAB1).

Storage: Store protected from light and moisture for no longer than 1 year.

EUROPEAN PEONY ROOT

Mode of Administration: European Peony root is administered as a tincture. European Peony flowers are used as an inactive ingredient in cough and fumigant teas and as a coloring agent in cough syrup.

How Supplied: Forms of commercial pharmaceutical preparations include drops and compound preparations.

Daily Dosage: Tincture: 30 to 50 drops daily.

Storage: Store protected from light and moisture for no longer than 1 year.

LITERATURE

Caesar W, Die Pfingstrose. In: DAZ 130(23):1339. 1990.

Hänsel R, Keller K, Rimpler H, Schneider G (Hrsg.), Hagers Handbuch der Pharmazeutischen Praxis, 5. Aufl., Bde 4-6 (Drogen), Springer Verlag Berlin, Heidelberg, New York, 1992-1994.

Hikino H, Economic and Medicinal Plant Research, Vol I., Academic Press UK 1985.

Lewin L, Gifte und Vergiftungen, 6. Aufl., Nachdruck, Haug Verlag, Heidelberg 1992.

Madaus G, Lehrbuch der Biologischen Arzneimittel, Bde 1-3, Nachdruck, Georg Olms Verlag Hildesheim 1979.

Roth L, Daunderer M, Kormann K, Giftpflanzen, Pflanzengifte, 4. Aufl., Ecomed Fachverlag Landsberg Lech 1993.

Teuscher E, Lindequist U, Biogene Gifte - Biologie, Chemie, Pharmakologie, 2. Aufl., Fischer Verlag Stuttgart 1994.

Wichtl M (Hrsg.), Teedrogen, 4. Aufl., Wiss. Verlagsges. Stuttgart 1997.

European Sanicle

Sanicula europaea

DESCRIPTION

Medicinal Parts: The medicinal parts are the fresh flowering herb and the basal leaves collected during the flowering season and dried.

Flower and Fruit: The white or reddish inflorescences form a cyme with small head-like umbels with 4 to 6 linear bracts. The calyx is 5-tipped and there are 5 petals. The androgynous florets are in the center of the small umbel surrounded by 10 to 20 male florets. The ribless fruit is densely covered with barbed thorns and almost globular, with long styles that curve downwards. The mericarps are distinctly domed and almost flat at the narrow groove. There are numerous oil lines.

Leaves, Stem and Root: The perennial plant grows 20 to 40 cm high. The short rhizome is solid, horizontal, multi-segmented, broken off and covered in thick fibers. It has scales formed by leaf stalk remnants at the neck and has a number of segments. The stem is usually undivided, erect, grooved, and has only 1 to 2 sessile leaves. The leaves are basal, long-petioled, and palmate with 5 lobes. The tips are 3-lobed. The lateral tips are divided in 2 and especially glossy underneath.

Characteristics: The taste is slightly salty, bitter and dry.

Habitat: The plant is indigenous to Europe, Asia Minor, the Caucasus, western Siberia, northern Africa, and in the mountains of tropical Africa.

Production: European Sanicle consists of the dried, above-ground parts of Sanicula europaea, which is collected in the wild.

Not to be Confused With: Commercially, the herb may be mixed with leaves of Cardamine enneaphylos. In some areas, Astrantia major is labeled as sanicle and used accordingly in folk medicine.

Other Names: Poolroot, Self-Heal, Sanicle

ACTIONS AND PHARMACOLOGY

COMPOUNDS

Triterpene saponins (up to 13%): including among others, acyl-saniculosides A-D, aglycones including A1-barrigenol, R1-barrigenol, barringtogenol

Caffeic acid derivatives: rosmarinic acid, chlorogenic acid

Flavonoids: chief components rutin, isoquercitrin, astragalin

EFFECTS

The drug has a mild astringent and expectorant effect. It also reduces edema in animal experiments. The saponin complex has been shown to be antimicrobial and antifungal.

INDICATIONS AND USAGE

Approved by Commission E:

■ Cough/bronchitis

European Sanicle is used for mild inflammation of the mucous membranes of the respiratory tract.

Unproven Uses: Past external uses in folk medicine have included wounds and contusions, and European Sanicle has been used internally for stomach inflammations and bloody vomiting, among other applications.

Homeopathic Uses: The primary application of European Sanicle in homeopathy is for diarrhea.

PRECAUTIONS AND ADVERSE REACTIONS

No health hazards or side effects are known in conjunction with the proper administration of designated therapeutic dosages.

DOSAGE

Mode of Administration: Comminuted drug for decoctions and other preparations for oral application.

How Supplied: Commercial pharmaceutical preparations include juices, tablets and compound preparations.

Preparation: No information is available.

Daily Dosage: The average daily dose is 4 to 6 g of the herb.

Homeopathic Dosage: 5 drops, 1 tablet or 10 globules every 30 to 60 minutes (acute) or 1 to 3 times daily (Chronic); parenterally: 1 to 2 ml sc acute: 3 times daily: chronic once a day (HAB34).

Storage: The drug must be kept in sealed containers, protected from light.

LITERATURE

Engel S, Horn K, Phytodermatosen durch Dictamnus albus, Sanicula europaea und Philodendron consanguineum. In: Dermat Mschr 158(1):22-27. 1972.

Hänsel R, Keller K, Rimpler H, Schneider G (Hrsg.), Hagers Handbuch der Pharmazeutischen Praxis, 5. Aufl., Bde 4-6 (Drogen), Springer Verlag Berlin, Heidelberg, New York, 1992-1994.

Hiller K et al., PA 24:178. 1969.

Hiller K et al., PA 22:220-221. 1967.

Madaus G, Lehrbuch der Biologischen Arzneimittel, Bde 1-3, Nachdruck, Georg Olms Verlag Hildesheim 1979.

European Water Hemlock

Cicuta virosa

DESCRIPTION

Medicinal Parts: The medicinal part is the rhizome with roots.

Flower and Fruit: The flower is a white umbelliferous blossom with distinct calyx tips. The petals have indented tips. The style cushion is flat. The fruit is brown-yellow, 2.5 mm by 3 mm, and has dark-brown stripes.

Leaves, Stem and Root: The plant grows to a height of 30 to 120 cm. The leaves are 2- to 3-pinnate. The leaflets are lanceolate and sharply serrate. The whole plant is glabrous. The rhizome is tuberous, fleshy and hollow. The stem is erect, round, hollow, glabrous, branched above, and forms adventitious roots at the nodes.

Characteristics: The rhizome has a bad odor and is extremely poisonous.

Habitat: The plant is indigenous to Europe and Asia.

Other Names: Cowbane

ACTIONS AND PHARMACOLOGY

COMPOUNDS

Polyynes: including cicutoxin (0.07-0.2% in the fresh rhizome tuber), isocicutoxin, cicutol, cicudiole, falcarindiol

Furanocoumarins

Alkyl phthalides

EFFECTS

No information is available.

INDICATIONS AND USAGE

Homeopathic Uses: The drug is used in homeopathic dilutions for migraine, painful menstruation, worm infestation and inflammation of the skin.

PRECAUTIONS AND ADVERSE REACTIONS

The freshly harvested root stock is extremely poisonous due to its cicutoxin content. The plant itself is weakly poisonous.

OVERDOSAGE

Two to 3 gm of the root stock are said to be fatal for an adult. The toxicity of the drug declines through dehydration and storage. Symptoms of poisoning, following the initial stupor and nausea, include severe tonic-clonic spasms, unconsciousness, canosis and extremely widened pupils. Death occurs through asphyxiation at the peak of a convulsive attack or through heart failure.

Forced diuresis, hemodialysis and hemoperfusion are initiated as treatment for poisonings. Gastric lavage should only be carried out under anesthetic because of the danger of convulsion. Benzodiazepine or barbiturates are used to lessen the effects of the spasms.

DOSAGE

Mode of Administration: The drug is used topically and internally as a dilution of the mother tincture.

LITERATURE

Bilia AR, Ctalano S, Fontana C, Morelli I, Palme E, A new saponin from Potentilla tormentilla. In: PM 58(7)23. 1992.

Strauss U, Wittstock U, Schubert R, Teuscher E, Jung S, Mix E, Cicutoxin from Cicuta virosa—a new and potent potassium channel blocker in T lymphocytes. Biochem Biophys Res Commun, 219:332-6. 1996.

Wittstock U, Hadacek F, Wurz G, Teuscher E, Greger H, Polyacetylenes from water hemlock, Cicura virosa. In: PM 61(5):439-445. 1995.

Wittstock U, Lichtnow KH, Teuscher E, Effects of cicutoxin and related polyacetylenes from cicuta virosa on neuronal action potentials: a comparative study on the mechanism of the convulsive action. In: PM 63(2):120-124. 1997.

Wittstock U, Lichtnow KH, Teuscher E, Effects of polyacetylenes from Cicuta virosa on the electrical activity of molluscan giant neurones. In: PM 61(Abstracts of 43rd Ann Congr):84. 1995.

Wittstock U, Wurz G, Hadacek F, Greger H, Teuscher E, Biocative polyacetylens from Cicuta virosa. In: PM 58(7)22. 1992.

Further information in:

Frohne D, Pfänder HJ: Giftpflanzen - Ein Handbuch für Apotheker, Toxikologen und Biologen, 4. Aufl., Wiss. Verlagsges. mbH Stuttgart 1997.

Kern W, List PH, Hörhammer L (Hrsg.), Hagers Handbuch der Pharmazeutischen Praxis, 4. Aufl., Bde 1-8, Springer Verlag Berlin, Heidelberg, New York, 1969.

Lewin L, Gifte und Vergiftungen, 6. Aufl., Nachdruck, Haug Verlag, Heidelberg 1992.

Madaus G, Lehrbuch der Biologischen Arzneimittel, Bde 1-3, Nachdruck, Georg Olms Verlag Hildesheim 1979.

Roth L, Daunderer M, Kormann K, Giftpflanzen, Pflanzengifte, 4.Aufl., Ecomed Fachverlag Landsberg Lech 1993.

Teuscher E, Lindequist U, Biogene Gifte - Biologie, Chemie, Pharmakologie, 2. Aufl., Fischer Verlag Stuttgart 1994.

Teuscher E, Biogene Arzneimittel, 5. Aufl., Wiss. Verlagsges. mbH Stuttgart 1997.

Evening Primrose

Oenothera biennis

TRADE NAMES

Evening Primrose Oil Capsules (available from numerous manufacturers), Mega Primrose Oil, Oil of Evening Primrose, Original Primrose for Women, Royal Brittany Evening Primrose Oil

DESCRIPTION

Medicinal Parts: The medicinal parts are the fatty oil extracted from the ripe seeds and the fresh plant gathered at the beginning of the flowering season.

Flower and Fruit: The fragrant flowers are 2 to 3 cm long and are solitary in the leaf axils. The open ones are lower than the buds. The sepals are lanceolate, acuminate, turned down, thin, more or less pale green and smooth on the outside with a few scattered hairs. The petals are obovate. The ovary is inferior. The style has a 4-sectioned stigma. The fruit is a linear-oblong, quadrangular, downy-villous capsule that's up to 3 cm long. The seeds are 1.5 mm long, dark gray to black with irregular sharp edges.

Leaves, Stem and Root: This biennial grows up to 1 m and has a spindle-shaped, fleshy, turnip-like root, which produces leaf rosettes in the first year. The stem is erect, unbranched or branched higher up and angular. The ovary is a capsule covered in short glandular hairs, with simple, light hairs on the purple papilla. The cauline leaves are short-petioled or sessile, often hanging, oblong-lanceolate, pointed, irregular and finely dentate.

Characteristics: The flowers are fragrant and open in the evening.

Habitat: Originally indigenous to North America, it is now naturalized throughout most of Europe and parts of Asia.

Production: Evening Primrose oil is the fatty seed oil of Oenothera biennis. The oil is extracted by means of a cold-extraction process, which involves hexane in steel or glass-lined tanks. The extract is washed and the solvent removed using low pressure.

Other Names: Fever Plant, King's Cureall, Night Willow-herb, Scabish, Sun Drop

ACTIONS AND PHARMACOLOGY

COMPOUNDS

Fatty oil: chief fatty acids linoleic acid (65-80%), gamma-linolenic acid (8-14%), oleic acid (6-11%), palmitic acid (7-10%)

EFFECTS

Gamma-linolenic acid (a component in Evening Primrose oil) is converted to dihomo-gamma-linolenic acid and then to prostaglandin E1 (PGE1) in-vivo by the enzyme delta-6-desaturase. PGE1 has anti-inflammatory and cell membrane stabilizer activity in the body. Evening Primrose oil supplements provide increased levels of dihomo-gamma-linolenic acid in the blood of people with a deficiency of the enzyme delta-6-desaturase. Gamma-linolenic acid is also a component in breast milk, but is not added to infant formulas. It has been postulated that gamma-linolenic acid may be beneficial to neural development in breast-fed infants (Newall, 1996).

A review of the literature involving human trials shows that EPO has not been effective in the treatment of atopic asthma, weight loss, atopic dermatitis, arthritis, attention deficit disorder, diabetes or premenstrual syndrome. Animal studies have demonstrated benefits in treating hypertension, thrombosis, hypercholesterolemia and platelet aggregation.

CLINICAL TRIALS

Mastalgia

A retrospective study covering seven years involving 566 women with cyclical breast pain (mastalgia) was performed. Most women were first treated with Vitamin B-6 (pyridoxine HCL) 100 mg daily for a 3-month period. Those that did not respond were given 3 g of Evening Primrose Oil (EPO) daily for a one-month period followed by 2 g daily for an additional two months. Other women were given the Evening Primrose oil regimen as first-line treatment. 58% of the pyridoxine/EPO treatment group reported pain relief and 59% of the EPO first-line group reported relief. The author concluded that good responses can be obtained from products devoid of significant side effects, such as EPO and Vitamin B-6 as a first line treatment (McFayden, 1992). Tamoxifen and danazol should be reserved for those patients who do not respond to EPO or pyridoxine.

Premenstrual Syndrome

A meta-analysis of 7 placebo-controlled trials involving the use of EPO for the treatment of premenstrual syndrome (PMS) was carried out in 1996. The authors note that two well-constructed studies in the group failed to show any statistically relevant beneficial effects with EPO in treating PMS symptoms. The scoring in the remaining studies was not consistent and therefore the authors were not able to pool the results for statistical analysis (Budeiri, 1996).

INDICATIONS AND USAGE

Unproven Uses: Evening Primrose oil is used for neurodermatitis, premenstrual syndrome and as a dietary aid. The drug is also used to treat hyperactivity in children, high cholesterol levels, menopausal hot flashes and mastalgia.

Capsules containing 500 mg of Evening Primrose oil have been approved for use in Germany, in the treatment of and to relieve the symptoms of atopic eczema.

PRECAUTIONS AND ADVERSE REACTIONS

There are case reports of seizures in schizophrenic patients that were being treated with Evening Primrose oil along with phenothiazine medications. Practitioners should be aware that Evening Primrose oil has a potential to lower the seizure threshold in patients with seizure disorders or those being treated with drugs that lower the seizure threshold.

DOSAGE

Mode of Administration: Evening Primrose oil is available in capsules for oral administration.

How Supplied:
Capsules—500 mg, 1300 mg.

Most commercial products (capsules) are standardized for gamma linolenic acid content of 9%.

Daily Dosage: Treatment with Evening Primrose oil may require up to 3 months duration before positive results are attained for all indications listed below (Newall, 1996).

Atopic eczema

Adult—6 to 8 grams daily in divided doses

Pediatric—2 to 4 grams daily in divided doses

Mastalgia (breast pain)

3 to 4 grams daily in divided doses

Storage: Evening Primrose oil is rinsed in nitrogen and stored in cooled tanks lined with polyethylene. Commercial products should be stored at room temperature in an area that is dry and not in direct sunlight.

LITERATURE

Berth-Jones J, Placebo controlled trial of essential fatty acid supplementation in atopic dermatitis. In: Lancet 341:1557-1560. 1993.

Budeiri D, Li Wan Po A, Dornan JC, Is Evening Primrose oil of value in the treatment of premenstrual syndrome? Control Clin Trials 17:60-68. 1996.

Haslett C et al., (1983) Int J Obesity 7(6):549.

Horrobin DF, (1983) J Reprod Med 28(7):465.

Ihrig M, Blume H, Nachtkerzenöl-Präparate: Ein Qualitätsvergleich. In: PZ 139(9):668. 1994.

Ippen H, Gamma-Linolensäure besser aus Nachtkerzen- oder aus Borretschöl? In: ZPT 16(3):167-170. 1995.

McFayden IJ, Forrest AP, Chetty U, Cyclical breast pain - some observations and the difficulties in treatment. BJCP 46:161-164.1992.

Midwinter RE et al., (1982) Lancet I, 339.

Pye J K et al., (1985) Lancet II, 373.

Seaman GVF et al., (1979) Lancet I: 1139.

Ten Hoor F, (1980) Nutr Metab 24(Suppl. 1):162.

Willuhn G, Phytopharmaka in der Dermatologie. In: ZPT 16(6):325-342. 1995.

Wright S, Burton JL, (1982) Lancet II, 1120.

Further information in:

Hänsel R, Keller K, Rimpler H, Schneider G (Hrsg.), Hagers Handbuch der Pharmazeutischen Praxis, 5. Aufl., Bde 4-6 (Drogen), Springer Verlag Berlin, Heidelberg, New York, 1992-1994.

Madaus G, Lehrbuch der Biologischen Arzneimittel, Bde 1-3, Nachdruck, Georg Olms Verlag Hildesheim 1979.

Newall CA, Anderson LA & Phillipson JD, Herbal Medicines. The Pharmaceutical Press, London, 110-113.1996.

Schulz R, Hänsel R, Rationale Phytotherapie, Springer Verlag Heidelberg 1996.

Steinegger E, Hänsel R, Pharmakognosie, 5. Aufl., Springer Verlag Heidelberg 1992.

Teuscher E, Biogene Arzneimittel, 5. Aufl., Wiss. Verlagsges. Stuttgart 1997.

Wagner H, Wiesenauer M, Phytotherapie. Phytopharmaka und pflanzliche Homöopathika, Fischer-Verlag, Stuttgart, Jena, New York 1995.

Eyebright

Euphrasia officinalis

TRADE NAMES

Eyebright (Available from numerous manufacturers) Eyebright Herb, Herbal Eyebright, NuVeg Eyebright

DESCRIPTION

Medicinal Parts: The medicinal part is the flowering plant.

Flower and Fruit: White, bluish or reddish-violet flowers are in spike-like inflorescence in the axils of the upper leaves. The calyx has 4 tips and is glabrous to short bristly. The corolla is bilabiate and is 8 to 12 mm long. The upper lip is domed, helmet-like and revolute at the tips. The lower lip has 9 dark violet long stripes. There are 4 stamens and 1 superior ovary. The fruit is a narrow, oblong capsule with a ciliate edge. The seeds are numerous and grooved.

Leaves, Stem and Root: The plant is about 30 cm high. It is annual. The stem is rigid, erect, lightly branched below. The leaves are opposite, sessile and grass-green. They are ovate or oblong-ovate and twice as long as wide. The involucral bracts have 4 to 7 teeth.

Characteristics: Eyebright is odorless and has a bitter and salty taste. It is semi-parasitic.

Habitat: Europe.

Production: Eyebright consists of the whole plant of Euphrasia officinalis gathered during flowering season. Eyebright herb consists of the fresh or dried, above-ground parts of Euphrasia officinalis.

Other Names: Euphrasia

ACTIONS AND PHARMACOLOGY

COMPOUNDS

Iridoide monoterpenes: aucubin, catalpol, euphroside, ixoroside, veronicoside, verproside, mussaenoside, ladroside

Lignans: dehydrodiconiferyl-4-beta-D-glucoside

Flavonoids: including apigenin-, chrysoeriol- and luteolin-7-O-galactosides and -rhamnogalactosides

Tannins

EFFECTS

No documentation available.

INDICATIONS AND USAGE

Unproven Uses: Eyebright preparations are used externally as lotions, poultices, and eye-baths, for eye complaints associated with disorders and inflammation of the blood vessels, inflammation of the eyelids and conjunctiva, as a preventive measure against mucus and catarrh of the eyes. In folk medicine, Eyebright is used for blepharitis, conjunctivitis, styes, eye fatigue symptoms, functional eye disorders of muscular and nervous origin, coughs and hoarseness.

The efficacy of the herb for its claimed uses is not documented.

PRECAUTIONS AND ADVERSE REACTIONS

Health risks or side effects following the proper administration of designated therapeutic dosages are not recorded.

DOSAGE

Mode of Administration: Since the efficacy of the claimed uses is undocumented, and external eye application is not absolutely hygienic, therapeutic use cannot be recommended.

Preparation: To prepare a tea, add 2 to 3 gm of finely cut drug to boiling water; strain after 5 to 10 minutes.

Decoction — 2%.

Daily Dosage: A decoction is used 3 to 4 times daily for eye rinses.

LITERATURE

Harkiss KJ, Timmins P, (1973) Planta Med 23:342.

Luczak S, Swiatek L, Plantes Med Phytothér 24:66. 1990.

Salama O et al., PH 20:2603. 1981.

Salama O, Sticher O, (1983) Planta Med 47:90.

Sicher O, Salama O, PM 39:269. 1980.

Sicher O, Salama O, PM 42:122. 1981.

Further information in:

Kern W, List PH, Hörhammer L (Hrsg.), Hagers Handbuch der Pharmazeutischen Praxis, 4. Aufl., Bde 1-8, Springer Verlag Berlin, Heidelberg, New York, 1969.

Madaus G, Lehrbuch der Biologischen Arzneimittel, Bde 1-3, Nachdruck, Georg Olms Verlag Hildesheim 1979.

Wagner H, Wiesenauer M, Phytotherapie. Phytopharmaka und pflanzliche Homöopathika, Fischer-Verlag, Stuttgart, Jena, New York 1995.

Wichtl M (Hrsg.), Teedrogen, 4. Aufl., Wiss. Verlagsges. Stuttgart 1997.

Fagopyrum esculentum

See Buckwheat

False Schisandra

Kadsura japonica

DESCRIPTION

Medicinal Parts: The fruit of the plant is considered to have medicinal value, but efficacy has not been documented.

Flower and Fruit: Single axillary flowers on up to 4 cm long, purple stems; there are 9 to 15 white, reddish or yellow tepals. Male flowers have numerous stamens; female flowers have numerous carpels and a superior ovary. The fruit is a berry-like, globose aggregate fruit.

Leaves, Stem and Root: This dioecious climbing shrub has leaves that are 6 to 11 cm long, elliptical to lanceolate, simple, pergament-like with a slightly crenate margin.

Habitat: Indigenous to Japan.

Production: False Schisandra fruit are the dried fruits of Kadsura japonica. They are collected in the wild.

Not to be Confused With: Schisandra chinensis

Other Names: Kadsura fruit

ACTIONS AND PHARMACOLOGY

COMPOUNDS

Volatile oil: including germacrene C

Lignans: dibenzo[a,c]cyclooctene lignans, including binan-kadsurin-A-ester

EFFECTS

Although clinically unsubstantiated, False Schisandra fruit is credited in classical Chinese-Tibetan medicine with an efficacy analogous to that of Schisandra fruit. That drug exhibits liver-protective, inflammation- and tumor-inhibiting, neuroleptic and anti-convulsive effects, as well as a non-specific enhancement of physical performance ability. Experimental documentation regarding analogous efficacy of kadsura fruit has not been forthcoming, however.

INDICATIONS AND USAGE

Unproven Uses: The fruit is used for chronic coughs and asthma, chronic diarrhea, enuresis, spermatorrhoea, night sweats and insomnia.

Chinese Medicine: The fruit is used as an analgesic for pains in the bones, ligaments, stomach and during menstruation, as well as for spontaneous, painful local swellings.

DOSAGE

Preparation: Before being dried and cut, the fruits are simmered in vinegar.

Daily Dosage: 1.5 to 6 g

Chinese Dosage: 9 to 15 g drug daily

PRECAUTIONS AND ADVERSE REACTIONS

No health hazards are known in conjunction with the proper administration of designated therapeutic dosages.

LITERATURE

Hänsel R, Keller K, Rimpler H, Schneider G (Ed), Hagers Handbuch der Pharmazeutischen Praxis, 5. Aufl., Bde 4 - 6 (Drogen), Springer Verlag Berlin, Heidelberg, New York, 1992-1994.

False Unicorn Root

Veratrum luteum

DESCRIPTION

Medicinal Parts: The medicinal part is the root.

Flower and Fruit: The flowers are numerous, greenish-white, without covering leaves. They are dioecious and arranged in terminal racemes of 15 cm with nod-like feathers. The petals are narrow and shorter than the stamens, while the filaments taper to a point. The anthers are terminal and 2-lobed. The petals of the female flowers are linear, the stamens short, and the ovary ovate, deltoid and grooved. The stigmas are oblong, have 3 grooves and open upward. The fruit is numerous and capsule-like, compressed and acute.

Leaves, Stem and Root: The plant is a perennial with a strong leafy stem 30 to 90 cm high. The stem is undivided, smooth and angular. The foliage leaves are alternate; the lower ones spatulate and the upper ones lanceolate. The basal leaves are 20 cm long, 1.25 cm wide, narrow and whorled at the base. The rhizome is tuberous and stunted. It is approximately 1.25 cm long.

Characteristics: False Unicorn Root has a bitter taste.

Habitat: The plant grows in the Mississippi Delta region.

Production: False Unicorn Root is the rhizome of Veratrum luteum.

Other Names: Starwort, Helonias Root, Blazing Star, Fairy-Wand

ACTIONS AND PHARMACOLOGY

COMPOUNDS

Steroid saponins: (mixture is referred to as chamaelirin, ca. 10%), aglycone diosgenin

EFFECTS

Oxytocic, diuretic, anthelmintic

INDICATIONS AND USAGE

Unproven Uses: False Unicorn Root is used for menstrual disturbances, dysmenorrhea and pregnancy complaints.

PRECAUTIONS AND ADVERSE REACTIONS

General: No health hazards or side effects are known in conjunction with the proper administration of designated therapeutic dosages. The appearance of gastric complaints is conceivable with the drug, due to the high saponin content, particularly in cases of overdosage.

Pregnancy: Not to be used during pregnancy.

LITERATURE

Atta-Ur-Rahman, Ali RA, Choudhary MI, New steroidal alkaloids from rhizomes of Veratrum album. In: JNP 55:565-570. 1992.

Hegnauer R, Chemotaxonomie der Pflanzen, Bde 1-11: Birkhäuser Verlag Basel, Boston, Berlin 1962-1997 (unter Chamaelirium luteum (L.) GRAY).

Madaus G, Lehrbuch der Biologischen Arzneimittel, Bde 1-3, Nachdruck, Georg Olms Verlag Hildesheim 1979 (unter Helionas dioica).

Wagner H, Wiesenauer M, Phytotherapie. Phytopharmaka und pflanzliche Homöopathika, Fischer-Verlag, Stuttgart, Jena, New York 1995.

Fennel

Foeniculum vulgare

DESCRIPTION

Medicinal Parts: The medicinal parts are the Fennel oil extracted from the ripe fruit and the dried ripe fruit and Fennel seeds of Foeniculum vulgare.

Flower and Fruit: The inflorescence is fairly large umbels almost 15 cm across on very irregular rays. The flowers are fairly small and usually androgynous. The petals are a rich yellow, broadly ovate and have an involute lobe at the tip. The style is very short and almost wart-like. The fruit is glabrous, brownish or greenish-gray. They are 6 to 10 mm long, somewhat cylindrical with blunt ribs and strongly domed.

Leaves, Stem and Fruit: The plant is biennial to perennial, about 80 to 150 cm high, glabrous, sea-green to glaucous and has a strong spicy smell. The stem is erect, round, glabrous, smooth and filled with latex. The lower leaves are petiolate and have long sheaths.

Characteristics: Fennel has a spicy aroma.

Habitat: Fennel is indigenous to the Mediterranean region, has spread to England, Germany, South Tyrol and Argentina. Fennel is also found today in Iran, India and China.

Production: Fennel oil is the essential oil obtained from the dried, ripe fruits of Foeniculum vulgare by steam distillation. Fennel seed consists of the dried, ripe fruits of Foeniculum vulgare.

Other Names: Large Fennel, Sweet Fennel, Wild Fennel, Fenkel, Bitter Fennel

ACTIONS AND PHARMACOLOGY

COMPOUNDS: FENNEL OIL

When extracted from bitter fennel the chief components are:

Trans-anethols (50-75%)

Fenchone (12-33%)

Estragole (2-5%)

Additional components are - alpha-pinenes, camphene, p-cymene, myrcene, limonene, alpha- and beta-phellandrene, gamma-terpenes, terpinols, cis-ocimene

When extracted from sweet fennel the chief components are:

Trans-anethole (80-90%)

Fenchone (1-10%)

Estragole (3-10%)

Additional components are - alpha-pinenes, camphene, p-cymene, myrcene, limonene, alpha- and beta-phellandrene, gamma-terpenes, terpinols, gamma-fenchen

EFFECTS: FENNEL OIL

Stimulation of gastrointestinal motility; in higher concentrations, antispasmodic; experimentally, anethole and fenchone have shown a secretolytic action on the respiratory tract. In vitro, it is antimicrobial.

COMPOUNDS: FENNEL SEED

Volatile oil

With bitter fennel the chief components are:

Trans-anethole (50-75%)

Fenchon (12-33%)

Estragole (2-5%)

Additional components - alpha-pinenes, camphene, p-cymene, myrcene, limonene, alpha- and beta-phellandrene, gamma-terpenes, terpinols cis-ocimene

With sweet fennel the chief components are:

Trans-anethole (80-90%)

Fenchon (1-10%)

Estragole (3-10%)

Additional components - alpha-pinenes, camphene, p-cymene, myrcene, limonene, alpha- and beta-phellandrene, gamma-terpenes, terpinols, gamma-fenchen

Hydroxycoumarins (traces): umbelliferone, scopoletine, osthenol, scoparin, Furocoumarins traces) including bergapten, columbianetin, psoralen, xanthotoxin

Pyranocoumarins

Flavonoids

Fatty oil

EFFECTS: FENNEL SEED

The seed promotes gastrointestinal motility. In higher concentrations, Fennel has an antispasmodic effect. Experimentally, anethole and fenchone have been shown to have a secretolytic effect in the respiratory tract of frogs. Aqueous Fennel extracts raised the mucociliary activity of the ciliary epithelium.

INDICATIONS AND USAGE

FENNEL OIL

Approved by Commission E:

- Cough
- Bronchitis
- Dyspeptic complaints

Unproven Uses: Peptic discomforts, such as mild, spastic disorders of the gastrointestinal tract, feeling of fullness, flatulence; catarrh of the upper respiratory tract. Fennel honey is used for catarrh of the upper respiratory tract in children.

PRECAUTIONS AND ADVERSE REACTIONS

General: Health risks or side effects following the proper administration of designated therapeutic dosages are not recorded. Allergic reactions following intake of Fennel have been only very rarely observed. Cross Sensitivity among patients with celery allergy appear to be possible.

Pregnancy: Preparations, excluding the drug itself and tea infusions are not to be administered during pregnancy.

Pediatric Use: Preparations, excluding the drug itself and tea infusions are not to be administered to small children.

DOSAGE

FENNEL OIL

Mode of Administration: Essential oil and galenic preparations for internal use.

Note: Diabetics must check the sugar content of available preparations.

Daily Dosage: 0.1 to 0.6 ml of Fennel oil

Duration of administration: Maximum of 2 weeks.

FENNEL SEED

Mode of Administration: Crushed or ground seeds for teas, tea-like products, as well as other galenic preparations for internal use.

Daily Dosage: 5 to 7 gm of drug

LITERATURE

Betts TJ, J Pharm Pharmacol 20:469-472 et 61S-64S. 1968.

Czygan FC, ZPT 8:82. 1987.

El-Khrisy EAM et al., (1980) Fitoterapia 51:273.

Forster HB et al., (1980) Planta Med 40(4):309.

Gershbein LL, (1977) Food Cosmet Toxicol 15(3):173.

Harborne JB, Williams CE, (1972) Phytochemistry 11:1741.

Harries N et al., (1978) J Clin Pharm 2:171.

Hiller K, Pharmazeutische Bewertung ausgewählter Teedrogen. In: DAZ 135(16):1425-1440. 1995.

Karlsen J et al., (1969) Planta Med 17:281.

Karlsen J et al., PM 17:281-293. 1969.

Kunzemann J, Hermann K, (1977) Z Lebensm Unters Forsch 164:194.

Massoud H, Study on the essential oil in seeds of some fennel cultivars under egyptian environmental conditions. In: PM 58(7):A681. 1992.

Parzinger R, Fenchel. In: DAZ 136(7):529-530. 1996.

Rothbacher H, Kraus A, (1970) Pharmazie 25:566.

Shah CS et al., PM 18:285-295. 1970.

Stahl E, (1980) Dtsch Apoth Ztg 45:2324.

Trenkle K, PA 27:319-324. 1972.

Further information in:

Hänsel R, Keller K, Rimpler H, Schneider G (Hrsg.), Hagers Handbuch der Pharmazeutischen Praxis, 5. Aufl., Bde 4-6 (Drogen), Springer Verlag Berlin, Heidelberg, New York, 1992-1994.

Leung AY, Encyclopedia of Common Natural Ingredients Used in Food, Drugs and Cosmetics, John Wiley & Sons Inc., New York 1980.

Madaus G, Lehrbuch der Biologischen Arzneimittel, Bde 1-3, Nachdruck, Georg Olms Verlag Hildesheim 1979.

Schulz R, Hänsel R, Rationale Phytotherapie, Springer Verlag Heidelberg 1996.

Steinegger E, Hänsel R, Pharmakognosie, 5. Aufl., Springer Verlag Heidelberg 1992.

Teuscher E, Biogene Arzneimittel, 5. Aufl., Wiss. Verlagsges. mbH Stuttgart 1997.

Wagner H, Wiesenauer M, Phytotherapie. Phytopharmaka und pflanzliche Homöopathika, Fischer-Verlag, Stuttgart, Jena, New York 1995.

Wichtl M (Hrsg.), Teedrogen, 4. Aufl., Wiss. Verlagsges. Stuttgart 1997

Fenugreek

Trigonella foenum-graecum

TRADE NAME

Fenugreek Seed (from various manufacturers) Premium Fenugreek Seed

DESCRIPTION

Medicinal Parts: The medicinal parts are the ripe, dried seeds.

Flower and Fruit: The 0.8 to 1.8 cm long flowers are solitary or in pairs in the leaf axils. They are almost sessile. The calyx tube is membranous and usually longer than the lanceolate tips. The corolla is usually pale yellow, occasionally darker or violet and about double the length of the calyx. The wings are about half as long as the standard and the carina is very obtuse, round and barely longer than the calyx. The fruit is a 2.5 to 10 cm long and 0.5 to 1 cm wide, erect, leaning, linear and appressed pubescent pod with a long lip. The 4 to 20 seeds are flattened, divided into 2 uneven halves by a deep groove, ovate to di-shaped, yellow-brown, or brown-red and very hard when dry.

Leaves, Stem and Root: The plant is an annual, 10 to 50 cm high herb with a long vertical taproot. The stem is sturdy, round, erect or decumbent and branched. The leaves are trifoliate and the petioles are 0.5 to 2 cm long. The leaflets are 1 to 3 cm long, obovate to oblong-lanceolate, obtusely deltoid to rounded. The stipules are fairly large, membranous, ovate, acute and more or less softly pubescent.

Habitat: The species is common all over the Mediterranean region as far as India and China and southward as far as Ethiopia. The main regions of cultivation are southern France, Turkey, northern Africa, India and China.

Production: Fenugreek consists of the ripe, dried seed of Trigonella foenum-graecum.

Other Names: Greek Hay Seed, Bird's Foot

ACTIONS AND PHARMACOLOGY

COMPOUNDS

Mucilages (25-45%, mannogalactans)

Proteins (25-30%)

Proteinase inhibitors

Steroid saponins (1.2-1.5%): including trigofoenosides A to G (to some extent bitter), aglycones including diosgenin, yamogenin, gitogenin, smilagenin, tigogenin, yuccagenin

Steroid saponin-peptide ester: including foenugraecin

Sterols: chief constituents 24xi-ethyl-cholest-5-en-3beta-ole (65%), sterols that are to some extent estered

Flavonoids: including isoorientin, isovitexin, orientin, orientin arabinoside, isoorientin arabinoside, saponaretin, vicenin-1, vincenin-2, vitexin

Trigonelline (coffearin, N-methylbetaine of the nicotinic acid, 0.4%)

Volatile oil (0.01%): aroma bearer 3-hydroxy-4,5-dimethyl-2(5H)-furanone

EFFECTS

Externally, the drug acts as an emollient. Internally, Fenugreek reduces blood sugar, but the mode of action is unclear. In addition, a lipid-lowering effect attributed to the saponin fraction has been proven as well as a hydrogogic effect. There is no indication of a lactation-promoting effect.

INDICATIONS AND USAGE

Approved by Commission E:

- Loss of appetite
- Inflammation of the skin

Unproven Uses: Internal uses include upper respiratory catarrh, diabetes, and to increase milk production. Externally, the drug is used as poultice for local inflammation, ulcers, and eczema.

Chinese Medicine: The drug is used to treat cold pain in the lower abdomen, impotence, and hernia (said to be due to cold 'chi').

Indian Medicine: The drug is used for fever, vomiting, anorexia, coughs, bronchitis, and colitis.

CONTRAINDICATIONS

The drug should not be used during pregnancy.

PRECAUTIONS AND ADVERSE REACTIONS

General: Health risks or side effects following the proper administration of designated therapeutic dosages are not recorded. Sensitization is possible through repeated external administration of the drug.

Drug Interactions: Fenugreek has hypoglycemic effect. There is a potential for the herb to interact with hypoglycemic drugs that are used to treat diabetes resulting in an exaggerated hypoglycemic effect.

DOSAGE

Mode of Administration: Whole and powdered drug is available in the form of teas and compound preparations.

How Supplied:

Capsules — 575 mg, 610 mg, 626 mg

Preparation: To prepare a tea, leave 0.5 gm drug to steep in cold water for 3 hours, then strain; the tea may be sweetened with honey. A poultice is prepared as a thick paste made from the powdered seeds: add 50 gm of powdered drug to 1/4 liter of boiling water for 5 minutes. To make a cold maceration, soak 0.5 gm of drug in cold water, then filter.

Daily Dose: The daily internal dose of the drug is 6 gm. One cup of the tea may be taken several times a day. For loss of appetite, take 2 gm of cut drug with fluid 3 times daily, before meals. The cold maceration can be drunk several times a day.

LITERATURE

Abdo MS, Al-Khafawi AA, (1969) Planta Med 17:14.

Adamska M, Lutomski J, (1971) Planta Med 20:224.

Al-Meshal IA et al., (1985) Fitoterapia 56 (4):232.

Ali L et al., Characterization of the hypoglycemic effect of Trigonella foenum graecum seed. In: PM 61(4):358-360. 1995.

Bohlmann MB et al., (1974) Phytochemistry 13:1513.

Girardon P et al., (1985) Planta Med 51 (6):533.

Girardou P et al., PM 51:533. 1985.

Gupta RK, Jain DC, Thakur RS, PH 23:2605. 1984.

Gupta RK, Jain DC, Thakur RS, PH 24:2399. 1986.

Gupta RK, Jain DC, Thakur RS, PH 25:2205. 1986.

Hardman R et al., (1980) Phytochemistry 19:698.

Ribes G et al., (1986) Ann Nutr Metab. 28:37.

Ribes G et al., (1986) Phytother Res 1(1):40.

Ribes G et al., (1986) Proc. Soc Exp Biol Med 183:159.

Sood AR et al., (1976) Phytochemistry 15:351.

Weder JK, Heußner K, Z Lebensm Untersuch Forsch 193:242 et 321. 1991.

Further information in:

Chan, EH et al., (Eds.), Advances in Chinese Medicinal Materials Research, World Scientific Pub. Co. Singapore 1985.

Hänsel R, Keller K, Rimpler H, Schneider G (Hrsg.), Hagers Handbuch der Pharmazeutischen Praxis, 5. Aufl., Bde 4-6 (Drogen), Springer Verlag Berlin, Heidelberg, New York, 1992-1994.

Leung AY, Encyclopedia of Common Natural Ingredients Used in Food Drugs and Cosmetics, John Wiley & Sons Inc., New York 1980.

Madaus G, Lehrbuch der Biologischen Arzneimittel, Bde 1-3, Nachdruck, Georg Olms Verlag Hildesheim 1979.

Steinegger E, Hänsel R, Pharmakognosie, 5. Aufl., Springer Verlag Heidelberg 1992.

Teuscher E, Biogene Arzneimittel, 5. Aufl., Wiss. Verlagsges. mbH Stuttgart 1997.

Wichtl M (Hrsg.), Teedrogen, 4. Aufl., Wiss. Verlagsges. Stuttgart 1997.

Ferula foetida

See Asa Foetida

Ferula gummosa

See Galbanum

Ferula sumbul

See Sumbul

Fever Bark

Alstonia constricta

DESCRIPTION

Medicinal Parts: The medicinal parts are the bark of the root and trunk.

Flower and Fruit: The flowers are creamy white and star-shaped.

Leaves, Stem and Root: Alstonia are evergreen trees, which grow to a height of 15 m. The leaves are glossy, oblong and petiolate. The tree has a 2 to 7 cm rusty-brown, rugose periderm, which is deeply fissured. The inner surface is yellowish brown and coarsely striated longitudinally, fracture fibrous.

Characteristics: The tree is a protected species in some countries. The taste is very bitter; the odor is slightly aromatic.

Habitat: Alstonia constricta is indigenous to Australia; Alstonia scholaris is indigenous to India and the Philippines.

Production: Alstonia bark is the trunk and branch bark of Alstonia constricta.

Other Names: Australian Quinine, Australian Febrifuge, Alstonia Bark, Devil Tree, Dita Bark, Pale Mara, Devil's Bit, Australian Fever Bush, Pali-Mara

ACTIONS AND PHARMACOLOGY

COMPOUNDS

Indole alkaloids: including reserpine, deserpidine, alstonine, tetrahydroalstonine, alstonidine, yohimbine

EFFECTS

The drug is said to be a febrifuge, antispasmodic and antihypertensive. The antihypertensive effect is due to the reserpine and echitamin content.

INDICATIONS AND USAGE

Unproven Uses: The drug is used as a febrifuge and stimulant and for its reserpine content. In the past, it was used to treat rheumatism.

Chinese Medicine: In the Far East, Fever Bark is used for diarrhea and malaria. It has also been used as a uterine stimulant.

PRECAUTIONS AND ADVERSE REACTIONS

No health hazards or side effects are known in conjunction with the proper administration of designated therapeutic dosages. Due to the presence of pharmacologically active indole alkaloids of the beta-carbolin type, side effects may resemble those of Rauwolfia. Symptoms of poisoning following the intake of higher dosages are conceivable.

DOSAGE

Mode of Administration: The forms available are powder, liquid extract, infusion and tincture. Up-to-date information on usage is not available.

Preparation: Fever Bark is available as an infusion, 1:20, a tincture, 1:8 or 1:10 and as a liquid extract, 1:1.

Daily Dosage: The average daily dose of the infusion is 15 to 20 ml; tincture, 2 to 4 ml; liquid extract, 4 to 8 ml.

LITERATURE

Atta-ur-Rahman AM, et al., (1985) Phytochemistry 24:2771.

Chopra RN, et al., (Eds.) Chopra's Indigeneous Drugs of India, Vol 1, Dhur and Sons Calcutta 1938.

Goyal H, et al., (1981) J Res Ayur Siddha. 2 (3):286.

Khan I, Qureshi Z, (1967) J Pharm Pharmacol 19:815.

Kucera MV, et al., (1973) Afric J Pharm Pharm Sci: 3228.

Oliver-Bever B (Ed.), Medicinal Plants of Tropical West Africa, Cambridge University Press Cambridge, London 1986.

Sharp TM, (1934) J Chem Soc 287.

Further information in:

Kern W, List PH, Hörhammer L (Hrsg.), Hagers Handbuch der Pharmazeutischen Praxis, 4. Aufl., Bde. 1-8, Springer Verlag Berlin, Heidelberg, New York, 1969.

Feverfew

Tanacetum parthenium

TRADE NAMES

Feverfew (available from numerous manufacturers), Feverfew Extract, Herbal Sure Feverfew, NuVeg Feverfew Leaf, Premium Feverfew Leaf, Feverfew Traditional Herb, Standardized Feverfew Extract, Feverfew Leaf, Mygrafew

DESCRIPTION

Medicinal Parts: The medicinal parts are the herb of the plant.

Flower and Fruit: The 5 to 20 composite flower heads are in a dense corymb. The epicalyx has a diameter of 6 to 8 mm. The lingual florets are white and female. The ray florets are 2.5 to 7 mm. The achenes are 1.2 to 1.5 mm and 5- to 8-ribbed.

Leaves, Stem and Root: The plant is a strongly aromatic perennial. The leaves are pinnatisect to pinnatifid and yellowish-green. The basal and lower cauline leaves are more or less ovate with 3 to 7 oblong-elliptical to ovate segments, which are subpinnately divided. They are crenate or entire-margined.

Habitat: The plant originated in southeastern Europe and is now found all over Europe, Australia and North America.

Production: Feverfew leaves are the leaves of Tanacetum parthenium. The plant is cut before full flowering. It is dried in thin layers in the shade, at temperatures not exceeding 35° C.

Other Names: Featherfew, Featherfoil, Midsummer Daisy

ACTIONS AND PHARMACOLOGY

COMPOUNDS

Volatile oil (0.75%): chief constituents are L-camphor, trans-chrysanthyl acetate, including, camphene, p-cymene, gamma-terpinene, D-germacrene, linalool, borneol, terpinenes-4-ol

Sesquiterpene lactones: especially parthenolide, and also 3-beta-hydroxy-parthenolide, costunolid, reynosin, 8-beta-hydroxy-reynosin, tanaparthin-alpha-peroxide, canin, artecanin, secotanapartholide A

Flavonoids: including apigenin-7-0-glucuronide, chrysoeriol-7-0-glucuronide, luteolin-7-0-glucuronide, luteolin-7-0-glucoside, tanetin

Polyynes: presumably only in fresh plants

EFFECTS

Sesquiterpene lactones, especially parthenolide, are the active compounds in Feverfew (Groenewegen, 1986; Sumner, 1992). Parthenolide, although a key determinant of biological activity for Tanacetum parthenium leaf extracts, is not the sole pharmacologically active constituent (Brown, 1997). Other sespuiterpene lactones such as 3-beta-hydroxy-parthenolide, secotanapartholide A, canin and artecanin, contain an alpha-methylene butyrolactone unit responsible for anti-secretory (anti-inflammatory) activity (Groenewegen, 1986). Physiochemical methods were used to measure partholide in several purported commercial Feverfew products. The results found a wide variation in partholide content and in some products, partholide was not detected (Heptinstall, 1992).

Crude chloroform extracts of fresh Feverfew leaves (rich in sesquiterpene lactones) and of commercially available powdered leaves (lactone-free) produce a dose-dependent inhibition of thromboxane B2 and leukotriene B4 (eicosanoids) for an anti-inflammatory effect (Sumner, 1992). Anti-inflammatory properties of Feverfew also consist of inhibition of cellular phospholipases, which prevents release of arachidonic acid (Makheja, 1982). Parthenolide and chrysanthenyl acetate have also been shown to inhibit prostaglandin synthetase (Pugh, 1988). Extracts of Feverfew also inhibit granule secretion in blood platelets and polymorphonuclear leukocytes (Heptinstall, 1985).

Major flavonol and flavone methyl ethers (tanetin) of the herb inhibit the major pathways of arachidonate metabolism in leukocytes (Williams, 1999).

Feverfew extract and parthenolide inhibit human blood aggregation and serotonin (5-HT) secretion by platelets (Groenewegen, 1990). The extract does this through neutralizing cellular sulfhydryl-affecting substances, which are properties of monocyte adherence (Krause, 1990). The chloroform extract of the Feverfew leaf contains an unidentified substance capable of producing a selective, open-channel block of voltage-dependent potassium channels, which results in an anti-spasmodic effect (Barsby, 1993). Feverfew extract inhibited anti-IgE-induced histamine release in a unique way, which concludes that Feverfew extract contains a novel type of mast cell inhibitor (Hayes, 1987).

CLINICAL TRIALS

The efficacy of dried Feverfew leaves for migraine prophylaxis was assessed in a randomized, placebo-controlled, double-blind, cross-over study. The study consisted of 72 patients with classic or common migraine headaches for over 2 years. The effect of 1 capsule daily of Feverfew was determined by the use of diary cards and visual analogue scores. Duration of treatment was 4 months. After this time, Feverfew was associated with a reduction in number and severity of attacks in each 2-month period. The degree of vomiting was also reduced in the Feverfew treatment group. A significant improvement in the visual analogue scale was also observed in the Feverfew treatment group (Murphy, 1988).

Patients already taking Feverfew for migraine prophylaxis were randomized in a double-blind, placebo-controlled trial. The placebo groups had a significant increase in the frequency and severity of headache, nausea and vomiting with the emergence of untoward effects during the early months of treatment. There was no change in the frequency or severity of symptoms of migraine in the Feverfew treatment group, thus suggesting that Feverfew may be taken prophylactically to prevent attacks of migraines (Johnson, 1985).

A double-blind, placebo-controlled study evaluated the use of dried chopped Feverfew (70-86 mg) in patients with symptomatic rheumatoid arthritis. There were 41 patients involved in the study, and they were observed during a 6-week period. Variables assessed in the study included stiffness, pain (visual analogue scale), grip strength, articular index, full blood count, erythrocyte sedimentation rate, urea, creatinine, C reactive protein, complement breakdown products, rheumatoid factor titre, immunoglobulins (IgG, IgA, IgM), functional capacity, and patient and observer global opinions. There were no important differences in clinical or laboratory variables between the groups during the study period (Pattrick, 1989).

INDICATIONS AND USAGE

Feverfew is used mainly for migraine, arthritis, rheumatic diseases and allergies.

Unproven Uses: In folk medicine, Feverfew is used for cramps, as a tonic, a stimulant, a digestive agent and a blood purifier. Other uses in folk medicine include migraine prophylaxis, digestion problems, intestinal parasites and gynecological disorders. The herb is also used as a wash for inflammation and wounds, as a tranquilizer, an antiseptic, and following tooth extraction as a mouthwash. The infusion is used for dysmenorrhea. In post-natal care, Feverfew is used to reduce lochia. The drug is used externally as an antiseptic and insecticide.

CONTRAINDICATIONS

The herb is not to be used during pregnancy or during breast-feeding.

PRECAUTIONS AND ADVERSE REACTIONS

General: No health hazards or side effects are known in conjunction with the proper administration of designated therapeutic dosages. The drug has a high potential for sensitization via skin contact. Feverfew has been known to cross-react with Tansy, Yarrow, Marguerite, Aster, Sunflower, Laurel and Liverwort (Schmidt, 1986). A post-Feverfew syndrome has been reported in about 10% of migraine patients who abruptly stopped taking Feverfew. Rebound headaches, insomnia, muscle stiffness, joint pain, fatigue, nervousness and tension have occurred (Miller, 1998).

Gastrointestinal: Gastrointestinal irritation and abdominal pain or heartburn have been reported (Johnson, 1985; Murphy, 1988; O'Hara, 1998). Glossitis and stomatitis are significant problems if they do occur (Brown, 1996). The occurrence of glossitis and stomatitis with encapsulated products has not been shown to be more common than placebo (Johnson, 1985; Murphy, 1988).

Skin: There are reports of allergic dermatitis on exposure to the leaves and petals of Feverfew (Schmidt, 1986). Two elderly individuals suffering from acute recurrent photodermatitis were shown to be allergic to Feverfew (Mensing, 1985). Eczema was reported in greenhouse workers exposed to various members of the Compositae family, including Feverfew (Paulsen, 1998). A recent investigation does not support the theory of airborne sesquiterpine lactone-containing plant parts, or of direct release of sesquiterpene lactones from living plants as the only explanations for airborne Compositae dermatitis (Christensen, 1999).

Musculoskeletal: Feverfew contains sesquiterpenes (parthenolide and cynaropicrin), which have been shown to induce toxic and irreversible inhibition of smooth muscle contractility when there are high concentrations in the tissue (Hay, 1994).

Drug Interactions: Although reports are sketchy, and most involve animal subjects and *in vitro* research, there is a strong possibility that Feverfew may interact with thrombolytics, anticoagulants and platelet aggregation. The mechanism of action is believed to be inhibition of arachidonic acid, which is a precursor for prostaglandins that are involved in the clotting mechanism.

DOSAGE

Mode of Administration: Feverfew preparations are used both internally and externally.

How Supplied:

Capsules — 80 mg, 380 mg, 384 mg, 400 mg, 500 mg, 1000 mg

Tablets — 12mg (standardized to 600 mcg sesuiterpine lactone content)

Preparation: To make an infusion, use 2 teaspoonfuls of the drug per cup, allow to draw for 15 minutes. To make a strong infusion, double the amount and allow to draw for 25 minutes.

Daily Dosage:

Capsules — 200 to 250 mg daily for the treatment of migraines; the usual standardization level is 0.2% parthenolide content (Brown, 1996). Freshly dried powdered Feverfew of 25 mg is approximately equal to 0.1 mg of sesquiterpine lactones (SL) (Mervyn,1986).

Fresh leaf — 1 to 3 leaves (25 to 75 mg) once or twice daily has been recommended (Johnson et al, 1985; O'Hara, 1998).

Unproven uses — 3 cups of the infusion are taken per day. The stronger infusions are used for washes.

Storage: Store the herb in sealed containers.

LITERATURE

Abad MJ, Berjemo P, Villar A, Phytother Res 9:79-92. 1995.

Anderson D, Jenkinson PC, Dewdney RS, Blower SD, Johnson ES, Kadam NP, Human Toxicol 7:145-152. 1988.

Anonym, Naturmedizin: Mutterkraut gegen Migräne. In: DAZ 137(28):2424. 1997.

Awang DVC, Dawson BA, Kindack DG, Crompton CW, Heptinstall S, JNP 54:1516-1521. 1991.

Barsby RW, Knight DW, McFadzean I, A chloroform extract of the herb Feverfew blocks voltage-dependent potassium currents recorded from single smooth muscle cells. J Pharm Pharmacol 1993 Jul;45(7):641-5.

Berry MI, (1984) Pharm J 232:611.

Bohlmann F, Arndt C, Bornowski H, Kleine KM, Herbst P, Chem Ber 97, 1179-1192. 1964.

Bohlmann F, Zdero C, (1982) Phytochemistry 21(10):2543.

Brown AMG et al., Inhibition of human neutrophils by aqueous and organic extracts of Tanacetum ssp. In: PM 62, Abstracts of the 44th Ann Congress of GA, 66. 1996.

Brown AM, Edwards CM, Davey MR et al., Pharmacological activity of Feverfew (Tanacetum parthenium (L.) Schultz-Bip): assessment by inhibition of human polymorphnuclear leukocyte chemiluminescence in-vitro. J Pharm Pharmacol 1997 May;49(5):558-61.

Christensen LP; Jakobsen HB; Paulsen E et al. Airborne Compositae dermatitis: monoterpenes and no parthenolide are released from flowering Tanacetum parthenium (feverfew) plants. Arch Dermatol Res 1999 Jul-Aug;291(7-8):425-31.

Collier HOJ et al., (1980) Lancet II:922.

Deweerdt CJ, Bootsma HPR, Hendricks H, Herbal medicines in migraine prevention. In: Phytomedicine 3(3):225-230. 1996.

Govindachari TR et al., (1964) Tetrahedron 21(6):1509.

Groenewegen WA, Heptinstall S, A comparison of the effects of an extract of Feverfew and parthenolide, a component of Feverfew, on human platelet activity in-vitro. J Pharm Pharmacol 1990 Aug;42(8):553-557.

Groenewegen WA, Heptinstall S, Lancet, No 8471, 44-45. 1986.

Groenewegen WA, Knight DW, Heptinstall S. J Pharm Pharmacol 1986 Sep;38(9):709-712.

Groenewegen WA, Knight DW, Heptinstall S, Progr Med Chem 29:217-238. 1992.

Guin JD, Skidmore G, Arch Derm 123:500-503. 1987.

Hay AJ, Hamburger M, Hostettmann K et al., Toxic inhibition of smooth muscle contractility by plant-derived sesquiterpenes caused by their chemically reactive alpha-methylenebutyrolactone functions. Br J Pharmacol 1994;112:9-12.

Hayes NA, Foreman JC, J Pharm Pharmacol 1987 Jun;39(6):466-70.

Heptinstall S et al., (1985) Lancet I:1071.

Heptinstall S, Awang DVC, Dawson BA, Kindack D, Knight DW, May J, J Pharm Pharmacol 44:391-395. 1992.

Heptinstall S, Groenewegen WA, Spangenberg P, Lösche W, J Pharm Pharmacol 39:459-456. 1984.

Heptinstall S, Groenewegen WA, Spangenberg P, Lösche W, J Pharm Pharmacol 39:459-465. 1987.

Heptinstall S, Groenewegen WA, Spangenberg P, Lösche W, J Pharm Pharmacol 39:459-465. 1987.

Heptinstall S, J R Soc Med 81:373. 1988.

Heptinstall S, White A, Williamson L, Mitchell J, Extracts of Feverfew inhibit granule secretion in the blood platelets and polymorphonuclear leukocytes. Lancet 1985 May 11;1(8437):1071-4.

Hylands PJ, Hylands DM, Dev Drugs Mod Med 100-104. 1986.

Johnson ES, Kadam NP, Hylands DM et al., Efficacy of Feverfew as prophylactic treatment of migraine. Brit Med J 1985 Aug 31;291(6495) 291:569.

Krause S, Arese P, Heptinstall S, Losche W, Influence of substances affecting cell sulfhydryl/disulfide status on ahderence of human monocytes. Arzneimittelforschung 1990 Jun;40(6):689-92.

Lösche W, Mazurov AV et al., An extract of Feverfew inhibits interaction of human platelets with collagen substrates. Thromb Res. 1987; 48(5):511-518.

Lösche W, Mazurov AV, Heptinstall S, Groenewegen WA, Repin VS, Till U, Throm Res 48:511-518. 1978.

Lösche W, Mazurow AV, Voyno-Yasenetskaja TA, Groenewegen WA, Heptinstall, Repin VS, Folia Haematol 115:181184. 1988.

Lösche W, Michel E, Heptinstall S, Krause S, Groenewegen WA, Pescarmona GP, Thielmann K, Plant Med 54:381-384. 1988.

Makheja AN, Bailey JM, (1981) Lancet II:1054.

Makheja AN, Bailey JM, A platelet phospholipase inhibitor from the medicinal herb Feverfew (Tanacetum parthenium). Prostaglandins Leukot Med 1982 Jun;8(6):653-60.

Makheja AN, Bailey JM, Prostaglandins Leukot Med 8:653-660. 1982.

Mensing H, Kimmig W & Hausen BJ, Airborne contact dermatitis. Hautarzt 1985; 36:398-402.

Mervyn L, Standardized Feverfew preparations. Lancet 1986; 1:209.

Miller LG, Herbal medicinals: selected clinical considerations focusing on known or potential drug-herb interactions. Arch Intern Med 1998; 158:2200-2211.

Mitchell JC, Geissman TA, Dupuis G, Towers GHN, Invest Dermatol 56:98-101. 1971.

Murphy JJ, Heptinstall S, Mitchell JRA, Randomized double-blind placebo-controlled trial of Feverfew in migraine prevention. Lancet 1988 Jul 23;2(8604):189-192.

O'Hara MA, Kiefer D, Farrell K et al., A review of 12 commonly used medicinal herbs. Arch Fam Med 1998; 7:523-536.

Pattrick M, Heptinstall S, Doherty M, Feverfew in rheumatoid arthritis: a double-blind, placebo-controlled study. Ann Rheum Dis 1989 Jul;48(7):547-9.

Paulsen E. Occupational dermatitis in Danish gardeners and greenhouse workers (II). Etiological factors. Contact Dermatitis 1998 Jan;38(1):14-9.

Pugh WJ, Sambo K, Prostaglandin synthetase inhibitors in Feverfew. J Pharm Pharmacol 1988 Oct;40(10):743-5.

Romo de Viva A, Jiminez H, (1965) Tetrahedron 21(7):1742.

Schmidt RJ, Plant dermatitis. Compositae. Clin Dermatol 1986 Apr-Jun;4(2):46-61.

Sumner H, Salan U, Knight D, Hoult J, Inhibition of 5-lipoxygenase and cyclo-oxygenase in leukocytes by feverfew. Involvement of sesquiterpene lactones and other components. Biochem Pharmacol 1992Jun 9;43(11):2313-20.

Voyna-Yasenetskaja TA, Lösche W, Groenewegen WA, Heptintall S, Repin VS, Till U, J Pharm Pharmacol 40:501-502. 1988.

Warren RG, Austr J Pharm 67:475. 1986.

Williams CA, Harborne JB, Geiger H, Hoult JR, The flavonoids of Tanacetum parthenium and T. vulgare and their anti-inflammatory properties. Phytochemistry 1999 Jun;51(3):417-23.

Williams CA, Hoult JR, Harborne JB et al., A biologically active lipophilic flavonol from Tanacetum parthenium. Phytochemistry 1995 Jan;38(1):267-70.

Willuhn G, Parthenolid - Sesquiterpenlacton zur Migräneprophylaxe. In: DAZ 133(37):3292. 1993.

Further information in:

Hausen B, Allergiepflanzen, Pflanzenallergene, ecomed Verlagsgesellsch. mbH, Landsberg 1988.

Kern W, List PH, Hörhammer L (Hrsg.), Hagers Handbuch der Pharmazeutischen Praxis, 4. Aufl., Bde. 1-8, Springer Verlag Berlin, Heidelberg, New York, 1969.

Schulz R, Hänsel R, Rationale Phytotherapie, Springer Verlag Heidelberg 1996.

Teuscher E, Lindequist U, Biogene Gifte - Biologie, Chemie, Pharmakologie, 2. Aufl., Fischer Verlag Stuttgart 1994.

Wagner H, Wiesenauer M, Phytotherapie. Phytopharmaka und pflanzliche Homöopathika, Fischer-Verlag, Stuttgart, Jena, New York 1995.

Ficus carica

See Figs

Field Scabious

Knautia arvensis

DESCRIPTION

Medicinal Parts: The medicinal parts are the leafy stem including the flower heads and the fresh aerial parts of the flowering plant.

Flower and Fruit: The flat-domed, composite flowers are on long, pubescent, glandular or non-glandular pedicles. The androgynous heads are 2 to 4 cm in diameter and contain 85 to 100 florets. The female capitula are smaller and contain 55 to 60 florets. The florets are blue-lilac, occasionally red-lilac or yellowish-white to pure white. The lateral florets are ray-like. The 2- to 3-rowed involucre bracts are lanceolate, compressed and long-haired. The edge of the calyx has 8 to 16 bristles. The corolla is fused and 4 tipped. There are 4 stamens and 1 inferior ovary. The fruit is a nutlet 5 to 6 mm long and about 2 mm wide. The fruit is thickly covered in vertical hairs.

Leaves, Stem and Root: The plant is perennial and 30 to 150 cm high. The rhizome is branched and has a strong taproot. The rhizome produces a flowering stem from the leaf rosette, which survives the winter. The stem is erect, lightly branched and has short gray hairs. The leaves are opposite, gray-green and matte. The lower ones are petioled, oblong and entire-margined. The upper leaves are sessile, pinnatisect and have lanceolate tips.

Habitat: The plant is found all over Europe except the Arctic. It is also found in the Caucasus and western Siberia.

Production: Field Scabious herb consists of the leafy stems and flower heads and also occasionally the root of Knautia arvensis.

Other Names: Devil's Bit, Seabridge

ACTIONS AND PHARMACOLOGY

COMPOUNDS

Triterpene saponins: knautioside (1.1-1.7%)

Steroids: sterols, including beta-sitosterol glucoside, knautiosides A and B

Iridoide monoterpenes: including dipsacan

Flavonoids: including leucanthoside, luteoloside

Tannins

EFFECTS

The drug is said to have an astringent, antiseptic, expectorant and even purgative effect. None of these effects have been proven.

INDICATIONS AND USAGE

Unproven Uses: The drug is used for chronic skin diseases, eczema, anal fissures, pruritus ani, urticaria, scabies, favus, and for the cleansing and healing of ulcers. It is also used to treat coughs and throat complaints, as well as cystitis.

Homeopathic Uses: Field Scabious is used in homeopathic remedies to treat respiratory tract inflammations and poor digestion.

PRECAUTIONS AND ADVERSE REACTIONS

No health hazards or side effects are known in conjunction with the proper administration of designated therapeutic dosages.

DOSAGE

Mode of Administration: Decoction and infusion preparations are used both internally and externally.

Preparation: For preparation of the drug, use approximately 30 gm infusion or decoction, add to 1 liter of hot water, strain and cool.

Daily Dosage: For chronic eczema, add 4 teaspoonfuls to 2 glasses of water, leave to draw for 10 minutes and drink during the course of the day.

Homeopathic Dosage: 5 drops, 1 tablet or 10 globules every 30 to 60 minutes (acute) or 1 to 3 times daily (chronic); parenterally: 1 to 2 ml s.c., acute: 3 times daily; chronic: once a day (HAB1).

LITERATURE

Hänsel R, Keller K, Rimpler H, Schneider G (Hrsg.), Hagers Handbuch der Pharmazeutischen Praxis, 5. Aufl., Bde 4-6 (Drogen), Springer Verlag Berlin, Heidelberg, New York, 1992-1994.

Madaus G, Lehrbuch der Biologischen Arzneimittel, Bde 1-3, Nachdruck, Georg Olms Verlag Hildesheim 1979.

Figs

Ficus carica

DESCRIPTION

Medicinal Parts: The medicinal parts are the fruit and the tree sap latex.

Flower and Fruit: In its known form, the fig is neither a fruit nor a flower. It is a hollow, fleshy receptacle enclosing numerous flowers, which are never exposed to sunlight, but nevertheless develop fully and produce seeds. The inflorescence is hidden in the body of the fruit. The edge of the pear-shaped receptacle is curved inwards forming an almost closed hollow space. The numerous fertile and sterile florets are on the inner surface. When it ripens, the receptacle enlarges and the one-seeded fruit becomes embedded in it. It appears as a single purple-brown fruit.

Leaves, Stem and Root: Ficus carica is a deciduous, heavily branched tree growing to 4 m or more. The leaves are downy beneath and are 10 to 20 cm long, broad-ovate to orbicular with 3 to 5 deep lobes.

Habitat: Indigenous to Asia Minor, Syria and Iran. It is cultivated or grows wild in many subtropical regions.

Production: Figs consists of the dried fruits of Ficus carica.

ACTIONS AND PHARMACOLOGY

COMPOUNDS

Furanocoumarins: including psoralen, bergaptene

Fruit acids: citric acid, malic acid

Monosaccharides/oligosaccharides (approximately 50%), to some extent transformed into inverted sugar

Mucilages

Pectin

Vitamin B and C

EFFECTS

No information is available

INDICATIONS AND USAGE

Unproven Uses: Fig preparations are used as a laxative.

Chinese Medicine: In China, figs are used for dysentery and enteritis.

PRECAUTIONS AND ADVERSE REACTIONS

No health hazards or side effects are known in conjunction with the proper administration of designated therapeutic dosages.

LITERATURE

Kern W, List PH, Hörhammer L (Hrsg.), Hagers Handbuch der Pharmazeutischen Praxis, 4. Aufl., Bde. 1-8, Springer Verlag Berlin, Heidelberg, New York, 1969.

Siewek F et al. (1985) Z NaturForsch 40 (1/2): 8.

Teuscher E, Biogene Arzneimittel, 5. Aufl., Wiss. Verlagsges. mbH Stuttgart 1997.

Figwort

Scrophularia nodosa

DESCRIPTION

Medicinal Parts: The medicinal parts of the plant are the dried herb harvested before flowering, the herb with the root, and the root alone.

Flower and Fruit: The reddish-brown or greenish-yellow flowers are in terminal panicles. The calyx has 5 segments, with ovate, narrow-tunicate margined cusps. The corolla is a bilabiate, swollen, almost globular tube. The upper lip is divided into 2 and the lower lip is 3-lobed with revolute lobes. There are 4 stamens and 1 superior ovary. The fruit is an ovate, many-seeded, and pointed green capsule.

Leaves, Stem and Root: The perennial plant grows from 50 to 100 cm high. The root capitula have ovate, tuberous nodes. The stem is erect, sharply quadrangular, often purple, glabrous, and has a row of hairs at the nodes. The leaves are crossed opposite, dark green, oblong, double serrate and often cordate at the base.

Habitat: The plant is indigenous to Europe, central Asia, and North America.

Other Names: Throatwort, Carpenter's Square, Kernelwort, Heal-All Scrofula Plant, Rosenoble

ACTIONS AND PHARMACOLOGY

COMPOUNDS

Iridoides: including monoterpenes

Flavonoids: including among others, diosmin

Tannins

Saponins

EFFECTS

Figwort has a diuretic and mildly laxative effect. (No new research is available.)

INDICATIONS AND USAGE

Unproven Uses: External uses as folk remedies have included skin rashes, venereal warts, hemorrhoids, lacrimation and earache. According to English sources, the plant was used as a remedy for rabies.

Homeopathic Uses: The drug is used for low resistance, chronic tonsillitis, and tonsillar hypertony as well as for lymphedema.

PRECAUTIONS AND ADVERSE REACTIONS

No health hazards or side effects are known in conjunction with the proper administration of designated therapeutic dosages.

DOSAGE

Preparation: Homeopathic preparations of the mother tincture are derived from the whole Figwort plant in dilutions.

Homeopathic Dosage: 15 to 20 drops to be taken orally 3 times daily. Scrophularia nodosa can be administered by injection for long-term treatment

LITERATURE

Inouye H et al., (1974) Planta Med 25:285.

Jerznanowska Z, Pijewska L, (1954) Acta Polon. Pharm 11:1.

Kato Y, (1946) Folia Pharmacol Jap. 42:37 (via CA 47:1843)

Pauli GF, Ofterdinger-Daegel, S, Teborg D, Digitalis, Scrophularia & Co. In: DAZ 135(2):111.1995.

Pethes E et al., (1973) Herba Hung 12:101.

Swann K, Melville C, (1972) J Pharm Pharmacol 24:170P.

Weinges K, Von der Eltz H, (1978) Justus Liebigs Ann Chem 1968.

Further information in:

Fernandez MA, Garcia MD, Saenz MT Antibacterial activity of the phenolic acids fractions of Scrophularia frutescens and Scrophularia sambucifolia. J Ethnopharmacol, 53:11-4, Jul 26 1996.

Fernandez MA, Garcia MD, Saenz MT Anti-inflammatory effects of different extracts and harpagoside isolated from Scrophularia frutescens L. Farmaco, 53:443-6, Jun 1996.

Fernandez MA, Garcia MD, Saenz MT Gas chromatographic determination of chlorothalonil in leaves and roots of Scrophularia and in soil. J AOAC Int, 53:587-8, Mar-Apr 1996.

Hegnauer R, Chemotaxonomie der Pflanzen, Bde 1-11: Birkhäuser Verlag Basel, Boston, Berlin 1962-1997.

Kern W, List PH, Hörhammer L (Hrsg.), Hagers Handbuch der Pharmazeutischen Praxis, 4. Aufl., Bde 1-8: Springer Verlag Berlin, Heidelberg, New York, 1969.

Madaus G, Lehrbuch der Biologischen Arzneimittel, Bde 1-3, Nachdruck, Georg Olms Verlag Hildesheim 1979.

Wagner H, Wiesenauer M, Phytotherapie. Phytopharmaka und pflanzliche Homöopathika, Fischer-Verlag, Stuttgart, Jena, New York 1995.

Filipendula ulmaria

See Meadowsweet

Fish Berry

Anamirta cocculus

DESCRIPTION

Medicinal Parts: The medicinal part of the plant is the ripe, dried fruit.

Flower and Fruit: The plant's petiolate inflorescences are panicle-like, 16 to 40 cm long and usually inserted in the stem. Male flowers are occasionally axillary. The two outer petals are smaller and about 1 mm long. The inner ones are whitish or yellowish-green, broad-elliptoid, 2 to 3 mm long, in 2 alternating, triple whorls and are imbricate. The synandria are formed from a short-stemmed, globose cluster of about 30 to 35 anthers. The pollen is round and tricolporate. The female flowers have 3 tepals as well as small staminoids. The 3 or 4 carpels are set sideways on a central, erect fruit axis that becomes conically oblong when the fruit ripens. The style is inserted in the side and the stigma is turned back. The drupes are globose to reniform, 9 to 11 mm long, glabrous, and sit on the short, spreading branches of the fruit axis. The fruit is about 1 cm long, blackish, and contains a horseshoe-shaped seed.

Leaves, Stem and Root: Anamirta cocculus are hardy, woody lianas with ash-gray to straw-yellow striped bark. The leaves are ovate to cordate. The leaf blade is 16 to 28 cm long and 10 to 24 cm wide and coriaceous. The main veins are arranged in palmate fashion at the base with parallel secondary veins. The 6 to 18 cm petiole is thickened at both ends.

Characteristics: The fruit shell is tasteless, the seed is bitter and oily.

Habitat: The plant grows in India, Sri Lanka and Malaysia.

Production: Fish Berry seeds are the fruit of the false myrtle Anamirta cocculus. They are collected in the wild and sun-dried after harvesting.

Other Names: Levant Nut, Crow Killer, Fish Killer, Indian Berry, Cocculus Indicus

ACTIONS AND PHARMACOLOGY

COMPOUNDS

Sesquiterpens: picrotoxin, a mixture of picrotoxinine and its by product picrotin, picrotoxin acid methyl ester

Isoquinoline alkaloids: menispermine, paramenispermine

Fatty oil

EFFECTS

The effect of the drug is due to the picrotoxin content. Picrotoxin paralyzes presynaptic blocking mechanisms and, like strychnine, has an analeptic effect in low doses. The central ends of the parasympathetic nerves are stimulated, as is the medulla oblongata. Breathing frequency is initially increased and subsequently decreased. The pulse slows due to the stimulation of the vagus and an increase in blood pressure. Central nervous system-stimulated vomiting along with an increase in perspiration and saliva are probably also due to the action of picrotoxin.

INDICATIONS AND USAGE

Unproven Uses: In the past, the drug was used as an insecticide in powder form for scabies. Its use against skin parasites and lice, while not substantiated, seems plausible. It was also used in cases of barbituric acid poisoning. In more recent times, it has been used in the treatment of peripheral and vestibular nystagmus, and in both long and short-term therapy for peripherally based dizziness as well as travel sickness.

Indian Medicine: The seeds have been used externally in India and on the Malaysian archipelago for gout, skin diseases and parasites. The tender leaves are used as a contracting agent for the womb after birth.

Homeopathic Uses: The drug is used for nervous exhaustion, attacks of dizziness, cramps, paralysis, dysmenorrhea and occipital headaches. Efficacy has not been proven.

PRECAUTIONS AND ADVERSE REACTIONS

The drug is very poisonous. Mild poisonings cause headache, dizziness, nausea, coordination disturbances, general depression and spastic twitching.

OVERDOSAGE

With high dosages, the symptoms above are followed by frequent vomiting, sleepiness and tonic-clonic spasms. Death follows, often not until days later, through asphyxiation and heart failure. Two to three Cocculus kernels can be fatal.

Treatment consists of inducing vomiting and/or gastric lavage, purging with sodium sulphate, instillation of activated charcoal and forced diuresis. The spasms should be suppressed with diazepam, but only as much as is absolutely necessary. In case of fever, the patient should be wrapped in ice packs, administered high-caloric infusions and possibly given oxygen respiration. Phenothiazines and analeptics should be avoided.

DOSAGE

Mode of Administration: In combination preparations.

How Supplied: Commercial preparations include ampules, drops and tablets.

Preparation: Liquid extract is prepared using a 1:1 ratio of the drug and 90% ethanol A mixture of the extract and coconut oil is prepared using a ratio of 1:8

Tincture: 1:10 tincture: 70% ethanol

Unguetum cocculi: 125 g extract plus 650 g coconut oil plus 50 g beeswax and 250 g paraffin

Picrotoxin extraction is made using special procedures; maximum yield 1.5%

Daily Dosage: One to 5 mg can be taken by healthy patients who do not experience side effects. For peripheral states of dizziness: 1 mg to 5 mg (picrotoxin) slow intravenous infusion. As a long-term treatment: 1 mg suppositories for 3 weeks.

Homeopathic Dosage: 5 drops, 1 tablet or 10 globules every 30 to 60 minutes (for acute conditions), or 1 ml twice a week sc or ointment 1 or 2 times daily for chronic conditions.

Storage: Because they are poisonous, preparations should be secured in tightly closed containers, protected from light and unauthorized access.

LITERATURE

Frohne D, Pikrotoxin - Renaisssance eines ''obsoleten'' pflanzlichen Arzneistoffes. In: ZPT 10(3):101. 1989.

Hänsel R, Keller K, Rimpler H, Schneider G (Hrsg.), Hagers Handbuch der Pharmazeutischen Praxis, 5. Aufl., Bde 4-6 (Drogen), Springer Verlag Berlin, Heidelberg, New York, 1992-1994.

Hoppe HA, (1975-1987) Drogenkunde, 8. Aufl., Bde 1-3, W. de Gruyter Verlag, Berlin, New York.

Lewin L, Gifte und Vergiftungen, 6. Aufl., Nachdruck, Haug Verlag, Heidelberg 1992.

Madaus G, Lehrbuch der Biologischen Arzneimittel, Bde 1-3, Nachdruck, Georg Olms Verlag Hildesheim 1979.

Roth L, Daunderer M, Kormann K, Giftpflanzen, Pflanzengifte, 4. Aufl., Ecomed Fachverlag Landsberg Lech 1993.

Steinegger E, Hänsel R, Pharmakognosie, 5. Aufl., Springer Verlag Heidelberg 1992.

Teuscher E, Biogene Arzneimittel, 5. Aufl., Wiss. Verlagsges. mbH Stuttgart 1997.

Teuscher E, Lindequist U, Biogene Gifte - Biologie, Chemie, Pharmakologie, 2. Aufl., Fischer Verlag Stuttgart 1994.

Wagner H, Wiesenauer M, Phytotherapie. Phytopharmaka und pflanzliche Homöopathika, Fischer-Verlag, Stuttgart, Jena, New York 1995.

Flax

Linum usitatissimum

TRADE NAMES

Bio flax, Flaxseed Oil, New Energy

DESCRIPTION

Medicinal Parts: The medicinal parts are the stem as a sterile linen thread, the oil extracted from the seeds, the dry ripe seeds, the linseed cakes and the fresh flowering plant.

Flower and Fruit: The flowers are panicle-like loose cymes on long peduncles in the leaf axils of the upper part of the stem. They have 5 ovate, acuminate, finely ciliate sepals and 5 obovate petals, which are sky blue and longer than the sepals. There are 5 stamens fused at the base and 1 ovary. The fruit is an almost globular, 6 to 8 mm long capsule on an erect or slightly bent stem. The seeds are flat, brown and glossy.

Leaves, Stem and Root: The plant is an annual and grows from 20 to 150 cm high. The root is short, fusiform and light yellow. The stem is unbranched, erect or ascending in short curves. The leaves are smooth edged, gray-green, sessile and almost awn-like acuminate.

Characteristics: The plant flowers only in the morning.

Habitat: The plant is cultivated in temperate and tropical regions the world over.

Production: Flaxseed consists of the dried, ripe seed of the collective variations of Linum usitatissimum as well as its preparations. The various cultivars of Linum usitatissimum are equally acceptable for the indications listed. The plant is cultivated. The ripe seeds are recovered from the capsules by threshing. The oil contained within the seeds is perishable. Processing of the seeds should take place by cold pressing at a temperature below 40° C.

Not to be Confused With: Lolium temulentum and weed seeds.

Other Names: Flaxseed, Lint Bells, Winterlien, Linseed

ACTIONS AND PHARMACOLOGY

COMPOUNDS

Mucilages (3-10%, in the epidermis, high swelling capacity): including arabinoxylans, galactans, rhamnogalacturonans

Cyanogenic glycosides (0.05-0.1%): linustatin and neolinustatin (yielding under optimal conditions 30-50 mg HCN per 100 gm)

Fatty oil (30-45%): chief fatty acids linolenic acid (40-70%), linoleic acid (10-25%), oleic acid (13-30%)

Proteins (20-27%)

Lignans: secoisolariciresinol-diglucoside

Phenylpropane derivatives: including among others, linusitamarine

EFFECTS

The bulk material and mucins (swelling agent and mucilage) are responsible for the laxative effect.

In animal experiments a reduction of cholesterol levels in the liver was observed (due to the unsaturated fatty acids). A blood sugar lowering effect was also proven. The antitumoral effect is attributed to the lignans (lignans are antimycotic, anti-oxidative and anti-estrogenic).

Toxic principle: there is a discussion on the toxic effect of the cyanogenic glycosides in the drug which may cause prussic acid poisoning in humans. However, neither high single doses nor chronic intake of linseed have caused any signs of poisoning in humans.

INDICATIONS AND USAGE

Approved by Commission E:

■ Constipation

■ Inflammation of the skin

Unproven Uses: Internally, Flax is used for irritable colon, diverticulitis and as mucilage for gastritis and enteritis. A decoction is used for bladder catarrh and inflammation, gastritis.

Externally, Flaxseed is used for removing foreign bodies from the eye. A single Flaxseed is moistened and placed under the eyelid, the foreign body should stick to the mucous secretion of the seed; as cataplasm for local skin inflammation.

Indian Medicine: Flax is used in India as a tea for coughs, bronchial conditions, urethritis, diarrhea and gonorrhea; externally for skin infections. The seeds are also used in Indian veterinary medicine.

CONTRAINDICATIONS

Flaxseed is contraindicated in the following conditions: ileus, stricture of the esophagus and in the gastrointestinal area, acute inflammatory illnesses of the intestine, of the esophagus and of the stomach entrance.

PRECAUTIONS AND ADVERSE REACTIONS

General: No health hazards or side effects are known in conjunction with the proper administration of designated therapeutic dosages. The use of large quantities of the drug as a laxative with too little fluid intake can lead to an ileus. The cyanogenic glycosides present no danger with the intake of therapeutic dosages; the glycosides are broken down only to a limited extent in the body. An elevation in the concentration of cyanide ions and of the detoxification product thiocyanic acid in the blood could not be demonstrated.

It is recommended that if flaxseed is taken for inflammatory bowel conditions, that the flaxseed be preswollen before use (Bisset & Wichtl, 1994).

Drug Interactions: The absorption of other drugs taken simultaneously may be delayed.

Food Interactions: The absorption of Flaxseed oil is facilitated when taken with food.

DOSAGE

Mode of Administration: Internally, the cracked or coarsely ground seed, in which only the cuticle and mucilage epidermis are damaged is used. Linseed gruel and other galenic preparations are also available for internal use. Externally, as linseed meal or linseed expellent.

How Supplied:

Capsules — 1000 mg, 1300 mg

Oil

Seeds (whole or crushed)

Powder

Preparation: To prepare a demulcent for use in gastritis and enteritis, allow 5 to 10 gm of whole seeds to stand in cold water for 20 to 30 minutes, then pour off the liquid (Bisset & Wichtl, 1994).

Daily Dosage:

Constipation — 1 dessertspoon of whole or bruised (not ground) seed with at least 150 ml of liquid 2 to 3 times daily.

Lower Cholesterol — 35 to 50 gm daily of the crushed seeds. May be incorporated into muffins or breads (Arjmandi et al, 1998).

Decrease platelet aggregation — 1 to 2 tablespoonfuls flaxseed oil daily (Allman et al, 1995).

Gastritis and enteritis — 2 to 4 tablespoons of milled linseed prepared as recommended above (the seeds should not be taken in the dry state, should be pre-hydrated.)

External — 30 to 50 gm Flaxseed flour for a hot moist cataplasm or compress.

Storage: Flaxseed oil must be processed and stored properly (see ''Production'' above). Flaxseed meal is less vulnerable to rancidity when exposed to light and heat than the processed oil. The seeds should be protected from light and stored in a sealed container. The oil should also be protected from light and should be refrigerated.

LITERATURE

Allman MA, Pena MM & Pang D: Supplementation with flaxseed oil versus sunflower seed oil in healthy young men consuming a low fat diet: effects on platelet composition and function. In: Eur J Clin Nutr 49(3):169-178, 1995.

Anonym, Leinöl als diätetisches Adjuvans. In: DAZ 135(16):1501. 1995.

Anonym, Leinsamen (Semen Lini) ist ungiftig. In: ZPT 5:770. 1984.

Anonym, Pharmaceutical Care:''Den Mißbrauch von Laxanzien vermeiden helfen.'' In: DAZ 135(20):1867-1868. 1995.

Arjmandi BH, Khan DA, Juma S et al., Whole flaxseed consumption lowers serum LDL-cholesterol and lipoprotein(a) concentrations in postmenopausal women. In: Nutr Res 18(7):1203-1214, 1998.

Bisset NG & Wichtl M (eds): Lini semen. Herbal Drugs and Phytopharmaceuticals: A Handbook for Practice on a Scientific Basis. Medpharm Scientific Publishers, CRC Press, Stuttgart, Germany, pp 298-300, 1994.

Curry CE, (1982) Laxative products. In: Handbook of Nonprescription Drugs, Am Pharmac Assoc, Washington, S 69-92.

Ecker-Schlipf B, Östrogensubstitution mit Leinsamen und Sojamehl. In: DAZ 131(19):953. 1991.

Hiller K, Pharmazeutische Bewertung ausgewählter Teedrogen. In: DAZ 135(16):1425-1440. 1995.

Schiebel-Schlosser G, Leinsamen - die richtige Wahl. In: PTA 8(4):300. 1994.

Schulz V, (1984) Clinical Pharmacokinetics of Nitroprusside, Cyanide, Thiosulphate and Thiocyanate. Clinical Pharmacokinetics 9:239-251.

Schulz V, Löffler A, Gheorghiu Th, (1983) Resorption von Blausäure aus Leinsamen. Leber Magen Darm 13:10-14.

Sewing KFR, (1986) Obstipation. In: Fülgraff G, Palm D (Hrsg) Pharmakotherapie, Klinische Pharmakologie, 6. Auflage. Fischer, Stuttgart, S 162-168.

Further information in:

Frohne D, Pfänder HJ, Giftpflanzen - Ein Handbuch für potheker, Toxikologen und Biologen, 4. Aufl., Wiss. Verlags-Ges Stuttgart 1997.

Hänsel R, Keller K, Rimpler H, Schneider G (Hrsg.), Hagers Handbuch der Pharmazeutischen Praxis, 5. Aufl., Bde 4-6 (Drogen), Springer Verlag Berlin, Heidelberg, New York, 1992-1994.

Lewin L, Gifte und Vergiftungen, 6. Aufl., Nachdruck, Haug Verlag, Heidelberg 1992.

Madaus G, Lehrbuch der Biologischen Arzneimittel, Bde 1-3, Nachdruck, Georg Olms Verlag Hildesheim 1979.

Roth L, Daunderer M, Kormann K, Giftpflanzen, Pflanzengifte, 4. Aufl., Ecomed Fachverlag Landsberg Lech 1993.

Schulz R, Hänsel R, Rationale Phytotherapie, Springer Verlag Heidelberg 1996.

Steinegger E, Hänsel R, Pharmakognosie, 5. Aufl., Springer Verlag Heidelberg 1992.

Teuscher E, Biogene Arzneimittel, 5. Aufl., Wiss. Verlagsges. Stuttgart 1997.

Teuscher E, Lindequist U, Biogene Gifte - Biologie, Chemie, Pharmakologie, 2. Aufl., Fischer Verlag Stuttgart 1994.

Wagner H, Wiesenauer M, Phytotherapie. Phytopharmaka und pflanzliche Homöopathika, Fischer-Verlag, Stuttgart, Jena, New York, 1995.

Wichtl M (Hrsg.), Teedrogen, 4. Aufl., Wiss. Verlagsges. Stuttgart 1997.

Foeniculum vulgare

See Fennel

Fool's Parsley

Aethusa cynapium

DESCRIPTION

Medicinal Parts: The medicinal parts are the entire fresh plant and the dried aerial parts (herb).

Flower and Fruit: The plant has white long-stemmed umbels with many florets and no involucre. The calyx has 5 fused sepals. There are 5 white, sometimes reddish, obcordate, irregular petals. The flowers have 5 stamens and a 2-valved ovate ovary. The fruit is a 3 to 5 mm wide, globose schizocarp, straw yellow when ripe with red-brown stripes; it opens easily. Each section has 5 triangular ribs with 1 or 2 oil grooves in the hollow and 2 in the joints.

Leaves, Stem and Root: The plant is a leafy, 60 cm high annual or biennial plant. The root is thin, spindle-shaped and whitish. The stem is erect, round, grooved, hollow, glabrous and usually forked with a bluish bloom, which rubs off when handled. The leaves are glossy, dark green above and light green beneath. Leaflets are serrate with a triangular outline and double to treble pinnatifid. They give off an unpleasant garlic odor when rubbed.

Characteristics: The plant is poisonous. The plant can be mistaken for Parsley because of its similar appearance, but the plant is poisonous and can have fatal consequences. This similarity has resulted in its being given the name Fool's Parsley. It also bears a resemblance to Hemlock, though it is not as poisonous.

Habitat: The plant is indigenous to northern and central Europe, introduced into North America; cultivated and used as an ornamental plant for meadows in southern Germany.

Not to be Confused With: Young garden parsley is very similar. However, it differs in the glossiness of the underside surface of the leaf and pungent, burning, garlic-like smell of the leaves when rubbed.

Other Names: Dog Poison, Fool's-Cicely, Small Hemlock, Dog Parsley, Lesser Hemlock

ACTIONS AND PHARMACOLOGY

COMPOUNDS

Polyynes: (only in freshly-harvested leaves) including aethusin, aethusanol A, aethusanol B

Flavone glycosides: including rutoside, narcissine, camphor oil-3-glucorhamnoside

Ascorbic acid

EFFECTS

No information is available.

INDICATIONS AND USAGE

Unproven Uses: Fool's Parsley has been used for gastrointestinal complaints in children, infantile cholera, summer diarrhea and convulsions.

Homeopathic Uses: Aethusa cynapium is used for milk intolerance in children, pylorus cramp, acute diarrhea with vomiting and poor concentration (HAB1).

PRECAUTIONS AND ADVERSE REACTIONS

Fool's Parsley is considered a toxic plant. The older literature contains descriptions of poisonings, sometimes fatal, occurring as a result of confusing garden parsley with the freshly harvested drug. Probably, however, these had to do with poisonings by spotted hemlock. Caution should nevertheless be exercised.

DOSAGE

Mode of Administration: The juice of the fresh drug is used in poultices; also available as alcoholic extracts.

Homeopathic Dosage: 5 to 10 drops, 1 tablet or 5 to 10 globules, 1 to 3 times daily; injection solution 1 ml twice weekly sc (HAB1).

LITERATURE

Bohlmann F, et al., Chem Ber 93:981. 1968.

Bohlmann F, et al., Chem Ber 88:1245. 1960.

Teuscher E, et al., PA 45:537. 1990.

Further information in:

Frohne D, Pfänder HJ, Giftpflanzen - Ein Handbuch für Apotheker, Toxikologen und Biologen, 4. Aufl., Wiss. Verlags-Ges Stuttgart 1997.

Hänsel R, Keller K, Rimpler H, Schneider G (Hrsg.), Hagers Handbuch der Pharmazeutischen Praxis, 5. Aufl., Bde 4 - 6 (Drogen), Springer Verlag Berlin, Heidelberg, New York, 1992-1994.

Lewin L, Gifte und Vergiftungen, 6. Aufl., Nachdruck, Haug Verlag, Heidelberg 1992.

Madaus G, Lehrbuch der Biologischen Arzneimittel, Bde 1-3, Nachdruck, Georg Olms Verlag Hildesheim 1979.

Roth L, Daunderer M, Kormann K, Giftpflanzen, Pflanzengifte, 4. Aufl., Ecomed Fachverlag Landsberg Lech 1993.

Teuscher E, Lindequist U, Biogene Gifte - Biologie, Chemie, Pharmakologie, 2. Aufl., Fischer Verlag Stuttgart 1994.

Forget-Me-Not

Myosotis arvensis

DESCRIPTION

Medicinal Parts: The medicinal part is the flowering plant.

Flower and Fruit: The blue flowers are in leafless racemes. The calyx is fused and leaf-like with 5 tips. The corolla is shaped like a stemmed plate, has 5 tips, and is glabrous with yellow scales in the tube. The tube is enclosed in the calyx. There are 5 stamens and a 4-valvular ovary. The fruit stems are twice as long as the caylx and stand out. The calyx is closed when the fruit ripens. The fruit is composed of 4 nutlets.

Leaves, Stem and Root: The plant is leafy and grows from 15 to 40 cm high. The stem is erect or ascendent and pubescent. The leaves are alternate. The lower leaves are petiolate and oblong-obovate, the upper ones sessile and lanceolate to lanceolate-oblong.

Habitat: The plant grows in Europe.

Production: Forget-Me-Not is the flowering plant Myosotis arvensis.

ACTIONS AND PHARMACOLOGY

COMPOUNDS

Pyrrolizidine alkaloids

Caffeic acid derivatives: rosmarinic acid

EFFECTS

No information is available.

INDICATIONS AND USAGE

Unproven Uses: Forget-Me-Not is used in the treatment of respiratory disorders and nose bleeds.

PRECAUTIONS AND ADVERSE REACTIONS

Hepatotoxicity and carcinogenicity are possible consequences when taken internally, due to the presence of pyrrolizidine alkaloids with 1,2-unsaturated necic parent substances. Therefore, the drug should not be taken internally.

DOSAGE

Mode of Administration: The herb is administered ground and as an extract for external use.

LITERATURE

Kern W, List PH, Hörhammer L (Hrsg.), Hagers Handbuch der Pharmazeutischen Praxis, 4. Aufl., Bde. 1-8, Springer Verlag Berlin, Heidelberg, New York, 1969.

Madaus G. Lehrbuch der Biologischen Arzneimittel, Bde 1-3, Nachdruck, Georg Olms Verlag Hildesheim 1979.

Fragaria vesca

See Strawberry

Frangula

Rhamnus frangula

DESCRIPTION

Medicinal Parts: The medicinal parts are the dried bark of the trunk and branches and the fresh bark of the trunk and branches.

Flower and Fruit: The flowers are in 2 to 10 axillary blossomed cymes on pedicles that are 1 to 3 times as long. The flowers are greenish white, infundibular, 3 to 4 mm long with 5 sepals and 5 petals, which are initially pubescent. The sepals are 3 mm long, oblong-triangular and acute. The petals are whitish, erect and stemmed. The petals enclose the stamens. The stamens are somewhat shorter than the petals and have large anthers and short filaments. The fruit is a globular, initially green, later red when ripe. The black-purple drupe is about 8 cm wide containing 2 to 3 seeds. The seeds are wide, flat triangular-lentil-shaped with a longer, very narrow groove.

Leaves, Stem and Root: The plant is a thornless, 1 to 3 m high bush or a 7 m high weedy tree. The branches are piled on the boughs and densely foliated. The bark is initially green later gray-brown and covered in gray-white lenticles. The leaf buds are pubescent. The leaves are thin, soft when young later becoming stiffer. They are broadly elliptical to obovate and about 3.5 to 5 cm long. The leaves are usually entire-margined and pubescent on the ribs of the under surface.

Characteristics: The heartwood is bright yellow-red. The odor is somewhat foul and the taste is disgustingly bitter.

Habitat: The plant is indigenous to all of Europe, Western Asia, Asia Minor and the Caucasus; it has spread to the wild in North America.

Production: Frangula bark consists of the dried bark of the trunks and branches of Rhamnus frangula. The bark is peeled in May and June, then either dried and stored for 1 year to dry or heated for 1 hour at 100° C.

Other Names: Buckthorn, Frangula, Alder Buckthorn, Black Alder, Dog Wood, Black Dogwood, Black Alder Tree, European Black Alder, Black Alder Dogwood, Arrow Wood, European Buckthorn, Persian Berries, Alder Dogwood

ACTIONS AND PHARMACOLOGY

COMPOUNDS

Anthracene derivatives (4 to 6%): anthranoids, chief components glucofrangulin A, glucofrangulin A-diacetate (estered at rhamnose remnant), as well as frangulin A, frangulin C

Naphthalene derivatives: naphthoquinones

Peptide alkaloids (traces): including frangulanine

EFFECTS

The bark contains anthracene derivatives and their aglycones which have an anti-absorptive and hydrogogic effect. The anthracene derivatives induce active secretion of electrolytes and water in the intestinal lumina and inhibit the absorption of electrolytes and water from the colon by stimulating propulsive contractions. This results in accelerated intestinal passage time. In this manner, the increased water and subsequent volume of the intestinal content raise pressure and stimulate intestinal peristalsis.

INDICATIONS AND USAGE

Approved by Commission E:

■ Constipation

Unproven Uses: Frangula bark is used to ease bowel evacuation in the case of anal fissures, hemorrhoids and after rectal-anal surgery. It may also be used in preparation for exploratory surgery of the gastrointestinal tract.

Homeopathic Uses: Rhamnus frangula is used for weak digestion with a tendency to diarrhea.

CONTRAINDICATIONS

The drug is not to be used with intestinal obstruction, acute inflammatory intestinal diseases, appendicitis or with children under 12 years of age. The drug is not to be administered during pregnancy or while nursing.

PRECAUTIONS AND ADVERSE REACTIONS

General: Long-term use leads to loss of electrolytes, especially potassium ions. This may lead to hyperaldosteronism, inhibition of intestinal motility and enhancement of the effect of cardioactive steroids, which may lead to arrhythmias. Nephropathies, edema and accelerated bone deterioration are possible after long term use.

The question of an increased incidence of carcinoma of the colon following long-term administration of anthracene drugs has not yet been fully clarified. Recent studies show no definite connection between the administration of anthracene drugs and the frequency of carcinoma of the colon.

Pregnancy: Not to be used during pregnancy.

OVERDOSAGE

Vomiting and spasmodic gastrointestinal complaints could occur as side effects to the drug's purgative effect or with overdosages.

DOSAGE

Mode of Administration: Frangula Bark is available in solid pharmaceutical form and in commercial compounded preparations for oral intake. It is also available parenterally for homeopathic use.

Preparations:

Tea — scald 2 gm finely cut drug and strain after 15 minutes. The drug may also be left to steep in cold water for 12 hours.

Dry extract — percolation of 100 gm bark with methanol, after 1 day 400 gm to 500 gm percolate are extracted. The liquids (percolate and pressed juice) are left to stand for 8 days at 2 to 8° C before being filtered and dried. The glucofrangulin content must be stabilized at 15 to 17%.

Daily Dosage: 20 mg to 180 mg hydroxyanthracene derivatives

Tea — 1 cup mornings and evenings

The correct dosage for each individual is the smallest dosage necessary to maintain a soft stool. Frangula bark should not be used continuously for more than 1 or 2 weeks.

Homeopathic Dosage: from D3: 5 drops, 1 tablet or 10 globules every 30 to 60 minutes (acute) or 1 to 3 times daily (chronic); parenterally: 1 to 2 ml sc acute: 3 times daily; chronic: once a day (HAB1)

Storage: Frangula may be stored for at least 1 year if protected from light and moisture.

LITERATURE

Anonym, Abwehr von Arzneimittelrisiken, Stufe II. In: DAZ 136(38):3253-2354. 1996.

Anonym, Pharmaceutical Care: ''Den Mißbrauch von Laxanzien vermeiden helfen''. In: DAZ 135(20):1867-1868. 1995.

Demirezer LÖ, Glucofrangulinanthrone A/B, deren Oxidationsformen und davon abgeleitete Zuckerester aus Rhamnus-Arten. In: Dissertation Universität Frankfurt/Main. 1991.

Helmholz H, Ruge A, Piasecki A, Schröder S, Westendorf J, Genotoxizität der Faulbaumrinde. In: PZ 138(43):3478. 1993.

Pailer M, Haslinger E, (1972) Monatsh. Chem 103:1399.

Sydiskis RJ, Owen DG, Lohr JL, Rosler KHA, Blosmster RN, Inactivation of enveloped viruses by anthraquinones extracted from plants. In: Antimicrob Agents Chemother 35:2463-2466. 1991.

Van Os FHL, (1976) Pharmacology 14(Suppl 1)7:18.

Wagner H et al., (1978) Planta Med 33:53.

Further information in:

Frohne D, Pfänder HJ, Giftpflanzen - Ein Handbuch für Apotheker, Toxikologen und Biologen, 4. Aufl., Wiss. Verlagsges. mbH Stuttgart 1997.

Hänsel R, Keller K, Rimpler H, Schneider G (Hrsg.), Hagers Handbuch der Pharmazeutischen Praxis, 5. Aufl., Bde 4-6 (Drogen): Springer Verlag Berlin, Heidelberg, New York, 1992-1994.

Leung AY, Encyclopedia of Common Natural Ingredients Used in Food, Drugs and Cosmetics, John Wiley & Sons Inc., New York 1980.

Roth L, Daunderer M, Kormann K, Giftpflanzen, Pflanzengifte, 4. Aufl., Ecomed Fachverlag Landsberg Lech 1993.

Schulz R, Hänsel R, Rationale Phytotherapie, Springer Verlag Heidelberg 1996.

Steinegger E, Hänsel R, Pharmakognosie, 5. Aufl., Springer Verlag Heidelberg 1992.

Teuscher E, Lindequist U, Biogene Gifte - Biologie, Chemie, Pharmakologie, 2. Aufl., Fischer Verlag Stuttgart 1994.

Teuscher E, Biogene Arzneimittel, 5. Aufl., Wiss. Verlagsges. mbH Stuttgart 1997.

Wagner H, Wiesenauer M, Phytotherapie. Phytopharmaka und pflanzliche Homöopathika, Fischer-Verlag, Stuttgart, Jena, New York 1995.

Wichtl M (Hrsg.), Teedrogen, 4. Aufl., Wiss. Verlagsges. Stuttgart 1997.

Frankincense

Boswellia carteri

DESCRIPTION

Medicinal Parts: The medicinal part of the tree is the resin gum exuded when incisions are made in the bark of the trunk.

Flower and Fruit: The flowers are solitary on short stalks and single axillary inflorescences. The calyx is small, 5-toothed and perennial. The corolla has 5 elongated petals, and there are 5 stamens. The long anthers fall early. The fruit is a capsule divided into 3 parts with a seed in each section. The seeds are surrounded by a wide membranous leaf.

Leaves, Stem and Root: Boswellia carteri is a richly foliated tree whose leaves alternate unevenly on the branches to the tips. The 10 pairs and one leaflet are short-stalked, elongated, blunt, serrate, finely pubescent and mostly alternate. The base of the leaf is a fleshy cup-shaped disc that is larger than the corolla. The plant grows on few roots, which appear to be fused with the stony soil via an inert mass.

Habitat: Boswellia carteri is found in Somalia and parts of Saudi Arabia.

Production: (Indian) Frankincense or Olibanum is the hardened gum resin of Boswellia carteri, which exudes when incisions are made in the trunk. It is collected after being allowed to harden in the open air for about three weeks.

Not to be Confused With: The exuded gum resin of the trunk of Boswellia serrata also is called Frankincense or Olibanum.

Other Names: Olibanum

ACTIONS AND PHARMACOLOGY

COMPOUNDS

Volatile oil (5-9%): chief components 1-octyl acetate (share 60%), 1-octanol (share 12.7%), including as well alpha-pinene (3.5%), incensol (2.7%)

Resins (60%): components including among others alpha-boswellic acid, beta-boswellic acid, methyl ester of 3-acetyl-β-boswellic acid

Mucilages (12-20%)

EFFECTS

Externally, Frankincense can cause mild irritation of the skin. Internally, it is a mild carminative.

INDICATIONS AND USAGE

The drug is considered obsolete for medicinal use because its mode of action has not been documented. In vitro, the alpha and beta boswellic acids showed antimicrobial activity and inhibited the complementary system. The mucin, triterpene and essential oil content make application for respiratory conditions and its use for wounds seem plausible.

PRECAUTIONS AND ADVERSE REACTIONS

The drug is considered obsolete, even though no health hazards or side effects are known in conjunction with the proper administration of designated therapeutic dosages.

DOSAGE

Preparation: The Frankincense resin is obtained by tapping the bark and leaving the exudate for about three months, during which time it hardens slightly, allowing the resin to be collected.

LITERATURE

Ammon HPT, Entzündliche Darmerkrankungen: Weihrauch bei Colitis ulcerosa, siehe auch folgenden Artikel. In: DAZ 137(3):125. 1997.

Ammon HPT, Hemmstoffe der Leukotrienbiosynthese. In: DAZ 137(3):139-40. 1997.

Ammon HPT, Weihrauch - ein neuer Weg in der Therapie der Entzündungen. In: DAZ 132(45).2442. 1991.

Ammon S, Ein pflanzliches Antirheumaticum. In: DAZ 131(19):972. 1991.

Ammon T, Lipoxygenasehemmer aus Weihrauch. In: DAZ 133(37):3295. 1993.

Anonym, Weihrauchtherapie. In: DAZ 134(4):324-325. 1995.

Hoernlein RF et al., Die Hemmung der 5-Lipoxygnesae durch Acetyl-11-keto-β-Boswelliasäure (AKBA): Struktur-Wirkungsbeziehungen. In: 8. Frühjahrstagung der DPhG, Salzau, Abstracts, in PUZ 25(3):140. 1996.

Kern W, List PH, Hörhammer L (Hrsg.), Hagers Handbuch der Pharmazeutischen Praxis, 4. Aufl., Bde. 1-8, Springer Verlag Berlin, Heidelberg, New York, 1969.

Kreymeier J, Rheumatherapie mit Phytopharmaka. In: DAZ 137(8):611-613. 1997.

Madaus G, Lehrbuch der Biologischen Arzneimittel, Bde 1-3, Nachdruck, Georg Olms Verlag Hildesheim 1979.

Martinetz D, Der Indische Weihrauch - neue Aspekte eines alten Harzes. In: ZPT 13(4):121. 1992.

Müller-Bohn T, Chemie und Pharmakologie des Weihrauchs: Boswelliasäuren gegen chronische Polyarthritis und Colitis ulcerosa. In: DAZ 136(48):4324-4325. 1996.

Pfister-Hotz G, Phytotherapie in der Geriatrie. In: ZPT 18(3):165-162. 1997.

Rall B et al., Boswellic acids and protease activity (s.auch folgende Abstracts). In: PM 61(Abstracts of 43rd Ann Congr):105. 1995.

Wagner H, Wiesenauer M, Phytotherapie. Phytopharmaka und pflanzliche Homöopathika, Fischer-Verlag, Stuttgart, Jena, New York 1995.

Wasielewski S, Maligne G, Weihrauchextrakt bei bösartigen Hirntumoren. In: DAZ 137(26):2250-2251. 1997.

Fraxinus excelsior

See Ash

Fraxinus ornus

See Manna

French Tarragon

Artemisia dracunculus

DESCRIPTION

Medicinal Parts: The medicinal parts are the dried aerial parts of the plant.

Flower and Fruit: The flowers are drooping, almost globular and 2 to 3 mm across. They are whitish, later reddish, and clustered in loose panicles. The sepals of the epicalyx are oblong-elliptic and mostly green; the inner ones are ovate with a broad membranous edge. The ray florets are female. The disc florets are androgynous and infertile. The corolla is yellow with a glabrous receptacle.

Leaves, Stem and Root: The plant is a glabrous, 60- to 120-cm high herbaceous perennial. There are numerous stems, which are bushily branched with flowering branches at the top. The leaves are simple, lanceolate-linear, 2 to 10 cm by 2 to 10 mm, thorn-tipped, entire or slightly serrate, and somewhat glossy.

Characteristics: The odor is aromatic and intense.

Habitat: The plant is indigenous to Germany, Russia and southern Europe.

Production: French Tarragon leaves or herbs are picked when in bloom and carefully dried.

Other Names: Little Dragon, Mugwort, Estragon

ACTIONS AND PHARMACOLOGY

COMPOUNDS

Volatile oil of complex, variety-specific composition (0.25-3.1%): chavicol methyl ether dominates in German species, accompanied by ocimene, myrcene, alpha-pinene, beta-pinene, camphene, limonene, linalool

Flavonoids: including quercetin and patuletin glycosides

Hydroxycoumarins: including herniarin, scopoletin

Isocoumarins: including artemidin

Polyynes

EFFECTS

The essential oil of the drug is an appetite stimulant.

INDICATIONS AND USAGE

Unproven Uses: French Tarragon is used as an appetite stimulant.

PRECAUTIONS AND ADVERSE REACTIONS

No health hazards or side effects are known in conjunction with the proper administration of designated therapeutic dosages.

DOSAGE

Mode of Administration: Both the fresh and dried plant is used, mostly as a culinary herb.

LITERATURE

Balza F, Jamieson L, Towers GHN, Chemical constituents of the aerial parts of Artemisia dracunculus. In: JNP 48:339. 1985.

Greger H, Bohlmann F, Zdero Ch, Neue Isocumarine aus Dracunculus. In: PH 16:795. 1977.

Hänsel R, Keller K, Rimpler H, Schneider G (Hrsg.), Hagers Handbuch der Pharmazeutischen Praxis, 5. Aufl., Bde 4-6 (Drogen). Springer Verlag Berlin, Heidelberg, New York, 1992-1994.

Lakupovic J, Tan RX, Bohlmann F, Jia ZJ, Huneck S, Acetylenes and other constituents from Artemisia dracunculus. In: PM 57:450. 1992.

Marco JA et al., Sesquiterpenes lactones from Artemisia species. In: PH 32:460. 1993.

Schormüller B, In: Schormüller J: Alkaloidhaltige Genuβmittel, Gewürze, Kochsalz, Springer Verlag, Berlin, Heidelberg, New York. 1970.

Thieme H, Nguyen TT, PA 27:255-265. 1972.

Vostrowsky O et al., Über die Komponenten des ätherischen Öls aus Estragon (Artemisia dracunculus L.). In: Z Lebensm Untersuch Forsch 173:365-367. 1981.

Fringetree

Chionanthus virginicus

DESCRIPTION

Medicinal Parts: The medicinal part is the dried root or tree bark.

Flower and Fruit: The tree bears long peduncles of white, snowdrop-like flowers with fringed petals the same size as magnolia flowers. The flowers are androgynous, but on some stalks the flowers are almost exclusively male or female. The calyx is short and consists of four parts. The four petals are fused at the base. They are initially green but turn snow white and extend about 2.5 cm. Two stamens are enclosed in the short tube. The fruit is 1.5 to 2 cm across, dark blue to black, and oval and with a hard stone.

Leaves, Stem and Root: Fringetree is a deciduous shrub or tree up to 10 m tall. The leaves are smooth or downy, oblong or oval, 7.5 to 20 cm long and opposite. The root bark is about 3 mm thick and consists of irregular, quilled pieces up to about 8 cm long. The exterior of the bark is dull brown with concave scars. The inner surface is smooth and buff colored. The fracture is short and dense with projecting bundles of stone cells.

Characteristics: Fringetree is almost odorless and very bitter. The bark is so dense that, unlike most other barks, it sinks in water.

Habitat: Fringetree grows in the central and southern U.S. and also in eastern Asia.

Production: Fringetree root bark is the root bark of Chionanthus virginicus.

Other Names: Gray Beard Tree, Old Man's Beard, Poison Ash, Snowflower, White Fringe, Chionanthus, Snowdrop Tree

ACTIONS AND PHARMACOLOGY

COMPOUNDS

Lignane glycosides: phillyrin (chioanthine)

Saponins

EFFECTS

Fringetree, because of its saponin content, is said to have hepatic, cholagogue, diuretic and tonic effect.

INDICATIONS AND USAGE

Unproven Uses: Fringetree is used in treatment of the liver and gallbladder conditions (including gallstones). North American folk uses include jaundice, hepatatrophy, wounds and ulcers.

Homeopathic Uses: Although mention is made of significant homeopathic use, no details are given.

PRECAUTIONS AND ADVERSE REACTIONS

No health hazards or side effects are known in conjunction with the proper administration of designated therapeutic dosages.

DOSAGE

Mode of Administration: Liquid extract and preparations are administered internally.

LITERATURE

Kern W, List PH, Hörhammer L (Hrsg.), Hagers Handbuch der Pharmazeutischen Praxis, 4. Aufl., Bde. 1-8, Springer Verlag Berlin, Heidelberg, New York, 1969.

Madaus G, Lehrbuch der Biologischen Arzneimittel, Bde 1-3, Nachdruck, Georg Olms Verlag Hildesheim 1979.

Steinegger E, Jacober H, Pharm Acta Helv 34:585. 1959.

Frostwort

Helianthemum canadense

DESCRIPTION

Medicinal Parts: The medicinal part is the herb.

Flower and Fruit: The plant flowers twice each season, once early and again near the end. The first flowers are flat with large, bright yellow petals. The second flowers are in terminal clusters.

Leaves, Stem and Root: The plant is a perennial that grows 3 to 6 cm high and has a simple, erect and sparsely branched white stem. The few branches are slender and purplish-green with opposite leaves and leaf scars. The leaves are linear, up to 1.5 cm long, grayish-green and downy.

Characteristics: The taste is astringent and bitter. The plant is odorless.

Habitat: Frostwort is indigenous to the eastern U.S., but is now also found in Europe.

Production: Frostwort is the aerial part of Helianthemum canadense.

Other Names: Frost Plant, Frostweed, Rock-Rose, Sun Rose

ACTIONS AND PHARMACOLOGY

COMPOUNDS

Tannins

Glycoside: helianthinin

The constituents of the drug have not been fully investigated.

EFFECTS

Frostwort is astringent and tonic.

INDICATIONS AND USAGE

The herb is used internally for digestive disorders and externally for ulcers.

PRECAUTIONS AND ADVERSE REACTIONS

Health risks or side effects following the proper administration of designated therapeutic dosages are not recorded.

DOSAGE

Mode of Administration: Frostwort is administered as a liquid extract.

LITERATURE

Kern W, List PH, Hörhammer L (Hrsg.), Hagers Handbuch der Pharmazeutischen Praxis, 4. Aufl., Bde. 1-8, Springer Verlag Berlin, Heidelberg, New York, 1969.

Madaus G, Lehrbuch der Biologischen Arzneimittel, Bde 1-3, Nachdruck, Georg Olms Verlag Hildesheim 1979.

Wagner H, Wiesenauer M, Phytotherapie. Phytopharmaka und pflanzliche Homopathika, Fischer-Verlag, Stuttgart, Jena, New York 1995.

Fucus vesiculosus

See Bladderwrack

Fumaria officinalis

See Fumitory

Fumitory

Fumaria officinalis

DESCRIPTION

Medicinal Parts: The medicinal parts are the dried herb and the aerial parts of the fresh flowering plant.

Flower and Fruit: The short pedicled flowers are in erect, dense, terminal racemes opposite the leaves and are 5 to 8 mm long. The outer petals are rounded at the front and are crimson to pink. But like the inner petals they are dark-red to black at the tip and have a green keel. The fruit, which appears in the flowering season, is nut-like, globular, slightly flattened at the side, green and has a dent in the top.

Leaves, Stem and Root: The plant is 10 to 50 cm high and has a tender, erect, angular, branched, hollow and glabrous stem which, like the leaves, is bluish green. The leaves are alternate and divided into 3-pinnate sections. They are petiolate, double pinnate, soft with petioled palmate or pinnatifid pinna.

Characteristics: The herb has a bitter, salty taste.

Habitat: The plant is indigenous to the Mediterranean region to northern Africa and in all of Europe and Siberia. The herb has been introduced into North and South America.

Production: Common Fumitory herb consists of the dried, above ground parts of Fumaria officinalis, gathered during the flowering season.

Not to be Confused With: The very similar species F. vaillanti and F. schleicheri.

Other Names: Earth Smoke, Hedge Fumitory, Beggary, Fumus, Vapor, Wax Dolls

ACTIONS AND PHARMACOLOGY

COMPOUNDS

Flavonoids: including rutin

Hydroxycinnamic acid derivatives: including caffeoylmalic acid

Isoquinoline alkaloids: some of them include -

Protoberberine-type: including (-)-scoulerine

Protopine-type: including protopine; main alkaloid

Spirobenzylisoquinoline-type: fumaricine, (+)-fumariline

Indenobenzazepine-type: including fumaritine, fumarofine

Organic acids: fumaric acid

EFFECTS

Fumitory has a light, antispasmodic effect on the bile ducts and the gastrointestinal tract. It is also amphicholeretic.

INDICATIONS AND USAGE

Approved by Commission E:

■ Liver and gallbladder complaints

Spastic discomfort in the area of the gallbladder and bile ducts, as well as the gastrointestinal tract.

Unproven Uses: In folk medicine, the herb has been used for skin diseases, constipation, cystitis, arteriosclerosis, rheumatism, arthritis, as a blood purifier, hypoglycemia and for infections.

Homeopathic Uses: for chronic, itching eczema resulting from liver disease.

PRECAUTIONS AND ADVERSE REACTIONS

Health risks or side effects following the proper administration of designated therapeutic dosages are not recorded.

DOSAGE

Mode of Administration: Comminuted drug and its galenic preparations for internal use.

Preparation: To prepare an infusion, pour boiling water over 2 to 3 gm drug and strain after 20 minutes.

Daily Dosage: 6 gm of drug. Infusions for gallbladder complaints, drink 1 warm cup 30 minutes before meals.

Pressed juice—2 to 3 teaspoons (2.4 to 3.5 gm drug) daily as a cold or hot infusion.

Grated fresh plant—1 teaspoon 3 times daily (about 50% plant material).

Homeopathic Dosage: 5 drops, 1 tablet or 10 globules every 30 to 60 minutes (acute) or 1 to 3 times daily (chronic); parenterally: 1 to 2 ml sc acute: 3 times daily; chronic: once a day (HAB34).

Storage: Protect from light and moisture.

LITERATURE

Duke JA, (1985) Die amphocholeretische Wirkung der Fumaria officinalis. Z Allg Med 34: 1819.

Hahn R, Nahrstedt A, High Content of Hydroxycinnamic Acids Esterified with (+)-D-Malic-Acid in the Upper Parts of Fumaria officinalis. In: PM 59(2):189. 1993.

Mardirossian ZH et al., PH 22:759. 1983.

Willaman JJ, Hui-Li L (1970) Lloydia 33 (3A): 1.

Further information in:

Hänsel R, Keller K, Rimpler H, Schneider G (Hrsg.), Hagers Handbuch der Pharmazeutischen Praxis, 5. Aufl., Bde 4-6 (Drogen), Springer Verlag Berlin, Heidelberg, New York, 1992-1994.

Madaus G, Lehrbuch der Biologischen Arzneimittel, Bde 1-3, Nachdruck, Georg Olms Verlag Hildesheim 1979.

Roth L, Daunderer M, Kormann K, Giftpflanzen, Pflanzengifte, 4. Aufl., Ecomed Fachverlag Landsberg Lech 1993.

Teuscher E, Lindequist U, Biogene Gifte - Biologie, Chemie, Pharmakologie, 2. Aufl., Fischer Verlag Stuttgart 1994.

Wichtl M (Hrsg.), Teedrogen, 4. Aufl., Wiss. Verlagsges. Stuttgart 1997.

Galanthus nivalis

See Snowdrop

Galbanum

Ferula gummosa

DESCRIPTION

Medicinal Parts: The medicinal part is the oily gum-resin.

Two types of Galbanum are used: Levant or Soft Galbanum is more viscous and often contains small root pieces. Persian or Hard Galbanum sometimes contains pieces of stem and is friable in texture.

Flower and Fruit: The plant bears yellowish-white flowers in a few flat umbels. The fruit is thin and flat. The seeds are glossy.

Leaves, Stem and Root: Ferula gummosa is a perennial plant with a firm, smooth and hollow stem that grows up to 1.75 m tall. The leaflets are glossy, ovate, wedge-shaped and have sharply serrate margins.

Characteristics: The gum-resin occurs in translucent, yellowish or bluish-green masses of tears. Soft Galbanum (Levant) is more viscous and may contain small pieces of root. Hard Galbanum (Persian) is friable and may contain pieces of stem. The odor is similar to musk or turpentine.

Habitat: The plant is found in central Asia, Iran, the Mediterranean region and also at the Cape of Good Hope.

Production: Galbanum is the resin from the roots and trunk of Ferula gummosa and other related varieties. The exuding resin is collected from the pith without wounding the plant.

ACTIONS AND PHARMACOLOGY

COMPOUNDS

Resinous substances (60%): chiefly galbaresenic acid and galbanic acid

Mucilages (40%)

Volatile oil (10-20%): including among others, alpha-pinenes, beta-pinenes, myrcene, cadinenes, guaiazulene, aroma bearer undecatriene

EFFECTS

The drug acts as stimulant, expectorant, and vulnerary. In vitro an antimicrobial effect has been proven.

INDICATIONS AND USAGE

Unproven Uses: Internally, Galbanum is used for digestive disorders and flatulence; externally it is used in the treatment of wounds.

PRECAUTIONS AND ADVERSE REACTIONS
Health risks or side effects following the proper administration of designated therapeutic dosages are not recorded.

DOSAGE
Mode of Administration: Preparations for internal and external use.

LITERATURE
Kern W, List PH, Hörhammer L (Hrsg.), Hagers Handbuch der Pharmazeutischen Praxis, 4. Aufl., Bde 1-8, Springer Verlag Berlin, Heidelberg, New York, 1969.

Galega officinalis
See Goat's Rue

Galeopsis segetum
See Hempnettle

Galipea officinalis
See Angostura

Galium aparine
See Cleavers

Galium odoratum
See Sweet Woodruff

Galium verum
See Lady's Bedstraw

Gambir
Uncaria species

DESCRIPTION
Medicinal Parts: The medicinal parts are the leaves and young shoots of the plant.

Flower and Fruit: The flowers are single or in loose, globose inflorescences. The flowers are fused and grow in fives. The corolla is funnel-shaped, the 2-part ovary is inferior. The fruit is a loculicidal capsule opening on 2 sides. The seeds are long-winged at both ends.

Leaves, Stem and Root: This woody liana or climbing shrub has leaves that are opposite and short-petiolate. Young branches are 4-sided or orbicular and have pairs of stipules. Using Uncaria gambir as a prototype, the calyx is 5-tipped, the corolla light purple. The leaves are 6 to 11 mm long with a 1 to 2 cm long petiole, coriaceous, lanceolate to oval, entire, pubescent at the veins. After the leaf-axillary flower branches drop, a barbed tendril, which is 1 to 2 cm long and woody, is formed.

Habitat: Indonesia and Malaysia

Production: Yellow catechu is the dried aqueous extract of the leaves and young shoots of Uncaria gambir. Cultivated stock is harvested, then the leaves and shoots are boiled with water to form a decoction that is pressed and evaporated to the consistency of syrup. The resulting lumps are dried in the sun.

Not to be Confused With: Acacia

Other Names: Yellow Catechu

ACTIONS AND PHARMACOLOGY
COMPOUNDS
Catechin tannins (20 to 50%): among them gambirines A1 to A3 (astringently active flavanol dimers)

Flavanols (10 to 50%): particularly (+)-catechin, gambirines B1 to B3 (dimers)

Indole alkaloids of the beta-carboline type (presumably only traces in the drug): including gambirtanine, dihydrogambirtanine

EFFECTS
The drug is astringent in effect because of the tannins it contains, which are also said to exhibit antibacterial and algicidal efficacy. The flavonoid fraction (cyanidanol = (+)-catechin) is said to be hepatoprotective in effect.

INDICATIONS AND USAGE
Unproven Uses: Catechu tincture is used in folk medicine for diarrhea, nausea and gastrointestinal disturbances. Decoction is used for ulcers of the stomach and oral mucosa, and also asthma. The effect for diarrhea appears plausible because of the tannin content.

PRECAUTIONS AND ADVERSE REACTIONS
No health hazards are known in conjunction with the proper administration of designated therapeutic dosages.

DOSAGE

Mode of Administration: Whole and powdered drug for internal use.

Preparation: Tincture: 200 g drug (pounded), 50 g cut cinnamon to 1 liter 45% ethanol, macerated (BP88)

Daily Dosage: 0.5 to 2 g drug; Catechu Tincture: 2.5 to 5 ml

LITERATURE

Balz JP, Das NP, Uncaria elliptica a major source of rutin. Planta Med, 25:174-7, 1979 Jun.

Blaschek W, Hänsel R, Keller K, Reichling J, Rimpler G, Schneider G (Eds), Hagers Handbuch der Pharmazeutischen Praxis. Folgeb nde 1 und 2. Drogen A-Z. Springer. Berlin, Heidelberg 1998.

Chang CC, Tung LH, Chen RR, Chiueh CC, A study on the antihypertensive action of uncarine A, an alkaloid of Uncaria formosana used in Chinese herb medicine. Taiwan I Hsueh Hui Tsa Chih, 25:61-9, 1979 Feb.

Chang P, Koh YK, Geh SL, Soepadmo E, Goh SH, Wong AK, Cardiovascular effects in the rat of dihydrocorynantheine isolated from Uncaria callophylla. J Ethnopharmacol, 25:213-5, 1989 Apr.

Endo K, Oshima Y, Kikuchi H, Koshihara Y, Hikino H, Hypotensive principles of Uncaria hooks. Planta Med, 25:188-90, 1983 Nov.

Haginiwa J, Sakai S, Takahashi K, Taguchi M, Shujiro S, Studies of plants containing indole alkaloids. I. Alkaloids in Uncaria genus. Yakugaku Zasshi, 25:575-8, 1971 May.

Law KH, Das NP, Initiation and maintenance of callus tissue culture of Uncaria elliptica for flavonoid production. Prog Clin Biol Res, 25:67-70, 1988.

Lin CC, Lin JM, Chiu HF, Studies on folk medicine 'thang-kau-tin' from Taiwan. (I). The anti-inflammatory and liver-protective effect. Am J Chin Med, 57:37-50, 1992.

Lin JM, Lin CC, Chen MF, Ujiie T, Takada A, Studies on Taiwan folk medicine, thang-kau-tin (II): Measurement of active oxygen scavenging activity using an ESR technique. Am J Chin Med, 57:43-51, 1995.

Mimaki Y, Toshimizu N, Yamada K, Sashida Y, Anti-convulsion effects of choto-san and chotoko (Uncariae Uncis cam Ramlus) in mice, and identification of the active principles. Yakugaku Zasshi, 57:1011-21, 1997 Dec.

Yamanaka E, Kimizuka Y, Aimi N, Sakai S, Haginiwa J, Studies of plants containing indole alkaloids. IX. Quantitative analysis of tertiary alkaloids in various parts of Uncaria rhynchophylla MIQ. Yakugaku Zasshi, 25:1028-33, 1983 Oct.

Yano S, Horiuchi H, Horie S, Aimi N, Sakai S, Watanabe K, Alkaloids from the leaves of Uncaria homomalla. Planta Med, 57:749-52, 1980 Sep.

Yano S, Horiuchi H, Horie S, Aimi N, Sakai S, Watanabe K, Alkaloids of Uncaria pteropoda. Isolation and structures of pteropodine and isopteropodine. J Chem Soc Perkin 1, 57:2245-9, 1966.

Yano S, Horiuchi H, Horie S, Aimi N, Sakai S, Watanabe K, Ca2+ channel blocking effects of hirsutine, an indole alkaloid from Uncaria genus, in the isolated rat aorta. Planta Med, 57:403-5, 1991 Oct.

Yano S, Horiuchi H, Horie S, Aimi N, Sakai S, Watanabe K, Gambirine, a new indole alkaloid from Uncaria gambier roxb. Tetrahedron Lett, 57:1571-4, 1967 Apr.

Yano S, Horiuchi H, Horie S, Aimi N, Sakai S, Watanabe K, Studies on flavonoid metabolism. Biosynthesis of (+)-14Ccatechin by the plant Uncaria gambir Roxb. Biochem J, 57:73-7, 1967 Oct.

Yano S, Horiuchi H, Horie S, Aimi N, Sakai S, Watanabe K, Studies on Uncaria alkaloid. XXI. Separation of rhynchophylline and corynoxeine (author's transl.). Yakugaku Zasshi, 57:758-9, 1975 Jun.

Yano S, Horiuchi H, Horie S, Aimi N, Sakai S, Watanabe K, The antihypertensive effect of Uncaria rhynchophylla in essential hypertension (author's transl.). Taiwan I Hsueh Hui Tsa Chih, 57:749-52, 1980 Sep.

Zhu M, Bowery NG, Greengrass PM, Phillipson JD, Application of radioligand receptor binding assays in the search for CNS active principles from Chinese medicinal plants. J Ethnopharmacol, 57:153-64, 1996 Nov.

Gamboge

Garcinia hanburyi

DESCRIPTION

Medicinal Parts: The medicinal part of the tree is the resin extracted from the plant.

Leaves, Stem and Root: The tree grows to about 15 m and has a diameter of about 30 cm. The bark is usually in the form of cylindrical sticks, deep orange-brown and opaque. The transverse fracture is smooth and almost conchoidal.

Characteristics: The taste is innocuous at first, then becomes very acrid and causes an unpleasant stinging sensation shortly after being placed in the mouth. The powder is highly sternutatory.

Habitat: The plant is indigenous to Indochina and Sri Lanka.

Production: Gamboge is the gum-resin from the trunk of Garcinia hanburyi harvested from trees that are at least ten years old.

Other Names: Camboge, Gutta Cambodia, Gutta Gamba, Gummigutta, Tom Rong, Gambodia

ACTIONS AND PHARMACOLOGY

COMPOUNDS

Resins (70-75%): consisting mainly of yellow or red-colored benzophenones and xanthones, including morellic acid, isomorellic acid, alpha-gambogic acid (alpha-guttic acid)

Mucilages (25-30%)

EFFECTS

The drug's mucilage content produces a strong laxative effect. The beta gutteriferine componant acts as a strong irritant to intestinal mucous membranes and also exhibits antimicrobial properties.

INDICATIONS AND USAGE

Unproven Uses: Gamboge is used for the treatment of digestive disorders, in particular constipation, and is used in combination with other laxatives.

PRECAUTIONS AND ADVERSE REACTIONS

As little as 0.2 g of the drug can lead to abdominal pain and vomiting.

OVERDOSAGE

Fatalities have been observed with administration of 4 g.

DOSAGE

No information is available in the literature.

LITERATURE

Hegnauer R, Chemotaxonomie der Pflanzen, Bde 1-11, Birkhäuser Verlag Basel, Boston, Berlin 1962-1997.

Kern W, List PH, Hörhammer L (Hrsg.), Hagers Handbuch der Pharmazeutischen Praxis, 4. Aufl., Bde. 1-8, Springer Verlag Berlin, Heidelberg, New York, 1969.

Lewin L, Gifte und Vergiftungen, 6. Aufl., Nachdruck, Haug Verlag, Heidelberg 1992.

Lu GB et al., (1984) Yao Hsueh Husueh Pao 19 (8): 636.

Wagner H, Wiesenauer M, Phytotherapie. Phytopharmaka und pflanzliche Homöopathika, Fischer-Verlag, Stuttgart, Jena, New York 1995.

Garcinia hanburyi

See Gamboge

Garden Cress

Lepidium sativum

DESCRIPTION

Medicinal Parts: The medicinal part is the fresh or dried herb harvested during or shortly after the flowering season.

Flower and Fruit: The racemes are terminal or axillary. The sepals are elliptical, 1 to 1.5 mm long and bristly downy. The petals are longer than the calyx, white or reddish, oblong-spatulate and indistinctly stemmed. The anthers are often violet. The fruit is a compressed, orbicular-ovate, 5 to 6 mm long, clearly winged small pod on an erect stem. The seeds are ovate, almost smooth and red-brown.

Leaves, Stem and Root: Garden Cress is a 20 to 40 cm high herb with a glabrous bluish bloom. The stem is erect, round and branched. The leaves are light green and thin. The basal leaves are usually lyrate-pinnatesect. The lower cauline leaves are usually doubly or singly pinnatesect. All leaves have dentate to prickly segments.

Characteristics: Garden Cress has a radish-like taste. The seeds have a slimy skin and swell in water.

Habitat: The herb is grown worldwide.

Production: Garden Cress is the fresh plant (aerial part) of Lepidium sativum, harvested during the flowering season or shortly afterward. The fresh herb has a spicy odor. It is rarely dried, either naturally or artificially, since the fresh plant is used most often.

Not to be Confused With: Adulterations rarely occur, since it is usually cultivated.

ACTIONS AND PHARMACOLOGY

COMPOUNDS: IN THE FRESH FOLIAGE

Glucosinolates: chief components glucotropaeolin, yielding benzyl isothiocyanate (benzyl mustard oil) and its autolysis products (including benzyl cyanide, 3-phenyl propionitrile, benzaldehyde) when the plant is bruised

Ascorbic acid (vitamin C, 37%)

COMPOUNDS: IN THE SEEDS

Glucosinolates (3.5 to 5.3%): glucotropeolin

Cucurbitacins

Cardiac steroids (cardenolides)

EFFECTS

The antibacterial action of Garden Cress has been demonstrated in various tests. It was completely inhibitory in the case of 3 microorganisms, although the antibacterial characteristics depended largely on the age of the plants used. An antiviral effect against the encephalitis virus *Columbia SH*, was demonstrated in tests on mice. Its diuretic action has not been proven through experiments.

INDICATIONS AND USAGE

Unproven Uses: The herb is used for coughs, vitamin C deficiency, constipation, poor immunity and as a diuretic.

Indian Medicine: Garden Cress is used for vitamin C deficiency, liver disease, asthma, hemorrhoids and as an abortifacient.

PRECAUTIONS AND ADVERSE REACTIONS

No health hazards or side effects are known in conjunction with the proper administration of designated therapeutic dosages. The mustard oil contained in Garden Cress can cause skin blisters and necrosis in higher concentrations. It is sometimes misused as an abortifacient because the internal administration of mustard oil causes severe anemia of the internal organs.

DOSAGE

Mode of Administration: Garden Cress is administered as a freshly cut herb in oral preparations.

LITERATURE

Hänsel R, Keller K, Rimpler H, Schneider G (Hrsg.), Hagers Handbuch der Pharmazeutischen Praxis, 5. Aufl., Bde 4-6 (Drogen), Springer Verlag Berlin, Heidelberg, New York, 1992-1994.

Iori R, Rollin P, Streicher H, Thiem J, Palmieri S, The myrosinase-glucosinolate interaction mechanism studied using some synthetic competitive inhibitors. FEBS Lett, 385:87-90, 1996 Apr 29.

Rao KV, Beach JW, Streptonigrin and related compounds. 5. Synthesis and evaluation of some isoquinoline analogues. J Med Chem, 19:1871-9, 1991 Jun.

Ugazio G et al., co-toxicological study conducted with a battery of biological and phytological tests on sediments carried out on a series of 24 tributaries of the Po in 1994 and 1995. G Ital Med Lav Ergon, 19:10-6, 1997 Jan-Mar.

Garlic

Allium sativum

TRADE NAMES

Garlic (available from numerous manufacturers), Garlicin, Garlique, Garlic Oil, Garlic Power, Triple Garlic, High Potency Garlic Oil, Garlic Odorless, Chinese Tian Shan Garlic, Deodorized Garlic, Kyolic Reserve Aged Garlic Extract, Odor Free Concentrated Garlic, Aged Garlic Extract, Kyolic Hi-Po Formula, High Alicin Garlic, Standardized Garlic, Natural Garlic Oil

DESCRIPTION

Medicinal Parts: The medicinal parts are the whole fresh bulb, the dried bulb and the oil of garlic.

Flower and Fruit: The plant consists of a cluster of long flowers where the floral axis terminates in a single flower and contains few florets (small flowers or buds). There are numerous 1 cm deciduous bulbs capable of producing new plants, which shed simultaneously. The flowers usually remain in bud form and often do not produce any seed. The petals are reddish or greenish-white and longer than the stamens. The anthers of the middle stamens are spread at the base and have fan-shaped tips.

Leaves, Stem and Root: Allium sativum is a perennial plant that grows 25 to 70 cm high. The plant contains an erect, rigid or curved stem, which is leafy in the middle. The leaves are flat, 4 to 25 mm, straight and broad, with a wedge-shaped tip; they can be rough or smooth-edged. The sheath, or lower part of the leaf surrounding the stem, is pointed and longer than the flower cluster. The garlic bulb is usually a compound bulb, and the secondary bulbs are oval in shape. The bulb skin color is either silky white or green.

Habitat: Central to southern Asia is considered the region of origin; garlic has been introduced to the Mediterranean with cultivation worldwide.

Production: Garlic bulbs, either fresh or carefully dried, consist of the main bulb with several secondary bulbs (cloves). Garlic may be harvested in September and October when the leaves and bulbs are dry.

Other Names: Poor Man's Treacle, Clove Garlic, Common Garlic, Allium, Stinking Rose

ACTIONS AND PHARMACOLOGY

COMPOUNDS

Alliins (alkylcysteine sulfoxides): in particular allylalliin, propenyl alliin and methylalliin (including their gamma-glutamyl conjugates. Once cut, the alliin in the freshly harvested bulbs is converted to allicin (diallyl-disulphide-mono-S-oxide). Bulbs that have been dried and then re-moistened, ferment into alliaceous oils. These oils are oligosulfides, ajoens (dialkyl-trithiaalkane-monoxides) and vinyl dithiins.

Fructosans (polysaccharides)

Saponins

EFFECTS

The alliin in the drug is antimicrobial, lipid-reducing, anti-oxidative and fibrinolytic. The antibacterial, antimycotic and lipid-reducing effects have been well-documented. Inhibition of thrombocyte aggregation, increased bleeding time and clotting time, and enhancement of fibrinolytic activity have been demonstrated in clinical trials.

A study of the lipid-lowering effect with isolated hepatocytes suggest that garlic extracts are responsible for early inhibition of sterol synthesis due to their sulfur-containing compounds. Alliin, the main sulfur-containing compound of garlic, when coverted to allicin, exerts inhibitory effects on key enzymes in cholesterol biosynthesis, including HMG CoA reductase (Gebhardt, 1993; Gebhardt, 1996).

Garlic tablets studied *in vitro* were found to enhance natural killer (NK) cells, which are an important part of the immune system in fighting cancers, viruses and certain bacteria. Antioxidative effects of garlic, determined by an increase in intracellular glutathione (GSH) levels, are responsible for decreasing poor cellular function and premature aging. Antiviral activity was also noted *in vitro* with garlic tablets (See, 1999).

Ajoen is the antithrombotic compound that inhibits fibrinogen receptors on platelets (Robbers, 1996). The allicin and oligosulfides in garlic oil have antiplatelet activity through inhibition of adenosine diphosphate, collagen and beta-thromboglobulin release after collagen stimulation. The compounds also exert antithrombotic effects through inhibition of platelet thromboxane formation (Bordia, 1998; Legnani 1993).

CLINICAL TRIALS

A randomized, placebo-controlled, double-blind study involving 42 outpatients was conducted over a 12-week period to assess the effects of standardized garlic powder tablets on serum lipids and lipoproteins, glucose and blood pressure. Standardized garlic powder administered 900 mg daily produced a significantly greater reduction in serum total cholesterol (262+/- 34mg/dL to 247 +/-40mg/dL with garlic compared to 276+/-34mg/dL to 274+/- 29mg/dL with placebo). Low-density lipoprotein cholesterol (LDL-C) was significantly reduced with garlic treatment by 11% compared to 3% with placebo treatment. No significant change was demonstrated in high-density lipoprotein cholesterol, triglycerides, serum glucose, blood pressure and other monitored parameters (Jain, 1993).

The lipid-lowering effect of garlic powder tablets was tested by administering a dose of 900 mg daily (equivalent to approximately 2.7 grams or 1 clove of fresh garlic daily) to 28 outpatients with hypercholesterolemia. After 12 weeks of treatment, there were no significant lipid or lipoprotein changes in either the placebo- or garlic-treated groups (Isaacsohn, 1998).

A 5 mg dose of steam distilled garlic oil was administered twice daily to 25 outpatients with moderate hypercholesterolemia in a randomized, double-blind, placebo-controlled trial. The hypocholesterolemic effect of garlic oil was determined after a 12-week period. The commercial garlic oil preparation did not have a significant effect on serum lipoproteins, cholesterol absorption or cholesterol synthesis (Berthold, 1998).

Note: There are contradicting results regarding the lipid-lowering effect of garlic, which may be attributed to lack of manufacturing standardization of the products used in the studies. The fresh garlic may contain higher amounts of the active ingredient, allicin, which is inactivated upon cooking.

INDICATIONS AND USAGE

Approved by Commission E:

- Arteriosclerosis
- Hypertension
- Raised levels of cholesterol

Garlic is used internally as an adjuvant to dietetic measures for elevated lipid levels. The herb is also used for prevention of age-related vascular changes and arteriosclerosis.

Unproven Uses: In folk medicine, garlic is utilized internally for inflammatory respiratory conditions, whooping cough and bronchitis. Garlic is also used for gastrointestinal ailments, particularly digestive disorders with flatulence and gastrointestinal spasms. Other uses consist of menstrual pains, treatment of diabetes, and as a tonic for diverse illnesses and debilities. Externally, garlic is used for corns, warts, calluses, otitis, muscle pain, neuralgia, arthritis and sciatica.

Indian Medicine: Garlic is used in bronchitis, constipation, joint pain and fever.

Homeopathic Uses: Garlic is used in conditions such as inflammation of the upper respiratory tract, digestive complaints and muscle rheumatism in the lumbar region.

PRECAUTIONS AND ADVERSE REACTIONS

General: Adverse effects such as headache, myalgia, fatigue and vertigo have been seen with therapeutic doses of garlic (Holzgartner, 1992).

Allergic Reactions: Frequent contact with the drug may result in allergic reactions such as contact dermatitis and asthma (Asero, 1998; Lee, 1991).

Burns: Garlic associated partial thickness burns and necrosis have been reported in several case studies in which the herb remained in contact with the skin for a minimum of 6 to 18 hours (Roberge, 1997; Garty, 1993; Parish, 1987).

Gastrointestinal: Abdominal discomfort, nausea, vomiting, diarrhea and a feeling of fullness have occurred with garlic therapy (Holzgartner, 1992; Berthold, 1998)

Hematologic: A significant decrease in hematocrit values and plasma viscosity have been associated with the administration of garlic powder (Jung, 1991). There has been risk of postoperative bleeding with TURP (trans-urethral resection of prostate) or mammaplasty surgery (Burnham, 1995;

German, 1995). Also, spontaneous spinal epidural hematoma has been reported with garlic (Rose, 1990).

Hypersensitivity: Occupational asthma induced by inhalation and ingestion of garlic has been observed (Lybarger, 1982).

Ocular: The alliin, S-alkyl cysteine sulfoxide, which decomposes into a variety of thiosulfinates and polysulfides via allinase upon extraction (crushing), produces a lacrimation effect (Augusti, 1996).

Olfactory: Garlic therapy is associated with body odor or halitosis (Berthold, 1998).

Nursing: Not to be used while nursing.

Drug Interactions: Concomitant use of garlic with anticoagulants such as coumadin and antiplatelets such as aspirin and dipyridamole could increase the risk of bleeding due to the effect of garlic on platelet aggregation and fibrinogen. (Agerwal, 1996; Bordia, 1998; Legnani, 1993; Newall, 1996; Robbers, 1996). NSAID's, such as indomethacin, could increase bleeding time by decreasing platelet aggregation (Agerwal, 1996; Bordia, 1998; Legnani, 1993).

DOSAGE

Mode of Administration: The minced bulb and preparations are for internal use and external treatment. Garlic oil maceration or garlic oil resulting from steam distillation is widely available.

How Supplied:

Capsules — 3 mg, 100 mg, 270 mg (total allicin 5000 mcg), 300 mg, 500 mg, 580 mg (total allicin 3 mg), 600 mg (total allicin 2500 mcg or standardized to 500 mcg allicin), 1000 mg, 1500 mg, 5000 mg

Dried powder

Oil macerations

Tablets — 300 mg, 400 mg (total allicin 3 mg), 500 mg, 600 mg (total allicin 5000 mcg), 810 mg

Preparation: Garlic oil maceration — Bulbs are homogenized and stirred in fatty oil (1:1) for 48 hours, then filtered.

Solid garlic extract — An extraction of the chopped bulbs with ethanol or methanol is allowed to evaporate.

Aqueous extract — Fresh bulbs are macerated in cold water (1:1).

Fermented garlic — The minced drug is soaked over a long duration in a water-ethanol mixture, volatile agents escape, and the garlic becomes odorless. Steam distillations and tinctures are also possible.

Daily Dosage:

General — The average daily dose is 4 gm of fresh garlic or 8 mg of essential oil. One fresh garlic clove, 1 to 2 times daily.

Arteriosclerosis — Daily doses of 600-800 mg of garlic powder and dried garlic have been shown to be effective (Harenberg, 1988; Kiesewetter, 1991).

Hyperlipidemia — A total daily dose of 600-900 mg of garlic powder (standardized to 1.3% of alliin content) has been shown effective (Holzgartner, 1992; Isaacsohn, 1998; Mader, 1990; Simons, 1995).

Hypertension — The effective dose is garlic powder taken 200-300 mg three times daily (Auer, 1990; Sigagy, 1994).

External — Fresh garlic applied to the skin as an antimicrobial dressing should not be left for more than a few hours due to case reports of burns (Garty, 1993; Parish, 1987; Roberge, 1997).

Homeopathic Dosage: 5 drops, 1 tablet or 10 globules every 30 to 60 minutes (acute) or 1 to 3 times daily (chronic); parenterally: 1 to 2 times daily sc; ointment 1 to 2 times daily (HAB1)

Storage: Garlic should be hung in plaits in a dry place.

LITERATURE

Agarwal KC, Therapeutic actions of garlic constituents. Med Res Rev 1996; 16(1):111-124.

Anonym, Knoblauch, Blockade der Cholesterinsynthese in der Leber. In: DAZ 134(45):4468. 1994.

Apitz-Castro R et al., (1983) Thromb Res 32:155.

Asero R, Mistrello G, Roncarolo D et al., A case of garlic allergy. J Allergy Clin Immunol 1998 Mar;101(3):427-8.

Augusti KT, Therapeutic values of onion (Allium cepa L.) and garlic (Allium sativum L.). Indian J Exp Biol 1996 Jul;34(7):634-40.

Augusti KT, Benaim ME, (1974) Clin Chim Acta 60:121.

Augusti KT, Mathew PT, (1974) Experientia 30:468.

Block E et al., (1984) J Am Chem Soc 106:8295.

Berthold HK, Sudhop T, von Bergmann K, Effect of garlic oil preparation on serum lipoproteins and cholesterol metabolism: a randomized controlled trial. JAMA 1998 Jun 17;279(23):1900-2.

Bordia A et al., Effect of garlic (Allium sativum) on blood lipids, blood sugar, fibrinogen and fibrinolytic activity in patients with coronary artery disease. Prostaglandins Leukot Essent Fatty Acids. 1998 Apr;58(4):257-63.

Brahmachar MD, Augusti KT, (1962) J Pharm Pharmacol 14: 254 and 617.

Burnham BE, Garlic as a possible risk for postoperative bleeding. Plast Reconstr Surg 1995 Jan;95(1):213.

Chaudhuri BN et al., (1984) Biomed Biochim Acta 41:1045.

Garty BZ, Garlic Burns. Pediatrics 1993 Mar;91(3):658-9.

Gebhardt R, Multiple inhibitory effects of garlic extracts on cholesterol biosynthesis in hepatocytes. Lipids 1993;28:613-619.

Gebhardt R, Beck H, Differential inhibitory effects of garlic-derived organosulfur compounds on cholesterol biosynthesis in primary rat hepatocyte cultures. Lipids 1996 Dec;31(12):1269-76.

German K, Kumar U, Blackford HN, Garlic and the risk of TURP bleeding. Br J Urol 1995 Oct;76(4):518.

Harenberg J, Giese C, Zimmermann R, Effect of dried garlic on blood coagulation, fibrinolysis, platelet aggregation and serum cholesterol levels in patients with hyperlipoproteinemia. Atherosclerosis 1988 Dec;74(3):247-9.

Holzgartner H, Schmidt U, Kuhn U, Comparison of the efficacy and tolerance of a garlic preparation vs. bezafibrate. Arzneimittelforschung 1992 Dec;42(12):1473-7.

Ide N et al., Aged garlic extract and its constituents inhibit Cu+-induced oxidative modification of low density lipoproteins.PM (1997) 63(3):263-264.

Imai J et al., Antioxidant and radical scavenging effects of aged garlic extracts and its constituents. PM (1994) 60(5):417.

Isaacsohn JL, MoserM, Stein EA et al., Garlic powder and plasma lipids and lipoproteins: a multicenter, randomized, placebo-controlled trial. Arch Intern Med 1998 Jun 8;158(11):1189-94.

Jain AK, Vargas R, Gotzkowsky S, McMahon FG, Can garlic reduce levels of serum lipids? A controlled clinical study. Am J Med (1993) 94:632-635.

Jain RC, Vyas CR, (1974) Brit Med J 2:730.

Jung EM, Jung F, Mrowietz C et al., Influence of garlic powder on cutaneous microcirculation. A randomized placebo-controlled double blind cross-over study in apparently healthy subjects. Arzneimittelforschung 1991 Jun;41(6):626-30.

Jung F, Kiesewetter H, Mrowietz C, Pindur G, Heiden M, Miyashita C, Wenzel E, (1989) Akutwirkungen eines zusammengesetzten Knoblauchpräparates auf die Fließfähigkeit des Blutes. ZPT 10(3):87.

Kabelik J, (1970) Pharmazie 25:266.

Kiesewetter H, Jung F, Pindur G et al., Effect of garlic on thrombocyte aggregation, microcirculation, and other risk factors. Int J Clin Pharmacol Ther Toxicol 1991 Apr;29(4):151-5.

Koch HP, Der lange Weg zum ''geruchlosen Knoblauch.'' PUZ (1996) 25(4):186-191.

Koch HP, Epidemiologie der Knoblauchforschung. DAZ (1992)132(40):2103.

Koch HP, Hormonwirkungen bei Allium-Arten. ZPT (1992)13(6):177.

Koch HP, Metabolismus und Pharmakokinetik der Inhatsstoffe des Knoblauchs. Was wissen wir darüber? ZPT (1992) 13(3):83.

Koch HP, Saponine in Knoblauch und Küchenzwiebel. In: DAZ 133(41):3733. 1993.

Koch HP, Wie ''sicher'' ist Knoblauch? Toxische, allergische und andere unerwünschte Nebenwirkungen. DAZ (1992) 132(27):1419.

Koch B, In: Koch HP, Lawson LD: Garlic - The Science and Therapeutic Application of Allium sativum L. and Related Species, Williams & Wilkins, Baltimore. 1996.

Kubitschek J, Knoblauch blockiert Cholesterolsynthese in der Leber. ZPT (1995) 16(2):74, s. auch (3):146.

Lawson LD, Wang ZJ, Pre-hepatic fate of the organosulfur compounds derived from garlic (Allium sativum). PM (1993) 59(7)88.

Lee TY, Lam TH, Contact dermatitis due to topical treatment with garlic in Hong Kong. Contact Dermatitis 1991 Mar;24(3):193-6.

Legnani C, Frascaro M, Guazzaloca G et al., Effects of a dried garlic preparation on fibrinolysis and platelet aggregation in healthy subjects. Arzneimittelforschung 1993 Feb;43(2):119-22.

Lybarger JA, Gallagher JS, Pulver DW et al., Occupational asthma induced by inhalation and ingestion of garlic. J Allergy Clin Immunol 1982 May;69(5):448-54.

Mader FH, Treatment of hyperlipidemia with garlic-powder tablets. Evidence from the German Association of General Practitioners' multicenter placebo-controlled double-blind study. Arzneimittelforschung 1990 Oct;40(10):1111-6.

Mütsch-Eckner M, Erdelmeier CAJ, Sticher O, A novel amino acid glycoside and three amino acids from Allium sativum. JNP (1993) 56(6):864.

Nagae S et al., Pharmacokinetics of the garlic compound S-allylcystein. PM (1994) 60(3):241.

Newall CA, Anderson LA, Philpson JD, Herbal Medicine: A Guide for Healthcare Professionals. London, UK: The Pharmaceutical Press, 1996.

Parish RA, McIntire S, Heimbach DM, Garlic burns: a naturopathic remedy gone awry. Pediatr Emerg Care 1987 Dec;3(4):258-60.

Reuter HD, 6. Kongreß der Gesellschaft für Phytotherapie:Satelliten-Symposium ''International Garlic Research''. ZPT (1996) 17(1):13-25.

Reuter HD, Chemie, Pharmakologie und medizinische Anwendung von Knoblauch. ZPT (1989) 10(4):124.

Reuter HD, II. Internationales Knoblauch-Symposium. ZPT (1991)12(3):83.

Robbers JE, Speedie MK, Tyler VE, Pharmacognosy and Pharmacobiotechnology. Baltimore, MD: Williams & Wilkins, 1996.

Roberge RJ, Leckey R, Spence R, Krenzelok EJ, Garlic burns of the breast. Am J Emerg Med 1997 Sep;15(5):548.

Rose KD, Croissant PD, Parliament CF, Levin MB. Spontaneous spinal epidural hematoma with associated platelet dysfunction from excessive garlic consumption: a case report. Neurosurgery 1990;26:880-82.

Schiewe FP, Hein T, Knoblauch bei Hyperlipidämie. ZPT (1995)16(6):343-348.

Schoetan A et al., (1984) Experientia 40(3):261.

See, D, Gurnee K, LeClair, M, An in vitro screening study of 196 natural products for toxicity and efficacy. JANA 1999 Winter;2(1):25-39.

Sendl A, Phytotherapie: Bärlauch und Knoblauch im Vergleich. DAZ (1993)133(5):392.

Siegers CP, Neues zur arteriosklerotischen Wirkung des Knoblauchs. ZPT (1993)14(1):21.

Simons LA, Balasubramaniam S, von Konigsmark M et al., On the effect of garlic on plasma lipids and lipoproteins in mild hypercholesterolemia. Atherosclerosis 1995 Mar;113(2):219-25.

Walper A et al., Effizienz einer Diätempfehlung und einer zusätzlichen Phytotherapie mit Allium sativum bei leichter bis mäβiger Hypercholesterinämie. Medwelt (1994) 45(7/8):327.

Wenkert E et al., (1971) Experientia 28:377.

Whitaker JR, (1976) Adv Food Res 22:73.

Wichtl M, Pflanzliche Pille für die ewige Jugend. DAZ (1991)131(17):837.

Further information in:

Chan H, But P, Pharmacology and Applications of Chinese Materia Medica Vol 1, World Scientific, Singapore 1986.

Frohne D, Pfänder HJ, Giftpflanzen - Ein Handbuch für Apotheker, Toxikologen und Biologen, 4. Aufl., Wiss. Verlags-Ges Stuttgart 1997.

Hänsel R, Keller K, Rimpler H, Schneider G (Hrsg.), Hagers Handbuch der Pharmazeutischen Praxis, 5. Aufl., Bde 4-6 (Drogen), Springer Verlag Berlin, Heidelberg, New York, 1992-1994.

Hausen BM, Allergiepflanzen - Pflanzenallergene, Ecomed Fachverlag Landsberg Lech 1988.

Madaus G, Lehrbuch der Biologischen Arzneimittel, Bde 1-3, Nachdruck, Georg Olms Verlag Hildesheim 1979.

Schulz R, Hänsel R, Rationale Phytotherapie, Springer Verlag Heidelberg 1996.

Steinegger E, Hänsel R, Pharmakognosie, 5. Aufl., Springer Verlag Heidelberg 1992.

Tang W, Eisenbrand G, Chinese Drugs of Plant Origin, Springer Verlag Heidelberg 1992.

Teuscher E, Biogene Arzneimittel, 5. Aufl., Wiss. Verlagsges. Stuttgart 1997.

Wagner H, Wiesenauer M, Phytotherapie. Phytopharmaka und pflanzliche Homöopathika, Fischer-Verlag, Stuttgart, Jena, New York 1995.

Gaultheria procumbens

See Wintergreen

Gelidium amansii

See Agar

Gelsemium sempervirens

See Yellow Jessamine

Genista tinctoria

See Dyer's Broom

Gentiana lutea

See Yellow Gentian

Geranium maculatum

See Cranesbill

Geranium robertianum

See Herb Robert

German Chamomile

Matricaria Recutita

TRADE NAMES

Chamomile Flowers (available from numerous manufacturers), Standardized Chamomile Extract, Wild Chamomile, Kid Chamomile

DESCRIPTION

Medicinal Parts: The medicinal parts consist of the entire flowering herb or only the flowers.

Flower and Fruit: The flower heads are terminal and long-pedicled. The flower is white with a yellow center. The margin flowers are obtuse with a tunicate margin. The ray florets are white, linguiform, female and 3-toothed. The disc florets are tubular, androgynous, 5-toothed, with a hollow receptacle.

Leaves, Stem and Root: The plant is a 20 to 40 cm high herb with an erect, glabrous stem, which is branched above. The leaves are 2 to 3 pinnatisect and have a narrow thorny tip.

Characteristic: The receptacle of the compound head of German Chamomile is hollow which distinguishes it from other types of chamomile.

Habitat: German Chamomile is indigenous to Europe and northwest Asia, naturalized in North America and elsewhere.

Production: German Chamomile consists of the fresh or dried flower heads of Matricaria recutita and their preparations.

Other Names: Pin Heads, Chamomilla, Chamomile, Single Chamomile, Hungarian Chamomile

ACTIONS AND PHARMACOLOGY

COMPOUNDS

Volatile oil (0.4-1.5%): chief components (-)-alpha-bisabolol (levomenol), bisabolol oxide A, bisabolol oxide B, bisabololone oxide A, beta-trans-farnesene, trans-en-yne-dicycloether (polyyne spiroether, adjoining cis-en-yn-dicycloether), chamazulene (blue in color, arising from the non-volatile proazulene matricin after steam distillation), spathulenol

Flavonoids: flavone glycosides; aglycones apigenin, luteolin, chrysoeriol, chief glycosides apigenin-7-O-glucoside, apigenin glucoside acetate, - flavonol glycosides, aglycones including quercetin, isorhamnetin, patuletin, for example rutin, hyperoside

Unbound, Highly Methoxylized Flavonoids: jaceidinem chrysospenol, chrysosplenetin

Hydroxycoumarins: including umbelliferone, herniarin

Mucilages: (10% in the mucilage ribs, fructans) including rhamanogalacturonane

EFFECTS

Gastrointestinal Effects

The proteolytic activity of pepsin is reduced by (-)-alpha-bisabolol in the gastrointestinal tract (Isaac, 1975). The (-)-alpha-bisabolol exerts a protective effect from gastric toxicity produced by acetylsalicylic acid (Torrado, 1995).

Anti-Inflammatory Effects

Chamazulene exerts anti-inflammatory effects through inhibition of leukotriene B4 formation (Safayhi, 1994). The en-yne dicycloether inhibits degranulation of mast cells to prevent histamine release (Miller, 1996). Apigenin, a flavonoid, effectively blocks intercellular adhesion molecule-1 upregulation and leukocyte adhesion in response to cytokines. This activity is through a mechanism unrelated to free radical scavenging or leukocyte formation (Panes, 1996).

Antioxidant Effects

Chamazulene, a volatile oil, exerts antioxidant effects through inhibition of lipid peroxidation (Rekka, 1996). Chamazulene also blocks chemical peroxidation of arachidonic acid for antioxidant and anti-inflammatory effects (Safayhi, 1994).

Antineoplastic Effects

Apigenin applied topically has effects on skin tumorigenesis through inhibition of skin papillomas and a tendency to decrease the conversion of papillomas to carcinomas (Li, 1996; Wei, 1990). Apigenin inhibits UV-induced tumorigenesis when applied topically via G2/M and G1 cell-cycle arrest in keratinocytes (Lepley, 1996; Lepley, 1997). The chemoprevention mechanisms occur through inhibition of the mitotic kinase activity, perturbation of cyclin B1 levels, and inhibition of protein kinase C (Lepley, 1996; Lin, 1997). Apigenin suppresses transcriptional activation of cyclooxygenase-2 and inducible nitric oxide synthase in macrophages, which is important for the prevention of carcinogenesis and inflammation (Liang, 1999).

Anxiolytic Effects

Flavonoids are CNS-active molecules and the chemical modification of the flavone nucleus dramatically increases the anxiolytic potency (Paladini, 1999). Apigenin is a ligand for the central benzodiazepine receptors exerting anxiolytic and slight sedative effects (Viola, 1995).

Miscellaneous Effects

Apigenin has been associated with an increase in atrial rate as a result of a reduction in noradrenaline uptake and a reduction in monoamine oxidase activity (Lorenzo, 1996). The herb exerts antibacterial and drying effects on weeping wound areas, which increase healing (Glowania, 1987). Chamomile oil has antimicrobial activity against some skin pathogens such as *Staphylococcus* and *Candida* species (Aggag, 1972).

CLINICAL TRIALS

A Phase III, double-blind, placebo-controlled trial evaluated chamomile mouthwash for prevention of 5-fluorouracil(5-FU) chemotherapy induced oral mucositis. There were 164 patients included in the study at the time of their fist cycle of 5-FU based chemotherapy, All patients received oral cryotherapy for 30 minutes with each dose of 5-FU. Chamomile mouthwash was administered three times daily for 14 days in the treatment group. Stomatitis scores determined by health care providers and by patients suggested no difference of stomatitis between the chamomile and placebo-treatment group (Fidler, 1996).

The efficacy of Kamillosan cream (topical chamomile cream) was compared to steroidal (0.25% hydrocortisone, 0.75% fluocortin butyl ester) and non-steroidal (5% bufexamac) deramatologic agents for the maintenance therapy of eczematous disease. There were 161 patients suffering from inflammatory dermatoses on hands, forearms, and lower legs included in the study. The patients had initially been treated with 0.1% difluocortolone valerate. The Kamillosan cream was slightly less effective as 0.25% hydrocortisone and superior to 5% bufexamac and 0.75% fluocortin butyl ester (Aertgeerts, 1985).

INDICATIONS AND USAGE

Approved by Commission E:

- Cough/bronchitis
- Fevers and colds
- Inflammation of the skin
- Inflammation of the mouth and pharynx
- Tendency to infection
- Wounds and burns

Chamomile is used internally for inflammatory diseases of the gastrointestinal tract associated with gastrointestinal spasms, irritation of the oral pharygeal mucous membrane and upper respiratory tract. Externally, the drug is used for skin and mucous membrane inflammations, pulpitis, gingivitis, respiratory catarrh, and ano-genital inflammation.

Unproven Uses: In Folk medicine, the herb is used internally for diarrhea and flatulence. The herb is used externally for furuncles, hemorrhoids, abscesses, and acne.

Homeopathic Uses: The herb is used for inflammation and cramps in the gastrointestinal tract, teething symptoms, severe pain, inflammation of the upper respiratory tract, and dysmenorrhea.

CONTRAINDICATIONS

Chamomile should not be taken by anyone with a known allergy to its components or other members of the Compositae family (eg, arnica, yarrow, feverfew, tansy, artemesia) (Hausen, 1996). A case report indicates chamomile may precipitate severe anaphylactic reactions in patients with hay fever and bronchial asthma caused by a variety of pollens (grass, olive, and mugwort) (Subiza, 1989).

PRECAUTIONS AND ADVERSE REACTIONS

Anaphylactic Reactions: Ingestion of chamomile-tea infusion has precipitated an anaphylactic reaction in an 8 year old male with hay fever and broncial asthma caused by a variety of pollens (Subiza, 1989).

Contact Dermatitis: Chamomile, a Compositae plant, is associated with allergic contact dermatitis (Hausen, 1996; Pereira, 1997; Rodriguez-Serna, 1998).

Allergic Conjunctivitis: Chamomile tea eye washing to treat ocular reactions has induced allergic conjunctivitis with lid angioedema (Subiza, 1990).

Drug Interactions:

Coumarin Anticoagulants — Due to the content of hydroxycoumarins in chamomile, there may be an additive effect when taken with warfarin.

Alcohol/Benzodiazepines — Chamomile has week anxiolytic properties at benzodiazepine receptor sites, thus concomitant use of alcohol and benzodiazepines should be avoided.

DOSAGE

Mode of Administration: Liquid and solid preparations are available for external and internal application.

How Supplied:

Capsule — 125 mg, 350 mg, 354 mg

Liquid — 1:4

Oil — 100%

Preparation: An infusion for internal use is prepared by pouring boiling water (150 ml) over 3 gm of chamomile, cover for 5 to 10 minutes and strain. (1 teaspoonful = 1 gm drug).

An infusion for external poultice application is prepared by pouring one and one-half cups of hot water over 2 dessertspoons of the drug, cover, leave to draw for 15 minutes and then strain. Ointments and gels are available in strengths of 3 to 10%.

Daily Dosage: An internal single dose is approximately 3 gm as an infusion. Liquid extract 1-4 ml or 1 cup of freshly made tea is administered 3-4 times daily. Externally as a bath additive, 50 gm is added to 1 Liter of water or 6 gm of drug for a steam bath. Washes and gargles may be administered several times a day.

Homeopathic Dosage: Internally, the herb is given as 5-10 drops, 1 tablet, or 5-10 globules. Externally, dilute 1 dessertspoon with 250 ml water and use 2-3 times daily in poutices or washes (HAB1).

LITERATURE

Achterrath-Tuckerman U et al., (1980) Planta Med 39(1):38.

Aertgeerts P, Albring M, Klaschka F, Nasemann T, Patzelt-Wenczler R, Rauhut K, Weigl B, (1985) Vergleichende Prüfung von Kamillosan(Creme gegenüber steroidalen (0,25 % Hydrocortison, 0,75 % Bluocortinbutylester) und nichtsteroidalen

(5 % Bufexamac) Externa in der Erhaltungstherapie von Ekzemerkrankungen. Z Hautkr 60:270-277.

Aggag M, Yousef R. Study of antimicrobial activity of chamomile oil. Planta Med 1972 Sep;22(2):140-4.

Albring M, Albrecht H, Alcorn G, Lücker PW, (1983) The measuring of the anti-inflammatory effect of a compound of the skin of volunteers. Meth Find Exp Clin Pharmacol 5:75-77.

Ammon HPT, Kaul R, (1992) Pharmakologie der Kamille und ihrer Inhaltsstoffe. Dtsch Apoth Z 132(SuppI 27):3-26.

Dorsch W, Neues über antientzündliche Drogen. In: ZPT 14(1):26. 1993.

Fidler R, Loprinzi C, O'Fallon J et al. Prospective evaluation of a chamomile mouthwash for prevention of 5-FU-induced oral mucositis. Cancer 1996 Feb 1;77(3):522-5.

Füller E et al., Anti-inflammatory activity of Chamomilla polysaccharides. In: PM 59(7)66. 1993.

Füller E, Franz G, Neues von den Kamillenpolysacchariden. In: DAZ 133(45):4224. 1993.

Gasic O et al., (1983) Fitoterapia 2:51.

Glowania HJ; Raulin C; Swoboda M. Effect of chamomile on wound healing—a clinical double-blind study. Z Hautkr 1987 Sep 1;62(17):1262, 1267-71.

Habersang S, (1979) Planta Med 37(2):115.

Hausen HM, Busker E, Carle R, (1984) Über das Sensibilierungsvermögen von Compositenarten. VII. Experimentelle Untersuchungen mit Auszügen und Inhaltsstoffen von Chamomilla recutita L. Rauschert und Anthemis cotula L. Planta Med 50:229-234.

Heilmann J, Kamillenflavonoide: Nur Aglyka dringen in die Haut ein. In: DAZ 133(37):3296. 1993.

Isaac D, (1980) Die Kamillentherapie - Erfolg und Bestätigung. Dtsch Apoth Ztg 120:567-570.

Isaac O, (1979) Planta Med 35(2):3, 118.

Isaac O; Thiemer K. Biochemical studies on camomile components/III. In vitro studies about the antipeptic activity of (-)-alpha-bisabolol. Arzneimittelforschung 1975 Sep;25(9):1352-4.

Jakovlev V et al., (1979) Planta Med 35(2):3.

Jakovlev V et al., (1983) Planta Med 49(2):67.

Jakovlev V, Isaac O, Flaskamp E, (1983) Pharmakologische Untersuchungen von Kamillen-Inhaltsstoffen. VI. Untersuchungen zur antiphlogistischen Wirkung von Chamazulen und Matricin. Planta Med 49:67-73.

Jakovlev V, Isaac O, Flaskamp E, Pharmakologische Untersuchungen von Kamilleninhaltsstoffen VI. Untersuchungen zur antiphlogistischen Wirkung von Chamazulen und Matricin. In: PM 49:67. 1983.

Jenss H, (1985) Zur Problematik funktioneller Magen-Darm-Krankheiten am Beispiel des Colon irritabile. In: Oepen I (Hrsg) An den Grenzen der Schulmedizin, eine Analyse umstrittener Methoden. Deutscher Ärzte-Verlag Köln, S 197-212.

Lepley DM; Pelling JC. Induction of p21/WAF1 and G1 cell-cycle arrest by the chemopreventive agent apigenin. Mol Carcinog 1997 Jun;19(2):74-82.

Lepley DM; Li B; Birt DF; Pelling JC. The chemopreventive flavonoid apigenin induces G2/M arrest in keratinocytes. Carcinogenesis 1996 Nov;17(11):2367-75.

Li B; Pinch H; Birt DF. Influence of vehicle, distant topical delivery, and biotransformation on the chemopreventive activity of apigenin, a plant flavonoid, in mouse skin. Pharm Res 1996 Oct;13(10):1530-4.

Liang YC; Huang YT; Tsai SH et al. Suppression of inducible cyclooxygenase and inducible nitric oxide synthase by apigenin and related flavonoids in mouse macrophages. Carcinogenesis 1999 Oct;20(10):1945-52.

Lin JK; Chen YC; Huang YT; Lin-Shiau SY. Suppression of protein kinase C and nuclear oncogene expression as possible molecular mechanisms of cancer chemoprevention by apigenin and curcumin. J Cell Biochem Suppl 1997;28-29:39-48.

Lorenzo PS; Rubio MC; Medina JH; Adler-Graschinsky E. Involvement of monoamine oxidase and noradrenaline uptake in the positive chronotropic effects of apigenin in rat atria. Eur J Pharmacol 1996 Sep 26;312(2):203-7.

Maiche AG, Gröhn P, Mäki-Hokkonen H, (1991) Effect of chamomile cream and almond ointment of acute radiation skin reaction. Acta Oncol 30:395-396.

Miller Th, Wittstock U, Lindequist U, Teuscher E, Effects of some components of the essential oil of chamomile, Chamomilla recutita, on histamine release from mast cells. Planta Med 1996 Feb;62(1):60-61.

Nissen HP, Blitz H, Kreysel HW, (1988) Profilometrie, eine Methode zur Beurteilung der therapeutischen Wirksamkeit von Kamillosan-Salbe. Z Hautkr 63:184-190.

Paladini AC; Marder M; Viola H et al. Flavonoids and the central nervous system: from forgotten factors to potent anxiolytic compounds. J Pharm Pharmacol 1999 May;51(5):519-2.

Panes J; Gerritsen ME; Anderson DC et al. Apigenin inhibits tumor necrosis factor-induced intercellular adhesion molecule-1 upregulation in vivo. Microcirculation 1996 Sep;3(3):279-86.

Pereira F; Santos R; Pereira A. Contact dermatitis from chamomile tea. Contact Dermatitis 1997 Jun;36(6):307.

Rekka EA; Kourounakis AP; Kourounakis PN. Investigation of the effect of chamazulene on lipid peroxidation and free radical processes. Res Commun Mol Pathol Pharmacol 1996 Jun;92(3):361-4.

Redaelli C et al., (1981) J Chrom. 209:110.

Redaelli C et al., (1981) Plant Med 42:288.

Rodriguez-Serna M; Sanchez-Motilla JM; Ramon R; Aliaga A. Allergic and systemic contact dermatitis from Matricaria chamomilla tea.Contact Dermatitis 1998 Oct;39(4):192-3.

Safayhi H et al., Chamazulene: an antioxidant-type inhibitor of leukotriene B4 formation. In: PM 60(5):410. 1994.

Schilcher H, (1987) Die Kamille. Handbuch für Ärzte, Apotheker und andere Naturwissenschaftler. Wissenschaftliche Verlagsgesellschaft, Stuttgart Ammon HPT, Sabieraj J, Kaul R, Kamille - Mechanismus der antiphlogistischen Wirkung von Kamillenextrakten und -inhaltsstoffen. In: DAZ 136(22):1821-1834. 1996.

Sorkin B, Untersuchungen zur Wirksamkeit von Kamille am Menschen. In: Seifen, Öle, Fette, Wachse 108(1):9-10. 1982.

Subiza J; Subiza JL; Hinojosa M et al. Anaphylactic reaction after the ingestion of chamomile tea: a study of cross-reactivity with other composite pollens. J Allergy Clin Immunol 1989 Sep;84(3):353-8.

Subiza J, Subiza JL, Alonso M et al. Allergic conjunctivitis to chamomile tea. Ann Allergy 1990 Aug;65(2):127-32.

Szelenyi I et al., (1979) Planta Med 35(3):218.

Torrado S; Torrado S; Agis A et al. Effect of dissolution profile and (-)-alpha-bisabolol on the gastrotoxicity of acetylsalicylic acid. Pharmazie 1995 Feb;50(2):141-3.

Vilagines P et al., (1985) C R Acad Sci (III)301(6):289.

Viola H; Wasowski C; Levi de Stein M et al. Apigenin, a component of Matricaria recutita flowers, is a central benzodiazepine receptors-ligand with anxiolytic effects. Planta Med 1995 Jun;61(3):213-6.

Wei H, Tye L, Bresnick E, Birt D. Inhibitory effect of apigenin, a plant flavonoid, on epidermal ornithine decarboxylase and skin tumor promotion in mice. Cancer Res 1990 Feb 1;50(3):499-502.

Further information in:

Hänsel R, Keller K, Rimpler H, Schneider G (Hrsg.), Hagers Handbuch der Pharmazeutischen Praxis, 5. Aufl., Bde 4-6 (Drogen), Springer Verlag Berlin, Heidelberg, New York, 1992-1994 (unter Chamomilla recutita).

Hausen B, Allergiepflanzen, Pflanzenallergene, ecomed Verlagsgesellsch. mbH, Landsberg 1988 (unter Chamomilla recutita).

Leung AY, Encyclopedia of Common Natural Ingredients Used in Food, Drugs and Cosmetics, John Wiley & Sons Inc., New York 1980.

Madaus G, Lehrbuch der Biologischen Arzneimittel, Bde 1-3, Nachdruck, Georg Olms Verlag Hildesheim 1979.

Schulz R, Hänsel R, Rationale Phytotherapie, Springer Verlag Heidelberg 1996.

Steinegger E, Hänsel R, Pharmakognosie, 5. Aufl., Springer Verlag Heidelberg 1992.

Teuscher E, Biogene Arzneimittel, 5. Aufl., Wiss. Verlagsges. Stuttgart 1997.

Wagner H, Wiesenauer M, Phytotherapie. Phytopharmaka und pflanzliche Homöopathika, Fischer-Verlag, Stuttgart, Jena, New York 1995.

Wichtl M (Hrsg.), Teedrogen, 4. Aufl., Wiss. Verlagsges. Stuttgart 1997.

German Ipecac

Cynanchum vincetoxicum

DESCRIPTION

Medicinal Parts: The medicinal parts of the plant are the leaves or rhizome with the attached roots.

Flower and Fruit: The plant has small white flowers in peduncled cymes, 5 sepals and a wheel-shaped corolla. There is a 5-lobed secondary corolla. There are 5 stamens whose anthers are fused to a 5-sectioned wreath. The 2 superior ovaries have a common stigma. The fruit is a 5 cm long, glabrous, striped, clavate follicle. The seeds have silky tufts of hair.

Leaves, Stem and Root: The plant grows from 30 to 100 cm. The underground creeping rhizome has heavily branched runners. The stem is unbranched, thin and erect. The leaves are opposite, short petioled, ovate to oblong and entire-margined.

Characteristics: The fresh rhizome has an intensive odor. The taste is sweet, then bitter-hot. It is poisonous.

Habitat: The plant is indigenous to Europe.

Production: German Ipecac herb and rhizome are the leaves and rhizome (including attached roots) of Cynanchum vincetoxicum. The subterranean rhizome, including parts of the roots, are dug up in autumn, cleaned and quickly dried at temperatures of up to 50° C.

ACTIONS AND PHARMACOLOGY

COMPOUNDS

Saponin-like 15-oxasteroide glycosides (mixture termed vincetoxin): aglycones including hirundigenin, anhydrohirundigenin, vincetogenin

Isoquinoline alkaloids: including tylophorine

EFFECTS

The drug has diuretic, diaphoretic, digestive and emmenagogic effects. The alkaloids have an antitumoral effect, and the chloroform extract has an antimicrobial effect.

INDICATIONS AND USAGE

Unproven Uses: The drug was formerly used as a diuretic, diaphoretic and emetic, and for the treatment of kidney complaints, edema, the plague, snake bite and dysmenorrhea. Today, it is used in the treatment of digestive and kidney disorders and for dysmenorrhea. The poultices heal swellings and bruising. The drug can also be found in homeopathic preparations.

PRECAUTIONS AND ADVERSE REACTIONS

According to older scientific literature, "vincetoxin" in high dosages causes vomiting, apnea and cardiac paralysis in animal experiments. Seed extracts led to advancing paralysis of the central nervous system. Poisonings of humans have not been found in recent reports.

DOSAGE

Mode of Administration: As an infusion, powdered drug, alcoholic extract and homeopathic dilution.

Preparation: The drug is prepared as an infusion.

Daily Dosage: The infusion should be administered under medical supervision.

LITERATURE

Frohne D, Pfänder HJ, Giftpflanzen - Ein Handbuch für Apotheker, Toxikologen und Biologen, 4. Aufl., Wiss. Verlagsges. mbH Stuttgart 1997.

Hänsel R, Keller K, Rimpler H, Schneider G (Hrsg.), Hagers Handbuch der Pharmazeutischen Praxis, 5. Aufl., Bde 4-6 (Drogen), Springer Verlag Berlin, Heidelberg, New York, 1992-1994.

Kennard O et al., Tetrahedron Letters 3799-3804. 1968.

Lewin L, Gifte und Vergiftungen, 6. Aufl., Nachdruck, Haug Verlag, Heidelberg 1992.

Madaus G, Lehrbuch der Biologischen Arzneimittel, Bde 1-3, Nachdruck, Georg Olms Verlag Hildesheim 1979.

Roth L, Daunderer M, Kormann K, Giftpflanzen, Pflanzengifte, 4. Aufl., Ecomed Fachverlag Landsberg Lech 1993.

Steinegger E, Hänsel R, Pharmakognosie, 5. Aufl., Springer Verlag Heidelberg 1992.

Teuscher E, Lindequist U, Biogene Gifte - Biologie, Chemie, Pharmakologie, 2. Aufl., Fischer Verlag Stuttgart 1994.

German Sarsaparilla

Carex arenaria

DESCRIPTION

Medicinal Parts: The medicinal part is the dried rhizome.

Flower and Fruit: The inflorescence is somewhat hanging and consists of 6 to 16 ovoid, 1 cm long, terminal, straight, greenish spikes. The lower ones are female; the middle ones are female at the base and male at the tip. The upper ones are only male. These are simple greenish unisexual flowers without a corolla. They have 1 husk with an ovary surrounded by a tubular-like involucre. The style has 2 stigmas, 3 stamens and a fruit oval. It is somewhat acute at both ends, and the tube has a winged edge. The flowers form many blossomed spikelets, which in turn form a terminal, oblong ear. The middle spikelets contain male flowers at the tip and female flowers at the base. The upper spikelets are male.

Leaves, Stem and Root: German Sarsaparilla is a 15 to 45 cm high plant with a 2 to 5 mm thick, horizontally creeping rhizome, which produces extremely long runners. The plant has black-brown basal leaves, which break up into long fibers. The stem is sturdy, upright and about 1 mm thick. It is sharply triangular, rough above, and surrounded by brown leaf sheaths at the base. The leaves are linear and usually grooved. The lamina are rigid and gradually tapering forward to the involute tip. The roots form such a thick mass that they prevent water from getting in and thus prevent the washing away of dykes and dams.

Characteristics: The rootstock has an aromatic-turpentine odor.

Habitat: The plant grows in Europe mainly on the Atlantic, Baltic and southern Scandinavian coasts as far as central Germany. It was introduced to the American Atlantic coast.

Production: German Sarsaparilla consists of the dried, underground parts of Carex arenaria. The root is dug up in March and April, dried and cut into pieces for sale.

Not to be Confused With: Other Carex varieties

Other Names: Red Sedge, Sand Sedge, Red Couchgrass, Sea Sedge

ACTIONS AND PHARMACOLOGY

COMPOUNDS

Saponins

Volatile oil: contents include methyl salicylate and cineol

Flavonoids: including tricine

Tannin: (8 to 10%, catechin tannins)

EFFECTS

There are no studies available on efficacy. The main constituents, saponins, essential oil and flavones, as well as the tannins, are most likely responsible for the effect.

INDICATIONS AND USAGE

Unproven Uses: There are no documented indications to date. In folk medicine, preparations of German Sarsaparilla are used for the prevention of gout, rheumatism, inflammation of the joints, for skin ailments and as a diaphoretic and diuretic; further, for venereal disease, flatulence, colic, liver disorders, diabetes, edema, lung tuberculosis and amenorrhea.

PRECAUTIONS AND ADVERSE REACTIONS

No health hazards or side effects are known in conjunction with the proper administration of designated therapeutic dosages.

DOSAGE

Mode of Administration: Since the efficacy for the claimed uses are not documented, a therapeutic application cannot be recommended. The cold maceration and the decoction are used in folk medicine.

Preparation: A decoction is prepared by adding 3 gm drug to 1 cup water. A cold maceration is made by adding 2 teaspoonfuls drug to 1/4 liter water.

Daily Dosage: The average daily dose is 3 gm drug as a decoction. The cold maceration is dosed 1 cup, 2 to 3 times daily.

LITERATURE

Hänsel R, Keller K, Rimpler H, Schneider G (Hrsg.), Hagers Handbuch der Pharmazeutischen Praxis, 5. Aufl., Bde 4-6 (Drogen), Springer Verlag Berlin, Heidelberg, New York, 1992-1994.

Madaus G, Lehrbuch der Biologischen Arzneimittel, Bde 1-3, Nachdruck, Georg Olms Verlag Hildesheim 1979.

Germander

Teucrium chamaedrys

DESCRIPTION

Medicinal Parts: The medicinal part is the herb collected during the flowering season.

Flower and Fruit: The flowers are 10 to 12 mm long and are erect. They are arranged on long pedicles in 1-to-6 blossomed, false racemes inclined to one side. The calyx is tubular-campanulate, often tinged with red-violet and is pubescent. The corolla is usually carmine red, occasionally white. The stamens and styles are exserted. The nutlet is ovoid, 1.5 to 2 cm long, smooth, finely reticulate and has a large, circular, attaching surface.

Leaves, Stem and Root: The plant is a subshrub with a short-lived main root from which grow long-reaching, branched, thin woody roots and a stem-producing runner. The stems are usually erect and branched. The older branches are decumbent; the younger ones erect, tough, round and lanate. The branches are occasionally covered in glandular hairs, which are often red-violet. The leaves are in close pairs and are always covered in teeth. They are summer-green and have distinctly protruding pinnatifid ribs.

Habitat: The plant is indigenous to the Mediterranean region as far as Anatolia and the Urals.

Production: Germander is the aerial part of Teucrium chamaedrys.

ACTIONS AND PHARMACOLOGY

COMPOUNDS

Volatile oil (0.07%): chief components beta-caryophyllene (20%), humulene (15%)

Iridoide monoterpenes: including among others, harpagide, acetyl harpagide

Diterpenes: including among others, teugin, teuflin, teuflidin, dihydroteugin, teucrin A, B, E, F, G, marrubiin

Caffeic acid derivatives: including among others, teucroside

Flavonoids: including among others, cirsiliol, cirsimaritin, luteolin

EFFECTS

The drug, which contains strong amaroids, is said to have a cholagogic effect, but this has not been scientifically proven. The toxic principle is therefore unknown. Higher doses or poisoning results in hepatitis-like symptoms, which may include liver cell necrosis.

INDICATIONS AND USAGE

Unproven Uses: Germander is used as a digestive aid, as a rinse for gout, as weight-loss aid and for fever.

CONTRAINDICATIONS

The drug is highly toxic and should not be used (see PRECAUTIONS).

PRECAUTIONS AND ADVERSE REACTIONS

Liver cell necrosis has been observed following intake of the drug. Symptoms include jaundice and an elevated level of aminotransferase in the blood. One case of death has been recorded. For that reason, the drug is not to be administered.

DOSAGE

Mode of Administration: Germander is occasionally used in tea mixtures (see PRECAUTIONS).

Daily Dosage: Dosages of more than 600 mg daily can cause toxic effects.

LITERATURE

Chialva F et al., J High Res Chromatogr Chromatogr Commun 5:182. 1982.

Fikenscher LH, Hegnauer R, Plant Med Phytother 3(3):183.

Malakov PY et al., PH 24:301-303. 1985.

Reinbold AM, Popa PD, (1974) Khim Prir Soedin. 589.

Rodriguez MC et al., (1984) Phytochemistry 23(7):1467.

Rodriguez MC et al., PH 23:2960-2961. 1984.

Rovesti P, (1957) Ind Perf. 12:334.

Savona G et al., PH 21:721-723. 1982.

Sticher O, Lahloub MF, (1982) Planta Med 30:124.

Further information in:

Frohne D, Pfänder HJ, Giftpflanzen - Ein Handbuch für Apotheker, Toxikologen und Biologen, 4. Aufl., Wiss. Verlags-Ges. Stuttgart 1997.

Hänsel R, Keller K, Rimpler H, Schneider G (Hrsg.), Hagers Handbuch der Pharmazeutischen Praxis, 5. Aufl., Bde 4-6 (Drogen): Springer Verlag Berlin, Heidelberg, New York, 1992-1994.

Geum rivale

See Water Avens

Geum urbanum

See Bennet's Root

Giant Milkweed

Calotropis gigantea

DESCRIPTION

Medicinal Parts: The medicinal parts of the plant are the bark and roots.

Flower and Fruit: The flowers are arranged in umbels. The flower structures are arranged in fives. The corolla is fused and campanulate, 3 to 5 cm wide and split up to two-thirds of the length. The lobes are greenish with purple tips. The paracorolla is composed of 5 cap-like points. The 5 stamens and the 2 styles are fused to a stemmed gynostegium and the pollen sticks together to form to a pollinium. The sepals are ovate and the ovary superior. The fruit is a swollen follicle, 9 to 10 cm long and turned back. The seeds have a silky tuft of hair.

Leaves, Stem and Root: Calotropis gigantea is a shrub, occasionally tree-like, which grows up to 3 m high. The leaves are sessile with the base clasping the stem, fleshy, 10 to 20 cm long and 4 to 10 cm wide, elongate-ovate or elliptical. The stem is woody.

Habitat: India, China, and Malaysian archipelago

Other Names: Giant Swallow Root, Swallow Wort, Crown Flower

ACTIONS AND PHARMACOLOGY

COMPOUNDS

Cardioactive steroid glycosides (cardenolids): calotropin, calactin and uscharidin

Steroids: sterols, including beta-sitosterol, taraxasterol

EFFECTS

The drug contains cardioactive cardenolide glycosides and exhibits an emetic-cathartic effect resembling that of Ipecacuanha. The calotropin demonstrates anti-tumor qualities against human epidermoid carcinoma cells of the nasopharynx, *in vitro.*

INDICATIONS AND USAGE

Unproven Uses: Giant Milkweed has been used for dysentery, vomiting, toothache, syphilis, convulsions, warts, leprosy and digestion problems.

Indian Medicine: Preparations are used for skin conditions, intestinal worms, coughs, ascites and anasarca.

Homeopathic Uses: Calotropis gigantea is used for obesity.

PRECAUTIONS AND ADVERSE REACTIONS

No health hazards are known in conjunction with the proper administration of designated therapeutic dosages.

OVERDOSAGE

Higher dosages cause severe mucous membrane irritation, characterized by vomiting and diarrhea, as well as bradycardia and convulsions, sometimes leading to death. It is not known whether those compounds found in the plant that belong chemically to the cardioactive steroid glycoside group are indeed cardioactive, because of their unusual structure (the sugar remnant is bound to the aglycone both as a glycoside and as an ether). Mucilaginous drinks are recommended to treat the symptoms of inflammation; morphine and atrophine for treating pain.

DOSAGE

Mode of Administration: Whole and cut drug preparations for internal use.

Daily Dosage: As an emetic: 2 to 4 gm; As a diaphoretic and expectorant: 200 to 600 mg.

Homeopathic Dosage: (from D4) 5 to 10 drops, 1 tablet, 5 to 10 globules, 1 to 3 times daily or from D6 1 ml injection solution sc. twice weekly (HAB1).

LITERATURE

Hänsel R, Keller K, Rimpler H, Schneider G (Ed), Hagers Handbuch der Pharmazeutischen Praxis, 5. Aufl., Bde 4 - 6 (Drogen), Springer Verlag Berlin, Heidelberg, New York, 1992-1994.

Kiuchi F, Fukao Y, Maruyama T, Obata T, Tanaka M, Sasaki T, Mikage M, Haque ME, Tsuda Y, Cytotoxic principles of a

Bangladeshi crude drug, akond mul (roots of Calotropis gigantea L.). Chem Pharm Bull (Tokyo), 46:528-30, 1998 Mar.

Sen S, Sahu NP, Mahato SB, Flavonol glycosides from Calotropis gigantea. Phytochemistry, 232:2919-21, 1992 Aug.

Sengupta A, Bhattacharya D, Pal G, Sinha NK, Comparative studies on calotropins DI and DII from the latex of Calotropis gigantea. Arch Biochem Biophys, 232:17-25, 1984 Jul.

Gillenia trifoliata

See Indian Physic

Ginger

Zingiber officinale

TRADE NAMES

Ginger Root (available from numerous manufacturers,) Ginger Kid, Alcohol Free Ginger Root, Ginger Power, Caffeine-Free Ginger Root, Quanterra Stomach Comfort

DESCRIPTION

Medicinal Parts: The medicinal part is the root.

Flower and Fruit: The flower scape grows directly from the root and terminates in a long, curved spike. A white or yellow flower grows from each spike.

Leaves, Stem and Root: Ginger is a creeping perennial on a thick tuberous rhizome, which spreads underground. In the first year, a green, erect, reed-like stem about 60 cm high grows from this rhizome. The plant has narrow, lanceolate to linear-lanceolate leaves 15 to 30 cm long, which die off each year.

Characteristics: The fracture is short and fibrous. The odor and taste are characteristic, aromatic and pungent.

Habitat: The plant is indigenous to southeastern Asia, and is cultivated in the U.S., India, China, the West Indies and tropical regions.

Production: Ginger root consists of the peeled, finger-long, fresh or dried rhizome of Zingiber officinale.

ACTIONS AND PHARMACOLOGY

COMPOUNDS

Volatile oil (2.5-3.0%): chief components vary greatly, depending upon country of origin: (-)-zingiberene and ar-curcumene, beta-bisabolene and ar-curcumene, neral and geranial, D-camphor, beta-phellandrene, geranial, neral and linalool, (E)-alpha-farnesene, important as aroma carrier zingiberol (mixture of cis- and trans-beta-eudesmol)

Aryl alkanes

Gingerols: chief components [6]-gingerol (pungent substances), [8]-gingerol, [10]-gingerol

Shogaols: chief components [6]-shogaol (pungent substane), [8]- shogaol, [10]- shogaol (artifacts formed during storage, arising from the gingerols)

Gingerdiols

Diarylheptanoids: including among others, gingerenone A and B

Starch (50%)

EFFECTS

Compounds isolated from the Ginger rhizome have been studied in numerous in vitro and animal experiments. Other studies show that Ginger root is positively inotropic, antithrombotic; has anti-oxidant, anti-migraine and anti-lipidemic effects, and promotes secretion of saliva, gastric juices and bile.

Anti-Emetic Effects

The components in Ginger that are responsible for the anti-emetic effect are thought to be the gingerols and shogaols.The mechanism of action is not due to a nystagmus response or vestibular stimulation (Holtmann, 1989). In contrast to most anti-emetic medications that act on the CNS, the anti-emetic effect of Ginger is thought to be due to local gastrointestinal actions (Mowrey & Clayton, 1982).

Anti-Inflammatory Effects

The anti-inflammatory effect of Ginger is thought to be due to inhibition of cyclooxygenase and 5-lipoxygenase, results in reduced leukotriene and prostaglandin synthesis (Kiuchi, 1992; Srivastava & Mustafa, 1992).

Miscellaneous Effects

In humans, Ginger increases the tone and peristalsis of the intestine (Bisset, 1994; Iwu, 1993). The root of Zingiber officinale has also shown immune system stimulation (Chang, 1995) and platelet aggregation inhibitory activity (Verma, 1993).

CLINICAL TRIALS

Motion Sickness

One double-blind, randomized, non-placebo controlled study compared the effectiveness of Ginger and six other commonly used non-herbal drugs (scopolamine, dimenhydrinate with caffeine, cyclizine, cinnarizine, cinnarizine with domperidone, meclizine with caffeine) in 1489 participants during whale-watching voyages off the coast of Norway. 78.3% of those that took 500 mg of Ginger root 2 hours prior to a boat trip were symptom-free for the 6-hour duration. The incidence of severe vomiting did not differ in a statistically significant way between Ginger and any of the other test groups (Schmid, 1994).

Postoperative Nausea and Vomiting

A double-blind, placebo-controlled study involving 120 females that underwent gynecologic outpatient surgery was performed. The participants were randomly given either 1 gm of powdered Ginger root or 10 mg of metoclopramide orally and evaluated for incidence of postoperative nausea and vomiting. Ten percent of the patients in the Ginger group had one or more episodes of vomiting. 17.5% of the metoclopramide arm and 22.5% of the placebo group had one or more episodes of vomiting. Fifteen percent of the Ginger group and 32.5% of the metoclopramide group required antiemetic treatment compared to 37.5% of the placebo group. The authors concluded that the Ginger group had a statistically significant lower incidence of nausea and vomiting when compared to placebo (Phillips, 1993).

INDICATIONS AND USAGE

Approved by Commission E:

- Loss of appetite
- Travel sickness
- Dyspeptic complaints

Unproven Uses: In folk medicine, Ginger is used as a carminative, expectorant, and astringent.

Chinese Medicine: In China, Ginger is used to treat colds, nausea, vomiting and shortness of breath.

Indian Medicine: Indian medicine uses include anorexia, dyspeptic symptoms and pharyngitis.

CONTRAINDICATIONS

The German Commission E contraindicates the use of Ginger in morning sickness associated with pregnancy. Most research provides evidence that Ginger can be used and is effective in the treatment of morning sickness. It is recommended that excessive doses are avoided for this purpose (see PRECAUTIONS and ADVERSE REACTIONS).

Because of its cholagogic effect, the drug should not be taken in the presence of gallstone conditions except after consultation with a physician.

Ginger has been found to inhibit thromboxane synthesis, therefore it should not be used by patients who are at risk for hemorrhage (Bracken, 1991)

PRECAUTIONS AND ADVERSE REACTIONS

General: No health hazards or side effects are known in conjunction with the proper administration of designated therapeutic dosages.

It has been reported that administration of 6 grams of dried powdered Ginger has been shown to increase the exfoliation of gastric surface epithelial cells in human subjects. It is postulated that this action may possibly lead to ulcer formation. Therefore, it is recommended that dosages on an empty stomach be limited to 6 grams (Desai, 1990).

There have been reports that Ginger can cause hypersensitivity reactions resulting in dermatitis. Large overdoses can cause central nervous system depression and cardiac arrhythmias.

Pregnancy: A study in 27 pregnant patients with hyperemesis gravidarum (persistent vomiting occurring prior to the 20th week of pregnancy and requiring hospitalization) found that 1 gram per day (250 milligrams 4 times a day) for 4 days caused no adverse effects. One spontaneous abortion occurred; a causal relationship between the abortion and the use of Ginger was not determined. All infants were normal (Fischer-Rasmussen, 1990).

Drug Interactions: More than one in-vitro study confirms an antithrombotic effect. It is recommeded that patients taking anticoagulants or those with bleeding disorders avoid the use of large doses of Ginger.

OVERDOSAGE

According to research, the LD50 of 6-gingerol and 6-shogaol is set between 250 and 680 mg/kg. (Fulder & Tenne, 1991; Suekawa et al, 1984.) Toxicity tests in mice using a Ginger extract via lavage resulted in no mortality or adverse effects in doses up to 2.5 g/kg over a 7 day period. When the dose was increased to between 3 and 3.5 g/kg, a 10% to 30% mortality rate was reported (Macola, 1989.)

Overdosage may cause cardiac arrhythmia and CNS depression (Iwu, 1993).

DOSAGE

Mode of Administration: Comminuted rhizome and dry extracts for teas and other galenic preparations for internal use. The powdered drug is used in some stomach preparations.

How Supplied:

Capsules — 100 mg, 400 mg, 420 mg, 460 mg, 470 mg, 500 mg, 550 mg, 1000 mg

Chewable Tablets — 67.5 mg

Fluid Extract — 1:1

Liquid — 1:4

Oil — 100%

Tea Bags

Preparation: To prepare an infusion, pour boiling water over 0.5 to 1 g drug and strain after 5 minutes (1 teaspoonful = 3 g drug).

Daily Dosage:

ANTI-EMESIS

Capsules/Powder — 0.5 to 2 grams (Bisset,1994; Schmid et al, 1994)

CHEMOTHERAPY-INDUCED NAUSEA AND VOMITING

All dosage forms — 1.5 grams (Myer et al, 1995).

DYSPEPSIA

Capsules/Powder — 2 to 4 grams/day

HYPEREMESIS GRAVIDARUM

Capsules/Powder — 1 gram/day given for 4 days (Fischer-Rasmussen et al, 1990).

MOTION SICKNESS

Capsules/Powder — 1 gram to be taken 30 minutes before travel; for continuing symptoms, 0.5 to 1 gram every 4 hours (Muller & Clauson, 1997).

POSTOPERATIVE NAUSEA AND VOMITING

Capsules/Powder — 0.5 to 2 gram daily

RHEUMATOID ARTHRITIS, OSTEOARTHRITIS

Powder — 1 to 2 grams/day (Srivastava & Mustafa, 1992).

Storage: Powdered Ginger root should be stored in a cool, dry place protected from light. Powdered Ginger should not be stored in plastic containers.

LITERATURE

Bisset NG (ed), Herbal Drugs and Phytopharmaceuticals; a Handbook for Practice on a Scientific Basis. Medpharm Scientific Publishers, Stuttgart and CRC Press, Boca Raton, 1994.

Bone ME, Wilkinson DJ, Young JR et al., Ginger root- a new antiemetic. The effect of ginger root on postoperative nausea and vomiting after major gynecological surgery. Anaesthesia 45:669-71. 1990.

Bracken J, Ginger as an antiemetic: possible side effects due to its thromboxane synthetase activity. Anaesthesia; 46:705-706. 1991.

Chang CP, Chang JY, Wang FY et al., The effect of Chinese medicinal herb Zingiberis rhizoma extract on cytokine secretion by human peripheral blood mononuclear cells. J Ethnopharmacol 48:13-19. 1995.

Chen CC, Ho CT, J Agric Food Chem 36:322. 1988.

Denyer CV, Jackson P, Loakes DM, Isolation of antirhinoviral sesquiterpenes from ginger (Zingiber officinale). In: JNP 57(5):658-662. 1994.

Desai HG, Kalro RH & Choksi AP, Effect of ginger & garlic on DNA content of gastric aspirate. Ind J Med Res 92:139-41, 1990.

Erler J et al., Z Lebensm Unters Forsch 186:231. 1988.

Fintelmann V, Phytopharmaka in der Gastroenterologie. In: ZPT 15(3):137. 1994.

Fischer-Rasmussen W, Kjaer S, Dahl C et al., Ginger treatment of hyperemesis gravidarum. Eur J Obstet Gynecol Reprod Biol 38:19-24. 1990.

Fulder S & Tenne M, Ginger as an anti-nausea remedy in pregnancy; the issue of safety. Herbalgram 1991; 38(Fall):47-50.

Gujral S et al., (1978) Nutr Rep Int 17:183.

Harvey DJ, J Chromatogr 212:75. 1981.

Iwu MM (ed), Handbook of African Medicinal Plants. CRC Press, Boca Raton, FL, 1993.

Hikino H, In: Economic, Medicinal Plant Research, Vol. 1, Acadamic Press UK 1985.

Kasahara Y, Hikino H, (1983) Shoyakugaku Zasshi 37:73.

Kawai T et al., Anti-emtic principles of Magnolia obovata bark and Zingiber officinale rhizome. In: PM 60:17. 1994.

Kikuchi F et al., (1982) Chem Pharm Bull 30. 754.

Kikuzaki H, Kobayashi M, Nakatani N, Constituents of Zingiberaceae. 4. Diarylheptanoids from Rhizomes of Zingiber officinale. In: PH 30: 3947. 1991.

Kikuzaki H, Kobayashi M, Nakatani N, Diarylheptanoids from rhizomes of Zingiber officinale. In: PH 30(11):3647-3651. 1991.

Kikuzaki H, Tsai SM, Nakatani N, Gingerdiol related compounds from the rhizomes of Zingiber officinale. In: PH 31(5):1783-1786. 1992.

Kiuchi F, Iwakami S, Shibuya M et al., Inhibition of prostaglandin and leukotriene biosynthesis by gingerols and diarylheptanoids. Chem Pharm Bull 40(2):387-391. 1992.

Macolo N, Jain R, Jain SC et al., Ethnopharmacologic investigation of ginger (Zingiber officinale). J Ethnopharmacol 27:129-40, 1989.

Marles RJ, Kaminski J, Arnason JT, Pazos-Sanou L, Heptinstall S, Fischer NH, Crompton CW, Kindack DG, A bioassay for inhibition of serotonin release from bovine platelets. In: JNP 55:1044-1056. 1992.

Mikawa U et al., Delayed-type allergy-controlling agents containing gingerones. In: Patent Jap. 1988.

Mowrey DB, Clayson DE, (1982) Lancet II, 655.

Muller JL & Clauson KA., Pharmaceutical considerations of common herbal medicine. Am J Managed Care 1997; 3:1753-1770. 1997.

Nagabhushan M, Amonkar AJ, Bhide SV, Mutagenicity of gingerol and shoagol and antimutagenicity in zingerone in Salmonella/microsme assay. In: Cancer-Lett (Shannon Irel) 36(2)221-233. 1987.

Narasimhan S, Govinarajan VS, (1978) J Food Tech 13:31.

Phillips S, Ruggier R & Hutchinson SE., Zingiber officinale (ginger) - an antiemetic for day case surgery. Anaesthesia 48:715-717. 1993.

Saller R, Hellenbrecht D, Zingiber officinale. In: Tägl Praxis 33(3):629. 1992.

Suekawa M et al., (1984) J Pharmacobio-Dyn 7 (11):836.

Sugaya A et al., (1975) Shoyakugaku Zasshi 29:160.

Further information in:

Chan H, But P, Pharmacology, Applications of Chinese Materia Medica, Vol 1, World Scientific Singapore 1986.

Kern W, List PH, Hörhammer L (Hrsg.), Hagers Handbuch der Pharmazeutischen Praxis, 4. Aufl., Bde 1-8: Springer Verlag Berlin, Heidelberg, New York, 1969.

Leung AY, Encyclopedia of Common Natural Ingredients Used in Food, Drugs, Cosmetics, John Wiley & Sons Inc., New York 1980.

Madaus G, Lehrbuch der Biologischen Arzneimittel, Bde 1-3, Nachdruck, Georg Olms Verlag Hildesheim 1979.

Roth L, Daunderer M, Kormann K, Giftpflanzen, Pflanzengifte, 4. Aufl., Ecomed Fachverlag Landsberg Lech 1993.

Schmid R, Schick T, Steffen R et al., Comparison of seven commonly used agents for prophylaxis of seasickness. J Trav Med 1:203-206. 1994.

Srivastava KC & Mustafa T, Ginger (Zingiber officinale) in rheumatism and musculoskeletal disorders. Med Hypotheses 39:342-348. 1992.

Steinegger E, Hänsel R, Pharmakognosie, 5. Aufl., Springer Verlag Heidelberg 1992.

Suekawa M, Ishige A, Yuasa K et al., Pharmacological studies on ginger. I. Pharmacological actions of pungent constituents, (6)-gingerol and (6)-shogoal. J Pharm Dyn 7:836-848. 1984.

Teuscher E, Biogene Arzneimittel, 5. Aufl., Wiss. Verlagsges. Stuttgart 1997.

Wagner H, Wiesenauer M, Phytotherapie. Phytopharmaka und pflanzliche Homöopathika, Fischer-Verlag, Stuttgart, Jena, New York 1995.

Wichtl M (Hrsg.), Teedrogen, 4. Aufl., Wiss. Verlagsges. Stuttgart 1997.

Ginkgo

Ginkgo biloba

TRADE NAMES

Ginkgo Biloba (available from numerous manufacturers and as a combination product), Bioginkgo, Gincosan, Ginexin Remind, Ginkai, Ginkoba, Ginkgo Go!, Ginkgold, Ginkgo Power, Ginkgoba, Ginkgo Leaf, Quanterra Mental Sharpness, Ginko Biloba Premium Extract, Gingko Biloba Extract, Activated Ginkgo, Nuveg Ginkgo Power, Time Release Ginkgo Power, Senior Ginkgo Power, Herbal Sure Maximum Strength Gingko Biloba

DESCRIPTION

Medicinal Parts: The medicinal parts are the fresh or dried leaves, and the seeds separated from their fleshy outer layer.

Flower and Fruit: The tree flowers for the first time when it is between 20 and 30 years old. The flowers are dioecious. They are in the axils of the lower leaves of the current year's short shoots. The male flowering parts are attached to short catkins. The female flowers have longer pedicles and are at the end of a leafless branch. Fertilization occurs months after pollination by spermatozoids, although usually only one ovule is fully formed. The light green or yellowish seeds, incorrectly called fruit, later become fleshy and plum-like. They have a diameter of 2.5 to 3 cm, and each contains a two-edged edible nut.

Leaves, Stem and Root: Ginkgo biloba is a 30 to 40 m high dioecious tree with a girth of about 4 m. The trees can live for hundreds of years. The bark is light to dark brown with rough grooves and reticulate fissures. The leaves are fan-shaped with bifurcated ribs and glabrous. They are fresh green to golden yellow in autumn. The female trees are pointed and pyramid-shaped; the male trees are broad and sparer.

Characteristics: The seeds smell like butyric, capric or valeric acid when ripe.

Habitat: Ginkgo is indigenous to China, Japan and Korea, and is also found in Europe and the U.S.

Production: The leaves are harvested either mechanically or by hand from plantations or in the wild. The leaves are then dried and pressed into balls. A dry extract from the dried leaf of Ginkgo biloba is manufactured using acetone/water and subsequent purification steps without addition of concentrates or isolated ingredients.

Other Names: Maidenhair-Tree

ACTIONS AND PHARMACOLOGY

COMPOUNDS

Flavonoids (0.5-1.8%): including monosides, biosides and triosides of quercetin, isorhamnetins, 3-O- methylmyristicins, and kaempferol, to some extent estered with p-coumaric acid

Biflavonoides (0.4-1.9%): for example, amentoflavone, bilobetin, 5-methoxybilobetin, ginkgetin, isoginkgetin

Proanthocyanidins (8-12%)

Trilactonic diterpenes (0.06-0.23%): ginkgolide A, B, C

Trilactonic sesquiterpene bilabolids (0.04-0.2%)

EFFECTS

Ginkgolide B is a potent inhibitor of platelet-activating factor (PAF), which is important for the induction of arachidonate-independent platelet aggregation. Ginkgolide B blocks the binding to PAF to its receptor resulting in an antagonistic effect (Chung, 1987). This effect will inhibit PAF-induced bronchoconstriction and airway hyperactivity, along with T-lymphocyte proliferation and cytokine production. PAF induces inflammation and changes in vascular permeability (Braquet, 1989; Della Loggia, 1993).

Ginkgo biloba exerts ischemic protective and antioxidant effects through the flavonoids. This occurs through a free scavenger action and prevention of lipid peroxidation. Lipid peroxidation is involved in producing tissue and vascular damage, and neuronal loss, which may lead to dementia (Dorman, 1992; Koc, 1995; Otamiri, 1989). The herb also reduces neutrophil infiltration and increases blood flow to prevent the progression of dementia ischemia. The antioxidant and membrane-stablizing activity increases cerebral hypoxia tolerance (Koltringer, 1989; Otamiri, 1989).

Other effects consist of spasmolytic properties through direct action on alpha-adrenoceptors and smooth muscle relaxing properties via the signal transduction pathway, intracellular cAMP, antagonism of the adrenergic nervous system and hyperpolarization (Hellegouarch, 1985; Struillon, 1995).

CLINICAL TRIALS

Dementia

A placebo-controlled, double-blind, randomized trial with a particular extract of Ginkgo biloba (EGb 761) was conducted to assess the efficacy and safety in Alzheimer's disease and multi-infarct dementia. Alzheimer's Disease Assessment Scale-Cognitive subscale (ADAS-Cog), Geriatric Evaluation by Relative's Rating Instrument (GERRI) and Clinical Global Impression of Change (CGIC) were used to evaluate the response in 309 patients over a 52-week period. EGb 120 mg daily was safe and was shown to stabilize or improve cognitive performance and the social functioning of demented patients for 6 months to 1 year (Le Bars, 1998).

Peripheral Occlusive Arterial Disease

The clinical efficacy of Ginkgo biloba special extract (EGb 761) was demonstrated in 111 patients with peripheral occlusive arterial disease (POAD) in Fontaine stage IIb and intermittent claudication. The mean pain-free walking distances were very similar at the beginning of the treatment period. After 8, 16 and 24 weeks, the EGb treatment group was significantly better than the placebo group with maximum walking distance and relative increases of the pain-free walking distance. The doppler indices remained nearly unchanged during the coarse of therapy (Peters, 1998).

Equilibrium Disorders

An open, controlled study consisted of 44 patients complaining of vertigo, dizziness or both, caused by vascular vestibular disorders. The patients were randomly treated with extract of Ginkgo biloba (EGb 761) 80 mg twice daily or with betahistine dihydrochloride (BI) 16 mg twice daily for 3 months. A complete neuro-otologic and equilibrimetric examination was performed at baseline and after 3 months of treatment, including an evaluation of clinical findings. Dizziness and vertigo improved in 64.7% of patients in the BI treatment group and in 65% of those in the EGb 761 treatment group in the first month of therapy. No significant changes were observed in cranial scans for patients with a 'central' cranial pattern or with the equilibrium score. EGb 761 induced a slight decrease of saccadic delay and considerably increased saccadic velocities while BI improved saccadic accuracy but did not modify delay. EGb 761 improved smooth pursuit gain three times more than BI. Both drugs asymmetrically reduced nystagmus maximum velocity and improved the sinusoidal vestibulo-ocular reflex. BI considerably reduced, whereas EGb 761 considerably improved, visuovestibular ocular reflex (Cesarani, 1998).

INDICATIONS AND USAGE

Approved by Commission E:

- Symptomatic relief of organic brain dysfunction
- Intermittent claudication
- Vertigo (vascular origin)
- Tinnitus (vascular origin)

The Commission E approvals listed are limited to special standard extracts of Ginkgo.

Unproven Uses: The drug is used for disturbed brain functions that result in dizziness and headache with emotional lability and anxiety. Ginkgo has been demonstrated to improve concentration and memory deficits as a result of peripheral arterial occlusive disease.

Chinese Medicine: Among traditional Chinese uses for Ginkgo biloba are asthma, tinnitus, hypertonia and angina pectoris.

Homeopathic Uses: Homeopathy includes tonsillitis and cephalgia among the indications for use of Ginkgo.

CONTRAINDICATIONS

The drug is contraindicated in patients known to be hypersensitive to Ginkgo biloba preparations.

Patients with known risk factors for intracranial hemorrhage (systematic arterial hypertension, diabetes amyloid senile plaques) should avoid the use of Ginkgo biloba due to a recent case report of subarachnoid hemorrhage associated with the herb (Vale, 1998).

PRECAUTIONS AND ADVERSE REACTIONS

General: Health risks or side effects following the proper administration of designated therapeutic dosages are not recorded. Mild gastrointestinal complaints could occur as side effects (Cohen, 1998). Also, blood pressure problems, allergic reactions and phlebitis have occasionally been documented after parenteral administration. Allergic skin reactions have been observed on extremely rare occasions. The possible hypersensitivity reactions consist of occurrence of spasms and cramps and, in cases of acute toxicity, atonia and adynamia.

Fertility: Ginkgo has adverse effects on oocytes (Ondrizek, 1999):

Hematologic Effects: Spontaneous bilateral subdural hematomas, subarachnoid hemorrhage and an increase in bleeding time have been associated with chronic Ginkgo biloba ingestion (Rowin, 1996; Vale, 1998).

Drug Interactions: Antithrombolytic Agents (anticoagulants, antiplatelets and aspirin) — Spontaneous bleeding has been associated with the herb due to its potent inhibitory effect on the platelet-activating factor (PAF). Case reports involving the herb associated with subarachnoid hemorrhage and intracerebral hemorrhage suggests an additional risk of intracerebral hemorrhage with the use of thrombolytic therapy (Matthews, 1998; Rowin, 1996; Vale, 1998).

DOSAGE

Mode of Administration: Ginkgo is available in liquid or solid pharmaceutical forms, for oral intake and parenterally for homeopathic use.

How Supplied:

Capsules—30 mg, 40 mg, 50 mg, 60 mg, 100 mg, 120 mg, 260 mg, 400 mg, 420 mg, 440 mg, 450 mg, 500 mg

Extract—50:1

Liquid—40mg/5mL

Tablets—30 mg, 40 mg, 60 mg, 80 mg, 120 mg, 260 mg

Daily Dosage: Ginkgo biloba extract should be standardized to contain 24% flavone and 6% terpene lactones: 40 to 80 mg three times a day (van Beek, 1998). Studies have demonstrated efficacy with 120 mg daily in 2 to 3 divided doses for dementia, peripheral arterial occlusive disease and for equilibrium disorders like tinnitus or vertigo (Cesarani, 1998; Le Bar, 1998; Peters, 1998).

Chinese Medicine: In traditional Chinese medicine, the daily dose is 3 to 6 g of leaves as an infusion.

Homeopathic Dosage: 5 drops, 1 tablet or 10 globules every 30 to 60 minutes (acute) or 1 to 3 times daily (chronic); parenterally: 1 to 2 ml acute, 3 times daily; chronic: once a day (HAB1).

Storage: Ginkgo must be protected from light and moisture.

LITERATURE

American Psychiatric Association (Ed.), DSM-IV. Diagnostic and Statistical Manual of Mental Disorders, 4th Ed. R. R. Donnelly & Sons Company 1994.

Amling R, Phytotherapeutika in der Neurologie. In: ZPT 12(1):9. 1991.

Anonym, Ginkgo und Crataegus. In: DAZ 137(20):1751-1753. 1997.

Anonym, Phytopharmaka für ältere Menschen: Ginkgo, Kava, Hypericum und Crataegus. In: DAZ 135(5):400-402. 1995.

Anonym, Psycho-Phytos: Ginkgo, Johanniskraut und Kava-Kava. In: DAZ 135(18):1632-1634. 1995.

Bach D, Behandlung der benignen Prostatahypertrophie. In: ZPT 17(4):209-218. 1996.

Bauer R, Zschocke S, Medizinische Anwendung von Ginkgo biloba Geschichtliche Entwicklung. In: ZPT 17(5):275-283. 1996.

Beske F, Kunczik T, (1991) Frühzeitige Therapie kann Milliarden sparen. Der Kassenarzt 42:36-42.

Blaha L, (1989) Differential diagnose der zerebralen Insuffizienz in der Praxis. Geriatrie und Rehabilitation 2,1:23-28.

Braquet P (Ed.), Ginkgolides. Chemistry, Biology, Pharmacology and Clinical Perspectives. Vol I. JR Prous Science, Barcelona 1988.

Braquet P (Ed.), Ginkgolides. Chemistry, Biology, Pharmacology and Clinical Perspectives. Vol II, JR Prous Science, Barcelona 1989.

Brüchert E, Heinrich SE, Ruf-Kohler P, (1991) Wirksamkeit von LI 1370 bei älteren Patienten mit Hirnleistungsschwäche. Münch Med Wschr 133(Suppl 1):9-14.

Bundesgesundheitsamt, (1991) Empfehlungen zum Wirksamkeitsnachweis von Nootropika im Indikationsbereich ''Demenz'' (Phase III). Bundesgesundheitsblatt 7:342-350.

Burkard G, Lehrl S, (1991) Verhältnis von Demenzen vom Multiinfarkt- und vom Alzheimertyp in ärztlichen Praxen. Münch Med Wschr 133(Supp. 1):38-43.

Caesar W, Alles über Ginkgo. In: DAZ 134(44):4363. 1994.

Cesarani A, Meloni F, Alpini D et al., Ginkgo biloba (EGb 761) in the treatment of equilibrium disorders. Adv Ther 1998 Sep-Oct;15(5):291-304.

Chung KF, Dent G, McCusker M et al., Effect of a ginkgolide mixture (BN 52063) in antagonising skin and platelet responses to platelet activating factor in man. Lancet 1987 Jan 31;1(8527):248-51.

Cohen AJ & Bartlick B: Ginkgo biloba for antidepressent-induced sexual dysfunction. J Sex Marital Ther 1998; 24:139-143.

Della Loggia R, Sosa S, Tubaro A, Bombardelli E, Anti-inflammatory activity of Ginkgo biloba flavonoids. In: PM 59 (1992), A588.

Deutsches Institut für medizinische Dokumentation und Information (Hrsg.), ICD-10. Internationale und statistische Klassifikation der Krankheiten und verwandter Gesundheitsprobleme. 10. Revision. Bd 1. Urban & Schwarzenberg, München Wien Baltimore 1994.

Dfeudis FV, Ginkgo biloba extract (EGb 761): Pharmacological activities and clinical applications. In: Elsevier Editions Scientifiques Paris. 1991.

Dingermann T, Phytopharmaka im Alter: Crataegus, Ginkgo, Hypericum und Kava- Kava. In: PZ 140(23):2017-2024. 1995.

Dorman D, Cote L, Buck W, Effects of an extract of Gingko biloba on bromethalin-induced cerebral lipid peroxidation and edema in rats. Am J Vet Res 1992 Jan;53(1):138-42.

Dorn M, Bräunig B, Gross HD, Ginkgo-Dragees bei zerebraler Leistungsschwäche. In: ZPT 12(6):180. 1991.

Ermini-Fünfschilling D, (1992) Möglichkeiten und Grenzen eines Gedächtnistrainings mit Patienten bei beginnender Demenz. Z Moderne Geriatrie 12:459-456.

Gräßel E, (1989) Vergleich zweier Personengruppen bezüglich der Auswirkungen des mentalen Trainings (''Gehirn-Jogging'') auf die Selbsteinschätzung der Leistungsfähigkeit in Abhängigkeit von der Trainingszeit (Tageszeit der Trainingsdurchführung). Geriatrie & Rehabilitation 2,1:44-46.

Hartmann A, Schulz V (Hrsg.), (1991) Ginkgo biloba, Aktuelle Forschungsergebnisse 1990/91. Münch Med Wschr 133:1-64.

Hellegouarch A, Baranes J, Clostre F et al., Comparison of the contractile effects of an extract of Ginkgo biloba and some neurotransmitters on rabbit isolated vena cava. Gen Pharmacol 1985; 16:129-132.

Hopfenmüller W, (1994) Nachweis der therapeutischen Wirksamkeit eines Ginkgo biloba-Spezialextraktes. Metaanalyse von 11 klinischen Studien bei Patienten mit Hirnleistungsstörungen im Alter Arzneim Forsch/Drug Res 44:1005-1013.

Israel L, Dell'Accio E, Martin G, Hugonot R, (1987) Extrait de Ginkgo biloba et exercices d'entra nement de la memoire. Evaluation comparative chez personnes (gées ambulatoiRes Psychologie Médicinale 19(8):1431-1439.

Joyeux M et al., Comparative antilipoperoxidant, antinecrotic and scavenging properties of terpenes and biflavones from Ginkgo and some flavonoids. In: PM 61(2):126-129. 1995.

Kanowski S, (1991) Klinischer Wirksamkeitsnachweis bei Nootropika. Münch Med Wschr 133:5-8.

Kanowski S, Herrmann WM, Stephan K, Wierich W, Hörr R, (1995) Proof of efficacy of the Ginkgo biloba special extract EGb 761 in outpatients suffering from primary degenerative dementia of the Alzheimer type and multi-infarct dementia. Pharmacopsychiatry 4:149-158.

Kleijnen J, Knipschild P, (1992a) Ginkgo biloba for cerebral insufficiency. Br J Clin Pharmac 35:352-358.

Kleijnen J, Knipschild P, (1992b) Ginkgo biloba. Lancet, 1136-1139.

Koalik F et al., (1992) Kombinierte Anwendung von nootroper Therapie und kognitivem Training bei chronischen organischen Psychosyndromen. Neuropsychiatrie 6:47-52.

Koc R, Akdemir H, Kurtsoy A et al., Lipid peroxidation in experimental spinal cord injury. Comparison of treatment with Ginkgo biloba, TRH and mehtylprednisolone. Res Exp Med (Berl) 1995;195(2):117-23.

Koltringer P, Eber O, Lind P et al., Mikrozirkulation und Viskoelastizitaet des Vollblutes unter Ginkgo-biloba extrakt. Eine plazebokonntrollierte, randomisierte Douppelblind-Studie. Perfusion 1989; 1:28-30.

Krieglstein J, Neuroprotective properties of Ginkgo biloba-constituents. In: ZPT 15(2):92-96. 1994.

Kurz A, Ginkgo biloba bei Demenzerkrankungen. In: Loew D, Rietbrock N (Hrsg.), Phytopharmaka. Steinkopff Verlag, Darmstadt 1995, S 145-149.

Le Bars PL, Katz MM, Berman N et al., A placebo-controlled, double-blind, randomized trial of an extract of Ginkgo biloba for dementia. North American EGb Study Group. JAMA 1997 Oct 22-29;278(16):1327-32.

Matthews MK, Association of Ginkgo biloba with intracerebral hemorrhage. Neurology 1998;50:1933-4.

Nieder M, (1991) Pharmakokinetik der Ginkgo-Flavonole im Plasma. Münch Med Wschr 133:61-62.

Oberpichler-Schwenk H, Krieglstein J, (1992) Pharmakologische Wirkungen von Ginkgo-biloba-Extrakt und -Inhaltsstoffen. Pharmazie in unserer Zeit 21:224-235.

Ondrizek RR, Chan PJ, Patton WC, King A. An alternative medicine study of herbal effects on the penetration of zona-free hamster occytes and the integrity of sperm deoxyribonucleic acid. Fertil Steril 1999 Mar;71(3):517-22.

Otamiri T, Tagesson C: Ginkgo biloba extract prevents mucosa damage associated with small-intestinal ischaemia. Scand J Gastroenterol 1989; 24:666-670.

Peters H, Kieser M, Holscher U. Demonstration of the efficacy of Ginkgo biloba special extract EGb 761 on intermittent claudication—a placebo-controlled, double-blind multicenter trial. Vasa 1998 May;27(2):106-10.

Pfister-Hotz G, Phytotherapie in der Geriatrie. In: ZPT 18(3):165-162. 1997.

Riederer P, Laux G, Pöldinger W (Hrsg.), Neuropsychopharmaka. Band 5: Parkinsonmittel und Nootropika. Springer Verlag, Wien Noew York 1992, S. 161-324.

Rosenblatt M, Mindel J, Spontaneous bilateral hyphema associated with ingestion of Ginkgo biloba extract. N Engl J Med. 1997 Apr 10; 336(15):1108.

Rowen J, Lewis S, Spontaneous bilateral subdural hematomas associated with chronic Ginkgo biloba ingestion. Neurology 1996 Jun;46(6):1775-6.

Rupalla K, Oberpichler-Schwenk H, Krieglstein J, Neuroprotektive Wirkungen des Ginkgo-biloba-Extrakts und seiner Inhaltsstofe. In: Loew D, Rietbrock N (Hrsg.) Phytopharmaka in Forschung und klinischer Anwendung. Steinkopff Verlag, Darmstadt 1995, S 17-27.

Schilcher H, Ginkgo biloba L. In: ZPT 9:119. 1998.

Schmid M, Schmoll H (Hrsg.), Ginkgo. Wissenschaftliche Verlagsgesellschaft mbH Stuttgart 1994.

Schmid B, In: Schmid, Schmoll gen. Eisenwert: Ginkgo, Ur-Baum und Arzneipflanze, Mythos, Dichtung und Kunst. 1994.

Schwabe U, Paffrath D (Hrsg.), Arzneiverordnungsreport '95. Gustav Fischer Verlag, Stuttgart Jena 1995, S 214-224, 373-374.

Sowers S, Weary PE, Collins OD, Cnoley EP, Ginkgo tree dermatitis. In: Arch Dermatol 81:452-456. 1965.

Spegg H, Ginkgo biloba - ein Baum aus Urzeiten, ein Phytopharmakon mit Zukunft. In: PTA 4(12):576. 1990.

Sprecher E, Pflanzliche Geriatrika. In: ZPT 9(2):40. 1988.

Sticher O, (1993) Ginkgo biloba - Ein modernes pflanzliches Arzneimittel. Vierteljahresschrift der Naturforschenden Gesellschaft in Zürich 138/3:125-168.

Sticher O, Hasler A, Meier B, Ginkgo biloba - Eine Standortbestimmung. In: DAZ 131(36):1827. 1991.

Sticher O, Quality of Ginkgo preparations. In: PM 59(1):2-11. 1993.

Struillon L, Cohen Y, Vilde JL et al., Ginkgo biloba extract EGb 761 is not active against Mycobacterium avium infection in C57BL/6 mice. Antimicrob Agents Chemother 1995; 39:1013-1014.

Vale, S, Subarachnoid hemorrhage associated with Ginkgo biloba. Lancet 1998 Jul 4;352(9121):36.

Vesper J, Hänsgen KD, (1994) Efficacy of Ginkgo biloba in 90 Outpatients with Cerebral Insufficiency Caused by Old Age. Phytomedicine 1:9-16.

Volz HP, Hänsel R, (1994) Ginkgo biloba - Grundlagen und Anwendung in der Psychiatrie. Psychopharmakotherapie 1:70-76.

Volz HP, Hänsel R, (1994) Kava-Kava und Kavain in der Psychopharmakotherapie. Psychopharmakotherapie 1:33-39.

Vorberg G, Schenk N, Schmidt U, (1989) Wirksamkeit eines neuen Ginkgo-biloba- Extraktes bei 100 Patienten mit zerebraler Insuffizien. Z Herz & plus; Gefäße 9:396-401.

Wichtl M, Pflanzliche Geriatrika. In: DAZ 132(30):1576. 1992.

Woerdenberg HJ, Van Beek TA, Ginkgo biloba. In: DeSmet PAGM, Keller K, Hansel R, Chandler RF ed., Adverse Effects of Herbal Drugs. Springer-Verlag Berlin Heidelberg 1997; 3:51-66.

FURTHER INFORMATION IN:

Hänsel R, Keller K, Rimpler H, Schneider G (Hrsg.), Hagers Handbuch der Pharmazeutischen Praxis, 5. Aufl., Bde 4-6 (Drogen), Springer Verlag Berlin, Heidelberg, New York, 1992-1994.

Madaus G, Lehrbuch der Biologischen Arzneimittel, Bde 1-3, Nachdruck, Georg Olms Verlag Hildesheim 1979.

Schulz R, Hänsel R, Rationale Phytotherapie, Springer Verlag Heidelberg 1996.

Steinegger E, Hänsel R, Pharmakognosie, 5. Aufl., Springer Verlag Heidelberg 1992.

Tang W, Eisenbrand G, Chinese Drugs of Plant Origin, Springer Verlag Heidelberg 1992.

Teuscher E, Biogene Arzneimittel, 5. Aufl., Wiss. Verlagsges. mbH Stuttgart 1997.

Wagner H, Wiesenauer M, Phytotherapie. Phytopharmaka und pflanzliche Homöopathika, Fischer-Verlag, Stuttgart, Jena, New York 1995.

Wichtl M (Hrsg.), Teedrogen, 4. Aufl., Wiss. Verlagsges. Stuttgart 1997.

Ginkgo biloba

See Ginkgo

Ginseng

Panax ginseng

TRADE NAMES

Ginseng (available from numerous manufacturers), Ginsana, Gin Zip, Chinese Red Panax Ginseng, Manchurian Ginseng, Premium Blend Korean Ginseng, Ginseng Complex, Korean Ginseng, Siberian Ginseng, Korean Ginseng Extract, Korean White Ginseng, The Ginseng Solution, Herbal Sure Korean Ginseng, American Ginseng Root, Korean Ginseng Root, Standardized Siberian Ginseng Root, Natural Ginseng, Ginseng Up, Herbal Sure Chinese Red Ginseng, Siberian Ginseng Power Herb, Time Release Korean Ginseng Power, American Ginseng, Chinese Red Panax, Concentrated Ginseng Extract, Eleuthero Ginseng Root, Siberian Ginseng Root, Korean White Ginseng Root, Centrum Ginseng, Gin-Action, Ginsai, Ginseng Concentrate, Ginseng Manchurian, Ginseng Natural, Ginseng Power Max 004X G-Sana, Lynae Ginse-Cool, Power Herb Korean Ginseng

DESCRIPTION

Medicinal Parts: The medicinal part is the dried root.

Flower and Fruit: The inflorescence is simple or branched with 1 to 3 umbels of 15 to 30 flowers. The flowers are androgynous and have greenish-yellow corollas. The ovary is inferior. The fruit is a pea-sized, globular to reniform, scarlet, smooth and glossy drupe, which contains 2 seeds.

Leaves, Stem and Root: The plant is a perennial, and stands erect from 30 to 80 cm high. It has a smooth, round stem and bears terminal whorls of 3 to 5 palmate leaves. The leaflets are thin, finely serrate, gradually acuminate, 7 to 20 cm long and 2 to 5 cm wide. The rhizome tapers at the ends and is often palmate at the tip, giving it a human-like form.

Habitat: Panax ginseng is indigenous to China. It is cultivated in China, Korea, Japan and Russia.

Production: Ginseng root consists of the dried main and lateral root and root hairs of Panax ginseng.

Other Names: Five-fingers, Red berry, American Ginseng, Chinese Ginseng, Korean Ginseng, Oriental Ginseng

ACTIONS AND PHARMACOLOGY

COMPOUNDS

Triterpene saponins

Aglycone (20S)-protopanaxadiol: including ginsenoside Ra1, Ra2, Ra3, Rb1, Rb2, Rb3, notoginsenoside R4, Rs1, Rs2, Rs3, Rs4, malonylginsenoside Rb1, Rc, Rd

Aglycone (20S)-protopanaxytriol: including ginsenoside Re, Rf, Rg1, notoginsenoside R1

Aglycone oleanolic acid: including ginsenoside Ro, chikusetsusasaponin-V Rb1, Rb2, Rc, Rd, Re, Rg1

Water-soluble polysaccharides: panaxane A to U

Polyynes: including falcarinol (panaxynol), falcarintriol (panaxytriol), examples estered with acetic acid or linolenic acid

EFFECTS

The main active component in Ginseng consists of the ginsenosides, a diverse group of steroidal saponins. There are twenty-five ginsenosides that have been separated and detected based on the sugar unit sequences and aglycone moieties (Attele, 1999; Fuzzati, 1999; Wang, 1999). The ginsenosides demonstrate the ability to target a myriad of tissues, producing a variety of pharmaceutical responses quite different from one another. A single ginsenoside may initiate multiple or opposing actions in the same tissue, thus making the overall phamacology of ginseng complex (Attele, 1999).

Cognitive Function Effects

The loss of nicotinic receptor binding has been associated with age-related cognitive impairments. Nicotinic receptor stimulation of the central nervous system is beneficial for neuroprotection against age associated cognitive disorders. A non-ginsenoside component of the herb has demonstrated affinity for the nicotinic receptor. This binding of the compound to the receptor results in nicotinic activity (Lewis, 1999). Ginsenoside-Rg2 and -Rg3 block nicotinic acetylcholine and gamma-aminobutyric acid receptors. This results in an inhibitory effect of the acetylcholine-evoked secretion of catecholamines. (Tachikawa, 1999). These different effects of Panax gingseng contribute to the variety of pharmacological effects.

Antineoplastic Effects

A protopanaxadiol component of Ginseng was shown to inhibit proliferation of pulmonary adenocarcinoma cells resistant to cisplatin (Lee, 1999). Ginsenoside-Rs4 and -Rs3 elevates protein levels of p53 and p21WAF1, which are associated with the induction of apoptosis in human hepatoma cells (Kim, 1999). Ginsenoside Rh2 induces apoptotic cell death in the glioma cell line through activation of caspase and production of oxygen species (Kim, 1999).

Antioxidant Effects

The antioxidant effects of Ginseng protect against oxidative DNA and protein (globin) damage caused by free radicals (Lee, 1998). Antioxidant activity of the herb also provides a hepatoprotective effect by increasing hepatic gluathione peroxidase activity (Voces, 1999). Antioxidant intervention by Ginseng is exerted by weak radical scavenging activity and stimulation of endothelial nitric oxide synthase in cardiac tissue (Maffei, 1999).

Antiplatelet Effects

The antiplatelet components consist of panaxynol and ginsenosides Ro, Rg1, and Rg2 in the diethyl ether and 1-butanol fractions of the herb. Panaxynol inhibits the aggregation, release reaction, and thromboxane formation in platelets while ginsenosides Ro, Rg1, and Rg2 suppress the release reaction only (Kuo, 1990; Teng, 1989).

Antiviral Effects

Ginseng induces production of interferon, enhances natural killer cell and antibody dependent cytotoxic activities, and stimulates cell mediated immunity (Singh, 1983; Singh, 1984).

Decrease in Alcohol Levels

The effect of ginseng in the reduction of blood ethanol levels may be attributed to different mechanisms. Ginseng increases alcohol dehydrogenase and aldehyde dehydrogenase activity at high concentrations due to an augmented induction of the microsomal ethanol oxidizing system. Ginseng enhances blood alcohol clearance in man (Lee, 1987). The ginsenosides also reduce plasma ethanol by a delay in gastric emptying time (Koo, 1999).

Hypolipidemic/Cardiac Effects

Ginseng saponins activate lipoprotein lipase, an enzyme that reduces chylomicrons and very low-density lipoproteins, and results in a decrease of triglycerides and cholesterol (Inoue, 1999). The ginsenosides demonstrate negative chronotropic effects and positive and negative inotropic effects on the heart (Wu, 1988). The anti-arrhythmic properties of Rg1 consist of prolonged ventricular refractoriness and repolarization, and increased ventricular fibrillation threshold (Wu, 1995).

Miscellaneous Effects

Stimulation of corticotrophin secretion and increased hepatic ribonucleic acid (RNA) and protein synthesis are effects of the saponin glycosides in Ginseng. Panax ginseng is comprised of at least 28 different saponin glycosides, which contain nuclei resembling those of steroids (Punnonen, 1980). The ginsenosides also stimulate insulin release and increase insulin receptors to exert a hypoglycemic effect (Guodong, 1987). Ginseng also decreases blood sugar through glucose metabolism related to adrenergic receptors. Ginseng decreases lactic acid and stimulates other respiratory enzymes in the electron transport chain to promote aerobic oxidation (Yao, 1990). The saponins have shown enhancement of erectile capacity mediated by endothelium-derived relaxing factor and peripheral neurophysiologic enhancement (Choi, 1999; Choi, 1995).

CLINICAL TRIALS

Cognitive Function

A randomized, double-blind, placebo-controlled study was conducted to evaluate the effect of Ginseng on cognitive function over an 8-week period. There were 112 healthy volunteers over 40 years of age. The primary outcome was the change in score on each cognitive test, evaluated at baseline, and again at 8 weeks. Oral standardized ginseng 400 mg daily was significantly better compared to placebo with abstract thinking and a tendency toward faster simple reaction times. There was no difference between the groups with regard to concentration, memory, or subjective experience (Sorenson, 1996).

Hypoglycemic

The effect on blood glucose with Ginseng was demonstrated in a double-blind, placebo-controlled study including 36 newly diagnosed Type 2 diabetic patients. Ginseng 200 mg daily improved glycated hemoglobin, serum aminoterminal-propetptide concentration and physical activity after 8 weeks of therapy. Ginseng 100 mg and 200 mg daily dose elevated mood, improved psychophysical performance, and reduced fasting blood glucose and weight (Sotaniemi, 1995).

Antiviral

The properties of a standardized extract of ginseng root for inducing a higher immune response in vaccination against influenza were evaluated in 227 volunteers. The placebo-controlled, randomized, double-blind study was conducted over a 12-week period. Oral standardized ginseng extract 100 mg daily was given over the entire 12-week period, with anti-influenza polyvalent vaccination given to all volunteers at week 4. There were significantly fewer cases of influenza or the common cold in the ginseng-treatment group, and significantly higher antibody titers and natural killer cell levels at 8 and 12 weeks in the ginseng treatment group (Scaglione, 1996).

INDICATIONS AND USAGE

Approved by Commission E:

- Lack of stamina

Ginseng is used internally for fatigue and debility, and for a decrease capacity for work and concentration.

Unproven Uses: In Folk medicine, Ginseng is used for loss of appetite, cachexia, anxiety, impotence and sterility, neuralgia and insomnia.

Chinese Medicine: In Chinese medicine, Ginseng is used for hemoptysis, gastric disturbances, and vomiting.

Homeopathic Uses: Ginseng is used for rheumatism and debility.

PRECAUTIONS AND ADVERSE REACTIONS

General: Caution should be taken in patients with cardiovascular disease or diabetes. Hypertension resulting from Ginseng Abuse Syndrome is associated with prolonged high dose Ginseng with concomitant use of caffeine (Siegel, 1979; Siegel, 1980). General adverse effects include insomnia, epistaxis, headache, nervousness, and vomitting.

Mastalgia: Mastalgia with diffuse breast nodularity has been reported with Ginseng use (Palmer, 1978).

Vaginal Bleeding: Oral Ginseng and Ginseng face cream have been associated with post menopausal vaginal bleeding (Greenspan, 1983; Hopkins, 1988).

Pregnancy/Lactation: Maternal use of Ginseng has been associated with neonatal androgenization, thus it is not recommended for use during pregnancy or lactation (Awang, 1991).

Drug Interactions:

Diabetic Agents/Insulin — Caution should be taken when taking an antidiabetic agent or insulin to lower blood glucose because Ginseng has been shown to have hypoglycemic effects (See EFFECTS and CLINICAL TRIALS).

Warfarin/NSAIDS/Antiplatelet Agents — A case report of a 47-year old male with a mechanical valve in the aortic position taking warfarin had a decrease in the INR 2 weeks after initiating Ginseng therapy. The INR returned to normal 2 weeks after discontinuation of warfarin (Awang, 1991). Due to the antiplatelet effect of Ginseng, avoid concomitant use with antiplatelet agents or NSAIDS.

Phenelzine (MAOI) — Headache, tremors, and mania have been reported with concomitant use of phenelzine and Ginseng (Jones, 1987).

Loop Diuretics — Germanium, present in most Ginseng products, was reported to cause loop diuretic resistance in a 63 year old male with glomerulonephritis. Germainium causes nephrotoxicity in the nephron segment where loop diuretics work (Becker, 1996).

OVERDOSAGE

Massive overdosages can bring about Ginseng Abuse Syndrome, which is characterized by hypertension, insomnia, hypertonia and edema.

DOSAGE

Mode of Administration: Comminuted drug infusions, powder and galenic preparations for internal use. Various standardized preparations containing Ginseng root are available.

How Supplied:

Capsules — 100mg, 150mg, 200mg, 250mg, 404mg, 405mg, 410mg, 424mg, 470mg, 500mg, 505mg, 535mg, 560mg, 1000mg, 1250mg

Liquid — 300mg/ml

Tablet — 350mg, 500mg

Preparation: To make an infusion, pour boiling water over 3 gm comminuted drug and strain after 5 to 10 minutes.

Daily Dosage: The average daily dosage is 1 to 2 gm root. The infusion may be taken 3 to 4 times a day over 3 to 4 weeks.

Cognitive Function — Oral standardized Ginseng 400 mg daily was effective in improving cognitive function (Sorenson, 1996).

Hypoglycemic Effects — Dosage of 100-200 mg of oral standardized Ginseng has been effective in Type 2 diabetic patients (Sotaniemi, 1995).

Antiviral — Studies have proven efficacy in addition vaccination with 100-200 mg daily of oral standardized Ginseng extract (Scaglione, 1996).

Erectile Dysfunction — Korean Red Ginseng given orally as 600 mg three times daily has been effective (Choi, 1995).

Physical and Psychological Performance Capacity (lack of stamina) — Ginsana given 100 mg twice daily has improved oxygen capacity, reduction of maximum stress frequency, increase in ling function parameters and shortened reaction time to visual stimulants after 11 weeks (Forgo, 1985).

Homeopathic Dosage: 5 drops, 1 tablet, 5 to 10 globules or 1 mL injection solution sc twice weekly.

LITERATURE

Anonym, Kann Ginseng die Leistungsfähigkeit erhöhen? In: DAZ 132(12):XLVIII. 1992.

Anonym, Mythos-Tonikum-Arzneimittel. Ginsengextrakt bei Atemwegserkrankungen. In: DAZ 134(26):2461. 1994.

Attele AS; Wu JA; Yuan CS. Ginseng pharmacology: multiple constituents and multiple actions. Biochem Pharmacol 1999 Dec 1;58(11):1685-93.

Avakian EV et al., (1984) Planta Med 50:151.

Awang DV. Maternal use of ginseng and neonatal androgenization. JAMA 1991 Jul 17;266(3):363.

Baldwin CA et al., (1986) Pharm J 237:583.

Bauer R, Neues von ''immunmodulierenden Drogen'' und ''Drogen mit antiallergischer und antiinflammatorischer Wirkung''. In: ZPT 14(1):23-24. 1993.

Becker BN; Greene J; Evanson J et al. Ginseng-induced diuretic resistance. JAMA 1996 Aug 28;276(8):606-7.

Blasius H, Phytotherapie: Adaptogene Wirkung von Ginseng. In: DAZ 135(23):2136-2138. 1995.

Caesar W, Ginsengwurzel in Europa. Eine alte Geschichte. In: DAZ 131(19):935. 1991.

Choi H, Seong D, Rha K. Clinical efficacy of Korean red ginseng for erectile dysfunction. Int J Impot Res 1995 Sep;7(3):181-6.

Choi Y, Rha K, Choi H. In vitro and in vivo experimental effect of Korean red ginseng on erection. J urol 1999 Oct;162(4):1508-11.

Forgo I, Schimert G. Zur Frage der Wirkungsdauer des standardisierten Ginseng-Extraktes G 115 bei gesunden Leistungssportiern. Notabene medici 1985 9:636-649.

Fulder SJ, (1981) Am J Chin Med 9:112.

Fuzzati N; Gabetta B; Jayakar K et al. Liquid chromatography-electrospray mass spectrometric identification of ginsenosides in Panax ginseng roots. J Chromatogr A 1999 Aug 27;854(1-2):69-79.

Greenspan EM. Ginseng and vaginal bleeding. JAMA 1983 Apr 15;249(15):2018.

Guodong L, Zhongqui L. Effects of ginseng saponins on insulin release from isolated pancreatic islets of rats. Chin J Integr Trad Western Med 1987;7:326.

Hansen L, Boll PM, (1986) Phytochemistry 25(2):285.

Hirakura K, Morita M, Nakajima K, Ikeya Y, Mitsuhashi H, Polyacetylenes from them roots of Panax ginseng. In: PH 30:3327-3333. 1991.

Hopkins M, Androff L, Benninghoff A. Ginseng face cream and unexplained vaginal bleeding. Am J Obstet Gynecol 1988,159:1121-1122.

Hyo-Won B, Il-Heok K, Sa-Sek H, Byung-Hun H, Mun-Hae H, Ze-Hun K, Nak-Du K, (1987) Roter Ginseng. Schriftenreihe des Staatlichen Ginseng-Monopolamtes der Republik Korea.

Inoue M; Wu CZ; Dou DQ et al. Lipoprotein lipase activation by red ginseng saponins in hyperlipidemia model animals. Phytomedicine 1999 Oct;6(4):257-65.

Jones BD; Runikis AM. Interaction of ginseng with phenelzine. J Clin Psychopharmacol 1987 Jun;7(3):201-2.

Kim HE, Oh JH, Lee SK, Oh YJ. Ginsenoside RH-2 induces apoptotic cell death in rat C6 glioma via a reactive oxygen and caspase dependent but Bcl-X(L)-independent pathway. Life Sci 1999;65(3):PL33-40.

Kim SE; Lee YH; Park JH; Lee SK. Ginsenoside-Rs3, a new diol-type ginseng saponin, selectively elevates protein levels of p53 and p21WAF1 leading to induction of apoptosis in SK-HEP-1 cells. Anticancer Res 1999 Jan-Feb;19(1A):487-91.

Kim SE; Lee YH; Park JH; Lee SK. Ginsenoside-Rs4, a new type of ginseng saponin concurrently induces apoptosis and selectively elevates protein levels of p53 and p21WAF1 in human hepatoma SK-HEP-1 cells. Eur J Cancer 1999 Mar;35(3):507-11.

Kitigawa I, (1983) Yaligali Zasshi 103:612.

Konno C et al., (1984) Planta Med 50(5):434.

Koo MW. Effects of ginseng on ethanol induced sedation in mice. Life Sci 1999;64(2):153-60.

Kuo SC; Teng CM; Lee JC et al. Antiplatelet components in Panax ginseng. Planta Med 1990 Apr;56(2):164-7.

Lee FC; Ko JH; Park JK; Lee JS. Effects of Panax ginseng on blood alcohol clearance in man. Clin Exp Pharmacol Physiol 1987 Jun;14(6):543-6.

Lee BM, Lee SK, Kim HS. Inhibition of oxidative DNA damage, 8-OhdG, and carbonyl contents in smokers treated with antioxidants (vitamin E, vitamin C, beta-carotene and red ginseng). Cancer Lett 1998 Oct 23;132(1-2):219-27.

Lee SJ; Sung JH; Lee SJ et al. Antitumor activity of a novel ginseng saponin metabolite in human pulmonary adenocarcinoma cells resistant to cisplatin. Cancer Lett 1999 Sep 20;144(1):39-43.

Lewis R; Wake G; Court G et al. Non-ginsenoside nicotinic activity in ginseng species. Phytother Res 1999 Feb;13(1):59-64.

Maffei F, Carini M, Aldini G, et al. Panax ginseng administration in the rat prevents myocardial ischemia-reperfusion damage induced by hyperbaric oxygen: evidence for an antioxidant intervention. Planta Med 1999 Oct;65(7):614-9.

Matsuda H et al., (1986) Chem Pharm Bull 34(3):1153.

Obermeier A, (1980) Zur Analytik der Ginseng- und Eteutherococcusdroge. Dissertation Ludwig-Maximilians-Universität München.

Palmer BV, Montgomery ACV, Monteiro JC. Ginseng und mastalgia. BMJ 1978;1:1284.

Petkov VD et al., Memory effect of standardized extracts of Panax ginseng(G 115), Ginkgo biloba(GK 501) and their combination Gincosan (PHL-00701). In: PM 59(2).106. 1993.

Pfister-Hotz G, Phytotherapie in der Geriatrie. In: ZPT 18(3):162-165. 1997.

Ploss E, (1988) Panax Ginseng C. A. Meyer. Wissenschaftlicher Bericht. Kooperation Phytopharmaka, Köln Bonn Frankfurt Bad Homburg.

Punnonen R; Lukola A. Oestrogen-like effect of ginseng. Br Med J 1980 Oct 25;281(6248):1110.

Ro JY; Ahn YS; Kim KH. Inhibitory effect of ginsenoside on the mediator release in the guinea pig lung mast cells activated by specific antigen-antibody reactions. Int J Immunopharmacol 1998 Nov;20(11):625-41.

Scaglione F; Cattaneo G; Alessandria M et al. Efficacy and safety of the standardised Ginseng extract G115 for potentiating vaccination against the influenza syndrome and protection against the common cold. Drugs Exp Clin Res 1996;22(2):65-72.

Siegl RK, (1979) Ginseng abuse syndrome - problems with the panacea. J Amer Assoc 241:1614-1615.

Siegl RK, (1980) Ginseng and the high blood pressure. J Am Med Assoc 243:32.

Singh VK, George CX, Singh N, et al. Combined treatment of mice with Panax ginseng extract and interferon inducer. Amplification of host resistance to Semliki forest virus. Planta Med. 1983 Apr;47(4):234-6.

Singh VK, Agarwal SS, Gupta BM. Immunomodulatory activity of Panax ginseng extract. Planta Med 1984 Dec;50(6):462-5.

Sonnenborn U, Proppert Y, (1990) Ginseng (Panax ginseng C.A. Meyer). Z Phytotherapie 11:35-49.

Sorensen H, Sonne J. A double-masked study of the effects of ginseng on cognitive functions. Curr Ther Res 1996;57:959-68.

Sotaniemi E, Haapakoski E, Rautio A. Ginseng therapy in non-insulin-dependent diabetic patients. Diabetes Care 1995 Oct;18(10):1373-5.

Sprecher E, Pflanzliche Geriatrika. In: ZPT 9(2):40. 1988.

Sprecher E, Phytotherapeutika als Wunderdrogen? Versuch einer Bewertung. In: ZPT 10(1):1. 1989.

Tachikawa E; Kudo K; Harada K et al. Effects of ginseng saponins on responses induced by various receptor stimuli. Eur J Pharmacol 1999 Mar 12;369(1):23-32.

Takahashi M, Yoshikura M, (1966) Yakugaku Zasshi 86:1051 and 1053.

Teng CM; Kuo SC; Ko FN et al. Antiplatelet actions of panaxynol and ginsenosides isolated from ginseng. Biochim Biophys Acta 1989 Mar 24;990(3):315-20.

Voces J, Alvarez A, Vila L, et al. Effects of administration of the standardized Panax ginseng extract G115 on hepatic antioxidant function after exhaustive exercise. Comp Biochem Physiol C Pharmacol Toxicol Endocrinol 1999 Jun;123(2):175-84.

Wang B, Yang M, Jin Y, Liu P. Studies on the mechanism of ginseng polypeptide induced hypoglycemia. Yao Hsueh Hsueh Pao 1990;25(10):727-31.

Wang X; Sakuma T; Asafu-Adjaye E. Determination of ginsenosides in plant extracts from Panax ginseng and Panax quinquefolius L. by LC/MS/MS. Anal Chem 1999 Apr 15;71(8):1579-84.

Wichtl M, Pflanzliche Geriatrika. In: DAZ 132(30):1576. 1992.

Wu JX; Chen JX. Negative chronotropic and inotropic effects of Panax notoginseng saponins. Chung Kuo Yao Li Hsueh Pao 1988 Sep;9(5):409-12.

Wu W; Zhang XM; Liu PM et al. Effects of Panax notoginseng saponin Rg1 on cardiac electrophysiological properties and ventricular fibrillation threshold in dogs. Chung Kuo Yao Li Hsueh Pao 1995 Sep;16(5):459-63.

Youn YS, (1987) Analytisch vergleichende Untersuchungen von Ginsengwurzeln verschiedener Provenienzen. Dissertation Freie Universität Berlin.

Further information in:

Chan, EH et al., (Eds) Advances in Chinese Medicinal Materials Research, World Scientific Pub. Co. Singapore 1985.

Frohne D, Pfänder HJ, Giftpflanzen - Ein Handbuch für potheker, Toxikologen und Biologen, 4. Aufl., Wiss. Verlagsges. mbH Stuttgart 1997.

Hänsel R, Keller K, Rimpler H, Schneider G (Hrsg.), Hagers Handbuch der Pharmazeutischen Praxis, 5. Aufl., Bde 4-6 (Drogen), Springer Verlag Berlin, Heidelberg, New York, 1992-1994.

Madaus G, Lehrbuch der Biologischen Arzneimittel, Bde 1-3, Nachdruck, Georg Olms Verlag Hildesheim 1979.

Roth L, Daunderer M, Kormann K, Giftpflanzen, Pflanzengifte, 4. Aufl., Ecomed Fachverlag Landsberg Lech 1993.

Schulz R, Hänsel R, Rationale Phytotherapie, Springer Verlag Heidelberg 1996.

Steinegger E, Hänsel R, Pharmakognosie, 5. Aufl., Springer Verlag Heidelberg 1992.

Tang W, Eisenbrand G, Chinese Drugs of Plant Origin, Springer Verlag Heidelberg 1992.

Teuscher E, Biogene Arzneimittel, 5. Aufl., Wiss. Verlagsges. mbH Stuttgart 1997.

Wagner H, Wiesenauer M, Phytotherapie. Phytopharmaka und pflanzliche Homöopathika, Fischer-Verlag, Stuttgart, Jena, New York 1995.

Glechoma hederacea

See Ground Ivy

Globe Flower

Trollius europaeus

DESCRIPTION

Medicinal Parts: The medicinal part is the whole fresh plant.

Flower and Fruit: Every branch of the stem bears a solitary, terminal flower. They are up to 5 cm in diameter, globular and have no calyx. The flowers usually have 10 perianth segments. The petals are lemon yellow. The outer petals are occasionally green underneath. They are bent. The stamens are approximately 12 mm long and have a 0.5 to 5 mm long appendage.

Leaves, Stem and Root: The plant is 10 to 70 cm high and glabrous. The stem is hollow, smooth and branched upward. The basal leaves are long-petioled and 3 to 5 lobed. The lobes are cuneate and more or less deeply indented and serrate. The cauline leaves are smaller and more or less sessile.

Habitat: The plant is indigenous to northern and central Europe.

Production: Globe flowers are the flowers of Trollius europaeus.

Other Names: Globe Ranunculus, Globe Crowfoot, Globe Trollius

ACTIONS AND PHARMACOLOGY

COMPOUNDS

Ranunculin: protoanemonine-forming substance in the freshly harvested plant that changes enzymatically when the plant is cut into small pieces. The pungent, volatile protoanemonine quickly dimerizes to the non-mucous membrane irritating anemonine. When dried, the plant is not capable of protoanemonine formation.

Flavonoids

Carotinoids: including neoxanthine (trollixanthine), xanthophyll epoxide

Ascorbic acid (vitamin C)

EFFECTS

No information is available.

INDICATIONS AND USAGE

Unproven Uses: Formerly, the plant was used to treat scurvy. It loses most of its active properties on drying.

PRECAUTIONS AND ADVERSE REACTIONS

No health hazards or side effects are known in conjunction with the proper administration of designated therapeutic dosages. Extended skin contact with the freshly harvested, bruised plant can lead to blisters and cauterizations due to the resulting protoanemonine formation, which is severely irritating to skin and mucous membranes.

If taken internally, severe irritation to the gastrointestinal tract, combined with colic and diarrhea, as well as irritation of the urinary drainage passages, are possible. Because of the very low level of protoanemonine-forming substances in the plant, the danger of poisoning is quite low.

DOSAGE

Mode of Administration: The drug is obsolete.

LITERATURE

Kern W, List PH, Hörhammer L (Hrsg.), Hagers Handbuch der Pharmazeutischen Praxis, 4. Aufl., Bde. 1-8: Springer Verlag Berlin, Heidelberg, New York, 1969.

Roth L, Daunderer M, Kormann K, Giftpflanzen, Pflanzengifte, 4. Aufl., Ecomed Fachverlag Landsberg Lech 1993.

Glycine soja

See Soybean

Glycyrrhiza glabra

See Licorice

Gnaphalium uliginosum

See Cudweed

Goa Powder

Andira araroba

DESCRIPTION

Medicinal Parts: The medicinal part is the dried and pulverized latex of the trunk and branches.

Flower and Fruit: Andira araroba is a large smooth tree whose yellowish wood has vertically running channels and spaces. The latex collects increasingly in these spaces as the tree ages. The bark forms in long flat pieces about 3 mm thick and is grayish-white and fissured externally. The inner surface is brownish and striated. The fracture is laminated with yellow fibers.

Characteristics: The taste is mucilaginous and bitter, and the odor is slight but disagreeable.

Habitat: The tree grows in Brazil.

Production: Goa powder is exuded from the nuclear cavity of Andira araroba. The exuded substance is purified by recrystalization in benzol, thus producing raw chrysarobin.

Other Names: Araroba, Bahia Powder, Brazil Powder, Chrysatobine, Crude Chrysarobin, Ringworm Powder

ACTIONS AND PHARMACOLOGY

COMPOUNDS

Anthrone derivatives: in particular chrysophanolanthrone, dehydroemodine anthrone monomethyl ether, emodine anthrone monomethyl ether, dimerics of these compounds

EFFECTS

The powder is a strong reducing agent. It causes severe erythema upon contact with the skin. It inhibits glucose-6-phosphate-dehydrogenization in psoriatic skin conditions. The drug easily absorbs through the skin.

INDICATIONS AND USAGE

Unproven Uses: Goa Powder is used for psoriasis in chrysarobin ointments and for various kinds of dermatomycosis. It has been widely replaced by synthetic anthranol, which is also used in the treatment of psoriasis.

PRECAUTIONS AND ADVERSE REACTIONS

The drug is severely irritating to skin and mucous membranes (redness, swelling, pustules and conjunctivitis, even without eye contact). Internal administration leads to vomiting, diarrhea and kidney inflammation (with as little as 0.01 g). External administration on large skin areas could cause resorptive poisonings.

DOSAGE

Mode of Administration: Goa Powder is administered topically in emulsion form, but has largely been replaced by the synthetic anthranol cignolin.

LITERATURE

Anonym, Abwehr von Arzneimittelrisiken, Stufe II. In: DAZ 136(38):3253-2354. 1996.

BGA, Arzneimittelrisiken: Anthranoide. In: DAZ 132(21):1164. 1992.

Müller K, Wiegrebe W, Psoriasis und Antipsoriatika. In: DAZ 137(22):1893-1902. 1997.

Further information in:

Kern W, List PH, Hörhammer L (Hrsg.), Hagers Handbuch der Pharmazeutischen Praxis, 4. Aufl., Bde. 1-8, Springer Verlag Berlin, Heidelberg, New York, 1969.

Lewin L, Gifte und Vergiftungen, 6. Aufl., Nachdruck, Haug Verlag, Heidelberg 1992.

Thomson RH, Naturally Occurring Quinones, 2nd Ed., Academic Press New York 1971.

Goat's Rue

Galega officinalis

DESCRIPTION

Medicinal Parts: The medicinal parts are the leaves collected at the beginning of the flowering season and dried, as well as the tips of the flowering branches.

Flower and Fruit: The plant's long-peduncled, axillary racemes are made up of numerous 1 cm long, slightly inclined florets. The petals are bluish-white and short stemmed. The filaments are fused. The fruit is a round, indented pod that grows 2 to 3 cm long and 2 to 3 mm thick, and contains many seeds.

Leaves, Stem and Root: The strong, bright green shrub has numerous 40 cm to 1 m high, erect, branched, hollow stems. It has a divided rhizome with brown fibers sprouting numerous erect, corrugated, round, tall stems. The leaves are odd-pinnate; the leaflets are 1.5 to 4 cm long and 4 to 16 mm wide, elliptical to lanceolate and thorny-tipped with a rich green upper surface and a lighter undersurface.

Characteristics: The plant is odorless unless bruised, whereupon it emits a disagreeable smell, which probably gave rise to the common name Goat's Rue.

Habitat: Goat's Rue grows wild throughout Europe and Asia.

Production: Goat's Rue herb consists of the dried, above-ground parts of Galega officinalis, harvested during the flowering season.

Other Names: Italian Fitch, French Lilac

ACTIONS AND PHARMACOLOGY

COMPOUNDS

Guanidine derivatives: galegine, 4-hydroxygalegine

Quinazoline alkaloids: (+)-peganine

Lectins

Flavonoids: including galuteolin

EFFECTS

The herb contains galegin, which affects blood sugar. *In vitro*, an inhibiting effect on the glucose transport of human epithelium cells has been demonstrated. The reported blood sugar-lowering effect of Goat's Rue herb on humans has not been documented, nor have the reported aggregation-inhibiting, lactagogic and diuretic effects.

INDICATIONS AND USAGE

Unproven Uses: Preparations of Goat's Rue herb are used as a diuretic, and also as supportive therapy for diabetes.

PRECAUTIONS AND ADVERSE REACTIONS

General: Health risks or side effects following the proper administration of designated therapeutic dosages have not been recorded.

Poisonings have only been observed in animals, and then only following the intake of large quantities of the plant. Sheep reportedly experienced salivation, spasms, paralyses and death through asphyxiation following ingestion of inordinate amounts.

Drug Interactions: A possible interaction exists with hypoglycemic medication. Goat's Rue should not be used by diabetics currently maintained with commercial pharmaceutical hypoglycemics.

DOSAGE

Mode of Administration: Since the efficacy for the claimed uses is not documented, therapeutic application cannot be recommended. Goat's Rue cannot be recommended for diabetes mellitus because of the severity of the disease and the availability of effective therapeutic alternatives.

Preparation: To prepare an infusion, pour boiling water over 2 gm of ground drug and strain after 5 to 10 minutes.

Liquid Extract — Drug 1:1

Tincture — 1:10 45% ethanol

LITERATURE

Barthel A, Reuter G, PA 23:26. 1968.

Reuter G, Flora 154:136. 1964.

Schreiber K, Pufahl K, Bräuninger H, Liebigs Ann Chem 671:142. 1964.

Further information in:

Frohne D, Pfänder HJ, Giftpflanzen - Ein Handbuch für Apotheker, Toxikologen und Biologen, 4. Aufl., Wiss. Verlagsges. mbH Stuttgart 1997.

Kern W, List PH, Hörhammer L (Hrsg.), Hagers Handbuch der Pharmazeutischen Praxis, 4. Aufl., Bde. 1-8, Springer Verlag Berlin, Heidelberg, New York, 1969.

Lewin L, Gifte und Vergiftungen, 6. Aufl., Nachdruck, Haug Verlag, Heidelberg 1992.

Madaus G, Lehrbuch der Biologischen Arzneimittel, Bde 1-3, Nachdruck, Georg Olms Verlag Hildesheim 1979.

Poisonous Plants in Britain and Their Effects on Animals and Man, Ministry of Agriculture Fisheries and Food, HMSO, UK 1984.

Roth L, Daunderer M, Kormann K, Giftpflanzen, Pflanzengifte, 4. Aufl., Ecomed Fachverlag Landsberg Lech 1993.

Steinegger E, Hänsel R, Pharmakognosie, 5. Aufl., Springer Verlag Heidelberg 1992.

Teuscher E, Lindequist U, Biogene Gifte - Biologie, Chemie, Pharmakologie, 2. Aufl., Fischer Verlag Stuttgart 1994.

Golden Ragwort

Senecio aureus

DESCRIPTION

Medicinal Parts: The medicinal parts are the fresh plant harvested during the flowering season and the dried herb.

Flower and Fruit: The few capitula are in a loose, many-blossomed corymb that is up to 2.5 cm wide. They are surrounded by a double involucre and consist of 8 to 12 yellow lingual, female florets. There are also numerous androgynous, tubular ray florets, which are somewhat darker.

Leaves, Stem and Root: The perennial plant grows up to 60 cm tall. The rhizome is 2 to 5 cm thick, has numerous thread-like roots, and produces an erect or ascending stem. The root bark is hard and blackish. It surrounds a ring of whitish, woody bundles and a large, dark, central pith. The stem is fluffy-haired when young, later glabrous, and bears alternate leaves. The basal leaves grow up to 15 cm long. They are long-petioled, simple, round, and reniform with a cordate base. The cauline leaves are shorter, incised and pinnatifid, becoming bracts.

Characteristics: The herb has a bitter and astringent taste. The smell is slightly acrid.

Habitat: The plant is indigenous to North America.

Other Names: Squaw Weed, Golden Senecio, Golden Groundsel, Ragwort, Coughweed, Cocash Weed, Grundy Swallow, Life Root

ACTIONS AND PHARMACOLOGY

COMPOUNDS

Pyrrolizidine alkaloids: chief alkaloids are floridanine, florosenine, otosenine

Sesquiterpenes of the eremophilane-type: including among others, ligularenolide, tetrahydroligularenolide, dehydrofukinone, trans-9-oxofuranoeremophilane

Flavonoids: including among others, kaempferol-3-O-glucosyl acetate, quercetin-3-O-glucosyl acetate

EFFECTS

The active agents are seneciionin (aurein), other alkaloids, and resins. The drug has menstruation stimulant, diuretic, and astringent properties, although the mode of action has not been documented. The pyrrolizidine alkaloids are hepatotoxic and carcinogenic.

INDICATIONS AND USAGE

Unproven Uses: Life Root is used for loss of blood (bleeding) and menopausal symptoms.

PRECAUTIONS AND ADVERSE REACTIONS

Life Root should not be taken internally. Hepatotoxicity and carcinogenicity are possible due to the pyrrolizidine alkaloids and 1,2-unsaturated necic parent substances.

DOSAGE

Mode of Administration: Internal use of Life Root is not recommended.

Daily Dosage: The traditional average daily dose of the drug as a liquid extract is 4 g taken 3 to 4 times daily. (See Precautions and Adverse Reactions.)

LITERATURE

Hänsel R, Keller K, Rimpler H, Schneider G (Hrsg.), Hagers Handbuch der Pharmazeutischen Praxis, 5. Aufl., Bde 4-6 (Drogen): Springer Verlag Berlin, Heidelberg, New York, 1992-1994.

Nachmann RJ, PH 22:780-782. 1983.

Resch JF et al., PM 47:255. 1983.

Röder E et al., (1983) Planta Med 49:57.

Röder E, DAZ 132:2427. 1992.

Zalkow LH et al., (1979) J Chem Soc Perkin Trans. 1:1542.

Golden Shower Tree

Cassia fistula

DESCRIPTION

Medicinal Parts: The medicinal parts of the plant are the bark, fruit and seeds.

Flower and Fruit: The flowers are in loose, hanging, 30 to 50 cm long racemes. There are 5 pale yellow, ovate petals. The diameter of the corolla is approximately 3.8 cm. The calyx is deeply divided and 5-toothed. There are 10 stamens. The fruit is a legume, 30 to 60 cm long, hanging and indehiscent.

Leaves, Stem and Root: Cassia fistula is a tree, that grows up to 9 m high. The leaves are 20 to 40 cm long, 4- to 8-paired pinnate. The leaf spindle is hairy and the leaflet is petiolate, ovate to oval, acuminate, 5 to 12 cm long, 4 to 9 cm wide and silvery haired underneath. The young bark is smooth and greenish-gray. Older bark is dark brown and rough.

Habitat: India, Africa and South America

Production: Cassia pods are the dried ripe fruit of Cassia fistula.

Not to be Confused With: Very occasionally the tree has been confused with South American Cassia species.

Other Names: Canafistula, Indian Laburnum, Pudding Pipe Tree, Purging Cassia

ACTIONS AND PHARMACOLOGY

COMPOUNDS

Anthracene derivatives (1% in the mesocarp): sennosides, fistulinic acid

Monosaccharides/oligosaccharides (50%): particularly saccharose

Fruit acids: citric acid

Steroids: sterols (in the seeds), including beta-sitosterol

Fatty oil (in the seeds)

EFFECTS

The anthracene derivatives have a laxative effect. Preparations from the fruit have demonstrated antimicrobial and antiviral effects in vitro.

INDICATIONS AND USAGE

Indian Medicine: Golden Shower Tree is used for flatulence, constipation, fever, anorexia, gout, jaundice, itching and skin conditions. Efficacy for constipation is plausible because of the anthranoid content; the other indications have not been proven.

CONTRAINDICATIONS

The drug is contraindicated with ileum, acute-inflammatory diseases of the intestine and appendicitis. It is also contraindicated for children under 12 years of age and for women during pregnancy or while nursing.

PRECAUTIONS AND ADVERSE REACTIONS

No health hazards are known in conjunction with the proper administration of designated therapeutic dosages. The question of the increase in probability of the appearance of carcinomas in the colon following long-term administration of Anthracene drugs has not yet been fully clarified. Recent studies, however, have revealed no connection between the administration of Anthracene drugs and the frequency of carcinomas of the colon.

OVERDOSAGE

In the case of overdose, cramp-like gastrointestinal complaints could occur as a side effect of the laxative effect of the drug. Prolonged administration leads to loss of electrolytes, particularly of potassium ions, which in turn leads to aldosteronism, albuminuria, hematuria, inhibition of intestinal motility, muscle weakness, enhancement of the effect of cardioactive steroids and an influence upon the effect of antiarrhythmics. In rare cases, administration of the drug may lead to cardiac arrhythmia, nephropathy, edema and accelerated osteoclasis.

DOSAGE

Mode of Administration: Whole drug preparations are for internal use.

Preparation: To prepare an extract, use pulp and distilled water in a 1:1 ratio, macerate, then exhaustively percolate with distilled water and filter. Evaporate to a soft extract.

Daily Dosage: 4 to 8 gm of fruit pulp

LITERATURE

el-Saadany SS, el-Massry RA, Labib SM, Sitohy MZ, The biochemical role and hypocholesterolaemic potential of the legume Cassia fistula in hypercholesterolaemic rats. Nahrung, 35:807-15, 1991.

Espósito Avella M, Díaz A, de Gracia I, de Tello R, Gupta MP, Evaluation of traditional medicine: effects of Cajanus cajan L. and of Cassia fistula L. on carbohydrate metabolism in mice. Rev Med Panama, 16:39-45, 1991 Jan.

Espósito Avella M, Díaz A, de Gracia I, de Tello R, Gupta MP, Studies on the possibilities to infect the cells of callus of Cassia fistula by an animal virus & induce production of interferon-like antiviral factor(s). Indian J Exp Biol, 16:349-55, 1981 Apr.

Hänsel R, Keller K, Rimpler H, Schneider G (Ed), Hagers Handbuch der Pharmazeutischen Praxis, 5. Aufl., Bde 4 - 6 (Drogen), Springer Verlag Berlin, Heidelberg, New York, 1992-1994.

Goldenseal

Hydrastis canadensis

TRADE NAMES

Golden Seal, Goldenseal (Available from numerous manufacturers), Goldenseal Power, Golden Seal Herb, Golden Seal Root, Golden Seal Plus, Goldenseal Root Alcohol Free, Herbal Sure Goldenseal Root

DESCRIPTION

Medicinal Parts: The medicinal parts are the air-dried rhizome with the root fibers.

Flower and Fruit: The flower is small, solitary, terminal and erect. It has 3 small greenish white petals which drop as soon as they come out. The fruit is a group of small, fleshy, oblong carmine berries with 1 or 2 hard, black and glossy seeds. The fruit is similar to the raspberry but is not edible.

Leaves, Stem and Root: The plant is a low herbaceous perennial about 30 cm high. It has a horizontal bright yellow, knotty and twisted rhizome about 0.6 to 1.8 cm thick out of which the root fibers grow. It is folded longitudinally and encircled by old leaf scars. The fracture is short and shows a dark, yellow cut surface, thick bark, large pith and broad medullary rays. The flowering stem appears in spring and is erect, cylindrical, downward pubescent, 15 to 30 cm tall and has a few short brown scales at the base. It bears 2 clearly ribbed, dark green and pubescent, cauline leaves. The lower one is sessile the upper one petiolate, round and divided into 7 lobes and finely serrate. There is also a root leaf on a long petiole, which is similar to the cauline leaves but larger.

Characteristics: The taste is very bitter, the smell is strong, characteristic and disagreeable.

Habitat: Indigenous to the U.S., cultivated elsewhere.

Production: Goldenseal root is the rhizome of Hydrastis canadensis. The root is dug up in the autumn and dried.

Not to be Confused With: Goldenseal is often adulterated with Bloodroot.

Other Names: Orange Root, Yellow Root, Yellow Puccoon, Ground Raspberry, Wild Curcuma, Turmeric Root, Indian Dye, Eye Root, Eye Balm, Indian Paint, Jaundice Root, Warnera, Indian Plant

ACTIONS AND PHARMACOLOGY

COMPOUNDS

Isoquinoline alkaloids: chief alkaloids hydrastine (1.5 to 4%), berberine (0.5 to 6%), (-)-canadine (0.5%)

Starch

EFFECTS

Many of the studies that have been conducted focus on the berberine and hydrastine componants that are found not only in Goldenseal, but also in numerous other herbs commonly used in Chinese and Indian medicine. The effects reported here focus on these componants and not necessarily the Goldenseal in it's raw form.

Berberine sulfate has been shown to inhibit the growth of *Entamoeba histolytica, Giardia lamblia* and *Trichomonas vaginalis, in vitro.* The parasites all exhibited morphological changes after exposure to berberine sulfate (Kaneda, 1991). In one experiment by Swab et al (1981), berberine hydrochloride reduced the cholera toxin-induced secretion of water, sodium and chloride in perfused rat ileum. Berberine was also found to inhibit the intestinal secretory response of *Vibrio cholerae* and *Escherichia coli* enterotoxins without causing histological damage to the intestinal mucosa (Sack, 1982). Berberine is also active against other intestinal infections that cause aute diarrhea such as *Shigella dysenteriae, Salmonella paratyphi* and various *Klebsiella species.* Berberine sulfate has been shown to block the adherence of *Streptococcus pyrogenes* and *E. coli* to host cells, possibly explaining it's mechanism of action against numerous pathogens (Sun, 1988).

Berberine was found to be the active constituent in an extract of Hydrastis canadensis root that demonstrated activity against a multiple drug-resistant strain of *Mycobacterium tuberculosis* (Gentry, 1998). Berberine also inhibits *Helicobacter pylori* (Bae, 1998).

Berberine has a long history of use for eye infections. In one study that looked at effectiveness in treating trachoma, berberine was more effective than sulfacetamide in eradicating *Chlamydia trachomatis* from the eye and preventing relapse of symptoms (Babbar, 1982; Mohan, 1982).

Berberine has a choleretic (bile-stimlating) effect and has been shown to lower bilirubin levels (Chan, 1977).

Berberine inhibited the effects of tumor promotors on the skin using a mouse model (Nishino, 1986). There is evidence that berberine also has a direct tumor killing effect and has the ability to stimulate production of white blood cells (Zhang, 1990; Liu, 1991).

Berberine has hypotensive, antisecretory and sedative effects. The mechanism for these effects may be explained by the fact that berberine has platelet alpha 2 adrenoceptor agonist activity that is similar to that of clonidine (Hui, 1984).

CONTRAINDICATIONS

Goldenseal is contraindicated in pregnancy.

Goldenseal is contraindicated in people with glucose-6-phosphate-dehydrogenase deficiency (Chan, 1993).

INDICATIONS AND USAGE

Unproven Uses: Goldenseal is used as an antiseptic externally on wounds and *herpes labialis.* It is also used for gastritis and as an astringent. The berberine componant is used to treat acute diarrhea caused by numerous gastrointestinal pathogens. Berberine is also used as an adjunct treatment in various cancers and in neutropenia resulting from radiation and chemotherapy. Berberine has been used to treat trachoma, gastric ulcers and gallbladder disease.

Homeopathic Uses: In homeopathic dilutions, Hydrastis canadensis is used for the treatment of irregular menstruation, digestive problems and bronchitis.

PRECAUTIONS AND ADVERSE REACTIONS

General: If taken over an extended period, the drug can bring about digestive disorders, mucous membrane irritation, constipation, excitatory states, hallucinations and occasionally deliria.

Pregnancy: Goldenseal should not be taken during pregnancy.

Drug Interactions: Berberine has an antagonistic effect on the anticoagulant activity of heparin (Preininger, 1975).

There have been reports of decreased vitamin B absorption with higher doses of Goldenseal (Tierra, 1980).

Drug/Laboratory Interactions: At one time it was believed that Goldenseal could mask the detection of tetrahydrocannabinol (THC/Marijuana) in illicit drug urinalysis. This effect has since been disproved (Mikkelsen & Ash, 1988).

OVERDOSAGE

The LD50 for berberine in rats was found to be greater than 1,000 mg/kg of body weight making the toxicity of this componant in Goldenseal very low (Haldon, 1975). The hydrastine componant appears to be the toxic compound in Goldenseal. High doses result in strychnine-like convulsions and gastrointestinal relaxation (Osol & Garrar, 1955). Other effects of overdose that have been reported include difficulty in breathing, bradycardia and central paralysis.

Following stomach and intestinal emptying (inducement of vomiting, gastric lavage with burgundy-colored potassium permanganate solution, sodium sulfate) the treatment for poisonings consists of the instillation of activated charcoal and shock prophylaxis (quiet, warmth). The treatment of spasms with diazepam (I.V.), electrolyte substitution and the countering of any acidosis imbalance that may appear with sodium bicarbonate infusions may be necessary. In the event of shock, plasma volume expanders should be infused. Intubation and oxygen respiration may also be required.

DOSAGE

Daily Dosage:

Extract — Standardized extract (5% hydrastine) 250-500 mg 3 times daily (Werbach & Murray, 1994)

Fluid extract — 1/4 to 1 teaspoonful (1.25-5 ml) (Grieve, 1971)

Solid extract — 325-520 mg (Grieve, 1971)

Local antiseptic — 1 teaspoonful powder steeped in 1 cup boiling water for 15 minutes. Swish around the mouth or gargle for mouth or throat sores (Tyler, 1997).

Travelers diarrhea — One capsule (500-1000 mg root) 3 times daily (Tyler, 1997)

Storage: Store at room temperature. Avoid moisture, high temperatures and direct light.

LITERATURE

Babbar OP, Chhatwal VK, Ray IB et al: Effect of berberine chloride eye drops on clinically positive trachoma patients. Ind J Med Res 76(suppl):83-88. 1982.

Bae EA, Han MJ, Kim NJ et al: Anti-helicobacter pylori activity of herbal medicines. Biol Pharmaceut Bull 21(9):990-992. 1998.

Chan MY: The effect of berberine on bilirubin excretion in the rat. Comp Med East West 5:161-168. 1977.

Galefi C et al., Canadinic acid: an alkaloid from Hydrastis canadensis. In: PM 63(2):194. 1997.

Gentry EJ, Jampani HB, Keshavarz-Shokri A et al: Antitubercular natural products: berberine from the roots of commercial Hydrastis canadensis powder. J Nat Prod 61(10):1187-1193. 1998.

Gleye J et al., (1974) Phytochemistry 13:675.

Grieve M: A Modern Herbal. Dover Publications, Inc, New York, New York, p 362-364. 1971.

Haginiwa J, Harada M, (1962) Yakugaku Zasshi 82:726.

Haldon B: Toxicity of berberine sulfate. Acta Pol Pharm 32:113-120. 1975.

Hui K, Yu J, Chan W, Tse E: Interaction of berberine with human platelet alpha 2 adrenoceptors. Life Sci 49(4): 315-24. 1991.

Kaneda Y, Torii M & Tanaka T: In vitro effects of berberine sulfate on the growth of Entamoeba histolytica, Giardia lamblia and Tricomonas vaginalis. Ann Trop Med Parasitol 85:417-425. 1991.

Kern W, List PH, Hörhammer L (Hrsg.), Hagers Handbuch der Pharmazeutischen Praxis, 4. Aufl., Bde 1-8, Springer Verlag Berlin, Heidelberg, New York, 1969.

Leung AY, Encyclopedia of Common Natural Ingredients Used in Food, Drugs and Cosmetics, John Wiley & Sons Inc., New York 1980.

Lewin L, Gifte und Vergiftungen, 6. Aufl., Nachdruck, Haug Verlag, Heidelberg 1992.

Liu CX et al: Studies on plant resources, pharmacology and clinical treatment with berbamine. Phytother Res 5:228-230. 1991.

Madaus G, Lehrbuch der Biologischen Arzneimittel, Bde 1-3, Nachdruck, Georg Olms Verlag Hildesheim 1979.

Mikkelsen SL & Ash KO: Adulterants causing false negatives in illicit drug testing. Clin Chem 34:2333-2336. 1988.

Mohan M, Pant CR, Angra SK et al: Berberine in trachoma. Ind J Opthalmol 30:69-75. 1982.

Nishino H, Kitagawa K, Fujiki H et al: Berberine sulfate inhibits tumor-promoting activity of teleocidin in two stage carcinogenesis on mouse skin. Oncology 43:131-134. 1986.

Osol A & Farrar CG (eds): The Dispensatory of the United States of America, 25th ed. JB Lippincott Company, Philadelphia, PA, USA, pp 660-661. 1955.

Preininger V: The pharmacology and toxicology of the Papaveraceae alkaloids, in Manske RHF & Holmes HL (eds): The Alkaloids, Vol. 15. Academic Press, p 239. 1975.

Roth L, Daunderer M, Kormann K, Giftpflanzen, Pflanzengifte, 4. Aufl., Ecomed Fachverlag Landsberg Lech 1993.

Sack RB & Froehlich JL: Berberine inhibits intestinal secretory response of Vibrio cholerae toxins and Escherichia coli enterotoxins. Infect Immun 35:471-475. 1982.

Steinegger E, Hänsel R, Pharmakognosie, 5. Aufl., Springer Verlag Heidelberg 1992.

Sun D, Courtney HS & Beachey EH: Berberine sulfate blocks adherence of Streptococcus pyogenes to epithelial cells, fibronectin, and hexadecane. Antimicrob Agents Chemother 32:1370-1374. 1988.

Swabb EA, Tai YH & Jordan L: Reversal of cholera toxin-induced secretion in rat ileum by luminal berberine. Am J Physiol 1981; 241:G248-252.

Tierra M: The Way of Herbs. Unity Press, Santa Cruz, CA, USA, 1980.

Tyler VE: The Honest Herbal. George F Stickley Company, Philadelphia, PA, USA, pp 111-112. 1982.

Tyler VE: Golden Seal: can this herb boost immunity. Prevention July:68-70. 1997.

Wagner H, Wiesenauer M, Phytotherapie. Phytopharmaka und pflanzliche Homöopathika, Fischer-Verlag, Stuttgart, Jena, New York 1995.

Zhang RX, Dougherty DV & Rosenblum ML: Laboratory studies of berberine used alone and in combination with 1,3-bis(2-chloroethyl)-1-nitrosourea to treat malignant brain tumors. Chinese Med J 103:658-665. 1990.

Goldthread

Coptis trifolia

DESCRIPTION

Medicinal Parts: The medicinal parts are the rhizome and sometimes the stems and leaves.

Flower and Fruit: The solitary flowers are small and white, and are arranged on leafless scapes.

Leaves, Stem and Root: Goldthread is a perennial plant in bushes of up to 15 cm with yellowish, scaly leaves at the base and long-petioled, obovate, evergreen leaves. The rhizome is thread-like, golden yellow with a matte surface and very small roots.

Characteristics: Goldthread has a very bitter taste and slight odor.

Habitat: Coptis trifolia is indigenous to India and Coptis groenlandica, which is also used, is indigenous to Greenland and Iceland.

Production: Goldthread rhizome is the rhizome of Coptis trifolia.

Other Names: Mouth Root, Cankerroot, Yellowroot, Coptis, Coptide, Coptis Groenlandica

ACTIONS AND PHARMACOLOGY

COMPOUNDS

Isoquinoline alkaloids (6 to 9%): including coptin, berberine

EFFECTS

The herb is a bitter tonic.

INDICATIONS AND USAGE

Unproven Uses: Goldthread is used in digestive disorders.

PRECAUTIONS AND ADVERSE REACTIONS

General: Health risks or side effects following the proper administration of designated therapeutic dosages are not recorded.

Berberine has a mutagenic effect upon yeast cells and in the Ames test (intercalation into the DNA), although that does not necessarily mean a mutagenic effect for the drug when administered to humans.

Pregnancy: Not to be used during pregnancy.

DOSAGE

Mode of Administration: Internally as a powdered drug or a liquid extract.

LITERATURE

Hegnauer R Chemotaxonomie der Pflanzen. Bde 1-11, Birkhäuser Verlag Basel, Boston, Berlin 1962-1997.

Kern W, List PH, Hörhammer L (Ed), Hagers Handbuch der Pharmazeutischen Praxis. 4. Aufl., Bde. 1-8, Springer Verlag Berlin, Heidelberg, New York 1969.

Gossypium herbaceum

See Levant Cotton

Gossypium hirsutum

See Cotton

Gotu Kola

Centella asiatica

TRADE NAMES

Gotu Kola (available from numerous manufacturers and as a combination product), Gotu Kola Herb, Wild Countryside Gotu Kola, Natural Herbal Gotu Kola, Alcohol Free Gotu Kola Herb

DESCRIPTION

Medicinal Parts: The medicinal parts are the dried above-ground parts, the fresh and dried leaves and stem.

Flower and Fruit: The pedicles are 1.2 to 4 cm long. The sepals of the epicalyx are oval to circular, with a membranous border. They are about 2.5 to 3 mm long and 1.5 to 2.5 mm wide. The umbels have 2 or 3 sessile or short-pedicled florets. The petals are white, to purple or pink. The calyx is not generally dentate. The fruit is oval to globular in shape, and has a diameter of 2 to 5 mm. The mericarps are clearly flattened at the sides and usually have 7 to 9 ribs and are raised rugose.

Leaves, Stem and Root: Centella asiatica is a tender umbel plant, which has numerous creeping stems. The stems have roots at the nodes, which are smooth. The circular-reniform leaves are 2 to 6 cm long and 1.5 to 5 wide, with a crenate margin and 5 to 9 ribs. The petioles are 3 to 30 cm long.

Characteristics: Gotu Kola is almost tasteless and odorless.

Habitat: The plant is indigenous to southeast Asia, India, Sri Lanka, parts of China, the western South Sea Islands, Madagascar, South Africa, southeast U.S., Mexico, Venezuela, Columbia, and eastern South America.

Production: Hydrocotyle herb is the aerial part of Centella asiatica. The plant is gathered throughout the year and dried in the sun.

Other Names: Indian Pennywort, Marsh Penny, Indian Hydrocotyle, White Rot, Thick-leaved Pennywort, Hydrocotyle

ACTIONS AND PHARMACOLOGY

COMPOUNDS

Triterpene acids: including asiatic acid, madecassic acid (6-hydroxy asiatic acid), terminolic acid

Triterpene acid ester from oligosaccharides (pseudosaponins): including asiaticoside, asiaticoside A, asiaticoside B

Volatile oil (0.1%)

EFFECTS

The main constituents of the drug are triterpene acids and their sugar residues (asiaticoside and madegassoside).

Anti-Inflammatory Effects

Anti-inflammatory effects exerted by extracts of Centella asiatica were demonstrated by a reduction of acute radiation reaction in rats (Chen, 1999).

Anti-Neoplastic Effects

Cytotoxic and antitumor effects of Centella asiatica involve direct action on DNA synthesis. The development of solid and ascites tumors was decreased by the herb (Babu, 1985).

Ulcer-protective Effects

Asiaticoid (suspended in propylene glycol) administered orally to rats, significantly reduced the formation of stress-induced ulcers (Ravokatra, 1993). An extract of the herb also significantly inhibited gastric ulceration induced by cold and restraint stress in animal models. The dose dependent reduction of gastric ulceration was associated with a dose dependent increase of the GABA level in the brain (Chatterjee, 1992).

Vascular/Venous Tone Effects

Ethanol extracts of Centella asiatica, *in vitro*, had a remarkable enhancement of fibroblast cell attachment and tissue plasminogen activator (Kim, 1993). Varicose veins are associated with increased uronic acid and lysosomal enzymes involved with mucopolysaccharide (beta-glycuronidase, beta-N-acetylglucosaminidase) metabolism. Total triterpenic fraction of Centella asiatica (TTFCA) decreases uronic acid, beta-glycuronidase, beta-N-acetylglucosaminidase, and arysulfatase in the connective tissue and vascular wall (Arpaia, 1990).

Wound Healing Effects

Asiaticoside facilitates wound healing through an increase in peptidic hydroxyproline content, tensile strength, collagen synthesis, angiogenesis and epithelialization, as shown in animal models (Bonte, 1994; Maquart, 1990; Shukla, 1999). Asiatic acid and madecassic have also demonstrated an increase in peptidic hydroxyproline showing an increased remodeling of the collagen matrix (collagen synthesis) in wounds (Bonte, 1994; Maquart, 1999). Asiaticoside also induces enzymatic and non-emzymatic antioxidants, namely superoxide dismutase, catalase, glutathione peroxidase, vitamin E, and ascorbic acid in newly formed tissue (initial stage of wound healing) (Shukla, 1999).

CLINICAL TRIALS

Chronic Venous Insufficiency

A randomized, double-blind, placebo-controlled study evaluated the efficacy of a titrated extract of Centella asiatica in treating chronic venous insufficiency. Ninety-four patients with chronic venous insufficiency were included in the study. The asiaticoid mixture, administered as 60 mg daily and 120 mg daily for 2 months, led to significant improvement in subjective (heaviness in the legs, pain in standing up, edema) and objective (plethysmographic measurements of vein tone) parameters compared to placebo (Pointel, 1987).

Venous Hypertension

The effect of an extract of Centella asiatica with capillary filtration and ankle edema was evaluated in patients with venous hypertension. Sixty-two patients were included in the study and administered either placebo or the extract as 60 mg or 30 mg three times daily. Capillary filtration rate and ankle edema both significantly improved in a dose-dependent manner in the extract-treatment groups. The subjective symptoms (swelling, sensation, restless lower extremity, pain and cramps, and tiredness) were significantly improved in the extract-treatment groups, with no change in the placebo-treatment group (Belcaro, 1990).

INDICATIONS AND USAGE

Unproven Uses: The drug is used internally for rheumatism and skin diseases. Externally, the drug is used for poorly healing wounds, leprosy sores, and post-operative scarring. In Asia, the drug is used to enhance urination, for physical and mental exhaustion, diarrhea, eye diseases, inflammations, asthma, and high blood pressure.

Indian Medicine: The drug is used for skin diseases, syphilis, rheumatism, and leprosy. Gotu kola is also used for the treatment of mental illness, epilepsy, hysteria, and for dehydration.

Chinese Medicine: The herb is used for dysentery and summer diarrhea, vomiting, jaundice, urinary calculi, epistaxis and scabies.

Homeopathic Uses: Gotu Kola is used for skin diseases associated with itching and swelling and inflammation of the uterus.

PRECAUTIONS AND ADVERSE REACTIONS

Allergic Contact Dermatitis: Although there have been case reports of allergic contact dermatitis due to Centella asiatica, the plant's sensitizing capacity is considered low (Bilbao, 1995; Danese, 1994; Gonzalo, 1996; Hausen, 1993).

DOSAGE

Mode of Administration: Gotu Kola is available in liquid or solid pharmaceutical forms, for oral intake. Gotu Kola is also available parenterally for homeopathic use.

How Supplied:

Capsules — 400 mg, 435 mg, 439 mg, 440 mg, 450 mg, 500 mg

Liquid — 1:1; 250 mg/ml

Daily Dosage: 0.6 gm of dried leaves or infusion taken 3 times daily; normal single dose is 0.33 to 0.68 gm.

Varicose Veins — Centella asiatica extract administered as 60 mg daily has shown improvement (Arpaia, 1990).

Venous Hypertension — Total triterpenic fraction of centella asiatica (TTFCA) tablets have demonstrated improvement of venous hypertension at doses of 30 mg given three times daily or 60 mg given three times daily (Belcaro, 1990).

Chronic Venous Insufficiency — Titrated extract of Centella asiatica (TECA) administered as 120 mg daily and 60 mg daily have demonstrated efficacy in chronic venous insufficiency (Pointel, 1987).

Homeopathic Dosage: 5 to 10 drops, 1 tablet, 5 to 10 globules or 1 ml injection solution sc twice weekly; ointment 1 to 2 times daily (HAB1).

Storage: Store in a cool, dry place and in well-sealed containers.

LITERATURE

Asakawa Y et al., (1982) Phytochemistry 21(10):2590.

Allegra G et al., (1981) Clin Terap. 99:507.

Arpaia MR, Ferrone R, Amitrano M, Nappo C, Leonardo G, del Guercio R, Effects of Centella asiatica extract on mucopolysaccharide metabolism in subjects with varicose veins. Int J Clin Pharmacol Res, 10:229-33, 1990

Babu TD, Kuttan G, Padikkala J, Cytotoxic and anti-tumour properties of certain taxa of Umbelliferae with special reference to Centella asiatica (L.) Urban. J Ethnopharmacol, 48:53-7, 1995 Aug 11.

Belcaro GV; Rulo A; Grimaldi R. Capillary filtration and ankle edema in patients with venous hypertension treated with TTFCA. Angiology 1990 Jan;41(1):12-8.

Belcaro GV; Grimaldi R; Guidi G. Improvement of capillary permeability in patients with venous hypertension after treatment with TTFCA. Angiology 1990 Jul;41(7):533-40.

Bilbao I; Aguirre A; Zabala R et al. Allergic contact dermatitis from butoxyethyl nicotinic acid and Centella asiatica extract. Contact Dermatitis 1995 Dec;33(6):435-6.

Bonte F; Dumas M; Chaudagne C; Meybeck A, Influence of asiatic acid, madecassic acid, and asiaticoside on human collagen I synthesis. Planta Med 1994 Apr;60(2):133-5.

Bossé JP et al., (1979) Ann Plastic Surg 3(1):13.

Brevoort P, Der Heilpflanzenmarkt der USA - Ein Überblick. In: ZPT 18(3):155-162. 1997.

Castellani C et al., Boll Chim Farm 120:570-605. 1981.

Chatterjee TK; Chakraborty A; Pathak M; Sengupta GC. Effects of plant extract Centella asiatica (Linn.) on cold restraint stress ulcer in rats. Indian J Exp Biol 1992 Oct;30(10):889-91.

Chen YJ; Dai YS; Chen BF et al. The effect of tetrandrine and extracts of Centella asiatica on acute radiation dermatitis in rats. Biol Pharm Bull 1999 Jul;22(7):703-6.

Danese P; Carnevali C; Bertazzoni MG. Allergic contact dermatitis due to Centella asiatica extract. Contact Dermatitis 1994 Sep;31(3):201.

Di Carlo FI et al., (1964) J Reticuloendothelial Soc 1:224.

Dutta T, Basu UP, (1968) Ind J Exp Biol 6(3):181.

Dutta T, Basu UP, (1967) Ind J Chem 5:586.

Dutta T, Basu UP, Bull Nat Inst Sci India 37:178-184. 1968.

Gonzalo Garijo MA, Revenga Arranz F, Bobadilla Gonzalez P, Allergic contact dermatitis due to Centella asiatica: a new case. Allergol Immunopathol (Madr), 24:132-4, 1996 May-Jun.

Grimaldi R et al., Pharmacokinetics of the total triterpenic fraction of Centella asiatica after single and multiple administrations to healthy volunteers. A new assay for asiatic acid. J Ethnopharmacol, 24:235-41, 1990 Feb.

Hänsel R, Keller K, Rimpler H, Schneider G (Hrsg.), Hagers Handbuch der Pharmazeutischen Praxis, 5. Aufl., Bde 4-6 (Drogen), Springer Verlag Berlin, Heidelberg, New York, 1992-1994.

Hausen B, Allergiepflanzen, Pflanzenallergene, ecomed Verlagsgesellsch. mbH, Landsberg 1988.

Hausen BM. Centella asiatica (Indian pennywort), an effective therapeutic but a weak sensitizer. Contact Dermatitis 1993 Oct;29(4):175-9.

Kim YN; Park YS; Kim HK et al. Enhancement of the attachment on microcarriers and tPA production by fibroblast cells in a serum-free medium by the addition of the extracts of Centella asiatica. Cytotechnology 1993;13(3):221-6.

Madaus G, Lehrbuch der Biologischen Arzneimittel, Bde 1-3, Nachdruck, Georg Olms Verlag Hildesheim 1979.

Maquart FX, Bellon G, Gillery P, Wegrowski Y, Borel JP, Stimulation of collagen synthesis in fibroblast cultures by a triterpene extracted from Centella asiatica. Connect Tissue Res, 24:107-20, 1990.

Maquart FX; Chastang F; Simeon A et al., Triterpenes from Centella asiatica stimulate extracellular matrix accumulation in rat experimental wounds. Eur J Dermatol 1999 Jun;9(4):289-96.

Montecchio GP, Samaden A, Carbone S, Vigotti M, Siragusa S, Piovella F, Centella asiatica Triterpenic Fraction (CATTF) reduces the number of circulating endothelial cells in subjects with post phlebitic syndrome. Haematologica, 48:256-9, 1991 May-Jun.

Pointel JP; Boccalon H; Cloarec M et al., Titrated extract of Centella asiatica (TECA) in the treatment of venous-insufficiency of the lower limbs. Angiology 1987 Jan;38(1 Pt 1):46-5.

Rao PS, Seshardri TR, (1969) Curr. Sci 38:77.

Ravokatra A; Loiseau A; Ratsimamanga-Urverg S et al., Action of asiaticoside (pentacyclic triterpene) extracted from Hydrocotyle madagascariensis on duodenal ulcers induced with mercaptoethylamine in male Wistar rats. C R Acad Sci Hebd Seances Acad Sci D 1974 Apr 29;278(18):2317-21.

Roth L, Daunderer M, Kormann K, Giftpflanzen, Pflanzengifte, 4. Aufl., Ecomed Fachverlag Landsberg Lech 1993.

Shukla A; Rasik AM; Jain GK et al. In vitro and in vivo wound healing activity of asiaticoside isolated from Centella asiatica. J Ethnopharmacol 1999 Apr;65(1):1-11.

Shukla A; Rasik AM; Dhawan BN. Asiaticoside-induced elevation of antioxidant levels in healing wounds. Phytother Res 1999 Feb;13(1):50-4.

Steinegger E, Hänsel R, Pharmakognosie, 5. Aufl., Springer Verlag Heidelberg 1992.

Suguna L, Sivakumar P, Chandrakasan G, Effects of Centella asiatica extract on dermal wound healing in rats. Indian J Exp Biol, 24:1208-11, 1996 Dec

Tang W, Eisenbrand G, Chinese Drugs of Plant Origin, Springer Verlag Heidelberg 1992.

Vecchaio AD et al., (1984) Farm Ed Prat 39(10):355.

Wagner H, Wiesenauer M, Phytotherapie. Phytopharmaka und pflanzliche Homöopathika, Fischer-Verlag, Stuttgart, Jena, New York 1995.

Goutweed

Aegopodium podagraria

DESCRIPTION

Flower and Fruit: The flowers range from 50 to 100 cm. They have large white or reddish double umbels that are usually androgynous. The flowers have no involucre and no calyx. The petals are white or pink, about 1.5 mm long, obcordate and cuneate at the base. The fruit is oblong and brownish with pale veins. The fruit is slightly pressed in at the sides, unwinged, unstriped, with a 3 mm-long mericarp.

Leaves, Stem and Root: The stem is erect, angular, grooved, hollow, glabrous and branched. The lower leaves are double trifoliate, and the upper leaves trifoliate. The leaflets are ovate and crenate-serrate.

Characteristics: Propagates via underground runners.

Habitat: Indigenous to Europe (not Spain), West Asia.

Production: Goutweed is the aerial part of Aegopodium podagraria.

Other Names: Goutwort, Ground Elder, Gout Herb, Herb Gerard(e), Jack-Jump-About, Goatweed, Ashweed, Achweed, English Masterwort, Pigweed, Eltroot, Bishop's Elder, Weyl Ash, White Ash, Bishopsweed, Bishopswort.

ACTIONS AND PHARMACOLOGY

COMPOUNDS

Volatile oil

Polyynes: only in freshly-harvested leaves

Flavonol glycosides: including hyperoside, isoquercitrin

Caffeic acid derivatives: including chlorogenic acid

Ascorbic acid

EFFECTS

No information available.

INDICATIONS AND USAGE

Unproven Uses: The herb is used internally as an infusion for gout and rheumatic diseases. It is used externally in macerations for poultices and baths for hemorrhoids, gout and rheumatic diseases, as well as for kidney and bladder disorders and intestinal disorders.

PRECAUTIONS AND ADVERSE REACTIONS

No health hazards or side effects are known in conjunction with the proper administration of designated therapeutic dosages.

DOSAGE

Mode of Administration: Internally as a tea; externally, the fresh herb is squeezed for poultices.

Daily Dosage: There is no exact dosage. A daily recommended dose consists of 1 to 2 dessertspoonfuls (30ml) of the juice of the fresh plant.

LITERATURE

Bohlmann F et al., Chem Ber 93, 981. 1968.

Hänsel R, Keller K, Rimpler H, Schneider G (Hrsg.), Hagers Handbuch der Pharmazeutischen Praxis, 5. Aufl., Bde 4-6 (Drogen), Springer Verlag Berlin, Heidelberg, New York, 1992-1994.

Harborne JB, Williams CA, PH 11(5):1741-1750. 1972.

Schneider V, Ernähr-Umschau 31(2):54-57. 1984.

Grains-of-Paradise

Aframomum melegueta

DESCRIPTION

Medicinal Parts: The medicinal parts are the ripe seeds.

Flower and Fruit: The flowers are solitary, mauve and wax-like. The fruit is 10 cm long, pear-shaped and scarlet. The seeds are small, hard, shiny, reddish-brown and oyster-shaped. They have an aromatic and pungent taste and smell.

Leaves, Stem and Root: Aframomum melegueta is a reed-like plant, 1 to 2.5 m high. The leaves are long and narrow.

Habitat: The plant is indigenous to tropical West Africa.

Not to be Confused With: The seeds can be mistaken for peppercorns.

Other Names: Guinea Grains, Melegueta Pepper, Mallaguetta Pepper

ACTIONS AND PHARMACOLOGY

COMPOUNDS

Volatile oil

Pungent substances: including hydroxyphenylalkanones and hydroxyphenylalkanoles

Tannins

Starch

Fatty oil

EFFECTS

The seed is a stimulant.

INDICATIONS AND USAGE

Unproven Uses: Grains-of-Paradise was used as a stimulant. Now it is obsolete as a drug.

PRECAUTIONS AND ADVERSE REACTIONS

No health hazards or side effects are known in conjunction with the proper administration of designated therapeutic dosages.

OVERDOSAGE

Due to the constituent pungent substances, the intake of larger dosages may lead to irritation of the stomach and the urinary tract.

LITERATURE

Connell WD, J Chem 23:369. 1970.

Hoppe HA, (1975-1987) Drogenkunde, 8. Aufl., Bde 1-3, W. de Gruyter Verlag, Berlin, New York.

Kern W, List PH, Hörhammer L (Hrsg.), Hagers Handbuch der Pharmazeutischen Praxis, 4. Aufl., Bde. 1-8, Springer Verlag Berlin, Heidelberg, New York, 1969.

Grape

Vitis vinifera

TRADE NAMES

Grape Seed Extract (Available from numerous manufacturers), Red Wine Extract, Grape Seed, Activin, Dr. Masquelier's Authentic OPC

DESCRIPTION

Medicinal Parts: The medicinal parts are the leaves, the fruit and the juice.

Flower and Fruit: The flowers are in compound compact panicles. The petals are about 5 mm long and droop like the sepals. The fruit is oblong to globular, 6 to 22 mm long, dark blue-violet, red, green or yellow, juicy, sweet or sour. The seeds are pear-shaped, with hard skin and two long dimples on the side.

Leaves, Stem and Root: The vine is a 30 cm high climber with deep, heavily-branched roots and a woody trunk. The trunk has striped, loose bark. The brown-red to brown-yellow branches are glabrous or slightly downy and finely grooved. The leaves are orbicular, generally in 3 to 5 lobes or blades. They are deeply notched at the stem. The upper surface of the leaves is glabrous, the under surface is lanate.

Habitat: The plant is indigenous to southern Europe and western Asia and is cultivated today in all temperate regions of the world.

Production: Vine leaves are the foliage leaves of Vitis vinifera.

ACTIONS AND PHARMACOLOGY

COMPOUNDS

Flavonoids (4 to 5%): including, kaempferol-3-O-glucosides, quercetin-3-O-glucosides

Tannins: procyanidolic oligomers (proanthocyanidins), including constituent monomers of catechin epicatechin

Non-flavonoids (Stilbenes): resveratrol and viniferins

Fruit acids: including, tartaric acid, malic acid, succinic acid, citric acid, oxalic acid

Phenylacrylic acid derivatives: p-cumaroyl acid, caffeoyl acid, feruloylsuccinic acid

EFFECTS

Antiatherosclerotic Effects: The oxidation of low-density lipoproteins (LDL) by free radicals is associated with the initiation of atherosclerosis. Proanthocyanidin decreases the number of LDL-positive macrophage-derived foam cells in atherosclerotic lesions. The compound also inhibits the oxidation of cholesteryl linoleate in LDL to exert a reduction in atherosclerosis of the aorta (Nuttall, 1998, Yamakoshi, 1999).

Anticarcinogenic/Antitumor: Chemoprotective properties of proanthocyanidins include activity against free radicals and oxidative stress (Ye, 1999). The anti-tumor-promoting acitvity due to strong antioxidant effects of the compound has been demonstrated in animal models (Zhao, 1999).

Antioxidant Effects: Proanthocyanidin from the Grape Seed extract exerts a concentration-dependent inhibition of oxygen free radicals. In one study, the antioxidant effect of proanthocyanidin was more potent compared to vitamin C and vitamin E succinate (Bagchi, 1997). The compound also inhibits peroxidation of phosphatidylcholine liposomes (Plumb, 1998).

Hair Growth: Proanthocyanidins extracted from Grape Seeds promote proliferation of hair follicle cells, and possess remarkable hair-cycle converting activity from the telogen phase to the anagen phase. Epicatechin and catechin are the constitutive monomers inducing the degree of polymerization inducing hair growth (Takahashi, 1998).

Hepatoprotective Effects: Proanthocyanidin has been shown to significantly attenuate acetaminophen induced hepatic DNA damage, apoptosic and necrotic cell death of liver cells. The component also antagonizes acetaminophen induced changes in bcl-X1 expression (Ray, 1999).

Ischemia Prevention: Maintenance of microvascular injury by procyanidins occurs through the scavenger effect of reactive oxygen species (Maffei Facino, 1994). Procyanidins also reduce ventricular contraction in a dose-dependent fashion. Procyandins decrease coronary perfusion pressure and improve cardiac mechanical performance. (Maffei Facino R, 1996).

Vascular Effects: Procyanidins isolated from Grape Seed stabilizes capillary walls and prevents increases in permeability which inhibits edema (Robert, 1990; Zafirov, 1990). Overproduction of hyaluronan content associated with pathologic venous walls, in particular vein-lymphatic edema, is decreased by procyanidolic oligomers (Drubaix, 1997). Procyanidolic oligomers cross-link collagen fibers, resulting in reinforcement of the natural cross-linking of collagen that forms the collagen matrix of vascular connective tissue (Tixier et al, 1984). The vascular activity of procyanidin has positive effects on diabetic retinopathy, night vision and ocular stress (Boissin, 1988; Corbe, 1988; Soyeux, 1987).

CLINICAL TRIALS

Peripheral Venous Insufficiency

The efficacy of Grape Seed extract was evaluated for the treatment of venous insufficiency and symptoms due to hormonal supplementation. Grape Seed extract (150 mg twice daily) was administered to 4,729 patients in an open-label study. Peripheral venous insufficiency was evaluated 45 and 90 days after treatment. The efficacy score was based on symptoms of nocturnal cramps, paresthesias, sensation of warmth, cyanosis and edema. The sensation of heaviness in the legs decreased in 57% of cases by day 45 and 89.4% by day 90. In addition, the improvement of symptoms occurred in 66% of cases by day 45 and 79-83% of cases by day 90 (Henriet, 1993).

Ocular Effects

A lower resistance to glare and alteration of scotopic vision are associated with retinal pathology related to age, fatigue and stress. The effect of procyanidolic oligomers (PCO) on light vision and chorioretinal circulation was determined in 100 subjects. PCO (Endotelon) was administered in tablets of 50 mg four times daily for five weeks. Improvements in visual adaptation to low luminances and visual performances after glare, as measured by a nyctometer were significant (Corbe, 1988).

Postoperative Edema

The effect of PCO from Grape Seed extract was shown to have protective effects on the postoperative edema compared to placebo in a double-blind, placebo-controlled study. Thirty-two female patients undergoing a facelift were administered either 300 milligrams Grape Seed extract or placebo daily over the 5 days preceding the operation, and postoperatively from days 2 to 6. Prophylactic decrease in postoperative facial edema was the main efficacy criteria. The Grape Seed extract cohort scored significantly better than placebo against postoperative facial swelling (Baruch, 1984).

INDICATIONS AND USAGE

Unproven Uses: In Folk medicine, Grape preparations are used in venous diseases and blood circulation disorders.

Indian Medicine: Grape is used for headache, dysuria, scabies, skin diseases, gonorrhea, hemorrhoids and vomiting.

PRECAUTIONS AND ADVERSE REACTIONS

General: No health hazards or side effects are known in conjunction with the proper administration of designated therapeutic dosages. A reversible inhibition of intestinal enzyme activity (alkaline phosphatase, sucrase and dipeptidyl peptidase) was demonstrated in animal models (Tebib, 1994).

DOSAGE

How Supplied:

Capsule—25 mg, 30 mg, 50 mg, 60 mg, 500 mg

Tablet—50 mg

Daily Dosage: Grape Seed extract has been used for preventive therapy with 50 mg daily and treatment doses of 150-600 mg daily in divided doses (Arne, 1982; Baruch, 1984; Corbe; 1988; Delacroix, 1981; Henriet, 1993; Nuttall, 1998; Soyeux, 1987).

LITERATURE

Arne JL: Contribution to the study of procyanidolic oligomers: Endotelon in diabetic retinopathy. Gaz Med France 1982; 89(30):3610-3614.

Bagchi D; Garg A; Krohn RL et al. Oxygen free radical scavenging abilities of vitamins C and E, and a grape seed proanthocyanidin extract in vitro. Res Commun Mol Pathol Pharmacol 1997 Feb;95(2):179-89.

Baruch. Effect of Endotelon in postoperative edema. Results of a double-blind study versus placebo in 32 female patients. Ann Chir Plast Esthet 1984;29(4):393-5.

Bavaresco L; Fregoni C; Cantu E; Trevisan M. Stilbene compounds: from the grapevine to wine. Drugs Exp Clin Res 1999;25(2-3):57-63.

Boissin JP; Corbe C; Siou A. Chorioretinal circulation and dazzling: use of procyanidol oligomers (Endotelon). Bull Soc Ophtalmol Fr 1988 Feb;88(2):173-4, 177-9.

Corbe C; Boissin JP; Siou A. Light vision and chorioretinal circulation. Study of the effect of procyanidolic oligomers (Endotelon). J Fr Ophtalmol 1988;11(5):453-60.

Delacroix P: Double-blind trial of endotelon in chronic venous insufficiency. Rev Med 1981;27-28:1793-1802.

Drubaix I; Maraval M; Robert L; Robert AM. Hyaluronic acid (hyaluronan) levels in pathological human saphenous veins. Effects of procyanidol oligomers. Pathol Biol (Paris) 1997 Jan;45(1):86-91.

Henriet JP. Veno-lymphatic insufficiency. 4,729 patients undergoing hormonal and procyanidol oligomer therapy. Phlebologie 1993 Apr-Jun;46(2):313-25.

Kern W, List PH, Hörhammer L (Hrsg.), Hagers Handbuch der Pharmazeutischen Praxis, 4. Aufl., Bde 1-8: Springer Verlag Berlin, Heidelberg, New York, 1969.

Maffei Facino R, Carini M, Aldini G, et al. Free radicals scavenging action and anti-enzyme activities of procyanidines from Vitis vinifera. A mechanism for their capillary protective action. Arzneimittelforschung 1994 May;44(5):592-601.

Maffei Facino R, Carini M, Aldini G, et al. Procyanidines from Vitis vinifera seeds protect rabbit heart from ischemia/ reperfusion injury: antioxidant intervention and/or iron and copper sequestering ability. Planta Med 1996 Dec;62(6):495-502.

Nutall SL, Kendall MJ, Bombardelli E et al: An evaluation of the antioxidant activity of a standardized grape seed extract, Leucoselect(R). J Clin Pharm Ther 1998; 23:385-389.

Plumb GW; De Pascual-Teresa S; Santos-Buelga C et al. Antioxidant properties of catechins and proanthocyanidins: effect of polymerisation, galloylation and glycosylation. Free Radic Res 1998 Oct;29(4):351-8.

Ray SD, Kumar MA, Bagchi D. A novel proanthocyanidin IH636 grape seed extract increases in vivo Bcl-XL expression and prevents acetaminophen-induced programmed and unprogrammed cell death in mouse liver. Arch Biochem Biophys 1999 Sep 1;369(1):42-58.

Robert L; Godeau G; Gavignet-Jeannin C et al. The effect of procyanidolic oligomers on vascular permeability. A study using quantitative morphology. Pathol Biol (Paris) 1990 Jun;38(6):608-16.

Soyeux A; Seguin JP; Le Devehat C; Bertrand A. Endotelon. Diabetic retinopathy and hemorheology (preliminary study). Bull Soc Ophtalmol Fr 1987 Dec;87(12):1441-4.

Takahashi T; Kamiya T; Yokoo Y. Proanthocyanidins from grape seeds promote proliferation of mouse hair follicle cells in vitro and convert hair cycle in vivo. Acta Derm Venereol 1998 Nov;78(6):428-32.

Tebib K, Rouanet JM, Besancon P. Effect of grape seed tannins on the activity of some rat intestinal enzyme activities. Enzyme Protein 1994-95;48(1):51-60.

Tixier JM; Godeau G; Robert AM; Hornebeck W. Evidence by in vivo and in vitro studies that binding of procyagenols to elastin affects its rate of degradation by elastases. Biochem Pharmacol 1984 Dec 15;33(24):3933-9.

Yamakoshi J; Kataoka S; Koga T; Ariga T. Proanthocyanidin-rich extract from grape seeds attenuates the development of aortic atherosclerosis in cholesterol-fed rabbits. Atherosclerosis 1999 Jan;142(1):139-49.

Ye X; Krohn RL; Liu W et al. The cytotoxic effects of a novel IH636 grape seed proanthocyanidin extract on cultured human cancer cells. Mol Cell Biochem 1999 Jun;196(1-2):99-108.

Zafirov D; Bredy-Dobreva G; Litchev V et al. Antiexudative and capillaritonic effects of procyanidines isolated from grape seeds (V. Vinifera). Acta Physiol Pharmacol Bulg 1990;16(3):50-4.

Zhao J, Wang J, Chen Y, Agarwal R. Anti-tumor-promoting activity of a polyphenolic fraction isolated from grape seeds in the mouse skin two-stage initiation-promotion protocol and identification of procyanidin B5-3′-gallate as the most effective antioxidant constituent. Carcinogenesis 1999 Sep;20(9):1737-4.

Gratiola officinalis

See Hedge-Hyssop

Gray Wallflower

Erysimum diffusum

DESCRIPTION

Medicinal Parts: The medicinal part is the plant's radish.

Flower and Fruit: The flowers are in densely flowered racemes. The 4 sepals are upright and gray-haired, the 4 petals yellow, long-petiolate, pubescent on the lower surface and 8 to 14 mm long. There are 2 short and 4 long stamens; the ovary is superior with 4 fused carpels. The fruit is a 3.5 to 8 cm long, approximately 1 mm wide, 4-sided, appressed pubescent, dehiscent pod that opens on 2 sides. The seeds are elongate with a diameter of approximately 1 to 1.5 mm.

Leaves, Stem and Root: Gray Wallflower is a herbaceous biennial or perennial upright that grows up to 1.2 m high. The leaves are alternate. The lower ones are petiolate, 1 to 8 mm wide, gray-haired, narrow, linear-lanceolate, entire or dentate; the middle and upper ones are sessile. The stem is edged, covered in jointed hairs and branched in larger plants. The root is thin, spindle-shaped and branched.

Habitat: The plant is indigenous to the Commonwealth of Independent States and Hungary.

Production: The gray-leaved wild radish is collected during the flowering season of the two-year-old plants of Erysimum diffusum and dried after harvesting at a maximum temperature of 40° C.

ACTIONS AND PHARMACOLOGY

COMPOUNDS

Cardioactive steroid glycosides (cardenolids, 1 to 3%): chief component erysimoside (primary glycoside, aglycone k-strophanthidin, 0.6%)

Helveticoside (secondary glycoside)

Canescine

Cheirotoxin

Erycanoside

EFFECTS

The drug contains cardioactive glycosides of the cardenolide type with k-strophantidin as the aglycone. It is accordingly positively inotropic and negatively chronotropic in its effect.

INDICATIONS AND USAGE

Unproven Uses: The drug was used in the past for cardiac insufficiency (NYHA I and II), but can no longer be recommended.

PRECAUTIONS AND ADVERSE REACTIONS

No health hazards are known in conjunction with the proper administration of designated therapeutic dosages.

Although poisonings among humans are both unknown and unlikely, due to the difficulties accompanying resorption of the glycosides, the possibility of a poisoning resulting from either high dosages of the drug or its glycosides through peroral administration is not to be completely ruled out.

DOSAGE

How Supplied: capsules; tablets.

Storage: Drug should be stored in a tightly sealed, secure container.

LITERATURE

Hänsel R, Keller K, Rimpler H, Schneider G (Ed.), Hagers Handbuch der Pharmazeutischen Praxis, 5. Aufl., Bde 4 - 6

(Drogen), Springer Verlag Berlin, Heidelberg, New York, 1992-1994.

Great Burnet

Sanguisorba officinalis

DESCRIPTION

Medicinal Parts: The medicinal parts of the plant are the fresh aerial parts, the dried herb, the rhizomes and roots.

Flower and Fruit: The composite heads are ovate-oblong, approximately 1 to 2 cm long and consist of 5 to 10 usually androgynous flowers. The calyx has 4 dark red-brown tips, 4 stamens with stiffly patent red filaments and yellow anthers. The smooth, spike-like, quadrangular fruit calyx has 1 carpel and 1 style and is narrowly winged. The fruit is a nut enclosed in the perigone tube.

Leaves, Stem and Root: Great Burnet is a semi-rosette shrub with a strong dark brown root that produces thick fibers and a short rhizome. The stems are erect, angular, glabrous, and bifurcated. The rosette leaves are 20 to 40 cm long and consist of 7 to 15 ovate leaflets, which are cordate at the base and blue-green beneath. There are only a few cauline leaves, which taper towards the top.

Characteristics: The brown-red composite head is characteristic for this plant.

Habitat: The plant is widespread in the northern, temperate regions of Europe, temperate Asia, and North America.

Production: Great Burnet is the Sanguisorba officinalis plant in flower. The fresh aerial parts are collected in the wild during the flowering season. The rhizomes and roots are harvested in autumn, then washed and dried.

ACTIONS AND PHARMACOLOGY

COMPOUNDS

Flavonoids: including among others, rutin, flavonoid sulfates

Tannins: including ellagitannins, sanguinarine H-11, casuarinin

Triterpene glycosides: aglycones pomolic acid, tormentolic acid, including among others, ziyuglycosides I and II (sanguisorbin), betulinic acid, ursolic acid

Sterols: including beta-sitosterol

EFFECTS

The drug has been credited with decongestant, astringent and diuretic properties, but no investigation into effects has been carried out.

INDICATIONS AND USAGE

Unproven Uses: The drug is used internally for female disorders, menorrhagia during menopause, hot flushes, dysentery, enteritis, diarrhea, bladder restraint, hemorrhoids, phlebitis, and varicose veins. Externally, Great Burnet is used in plaster for wounds and ulcers. Folk medicine uses included administration of the plant latex as a remedy for pulmonary tuberculosis.

Chinese Medicine: The Chinese use Great Burnet as an astringent and hemostyptic for nosebleeds, dysentery, reptile bites and bloody coughs.

Homeopathic Uses: Among uses in homeopathy are uterine bleeding, varicose veins and diarrhea.

PRECAUTIONS AND ADVERSE REACTIONS

No health hazards or side effects are known in conjunction with the proper administration of designated therapeutic dosages.

DOSAGE

Mode of Administration: The drug is used internally and externally. It is available in ground form and is used as an extract, juice or tea. A plaster is used externally.

Homeopathic Dosage: 5 drops, 1 tablet or 10 globules every 30 to 60 minutes (acute) or 1 to 3 times a day (chronic); parenterally: 1 to 2 ml sc acute: 3 times daily; chronic: once a day (HAB34).

LITERATURE

Bastow KF et al., Inhibition of DNA topoisomerase by sanguiin H-6, a cytotoxic dimeric ellagitannin from Sanguisorba officinalis. In: PM 59(3):240. 1993.

Chang, EH et al. (Eds), Advances in Chinese Medicinal Materials Research, World Scientific Pub. Co. Singapore 1985.

Hänsel R, Keller K, Rimpler H, Schneider G (Hrsg.), Hagers Handbuch der Pharmazeutischen Praxis, 5. Aufl., Bde 4-6 (Drogen), Springer Verlag Berlin, Heidelberg, New York, 1992-1994.

Kaneta M et al., Agric Biol Chem 43:657. 1979.

Kashiwada Y, Nonaka GI, Niskioka I, Chang JJ, Lee KH, Antitumor agents, 129. Tannins and related compounds as selective cytotoxic agents. In: JNP 55:1033-1043. 1992.

Kosuga T et al., (1981) Yakugaku Zasshi 101(6):501.

Kosuga T et al., (1984) Chem Pharm Bull 32(11):448.

Madaus G, Lehrbuch der Biologischen Arzneimittel, Bde 1-3, Nachdruck, Georg Olms Verlag Hildesheim 1979.

Nonaka GI et al., (1982) J Chem Soc Perkin Trans. 10(4):1067.

Nonaka GI et al., (1984) Chem Pharm Bull 32(2):483.

Reher G et al., PH 31:3909-3914. 1992.

Sunstar Inc. (1980) Pat. JP 80/120509 Japan.

Tanaka T et al., (1983) Phytochemistry 22(11):2575.

Tanaka T et al., (1984) Chem Pharm Bull 32(1):117.

Tanake T et al., (1985) J Chem Res (S)6:176.

Yosioka I et al., Chem Pharm Bull 19:1700. 1971.

Greater Bindweed

Calystegia sepium

DESCRIPTION

Medicinal Parts: The medicinal parts are the whole flowering plant and the root.

Flower and Fruit: The solitary white flowers are about 5 cm long, the pedicle is quadrangular. Under the calyx there are 2 cordate, pointed, red-bordered bracts, which extend to cover the calyx. There are 5 sepals. The corolla is fused and conical. There are 5 stamens and 1 superior ovary. The fruit is a capsule.

Leaves, Stem and Root: The plant is about 10 to 30 cm high and has a creeping rhizome. The stem is angular, glabrous and twining. The leaves are alternate, petiolate, cordate or arrow-shaped. The base of the leaves are acuminate, and they often have dentate lobes. Most twining plants seem to follow the course of the sun and bind round a support from left to right. But the Bindweed will always twine against the sun, confounding all attempts to train it, even dying in the process.

Characteristics: The flowers close in damp weather.

Habitat: The plant is indigenous to Europe and eastern U.S.

Production: The upper part of the herb is harvested during the flowering season and dried at temperatures of no more than 40° C in a well-aired place.

Other Names: Devil's Vine, Hedge Lily, Lady's Nightcap, Rutland Beauty, Hedge Convolvulus, Old Man's Night Cap, Bearbind

ACTIONS AND PHARMACOLOGY

COMPOUNDS

Glycoretines: polymeric, resinous glycosides of hydroxy fatty acids (C12-C16) with oligosaccharides; the hydroxyl groups have been esterified with acetic, propionic, isobutyric and valeric acids, among others

Tannins

EFFECTS

The drug has a powerful effect; activity in the smooth muscle area is stimulated, intestinal peristalsis is increased, and there is an increase in bile production.

INDICATIONS AND USAGE

Unproven Uses: Greater Bindweed is used for fevers, urinary tract diseases, as a purgative for constipation and to increase the production of bile.

PRECAUTIONS AND ADVERSE REACTIONS

No health hazards or side effects are known in conjunction with the proper administration of designated therapeutic dosages. It is conceivable that an overdose of the drug would trigger intestinal colic.

DOSAGE

Mode of Administration: The pressed juice, powdered root and an infusion are used internally. The drug is rarely used anymore due to its strong intestinal effects.

Preparation: An infusion is prepared by adding 1 to 2 teaspoons of cut drug per cup of water.

LITERATURE

Asano N, Kato A, Oseki K, Kizu H, Matsui K, Calystegins of Physalis alkekengi var. francheti (Solanaceae). Structure determination and their glycosidase inhibitory activities. Eur J Biochem, 14:369-76, 1995.

Kern W, List PH, Hörhammer L (Hrsg.), Hagers Handbuch der Pharmazeutischen Praxis, 4. Aufl., Bde 1-8, Springer Verlag Berlin, Heidelberg, New York, 1969.

Peumans WJ, Winter HC, Bemer V, Van Leuven F, Goldstein IJ, Truffa-Bachi P, Van Damme EJ, Isolation of a novel plant lectin with an unusual specificity from Calystegia sepium. GlycoconJ J, 14:259-65, 1997.

Roth L, Daunderer M, Kormann K Giftpflanzen, Pflanzengifte. 4. Aufl., Ecomed Fachverlag Landsberg / Lech 1993.

Van Damme EJ, Barre A, Verhaert P, Rouge P, Peumans WJ, Molecular cloning of the mitogenic mannose/maltose-specific rhizome lectin from Calystegia sepium. FEBS Lett, 14:352-6, 1996.

Greek Sage

Salvia triloba

DESCRIPTION

Medicinal Parts: The medicinal part of the plant is the leaf.

Flower and Fruit: The flowers are in false whorls of 2 to 6 blossoms. The calyx is campanulate, dentate, 5 to 8 mm long, often purple and pubescent. The corolla is 16 to 25 mm long, typically lilac or pink but occasionally white.

Leaves, Stem and Root: Salvia triloba grows as a semi-shrub, up to 1.2 m high. The leaves are petiolate and tomentose. The lamina is simple or pinnatifid with 1 to 2 pairs of lateral leaf sections and a large elongate-ovate end section. The stem is square, appressed pubescent, grayish-white beneath and green above.

Habitat: The plant is indigenous to Greece, the Commonwealth of Independent States, Albania, Turkey and Cyprus. Various species are particularly widespread in the Mediterranean region.

Production: Greek Sage leaves are the dried leaves of Salvia triloba, which are harvested once a year if collected in the wild and three times a year when cultivated.

Other Names: Three-Lobed Sage, Turkish Sage

ACTIONS AND PHARMACOLOGY

COMPOUNDS

Volatile oil (1.5 to 3.5%): chief component 1.8-cineole (40 to 67%), camphor (2 to 25%), thujone (5 to 6%), including as well camphene, beta-caryophyllene, myrcene, alpha-pinene, beta-pinene

Flavonoids: including 7-O-glucosides and 7-O-glucuronides of apigenin, chrysoeriol, hispidulin, luteolin, 6-methyl luteolin, as well as salvigenin, jaceosidin

Caffeic acid derivatives: rosmarinic acid (1.0 to 2.5%)

Diterpenes: including carnosol (0.5%)

Triterpenes (8%): ursolic acid, oleanolic acid

EFFECTS

The chief active ingredient (cineole) of the drug's essential oil has an antimicrobial effect. The combined action of the essential oil and the tannins is antiseptic and anti-inflammatory, particularly in the region of the mouth and throat. Decoctions and infusions of the leaves exhibit antihypertensive, spasmolytic and blood sugar-reducing effects in animal experiments, during which the plasma insulin levels remain unchanged. The hypoglycemic effect is traced to the inhibition of intestinal glucose resorption. A sedative effect has also been described.

INDICATIONS AND USAGE

Unproven Uses: Salvia triloba is used internally for diabetes in Israel and Cyprus, and elsewhere for cardiac symptoms, lung complaints, colds, coughs, nervousness and digestion problems. Externally it is used to treat skin damage.

PRECAUTIONS AND ADVERSE REACTIONS

No health hazards are known in conjunction with the proper administration of designated therapeutic dosages.

DOSAGE

Mode of Administration: Aqueous decoctions and infusions prepared from the whole, cut and powdered drug are used internally. The fresh cut leaves are applied topically.

Preparation: The literature contains no detailed descriptions.

Storage: Store tightly sealed and protected from light.

LITERATURE

Hänsel R, Keller K, Rimpler H, Schneider G (Ed), Hagers Handbuch der Pharmazeutischen Praxis, 5. Aufl., Bde 4 - 6 (Drogen), Springer Verlag Berlin, Heidelberg, New York, 1992-1994.

Ulubelen A, Ozturk S, Isildatici S, A new flavone from Salvia triloba L.f (Labiatae). J Pharm Sci, 57:1037-8, 1968 Jun.

Green Hellebore

Helleborus viridis

DESCRIPTION

Medicinal Parts: The drug derived from the plant's rhizome and roots is obsolete in medicine today.

Flower and Fruit: There are 2 to 3 flowers with a diameter of 4 to 7 cm and 5 ovate, grass-green, broad flower bracts. The petals are in the form of petaloid honey glands, and there are numerous stamens. The ovary is superior with the carpels only fused at the base. The fruit is a 25 to 28 mm long follicle with beak. The seeds have a narrow longitudinal strip with a ring at the end.

Leaves, Stem and Root: This herbaceous perennial grows upright, up to 40 cm high. There are 2 basal, long-petioled leaves; the lamina is divided like a foot into 7 to 13 sections that are narrow-lanceolate, serrate and dark green. The stem is upright, branching higher up and leafless to that point. The cauline leaves are similar to the basal ones but sessile and smaller. The rhizome is usually branched.

Habitat: The various species of Hellebore grow mainly in mountainous regions of Europe and North America. The plant is most commonly found in the Alps; Helleborus viridis is found growing as far north as northwest France.

Production: Green Hellebore root is the dried rhizome with roots of Helleborus viridis.

Not to be Confused With: Adulteration and mistaken identity can occur with Hellebori nigri rhizoma, Actaea spicata, Adonis vernalis, Trollius europaeus and Eupatorium cannabium.

Other Names: Bear's Foot

ACTIONS AND PHARMACOLOGY

COMPOUNDS

Cardioactive steroid glycosides (bufadienolids, 0.5 to 1.5%): chief component hellebrin, including deglucohellebrin

Alkaloids of unknown structure: celliamine, sprintillamine, sprintilline

Steroid saponins

EFFECTS

The steroid saponin mixture helleborin is severely toxic and irritating to mucous membranes (ptarmic). It exhibits digitalis-like effects through the cardioactive glycosides it contains (hellebrin). The alkaloids it contains produce an excitation of the motor centers, eventually leading to convulsions and respiratory failure and triggering bradycardia in the heart and a negatively inotropic effect.

INDICATIONS AND USAGE

Unproven Uses: The drug is obsolete today because the risks of use are considered too high, given that efficacy for previously accepted indications has not yet been proven.

Previous uses in folk medicine included nausea, constipation and worm infestation. Root preparations were used also for heart failure and as a diuretic. Helleborus viridis was employed as a laxative according to Hager (around 1930) and was important in homeopathic medicine.

Homeopathic Uses: Helleborus viridis is used for diarrhea.

PRECAUTIONS AND ADVERSE REACTIONS

The drug is not to be administered in allopathic medicine. No risks are known in connection with the administration of homeopathic dosages of the drug.

OVERDOSAGE

The mucous membrane-irritating effect of the saponins appears to play the largest role in poisonings with the drug, resulting in scratchiness in mouth and throat, salivation, nausea, vomiting, diarrhea, dizziness, shortness of breath, and possible convulsions and asphyxiation. The ingestion of very large dosages leads to disorders of cardiac function (cardiac arrhythmias).

Following gastrointestinal emptying (gastric lavage, sodium sulfate) and the administration of activated charcoal, the treatment for poisonings consists of the treatment of spasms with diazepam (i.v.), electrolyte substitution and the countering of any acidosis that may appear through sodium bicarbonate infusions. Intubation and oxygen respiration may also be required.

Cases of fatal poisonings are known among animals who fed on the leaves of the plant.

DOSAGE

Mode of Administration: Whole, cut and powdered drug.

Daily Dosage: 1 g drug; maximum single dosage: 0.2 g drug.

Homeopathic Dosage: 5 drops, 1 tablet or 10 globules every to 30 to 60 minutes (acute) and 1 to 3 times daily (chronic); parenterally: 1 to ml sc acute, 3 times daily; chronic: once a day (HAB34).

Storage: Store securely.

LITERATURE

Hänsel R, Keller K, Rimpler H, Schneider G (Ed.), Hagers Handbuch der Pharmazeutischen Praxis, 5. Aufl., Bde 4 - 6 (Drogen), Springer Verlag Berlin, Heidelberg, New York, 1992-1994.

Johnson CT, Routledge JK, Suspected helleborus viridis poisoning of cattle. Vet Rec, 89:202, 1971 Aug 14.

Green Tea

Camellia sinensis

TRADE NAMES

Green Tea Leaf (available from numerous manufacturers and as a combination product,) Green Tea Extract, Green Tea, Standardized Green Tea Extract, Green Tea Power, Chinese Green Tea Bags, Green Tea Power Caffeine Free

DESCRIPTION

Medicinal Parts: The medicinal parts are the very young downy leaves, from which green or black tea is prepared according to the treatment being given.

Flower and Fruit: The flowers grow short-pedicled and singly or in clusters of a few flowers in the leaf axils. They are white or pale pink and have a diameter of 3 to 5 cm. The flowers have between 5 and 7 sepals and petals at a time. The petals are fused at the base with the numerous stamens. The ovary has 3 chambers. The fruit is a greenish-brown, woody capsule with a diameter of 1 to 1.5 cm and contains 1 to 3 smooth brown seeds.

Leaves, Stem and Root: The plant is an evergreen, heavily-branched shrub. The leaves are glossy dark green, alternate, short-petiolate, coreacious, lanceolate or elongate-ovate and roughly serrate. The young leaves appear silver because of the covering of downy hairs on the surface.

Habitat: The plant does not originate in the wild. It was originally cultivated in China and is grown as a tea plant today in India, China, Sri Lanka, Japan, Indonesia, Kenya, Turkey, Pakistan, Malawi and Argentina.

Production: Tea leaves are the fermented and/or dried leaves of Camellia sinensis. Harvesting takes place under stringent quality control. Green Tea is produced by steaming the fresh-cut leaf. Black Tea is produced by allowing the leaves to oxidize. During oxidation, enzymes present in the tea convert many of the polyphenolic therapeutic substances to less active compounds. Oxidation does not occur with Green Tea because the steaming process inactivates the enzymes responsible for oxidation. The anti-oxidant activity of Green Tea is six times greater than that of Black Tea.

Other Names: Black Tea, Chinese Tea, Green Tea

ACTIONS AND PHARMACOLOGY

COMPOUNDS

Purine alkaloids (methyl xanthines): caffeine (previously referred to as theine or teine; depending upon the development stage of the leaves, 2.9-4.2%, content declining with age), theobromine (0.15-0.2%), theophylline (0.02-0.04%)

Triterpene saponins (theafolia saponins): aglycones including among others, barringtogenol C, R1-barringenol

Catechins: in unfermented (green) tea 10-25%, with fermentation partially changing over into oligomeric quinones with tannin character, into theaflavine, theaflavin acid, thearubigene, or into non-water soluble polymeric- flavonoids: including, among others, quercetin, kaempferol, myrecetin

Flavonoids: including quercetin, kaempferol, myricetin

Caffeic acid derivatives: including among others, chlorogenic acid, theogallin

Anorganic ions: high fluoride content (130-160 mg/kg), potassium and aluminum ions

Volatile oil: chief components linalool, in fermented tea also 2-methyl-hept-2-en-6-on, alpha-ionon and beta-ionon, more than 300 volatile compounds are involved in tea aroma

EFFECTS

The caffeine in the drug has a centrally stimulating and antidepressive effect (adenosine antagonism.) Adenosine antagonism leads to dilation of the renal vessels with a consecutive increase of the rate of filtration (diuresis). Caffeine is positively inotropic, promotes the secretion of gastric juices, glycolysis and lipolysis. In animal tests, bradykinin and prostaglandin antagonism caused a capillary sealing and anti-inflammatory effect.

An antidiarrheal effect can be attributed to a combination of the tannin effect and the fact that doses of 400 mg polyphenols administered three times daily promotes the growth of *Lactobacillis* and *Bifidobacter* species while inhibiting the growth of *Clostridium perfringens* and *Clostridium difficile* (Yamamoto, 1997).

There is clinical evidence that Green Tea has cancer preventive effects. The types of cancer that Green Tea has been shown to prevent as demonstrated in well controlled clinical studies include cancers of the pancreas, colon, small intestine, stomach, breast and the lung.

Green Tea mouthwashes have been shown to inhibit the growth of cavity-associated bacteria such as *Streptococcus mutans, Streptococcus salivarius* and *Escherichia coli* (Rasheed 1998; Haider, 1998).

CLINICAL TRIALS

Cancer Treatment/Prevention

A large (n = 2226) case-control study was conducted in China, where recently diagnosed cancer cases (pancreatic, colon and rectum) among residents between the ages of 30 and 74 years were included. Controls (n = 1552) were selected and matched to cases by age and gender and adjustments were made for age, income, education and cigarette smoking. As tea consumption increased, the incidence of all three cancers decreased. Women with the highest tea consumption (> or = 200 g/month) had a 33% reduced risk for colon cancer, 43% reduced risk of rectal cancer and 47% reduction in the risk for pancreatic cancer (p= 0.07, 0.001 and 0.008 respectively). For men who consumed > or = 300 g/month of Green Tea, the risk of colon cancer was reduced by 18%, for rectal cancer there was a 43% reduction of risk and for pancreatic cancer the risk reduction was 47% (p= 0.38, 0.04 and 0.04 respectively) (Ji, 1997).

A two-part case control study of 472 Japanese women with stage I, II or III breast cancer was conducted. The first part of the study assessed the association between consumption of Green Tea prior to clinical cancer and the number of axillary lymph node metastases for premenopausal women or the increased expression of progesterone receptor and estrogen receptor among postmenopausal women with stage I or II cancer. The second part of the study investigated the recurrence rate of those with stage I or II breast cancer in relation to the amount of Green Tea consumption. There was an inverse relationship between the amount of Green Tea consumption and the rate of cancer recurrence. The recurrence rate was 16.7% for those that consumed > or = 5 cups/day and 24.3% among those consuming < or = 4 cups/day (p < 0.05). The authors concluded that increased consumption of Green Tea prior to clinical cancer onset is significantly associated with improved prognosis of stage I and II breast cancer, and that this association may be related to a modifying effect of Green Tea on the clinical characteristics of the disease (Nakachi, 1998).

Dental Caries Prevention

An extract of oolong tea (semifermented tea leaves of Camellia sinensis) containing polymerized polyphenols in 0.2% ethanol was administered to 35 volunteers between 18 and 29 years of age to test the inhibitory effect of the extract on dental plaque deposition. The study was repeated 1 week after the first trial using 0.2% ethanol without the tea extract. The oolong tea cohort showed significant inhibition of plaque deposition (Ooshima, 1994).

In another study, it was demonstrated that total inhibition of *Streptococcus mutans* was possible after exposure to a 0.1%

infusion of Chinese Green Tea polyphenols (CTP) for 5 minutes. Plaque Index and Gingival Index decreased significantly ($p < 0.001$) after a 0.2% CTP rinse and brush regimen was used by the study participants. The authors conclude that CTP is an effective agent to prevent dental caries (Chung, 1993).

INDICATIONS AND USAGE

Though no Commission E monograph is available for Green Tea, there is clinical evidence that Green Tea is likely to be useful as a cancer preventive and as a preventive for dental caries.

Unproven Uses: Internal application: Green Tea is used for stomach disorders, migraine, symptoms of fatigue, vomiting and diarrhea when taken as a beverage. It can be used to increase performance (stimulant effect).

Homeopathic Uses: Camellia sinensis is used for cardiac and circulatory conditions, headaches, states of agitation, states of depression and stomach complaints.

Indian Medicine: In India, tea preparations are used for diarrhea, loss of appetite, hyperdipsia, migraine, cardiac pain, fever and fatigue.

Chinese Medicine: In China Green Tea is used to treat migraine, nausea, diarrhoea resulting from malaria and digestion problems. It is also used as a cancer preventive.

PRECAUTIONS AND ADVERSE REACTIONS

General: No health hazards are known in conjunction with the proper administration of designated therapeutic dosages. Side effects of tea consumption are possible with persons who have sensitive stomachs, chiefly due to the chlorogenic acid and tannin content. Hyperacidity, gastric irritation, reduction of appetite, as well as obstipation or diarrhea, could be the result of intense tea consumption. These side effects can be generally avoided by the addition of milk (reduction of the chlorogenic acid and other tannins).

Care should be taken with patients that have weakened cardiovascular systems, renal diseases, thyroid hyperfunction, elevated susceptibility to spasm and certain psychic disorders, such as panicky states of anxiety. With long-term intake of dosages above 1.5 g caffeine per day, non-specific symptoms occur, such as restlessness, irritability, sleeplessness, palpitation, vertigo, vomiting, diarrhea, loss of appetite and headache.

Pregnancy: Pregnant women should not exceed a dosage of 300 mg per day (5 cups of tea spread out over the course of a day).

Nursing Mothers: Infants whose nursing mothers consume beverages containing caffeine could suffer from sleep disorders.

Children: There have been reports of microcytic anemia in infants that were fed an average of 250 ml Green Tea daily. This effect may possibly be due to impairment of iron metabolism (Merhav, 1985).

Drug Interactions: The resorption of alkaline medications can be delayed because of chemical bonding with the tannins.

OVERDOSAGE

Overdosage (quantities corresponding to more than 300 mg caffeine, or 5 cups of tea as a beverage) can lead to restlessness, tremor and elevated reflex excitability. The first signs of poisoning are vomiting and abdominal spasm. Fatal poisonings are not possible with tea beverages.

DOSAGE

Mode of Administration: Green Tea is administered as an infusion or in capsule form for internal use.

How Supplied: The usual concentration of total polyphenols in dried Green Tea leaf is around 8% to 12%. One cup of Green Tea normally contains 50 to 100 milligrams polyphenols (Murray & Pizzorno, 1998; Yamamoto, 1997).

Capsules — 100 mg, 150 mg, 175 mg, 333 mg, 383 mg, 500 mg

Liquid — 1:1

Tablets — 100 mg

Dried extract (instant tea) — Processed using steam extraction followed by drying

Filter tea bags — Available commercially containing 1.8 to 2.2 gm tea

Preparation: To prepare a tea, boiling water is poured over a heaped teaspoon of leaf tea, a level teaspoon of crushed leaves or a tea bag and left to draw for 3 to 10 minutes as required. The caffeine is almost completely drawn after approximately 3 minutes. The tannin-containing substance (and with it the antidiarrheal action) increases when the tea is left to brew.

Daily Dosage: A daily dose of 300 to 400 mg of polyphenols is typical. The amount of polyphenols in 3 cups of Green Tea is between 240 and 320 mg.

Homeopathic Dosage: 5 to 10 drops, 1 tablet or 5 to 10 globules 1 to 3 times daily or 1 ml injection solution sc twice weekly (HAB1).

Storage: Store tightly sealed and dried; store separately from other chemicals and aromatic substances.

LITERATURE

Anonym, Grüner Tee schützt vor Krebs. In: DAZ 137(24):2045. 1997.

Büechi S, Antivirale Saponine, pharmakologische und klinische Untersuchungen. In: DAZ 136(2):89-98. 1996.

Graham B, In: Graham HN: Tea: The Plant and Its Manufacture, Chemistry, and Consumption of the Beverage. In: The Methylxanthine Beverages and Foods: Chemistry, Consumption, and Heath Effects, Alan R. Liss, New York, S.29-74. 1984.

Haslam E, Natural polyphenols (vegetable tannins) as drugs: possible modes of action. In: JNP 59(2):205-215. 1996.

Imai K, Nakachi K, Cross sectional study of effects of drinking Green Tea on cardiovascular and liver disease. In: Brit Med J 310:693-696. 1995.

Jain AK, Shimoi K, Nakamura Y, Kada T, Hana Y, Tomita J, Crude tea extracts decrease the mutagenic activity of N-methyl-N'-nitro-N-nitrosoguanidine in-vitro and in gastric tract of rats. In: Mutat Res 210(1)1-8. 1989.

Ji BT, Chow WH, Hsing AW et al., Green Tea consumption and the risk of pancreatic and colorectal cancer. Int J Cancer 70(3):255-258. 1997.

John TJ, Mukundan P, Antiviral property of tea. In: Curr Sci 47:159. 1978.

Ludewig R, (1995) Schwarzer und Grüner Tee als Genuβ- und Heilmittel. Dtsch Apoth Z 135:2203-2218.

Murray MT & Pizzorno: Camellia Sinensis (green tea), in A Textbook of Natural Medicine. Churchill Livingstone, pp 625-627. 1998.

Nakachi K, Suemasu K, Suga K, Takeo T, Imai K, Higashi Y. Influence of drinking Green Tea on breast cancer malignancy among Japanese patients. In: Jpn J Cancer 89(3): 254-61. Mar, 89.

Rasheed A & Haider M, Antibacterial activity of Camellia sinensis extracts against dental caries. Arch Pharm Res 21:348-352. 1998.

Scholz E, Camellia sinensis (L.) O. KUNTZE. Der Teestrauch. In: ZPT 16(4):231-250. 1995.

Schröder B, In: Schröder R: Kaffee, Tee und Kardamom, Ulmer-Verlag, Stuttgart. 1991.

Sur P, Ganguly DK, Tea root extract (TRE) as an antineoplastic agent. In: PM 60(2):106. 1994.

Yamamoto T, Juneja LR, Chu DC et al., Chemistry and Applications of green tea. CRC Press, Boca Raton, FL, USA, 1997.

Yoshizawa S et al., (1987) Phytother Res 1(1):44.

Further information in:

Hänsel R, Keller K, Rimpler H, Schneider G (Hrsg.), Hagers Handbuch der Pharmazeutischen Praxis, 5. Aufl., Bde 4-6 (Drogen): Springer Verlag Berlin, Heidelberg, New York, 1992-1994.

Leung AY, Encyclopedia of Common Natural Ingredients Used in Food, Drugs, Cosmetics, John Wiley & Sons Inc., New York 1980.

Lewin L, Gifte und Vergiftungen, 6. Aufl., Nachdruck, Haug Verlag, Heidelberg 1992.

Oliver-Bever B (Ed.), Medicinal Plants of Tropical West Africa, Cambridge University Press, Cambridge 1986.

Roth L, Daunderer M, Kormann K, Giftpflanzen, Pflanzengifte, 4. Aufl., Ecomed Fachverlag Landsberg Lech 1993.

Steinegger E, Hänsel R, Pharmakognosie, 5. Aufl., Springer Verlag Heidelberg 1992.

Teuscher E, Lindequist U, Biogene Gifte - Biologie, Chemie, Pharmakologie, 2. Aufl., Fischer Verlag Stuttgart 1994.

Teuscher E, Biogene Arzneimittel, 5. Aufl., Wiss. Verlagsges. Stuttgart 1997.

Wagner H, Wiesenauer M, Phytotherapie. Phytopharmaka und pflanzliche Homöopathika, Fischer-Verlag, Stuttgart, Jena, New York 1995.

Wichtl M (Hrsg.), Teedrogen, 4. Aufl., Wiss. Verlagsges. Stuttgart 1997.

Grindelia camporum

See Gumweed

Ground Ivy

Glechoma hederacea

DESCRIPTION

Medicinal Parts: The medicinal parts are the herb collected during the flowering season and dried, the fresh aerial parts collected during the flowering season, and the whole plant.

Flower and Fruit: The flowers are in 2- to 6-blossomed false whorls in the axils of the foliage leaves. The individual flowers are 1 to 2 cm long with distinct pedicles and bracteoles that are 1 to 1.5 mm long. The calyx is bilabiate and tubular, with 5 tips. The bilabiate corolla is 15 to 22 mm long, usually blue-violet but occasionally red-violet or white. The fruit is a nut of about 2 mm.

Leaves, Stem and Root: This perennial herb grows 15 to 60 cm high and has a creeping main stem, which roots at the lower nodes and keeps its leaves in winter. The quadrangular stem is up to 2 mm thick and often tinged with blue-violet, as are the petioles. The leaves are crossed opposite, long-petioled, reniform to broadly cordate, crenate; dark green above and paler green beneath.

Characteristics: The plant has a mild unpleasant smell; the taste is hot and bitter.

Habitat: Ground Ivy is a common wild plant in Europe.

Production: Ground Ivy is the aboveground part of Glechoma hederacea, gathered when in flower (from April to June). It is air-dried in the shade to keep loss of the essential oil to a minimum.

Other Names: Alehoof, Gill-Go-over-the-Ground, Lizzy-Run-up-the-Hedge, Gill-to-by-the-Hedge, Robin-Run-in-the-Hedge, Catsfoot, Hedgemaids, Tun-Hoof, Haymaids, Turnhoof, Creeping Charlie, Cat's-Paw

ACTIONS AND PHARMACOLOGY

COMPOUNDS

Volatile oil (traces): chief components (-)-pinocarvone, (-)-menthone, (+)-pulegone, also including germacran D, germacran B, cis-ocimene

Sesquiterpenes: glechomafuran, glechomanolide

Hydroxy fatty acid: 9-hydroxy-10-trans, 12-cis-octadecadiendic acid

Caffeic acid derivatives: rosmaric acid

Flavonoids: including cymaroside, cosmosyin, hypersoside isoquercitrin

EFFECTS

The drug is said to be an anti-inflammatory, which is believed to be due to the tripterpen content. No detailed information is available.

INDICATIONS AND USAGE

Unproven Uses: In folk medicine, the drug is used internally for inflammation of gastrointestinal mucous membranes and diarrhea. Ground Ivy is also used for mild respiratory complaints of the upper bronchia; in the symptomatic treatment of coughs; and as a diuretic in cases of bladder and kidney stones. Externally, the drug is used for the treatment of poorly healing wounds, ulcers and skin diseases. In Italy, it is used for arthritis and rheumatism.

Chinese Medicine: Ground Ivy is used to treat carbuncles, erysipelas, lower abdominal pain, scabies, scrofulous, irregular menstruation, coughs, dysentery and jaundice. Efficacy has not, however, been proven for these indications.

Homeopathic Uses: Uses in homeopathy include diarrhea and hemorrhoids.

PRECAUTIONS AND ADVERSE REACTIONS

Health risks or side effects following the proper administration of designated therapeutic dosages are not recorded. Fatal poisonings were observed among horses following intake of large quantities of the fresh plant. Mice who were fed solely on the plant died after 3 to 4 days.

DOSAGE

Mode of Administration: The drug is used internally as well as externally.

Preparations: The liquid extract (1:1) is prepared by using 25% ethanol.

Daily Dosage: The normal single daily dose of the dried drug is 2 to 4 gm internally; externally, crushed leaves are placed on the affected areas.

Homeopathic Dosage: 5 drops, 1 tablet or 10 globules every 30 to 60 minutes (acute) or 1 to 3 times daily (chronic); parenterally: 1 to 2 ml sc acute, 3 times daily; chronic: once a day; suppositories: 1 suppository 2 to 3 times daily (chronic and acute) (HAB34)

Storage: Ground Ivy should be stored where it is not exposed to light.

LITERATURE

Barberan FAT, (1986) Fitoterapia 57(2):67.

Bohinc P, Korbar-Smid J, Cicerov-Cergol M, Über die kardiotonischen Substanzen des Gnadenkrautes - Gratiola officinalis. In: Sci Pharm 47:108-113. 1979.

Hänsel R, Keller K, Rimpler H, Schneider G (Hrsg.), Hagers Handbuch der Pharmazeutischen Praxis, 5. Aufl., Bde 4-6 (Drogen), Springer Verlag Berlin, Heidelberg, New York, 1992-1994.

Lewin L, Gifte und Vergiftungen, 6. Aufl., Nachdruck, Haug Verlag, Heidelberg 1992.

Madaus G, Lehrbuch der Biologischen Arzneimittel, Bde 1-3, Nachdruck, Georg Olms Verlag Hildesheim 1979.

Mascolo N et al., (1987) Phytother Res 1(1):28.

Roth L, Daunderer M, Kormann K, Giftpflanzen, Pflanzengifte, 4. Aufl., Ecomed Fachverlag Landsberg Lech 1993.

Sevenet T, Looking for new drugs: what criteria? J Ethnopharmacol, 32:83-90, Apr 1991.

Ground Pine

Ajuga chamaepitys

DESCRIPTION

Flower and Fruit: The plant has 2 to 4 flowers at each node. The petals are 4 to 6 mm. The tips of the petals are as long as or shorter than the tube. The corolla is yellow with red or purple markings, rarely entirely purple. The lower lip is entire, and the stamens are exerted. The filaments are hairy. The mericarps are 2 to 5 mm long, obovate and reticulate-wrinkled with a pitted surface.

Leaves, Stem and Root: Ground Pine is an annual or short-lived perennial. The stem is 5 to 30 cm long. It is usually heavily branched, glabrous to densely villous. The leaves are 3-partite with linear segments. They are 0.5 to 4 mm wide. The segments are sometimes 3-pinnatifid. The bracts are similar to the leaves.

Habitat: Sandy, stony areas of southern Britain and parts of Europe.

Other Names: Yellow Bugle

ACTIONS AND PHARMACOLOGY

COMPOUNDS

Volatile oil

Diterpene bitter principles

Caffeic acid derivatives: including rosemary acid

EFFECTS

Emmenagogue (stimulates menstrual flow), stimulant, diuretic.

INDICATIONS AND USAGE

Unproven Uses: Ground Pine is used for gout, rheumatism and gynecological disorders.

PRECAUTIONS AND ADVERSE REACTIONS

No health hazards or side effects are known in conjunction with the proper administration of designated therapeutic dosages.

DOSAGE

Mode of Administration: Ground Pine is available in compounded preparations as a liquid extract for internal use.

LITERATURE

Camps F, et al., (1985) An Quim 81C(1):74-75.

Kooiman P, (1972) Acta Bot Nederl 21(4):417.

Groundsel

Senecio vulgaris

DESCRIPTION

Medicinal Parts: The medicinal part is the herb collected during the flowering season.

Flower and Fruit: The yellow composite flowers are in compact cymes. The small capitula have tubular florets but no lingual ones. The bract calyx is globose. The involucre and the very short outer bracts have black tips. The fruit is 1.2 to 2 mm long and densely downy. The pappus, which is 3 times as long as the fruit, is silky and pure white.

Leaves, Stem and Root: Groundsel grows from about 10 to 30 cm high. It is annual, biennial or occasionally perennial. The plant has a thin, fusiform, pale root, which is densely covered in lateral roots. The stem is erect, simple or branched. The leaves are glabrous or cobweb-lanate and pinnatisect. The lower leaves narrow to the petiole; the upper ones are slit at the base and clasping. The tips are detached, oblong, obtuse and unevenly acute dentate.

Habitat: The plant is common in all of Europe, northern and central Asia, northern Africa and has been introduced into various other parts of Africa as well as Australia and the Americas.

Production: Groundsel is the flowering plant of Senecio vulgaris. The herb is gathered in uncultivated regions and dried in the shade.

Other Names: Grundy Swallow, Ground Glutton, Simson

ACTIONS AND PHARMACOLOGY

COMPOUNDS

Pyrrolizidine alkaloids (up to 0.16% in the fresh foliage): chief alkaloids are senecionine, seneciphylline

Flavonoids: including among others, isorhamnetin-3-O-glucosides, isorhamnetin-3-O-rutinosides, isorhamnetin-3-monosulphate

Volatile oil (traces)

EFFECTS

The toxic principles of the drug are the pyrrolizidine alkaloids, which are hepatotoxic and carcinogenic. Use of Groundsel for worm infestation can be explained by the high toxicity of the drug.

INDICATIONS AND USAGE

Unproven Uses: Internal use of Groundsel is not recommended because, similar to S. jacoboeae, it contains toxic and carcinogenic pyrrolizidine alkaloids. Prior uses have included the treatment of worm infestations, colic and epilepsy. The pressed juice has been used for dysmenorrhea, epilepsy, and as a styptic in dentistry.

PRECAUTIONS AND ADVERSE REACTIONS

Groundsel should not be taken internally because hepatotoxicity and carcinogenicity are possible due to the pyrrolizidine alkaloids with 1,2-unsaturated necic parent substances in its makeup.

DOSAGE

Mode of Administration: Internal use of Groundsel is not advised.

LITERATURE

Bull LB et al. in: The Pyrrolizidine Alkaloids, Pub. Wiley NY 1968.

Mansour RMA, Saleh, NAM (1981) Phytochemistry 20:1180.

Qualls CW, Segall H J (1978) J Chrom. 15:202.

Toppel G, Hartmann T (1986) Planta Med 6:25P.

Van Borstel K et al., PH 28:1635-1638. 1989.

Van Dooren Bos R et al., (1981) Planta Med 42:385.

Further information in:

Hänsel R, Keller K, Rimpler H, Schneider G (Hrsg.), Hagers Handbuch der Pharmazeutischen Praxis, 5. Aufl., Bde 4-6

(Drogen): Springer Verlag Berlin, Heidelberg, New York, 1992-1994.

Madaus G, Lehrbuch der Biologischen Arzneimittel, Bde 1-3, Nachdruck, Georg Olms Verlag Hildesheim 1979.

Teuscher E, Lindequist U, Biogene Gifte - Biologie, Chemie, Pharmakologie, 2. Aufl., Fischer Verlag Stuttgart 1994.

Guaiac

Guaiacum officinale

DESCRIPTION

Medicinal Parts: The primary medicinal part is the resin of the heartwood, which is used for various preparations. The wood also has some medicinal properties.

Flower and Fruit: The pale blue star-shaped flowers are in false umbels with 6 to 10 blooms that have 2 cm long pedicles. There are 5 sepals, 5 petals, 10 stamens and a bilocular ovary. The fruit is a bilocular, cordate capsule that is compressed at the side and contains a long and hard seed, in each chamber.

Leaves, Stem and Root: Guaiacum officinale is an evergreen tree that grows to 13 m high and has a greenish-brown, usually twisted trunk covered in furrowed bark. The heartwood is greenish brown and heavier than water, with an aromatic taste. The opposite leaves are short-petioled, coriaceous and di- to tri-pinnate. The leaflets are ovate or oblong, obtuse and entire-margined.

Characteristics: The shavings turn green on exposure to the air and blue-green in the presence of nitrogen.

Habitat: The plant grows in Florida, on the Antilles, in Guayana, Venezuela and Columbia. It is closely related to Guaiacum sanctum, which grows in the Bahamas and southern Florida.

Production: Guaiac wood consists of the heartwood and sapwood of Guaiacum officinale and/or Guaiacum sanctum.

Other Names: Guaiacum, Lignum Vitae, Pockwood

ACTIONS AND PHARMACOLOGY

COMPOUNDS

Triterpene saponins: aglycone oleanolic acid

Resin: containing, among others, the lignans (-)-guaiaretic acid, dihydroguajaretic acid, guaiacin

Isoguajacin: alpha-guaiaconic acid, tetrofuroguaiacine A and B

Volatile oil: chief components sesquiterpene alcohols; such as guaiole, which changes into quaiazulene with steam distillation

EFFECTS

Guaiacum officinale is fungistatic because of its saponin content.

INDICATIONS AND USAGE

■ Rheumatism

Guaiac is used as supportive therapy for rheumatic complaints.

Unproven Uses: Although folk medicine use has declined, it is used for respiratory complaints, skin disorders and syphilis in the Caribbean.

PRECAUTIONS AND ADVERSE REACTIONS

Health risks or side effects following the proper administration of designated therapeutic dosages are not recorded. High dosages of the drug can lead to diarrhea, gastroenteritis and intestinal colic. Skin rashes have also been observed following intake of the drug.

DOSAGE

Mode of Administration: The comminuted wood is used for decoctions and other galenic preparations for internal use. The essential oil, known as guaiac wood oil, must be evaluated separately.

How Supplied: Forms of commercial pharmaceutical preparations include drops, ointments and compound preparations.

Preparation: To make an infusion, use 1.5 g drug in 1 cup cold water (150 ml). Slowly bring to a boil, remove from heat and let steep, then strain after 15 minutes.

Daily Dosage: The average daily dose is 4 to 5 g of the drug. When using a tincture (Guajaci Ligni Tinctura), 20 to 40 drops make a single dose.

LITERATURE

Ahmad VU, Bano N, Bano S, PH 23:2612-2616. 1984.

Ahmad VU, Bano N, Bano S, PH 25:951-952. 1986.

King FE, Wilson JG, (1964) J Chem Soc:4011-4024.

King FE, Wilson JG, J Chem Soc:1572-1580. 1965.

Kratochvil JF et al., (1971) Phytochem 10:2529.

Majuinder PL, Bhattacharya M, (1974) Chem Ind 77.

Schrecker AW, (1957) J Am Chem Soc 79:3823.

Further information in:

Hänsel R, Keller K, Rimpler H, Schneider G (Hrsg.), Hagers Handbuch der Pharmazeutischen Praxis, 5. Aufl., Bde 4-6 (Drogen), Springer Verlag Berlin, Heidelberg, New York, 1992-1994.

Lewin L, Gifte und Vergiftungen, 6. Aufl., Nachdruck, Haug Verlag, Heidelberg 1992.

Madaus G, Lehrbuch der Biologischen Arzneimittel, Bde 1-3, Nachdruck, Georg Olms Verlag Hildesheim 1979.

Roth L, Daunderer M, Kormann K, Giftpflanzen, Pflanzengifte, 4. Aufl., Ecomed Fachverlag Landsberg Lech 1993.

Teuscher E, Biogene Arzneimittel, 5. Aufl., Wiss. Verlagsges. mbH Stuttgart 1997.

Guaiacum officinale

See Guaiac

Guar Gum

Cyamopsis tetragonoloba

DESCRIPTION

Medicinal Parts: The whole plant has medicinal properties.

Flower and Fruit: The flowers are in axillary, 6- to 30-flowered racemes. The structures of the flowers are arranged in fives. The sepals are fused and hairy on the outside; the lower calyx teeth are longer than the upper ones. The corolla is butterfly-shaped (flag, 2 wings, keel formed from 2 fused petals), small and reddish; there are 10 stamens. The fruit developing from a carpel is an upright, 3.8 to 5 cm long, sparsely haired legume with 5 to 6 seeds; these have a very well-developed, slimy endosperm.

Leaves, Stem and Root: Cyamopsis tetragonoloba is an annual herb, which grows up to 60 cm high. The leaves are alternate, triple-pinnate; the leaflets are broad-elliptical, acuminate, dentate, pubescent on both surfaces. They measure 3.8 to 7.5 cm long and 1.2 to 5 cm wide. The petiole is 2.5 to 3.8 cm long, while the stipules are 6 to 10 mm long. The root and root tuber have symbiotic bacteria, which bonds nitrogen from the air.

Habitat: The plant is native to the Indian subcontinent. It originated from India, Australia, South Africa and the U.S.

Production: Guar Gum is the powder extracted by milling from the endosperm of Cyamopsis tetragonoloba. A dry or wet milling process separates the endosperm from the seed shell.

Other Names: Aconite Bean, Calcutta Lucerne, Guar, Clusterbean

ACTIONS AND PHARMACOLOGY

COMPOUNDS

Water-soluble polysaccharides: galactomannans (85%)

Proteins (2 to 5%)

Saponins (0.1%)

EFFECTS

Clusterbean or Guar Gum causes a lowering of postprandial serum glucose values through (among other things) the influence of the hydrocolloid guar upon glucose resorption (delaying of stomach emptying into the duodenum), a reduction of glucosuria, improvement of the HBA1 value and leveling of the blood sugar profile. A lipid-lowering effect has also been demonstrated.

INDICATIONS AND USAGE

Unproven Uses: Internal application: Guar Gum has been used for diabetes mellitus, for postprandial hyperglycemia and glucosuria, and for hyperlipoproteinemia. It has also been used to regulate digestion.

Indian Medicine: Night blindness, dyspeptic complaints, anorexia, constipation and agalactia have all been treated with Guar Gum.

CONTRAINDICATIONS

Contraindicated in diseases of esophagus, stomach and intestine, which might hinder passage of the chyme.

PRECAUTIONS AND ADVERSE REACTIONS

No health hazards are known in conjunction with the proper administration of designated therapeutic dosages of the drug, nor with its use as a pharmaceutical vehicle. Possible side effects, particularly at the beginning of treatment, might include feelings of fullness, nausea, wind and diarrhea. Symptoms of hypoglycemia (outbreaks of sweating, vertigo, ravenous hunger) and resorption difficulties involving vitamins, minerals and medications (such as contraceptives!) have been observed, although rarely. Inadequate intake of fluids could lead to the danger of bolus formation.

DOSAGE

Mode of Administration: Powdered drug, granules and tablets for internal use.

Daily Dosage: Commercial pharmaceutical preparation with one dose of 5 gm per tablet or granules, 3 times daily.

Storage: Keep Guar Gum sealed tightly.

LITERATURE

Hänsel R, Keller K, Rimpler H, Schneider G (Ed.), Hagers Handbuch der Pharmazeutischen Praxis, 5. Aufl., Bde 4 - 6 (Drogen), Springer Verlag Berlin, Heidelberg, New York, 1992-1994.

Guarana

Paullinia cupana

TRADE NAME

Guarana (available from numerous manufacturers), Guarana Seed

DESCRIPTION

Medicinal Parts: The medicinal parts are the peeled, dried, roasted and pulverized seeds, formed into a thick paste with water.

Flower and Fruit: The usually unisexual flowers are inconspicuous, yellow to whitish and fragrant. They are in 30 long panicles, which only produce female or male flowers at any one time. The fruit is a hazelnut-sized, deep yellow to red-orange 3-sectioned capsule, which bursts open when ripe and releases 1 purple-brown to black seed in a cup-like aril.

Leaves, Stem and Root: The plant is a woody, evergreen perennial vine up to 10 m long, which climbs through the jungle. It is bushier in its cultivated form. The leaves are large, palmate, coriaceous, distinctly ribbed and roughly crenate-serrate.

Characteristics: A paste is formed from the pulverized and roasted seeds, formed into rolls or bars and dried. The taste is astringent, bitter then sweet, and the odor is reminiscent of chocolate.

Habitat: The plant is indigenous to the Amazon basin and has been introduced into other rain forests. The main area of cultivation is between Maues and Manau in Brazil.

Production: Guarana seeds are the seeds of Paullinia cupana. A preparation is also made from the ground seeds. Over a period of approximately 75 days, the pollinated flower develops a ''ripe'' guarana raceme, which is harvested by hand from October to December. Seeds (up to 80 per raceme) are taken out of the capsule shells, soaked for a time in water and then finally separated from the arillus. Subsequent to being dried in the sun, the seeds are roasted for 2 to 3 hours in special clay ovens. Once they have cooled, the parchment-like shell is removed and the seeds are ground down. Following this, the resulting paste is smoked over aromatic charcoal. The final product is dark brown in color and in stick form.

Other Names: Brazilian Cocoa, Guarana Bread, Paullinia

ACTIONS AND PHARMACOLOGY

COMPOUNDS

Purine alkaloids: chief alkaloid caffeine (3.6-5.8%), in addition, small amounts of theophylline and theobromine

Tannins (12%): oligomeric proanthocyanidins, condensed tannins

Cyanolipides: including among others, 2,4-dihydroxy-3-methylene-butyronitrile

Saponins

Starch (30%)

Proteins (15%)

EFFECTS

Guarana produces a stimulating effect, due to the presence of purines (caffeine, theobromine, theophylline). Caffeine is centrally stimulating, has a positive inotropic and, in high concentrations, has a positive chronotropic cardiac effect. It relaxes the vascular muscles (with the exception of cerebral vessels that constrict) and the bronchial tube.

Caffeine works as a short-term diuretic and increases gastric secretion. Furthermore, it increases the release of catecholamines. Inhibition of blood platelet aggregation has been observed.

INDICATIONS AND USAGE

Unproven Uses: Guarana is used as a tonic for fatigue and to quell hunger and thirst, for headache and dysmenorrhoea, digestion problems, fever and as a diuretic. Its effect in stimulating the circulation, heart and diuresis can be explained by the caffeine content.

Homeopathic Uses: Headache

PRECAUTIONS AND ADVERSE REACTIONS

General: No health hazards or side effects are known in conjunction with the proper administration of designated therapeutic dosages. Quantities corresponding to up to 400 mg caffeine per day (7 to 11 gm of the herb), spread out over the day, are toxicologically harmless to a healthy adult habituated to caffeine, through regular consumption of coffee or black tea.

One must remember that the quantities of caffeine considered harmless are calculated to include all of the foodstuffs and beverages containing the substance (including coffee, tea, cola, etc.). Caution is advised for patients with sensitive cardiovascular systems, renal diseases, hyperthyroidism, increased tendency to spasms and certain psychic disorders such as panic anxiety.

Drug Interactions: The diuretic action of Guarana may lead to hypokalemia with excessive use. Hypokalemia may increase digoxin toxicity.

Pregnancy: Pregnant women should avoid caffeine, and under no circumstances exceed a dosage of over 300 mg per day.

Nursing Mothers: Infants whose nursing mothers consume caffeine products could suffer from sleeping disorders.

OVERDOSAGE

The first symptoms of poisoning are dysuria, vomiting and abdominal spasms.

DOSAGE

Mode of Administration: The seeds of Paullinia cupana are grated and taken directly as powder or diluted in water or juice as a drink. It is not in use as a drug. It is available in various medicinal preparations.

How Supplied:
Capsules — 200 mg

Liquid — 1:1

Tablets — 800 mg, 1000 mg

Daily Dosage: Average single dose: 1 gm of the powder

Homeopathic Dosage: 5 drops, 10 globules every 30 to 60 minutes (acute) or 1 to 3 times a day (chronic); parenterally: 1 to 2 ml sc, acute: 3 times daily; chronic: once a day (HAB34)

LITERATURE

Frohne D, Guaraná; - der neue Muntermacher. In: DAZ 133(3):218. 1993.

Hänsel R, Keller K, Rimpler H, Schneider G (Ed.), Hagers Handbuch der Pharmazeutischen Praxis, 5. Aufl., Bde 4-6 (Drogen), Springer Verlag Berlin, Heidelberg, New York, 1992-1994.

Katzung W, Guaraná; - ein Naturprodukt mit hohem Coffeingehalt. In: Med Mo Pharm 16(11):330-333. 1993.

Leung AY, Encyclopedia of Common Natural Ingredients Used in Food, Drugs and Cosmetics, John Wiley & Sons Inc., New York, 1980.

Steinegger E, Hänsel R, Pharmakognosie, 5. Aufl., Springer Verlag Heidelberg 1992.

Teuscher E, Biogene Arzneimittel, 5. Aufl., Wiss. Verlagsges. Stuttgart 1997.

Wichtl M (Ed.), Teedrogen, 4. Aufl., Wiss. Verlagsges. Stuttgart 1997.

Gum Arabic

Acacia senegal

DESCRIPTION

Medicinal Parts: The latex from the trunk and branches is the medicinal part of the plant.

Flower and Fruit: The inflorescences, which grow from the leaf axils, are up to 10 cm long. The flowers are white and grow in cylindrical, dense spikes. The calyx is cup-shaped with 5 sepals. The 5 petals are lanceolate. The numerous stamens are long and fused at the base. The pods are about 10 cm long and contain 5 to 6 shiny brown seeds.

Leaves, Stem and Root: Acacia senegal is up to 6 m tall with a 12 to 25 cm thick, slightly leaning trunk, which has knotty branches and a thin crown. The sapwood is white and the heartwood is black. The bark is fibrous, gray on the outside and rust-colored on the inside. The leaves are double abruptly pinnate. The leaflets are in 10 to 15 pairs, narrow, gray-green, up to 5 mm long, opposite and very short-petioled. There are 2 to 3 stipules, which have formed into thorns, and are covered on the upper surface with yellow, fleshy glands.

Habitat: Acacia senegal is found in the tropical Savannah belt of Africa, in the southern Sahara (Senegal, Gambia), in Arabia, Beludschistan and Sind. Grown in forest-like conditions in the western and southwestern Sahara region (Senegal, Gambia, Ivory Coast, northern Dahomey and northern Nigeria).

Production: Acacia gummi, the latex, is the result of a wound infection of the tree, which has occurred naturally or has been induced. The incised bark is removed in strips of approximately 4 cm by 60 cm. The liquid discharge dries to form a hard, glazed substance, which is collected on a weekly basis. The latex is harvested from trees, ranging from 3 to 12 years old.

Not to be Confused With: According to DAB 10 (EUR), USP XXII, only latex from Acacia senegal or other African varieties are officially recognized. In other words, Asian, Australian and American latex are not official.

Other Names: Acacia, Cape Gum, Egyptian Thorn, Gum Acacia, Gum Senegal

ACTIONS AND PHARMACOLOGY

COMPOUNDS

Colloidally soluble polysaccharides: especially Arabic acid (acidic arabinogalactan)

Glycoproteins

EFFECTS

No information is available.

INDICATIONS AND USAGE

Unproven Uses: Acacia gummi is used in the preparation of emulsions. The drug is used as a mild stimulant and to impede absorption. It is also used for the treatment of catarrh and diarrhea. Acacia is often a constituent of cough drops. It is also used in veterinary medicine for mild diarrhea in small animals, foals and calves.

PRECAUTIONS AND ADVERSE REACTIONS

No health hazards or side effects are known in conjunction with the proper administration of designated therapeutic dosages.

DOSAGE

Mode of Administration: Acacia is used as a pharmaceutical aid and is also administered internally in combination preparations.

Storage: The drug should be stored in tightly closed containers.

LITERATURE

Beuscher N, Bodinet C, Willigmann I, Harnischfeger G, Biological activity of Baptisia tinctoria extracts. In: Inst. für Angew. Botanik der Univ. Hamburg, Angewandte Botanik, Berichte 6, 46-61. 1997.

Randall RC, Phillips GO, Williams PA, Food Hydrocolloids 3:65-75, 1989.

Further information in:

Berger F, Handbuch der Drogenkunde, W Maudrich Verlag Wien 1964.

Hänsel R, Keller K, Rimpler H, Schneider G (Hrsg.), Hagers Handbuch der Pharmazeutischen Praxis, 5. Aufl., Bde 4-6 (Drogen): Springer Verlag Berlin, Heidelberg, New York, 1992-1994.

Steinegger E, Hänsel R, Pharmakognosie, 5. Aufl., Springer Verlag Heidelberg 1992.

Teuscher E, Biogene Arzneimittel, 5. Aufl., Wiss. Verlagsges. Stuttgart 1997.

Gumweed

Grindelia camporum

DESCRIPTION

Medicinal Parts: The medicinal parts are the flowering branches and the dried leaves.

Flower and Fruit: Gumweed has a number of individual composite heads, each with a diameter of 2 to 3 cm, at the end of leafy stems. The involucral bracts are 3 to 8 mm by 0.5 to 1 mm, with very viscid, cylindrical, deflected apexes. If present, the ligules are 7 to 15 mm long and yellow to orange-yellow. The inner florets are yellow. The achaenes are 2 to 3 mm, oblong and brown. The 2 to 8 pappus-awns are 3 to 5 mm long and usually finely serrulate.

Leaves, Stem and Root: The plant is an erect biennial or perennial herb or small bush that grows up to 1 m high, often branched above. The alternate leaves are 3 to 7 cm long, triangular to ovate-oblong, clasping, resinous-punctate, serrate-crenate or entire-margined, and light green. They break off easily when dry.

Habitat: The plant grows in the Southwestern U.S. and in Mexico.

Production: Gumweed herb consists of the dried tops and leaves of Grindelia robusta and/or Grindelia squarrosa, which are gathered during flowering season.

Other Names: August Flower, Grindelia, Rosin Weed, Tar Weed

ACTIONS AND PHARMACOLOGY

COMPOUNDS

Diterpene acids: grindelic acid, hydroxygrindelic acid, 6-oxogrindelic acid. 7alpha,8alpha-epoxygrindelic acid

Volatile oil: including, among others, borneol, bornyl acetate, camphene, camphor, myrcene, alpha- and beta-pinene

Polyynes: including matricarianol, matricarianolacetate

Saponins

Tannins

Flavonoids: including kaempferol-3,7-dimethyl ether, kaempferol-3-dimethyl ether, luteolin, quercetin, quercetin-3,3′-dimethyl ether

EFFECTS

In vitro, the drug has an antimicrobial, fungistatic and spasmolytic effect caused by the resin, which contains diterpenes, and the phenol carbolic acids. An antibacterial effect has also been demonstrated in vitro. In addition, an inflammation-inhibiting effect has been proven.

INDICATIONS AND USAGE

Approved by Commission E:

- Cough
- Bronchitis

Unproven Uses: Gumweed is also used for infections in the mucous membranes of the upper respiratory tract.

PRECAUTIONS AND ADVERSE REACTIONS

Health risks following the proper administration of designated therapeutic dosages are not recorded. Side effects listed in older scientific literature (Lewin) include gastric irritation and diarrhea. Large dosages, however, are said to have a poisonous effect.

DOSAGE

Mode of Administration: Comminuted herb for teas and other galenic preparations for internal use.

Preparation: The tincture is prepared in a 1:10 or 1:5 concentration with 60% to 80% ethanol (v/v).

Daily Dosage: The recommended dosage is 4 to 6 g of drug or 3 to 6 g Gumweed liquid extract. If using the tincture, the dosage is 1.5 to 3 ml.

LITERATURE

Hegnauer R, Chemotaxonomie der Pflanzen, Bde 1-11, Birkhäuser Verlag Basel, Boston, Berlin 1962-1997.

Kern W, List PH, Hörhammer L (Hrsg.), Hagers Handbuch der Pharmazeutischen Praxis, 4. Aufl., Bde. 1-8, Springer Verlag Berlin, Heidelberg, New York, 1969.

Lewin L, Gifte und Vergiftungen, 6. Aufl., Nachdruck, Haug Verlag, Heidelberg 1992.

Madaus G, Lehrbuch der Biologischen Arzneimittel, Bde 1-3, Nachdruck, Georg Olms Verlag Hildesheim 1979.

Mascolo, N et al., (1987) Phytother Res 1(1):28.

Schimmer O, Egersdörfer S, Grindelia-Arten - Die Grindelie. In: ZPT 9(3):86. 1988.

Timmermann B et al., (1985) Phytochemistry 24(5):1031.

Wagner H, Wiesenauer M, Phytotherapie. Phytopharmaka und pflanzliche Homöopathika, Fischer-Verlag, Stuttgart, Jena, New York 1995.

Guraea rusbyi

See Cocillana Tree

Haematoxylon campechianum

See Logwood

Hagenia abyssinica

See Kousso

Hamamelis virginiana

See Witch Hazel

Haronga

Haronga madagascariensis

DESCRIPTION

Medicinal Parts: The medicinal parts of the tree are the leaves and bark.

Flower and Fruit: The inflorescences are richly blossomed, terminal and umbel-like, with a diameter of about 20 cm. The flowers are small and white; they have 5 sepals, 5 petals, 4 stamens and a fanned ovary with 2 ovules per section. The fruit is a roundish, reddish drupe. The seeds (approximately 10) are cylindrical and have black glandular hairs and a reticulate surface structure.

Leaves, Stem and Root: Haronga madagascariensis is a small evergreen tree that grows up to 8 m high with a heavily branched crown. It has opposite, elliptical-oval leaves, which are rounded to cordate at the base and dotted black. The upper surface is dark green. The lower surface has red-brown hairs.

Habitat: The plant originated in Madagascar and east Africa; it grows in many areas throughout tropical Africa.

Production: Haronga is a collective term for extracts from the leaves and bark of the trunk and branches of Haronga madagascariensis, as well preparations made from those components. The leaves are collected and then air-dried whole; the bark is peeled and also air-dried.

ACTIONS AND PHARMACOLOGY

COMPOUNDS

Anthracene derivatives: including harunganin, madagascin, madagascinanthrone, haronginanthrone, chrysophanol, physcione, hypericin, pseudohypericin, madagascarine

Volatile oil (traces)

Oligomeric procyanidins

Flavonoids (in the leaves): including quercetin-3-O-arabinsoide, quercetin-3-O-xyloside, quercitrin

EFFECTS

Haronga has a digestion regulatory effect through stimulation of the excretory function of the pancreas and gastric juice secretion. In animal experiments, it has demonstrated a choleretic, cholecystokinetic and antihepatoxic effect. An antimicrobial effect has also been observed.

INDICATIONS AND USAGE

Approved by Commission E:

■ Dyspeptic complaints

Unproven Uses: Haronga is used for mild exocrine pancreatic insufficiency. Internal uses of the bark and leaves in folk medicine include constipation, diarrhea, liver and gallbladder conditions, worm infestations, gonorrhea, hemorrhoids, menstrual disturbances and puerperal fever. The bark is used externally for eczema. The effect for the external application seems plausible because of the drug's antibacterial effect.

CONTRAINDICATIONS

The drug is not to be used in patients with acute pancreatitis, severe liver function disorders, gallstone illnesses, obstruction of the biliary ducts, gallbladder empyema or ileus.

PRECAUTIONS AND ADVERSE REACTIONS

Health risks or side effects following the proper administration of designated therapeutic dosages are not recorded. Photosensitization in fair-skinned people can be caused by hypericin and pseudohypericin, but is unlikely due to the small size of therapeutic dosages.

DOSAGE

Mode of Administration: As comminuted Haronga bark with leaves for decoctions, extracts and other preparations.

How Supplied: Forms of commercial pharmaceutical reparations include drops, tablets and compound preparations.

Preparation: Extracts are standardized to 0.1% chrysophanic acid derivatives; tinctures are standardized to 0.01% chrysophanic acid derivatives.

Daily Dosage: The average daily dose is 7.5 to 15 mg of an aqueous-alcoholic dry extract corresponding to 25 to 50 mg drug.

LITERATURE

Baldi A et al., Polyphenols from Harungana madagascarienis. In: PM 58(7)91. 1992.

Buckley DG et al., Aust J Chem 25:843-855. 1972.

Fisel J et al., DAZ 106:1053-1060. 1966.

Gehrmann B, Analytische Studie an Harungana madagascariensis Lam. ex Poir. In: Dissertation Universität Hamburg. 1989.

Hänsel R, Keller K, Rimpler H, Schneider G (Hrsg.), Hagers Handbuch der Pharmazeutischen Praxis, 5. Aufl., Bde 4-6 (Drogen), Springer Verlag Berlin, Heidelberg, New York, 1992-1994.

Messerschmidt W, DAZ 106:1209-1211. 1966.

Steinegger E, Hänsel R, Pharmakognosie, 5. Aufl., Springer Verlag Heidelberg 1992.

Haronga madagascariensis

See Haronga

Harpagophytum procumbens

See Devil's Claw

Hartstongue

Scolopendrium vulgare

DESCRIPTION

Medicinal Parts: The medicinal part is the frond.

Flower and Fruit: Two rows of large sporangia lie almost horizontally on the under surface of the fronds, with a long film stretching toward the margin.

Leaves, Stem and Root: The evergreen plant is a fern with long, wide, simple, short-petioled dark green fronds. They are arranged in clusters and are broad linear-lanceolate, 2-lobed cordate at the base and acuminate higher up, with a sinuate margin. The stem is covered in brown, almost hair-like scales. The root is bushy, short and sturdy.

Habitat: The plant is indigenous to almost all of Europe, North America, northern Africa, and eastern Asia.

Production: Hartstongue is the aerial part of Scolopendrium vulgare.

Other Names: Hind's Tongue, Horse Tongue, Buttonhole, God's-Hair

ACTIONS AND PHARMACOLOGY

COMPOUNDS

Tannins

Mucilages

Flavonoids: including among others, kaempferol-7-rhamnoside-3-coffeoyl-7-diglucoside

Thiaminase (probably present only in the fresh plant)

Monosaccharides/oligosaccharides: saccharose, invert sugar

EFFECTS

Hartstongue is a diuretic and has a mild laxative effect.

INDICATIONS AND USAGE

Unproven Uses: Hartstongue is used in folk medicine for digestive disorders, urinary tract diseases, and spleen and liver complaints.

PRECAUTIONS AND ADVERSE REACTIONS

No health hazards or side effects are known in conjunction with the proper administration of designated therapeutic dosages.

DOSAGE

Mode of Administration: Hartstongue is used internally as an infusion.

LITERATURE

Hegnauer R, Chemotaxonomie der Pflanzen, Bde 1-11: Birkhäuser Verlag Basel, Boston, Berlin 1962-1997.

Kern W, List PH, Hörhammer L (Hrsg.), Hagers Handbuch der Pharmazeutischen Praxis, 4. Aufl., Bde 1-8: Springer Verlag Berlin, Heidelberg, New York, 1969 (unter Phyllitis scolopendrium).

Madaus G, Lehrbuch der Biologischen Arzneimittel, Bde 1-3, Nachdruck, Georg Olms Verlag Hildesheim 1979.

Heartsease

Viola tricolor

DESCRIPTION

Medicinal Parts: The medicinal parts are the dried aerial parts, the fresh aerial parts of the flowering plant and the whole plant.

Flower and Fruit: The solitary, long-pedicled flower is yellow or tricolored. It has 5 lanceolate, acute and uneven sepals with an appendage and 5 uneven petals, the largest of which is spurred. The 5 stamens also have an appendage at the tip. There are 3 fused superior ovaries. The fruit is an ellipsoid, obtusely angular capsule, which bursts open at 3 points. The seeds are pear-shaped and yellow.

Leaves, Stem and Root: Heartsease is annual to perennial and grows about 30 cm high. The shoots are usually yellowish green, glabrous or covered in scattered hairs. The stem is erect, angular, unbranched or branched, glabrous or short-haired. It has short internodes below and longer ones above. The leaves are alternate, glabrous, or short-haired. The lower leaves are cordate; the upper ones are oblong-elliptical. The stipules are lyrate-pinnatesect and have a large, crenate terminal tip.

Characteristics: The plant is odorless and the taste slimy-sweetish.

Habitat: The plant is indigenous to temperate Eurasia, from the Mediterranean to India and as far as Ireland. It is cultivated in Holland and France.

Production: Viola herb consists of the dried, above-ground parts of Viola tricolor, mainly of the subspecies vulgaris and subspecies arvensis, harvested at flowering season. The herb is cultivated predominantly in central Europe. The flowering above-ground parts are harvested in the summer months and carefully dried on a well ventilated floor or at 45° C to 50° C. Two to three harvests per year are possible.

Other Names: European Wild Pansy, Johnny-Jump-Up, Wild Pansy

ACTIONS AND PHARMACOLOGY

COMPOUNDS

Flavonoids (0.2-0.4%): including among others rutin (violaquercitrin, 23%), luteolin-7-O-glucosides, scoparin, saponarine, violanthin, vicinein-2, vitexin

Phenol carboxylic acid: salicylic acid (0.06-0.3%), violutoside (violutin, glucoarabinoside of the methyl salicylate)

Mucilage (10%)

Tannins (2-5%)

Hydroxycoumarins: umbelliferone

Triterpene saponins (speculated)

EFFECTS

The drug has soothing, salve-like effects due to its mucin content; in animal experiments oral administration brought about an improvement of eczema-like skin conditions after long-term use. The antisporiatic effect attributed to the drug may be explained by the saponin content, as can its use for catarrh of the upper respiratory tract. In vitro the drug is hemolytic and increases chloride elimination in the urine.

INDICATIONS AND USAGE

Approved by Commission E:

- Inflammation of the skin

Unproven Uses: External uses include mild seborrheic skin diseases, cradle cap in children and various skin disorders, including wet and dry exanthema, eczema, *Crusta lactea*, acne, impetigo and *Pruritus vulvae*. The plant is used internally as a mild laxative for constipation and as an auxiliary agent to promote metabolism.

Historic uses of Heartsease include the treatment of respiratory catarrh, throat inflammation, whooping cough and feverish colds.

Homeopathic Uses: The drug is used for eczema and inflammation of the urinary tract.

PRECAUTIONS AND ADVERSE REACTIONS

No health hazards or side effects are known in conjunction with the proper administration of designated therapeutic dosages.

DOSAGE

Mode of Administration: Whole, cut and powdered drug is available for infusions, decoctions and other galenic preparations. It is also available in ointments and shampoos for external use.

Preparation: To make a tea, pour 1 cup of scalding water over 1 dessertspoonful of drug. An infusion for internal use is prepared using 5 to 10 gm drug per 1 liter of water. A decoction for internal use is prepared by adding 1.5 gm drug to 1 cup water. The drug is also used as a bath additive.

Daily Dosage: A cup of tea should be taken 3 times daily after meals. The dose for the infusion is 1 dessertspoonful 3 times daily. The dose for the powdered drug is 1/2 teaspoonful in hot sugar water 3 times daily.

Homeopathic Dosage: 5 drops, 1 tablet or 10 globules every 30 to 60 minutes (acute) or 1 to 3 times daily (chronic); parenterally: 1 to 2 ml sc, acute: 3 times daily; chronic: once a day (HAB1).

Storage: Heartsease must be kept stored away form light sources, and if possible, from moisture in well-sealed containers.

LITERATURE

Hörhammer L et al., (1965) Tetrahedron Letters 1707.

Komorowski T et al., Herba Pol 29:5. 1983.

Mánez S, Villar A, PA 44:250. 1988.

Molnár P et al., PH 25:195. 1986.

Further information in:

Fenaroli's Handbook of Flavor Ingredients, Vol. 1, 2nd Ed., CRC Press 1975

Hänsel R, Keller K, Rimpler H, Schneider G (Hrsg.), Hagers Handbuch der Pharmazeutischen Praxis, 5. Aufl., Bde 4-6 (Drogen): Springer Verlag Berlin, Heidelberg, New York, 1992-1994.

Leung AY, Encyclopedia of Common Natural Ingredients Used in Food, Drugs, Cosmetics, John Wiley & Sons Inc., New York 1980.

Steinegger E, Hänsel R, Pharmakognosie, 5. Aufl., Springer Verlag Heidelberg 1992.

Teuscher E, Biogene Arzneimittel, 5. Aufl., Wiss. Verlagsges. Stuttgart 1997.

Wagner H, Wiesenauer M, Phytotherapie. Phytopharmaka und pflanzliche Homöopathika, Fischer-Verlag, Stuttgart, Jena, New York 1995.

Wichtl M (Hrsg.), Teedrogen, 4. Aufl., Wiss. Verlagsges. Stuttgart 1997.

Heather

Calluna vulgaris

DESCRIPTION

Medicinal Parts: The medicinal parts are the complete herb with leaves, the flowers, and the growing shoots of the plant that are collected and dried when the plant is in bloom, as well as the fresh aerial parts collected at the same time.

Flowers and Fruit: The inflorescence is turned to one side, dense and hanging. The short-pedicled flowers are nodding, pale-violet-pink and occasionally white; they have 4 small, oval, fringed bracts. The calyx has 4 violet-pink, glossy and petaloid sepals, which have the consistency of straw. The 8 stamens form a brown-red club. The superior ovary has 4 sections, and the style is larger than the calyx. The style has a thick, button-like, 4-knobbed stigma. The fruit capsule is globose, 1.5 mm long and 4 sectioned. The fruit is covered in thick white bristles and is many-seeded. The dividing walls break off easily.

Leaves, Stem and Root: Calluna vulgaris is a dwarf shrub, 0.2 to 1 m high with decumbent, rooting shoots and ascending branches. The small stems are thin, gray-brown, heavily branched and have numerous upright branches. The leaves are linear-lanceolate, in groups of 4 rows. They are imbricate, 1 to 3.5 mm long, revolute, sessile and have 2 mm long points at the base. The margins are glandular with downward-pointing spurs.

Habitat: With the exception of a few Mediterranean islands, the plant is distributed throughout most of Europe, Russia and Asia Minor, as well as on the Atlantic coast of North America.

Production: The herb is harvested from July to October and dried.

Not to be Confused With: Erica tetralix.

Other Names: Ling

ACTIONS AND PHARMACOLOGY

COMPOUNDS

Flavonoids: including kempferol, quercetin, myricetin, taxifolin, and the glycosides of each, as well as callunin

Catechin tannins (3-7%): (+)-catechin, (-)-epicatechin

Oligomeric proanthocyanidins

Caffeic acid derivatives: including chlorogenic acid

Phenols: orcin, orcinol

Triterpenes: including ursolic acid (2.5%)

Steroids: beta-sitosterol

Hydroquinone glycosides: including arbutin

EFFECTS

Heather is said to be diuretic, antimicrobial, cholagogic and antirheumatic. It is also used as an agent for wound healing. However, these effects have not yet been documented.

INDICATIONS AND USAGE

Unproven Uses: Preparations of Heather and/or Heather flowers are used as a diuretic for diseases and ailments of the kidneys and the lower urinary tract, and for enlargement of the prostate. They are also used for gastrointestinal disorders, colic, liver and gallbladder disease, gout, rheumatism, respiratory complaints, insomnia, agitation and wounds.

The efficacy for the claimed uses is not documented.

PRECAUTIONS AND ADVERSE REACTIONS

No health hazards or side effects are known in conjunction with the proper administration of designated therapeutic dosages.

DOSAGE

Mode of Administration: Whole, cut and powdered forms are available for internal and external use.

Preparation: A decoction is prepared by adding 1.5 gm of the drug to 1/4 liter of water and then boiling for 3 minutes. For a bath additive, 500 gm of the drug is boiled in a few liters of water, strained and added to the bath. A liquid extract 1:1 is also used.

Daily Dosage: The average daily dose of the decoction is 3 cups daily between meals; the dose for the liquid extract is 1 to 2 teaspoonfuls daily.

Externally, the drug is added to full baths.

Storage: Heather should be stored in well-dried, sealed containers.

LITERATURE

Hänsel R, Keller K, Rimpler H, Schneider G (Hrsg.), Hagers Handbuch der Pharmazeutischen Praxis, 5. Aufl., Bde 4-6 (Drogen): Springer Verlag Berlin, Heidelberg, New York, 1992-1994.

Jaläl MAF, Read DJ, Haslam E, Phenolic composition and its seasonal variation in Calluna vulgaris. In: PH 21(6):1397. 1982.

Madaus G, Lehrbuch der Biologischen Arzneimittel, Bde 1-3, Nachdruck, Georg Olms Verlag Hildesheim 1979.

Mantilla JLG, Vieitez E, An Edafol Agrobiol 34:765-774. 1975.

Simon A et al., Further flavonoid glycosides from Calluna vulgaris. In: PH 32:1045. 1993.

Simon A et al., Two flavonol 3-[triacetylarabinosyl(1-6) glucosides] from Calluna vulgaris. In: PH 33:1237. 1993.

Hedera helix

See English Ivy

Hedge Mustard

Sisymbrium officinale

DESCRIPTION

Medicinal Parts: The medicinal parts are the fresh, flowering herb and the fresh aerial parts of the flowering plant.

Flower and Fruit: The inflorescences at the end of the stems and branches have no bracts and are initially umbelliferous-racemous, later stretching into spikes. The pedicles are thin and approximately 1.5 cm long, bearing the small flowers. The 4 sepals are 1.5 to 2.5 mm long, erect, pubescent and narrowly elliptical. The petals are pale yellow and 3 to 4 mm long. The stamens have 0.5 to 0.5 mm long anthers. The fruit is a pubescent pod appressed to the axis of the infructescence. The fruits are 1 to 1.5 cm long and 1 to 1.5 mm thick. The almost-smooth seeds are about 1 mm long, ovate, compressed and unwinged with reddish, yellow-brown seed-skins.

Leaves, Stem and Root: The plant is an annual or biennial, 30 to 60 cm high, and has a thin taproot. The stem is branched, round, leafy and covered in scattered patent hairs. The basal leaves and lower cauline leaves are petiolate-pinnatifid with 3 to 9 segments. The upper leaves are oblong-lanceolate, simple or with 2 to 4 lateral segments, and often hastate and pubescent.

Habitat: The herb is found mainly in temperate Europe, but it also grows as far as northern Africa and eastern Siberia.

Production: Hedge Mustard is the fresh flowering herb of Sisymbrium officinale.

Other Names: Singer's Plant, St. Barbara's Hedge Mustard, English Watercress, Erysimum, Thalictroc

ACTIONS AND PHARMACOLOGY

COMPOUNDS

Cardioactive steroid glycosides (cardenolides, 0.05% in the tips of the foliage): including among others corchorosid A and helveticosid

Glucosinolates: chiefly sinigrin (allylglucosinolates) and gluconapin (3-butenylglucosinolates), releasing through cell destruction the volatile mustard oil allylisothiocyanate and 3-butenylisothiocyanate

Vitamins: ascorbic acid (vitamin C, up to 0.2 % in the fresh foliage)

EFFECTS

Hedge mustard contains cardio-active steroids (cardenolids) and is said to be spasmolytic and analgesic. Its use for pharyngitis and laryngitis as well as severe hoarseness may be due to the mustard oils.

INDICATIONS AND USAGE

Unproven Uses: In folk medicine, the drug is used for laryngitis and pharyngitis, severe hoarseness including loss of voice, chronic bronchitis and inflammation of the gallbladder.

PRECAUTIONS AND ADVERSE REACTIONS

No health hazards or side effects are known in conjunction with the proper administration of designated therapeutic dosages.

OVERDOSAGE

It is conceivable that overdosage would have digitalis-like effects. These include queasiness, vomiting, diarrhea, headache and cardiac rhythm disorders. Cases of poisonings have not, however, been recorded.

DOSAGE

Daily Dosage: The average daily internal dose of the drug is 0.5 to 1.0 gm, which would be equal to 3 to 4 cups daily of an infusion. It takes between 6 and 8 g of drug to make 1 g extract.

Externally, the infusion is used as a gargle or mouthwash, several times daily.

LITERATURE

Bachelard HS, Trikojus VM, (1963) Austral. J Biol Sci 16: 147.

Ockendon JG, Buczki ST, (1979) Trans Brit Mycol Soc 72:156.

Schultz OE, Gmelin R, Naturforsch Z, 7b:500-506. 1952.

Further information in:

Hänsel R, Keller K, Rimpler H, Schneider G (Hrsg.), Hagers Handbuch der Pharmazeutischen Praxis, 5. Aufl., Bde 4-6 (Drogen): Springer Verlag Berlin, Heidelberg, New York, 1992-1994.

Roth L, Daunderer M, Kormann K, Giftpflanzen, Pflanzengifte, 4. Aufl., Ecomed Fachverlag Landsberg Lech 1993.

Teuscher E, Lindequist U, Biogene Gifte - Biologie, Chemie, Pharmakologie, 2. Aufl., Fischer Verlag Stuttgart 1994.

Hedge-Hyssop

Gratiola officinalis

DESCRIPTION

Medicinal Parts: The medicinal parts are the herb and roots. (In contrast to what its name suggests, Hedge-Hyssop is not a member of the Hyssop family, even though it has a similarly bitter taste.)

Flower and Fruit: The pedicled flowers are arranged singly in the axils of the upper leaf pairs and are a pale red or yellowish-white. The calyx is only fused at the base and has 5 tips. The corolla has a distinct tube and a bilabiate border. The upper lip is margined, and the lower lip is divided into 3. There are 4 stamens, 2 sterile and 2 fertile, and 1 superior ovary. The fruit has 4 lids, which burst open.

Leaves, Stem and Root: The plant is a perennial that grows 15 to 30 cm high. The stem grows from a creeping scaly rhizome. It is erect and becomes glabrous and quadrangular higher up. The leaves are opposite, lanceolate, weakly serrate, smooth and pale green.

Characteristics: The plant is poisonous and has a bitter taste.

Habitat: The herb is indigenous to western and central Asia, as well as southern Europe.

Production: Hedge-Hyssop is the herb of Gratiola officinalis, which is harvested shortly before flowering. The upper portion of the stem is cut down, then dried in thin layers in the shade at temperatures not exceeding 45° C.

Other Names: Gratiola

ACTIONS AND PHARMACOLOGY

COMPOUNDS

Cucurbitacins: gratiogenin, 16-hydroxygratiogenin, cucurbitacins E, I, the glycosides gratiogenin-3beta-D-glucoside, gratioside (gratiolin, gratiogenindiglucoside), elaterinide, desacetylelaterinide

Saponins

Lignans

Flavonoids

EFFECTS

The glycosides are said to be cardiotonic. The cucurbaticins, especially elaterinide, cause a reduction of the contraction power of cardiac muscle, a lowering of cardiac frequency and a distinct increase in coronary flow. Elaterinide has a laxative effect. The drug is a strong purgative; it eliminates intestinal parasites and increases micturation.

INDICATIONS AND USAGE

Unproven Uses: The herb was formerly used as a purgative and for treating the liver. In folk medicine, it is used as purgative and emetic for gout, liver complaints and constipation, as well as for chronic skin conditions. The drug is only to be taken under medical supervision of a doctor because of its toxicity.

Homeopathic Uses: Uses in homeopathy include stomach colic and bladder and kidney conditions.

PRECAUTIONS AND ADVERSE REACTIONS

Health risks or side effects following the proper administration of designated therapeutic dosages are not recorded. Nonetheless, the drug is extremely poisonous. It is severely irritating to mucous membranes due to the cucurbitacin and cucurbitacin glycosides content, out of which cucurbitacins are released in watery environments.

OVERDOSAGE

The intake of toxic dosages leads to vomiting, bloody diarrhea, colic, kidney irritation and initially to elevated diuresis, then to anuria. Very high dosages lead to spasm, paralysis and circulatory collapse. Fatalities are seen only rarely. Following gastric lavage, the treatment for poisonings should proceed symptomatically.

DOSAGE

Mode of Administration: Hedge-Hyssop is most effective in alcoholic extracts, but it also is used in infusions and in homeopathic dilutions. Today, it is rarely used in folk medicine.

Daily Dosage: A single dose of tea is noted as containing 0.3 g drug.

Homeopathic Dosage: 5 drops, 1 tablet or 10 globules every 30 to 60 minutes (acute) or 1 to 3 times daily (chronic); parenterally: 1 to 2 ml sc acute, 3 times daily; chronic: once a day (HAB1).

LITERATURE

Bohinc P, Korbar-Smid J, Cicerov-Cergol M, Über die kardiotonischen Substanzen des Gnadenkrautes - Gratiola officinalis. In: Sci Pharm 47:108-113. 1979.

Kern W, List PH, Hörhammer L (Hrsg.), Hagers Handbuch der Pharmazeutischen Praxis, 4. Aufl., Bde. 1-8, Springer Verlag Berlin, Heidelberg, New York, 1969.

Lewin L, Gifte und Vergiftungen, 6. Aufl., Nachdruck, Haug Verlag, Heidelberg 1992.

Madaus G, Lehrbuch der Biologischen Arzneimittel, Bde 1-3, Nachdruck, Georg Olms Verlag Hildesheim 1979.

Müller A, Wichtl M, Herzwirsamkeit des Gnadenkrautes (Gratiola officinalis). In: Pharm Ztg 124(37):1761-1766. 1979.

Roth L, Daunderer M, Kormann K, Giftpflanzen, Pflanzengifte, 4. Aufl., Ecomed Fachverlag Landsberg Lech 1993.

Teuscher E, Lindequist U, Biogene Gifte - Biologie, Chemie, Pharmakologie, 2. Aufl., Fischer Verlag Stuttgart 1994.

Helianthemum canadense

See Frostwort

Helianthus annuus

See Sunflower

Helichrysum arenarium

See Immortelle

Helleborus niger

See Black Hellebore

Helleborus viridis

See Green Hellebore

Hemlock

Conium maculatum

DESCRIPTION

Medicinal Parts: The medicinal parts of the plant are the fresh flowering foliage, the branches and the dried leaves.

Flower and Fruit: The plant has white flowers in 10 to 20 rayed umbels. The 3 to 5 triangular to lanceolate bracts are acuminate; 3 to 6 small bracts only on the outside of the small umbels. The blossoms have 1.5 mm white petals. The fruit is ovate with undulating veins. Deep indentations on the mericarp on the seam side—with no oil marks in the indentations—are a unique feature.

Leaves, Stem and Root: The plant can be annual or perennial; it grows up to 2 m high. The stem is erect, tubular, hollow, round and finely grooved. It is branched above, glabrous with brownish-red marks below. The leaves are a glossy dark green, 3-pinnate. The root is whitish and fusiform or branched.

Characteristics: When wilting, the highly poisonous herb smells of mice. It tastes disgustingly salty and pungent. The stem has distinctive red marks.

Habitat: The plant is indigenous to Europe and the temperate zones of Asia, North Africa, and North and South America.

Production: Hemlock is the fresh or dried leaves and the flowering branch tips of Conium maculatum. They are gathered from June to September in the second year of grown and air-dried in a shaded, open location.

Not to be Confused With: Hemlock may be confused with water hemlock, canine parsley, wild chervil and with tuberous chervil.

Other Names: Cicuta, Poison Parsley, Poison Root, Poison Snakeweed, Spotted Crowbane, Spotted Hemlock, Spotted

Parsley, Water Parsley, Winter Fern, Herb Bennet, Spotted Corobane, Musquash Root, Beaver Poison, Kex, Kecksies

ACTIONS AND PHARMACOLOGY

COMPOUNDS

Piperidin alkaloids: main alkaloid coniine, including, among others, N-methyl coniine, gamma-coniceine

The piperidin alkaloids are volatile and are likely to be present in toxicologically harmful quantities only in the freshly harvested plant, particularly in its berries, and in the freshly dried plant.

Polyynes: including falcarinol, falcarindiol

Furanocoumarins: including bergaptene, xanthotoxin

EFFECTS

The plant is poisonous. The effects of the drug are caused by coniine in particular. Toxic doses given to mice, rats, guinea pigs and cats provoked the autonomous ganglion, clonic and tonal contractions of individual limbs, cramps and eventually, paralysis. Small doses given to mice led to blood pressure reduction in the short term. Higher doses resulted in a rise in blood pressure. Smaller doses stimulated respiration in cats, while higher doses impeded or slowed down the initial stimulus. In isolated guinea pig ileum, coniine brought on contractions. In isolated perfused rabbit hearts, coniine was negatively inotropic while a stable heart beat was maintained. With anesthetized cats, a suppression of the muscle contraction reflex took place. Feeding or injecting lethal doses of coniine into cows, horses, pigs, sheep and hamsters was initially stimulating, producing twitching of the eyes and ears, which was followed by muscular debility, collapse, limpness and death through paralysis. Coniine absorbed through the skin and mucous membranes is stimulating at first, then causes gradual paralysis of the spinal cord and blockage of the medulla oblongata. Nicotine-like receptors are at first activated, then paralyzed.

INDICATIONS AND USAGE

Unproven Uses : Use is inadvisable due to the uncontrollable amounts of coniine. Formerly, in folk medicine, the drug was used internally for neuralgia, rheumatism of the muscles and joints, stiffness of the neck, tetanic and epileptic cramps, bronchial spasms and pylori spasms. Externally, the drug was used as an ointment for coughs, asthma, sciatica, backache and neuralgia.

Homeopathic Uses: Swollen glands, pareses, calcification of cerebral vessels and depressive moods are considered to be indications for use in homeopathy.

PRECAUTIONS AND ADVERSE REACTIONS

General: The drug is severely poisonous and use is not advised.

Pregnancy: The drug has a teratogenic effect with chronic intake.

OVERDOSAGE

Symptoms of poisoning following intake of toxic quantities (corresponding to 150 mg coniine, approximately 10 g of the freshly dried berries, approximately 30 g of the freshly dried leaves) include burning of the mouth, scratchy throat, salivation, rolling of the eyes, visual disorders and weakness in the legs. Lethal dosages (corresponding to approximately 500 mg coniine) cause glossoplegia, mydriasis, pressure in the head, dizziness, nausea, vomiting, diarrhea, loss of orientation, rising central paralysis, dyspepsia and cyanosis. Death ultimately results through central asphyxiation, in the cases of very high dosages, and also through curare-like paralysis of the breathing musculature.

Following stomach and intestinal emptying (gastric lavage, sodium sulfate) and the administration of activated charcoal, plasma volume expanders and sodium bicarbonate infusions should be given in case of shock or to restore acidosis balance. If necessary, intubation and respiration should be carried out.

DOSAGE

Mode of Administration: Hemlock is obsolete and strongly advised against as an internal drug because of the danger of poisoning. Homeopathic dilutions and ointments containing hemlock are used externally.

How Supplied: Liquid rubs, ointments.

Daily Dosage: Use is discouraged, but the maximum single dose mentioned for internal use is 0.3 g, not to exceed 1.5 g, per day. The standard single dose is 0.1 g.

Homeopathic Dosage: 5 drops, 1 tablet or 10 globules every 30 to 60 minutes (acute) or 1 to 3 times daily (chronic); parenterally: 1 to 2 ml sc acute, 3 times daily; chronic: once a day; ointment 1 to 2 times daily (HAB34).

Storage: Hemlock should be stored above caustic lime, well dried, in closed containers and kept for no more than one year.

LITERATURE

Cromwell BT, Biochem J 64:259-266. 1956.

Kreitmair H, PA 3:565-566. 1948.

Madaus S, Schindler H, Arch Pharm 276:280-290. 1938.

Roberts MF, (1975) Phytochemistry 14:2395.

Roberts MF, (1980) Planta Med 39:216.

Seeger R, Neumann HG, DAZ-Giftlexikon Coniin. In: DAZ 131(13):720. 1991.

Further information in:

Frohne D, Pfänder HJ, Giftpflanzen - Ein Handbuch für Apotheker, Toxikologen und Biologen, 4. Aufl., Wiss. Verlagsges. mbH Stuttgart 1997.

Hänsel R, Keller K, Rimpler H, Schneider G (Hrsg.), Hagers Handbuch der Pharmazeutischen Praxis, 5. Aufl., Bde 4-6 (Drogen), Springer Verlag Berlin, Heidelberg, New York, 1992-1994.

Lewin L, Gifte und Vergiftungen, 6. Aufl., Nachdruck, Haug Verlag, Heidelberg 1992.

Madaus G, Lehrbuch der Biologischen Arzneimittel, Bde 1-3, Nachdruck, Georg Olms Verlag Hildesheim 1979.

Roth L, Daunderer M, Kormann K, Giftpflanzen, Pflanzengifte, 4. Aufl., Ecomed Fachverlag Landsberg Lech 1993.

Teuscher E, Lindequist U, Biogene Gifte - Biologie, Chemie, Pharmakologie, 2. Aufl., Fischer Verlag Stuttgart 1994.

Teuscher E, Biogene Arzneimittel, 5. Aufl., Wiss. Verlagsges. mbH Stuttgart 1997.

Hemp Agrimony

Eupatorium cannabinum

DESCRIPTION

Medicinal Parts: The medicinal part is the flowering herb.

Flower and Fruit: The flowers are in compact, terminal, umbrella-like umbels. They are small dull pink tubular androgynous flowers whose corolla tube has a 5-tipped edge. The epicalyx is cylindrical and consists of a few bracts. The edge of the calyx consists of yellowish hairs. The style is divided in two parts and shows above the flower. The corolla is covered in resinous spots. The angular fruit bears a crown of hair and is dirty white.

Leaves, Stem and Root: The plant is a small perennial herb 75 to 150 cm high. The rhizome is woody and has stems growing from it, which have short axillary branches. The stems are erect, reddish, pubescent and resinous below. The root leaves are long-petioled. The opposite cauline leaves are short-petioled, trifoliate and serrate and covered in resinous spots.

Habitat: Hemp Agrimony grows in damp regions of Europe.

Production: Hemp Agrimony is the flowering herb of Eupatorium cannabium.

Other Names: Holy Rope, St. John's Herb, Sweet-Smelling Trefoil, Water Maudlin

ACTIONS AND PHARMACOLOGY

COMPOUNDS

Caffeic acid ester: chlorogenic acid

Immunostimulating polysaccharides (heteroxylans)

Pyrrolizidine alkaloids: including echinatine, supinine, eucanecine, amabiline, lycopsamin, intermedin

Sesquiterpene lactones: including eupatoriopicrin, eupatolid

EFFECTS

Eupatorin is said to be cytotoxic and has an immune-stimulating effect. It is also a bitter tonic.

INDICATIONS AND USAGE

Unproven Uses: The herb is used for disorders of the liver and gallbladder and for fevers.

Homeopathic Uses: Eupatorium cannabinum is used to treat illnesses of the respiratory organs.

PRECAUTIONS AND ADVERSE REACTIONS

Because of the pyrrolizidine alkaloid content with 1,2-unsaturated necic parent substances, hepatotoxicity and carcinogenicity are likely consequences of internal use. Therefore the drug should not be taken internally. Sensitization after skin contact with the plant has been reported.

DOSAGE

Mode of Administration: The herb is used topically as an alcoholic extract, as a tea, and as an inhalation for the treatment of colds.

LITERATURE

Anonym, Positive Auswirkungen von Olivenöl auf den Blutdruck. In: ZPT 12(1):13. 1991.

Antibiotika und Immunabwehr. In: Symbiose 4(2):20. 1992.

Elsässer-Beile U, Willenbacher W, Bartsch HH, Gallati H, Schulte Mönting J, Kleist von S et al., Cytokine production in leukocyte cultures during therapy with echinacea extract. In: J Clin Lab Analysis 10(6):441-445. 1996.

Hendriks H et al., (1983) Pharm Weekblad 5:281.

Pederson E (1975) Phytochemistry 14:2086.

Röder E, Pyrrolizidinhaltige Arzneipflanzen. In: DAZ 132(45):2427-2435. 1992.

Vollmar A et al., (1986) Phytochemistry 25(2):377.

Winterhoff H, Gumbinger HG, Pharmakologische Untersuchungen mit Pflanzenextrakten. Probleme und Lösungsmöglichkeit. In: DAZ 130(49):2668. 1990.

Woerdenbag HJ et al., (1987) Phytother Res 2(2):76.

Further information in:

Kern W, List PH, Hörhammer L (Hrsg.), Hagers Handbuch der Pharmazeutischen Praxis, 4. Aufl., Bde 1-8, Springer Verlag Berlin, Heidelberg, New York, 1969.

Madaus G, Lehrbuch der Biologischen Arzneimittel, Bde 1-3, Nachdruck, Georg Olms Verlag Hildesheim 1979.

Roth L, Daunderer M, Kormann K, Giftpflanzen, Pflanzengifte, 4. Aufl., Ecomed Fachverlag Landsberg Lech 1993.

Teuscher E, Lindequist U, Biogene Gifte - Biologie, Chemie, Pharmakologie, 2. Aufl., Fischer Verlag Stuttgart 1994.

Wagner H, Wiesenauer M, Phytotherapie. Phytopharmaka und pflanzliche Homöopathika, Fischer-Verlag, Stuttgart, Jena, New York 1995.

Hempnettle

Galeopsis segetum

TRADE NAMES

Hempnettle is available from numerous manufacturers.

DESCRIPTION

Medicinal Parts: The medicinal part is the flowering herb.

Flower and Fruit: The large, pale yellow, bilabiate flowers are in false whorls on the branch ends. The calyx is evenly 5-dentate and covered in patent glandular hairs. The upper lip of the corolla is domed, finely dentate and pubescent. The lateral tips of the 3-lobed lower lip are wide, obtuse and have 1 hollow erect tooth at either side of the base. The stamen halves are horizontal. The fruit is smooth.

Leaves, Stem and Root: The herb grows 15 to 100 cm high. The stem is erect, heavily branched and downy, with unthickened nodes. The leaves are ovate and serrate. The lower ones are long petioled, the upper are short petioled.

Habitat: Hempnettle is found in southern and central Europe.

Production: Hempnettle consists of the aboveground parts of Galeopsis segetum Necker (synonym Galeopsis ochroleuca Lamarck) and is gathered in the wild during the flowering season.

ACTIONS AND PHARMACOLOGY

COMPOUNDS

Iridoide monoterpenes: including harpagide, 8-O-acetylharpagide, antirrinoside, 5-O-glucosylantirrinoside

Silicic acid (to some extent water-soluble)

Tannins

Flavonoids

EFFECTS

The herb acts as expectorant, due to its saponin content, and as an astringent because of the tannins, silicic acid, iridoids and antirrhinoside.

INDICATIONS AND USAGE

Approved by Commission E:

- Cough
- Bronchitis

Unproven Uses: In folk medicine, the herb is used for pulmonary afflictions and as a diuretic.

PRECAUTIONS AND ADVERSE REACTIONS

Health risks or side effects following the proper administration of designated therapeutic dosages are not recorded.

DOSAGE

Mode of Administration: Ground and cut herb for teas and other galenic preparations for internal use.

Preparation: To prepare an infusion, pour boiling water over 2 g of comminuted drug, strain after 5 minutes.

Daily Dosage: Average daily dose: 6 g drug. One cup of the infusion may be taken several times daily and, if preferred, sweetened with honey.

LITERATURE

Junod-Busch U, Dissertation ETH Zürich. 1976.

Kern W, List PH, Hörhammer L (Hrsg.), Hagers Handbuch der Pharmazeutischen Praxis, 4. Aufl., Bde. 1-8, Springer Verlag Berlin, Heidelberg, New York, 1969.

Madaus G, Lehrbuch der Biologischen Arzneimittel, Bde 1-3, Nachdruck, Georg Olms Verlag Hildesheim 1979.

Tomas-Barberan FA et al., PH 30:3311. 1991.

Steinegger E, Hänsel R, Pharmakognosie, 5. Aufl., Springer Verlag Heidelberg 1992.

Wichtl M (Hrsg.), Teedrogen, 4. Aufl., Wiss. Verlagsges. Stuttgart 1997.

Henbane

Hyoscyamus niger

DESCRIPTION

Medicinal Parts: The medicinal parts are the dried leaves or the dried leaves with the flowering branches, the dried seeds and the whole fresh flowering plant.

Flower and Fruit: The flowers are in almost sessile terminal, one-sided leafy and revolute spikes. The calyx is jug-shaped, 5-tipped and does not drop. The corolla is funnel-shaped, 5-lobed, dirty yellow with violet veins and dark violet in the tube. The flower has 1 superior ovary and 5 stamens. The fruit is a swollen pixidium with up to 200 seeds. The seeds are gray-brown, pitted, slightly reniform, compressed, 1 to 1.3 mm long and 1 mm wide.

Leaves, Stem and Root: The plant is erect and grows up to 80 cm high. It is an herb with simple leaves. The root is fusiform and turnip-like at the top. The stem is erect and sticky-villous. The leaves are oblong, roughly crenate-dentate and gray-green. The basal leaves are petiolate, and the cauline leaves are stem clasping.

Characteristics: Henbane has a strong, distinctive odor. The plant is poisonous.

Habitat: The plant is indigenous to Europe, western and northern Asia, and northern Africa. It has been introduced to eastern Asia, North America and Australia.

Production: Henbane leaf consists of the dried leaves or the dried leaves and flowering tops of Hyoscyamus niger, harvested from cultures or in the wild when in bloom and dried mechanically or in the sun. Henbane seeds are the seeds of Hyoscyamus niger.

Other Names: Devil's Eye, Fetid Nightshade, Stinking Nightshade, Hen Bell, Hogbean, Jupiter's Bean and Poison Tobacco

ACTIONS AND PHARMACOLOGY

COMPOUNDS: HENBANE LEAF

Tropane alkaloids (0.05- 0.28%): chief alkaloid (-)-hyoscyamine, under storage conditions changing over to some extent into atropine, and scopolamine

Flavonoids: including, among others, rutin

COMPOUNDS: HENBANE SEED

Tropane alkaloids (0.05-0.3%): chief alkaloid (-)-hyoscyamine, under storage conditions changing to some extent into atropine, and scopolamine

Fatty oil

EFFECTS: HENBANE LEAF AND SEED

Main active agents: Alkaloids, flavonids. Henbane preparations produce a parasympatholytic or anticholinergic effect by competitive inhibition of acetylcholine. This inhibition affects the muscarinic action of acetylcholine but not its nicotine-like effects on ganglia and motor end plates.

Henbane preparations exert peripheral actions on the autonomic nervous system and on smooth muscle, as well as the central nervous system. Because of their parasympatholytic properties, they cause relaxation of organs containing smooth muscle, particularly in the region of the gastrointestinal tract. Furthermore, they relieve muscular tremors of central nervous origin.

The spectrum of actions of Hyoscyamus niger additionally includes a sedative effect.

INDICATIONS AND USAGE

HENBANE LEAF

Approved by Commission E:

■ Dyspeptic complaints

Unproven Uses: Preparations of henbane oil are used for the treatment of scar tissue.

In folk medicine, Henbane is used internally for various pain syndromes, in particular toothache and facial pain, painful ulcers and tumors, stomach cramps and lower abdominal pain. Externally, henbane oil is used for the treatment of scar tissue.

It has been used for hundreds of years in so-called witches' ointments, as a repellent against mice and rats, as stunning agent for fish and to increase the narcotic effect of beer.

Indian Medicine: Used for toothache, bleeding gums and nose, orchitis, dysmenorrhea, worm infestation, black vomit, asthma, diverse pain syndromes and meningitis.

HENBANE SEED

Approved by Commission E:

■ Dyspeptic complaints

Unproven Uses: Internal application: Spasms of the gastrointestinal tract; preparations of Henbane oil are used for the treatment of scar tissue.

In folk medicine, Henebane was formerly used as a fumigant for asthma and toothache.

Chinese Medicine: Used for convulsions, psychoses, joint pains, stomach pains, asthma, chronic dysentery and diarrhea.

CONTRAINDICATIONS

HENBANE LEAF AND SEED

Tachycardiac arrhythmias, prostatic adenoma, angle-closure glaucoma, acute pulmonary edema, mechanical stenoses in the area of the gastrointestinal tract, megacolon.

PRECAUTIONS AND ADVERSE REACTIONS

HENBANE LEAF AND SEED

General: No health hazards are known in conjunction with the proper administration of designated therapeutic dosages. Skin reddening, dryness of the mouth, tachycardiac arrhythmias, mydriasis (the 4 early warning symptoms of a poisoning), accommodation disorders, heat build-up through decline in sweat secretion, miction disorders and obstipation can occur as side effects, particularly with overdoses.

Drug Interactions: Enhancement of anticholinergic action by tricyclic antidepressants, amantadine, antihistamines, phenothiazines, procainamide and quinidine.

OVERDOSAGE

HENBANE LEAF AND SEED

Because of the high content of scopolamine in the drug, poisonings lead at first to somnolence, but then also, after the intake of very high dosages, to central excitation (restlessness, hallucinations, deliria, and manic episodes), followed by exhaustion and sleep. Lethal dosages carry with them the danger of asphyxiation (for adults starting at 100 mg atropine, with an alkaloid-rich drug at 30, considerably less for children). Severe poisonings are particularly conceivable in connection with the misuse of the drug as an intoxicant. Treatment for poisonings include gastric lavage, temperature-lowering measures with wet cloths (no antipyretics!), oxygen respiration for respiratory distress, intubation, parenteral physostigmine salts as an antidote, diazepam for spasms and chlorpromazine for severe excitation.

DOSAGE

HENBANE LEAF

Mode of Administration: Standardized Henbane powder and galenic preparations for internal application.

Daily Dosage: The average single dose is 0.5 gm of standardized Henbane powder corresponding to 0.25 to 0.35 mg total alkaloid. Maximum daily dose is 3.0 gm of standardized Henbane powder corresponding to 1.5 to 2.1 mg total alkaloid, calculated as hyoscyamine.

Storage: Keep protected from light in tightly sealed containers.

HENBANE SEED

Mode of Administration: The drug is available as an emulsion or powder.

Storage: Should be stored separate from other medicines.

LITERATURE

HENBANE LEAF

Frohne D, Pfänder HJ, Giftpflanzen - Ein Handbuch für Apotheker, Toxikologen und Biologen, 4. Aufl., Wiss. Verlags-Ges. Stuttgart 1997.

Hänsel R, Keller K, Rimpler H, Schneider G (Hrsg.), Hagers Handbuch der Pharmazeutischen Praxis, 5. Aufl., Bde 4-6 (Drogen), Springer Verlag Berlin, Heidelberg, New York, 1992-1994.

Kraft K, Europäische Rauschdrogen. In: ZPT 17(6):343-355. 1996.

Lewin L, Gifte und Vergiftungen, 6. Aufl., Nachdruck, Haug Verlag, Heidelberg 1992.

Madaus G, Lehrbuch der Biologischen Arzneimittel, Bde 1-3, Nachdruck, Georg Olms Verlag Hildesheim 1979.

Roth L, Daunderer M, Kormann K, Giftpflanzen, Pflanzengifte, 4. Aufl., Ecomed Fachverlag Landsberg Lech 1993.

Sharova EG et al., Khim Prir Soedin (1):126. 1977.

Steinegger E, Hänsel R, Pharmakognosie, 5. Aufl., Springer Verlag Heidelberg 1992.

Teuscher E, Lindequist U, Biogene Gifte - Biologie, Chemie, Pharmakologie, 2. Aufl., Fischer Verlag Stuttgart 1994.

Teuscher E, Biogene Arzneimittel, 5. Aufl., Wiss. Verlagsges. Stuttgart 1997.

Wagner H, Wiesenauer M, Phytotherapie. Phytopharmaka und pflanzliche Homöopathika, Fischer-Verlag, Stuttgart, Jena, New York 1995.

Wellen BJ, Zur Geschichte des Bilsenkrautes. Eine pharmaziehistorische Untersuchung besonders zu Hyoscyamus niger L. In: Dissertation Universität Marburg. 1986.

HENBANE SEED

Frohne D, Pfänder HJ, Giftpflanzen - Ein Handbuch für Apotheker, Toxikologen und Biologen, 4. Aufl., Wiss. Verlags-Ges. Stuttgart 1997.

Hänsel R, Keller K, Rimpler H, Schneider G (Hrsg.), Hagers Handbuch der Pharmazeutischen Praxis, 5. Aufl., Bde 4-6 (Drogen), Springer Verlag Berlin, Heidelberg, New York, 1992-1994.

Lewin L, Gifte und Vergiftungen, 6. Aufl., Nachdruck, Haug Verlag, Heidelberg 1992.

Madaus G, Lehrbuch der Biologischen Arzneimittel, Bde 1-3, Nachdruck, Georg Olms Verlag Hildesheim 1979.

Roth L, Daunderer M, Kormann K, Giftpflanzen, Pflanzengifte, 4. Aufl., Ecomed Fachverlag Landsberg Lech 1993.

Tattje DHE et al., Zusammensetzung der etherischen Öle von Laurus nobilis, L. nobilis var. angustifolia und L. azorica. In: PM 44:116-119. 1982.

Teuscher E, Lindequist U, Biogene Gifte - Biologie, Chemie, Pharmakologie, 2. Aufl., Fischer Verlag Stuttgart 1994.

Henna

Lawsonia inermis

DESCRIPTION

Medicinal Parts: The medicinal parts are the pulverized leaves, the fruit and the bark.

Flower and Fruit: The flowers are in small impressive groups of 4 panicles and yellowy-white to brick-red. The calyx is top-shaped, later bowl-shaped without appendages. The petals are thick, very wrinkled, yellowish-white to brick-red. The stamens are arranged in pairs. The fruit is an indehiscent or a fibrously torn berry. The seeds are small and angular, and the seed skin is spongy at the tip.

Leaves, Stem and Root: Henna is a deciduous, 2 to 6 m high shrub with partly thorny, short shoots and opposite paired, narrowly acuminate lanceolate leaves.

Habitat: Found in Egypt, India, the Middle East, Kurdistan and Iran.

Production: Henna is the aerial part of Lawsonia inermis.

Other Names: Alcanna, Egyptian Privet, Jamaica Mignonette, Mignonette Tree, Reseda, Henne, Mehndi, Mendee, Smooth Lawsonia

ACTIONS AND PHARMACOLOGY

COMPOUNDS

Naphthalene derivatives (1,4-naphthaquinones): in particular lawsone (2-hydroxy-1,4-naphthaquinone), arising during dehydration of the leaves out of the precursor 1,2,4-trihydroxy-naphthalen-4-beta-D-glucoside

Tannins

EFFECTS

The drug is an astringent and a diuretic, and has an antibacterial effect.

INDICATIONS AND USAGE

Unproven Uses: The drug is used externally for eczema, scabies, fungal infections and ulcers. It is also used for amebic dysentery and gastrointestinal ulcers. In African folk medicine, it is used as an abortifacient. The drug is also contained in facial and hair lotions and is used to treat dandruff.

Indian Medicine: Henna root preparations are used to treat leprosy, skin diseases, amenorrhea and dysmenorrhea. Henna leaves are used to treat wounds, ulcers, dysuria, coughs, bronchitis, one-sided headache, rheumatism and anemia. The flowers are used for headache, fever and acute psychosis. Henna seeds are used to treat intermittent fever, diarrhea and dysentery.

PRECAUTIONS AND ADVERSE REACTIONS

Health risks or side effects following the proper administration of designated therapeutic dosages are not recorded. Stomach complaints are possible due to the tannin content.

DOSAGE

Mode of Administration: Henna is used rarely for internal use in ground form or as an infusion. Henna is applied externally as an ingredient in hair and skin lotions.

Daily Dosage: For internal use, 3 gm of powder leaves to be taken daily, for amebiasis and ulcers.

LITERATURE

Bardwaj DK et al., (1978) Phytochemistry 17:1440.

Karawya MS et al., (1969) Lloydia 32:76.

Kern W, List PH, Hörhammer L (Hrsg.), Hagers Handbuch der Pharmazeutischen Praxis, 4. Aufl., Bde. 1-8, Springer Verlag Berlin, Heidelberg, New York, 1969.

Mahmood ZF et al., (1983) Fitoterapia 4:153.

Teuscher E, Biogene Arzneimittel, 5. Aufl., Wiss. Verlagsges. mbH Stuttgart 1997.

Wichtl M (Hrsg.), Teedrogen, 4. Aufl., Wiss. Verlagsges. mbH Stuttgart 1997.

Hepatica nobilis

See American Liverleaf

Heracleum sphondylium

See Hogweed

Herb Paris

Paris quadrifolia

DESCRIPTION

Medicinal Parts: The medicinal part is the whole fresh plant when the fruit begins to ripen.

Flower and Fruit: The flowers are solitary and terminal. The sepals are lanceolate, acuminate, 3-veined and 4 times as wide as the linear-awl-shaped petals. The stamens are thread-like to awl-shaped and bear linear anthers in the middle. The ovary has 5 thread-like stigmas, both of which are purple-brown. The fruit is a blue-black globular berry the size of a small cherry.

Leaves, Stem and Root: The 15 to 30 cm high plant is a perennial herb with a creeping, fleshy rhizome. The stem is erect, round, unbranched and crowned by 4 acuminate leaves. The leaves are whorled, almost obovate, acute, entire-margined and glabrous. The leaves have 3 to 5 ribs. They are dark green and matte above, pale and slightly glossy beneath.

Characteristics: The plant has an unpleasant smell and is poisonous.

Habitat: The plant is indigenous to Europe and Asian Russia.

Production: Herb Paris is the fresh plant of Paris quadrifolia, when the fruit is ripe.

Not to be Confused With: Poisoning can occur in children when they confuse the fruit of the Herb Paris plant with that of blueberries.

Other Names: One Berry

ACTIONS AND PHARMACOLOGY

COMPOUNDS

Steroid saponins: chief components are pennogenin triglycoside, pennogenin tetraglycoside, and their bisdemosidic precursors (26-O-glucosides), including 1-dehydrotrillenogenin

EFFECTS

The active agents are the saponins (which irritate mucous membranes), paristyphnin, paridin, citric acid and pectin. The parissaponins are local irritants as well as absorptive when taken orally. The main toxin is paristyphnin, which, when taken orally, leads to miosis and can consequently cause paralysis of the respiratory system.

INDICATIONS AND USAGE

Homeopathic Uses: Herb Paris is used as a homeopathic remedy for headaches, neuralgia, nervous tension, dizziness, palpitations and migraine.

PRECAUTIONS AND ADVERSE REACTIONS

The drug is considered poisonous. Symptoms of poisoning following intake of the berries include nausea, vomiting, diarrhea, miosis and headache. However, no serious poisonings have been recorded in this century.

DOSAGE

Mode of Administration: Herb Paris is available in homeopathic dilutions.

LITERATURE

Frohne D, Pfänder HJ, Giftpflanzen - Ein Handbuch für Apotheker, Toxikologen und Biologen, 4. Aufl., Wiss. Verlags-Ges. Stuttgart 1997.

Kern W, List PH, Hörhammer L (Hrsg.), Hagers Handbuch der Pharmazeutischen Praxis, 4. Aufl., Bde. 1-8, Springer Verlag Berlin, Heidelberg, New York, 1969.

Lewin L, Gifte und Vergiftungen, 6. Aufl., Nachdruck, Haug Verlag, Heidelberg 1992.

Madaus G, Lehrbuch der Biologischen Arzneimittel, Bde 1-3, Nachdruck, Georg Olms Verlag Hildesheim 1979.

Nohara T et al., Chem Pharm Bull 30:1851. 1982.

Roth L, Daunderer M, Kormann K, Giftpflanzen, Pflanzengifte, 4. Aufl., Ecomed Fachverlag Landsberg Lech 1993.

Teuscher E, Lindequist U, Biogene Gifte - Biologie, Chemie, Pharmakologie, 2. Aufl., Fischer Verlag Stuttgart 1994.

Herb Robert

Geranium robertianum

DESCRIPTION

Medicinal Parts: The medicinal parts of the plant are the fresh or dried aerial parts collected during the flowering season, as well as the whole fresh or dried plant.

Flower and Fruit: The peduncles are usually distinctly longer than the bracts and the 2.2 to 7 mm long, permanently erect pedicles. The flowers are longer than their pedicles. There are 5 separate sepals and 5 petals. The sepals are erect when they first bloom and hang when the fruit matures. The petals have long stems. There are 10 stamens and 5 ovaries with long styles, which form an upward curve when mature. The fruit is circular and 2 cm long, with 3 mm long protruding, reticulate, glabrous or pubescent fruit lobes which are upward horizontally wrinkled. These permanently enclose the smooth, finely spotted seeds. The fruit lobes burst off from the central column without the awn.

Leaves, Stem and Root: Geranium robertianum is a 20 to 40 cm high annual or hardy annual with a weak, branched tap root and a long hypocotyl. The stems are heavily branched, usually red, and glandular-haired. The leaves are 3- to 5-sectioned compound leaves with petiolate, entire-margined to double-pinnasect leaflets.

Characteristics: Herb Robert has an unpleasant smell often associated with goats or bugs.

Habitat: The plant is indigenous to the area stretching from Europe to China and Japan; to Africa southward as far as Uganda; to the Atlantic seaboard of North America; and the temperate areas of South America.

Production: Herb Robert is the aerial parts of Geranium robertianum, which are gathered between May and October in uncultivated regions, then dried in the open air in the shade.

Not to be Confused With: The herbs of Geranium palustre and Geranium pratense are frequently used as an adulteration.

Other Names: Dragon's Blood, Storkbill, Wild Crane's-Bill

ACTIONS AND PHARMACOLOGY

COMPOUNDS

Flavonoids: including rutin, quercetin-3-O-rhamnogalactoside, kaempferol-3-O-rhamnoglucoside, hyperoside

Tannins: geraniin, isogeraniin, beta-penta-O-galloylglucose

EFFECTS

The drug has the following effects:

Antiviral: The extract of the fresh herb, including rhizome, has been shown to have a mild antiviral effect against the *vesicular stomatitis virus*. In another study, however, the aqueous solution of the ethanol extract was not shown to have an antiviral effect against the polio virus Type 1, measles, coxsachie-B2, adeno- or Semliki forest virus.

Antimicrobial: The fraction of an extract produced with 80% ethanol was shown to have an inhibitory effect on the growth of Escherichia coli, Pseudomonas aeruginosa and Staphylococcus aureus. In the serial dilution test, growth of Microsporum canis and Trichophyton mentagrophytes was completely stunted.

Hypotensive effect: Effects have only been described in general reviews.

INDICATIONS AND USAGE

Unproven Uses: The drug is used internally for functional impairment of the liver and gallbladder, inflammatory conditions of gallbladder and its ducts, inflammation of the kidney and bladder, and calculosis. Folk medicine uses have also included internal use of the drug for diarrhea. In addition, washed fresh leaves are chewed or prepared as an infusion or decoction used as a mouthwash or gargle for inflammatory conditions of the oral mucous membrane. External application is used to treat poorly healing wounds. These uses appear plausible because of the tannins.

PRECAUTIONS AND ADVERSE REACTIONS

Health risks or side effects following the proper administration of designated therapeutic dosages are not recorded.

DOSAGE

Mode of Administration: The drug is used internally as well as externally.

Preparation: To prepare an infusion, add 1 dessertspoonful of drug to 1/2 liter of cold water. Bring to a boil and leave to steep.

Daily Dosage: Internally, the average single dose of the drug is 1.5 g; drink 2 to 3 cups of the infusion daily, between meals.

LITERATURE

Haddock EA et al., J Chem Soc Perkin Trans 1:2535-2545. 1982.

Hänsel R, Keller K, Rimpler H, Schneider G (Hrsg.), Hagers Handbuch der Pharmazeutischen Praxis, 5. Aufl., Bde 4-6 (Drogen), Springer Verlag Berlin, Heidelberg, New York, 1992-1994.

Karnig T, Bucar-Stachel J, PM 57:292-293. 1991.

Madaus G, Lehrbuch der Biologischen Arzneimittel, Bde 1-3, Nachdruck, Georg Olms Verlag Hildesheim 1979.

Herniaria glabra

See Rupturewort

Hibiscus

Hibiscus sabdariffa

DESCRIPTION

Medicinal Parts: The medicinal parts of the plant are the flowers.

Flower and Fruit: The flowers are solitary, axillary and almost sessile. The calyx is red, the corolla is yellow, and the anthers are blood red. The fruit is a 2 cm long, ovoid, many-seeded capsule.

Leaves, Stem and Root: Hibiscus is a 0.15 to 1 m bushy annual that is branched from the base. The stems are reddish, almost glabrous. The basal leaves are undivided and ovate; the cauline leaves are 3-lobed and 7.5 to 10 cm wide. The lobes are 2.5 cm wide and crenate.

Habitat: Hibiscus sabdariffa originally came from the area around the source of the Niger. It grows worldwide in the tropics and is cultivated in Europe.

Production: Hibiscus flowers consist of the calyces of Hibiscus sabdariffa (sabdariffa ruber variety).

Other Names: Guinea Sorrel, Jamaica Sorrel, Red Sorrel, Roselle

ACTIONS AND PHARMACOLOGY

COMPOUNDS

Fruit acids (15-30%): in particular hibiscus ((+)-allohydroxy citric acid lacton), additionally lemons, malic acid, tartaric acid

Anthocyans (intensive red): including delphinidin-3-xyloglucoside, delphinidin-3-glucoside, cyanidin-3-xyloglucoside

Flavonoids: including gossypetin

Mucilages: rhamnogalacturonans, arabinogalactans, arabinans

EFFECTS

Hibiscus tea has a laxative effect due to the high content of poorly absorbable fruit acids.

Aqueous extracts of hibiscus leaves have a relaxant effect on the uterus musculature. The drug also has a hypotensive effect.

INDICATIONS AND USAGE

Unproven Uses: Hibiscus flowers are used for loss of appetite, for colds that affect the respiratory tract and stomach, to dissolve phlegm, as a diuretic and gentle laxative, and for disorders of circulation.

Chinese Medicine: Preparations of the plant are used to treat carbuncles, swelling and inflammation of the skin, scalding, conjunctivitis and *herpes zoster*.

PRECAUTIONS AND ADVERSE REACTIONS

Health risks or side effects following the proper administration of designated therapeutic dosages are not recorded.

DOSAGE

Mode of Administration: Hibiscus sabdariffa is available as a tea preparation.

Preparation: To make a tea, pour boiling water over 1.5 gm comminuted drug and strain after 5 to 10 minutes.

LITERATURE

Franz M, Franz G, Hibiscus sabdariffa - Hibiscusblüten. In: ZPT 9(2):63. 1988.

Kern W, List PH, Hörhammer L (Hrsg.), Hagers Handbuch der Pharmazeutischen Praxis, 4. Aufl., Bde. 1-8, Springer Verlag Berlin, Heidelberg, New York, 1969.

Menβen HG, Staesche K, DAZ 114:1211. 1974.

Müller BM, Franz G, PM 58:60. 1992.

Steinegger E, Hänsel R, Pharmakognosie, 5. Aufl., Springer Verlag Heidelberg 1992.

Teuscher E, Biogene Arzneimittel, 5. Aufl., Wiss. Verlagsges. mbH Stuttgart 1997.

Wichtl M (Hrsg.), Teedrogen, 4. Aufl., Wiss. Verlagsges. Stuttgart 1997.

Hibiscus sabdariffa

See Hibiscus

High Mallow

Malva sylvestris

DESCRIPTION

Medicinal Parts: The medicinal parts are the dried flowers, the dried leaves and the whole of the flowering fresh plant.

Flower and Fruit: The bright purple flowers with long dark stripes are clustered in leaf axils. They have 3 epicalyx leaves, 5 sepals and 5 petals that are much longer than the calyx and have a deep margin. The numerous stamens are fused to a 10 to 12 mm column. The fruit stems are erect or slanted to one side. The ovaries are made up of a ring of 9 to 11 carpels. The fruit is a 7 to 9 mm wide and 2 mm thick disc, which breaks up into mericarps. These are glabrous or covered in a few scattered hairs, sharply angular and punctate.

Leaves, Stem and Root: Malva sylvestris is a biennial or perennial leafy herb 0.3 to 1.2 m high. The stems are branched, prostrate to curved, ascending, slightly woody and roughly pubescent. The leaves are alternate, long-petioled, reniform-orbicular, 5-lobed and crenate-serrate.

Characteristics: High Mallow has a 3-leaved epicalyx (compare with Althaea officinalis).

Habitat: The plant probably originated in the southern European-Asia region. Today the tree can be found in subtropical and temperate latitudes of both hemispheres.

Production: Blue Mallow flower and leaves consist of the dried flowers of Malva sylvestris and/or Malva sylvestris sps. Mauritiana, Ascherson and Graebner, as well as its preparations. High Mallow leaves are harvested from June to the beginning of September and dried in thin layers in the shade. High Mallow flowers are harvested without the pedicles from the end of June to October and are dried in layers in the shade.

Not to be Confused With: Other varieties of Malvae, the leaves of Althaea officinalis.

Other Names: Mallow, Blue Mallow, Mauls, Cheeseflower

ACTIONS AND PHARMACOLOGY

COMPOUNDS: MALVA LEAF

Flavonoids: including among others hypolaetin-3-glucoside, gossypetin-3-glucoside; also flavonoid sulfates including among others gossypetin-8-O-beta-D-glucuronide-3-sulfate

Mucilages: 6-8% (galacturonorhamane and arabinogalactans)

COMPOUNDS: MALVA FLOWER

Anthocyans: including among others malvin

Mucilages: 10% (galacturonorhamane and arabinogalactane)

EFFECTS: MALVA LEAF AND FLOWER

Leaf: Main active principles - polysaccharides, flavonoids, tannins; Flower: Main active principles - polysaccharides, flavonoids.

The drug has a mucous membrane-protective effect; it relieves irritation because of the high level of mucilaginous material.

INDICATIONS AND USAGE

MALVA FLOWER

Approved by Commission E:

- Cough
- Bronchitis
- Inflammation of the mouth and pharynx

Unproven Uses: In folk medicine, the drug is used internally for bronchial catarrh, gastroenteritis, bladder complaints, and it is used externally for wounds. Externally, it is used as a poultice and bath additive for wound treatment.

MALVA LEAF

Approved by Commission E:

- Cough
- Bronchitis
- Inflammation of the mouth and pharynx

Unproven Uses: In folk medicine, the drug is used as poultices and bath additives for wounds.

PRECAUTIONS AND ADVERSE REACTIONS

MALVA LEAF AND FLOWER

No health hazards or side effects are known in conjunction with the proper administration of designated therapeutic dosages.

DOSAGE

MALVA FLOWER

Mode of Administration: High Mallow flowers are in various tea mixtures as an inactive ingredient.

Preparation: To prepare an infusion, 1.5 to 2 gm of comminuted drug is added to cold water and boiled or scalded and strained after 10 minutes.

Daily Dosage: The average daily dose is 5 gm of the drug. Tea: Drink 2 to 3 times a day.

Storage: The drug should be protected from light, moisture and insects.

MALVA LEAF

Mode of Administration: Comminuted herb for teas and other preparations are for internal use.

Daily Dosage: The average daily dose is 5 gm of the drug. Tea: drink 2 to 3 times a day.

Preparation: To prepare an infusion, pour 150 ml of boiling water over 3 to 5 gm of the drug (about 2 teaspoonfuls) and leave to draw for 2 to 3 hours; stir occasionally.

Storage: The drug should be protected from light, moisture and insects.

LITERATURE

MALVA LEAF AND FLOWER

Classen B, Amelunxen F, Blaschek W, Analytical and structural investigations of the mucilage of Malva species. In: PM 59(7)14. 1993.

Classen B, Amelunxen F, Blaschek W, Malva sylvestris - Mikroskopische Untersuchungen zur Entstehung von Schleimbehältern. In: DAZ 134(38):3597. 1994.

Hänsel R, Keller K, Rimpler H, Schneider G (Hrsg.), Hagers Handbuch der Pharmazeutischen Praxis, 5. Aufl., Bde 4-6 (Drogen), Springer Verlag Berlin, Heidelberg, New York, 1992-1994.

Madaus G, Lehrbuch der Biologischen Arzneimittel, Bde 1-3, Nachdruck, Georg Olms Verlag Hildesheim 1979.

Papageorgiou VP, (1980) Planta Med 38 (3):193.

Schneider K, Ullmann V, Kubelka W, Malvaceen-Schleimdrogen. Zur Bestimmung des Quellungsfaktors. In: DAZ 130(42):2303. 1990.

Steinegger E, Hänsel R, Pharmakognosie, 5. Aufl., Springer Verlag Heidelberg 1992.

Teuscher E, Biogene Arzneimittel, 5. Aufl., Wiss. Verlagsges. Stuttgart 1997.

Wagner H, Wiesenauer M, Phytotherapie. Phytopharmaka und pflanzliche Homöopathika, Fischer-Verlag, Stuttgart, Jena, New York, 1995.

Wichtl M (Hrsg.), Teedrogen, 4. Aufl., Wiss. Verlagsges. Stuttgart 1997.

Hippophaë rhamnoides

See Sea Buckthorn

Hogweed

Heracleum sphondylium

DESCRIPTION

Medicinal Parts: The medicinal parts are the dried roots, the herb collected in the flowering season and dried, the fruit, the fresh herb and the whole fresh flowering plant.

Flower and Fruit: The flowers are 15 to 30 rayed, flat umbels with no involucre. The numerous epicalyx leaves are lanceolate and densely pubescent. The petals have a cordate margin with indented lobes. They are irregular, often pubescent on the outside, whitish or greenish, green-yellow or yellowish and sometimes pink. The fruit is compressed, flat, 8 mm long and 5 mm wide, roundish-oval and brownish yellow. The fruit has 10 ribs and oil grooves.

Leaves, Stem and Root: The plant grows from 80 to 150 cm high, is biennial to perennial and has a strong tuberous, whitish-yellow root. The stem is erect, angular, grooved, hollow, stiff-haired and branched above. The leaves are large and odd-pinnate, with 1 to 3 pairs of leaflets. The leaflets are large, ovate and lobed to pinnate. There is a 3-lobed terminal leaflet. The basal leaves are very large and have grooved petioles, which gradually merge into leaf sheaths. The basal and stem foliage are clasping.

Characteristics: There is hot, yellow latex in the stem. The leaf umbel is fragrant.

Habitat: Heracleum sphondylium is found in most of Europe and in western and northern Asia. Subspecies are found mainly in northwestern Europe, eastern and central Europe, and in the Mediterranean region.

Production: Hogweed is the aerial part of Heracleum sphondylium collected between June and August and dried.

Other Names: Masterwort

ACTIONS AND PHARMACOLOGY

COMPOUNDS

Furocoumarins (0.5-0.6%): in particular bergaptene, isopimpinellin, pimpinellin, isobergaptene, sphondin

Volatile oil: including those containing n-octylacetate

EFFECTS

Hogweed is considered a mild expectorant; however, this has not been scientifically proven. A phototoxic effect should be expected after administration.

INDICATIONS AND USAGE

Unproven Uses: In folk medicine, the drug is used to relieve muscle cramps, stomach disorders, digestion problems, diarrhea, gastrointestinal catarrh and diarrhea following a cold. The furocoumarin methoxsalin is used in the treatment of psoriasis.

PRECAUTIONS AND ADVERSE REACTIONS

Phototoxic effects must be avoided following intake of the drug due to its furocoumarin content. For that reason, UV-radiation and solaria should be avoided after its administration. The same danger exists following contact with the freshly bruised plant.

DOSAGE

Mode of Administration: An infusion is used internally.

Preparation: To make an infusion, add 3 teaspoonfuls of herb to 2 glasses of cold water and allow to draw for 8 hours.

Daily Dosage: The preparation should be drunk throughout the day.

LITERATURE

Baerheim Svendsen A et al., PM 7:113-117. 1959.

Frohne D, Pfänder HJ: Giftpflanzen - Ein Handbuch für Apotheker, Toxikologen und Biologen, 4. Aufl., Wiss. Verlagsges. mbH Stuttgart 1997.

Hänsel R, Keller K, Rimpler H, Schneider G (Hrsg.), Hagers Handbuch der Pharmazeutischen Praxis, 5. Aufl., Bde 4-6 (Drogen), Springer Verlag Berlin, Heidelberg, New York, 1992-1994.

Madaus G: Lehrbuch der Biologischen Arzneimittel, Bde 1-3, Nachdruck, Georg Olms Verlag Hildesheim 1979.

Ognyanov I et al., PM 14:19-21. 1966.

Roth L, Daunderer M, Kormann K: Giftpflanzen, Pflanzengifte, 4.Aufl., Ecomed Fachverlag Landsberg Lech 1993.

Teuscher E, Lindequist U: Biogene Gifte - Biologie, Chemie, Pharmakologie, 2. Aufl., Fischer Verlag Stuttgart 1994.

Holly

Ilex aquifolium

DESCRIPTION

Medicinal Parts: The medicinal parts are the dried foliage leaves, the fresh leaves, the young leafy branches with the ripe berries and the flowers of the branch tips with the leaves.

Flower and Fruit: Because of the shrinking of the one sex, the flowers are usually dioecious. The inflorescence is a 1 to 3 flowered axillary cyme. They are white. The calyx is small and has 4 to 5 tips. The 5-petalled corolla is rotate. The ovary is superior. There are 4 to 5 stamens. The coral red fruit is a 4-sectioned, sessile, berry-like, pea-sized drupe with 4 to 5 seeds.

Leaves, Stem and Root: The plant is a 10 m high evergreen bush or tree with smooth, dark, gray-brown bark. The bark on the younger branches is green and glossy. The branches and foliage are glabrous. The leaves are alternate, coriaceous, stiff, ovate or elliptical and acute. The lower ones are thorny denate, the upper ones entire-margined.

Characteristics: The flowers have a weak pleasant scent. The berries are poisonous to children.

Habitat: The plant is found in central Europe, North America and eastern Asia.

Production: Holly leaves and fruits are the leaves and fruits of Ilex aquifolium.

Other Names: Hulver Bush, Holm, Hulm, Holme Chase, Holy Tree, Christ's Thorn, Hulver Tree

ACTIONS AND PHARMACOLOGY

COMPOUNDS

Saponins

Nitrile glycosides: menisdaurin, not cyanogenic

Flavonoids: including, among others, rutin, kaempferol and quercetin glycosides

Caffeic acid derivatives: chlorogenic acid

Sterols: beta-sitosterol, stigmasterol

Triterpenes: alpha-amyrin, alpha-amyrinester, beta-amyrin, ursolic acid

Purine alkaloids: only traces of theobromine

EFFECTS

No information is available.

INDICATIONS AND USAGE

Unproven Uses: Holly is used as a diuretic. Also used for coughs, digestive disorders and jaundice.

In folk medicine, Holly is used for fever, chronic bronchitis, constipation, rheumatism and gout.

Homeopathic Uses: Ilex aquifolium is used for conjunctivitis.

PRECAUTIONS AND ADVERSE REACTIONS

No health hazards or side effects are known in conjunction with the proper administration of designated therapeutic dosages.

OVERDOSAGE

The intake of more than 5 berries can lead to nausea, vomiting and diarrhea. Fatal gastrointestinal inflammation is said to have taken place following the ingestion of very large quantities (20 to 30 berries) (Lewin). Stomach emptying and the administration of activated charcoal should therefore be carried out with the intake of more than 10 berries. Further treatment should proceed according to symptoms. Poisonings have not been reported in recent times.

DOSAGE

Mode of Administration: As a tea and alcoholic extract for internal use.

Homeopathic Dosage: 5 drops, 1 tablet or 10 globules every 30 to 60 minutes (acute) or 1 to 3 times daily (chronic); parenterally: 1 to 2 ml sc acute, 3 times daily; chronic: once a day (HAB34).

LITERATURE

Catalano S, Marsili A, Morelli J, Pistelli L, Constituents of the leaves of Ilex aquifolium. In: PM 33:416. 1978.

Frohne D, Pfänder HJ, Giftpflanzen - Ein Handbuch für Apotheker, Toxikologen und Biologen, 4. Aufl., Wiss. Verlags-Ges Stuttgart 1997.

Hänsel R, Keller K, Rimpler H, Schneider G (Hrsg.), Hagers Handbuch der Pharmazeutischen Praxis, 5. Aufl., Bde 4-6 (Drogen), Springer Verlag Berlin, Heidelberg, New York, 1992-1994 (unter Ilex paraguariensis).

Lassere B et al., (1983) Naturwissenschaft 70:95.

Lewin L, Gifte und Vergiftungen, 6. Aufl., Nachdruck, Haug Verlag, Heidelberg 1992.

Madaus G, Lehrbuch der Biologischen Arzneimittel, Bde 1-3, Nachdruck, Georg Olms Verlag Hildesheim 1979.

Poisonous Plants in Britain and Their Effects on Animals and Man, Ministry of Agriculture Fisheries and Food, Pub; HMSO UK 1984.

Roth L, Daunderer M, Kormann K, Giftpflanzen, Pflanzengifte, 4. Aufl., Ecomed Fachverlag Landsberg Lech 1993.

Teuscher E, Lindequist U, Biogene Gifte - Biologie, Chemie, Pharmakologie, 2. Aufl., Fischer Verlag Stuttgart 1994.

Hollyhock

Alcea rosea

DESCRIPTION

Medicinal Parts: The medicinal parts are the dried flowers of plants bearing dark purple flowers.

Flower and Fruit: Six to 10 cm flowers sit in the axils of the cauline leaves singly or in groups of 2 or 4, with the upper ones forming long spikes. Sepals of the epicalyx are broadly triangular and sharp-edged. The epicalyx is significantly shorter than the calyx and both are gray-green haired.

Leaves, Stem and Root: Hollyhock is a biennial plant. In the second year it produces a spire-like, hairy stem up to 3 m tall. The leaves are cordate-orbicular to rhomboid, weakly 3- to 5-lobed and slightly scabrid-setulose. The sepals are epiclyx-subacute and triangular. The flowers are found in the leaf axils with short peduncles. The petals are 30 to 50 mm, contiguous, usually pink but sometimes white or violet. The mericarps are 7 mm long. The dorsal face has a deep, narrow furrow with rugose angles produced into parallel wings. The lateral faces are appressed-setose.

Habitat: The plant was originally indigenous to southwest and central Asia. A few species were probably introduced into southeast central Europe as ornamental plants and then spread in the wild. Hollyhock is now widely cultivated in Europe and temperate regions of Asia. The main suppliers of the drug are Belgium, Hungary, Bulgaria, former Yugoslavia, Rumania, Albania.

Production: Hollyhock flower consists of the flowers of Alcea rosea as well as their preparations. The flowers are harvested when not quite in full bloom on plants with over 2 to 3 years of growth, then air-dried at 35°C.

Other Names: Althea Rose, Malva Flowers, Rose Mallow

ACTIONS AND PHARMACOLOGY

COMPOUNDS

Mucilages (acetylated galacturonorhamane)

Anthocyans (termed althaein): delphinidine- and malvidine-mono glycosides

EFFECTS

No information is available.

INDICATIONS AND USAGE

Unproven Uses: The herb, roots and seeds have been used internally and externally for treating coughs and lung diseases. The Hollyhock's flower is used as mucilage for prophylaxis and therapy of diseases and discomforts of the respiratory, gastrointestinal and urinary tracts, and to relieve fever and thirst. Other folk uses include external application for skin inflammations and ulcers. Infusions and decoctions made with the flowers have been used as a gargle for oral and pharyngeal inflammation.

PRECAUTIONS AND ADVERSE REACTIONS

No health hazards or side effects are known in conjunction with the proper administration of designated therapeutic dosages.

DOSAGE

Mode of Administration: Administered internally as a mucilage for respiratory, gastrointestinal and urinary tract discomforts and diseases, and to relieve fever and thirst. External applications include use for skin inflammations and ulcers. Infusions and decoctions, often with added herbs, are used as a gargle for oral and pharyngeal inflammation.

How Supplied: Whole, cut and powdered drug.

Preparation: To prepare as a tea, use 1 to 2 g of the drug per teacup. For a mouthwash, boil 1.5 g drug with 100 ml water.

LITERATURE

Hänsel R, Keller K, Rimpler H, Schneider G (Hrsg.), Hagers Handbuch der Pharmazeutischen Praxis, 5. Aufl., Bde 4-6 (Drogen), Springer Verlag Berlin, Heidelberg, New York, 1992-1994 (unter Alcea rosea).

Steinegger E, Hänsel R, Pharmakognosie, 5. Aufl., Springer Verlag Heidelberg 1992 (unter Alcea rosea).

Teuscher E, Biogene Arzneimittel, 5. Aufl., Wiss. Verlagsges. Stuttgart 1997.

Honeysuckle

Lonicera caprifolium

DESCRIPTION

Medicinal Parts: The medicinal parts are the flowers, the seeds and the leaves.

Flower and Fruit: The flowers are in sixes directly on the upper leaf pair. There are sometimes whorls of 6 in the next 1 or 2 leaf pairs. The corolla has a tight, 25 to 28 mm long tube and a bilabiate margin. It is yellowish-white, often red-tinged, glabrous inside and glandular outside. The ovary is jug-shaped. The fruit is a berry. They are ellipsoid, 8 mm long and coral red. The seeds are ellipsoid, flattened, longitudinally grooved and 4 mm long.

Leaves, Stem and Root: Honeysuckle is an up to 4 m high, deciduous, clockwise-climbing shrub. The foliage leaves are short-petioled, elliptical or obovate, blunt, entire, glabrous, blue-green beneath and 4 to 10 cm by 3.5 to 6 cm. The leaves are shortly fused in pairs, but the upper ones are fused to an oval or circular leaf through which the stem grows. They are short-petioled and elliptical. The lower leaves are paired.

Habitat: The plant grows in the northern temperate zones as far as the northern edges of the subtropics and is cultivated extensively.

Production: Honeysuckle flowers and leaves are from Lonicera caprifolium.

Other Names: Goat's Leaf, Woodbine

ACTIONS AND PHARMACOLOGY

COMPOUNDS

Saponins

Further constituents are largely unknown; iridoide monoterpenes have been demonstrated in the rind including among others loganin (extremely bitter), that possibly also occurs in the drug.

EFFECTS

The main active principles are saponin and luteolin. The drug has a laxative and diaphoretic effect.

INDICATIONS AND USAGE

Unproven Uses: The drug is used for digestive disorders, malignant tumors and as a diaphoretic agent. It is rarely used today.

PRECAUTIONS AND ADVERSE REACTIONS

No health hazards or side effects are known in conjunction with the proper administration of designated therapeutic dosages.

OVERDOSAGE

Because of the saponin content, irritation of the gastrointestinal tract and possibly of the kidneys, urinary passages and urinary bladder are possible in the event of overdosage. Case studies are not known. (The berries of the red honeysuckle are considered poisonous. Intakes above 10 berries are said to trigger nausea, vomiting and tachycardia, elevated body temperature, exanthemas and cyanosis.)

DOSAGE

Mode of Administration: The drug is obsolete.

LITERATURE

Frohne D, Pfänder HJ, Giftpflanzen - Ein Handbuch für Apotheker, Toxikologen und Biologen, 4. Aufl., Wiss. Verlags-Ges Stuttgart 1997.

Kern W, List PH, Hörhammer L (Hrsg.), Hagers Handbuch der Pharmazeutischen Praxis, 4. Aufl., Bde. 1-8, Springer Verlag Berlin, Heidelberg, New York, 1969.

Roth L, Daunderer M, Kormann K, Giftpflanzen, Pflanzengifte, 4. Aufl., Ecomed Fachverlag Landsberg Lech 1993.

Teuscher E, Lindequist U, Biogene Gifte - Biologie, Chemie, Pharmakologie, 2. Aufl., Fischer Verlag Stuttgart 1994.

Hops

Humulus lupulus

DESCRIPTION

Medicinal Parts: The medicinal parts are the glandular hairs separated from the infructescence, the whole dried female flowers, the fresh cones (preferably with few seeds) collected before the seeds ripen and the fresh or dried female inflorescence.

Flower and Fruit: The male flowers are yellowish-greenish, inconspicuous and about 5 mm in diameter. The female flowers are in richly blossomed, heavily branched inflorescence. The ovary, which has 2 long downy stigma, is surrounded at the base by a round compressed nutlet. A yellowish fruit cone grows from the female flower. The inside of the bracts is covered with small, glossy, light yellow glandular scales, which contain hop bitter (Lupulin).

Leaves, Stem and Root: The hop plant is a perennial. The annual shoots reach a height of 6 m (12 m when cultivated). The stems are pencil-thick, green and do not turn woody. They are covered in 6 rows of climbing barbs. The leaves are 3 to 5 lobed, serrate and opposite.

Characteristics: Lupulin has a very strong odor and an extremely bitter taste.

Habitat: Indigenous to Europe, cultivated in Asia, U.S. and elsewhere.

Production: Hop cones consist of the whole dried female inflorescence of Humulus lupulus. After the harvest, the hops are dried on racks at temperatures of 30 to 60° C.

ACTIONS AND PHARMACOLOGY

COMPOUNDS

Acylphloroglucinols (10%)

Alpha-bitter acids: including, among others, humulone, cohumulone, adhumulone

Beta-bitter acids: including, among others, lupulone, colupulone, adlupulone

Volatile oil (0.3-1.0%): very complex in makeup, chief components myrcene, humulene, beta-caryophyllene, undecane-2-on, furthermore 2-methyl-but-3-en-ol (particularly following storage, as breakdown product of the acylphloroglucinols)

Resins (oxidation products of the bitter acids)

Phenolic acid: including, among others, ferulic acid, caffeic acid and their derivatives, for example, chlorogenic acid

Tannins: oligomeric proanthocyanidines

Flavonoids: including, among others, xanthohumole

EFFECTS

The drug is a sedative and therefore has sleep-inducing effect. This effect, however, strongly depends on the quality of the extract used.

In animal experiments, the 2-methyl-3-buten-2-ol exhaled by the plant caused a long and deep narcotic sleep after a short period of excitation.

The hop bitter acids are antibacterial and antimycotic. They stimulate the secretion of gastric juices. In animal experiments, a strong spasmolytic effect on the smooth muscle of the intestinal tract has been reported.

An estrogenic principle is considered plausible.

INDICATIONS AND USAGE

Approved by Commission E:

■ Nervousness and insomnia

Unproven Uses: Used as a bitter and stomachic to stimulate the appetite and increase the secretion of gastric juices.

In folk medicine, Hops has been used internally for nerve pain, priapism, inflammation of the intestinal mucous membrane and tension headaches and used externally for ulcus cruris, ulcers and skin abrasions.

Homeopathic Uses: Humulus lupulus is found in preparations for treating nervousness and insomnia.

PRECAUTIONS AND ADVERSE REACTIONS

No health hazards or side effects are known in conjunction with the proper administration of designated therapeutic dosages. The fresh plant has a sensitizing effect (hop-picker's disease), which may occur, more rarely, with the dust of the drug as well.

DOSAGE

Mode of Administration: Comminuted drug, powdered drug or dry extract powder for infusions or decoctions or other preparations; liquid and solid preparations for internal use and externally for bath additives.

Hops is often found in combination with other sedatives.

How Supplied:

Liquid extract — drug: 1:1 45% ethanol (V/V) (BHP83).

Tincture — drug 1:5 60% ethanol (V/V) (BHP83)

Preparation: To prepare an infusion, boiling water is poured over the ground hop cones and left to draw for 10 to 15 minutes (1 teaspoonful is equal to 0.4 gm drug).

Daily Dosage: For most indications, a single dose of 0.5 gm is given.

To promote sleep, a single dose of 1 to 2 gm drug is given; liquid extract: single dose: 0.5 to 2 ml; tincture: single dose: 1 to 2 ml.

Tea: 1 cup before bedtime for 2 to 3 days.

Homeopathic Dosage: 5 drops, 1 tablet or 10 globules every 30 to 60 minutes (acute) or 1 to 3 times daily (chronic); parenterally: 1 to 2 ml sc acute, 3 times daily; chronic: once a day (HAB1).

Storage: Protect from light and moisture in well-sealed containers.

LITERATURE

Bravo L et al., (1974) Boll Chim Farm:306.

Caujolle F et al., (1969) Agressologie 10:405.

Field JA et al., Determination of essential oils in hops by headspace solid- phase microextraktion. In: J Agric Food Chem 44(7):1768-1772. 1996.

Fintelmann V, Klinisch-ärztliche Bedeutung des Hopfens. In: ZPT 13(5):165. 1992.

Ganzer BM, Hopfen: nicht nur für die Bierbrauerei. In: PZ 137(38):2824. 1992.

Hänsel R et al., (1982) Planta Med 45(4):224.

Hänsel R, Pflanzliche Beruhigungsmittel Möglichkeiten und Grenzen der Selbstmedikation. In: DAZ 135(32):2935-2943. 1995.

Hänsel R, Wagener HH, (1967) Versuche, sedativ-hypnotische Wirkstoffe im Hopfen nachzuweisen. Arzneim Forsch/Drug Res 17:79-81.

Hartley RD, (1968) Phytochemistry 7:1641.

Hartley RD, Fawcett CH, (1968) Phytochemistry 7:1395.

Hölzl J, Inhaltsstoffe des Hopfens (Humulus lupulus L.). In: ZPT 13(5):155. 1992.

Kumai A, Okamoto R, (1984) Toxicol Lett 21(2):203.

Moir M et al., (1980) Phytochemistry 19(10):2201.

Orth-Wagner S, Ressin WJ, Friedrich I, Phytosedativum gegen Schlafstörungen. In: ZPT 16(3):147-156. 1995.

Schmalreck AF et al., (1975) Can J Microbiol 21:205.

Schulz V, Hübner WD, Ploch M, Klinische Studien mit Psycho-Phytopharmaka. In: ZPT 18(3):141-154. 1997.

Stevens JF, Ivancic M, Hsu VL, Deinzer ML, Prenylflavonoids from Humulus lupulus. In: PH 44(8):1575-1585. 1997.

Stocker HR, (1967) Sedative und hypnogene Wirkung des Hopfens. Schweizer Brauerei Rundschau 78:80-89.

Tobe H, Muraki Y, Kitamura K, Komiyama O, Sato Y, Sugioka T, Maruyama HB, Matsuda E, Nagai M, Bone resorption inhibitors from hope extract. In: Biosc Biotech Biochem 61(1):158-159. 1997.

Wohlfart R, (1983) Dtsch Apoth Ztg 123:1637.

Wohlfart R, Hänsel R, Schmidt H, (1983) Nachweis sedativ-hypnotischer Wirkstoffe im Hopfen. 4. Mittlg. Die Pharmakologie des Hopfeninhaltsstoffes 2-Methyl-3-buten-2-ol. Planta Med 48:120-123.

Wohlfart R, Wurm G, Hänsel R, Schmidt H, (1983) Der Abbau der Bittersäuren zum 2-Methyl-3-buten-2-ol, einem Hopfeninhaltsstoff mit sedativ-hypnotischer Wirkung. Arch Pharmaz 315:132-137.

Further information in:

Hänsel R, Keller K, Rimpler H, Schneider G (Hrsg.), Hagers Handbuch der Pharmazeutischen Praxis, 5. Aufl., Bde 4-6 (Drogen), Springer Verlag Berlin, Heidelberg, New York, 1992-1994.

Lewin L, Gifte und Vergiftungen, 6. Aufl., Nachdruck, Haug Verlag, Heidelberg 1992.

Madaus G, Lehrbuch der Biologischen Arzneimittel, Bde 1-3, Nachdruck, Georg Olms Verlag Hildesheim 1979.

Roth L, Daunderer M, Kormann K, Giftpflanzen, Pflanzengifte, 4. Aufl., Ecomed Fachverlag Landsberg Lech 1993.

Schulz R, Hänsel R, Rationale Phytotherapie, Springer Verlag Heidelberg 1996.

Steinegger E, Hänsel R, Pharmakognosie, 5. Aufl., Springer Verlag Heidelberg 1992.

Teuscher E, Biogene Arzneimittel, 5. Aufl., Wiss. Verlagsges. Stuttgart 1997

Wagner H, Wiesenauer M, Phytotherapie. Phytopharmaka und pflanzliche Homöopathika, Fischer-Verlag, Stuttgart, Jena, New York 1995.

Wichtl M (Hrsg.), Teedrogen, 4. Aufl., Wiss. Verlagsges. Stuttgart 1997.

Hordeum distichon

See Barley

Horehound

Marrubium vulgare

DESCRIPTION

Medicinal Parts: The medicinal parts are the dried flowering branches, the fresh aerial parts of the flowering plant and the whole plant.

Flower and Fruit: The small, white 5 to 7 mm long, labiate globular flowers are sessile. There are 6 to 8 richly flowered false whorls that are 1.5 to 2 cm long on each stem. The calyx is tubular, white and tomentose with 10 awl-shaped tips, which are curved back in a hook. The corolla is white and downy. The fruit is an ovate, 1.5 to 2 mm long, obtusely triangular, smooth, gray-brown with darker marbling or light brown nut.

Leaves, Stem and Root: The plant is a perennial herb with a fusiform root and a multi-headed, often woody, root crown. The stems are erect, branched, obtusely quadrangular, and about 40 to 60 cm high and 7 mm thick at the base. The branches are curved, spreading out, obtusely quadrangular, and loosely downy, like the leaves. The leaves are tomentose-downy, petiolate, orbicular and unevenly crenate. They have distinct veins on the underside and are wrinkled.

Characteristics: The leaves smell tangy when rubbed and contain musk juice, which taste bitter and hot.

Habitat: The plant is indigenous to the Mediterranean region to central Asia. It has become established in central Europe; introduced to America, South Africa and Australia.

Production: Horehound herb consists of the fresh or dried, above-ground parts of Marrubium vulgare as well as their preparations. The plant is harvested during the flowering season from June to August. Fast drying is recommended.

Other Names: Houndsbane, Marrubium, White Horehound

ACTIONS AND PHARMACOLOGY

COMPOUNDS

Diterpene bitter principles: chief components marrubiin (0.1-1.0%), premarrubiin (0.1%)

Caffeic acid derivatives: including among others chlorogenic acid, cryptochlorogenic acid

Flavonoids: including among others chrysoeriol, vicenin II, lactoyl flavones, for example luteolin-7-lactate, apigenin-7-lactate

Volatile oil (traces): including among others camphene, p-cymene, fenchene

EFFECTS

The bitter ingredients act as a gastric juice stimulant; marrubinic acid acts as a choleretic. In animal experiments, a significant increase of bile secretion was observed after administration of marrubinic acid and its salt. The main active principles, essential oil, diterpene-amaroids, tannins and flavonoids indicate that the drug would probably stimulate gastric juice secretion.

INDICATIONS AND USAGE

Approved by Commission E:

- Dyspeptic complaints
- Loss of appetite

Unproven Uses: The drug is used for dyspepsia, loss of appetite, bloating and flatulence, and respiratory catarrh. In folk medicine, it is used internally for acute and chronic bronchitis, whooping cough, asthma, tuberculosis, pulmonary catarrh, respiratory infections, diarrhea, jaundice, debility and painful menstruation, and as a laxative in higher doses; externally for skin damage, ulcers and wounds, and as a gargle for mouth and throat infections.

Homeopathic Uses: Inflammation of the respiratory tract.

PRECAUTIONS AND ADVERSE REACTIONS

General: No health hazards or side effects are known in conjunction with the proper administration of designated therapeutic dosages.

Pregnancy: Not to be used during pregnancy.

DOSAGE

Mode of Administration: Comminuted herb, freshly pressed plant juice and other galenic preparations for internal use.

Preparation: To prepare an infusion, pour boiling water over 1 to 2 gm of the drug; strain after 10 minutes. For a liquid extract, prepare as a (1:1) dilution with ethanol (20%).

Daily Dosage: The average daily dose is 4.5 gm of the drug; 30 to 60 ml pressed juice.

The infusion dosage is 1 to 2 gm of the drug taken up to 3 times daily. The liquid extract dosage is 2 to 4 ml 3 times daily.

Homeopathic Dosage: 5 drops, 1 tablet or 10 globules every 30 to 60 minutes (acute) or 1 to 3 times daily (chronic); parenterally: 1 to 2 ml sc acute, 3 times daily; chronic: once a day (HAB1).

LITERATURE

Bartarelli IM, (1966) Boll Chim Farm 105:787.

Brieskorn CH, Feilner K, (1968) Phytochemistry 7:485.

Busby MC et al., (1983) Proc R IR Acad Sect B 83:1.

Cahen R, (1970) C R Soc Biol 164:1467.

Henderson MS, McCrindle R, (1969) J Chem Soc Chem Comm 15:2014.

Karryev MO et al., (1976) Izv Akad Nauk Turkm Ser Biol 3:86.

Mascolo N et al., (1987) Phytother Res 1(1):28.

Nicholas HJ, (1964) J Pharm Sci 53:895.

Pandler WW, Wagner S, (1963) Chem Ind 42:1693.

Popa DP et al., (1968) Khim Prir Soedin 4(6):345.

Popa DP et al., (1974) Rastit Resur 10(3):365.

Popa DP, Salei LA, (1973) Rastit Resur 9(3):384.

Further information in:

Hänsel R, Keller K, Rimpler H, Schneider G (Hrsg.), Hagers Handbuch der Pharmazeutischen Praxis, 5. Aufl., Bde 4-6 (Drogen), Springer Verlag Berlin, Heidelberg, New York, 1992-1994.

Leung AY, Encyclopedia of Common Natural Ingredients Used in Food, Drugs and Cosmetics, John Wiley & Sons Inc., New York 1980.

Madaus G, Lehrbuch der Biologischen Arzneimittel, Bde 1-3, Nachdruck, Georg Olms Verlag Hildesheim 1979.

Roth L, Daunderer M, Kormann K, Giftpflanzen, Pflanzengifte, 4. Aufl., Ecomed Fachverlag Landsberg Lech 1993.

Steinegger E, Hänsel R, Pharmakognosie, 5. Aufl., Springer Verlag Heidelberg 1992.

Teuscher E, Biogene Arzneimittel, 5. Aufl., Wiss. Verlagsges. Stuttgart 1997.

Wichtl M (Hrsg.), Teedrogen, 4. Aufl., Wiss. Verlagsges. Stuttgart 1997.

Horse Chestnut

Aesculus hippocastanum

TRADE NAMES

Horse Chestnut (available from numerous manufacturers), Horse Chestnut-Power, Venastat, Standardized Horsechestnut Extract

DESCRIPTION

Medicinal Parts: The medicinal parts are the dried Horse Chestnut leaves, the oil extracted from the peeled fruit capsules (seeds) and dried chestnut seeds.

Flower and Fruit: The white flowers are in stiffly upright panicles gradually thickening near the distal end. Most of the flowers are male, but a few are female or androgynous. The calyx is fused and bell-shaped with 5 irregular tips. The petals are 10 to 15 mm long with a yellow spot, which turns red. There are 3 upward petals and 2 downward, which are folded at the edge. The flower is ciliate and cordate (heart shaped) at the base and contains 7 S-shaped, bending stamens with red anthers that are longer than the petals. The ovary is 3-valved, superior and velvety. The fruit capsules are green and globular with soft spines and fine hairs. There are 1 to 3 red-brown seeds (Chestnuts) within the capsules, which are shiny brown with a yellowish gray-brown navel and a tough shell.

Leaves, Stem and Root: The seasonal tree is up to 35 m high; it includes a large regular crown and widely spread roots. The trunk is initially smooth but later has thinly scaled, peeling and fissured bark. The young twigs are yellowish to red-brown and are initially covered with brown hairs. The buds gradually thicken near the distal end and are extremely sticky with dark red bud scales to protect the seed plant bud. The leaves are long, 5 to 7 palmate, with a 20 cm long grooved petiole. The leaflets are initially red-haired, 20 cm long, cuneate-obovate, acute and dentate. The leaflets are rich green above and beneath are light green.

Habitat: Although the herb is indigenous to the mountains of Greece, Bulgaria, the Caucasus, northern Iran and the Himalayas, it is cultivated elsewhere, especially in northern Europe including the British Isles, Denmark, Scandinavia and Russia (Narva and St. Petersburg).

Production: Horse Chestnut leaf consists of the fresh or dried leaf of Aesculus hippocastanum. A dry extract is manufactured from Horse Chestnut seeds standardized to a content of 16-20% triterpene glycosides (calculated as anhydrous aescin).

Not to be Confused With: The leaves of the Horse Chestnut are commonly confused with those of Sweet Chestnut.

Other Names: Spanish Chestnut, Buckeye, Common Horse Chestnut, Conqueror Tree

ACTIONS AND PHARMACOLOGY

COMPOUNDS: HORSE CHESTNUT LEAF

Triterpene saponins

Hydroxycoumarins: chief component is aesculin, in addition fraxin and scopolin

Flavonoids: including rutin, quercitrin, and isoquercitrin

Tannins

EFFECTS: HORSE CHESTNUT LEAF

The main active principles of the anti-exudative effect and improvement of venous tone are hydroxycoumarins (aesculin and fraxin), triterpene saponins in the petioles and leaf veins, flavonoids and a rich supply of tannins. Although the drug is said to have an anti-exudative effect and improve venous tone, there is a lack of clinical data to support the efficacy.

COMPOUNDS: HORSE CHESTNUT SEEDS

Triterpene saponins (3-5%): The triterpene saponine mixture known as aescin (also escin) consists of diacylated tetra-and pentahydroxy-beta-amyrin compounds.The compounds bear a glucuronic acid remnant substituted with 2 monosaccharide remnants in position 3 at the OH-group. Aglycones, protoescigenin and barringtogenol C, are bonded like esters onto the OH-group at position 21 with either angelic or tiglic acid, or with either alpha-methyl butyric or isobutyric acid remnants. The OH-group in position 22 (beta-escin) or 28 (cryptoescin) is acetylated, and both positional isomeric compounds remain in equilibrium though migration of the acetyl remnant.

Flavonoids: in particular biosides and triosides of the quercetins

Oligosaccharides: including 1-kestose, 2-kestose, stachyose

Polysaccharides: starch (50%)

Oligomeric proanthocyanidins, condensed tannins: (only in the seed-coat)

Fatty oil (2-3%)

EFFECTS: HORSE CHESTNUT SEEDS

As found in different animal tests and preclincal investigations, the principal ingredient of Horse Chestnut seed extract, triterpene glycoside mixture (aescin), has an anti-exudative, vascular tightening effect, and reduction of vascular permeability which result in an antiedemic effect. The vein-toning properties of the Horse Chestnut extract also demonstrated improvement of venous return flow. A significant reduction of transcapillary filtration was seen in a placebo-controlled human pharmacological trial (Bisler, 1986). Significant improvement in the symptoms of chronic venous insufficiency was demonstrated in diverse, randomized, double-blind and cross-over studies (Calabrese, 1993; Steiner, 1990).

There are indications that Horse Chestnut seed extract reduces the activity of lysosomal enzymes, which increases in chronic pathological conditions of the veins. The enzymes will break down glycoacalyx (mucopolysaccharides) in the region of the capillary walls, allowing proteins to leak into the interstitium. The activity of the enzymes is reduced by the aescin and so the breakdown of glycoacalyx is also inhibited. The transcapillary filtration of low-molecular proteins, electrolytes and water into the interstitium is inhibited through a reduction of vascular permeability by the aescin.

CLINICAL TRIALS

The efficacy and safety of Horse Chestnut seed extract, given as Venostasin retard (50mg aescin) twice daily, was compared to mechanical compression involving bandages and stockings in a randomized, placebo-controlled clinical study. The study consisted of 240 patients with chronic venous insufficiency over a 12-week period. The results determined a similar decrease of lower leg volume of approximately 25% and noted compression treatment is uncomfortable, not convenient and subject to poor compliance (Diehm, 1996).

Venostasin retard was administered to 52 pregnant women with edema due to venous insufficiency in a placebo-controlled, double-blind, cross-over study. A significant reduction of edema and greater resistance to edema provocation was demonstrated in the Venostasin retard group. There were also less severe symptoms of pain, fatigue, swelling and itching with patients receiving Venostasin retard therapy (Steiner, 1990).

A randomized, placebo-controlled, double-blind study was conducted on 40 patients with venous edema in chronic deep vein incompetence to determine the edema-reducing effect of Horse Chestnut seed extract. The edema reduction effect and reduction of leg volume with edema provocation of the Horse Chestnut seed extract were both statistically significant (Diem, 1992).

INDICATIONS AND USAGE

HORSE CHESTNUT LEAF

Unproven Uses: Eczema, superficial and deep varicose veins, leg pains, phlebitis, hemorrhoids, pains before and during menstruation. In folk medicine, the leaves are used as a cough remedy, as well as for arthritis and rheumatism.

HORSE CHESTNUT SEEDS

Approved by Commission E:

■ Venous conditions (chronic venous insufficiency)

Treatment of symptoms found in pathological conditions of the veins of the legs (chronic venous insufficiency), for example pain and a sensation of heaviness in the legs, nocturnal cramps in the calves, pruritis and swelling of the legs.

Unproven uses: Horse Chestnut seeds are used for symptoms of post-traumatic and post-operative soft tissue swelling. Further indications are painful injuries, sprains, bruising, pain syndrome of the spine, edema, rheumatic disease and varicose veins.

Homeopathic Uses: Homeopathic treatments include hemorrhoids, lumbar and low back pain, venous back pressure.

PRECAUTIONS AND ADVERSE REACTIONS

HORSE CHESTNUT LEAF

General: Health risks or side effects following the proper administration of designated therapeutic dosages are not recorded. One case of liver damage following intramuscular administration of an extract of the drug (origin details of the drug uncertain) is known.

Drug Interactions: Horse Chestnut leaf has a coumarin componant and may interact with warfarin, salicylates and other drugs with anti-coagulant properties.

HORSE CHESTNUT SEEDS

Health risks following the proper administration of designated therapeutic dosages are not recorded. Susceptible patients may nevertheless experience mucous membrane irritations of the gastrointestinal tract (e.g. nausea) following intake of the drug; decrease in kidney function with pre-existing renal insufficiency and acute nephrotoxicity. Hepatotoxicity and urticaria have also been observed. I.V administration of aescin can lead to anaphylactic reactions.

OVERDOSAGE

HORSE CHESTNUT SEEDS

The intake of larger quantities of Horse Chestnut seeds (in one case of a child with 5 seeds) can bring about vomiting, diarrhea, severe thirst, reddening of the face, enlargement of pupils, vision and consciousness disorders. Following stomach and intestinal emptying (gastric lavage, sodium sulfate) and the administration of activated charcoal, therapy for poisonings consists of diazepam for spasms, atropine for colic, electrolyte replenishment and sodium bicarbonate infusions for any acidosis that may arise. Intubation and oxygen respiration may also be necessary.

DOSAGE

HORSE CHESTNUT LEAF

Mode of Administration: Extracts of the drug are contained in "vein teas" or "hemorrhoid teas," as well as in pharmaceutical preparations for the treatment of venous symptoms.

Preparation: One ampule corresponds to 4 mg flavones in 0.9% NaCl.

Daily Dosage:
Infusion (as a tea)—Pour boiling water over 1 tsp. of finely cut drug and strain after 5 to 10 minutes (1tsp = 1 gm drug).

Intravenously—1 to 2 ampules daily.

Intramuscularly—1 ampule daily.

HORSE CHESTNUT SEEDS

Mode of Administration: Available in liquid and solid preparations for internal use; semi-solid preparations for external use; and parenterally for homeopathic use.

How Supplied:
Ampules

Capsules — 250 mg, 300 mg, 485 mg

Coated tablets

Drops

Ointment/Gels

Tablets

Tincture

Preparation: Stabilized extract of Horse Chestnut (5:1) is standardized for aescin; tincture of Horse Chestnut 1:1 with 75% ethanol; isolated aescin.

Daily Dosage:
Intravenous—Doses of 5 mg once or twice daily of aescin as the sodium salt has been used for treatment or prevention of post-traumatic edema and potoperative edema. The maximum daily dose is 20 mg (Brandt, 1992/1993).

Oral—Aescin from encapsulated standardized extracts are initially given at doses of 10 mg (Chandler, 1993). The encapsulated standardized extract has been used for the treatment of postoperative or traumatic edema, hemorrhoids or symptoms due to varicose veins in doses providing 40 to 120 mg of aescin per day (Schlesser, 1991). Aescin (escin) 100 mg corresponding to 250-312.5 mg extract may be administered twice daily in delayed-release form.

Tincture—For the treatment of painful hemorrhoids, a dose of 1:10 tincture is 0.6 ml (Reynolds, 1977).

Topical—A 1 to 2% gel is applied topically several times daily for soft tissue injuries, bruises and symptomatic relief of varicose veins (Fachinfo Reparil (R)- Sportgel 1994; Fachino Opijo (R) N gel, 1991; Calabrese & Preston 1993).

Homeopathic Dosage: 5 drops, 1 tablet or 10 globules every 30 to 60 minutes (acute) and 1 to 3 times daily (chronic); parenterally: 1 to 2 ml 3 times daily sc; ointment 1 to 2 times daily (HAB1).

Storage: The herb should be stored in a dry and dark place.

LITERATURE

Aizawa X, Fukui, Yamada K, Kogo H, Aescin, antiinflammatory action of Aescin (1, intravenous injection). In: Pharmacometrics (Tokyo) 8:211. 1974.

Alter H, (1973) Zur medikamentösen Therapie der Varikosis. Z Allg Med 49(17):1301-1304.

Annoni F, Mauri A, Marincola Resele LF, (1979) Venotonic activity of Escin on the human saphenous vein. Arzneim Forsch/Drug Res 29:672.

Arnold M, Przerwa M, Die therapeutische Beeinflußbarkeit experimentell erzeugter Ödeme. In: Arzneim Forsch 26:402-409. 1976.

Auster F, Wirkung eines Roßkastanienpräparates auf die Resistenz der Hautkapillaren. In: Pharmazie 11:726-730. 1956.

Bisler H, Pfeifer R, Klüken N, Pauschinger P, (1986) Wirkung von Roßkastaniensamenextrakt auf die transkapilläre Filtration bei chronischer venöser Insuffizien. Z Dtsch Med Wschr 111: 1321-1328.

Brandt D (ed.): Reparil (R) -Ampoules. In: MDR, MIMS Desk Reference Vol 28. MIMS, Pretoria, 1992/93.

Büechi S, Antivirale Saponine, pharmakologische und klinische Untersuchungen. In: DAZ 136(2):89-98. 1996.

Calabrese C, Preston P, Report of the results of a double-blind, randomized, single-dose trial of a topical 2% escon gel versus placebo in the acute treatment of experimentally-induced hematoma volunteers. Planta Med 59:394-397. 1993.

Chandler RF, Herbal Medicine: Horse Chestnut. Can Pharm J 1993; 126:297-306.

Comaish JS, Kersey PJ, Contact dermatitis to extract of horse chestnut (esculin). Contact Dermatitis 1980 Jan;6(2):150-1.

Daub B, Chronische Veneninsuffizienz: Roβkastanienextrakt oder Kompressionsstrumpf - gleiche Wirkung. In: DAZ 136(12):946. 1996.

De Smet PA, Van den E, Lesterhuis W, Hepatotoxicity associated with herval tablets. BJM 1996; July 13, 313:92.

Diehm C, Vollbrecht D, Amendt K, Comberg HU, Medical edema protection-clinical benefit in patients with chronic deep vein incompetence. A placebo controlled double blind study. Vasa 21 (2):199-92.1992.

Diehm C, Trampisch HJ, Lange S, Schmidt C, Comparison of leg compression stocking and oral horse-chestnut seed extract in patients with chronic venous insufficiency. Lancet Feb 3;347:292-294. 1996.

Ehringer H, Objektivierbare Venentonisierung nach oraler Gabe eines Kombinationspräparates mit Roβkastanienextrakt. In: Arzneim Forsch 18:432. 1968.

Escribano MM, Munoz-Bellido FJ, Velazquez E et al., Contact urticaria due to aescin. Contact Dermatitis 1997 Nov:37(5):233.

Fachinformation: Opino (R) N gel, Aescin. Toponwerke GmbH & Co, KG, Koeln, 1991.

Fachinformation: Reparil (R)- Sportgel, Aescin, Diethylamin-salicylat. Madaus AG, Koeln, 1994.

Felix W, Schneider E, Schmidt A, Grimm G, Vasoaktive Wirkung von alpha-Aescin. In: Fischer H (Hrsg) Ergebnisse der Angiologie: Chronische Veneninsuffizienz. Pathogenese und medikamentöse Therapie, Schattauer, Stuttgart, 30:93-105. 1984.

Felix W, Spektrum Venenmittel. In: Arzneimitteltherapie heute. Bd. 45. Spektrum Venenmittel. Aesopus Verlag Zug S 29. 1986.

Felix W, Wirkungsmechanismen der internen Therapie mit "Venopharmaka". In: Dt med J 21:458-465. 1970.

Fink Serralde C, Dreyfus Cortes GO, Colo Hernandesz, Marquez Zacarias LA, (1975) Valoracion de la escina pura en el tratamiento del sindrome des estasis venosa cronica. Münch Med Wschr (mex. Ausgabe) 117(1):41-46.

Fischer H, Pflanzliche Venentherapeutica. In: Therapiewoche 34:4101-4106. 1984.

Fricke U, (1995) Venenmittel. In: Schwabe U, Paffrath D (Hrsg), Arzneiverordnungs-Report '95. Gustav Fischer Verlag Stuttgart, Jena, S 421-430.

Friederich HC, Vogelsberg H, Neiss A, (1978) Ein Beitrag zur Bewertung von intern wirksamen Venenpharmaka. Z Hautkrankheiten 53(11):369-374.

Girerd I, DiPasquale, Steinetz G, Beach BG, Pearl VLW, The anti-edema properties of aescin. In: Arch internat Pharmacodyn Thér, Bruxelles 133:127-137. 1961.

Hampel H, Hofrichter G, Liehn HD, Schlemmer W, Zur Pharmakologie der Aescin-Isomere unter besonderer Berücksichtigung von alpha-Aescin. In: Arzneim Forsch 20:209-215. 1970.

Hellberg K, Ruschewski W, de Vivie R, Drug induced acute renal failure after heart surgery. Thoraxchir Vask Chir 1975 Aug;23(4):396-9.

Hitzenberger G, (1989) Die therapeutische Wirksamkeit des Roβkastaniensamenextraktes. Wien Med Wschr 139(17):385-389.

Hübner G, Wray V, Nahrstedt A, Flavonolglycosides in Aesculus hippocastanum L.: Isolation, structure elucidation and quantification. In: PM 62, Abstracts of the 44th Ann Congress of GA, 139. 1996.

Jacker HJ, Zur Pharmakologie der Roβkastanie. In: PZH 116(9):959-968. 1977.

Konoshima T, Lee KH, (1986) J Nat Prod 49(4):650.

Kreysel HW, Nissen HP, Enghofer E, A possible role of lysosomal enzymes in the pathogenesis of varicosis and the reduction in their serum activity by Venostasin. Vasa 12(4):377-82. 1983.

Locks H, Baumgartner H, Konzett H, (1974) Zur Beeinflussung des Benentonus durch Roβkastanienextrakte. Arzneim Forsch 24:1347.

Lohr E, Garanin G, Jesau P, Fischer H, (1986) Ödemprotektive Therapie bei chronischer Veneninsuffizienz mit Ödemneigung. Münch Med Wschr 128:579-581.

Longiave D, Omini C, Nicosia S, Berti F, (1978) The Mode of Action of Escin on Isolated Veins, Relationship with PGF2. Pharmacol Res 10:145.

Lorenz D, Marek ML, (1960) Das therapeutisch wirksame Prinzip der Roβkastanie (Aesculus hippocastanum). Arzneim Forsch 10:263-272.

Marshall M, Dormandy JA, (1987) Oedema of long distant flights. Phlebol 2:123-124.

Marshall M, Loew D, (1994) Diagnostische Maβnahmen zum Nachweis der Wirksamkeit von Venentherapeutika. Phlebol 23:85-91.

Marshall M, Wüstenberg P, Klinik und Therapie der chronischen venösen Insuffizienz. In: Klinik und Therapie der chronischen venösen Insuffizienz, Braun Fachverlage, Karlsruhe 1994.

Neiss A, Böhm C, (1976) Zum Wirksamkeitsnachweis von Roβkastaniensamenextrakt beim varikösen Symptomenkomplex. Münch Med Wschr 7:213-216.

Pauschinger P, (1987) Klinisch experimentelle Untersuchungen zur Wirkung von Roβkastaniensamenextrakt auf die transkapilläre Filtration und das intravasale Volumen an Patienten mit chronisch venöser Insuffizien. Z Phlebol Proktol 16:57-61.

Preziosi P, Manca P, (1965) Arzneim Forsch 15:404.

Proserpio G et al., (1980) Fitoterapia 2:113.

Rao GS et al., (1974) J Pharm Sci 63:471.

Reynolds JEF, Martindale: The Extra Pharmacopoeia. Pharmaceutical Press, London, 1998.

Rothkopf M, Vogel G, Neue Befunde zur Wirksamkeit und zu Wirkungsmechanismen des Roβkastanien-Saponins Aescin. In: Arzneim Forsch 26:225-235. 1976.

Rothkopf M, Vogel G, Lang W, Leng E, Animal experiments on the question of the renal toleration of the horse chestnut saponin aescin. Arzneimittelforschung 1977;27(3):598-605.

Rudofsky G, Neiβ A, Otto K, Seibel K, (1986) Ödemprotektive Wirkung und klinische Wirksamkeit von Roβkastaniensamenextrakt im Doppelblindversuch. Phlebol Proktol 15:47-54.

Schlesser JL (ed.), Drugs Available Abroad. Gale Research Inc, Detroit, MI, 1991.

Simini B, Horse-chestnut seed extract for chronic venous insufficiency (letter;comment). Lancet 1996 Apr 27;347 (9009):1182-3.

Steiner M, Hillemanns HG, (1986) Untersuchung zur ödemprotektiven Wirkung eines Venentherapeutikums. Münch Med Wschr 31:551-552.

Steiner M, Untersuchung zur ödemvermindernden und ödemprotektiven Wirkung von Roβkastanienextrakt. In: Phlebol Proktol 19:239-242. 1990.

Steiner M, Hillemanns HG, Venostasin retard in the management of venous problems during pregnancy. Phlebology 5:41-44. 1990.

Vayssairat M et al., Horse-chestnut seed extract for chronic venous insufficiency. In: Lancet 347(9009):182-183. 1996.

Vogel G, Aesculus hippocastanum L. - Die Roβkastanie. In: ZPT 10:102 - 106. 1989.

Vogel G, Marek ML, Stoeckert J, Weitere Untersuchungen zum Wirkungsmechanismus des Roβkastanien-Saponins Aescin. In: Arzneim Forsch 13:59. 1963.

Further information in:

Chan, EH et al. (Ed.), Advances in Chinese Medicinal Materials Research, World Scientific Pub. Co. Singapore 1985.

Frohne D, Pfänder HJ, Giftpflanzen - Ein Handbuch für Apotheker, Toxikologen und Biologen, 4. Aufl., Wiss. Verlagsges. mbH Stuttgart 1997.

Hänsel R, Keller K, Rimpler H, Schneider G (Hrsg.), Hagers Handbuch der Pharmazeutischen Praxis, 5. Aufl., Bde 4-6 (Drogen), Springer Verlag Berlin, Heidelberg, New York, 1992-1994.

Madaus G, Lehrbuch der Biologischen Arzneimittel, Bde 1-3, Nachdruck, Georg Olms Verlag Hildesheim 1979.

Roth L, Daunderer M, Kormann K, Giftpflanzen, Pflanzengifte, 4. Aufl., Ecomed Fachverlag Landsberg Lech 1993.

Schulz R, Hänsel R, Rationale Phytotherapie, Springer Verlag Heidelberg 1996.

Steinegger E, Hänsel R, Pharmakognosie, 5. Aufl., Springer Verlag Heidelberg 1992.

Teuscher E, Lindequist U, Biogene Gifte - Biologie, Chemie, Pharmakologie, 2. Aufl., Fischer Verlag Stuttgart 1994.

Teuscher E, Biogene Arzneimittel, 5. Aufl., Wiss. Verlagsges. mbH Stuttgart 1997.

Wagner H, Wiesenauer M, Phytotherapie. Phytopharmaka und pflanzliche Homöopathika, Fischer-Verlag, Stuttgart, Jena, New York 1995.

Wichtl M (Hrsg.), Teedrogen, 4. Aufl., Wiss. Verlagsges. Stuttgart 1997.

Horsemint

Monarda Punctata

DESCRIPTION

Medicinal Parts: The medicinal part is the herb.

Flower and Fruit: The flowers grow in axillary whorls. They are bilabiate. The corolla is yellow with red spots. The 2 stamens and the sessile bracts are yellow and purple.

Leaves, Stem and Root: The plant is a perennial and grows up to 90 cm high with a branched, round stem. The leaves are opposite, lanceolate and downy.

Characteristics: The taste is pungent and bitter; the odor reminiscent of thyme.

Habitat: The plant is indigenous to the eastern and central U.S.

Other Names: Spotted Monarda, Monarda Lutea, Wild Bergamot

ACTIONS AND PHARMACOLOGY

COMPOUNDS

Volatile oil: including among others thymol (20%), thymol methyl ether, thymol hydroquinone; in Monarda punctata varieties, maritima including also gamma-terpinene, geranylformate, nerylformate

EFFECTS

The drug has carminative, stimulant and emmenagogic effects.

CONTRAINDICATIONS

The drug is not to be used during pregnancy.

INDICATIONS AND USAGE

Unproven Uses: The drug is used for digestive disorders, flatulence and dysmenorrhea.

Indian Medicine: American Indians use the drug for inflammations, rheumatism and backache.

PRECAUTIONS AND ADVERSE REACTIONS

No health hazards or side effects are known in conjunction with the proper administration of designated therapeutic dosages. (Oil from the plant, however, is only to be administered externally. Even then, because it raises blisters in its pure form, it should be diluted with olive oil before application.)

DOSAGE

Mode of Administration: Ground drug used as an infusion.

LITERATURE

Kern W, List PH, Hörhammer L (Hrsg.), Hagers Handbuch der Pharmazeutischen Praxis, 4. Aufl., Bde. 1-8, Springer Verlag Berlin, Heidelberg, New York, 1969.

Horseradish

Armoracia rusticana

DESCRIPTION

Medicinal Parts: The medicinal part of the plant is the fresh or dried horseradish root.

Flower and Fruit: The inflorescence is made up of numerous, richly flowered racemes (cymes). The fragrant flowers are on 5 to 7 mm long, upright pedicles. The sepals are 2.5 to 3 mm long, broadly ovate, with a membranous white margin. The white petals are 5 to 7 mm long and broadly obovate. The inner stamens are 2.5 mm long; the outer ones 1.5 mm long. The stigma is broad, round and gently 2-lobed. The small pods are on 20 mm long, upright spreading stems. They are globose to obovate and 4 to 6 mm long. The seeds are smooth.

Leaves, Stem and Root: The plant is 40 to 120 cm high. It is a sturdy and glabrous perennial. The root is quite thick and woody. In cultivated varieties, it is thick and fleshy with numerous root heads, which are light yellowish-white and have horizontal underground runners. The sometimes solitary stems are upright, branched above, grooved and hollow. The leaves are long-petioled, oblong-ovate, cordate at the base, 30 to 100 cm long and unevenly crenate. The lower cauline leaves have shorter petioles and are lobed or comb-shaped pinnate with linear-oblong, entire-margined or serrate sections. The upper cauline leaves with narrowed bases are sessile, oblong or lanceolate, unevenly crenate to serrate and obtuse. The uppermost leaves are linear or almost entire-margined.

Characteristics: The rootstock has an odor that is strong and irritating, and a sharp, burning taste.

Habitat: The plant is indigenous to the Volga-Don region but has spread to almost all of Europe and other parts of the world.

Production: Horseradish consists of the fresh or dried, peeled or unpeeled roots of Armoracia rusticana.

Other Names: Mountain Radish, Red Cole, Great Raifort

ACTIONS AND PHARMACOLOGY

COMPOUNDS

Glucosinolates sinigrin and gluconasturtin: The freshly harvested root contains the glucosinolates sinigrin (0.3%) and gluconasturtin, which release enzymatically triggered (myrosinase) allyl mustard oil (up to 90%) and a little 2-phenyl mustard when the root is cut up. The dehydrated root contains both of these mustard oils.

EFFECTS

Horseradish works antimicrobially against gram-positive and gram-negative pathogens, and is hyperemic on skin and mucous membranes and carcinostatic (due to the mustard oils). Horseradish demonstrated an antispasmodic effect in animal experiments.

INDICATIONS AND USAGE

Approved by Commission E:

- Cough/Bronchitis
- Infections of the urinary tract

Unproven Uses: Internally, Horseradish is used to treat inflammation of the respiratory tract and as supportive therapy for infections of the urinary tract. Externally, the drug is used for inflammation of the respiratory tract and for hyperemic treatment for minor muscle aches. In folk medicine, horseradish is administered for influenza, respiratory ailments, digestion, gout, rheumatism, and liver and gallbladder disorders.

Homeopathic Uses: Uses in homeopathy include eye inflammations, upper respiratory tract inflammations and upper abdominal colic.

CONTRAINDICATIONS

Because of the mucous membrane-irritating effect of the mustard oils, the intake of the drug should not be carried out in the presence of stomach or intestinal ulcers or in patients with a history of kidney disease.

PRECAUTIONS AND ADVERSE REACTIONS

General: No health hazards or side effects are known in conjunction with the proper administration of designated therapeutic dosages.

Pediatric Use: Preparations of horseradish should not be administered to children under 4 years of age.

DOSAGE

Mode of Administration: Fresh or dried root that has been cut or ground, freshly pressed juice or other galenic preparations for internal or external applications.

Daily Dose: The average dose for internal use is 20 g of fresh root; for external use, ointments and gels with a maximum of 2% mustard oils may be used.

Homeopathic Dosage: 5 drops, 1 tablet or 10 globules every 30 to 60 minutes (acute) or 1 to 3 times daily (chronic); parenterally: 1 to 2 ml 3 times daily sc (HAB34). The mother tincture and first decimal dilution to be taken diluted with water.

Storage: Fresh roots should be buried in soil or sand.

LITERATURE

Hänsel R, Keller K, Rimpler H, Schneider G (Hrsg.), Hagers Handbuch der Pharmazeutischen Praxis, 5. Aufl., Bde 4-6 (Drogen), Springer Verlag Berlin, Heidelberg, New York, 1992-1994.

Lewin L, Gifte und Vergiftungen, 6. Aufl., Nachdruck, Haug Verlag, Heidelberg 1992.

Simon JE, Chadwick AF, Craker LE (Eds), Herbs. An Indexed Bibliography 1971-80. Archon Books, USA 1984.

Stoll A, Seebeck E, Helv Chim Acta 31:1432-1434. 1948.

Teuscher E, Lindequist U, Biogene Gifte - Biologie, Chemie, Pharmakologie, 2. Aufl., Fischer Verlag Stuttgart 1994.

Teuscher E, Biogene Arzneimittel, 5. Aufl., Wiss. Verlagsges. Stuttgart 1997.

Wagner H, Wiesenauer M, Phytotherapie. Phytopharmaka und pflanzliche Homöopathika, Fischer-Verlag, Stuttgart, Jena, New York, 1995.

Horsetail

Equisetum arvense

TRADE NAMES

Alcohol Free Horsetail, Horsetail, Horsetail Grass, Wild Countryside Springtime Horsetail

DESCRIPTION

Medicinal Parts: The medicinal parts are the dried green, sterile shoots and fresh sterile shoots.

Flower and Fruit: Horsetail appears in two forms during the year. From March to April the red-brown to straw yellow simple stem develops with leaves arranged in a number of levels on the stem in whorls. The leaves are brown, fused to a sheath at the lower level with black-tipped, dry sporangia cones at the tip sprinkling greenish spore powder. In May and June there is a sterile summer form with 10 to 14 cm high stems and numerous branches that are arranged in whorls at the nodes. The stem and branches are deeply grooved, usually square and rough.

Habitat: Horsetail grows throughout Europe. It grows in Asia as far south as Turkey and Iran. The plant is also found in the Himalayas, central and north China and Japan.

Production: Horsetail consists of the fresh or dried, green, sterile stems of Equisetum arvense harvested in the summer. The herb is collected in the wild and air-dried.

Not to be Confused With: Other Equisetum species.

Other Names: Bottle-Brush, Corn Horsetail, Dutch Rushes, Field Horsetail, Horse Willow, Horsetail Grass, Horsetail Rush, Paddock-Pipes, Pewterwort, Scouring Rush, Shave Grass, Toadpipe

ACTIONS AND PHARMACOLOGY

COMPOUNDS

Flavonoids: (0.6 to 0-9%): apigenin-5-0-glucoside, genkwanin-5-O-glucoside, kaempferol-3,7-di-O-glucoside, kaempferol-3-O-(6′-O-malonyl-glucoside)-7-O-glucoside, kaempferol-3-O-sophoroside, luteolin-5-O-glucoside, quercetin-3-O-glucoside

Caffeic acid ester (up to 1%): including chlorogenic acid, dicoffeoyl-meso-tartaric acid

Silicic acid (5 to 7.7%): to some extent water-soluble

Pyridine alkaloids: nicotine (traces), palustrine (in the gamatophytes and in the rhizome styrolpyrone glucosides, including equisetumpyrone)

EFFECTS

Horsetail has a mild diuretic and spasmolytic action in animal tests. The flavonoids and silicic acid contribute to the astringent effect.

INDICATIONS AND USAGE

Approved by Commission E:

- Infections of the urinary tract
- Kidney and bladder stones
- Wounds and burns

Internal preparations are used for post-traumatic and static edema, flushing-out therapy for bacterial and inflammatory diseases of the lower urinary tract and renal stones. It is used externally as a supportive treatment for poorly healing wounds.

Unproven Uses: In folk medicine, Equisetum arvense is used for tuberculosis, as a catarrh in the kidney and bladder regions, as a hematostatic for profuse menstruation, nasal, pulmonary and gastric hemorrhages, for brittle fingernails and loss of hair, for rheumatic diseases, gout, poorly healing wounds and ulcers, swelling and fractures and for frostbite.

CONTRAINDICATIONS

Horsetail is contraindicated in patients who have edema due to impaired heart and kidney function.

PRECAUTIONS AND ADVERSE REACTIONS

Health risks or side effects following the proper administration of designated therapeutic dosages are not recorded.

A doctor should be consulted when the drug is utilized as a bath additive in cases of major skin lesions, acute skin lesions of unknown origin, major feverish and infectious diseases, cardiac insufficiency and hypertonia.

DOSAGE

Mode of Administration: Comminuted herb for infusions and other galenic preparations are available for oral administration. Comminuted herb for decoctions and other galenic preparations are used externally.

Preparation: To make a tea, pour 200 ml boiling water over 2 to 3 gm drug and boil for 5 minutes. Strain after 10 to 15 minutes. To make an infusion, use 1.5 gm drug per 1 cup water. A liquid extract is prepared in a 1:1 ratio in 25% alcohol.

Daily Dosage: Daily dose of Horsetail is 6 g drug. The drug should be administered with plenty of fluids.

The internal dosages are as follows:

Infusion — 2 to 4 g

Liquid extract — 1 to 4 ml 3 times daily

Tea — 2-3 g per cup repeatedly during the day between mealtimes

External use:

Compresses: 10 g drug to 1 liter

Homeopathic Dosage: 5 drops, 1 tablet or 10 globules every 30 to 60 minutes (acute) or 1 to 3 times a day (chronic); parenterally: 1 to 2 ml sc 3 times daily (HAB1).

Storage: Horsetail must be protected from light in well-sealed containers.

LITERATURE

Beckert C, Veit M, Styrylpyrone im Schachtelhalm. In: DAZ 137(28):2474-2475. 1997.

Eugster C, Heterocycles 4:51. 1976.

Gibelli C, (1931) Arch Int Pharmacodyn 41:419.

Hiller K, Pharmazeutische Bewertung ausgewählter Teedrogen. In: DAZ 135(16):1425-1440. 1995.

Karrer P et al., Helv Chim Acta 32:2397-2399. 1949.

Pohl RW, (1955) Am Fern J 45:95.

Sökeland J, Phytotherapie in der Urologie. In: ZPT 10(1):8. 1989.

Veit M, Problem bei der Bewertung pflanzlicher Diuretika. Als Beispiel Schachtelhalmkraut DAB 10 (Equiseti herba). In: ZPT 15(6):331-341. 1994.

Veit M et al., Flavonoids of the Equisetum hybrids in the subgenus Equisetum. In: PM 58(7)97. 1992.

Further information in:

Hänsel R, Keller K, Rimpler H, Schneider G (Hrsg.), Hagers Handbuch der Pharmazeutischen Praxis, 5. Aufl., Bde 4-6 (Drogen), Springer Verlag Berlin, Heidelberg, New York, 1992-1994.

Madaus G, Lehrbuch der Biologischen Arzneimittel, Bde 1-3, Nachdruck, Georg Olms Verlag Hildesheim 1979.

Steinegger E, Hänsel R, Pharmakognosie, 5. Aufl., Springer Verlag Heidelberg 1992.

Teuscher E, Biogene Arzneimittel, 5. Aufl., Wiss. Verlagsges. mbH Stuttgart 1997.

Wagner H, Wiesenauer M, Phytotherapie. Phytopharmaka und pflanzliche Homöopathika, Fischer-Verlag, Stuttgart, Jena, New York 1995.

Wichtl M (Hrsg.), Teedrogen, 4. Aufl., Wiss. Verlagsges. Stuttgart 1997.

Hound's Tongue

Cynoglossum officinale

DESCRIPTION

Medicinal Parts: The medicinal parts are the aerial and root of the herb.

Flower and Fruit: The flowers are on short, bent pedicles, which grow to 1 cm after flowering. The corolla is cup-shaped and larger than the calyx. The corolla is initially dark violet, then dull brown. It is occasionally white with thickened, velvety purple or light red, tubular scales. The nutlets are flat, ovoid and light brown. They are 5 to 7 mm wide, thickened at the edge and covered with barbs.

Leaves, Stem and Root: The plant is a biennial. The taproot is 10 to 30 cm long and up to 1.5 cm thick. It is reddish colored with a few fibers. The shoots are gray-green and smell of mice. The stems are usually rigidly erect, angular, hairy and heavily foliated. They are 30 to 80 cm high and up to 1 cm thick. The lower leaves are in rosettes, which form a tough, coriaceous sheath at the base. The upper leaves are sessile and clasping.

Habitat: Especially common in Germany and Switzerland, now also found in the U.S. in areas where Germans and Swiss settled.

Production: Hound's Tongue herb consists of the above-ground parts of Cynoglossum officinale. Hound's Tongue root is the root of Cynoglossum officinale. The root is gathered in the second spring and then dried.

Other Names: Dog's Tongue, Dog-Bur, Gypsy Flower, Sheep-Lice, Woolmat

ACTIONS AND PHARMACOLOGY

COMPOUNDS: HOUND'S TONGUE HERB

Pyrrolizidine alkaloids (0.7 to 1.5%): main alkaloids heliosupine, echinatine, also 7-angeloylheliotridine, acetylheliosupine

EFFECTS:

No information is available.

COMPOUNDS: HOUND'S TONGUE ROOT

Pyrrolizidine alkaloids: main alkaloids presumably, as in the plant, heliosupine and echinatine

Tannins

EFFECTS: HOUND'S TONGUE ROOT

The root has antidiarrheal and wound-healing effects. It is both toxic and carcinogenic.

According to previous reports, cynoglossin has a paralyzing effect on the peripheral nerve ends of frogs. The substances consolicin and consolidin have a paralyzing effect on the CNS, which is 3 times stronger than the effect of cynoglossin. The toxicity should disappear with storage.

INDICATIONS AND USAGE

HOUND'S TONGUE HERB

Unproven Uses: Preparations of Hound's Tongue have been used as an antidiarrheal and an expectorant. The effectiveness of the herb for the claimed applications is not documented.

CYNOGLOSSUM ROOT

Unproven Uses: In the past, it was used as an analgesic both internally and externally, as a cough sedative and for diarrhea. The root is used externally in the treatment of wounds.

PRECAUTIONS AND ADVERSE REACTIONS

HOUND'S TONGUE HERB AND ROOT

WARNING: The traditional folk medicinal preparations should not be used!

Because of its high pyrrolizidine alkaloid content with 1,2-unsaturated necine parent substances, the drug is both hepatotoxic and hepatocarcinogenic in effect. The drug should under no circumstances be taken internally.

DOSAGE

HOUND'S TONGUE HERB AND ROOT

See Warning above regarding internal use.

Storage: The herb should be protected from light and kept dry above annealed calcium chloride in air-tight, sealed glass or chalk containers, with the possible addition of a few drops of chloroform or carbon tetrachloride as an insecticide. It should be renewed annually.

LITERATURE

HOUND'S TONGUE HERB

Frohne D, Pfänder HJ: Giftpflanzen - Ein Handbuch für Apotheker, Toxikologen und Biologen, 4. Aufl., Wiss. Verlagsges. mbH Stuttgart 1997.

Kern W, List PH, Hörhammer L (Hrsg.), Hagers Handbuch der Pharmazeutischen Praxis, 4. Aufl., Bde 1-8, Springer Verlag Berlin, Heidelberg, New York, 1969.

Knight AP, Kimberling CV, Stermitz FR, Roby MR, Cynoglossum officinale (hounds-tongue) - a cause of pyrrolizidine-alkaloid poisoning in horse. In: J Am Vet Med Assoc 185(6):647-650. 1984.

Lewin L, Gifte und Vergiftungen, 6. Aufl., Nachdruck, Haug Verlag, Heidelberg 1992.

Mattocks AR, Pigott CD, Pyrrolizidine lakloids from Cynoglossum germanicum. In: PH 29(9):2871. 1990.

Steinegger E, Hänsel R, Pharmakognosie, 5. Aufl., Springer Verlag Heidelberg 1992.

Teuscher E, Lindequist U, Biogene Gifte - Biologie, Chemie, Pharmakologie, 2. Aufl., Fischer Verlag Stuttgart 1994.

HOUND'S TONGUE ROOT

Kern W, List PH, Hörhammer L (Hrsg.), Hagers Handbuch der Pharmazeutischen Praxis, 4. Aufl., Bde 1-8, Springer Verlag Berlin, Heidelberg, New York, 1969.

Knight AP, Kimberling CV, Stermitz FR, Roby MR, Cynoglossum officinale (hounds-tongue) - a cause of pyrrolizidine-alkaloid poisoning in horse. In: J Am Vet Med Assoc 185(6):647-650. 1984.

Mattocks AR, Pigott CD, Pyrrolizidine lakloids from Cynoglossum germanicum. In: PH 29(9):2871. 1990.

Houseleek

Sempervivum tectorum

DESCRIPTION

Medicinal Parts: The medicinal parts are the fresh leaves before flowering and their juice.

Flower and Fruit: The pink or red flowers are in cymes on their own peduncles, which are about 22 cm high. The individual flowers are short-pedicled and splayed in a star shape. The 12 sepals and petals are twice as long as the calyx. The 24 stamens are in 2 circles. There are 24 ovaries. The small fruit is many-seeded and fused at the base.

Leaves, Stem and Root: The green succulent leaves grow directly from the perennial fibrous root and form a dense, obovate, basal rosette 5 to 10 cm in diameter. They are fleshy and juicy, flat, 2.5 to 5 cm long. The purple leaves are sessile-oblong with a ciliate margin and are often in carpets of tufts.

Habitat: The plant is indigenous to central and southern Europe and now grows wild in northern Europe, northern Africa, and western Asia.

Other Names: Jupiter's Eye, Jupiter's Beard, Thor's Beard, Bullock's Eye, Sengreen, Ayron, Ayegreen, Aaron's Rod, Hens and Chickens, Liveforever, Thunder Plant

ACTIONS AND PHARMACOLOGY

COMPOUNDS

Fruit acids: L(-)-malic acid, isocitric acid, succinic acid

Tannins

Mucilage

EFFECTS

The active agents are the leaves containing tannin, bitter substances, sugar, and mucous. Results of research carried out to date point to a possible liver-protective and anti-oxidative effect. There are no studies available for the astringent, diuretic and antiseptic effects attributed to the drug.

INDICATIONS AND USAGE

Unproven Uses: Houseleek is used internally to relieve severe diarrhea. Folk medicine uses include dysentery, dysmenorrhea and amenorrhea, impairment of hearing and fever, worm infestation, uterine neuralgia, tonsillitis, headache and toothache. Externally, the drug is used for burns, wounds, ulcers and swelling caused by insect bites, open wounds, sore nipples, corns, inflammation of the throat, hemorrhoids, eczema, stomatitis, oral fungal infections and inflammation of mucous membranes and for the treatment of itchy and burning skin parts. A gargle of diluted juice made from the leaves is used for stomatitis.

PRECAUTIONS AND ADVERSE REACTIONS

No health hazards or side effects are known in conjunction with the proper administration of designated therapeutic dosages.

DOSAGE

Mode of Administration: Houseleek is used internally as a decoction. Freshly pressed leaves and their juice is used externally.

Preparation: To prepare an infusion, allow 15 g of the drug to steep in 1000 ml water for 10 minutes. Poultices are prepared using crushed fresh leaves. A compress is made by soaking a cloth in plant juice that has been diluted with water. Gargles are prepared using plant juice diluted with water and sweetened with honey. The pure plant juice is used for ear drops.

Daily Dosage: Infusion dosage is 1 cup every 3 hours.

LITERATURE

Kern W, List PH, Hörhammer L (Hrsg.), Hagers Handbuch der Pharmazeutischen Praxis, 4. Aufl., Bde 1-8: Springer Verlag Berlin, Heidelberg, New York, 1969.

Madaus G, Lehrbuch der Biologischen Arzneimittel, Bde 1-3, Nachdruck, Georg Olms Verlag Hildesheim 1979.

Humulus lupulus

See Hops

Hwema Bark

Corynanthe pachyceras

DESCRIPTION

Medicinal Parts: The medicinal part of the plant is the bark.

Flower and Fruit: The inflorescence is an apical, up to 10-cm long panicle. The calyx has 4 short tips. The corolla tube is white and urn-shaped with 4 narrow, approximately 2-mm long lobes. The lobes have globular appendages, with 4 stamens and a 2-chambered ovary. The fruit is a 7 to 10 mm long and 2 to 4 mm wide, loculicidal capsule, which is black when ripe, with numerous double slit winged seeds.

Leaves and Trunk: Corynanthe pachyceras is a tree that grows up to 20 m high. The leaves are opposite, with simple lamina that are paper-like. The lamina grow from 15 to 25 cm long and 5 to 7 cm wide. They are elongate-ovate with approximately 12 mm long stipules. The branches are glabrous and the trunk bark is dark green to reddish brown.

Habitat: Tropical Africa

Production: Hwema bark is the dried bark of Corynanthe pachyceras. It is dried in the sun or drying cupboard with circulating air at temperatures less than 70° C after harvesting.

Not to be Confused With: Incorrect identification can occur with Cinchonae cortex and sometimes with Yohimbe Cortex.

ACTIONS AND PHARMACOLOGY

COMPOUNDS

Indole alkaloids of the beta-carboline and oxindole type: chief alkaloids corynanthine (1.2%) and corynantheidine, including as well, corynanthidine (alpha-yohimbine), beta-yohimbine, corynantheine, dihydrocorynantheine, corynoxine, corynoxeine

EFFECTS

The alkaloid-containing drug (yohimbine-corynantheine type) affects the CNS by inhibiting motility in animal experiments. The drug is spasmolytic, blood pressure reducing and also mildly analgesic and locally anesthetic in effect.

INDICATIONS AND USAGE

Unproven Uses: In folk medicine, Hwema Bark preparations are used for fever and malaria (infusion), leprosy (decoction), colds, and to lower blood pressure (dry extract).

PRECAUTIONS AND ADVERSE REACTIONS

No health hazards are known in conjunction with the proper administration of designated therapeutic dosages. The LD50 in mice was determined to be 4.9 mg dry extract/kg body weight, I.V. The symptoms observed included convulsions and dyspnea.

OVERDOSAGE

Overdoses among humans could conceivably lead to signs of poisoning.

DOSAGE

Mode of Administration: Whole and cut drug, liquid and solid preparations for internal use; solid preparations for external use.

Preparation: To prepare a dry extract (10:1), the bark powder is succussed for 30 minutes at 95°C with a 10-fold amount of isotonic Nacl solution. It is filtered after cooling and the solution is concentrated to double the weight of the drug. Freeze-drying follows a 48-hour clarification period. This produces a brown powder. Drug:native dry extract is 10:1.

Daily Dosage: Dry extract — 200 mg 1 to 4 times daily.

How Supplied: Tablets, capsules, suppositories and drink ampules.

Storage: Hwema Bark should be stored in a dry place.

LITERATURE

Hänsel R, Keller K, Rimpler H, Schneider G (Ed) Hagers Handbuch der Pharmazeutischen Praxis. 5. Aufl., Bde 4 - 6 (Drogen), Springer Verlag Berlin, Heidelberg, New York, 1992-1994

Hydnocarpus species

See Chaulmoogra

Hydrangea

Hydrangea arborescens

DESCRIPTION

Medicinal Parts: The medicinal parts are the dried rhizome and the roots.

Flower and Fruit: The inflorescence is flat cymes of umbels with creamy white flowers. They are androgynous or completely sexless and have inferior ovaries. The fruit is a schizocarp or capsule.

Leaves, Stem and Root: Hydrangea is a marsh plant, a bush up to 3 m high whose leaves are only pubescent on the veins of the undersides. The petiole is 2 to 5 cm long. The leaves are simple or lobed and opposite. There are no stipules. The bark is rough and tends to peel off. The roots are of various lengths and widths. They are pale gray on the outside and solid with a slight splitting structure.

Habitat: Indigenous to the eastern U.S. as far south as Florida.

Production: Hydrangea root is the root of Hydrangea arborescens.

Other Names: Seven Barks

ACTIONS AND PHARMACOLOGY

COMPOUNDS

Saponins

Flavonolids: including, among others, rutin

Volatile oil

Isocoumarin derivatives: including, among others, hydrangenol

EFFECTS

The drug has a diuretic effect.

INDICATIONS AND USAGE

Unproven Uses: Hydrangea is used in the treatment of conditions of the urinary tract, particularly bladder and kidney stones.

PRECAUTIONS AND ADVERSE REACTIONS

No health hazards or side effects are known in conjunction with the proper administration of designated therapeutic dosages. According to information in older medical literature, the intake of larger dosages can lead to dizziness, feelings of constriction in the chest and central nervous system disorders. The plant has a weak potential for sensitization (chief allergen hydrangenol).

DOSAGE

Mode of Administration: As a liquid extract, in compounded preparations.

LITERATURE

Bate-Smith EC, (1978) Phytochemistry 17:267.

Der Mardirossian A et al., (1976) J Toxicol Environ Health 1: 939.

Frohne D, Pfänder HJ, Giftpflanzen - Ein Handbuch für Apotheker, Toxikologen und Biologen, 4. Aufl., Wiss. Verlags-Ges. Stuttgart 1997.

Hausen B, Allergiepflanzen, Pflanzenallergene, ecomed Verlagsgesellsch. mbH, Landsberg 1988.

Kern W, List PH, Hörhammer L (Hrsg.), Hagers Handbuch der Pharmazeutischen Praxis, 4. Aufl., Bde 1-8, Springer Verlag Berlin, Heidelberg, New York, 1969.

Leung AY, Encyclopedia of Common Natural Ingredients Used in Food, Drugs and Cosmetics, John Wiley & Sons Inc., New York 1980.

Lewin L, Gifte und Vergiftungen, 6. Aufl., Nachdruck, Haug Verlag, Heidelberg 1992.

Madaus G, Lehrbuch der Biologischen Arzneimittel, Bde 1-3, Nachdruck, Georg Olms Verlag Hildesheim 1979.

Roth L, Daunderer M, Kormann K, Giftpflanzen, Pflanzengifte, 4. Aufl., Ecomed Fachverlag Landsberg Lech 1993.

Hydrangea arborescens

See Hydrangea

Hydrastis canadensis

See Goldenseal

Hyoscyamus niger

See Henbane

Hypericum perforatum

See St. John's Wort

Hypoxis rooperi

See African Potato

Hyssop

Hyssopus officinalis

TRADE NAMES

Hyssop (available from numerous manufacturers and as combination product), Hyssop Herb

DESCRIPTION

Medicinal Parts: The medicinal parts are the leaves, the flower tips and the essential oil.

Flower and Fruit: The dark-blue bilabiate flowers are medium-sized false whorls in one-sided, terminal, leafy racemes. The calyx is downy, 5-tipped and glabrous inside. There are 4 stamens, which are turned away from each other and extend far above the perianth. The style is very long.

Leaves, Stem and Root: The plant is an evergreen subshrub about 60 cm high. The stem is erect, quadrangular, shrubby and branched. The leaves are sessile, lanceolate, acute, entire-margined, punctate, glabrous, dark green and paler beneath.

Characteristics: The plant has a weak sweetish smell. The taste is bitter.

Habitat: The plant is indigenous to southern Europe and grows wild in the Mediterranean region. It is cultivated elsewhere.

Production: Hyssop herb consists of the fresh or dried aboveground parts of Hyssopus officinalis. Hyssop oil consists of the essential oil of Hyssopus officinalis, obtained by steam distillation.

ACTIONS AND PHARMACOLOGY

COMPOUNDS

In the foliage:

Volatile oil

Tannins

Bitter principles: including, among others, marubiin

Flavonoids: glycosides of hesperidin and diosmetin

In the volatile oil:

Chief components: 1-pinocamphone, isocamphone, pinocarvone, alpha- and beta-pinene

EFFECTS

1-pinocamphone and isopinocamphone are the toxically active constituents of the drug. The oil has an antimicrobial and anthelmintic effect. Extracts of the leaves are antimicrobial, antiviral (*herpes simplex*) and mildly spasmolytic.

INDICATIONS AND USAGE

Unproven Uses: Preparations of Hyssop herb are used for the gentle stimulation of circulation, for intestinal catarrhs, for diseases of the respiratory tract, colds, chest and lung ailments.

PRECAUTIONS AND ADVERSE REACTIONS

General: No health hazards are known in conjunction with the proper administration of designated therapeutic dosages. Isolated cases of tonic-clonic spasms have been observed among adults after intake of 10 to 30 drops of the volatile oil over a number of days (2 to 3 drops for children).

Pregnancy: Not to be used during pregnancy.

DOSAGE

Mode of Administration: Hyssop herb preparations are available as capsules for internal use.

How Supplied:
Capsules — 445 mg

LITERATURE

Joulain D, (1979) Riv Ital Ess Prof Piante Off Ar Sap Cosm 48:479.

Kern W, List PH, Hörhammer L (Hrsg.), Hagers Handbuch der Pharmazeutischen Praxis, 4. Aufl., Bde. 1-8, Springer Verlag Berlin, Heidelberg, New York, 1969.

Leung AY, Encyclopedia of Common Natural Ingredients Used in Food, Drugs and Cosmetics, John Wiley & Sons Inc., New York 1980.

Madaus G, Lehrbuch der Biologischen Arzneimittel, Bde 1-3, Nachdruck, Georg Olms Verlag Hildesheim 1979.

Opdyke DLJ, (1978) Food Cosmet Toxicol 16 (Suppl. 1):787.

Hyssopus officinalis

See Hyssop

Iberis amara

See Bitter Candytuft

Iceland Moss

Cetraria islandica

DESCRIPTION

Medicinal Parts: The medicinal part is the dried thallus commonly known as Iceland Moss.

Flower and Fruit: Cetraria islandica is a lichen that grows on the ground and has a stiff, curling thallus. The thallus is from 2 to 6 cm high, erect, dichotomously branched, with a 1 to 10 cm wide section. The upper surface is olive-brown-green or brown, the underside is whitish to light brownish. The margins are covered in 0.5 mm long papilla, which contain the reproductive parts.

Characteristics: Iceland Moss tastes bitter, and when wet, has a smell reminiscent of seaweed.

Habitat: Grows in the boreal, alpine and Arctic regions of the Northern Hemisphere and in some regions of the Southern Hemisphere.

Production: Iceland Moss consists of the dried thallus of Cetraria islandica as well as its preparations. It is collected in the wild, then air-dried, moistened, cut and re-dried.

Other Names: Iceland Lichen, Cetraria, Eryngo-Leaved Liverwort

ACTIONS AND PHARMACOLOGY

COMPOUNDS

Mucilages, glucans (50%): lichenan (lichenan), isolichenan (isolichenan)

Aromatic lichen acids (2-3%): fumarprototcetraric acid, protocetraric acid, cetraric acid

Aliphatic lichen acids (1.0-1.5%): esp. protolichesteric acid

EFFECTS

The bitter organic acids have an antibiotic effect. It is also a demulcent and a mild antimicrobial.

The drug has an demulcent effect due to the sesquitering action of the polysaccharides. An ethanol precipitation of the aqueous extract containing lichenan and isolichenan demonstrated an antitumoural effect in animal tests.

INDICATIONS AND USAGE

Approved by Commission E:

- Cough/bronchitis
- Dyspeptic complaints
- Inflammation of the mouth and pharynx
- Loss of appetite

Unproven Uses: Iceland Moss is also used for irritation of the oral and pharyngeal mucous membranes; loss of appetite and gastroenteritis (the bitter organic acids). In folk medicine, the drug has been used for lung disease, kidney and bladder complaints, gastric conditions, nausea and vomiting (in particular in pregnancy and with migraine), bronchitis, whooping cough and diarrhea. It is also used externally for poorly healing wounds.

Homeopathic Uses: Cetraria islandica is used to treat bronchitis.

PRECAUTIONS AND ADVERSE REACTIONS

No health hazards or side effects are known in conjunction with the proper administration of designated therapeutic dosages. In rare cases, external administration of the drug led to sensitization.

DOSAGE

Mode of Administration: Comminuted thallus for infusions and other galenic formulations for internal use; comminuted thallus preferably for cold maceration and other bitter-tasting preparations for internal use.

Preparation: To prepare an infusion, pour boiling water over 1.5 to 2.5 gm of comminuted drug and strain after 10 minutes (1 teaspoonful = 1.3 gm of drug); infusion may be sweetened.

Daily Dosage: The average daily dose is 4 to 6 gm. Single dose: 1.5 g drug in a teacup.

Homeopathic Dosage: 5 drops, 1 tablet, 10 globules every 30 to 60 minutes (acute) or 1 to 3 times daily (chronic); parenterally: 1 to 2 ml sc acute: 3 times daily; chronic: once daily (HAB1).

Storage: Store in the dark and well-sealed containers.

LITERATURE

Anonym, Niedere Pflanzen ganz groβ - 39. Jahrestagung der Gesellschaft für Arzneipflanzenforschung in Saarbrücken. In: DAZ 131(37):1899.

Pengsuparp Th, et al., Mechanistic evaluation of new plant-derived compounds that inhibit HIV-1 reverse transcriptase. In: JNP 58(7):1024-1031. 1995.

Wunderer H, Zentral und peripher wirksame Antitussiva: eine kritische Übersicht. In: PZ 142(11):847-852. 1997.

Further information in:

Fenaroli's Handbook of Flavor Ingredients, Vol. 1. 2nd Ed. Pub. CRC Press Boca Raton 1975.

Hänsel R, Keller K, Rimpler H, Schneider G (Hrsg.), Hagers Handbuch der Pharmazeutischen Praxis, 5. Aufl., Bde 4-6 (Drogen): Springer Verlag Berlin, Heidelberg, New York, 1992-1994 (unter Cetraria).

Steinegger E, Hänsel R, Pharmakognosie, 5. Aufl., Springer Verlag Heidelberg 1992.

Teuscher E, Biogene Arzneimittel, 5. Aufl., Wiss. Verlagsges. Stuttgart 1997.

Wichtl M (Hrsg.), Teedrogen, 4. Aufl., Wiss. Verlagsges. Stuttgart 1997.

Ignatius Beans

Strychnos ignatii

DESCRIPTION

Medicinal Parts: The medicinal parts are the ripe seeds and the dried root bark.

Flower and Fruit: The flowers are in dense, axillary thyrses. Their parts are arranged in fives. They are greenish-white, pubescent and have a 2-valved superior ovary. The fruit is a golden-yellow berry. The berry is up to 13 cm wide and has a hard exocarp. The fruit pulp is yellow and contains up to 40 seeds. The seeds are 2 to 3 cm long by 2 cm wide, oval or rounded-angular, obtuse and very hard.

Leaves, Stem and Root: The plant is a climbing shrub with hooked stems that are up to 20 m long. The truck is up to 10 cm thick. It is occasionally a small tree. It bears leaves that are up to 25 cm long, broad-ovate, opposite and short-petioled.

Habitat: The plant is common all over southeastern Asia and is cultivated there; especially in Vietnam and the Philippines.

Production: Ignatius beans are the seeds of Strychnos ignatii.

Not to be Confused With: The seeds of S. Ianata and S. multiflora were once treated in the same manner as Ignatii seeds.

ACTIONS AND PHARMACOLOGY

COMPOUNDS

Indole alkaloids (2.5-5.6%): chief alkaloid strychnine (share 45-60%), in addition, above all, brucine, further including, among others, 12-hydroxystrychnine, alpha-colubrine, icajine, vomicine, novacine. There are also chemical strains for which brucine predominates, and others in which strychnine occurs only in traces.

Fatty oil

EFFECTS

The drug, which contains strychnine and brucine, is psychoanaleptic (see Nux Vomica).

INDICATIONS AND USAGE

Unproven Uses: Preparations made of the Ignatius Bean are used to treat faintness. Therapeutic use as a bitter or tonic is not recommended.

Homeopathic Uses: The drug is used for nervous disorders, cramps in hollow organs and muscles, and depressive states.

PRECAUTIONS AND ADVERSE REACTIONS

The drug is severely toxic due to the strychnine content and should not be administered in allopathic medicine.

OVERDOSAGE

Symptoms of poisoning can occur after ingestion of one bean. Strychnine doses of as little as 1.5 mg (30-50 mg of the drug) initially cause restlessness, feelings of anxiety, heightening of sense perception, enhanced reflexes, equilibrium disorders and painful stiffness of the neck and back musculature. Later, twitching, tonic spasms of the masseter and neck musculature, and finally, painful convulsions of the entire body are triggered by visual or tactile stimulation. Dyspnea comes following spasm of the breathing musculature. Death occurs through suffocation or exhaustion. The lethal dosage for an adult is approximately 50 mg strychnine (1-2 gm of the drug). Chronic intake of subconvulsive dosages can also lead to death under similar conditions after a period of weeks. This is due to an accumulation of drug in the body, particularly in those who have liver damage.

Following the administration of a watery suspension of activated charcoal, the therapy for poisoning consists of keeping external stimulation to a minimum through placement in a quiet, warm, darkened room. Convulsions should be treated with dosages of diazepam or barbital (i.v.). High-calorie glucose infusions should also be given. Intubation and oxygen respiration may also be required. Gastric lavage should be avoided, due to the danger of triggering convulsions. Analeptics or phenothiazines should not be administered. Because of the possibility of unwanted effects occurring in conjunction with the administration of therapeutic dosages, one should forgo any administration of the drug.

DOSAGE

Mode of Administration: It is used in the manufacture of strychnine and brucine.

Daily Dosage: If the drug is taken internally, the maximum single dose is 0.1 gm; the maximum daily dosage is 0.3 gm.

Homeopathic Dosage: from D4: 5 drops, 1 tablet or 10 globules every 30 to 60 minutes (acute) or 1 to 3 times daily (chronic); parenterally: 1 to 2 ml sc, acute: 3 times daily; chronic: once a day (HAB1).

Storage: Mark the container as ''poisonous'' and keep tightly sealed; protect the drug from cool air and light.

LITERATURE

Bisset NG, Phillipson JD, JNP 39:263. 1976.

Hänsel R, Keller K, Rimpler H, Schneider G (Hrsg.), Hagers Handbuch der Pharmazeutischen Praxis, 5. Aufl., Bde 4-6 (Drogen): Springer Verlag Berlin, Heidelberg, New York, 1992-1994.

Lewin L, Gifte und Vergiftungen, 6. Aufl., Nachdruck, Haug Verlag, Heidelberg 1992.

Madaus G, Lehrbuch der Biologischen Arzneimittel, Bde 1-3, Nachdruck, Georg Olms Verlag Hildesheim 1979.

Marini-Bettolo GB, Advances in the research of curare and Strychnos. In: Rend Accad Naz 40:1975-1976, 1-2, 61-76. 1977.

Roth L, Daunderer M, Kormann K, Giftpflanzen, Pflanzengifte, 4. Aufl., Ecomed Fachverlag Landsberg Lech 1993.

Teuscher E, Lindequist U, Biogene Gifte - Biologie, Chemie, Pharmakologie, 2. Aufl., Fischer Verlag Stuttgart 1994.

Wagner H, Wiesenauer M, Phytotherapie. Phytopharmaka und pflanzliche Homöopathika, Fischer-Verlag, Stuttgart, Jena, New York 1995.

Ilex aquifolium

See Holly

Ilex paraguariensis

See Maté

Illicium verum

See Star Anise

Immortelle

Helichrysum arenarium

DESCRIPTION

Medicinal Parts: The medicinal parts are the composite heads and the whole of the flowering plant.

Flower and Fruit: The small orange flowers are in dense clustered cymes. The bracts are dry-membranous and usually lemon-yellow. All the florets are tubular and funnel-shaped. The fruit is pentangular with a tuft of hair.

Leaves, Stem and Root: The plant grows from 10 to 30 cm high. The stem is erect, unbranched and gray-tomentose. The leaves are alternate. The lower leaves are spatulate and the upper ones lanceolate, acute and as gray-tomentose as the stem.

Characteristics: Immortelle has a weak aroma.

Habitat: The plant grows in Europe and the U.S.

Production: Immortelle consists of the dried flowers of Helichrysum arenarium gathered shortly before fully unfolding.

Not to be Confused With: Confusion can arise with the capitula of Helichrysum stoechas and Helichrysum augustifolium.

Other Names: Common Shrubby Everlasting, Eternal Flower, Goldilocks, Yellow Chaste Weed

ACTIONS AND PHARMACOLOGY

COMPOUNDS

Flavonoids: in particular isosalipurposide (intensive yellow chalcone glycoside), naringenin-5-glucosyl-glucoside, helichrysin A and B (C-2-enantiomeric narigenin-5-O-glucosides, B-salipurposide)

Phthalides: including 5-methoxy-7-hydroxy-phthalides and their monoglucoside

Alpha-pyrone derivatives: arenole, homoarenole

Sesquiterpene bitter principles

Volatile oil (traces)

Caffeic acid derivatives

EFFECTS

The drug has antibacterial principles, and is mildly choleretic and mildly spasmolytic.

INDICATIONS AND USAGE

Approved by Commission E:

■ Dyspeptic complaints

Unproven Uses: The drug is used as an adjunct in the treatment of chronic cholecystitis and gallbladder complaints with accompanying cramps. In folk medicine, it is used as a diuretic and for jaundice, gout, rheumatism, kidney complaints and dropsy.

CONTRAINDICATIONS

Because of the bile-stimulating effect of the drug, it is not to be administered when there is biliary obstruction. The presence of gallstone illnesses can lead to colic.

PRECAUTIONS AND ADVERSE REACTIONS

Health risks or side effects following the proper administration of designated therapeutic dosages are not recorded.

DOSAGE

Mode of Administration: Immortelle is used as a comminuted herb for infusions and other galenic preparations for internal use. Pharmaceutical cholagogues contain extracts of the drug. It is an inactive ingredient in many tea specialties.

How Supplied: Forms of commercial pharmaceutical preparations include teas, drops and compound preparations.

Preparation: To make an infusion, pour boiling water over 2 teaspoonfuls of the drug (3 to 4 g). Allow to stand for 10 minutes and then strain. Drink throughout the day and make a fresh batch daily.

Daily Dosage: The average daily dose is 3 g of drug.

Storage: Store Immortelle protected from light and moisture.

LITERATURE

Derkach AI et al., Chem Nat Comp 6:722. 1986.

Kern W, List PH, Hörhammer L (Hrsg.), Hagers Handbuch der Pharmazeutischen Praxis, 4. Aufl., Bde. 1-8, Springer Verlag Berlin, Heidelberg, New York, 1969.

Leung AY, Encyclopedia of Common Natural Ingredients Used in Food, Drugs and Cosmetics, John Wiley & Sons Inc., New York 1980.

Madaus G, Lehrbuch der Biologischen Arzneimittel, Bde 1-3, Nachdruck, Georg Olms Verlag Hildesheim 1979.

Mericli AH et al., Sci Pharm 54:363. 1986.

Teuscher E, Biogene Arzneimittel, 5. Aufl., Wiss. Verlagsges. mbH Stuttgart 1997.

Wichtl M (Hrsg.), Teedrogen, 4. Aufl., Wiss. Verlagsges. Stuttgart 1997.

Impatiens biflora

See Jewel Weed

Impomoea hederacea

See Morning Glory

Indian Hemp

Apocynum cannabinum

DESCRIPTION

Medicinal Parts: The medicinal parts are the root and the juice obtained from the fresh plant.

Flower and Fruit: The small whitish-green, occasionally pink to violet flowers are on pods that grow to 2 to 4 mm in length. The calyx is deeply lobed and half as long as the corolla. The petals are oblong-lanceolate. The tufts of hair on the seeds are 2 to 3 cm long.

Leaves, Stem and Root: Indian Hemp is a perennial up to 2 m tall. It has an erect stem, which branches at the top. The whole plant is glabrous or downy. The short-petioled leaves are 5 to 11 cm long, yellowish-green and oblong or oblong-ovoid. The tips of the leaves are initially rounded and then terminate abruptly in a thorny tip.

Characteristics: The plant has an acrid taste and is to a certain degree poisonous.

Habitat: The plant is found mostly in the U.S. and Canada.

Not to be Confused With: Indian Hemp (Cannabis indica), though both species contain latex and their tough, fibrous bark can be used as a substitute for hemp, hence the name.

Production: Indian Hemp root is the root of Apocynum cannabinum, which is gathered (and sometimes dried), in autumn. The plant is cultivated as a crop in Germany and Russia.

Other Names: Bitterroot, Catchfly, Dogbane, Fly-Trap, Honeybloom, Milk Ipecac, Milkweed, Mountain Hemp, Wallflower, Wild Cotton, Canadian Hemp

ACTIONS AND PHARMACOLOGY

COMPOUNDS

Cardioactive steroid glycosides (cardenolids): in particular cymarin, k-strophantoside, apocannoside, cynocannoside

EFFECTS

The high content of cardenolide glycosides causes bradycardia and increased contraction of the heart. Blood pressure is lowered, and rebound vagotonia hypertension can occur. The drug increases diuresis and stimulation of the vasomotor centers. It causes more severe irritation of the intestinal mucous membrane than digitalis and strophantus preparations. It has a lower therapeutic effect on atrial fibrillation than digitalis.

Cardenollide glycoside cymine has an effect that is similar but generally weaker than glycoside strophantine, with the exception of the stronger diuretic effect in edema. It is less cumulative.

INDICATIONS AND USAGE

Unproven Uses: The juice of the fresh plant is used in the treatment of condylomatosis and warts. American Indians use the roots for asthma, dropsy, coughs, syphilis and rheumatism. In folk medicine, the root is used to strengthen weak heart muscles following pneumonia, valvular insufficiency and senile heart. It is also used as a diuretic.

Homeopathic Uses: Homeopathic uses include cardiac insufficiency, renal inflammation with edema, and vomiting with diarrhea.

PRECAUTIONS AND ADVERSE REACTIONS

The drug should be administered only by someone who is expert in its use. Topical irritation of the mucous membrane of the alimentary canal, accompanied by nausea and vomiting, is more common than in other drugs containing cardenolid glycosides. Vomiting and gastrointestinal irritations can occur, even with the administration of therapeutic doses of the drug because of the mucous membrane-irritating resin fraction.

OVERDOSAGE

For possible symptoms of overdose and treatment of poisonings see Digitalis folium. Despite the strong efficacy of the drug's cardioactive steroid glycosides in parenteral application, serious poisoning in the course of peroral administration is unlikely, due to the low resorption rate.

DOSAGE

Daily Dosage: The average daily dose of the liquid extract is 10 to 30 drops to be taken 3 times daily or 0.3 to 0.6 ml. of a 1:10 tincture.

Homeopathic Dosage: 5 drops, 1 tablet or 10 globules every 30 to 60 minutes (acute) or every 1 to 3 days (chronic); Parenterally: 1 to 2 ml 3 times daily sc (HAB1).

Storage: Store in secure area as the drug is poisonous.

LITERATURE

Belkin M et al., (1952) J Nat Cancer Inst 13:742.

Desruelles J et al., Therapie 28:103-113. 1973.

Kupchan SM et al., J Med Chem 7:803-805. 1964.

Further information in:

Hänsel R, Keller K, Rimpler H, Schneider G (Hrsg.), Hagers Handbuch der Pharmazeutischen Praxis, 5. Aufl., Bde 4-6 (Drogen): Springer Verlag Berlin, Heidelberg, New York, 1992-1994.

Lewin L, Gifte und Vergiftungen, 6. Aufl., Nachdruck, Haug Verlag, Heidelberg 1992.

Madaus G, Lehrbuch der Biologischen Arzneimittel, Bde 1-3, Nachdruck, Georg Olms Verlag Hildesheim 1979.

Roth L, Daunderer M, Kormann K, Giftpflanzen, Pflanzengifte, 4. Aufl., Ecomed Fachverlag Landsberg Lech 1993.

Teuscher E, Lindequist U, Biogene Gifte - Biologie, Chemie, Pharmakologie, 2. Aufl., Fischer Verlag Stuttgart 1994.

Teuscher E, Biogene Arzneimittel, 5. Aufl., Wiss. Verlagsges. Stuttgart 1997.

Wagner H, Wiesenauer M, Phytotherapie. Phytopharmaka und pflanzliche Homöopathika, Fischer-Verlag, Stuttgart, Jena, New York 1995.

Indian Nettle

Acalypha indica

DESCRIPTION

Medicinal Parts: The medicinal part of the plant is the whole flowering plant.

Flower and Fruit: The inflorescence is spike-like, has 3 to 7 female flowers below, which consist only of a 3-carpeled-ovary with 3 styles. The male flowers are above these with 4 sepals and 8 stamens. On the tips of the young flower shoots are T-shaped, hairy structures approximately 2 mm wide with 2 side openings. The fruit is a 3-chambered capsule with 3 gray-brown seeds of approximately 1 mm diameter.

Leaves, Stem and Root: Indian nettle is an annual, upright, nettle-like diclinous, monoecious herb, which grows up to 60 cm high. The leaves are alternate, long-petiolate, round to rhomboid, 2 to 6 cm long, 1.5 to 5 cm wide narrowing to the petiole. They are matte above, glossy beneath with strongly protruding ribs, dentate at the front and smooth toward the base. The margin, petiole and ribs are weakly pubescent with 2 awl-like stipules. The stem is usually unbranched and pubescent. The main root is unbranched with thin secondary roots.

Habitat: The plant comes from India, Indochina and Ethiopia.

Other Names: Cat's Nettle

Production: Indian nettle is the whole fresh plant of Acalypha indica collected during the flowering season and dried.

ACTIONS AND PHARMACOLOGY

COMPOUNDS

Cyanogenic glycosides: acalyphin (0.3%, 3-cyanopyridone derivative)

Tannins: including tri-O-methyl ellagic acid

Volatile oil

EFFECTS

The drug is hemostyptic and antibacterial in effect (cyanogenic glucoside acalyphine). In vitro, proof of an acceleration of blood coagulation exists, which is due to the high levels of calcium salts. The leaf latex is said to have emetic and expectorant effects upon children. When administered as a suppository for constipation, it is said to immediately relax the contracted anal sphincter.

INDICATIONS AND USAGE

Unproven Uses: Internally used for worm infestation and constipation, for pregnant women, also for upset stomach and bronchitis. Externally used for eczema and skin rashes, ear ache (decoction), tumors (juice), as well as for cuts and other wounds, and also for inflammation of the joints (cut leaves and stems).

Indian Medicine: Preparations are used for ulcers, changes to the skin, bronchitis, constipation, croup and earache.

PRECAUTIONS AND ADVERSE REACTIONS

No health hazards or side effects other than possible gastric irritation are known in conjunction with the proper administration of designated therapeutic dosages. Dermatitis has been observed following skin contact with the latex of the fresh plant. Cyanide poisonings from the drug are unlikely, due to the relatively low levels of cyanogenic glycoside content and the lack of stimuli leading to ingestion.

OVERDOSAGE

In animal experiments (rabbits), administration of large quantities of the drug led to gastrointestinal inflammation and to a change in blood color to chocolate-brown, indicating the presence of additional toxic substances.

DOSAGE

Mode of Administration: Liquid preparations and other galenic preparations for internal use and liquid preparations for external use.

Preparation:

Decoction: 100 gm drug to 1 liter water
Extract: 1000 gm drug to 1000 ml 90% ethanol (V/V)
Infusion: 50 gm drug to 1 liter water
Juice: 800 gm drug to 800 ml water and 200 ml ethanol 90%
Tincture: 125 gm drug to 1000 ml ethanol 90% (V/V)

Daily Dosage:

Decoction — single dose: 15 to 30 ml

Extract — single dose: 0.3 to 2 ml

Infusion — single dose: 15 to 30 ml

Juice — single dose: 0.3 to 2 ml

Tincture — single dose: 2 to 4 ml

LITERATURE

Blaschek W, Hänsel R, Keller K, Reichling J, Rimpler G, Schneider G (Eds), Hagers Handbuch der Pharmazeutischen Praxis. Folgebände 1 und 2. Drogen A-Z. Springer. Berlin, Heidelberg 1998.

Senanayake N, Sanmuganathan PS, Acalypha indica induced haemolysis in G6PD deficiency. Ceylon Med J, 26:1996 Jan.

Senanayake N, Sanmuganathan PS, Acute intravascular haemolysis in glucose-6-phosphate dehydrogenase deficient patients following ingestion of herbal broth containing Acalypha indica. Trop Doct, 26:32, 1996 Jan.

Shanmugasundaram KR, Seethapathy PG, Shanmugasundaram ER, Anna Pavala Sindhooram - an antiatherosclerotic Indian drug. J Ethnopharmacol, 7:247-65, 1983 May.

Indian Physic

Gillenia trifoliata

DESCRIPTION

Medicinal Parts: The medicinal part is the dried and pulverized root bark.

Flower and Fruit: The flowers are white and tinged with red. They are arranged in a few loose, terminal panicles.

Leaves, Stem and Root: This perennial herb has irregular, cylindrical roots, which are usually transversely grooved and up to 15 cm long. The external surface is blackish, and the transverse section shows a thick, reddish bark, which easily separates from the white woody center. Sprouting from the root are a number of stems 60 to 90 cm high. The leaves and leaflets have various forms.

Characteristics: Indian Physic is odorless, but the plant has a pleasantly bitter taste.

Habitat: The plant is indigenous to the eastern U.S., and is cultivated in Europe and elsewhere.

Production: Indian Physic is the root bark of Gillenia trifoliata.

Other Names: Indian Hippo, Bowman's Root, American Ipecacuanha, Gillenia

ACTIONS AND PHARMACOLOGY

COMPOUNDS

Resins

Gillein (Gillenin)

The constituents of the drug have not been fully investigated.

EFFECTS

The drug is an expectorant, emetic and a "blood purifier."

INDICATIONS AND USAGE

Unproven Uses: The drug is used in the treatment of digestive disorders, particularly in cases in which a safe and reliable emetic is required. Folk medicine applications also include use with dyspepsia, dropsy, rheumatism and chronic constipation.

PRECAUTIONS AND ADVERSE REACTIONS

Health risks or side effects following the proper administration of designated therapeutic dosages are not recorded.

DOSAGE

Mode of Administration: The drug is available as a powder, an infusion or a tonic for internal use.

LITERATURE

Kern W, List PH, Hörhammer L (Hrsg.), Hagers Handbuch der Pharmazeutischen Praxis, 4. Aufl., Bde 1-8, Springer Verlag Berlin, Heidelberg, New York, 1969.

Indian Squill

Urginea indica

DESCRIPTION

Medicinal Parts: The parts used medicinally are the horizontal and vertically cut strips of the dried, middle, fleshy onion layers of the white flowering variety (which are collected after flowering) as well as the fresh, fleshy onion layers of the white and red varieties.

Flower and Fruit: The inflorescence is a 10 to 60 cm long, loose raceme with 4 to 30 flowers in the axils of the bracts, which usually drop before the flower. The peduncle is upright, up to 1 m high, cylindrical, ribbed, glabrous and reddish-brown. The pedicle is up to 3.5 cm long, splayed when in flower and upright when the fruit is ripe. The flowers are radial with 6 corolla-like tepals, which are 5 to 12 mm long, campanulate and reddish-green. There are 6 stamens, 3 fused carpels and a 3-chambered, superior ovary. The fruit is a capsule, 10 to 25 cm long, with 12 to 30 seeds. The seeds are clavate to elliptical with a diameter of 4 to 10 mm, dark brown to black, with orbicular, translucent wings.

Leaves, Stem and Root: Indian squill is a herbaceous perennial bulb plant that reaches up to 35 cm. The flowering varieties might reach up to 1 m high. The leaves are basal, in 2 rows, 13 to 35 cm long, 6 to 30 mm wide, linear to lanceolate or sword-shaped, flat, parallel-veined, glabrous and whorled at the base. The bulb is whitish, globose to ovoid with a diameter of 3 to 7 cm. The outer layer is membranous, the inner one fleshy.

Characteristics: The bulb tastes bitter; slimy.

Habitat: India and Sri Lanka

Production: Indian squill is the dried and cut bulb of Urginea indica freed from the outer layers shortly after harvesting. The bulbs are dug up, cleaned and cut into quarters. Then the core is removed and the remaining pieces are dried in the sun or over a fire until the weight is reduced by 80%.

Not to be Confused With: Because of the similarity in name, it can be confused with Scilla indica.

Other Names: South Indian Squill

ACTIONS AND PHARMACOLOGY

COMPOUNDS

Cardioactive steroid glycosides (bufadienolids, 0.1 to 1.5%): chief components proscillaridin A and scillaren A, including as well scillipheoside, scillarenine-bis-alpha-rhamnoside, scillicyanogenine glucoside, scillicyanosidine glucoside, scilliglaucosidine glucoside

Mucilages (50%, glucomannoxylans)

Steroids: sterols, including beta-sitosterol, campesterol, stigmasterol

EFFECTS
The drug's content levels of cardioactive glycosides explain the administration in the presence of cardiac insufficiency and cardio-conditioned edema formation. The expectorant may be due the drug's effect as a mild irritant of the gastrointestinal tract combined with an increase in secretions of the bronchial system. The drug's administration as an antirheumatic appears plausible, due to the skin-irritating effect of the oxalate raphides it contains.

INDICATIONS AND USAGE
Unproven Uses: For chronic bronchitis, asthma and cardiac insufficiency as a treatment of second choice in the case of hypersensitivity to digitalis.

Indian Medicine: For edema, digestion disturbances, menstruation disorders, worm infestation, chronic bronchitis, asthma, rheumatism and skin conditions.

CONTRAINDICATIONS
Neither the drug nor pure glycosides should be administered in the presence of first- and second-degree AV-Block, hypercalcemia, hypokalemia, hypertrophic cardiomyopathy, carotid sinus syndrome, ventricle tachycardia, thoracic aortic aneurysm, WPW syndrome.

PRECAUTIONS AND ADVERSE REACTIONS
General: No health hazards are known in conjunction with the proper administration of designated therapeutic dosages. Because of the limited therapeutic range of the cardioactive steroid glycosides, a number of patients receiving no more than therapeutic dosages might experience the following side effects: hypertonia in gastrointestinal area, loss of appetite, vomiting, diarrhea, headache and irregular pulse.

Drug Interactions: The simultaneous administration of arrhythmogenic substances (sympathomimetics, methyl xanthines, phosphodiesterase inhibitors, quinidine) increases the risk of cardiac arrhythmias. Contact with the latex of the fresh bulbs can lead to skin inflammation (Scilla dermatitis).

OVERDOSAGE
Overdose could lead to hypertonia in gastrointestinal area, loss of appetite, vomiting, diarrhea, headache and irregular pulse along with the following:

- heart: cardiac rhythm disorders as serious as life-threatening ventricular tachycardias, atrial tachycardias with atrioventricular block.

- CNS: dizziness, vision disorders, depressions, states of confusion, hallucinations, psychoses.

Lethal dosages lead to cardiac arrest or to asphyxiation. Because of the difficulties involved in standardizing the drug, the administration of pure glycosides is to be preferred (proscillaridin A).

The first-aid measures to be taken with poisonings are gastric lavage and instillation of activated charcoal. All other measures proceed according to the symptoms: careful potassium replacement for potassium loss; phenytoin as an antiarrhythmic for ectopic stimulation formation in the ventricle; lidocaine for ventricular extrasystole; atropine or orciprenaline for pronounced bradycardia. The prophylactic insertion of a cardiac pacemaker is recommended. Hemoperfusion for the elimination of the glycosides or cholestyramine administration for the interruption of the enterohepatic circulation are possible.

DOSAGE
Mode of Administration: Whole herb, cut drug, powdered drug and other galenic preparations for internal and external use.

Preparation: Liquid extract: 100 g drug are percolated with 70% ethanol and then evaporated to 850 ml; the rest is filled to 1000 ml again with 70% ethanol and filtered (BPC79).

Tincture: 100 gm drug is macerated with 1000 ml 60% ethanol (BPC79).

Acetic acid maceration: 100 gm drug is macerated with 1000 ml acetic acid in a closed vessel and then filtered. Finally the filtrate is heated and re-filtered after 7 days (BPC79).

Daily Dosage:

Drug: single dose: 60 to 200 mg; Tincture: 0.3 to 2 ml; Liquid extract: 0.06 to 0.2 ml; Acetic acid essence: 0.6 to 2 ml.

Storage: Store in a dry place and below 25°C.

LITERATURE
Hänsel R, Keller K, Rimpler H, Schneider G (Ed), Hagers Handbuch der Pharmazeutischen Praxis, 5. Aufl., Bde 4 - 6 (Drogen), Springer Verlag Berlin, Heidelberg, New York, 1992-1994

Inula britannica

See British Elecampane
(Xuan-Fu-Hua)

Inula helenium

See Elecampane

Ipecac

Cephaelis ipecacuanha

DESCRIPTION

Medicinal Parts: The medicinal parts are the pulverized roots of the 3-to-4-year-old plant, which have been dug up and dried quickly in the sun.

Flower and Fruit: The flowers are in terminal, capitulum-shaped inflorescences surrounded by 4 to 6 bracts. The individual florets have a 5-tipped calyx, ciliated at the tips with a white campanulate-conical, 5-tipped corolla. A bitter, dark purple, fleshy drupe develops from the 2-carpeled ovary.

Leaves, Stem and Root: Cephaelis ipecacuanha is a perennial, evergreen, leafy plant about 40 cm high with a 2 to 4 mm thick rhizome from which sprout numerous 20 cm long fibrous roots. Some of these roots develop into tubers. The green stem may be creeping or ascending, simple or branched. It is somewhat quadrangular, occasionally bears adventitious roots. The opposite leaves are entire-margined, and the leaf blade, narrows into the short petiole. There are stipules at the base of the leaf, which are slit like awls and fused together with the petiole-like leaf sheath.

Habitat: Indigenous to the sparser woods of Brazil; cultivated in India and on the Malaysian archipelago.

Production: Ipecac is the root of Cephaelis ipecacuanha. The subterranean parts of the 3-to-4-year-old plants are quickly dried in the sun and then cut into pieces of 5 to 10 cm in length.

Other Names: Ipecacuanha, Ipecacuanha Rio, Matto Grosso

ACTIONS AND PHARMACOLOGY

COMPOUNDS

Isoquinoline alkaloids of the emetine type (2-4%): chief alkaloids emetine and cephaelin

Starch (30 to 40%)

EFFECTS

Emetine hydrochloride and cephaelin hydrochloride, alkaloids contained in the drug, have a locally irritating effect on the gastric mucous membrane and are thus responsible for the reflex increase of bronchial secretions and the expectorant effect. The saponins probably support this effect.

The drug affects the sensory stomach nerves; it is secretory in small doses and emetic in larger doses. It is also spasmolytic and expectorant. It is partially effective in amoebic dysentery due to the action of the alkaloid emetin on the magna-form of the pathogen.

INDICATIONS AND USAGE

Unproven Uses: Ipecac is contained in expectorants and secretory preparations; it is used for amoebic dysentery, as a bronchial treatment and as an emetic in cases of poisoning. It is also used as an expectorant and to soothe and assist in coughing up of thick phlegm and in the treatment of croupous bronchitis in children.

Homeopathic Uses: Ipecae is used to treat bronchitis, asthma, whooping cough, gastrointestinal inflammations, disorders in blood pressure and bleeding of the mucous membranes.

PRECAUTIONS AND ADVERSE REACTIONS

General: No health hazards or side effects are known in conjunction with the proper administration of designated therapeutic dosages as an expectorant. Administration over extended periods can lead to myopathias. Frequent contact with the drug can trigger allergic reactions of the skin and the mucous membranes (''druggist's asthma,'' the allergen is a glycoprotein).

Pregnancy: Not to be used during pregnancy.

OVERDOSAGE

Higher dosages of the drug (1 to 2 gm) have a nauseate effect (therapeutically used as an emetic). Toxic dosages can lead to mucous membrane erosion in the gastrointestinal tract, tachycardia, drop in blood pressure and cardiac rhythm disorders, as well as disorders in respiratory function and possibly to convulsions, shock and coma.

Following intestinal emptying (sodium sulfate), the treatment for poisonings consists of the administration of generous amounts of liquids (warm tea), instillation of activated charcoal and shock prophylaxis (quiet, warmth), the treatment of spasms with diazepam (i.v.), electrolyte substitution and the countering of any acidosis imbalance that may appear through sodium bicarbonate infusions. In the event of shock, plasma volume expanders should be infused. Monitoring of kidney function is necessary. Intubation and oxygen respiration may also be required.

DOSAGE

Mode of Administration: Ipecac is used orally as a tincture, extract and fluid extract and in medicinal preparations with a standardized alkaloid content.

Preparation: Ipecac extract: After the alkaloids have been determined the powder is stabilized with lactose or dextrin (DAB10).

Tincture: 1 part root powder with 8 to 12 parts 70% ethanol (DAB10).

These preparations are stabilized to a standardized alkaloid content.

Dosage: Infusion 0.5%: 10 ml (adults)

Homeopathic Dosage: 5 drops, 1 tablet, 10 globules every 30 to 60 minutes (acute) or 1 to 3 times daily (chronic); parenterally: 1 to 2 ml sc acute: 3 times daily; chronic: once a day; suppositories: 2 to 3 times daily (chronic) (HAB1).

Storage: Store carefully in the dark in tightly sealed containers.

LITERATURE

Berrens L, Young E, (1963) Int. Arch All. Appl. Immunol. 22:51.

Garrettson LK, Ipecac home use- we need hope replaced with data- editoral comment. In: J Toxicol Clin Toxicol 29(4):515. 1991.

Kleinschartz W, Litovitz T, Overda GM, Bailey KM, Kuba A, The effect of milk on Ipecac-induced emesis. In: J Toxicol Clini Toxicol 29(4):505. 1991.

Kunkel N, Vergiftungen: Aktivkohle, Ipecacuanhasirup oder Magenspülung? In: DAZ 132(30):1587. 1992.

Nagakura N et al., Four tetrahydroisoquinoline-monoterpene glucosides from Cephaelis ipecacuanha. In: PH 32:761. 1993.

Wiegrebe W, Kramer WJ, Shamma M, The emetine alkaloids. In: JNP 47(3):397. 1984.

Further information in:

Hänsel R, Keller K, Rimpler H, Schneider G (Hrsg.), Hagers Handbuch der Pharmazeutischen Praxis, 5. Aufl., Bde 4-6 (Drogen), Springer Verlag Berlin, Heidelberg, New York, 1992-1994.

Leung AY, Encyclopedia of Common Natural Ingredients Used in Food, Drugs and Cosmetics, John Wiley & Sons Inc., New York 1980.

Lewin L, Gifte und Vergiftungen, 6. Aufl., Nachdruck, Haug Verlag, Heidelberg 1992.

Madaus G, Lehrbuch der Biologischen Arzneimittel, Bde 1-3, Nachdruck, Georg Olms Verlag Hildesheim 1979.

Roth L, Daunderer M, Kormann K, Giftpflanzen, Pflanzengifte, 4. Aufl., Ecomed Fachverlag Landsberg Lech 1993.

Steinegger E, Hänsel R, Pharmakognosie, 5. Aufl., Springer Verlag Heidelberg 1992.

Teuscher E, Lindequist U, Biogene Gifte - Biologie, Chemie, Pharmakologie, 2. Aufl., Fischer Verlag Stuttgart 1994.

Teuscher E, Biogene Arzneimittel, 5. Aufl., Wiss. Verlagsges. Stuttgart 1997.

Wagner H, Wiesenauer M, Phytotherapie. Phytopharmaka und pflanzliche Homöopathika, Fischer-Verlag, Stuttgart, Jena, New York 1995.

Wichtl M (Hrsg.), Teedrogen, 4. Aufl., Wiss. Verlagsges. Stuttgart 1997.

Ipomoea orizabensis

See Mexican Scammony Root

Ipomoea purga

See Jalap

Iporuru

Alchornea floribunda

DESCRIPTION

Medicinal Parts: The medicinal part of the plant is the bark.

Flower and Fruit: The female inflorescence is apical and up to 25 cm long; the male inflorescence is axillary and 10 to 25 cm long with pale green flowers. The ovary is 3-carpeled and fused. The fruit is a 3-chambered capsule with glossy brownish seeds.

Leaves, Stem and Root: Alchornea floribunda is a tree or shrub up to 4.5 m, occasionally up to 10 m high. The leaves are clustered at the end of the glabrous branches. They are short-petiolate, lanceolate to spatulate, 15 to 35 cm long, 6 to 13 cm wide, glabrous above and slightly downy beneath. The stipules are 3 to 9 mm long and downy.

Habitat: Tropical Africa, Amazon region

Production: Niando root is the fresh or dried root of Alchornea floribunda collected in the wild.

Other Names: Macochihua, Niando, Malan

ACTIONS AND PHARMACOLOGY

COMPOUNDS

Imidazole alkaloids (0.6 to 1.2%): alchornein (0.4%), isoalchornein (0.005%)

Tannins

EFFECTS

The drug has stimulating and hallucinogenic effect upon humans, due to the alkaloids it contains (chief active ingredient alchornein). An elevation in the sensitivity of the sympaticus to adrenaline was demonstrated in animal experiments. In comparison to atropine, alchorneine tartrate has a strong anticholinergic, vagolytic and peristalsis-inhibiting effect; in addition, it exhibits the action of a weak local anesthetic.

INDICATIONS AND USAGE

Unproven Uses: The drug can be used for respiratory and urinary tract infections and conditions of the gastrointestinal tract. The indigenous people of the Amazon have used the bark and roots of Iporuru for many different purposes for hundreds of years. One of the more popular preparations is an alcoholic bark tincture used to treat rheumatism, arthritis, colds and muscle pains. In Africa the drug is used frequently as an aphrodisiac and hallucinogen.

PRECAUTIONS AND ADVERSE REACTIONS

Nothing has been documented regarding side effects in connection with therapeutic administration.

OVERDOSAGE

The drug is considered severely toxic. High dosages in animal experiments led to severe excitation and spasms. Cases of death through exhaustion have been observed among humans following over-stimulation and hallucination.

DOSAGE

Mode of Administration: Whole herb and cut drug preparations for internal use.

Preparation: There are traditional preparations in the form of macerates or palm wine with the appropriate dosage.

LITERATURE

de Smet PA, Some ethnopharmacological notes on African hallucinogens. J Ethnopharmacol, 261: Drug Information Center, Royal Dutch Association for the Advancement of Pharmacy, The Hague, The Netherlands, 96.

Duke J, and Vasquez R, Amazonian Ethnobotanical Dictionary, CRC Press Inc., Boca Raton, FL, 1994.

Hänsel R, Keller K, Rimpler H, Schneider G (Ed), Hagers Handbuch der Pharmazeutischen Praxis, 5. Aufl., Bde 4 - 6 (Drogen), Springer Verlag Berlin, Heidelberg, New York, 1992-1994.

Raymond-Hamet Goutarel R, Are the stimulant effects of Alchornea floribunda Mueller Arg. in men due to yohimbine. C R Acad Sci Hebd Seances Acad Sci D, 261:3223-4, 1965 Oct 18.

Iris species

See Orris

Jaborandi

Pilocarpus microphyllus

DESCRIPTION

Medicinal Parts: The medicinal parts are the dried leaves.

Flower and Fruit: The numerous flowers are in terminal or axillary racemes that are up to 30 cm long and 0.5 cm wide. The pedicles are 0.1 to 1.5 mm long and have alternate bracts. The flowers have a diameter of 4 to 5 cm and are glabrous. The 5 sepals are free, broadly triangular to orbicular and coriaceous. The petals have forward-bending tips and are thinly coriaceous and somewhat translucent. The oval anthers have an oblong gland. The disc is 0.5 mm high and 1.3 to 1.5 mm in diameter. The ovary is 0.5 mm and extends past the disc with a head-like stigma. The mericarp has roundish, flattened, black-brown seeds.

Leaves, Stem and Root: The plant is a tree or shrub 3 to 7 m high with a trunk diameter of 3 to 7.5 cm. The branches are pubescent when young and glabrous when older. The leaves are alternate to opposite, odd-pinnate with 1 to 5 pairs of pinna. The pinna are sessile, elliptical, distinctly asymmetrical at the base and have an indented tip. The leaflets are dull green, up to 5 cm long and 3 cm wide, with entire, slightly recurved margins and an uneven base. The ribs are prominent on the upper surface and have visible oil cells.

Characteristics: The taste is bitter and the odor slightly aromatic.

Habitat: The plant grows in the northeastern part of Brazil.

Production: Jaborandi leaves are the dried leaves of Pilocarpus microphyllus.

Other Names: Arruda Brava, Arruda do Mato, Jamguarandi, Juarandi

ACTIONS AND PHARMACOLOGY

COMPOUNDS

Imidazole alkaloids (0.5-1.0%): chief alkaloid is (+)-pilocarpine, through drying and under storage conditions changing over to some extent into isopilocarpine, companion alkaloids including pilocarpidine, pilosine and others

Volatile oil (0.5%): chief components are limonene and undecanone

EFFECTS

The drug affects the parasympathetic system. It increases the secretion of saliva, sweat, gastric juices and tears, and stimulates the smooth muscle of the gastrointestinal tract, bronchi, bile duct and bladder.

INDICATIONS AND USAGE

Unproven Uses: Jaborandi has been used in the treatment of glaucoma. In folk medicine, it has been used for epilepsy, convulsions, gonorrhea, ischuria, as an anesthetic for mucous membranes, for fever, influenza, pneumonia, gastrointestinal inflammations, kidney disease, psoriasis, neurosis and poisoning.

PRECAUTIONS AND ADVERSE REACTIONS

General: No health hazards or side effects are known in conjunction with the proper administration of designated therapeutic dosages. The drug is used today as an industrial agent for the manufacture of pilocarpine, but is used medicinally only for homeopathic applications.

The incorrect administration of pilocarpine eyedrops can lead to poisoning through leakage into the nose or mouth. Symptoms include bradycardia, bronchial spasms, colics, collapse and possible cardiac arrest, convulsions, drop in blood pressure, dyspnea, nausea, severe salivation, strong secretion of sweat and vomiting.

Pregnancy: Jaborandi should not be used during pregnancy.

OVERDOSAGE

The lethal dose is approximately 60 mg of pilocarpine, corresponding to 5 to 10 gm of the drug. Individuals with cardiac and circulatory illnesses are particularly susceptible. Following stomach and intestinal emptying (gastric lavage, sodium sulphate), the treatment for poisonings consists of the instillation of activated charcoal with atropine and the use of diazepam in the case of spasms. Forced dialysis and the administration of plasma volume expanders can also be useful.

DOSAGE

Mode of Administration: Jaborandi is obsolete by itself as a drug.

LITERATURE

Craveiro AA et al., (1979) J Nat Prod 42:169.

Hänsel R, Keller K, Rimpler H, Schneider G (Hrsg.), Hagers Handbuch der Pharmazeutischen Praxis, 5. Aufl., Bde 4-6 (Drogen), Springer Verlag Berlin, Heidelberg, New York, 1992-1994.

Lewin L, Gifte und Vergiftungen, 6. Aufl., Nachdruck, Haug Verlag, Heidelberg 1992.

Madaus G, Lehrbuch der Biologischen Arzneimittel, Bde 1-3, Nachdruck, Georg Olms Verlag Hildesheim 1979.

Roth L, Daunderer M, Kormann K, Giftpflanzen, Pflanzengifte, 4. Aufl., Ecomed Fachverlag Landsberg Lech 1993.

Steinegger E, Hänsel R, Pharmakognosie, 5. Aufl., Springer Verlag Heidelberg 1992.

Tedeschi E, Kamionsky J, Fackler S, Sarel S, Isr J Chem 11:731-733. 1973.

Teuscher E, Lindequist U, Biogene Gifte - Biologie, Chemie, Pharmakologie, 2. Aufl., Fischer Verlag Stuttgart 1994.

Teuscher E, Biogene Arzneimittel, 5. Aufl., Wiss. Verlagsges. Stuttgart 1997.

Wagner H, Wiesenauer M, Phytotherapie. Phytopharmaka und pflanzliche Homöopathika, Fischer-Verlag, Stuttgart, Jena, New York, 1995.

Jack-in-the-Pulpit

Arisaema atrorubens

DESCRIPTION

Medicinal Parts: The medicinal part of the plant is the rhizome.

Flower and Fruit: The inflorescence (spadix) is yellowish-white, later brown, club-shaped and surrounded by a larger spathe. The spathe is greenish on the outside and white-striped with a weak purple-violet tinge on the inside. The fruit is a scarlet berry.

Leaves, Stem and Root: Jack-in-the-Pulpit is a herbaceous perennial rhizome, which extends up to 30 cm high. The leaves are basal and trifoliolate-digitate. The leaflets are ovoid, acuminate and entire. The rhizome is tuberous with hair-like roots at the top, shaped into a wreath.

Habitat: The plant is found in North America and China.

Production: Arisaema root is the fresh rhizome of Arisaema atrorubens.

ACTIONS AND PHARMACOLOGY

COMPOUNDS

Polysaccharides: starch

Pungent substances: structures are unknown (only in the fresh root)

EFFECTS

The pungent substances contained in the fresh drug are severely irritating to skin and mucous membranes, as well as being toxic. This toxicity is eliminated through dehydration and/or extended cooking. The dried or cooked root serves as a source of starch.

INDICATIONS AND USAGE

Unproven Uses: Preparations have been used for chronic bronchitis, asthma, colic, gastrointestinal disturbances, inflammation of the oral mucosa, rheumatism, for bumps, eye inflammations and abscesses (as a poultice) and as a contraceptive by the Hopi Indians.

PRECAUTIONS AND ADVERSE REACTIONS

General: No health hazards are known in conjunction with the proper administration of designated therapeutic dosages. The fresh rhizome is considered toxic. Internal administration leads to severe mucous membrane irritation and acute gastrointestinal inflammations, and skin inflammation.

Pregnancy: Contraindicated in pregnancy (used as a contraceptive in folk medicine).

DOSAGE

No information is available.

LITERATURE

Blaschek W, Hänsel R, Keller K, Reichling J, Rimpler G, Schneider G (Eds), Hagers Handbuch der Pharmazeutischen Praxis. Folgebände 1 und 2. Drogen A-Z. Springer. Berlin, Heidelberg 1998.

Jacob's Ladder

Polemonium caeruleum

DESCRIPTION

Medicinal Parts: The medicinal part is the herb.

Flower and Fruit: The numerous flowers grow in clusters at the end of the lateral branches. They are open, slightly hanging and have 5 sepals and 5 petals. The corolla is 2 to 2.5 cm, deep blue and has a short pollen tube. The stamens are enclosed in the tube and have yellow anthers.

Leaves, Stem and Root: The plant is a perennial. The plant is bright green and smooth. The upper section is covered in short glandular hairs. The rhizome is short and creeping, and the stem is 45 to 90 cm high, hollow and quadrangular. The leaves with numerous pairs of leaflets are 1.25 to 2.5 cm long. These are pinnate and alternate.

Habitat: The plant is indigenous to central and northern Europe.

Production: Jacob's Ladder is the aerial part of Polemonium caeruleum.

Other Names: Charity, English Greek Valerian

ACTIONS AND PHARMACOLOGY

COMPOUNDS

Triterpene saponins

Flavonoids

EFFECTS

All parts of the plant contain saponin, which has astringent, diaphoretic and hemolytic effects.

INDICATIONS AND USAGE

Unproven Uses: Jacob's Ladder is used for febrile and inflammatory conditions.

PRECAUTIONS AND ADVERSE REACTIONS

No health hazards or side effects are known in conjunction with the proper administration of designated therapeutic dosages.

DOSAGE

Mode of Administration: The ground drug is used as an infusion.

LITERATURE

Reznicek G et al., A new ester saponine from Polemonium caeruleum. In: PM 59(7)12. 1993.

Further information in:

Kern W, List PH, Hörhammer L (Hrsg.), Hagers Handbuch der Pharmazeutischen Praxis, 4. Aufl., Bde. 1-8, Springer Verlag Berlin, Heidelberg, New York, 1969.

Jalap

Ipomoea purga

DESCRIPTION

Medicinal Parts: The medicinal part is the root tuber.

Flower and Fruit: The flowers are single or in twos (occasionally in threes or fours), radial, with their structures grouped in fives. There are 5 narrow-lanceolate, purple-punctate sepals. The petals are fused to a 7 cm wide, funnel-shaped red corolla, and there are 5 stamens. The superior ovary is 2-chambered. The fruit is a capsule with 4 seeds.

Leaves, Stem and Root: This winding herb grows up to 4 m high. The leaves are alternate, up to 9 cm long and 5 cm wide, cordate, acuminate and entire. The stem is purple-tinged and glabrous. The rhizome is tuberously thickened, milky, approximately 5 cm long, with tuberous, thickened, secondary roots.

Habitat: Ipomoea purga grows in South and Central America, Mexico and Jamaica.

Production: Jalap resin (also known as jalap or Jalapae resina) is the resin of Ipomoea purga derived from alcoholic extraction of the jalap root powder. The tuberous, thickened secondary roots (black rhubarb tubers) of Ipomoea jalapae tuber are harvested from May to autumn and dried in the sun, on hot ash or over an open fire

Not to be Confused With: Jalap resin may be confused with Brazil jalap, Aloe, Orizaba jalap, colophonium, starch, dextrin and guaiac resin. Confusion can arise between Jalap tuber and Ipomoea orizabensis, Ipomoea operculata, Operculina turpethum, Convolvulus scammonia and Mirabilis jalapa.

ACTIONS AND PHARMACOLOGY

Ipomoea purga is a centuries-old purgative and vermifuge. It has also been used as an anthelmintic.

COMPOUNDS: JALAP RESIN

Glycoretines: convulvin (55%, non-ether-soluble), jalapin (7%, ether-soluble), convulvin and jalapin are mixtures made up of resinous glycosides of hydroxy-fatty acids (C12 to C16) with oligosaccharides, their hydroxyl groups estered to the fatty acid esters with, among others, acetic acid, propionic acid, iso-butyric acid, alpha-methylbutyric acid, tiglic acid and iso-valeric acid or n-valeric acid.

EFFECTS: JALAP RESIN

The drug has a drastic laxative effect due to the glycoretines it contains.

COMPOUNDS: JALAP TUBER

Resins (5 to 20%): glycoretines (see Jalap resin)

Polysaccharides: starch

EFFECTS: JALAP TUBER

The drug has a drastic laxative effect due to the glycoretines it contains.

INDICATIONS AND USAGE

JALAP RESIN

Unproven Uses: Used for constipation, colic and pain in the intestinal region, dysentery, colitis and rheumatism.

Homeopathic Uses: The drug is used for restlessness at night in children and diarrhea in homeopathic medicine.

JALAP TUBER

Unproven Uses: Jalap tuber is considered to be obsolete. In the past, it was used as a laxative and purgative.

PRECAUTIONS AND ADVERSE REACTIONS

JALAP RESIN

General: The drug's laxative effect frequently produces nausea, cramp-like pains and gastroenteritis.

Pregnancy: Administration is not advisable during pregnancy, particularly because of the possible teratogenic effect.

JALAP TUBER

General: Jalap tuber is to be used only under the supervision of an expert qualified in the appropriate use of this substance. The drug's laxative effect is frequently accompanied by nausea, cramp-like pains and gastroenteritis.

Pregnancy: The administration of jalap tuber is not advisable during pregnancy, particularly because of the possible teratogenic effect.

DOSAGE

JALAP RESIN

Preparation: There is no information in the literature.

Daily Dosage: 1.5 g drug; maximum single dosage: 0.1 to 0.3 g drug

Homeopathic Dosage: from D4: 5 drops, 1 tablet, 10 globules, every to 30 to 60 minutes (acute) and 1 to 3 times daily (chronic); parenterally: 1 to ml sc acute: 3 times daily; chronic once a day (HAB34).

Storage: Store securely in a tightly sealed container, protected from light.

JALAP TUBER

Mode of Administration: Whole, cut and powdered drug

Preparation: There is no information in the literature.

Daily Dosage: maximum 4.5 g drug; single dosage: maximum 1.5 g drug

Storage: Store protected from light in a secure, tightly sealed container.

LITERATURE

Hänsel R, Keller K, Rimpler H, Schneider G (Ed), Hagers Handbuch der Pharmazeutischen Praxis, 5. Aufl., Bde 4 - 6 (Drogen), Springer Verlag Berlin, Heidelberg, New York, 1992-1994.

Jamaica Dogwood

Piscidia piscipula

DESCRIPTION

Medicinal Parts: The medicinal part is the bark.

Flower and Fruit: The plant has blue to white flowers with white stripes out of which 4 pods with 4 longitudinal wings develop.

Leaves, Stem and Root: The plant is a tree or shrub up to 15 m high with compound leaves. The bark is 3 to 6 mm thick and dark gray-brown with thin, longitudinal and transverse ridges. It is roughish and wrinkled, and somewhat fissured. The fracture is tough, fibrous, showing blue-green or brownish-green patches.

Characteristics: The taste is bitter and acrid and the odor characteristic.

Habitat: The tree is indigenous to Central America and the northern parts of South America.

Production: Jamaica Dogwood is the root bark of Piscidia piscipula.

Other Names: Dogwood, Fish Poison Tree

ACTIONS AND PHARMACOLOGY

COMPOUNDS

Isoflavonoids: including among others jamaicine, ichthynone, the rotenoids rotenone, milleton, isomilletone

Tannins

EFFECTS

Research indicates that Jamaica Dogwood is mildly sedative and spasmolytic.

INDICATIONS AND USAGE

Unproven Uses: The drug is used for states of anxiety and fear and as a daytime sedative.

PRECAUTIONS AND ADVERSE REACTIONS

No health hazards or side effects are known in conjunction with the proper administration of designated therapeutic dosages.

DOSAGE

Mode of Administration: The drug and liquid extract are no longer in use. It has been used in some medicinal preparations.

LITERATURE

Aurousseau M et al., (1965) Ann Pharm Franc 23:251.

Heller W, Tamm C., (1975) Helv Chim Acta 58:974.

Nordal A et al., (1966) Acta Chem Scand 20:1431.

Pietta P, Zio C, (1983) J Chrom. 260:497.

Schwartz JSP et al., (1964) Tetrahedron 20:1317.

Stamm OA et al., (1958) Helv Chim Acta 41:2006.

Further information in:

Kern W, List PH, Hörhammer L (Hrsg.), Hagers Handbuch der Pharmazeutischen Praxis, 4. Aufl., Bde. 1-8, Springer Verlag Berlin, Heidelberg, New York, 1969.

Leung AY, Encyclopedia of Common Natural Ingredients Used in Food, Drugs and Cosmetics, John Wiley & Sons Inc., New York 1980.

Madaus G, Lehrbuch der Biologischen Arzneimittel, Bde. 1-3, Nachdruck, Georg Olms Verlag Hildesheim 1979.

Steinegger E, Hänsel R, Pharmakognosie, 5. Aufl., Springer Verlag Heidelberg 1992.

Wagner H, Wiesenauer M, Phytotherapie. Phytopharmaka und pflanzliche Homöopathika, Fischer-Verlag, Stuttgart, Jena, New York 1995.

Jambolan

Syzygium cumini

DESCRIPTION

Medicinal Parts: The medicinal parts are the dried bark, the dried seed kernels, the disintegrated kernels, the dried trunk bark and the macerated seeds.

Flower and Fruit: The flowers are in compound, triple panicles. They are sessile, whitish, fragrant, and are usually on older branches behind the leaves. The calyx tube is 4 to 6 mm long and twisted. The petals are hood-like. There are approximately 60 stamens, which are as long as the calyx tube. The drupe is initially pink, becoming black when ripe. The drupe is 1.2 to 3 cm long, globular to ovate, 1-valved, 1-seeded and edible. The seeds are subcylindrical, about 6 mm long and rather less in diameter. One end of the seed is truncated and has a central depression. Externally, they are hard, tough and blackish-brown; internally they are pinkish-brown.

Characteristics: The taste of the seeds is faintly astringent and aromatic; the odor is slight.

Habitat: The plant is indigenous to the east Indian Malayian region. It has spread as far as China and Australia and is cultivated on the Antilles.

Production: Jambolan seed consists of the dried seed of Syzygium cumini (syn. Syzygium jambolana). Because the commodity consists mostly of the dried, fallen apart cotyledons, they must be broken apart in order to produce the drug. Jambolan bark consists of the dried bark from the trunk of Syzygium cumini (syn Syzygium jambolana).

Other Names: Jambul, Jamum, Java Plum, Rose Apple

ACTIONS AND PHARMACOLOGY

COMPOUNDS: JAMBOLAN SEED

Fatty oil (3-5%): containing oleic acid, myristic acid, palmitic acid and linoleic acid, sterculiac acid and malvalic acid (cyclopropylidenic acids), among others, as well as vernolic acid (epoxy fatty acid)

Tannins (6%): including corilagin, 3,3′-Di-O-methyl ellagic acid, galloyl glucose

EFFECTS: JAMBOLAN SEED

Anti-inflammatory actions were demonstrated in animal experiments. Results of hypoglycemic and CNS experiments were not conclusive.

COMPOUNDS: JAMBOLAN BARK

Tannins: gallic and ellagic acid derivatives including 3,3′-Di-O-methyl ellagic acid

Steroids: sterols, including beta-sitosterol, beta-sitosterol glucoside

Triterpenes: betulinic acid, friedelin, friedelan-3-alpha-ole, epi-friedelanol, eugenin

Flavonoids: including myricetin, kempferol, quercetin, astragalin

EFFECTS: JAMBOLAN BARK

The bark has astringent effects because of the tannin content.

INDICATIONS AND USAGE

JAMBOLAN SEED

Unproven Uses: Jambolan seed is used for diabetes and in combination preparations for atonic and spastic constipation, diseases of the pancreas, gastric and pancreatic complaints, nervous disorders and as a diuretic.

JAMBOLAN BARK
Approved by Commission E:

- Diarrhea
- Inflammation of the mouth and pharynx
- Inflammation of the skin

Unproven Uses: Preparations are used internally for bronchitis, asthma, and dysentery, and externally for ulcers.

Indian Medicine: The drug is used for diabetes, leucorrhea, stomachache, fever, dysuria, and inflammation of the skin.

Homeopathic Uses: Syzygium cumini is used for diabetes.

PRECAUTIONS AND ADVERSE REACTIONS

JAMBOLAN SEED
No health hazards or side effects are known in conjunction with the proper administration of designated therapeutic dosages. Administration in the presence of diabetes mellitus is not recommended, due to the fact that the blood sugar-reducing effect is unproven.

JAMBOLAN BARK
No health hazards or side effects are known in conjunction with the proper administration of designated therapeutic dosages.

DOSAGE

JAMBOLAN SEED
Daily Dosage: A single dose is made up of 30 seeds (1.9 gm) in powdered form.

JAMBOLAN BARK
Mode of Administration: As a comminuted herb for decoctions and other galenic preparations for internal use (gargle, infusion) and local application (compresses).

Preparation: To make a decoction for internal and external use, place 1 to 2 teaspoonfuls of comminuted drug in about 150 ml cold water, bring to a boil, simmer for 5 to 10 minutes and strain.

Daily Dosage: The average daily dosage is 3 to 6 gm drug.

Homeopathic Dosage: 5 drops, 1 tablet or 10 globules every 30 to 60 minutes (acute) or 1 to 3 times a day (chronic); parenterally: 1 to 2 ml sc, acute: 3 times a day; chronic: once a day (HAB1).

LITERATURE

JAMBOLAN SEED
Bhatia IS et al., PM 28:346. 1975. Saeed MT et al., J Oil Technol Assoc India 19:86-88. 1991. Bhatia IS et al., PH 10:219. 1971. Desai HK et al., Ind J Chem 13:97-98. 1975.

Jain, SR, Sharma SN, (1967) Planta Med 15(4):439.

Linde H, (1983) Arch Pharm 316(11):971.

Mukherjee SK et al., (1963) Ind Med Gaz 3:97.

Nair AGR, Subramanian S, (1962) J Sci Ind Res India 21B, 437.

Shrothi, DS et al., (1963) Ind J Med Res 51:464.

Further information in:

Hänsel R, Keller K, Rimpler H, Schneider G (Hrsg.), Hagers Handbuch der Pharmazeutischen Praxis, 5. Aufl., Bde 4-6 (Drogen): Springer Verlag Berlin, Heidelberg, New York, 1992-1994.

Hoppe HA, (1975-1987) Drogenkunde, 8. Aufl., Bde 1-3: W de Gruyter Verlag, Berlin, New York.

Oliver-Bever B (Ed.), Medicinal Plants of Tropical West Africa, Cambridge University Press, Cambridge 1986.

JAMBOLAN BARK
Bhargava KK et al., Curr Sci 43:645-646. 1974.

Bhargava KK et al., Curr Sci 43:645. 1974.

Bhatia IS et al., PM 28:346. 1975.

Jain, SR, Sharma SN, (1967) Planta Med 15(4):439.

Kopanski L, Schnelle G, PM 54:572. 1988.

Linde H, (1983) Arch Pharm 316(11):971.

Mukherjee SK et al., (1963) Ind Med Gaz 3:97.

Nair AGR, Subramanian S, (1962) J Sci Ind Res India 21B, 437.

Sengupta D, Das PB, J Ind Chem Soc 42:255. 1965.

Shrothi DS et al., (1963) Ind J Med Res 51:464.

Further information in:

Hänsel R, Keller K, Rimpler H, Schneider G (Hrsg.), Hagers Handbuch der Pharmazeutischen Praxis, 5. Aufl., Bde 4-6 (Drogen): Springer Verlag Berlin, Heidelberg, New York, 1992-1994.

Hoppe HA, (1975-1987) Drogenkunde, 8. Aufl., Bde 1-3: W de Gruyter Verlag, Berlin, New York.

Oliver-Bever B (Ed.), Medicinal Plants of Tropical West Africa, Cambridge University Press, Cambridge 1986.

Japanese Atractylodes

Atractylodes japonica

DESCRIPTION

Medicinal Parts: The medicinal parts of the plant are the whole plant and roots.

Flower and Fruit: The composite flowers are surrounded by bracts. The capitulas are apical and upright, with a diameter of 1.5 to 2 cm. The calyx is double-rowed and double-pinnate. The lingual florets are in 7 or 8 rows, whitish and 1 to 1.2 cm long. The fruit is an achaene. The pappus is brownish and 8 to 9 mm long.

Leaves, Stem and Root: The plant is an upright, herbaceous perennial with a rhizome that extends up to 1 m high. The basal leaves wilt rapidly; the upper cauline leaves are alternate, small, usually simple and sessile. The lower leaves are long-petiolate, 8 to 10 cm long. The lamina is pergament-like, single pinnate with 3 to 5 elongate-elliptical leaflets. The apical leaflet is larger with short thorns on the margin. The rhizome is elongate, gnarled, 2 to 3 cm thick and up to 8 cm long.

Habitat: Japan.

Production: Japanese Atractylodes rhizome is the dried rhizome of Atractylodes japonica.

ACTIONS AND PHARMACOLOGY

COMPOUNDS

Volatile oil (1.5%): constituents not investigated

Sesquiterpenes: atractylon, atractylenolids I to III, eudesma-4 (14), 7(11)-dien-8-one

Polyynes: including diacetylatractylodiol, (4E, 6E, 12E)-tetradecatrien-8, 10-diin-1, 3-diolacetate

Water-soluble polysaccharides: atractan A, atractan B

EFFECTS

The furanosesquiterpenes isolated from the essential oil of the drug exhibit antimicrobial, hepatoprotective, mildly analgesic, antiphlogistic, tumor-inhibiting and antioxidative effects.

INDICATIONS AND USAGE

Unproven Uses: Japanese Atractylodes has been used for gastric complaints, inflammations, heavy sweating and as a diuretic.

Chinese Medicine: Preparations are used for loss of appetite, physical and mental exhaustion, diarrhea, edema, nausea and vomiting.

PRECAUTIONS AND ADVERSE REACTIONS

No health hazards are known in conjunction with the proper administration of designated therapeutic dosages.

DOSAGE

Mode of Administration: Whole herb, cut drug, powdered drug and liquid preparations for internal use.

Preparation: The powder is prepared in accordance with Jap XI. There is no information available on the preparation of the infusion.

Daily Dosage: Internally: single dose: 0.5 to 1.0 gm of powder; daily dose: 1.5 to 3.0 gm of powder

Infusion: single dose: 1 to 1.5 gm; daily dose: 3 to 5 gm

Storage: Should be tightly sealed.

LITERATURE

Blaschek W, Hänsel R, Keller K, Reichling J, Rimpler G, Schneider G (Eds), Hagers Handbuch der Pharmazeutischen Praxis. Folgebände 1 und 2. Drogen A-Z. Springer. Berlin, Heidelberg 1998.

Satoh K, Nagai F, Ushiyama K, Kano I, Specific inhibition of Na+,K(+)-ATPase activity by atractylon, a major component of byaku-Jutsu, by interaction with enzyme in the E2 state. Biochem Pharmacol (1997 Feb 21) 53(4):611-4.

Japanese Mint

Mentha arvensis var. piperascens

DESCRIPTION

Medicinal Parts: The medicinal parts are the dried aerial parts of the plant and the essential oil, which is extracted by steam distillation followed by partial removal of menthol and rectification.

Flower and Fruit: The flowers are in densely globular, sessile, 8- to 12-blossomed false whorls with small linear-lanceolate bracts. The inflorescence is leafy at the apex. The bracts are like the leaves, smaller above. The tepals are 1.5 by 2.5 mm, broadly campanulate and hairy. The corolla is lilac, white or, rarely, pink. The nutlets are pale brown.

Leaves, Stem and Root: Japanese Mint is a pubescent, fragrant perennial or occasionally annual that grows up to 60 cm. The stems are ascending or erect. The leaves are 15 to 70 mm by 10 to 40 mm, and are elliptic-lanceolate to broadly ovate, usually elliptical with the base narrowing to a petiole, and shallowly dentate.

Habitat: The plant is found in Europe as far north as the 65th latitude, in Asia (particularly in Siberia), the Caucasus, the Himalayas, China, Mongolia, Korea and Japan. It was probably introduced to North America.

Production: Mint oil consists of essential oil recovered from Mentha arvensis var. piperascens. The oil is obtained by steam distillation of the fresh, flowering herb, followed by partial removal of menthol and rectification.

Menthol is obtained from various species of Mentha, chiefly M. arvensis var. piperascens (from Japan), M. arvensis var. glabrata (from China) and M. piperata (from America). The product extracted from the first two is less valuable than the third, even though it contains a higher proportion of menthol.

ACTIONS AND PHARMACOLOGY

COMPOUNDS

Chief components: menthol (25-40%), menthone (15-30%), isomenthone (7-12%), limonene (7-12%), neomenthol (2-4%), menthyl acetate (1-5%), beta-caryophyllene (2-5%), piperitone (0.5-4%), alpha- and beta-pinene (2-4% each). The composition does not reflect the relationship of the components to one another in the plant. The volatile oil gained through steam distillation loses 30 to 50% of the menthol through winterization and rectification.

EFFECTS

Japanese Mint has carminative, cholagogic, antimicrobial and, possibly, secretolytic effects on the bronchial mucosa. It is also cooling to the skin.

INDICATIONS AND USAGE

Approved by Commission E:

- Common cold
- Cough/bronchitis
- Fevers and colds
- Inflammation of the mouth and pharynx
- Liver and gallbladder complaints
- Pain
- Tendency to infection

Unproven Uses: Internally, the herb is used for sensitivity to weather changes, breathing difficulties, flatulence, functional gastrointestinal and gallbladder disorders, and catarrhs of the upper respiratory tract. Externally, it is used for headaches, myalgia and neuralgic ailments. It is used both externally and internally for functional cardiac complaints.

Chinese Medicine: The herb is used for headaches, dyspeptic complaints, diarrhea and vomiting, toothaches and skin rashes.

Indian Medicine: The herb is used for joint pains, dyspeptic complaints, diarrhea and vomiting, coughs and asthma, headaches and toothaches, as well as general debility.

CONTRAINDICATIONS

Contraindications for the internal administration of the drug include occlusion of the biliary ducts, gallbladder inflammation and severe liver damage. Gallstone sufferers could experience colic due to the cholagogic effect.

PRECAUTIONS AND ADVERSE REACTIONS

General: No health hazards are known in conjunction with the proper administration of designated therapeutic dosages. The intake can lead to gastric complaints in susceptible patients. Volatile oils containing menthol can worsen the spasms of bronchial asthma. The volatile oil possesses a weak potential for sensitization due to its menthol content.

Pediatric Use: Preparations containing the oil should not be applied to the faces of infants or small children, particularly not in the nasal area (glottal spasm, bronchial spasm, asthma-like attacks, or even possible respiratory failure could occur).

OVERDOSAGE

Cases of poisoning are not recorded. The minimal lethal dosage of menthol is estimated to be 2 gm, although individuals have survived higher dosages (8 to 9 gm).

DOSAGE

Mode of Administration: The essential oil and other galenic preparations are available for internal and external application. Varieties are commercially available as Brazilian, Chinese, Indian and Japanese mint oil.

Daily Dosage: For internal use, the average daily dosage is 3 to 6 drops. When used as inhalation therapy, 3 to 4 drops are placed in hot water. To use externally, rub a few drops on the affected area.

In folk medicine, 2 drops are placed in a glass of water, tea or juice and taken once or twice a day. To make a heart poultice, 10 to 20 drops are placed on a compress, which is applied externally for 10 to 15 minutes. For headaches, 1 to 2 drops can be rubbed on the temples.

Storage: Store in air-tight containers protected from light; oils of different batches should not be mixed.

LITERATURE

Hänsel R, Keller K, Rimpler H, Schneider G (Hrsg.), Hagers Handbuch der Pharmazeutischen Praxis, 5. Aufl., Bde 4-6 (Drogen), Springer Verlag Berlin, Heidelberg, New York, 1992-1994.

Teuscher E, Biogene Arzneimittel, 5. Aufl., Wiss. Verlagsges. Stuttgart 1997.

Jasmine

Jasminum officinale

DESCRIPTION

Medicinal Parts: The medicinal parts of the plant are the fresh and dried flowers.

Flower and Fruit: The flowers are single or in 2 to 12 flowered, axillary cymes. The sepals are fused, with 5 awl-shaped, 6 to 8 mm long tips. The corolla is white. The corolla tube is 15 to 18 mm long with 8 to 9 mm long, ovate tips, which broaden like plates. There are 2 stamens. The fruit is a black berry.

Leaves, Stem and Root: Common jasmine is a procumbent or climbing shrub, that grows up to 5 m high. The leaves are opposite and 5 to 7 pinnatifid. The leaflets are elongate-lanceolate, acute, narrowing at the base, weakly pubescent on both surfaces with a ciliate margin. The branches are initially lightly pubescent, later becoming glabrous, slightly edged, green and cane-like.

Characteristics: The flowers are very fragrant.

Habitat: France, Italy, China, Japan, India, Morocco, Egypt

Production: Common jasmine flowers are the dried, fresh flowers of Jasminum officinale var. grandiflorum

Other Names: Royal Jasmine, Italian Jasmine, Catalonian Jasmine, Poet's Jasmine

ACTIONS AND PHARMACOLOGY

COMPOUNDS

Volatile oil

Pyrridine alkaloids: jasminine (presumably an artifact)

EFFECTS

No definitive data are available.

INDICATIONS AND USAGE

Chinese Medicine: Jasmine is used for hepatitis and abdominal pain in liver cirrhosis or dysentery.

Indian Medicine: Preparations are used for pain symptoms of the stomach, head, teeth and eyes, for leprosy, itching, skin disease and dysmenorrhea.

PRECAUTIONS AND ADVERSE REACTIONS

No health hazards are known in conjunction with the proper administration of designated therapeutic dosages.

DOSAGE

Preparation: Jasmine is available as a tea blend or oil.

LITERATURE

No data available

Jasminum officinale

See Jasmine

Jatamansi

Nardostachys jatamansi

DESCRIPTION

Medicinal Parts: The medicinal part of the plant is the rhizome.

Flower and Fruit: The flowers are in 1 to 5 capitula, which are usually surrounded by bracts. Their structures are in fives, the petals fused, the corolla tube 6 mm long and lightly pubescent on the inside. The fruit is crowned by pointed ovate calyx tips, which are covered in splayed white hairs.

Leaves, Stem and Root: This upright herbaceous perennial grows to a height reaching up to 60 cm high. The leaves are opposite, grow from the rhizome, are 15 to 20 cm long, 2.5 cm wide, spatulate and narrow toward the petiole. The cauline leaves are sessile, opposite, 2.5 to 7.5 cm long and narrow-ovate. The finger-thick, woody rhizome is covered with reddish brown fibers from the remains of the petioles.

Habitat: Nardostachys jatamansi is indigenous to China, India and Nepal.

Production: Jatamansi roots are the dried roots and rhizome of Nardostachys jatamansi. An essential oil is extracted from the rhizome.

Not to be Confused With: Selinum vaginatum

Other Names: Indian Nard, Indian Spikenard, Spikenard, Nard, Narrow-Leaved-Echinacea

ACTION AND PHARMACOLOGY

COMPOUNDS

Volatile oil (0.3 to 0.4%): including valeranone (jatamansone), nardosinone, calarene, beta-maaliene, maaliol, beta-ionone, 1(10)-aristelonone-(2), nardol, valerenal

EFFECTS

Valid data regarding the pharmacological efficacy of the drug have not yet become available. In animal experiments, a limiting effect upon convulsant thresholds and a reduction of motor coordination ability traceable to the sequiterpene ketone valeranone contained in the drug have been demonstrated. The authors conclude from this that the substance is anticonvulsive in effect without exhibiting neuroleptic characteristics. In addition, it manifests an antiulcerogenic effect.

INDICATIONS AND USAGE

Unproven Uses: In combination with cold water, the various oils are considered to be effective against nausea, stomachache, flatulence, liver problems, jaundice and kidney complaints, insomnia and headache. Externally, the oil is added to a steaming bath to treat inflammation of the uterus. The oils are also used in eye compounds and as poison antidotes.

Indian Medicine: Jatamansi is used for nervous headache, excitement, menopausal symptoms, flatulence, epilepsy and for pain in the intestinal region.

CONTRAINDICATIONS

Use of the drug is contraindicated during pregnancy.

PRECAUTIONS AND ADVERSE REACTIONS

No health hazards are known in conjunction with the proper administration of designated therapeutic dosages.

DOSAGE

Mode of Administration: Jatamansi root is used in the forms of a whole, cut or powdered drug for internal and external use.

How Supplied: Forms of commercial pharmaceutical preparations include capsules and compound preparations.

Daily Dosage:
Powder — 0.6 to 1.3 g drug as a single dose

Pure drug — 5 g of the drug 3 times daily with a cup of water

Liquid extract/tincture (1:10) — 1 wineglassful, 3 times daily (corresponds to approximately 2 g drug per single dose)

Infusion (1:40) — 1 wineglassful, 3 times daily (corresponds to approximately 2 g drug per single dose)

Storage: Seal tightly and store in a cool, dry place.

LITERATURE

Dixit VP, Jain P, Joshi SC, Hypolipidaemic effects of Curcuma longa L and Nardostachys jatamansi, DC in triton-induced hyperlipidaemic rats. Indian J Physiol Pharmacol, 32:299-304, 1988 Oct-Dec.

Hänsel R, Keller K, Rimpler H, Schneider G (Ed), Hagers Handbuch der Pharmazeutischen Praxis, 5. Aufl., Bde 4 - 6 (Drogen), Springer Verlag Berlin, Heidelberg, New York, 1992-1994.

Rucker G, Tautges J, Sieck A, Wenzl H, Graf E, Isolation and pharmacodynamic activity of the sesquiterpene valeranone from Nardostachys jatamansi. DC Arzneimittelforschung, 28:7-13, 1978.

Rucker G, Tautges J, Sieck A, Wenzl H, Graf E, Nardostachys jatamansi: a chemical, pharmacological and clinical appraisal. Spec Rep Ser Indian Counc Med Res, 28:1-117, 1978.

Jateorhiza palmata

See Colombo

Java Tea

Orthosiphon spicatus

DESCRIPTION

Medicinal Parts: The medicinal parts are the leaves and stem tips collected during the flowering season.

Flower and Fruit: The flowers usually are arranged in a whorl of 6 (occasionally 10) blooms. The calyx tube is short with an upright-curved upper lip. The corolla is blue to light violet. The corolla tube is about 2 cm long with a broad upper lip that has 3 indentations. The lower lip is narrow and ovate-lanceolate. The 4 stamens are blue and 2.5 to 3 cm long. The style is as long as the stamen, and the ovary has a disk. The fruit breaks up into 4 oval-oblong nutlets with bumpy surfaces.

Leaves, Stem and Root: The plant is a 40 to 80 cm high herb. The stem is quadrangular and glabrous to pubescent with crossed, opposite leaves. The leaves are about 75 mm long, usually short-petioled, ovate-lanceolate with an irregularly coarse, roughly serrate to dentate (or occasionally crenate) margin. The upper surface is brownish-green, the lower surface gray-green with strong, protruding ribs and glandular punctate markings. The plant resembles Peppermint.

Characteristics: The herb has a weak, unusual smell reminiscent of a cattle pen. The taste is salty, bitter and astringent.

Habitat: The plant is found in an area extending from tropical Asia to tropical Australia and is cultivated in those areas and elsewhere.

Production: Java Tea consists of the dried leaf and stem tips of Orthosiphon spicatus, which is harvested shortly before flowering. The leaves are then dried in a well-ventilated location.

Not to be Confused With: Confusion can arise with other Orthosiphon varieties and Eupatorium varieties from Java.

ACTIONS AND PHARMACOLOGY

COMPOUNDS

Volatile oil (0.02-0.06%): including among others beta-caryophyllene, alpha-humulene, caryophyllene-epoxide

Flavonoids: in particular more highly methoxylized examples (0.2%) including eupatorin, sinensetin, scutellarine tetramethyl ethers, salvigenin

Caffeic acid derivatives: including among others 2,3-dicoffeoyltartrate, rosmaric acid, 2-caffeoyl tartrate.

Diterpene ester: orthosiphole A to E, (diterpene dibenzoyl diacetyl ester of primarane type)

Triterpene saponins: (up to 4.5%): aglycone hederagenin

EFFECTS

Java Tea has been shown in human and animal tests to be a mild diuretic. The essential oil of the drug, which contains sesquiterpenes, is antimicrobial, antiphlogistic and possibly antitumoral.

INDICATIONS AND USAGE

Approved by Commission E:

- Infections of the urinary tract
- Kidney and bladder stones

Unproven Uses: In folk medicine, it is used for the above conditions and also for gout, rheumatism, hematuria and albuminuria.

CONTRAINDICATIONS

Use of the drug for irrigation therapy is contraindicated in the presence of edema resulting from reduced cardiac or renal activity.

PRECAUTIONS AND ADVERSE REACTIONS

No health hazards or side effects are known in conjunction with the proper administration of designated therapeutic dosages.

DOSAGE

Mode of Administration: Comminuted herb for infusions and other galenic preparations for internal use.

How Supplied: Forms of commercial pharmaceutical preparations include:

Capsules

Drops

Tablets

Preparation: To make an infusion (tea), pour 150 ml hot water over the drug and strain after 10 minutes.

Daily Dosage: The daily dosage ranges from 6 to12 g drug. Adequate fluid intake (at least 2 liters per day) is essential.

Storage: Java Tea should be stored in a tightly sealed container that protects it from light and moisture.

LITERATURE

Hänsel R, Keller K, Rimpler H, Schneider G (Hrsg.), Hagers Handbuch der Pharmazeutischen Praxis, 5. Aufl., Bde 4-6 (Drogen), Springer Verlag Berlin, Heidelberg, New York, 1992-1994.

Hiller K, Pharmazeutische Bewertung ausgewählter Teedrogen. In: DAZ 135(16):1425-1440. 1995.

Madaus G, Lehrbuch der Biologischen Arzneimittel, Bde 1-3, Nachdruck, Georg Olms Verlag Hildesheim 1979.

Proksch P, Orthosiphon aristatus (Blume) Miquel - der Katzenbart. In: ZPT 13(2):63. 1992.

Steinegger E, Hänsel R, Pharmakognosie, 5. Aufl., Springer Verlag Heidelberg 1992.

Takeda Y et al., Orthosiphol D and E, minor diterpenes from Orthosiphon stamineus. In: PH 33:411. 1993.

Teuber R, Neue Naturstoffe aus Orthosiphon stamineus Bentham. In: Dissertation Universität Marburg. 1986.

Teuscher E, Biogene Arzneimittel, 5. Aufl., Wiss. Verlagsges. Stuttgart 1997.

Wichtl M (Hrsg.), Teedrogen, 4. Aufl., Wiss. Verlagsges. Stuttgart 1997.

Jequirity

Abrus precatorius

DESCRIPTION

Medicinal Parts: The medicinal parts are the leaves, roots and seeds.

Flower and Fruit: The flowers are racemes of pink blossoms. The fruit is a pod with oval seeds, which are rounded at the ends. They are about 3 mm in diameter, hard, red and glossy, with a large black dot at one end. One variety has white seeds.

Leaves, Stem and Root: This deciduous climbing plant with compound leaves grows to about 4 m.

Characteristics: The plant is a protected species in some countries.

Habitat: The plant originated in India and is found today in all tropical regions of the world.

Other Names: Indian Licorice, Wild Licorice, Prayer Beads, Crab's Eyes, Gunga, Goonteh, Rati

ACTIONS AND PHARMACOLOGY

COMPOUNDS

Toxic lectins: abrine and isolectins.

EFFECTS

Jequirity is an irritant and abortifacient.

INDICATIONS AND USAGE

Unproven Uses: Jequirity was used for chronic conjunctivitis and as a contraceptive in folk medicine, but is no longer used for these purposes.

Indian Medicine: Jequirity is used for coughs as well as inflammations and conditions of the upper respiratory tract and lungs.

Chinese Medicine: The drug is used in hepatitis and bronchitis.

PRECAUTIONS AND ADVERSE REACTIONS

The drug is very poisonous because it contains the toxic lectin abrine and isolectins.

OVERDOSAGE

Severe poisonings among adults following the intake of one half to two seeds, as well as cases of death among children following the consumption of two seeds, have been recorded. Besides gastrointestinal emptying, counter-measures include, administration of large amounts of fluid, monitoring of the circulatory system, administration of anti-epileptic drugs and possibly artificial respiration.

LITERATURE

Desai VB, Rupawala EN, (1966) Ind J Pharm 29:235.

Desai VB, Sirsi M, (1966) Ind J Pharmac 28:340.

Dupaigne P, (1974) Plantes Med Phytother 8:104.

Karawya MS et al., (1981) Fitoterapia 4:175.

Ku SC et al., (1995) Planta Med 61:307.

Lin JY, Liu SV, (1986) Toxikon 24:757.

Lin JY et al., (1981) Toxikon 19:41.

Murray DR, Vairinhos F, (1982) Z Pflanzenphysiol 108:471.

Further information in:

Frohne D, Pfänder HJ, Giftpflanzen - Ein Handbuch für Apotheker, Toxikologen und Biologen, 4. Aufl., Wiss. Verlags-Ges Stuttgart 1997.

Kern W, List PH, Hörhammer L (Herausg.), Hagers Handbuch der Pharmazeutischen Praxis, 4. Aufl., Springer Verlag Berlin, Heidelberg, New York, 1969.

Roth L, Daunderer M, Kormann K, Giftpflanzen, Pflanzengifte - Vorkommen, Wirkung, Therapie, allergische Reaktionen, 3. Aufl., ecomed 1988.

Teuscher E, Lindequist U, Biogene Gifte - Biologie, Chemie, Pharmakologie, 2. Aufl., Fischer Verlag Stuttgart 1994.

Jewel Weed

Impatiens biflora

DESCRIPTION

Medicinal Parts: The medicinal part is the herb.

Flower and Fruit: The axillary flowers are orange-yellow with large reddish-brown spots. They have an irregular form. The sepal sac abruptly contracts to a spur of about 5 to 9 mm. The spur is bent 180 degrees to lie parallel with the sac. The fruit is an oblong capsule which, when ripe, bursts open at the slightest touch and spreads the seeds over large distances.

Leaves, Stem and Root: The plant is a glabrous, fleshy annual 20 to 180 cm high. The stems are simple or branched and have swollen nodes. The leaves are thin, ovate, with 5 to 12 (up to 14) teeth on each side and are often undulate. They are rich green.

Habitat: Impatiens is common in the temperate regions and in South Africa, but it grows mostly in the mountainous, tropical regions of Asia and Africa.

Production: Jewel Weed is the aerial part of Impatiens biflora.

Other Names: Wild Balsam, Balsam-Weed, Spotted Touch-Me-Not, Slipperweed, Silverweed, Wild Lady's Slipper, Speckled Jewels, Wild Celandine, Quick-in-the-Hand

ACTIONS AND PHARMACOLOGY

COMPOUNDS

Naphthalene derivatives: 1.4-naphthoquinone, in particular lawsone (2-hydroxy-1, 4- naphthoquinone), yielding from the precursor through drying of the leaves 1,2,4-trihydroxy-naphthalene-4-beta-D-glucoside

EFFECTS

Jewel Weed is a digestive, appetite stimulant and diuretic.

INDICATIONS AND USAGE

Unproven Uses: Jewel Weed is used for mild digestive disorders. In folk medicine the fresh plant is used as an ointment for hemorrhoids and the juice is used for removing warts.

PRECAUTIONS AND ADVERSE REACTIONS

No health hazards or side effects are known in conjunction with the proper administration of designated therapeutic dosages.

DOSAGE

Mode of Administration: Administered as the ground drug and as an infusion.

LITERATURE

Hegnauer R, Chemotaxonomie der Pflanzen, Bde 1-11, Birkhäuser Verlag Basel, Boston, Berlin 1962-1997.

Jimson Weed

Datura stramonium

DESCRIPTION

Medicinal Parts: The medicinal parts are the dried leaves or the dried leaves with the tips of the flowering branches. Occasionally the fruit, the ripe seeds and the fresh, aerial parts of the plant are used. Parts of the plant are regarded as poisonous.

Flower and Fruit: The flowers are large, white, solitary, terminal or in the branch bifurcations. The calyx has a long 5-edged and short 5-tipped tube. The corolla is funnel-shaped and folded with a short 5-sectioned border. There are 5 free stamens and 1 superior ovary. The fruit is a 5 cm long 4-valved capsule, which is densely thorny and walnut-sized. The numerous seeds are 3.5 mm long, flat, reniform and black.

Leaves, Stem and Root: The plant is an annual and grows to 1.2 m high. It has a simple or bifurcated, round, erect glabrous stem. The leaves are 20 cm long, long-petioled, ovate, dentate, glabrous and dark green.

Characteristics: The foliage has an unpleasant smell; the flowers are fragrant and poisonous.

Habitat: Jimson Weed is found in most temperate and subtropical parts of the world, probably originated in Central America.

Production: Jimson Weed leaf consists of the dried leaf, or the dried leaves and flowering tops of Datura stramonium. Jimson Weed seed consists of the ripe seed of Datura stramonium.

Other Names: Devil's Apple, Devil's Trumpet, Jamestown Weed, Mad-Apple, Nightshade, Peru-Apple, Stinkweed, Stinkwort, Stramonium, Thorn-Apple, Datura

ACTIONS AND PHARMACOLOGY

COMPOUNDS: JIMSON WEED LEAF

Tropane alkaloids (0.1-0.65%): chief alkaloids (-)-hyoscyamine, under drying conditions changing over to some extent into atropine and scopolamine (ratio 4:1), furthermore including, among others, apoatropine, belladonnine, tigloylmeteloidin

Flavonoids

Hydroxycoumarins: including, among others, umbelliferone, scopolin, scopoletin

Withanolide: including, among others, withastramonolide

COMPOUNDS: JIMSON WEED SEED

Tropane alkaloids (0.4-0.6%): chief alkaloids (-)-hyoscyamine, under drying conditions changing over to some extent into atropine, and scopolamine (ratio 4:1).

Indole alkaloids (β-carboline type): including, among others, fluorodaturin (very fluorescent).

Lectins

Fatty oil (15-45%)

Proteins (12-25%)

EFFECTS: JIMSON WEED LEAF AND SEED

The drug contains alkaloids (hyoscyamine, scopolamine) in extremely varying concentrations. The effect is anticholinergic and parasympatholytic (see Belladonna); the scopolamine fraction is more responsible for this effect.

INDICATIONS AND USAGE

JIMSON WEED LEAF AND SEED

Due to the inconsistent alkaloid content of the raw herb, the authors do not recommend use of non-standardized Jimson Weed products.

Unproven Uses: In folk medicine, Jimson Weed preparations have been used for asthma, convulsive cough, pertussis during bronchitis and influenza, for severe catarrh and as an expectorant. It was also used as a basic therapy for diseases of the autonomic nervous system. In the 18th century stramonium was first used for epileptic fits, and it was also used for hallucinogenic effect in magic and witch potions.

Homeopathic Uses: Used for infection with high temperatures, cramps and inflammations of the eyes.

Chinese Medicine: Used in Chinese medicine for general states of pain. It is smoked for asthma, dyspnea and coughs; externally for rheumatism.

CONTRAINDICATIONS

JIMSON WEED LEAF AND SEED

Glaucoma, suspicion of glaucoma, paralytic ileus, pyloric stenosis, enlarged prostate, tachycardic arrhythmias, acute pulmonary edema.

PRECAUTIONS AND ADVERSE REACTIONS

JIMSON WEED LEAF AND SEED

General: Patients with urine retention or coronoary sclerosis should not use Jimson Weed.

Drug Interactions: Jimson Weed will have an additive effect when taken with other anticholinergic medications.

OVERDOSAGE

JIMSON WEED LEAF AND SEED

The intake of very high dosages leads to central excitation (restlessness, compulsive speech, hallucinations, delirium, manic episodes), followed by exhaustion and sleep.

The 4 early warning symptoms of poisoning are skin reddening, dryness of the mouth, tachycardic arrhythmias and mydriasis. Accommodation disorders, heat build-up through decline in sweat secretion, miction disorders and severe constipation can occur as side effects, particularly with overdosages.

Lethal dosages (for adults starting at 100 mg atropine, depending upon atropine content, 15 to 100 g of the leaf drug, 15 to 25 g of the seed drug, considerably less for children) carry with them the danger of asphyxiation. Treatment for poisonings include stomach emptying, temperature-lowering measures with wet cloths (no antipyretics), oxygen respiration for respiratory distress, intubation, parenteral physostigmine salts as antidote, diazepam for spasms and chlorpromazine for severe excitation.

DOSAGE

JIMSON WEED LEAF

Daily Dosage: Stabilized leaf powder: 0.05 to 0.1 gm drug as a single dose up to 3 times a day; daily dose: 0.6 gm drug (ÖAB90); as a narcotic: 1 gm drug.

Homeopathic Dosage: from D4: 5 to 10 drops, 1 tablet or 5 to 10 globules 1 to 3 times a day or 1 ml injection solution sc twice weekly; eye drops 1 to 3 times a day (HAB1).

Storage: Keep carefully stored and protected from light.

JIMSON WEED SEED

Daily Dosage: Seeds: single oral dose: 0.05 gm; daily dose: 0.6 gm drug (EB6); seed tincture: single oral dose: 0.3 gm; daily dose: 3.0 gm (EB6).

Homeopathic Dosage: from D4: 5 to 10 drops, 1 tablet or 5 to 10 globules 1 to 3 times a day or 1 ml injection solution sc twice weekly; eye drops 1 to 3 times a day (HAB1).

Storage: Keep carefully stored and protected from light.

LITERATURE

JIMSON WEED LEAF AND SEED

Evans WC, PH 23:1717. 1984.

Friedmann M, Levin CE, J Agric Food Chem 37:998. 1989.

Itoh T et al., PH 17:971. 1978.

Kraft K, Europäische Rauschdrogen. In: ZPT 17(6):343-355. 1996.

Mechler E, Hann N, PM 42:102. 1981.

Mirazamatov RT et al., Khim Prir Soedin (3):381. 1986.

Sharova EG et al., Khim Prir Soedin (1):126. 1977.

Tursunova RL et al., Khim Prir Soedin (1):91. 1978.

Further information in:

Frohne D, Pfänder HJ, Giftpflanzen - Ein Handbuch für Apotheker, Toxikologen und Biologen, 4. Aufl., Wiss. Verlags-Ges. Stuttgart 1997.

Hänsel R, Keller K, Rimpler H, Schneider G (Hrsg.), Hagers Handbuch der Pharmazeutischen Praxis, 5. Aufl., Bde 4-6 (Drogen): Springer Verlag Berlin, Heidelberg, New York, 1992-1994.

Lewin L, Gifte und Vergiftungen, 6. Aufl., Nachdruck, Haug Verlag, Heidelberg 1992.

Madaus G, Lehrbuch der Biologischen Arzneimittel, Bde 1-3, Nachdruck, Georg Olms Verlag Hildesheim 1979.

Roth L, Daunderer M, Kormann K, Giftpflanzen, Pflanzengifte, 4. Aufl., Ecomed Fachverlag Landsberg Lech 1993.

Steinegger E, Hänsel R, Pharmakognosie, 5. Aufl., Springer Verlag Heidelberg 1992.

Teuscher E, Lindequist U, Biogene Gifte - Biologie, Chemie, Pharmakologie, 2. Aufl., Fischer Verlag Stuttgart 1994.

Teuscher E, Biogene Arzneimittel, 5. Aufl., Wiss. Verlagsges. Stuttgart 1997.

Wagner H, Wiesenauer M, Phytotherapie. Phytopharmaka und pflanzliche Homöopathika, Fischer-Verlag, Stuttgart, Jena, New York 1995.

Jojoba

Simmondsia chinesis

DESCRIPTION

Medicinal Parts: The medicinal part is the liquid Jojoba wax.

Flower and Fruit: The flowers are axillary. The male flowers are small and yellow and have no petals. The female flowers are usually solitary, inconspicuous and pale green. There may also be inflorescences in the form of panicles, umbels and cymes. Pollination is by wind. The fruit capsules contain 1 to 3 seeds although 1-seeded capsules are the most common. The seeds are approximately 2 cm long.

Leaves, Stem and Root: The plant is a heavily branched, evergreen dioecious bush. The male plants are larger, taller and less compact than the female. The desert variety develop taproots up to 3.6 m in length. The horizontal root branches reach from 60 to 90 cm in depth. The leaves are thick, coriaceous, blue-green, entire-margined and oblong. They are in pairs and depending on the dampness of the soil the leaves may remain on the bush for 2 to 3 periods of growth.

Characteristics: The oil from the fruit has a pleasant scent and taste.

Habitat: The plant is indigenous to areas extending from the Sonora dessert of the U.S. to northwest Mexico. It is cultivated in India and Israel.

Production: From the cultivation (of plants) in Mexico and in South America. Liquid Jojoba wax is a clear, light yellow, oily liquid, that is extracted from the seeds of Simmondsia chinesis.

ACTIONS AND PHARMACOLOGY

COMPOUNDS

Liquid wax exters: esters in position 9-10 simple unsaturated C20- and C22-fatty acids, chiefly gadolenic acid (20:1(9), make up 70% of the fatty acids) with the corresponding alcohols, chiefly eicosanol (20:1 (9)-OH) and docosenol (22:1 (9) OH)

EFFECTS

Active agents are the simple unsaturated C20/22 - fatty acids and alcohol.

Jojoba oil has a robust and stable constitution. It is used in skin care products as a carrier (substance) for oxidation sensitive substances (Vitamin A).

INDICATIONS AND USAGE

Skin care - cosmetics

PRECAUTIONS AND ADVERSE REACTIONS

No health hazards or side effects are known in conjunction with the proper external administration of designated therapeutic dosages. Jojoba wax is not suitable for internal use.

DOSAGE

Mode of Administration: In ointments and creams as a medium (or vehicle) for oxidation sensitive substances.

LITERATURE

Knoepfler NB et al., Agr Food Chem 6:118. 1958.

Miwa TK, J Am Oil Chem Soc 48:259. 1971.

Further information in:

Hänsel R, Keller K, Rimpler H, Schneider G (Hrsg.), Hagers Handbuch der Pharmazeutischen Praxis, 5. Aufl., Bde 4-6 (Drogen): Springer Verlag Berlin, Heidelberg, New York, 1992-1994.

Steinegger E, Hänsel R, Pharmakognosie, 5. Aufl., Springer Verlag Heidelberg 1992.

Teuscher E, Biogene Arzneimittel, 5. Aufl., Wiss. Verlagsges. Stuttgart 1997.

Juglans cinerea

See Butternut

Juglans regia

See Walnut

Jujube (Da-Zao)

Zyzyphus jujube

DESCRIPTION

Medicinal Parts: The medicinal part is the fruit. The Jujube berry is classed with raisins, dates and figs, and can be eaten fresh or dried.

Flower and Fruit: The flowers are small, pale yellow and solitary. The fruit is of variable size, depending on the origin, but is usually up to 3 cm long and 1.5 cm in diameter. The fruit is red, smooth and shiny when fresh, brownish-red and grooved when dried. It is pulpy and contains 1 or 2 acute, oblong seeds.

Characteristics: The taste of the fruit is sweet and mucilaginous.

Habitat: The plant grows in southern Europe, Africa, Middle East and the Far East.

Production: Jujube berries are the fruit of Zyzyphus jujube; Zyzyphus vulgaris is also used.

ACTIONS AND PHARMACOLOGY

COMPOUNDS

Triterpene saponins: zyzyphus saponins I, II and III, jujuboside-B, in the seeds jujuboside-A and -B, aglycone jujubogenine

Mucilage

Tannins (10%)

Flavonoids: including among others naringenin-6,8-di-C-glucosides, in the seeds spinosin (C-glycoflavone)

Isoquinoline alkaloids: oxonuciferin, nornuciferin

Peptide alkaloids: daechucyclopeptide, daechualkaloid-A

Triterpenes: betulinic acid, betulonic acid, maslinic acid, alphitolic acid and oleanolic acid

Hydroxycoumarins

Sugars: including among others saccharose, glucose, fructose, galactose

Fruit acids: including among others malic acid, tartaric acid

EFFECTS

Jujube is emollient, anti-allergenic and sedative. Zyzyphus vulgaris also has a hypotensive effect.

INDICATIONS AND USAGE

Unproven Uses: Jujube is used as a nutrient and tonic. It is also used as a prophylactic against liver disease and stress ulcers.

PRECAUTIONS AND ADVERSE REACTIONS

No health hazards or side effects are known in conjunction with the proper administration of designated therapeutic dosages.

LITERATURE

Ahn YS et al., (1982) Korean J Pharmacol 18 (1):17.

Cyong J et al., (1979) Proc Symp. Wakan-Yaku 12:1.

Cyong J, Hanabusa K, (1980) Phytochemistry 19:2747.

Cyong J, Takahashi M, (1982) Chem Pharm Bull 30:1081.

Hikino H, In: Economic, Medicinal Plant Research, Vol. 1, Acadamic Press UK 1985.

Ikram M et al., (1981) J Nat Prod 44:91.

Inoue O et al., (1978) J Chem Res 144.

Okamura N et al., (1981) Chem Pharm Bull 29:676, 3507.

Shibata S et al., (1970) Phytochemistry 9:677.

Woo WS et al., (1979) Phytochemistry 18:353.

Yagi A et al., (1978) Chem Pharm Bull 26:1798.

Further information in:

Hegnauer R, Chemotaxonomie der Pflanzen, Bde 1-11: Birkhäuser Verlag Basel, Boston, Berlin 1962-1997.

Kern W, List PH, Hörhammer L (Hrsg.), Hagers Handbuch der Pharmazeutischen Praxis, 4. Aufl., Bde 1-8: Springer Verlag Berlin, Heidelberg, New York, 1969.

Wagner H, Wiesenauer M, Phytotherapie. Phytopharmaka und pflanzliche Homöopathika, Fischer-Verlag, Stuttgart, Jena, New York 1995.

Wichtl M (Hrsg.), Teedrogen, 4. Aufl., Wiss. Verlagsges. Stuttgart 1997.

Juniper

Juniperus communis

TRADE NAMES

Juniper (available from numerous manufacturers and as combination product), Juniper Berry, Euro Quality Juniper Berries

DESCRIPTION

Medicinal Parts: The medicinal parts are the essential oil from the berry cones; the ripe, dried berry cones; the ripe fresh berry cones; the fresh or dried pseudo fruit or berry; and the ripe berry.

Flower and Fruit: The plant is usually dioecious, occasionally monoecious and occasionally bears androgynous flowers. The yellowish male flowers are in elliptical catkins consisting of numerous stamens in 3-segmented whorls in the leaf axils of young shoots. The greenish female flowers are almost ovoid and consist of 3 carpels. The carpels become fleshy and in the second year when ripe form pea-sized, globular, and dark-brown to violet, blue-frosted juniper berries. The berries ripen for 2 or 3 years so that blue (ripe) and green (unripe) berries are found on the same tree. The seeds are light brown, oblong-triangular. They are somewhat warty between the edges and have a hard shell.

Leaves, Stem and Root: Juniperus communis is a tree or shrub found in varying forms from 2 to 10 m in height. The bark is smooth and yellow-brown at first, later fissured, gray-black and peeling. The buds are covered in scale-like needles, which can be distinguished from the foliage needles by their length. The leaves are needles in whorls of 3 spreading from the branchlets. They are evergreen, stiff, pointed, prickly and sea green. The outer and inner membranes have thickened cell walls.

Characteristics: The berries have a tangy smell. The taste is tangy-sweet, then resinous and bitter.

Habitat: Europe, northern Africa, north Asia and North America.

Production: Juniper Berry is the ripe, fresh or dried spherical ovulate cone (berry) of Juniper communis as well as its preparations. The ripe berries are harvested from the end of August to the middle of September and then dried at room temperature and sorted.

Other Names: Juniper Berry, Ginepro, Enebro

ACTIONS AND PHARMACOLOGY

COMPOUNDS

Volatile oil (1-2%): make-up is very dependent upon the source of the drug, chief components monoterpene hydrocarbons, for example alpha-pinene, beta-myrcene, gamma-muurolen, sabinene, additionally including among others limonene, beta-elemene, beta-caryophyllene, beta-pinene, gamma-cadinene, terpinene-4-ol

Diterpenes

Catechin tannins

Flavonoids

Monosaccharides: inverted sugar (20 to 30%)

Oligomeric proanthocyanidins

EFFECTS

The diuretic effect is attributed to the essential oil content. The drug works to lower blood pressure and as an antidiabetic. In animal experiments a hypotensive, antidiabetic and antiexudative effect was proven. In vitro, an antiviral effect was also demonstrated.

In older studies a spasmogenic, expectorant and bronchospasmolytic effect has been described, for which there are no new data.

INDICATIONS AND USAGE

Approved by Commission E:

- Loss of appetite
- Dyspeptic complaints

Unproven Uses: Juniper is used externally for rheumatic symptoms (as a bath additive). In folk medicine it is used internally to regulate menstruation and to relieve menstrual pain, flushing out therapy for inflammatory diseases of the lower urinary tract, gout, arteriosclerosis, for severe irritation resulting from bronchitis and diabetes (ground juniper berries). It is often chewed for halitosis.

Homeopathic Uses: Juniperus communis is used for discharge disturbances of the efferent urinary tract and dyspeptic complaints.

CONTRAINDICATIONS

Contraindications for internal administration include pregnancy and inflammatory renal diseases.

PRECAUTIONS AND ADVERSE REACTIONS

General: No health hazards or side effects are known in conjunction with the proper administration of designated therapeutic dosages. Long-term internal administration or overdosage can bring about kidney irritation and kidney damage. External administration for large skin wounds, acute skin diseases, feverish diseases, cardiac insufficiency or hypertonia should only take place under the supervision of a doctor.

Pregnancy: Not to be used during pregnancy.

DOSAGE

Mode of Administration: Whole, crushed or powdered drug for infusions and decoctions, alcohol extracts, and in wine. Essential oil is used for oral application in liquid and solid medicinal forms. Combinations with other plant drugs in bladder and kidney teas and similar preparations may be useful. Juniper berry is also used as bath salts in the treatment of rheumatism.

How Supplied:

Capsules — 515 mg

Liquid — 1:1

Oil — 100%

Daily Dosage: The daily dose is 2 to 10 gm of the drug, corresponding to 20 to 100 mg of the essential oil. The duration of use should be limited to a maximum of 6 weeks. A 1:20 dilution infusion (0.5 gm in 1 teacup) may be taken 3 times daily. Tincture (1:5): 1 to 2 ml 3 times daily. Liquid extract: 2 to 4 ml 3 times daily.

For diabetes: 10 freshly ground berries to taken daily with water for 15 days; repeat after a month's break from treatment.

Homeopathic Uses: 5 drops, 1 tablet or 10 globules every 30 to 60 minutes (acute) or 1 to 3 times daily (chronic); parenterally: 1 to 2 ml sc acute, 3 times daily; chronic: once daily (HAB1).

Storage: Juniper should be protected from light.

LITERATURE

Chatzopoulou PS, Katsiotis ST, Study of the Essential Oil from Juniperus communis ''Berries'' (Cones)Growing in Greece. In: PM 59(6):554. 1993.

De Pascuale Teresa J, (1977) An Quim. 73(3):463.

Freidrich H, Engelshowe R, (1978) Planta Med 33:251.

Lamer-Zarawska E, Phytochemical studies on flavonoids and other compounds of juniper fruits (Juniperus communsi L.). In: Pol J Chem 54(2):213-219. 1980.

Mascolo N et al., (1987) Phytother Res 1(1):28.

Ramic S, Murko D, Chemical composition of fruit of Juniperus species. In: Archiv Farm 33(1):15-20. 1983.

Schilcher H, Boesel R, Effenberger ST Segebrecht S, Neuere Untersuchungsergebnisse mit aquaretisch, antibakteriell und prostatotrop wirksamen Arzneipflanzen. In: ZPT 10(3):77. 1989.

Schilcher H, Emmrich D, Koehler C, Gaschromatographischer Vergleich von ätherischen Wacholderölen und deren toxikologische Bedeutung. In: PZW 138(3/4)85. 1993.

Schilcher H, Heil BM, Nierentoxizität von Wacholderbeerzubereitungen. In: ZPT 15(4):205-213. 1994.

Schmidt M, Wacholderzubereitungen. Muβ die Monographie umgeschrieben werden? In: DAZ 135(14):1260-1264. 1995.

Sökeland J, Phytotherapie in der Urologie. In: ZPT 10(1):8. 1989.

Thomas AF, (1972) Helv Chim Acta 55:2429.

Thomas AF, (1972) Helv Chim. Acta 56:1800.

Further information in:

Frohne D, Pfänder HJ, Giftpflanzen - Ein Handbuch für Apotheker, Toxikologen und Biologen, 4. Aufl., Wiss. Verlags-Ges Stuttgart 1997.

Hänsel R, Keller K, Rimpler H, Schneider G (Hrsg.), Hagers Handbuch der Pharmazeutischen Praxis, 5. Aufl., Bde 4-6 (Drogen), Springer Verlag Berlin, Heidelberg, New York, 1992-1994.

Leung AY, Encyclopedia of Common Natural Ingredients Used in Food, Drugs and Cosmetics, John Wiley & Sons Inc., New York 1980.

Madaus G, Lehrbuch der Biologischen Arzneimittel, Bde 1-3, Nachdruck, Georg Olms Verlag Hildesheim 1979.

Roth L, Daunderer M, Kormann K, Giftpflanzen, Pflanzengifte, 4. Aufl., Ecomed Fachverlag Landsberg Lech 1993.

Steinegger E, Hänsel R, Pharmakognosie, 5. Aufl., Springer Verlag Heidelberg 1992.

Teuscher E, Biogene Arzneimittel, 5. Aufl., Wiss. Verlagsges. Stuttgart 1997.

Teuscher E, Lindequist U, Biogene Gifte-Biologie, Chemie, Pharmakologie, 2. Aufl., Fischer Verlag Stuttgart 1994.

Wagner H, Wiesenauer M, Phytotherapie. Phytopharmaka und pflanzliche Homöopathika, Fischer-Verlag, Stuttgart, Jena, New York 1995.

Wichtl M (Hrsg.), Teedrogen, 4. Aufl., Wiss. Verlagsges. Stuttgart 1997.

Juniperus communis

See Juniper

Juniperus sabina

See Savin Tops

Justicia adhatoda

See Malabar Nut

Kadsura japonica

See False Schisandra

Kalmia latifolia

See Mountain Laurel

Kamala

Mallotus philippinensis

DESCRIPTION

Medicinal Parts: The medicinal parts are the glands and hairs covering the fruit.

Flower and Fruit: The tree has dioecious flowers. The male flowers are in threes in the axils of the bracts, while the female flowers are on longer, heavily branched, lateral boughs. Both flowers are covered by rust-red matted hairs. The fruit is a 3-lobed, pea-sized capsule from which a red, mealy powder is obtained, which consists of minute glands and hairs.

Leaves, Stem and Root: Mallotus philippinensis is an 8 to 10 m high tree with a diameter of 90 to 120 cm. The bark of the slender branches is pale, and the younger ones are covered in rust-red matted hairs. The leaves are alternate and have articulate petioles, which are 2.5 to 5 cm long. The leaf blade is rusty tomentose, 8 to 15 cm long, ovate with two inconspicuous basal glands. It is entire-margined, coriaceous and glabrous above with very prominent ribs below.

Habitat: The plant is indigenous to India, Ethiopia, Saudi Arabia, China and Australia.

Production: Kamala fruit skins are from the fruits of Mallotus philippinensis, covered in hairs and glands. The fruit is collected in the uncultivated regions and cleaned.

Other Names: Kameela, Kamcela, Spoonwood, Röttlera Tinctoria

ACTIONS AND PHARMACOLOGY

COMPOUNDS

Phloroglucinol derivatives (red to yellow, 47 to 80%): chief constituents include rottlerin (ca. 1%), isorottlerin (ca. 0.1%), 3-hydroxyrottlerin, 3,4-dihydroxyrottlerin, methylene-bis-methyl phloroacetophenone and their resinous polymers, that arise through auto-oxidation

Bergenin

Tannins

EFFECTS

The drug has an anthelmintic and purgative effect.

INDICATIONS AND USAGE

Indian Medicine: Internally, Kamala is used to treat tape worm infestations (ascarides, rectal worms), constipation, kidney and bladder stones, leprosy lesions and as a contraceptive; externally for parasitic skin diseases and wound infections of the ear.

PRECAUTIONS AND ADVERSE REACTIONS

No health hazards or side effects are known in conjunction with the proper administration of designated therapeutic dosages.

DOSAGE

Mode of Administration: The drug is used orally as a powder or liquid extract.

Daily Dosage: For worms: adults: 6 to 12 gm drug in 2 to 3 portions at 30 minute intervals; young children: 1.5 gm drug; school children: 3 gm drug. Preparations can be sweetened with honey prior to administration.

Storage: Keep tightly sealed, dry and protected from light

LITERATURE

Kern W, List PH, Hörhammer L (Hrsg.), Hagers Handbuch der Pharmazeutischen Praxis, 4. Aufl., Bde. 1-8, Springer Verlag Berlin, Heidelberg, New York, 1969.

Lounasmaa M et al., (1975) Planta Med 28:16.

Widen CF, Puri HS, (1980) Planta Med 40:284.

Kava Kava

Piper methysticum

TRADE NAMES

Kava Kava (available from numerous manfacturers) Alcohol Free Kava Kava, Kava Kava Power, Kava Kava Premium, Kava Kava Root

DESCRIPTION

Medicinal Parts: The medicinal parts are the peeled, dried, cut rhizome, which has normally been freed from the roots, and the fresh rhizome with the roots.

Flower and Fruit: The plant has numerous small flowers in spike-like inflorescences 3 to 9 cm long.

Leaves, Stem and Root: The plant is a 2 to 3 m high, erect dioecious bush. The leaves are very large, measuring 13 to 28 cm by 10 to 22 cm. They have a deeply cordate base and 9 to 13 main ribs that are slightly soft on the undersurface. The stipules are large. The plant has a massive, 2 to 10 kg, branched and very juicy rhizome with many roots. They are blackish-gray on the outside and whitish on the inside. The fracture is mealy and somewhat splintery. The central portion is porous with irregularly twisted thin woody bundles, separated by broad medullary rays, forming meshes beneath the bark.

Characteristics: The taste is pungent and numbing, and the odor is reminiscent of lilac.

Habitat: The plant is indigenous to the South Sea Islands and is mainly cultivated there.

Production: Kava Kava rhizome consists of the dried rhizomes of Piper methysticum.

Other Names: Ava, Ava Pepper, Intoxicating Pepper, Kawa, Kawa Pepper, Tonga, Kew

ACTIONS AND PHARMACOLOGY

COMPOUNDS

Kava lactones (kava pyrones, 5-12%): chief components include (+)-kavain, dihydrokavain (marindinine), (+)-methysticin, dihydromethysticin, yangonine, desmethoxyyangonin

Chalcones: including flavokavin A and B

EFFECTS

The kava pyrones in the drug have centrally muscle-relaxing, anticonvulsive and antispasmodic effects. The herb also contains hypnotic/sedative, analgesic and psychotropic properties contributing to its use for anxiety and insomnia.

The centrally muscle-relaxing, analgesic and anticonvulsive action of the kava pyrones, kavain, dihydrokavain, dihydromethysticin and (+/-) kavain (synthetic kava pyrone) is attributed to the interaction with ion channels. The interaction consists of fast and specific inhibition of voltage-dependent sodium channels and reduction of currents through voltage-activated sodium and calcium channels (Friese, 1998; Gleitz, 1995; Gleitz, 1996; Schirrmacher, 1999). The paralysis effect of Kava on neuromuscular transmission and muscle contractility is similar to that of local anesthetics (Jameison, 1989; Singh, 1983). The lipid soluble extract (kava resin) decreases spontaneous motility and motor control (Jamieson, 1989).

The analgesic action of kavain, dihydrokavain, methysticin and dihydromethysticin is due to antinociceptive activities. Nalaxone (opiate antagonist) is ineffective in reversing the antinociceptive activities, thus indicating the analgesia produced from the compounds occurs via non-opiate pathways (Jameison, 1990; Jameison, 1989).

The lipid soluble components of kava do not interact with benzodiazepine binding sites, but do seem to potentiate the activity of GABA-A in the brain center for sedative effects (Davies, 1992; Jussofie, 1994). The psychotropic properties of Kava have been demonstrated by the inhibition of norepinephrine uptake by kavain, dihydromethysticin and the racemate (+/-) kavain (Seitz, 1997). One study did find that desmethoxyyangonin, methysticin, yangonin, dihydromethysticin, kihydrokavain and kavain reversibly inhibit MAO-B (Uebelhack, 1998). An increase of dopamine and serotonin by activation of neurons results in central nervous system effects (Fachinfo Antares 120(R), 1996).

A recent study investigated the antithrombotic activity of kava pyrones. Kavain exerts antithrombotic action on human platelets through the inhibition of cyclooxygenase (COX) as a primary target. This suppresses the generation of thromboxane (TXA2), which normally induces aggregation of platelets and exocytosis of ATP by its binding on TXA2 receptors (Gleitz, 1997).

CLINICAL TRIALS

A randomized, double-blind, placebo-controlled study was conducted with 101 outpatients suffering from anxiety of non-psychotic origin who met DSM-III-R criteria. Improvements in anxiety were seen after week 8 with a standardized Kava Kava extract (70% kava-pyrone). The study continued over a 25-week period with significant improvement based upon the Hamilton Anxiety Scale (HAMA), somatic and psychic anxiety, Clinical Global Impression, Self-Report Symptom Inventory and Adjective Mood Scale (Volz, 1997).

The anxiolytic effect of a special kava extract (70 mg of kava pyrones three times daily) was compared to two benzodiazepine preparations (oxazepam 15mg/day, bromazepam). The multi-center, double-blind study involved 172 patients. There was a therapeutically relevant reduction in the severity of anxiety according to the HAMA scale in all three groups. There wasn't a statistically significant difference between the three types of treatment in terms of reducing anxiety (Woelk, 1993).

A standardized Kava extract given 100 mg three times daily was compared to placebo in a randomized, double-blind study. The study included 58 patients with anxiety syndromes not caused by mental disorders. The HAMA overall score of anxiety symptoms revealed significant reduction in the Kava treatment group compared to placebo after 1 week of therapy. After 4 weeks of therapy, an even greater reduction in anxiety symptoms was seen with the Kava treatment group, with no adverse reactions (Lehmann, 1996).

INDICATIONS AND USAGE

■ Nervousness and insomnia

Kava Kava is used for nervous tension, stress and agitation.

Unproven Uses: In folk medicine, the herb is used as a sleeping agent and sedative; for asthma, rheumatism, dyspeptic symptoms, chronic cystitis, syphilis, gonorrhea and weight reduction.

Homeopathic Uses: Kava Kava is used for states of excitement and exhaustion. It is also used for gastritis and pain in the urethra.

CONTRAINDICATIONS

The drug is contraindicated in patients with endogenous depression because it increases the danger of suicide. It is also contraindicated during pregnancy and in nursing mothers. The herb is contraindicated in persons with endogenous depression, because there is an increased risk of suicide in this population.

PRECAUTIONS AND ADVERSE REACTIONS

General: No health hazards are known in conjunction with the proper administration of designated therapeutic dosages. Administration of the herb leads to rare cases of allergic reactions and gastrointestinal complaints. Slight morning tiredness can appear at the beginning of the therapy. Motor reflexes and judgment when driving may be reduced while taking the herb.

Central Nervous System: Dyskinesia and choreoathetosis of the limbs, trunk, neck and facial musculature have been reported secondary to the administration of kava (Schelosky, 1995; Spillane, 1997).

Endocrine: Following long-term use of high doses of Kava extract, weight loss was reported (Mathews, 1988).

Hepatotoxicity: Increase in gamma-glutamyl transferase (GGT) levels have been associated with high doses of Kava extract (Mathews, 1988). Two cases of acute hepatitis with an increase of liver enzymes were reported. Necrotizing hepatitis was determined after a liver biopsy, and upon discontinuation of Kava, liver tests normalized (Stahl, 1998).

Musculoskeletal: Minor inhibition of movement and impaired motor reflexes have been observed with the use of Kava (Jamieson, 1990).

Ocular: Increase in pupil diameter, reduction of the near point of accommodation and near point of convergence, and disturbance to the oculomotor balance have been reported with Kava (Garner, 1985). Eye irritation has been reported with the heavy consumption of Kava (Ruze, 1990).

Skin: Heavy chronic consumption of Kava is associated with a peculiar, scaly rash suggestive of ichthyosis (Ruze, 1990). A reversible, slight yellowing of the skin has been associated with long-term use of Kava. Sebotropic drug reactions resulting from Kava-Kava extract therapy has been reported (Jappe, 1998).

The drug should not be taken for longer than three months without a doctor's supervision.

Drug Interactions:

Alcohol — Concomitant use of Kava Kava with alcohol results in an increase in each other's hypnotic action. The alcohol also increases the possibility for kava toxicity (Jamieson, 1990).

Alprazolam — Kava used simutaneously with alprazolam has resulted in coma (Almeida, 1996).

CNS depressants, such as barbituates — The herb may potentiate the effectiveness of substances that act on the central nervous system.

Psychoactive agents — The intensity of psychoactive agents may be intensified with kava (Jamieson, 1990).

Dopamine — Kava Kava has been reported to antagonize the effect of dopamine. Patients with Parkinson's Disease taking levodopa should avoid the use of the herb (Baum, 1998; Cupp, 1999; Schelosky, 1995).

Pregnancy: The drug is contraindicated during pregnancy.

Nursing Mothers: The drug is contraindicated in nursing mothers.

OVERDOSAGE

Overdosage can result in disorders of complex movement, accompanied by undisturbed consciousness, later tiredness and tendency to sleep.

DOSAGE

Mode of Administration: Comminuted rhizome and other galenic preparations for oral use.

How Supplied:
Capsules — 100 mg, 125 mg, 128 mg, 150 mg, 250 mg, 390 mg, 400 mg, 425 mg, 455 mg, 500 mg

Liquid — 1:1, 1:2

Preparation: There are a number of different extraction recipes depending on the pharmaceutical companies.

Daily Dosage:
Capsules — The root extract is taken 150 mg to 300 mg twice daily, with a daily dosage of kava pyrones 50 to 240 mg (Herberg, 1996; Lehmann, 1996).

Tincture — The tincture is taken as 30 drops with water three times daily (Chavallier, 1996).

Infusion — Take 1/2 cup twice daily (Chavallier, 1996).

Note: The drug should be administered with food or liquid due to its lipid solubility (Fachinfo Antares 120 (R), 1996). The activity of the herb is enhanced when mixtures of the kava pyrones are taken instead of a single pyrone (Jamieson, 1989).

Homeopathic Dosage: The herb is taken as 5 to 10 drops, 1 tablet or 5 to 10 globules 1 to 3 times daily, or 1 ml injection solution sc twice weekly (HAB1).

Storage: The herb should be stored away from direct light, moisture and heat at room temperature.

LITERATURE

Almeida JC & Grimsley EW, Coma from the health food store: interaction between kava and alprazolam (letter). Ann Intern Med 1996; 125:940-941.

Backhaus C, Krieglstein J, (1992) Extract of kava and its methysticin constituents protect brain tissue against ischaemic damage in rodents. J Pharmacol 215:265-269.

Baum SS, Hill R, Rommelspacher H, Effect of kava extract and individual kavapyrones on neurotransmitter levels in the nucleus accumbens of rats. Prog Neuropsychopharmacol Biol Psychiatry 1998 Oct;22(7):1105-20.

Bhate H, Gerster G, Fracza E, (1989) Orale Prämedikation mit Zubereitungen aus Piper methysticum bei operativen Eingriffen in Epiduralanästhesie. Erfahrungsheilkunde 6:339-345.

Bhate H, Gerster G, Behandlung mit Phytotranquilizern vor der Narkose. Therapeutikon 1992 5:214-222.

Chavallier, A, The Encyclopedia of Medicinal Plants. DK Publishing Company, New York, New York, 1996.

Cupp MJ, Herbal remedies: adverse effects and drug interactions. Am Fam Physician 1999 Mar 1;59(5):1239-45.

Davies LP, Drew CA, Duffield P et al., Kava pyrones and resin: studies on GABAA, GABAB and benzodiazepine binding sites in rodent brain. Pharmacol Toxicol 1992 Aug;71(2):120-6.

Dingermann T, Phytopharmaka im Alter: Crataegus, Ginkgo, Hypericum und Kava-Kava. In: PZ 140(23):2017-2024. 1995.

Emser W, Bartylla K, (1991) Verbesserung der Schlafqualität. TW Neurol Psychiatr 5:636-642.

Fachinformation: Antares (R) 120, kava-kava extract. Krewel Meuselbach GmbH, Eitorf, 1996.

Fachinformation: Kavasporal (R) forte, kava-kava extract. Mueller Goeppingen Gmbh & Co KG, Goeppingen, 1996.

Friese J, Gleitz J, Kavain, dihydrokavain, and dihydromethysticin non-competitively inhibit the specific binding of [3H]-batrachotoxinin-A 20-alpha-benzoate to receptor site 2 of voltage-gated Na+ channels. Planta Med 1998 Jun;64(5):458-9.

Garner LF & Klinger JD, Some visual effects caused by the beverage kava. J Ethnopharmacol 1985; 13:307-311.

Geβner B, Cnota P, (1994) Untersuchung der Vigilanz nach Applikation von Kava-Kava-Extrakt, Diazepam oder Placebo. Z Phytother 15:30-37.

Gleitz J, Beile A, Wilkens P et al., Antithrombotic action of the kava pyrone (+)-kavain prepared from Piper methysticum on human platelets. Planta Med 1997 Feb;63(1):27-30.

Gleitz J et al., Kavain inhibits non-stereospecifically veratridine-activated Na+; channels. Planta Med 62(6):580-581. 1996.

Gleitz J, Friese J, Beile A et al., Anticonvulsive action of (+/-)-kavain estimated from its properties on stimulated synaptosomes and Na+ channel receptor sites. Eur J Pharmacol 1996 Nov 7;315(1):89-97.

Gleitz J, Beile A, Peters T et al., (+/-)-Kavain inhibits veratridine-activated voltage-dependent Na(+)-channels in synaptosomes prepared from rat cerebral cortex. Neuropharmacology 1995 Sep;34(9):1133-8.

Hänsel R, Beiersdorff HU, (1955) Arzneim Forsch 9:581.

Hänsel R, Kava-Kava (Piper methysticum G. Forster), in der modernen Arzneimittelforschung Portarit einer Arzneipflanze. In: ZPT 17(3):180-195. 1996.

Hänsel R, Pflanzliche Sedativa. In: ZPT 11(1):14. 1990.

Hänsel R, Woelk H, (1995) Spektrum Kava-Kava. 2. Auflage. Aesopus Verlag GmbH, Basel.

Herberg KW, Alltagssicherheit unter Kava-Kava-Extrakt, Bromazepam und deren Kombination. Z Allge Med 1996;72:973-977.

Herberg KW, (1991) Fahrtüchtigkeit nach Einnahme von Kava-Spezial-Extrakt WS 1490. Z Allge Med 67:842-846.

Jamieson DD, Duffield PH, The antinociceptive actions of kava components in mice. Clin Exp Pharmacol Physiol 1990 Jul;17(7):495-507.

Jamieson DD, Duffield PH, Cheng D et al., Comparison of the central nervous system activity of the aqueous and lipid extract of kava (Piper methysticum). Arch Int Pharmacodyn Ther 1989 Sep-Oct;301:66-80.

Jamieson DD, Duffield PH, Positive interaction of ethanol and kava resin in mice. Clin Exp Pharmacol Physiol 1990 Jul;17(7):509-14.

Jappe U, Franke I, Reinhold D et al., Sebotrophic drug reaction from kava-kava extract therapy: a new entity? J Am Acad Dermatol 1998; 38(1):104-106.

Johnson E, Frauendorf A, Stecker K, Stein U, (1991) Neurophysiologisches Wirkprofil und Verträglichkeit von Kava-Extrakt WS 1490. TW Neurol Psychiatr 5:349-354.

Jussofie A et al., Kavapyrone enriched extract from Piper methysticum as modulator of the GABA binding site in different regions of rat brain. Psychopharmacology (Berl). 1994 Dec;116(4):469-74.

Kinzler E, Krömer J, Lehmann, (1991) Wirksamkeit eines Kava-Spezial-Extraktes bei Patienten mit Angst-, Spannungs- und Erregungszuständen nicht-psychotischer Genese. Arzneim Forsch/Drug Res 41:584-588.

Lehmann E, Kinzler E, Friedemann J, Efficacy of a special Kava extract (piper methysticum) in patients with states of anxiety, tension and excitedness of non-mental origin - A double-blind placebo-controlled study of four weeks treatment. Phytomedicine 1996;2:113-119.

Mathews JD, Riley MD, Fejo L et al., Effects of the heavy usage of kava on physical health: summary of a pilot survey in an Aboriginal community. Med J Aust 1988; 148:548-555.

Münte TF, Heinze HJ, Matzke M, Steitz J, (1993) Effects of oxacepam and an extract of Kava roots (Piper methysticum) on event-related potentials in a word recognition task. Neuropsychobiology 27:46-53.

Norton SA & Ruze P, Kava dermopathy. J Am Acad Dermatol 1994; 31:89-97.

Ruze P, Kava-induced dermopathy: a niacin deficiency? Lancet 1990 Jun 16:335(8703):1442-1445.

Schelosky L, Raffauf C, Jendroska K et al., Kava and dopamine antagonism. J Neurol Neurosurg Psychiatry 1995 May;58(5):639-40.

Schirrmacher K, Busselberg D, Langosch JM et al., Effects of (+/-)-kavain on voltage-activated inward currents of dorsal root ganglion cells from neonatal rats. Eur Neuropsychopharmacol 1999 Jan;9(1-2):171-6.

Schmidt M, Kava-Kava. In: PTA 8(5):374. 1994.

Seitz U, Schule A, Gleitz J, [3H]-monoamine uptake inhibition properties of kava pyrones. Planta Med 1997 Dec;63(6):548-9.

Siegel RK, (1976) Herbal intoxication. Psychoactive effects from herbal cigarettes, tea and capsules. JAMA 236:473-476.

Singh YN, Effects of kava on neuromuscular transmission and muscle contractility. J Ethnopharmacol. 1983 May;7(3):267-76.

Smith RM, (1979) Tetrahedron 35(3):437.

Spree MH, Croy HH, Antares - ein standardisiertes Kava-Kava-Präparat mit dem Spezialextrakt KW 1491. Der Kassenarzt. 1992;17:44-51.

Stahl S, Ehret V, Dahm HH et al., Necrotizing hepatitis after taking herbal remedies. Dtsch Med Wochenschr 1998; 123(47):1410-1414.

Uebelhack R, Franke L, Schewe HJ, Inhibition of platelet MAO-B by kava pyrone-enriched extract from Piper methysticum Forster (kava-kava). Pharmacopsychiatry 1998 Sep;31(5):187-92.

Volz HP, Kieser M, Kava-Kava Extract WS 1490 versus Placebo in Anxiety Disorders - A Randomized Placebo-controlled 25-week Outpatients Trial. Pharmacopsychiatry 1997 Jan;30(1):1-5.

Volz HP, (1995) Die anxiolytische Wirksamkeit von Kava-Spezialextrakt WS 1490 unter Langzeittherapie - eine randomisierte Doppelblindstudie. Z Phytother Abstractband, S 9.

Volz HP, Hänsel R, (1994) Kava-Kava und Kavain in der Psychopharmakotherapie. Psychopharmakotherapie 1:33-39.

Warnecke G, Pfaender H, Gerster G, Gracza E, (1990) Wirksamkeit von Kawa-Kawa-Extrakt beim klimakterischen Syndrom. Z Phytother 11:81-86.

Woelk H et al., Behandlung von Angst-Patienten. Z Allgemeinmed 1993;10:271-277.

Further information in:

Hänsel R, Keller K, Rimpler H, Schneider G (Hrsg.), Hagers Handbuch der Pharmazeutischen Praxis, 5. Aufl., Bde 4-6 (Drogen), Springer Verlag Berlin, Heidelberg, New York, 1992-1994.

Lewin L, Gifte und Vergiftungen, 6. Aufl., Nachdruck, Haug Verlag, Heidelberg 1992.

Madaus G, Lehrbuch der Biologischen Arzneimittel, Bde 1-3, Nachdruck, Georg Olms Verlag Hildesheim 1979.

Roth L, Daunderer M, Kormann K, Giftpflanzen, Pflanzengifte, 4. Aufl., Ecomed Fachverlag Landsberg Lech 1993.

Schulz R, Hänsel R, Rationale Phytotherapie, Springer Verlag Heidelberg 1996.

Steinegger E, Hänsel R, Pharmakognosie, 5. Aufl., Springer Verlag Heidelberg 1992.

Teuscher E, Biogene Arzneimittel, 5. Aufl., Wiss. Verlagsges. Stuttgart 1997.

Wagner H, Wiesenauer M, Phytotherapie. Phytopharmaka und pflanzliche Homöopathika, Fischer-Verlag, Stuttgart, Jena, New York 1995.

Wichtl M (Hrsg.), Teedrogen, 4. Aufl., Wiss. Verlagsges. Stuttgart 1997.

Kelp

Laminaria hyperborea

DESCRIPTION

Medicinal Parts: The medicinal part is the stem-like part of the thallus.

Flower and Fruit: The plant fits the general description of brown algae. It is unsegmented to heavily segmented and can grow into plants many meters in length. The thallus is reminiscent of root, leaf or stem-like organs (in the case of *L. hyperborea* stem-like). The color is greenish-brown to reddish.

Habitat: The plant grows on the North Atlantic coast.

Production: Kelp consists of the dried, stem-like parts of the thallus of Laminaria hyperborea (syn. Laminaria cloustonii).

ACTIONS AND PHARMACOLOGY

COMPOUNDS

Salts of alginic acid (laminaric acid, 25%)

Iodine (to some extent organically bound, 0.3-0.45%)

Reserve carbohydrates: laminarin (47%), mannitol (5-6%), fucoidin, mannitol glucoside

EFFECTS

No information is available.

INDICATIONS AND USAGE

Unproven Uses: Preparations of kelp are used for the regulation of thyroid function.

PRECAUTIONS AND ADVERSE REACTIONS

No health hazards or side effects are known in conjunction with the proper administration of designated therapeutic dosages. The danger of induction or worsening of hyperthyroidism following internal administration of the drug exists with dosages above 150 µg iodide per day. In rare cases, it can lead to severe allergic reactions.

DOSAGE

No information is available.

LITERATURE

Chen FP, Soong YK, Hui YL, Successful treatment of severe uterine synechiae with transcervical resectoscopy combined with laminaria tent. Hum Reprod, 75:943-7, 1997 May.

Chiu KW, Fung AY, The cardiovascular effects of green beans (Phaseolus aureus) common rue (Ruta graveolens) and kelp (Laminaria Japonica) in rats. Gen Pharmacol, 75:859-62, 1997 Nov.

Drozhzhina VA, Petrishchev NN, Fedorov IuA, The enhancement of the physiological resistance of the periodontal tissues in white rats under the action of biologically active substances from Laminaria. Fiziol Zh Im I M Sechenova, 75:126-33, 1995 Dec.

Glatstein IZ, Pang SC, McShane PM, Successful pregnancies with the use of laminaria tents before embryo transfer for refractory cervical stenosis. Fertil Steril, 75:1172-4, 1997 Jun.

Jain JK, Mishell DR Jr, A comparison of misoprostol with and without laminaria tents for induction of second-trimester abortion. Am J Obstet Gynecol, 75:173-7, 1996 Jul.

Kern W, List PH, Hörhammer L (Hrsg.), Hagers Handbuch der Pharmazeutischen Praxis, 4. Aufl., Bde. 1-8, Springer Verlag Berlin, Heidelberg, New York, 1969.

Lin A, Kupferminc M, Dooley SL, A randomized trial of extra-amniotic saline infusion versus laminaria for cervical ripening. Obstet Gynecol, 75:545-9, 1995 Oct.

Nguyen MT, Hoffman DR, Anaphylaxis to Laminaria. J Allergy Clin Immunol, 75:138-9, 1995 Jan.

Read SM, Currie G, Bacic A, Analysis of the structural heterogeneity of laminarin by electrospray-ionisation-mass spectrometry. Carbohydr Res, 75:187-201, 1996 Feb 23.

Schneider D, Halperin R, Langer R, Caspi E, Bukovsky I, Abortion at 18-22 weeks by laminaria dilation and evacuation. Obstet Gynecol, 75:412-4, 1996 Sep.

Khat

Catha edulis

DESCRIPTION

Medicinal Parts: The medicinal parts of the tree are the leaves.

Flower and Fruit: The inflorescence is a cyme growing from the leaf axil. The flowers are radial and inconspicuous, with a fleshy disk and their structures are in fives. The calyx is 5-lobed and there are 5 elongate-oval, white-yellowish petals, 5 stamens, and 3 blunt stigmas. The fruit is 3-sided capsule with chamber containing 1, occasionally 2, seeds. The brownish seeds have a wing-like, whitish aril.

Leaves: Khat is an evergreen shrub or tree that reaches about 2 to 25 m high. The leaves are opposite on flowering branches. They are alternate, coriaceous, 3 to 12 cm long, oval to ovate and crenate or dentate. The upper surface of the leaves is wax-like glossy and olive green. The older leaves are occasionally red-violet.

Habitat: Ethiopia, Kenya, North Yemen, and northern Madagascar

Production: Khat or Arabian tea is the fresh leaves or shoots of Catha edulis. The leaves are harvested in the early morning, 5 to 8 years after planting. They are kept in banana leaves, paper or plastic to prevent it drying out.

Other Names: Abyssinian Tea, Arabian Tea, Somali Tea

ACTIONS AND PHARMACOLOGY

COMPOUNDS

Phenyl alkyl amines (0.3 to 0.9%): khatamine, in fresh leaves as chief effective agent (S)-(-)-cathinone (50% in young leaves, in fully-developed leaves only 2%), becoming dimers during dehydration, as well as (+)-norpseudoephedrine (cathine), (-)-norephedrine, merucathinone, pseudomerucathinone, (-)-formyl norephedrine

Sesquiterpene polyester alkaloids: cathaedulines K1 to K15

Catechin tannins

Volatile oil

EFFECTS

The alkaloid-containing drug (chief active ingredient cathinone) is centrally stimulating and indirectly sympathomimetic (amphetamine-like effect). In addition, the leaf preparations have ulcer-protective and insecticidal effects, and the drug's high tannin content makes it constipating.

INDICATIONS AND USAGE

Unproven Uses: Khat has been used for centuries in Islamic culture to improve communicative abilities, performance and to suppress feelings of hunger. The leaves can be chewed or administered as an infusion (Yemen) or paste (Ethiopia/Somalia). Khat leaves are said to have an aphrodisiac effect and are used for depression, headache, gonorrhea, gastric complaints, coughs, asthma and fever.

The medicinal use of Khat preparations is obsolete today.

PRECAUTIONS AND ADVERSE REACTIONS

The fresh shoot tips may lead to central excitation, suppression of appetite, widening of the pupils, increased motor activity, hypertonia and hyperthermia through the sympathomimetic effect of cathinone (the other constituents account for only approximately 10% of the effect) and its ability to bypass the blood-brain barrier. Moderate dosages (100 to 300 g of the fresh leaves) lead to a state of general well being, mental alertness and exaggerated self-regard. Physical ability is temporarily enhanced and the need for sleep is reduced. Depression and anxiety states can follow once the effect wears off. Diabetics could experience hyperglycemia. The tannin content of the drug leads to constipation and digestive disorders. Acute poisonings have not been recorded.

Chronic use can lead to such long-term ill effects as emaciation (through appetite suppression), increased susceptibility to infection, nervousness, insomnia and disturbances of the circadian rhythm. In addition, Khat preparations have been associated with ulcers in the digestive tract and liver and kidney damage. When the drug is used over periods of years, it can lead to personality disorders.

DOSAGE

Mode of Administration: Available as whole herb and powdered drug

Storage: Can be kept for several months deep-frozen

LITERATURE

Al-Ahdal MN, McGarry TJ, Hannan MA Cytotoxicity of Khat (Catha edulis) extract on cultured mammalian cells: effects on macromolecule biosynthesis. Mutat Res, 204:317-22, 1988 Feb

Al-Meshal IA, Tariq M, Parmar NS, Ageel AM Anti-inflammatory activity of the flavonoid fraction of khat (Catha edulis Forsk). Agents Actions, 19:379-80, 1986 Jan

Bálint GS, Bálint E Kath (Catha edulis) - a plant containing an amphetamine-like substançe Orv Hetil, 136:1063-6, 1995 May 14

Dhadphale M, Mengech A, Chege SW Miraa (catha edulis) as a cause of psychosis. East Afr Med J, 19:130-5, 1981 Feb

Geisshüsler S, Brenneisen R The content of psychoactive phenylpropyl and phenylpentenyl khatamines in Catha edulis Forsk. of different origin. J Ethnopharmacol, 19:269-77, 1987 May

Geisshüsler S, Brenneisen R The presumed neurotoxic effects of Catha edulis - an exotic plant now available in the United Kingdom. Br J Ophthalmol, 19:779-81, 1986 Oct

Hänsel R, Keller K, Rimpler H, Schneider G (Ed) Hagers Handbuch der Pharmazeutischen Praxis. 5. Aufl., Bde 4 - 6 (Drogen), Springer Verlag Berlin, Heidelberg, New York, 1992-1994

Kalix P Catha edulis, a plant that has amphetamine effects. Pharm World Sci, 18:69-73, 1996 Apr

Kalix P Hyperthermic response to (-)-cathinone, an alkaloid of Catha edulis (khat). J Pharm Pharmacol, 11:662-3, 1980 Sep

Nabil Z, Saleh M, Mekkawy H, Allah GA Effects of an extract of khat (Catha edulis) on the toad heart. J Ethnopharmacol, 18:245-56, 1986 Dec

Nencini P, Amiconi G, Befani O, Abdullahi MA, Anania MC Possible involvement of amine oxidase inhibition in the sympathetic activation induced by khat (Catha edulis) chewing in humans. J Ethnopharmacol, 11:79-86, 1984 Jun

Tariq M, Al-Meshal I, Al-Saleh A Toxicity studies on Catha edulis. Dev Toxicol Environ Sci, 11:337-40, 1983

Knautia arvensis

See Field Scabious

Knotweed

Polygonum aviculare

DESCRIPTION

Medicinal Parts: The medicinal parts are the herb, sometimes with the root, collected during the flowering season and dried, as well as the fresh aerial parts collected during the flowering season.

Flower and Fruit: The inflorescences are axillary cymes with 1 or a few flowers. The flowers are very small, short-pedicled, inconspicuous and green or red with white margins. The epicalyx has 5 bracts and is fused at the base. There are 5 stamens, and the superior ovary has 3 styles. The fruit is a nut, which is as long as the epicalyx and is matte brown with wrinkled stripes, ovate to almost elliptical and flattened on 3 sides.

Leaves, Stem and Root: The plant is a sturdy annual. The main stem is initially erect, up to 1 m high and heavily branched. It later becomes closely procumbent and spreads along the ground. The leaves are alternate, entire-margined, short-petioled with varying forms on the main and side shoots. They are broadly elliptical to linear-lanceolate, acute or obtuse. At the base of the leaves there is a scarious divided leaf sheath. The thin, fusiform, brownish roots produce a few hair-thin lateral roots.

Characteristics: The appearance depends on the location. It may also have an ascending stem.

Habitat: The plant is found in most temperate regions of the world.

Production: Knotweed herb consists of the dried herb, occasionally containing roots, of Polygonum aviculare, gathered during flowering season.

Other Names: Allseed Nine-Joints, Armstrong, Beggarweed, Bird's Tongue, Birdweed, Centinode, Cow Grass, Crawl-grass, Doorweed, Hogweed, Knotgrass, Ninety-Knot, Pig-rush, Pigweed, Red Robin, Sparrow Tongue, Swine's Grass, Swynel Grass

ACTIONS AND PHARMACOLOGY

COMPOUNDS

Flavonoids (0.1-1%): chief components are avicularin (quercetin-3-arabinoside), hyperoside, quercitrin, quercetin-3-galactoside, additionally including among others vitexin, isovitexin, rhamnazine bisulphate

Silicic acid (1%): partially water-soluble

Tannins

Hydroxycoumarins: umbelliferone, scopoletin

Lignans: aviculin

EFFECTS

Knotweed has astringent properties. In vitro, the flavonoid fraction is said to inhibit aggregation of human erythrocytes, probably by an effect on cyclo-oxigenase.

INDICATIONS AND USAGE

Approved by Commission E:

- Cough/bronchitis
- Inflammation of the mouth and pharynx

The herb is used as a mild catarrh of the respiratory tract for inflammatory changes to the oral and pharyngeal mucosa.

Unproven Uses: In folk medicine it is used as a supportive treatment for pulmonary disorders, as a perspiration inhibitor in cases of tuberculosis, as a diuretic, as a hemostatic in cases of hemorrhage and for skin disorders.

Chinese Medicine: In China, Knotweed is used for gonorrhoea, jaundice, skin defects, dysentery (red), itching and tapeworm in children.

Homeopathic Uses: In homeopathy, Polygonum aviculare is used for rheumatism of the fingers.

PRECAUTIONS AND ADVERSE REACTIONS

No health hazards or side effects are known in conjunction with the proper administration of designated therapeutic dosages.

DOSAGE

Mode of Administration: As a ground herb for teas and other galenic preparations for internal use and local application. The drug is a component of various pectoral and bronchial teas. The extract is found in standardized preparations of antitussives and diuretics.

Preparation: To make a tea, place 1.5 gm finely cut drug in cold water and bring to a simmer. Strain after 5 to 10 minutes (1 teaspoonful = 1.4 gm drug).

Daily Dosage: The daily dosage is 4 to 6 gm of drug.

Tea—As a supportive treatment for coughs and bronchial catarrh, drink 1 cup 3 to 5 times a day.

Infusion for external use—The daily dose is 5 g drug.

Homeopathic Dosage: 5 drops, 1 tablet or 10 globules every 30 to 60 minutes (acute) or 1 to 3 times daily (chronic); parenterally: 1 to 2 ml sc, acute: 3 times daily; chronic: once a day (HAB34)

LITERATURE

Hänsel R, Keller K, Rimpler H, Schneider G (Hrsg.), Hagers Handbuch der Pharmazeutischen Praxis, 5. Aufl., Bde 4-6 (Drogen), Springer Verlag Berlin, Heidelberg, New York, 1992-1994.

Haverland F, PA 18:59-87. 1963.

Madaus G, Lehrbuch der Biologischen Arzneimittel, Bde 1-3, Nachdruck, Georg Olms Verlag Hildesheim 1979.

Steinegger E, Hänsel R, Pharmakognosie, 5. Aufl., Springer Verlag Heidelberg 1992.

Wichtl M (Hrsg.), Teedrogen, 4. Aufl., Wiss. Verlagsges. Stuttgart 1997.

Kombe Seed

Strophanthus hispidus

DESCRIPTION

Medicinal Parts: The medicinal part of the plant is the ripe seed.

Flower and Fruit: The inflorescence is a many-blossomed, umbelliferous raceme. The flowers are radial and their structures are in fives. The sepals are 1.3 to 1 cm long and 0.1 to 1 cm wide. They are unevenly divided into five, the outer tips ovate, the inner ones lanceolate and densely pubescent. The corolla is tubular, with the upper part broadened into a cup shape. The margin is covered with 10 scales, 1.1 to 2 cm long with a diameter of 0.8 to 1.7 cm. The margin is white or yellow, with a purple spot in the shaft. There are 5 stamens and a 2-chambered, semi-inferior ovary. The fruit is a follicle, 24 to 48 cm long, 1.3 to 1.8 cm in diameter, dark brown, hard, grooved and white punctate with lenticles. The seeds are spindle-shaped, flat, 1 to 1.8 cm long, 2 to 3 mm wide, densely pubescent with an upright, 4 to 8 cm long tuft of hair.

Leaves, Stem and Root: Strophanthus hispidus is either a liana, up to 100 m long, or a shrub, up to 5 m high. The leaves are opposite. The petiole is 1 to 5 mm long, the lamina 15 to 22 cm long and 8 to 12 cm wide. They are simple, elliptical to obovate, acuminate, rounded at the base or cordate. The trunk has a diameter of up to 6 m and has dark gray bark. The branches are dark brown or almost black. The young branches are stiffly villous and punctate with lenticles.

Characteristics: The plant contains latex.

Habitat: West and Central Africa

Production: Brown Strophanthus seeds are the ripe seeds of Strophanthus hispidus freed from the bushel-like appendage. The seeds are first harvested after 3 years (first flowering). Then the fruit is picked, and the seeds are removed.

Not to be Confused With: Often confused in the past with Strophanthus kombe, S. sarmentosus and other Strophanthus species. Can also be confused with Alafia, Futumia, Kickxia and Holrrhena species.

Other Names: Arrow Poison

ACTIONS AND PHARMACOLOGY

COMPOUNDS

Cardioactive steroid glycosides (cardenolids, 4 to 8%): chief glycoside presumably k-strophanthoside (primary glycoside, strophanthidin glucosyl cymaroside) from which cymarin (strophantidin cymaroside) is formed through fermentation of the seeds

Saponins (0.2%)

Fatty oil (30%): chief fatty acids oleic acid, linoleic acid, palmitic acid and 9-hydroxy-delta12-octadecenoic acid

EFFECTS

The action mechanism of the drug is dependent upon the cardioactive cardenolide glycosides it contains (see S. kombé semen and strophantine effects).

INDICATIONS AND USAGE

Unproven Uses: Preparations of the herb have been used in the past for cardiac complaints.

Homeopathic Uses: In homeopathy, preparations are used for nervous cardiac complaints and cardiac insufficiency.

PRECAUTIONS AND ADVERSE REACTIONS

General: No health hazards are known in conjunction with the proper administration of designated therapeutic dosages.

Drug Interactions: The simultaneous administration of quinidine, calcium salts, saluretics, laxatives and glucocorticoids enhance effects and side effects. For symptoms of an acute poisoning and treatment, see Digitalis folium.

OVERDOSAGE

Nausea, vomiting, headache, stupor and cardiac arrhythmias could occur as side effects with parenteral administration of glycoside mixtures of the drug, particularly with overdoses.

DOSAGE

Mode of Administration: Communited drug, herb powder, liquid preparations for internal use.

Homeopathic Dosage: (from D4) 5 drops, 1 tablet, 10 globules every to 30 to 60 minutes, maximum 12 times daily (acute) and 1 to 3 times daily (chronic); parenterally: 1 to 2 ml sc., IV, IM, 3 times daily (acute) and once a day (chronic) (HPUS88).

LITERATURE

Hänsel R, Keller K, Rimpler H, Schneider G (Ed), Hagers Handbuch der Pharmazeutischen Praxis, 5. Aufl., Bde 4 - 6 (Drogen), Springer Verlag Berlin, Heidelberg, New York, 1992-1994

Kousso

Hagenia abyssinica

DESCRIPTION

Medicinal Parts: The medicinal parts are the leaves, the unripe fruit and the dried panicles of female flowers.

Flower and Fruit: The small flowers are large-branched, thickly glandular-haired panicles up to 0.5 m long. They are androgynous, male or female. The male flowers are greenish and have fertile stamens and hairy bracts. The female flowers are dark-red.

Leaves, Stem and Root: Hagenia abyssinica is tree that grows up to 6 m high with tuft-like, erect, pinnatifid leaves.

Habitat: The plant is indigenous to northeast Africa and is cultivated in Ethiopia.

Production: Kousso flowers are the flowers of Hagenia abyssinica.

Other Names: Cossoo, Kooso, Kosso

ACTIONS AND PHARMACOLOGY

COMPOUNDS

Acylphloroglucinols (kosotoxine): monomeric, dimeric, trimeric compounds, such as protocosin (trimeric); acyl residues are isobutyryl- isovaleryl- and alpha-metylbutyryl residues; representatives include, for example, cosin K6 and cosin K8 (monomerous), cusso toxin (dimerous), protocosin (trimerous)

Tannins

EFFECTS

Kousso is a vermifuge because of its complex mixture of aglyphloroglucinols, which has a taeiafugic effect. An antitumoral effect has also been described

INDICATIONS AND USAGE

Unproven Uses: This obsolete drug, which can no longer be procured, formerly was used to treat tapeworm infestation. Its efficacy depended on the composition of the drug.

PRECAUTIONS AND ADVERSE REACTIONS

Side effects include irritation of the gastrointestinal tract, salivation, nausea and diarrhea. A tendency toward fainting spells, headache and general weakness has been connected with the use of the drug during use as a tapeworm cure. Abortive effects have been described. The drug should no longer be administered in allopathic dosages.

OVERDOSAGE

Conditions of collapse and vision disorders have been observed with overdosages. The treatment for poisoning consists of gastrointestinal emptying (inducement of vomiting, gastric lavage with burgundy-colored potassium permanganate solution, sodium sulfate), installation of activated charcoal and shock prophylaxis (quiet, warmth). Diazepam (intravenous) should be used to treat spasms. Atropine and electrolyte substitution should be employed. Possible cases of acidosis should be countered with sodium bicarbonate infusions. In case of shock, plasma volume expanders should be administered. Monitoring of kidney function is essential. Intubation and oxygen respiration may also be necessary.

DOSAGE

Mode of Administration: The drug is obsolete in most countries.

LITERATURE

Kern W, List PH, Hörhammer L (Hrsg.), Hagers Handbuch der harmazeutischen Praxis, 4. Aufl., Bde. 1-8, Springer Verlag Berlin, Heidelberg, New York, 1969.

Lewin L, Gifte und Vergiftungen, 6. Aufl., Nachdruck, Haug Verlag, Heidelberg 1992.

Madaus G, Lehrbuch der Biologischen Arzneimittel, Bde 1-3, Nachdruck, Georg Olms Verlag Hildesheim 1979.

Metzner J et al., Antispastische Wirkung von Hagenia abyssinica. In: PM 47(4):240-241. 1983.

Roth L, Daunderer M, Kormann K, Giftpflanzen, Pflanzengifte, 4. Aufl., Ecomed Fachverlag Landsberg Lech 1993.

Schiemenz GP, Schroeder JM, Z Naturforsch 40B(5):669-680. 1985

Teuscher E, Lindequist U, Biogene Gifte - Biologie, Chemie, Pharmakologie, 2. Aufl., Fischer Verlag Stuttgart 1994. Metzner J et al Antispastische Wirkung von Hagenia abyssinica. Planta Med 47 (1983), 240-241

Woldemariam TZ, Fell AF, Linley PA, Chromatographic and spectroscopic studies on the constituents in male and female flowers of Hagenia abyssinica. J Pharm Biomed Anal, 8:859-65, 1990.

Woldemariam TZ, Fell AF, Linley PA, Bibby MC, Phillips RM, Evaluation of the anti-tumour action and acute toxicity of kosins from Hagenia abyssinica. J Pharm Biomed Anal, 10:555-60, 1992 Aug

Krameria triandra

See Rhatany

Labrador Tea

Ledum latifolium

DESCRIPTION

Medicinal Parts: The medicinal parts are the leaves and the flowering shoots.

Flower and Fruit: The flowers are in flat, terminal umbels. The calyx is small and has 5 tips. The 5-petalled corolla is white. The 10 stamens grow from the edge of a honey ring. The ovary is superior. The fruit is a 5-valvular capsule.

Leaves, Stem and Root: The evergreen, branched shrub grows to about 1.5 m. The young branches are gray or rust-colored. The 1.25 to 2.5 cm long leaves are alternate, short-petioled, entire-margined, and linear, have revolute margins, and are stiff, coriaceous, dark green above, rust-colored and woolly-downy underneath. L. palustre is larger, more regularly formed and has larger leaves.

Characteristics: It has a numbing, tangy aroma and is poisonous. It is a protected species.

Habitat: The plant grows in Greenland, Canada and the U.S. The very similar variety L. palustre is more common in northern Europe and northern Asia.

Production: Labrador herb is the aerial part of Ledum latifolium and L. palustre.

Other Names: St. James's Tea, Marsh Tea, Wild Rosemary

ACTIONS AND PHARMACOLOGY

COMPOUNDS

Volatile oil (0.9-2.6%): chief components sesquiterpenes, in particular ledol (ledum camphor, porst camphor) and palustrol, Japanese sources also yield ascaridol

Catechin tannins

Flavonoids: including among others hyperoside

Hydroglycosides: arbutin

EFFECTS

Internally mildly expectorant. Externally antiphlogistic (neither proven).

INDICATIONS AND USAGE

Unproven Uses: Labrador Tea has been used for respiratory conditions. Externally, it has been used for skin inflammation.

CONTRAINDICATIONS

The drug is contraindicated in pregnancy.

PRECAUTIONS AND ADVERSE REACTIONS

General: Initially, the drug causes severe gastrointestinal irritation (vomiting, gastroenteritis, diarrhea), due to its ledol content. Following absorption, the drug causes severe CNS excitation. This effect may lead to spasms and paralysis in some cases.

Pregnancy: Contraindicated. Poisonings in earlier times were seen in connection with its misuse for purposes of abortion.

OVERDOSAGE

Following gastrointestinal emptying (inducement of vomiting, gastric lavage with burgundy-colored potassium permanganate solution, sodium sulfate), and instillation of activated charcoal, the treatment of poisonings consists of treating spasms with diazepam (I.V.) and colic with atropine; electrolyte substitution and treating possible cases of acidosis with sodium bicarbonate infusions. Monitoring of kidney function is essential. Intubation and oxygen respiration may also be necessary.

DOSAGE

Mode of Administration: Labrador Tea is obsolete as a drug. It has been used as an extract in some bath additives and is also contained in homeopathic preparations.

LITERATURE

Frohne D, Pfänder HJ, Giftpflanzen - Ein Handbuch für Apotheker, Toxikologen und Biologen, 4. Aufl., Wiss. Verlags-Ges. Stuttgart 1997.

Kern W, List PH, Hörhammer L (Hrsg.), Hagers Handbuch der Pharmazeutischen Praxis, 4. Aufl., Bde. 1-8, Springer Verlag Berlin, Heidelberg, New York, 1969.

Lewin L, Gifte und Vergiftungen, 6. Aufl., Nachdruck, Haug Verlag, Heidelberg 1992.

Madaus G, Lehrbuch der Biologischen Arzneimittel, Bde 1-3, Nachdruck, Georg Olms Verlag Hildesheim 1979.

Roth L, Daunderer M, Kormann K, Giftpflanzen, Pflanzengifte, 4. Aufl., Ecomed Fachverlag Landsberg Lech 1993.

Teuscher E, Lindequist U, Biogene Gifte - Biologie, Chemie, Pharmakologie, 2. Aufl., Fischer Verlag Stuttgart 1994.

Wagner H, Wiesenauer M, Phytotherapie. Phytopharmaka und pflanzliche Homöopathika, Fischer-Verlag, Stuttgart, Jena, New York 1995.

Laburnum

Cytisus laburnum

DESCRIPTION

Medicinal Parts: The seeds are the medicinal parts.

Flower and Fruit: The flowers bow down in clusters of 10 to 30. There are 10 to 25 cm long racemes. The calyx is short, campanulate, pubescent and marked brown at the base. The anthers are orange. The pod is 5 to 8 cm by 8 to 9 cm, flat, lumpy and silky-haired with wings. The seeds are flat and dark brown.

Leaves, Stem and Root: Cytisus laburnum is a small shrub or tree that can occasionally grow up to 7 m high. It has light gray branches and smooth, dark green, initially erect branchlets. The alternate leaves are almost in rosettes on short shoots with 2 to 7 cm long petioles. The leaflets are elliptical to ovate, rounded or thorn tipped. They are glabrous above and light gray pubescent beneath.

Habitat: The plant is indigenous to mountainous regions of Europe. It is also cultivated worldwide.

Other Names: Golden Chain, Pea Tree, Bean Trifoil

ACTIONS AND PHARMACOLOGY

COMPOUNDS

Quinolizidine alkaloids (1-3%): main alkaloids (-)-cytisine (95%), as well as (-)-N-methylcytisine, epibaptifoline

Lectins

EFFECTS

No information is available.

INDICATIONS AND USAGE

Unproven Uses: Experiments in the use of cytisine as a pesticide (lice) have shown that in the necessary concentration the danger of poisoning is too high.

PRECAUTIONS AND ADVERSE REACTIONS

There are no indications for this drug. The drug is severely toxic. See Overdosage section.

OVERDOSAGE

Symptoms of poisoning include nausea, dizziness, salivation, pains in the mouth, in the throat and in the stomach area, outbreaks of sweat, headache as well as extended, severe, and sometimes bloody vomiting. If no vomiting occurs, excitatory states can come about from the centrally stimulating effect of the drug, with tonic-clonic spasms that later change over into paralyses. Anuria and uremia have also been observed. Death comes through asphyxiation.

Fifteen to 20 seeds or 3 to 4 unripe berries are considered fatal for an adult. While poisonings occur relatively frequently, cases of death have not been recorded in recent times. If no vomiting has occurred, poisonings are treated with gastric lavage, then through the administration of activated charcoal; spasms are to be treated with chlorpromazine or diazepam. In cases of asphyxiation, intubation and oxygen respiration are to be carried out.

LITERATURE

Frohne D, Pfänder HJ, Giftpflanzen - Ein Handbuch für Apotheker, Toxikologen und Biologen, 4. Aufl., Wiss. Verlagsges. mbH Stuttgart 1997.

Greinwald R, Untersuchungen zur chemotaxonomischen Bedeutung von Leguminosenalkaloiden und zum Alkaloidstoffwechsel in transformierten Geweben und Zellkulturen. In: Dissertation Universität Würzburg. 1988.

Gresser G, Der Besenginster - Cytisus scoparius (L.) LINK. In: ZPT 17(5):320-330. 1996.

Hänsel R, Keller K, Rimpler H, Schneider G (Hrsg.), Hagers Handbuch der Pharmazeutischen Praxis, 5. Aufl., Bde 4-6 (Drogen), Springer Verlag Berlin, Heidelberg, New York, 1992-1994.

Lewin L, Gifte und Vergiftungen, 6. Aufl., Nachdruck, Haug Verlag, Heidelberg 1992.

Madaus G, Lehrbuch der Biologischen Arzneimittel, Bde 1-3, Nachdruck, Georg Olms Verlag Hildesheim 1979.

Roth L, Daunderer M, Kormann K, Giftpflanzen, Pflanzengifte, 4. Aufl., Ecomed Fachverlag Landsberg Lech 1993.

Seeger R, Neumann HG, Cytisin. In: DAZ 132(7):303. 1992.

Teuscher E, Lindequist U, Biogene Gifte - Biologie, Chemie, Pharmakologie, 2. Aufl., Fischer Verlag Stuttgart 1994.

Teuscher E, Biogene Arzneimittel, 5. Aufl., Wiss. Verlagsges. mbH Stuttgart 1997.

Tschirch C, Kraus L, Goldregen-Alkaloid Cytisin. In: DAZ 132(47):2560. 1992.

Wagner H, Wiesenauer M, Phytotherapie. Phytopharmaka und pflanzliche Homöopathika, Fischer-Verlag, Stuttgart, Jena, New York 1995.

Lactuca virosa

See Lactucarium

Lactucarium

Lactuca virosa

DESCRIPTION

Medicinal Parts: The medicinal parts are the dried latex and the leaves.

Flower and Fruit: The composite flowers are in pyramid-shaped panicles. The capitula have a few florets. They are androgynous, pale yellow, lingual florets. The bracts are imbricate. The fruit is 4-lipped and black with a broad edge. It is glabrous at the tip. It has a whitish beak that is as long as the fruit, making the hair tuft look stemmed.

Leaves, Stem and Root: The plant is biennial, up to 1.2 m high, with a fusiform, pale root that produces the erect, branched and hollow stem. It is smooth, light green and sometimes has purple spots. The leaves are oblong to obovate, narrowed at the base, clasping and usually simple. They are thorny-tipped, lie horizontally and are thorny on the underside of the midrib.

Characteristics: The whole plant contains milky latex.

Habitat: The plant is indigenous to western and southern Europe and is cultivated in Germany, Austria, France and Scotland.

Production: Lactucarium leaves are the leaves of the aerial part of Lactuca virosa. They are gathered when in flower and then dried.

Not to be Confused With: L.sativa, L.serriola, L.quercina and Sonchus oleraceus.

Other Names: Prickly Lettuce, Strong-Scented Lettuce, Green Endive, Lettuce Opium, Acrid Lettuce, Poison Lettuce, Wild Lettuce

ACTIONS AND PHARMACOLOGY

COMPOUNDS

Sesquiterpene lactones: lactucin, lactucopicrin (lactupictin, intybin)

Triterpenes: including among others, taraxasterol, beta-amyrin

EFFECTS

The herb is supposed to have a narcotic effect. It is an analgesic and spasmolytic, and is said to act as a tranquilizer.

INDICATIONS AND USAGE

Unproven Uses: Medicines containing Lactucarium are used to treat whooping cough attacks. The drug is used for bronchial catarrh, asthma and urinary tract diseases. The oil of the seeds is used for arteriosclerosis and was also used as wheat germ oil.

Homeopathic Uses: Lactuca virosa is used for laryngitis, tracheitis with heavy coughing, for swelling of the liver and for urinary complaints.

PRECAUTIONS AND ADVERSE REACTIONS

No health hazards or side effects are known in conjunction with the proper administration of designated therapeutic dosages. The drug possesses a low potential for sensitization.

OVERDOSAGE

The following signs of poisoning can occur through overdosage or following intake of the fresh leaves, as in salads: outbreaks of sweating, acceleration of breathing, tachycardia, pupil dilation, dizziness, ringing in the ears, vision disorders, pressure in the head, somnolence, on occasion also excitatory states. The toxicity is, however, relatively low. Following gastrointestinal emptying (inducement of vomiting, gastric lavage with burgundy-colored potassium permanganate solution, sodium sulfate), as well as instillation of activated charcoal, the treatment of poisonings should proceed symptomatically.

DOSAGE

Mode of Administration: Due to its poison content, the drug is only administered under medical supervision. It is ground and used as an alcoholic extract and further processed in the pharmaceutical industry.

LITERATURE

Frohne D, Pfänder HJ, Giftpflanzen - Ein Handbuch für Apotheker, Toxikologen und Biologen, 4. Aufl., Wiss. Verlags-Ges Stuttgart 1997.

Huang ZJ et al., (1982) J Pharm Sci 71(2):270.

Kern W, List PH, Hörhammer L (Hrsg.), Hagers Handbuch der Pharmazeutischen Praxis, 4. Aufl., Bde. 1-8, Springer Verlag Berlin, Heidelberg, New York, 1969.

Lewin L, Gifte und Vergiftungen, 6. Aufl., Nachdruck, Haug Verlag, Heidelberg 1992.

Madaus G, Lehrbuch der Biologischen Arzneimittel, Bde 1-3, Nachdruck, Georg Olms Verlag Hildesheim 1979.

Marquardt P et al., (1976) Planta Med 30:68.

Rees S, Harborne J, (1984) Bot J Linn Soc 89(4):313.

Roth L, Daunderer M, Kormann K, Giftpflanzen, Pflanzengifte, 4. Aufl., Ecomed Fachverlag Landsberg Lech 1993.

Ruban G et al., (1978) Acta Crystalogr Sect B 34(4):1163

Teuscher E, Lindequist U, Biogene Gifte - Biologie, Chemie, Pharmakologie, 2. Aufl., Fischer Verlag Stuttgart 1994.

Lady Fern

Athyrium filix-femina

DESCRIPTION

Medicinal Parts: The medicinal part is the rhizome when gathered in spring or autumn.

Leaves, Stem and Root: Athyrium filix-femina is a 10- to 40-cm high fern. The pencil-thick, creeping rhizome is densely covered with dark-brown hairs. Numerous tomentose, long, branched, dark-brown root fibers sprout from the rhizome. The not-so-numerous leaves are in rigid, upright, double rows. They are coriaceous, glabrous, oblong-lanceolate or oblong, deeply pinnatifid and wintergreen. The petioles are semi-round, smooth and whitish. On the underside of the leaf tips there are 2 parallel rows of large groups of filmless sporangia, which are initially yellowish and later turn dark brown.

Habitat: Lady Fern is indigenous to Britain, parts of Europe and the U.S.

Other Names: Common Polypody, Brake Root, Rock Brake, Rock of Polypody, Oak Fern

ACTIONS AND PHARMACOLOGY

COMPOUNDS

Tannins (8%)

C-glucosyl flavones: including mangiferin

Phytoecdysones

Amaroids

Saponin: including the steroid saponin osladin

Essential oil

EFFECTS

The drug is a mild expectorant; a choleretic-type effect is questionable.

INDICATIONS AND USAGE

Unproven Uses: The drug is used for respiratory and gastrointestinal tract illnesses.

PRECAUTIONS AND ADVERSE REACTIONS

No health hazards or side effects are known in conjunction with the proper administration of designated therapeutic dosages.

DOSAGE

Mode of Administration: The drug is obsolete in German-speaking countries. However, Lady Fern is still found in commercial preparations as drops and tablets, as well as in preparations used in the religious system of anthroposophy.

Daily Dosage: In anthroposophic medicine, the usual dose to treat gastrointestinal illnesses is 1 to 2 tablets or 10 to 20 drops taken 3 times daily.

LITERATURE

Abraham H, Zucker und Süβstoff. In: PTA 7(10):744. 1993.

Anonym, Niedere Pflanzen ganz groβ - 39. Jahrestagung der Gesellschaft für Arzneipflanzenforschung in Saarbrücken. In: DAZ 131(37):1899.

Constantinescu E et al., (1966) Pharmazie 21:121.

Hegnauer R, Chemotaxonomie der Pflanzen, Bde 1-11, Birkhäuser Verlag Basel, Boston, Berlin 1962-1997.

Jizba J et al., (1971) Tetrahedron Lett 18:1329.

Kern W, List PH, Hörhammer L (Hrsg.), Hagers Handbuch der Pharmazeutischen Praxis, 4. Aufl., Bde 1-8, Springer Verlag Berlin, Heidelberg, New York, 1969.

Madaus G, Lehrbuch der Biologischen Arzneimittel, Bde 1-3, Nachdruck, Georg Olms Verlag Hildesheim 1979.

Lady's Bedstraw

Galium verum

DESCRIPTION

Medicinal Parts: The medicinal part is the dried herb.

Flower and Fruit: The small lemon-yellow flowers are in dense terminal panicles. The peduncle is very downy. The corolla is 2 to 3 mm wide, usually golden yellow, and smells strongly of honey. The border of the calyx is pointed, and the ovaries are bivalvular and inferior. The fruit is smooth, indehiscent, 1.5 mm long, glabrous and eventually black.

Leaves, Stem and Root: The true plant is a 30 to 100 cm high herbaceous perennial with a cylindrical, creeping rhizome that sprouts runners. The stem is ascending or erect, bluntly quadrangular with 4 vertical lines, downy or glabrous and rough. The leaves are in false whorls of 8 to 12. They are linear, dark green above, and gray and short-haired beneath.

Characteristics: The flowers have a strong honey fragrance.

Habitat: The plant grows throughout Europe (with the exception of Lapland and arctic Russia), as well as in Asia Minor, Iran and Syria.

Production: Lady's Bedstraw is the herb of Galium verum, collected during the flowering season and dried.

Other Names: Yellow Galium, Cheese Rennet, Curdwort, Maid's Hair, Yellow Cleavers, Petty Mugget, Cheese Renning

ACTIONS AND PHARMACOLOGY

COMPOUNDS

Iridoids: asperuloside, monotropein, scandoside, desacetylasperulosidic acid, asperulosidic acid, geniposidic acid, daphylloside

Rennin

Flavonoids : including rutin, isorutin, palustroside, cynaroside, quercetin-3-O-glucoside, quercetin-7-O-glucoside

Anthracene derivatives

Caffeic acid ester: chlorogenic acid

EFFECTS

No information is available.

INDICATIONS AND USAGE

Unproven Uses: Internally, the drug is used in folk medicine for swollen ankles and as a diuretic for bladder and kidney irritation. Externally, it is used for poorly healing wounds. The efficacy of this drug has not been proven.

PRECAUTIONS AND ADVERSE REACTIONS

Health risks or side effects following the proper administration of designated therapeutic dosages are not recorded.

DOSAGE

Mode of Administration: Currently obsolete but formerly the drug was used internally as a tea and topically in alcoholic extracts as a moist poultice.

Preparation: To prepare a tea or infusion, pour 250 ml of cold water over 2 heaping teaspoonfuls of the drug, bring to simmering point, simmer for 2 minutes and then allow to draw.

Daily Dosage: Internally, 2 to 3 cups of tea daily.

LITERATURE

Böjthe-Horvath K et al., PH 21:2917-2919. 1982.

Borisov MI et al., Rastit Resur 11:351. 1975.

Burnett AR, Thomsom RH, (1968) J Clin Soc (6):854.

Corrigan D et al., (1978) Phytochemistry 17:1131.

Hänsel R, Keller K, Rimpler H, Schneider G (Hrsg.), Hagers Handbuch der Pharmazeutischen Praxis, 5. Aufl., Bde 4-6 (Drogen), Springer Verlag Berlin, Heidelberg, New York, 1992-1994.

Mathé I et al., (1982) Planta Med 45:158.

Raynaud J, Mnajed H, (1972) C R Acad Sci Paris 274:1746.

Wichtl M (Hrsg.), Teedrogen, 4. Aufl., Wiss. Verlagsges. Stuttgart 1997.

Lady's Mantle

Alchemilla vulgaris

DESCRIPTION

Medicinal Parts: The medicinal part is the herb collected in the flowering season and dried.

Flower and Fruit: The plant has inflorescences of small, insignificant, yellow-green, many-flowered cymes. The perianth is 4-leaved. The flower has 4 stamens, 1 ovary and an inferior style. The fruit is enclosed in the calyx. The flowers are infertile.

Leaves, Stem and Root: Alchemilla vulgaris is a hardy, half-rosette shrub, which grows from 30 to 50 cm. It has a branched stem, which is villous to glabrous. The basal leaves are round, 7- to 9-lobed (dew cup); cauline leaves are short-petioled to sessile, 5- to 7-lobed, crenate or serrate and villous. Even the older leaves remain more or less folded.

Characteristics: Lady's Mantle is odorless and has an astringent taste.

Habitat: The plant grows in the Northern Hemisphere from North America, Greenland and Europe to the Mediterranean and Iceland; and Asia from the Caucasus and the Himalayas to Siberia.

Production: Lady's Mantle herb consists of the fresh or dried above-ground parts of Alchemilla vulgaris gathered at flowering time, as well as its preparations. It is produced mostly through cultivation.

Other Names: Bear's Foot, Leontopodium, Lion's Foot, Nine Hooks, Stellaria

ACTIONS AND PHARMACOLOGY

COMPOUNDS

Bitter principles

Flavonoids

Tannins

EFFECTS

Lady's Mantle herb has astringent properties, due to the presence of tannins. It has also been shown to inhibit tumor growth. In mice the total retardation of breast neoplasm-induced tumors was achieved using agrimoniin and the average life expectancy of the animals was increased. An extract of the drug hinders the enzymes elastase, trypsin and a-chymotrysin.

INDICATIONS AND USAGE

Approved by Commission E:

- Diarrhea

Unproven Uses: Lady's Mantle is used for mild and non-specific diarrhea and gastrointestinal disorders.

In folk medicine the drug is used internally for menopausal complaints, dysmenorrhea, gastrointestinal disorders, and as a gargle for mouth and throat inflammation. Externally, it is used for ulcers, eczema, skin rashes and as an additive in baths for the treatment of lower-abdominal ailments.

Homeopathic Uses: Alchemilla vulgaris is used for leucorrhea and for chronic diarrhea resulting from liver disease.

PRECAUTIONS AND ADVERSE REACTIONS

No health hazards or side effects are known in conjunction with the proper administration of designated therapeutic dosages.

DOSAGE

Mode of Administration: Lady's Mantle herb is administered as a cut herb for infusions and decoctions, as well as other galenic preparations for internal use.

Preparation: Tea: 2 to 4 gm drug to 150 ml hot water left to draw for 10 minutes. Prepare a fresh batch every day.

Daily Dosage: Lady's Mantle herb is administered in 2 to 4 gm single doses as an infusion; the average daily dose is 5 to 10 gm of herb. The tea is taken 3 times daily between meals.

Homeopathic Dosage: 5 drops, 1 tablet, 10 globules, every 30 to 60 minutes (acute) and 1 to 3 times daily (chronic); Parenterally: 1 to 2 ml 3 times daily sc; Ointment: Apply 1 to 2 times daily (HAB1).

LITERATURE

Dorne AJ et al., PH 25:65-68. 1986.

Filípek J, The effect of Alchemilla xanthochlora on lipid peroxidation and superoxide anion scavenging acticity. In: PA 47:717-718. 1992.

Geiger C, Rimpler H, PM 56:585-586. 1990.

Geiger C, Ellagitannine aus Alchemilla xanthochlora ROTHMALER und Potentilla erecta (L.) RAEUSCHEL. Beiträge zur Analytik und Strukturaufklärung. In: Dissertation Universität Freiburg. 1990.

Schimmer O, Felser C, Alchemilla xanthochlora ROTHM.- Der Frauenmantel. In: ZPT 13(6):207. 1993.

Schimmer O, Lindenbaum M, Tannins with antimutagenic properties in the herb of Alchemilla species and Potentilla anserina. In: PM 61(2):141-145. 1995.

Further information in:

Hänsel R, Keller K, Rimpler H, Schneider G (Hrsg.), Hagers Handbuch der Pharmazeutischen Praxis, 5. Aufl., Bde 4-6 (Drogen), Springer Verlag Berlin, Heidelberg, New York, 1992-1994.

Madaus G, Lehrbuch der Biologischen Arzneimittel, Bde 1-3, Nachdruck, Georg Olms Verlag Hildesheim. 1979.

Wagner H, Wiesenauer M, Phytotherapie. Phytopharmaka und pflanzliche Homöopathika, Fischer-Verlag, Stuttgart, Jena, New York. 1995.

Wichtl M (Hrsg.), Teedrogen, 4. Aufl., Wiss. Verlagsges. Stuttgart. 1997.

Laminaria hyperborea

See Kelp

Lamium album

See White Nettle

Larch

Larix decidua

DESCRIPTION

Medicinal Parts: The medicinal part is the outer bark separated from its outermost layer.

Flower and Fruit: The female flowers are cone-shaped, erect, 2 cm long, short-pedicled, round-ovate and encircled by scales at the base. The covering scales turn dark red when in bloom. The male catkins are sessile, about 1.5 cm long, sulfur yellow, ovoid-globular. The seeds are light brown, glossy with 13 mm long and 5 mm wide wings.

Leaves, Stem and Root: Larch is a deciduous tree that grows up to 54 m high tree (stunted at high altitudes) with a straight trunk, brown-red bark and pyramid-shaped, sparsely foliated crown. The main branches are horizontal and turned up at the tips. The secondary branches are hanging. The foliage is light green with delicate needles, arranged singly in spiral rows on long shoots and in bushels on short ones. They fall in autumn.

Habitat: The plant is indigenous to central Europe, cultivated in North America. It was first introduced to England in 1639.

Production: The balsam of Larix decidua is obtained by drilling into the trunks. The balsam contains up to 20% essential oil.

Other Names: European Larch, Common Larch

ACTIONS AND PHARMACOLOGY

COMPOUNDS

Volatile oil (14-15%): chief components: (-)-alpha-pinene (70%), Delta3-carene (10%) (-)-beta-pinene (6.5%), beta-pyrones (3%)

Resins: including among others oleoresin acids (50-65%): including among others laricinolic acid, alpha- and beta-laricinolic acid

EFFECTS

When used externally the drug has a hyperemic and antiseptic effect due the essential oil content. Its use for catarrhal infections of the upper respiratory tract also seems plausible.

INDICATIONS AND USAGE

Approved by Commission E:

- Fevers and colds
- Cough/bronchitis
- Tendency for infections
- Blood pressure problems
- Inflammation of the mouth and pharynx
- Rheumatism
- Common cold

Unproven Uses: The drug has been used to treat neuralgic discomforts and furuncles.

CONTRAINDICATIONS

Inhalation may cause acute inflammation of the airway passages.

PRECAUTIONS AND ADVERSE REACTIONS

No health hazards or side effects are known in conjunction with the proper external administration of designated therapeutic dosages.

OVERDOSAGE

Resorptive poisonings, such as kidney and central nervous system damage, are possible with large-area administration. Kidney damage is conceivable with internal administration.

DOSAGE

Mode of Administration: Available in form of ointments, gels, emulsions and oils.

Preparation: Liquid and semi-solid preparations 10 to 20%.

LITERATURE

Freudenberg K, Weinges K, (1959) Tetrahedron Letters 17:19.

Kern W, List PH, Hörhammer L (Hrsg.), Hagers Handbuch der Pharmazeutischen Praxis, 4. Aufl., Bde. 1-8: Springer Verlag Berlin, Heidelberg, New York, 1969.

Larix decidua

See Larch

Larkspur

Delphinium consolida

DESCRIPTION

Medicinal Parts: The medicinal parts are the seeds of the plant.

Flower and Fruit: The flowers are in short racemes and are blue, pink or purple. The petals are fused to a helmet-like form with a honey spur at the back, which reaches into the back of the 5 sepals. There is usually only 1 glabrous ovary, but numerous stamens. The fruit is a follicle with black, flattened seeds, which have sharp edges and a scarred surface.

Leaves, Stem and Root: The plant grows from 15 to 40 cm. Larkspur is an annual and has a thin stem that is sparsely branched from the middle. The leaves are alternate and divided into narrow linear sections. The lowers ones are petioled and the upper ones sessile.

Habitat: Europe, western U.S.

Production: Delphinium flower consists of the flowers of Delphinium consolida.

Not to be Confused With: the flowers of Delphinium oriental.

Other Names: Knight's Spur, Lark Heel, Lark's Claw, Lark's Toe, Staggerweed

ACTIONS AND PHARMACOLOGY

COMPOUNDS

Diterpene alkaloids: chief alkaloid delphinine

The presence of alkaloids has sometimes been described in the literature but they cannot always be found.

EFFECTS

No information is available.

INDICATIONS AND USAGE

Unproven Uses: Larkspur is obsolete. It is used only as an inactive ingredient in tea mixtures. Preparations of delphinium flower are sometimes used as a diuretic and vermifuge, as a sedative and an appetite stimulant. In folk medicine, Larkspur is used occasionally as a diuretic. It was formerly used as an anthelmintic.

PRECAUTIONS AND ADVERSE REACTIONS

Health risks or side effects following the proper administration of designated therapeutic dosages are not recorded.

OVERDOSAGE

Although the delphine has a paralyzing effect upon peripheral and motor nerve endings and the central nervous system, poisonings among humans by Delphinium consolida have never been observed.

Toxic dosages in animal experiments have led to death through asphyxiation (LD50 rabbits 1.5-3.0 mg/kg body weight, I.V.). Poisonings of animals with fatal results by Delphinium species are particularly frequent in the U.S.

DOSAGE

Mode of Administration: Since the efficacy of Delphinium and its preparations is not documented, a therapeutic administration cannot be recommended.

Preparation: Larkspur is found only in teas, often as an inactive ingredient.

LITERATURE

Atta-ur-Rahman AM, Nasreen A, Akhtar F, Shekhani MS, Clardy J, Parvez M, Choudhary MI, Antifungal diterpenoid alkaloids from Delphinium denudatum. J Nat Prod, 60:472-4, 1997 May.

Bhandary KK, Ramasubbu N, Joshi BS, Desai HK, Pelletier SW, Structure of delvestine: a norditerpenoid alkaloid from Delphinium vestitum Wall. Acta Crystallogr C, 59:1704-7, 1990 Sep 15.

Ding LS, Chen WX, Diterpenoid alkaloids from Delphinium kamaonense var. glabrescens. Yao Hsueh Hsueh Pao, 59:438-40, 1990.

Gheorgiu A et al., Ann Pharm Frnac 22 (1964), 49.

Manners GD, Panter KE, Pelletier SW, Structure-activity relationships of norditerpenoid alkaloids occurring in toxic larkspur (Delphinium) species. J Nat Prod, 59:863-9, 1995 Jun.

Yum L, Wolf KM, Chiappinelli VA, Description of a scale for rating the clinical response of cattle poisoned by larkspur. Am J Vet Res, 41:488-93, 1991 Mar.

Further information in:

Alkondon M, Pereira EF, Wonnacott S, Albuquerque EX, Blockade of nicotinic currents in hippocampal neurons defines methyllycaconitine as a potent and specific receptor antagonist. Mol Pharmacol, 41:802-8, 1992 Apr.

Kern W, List PH, Hörhammer L (Ed), Hagers Handbuch der Pharmazeutischen Praxis. 4. Aufl., Bde. 1-8, Springer Verlag Berlin, Heidelberg, New York 1969.

Olsen JD, Sisson DV, Toxicity of extracts of tall larkspur (Delphinium barbeyi) in mice hamsters rats and sheep. Toxicol Lett, 59:33-41, 1991 Apr.

Park JC, Desai HK, Pelletier SW Two new norditerpenoid alkaloids from Delphinium elatum var. 'black night'. J Nat Prod, 59:291-5, 1995 Feb.

Ralphs MH, Olsen JD, Comparison of larkspur alkaloid extract and lithium chloride in maintaining cattle aversion to larkspur in the field. J Anim Sci, 70:1116-20, 1992 Apr.

Siemion RS, Raisbeck MF, Waggoner JW, Tidwell MA, Sanchez DA, In vitro ruminal metabolism of larkspur alkaloids. Vet Hum Toxicol, 34:206-8, 1992 Jun.

Teuscher E, Lindequist U, Biogene Gifte - Biologie, Chemie, Pharmakologie. 2. Aufl., Fischer Verlag Stuttgart 1994.

Ulubelen A, Desai HK, Srivastava SK, Hart BP, Park JC, Joshi BS, Pelletier SW, Mericli AH, Mericli F, Ilarslan R, Diterpenoid alkaloids from Delphinium davisii. J Nat Prod, 59:360-6, 1996 Apr.

Yum L, Wolf KM, Chiappinelli VA, Nicotinic acetylcholine receptors in separate brain regions exhibit different affinities for methyllycaconitine. Neuroscience, 41:545-55, 1996 May.

Laurel

Laurus nobilis

DESCRIPTION

Medicinal Parts: The medicinal parts are the leaves, the fruit and the oil.

Flower and Fruit: The flowers are in axillary bushy umbels or short racemous panicles. They are dioecious, whitish-green with 4 petals fused at the base. The male flower usually has 10 to 12 stamens; the female has 4 staminoids. The ovary is short-stemmed with one chamber with a hanging ovule, a short style and a triangular obtuse stigma. The fruit develops on the stem into deep-black 2 cm long ovate berries.

Leaves, Stem and Root: Laurel is an evergreen shrub or up to 10 m high tree with smooth, olive green to black bark. The dark-green bay leaves are lanceolate and alternate, about 10 cm long and acuminate at both ends. They are short petioled and their margins are often sinuate and coriaceous.

Habitat: Laurel is indigenous to Mediterranean countries.

Production: Bay leaves are the leaves of Laurus nobilis. Bay berries are the fruits of Laurus nobilis.

Other Names: Sweet Bay, True Laurel, Bay, Roman Laurel, Noble Laurel, Daphne, Bay Laurel, Bay Tree, Grecian Laurel

ACTIONS AND PHARMACOLOGY

COMPOUNDS: LAUREL LEAF

Volatile oil (1-3%): chief components 1,8-cineol

Sesquiterpene lactones: dehydrocostuslactone, costunolide, furthermore eremanthin, laurenbiolide

Isoquinoline alkaloids: including, among others, reticulin

COMPOUNDS: LAUREL FRUIT

Volatile oil (1-4%): including, among others, 1,8-cineol, alpha- and beta-pinene, citral, methylcinnamat

Sesquiterpene lactones: dehydrocostuslactone, costunolid, furthermore eremanthin, laurenbiolide

Fatty oil (25-55%): chief fatty acids lauric, palmitic, oleic acid The green salve-like laurel oil is gained by pressing or cooking the berries. Besides fatty oil, it contains the components of the volatile oil and a large percentage of sesquiterpene lactones.

EFFECTS

Laurel leaves are externally rubefacient and allergenic because of the essential oil they contain. An antimicrobial, molluscidal and insect repellent effect has been demonstrated.

INDICATIONS AND USAGE

Unproven Uses: Both forms are used as a skin stimulant (rubefacient) and for rheumatic conditions.

PRECAUTIONS AND ADVERSE REACTIONS

No health hazards or side effects are known in conjunction with the proper administration of designated therapeutic dosages. The drug possesses a medium potential for sensitization.

DOSAGE

LAUREL LEAF

Mode of Administration: The essential oil is used in ointments and soaps.

LAUREL FRUIT

Mode of Administration: The mixture of essential and fatty oils, extracted through pressing, was formerly used in the treatment of furuncles; today Laurel is used externally in veterinary medicine, as an udder ointment.

LITERATURE

Hausen B, Allergiepflanzen, Pflanzenallergene, ecomed erlagsgesellsch. mbH, Landsberg 1988.

Hegnauer R, Chemotaxonomie der Pflanzen, Bde 1-11, Birkhäuser Verlag Basel, Boston, Berlin 1962-1997.

Hogg JW et al., (1974) Phytochemistry 13:868.

Kern W, List PH, Hörhammer L (Hrsg.), Hagers Handbuch der Pharmazeutischen Praxis, 4. Aufl., Bde 1-8, Springer Verlag Berlin, Heidelberg, New York, 1969.

Novak M, (1985) Phytochemistry 24(4):585.

Roth L, Daunderer M, Kormann K, Giftpflanzen, Pflanzengifte, 4. Aufl., Ecomed Fachverlag Landsberg Lech 1993.

Steinegger E, Hänsel R, Pharmakognosie, 5. Aufl., Springer Verlag Heidelberg 1992.

Tada H et al., (1976) Chem Pharm Bull 24:667.

Teuscher E, Lindequist U, Biogene Gifte - Biologie, Chemie, Pharmakologie, 2. Aufl., Fischer Verlag Stuttgart 1994.

Tori K et al., (1976) Tetrahedron Lett 5:387.

Laurus nobilis

See Laurel

Lavandula angustifolia

See English Lavender

Lavender Cotton

Santolina chamaecyparissias

DESCRIPTION

Medicinal Parts: The medicinal part of the plant is the herb.

Flower and Fruit: The yellow flower heads are 1 cm wide, almost semi-globular, long-pedicled, homogamous and without lingual florets. The corolla tube is compressed and somewhat winged, with a one-sided appendage. The fruit is glabrous.

Leaves, Stem and Root: The evergreen plant is a bushy, aromatic subshrub with brittle branches. There are 4 compact rows of small leaves that are narrow, linear, 2 to 3 cm wide, fleshy, obtuse, paired-pinate, gray-tomentose, and occasionally green.

Habitat: The plant is common in the Mediterranean region.

Characteristics: The plant has a strong scent similar to that of chamomile.

Production: Lavender Cotton is the aerial part of Santolina chamaecyparissias.

ACTIONS AND PHARMACOLOGY

COMPOUNDS

Volatile oil (1%): chief components artemisiaketone (3,5,6-trimethyl-1,5-heptadien-4-one, 65%), as well as myrcene, alpha-pinene

Alkaloids

EFFECTS

The drug has anti-inflammatory, digestive, stimulation of menstruation, and anthelmintic effects.

INDICATIONS AND USAGE

Unproven Uses: Lavender Cotton is used for digestive disorders, PMS, worm infestation, stomach complaints and also to treat jaundice.

PRECAUTIONS AND ADVERSE REACTIONS

No health hazards or side effects are known in conjunction with the proper administration of designated therapeutic dosages.

DOSAGE

Mode of Administration: The herb is used internally as an infusion, but medicinal use has generally ceased.

LITERATURE

Becchi M, Carrier M, (1980) Planta Med 38(3):267.

Giner R et al., (1986) Planta Med 6:83P.

Kern W, List PH, Hörhammer L (Hrsg.), Hagers Handbuch der Pharmazeutischen Praxis, 4. Aufl., Bde. 1-8: Springer Verlag Berlin, Heidelberg, New York, 1969.

Lawsonia inermis

See Henna

Ledum latifolium

See Labrador Tea

Lemna minor

See Duckweed

Lemon

Citrus limon

DESCRIPTION

Medicinal Parts: The medicinal parts are the juice, peel and oil of the fruit.

Flower and Fruit: Flowers are arranged singly or in short, sparsely flowered racemes, hermaphrodite or functionally male. The petals are suffused with purple on the outer surface. There are 25 to 40 stamens in coherent groups. The fruit is yellow when ripe and grows to 6.5 to 12.5 cm. It is 8-

to 10-locular, oblong or ovoid, with a broad, low, mamilliform projection at the apex. The rind is somewhat rough to almost smooth. The pulp is acidic.

Leaves, Stem and Root: Citrus limon is a small tree, growing only 3 to 6 m tall with twigs that are angular when young and soon become rounded and glabrous with stout axillary spines. The leaves are pale green, broadly elliptical, acute and serrate or crenate. The petiole has a flat wing or is merely margined and is distinctly articulated with the lamina.

Habitat: The tree is indigenous to northern India, cultivated in Mediterranean regions and worldwide in subtropical regions.

Production: Lemons are the fruit, lemon peel is the skin of the fruit and lemon oil the essential oil extracted from the skins of Citrus limon.

Other Names: Limon

ACTIONS AND PHARMACOLOGY

COMPOUNDS

Volatile oil in the fresh and dehydrated peel: chief components (+)-limonene in addition to citral (as an odor-bearer), n-nonanal, n-decanal, n-dodecanal, linalyl acetate, geranyl acetat, citronellyl acetat, methyl anthranilate; also in pressed oils, lipophilic flavinoids, including sinensetin, nobiletin and furocoumarins

Flavonoids: in particular the bitter neohesperidosides naringin and neohesperidin dyhydro chalcones, furthermore hesperidin, rutin and ericitrim

EFFECTS

The citroflavonoids in lemon affect vascular permeability and are anti-inflammatory, diuretic and a source of vitamin C.

INDICATIONS AND USAGE

Unproven Uses: Lemon is used as a source of vitamin C in cases of general low resistance, scurvy and colds. In folk medicine, lemon juice was recommended as a drink for fever, as a remedy for acute rheumatism and as an antidote to intoxicants, particularly opium. Additional traditional uses that are still recommended include sunburn, and as a quinine substitute for malaria or to reduce body temperature in typhus patients.

Indian Medicine: Uses in Indian medicine include as a remedy for shaking and heartburn.

PRECAUTIONS AND ADVERSE REACTIONS

No health hazards or side effects are known in conjunction with the proper administration of designated therapeutic dosages. There is a low potential for sensitization through skin contact with volatile oil.

DOSAGE

Mode of Administration: Lemon is used internally in the form of oil, tincture or fresh fruit.

LITERATURE

Calomme M et al., Inhibition of bacterial mutagenisis by Citrus flavonoids. In: PM 62(3):222-226. 1996.

Calomme M et al., PM 62:222. 1996.

Clavarano I, Essenze Deriv. Agrum 36:5. 1966.

Horowitz RM, Gentili B, Tetrahedron 19:773. 1963.

Paris R, (1977) Plant Med Phytother 11(Suppl):129.

Paris R, Delaveau P, (1977) Plant Med Phytother 11(Suppl):198.

Further information in:

Kern W, List PH, Hörhammer L (Hrsg.), Hagers Handbuch der Pharmazeutischen Praxis, 4. Aufl., Bde. 1-8, Springer Verlag Berlin, Heidelberg, New York, 1969.

Leung AY, Encyclopedia of Common Natural Ingredients Used in Food, Drugs and Cosmetics, John Wiley & Sons Inc., New York 1980.

Madaus G, Lehrbuch der Biologischen Arzneimittel, Bde 1-3, Nachdruck, Georg Olms Verlag Hildesheim 1979.

Oliver-Bever B (Ed.), Medicinal Plants of Tropical West Africa, Cambridge University Press Cambridge, London 1986.

Roth L, Daunderer M, Kormann K, Giftpflanzen, Pflanzengifte, 4. Aufl., Ecomed Fachverlag Landsberg Lech 1993.

Steinegger E, Hänsel R, Pharmakognosie, 5. Aufl., Springer Verlag Heidelberg 1992.

Tang W, Eisenbrand G, Chinese Drugs of Plant Origin, Springer Verlag Heidelberg 1992.

Teuscher E, Biogene Arzneimittel, 5. Aufl., Wiss. Verlagsges. mbH Stuttgart 1997.

Wichtl M (Hrsg.), Teedrogen, 4. Aufl., Wiss. Verlagsges. Stuttgart 1997.

Lemon Balm

Melissa officinalis

TRADE NAMES

Lemon Balm (available from numerous manufacturers and as combination product), Melissa Lemon Balm Herb, Quanterra Sleep

DESCRIPTION

Medicinal Parts: The medicinal parts are the oil extracted by distillation, the dried leaves, the fresh leaves and the whole plant.

Flower and Fruit: The small white bilabiate flowers are in 6 one-sided false whorls in the axils of the upper leaves. The calyx is campanulate, bilabiate, and it has a shortly dentate upper lip. The corolla tube is curved upward. The upper lip is slightly domed and divided in two parts, the lower lip is 3-lobed with an extended middle lobe. The flower has 4 stamens. The fruit is an oblong-ovate, 1.5 to 2 mm long and chestnut brown nutlet.

Leaves, Stem and Root: The plant is a perennial that grows up to 90 cm high, with an erect, quadrangular, branched and sparsely haired to glabrous stem. The leaves are petiolate and have an ovate to rhomboid, 2 to 6 cm long and 1.5 to 5 cm wide crenate leaf blade, which is shortly pointed at the end, and stunted or wedge-shaped at the base. It is usually only pubescent above or completely glabrous.

Characteristics: Before flowering, the taste and smell is lemon-like, later becoming astringent to balm-like and warming.

Habitat: The plant is indigenous to the east Mediterranean region and west Asia, and is cultivated in central Europe or established in the wild.

Production: Lemon balm is the fresh or dried leaves of Melissa officinalis as well as its preparations. The leaves are collected before flowering or before there is too much branching. Leaves and stem are separated and comminuted and dried quickly at temperatures between 30 to 40° C.

Not to be Confused With: Nepeta cataria. var. citriodora (lemon cat mint).

Other Names: Balm, Sweet Mary, Honey Plant, Cure-All, Dropsy Plant, Melissa

ACTIONS AND PHARMACOLOGY

COMPOUNDS

Volatile oil (0.02-0.8%): chief components geranial (citral a), neral (citral b), citronellal (together 40-75% of the volatile oil, aroma-carrier), furthermore, linalool, geraniol, geranylactetate, methyl citronellate, trans-β-ocimene, 1-Octen-3-ol, 6-methyl-5-heptene-2-on. beta-caryophyllene, caryophyllebepoxide, germacren D, eugenol

Glycosides: of the alcoholic or phenolic components of the volatile oil, for example eugenol glucoside

Caffeic acid derivatives: rosmaric acid (up to 4.7%)

Flavonoids: including among others cynaroside, cosmosiin, rhamnocitrin, isoquercitrin

Triterpene acids: including among others ursolic acid. Only the very fresh drug (maximum 6 months old) is usable as a sedative, because of the low volatile oil content and its high volatility; the requirements of the German-language medication texts do not take this into consideration (no minimum content requirement given).

EFFECTS

The drug has mild sedative and carminative, spasmolytic, antibacterial, antiviral, anti-oxidative and anti-hormonal effects.

INDICATIONS AND USAGE

Approved by Commission E:

■ Nervousness and insomnia

The drug is used for nervous agitation and sleeping problems.

Unproven Uses: In folk medicine, the drug is utilized as decoctions of the flowering shoots for nervous complaints, lower abdominal disorders, meteorism, nervous gastric complaints, hysteria and melancholia, chronic bronchial catarrh, nervous palpitations, vomiting, migraine, nervous debility, headache and high blood pressure. It is used externally for rheumatism, nerve pains and stiff necks (compress).

Homeopathic Uses: Melissa officinalis is used for menstrual irregularities.

PRECAUTIONS AND ADVERSE REACTIONS

No health hazards or side effects are known in conjunction with the proper administration of designated therapeutic dosages.

DOSAGE

Mode of Administration: Comminuted herb, herb powder, liquid extracts or dry extracts for teas and other galenic preparations; liquid and solid forms for internal and external use; combinations with other sedative and/or carminative herbs may be beneficial.

How Supplied:
Capsules — 395 mg

Preparation: To prepare an infusion pour one cup of hot water over 1.5 to 4.5 gm of the drug and strain after 10 minutes.

Daily Dosage: The average daily dose is 1.5 to 4.5 gm of drug.

Homeopathic Dosage: 5 drops, 1 tablet or 10 globules every 30 to 60 minutes (acute) or 1 to 3 times daily (chronic); parenterally: 1 to 2 ml sc acute, 3 times daily; chronic: once a day (HAB34).

Storage: Store in well-sealed, non-plastic containers, protected from light and moisture for up to 1 year.

LITERATURE

Auf'mkolk M, (1985) Endocrinology 116(5):1687.

Auf'mkolk M et al., (1984) Endocrinology 115(2):527.

Auf'mkolk M et al., (1984) Horm Metab Res 16(4):183.

Brieskorn CH, Krause W, (1974) Arch Pharm 307(8):603.

Buechner KH et al., (1974) Med Klein. 69(23):1032.

Chlabicz J et al., (1984) Pharmazie 39(11):770.

Cohen RA, Kucera LS, Herrmann EC Jr, Antiviral activity of Melissa officinalis (Limon Balm) extract. In: Proc Soc Exp Biol Med 117:431-434. 1964.

Czygan FC, Melisse - Objekt der Grundlagenforschung. In: DAZ 132(12):599. 1992.

De Jong CAG, (1978) Ned Tijdschr Geneeskd 112(3):82.

Enjalbert F et al., (1983) Fitoterapia 2:59.

Forster HB et al., (1980) Planta Med 40(4):309.

Hermann EC Jr., Kucera LS, Antiviral substances in plants of the mint family (Labiatae): II. Nontanninia polyphenols of Melissa officinalis. In: Proc soc Exp Bio Med 124:869. 1967.

Koch-Heitzmann I, Schultze W, 2000 Jahre Melissa officinalis. Von der Bienenpflanze zum Virustatikum. In: ZPT 9(3):77. 1988.

Kümel G, Stoll L, Brendel M, Herpes simplex. Therapie mit rezeptfreien Topika. In: DAZ 131(30):1609. 1991.

Kucera LS, Hermann EC Jr, (1967) Proc Soc Exp Biol Med 124:865 et 874.

Mohrig A, Melissenextrakt bei Herpes simplex - die Alternative zu Nucleosid-Analoga. In: DAZ 136(50):4575-4580. 1996.

Orth-Wagner S, Ressin WJ, Friedrich I, Phytosedativum gegen Schlafstörungen. In: ZPT 16(3):147-156. 1995.

Ozarowski A, (1982) Wiad 4:7.

Pertz H, Naturally occuring clavines: Antagonism/partial agonism at 5-HT2alpha receptors and antogonism at alpha1-adrenoceptors in blood vessel. In: PM 62(5)387-392. 1996.

Richter T, Melissa officinalis - Ein Leitmotiv für 1000 Jahre Medizingeschichte. In: DAZ 133(41):3723. 1993.

Sarer E, Kokdil G, Constitutents of the essential oil from Melissa officinalis. In: PM 57:89. 1991.

Schultze W, König WA, Hilker A, Richter R, Melissenöle. In: DAZ 135(7):557-577. 1995.

Thieme H, Kithe C, (1973) Pharmazie 28(1):69.

Uehleke B, Phytobalneologie. In: ZPT 17(1):26-43. 1996.

Vogt HJ, Tausch I, Wöbling RH, Kaiser PM (1991) Melissenextrakt bei Herpes simplex. Allgemeinarzt 14:832-841.

Wagner H, Sprinkmeyer L, (1973) Dtsch Apoth Z 113:1159.

Walz A, Melisse hilft heilen. In: DAZ 136(2):26. 1996.

Wolbling RH, Milbradt R, (1984) Therapiewoche 34(9):1193.

Zitiert nach: Koch- Heitzmann I, Schültze W, (1984) Melissa officinalis. Eine alte Arzneipflanze mit neue therapeutischen Wirkungen. Dtsch Apoth Z 124:2137-2145.

Further information in:

Hänsel R, Keller K, Rimpler H, Schneider G (Hrsg.), Hagers Handbuch der Pharmazeutischen Praxis, 5. Aufl., Bde 4-6 (Drogen), Springer Verlag Berlin, Heidelberg, New York, 1992-1994.

Leung AY, Encyclopedia of Common Natural Ingredients Used in Food, Drugs and Cosmetics, John Wiley & Sons Inc., New York 1980.

Madaus G, Lehrbuch der Biologischen Arzneimittel, Bde 1-3, Nachdruck, Georg Olms Verlag Hildesheim 1979.

Schulz R, Hänsel R, Rationale Phytotherapie, Springer Verlag Heidelberg 1996.

Steinegger E, Hänsel R, Pharmakognosie, 5. Aufl., Springer Verlag Heidelberg 1992.

Teuscher E, Biogene Arzneimittel, 5. Aufl., Wiss. Verlagsges. Stuttgart 1997.

Wagner H, Wiesenauer M, Phytotherapie. Phytopharmaka und pflanzliche Homöopathika, Fischer-Verlag, Stuttgart, Jena, New York 1995.

Wichtl M (Hrsg.), Teedrogen, 4. Aufl., Wiss. Verlagsges. Stuttgart 1997.

Lemon Verbena

Aloysia triphylla

DESCRIPTION

Medicinal Parts: The medicinal part is the oil of vervain as a distillate of the fresh twigs and the dried leaves and stems.

Flower and Fruit: The plant has numerous small flowers in panicle-like spikes. The hairy calyx is about 3 mm long with 4 tips. The petals are white or bluish, and fused to a 4 to 5 mm long funnel at the base. There are 2 short and 2 long stamens in the funnel.

Leaves, Stem and Root: Aloysia triphylla is an up to 3 m tall shrub. The branches are striate and scabrous. They bear leaves in whorls of 3 or 4 on the stem. The leaves are entire-margined, short-petioled, lanceolate and about 7 to 10 cm long. They have lateral veins almost at right angles to the midrib, and are dotted on the underside with oil-bearing glands.

Characteristics: The leaves have a lemony fragrance.

Habitat: The plant originated in Argentina, Chile and Peru, and is cultivated in most other warmer countries. Main countries of cultivation are Algeria, Chile, Israel and Morocco.

Production: Lemon Verbena leaves are the leaves and stems, in whole and ground form, of Aloysia triphylla. The shrubs are propagated by runners or cuttings. They are cut from the second year of growth, in the month of July, before flowering. The young lateral branches appear in October. They are dried rapidly in thin layers or bundles. The dried leaves are then stripped off. The harvest consists of approximately 10,000 kg of the leaf drug per hectare.

Other Names: Herb Louisa, Lemon-Scented Verbena

ACTIONS AND PHARMACOLOGY

COMPOUNDS

Volatile oil: main constituents are geraniol and neral

Flavonoids: including apigenin-, diosmetin- and luteolin-7-O-glucosides, in addition to mono-, di- and trimethoxyflavones, including eupatorin. (See Lippiae triphylla aetherolum.)

Iridoids: iridoid glycosides including geniposidic acid

EFFECTS

The leaves are considered to be antispasmodic, sedative and are a febrifuge. There are no up-to-date studies available.

INDICATIONS AND USAGE

Unproven Uses: In France, Lemon Verbena is used in the symptomatic treatment of digestive disorders, agitation and insomnia. The drug has also been used in the treatment of febrile hemorrhoids, varicose veins and impure skin. In Morocco it is also used for chills and constipation. Efficacy has not been proven in any of these areas. The plant is used as an inactive ingredient to improve the flavor in medicinal teas.

PRECAUTIONS AND ADVERSE REACTIONS

No health hazards or side effects are known in conjunction with the proper administration of designated therapeutic dosages.

DOSAGE

Mode of Administration: In France, the infusion is available in various restaurants under the name ''Vervaine oderante.'' Used in various medicinal preparations and tea mixtures.

Preparation: To prepare an infusion, use 5 to 29 g of the leaf per 1 liter of water.

Daily Dosage: Drink 2 to 5 cups of the infusion during the course of the day. In preparations with a high water content (such as instant teas), the daily dose equivalent should not exceed 10 g. The upper limit for daily dosages of powders and tinctures is 5 g.

Storage: The drug must be stored in sealed containers, protected from light and dampness.

LITERATURE

Breitweiser K, (1943) Pharmaz Ind 10:76.

Carnat A, Carnat AP, Chavignon O, Heitz A, Wylde R, Lamaison JL, Luteolin 7-diglucuronide the major flavonoid compound from Aloysia triphylla and Verbena officinalis. Planta Med, 61:490, 1995 Oct.

Hänsel R, Keller K, Rimpler H, Schneider G (Hrsg.), Hagers Handbuch der Pharmazeutischen Praxis, 5. Aufl., Bde 4-6 (Drogen), Springer Verlag Berlin, Heidelberg, New York, 1992-1994.

Killacky J et al., (1976) Planta Med 30:310.

Rimpler H, Sauerbier H, Biochem Syst Ecol 14:307-310. 1986.

Skalta H, Shammas G, PM 54:265. 1988.

Tomás-Barberán FA, Harborne JB, Self R, PH 26:2281-2284. 1987.

Torrent Marti MT, Rev R Acad Farm (Barcelona) 14:39-55. 1976.

Lemon-Wood

Schisandra sphenanthera

DESCRIPTION

Medicinal Parts: Medicinal properties are attributed to the fruit and seed of the plant.

Flower and Fruit: The flowers are in clusters with a few blossoms in the axils of the bracts. There are 5 to 8 tepals. The perigone of the male flowers has 5 to 8 sections and 11 to 19 stamens. The female flowers have a similar perigone and 30 to 50 ovaries. The fruit is elongate-elliptical, slim and hangs in aggregate clusters. The individual fruit is round, fleshy, brown-red to dark brown and berry-like.

Leaves, Stem and Root: The dioecious Schisandra sphenanthera has leaves that are alternate and arranged like whorls on short shoots. The petiole is 1 to 3 cm long. The lamina is dark green to brown, 5 to 11 cm long and 3 to 7 cm wide. It is ovate to elliptical, acute at both ends and serrate to dentate. The young branches are purple.

Habitat: The plant is indigenous to China.

Production: Southern schisandra fruit is the dried, ripe fruit of Schisandra sphenanthera.

ACTIONS AND PHARMACOLOGY

COMPOUNDS

Volatile oil

Ascorbic acid (vitamin C)

Lignans (in the seeds 2 to 10%): dibenzo[a,c]cyclooctene derivatives, including schizandrins A and B, schizandrols A and B, schizantherins A to E, additional lignans with other parent substances, including epigalbacin, anwulignan, ganschisandrin

Fatty oil (in the seeds)

EFFECTS

Various lignans have been isolated from the drug that are also present in Schisandra chinensis; some of the action mechanisms described there may also apply to Schisandra sphenanthera. (See Schisandra chinensis.)

INDICATIONS AND USAGE

Chinese Medicine: The plant is used for dyspnea, coughs caused by disturbance of lung function, dry mouth, thirst, spontaneous or night sweats, nocturia, insomnia, amnesia and anxiety states. Efficacy for these indications has not yet been proven.

PRECAUTIONS AND ADVERSE REACTIONS

No health hazards are known in conjunction with the proper administration of designated therapeutic dosages.

DOSAGE

Mode of Administration: Whole drug and preparations for internal use.

Preparation: To prepare Cuwuweizi powder, the drug is evaporated in the ratio of 1:5 with vinegar in closed containers until the surface turns black. The product is then ground to a powder.

Daily Dosage: The literature has no information.

LITERATURE

Hänsel R, Keller K, Rimpler H, Schneider G (Ed), Hagers Handbuch der Pharmazeutischen Praxis, 5. Aufl., Bde 4 - 6 (Drogen), Springer Verlag Berlin, Heidelberg, New York, 1992-1994.

Liu CS, Fang SD, Huang MF, Kao YL, Hsu JS, Studies on the active principles of Schisandra sphenanthera Rehd. et Wils. The structures of schisantherin A, B, C, D, E and the related compounds. Sci Sin, 21:483-502, 1978 Jul-Aug.

Lemongrass

Cymbopogon citratus

DESCRIPTION

Medicinal Parts: The medicinal parts are the dried leaves and the Lemongrass oil of Cymbopogon citratus and the citronella oil from Cymbopogon nardus.

CYMBOPOGON CITRATUS

Flower and Fruit: The flowers are 30 cm long and have false spikes with reddish brown sheaths 15 to 25 mm long. The racemes are 15 to 17 mm long. The sessile spikelet is 6 mm long and the upper spelts are 0.7 mm wide, lanceolate, narrowly winged, flattened at the back, slightly concave and ribless in the lower part. The stemmed spikelet is 4.5 mm long, and the lower spelt is 0.7 mm wide. Inflorescences are rarely formed on this variety.

Leaves, Stem and Root: Cymbopogon citratus is a perennial plant with a smooth and glabrous stalk up to 2 m. The leaf blade is linear, acuminate, up to 90 cm long and 5 mm wide and smooth on both sides. The leaf sheaths are round, glabrous and smooth. The ligule is paper-like and less than 1 mm long.

CYMBOPOGON NARDUS

Flower and Fruit: The inflorescence is very large and consists of a 1-meter long spike with numerous racemes up to 20 mm long and arranged in zigzag order. The sessile spike is 5 mm long. The lower spelt is oblong-lanceolate, usually flat, narrowly winged with 3 ribs. The awn, if there is one, is 5 mm long. The petiolar spike is 5 mm long, and the lower spelt lanceolate has 7 ribs.

Leaves, Stem and Root: Cymbopogon nardus is a perennial plant with a stalk that grows up to 2 to 2.5 m. It is smooth and glabrous. The leaf blade is up to 1 m long and 1.5 cm wide and usually light green. The upper surface is smooth, the lower surface and the margin are rough. The leaf sheaths are glabrous and yellowish-green. The basal leaf sheaths are also glabrous but green to reddish. The ligule is paper-like and about 1 mm long.

Characteristics: Cymbopogon species have essential oils in tube-like cells with corked walls.

Habitat: Citronella grass was originally indigenous to the tropics and the subtropics of the Old World. Today it is cultivated in Central and South America and Queensland, Australia.

Production: Lemongrass consists of the above-ground parts of Cymbopogon citratus. West Indian Lemongrass oil consists of the essential oil from Cymbopogon citratus. Citronella oil consists of the essential oil from Cymbopogon winterianus.

Other Names: Citronella, Fevergrass

ACTIONS AND PHARMACOLOGY

COMPOUNDS: LEMONGRASS LEAVES

Volatile oil (0.2-0.4%)

COMPOUNDS: LEMONGRASS LEAVES

Citral (65-86%)

Myrcene (12-20%)

COMPOUNDS: CITRONELLA OIL

Citronellal (32-45%)

Geraniol (12-25%)

Geranyl acetate (3-8%)

Citronellyl acetate (1-4%)

EFFECTS

In rats, i.v. administration of an infusion caused a drop in arterial pressure and a mild diuretic effect. The oral administration of an imprecise amount of extract caused a drop in temperature and tendency to lengthen intestinal passage time. Because of the small number of experiments carried out, a hypotensive action cannot be considered as conclusively proven. The essential oil has an antibacterial effect in animal tests; in higher doses, it has a sedative/analgesic effect.

INDICATIONS AND USAGE

Unproven Uses: Externally, Lemongrass is used for lumbago, neuralgic and rheumatic pain, sprains, and as a mild astringent. Internally, the herb is used for gastrointestinal symptoms and mild states of agitation.

Indian Medicine: Lemongrass is used for intestinal parasites, stomach complaints, flatulence, leprosy, bronchitis and fever.

PRECAUTIONS AND ADVERSE REACTIONS

The application of salves with the volatile oil upon the skin has led in rare cases to signs of allergy. A toxic alveolitis was observed in 2 cases following inhalation of the volatile oil.

DOSAGE

No information is available.

Storage: Store in air-tight containers protected from light.

LITERATURE

De Silva MG, Mfg Chemist 30:415-416. 1959.

Hänsel R, Keller K, Rimpler H, Schneider G (Hrsg.), Hagers Handbuch der Pharmazeutischen Praxis, 5. Aufl., Bde 4-6 (Drogen), Springer Verlag Berlin, Heidelberg, New York, 1992-1994.

Leung AY, Encyclopedia of Common Natural Ingredients Used in Food, Drugs and Cosmetics, John Wiley & Sons Inc., New York 1980.

Sarer E, Scheffer JJC, Svendsen AB, Composition of the essential oil of Cymbopogon citratus (DC.) STAPF cultivated in turkey. In: Sci Pharm 51:58. 1983.

Steinegger E, Hänsel R, Pharmakognosie, 5. Aufl., Springer Verlag Heidelberg 1992.

Teuscher E, Biogene Arzneimittel, 5. Aufl., Wiss. Verlagsges. mbH Stuttgart 1997.

Leonurus cardiaca

See Motherwort

Leonurus japonicus

See Chinese Motherwort

Lepidium sativum

See Garden Cress

Leptandra virginica

See Black Root

Lesser Celandine

Ranunculus ficaria

DESCRIPTION

Medicinal Parts: The medicinal part is the fresh herb.

Flower and Fruit: The golden yellow flowers have a diameter of 25 mm. The calyx usually has 3 sepals, the corolla 8 or more petals which are glossy and spread out in a star-shape. Since the petals are green underneath, the flowers are inconspicuous when closed. There are numerous stamens and ovaries. The fruit is 1-seeded and indehiscent.

Leaves, Stem and Root: The plant grows from 5 to 15 cm high. The stems are decumbent and bear bulbils in the leaf axils. The leaves, like the stems, are glabrous and fleshy. The lower ones are long-petioled, alternate and orbicular-cordate. The upper ones are 5-lobed. There are fleshy, cylindrical clavate tubers between the roots.

Characteristics: The herb has a hot, unpleasant taste and is toxic.

Habitat: The plant is found all over Europe, western Asia and northern Africa.

Production: Lesser Celandine is the fresh herb of Ranunculus ficaria.

Other Names: Pilewort, Figwort, Smallwort

ACTIONS AND PHARMACOLOGY

COMPOUNDS

The glycoside ranunculin as protoanemonine-forming agent: The freshly-harvested plant (0.06-0.35% of the fresh weight, of which only 3% of the overall content of the plant is contained in the leaves, 68% in the stalks, 25% in the blossoms) changes enzymatically when it is cut into small pieces, and probably also when it is dried, into the pungent, volatile protoanemonine that quickly dimerizes to non-mucus-membrane-irritating anemonine. When dried, the plant is not capable of protoanemonine-formation.

EFFECTS

Active agents are tannin, the alkaloids chelidonin and cholerytrin, the saponin fikarin and large quantities of vitamin C.

INDICATIONS AND USAGE

Unproven Uses: Lesser Celandine is used for scurvy, treatment of bleeding wounds, gums and swollen joints.

PRECAUTIONS AND ADVERSE REACTIONS

The dangers of irritation of the skin and mucus membranes are relatively low with pilewort. The consumption of small quantities of the fresh leaf sheaths (before blossoming; the stem should be discarded) as a springtime salad is unproblematic.

No health hazards or side effects are known in conjunction with the proper administration of designated therapeutic dosages of the dehydrated drug. Extended skin contact with the freshly-harvested, bruised plant can lead to blister formation and cauterizations which are difficult to heal due to the resulting protoanemonine, that is severely irritating to skin and mucus membranes.

If taken internally, severe irritation to the gastrointestinal tract, combined with colic and diarrhea, as well as irritations of the urinary drainage passages, are possible. Symptomatic treatment for external contact should consist of irrigation with diluted potassium permanganate solution; in case of internal contact, administration of activated charcoal should follow gastric lavage.

OVERDOSAGE

Death by asphyxiation following the intake of large quantities of protoanemonine-forming plants has been observed in animal experiments.

DOSAGE

Mode of Administration: Ground and as an extract. The drug extracts can be added to baths to treat hemorrhoids, warts and scratches.

LITERATURE

Bonora A et al., PH 26:2277. 1987.

Kolesnik et al., (1963) CA 59:7856.

Pourrat H, Pourrat A, (1966) Bull Soc Chim Franc 2410.

Pourrat H et al., (1979) Ann Pharm Franc 37:441.

Pourrat H et al., (1982) Ann Pharm Franc 40:373.

Ruijgrok HWL, PM 11:338-347. 1963.

Texier O et al., (1984) Phytochemistry 23(12):2903.

Further information in:

Hegnauer R, Chemotaxonomie der Pflanzen, Bde 1-11: Birkhäuser Verlag Basel, Boston, Berlin 1962-1997.

Kern W, List PH, Hörhammer L (Hrsg.), Hagers Handbuch der Pharmazeutischen Praxis, 4. Aufl., Bde 1-8: Springer Verlag Berlin, Heidelberg, New York, 1969.

Madaus G, Lehrbuch der Biologischen Arzneimittel, Bde 1-3, Nachdruck, Georg Olms Verlag Hildesheim 1979.

Roth L, Daunderer M, Kormann K, Giftpflanzen, Pflanzengifte, 4. Aufl., Ecomed Fachverlag Landsberg Lech 1993.

Teuscher E, Lindequist U, Biogene Gifte - Biologie, Chemie, Pharmakologie, 2. Aufl., Fischer Verlag Stuttgart 1994.

Lesser Galangal

Alpinia officinarum

DESCRIPTION

Medicinal Parts: The medicinal part of the plant is the rhizome.

Flower and Fruit: Galangal is a perennial plant. It is similar in appearance to the sword lily.

Leaves, Stem and Root: Lesser Galangal has a dark, reddish-brown, cylindrical rhizome about 1 to 2 cm in diameter and 3 to 6 cm long. The stem is marked at short intervals with raised rings, which are the scars of the leaf bases. Stems are up to 1.5 m with long narrow lanceolate leaves bearing racemes of orchid-shaped flowers, white and veined red. A fracture of the rhizome is hard and tough, showing a pale inside with a darker central column.

Characteristics: Lesser Galangal has a pungent and spicy taste. The odor is aromatic, rather like ginger.

Habitat: The plant is indigenous to China and entered Europe via India and Arabia in the Middle Ages.

Production: Lesser Galangal consists of the dried rhizome of Alpinia officinarum.

Not to be Confused With: The rhizome of Kaempferia galanga and other Alpina species

Other Names: Galanga, East India Root, Chinese Ginger, China Root, India Root, East India Catarrh Root, Gargaut, Colic Root, Catarrh Root, Galangal

ACTIONS AND PHARMACOLOGY

COMPOUNDS

Volatile oil: chief components-sesquiterpene hydrocarbons, sesquiterpene alcohols

Diarylheptanoids: mixture termed galangol, some of them pungent substances

Gingerole: phenyl alkanones, pungent substances

Starch

Tannin

Flavonoids: including galangin, galangin-3-methylether, kaempferide

EFFECTS

The plant is said to have antispasmodic, antiphlogistic and antibacterial properties.

INDICATIONS AND USAGE

Approved by Commission E:

- Dyspeptic complaints
- Loss of appetite

Unproven Uses: Folk medicine uses include painful upper abdominal syndrome of the Roemheld complex type, sluggish digestion, and for liver and gallbladder complaints. Additional uses include fevers and colds, cough/bronchitis, tendency for infections, and inflammation of the mouth and pharynx.

Chinese Medicine: The drug is used for pain, particularly stomach pain.

PRECAUTIONS AND ADVERSE REACTIONS

Health risks or side effects following the proper administration of designated therapeutic dosages are not reported.

DOSAGE

Mode of Administration: Comminuted drug and powder, as well as other galenic preparations for oral administration.

Preparation: Infusion - Pour boiling water over 0.5 to 1 g drug and strain after 10 minutes.

Daily Dosage: 2 to 4 g. The infusion dosage is 1 cup 30 minutes before meals.

LITERATURE

Collins KR, Pat EP 25649 (1981) Europe.

De Pooter HL, et al., PH 24:93. 1985.

Haraguchi H, et al., Antifungal activity from Alpinia galanga and the competition for incorporation of unsaturated fatty acids in cell growth. In: PM 62(4):308-313. 1996.

Haraguchi H, et al., PM 62:308. 1996.

Itokawa H, et al., (1987) Planta Med 53(1):32.

Mitsui S, et al., (1976) Chem Pharm Bull 24:2377.

Further information in:

Fenaroli's Handbook of Flavor Ingredients, Vol. 1, 2nd Ed., CRC Press, 1975.

Kern W, List PH, Hörhammer L (Hrsg.), Hagers Handbuch der Pharmazeutischen Praxis, 4. Aufl., Bde. 1-8, Springer Verlag Berlin, Heidelberg, New York, 1969.

Madaus G, Lehrbuch der Biologischen Arzneimittel, Bde 1-3, Nachdruck, Georg Olms Verlag Hildesheim 1979.

Steinegger E, Hänsel R, Pharmakognosie, 5. Aufl., Springer Verlag Heidelberg 1992.

Teuscher E, Biogene Arzneimittel, 5. Aufl., Wiss. Verlagsges. mbH Stuttgart 1997.

Wichtl M (Hrsg.), Teedrogen, 4. Aufl., Wiss. Verlagsges. Stuttgart 1997.

Levant Cotton

Gossypium herbaceum

DESCRIPTION

Medicinal Parts: The medicinal parts are the root bark, the fresh inner-root bark and the seeds.

Flower and Fruit: The yellow flowers have a dark red spot at the base of the petals. The calyx is 2 to 2.5 cm long. The bracts are broadly deltate-ovate to semicircular, usually at least as wide as long. Their margins have 6 to 8 acute or shortly acuminate teeth, usually less than 3 times as long as wide. The fruit is beak-shaped, terminally rounded, up to 18 mm long, with 3 to 4 chambers. The seeds, which are embedded in the hairs, are square with gray pubescense.

Leaves, Stem and Root: Gossypium herbaceum is an evergreen shrub 2 m high and 1 to 1.5 m wide. The few branches are glabrous to sparsely haired and foliated. The leaves are broadly cordate, coriaceous, reticulate, pubescent with undulate margins. They have a short tip and narrow base.

Habitat: The variety is indigenous to Asia and Africa. Today it is mainly cultivated in Egypt, China, India, Anatolia and the southern U.S.

Other Names: Cotton Root, Cotton

ACTIONS AND PHARMACOLOGY

COMPOUNDS

Volatile oil (traces): including with beta-bisabolol

Resinous substance: containing, among others, salicylic acid and 2,3-dihydroxybenzoic acid

Dimeric sesquiterpenes: (+)-gossypol, (+) -gossypol, p-hemigossypol in some strains presumably in very low quantities)

The drug has not been investigated in recent times.

EFFECTS

A histamine-releasing effect has been observed in vitro, in the lung tissue of pigs. The drug also appears to have emmenagogic, oxytocic and contraceptive (male) effects, but constituents have not yet been sufficiently investigated. The oxytocic effect, similar to that of secale, has been observed in animal experiments, making its use as a contraction stimulant seem plausible.

INDICATIONS AND USAGE

Unproven Uses: The drug has many indications in folk medicine, such as amenorrhea, dysmenorrhea, irregular menstruation, nausea, fever, headache, diarrhea and dysentery; as an oxytoxic, to expel the afterbirth, for urethritis, nerve inflammation, poor lactation, metrorrhagia, hemorrhage, menorrhagia and atonic amenorrhea, painful menstruation and climacteric complaints.

Chinese Medicine: Cotton is used in China as a male contraceptive.

Homeopathic Uses: The drug is used chiefly in gynecology to treat menstrual disturbances, menstrual bleeding, morning sickness and uterine bleeding.

PRECAUTIONS AND ADVERSE REACTIONS

General: Health risks or side effects following the proper administration of designated therapeutic dosages are not recorded.

Pregnancy: Cotton is not to be administered during pregnancy, except at delivery.

OVERDOSAGE

In animal studies, numerous poisonings, some of them fatal, have been observed following long-term feeding with large quantities of cotton seed press cakes.

DOSAGE

Mode of Administration: The drug is used as a decoction, liquid extract and tincture, as well as in combination with secale, hydrastis, chaemaelirium and leonurus.

Preparations: Tincture and liquid extract of 2 to 4 ml, liquid extract 20 to 40 drops per single dose.

Daily Dosage: The standard single dose to be taken internally is 2 g of the drug, or 10 g of a 20% decoction, i.e. 1 teaspoonful for a single-dose decoction. The dosage of the liquid extract administered during labor is a single dose of 1 to 2 level teaspoonfuls, with another similar dose given 2 to 4 times daily after the birth as a post-natal styptic.

Homeopathic Dosage: 5 drops, 1 tablet or 10 globules every 30 to 60 minutes (acute) or 1 to 3 times daily (chronic); parenterally: 1 to 2 ml sc acute, 3 times daily; chronic: once a day (HAB34).

Storage: Store Cotton in well-filled containers, protected from light and heat.

LITERATURE

Byzova MV, Kraev AS, Pozmogova GE, Skriabin KG, Molecular characteristics of chalcone synthase gene families from two cotton species using the polymerase chain reaction. Mol Biol (Mosk), 26:432-40, Mar-Apr1992.

Dai RX et al., (1978) Acta Biol Exp Sinica 11:27.

Dorsett PH et al., (1975) J Pharm Sci 64:1073.

Hamasaki Y, Tae HH, (1985) Biochim Biophys Acta 843(1):37.

Liu ZQ et al., In: Recent Advances in Fertility Regulation. Beijing 1980, Eds. C. C. Fen et al. Pub. S. A. Atar, Geneva 1981.

Qian SZ et al., (1980) Chin Med J 93:477.

Stipanovic RD et al., (1975) Phytochemistry 14:1077.

Further information in:

Hänsel R, Keller K, Rimpler H, Schneider G (Hrsg.), Hagers Handbuch der Pharmazeutischen Praxis, 5. Aufl., Bde 4-6 (Drogen), Springer Verlag Berlin, Heidelberg, New York, 1992-1994.

Hausen B, Allergiepflanzen, Pflanzenallergene, ecomed Verlagsgesellsch. mbH, Landsberg 1988.

Lewin L, Gifte und Vergiftungen, 6. Aufl., Nachdruck, Haug Verlag, Heidelberg 1992.

Madaus G, Lehrbuch der Biologischen Arzneimittel, Bde 1-3, Nachdruck, Georg Olms Verlag Hildesheim 1979.

Oliver-Bever B (Ed.), Medicinal Plants of Tropical West Africa, Cambridge University Press, Cambridge, London 1986.

Roth L, Daunderer M, Kormann K, Giftpflanzen, Pflanzengifte, 4. Aufl., Ecomed Fachverlag Landsberg Lech 1993.

Teuscher E, Lindequist U, Biogene Gifte - Biologie, Chemie, Pharmakologie, 2. Aufl., Fischer Verlag Stuttgart 1994.

Zheng MS, Zhang YZ Anti-HBsAg herbs employing ELISA technique. Chung Hsi I Chieh Ho Tsa Chih, 26:560-2 518, Sep1990.

Levisticum officinale

See Lovage

Liatris spicata

See Marsh Blazing Star

Licorice

Glycyrrhiza glabra

TRADE NAMES

Licorice Root (available from numerous manufacturers) Wild Countryside Licorice Root, Standardized Licorice, Licorice Power, Phyto Power, Licorice

DESCRIPTION

Medicinal Parts: The medicinal parts are the unpeeled, dried roots and the runners, the peeled dried roots, and the rhizome with the roots.

Flower and Fruit: The axillary inflorescences are upright, spike-like and 10 to 15 cm long. The individual flowers are 1 to 1.5 cm long, bluish to pale violet and short-pedicled. The calyx is short, bell-shaped and glandular-haired. The tips of the calyx are longer than the tube, and are pointed lanceolate. The petals are narrow, the carina petals are not fused, and they are pointed but not beaked. The fruit is a pod, 1.5 to 2.5 cm long, and 4 to 6 mm wide. It is erect and splayed, flat with thick sutures, glabrous, somewhat reticulate-pitted, and usually has 3 to 5 brown, reniform seeds.

Leaves, Stem and Root: The plant is a herbaceous perennial. It is 1 to 2 m high and has a long sturdy primary taproot. The taproot is 15 cm long and subdivides into 3 to 5 subsidiary roots, 1.25 m in length. There are several horizontal woody stolons which may reach 8 m. New stems are produced every year. They are sturdy, erect, branched either from the base or from further up, and are generally rough at the top. The foliage leaves are alternate, odd pinnate and 10 to 20 cm long. The leaflets are in 3 to 8 pairs. The stipules are very small and drooping.

Habitat: Individual varieties of Glycyrrhiza are found in different regions. Glycyrrhiza glanulifera is found in south-eastern Europe and western Asia. Glycyrrhiza pallida and violocea are found in Iraq. Glycyrrhiza typica is indigenous to southern Europe and southwest Asia.

Production: Licorice root consists of the peeled and un-peeled, dried roots and stolons of Glycyrrhiza glabra. Licorice juice is the extract of Glycyrrhiza glabra.

Other Names: Sweet Root, sweet wort

ACTIONS AND PHARMACOLOGY

COMPOUNDS: LICORICE EXTRACT

Triterpene saponins (3-15%): (according to DAB 1996, 4-6% in the adjusted Licorice extract, according to DAC 1995, 5-7% in the dry Licorice extract): chief components are glycyrrhetic acid (sweet-tasting, aglycone 18 beta-glycyr-rhetic acid, salts termed glycyrrizin)

Flavonoids: aglycones, including liquiritigenin, isoliquiri-tigenin (its chalcone), isolicoflavonol

Isoflavonoids: aglycones formononetin, glabren, glabridin, glabrol, 3-hydroxyglabrol, glycyrrhisoflavone

Cumestan derivatives: glycyrol, isoglycyrol, liqcoumarin

Hydroxycoumarins: including herniarin, umbelliferone, gly-cycoumarin, licopyranocumarin

Steroids: sterols, including beta-sitosterol, stigmasterol

The drug contains considerably more free flavonoid and isoflavonoid aglycones than the root drug does, due to the hydrolysis that takes place during the extraction procedure.

COMPOUNDS: LICORICE ROOT

Triterpene saponins (3-15%): chief components glycyrrhetic acid (sweet-tasting, aglycone 18beta-glycyrrhetic acid, salts termed glycyrrhizin), 18-alpha-glycrrhetic acid, glycyrrhetic acid methyl ester, glabric acid, glabrolide, uralenic acid

Flavonoids: aglycones including liquiritigenin, isoliquiritige-nin (its chalcone), isolicoflavonol, isoliquiritin, licoricidin

Isoflavonoids: aglycones formononetin, glabren, glabridin, glabrol, 3-hydroxyglabrol, glycyrrhisoflavone

Cumestan derivatives: glycyrol, isoglycyrol, liquocoumarin

Hydroxycoumarins: including herniarin, umbelliferone, gly-cycoumarin, licopyranocoumarin

Steroids: sterols, including beta-sitosterol, stigmasterol

Volatile oil (very little): with anethole, estragole, eugenol, hexanoic acid

EFFECTS: LICORICE EXTRACT AND ROOT

Anti-Inflammatory/Anti-platelet Effects

Glabridin exerts anti-inflammatory effects through inhibition of tyrosinase activity, superoxide anion production, and cyclooxygenase activity (Yokota, 1998). Licoricidin, a potent compound in the root, has an inhibitory effect on isoPAF(platelet-activating factor) acetyltransferase resulting in anti-inflammatory activity (Nagumo, 1999). Isoliquiritige-nin, an aldose reductase inhibitor, exerts anti-platelet effects through inhibition of cyclooxygenase, lipoxygenase, and peroxidase activity (Tawata, 1992). The anti-inflammatory effects of glycyrrhizin is attributed to its anti-thrombin action through inhibition of thrombin induced platelet aggregation (Francischetti, 1997).

Antiulcer Effects

Licorice has protective effects against gastric ulcers induced by aspirin (Dehpour, 1994). Licorice has the ability to release endogenous secretin, which is a potential mediator of the antiulcer actions (Shiratori, 1986). Carbenoxolone, a succinate derivative of glycyrrhetic acid, has been shown to accelerate the healing of ulcers (Barbara, 1979; Bianchi, 1985). Deglycyrrhizinated licorice is also effective for healing ulcers and lacks undesirable side effects seen with carbenoxolone (Morgan, 1982).

Antiviral/Antifungal Effects

Glycyrrhizin suppresses the secretion of hepatitis B virus (HBV) surface antigen (HbsAg) in patients with HBV. The compound is thought to bind to hepatocytes at a concentration able to modify the expression of HBV-related antigens on the hepatocytes and suppress sialylation of HbsAg (Sato, 1996). Glycyrrhizin stimulates interferon gamma produced by T-cells for an antiviral effect against influenza virus infection (Utsunomiya, 1997). Antiviral action of glycyrrhizin on the human immunodeficiency virus (HIV) occurs by inhibiting replication through interference with virus-cell binding and also suppression of giant cell formation (Ito, 1987; Nakashima, 1987). Glycyrrhizin induces CD4 T cells, which suppress type 2 cytokines produced by burn-associated type 2 T cells. This improves resistance to *Candida alibicans* associated with thermal injury (Utsunomiya, 1999).

Mineralcorticoid Effects

Licorice inhibits the enzyme 11-beta- hydroxysteroid dehydrogenase in the kidney, which leads to decreased transformation of cortisol into cortisone. The mineralocorticoid action of cortisol causes a decrease in serum potassium and an increase in serum sodium concentration resulting in retention of water, causing weight increase and hypertension (Palermo, 1996). Glycyrrhetic acid, the hydrolytic metabolite of glycerrhizic acid causes the inhibition of peripheral metabolism of cortisol and produces a pseudo-aldosterone-like effect (Heikens, 1995). Licorice induces high blood pressure also through inhibition of NADPH-dependent short chain dehydrogenase/reductase enzymes in the kidney (Duax, 1998).

Miscellaneous Effects

Glabridin has been shown to inhibit UVB induced pigmentation and erythema in skins of giunea pigs (Yokota, 1998). Isoliquiritin inhibits granuloma angiogenesis in a concentration dependent manner (Kobayashi, 1995). Glycyrrhizin has therapeutic effects on liver dysfunction associated with cytomegalovirus infection (Numazaki, 1994). Glycyrrhizin has complementary effects on intracelluar calcium mobilization to block neuromuscular transmission (Dezaki, 1995). Licorice exerts a choleretic effects through glycyrrhizin and other unknown components (Raggi, 1995).

CLINICAL TRIALS

Gastric Ulcer

A double-blind study involving thirty-four patients was conducted to compare carbenoloxalone and pirenzepine for treatment of a chronic gastric ulcer. Carbenoxalone was administered as 300 mg daily for 1 week followed by 150 mg daily for 5 weeks. Pirnzepine was administered as 150 mg daily for 6 weeks. There was no significant difference between the groups at the end of the treatment period with ulcers healed in 59% of the pirenzepine group and in 52% of the carbenoxolone group. The healing rates in this study do not compare well with reported treatment success rates of H2-receptor antagonists (Bianchi, 1985).

Peptic Ulcer

A randomized, single-blind trial compared the efficacy of deglycyrrhizinated licorice (Caved-S®) to cimetidine in 100 patients with peptic ulcer disease. The patients were administered either cimetidine 200 mg 3 times daily plus 400 mg at night or Caved-S plus antacid combination, 2 tablets to be chewed 3 times a day between meals. Caved-S® was as effective as cimetidine for healing peptic ulcers over 6 and 12 weeks but was slower in reducing night pain from peptic ulcer. The medications were equally effective and superior to placebo for the prevention of recurrences with peptic ulcers. Endoscopic evaluation showed healing of ulcers in 60% and 66% of the Caved-S and cimetidine groups, respectively at the end of 6 weeks. After 12 weeks, healing had occurred in 88% and 94%, respectively (Morgan et al, 1982).

Hepatitis

A retrospective study evaluated the long-term use of a glycyrrhizin-containing solution for prevention of hepatocellular carcinoma (HCC) in patients with chronic hepatitis C. One-hundred and ninety-two patients with chronic hepatitis C were included in the study. Stronger Neo-Minophagen C (SNMC), an intravenous solution containing 0.2% glycyrrhizin, 0.1% cysteine, and 2% glycine in physiologic solution, 100 milliliters (mL) daily was administered to 83 patients over an 8 week period, then followed by 2 to 7 times per week for 2 to 16 years (median 10.1 years). The other 109 patients were treated with other herbal remedies, such as vitamin K, for 1 to 16 years (median, 9.2 years). The 10-year rate occurrence of HCC were 7% in the SNMC treatment group and 12% respectively in the non-SNMC treatment group. The 15-year rate was 12% in the SNMC treatment group and 25% in the other treatment group (p=0.032). Elevated alanine aminotransferase (ALT), a characteristic of chronic hepatitis and a risk factor for the development of HCC normalized in 35.7% in the SNMC treatment group, which was significantly better than the 6.4% of the other treatment group (Arase et al, 1997).

INDICATIONS AND USAGE

LICORICE ROOT

Approved by Commission E:

■ Cough/bronchitis
■ Gastritis

Unproven Uses: The drug is used for catarrh of the upper respiratory tract as well as for gastric/duodenal ulcers. In folk medicine, the herb is used for appendicitis, constipation, and to increase milk production and micturation. The drug is also used as a treatment for epilepsy and inflammation of the gastrointestinal and urogenital tract. Externally, the herb is used for dermatoses.

Indian Medicine: Internally, the herb is used for gastric ulcers, headaches, bronchitis, eye diseases and sore throat. The drug is used externally for wounds and cuts.

Chinese Medicine: The herb is used for sore throats, carbuncles, spleen disorders, dry cough, and dehydration.

LICORICE EXTRACT

Unproven Uses: The drug is used for gastritis, gastric ulcers, ulcer prophylaxis, and viral liver inflammation.

CONTRAINDICATIONS

LICORICE ROOT AND FRUIT

Contraindications include chronic hepatitis, cholestatic diseases of the liver, cirrhosis of the liver, severe renal insufficiency, diabetes, arrythmias, hypertension, hypertonia, hypokalemia, and pregnancy. Tobacco use has been associated with licorice toxicity (Synhaivsky, 1980).

PRECAUTIONS AND ADVERSE REACTIONS

LICORICE ROOT AND EXTRACT

General: Intake of the herb over a prolonged period of time may result in hypokalemia, hypernatremia, edema, hypertension and cardiac complaints.

Endocrine: Pseudoaldosteronism reported with the use of licorice is attributed to glycyrrhetenic acid, the hydrolytic metabolite of glycerrhizic acid. Hypertension and hypokalemic metabolic alkylosis (e.g. lethargy, paresthesias, muscle cramps, headaches) are possible consequences of the hypermineralcorticoid effect of Licorice extracts. Retention of sodium and water and suppression of the renin-aldosterone system is associated with extracts of the root (Heikens, 1995; Seelen, 1996). Hypokalemic rhabdomyolysis, resulting in acute renal failure and profound deposition of calcium into the damaged skeletal and cardiac muscles was reported with glycyrrhizin use (Saito, 1994).

Drug Interactions: Furosemide/Thiazide Diuretics - Due to the additive effect of hypokalemia, the concomitant use of these medications with licorice is not recommended.

Digitalis Glycosides - Hypokalemia associated with the prolonged use of licorice may potentiate digitalis toxicity.

Anti-arrythmic Agents (procainamide, quinidine) - Hypokalemia and severe ventricular tachycardia of torsades de pointes type reported with licorice consumption may be potentiated with concomitant use of anti-arrythmic agents (Eriksson, 1999).

Corticosteroids - Concomitant use of licorice with corticosteroids potentiates effects due to the prolonged half-life of cortisol.

OVERDOSAGE

LICORICE ROOT AND EXTRACT

The intake of higher dosages (above 20 gm per day for the extract and above 50 gm per day for the root) over an extended period of time will lead to hypokalemia, hypernatremia, edemas, hypertension and cardiac complaints. In rare cases, myoglobinemia has resulted due to the mineralcorticoid (aldosterone-like) effect of the saponins (Heikens, 1995; Saito, 1994; Seelen, 1996). Preparations from the drug should not be administered for longer than 6 weeks. The complaints disappear after discontinuing the drug. (SEE PRECAUTIONS AND ADVERSE REACTIONS)

DOSAGE

LICORICE ROOT

Mode of Administration: Comminuted drug, drug powder, dry extracts for infusions, decoctions, liquid or solid forms for internal use. Various teas contain extracts of the drug, for example, bronchial teas, gastric teas, and laxative teas.

The drug should not be administered for more than 6 weeks (see side effects).

How Supplied:

Capsules — 100mg, 200mg, 400mg, 444mg, 445mg, 450mg, 500mg

Preparation: To prepare an infusion, use 1 to 1.5 gm of finely comminuted drug and add cold water. Bring to a boil, or pour the boiling water over the drug and allow to draw for 10 to 15 minutes and then strain (1 teaspoonful = 3 gm drug).

Daily Dosage: The average daily dose is 5 to 15 gm of the root, equivalent to 200 to 600 mg of glycyrrhizin. The drug is not to be taken longer than 6 weeks (SEE OVERDOSAGE). Succus liquiritiae: 0.5 to 1 gm for catarrhs of the upper respiratory tract and 1.5 to 3.0 gm for gastric/duodenal ulcers.

Tea - Drink one cup of tea after meals.

LICORICE EXTRACT

Mode of Administration: The drug is widely available in medicinal preparations, as tea or in drop form; the juice of licorice is found in liquorice edible goods and preparations.

Preparation: For preparation of tea, pour a cup of boiling water over 1 teaspoon of juice, leave to draw for 5 minutes.

Daily Dosage: Drink one cup of tea after each meal. The dosage for the drop form is 25 drops to be taken 4 times daily.

LITERATURE

Aikawa Y, Yoshiike T, Ogawa H, Effect of glycyrrhizin pain and HLA-DR antigen expression on CD8-positive cells in peripheral blood of herpes zoster patients in comparsion with other antiviral agents. In: Skin Pharmacol 3:268-271. 1990.

Amagaya S et al., J Pharmacobiodynamics 7 (12):923.

Anderson J, Smith WG, (1961) The antitussive activity of glycyrrhetinic acid and its derivatives. J Pharm Pharmacol

Arase Y, Ikeda K, Murashima N et al: The long term efficacy of glycyrrhizin in chronic hepatitis C patients.Cancer 1997; 79:1494-1500.

Baba M, Shigeta S, Antiviral activity of glycyrrhizin against varicella-zoster virus in vitro. In: Antiviral Res 7:99-106. 1987.

Barbara L; Belsasso E; Blasi A et al. Pirenzepine and carbenozolone in gastric ulcer. Preliminary results of a multicentre double-blind controlled clinical trial. Scand J Gastroenterol Suppl 1979;57:21-4.

Bardhan KD et al., (1978) Gut 19:779.

Bhardwaj DK et al., (1977) Phytochemistry 15:352.

Bhardwaj DK et al., (1977) Phytochemistry 16:401.

Bhardwaj DK, Singh R, (1977) Curr Sci 46:753.

Christensen SB et al., An antileishmanial chalcone from chinese licorice roots. In: PM 60(2):121. 1994.

Dehpour AR; Zolfaghari ME; Samadian T; Vahedi Y. The protective effect of liquorice components and their derivatives against gastric ulcer induced by aspirin in rats. J Pharm Pharmacol 1994 Feb;46(2):148-9.

Dezaki K; Kimura I; Miyahara K; Kimura M. Complementary effects of paeoniflorin and glycyrrhizin on intracellular Ca2+ mobilization in the nerve-stimulated skeletal muscle of mice. Jpn J Pharmacol 1995 Nov;69(3):281-4.

Duax WL; Ghosh D. Structure and mechanism of action and inhibition of steroid dehydrogenase enzymes involved in hypertension. Endocr Res 1998 Aug-Nov;24(3-4):521-9.

Eriksson JW; Carlberg B; Hillorn V. Life-threatening ventricular tachycardia due to liquorice-induced hypokalaemia. J Intern Med 1999 Mar;245(3):307-10.

Epstein MT et al., (1977) Brit Med J 19:488.

Fintelmann V, Moderne Phytotherapie am Beispiel gastroenterologischer Erkrankungen. In: ZPT 11(5):161. 1990.

Francischetti IM; Monteiro RQ; Guimaraes JA. Identification of glycyrrhizin as a thrombin inhibitor. Biochem Biophys Res Commun 1997 Jun 9;235(1):259-63.

Hattori T, Ikematsu Sh, Koito A, Matsushita Sh, Maeda Y, Hada M, Fujimaki M, Takatsuki K, Preliminary evidence for inhibitory effects of glycyrrhizin on HIV replication in patients with AIDS. In: Antiviral Res 11:255-262. 1989.

Hayashi H et al., Distribution patterns of saponine in different organs of Glycyrrhiza glabra. In: PM 59(4):351. 1993.

Hayashi Y et al., (1979) Yakuri to Chiryo 7:3861.

Heikens J, Fliers E, Endert E et al. Liquorice-induced hypertension: a new understanding of an old disease:case report and brief review. Neth J Med 1995; 47:230-234.

Inoue H, Saito K, Koshihara Y, Murota S, (1986) Inhibitory effect of glyzyrrhetinic acid derivatives of lipoxygenase and prostaglandin synthetase. Chem Pharm Bull 34:897.

Ito M, Nakashima H, Baba M, Pauwels R, De Clercq E, Shigeta S, Yamamoto N, Inhibitory effect of glycyrrhizin on the in vitro infectivity and cytopathic activity of the human immunodeficiency virus (HIV (HTLV-III/LAV). In: Antiviral Res 7:127-137. 1987.

Kato H; Kanaoka M; Yano S; Kobayashi M. 3-Monoglucuronyl-glycyrrhetinic acid is a major metabolite that causes licorice-induced pseudoaldosteronism. J Clin Endocrinol Metab 1995 Jun;80(6):1929-33.

Khaksa G et al., Anti-inflammatory and anti-nociceptive activity of disodium glycyrrhetinic acid hemiphthalate. In: PM 62(4):326-328. 1996.

Killacky J et al., (1976) Planta Med 30:310.

Kinoshita T et al., (1978) Chem Pharm Bull 26: 141 et 135.

Kiso Y et al., (1984) Planta Med 50:298.

Kobayashi S; Miyamoto T; Kimura I; Kimura M. Inhibitory effect of isoliquiritin, a compound in licorice root, on angiogenesis in vivo and tube formation in vitro. Biol Pharm Bull. 1995 Oct;18(10):1382-6.

Kumagai A, Takata M, (1978) Proc Symp Wakan-Yaku 11:73.

Miething H, Speicher-Brinker A, Hänsel R, Hochdruckflüssigchromatographische Untersuchungen der Flavonoidfraktion in Süßholzwurzeln und deren pharmazeutischen Zubereitungen. In: PZW 135(6):253. 1990.

Morgan AG, McAdam WAF, Pacsoo C et al: Comparison between cimetidine and Caved-S in the treatment of gastric ulceration, and subsequent maintenance therapy. Gut 1982; 23:545-551.

Nagumo S; Fukuju A; Takayama M et al. Inhibition of lysoPAF acetyltransferase activity by components of licorice root. Biol Pharm Bull 1999 Oct;22(10):1144-6.

Nakashima H; Matsui T; Yoshida O et al. A new anti-human immunodeficiency virus substance, glycyrrhizin sulfate; endowment of glycyrrhizin with reverse transcriptase- inhibitory activity by chemical modification. Jpn J Cancer Res 1987 Aug;78(8):767-71.

Neilsen I, Pedersen RS, (1984) Lancet 1:8389.

Nose M et al., A comparision of the antihepatotoxic activity between glycyrrhizin and glycerrhetinic acid. In: PM 60(2):136. 1994.

Numuzaki K, Umetsu M, Chiba S, Effects of glycyrrhizin in children with liver dysfunction assiciated with cytomegalovirus infections. In: Tohoku J Exp Med 172:147-153. 1994.

Palermo M; Shackleton CH; Mantero F; Stewart PM. Urinary free cortisone and the assessment of 11 beta-hydroxysteroid dehydrogenase activity in man. Clin Endocrinol (Oxf) 1996 Nov;45(5):605-11.

Raggi MA; Bugamelli F; Nobile L et al. The choleretic effects of licorice: identification and determination of the pharmacologically active components of Glycyrrhiza glabra. Boll Chim Farm 1995 Dec;134(11):634-8.

Rees WDW et al., (1979) Scand. J Gastroenterol. 14:605.

Saitoh T et al., (1976) Chem Pharm Bull 24:991.

Saitoh T et al., (1978) Chem Pharm Bull 26:752.

Saitoh T et al., (1976) Chem Pharm Bull 24:752 et 1242.

Sato H; Goto W; Yamamura J et al. Therapeutic basis of glycyrrhizin on chronic hepatitis B. Antiviral Res 1996 May;30(2-3):171-7.

Saito T; Tsuboi Y; Fujisawa G et al. An autopsy case of licorice-induced hypokalemic rhabdomyolysis associated with acute renal failure: special reference to profound calcium deposition in skeletal and cardiac muscle. Nippon Jinzo Gakkai Shi 1994 Nov;36(11):1308-14.

Seelen MA; de Meijer PH; Braun J et al. Hypertension caused by licorice consumption. Ned Tijdschr Geneeskd 1996 Dec 28;140(52):2632-5.

Synhaivsky A. Licorice, snuff, and hypokalemia. N Engl J Med 1980 Aug 21;303(8):463.

Segal R et al., (1985) J Pharm Sci 74 (1):79.

Shiratori K; Watanabe S; Takeuchi T. Effect of licorice extract (Fm100) on release of secretin and exocrine pancreatic secretion in humans. Pancreas 1986;1(6):483-7.

Suzuki H, Ohta Y, Takino T, Fujisawa K, Hirayama C, Effect of glycyrrhizin on biochemical test in patients with chronic hepatitis. Double blind trial. In: Asian Med J 26:423-438. 1983.

Takechi M, Tanaka Y, Structure-activity relationships of the synthetic methyl glycyrrhetate glycosides. In: PH 32: 1173. 1993.

Tamura Y, Nishikawa T, Yamada K, Yamamoto M, Kumagai A, (1979) Effects of glyzyrrhetinic acid and ist derivatives on Delta5-reductase in rat liver. Arzneimittel Forsch/Drug Res 29: 647.

Tanaka S et al., (1987) Planta Med 53 (1):5.

Tawata M; Aida K; Noguchi T et al. Anti-platelet action of isoliquiritigenin, an aldose reductase inhibitor in licorice. Eur J Pharmacol 1992 Feb 25;212(1):87-92.

Utsunomiya T; Kobayashi M; Herndon DN et al. Effects of glycyrrhizin, an active component of licorice roots, on Candida albicans infection in thermally injured mice. Clin Exp Immunol 1999 May;116(2):291-8.

Utsunomiya T; Kobayashi M; Pollard RB; Suzuki F. Glycyrrhizin, an active component of licorice roots, reduces morbidity and mortality of mice infected with lethal doses of influenza virus. Antimicrob Agents Chemother 1997 Mar;41(3):551-6.

Van Hulle C, (1970) Pharmazie 25:620.

Veit M, Wirkungen der Glycyrrhetinsäure auf den Steroidstoffwechsel. In: ZPT 14(1):43. 1993.

Watanabe Y, Watanabe K, (1980) Proc Symp Wakan-Yaku 13:16.

Yagura T et al., (1978) Proc Symp Wakan-Yaku 11:79.

Yamamura Y, Kawakami J, Santa T, Kotaki H, Uchino K, Sawada Y, Tanaka N, Iga T, Pharmacokinetic profile of glycyrrhizin in healthy volunteers by a new high-performance liquid chromatographic method. In: J Pharm Sci 81(10):1042-1046. 1992.

Yokota T; Nishio H; Kubota Y; Mizoguchi M. The inhibitory effect of glabridin from licorice extracts on melanogenesis and inflammation. Pigment Cell Res 1998 Dec;11(6):355-61.

Further information in:

Chang EH et al., (Eds), Advances in Chinese Medicinal Materials Research, World Scientific Pub. Co. Singapore 1985.

Frohne D, Pfänder HJ, Giftpflanzen - Ein Handbuch für Apotheker, Toxikologen und Biologen, 4. Aufl., Wiss. Verlags-Ges Stuttgart 1997.

Hänsel R, Keller K, Rimpler H, Schneider G (Hrsg.), Hagers Handbuch der Pharmazeutischen Praxis, 5. Aufl., Bde 4-6 (Drogen): Springer Verlag Berlin, Heidelberg, New York, 1992-1994.

Hikino H, Economic and Medicinal Plant Research, Vol I., Academic Press UK 1985.

Leung AY, Encyclopedia of Common Natural Ingredients Used in Food, Drugs and Cosmetics, John Wiley & Sons Inc., New York 1980.

Madaus G, Lehrbuch der Biologischen Arzneimittel, Bde 1-3, Nachdruck, Georg Olms Verlag Hildesheim 1979.

Roth L, Daunderer M, Kormann K, Giftpflanzen, Pflanzengifte, 4. Aufl., Ecomed Fachverlag Landsberg Lech 1993.

Schulz R, Hänsel R, Rationale Phytotherapie, Springer Verlag Heidelberg 1996.

Steinegger E, Hänsel R, Pharmakognosie, 5. Aufl., Springer Verlag Heidelberg 1992.

Tang W, Eisenbrand G, Chinese Drugs of Plant Origin, Springer Verlag Heidelberg 1992.

Teuscher E, Lindequist U, Biogene Gifte - Biologie, Chemie, Pharmakologie, 2. Aufl., Fischer Verlag Stuttgart 1994.

Wagner H, Wiesenauer M, Phytotherapie. Phytopharmaka und pflanzliche Homöopathika, Fischer-Verlag, Stuttgart, Jena, New York 1995.

Wichtl M (Hrsg.), Teedrogen, 4. Aufl., Wiss. Verlagsges. Stuttgart 1997.

Lilium candidum

See White Lily

Lilium martagon

See Martagon

Lily-of-the-Valley

Convallaria majalis

DESCRIPTION

Medicinal Parts: The medicinal parts are the dried flower tips and the dried inflorescence, the Lily-of-the-Valley herb, the dried root rhizome with the roots, the flowering aerial parts and the whole, fresh, flowering plant.

Flower and Fruit: The flowers are in racemes nodding to one side, usually with a triangular penduncle. The tips are hemispheric, campanulate, 6-petalled with ovoid revolute tips. The perigone is white or pink. The stamens are attached to the base of the perigone. The fruit is a bright red, globular berry with 2 blue seeds. The plant is autosterile.

Leaves, Stem and Root: The 15 to 20 cm high plant has 2 to 3 leaves at the tip of the runner-like, branched rhizome. The leaves are elliptoid and acute. They taper to a long, sharp petiole at the base, which is clasped by a membranous sheath.

Characteristics: Fragrant but poisonous (all parts).

Habitat: The plant is native to Europe and has been introduced into the U.S. and northern Asia.

Production: Lily-of-the-Valley herb consists of the dried, above-ground parts of Convallaria majalis (or closely related species), collected during the flowering season. The harvested parts of the plant must be dried quickly at a maximum temperature of 60°C.

Not to be Confused With: Lilly-of-the-Valley is easily confused with Polygonatum odoratum.

Other Names: May Lily, May Bells, Convallaria, Our Lady's Tears, Convall-Lily, Lily Constancy, Jacob's Ladder, Ladder-to-Heaven, Muguet

ACTIONS AND PHARMACOLOGY

COMPOUNDS

Cardioactive steroid glycosides (cardenolides): varying according to geographical source, chief glycoside convallatoxin (western and northwestern Europe), convalloside (northern and eastern Europe), or convallatoxin + convallatoxol (central Europe)

EFFECTS

Only older studies are available, which indicate the convallara glycosides are qualitatively similar to digitoxin and strophanthin. The studies show Lily-of-the-Valley to have the following effects:

Cardiac: The power and speed of cardiac muscle contraction is increased and there is a reduced relaxation time. The beat frequency is slowed, stimulation transfer is delayed and the ability of the chamber muscles to be stimulated is increased (positively inotropic, negatively chronotropic, negatively dromotropic and positively bathmotropic effect.)

Renal: In animal tests, the effect was natriuretic and diuretic.

Venous: In animal tests, Lily-of-the-Valley demonstrated a dose-dependent, veno-constrictive effect.

INDICATIONS AND USAGE

Approved by Commission E:

- Arrhythmia
- Cardiac insufficiency NYHA I and II
- Nervous heart complaints

Unproven Uses: The drug is used for mild cardiac insufficiency (stage I-II NYHA), heart insufficiency due to old age and chronic cor pulmonale. In folk medicine, Lily-of-the-Valley was also used for weak contractions in labor, epilepsy, dropsy, strokes and ensuing paralysis, conjunctivitis and leprosy. Use for these applications is no longer common because of the drug's toxic effect.

PRECAUTIONS AND ADVERSE REACTIONS

General: Health risks following the proper administration of designated therapeutic dosages are not recorded. Nausea, vomiting, headache, stupor, disorders of color perception and cardiac arrhythmias can occur as side effects, particularly with an overdosage.

Drug Interactions: The simultaneous administration of quinidine, digoxin, calcium salts, saluretics, laxatives and glucocorticoids enhances effects and side effects.

OVERDOSAGE

For symptoms of an acute poisoning and therapy, see Digitalis folium. The dangers of poisoning are relatively low with oral application, due to the poor absorbability of the glycosides.

DOSAGE

Mode of Administration: Comminuted herb, as well as galenic preparations for internal use; no longer considered safe because of the levels of toxins.

How Supplied: All information is based on stabilized Lilly-of-the-Valley powder as specified in the German pharmacopoeia. No other forms can be recommended. However, commercial pharmaceutical preparations are available as capsules, drops, solutions and tablets.

Preparation: Tincture 1:10; liquid extract: 1:1; dry extract: 4:1.

Daily Dosage: The average daily dose of the drug: 0.6 g of tincture; 0.6 g of liquid extract; 0.15 g of dried extract. The average single dose: 2 g of tincture; 0.2 g of liquid extract; 0.05 g of dry extract. In intravenous application, the full effective dose of convaltoxin is 0.4 to 0.6 mg, the prepared dose 0.2 to 0.3 mg.

Storage: The preparations should be stored in well-sealed containers and protected from light.

LITERATURE

Bleier W et al., (1965) Pharm Acta Helv 40:554.

Hölzl J, Franz C, PM 24:378. 1973.

Kopp B, Kubelka W, (1982) Planta Med 45:87.

Krenn L, Schlifelner L, Stimpfl T, Kopp B, HPLC separation and quantitative determination of cardenolides in Herba Convallariae. In: PM 58(7)A82. 1992.

Laufke R, (1958) Planta Med 6:237.

Loew D, Phytotherapie bei Herzinsuffizienz. In: ZPT 18(2):92-96. 1997.

Loew DA, Loew AD, Pharmakokinetik von herzglykosidhaltigen Pflanzenextrakten. In: ZPT 15(4):197-202. 1994.

Tschesche R et al., (1959) Naturwissensch. 46:109.

Tschesche R, in Pharmacognosy and Phytochemistry, Ed. H. Wagner and L. Hörhammer, Springer-Verlag Heidelberg, Berlin 1971.

Further information in:

Frohne D, Pfänder HJ, Giftpflanzen - Ein Handbuch für Apotheker, Toxikologen und Biologen, 4. Aufl., Wiss. Verlagsges. mbH Stuttgart 1997.

Hänsel R, Keller K, Rimpler H, Schneider G (Hrsg.), Hagers Handbuch der Pharmazeutischen Praxis, 5. Aufl., Bde 4-6 (Drogen), Springer Verlag Berlin, Heidelberg, New York, 1992-1994.

Lewin L, Gifte und Vergiftungen, 6. Aufl., Nachdruck, Haug Verlag, Heidelberg 1992.

Madaus G, Lehrbuch der Biologischen Arzneimittel, Bde 1-3, Nachdruck, Georg Olms Verlag Hildesheim 1979.

Roth L, Daunderer M, Kormann K, Giftpflanzen, Pflanzengifte, 4. Aufl., Ecomed Fachverlag Landsberg Lech 1993.

Schulz R, Hänsel R, Rationale Phytotherapie, Springer Verlag Heidelberg 1996.

Steinegger E, Hänsel R, Pharmakognosie, 5. Aufl., Springer Verlag Heidelberg 1992.

Teuscher E, Lindequist U, Biogene Gifte - Biologie, Chemie, Pharmakologie, 2. Aufl., Fischer Verlag Stuttgart 1994.

Teuscher E, Biogene Arzneimittel, 5. Aufl., Wiss. Verlagsges. mbH Stuttgart 1997.

Wagner H, Wiesenauer M, Phytotherapie. Phytopharmaka und pflanzliche Homöopathika, Fischer-Verlag, Stuttgart, Jena, New York 1995.

Lime

Citrus aurantifolia

DESCRIPTION

Medicinal Parts: The medicinal component is the bergamot oil extracted from the plant.

Flower and Fruit: The fragrant flowers are small and pure white. The fruit is about half the size of a lemon, with a smoother, thinner peel, a greenish-yellow color and sweet taste.

Leaves, Stem and Root: The evergreen tree is small, bent, thorny and normally only grows to a height of 2.5 m. The leaves are ovate-lanceolate and acuminate.

Habitat: Lime is indigenous to Southern Asia and is cultivated in the West Indies, semi-tropic areas of the U.S. and Central America.

Production: Limes and lemons are the fruit of Citrus aurantifolia.

Other Names: Limette, Italian Limetta, Adam's Apple

ACTIONS AND PHARMACOLOGY

COMPOUNDS

Volatile oil (in the fruit rind): containing, among others, citral, (+)-limonene, pinenes, alkanes, alkanols, alkanals, beta-bisabolene; also, in pressed oils, furocoumarins

Citric acid

Flavonoids: including hesperidine

EFFECTS

Lime acts as an antiscorbutic and refrigerant as well as a vitamin C supplement.

INDICATIONS AND USAGE

Lime is used as a source of vitamin C to treat scurvy and in cases of general low resistance.

PRECAUTIONS AND ADVERSE REACTIONS

No health hazards or side effects are known in conjunction with the proper administration of designated therapeutic dosages. There is a low potential for sensitization through skin contact with the juice of the fruit or with the volatile oil.

DOSAGE

Mode of Administration: Lime is used internally as a liquid extract of the fresh fruit.

LITERATURE

Kovats et al., Helv Chim Acta 46:2705. 1963.

Lund ED, Bryan WL, (1977) J Food Sci 42:385.

Natarajan S et al., (1976) Econ Bot 30:38.

Shaw PE, Coleman RL, (1971) J Agric Food Chem 19:1276.

Stanley et al., PH 6:585. 1967.

Strickler et al., Helv Chim Acta 49:2055. 1966.

Tatum JH, Berry RE, (1977) Phytochemistry 16:1091.

Wilson W, Shaw PE, (1977) J Agric Food Chem 25:211.

Further information in:

Kern W, List PH, Hörhammer L (Hrsg.), Hagers Handbuch der Pharmazeutischen Praxis, 4. Aufl., Bde. 1-8, Springer Verlag Berlin, Heidelberg, New York, 1969.

Leung AY, Encyclopedia of Common Natural Ingredients Used in Food, Drugs and Cosmetics, John Wiley & Sons Inc., New York 1980.

Roth L, Daunderer M, Kormann K, Giftpflanzen, Pflanzengifte, 4. Aufl., Ecomed Fachverlag Landsberg Lech 1993.

Linaria vulgaris

See Yellow Toadflax

Linden

Tilia species

DESCRIPTION

Medicinal Parts: The medicinal parts are the fresh and dried flowers.

Flower and Fruit: The yellowish-white flowers are arranged in clusters of 5 to 11. The calyx is 5-sepaled, oblong or ovate-lanceolate, acute and deep. The 5 petals are spatulate-lanceolate with crenate tips. There are numerous stamens and 1 superior ovary, which is almost globular and has silky-haired villi. The fruit is a 1-seeded, pear-shaped, indistinctly angular, thin-shelled nut. There is a tongue-shaped, parchment-like, greenish- or yellowish-white bract at the base of the flowers.

Leaves, Stem and Root: Linden is an impressive tree up to 25 m high with a large, closed crown. The bark is fissured, gray-brown or black-gray. The bark of the branches is smooth. The branchlets are olive-green, brown or brown-red with white warts. The leaves are long-petioled, uneven at the base and broadly cordate. They have a dark upper surface and are bluish-green beneath with rust-colored tufts of down in the vein axils.

Characteristics: The flowers have a strong, sweet fragrance and the fruit tastes slightly sweet, slimy and dry.

Habitat: The tree is common in northern temperate regions.

Production: Linden charcoal consists of the charcoal obtained from the wood of Tilia cordata and/or Tilia platyphyllos. Linden leaf consists of the dried leaf of Tilia cordata and/or Tilia platyphyllos. Silver Linden flower consists of the dried flowers of Tilia tomentosa (synonym Tilia argentea). Linden wood consists of the dried sapwood of Tilia cordata and/or Tilia platyphyllos. Linden flower consists of the dried flower of Tilia cordata and/or Tilia platyphyllos.

Not to be Confused With: Linden flower should not be confused with Tilia tometosa and Tilia x euchlora

Other Names: Lime, Linn Flowers

ACTIONS AND PHARMACOLOGY

COMPOUNDS: LINDEN CHARCOAL

Extremely adsorbent charcoals

EFFECTS: LINDEN CHARCOAL

No information is available.

COMPOUNDS: LINDEN LEAF

Flavonoids: including tiliroside, kempferol-3,7,-dirhamnoside, kempferol-3-O-glucoside-7-O-rhamnoside, linarine (acacetin-7-rutinoside), quercetin-3,7-di-O-rhamnoside, quercetin-3-O-glucoside-7-O-rhamnoside

Tannins

Mucilages

EFFECTS: LINDEN LEAF

The apparent diaphoretic effect has not been proven.

COMPOUNDS: SILVER LINDEN FLOWER

Flavonoids: including astragalin, isoquercitrin, kempferitrin, quercitrin, tiliroside, quercetin-3-O-glucoside-7-O-rhamnoside, kempferol-3-O-rhamnoside, kempferol-3-O-glucoside-7-O-rhamnoside, quercetin-rhamnoxyloside

Hydroxycoumarins: including, among others, calycanthoside, aesculin

Caffeic acid derivatives: chlorogenic acid

Mucilages

EFFECTS: SILVER LINDEN FLOWER

A possible sedative-anxiolytic effect and an anti-stress effect are under investigation. The flavone-like substances in the drug are thought to be responsible for these effects.

COMPOUNDS: LINDEN WOOD

Mucilages

Sterols: beta-sitosterol, stigmasterol, stigmastenol and their fatty acid esters

Triterpenes: squalene

EFFECTS: LINDEN WOOD

The diuretic, hypotensive, and choleretic effects ascribed to the drug are insufficiently documented. In animal experiments, an increase of bile secretion and a lowering of arterial pressure have been described. Aqueous extracts of the drug are antimicrobial.

COMPOUNDS: LINDEN FLOWER

Flavonoids (1%): including chief constituents astragalin, isoquercitrin, kempferol-3-O-rhamnoside, quercitrin, tiliroside (astragalin-6''-p-cumaroylester), including as well rutin, hyperoside, afzelin, kempferitrin

Mucilages(10%): arabino galactans with uronic acid share

Volatile oil (0.01-0.02%): including linalool, germacrene, geraniol, 1,8-cineole, 2-phenyl ethanol, phenyl ethyl benzoate, alkanes

Caffeic acid derivatives: chlorogenic acid

Tannins

EFFECTS: LINDEN FLOWER

The antitussive, astringent, diaphoretic, diuretic, sedative, and analgesic effects attributed to the drug have not yet been widely supported by experimental data. The toxic principle is unknown.

An alcoholic extract of the flowers is antimicrobial in vitro with the tannins, glycosides, and the essential oil the active components. Tilia flavonoids, which have not been described in detail, are anti-edemic in animal experiments. In addition, various experimental results point to a sedative effect. The diaphoretic effect is controversial. After steam inhalation with a lime flower additive, an improvement of the symptoms of uncomplicated colds was observed in comparison to a control group (only steam).

INDICATIONS AND USAGE

LINDEN CHARCOAL

Unproven Uses: Preparations of Linden charcoal are used internally for intestinal disorders and externally for ulcus cruris (leg ulcers).

LINDEN LEAF

Unproven Uses: Preparations of Linden leaf are used as a diaphoretic.

SILVER LINDEN FLOWER

Unproven Uses: Preparations of Silver Linden flower are used for catarrhs of the respiratory tract and as an antispasmodic, expectorant, diaphoretic and diuretic.

LINDEN WOOD

Unproven Uses: Preparations of Linden wood are used for diseases and ailments of the liver and gallbladder systems and for cellulitis.

LINDEN FLOWER

Approved by Commission E:

- Cough
- Bronchitis

Unproven Uses: The flowers are used for catarrh of the respiratory tract and as a diaphoretic for feverish colds and infectious diseases, where a sweating cure is needed. It is occasionally used as a diuretic, a stomachic, an antispasmodic and a sedative.

PRECAUTIONS AND ADVERSE REACTIONS

No health hazards or side effects are known in conjunction with the proper administration of designated therapeutic dosages.

DOSAGE

LINDEN FLOWER

Mode of Administration: The drug is available as a comminuted herb for teas, infusions, and other galenic preparations for internal use. The drug is a component of some standardized urologic, antitussive, and sedative preparations; it is also found in cold remedy tea mixtures.

Preparation: To make a tea, pour boiling water over 2 gm drug, or add the drug to cold water and boil briefly; steep 5 to 10 minutes and strain (1 teaspoonful = 1.8 gm drug).

Daily Dosage: The recommended daily dosage is 2 to 4 gm of drug.

LITERATURE

LINDEN LEAF

Kern W, List PH, Hörhammer L (Hrsg.), Hagers Handbuch der Pharmazeutischen Praxis, 4. Aufl., Bde. 1-8: Springer Verlag Berlin, Heidelberg, New York, 1969.

SILVER LINDEN FLOWER

Buchbauer G, Jirovetz L, Ätherisches Lindenblütenöl - Aromastoffanalyse. In: DAZ 132(15):748. 1992.

Further information in:

Fenaroli's Handbook of Flavor Ingredients, Vol. 1, 2nd Ed., CRC Press 1975.

Hegnauer R, Chemotaxonomie der Pflanzen, Bde 1-11: Birkhäuser Verlag Basel, Boston, Berlin 1962-1997.

Roth L, Daunderer M, Kormann K, Giftpflanzen, Pflanzengifte, 4. Aufl., Ecomed Fachverlag Landsberg Lech 1993.

LINDEN WOOD

Kern W, List PH, Hörhammer L (Hrsg.), Hagers Handbuch der Pharmazeutischen Praxis, 4. Aufl., Bde. 1-8: Springer Verlag Berlin, Heidelberg, New York, 1969.

LINDEN FLOWER
Buchbauer G, Jirovetz L, Ätherisches Lindenblütenöl-Aromastoffanalyse. In: DAZ 132(15):748. 1992.

Hildebrandt G, Engelbrecht P, Hildebrandt-Evers G, (1954) Physiologische Grundlagen für eine tageszeitliche Ordnung der Schwitzprozeduren. Z Klin Med 152:446-468.

Kram G, Franz G, PA 49:149. 1985.

Kram G, Franz G, PM 49:149. 1983.

Further information in:

Fenaroli's Handbook of Flavor Ingredients, Vol. 1, 2nd Ed., CRC Press 1975.

Kern W, List PH, Hörhammer L (Hrsg.), Hagers Handbuch der Pharmazeutischen Praxis, 4. Aufl., Bde. 1-8: Springer Verlag Berlin, Heidelberg, New York, 1969.

Madaus G, Lehrbuch der Biologischen Arzneimittel, Bde 1-3, Nachdruck, Georg Olms Verlag Hildesheim 1979.

Schulz R, Hänsel R, Rationale Phytotherapie, Springer Verlag Heidelberg 1996.

Steinegger E, Hänsel R, Pharmakognosie, 5. Aufl., Springer Verlag Heidelberg 1992.

Teuscher E, Biogene Arzneimittel, 5. Aufl., Wiss. Verlagsges. Stuttgart 1997.

Wichtl M (Hrsg.), Teedrogen, 4. Aufl., Wiss. Verlagsges. Stuttgart 1997.

Linum catharticum

See Mountain Flax

Linum usitatissimum

See Flax

Liquidambar orientalis

See Storax

Liriodendron tulipifera

See Tulip Tree

Lithospermum erytrorhizon

See Purple Gromwell
(Ying Zicao)

Lobaria pulmonaria

See Lungmoss

Lobelia

Lobelia inflata

DESCRIPTION

Medicinal Parts: The medicinal parts are the fresh and dried herb and the seeds.

Flower and Fruit: The flowers are on long pedicles in the leaf axils. They are pale violet-blue and lightly tinged with pale yellow. The fruit consists of an ovoid or flattened bilocular capsule containing numerous small, brown and reticulate seeds.

Leaves, Stem and Root: The plant is an erect annual or biennial herb 30 to 60 cm high. The stem is pubescent, angular, branching near the top. It contains an acrid latex. The leaves are pale green or yellowish, the lower ones are petiolate, the upper ones are sessile. They are alternate, ovate-lanceolate, 3 to 8 cm long, with a dentate margin and a finely pubescent lamina.

Characteristics: After chewing the leaves, the taste is similar to tobacco. The taste is acrid, the odor faintly irritant.

Habitat: The plant is indigenous to the regions in the north of U.S., Canada and Kamchatka. It is cultivated elsewhere.

Production: Lobelia is the aerial part of Lobelia inflata.

Other Names: Indian Tobacco, Pukeweed, Asthma Weed, Gagroot, Vomitwort, Bladderpod, Eyebright, Emetic Herb, Emetic Weed, Wild Tobacco and Vomitroot

ACTIONS AND PHARMACOLOGY

COMPOUNDS

Piperidine alkaloids (6%): chief alkaloids L-lobeline (alpha-lobeline); companion alkaloids including among others lobelanine, lobelanidine, norlobelanine, and isolobinine

EFFECTS

The main active principle is lobelin. The drug has a stimulating effect on the respiratory center but it is broken down too quickly in the body to be used as a respiratory analeptic.

INDICATIONS AND USAGE

Homeopathic Uses: Lobelia inflata is used only in homeopathy as an asthma treatment and also as an aid in curing addiction to smoking.

PRECAUTIONS AND ADVERSE REACTIONS

General: No health hazards or side effects are known in conjunction with the proper administration of designated therapeutic dosages.

Pregnancy: Not to be used during pregnancy.

OVERDOSAGE

Overdosage leads to dryness of the mouth, nausea, vomiting, diarrhea, abdominal pain, burning in the urinary passages, feelings of anxiety, dizziness, headache, shivering, respiratory difficulties, paraesthesias, outbreak of sweating, bradycardia, cardiac arrhythmias, somnolence and muscle twitching; death can occur through respiratory failure, accompanied by convulsions. 0.6 to 1 gm of the leaves are said to be toxic, 4 gm fatal.

Following gastrointestinal emptying (inducement of vomiting, gastric lavage with burgundy-colored potassium permanganate solution, sodium sulfate), instillation of activated charcoal, and shock prophylaxis (quiet, warmth), the therapy for poisonings consists of treating spasms with diazepam (i.v.), children with chloral hydrate (rectal); monitoring of ECG. Cardiac massage and artificial respiration may also be required.

DOSAGE

Mode of Administration: The drug is no longer used. It is a constituent in some homeopathic preparations.

LITERATURE

Chang, EH et al., (Eds): Advances in Chinese Medicinal Materials Research, World Scientific Pub. Co. Singapore 1985.

Gross D, (1971) Fortschr Chem Org Naturst 29:1.

Karawya MS et al., (1971) J Ass Off Ann Chem 54(6):1423.

Kern W, List PH, Hörhammer L (Hrsg.), Hagers Handbuch der Pharmazeutischen Praxis, 4. Aufl., Bde. 1-8, Springer Verlag Berlin, Heidelberg, New York, 1969.

Leung AY, Encyclopedia of Common Natural Ingredients Used in Food, Drugs and Cosmetics, John Wiley & Sons Inc., New York, 1980.

Lewin L, Gifte und Vergiftungen, 6. Aufl., Nachdruck, Haug Verlag, Heidelberg 1992.

Madaus G, Lehrbuch der Biologischen Arzneimittel, Bde 1-3, Nachdruck, Georg Olms Verlag Hildesheim 1979.

Roth L, Daunderer M, Kormann K, Giftpflanzen, Pflanzengifte, 4. Aufl., Ecomed Fachverlag Landsberg Lech 1993.

Schwarz HD, 100 Jahre Lobelin. In: ZPT 11(5):159. 1990.

Wagner H, Wiesenauer M, Phytotherapie. Phytopharmaka und pflanzliche Homöopathika, Fischer-Verlag, Stuttgart, Jena, New York, 1995.

Lobelia inflata

See Lobelia

Logwood

Haematoxylon campechianum

DESCRIPTION

Medicinal Parts: The medicinal part of the tree is the unfermented heartwood.

Flower and Fruit: The small yellow flowers grow in axillary racemes. There are 5 petals. The fruit is a flat pod, usually with 1 seed.

Leaves, Stem and Root: Haematoxylon campechianum is a 10 to 12 m high tree. The twisted branches are thorny, while the bark is rough and dark. The leaves have 4 pairs of small, smooth and cordate stipules whose tips point to the small trunk.

Habitat: The plant originated in the tropical regions of the U.S. and is cultivated in the Caribbean and other regions.

Production: Logwood is the wood from Haematoxylon campechianum. The cultivated trees are felled in their 11th year and the red heartwood is extracted.

Other Names: Bloodwood, H. lignum, Peachwood

ACTIONS AND PHARMACOLOGY

COMPOUNDS

Homoisoflavanes (neoflavane derivatives): to some extent in glycosidic bonds, changing over into the intensively red-colored, quinoide hematein through oxidation

Tannins

EFFECTS

Logwood has astringent properties, due to the isoflavone hematoxylin. An antiphlogistic effect has been proven in animal experiments and an antimicrobial effect in vitro. Hemateine and hematoxylin are said to inhibit the production of melanin in skin when used topically.

INDICATIONS AND USAGE

Unproven Uses: Folk medicine uses have included diarrhea and hemorrhage.

PRECAUTIONS AND ADVERSE REACTIONS
Health risks or side effects following the proper administration of designated therapeutic dosages are not recorded. However, internal administration of hematoxylin carried out in animal experiments led to elevated body temperature, vomiting, anuria, coma and death. Reports of these studies provided no information regarding dosage (Lewin).

DOSAGE
Mode of Administration: The drug is administered as an infusion and a liquid extract.

Daily Dosage: A single dose of a decoction equal to 1 g of drug is mentioned, but the number of times it could be taken daily was not specified.

LITERATURE
Kern W, List PH, Hörhammer L (Hrsg.), Hagers Handbuch der Pharmazeutischen Praxis, 4. Aufl., Bde. 1-8, Springer Verlag Berlin, Heidelberg, New York, 1969.

Lolium temulentum

See Taumelloolch

Lonicera caprifolium

See Honeysuckle

Loosestrife

Lysimachia vulgaris

DESCRIPTION
Medicinal Parts: The medicinal part is the dried herb.

Flower and Fruit: The flowers grow in long-peduncled racemes in the axils of the upper stem and in terminal, panicled inflorescence. The pedicle is about 1 cm long, downy and glandular-haired. The calyx is split almost to the base. The filaments are glandular-haired, usually fused to the middle with each other and in a tube containing the ovary. The seeds are triangular, covered thickly in long warts, whitish and 1.5 mm long.

Leaves, Stem and Root: The plant is a perennial and has underground runners, which produce new buds. The stem is erect, up to 1.5 m tall, branched, obtusely angular, leafy and thickly downy. The leaves are slightly downy with glandular hairs. The leaves are in whorls or opposite, rarely spiralled, up to 14 cm long and 3.5 cm wide, short petioled, tightly reticulate and red-glandular punctate.

Habitat: The plant is found in the temperate regions of Europe and Asia.

Production: Loosestrife is the aerial part of Lysimachia vulgaris.

Other Names: Yellow Willowherb

ACTIONS AND PHARMACOLOGY
COMPOUNDS
Flavonoids: glycosides of the myricetin, kaempferol and quercetin, including among others rutin

Steroids: beta-sitosterol, stigmasterol

The constituents of the drug have not been extensively investigated.

EFFECTS
Loosestrife has an astringent effect. The main active principle is rutin.

INDICATIONS AND USAGE
Unproven Uses: Loosestrife is used for scurvy, diarrhea and dysentery, as well as hemorrhages (nose bleeds and heavy menstrual blood flow) and wounds.

PRECAUTIONS AND ADVERSE REACTIONS
No health hazards or side effects are known in conjunction with the proper administration of designated therapeutic dosages.

DOSAGE
Mode of Administration: The herb is used externally in the powdered form.

LITERATURE
Hänsel R, Keller K, Rimpler H, Schneider G (Hrsg.), Hagers Handbuch der Pharmazeutischen Praxis, 5. Aufl., Bde 4-6 (Drogen), Springer Verlag Berlin, Heidelberg, New York, 1992-1994.

Lophophora williamsii

See Peyote

Lotus

Nelumbo nucifera

DESCRIPTION
Medicinal Parts: The medicinal parts are the roots, the seeds and the aerial parts of the flowering plant.

Flower and Fruit: The solitary flowers are 16 to 23 cm across, pink and scented. They grow above the leaves. The seeds are 1.7 by 1.3 cm and ovoid.

Leaves, Stem and Root: The rhizome is 10 to 20 cm long, stout and branching. It bears numerous scale-like leaves as well as foliage leaves. The foliage leaves are peltate and have no sinuses. The petioles are 1 to 2 cm long, the lamina are 30 to 100 cm in diameter and are almost circular, glossy and unwettable.

Habitat: The plant is indigenous to India.

Production: Lotus is the whole plant of Nelumbo nucifera.

ACTIONS AND PHARMACOLOGY

COMPOUNDS

Isoquinoline alkaloids: including,

benzyl isoquinoline type: armepavine, n-methyl coclaurine

aporphine type: roemerine (remerine), nuciferine, n-nornuciferine, nornuciferine, anonaine, liriodenine, asimilobin, lirinidin

proaporphine type: prunuciferine

Flavonoids: including hyperoside, isoquercitrin, nelumboside, quercetin glucuronide, camphor glucuronide

Tannins

EFFECTS

Active agents are the alkaloids nelumbin and roemerine in the leaves. The drug is an astringent.

INDICATIONS AND USAGE

Unproven Uses: The powdered beans are used in the treatment of digestive disorders, particularly diarrhea. The flowers are used as an astringent for bleeding.

Indian Medicine: Lotus is used for cholera, diarrhea, worm infestation, vomiting, states of exhaustion and intermittent fever.

PRECAUTIONS AND ADVERSE REACTIONS

No health hazards or side effects are known in conjunction with the proper administration of designated therapeutic dosages.

DOSAGE

Mode of Administration: Preparations of the plant are available in powder and liquid extract for internal use.

LITERATURE

Hegnauer R: Chemotaxonomie der Pflanzen, Bde 1-11, Birkhäuser Verlag Basel, Boston, Berlin 1962-1997.

Kern W, List PH, Hörhammer L (Hrsg.), Hagers Handbuch der Pharmazeutischen Praxis, 4. Aufl., Bde. 1-8, Springer Verlag Berlin, Heidelberg, New York, 1969.

Lovage

Levisticum officinale

DESCRIPTION

Medicinal Parts: The medicinal parts are the dried rhizome and roots, the cut, dried herb and the dried fruit.

Flower and Fruit: The flowers are in 8 to 20 rayed compound umbels. There is an involucre and epicalyx. There is no calyx. The orbicular petals are pale yellow and involute. The fruit is yellow-brown, 5 to 7 mm long, compressed, and has sharply keeled to winged ribs.

Leaves, Stem and Root: The plant is a sturdy perennial. It has a thick, spindle-shaped, branched root, which is brownish-yellow on the outside and whitish on the inside. The stem is erect, round, hollow, finely grooved, glabrous and up to 4 cm thick at the base. The leaves are rich green, glossy, coriaceous; the lower ones double pinnate, the upper ones simple-pinnate. The leaflets are broad and obovate.

Characteristics: The rubbed leaves give off an aromatic scent. The fruit is very fragrant.

Habitat: Lovage is indigenous to the Mediterranean region. It grows wild in the Balkans and northern Greece and is cultivated elsewhere.

Production: Lovage root consists of the dried rhizomes and roots of Levisticum officinale, as well as their preparations. Roots of 2-year-old plants are collected in autumn. It is important that the roots are not damaged during the drying process since this would result in a loss of the essential oil.

Not to be Confused With: Angelicae radix, Pastinacae radix or Pimpinellae radix.

Other Names: Lavose, Sea Parsley

ACTIONS AND PHARMACOLOGY

COMPOUNDS

Volatile oil (0.35-1.7%): chief components alkylphthalides (aroma-bearers), including among others 3-butylphthalide, ligusticumlactone (E- and Z-butylidenphthalides), E- and Z-ligustilide furthermore, including among others, alpha- and beta-pinene, beta-phellandrene, citronellal

Hydroxycoumarins: umbelliferone

Coumarin

Furocoumarins: bergaptene, apterin

Polyynes: including among others, falcarindiol (probably only in the fresh rhizome)

EFFECTS

Lovage has diuretic, sedative, antimicrobial and cholinergic properties.

The ligustilide-containing essential oil has an antispasmodic effect on smooth muscle.

The folk use for gastric complaints is probably based on the specific odor caused by phthalide as well as on the bitter taste, which increases saliva and gastric secretions.

INDICATIONS AND USAGE

Approved by Commission E:

- Infections of the urinary tract
- Kidney and bladder stones

Lovage is used for flushing-out therapy for inflammation of the lower urinary tract and flushing-out therapy for prevention of kidney gravel.

Unproven Uses: The folk medicine uses include dyspeptic complaints, such as indigestion, heartburn, feelings of fullness, flatulence, menstrual complaints. Lovage is also used as a secretolytic for respiratory catarrh.

CONTRAINDICATIONS

Because of the irritating effect of the volatile oil, the drug should not be administered in the presence of inflammation of the kidneys or of the urinary drainage passages, nor with reduced kidney function. No irrigation therapy is to be carried out in the presence of edema resulting from reduced cardiac and kidney function.

PRECAUTIONS AND ADVERSE REACTIONS

General: No health hazards or side effects are known in conjunction with the proper administration of designated therapeutic dosages. The drug possesses a low potential for sensitization. An elevation of UV-sensitivity among light-skinned people is possible (phototoxic effect of the furocoumarins).

Pregnancy: Not to be used during pregnancy.

DOSAGE

Mode of Administration: Comminuted herb and other galenic preparations for internal use.

Daily Dosage: 4 to 8 gm drug. Ample intake of liquid is essential. Tea: 2 to 4 gm drug to 1 cup, several times a day between meals.

Infusion: 1.5 gm per cup.

Storage: Protect from light and insects in well-sealed containers. The whole drug should be stored not longer than 18 months; the powdered drug, not longer than 24 hours.

LITERATURE

Albulescu D et al., (1975) Farmacia 23:159.

Bjeldanes LF, Kim I, (1977) J Org Chem 42:2333.

Fischer FC, Svendson AB, (1976) Phytochemistry 15:1079.

Gijbels MJ et al., (1981) Chromatographia 14(8):451.

Gijbels MJ et al., (1982) Planta Med 44:207.

Hänsel R, Keller K, Rimpler H, Schneider G (Hrsg.), Hagers Handbuch der Pharmazeutischen Praxis, 5. Aufl., Bde 4-6 (Drogen), Springer Verlag Berlin, Heidelberg, New York, 1992-1994.

Lawrence BM, (180) Perf Flav 5:29.

Leung AY, Encyclopedia of Common Natural Ingredients Used in Food, Drugs and Cosmetics, John Wiley & Sons Inc., New York 1980.

Madaus G, Lehrbuch der Biologischen Arzneimittel, Bde 1-3, Nachdruck, Georg Olms Verlag Hildesheim 1979.

Steinegger E, Hänsel R, Pharmakognosie, 5. Aufl., Springer Verlag Heidelberg 1992.

Teuscher E, Biogene Arzneimittel, 5. Aufl., Wiss. Verlagsges. Stuttgart 1997.

Teuscher E, Lindequist U, Biogene Gifte - Biologie, Chemie, Pharmakologie, 2. Aufl., Fischer Verlag Stuttgart 1994.

Vollmann C, Levisticum officinale - Der Liebstöckel. In: ZPT 9(4):128. 1988.

Yu SR, You SQ, (1984) Yao Hsueh Hsueh Pao 19(8):566.

Wichtl M (Hrsg.), Teedrogen, 4. Aufl., Wiss. Verlagsges. Stuttgart 1997.

Luffa

Luffa aegyptica

DESCRIPTION

Medicinal Parts: The medicinal part is the dried network of vascular bundles of the ripe cucumber-like plant. When dried, the dense vascular network that makes up the fruit becomes the Loofah, which is used to scrub and soften the skin.

Flower and Fruit: The plant bears solitary, yellow, female flowers, which are 5 to 10 cm wide and have an oblong, clavate calyx tube. The fruit is cylindrical or oblong-clavate. It is not ribbed, prickly or sharp-edged. It is somewhat tomentose, up to 40 cm long and 5 to 15 cm thick. The seeds are blackish, smooth and winged.

Leaves, Stem and Root: The plant is an annual climbing plant that grows from 3 to 6 m high. The stems are thin and pentangular. The leaves are cordate-indented, 15 to 30 cm long and wide and 3- to 7-lobed.

Habitat: The plant probably originated in India and was brought to Egypt in the Middle Ages. Today, it is cultivated in the tropical regions of the world.

Production: Luffa sponge consists of the dried fiber structure of the ripe cucumber-like fruits of Luffa aegyptica. The ripe fruit is freed of soft material by banging and washing.

ACTIONS AND PHARMACOLOGY

COMPOUNDS: LUFFA FRESH FRUIT

Triterpene saponins: including among others lucyoside A-M (aglycones including oleanolic acid, hederagenin 21-hydroxy-hederagenin, gypsogenin, arjunolic acid)

Cucurbitacins (the young fruits are eaten as salad)

Sterols: including delta5-sterols, delta7-sterols

Triterpenes (triterpene acids): including bryonolic acid (3%)

The luffa fungus (Luffa, Luffa aegyptica) is likely to be mostly free of soluble constituents and to consist chiefly of cellulose, hemicellulose and pectins.

EFFECTS

No information is available.

INDICATIONS AND USAGE

Unproven Uses: Preparations of Luffa sponge are used as a preventive for infections or colds, as a remedy for colds and nasal catarrhs, and for sinusitis and suppuration of the sinus.

Chinese Medicine: Luffa is used for coughs, chronic bronchitis, diseases of the spleen and paralyzing diseases.

Indian Medicine: Luffa is used for splenopathy, leprosy, syphilis, bronchitis, fever and hematuria.

PRECAUTIONS AND ADVERSE REACTIONS

No health hazards or side effects are known in conjunction with the proper administration of designated therapeutic dosages.

DOSAGE

No information is available.

LITERATURE

Hänsel R, Keller K, Rimpler H, Schneider G (Hrsg.), Hagers Handbuch der Pharmazeutischen Praxis, 5. Aufl., Bde 4-6 (Drogen), Springer Verlag Berlin, Heidelberg, New York, 1992-1994.

Luffa aegyptica

See Luffa

Lungmoss

Lobaria pulmonaria

DESCRIPTION

Medicinal Parts: The medicinal part is the lichen.

Flower and Fruit: Lobaria pulmonaria is a lichen, with deeply pinnatisect lobes with indented tips, measuring from 1.5 cm up to hand size. It is found on the trunks of old woodland trees and is browinsh-green or red-brown with a reticulate, punctate structure. It is tomentose and whitish-brown beneath and is covered with glabrous white spots on the margin and on the reticulate ridges.

Habitat: Lungmoss is found throughout Europe.

Production: Lungmoss is the whole lichen tissue of Lobaria pulmonaria. The lichen is gathered throughout the entire year. The minute roots in the subterranean part, along with any possible earth, are cleaned off (do not gather dry lichen, as they are mostly found on dead plants, and therefore are no longer effective).

Not to be Confused With: Common Lungwort, which is a plant.

Other Names: Oak Lungs, Lungwort

ACTIONS AND PHARMACOLOGY

COMPOUNDS

Lichen acids: including among others stictictic, norstictic, thelophoric acid, gyrophoric acid

Mucilages

EFFECTS

The drug has diaphoretic, expectorant, anti-inflammatory, and antimicrobial effects. The active agents exhibiting the antimicrobial effects are unknown.

INDICATIONS AND USAGE

Unproven Uses: As a result of the relaxing effect of Lungmoss on the respiratory tract, the drug is used for all chronic respiratory tract illnesses: bronchitis, coughs and asthma, as well as for irritable coughs and smoker's cough.

PRECAUTIONS AND ADVERSE REACTIONS

No health hazards or side effects are known in conjunction with the proper administration of designated therapeutic dosages.

DOSAGE

Mode of Administration: Lungmoss is available as dried lichen as a liquid extract for internal use. Lichen preparations can be bought as sweets, syrups or pastilles.

Storage: The drug should be stored in glass or porcelain containers, protected from light.

LITERATURE

Catalano S et al., (1976) Phytochemistry 15:22.

Kern W, List PH, Hörhammer L (Hrsg.), Hagers Handbuch der Pharmazeutischen Praxis, 4. Aufl., Bde. 1-8, Springer Verlag Berlin, Heidelberg, New York, 1969.

Madaus G, Lehrbuch der Biologischen Arzneimittel, Bde 1-3, Nachdruck, Georg Olms Verlag Hildesheim 1979.

Wagner H, Wiesenauer M, Phytotherapie. Phytopharmaka und pflanzliche Homöopathika, Fischer-Verlag, Stuttgart, Jena, New York 1995.

Lungwort

Pulmonaria officinalis

DESCRIPTION

Medicinal Parts: The medicinal parts are the dried herb and the fresh, aerial parts of the flowering plant.

Flower and Fruit: The blue, later blue-violet flowers are in terminal curled cyme-like inflorescences on flowering branches. The calyx is fused and has 5 tips. The corolla is fused to a tube and the 5 tips are rotate. There are 5 stamens and a 4-valved ovary with 1 style. There are both long and short-styled flowers. There are 5 tufts of hair at the entrance to the corolla tube. The fruit consists of 4 nuts 3.5 to 4 mm in length, glabrous when ripe, glossy brown to black, mildly keeled with a distinct displaced ring.

Leaves, Stem and Root: The plant grows from 15 to 30 cm high. The rhizome is quite thin and branched. First it produces flowering shoots and then the leaf rosettes. The shoots are fresh green and covered in glandular hairs. The stems are erect or ascending, slightly angular and pubescent. The rosette-like basal leaves that form after flowering are long petioled, cordate-ovate, acute, more long than wide with whitish spots. The cauline leaves are alternate, taper to a winged stem and are sharply pointed; only the lower ones have some pinnatifid ribs.

Characteristics: The taste is slightly bitter and slimy.

Habitat: The plant is common in many parts of Europe.

Production: Lungwort consists of the dried plant section of Pulmonaria officinalis and its effective pharmaceutical preparations. Lungwort is collected in uncultivated regions and air-dried.

Not to be Confused With: Lungwort is occasionally adulterated with other Pulmonaria species, particularly Pulmonaria mollis.

Other Names: Dage of Jerusalem, Common Lungwort

ACTIONS AND PHARMACOLOGY

COMPOUNDS

Allantoin

Caffeic acid derivatives: chlorogenic acid, rosmarinic acid

Flavonoids (0.3 to 0.5%): especially O-glycosides of the kaempferol and quercetin

Mucilages: polygalacturonane, arabinogalactans, rhamnogalacturonane

Silicic acid: more than 2.5% water-soluble silicic acid

Tannins

EFFECTS

The drug has an expectorant, soothing effect due to the mucilaginous polysaccharide and tannin content.

INDICATIONS AND USAGE

Unproven Uses: In folk medicine Lungwort is used internally for illnesses and conditions of the respiratory tract, gastrointestinal tract, kidney and efferent urinary tract; and externally in the treatment of wounds.

PRECAUTIONS AND ADVERSE REACTIONS

No health hazards or side effects are known in conjunction with the proper administration of designated therapeutic dosages.

DOSAGE

Mode of Administration: Lungwort is available as whole, cut and powdered drug for internal and external use. It is also available in commercial forms as syrup, juice, drops and in compounded preparations.

Preparation: To prepare a tea, 1.5 gm finely cut drug is put in cold water which is brought quickly to a boil or it is scalded with boiling water and strained after 5 to 10 minutes (1 teaspoon corresponds to approximately 0.7 gm drug).

Liquid extract: 1:1 with 25% ethanol. (V/V)

Daily Dosage: As bronchial tea it is drunk in sips throughout the day. It may be sweetened with honey.

Storage: Should be protected from light

LITERATURE

Brantner A, Kartnig Th, Flavonoid glycosides from aerial parts of Pulmonaria officinalis. In: PM 61(6):582. 1995.

Luthy J et al., (1984) Pharm Acta Helv 59(9/10):242.

Müller BM, Franz G, Polysaccharide aus Pulmonaria officinalis - Wertgebende Bestandteile der Droge? In: PZW 135(6):243-251. 1990.

Further information in:

Hänsel R, Keller K, Rimpler H, Schneider G (Hrsg.), Hagers Handbuch der Pharmazeutischen Praxis, 5. Aufl., Bde 4-6 (Drogen), Springer Verlag Berlin, Heidelberg, New York, 1992-1994.

Madaus G, Lehrbuch der Biologischen Arzneimittel, Bde 1-3, Nachdruck, Georg Olms Verlag Hildesheim 1979.

Roth L, Daunderer M, Kormann K, Giftpflanzen, Pflanzengifte, 4. Aufl., Ecomed Fachverlag Landsberg Lech 1993.

Steinegger E, Hänsel R, Pharmakognosie, 5. Aufl., Springer Verlag Heidelberg 1992.

Teuscher E, Biogene Arzneimittel, 5. Aufl., Wiss. Verlagsges. Stuttgart 1997.

Wichtl M (Hrsg.), Teedrogen, 4. Aufl., Wiss. Verlagsges. Stuttgart 1997.

Lupinus luteus

See Yellow Lupin

Lycium barbarum

See Lycium Berries (Go-Qi-Zi)

Lycium Bark (Di-Gu-Pi)

Lycium chinense

DESCRIPTION

Medicinal Parts: The medicinal parts of the plant are the fruit and root bark.

Flower and Fruit: The plant has 1 to 3 axillary, radial flowers. The calyx and petals are fused; the calyx is bilabial with a double-toothed upper lip and triple-toothed lower lip. The corolla is funnel-shaped, light purple or violet with a 5-lobed margin. There are 4 stamens, which are hairy at the base. The ovary is 2-chambered with 1 style. The fruit is a yellow-orange, elongate, sweet-tasting berry.

Leaves, Stem and Root: Lycium chinense is a shrub that grows up to 3 m high. The leaves are alternate, ovate-lanceolate to rhomboid, narrowing suddenly to the petiole, and bright green. The branches are cane-like, initially upright, then hanging down bow-like and thornless.

Habitat: The plant is native to eastern Asia, particularly to China and Japan.

Production: Lycium bark is the dried root bark of Lycium chinense or Lycium barbarum. Harvest begins in early spring or in late autumn when the roots are dug up and then peeled. The root bark is then cleaned and dried in the sun. Lycium leaves are the dried leaves of Lycium chinense.

Other Names: Chinese Matrimony Vine, Chinese Wolfberry

ACTIONS AND PHARMACOLOGY

COMPOUNDS: LYCIUM ROOT BARK

Polyamines: kukoamine A (spermidin-dihydrocaffeoyl-bisamide)

Dipeptides: Lyciumamide (N-benzoyl-L-phenylalanyl-L-phenylalaninol-acetate)

Cyclopeptides: lyciumin A, lyciumin B

Steroids: sterols, including beta-sitosterol, 5alpha-stigmastan-3,6-dione

Diterpenes: sugiol

EFFECTS: LYCIUM ROOT BARK

The methanolic root extract and the kukoamine A isolated from the plant are reported to have had significant antihypertensive effects in animal experiments. The isolated octapeptides lyciumines A and B are believed to inhibit the activity of renin and the angiotensin-converting enzyme. Experimental data confirming these results are not available.

COMPOUNDS: LYCIUM LEAVES

Steroids: withasteroids (0.1%), including withanolide A, withanolide B

Sterols: including beta-sitosterol and beta-sitosterol glucoside

EFFECTS: LYCIUM LEAVES

No experimental data regarding the pharmacological efficacy of the drug are available. In vitro experimental models have indicated that the steroid withanolide isolated from it may have immunosuppressive effect.

INDICATIONS AND USAGE

LYCIUM ROOT BARK

Unproven Uses: The root of the plant is used in fever and blood pressure-reducing medications. The berries are considered to provide a liver and kidney tonic.

Chinese Medicine: Used internally for fever, hyperhidrosis, thirst, coughs, nose bleeds, pulpitis, diabetes, hypertension, malaria and for black vomit. External uses include eczema and rheumatism. Efficacy for these indications has not yet been proven.

LYCIUM LEAVES

Unproven Uses: Preparations from the leave are used in folk medicine for whooping cough and paroxysmal cough (Iberian peninsula), as a mouthwash for toothache (Indonesia).

Chinese Medicine: Lycium leaf is used for inflammatory processes, such as rheumatism, and as a tea taken for pain.

Indian Medicine: Used for rheumatism.

PRECAUTIONS AND ADVERSE REACTIONS

LYCIUM ROOT BARK AND LEAVES

No health hazards are known in conjunction with the proper administration of designated therapeutic dosages.

CONTRAINDICATIONS

LYCIUM ROOT BARK

Contraindications include pregnancy, symptoms of the common cold and diarrhea.

LYCIUM LEAVES

Not to be used during pregnancy.

DOSAGE

LYCIUM ROOT BARK

Mode of Administration: Whole, cut and powdered drug preparations are administered internally and externally.

Storage: Store in a dry place.

LYCIUM LEAVES

Mode of Administration: Lycium leaf is administered as a tea or as an infusion for use as a gargle.

Daily Dosage: Drug/tea: 9 to 15 g or 6 to 12 g, depending on the literature source. For Whooping Cough, 1 cup of tea sipped throughout the day.

LITERATURE

Hänsel R, Keller K, Rimpler H, Schneider G (Ed), Hagers Handbuch der Pharmazeutischen Praxis, 5. Aufl., Bde 4 - 6 (Drogen), Springer Verlag Berlin, Heidelberg, New York, 1992-1994.

Kim HP, Kim SY, Lee EJ, Kim YC, Kim YC, Zeaxanthin dipalmitate from Lycium chinense has hepatoprotective activity. Res Commun Mol Pathol Pharmacol, 97:301-14, 1997 Sep.

Kim SY, Choi YH, Huh H, Kim J, Kim YC, Lee HS, New antihepatotoxic cerebroside from Lycium chinense fruits. J Nat Prod, 60:274-6, 1997 Mar.

Lycium Berries (Go-Qi-Zi)

Lycium barbarum

DESCRIPTION

Medicinal Parts: The medicinal part is the fruit.

Flower and Fruit: There are 1 to 3 axillary, radial flowers. The calyx and petals are fused; the calyx is bilabial with the upper lip double-toothed and the lower lip triple-toothed. The corolla is funnel-shaped, light purple or violet with a 5-lobed margin. There are 4 stamens, which are hairy at the base. The ovary is 2-chambered with 1 style. The fruit is a scarlet, elongate, sweet-tasting berry.

Leaves, Stem and Root: Lycium barbarum is a shrub, growing up to 3 m high. The gray-green leaves are alternate, lanceolate and gradually narrow to the petiole. The branches are cane-like, initially upright, then hanging down bow-like and often thorny.

Habitat: The shrub is indigenous to China and Mongolia.

Production: Barbary wolfberry fruits are the dried ripe fruit of Lycium barbarum. The fruit is harvested in summer or autumn. The whole fruit, with stem attached, is dried in the sun until the skin is hard and the fruit pulp is soft inside. After drying, the fruit stem is removed.

Other Names: Bastard Jasmine, Box Thorn, Common Matrimony Vine, Prickly Box, Tea Plant, Barbary, Tea Tree

ACTIONS AND PHARMACOLOGY

COMPOUNDS

Water-soluble polysaccharides

Glycoproteins

Carotinoids: particularly physalien (zeaxanthin dipalmitate)

EFFECTS

A possible immunostimulating and hypoglycemic effect has been described, The plant contains a mydriatic acting protein.

INDICATIONS AND USAGE

Unproven Uses: The drug is administered as a non-specific strengthening agent, due to the minerals and vitamins (particularly vitamin C) that it contains. Lycium barbarum is also used as a purgative and diuretic.

Chinese Medicine: The plant is used to treat weakness of the lumbar region and knee, liver and kidney disorders, diabetes, tinnitus, impaired hearing, poor sight, anemia, coughs, dizziness and excessive tear production.

Indian Medicine: Lycium barbarum is used for ascitis, anemia, menstruation disorders, toothache, scabies and bleeding hemorrhoids.

CONTRAINDICATIONS

Not to be used during pregnancy.

PRECAUTIONS AND ADVERSE REACTIONS

No health hazards are known in conjunction with the proper administration of designated therapeutic dosages.

DOSAGE

Mode of Application: Whole, cut and powdered drug.

Daily Dosage: Drug/tea: 6 to 12 g or 6 to 15 g, depending on the literature source.

Storage: Store in cool, dry place and in tightly sealed container.

LITERATURE

Hänsel R, Keller K, Rimpler H, Schneider G (Ed), Hagers Handbuch der Pharmazeutischen Praxis, 5. Aufl., Bde 4 - 6 (Drogen), Springer Verlag Berlin, Heidelberg, New York, 1992-1994.

Liu B, Effects of Lycium barbarum L and Drynaria fortunei, J Smith on in vitro attachment and growth of human gingival fibroblasts on root surfaces, Chung Hua Kou Chiang Hsueh Tsa Chih, 27:159-61, 190, 1992 May.

Lu CX, Cheng BQ, Radiosensitizing effects of Lycium barbarum polysaccharide for Lewis lung cancer, Chung Hsi I Chieh Ho Tsa Chih, 11:611-2, 582, 1991 Oct.

Ren B, Ma Y, Shen Y, Gao B, Protective action of Lycium barbarum L. (LbL) and betaine on lipid peroxidation of erythrocyte membrane induced by H_2O_2, Chung Kuo Chung Yao Tsa Chih, 20:303-4, inside cover, 1995 May.

Lycium chinense

See Lycium Bark (Di-Gu-Pi)

Lycoperdon species

See Puff Ball

Lycopersicon esculentum

See Tomato

Lycopodium clavatum

See Club Moss

Lycopus virginicus

See Bugleweed

Lysimachia nummularia

See Moneywort

Lysimachia vulgaris

See Loosestrife

Lythrum salicaria

See Purple Loosestrife

Ma-Huang

Ephedra sinica

DESCRIPTION

Medicinal Parts: The medicinal parts are the young canes collected in autumn and the dried rhizome with roots.

Flower and Fruit: The flowers are small and occasionally reduced to acuminate scales. They are fused in pairs at the base. They are unisexual, usually dioecious and sometimes monoecious. The male inflorescences consist of 2 to 24 blooms. The involucre is 2-lobed and fused to a tube. The fruit is a red, berry-like false fruit formed from the upper bract.

Leaves, Stem and Root: The plant is a 30 cm tall lightly branched subshrub with lengthened, cylindrical branches that are 1 to 2 mm in diameter. It is similar in appearance to Horsetail, and is sometimes twining and often has underground runners. The stem and branches are round with numerous vertical grooves of gray-green or bright green coloring. Very small leaves are occasionally reduced to pointed scales and are almost always fused at the base to form a sheath. They are reddish brown.

Habitat: Ephedra sinica grows mainly in Mongolia and the bordering area of China, Ephedra gerardiana is from India.

Production: Ma-Huang consists of the dried, young branchlets, harvested in the fall, of Ephedra sinica, Ephedra shennungiana, or other equivalent Ephedra species. It is mostly cultivated. The plant is harvested as late as possible after the last rain, but before the winter frost and is air-dried in the sun.

Not to be Confused With: Many similar species

Other Names: Desert Herb, Ephedrine

ACTIONS AND PHARMACOLOGY

COMPOUNDS

Alkaloids of the 2-aminophenylpropane type: main alkaloids L-(-)-ephedrine (1R,2S-(-)- ephedrine) and D-pseudoephedrine (1S,2S-(+)- ephedrine); lesser alkaloids L-norephedrine, D-norpseudoephedrine.

EFFECTS

The level of the active principles can fluctuate drastically. Ephedrine acts by indirectly stimulating the sympathomimetic and central nervous system. The herb is bacteriostatic, positively inotropic and positively chronotropic. In animal tests ephedrine acts as an antitussive.

INDICATIONS AND USAGE

Approved by Commission E:

- Cough/bronchitis

Unproven Uses: Ma-Huang is used for diseases of the respiratory tract with mild bronchospasms in adults and children over the age of six. Various indications include asthma, cardiovascular stimulation and as a CNS stimulant.

Chinese Medicine: The drug has been used for over 4000 years for severe febrile illnesses, bronchial asthma, joint symptoms, inability to perspire, coughing with dyspnea, edema and pains in the bones.

CONTRAINDICATIONS

Contraindications include states of anxiety and restlessness, high blood pressure, angle-closure glaucoma, cerebral perfusions, prostate adenoma with residual urine volume, pheochromocytoma and thyrotoxicosis.

PRECAUTIONS AND ADVERSE REACTIONS

General: Common side effects include headache, irritability, motor restlessness, nausea, sleeplessness, tachycardia, urinary disorders and vomiting. Higher dosages may result in blood pressure and cardiac rhythm disorders.

Dependence can develop with extended intake. Because of the danger of the development of tachyphylaxis and of dependence, the drug should only be administered for short periods.

Pregnancy: Ma-Huang should not to be used during pregnancy

Drug Interactions: Ephedra has an addictive effect on the CNS when used in conjunction with caffeine, decongestants and other central stimulants.

Cardiac heart glycosides or halothane: disturbance of heart rhythm.

Guanethidine: enhancement of the sympathomimetic effect.

MAO-inhibitors: potentiate the sympathomimetic action of ephedrine.

Secale alkaloid derivatives or oxytocin: development of high blood pressure.

OVERDOSAGE

Life-threatening poisonings are seen with very high dosages of the drug (over 100 gm, lethal dosage with oral administration corresponding to approximately 1 to 2 gm L-ephedrine). Symptoms of poisoning include severe outbreaks of sweating, enlarged pupils, spasms and elevated body temperature. Death following overdose is due to heart failure and asphyxiation. Following stomach emptying (gastric lavage with burgundy-colored potassium permaganate solution), therapy consists of the administration of activated charcoal and prophylaxis against shock. Spasms should be treated with diazepam, electrolyte substitution should be employed, and sodium bicarbonate infusions should be used to prevent acidosis. Intubation and oxygen respiration are also on occasion necessary.

DOSAGE

Mode of Administration: Ma-Huang is administered as a comminuted herb, as well as other galenic preparations for internal use.

Daily Dosage: For adults, the average single dose is 15 to 30 mg total alkaloid, calculated as ephedrine, for a total dose of 120 mg per day. When used in children, single doses of herb preparations corresponding to 0.5 mg total alkaloid per kg of body weight are employed. The recommended daily dosage for children is 2 mg.

Tea — Made with 1 to 4 gm, 3 times daily.

Ephedra tincture (1:1) — medium single dose 5 gm.

Ephedra extract — 1 to 3 ml 3 times daily.

Ephedra tincture (1:4) — 6 to 8 ml 3 times daily.

Storage: Ma-Huang must be protected from light.

LITERATURE

Gazaliev AM, Fazilov SD, Zhurinov MZ, Khim Prorod Soed 23:862-864. 1987.

Harada M, Nishimura M, J Pharm Dyn 4:691-699. 1981.

Further information in:

Hänsel R, Keller K, Rimpler H, Schneider G (Hrsg.), Hagers Handbuch der Pharmazeutischen Praxis, 5. Aufl., Bde 4-6 (Drogen), Springer Verlag Berlin, Heidelberg, New York, 1992-1994.

Madaus G, Lehrbuch der Biologischen Arzneimittel, Bde 1-3, Nachdruck, Georg Olms Verlag Hildesheim 1979.

Roth L, Daunderer M, Kormann K, Giftpflanzen, Pflanzengifte, 4. Aufl., Ecomed Fachverlag Landsberg Lech 1993.

Schulz R, Hänsel R, Rationale Phytotherapie, Springer Verlag Heidelberg 1996.

Steinegger E, Hänsel R, Pharmakognosie, 5. Aufl., Springer Verlag Heidelberg 1992.

Tang W, Eisenbrand G, Chinese Drugs of Plant Origin, Springer Verlag Heidelberg 1992.

Teuscher E, Lindequist U, Biogene Gifte - Biologie, Chemie, Pharmakologie, 2. Aufl., Fischer Verlag Stuttgart 1994.

Teuscher E, Biogene Arzneimittel, 5. Aufl., Wiss. Verlagsges. mbH Stuttgart 1997.

Wagner H, Wiesenauer M, Phytotherapie. Phytopharmaka und pflanzliche Homöopathika, Fischer-Verlag, Stuttgart, Jena, New York 1995.

Macrocystis pyrifera

See Brown Kelp

Madder

Rubia tinctorum

TRADE NAMES

Madder Whole Root (available from numerous manufactures and as combination product)

DESCRIPTION

Medicinal Parts: The medicinal part is the dried root.

Flower and Fruit: The small yellowish-green flowers are in loose, leafy, long-peduncled terminal or axillary cymes. The margin of the calyx is indistinct, 4 to 5 sectioned and has a tip which is curved inward. There are 5 stamens and an inferior ovary. The fruit is a black, pea-sized glabrous, smooth drupe containing 2 seeds.

Leaves, Stem and Root: The perennial plant grows from 60 to 100 cm high. The pencil-thick rhizome creeps widely underground. The stem is quadrangular with backward turning prickles at the edges. The stems are at times so thin that they are more descendent than erect. The leaves are in whorls, in fours below, in sixes above. They are oblong to lanceolate with 1 rib and are protrudingly reticulate beneath.

Habitat: The plant is indigenous to Southern Europe, Western Asia and North Africa and is cultivated elsewhere.

Production: Madder root consists of the dried root of Rubia tinctorum as well as its preparations.

Other Names: Dyer's Madder, Robbia

ACTIONS AND PHARMACOLOGY

COMPOUNDS

Anthracene derivatives (rubiadins, 2 to 4%): chief components alizarin, lucidin, pseudopurpurin (purpurin carboxylic acid), purpurin, rubiadin and the glucosides and/or the primerosides of these compounds.

EFFECTS

Madder root inhibits calcium oxalate crystallization in the kidney. Lucidin is the toxic principle and is mutagenic.

INDICATIONS AND USAGE

Unproven Uses: Madder root is used to dissolve kidney stones

PRECAUTIONS AND ADVERSE REACTIONS

Because of the possible carcinogenic effect of the rubiadins, the drug should not be administered.

DOSAGE

How Supplied:

Liquid — 1:4

LITERATURE

Anonym, Rubiae-tinctorum-radix-haltige Humanarzneimittel, Widerruf der Zulassung. In: DAZ 133(11):888. 1993.

BGA, Arzneimittelrisiken: Anthranoide. In: DAZ 132(21):1164. 1992.

Courchesne M, Brassard P, Identification and characterization of naturally occuring rubiadins. In: JNP 56(5):722. 1993.

Nung V N et al., (1971) Plant Med Phytother 5:177.

Schümann C, Apotheker und die Entwicklung der Färberei. In: PZ 140(39):3446-3451. 1995.

Westendorf J, Phytotherapie: Anthranoide in Arzneipflanzen. In: DAZ 133(25):2345. 1993.

Westendorf J, Poginskky B, Marquardt H, Marquardt H, The genotoxicity of Lucidin, a natural component of Rubia tinctorum L., and lucidinmethylether, a component of ethanolic Rubia extracts. In: Cell Biol Toxicol in press. 19.

Further information in:

Frohne D, Pfänder HJ, Giftpflanzen - Ein Handbuch für Apotheker, Toxikologen und Biologen, 4. Aufl., Wiss. Verlags-Ges. Stuttgart 1997.

Kern W, List PH, Hörhammer L (Hrsg.), Hagers Handbuch der Pharmazeutischen Praxis, 4. Aufl., Bde 1-8: Springer Verlag Berlin, Heidelberg, New York, 1969.

Madaus G, Lehrbuch der Biologischen Arzneimittel, Bde 1-3, Nachdruck, Georg Olms Verlag Hildesheim 1979.

Thomson RH, Naturally Occuring Quinones, 2nd Ed., Academic Press New York 1971.

Teuscher E, Lindequist U, Biogene Gifte - Biologie, Chemie, Pharmakologie, 2. Aufl., Fischer Verlag Stuttgart 1994.

Teuscher E, Biogene Arzneimittel, 5. Aufl., Wiss. Verlagsges. Stuttgart 1997.

Wagner H, Wiesenauer M, Phytotherapie. Phytopharmaka und pflanzliche Homöopathika, Fischer-Verlag, Stuttgart, Jena, New York 1995.

Magnolia

Magnolia glauca

DESCRIPTION

Medicinal Parts: The bark is the medicinal part.

Leaves, Stem and Root: The inner bark occurs in long, fibrous strips. The outer surface is rough, almost granular and pitted. The inner surface is striated but almost smooth. The fracture is short with the inner part tough and fibrous.

Habitat: The plant is indigenous to North America.

Production: Magnolia bark is the bark from the trunk and branches of Magnolia glauca.

Other Names: White Laurel, Beaver Tree, Swamp Sassafras, White Bay, Sweet Bay, Holly Bay, Indian Bark, Red Bay, Swamp Laurel

ACTIONS AND PHARMACOLOGY

COMPOUNDS

Neolignans: magnolol

Volatile oil

The constituents of the drug have not been widely investigated.

EFFECTS

Magnolia has diaphoretic, anti-inflammatory and stimulant effects. It is also a tonic.

INDICATIONS AND USAGE

Unproven Uses: The preparations are used for digestive disorders; used rarely, except in Oriental medicine.

PRECAUTIONS AND ADVERSE REACTIONS

No health hazards or side effects are known in conjunction with the proper administration of designated therapeutic dosages.

DOSAGE

Mode of Administration: Magnolia has been used internally as a powder or liquid extract.

LITERATURE

Hegnauer R, Chemotaxonomie der Pflanzen, Bde 1-11, Birkhäuser Verlag Basel, Boston, Berlin 1962-1997.

Kern W, List PH, Hörhammer L (Hrsg.), Hagers Handbuch der Pharmazeutischen Praxis, 4. Aufl., Bde. 1-8, Springer Verlag Berlin, Heidelberg, New York, 1969.

Yajara S, Nishiyori T, Kohda A, Nohra T, Nishioka I, Isolation and characterization of phenolic compounds from Magnolia cortex produced in China. In: Chem Pharm Bull Tokyo 39:2024. 1991.

Magnolia glauca

See Magnolia

Mahonia aquifolium

See Mountain Grape

Maidenhair

Adiantum capillus-veneris

TRADE NAMES

Oregon Grape (Berberis aquifolium variety available from numerous manufacturers) Oregon Grape Root

DESCRIPTION

Medicinal Parts: The dried fronds (Maidenhair) are used as a drug as well the dried herb with rhizome and roots (Maidenhair with roots).

Flower and Fruit: There are lumps of sporangia without a veil on the underside of the lateral lobes. The sporangia are square to reniform and later, dark brown.

Leaves, Stem and Root: Maidenhair is a hardy, up to 35 cm high plant with an aromatic lily fragrance. It has a creeping rhizome. The leaves are double-rowed, tender, glabrous and up to 50 cm long. They have a glossy black petiole and are covered with hairs at the base. The leaf-blade is ovate to oblong-ovate. The leaflets are light-green periolate. The pinnules have hair-like petioles. The veins of the sterile pinna terminate in teeth at the edge of the leaf.

Habitat: Southern Europe, Atlantic coast as far as Ireland, from the south to the southern Alpine valleys (Tessin, southern Tyrol).

Production: Maidenhair fern, which is gathered in June and dried, is the frond of Adiantum capillus-veneris.

Not to be Confused With: It has sometimes been observed that the drug has been made impure by an addition of bracken leaf fronds (Pteridium aquilinum).

Other Names: Venus Hair, Rock Fern, Hair of Venus, Five-Finger Fern, Maiden Fern

ACTIONS AND PHARMACOLOGY

COMPOUNDS

Flavonoids

Proanthocyanidins

Hydroxycinnamic acid ester

EFFECTS

The drug is an expectorant, beneficial in bringing up phlegm, and a demulcent.

INDICATIONS AND USAGE

Unproven Uses: In the middle ages, the drug was used for various illnesses of the respiratory tract, in the form of so-called pectoral teas and as a syrup for severe coughs. Because of its similarity to Maidenhair, the drug was used to treat a lack of hair growth and to promote dark hair color.

It is still taken as an infusion in Spain, Belgium and the Canary Islands to treat bronchitis, coughs and whooping cough, and also for painful and excessive menstruation.

PRECAUTIONS AND ADVERSE REACTIONS

General: No health hazards or side effects are known in conjunction with the proper administration of designated therapeutic dosages.

Pregnancy: Not to be used during pregnancy

DOSAGE

Mode of Administration: The drug is taken internally as a tea prepared from the ground or powdered drug.

Daily Dosage: The standard single dose is 1.5 gm of the drug to 1 cup of liquid per dose (average single dose)

Storage: Protect from light.

LITERATURE

Berti G et al., Tetrahedron Lett: 1-5. 1964.

Cooper-Driver G, Swain T, Bot J Linn Soc 74:1-21. 1977.

Imperato F, PH 21:2158-2159. 1982.

Imperator F, (1982) Phytochemistry 21(8):2158.

Jain SR, Sharma SN, (1967) Planta Med(4):439.

Twaij HAA et al., (1985) Indian J Pharmacol 17(1):73.

Malabar Nut

Justicia adhatoda

DESCRIPTION

Medicinal Parts: The medicinal parts are the dried foliage leaves, the flower collected in the flowering season, the dried bark of the trunk, branches and roots, and the fresh leaves.

Flower and Fruit: The flowers are in dense, 2.5 to 7.5 cm long peduncled, axillary spikes. The bracts are elliptical, and the bracteoles are oblong-lanceolate. The calyx is 1.5 cm long, glabrous or black pubescent, with 5 sections containing regular lanceolate segments. The corolla is white with red to purple bands. The corolla tube is 1.3 cm long and is cylindrical and pubescent inside of the lower half. The upper lip is convexly domed. The anthers are arrow-shaped and sometimes spurred at the base. The ovary is bivalvular with a 2-lobed stigma. The fruit is a 4-seeded, short-haired, longitudinally grooved capsule. The seeds are orbicular, glabrous, slightly bumpy-warty and 5 to 7 mm across.

Leaves, Stem and Root: The plant is an evergreen, unpleasant-smelling shrub 2.5 m high with numerous, usually opposite, branches. The bark is yellow. The leaves are 8 to 25 cm long, 2.5 to 8 cm wide, short-stalked, opposite, lanceolate to elliptical, tapering to an acute apex with entire margins. The leaf blade and petiole are finely pubescent.

Characteristics: The taste is bitter and the odor tea-like.

Habitat: Originally indigenous to northern India, the plant is now found in all the areas of Ayurveda medicine in India, Sri Lanka and the Maylan archipelago.

Production: Vasaca leaves are the leaves of Justicia adhatoda.

Other Names: Arusa, Adulsa

ACTIONS AND PHARMACOLOGY

COMPOUNDS

Quinazoline alkaloids: including vasicine and vasicinone

Volatile oil

EFFECTS

Mildly spasmolytic, bronchodilatory and expectorant

INDICATIONS AND USAGE

Unproven Uses: For acute and chronic bronchial infections, catarrh of the upper respiratory tract and tuberculosis as an expectorant and to alleviate coughs.

Indian Medicine: Justicia adhatoda is used as an expectorant and secretory agent.

Homeopathic Uses: Justicia adhatoda preparations are used for hay fever and acute inflammation of the upper respiratory tract.

CONTRAINDICATIONS

The drug is contraindicated in pregnancy.

PRECAUTIONS AND ADVERSE REACTIONS

General: No health hazards or side effects are known in conjunction with the proper administration of designated therapeutic dosages. Because of the vasicine content, the administration of large dosages can lead to excitatory states.

Pregnancy: Administration during pregnancy is to be avoided.

DOSAGE

Mode of Administration: Today, the extract of the leaves is only found in some combination preparations.

Daily Dosage: 1 to 2 gm as drug or liquid extract (1:1) with 40% ethanol (V/V)

Homeopathic Dosage: 5 drops, 1 tablet or 10 globules every 30 to 60 minutes (acute), and 1 to 3 times daily (chronic); Parenterally: 1 to 2 ml sc acute. 3 times daily; Chronic: once a day (HAB1).

LITERATURE

Brain KR, Thapa BB, J Chromatogr 258:183-188. 1988.

Cooper-Driver G, Swain T, Bot J Linn Soc 74:1-21. 1977.

Further information in:

Hänsel R, Keller K, Rimpler H, Schneider G (Hrsg.), Hagers Handbuch der Pharmazeutischen Praxis, 5. Aufl., Bde 4-6 (Drogen), Springer Verlag Berlin, Heidelberg, New York, 1992-1994.

Madaus G, Lehrbuch der Biologischen Arzneimittel, Bde 1-3, Nachdruck, Georg Olms Verlag Hildesheim 1979.

Male Fern

Dryopteris filix-mas

DESCRIPTION

Medicinal Parts: The medicinal parts are the dried fronds, the dried rhizome collected in autumn with the leaf bases, the fresh rhizome and the fresh aerial parts.

Flower and Fruit: On the underside of the leaflets there are 2 rows of sori, covered by kidney-shaped, red-brown film. The spores are dark brown.

Leaves, Stem and Root: The root is a crooked half-underground fleshy rhizome, covered in the remains of dark brown petioles, which produces long branched root fibers. The remains of the petioles are linear-lanceolate and tomentose with red-brown scales. The foliage grows in a crown, with fronds arranged in spirals, 60 cm to 1.5 m high. There are 2-pinnate, oblong-lanceolate, alternate, sessile leaflets, subdivided with round segments. The young fronds are rolled in spirals and thickly covered in hairs. They gradually open out as the fronds grow.

Habitat: The plant is found in the temperate zones of Europe, northern Asia and in North and South America.

Production: Male Fern leaf consists of the fresh or dried leaf of Dryopteris filix-mas. Male Fern herb consists of the fresh or dried above-ground parts of Dryopteris filix-mas. Male Fern rhizome consists of the fresh or dried rhizomes separated from the attached roots. The root-stock is collected in autumn and gently dried.

Not to be Confused With: The rhizomes of most European Dyopteris species.

Other Names: Aspidium, Bear's Paw Root, Fern, Knotty Brake, Male Shield Fern, Marginal Fern, Sweet Brake

ACTIONS AND PHARMACOLOGY

COMPOUNDS: MALE FERN RHIZOME

Acylphloroglucinoles (2%, mixtures termed raw filicin or filicin): in particular, flavaspidic acids, filicinic acids, paraspidin, desaspidin

Tannins

COMPOUNDS: MALE FERN LEAVES

Acylphloroglucinoles (0.2%, mixtures termed raw filicin or filicin): in particular, flavaspidic acids, filicinic acids, paraspidin, desaspidin

Flavonoids

EFFECTS

Male Fern herb has an anthelmintic effect and is strongly cytotoxic against band worms and liver flukes, although roundworm and oxyuris are resistant. It is also cell toxic, virostatic and antiviral. The pharmacological effect is largely due to the flavaspidic acid with filicic acids being the main active principle.

INDICATIONS AND USAGE

Unproven Uses: Preparations of Male Fern herb are used externally for rheumatism, sciatica, muscle pain, neuralgia, earache and toothache, for festering and poorly healing wounds, burns, hemorrhoids, for teething in infants, and sleep disorders, as well as internally for tapeworms and flukes.

Homeopathic Uses: Dryopteris filix-mas is used for weak sight and damage to the optic nerve.

CONTRAINDICATIONS

The drug should not be administered in the presence of anemia, cardiac, liver or kidney diseases or diabetes.

PRECAUTIONS AND ADVERSE REACTIONS

General: The following can occur even with therapeutic dosages: queasiness, nausea, severe headache, vomiting, diarrhea.

Pregnancy: The drug should not be used during pregnancy.

Pediatric Use: The drug should not be administered to children under 4 years.

Use in the Elderly: The drug should not be administered to elderly persons.

OVERDOSAGE

Overdosages in susceptible patients can lead to liver, cardiac and kidney damage as well as central nervous system disorders, psychoses and permanent injuries such as paralysis and visual disorders may be seen as a result of overdose.

Cases of death, particularly among children, have been observed following administration of Filmaron oil (10% solution of volatile extracts of the rhizomic drug in cooking oil).

DOSAGE

Mode of Administration: **Warning: Dosages may be toxic!** Due to the risks, internal application is not recommended; if possible other remedies should be used. Because the efficacy of the claimed applications is not documented, therapeutic usage is not recommended.

Preparation: Filix-mas extract: The percolate is completely freed from ether by steaming (maximum 50° C). It is made into a dried extract in a vacuum. The content is stabilized with high-fat cooking oil (DAB6)

Daily Dosage: The single and daily dose of Filix-mas extract is 6 to 8 gm for adults and 4 to 6 gm for children. In case of an unsuccessful cure, the treatment may only be repeated after an interim of a few weeks. The single and daily maximum dose of Filix-mas liquid extract is 3 gm. The maximum daily dosage of Aspidinolfilicium oil solution is 20 gm.

Homeopathic Dosage: 5 drops, 1 tablet or 10 globules every 30 to 60 minutes (acute) or 1 to 3 times daily (chronic); parenterally: 1 to 2 ml sc acute: 3 times daily; chronic: once a day (HAB1);

Storage: The drug is stored over adsorbant calcium for a maximum duration of 1 year, with a relative humidity below 0.05 in sealed containers away from light sources.

LITERATURE

Bottari F et al., (1972) Phytochemistry 11:2519.

Calderwood JM et al., J Pharm Pharmacol 21:55 S.

Frohne D, Pfänder HJ, Giftpflanzen - Ein Handbuch für Apotheker, Toxikologen und Biologen, 4. Aufl., Wiss. Verlagsges. mbH Stuttgart 1997.

Hänsel R, Keller K, Rimpler H, Schneider G (Hrsg.), Hagers Handbuch der Pharmazeutischen Praxis, 5. Aufl., Bde 4-6 (Drogen), Springer Verlag Berlin, Heidelberg, New York, 1992-1994.

Karl C, Pedersen PA, Müller G, Z Naturforsch 36C:607-610. 1981.

Leung AY, Encyclopedia of Common Natural Ingredients Used in Food, Drugs and Cosmetics, John Wiley & Sons Inc., New York 1980.

Roth L, Daunderer M, Kormann K, Giftpflanzen, Pflanzengifte, 4. Aufl., Ecomed Fachverlag Landsberg Lech 1993.

Teuscher E, Lindequist U, Biogene Gifte - Biologie, Chemie, Pharmakologie, 2. Aufl., Fischer Verlag Stuttgart 1994.

Widén CJ, Sarvela J, Britton OM, On the location and distribution of phloroglucinols (Filicins) in Ferns. In: Ann Bot Fennici 20:407. 1983.

Widén CJ, Vida G, Euw JV, Reichenstein T, Helv Chim Acta 54:2824-2850. 1971.

Mallotus philippinensis

See Kamala

Malus domestica

See Apple Tree

Malva sylvestris

See High Mallow

Manaca

Brunfelsia hopeana

DESCRIPTION

Medicinal Parts: The medicinal parts of Manaca are the roots and stem.

Flower and Fruit: The blue or white flowers are large, conical and very fragrant. The calyx is divided into 5 sections, with rounded lobes and 2 lips covering the bud. There are 4 fertile anthers, which fuse together above where they divide into 2 stigma-like lobes. The fruit is a fleshy or leathery capsule with numerous large seeds embedded in it.

Leaves, Stem and Root: Manaca is a shrub with obovate, deciduous leaves. The tough, woody roots are about 1.5 cm in diameter. They are yellow in the center and have a papery, pale brown epidermis. The stems have a small yellow medulla.

Habitat: Manaca grows in South America, the West Indies and Brazil.

Production: Manaca root is the root of Brunfelsia hopeana.

Other Names: Pohl, Vegetable Mercury

ACTIONS AND PHARMACOLOGY

COMPOUNDS

The active ingredients of the drug have not yet been adequately investigated. The spasmogenic brunfelsamidine (pyrrole-3-carboxamidine, identical with Nierembergia toxin) has been demonstrated in the related species Brunfelsia grandiflora.

EFFECTS

Diuretic and antirheumatic effect have been attributed to Manaca.

INDICATIONS AND USAGE

Unproven Uses: Manaca is used in the treatment of rheumatic conditions. In the past, folk medicine uses have included syphilis and scrofulosis.

PRECAUTIONS AND ADVERSE REACTIONS

No health hazards or side effects are known in conjunction with the proper administration of designated therapeutic dosages. In animal experiments, anxiety states, restlessness, increase in cardiac and pulmonary frequency, elevated salivation, vomiting, muscle tremors and tonic-clonic spasms were observed following intake of plant parts of Brunfelsia-species, as well as death.

DOSAGE

Mode of Administration: Liquid extract preparations for internal use.

LITERATURE

Frohne D, Pfänder HJ, Giftpflanzen - Ein Handbuch für Apotheker, Toxikologen und Biologen, 4. Aufl., Wiss. Verlags-Ges Stuttgart 1997.

Kern W, List PH, Hörhammer L (Hrsg.), Hagers Handbuch der Pharmazeutischen Praxis, 4. Aufl., Bde. 1-8, Springer Verlag Berlin, Heidelberg, New York, 1969.

Lloyd HA et al., Brunfeslamidine: A novel convulsant from the medicinal plant Brunfelsia grandiflora. In: Tetrahedron Letters 26(22):2623-2624. 1985.

Roth L, Daunderer M, Kormann K, Giftpflanzen, Pflanzengifte, 4. Aufl., Ecomed Fachverlag Landsberg Lech 1993.

Mandragora officinarum

See Mandrake

Mandrake

Mandragora officinarum

DESCRIPTION

Medicinal Parts: The medicinal parts are the dried underground part, the fresh herb and the root.

Flower and Fruit: The numerous flowers are on light green pedicles. They are glabrous on the outside. The corolla is light green to yellow. The calyx is lanceolate with a pointed tip, half as long as the 3 cm corolla. The hairs on the outside of the corolla have heads, which consist of 15 cells and sit on a tiny stem of 2 to 3 cm. The fruit is yellow, globular and extends with a diameter of 2 to 3 cm well beyond the calyx.

Leaves, Stem and Root: The plant has a thick, tuberous root and is almost stemless. The root is light brown on the outside, simple or branched, and up to 60 cm deep. The leaves are all the same size, pubescent, short petiolate, ovate-lanceolate. They have a disgusting smell.

Habitat: The plant is indigenous to the Mediterranean region and bordering frost-free regions.

Production: Mandrake root is the dried, underground part of Mandragora vernalis or M. officinarum. The plant is gathered in uncultivated regions.

Not to be Confused With: The roots of Atropa belladona, whose alkaloid pattern is similar.

Other Names: Mandragora, Satan's Apple

ACTIONS AND PHARMACOLOGY

COMPOUNDS: MANDRAGORA ROOT

Tropane alkaloids (0.4%): chief alkaloids (-)-hyoscyamine, under storage conditions changing over to some extent into atropine, and scopolamine

COMPOUNDS: MANDRAKE HERB

The leaves have hardly been investigated, but in view of the demonstrated toxicity, the same alkaloid mixture is to be assumed.

EFFECTS: MANDRAKE ROOT AND HERB

The action of the drug is mainly due to the anticholinergic effect of the main alkaloids (atropine, hyoscamin and scopolamine).

INDICATIONS AND USAGE

Unproven Uses: Mandragora is one of the oldest of the medicinal plants. In folk medicine, a tincture of Mandragora radix was used for stomach ulcers, colic, asthma, hay fever and whooping cough. Today, Mandrake is only used in homeopathy.

PRECAUTIONS AND ADVERSE REACTIONS

No health hazards are known in conjunction with the proper administration of designated therapeutic dosages. Skin reddening, dryness of the mouth, tachycardiac arrhythmias, mydriasis (the 4 early warning symptoms of a poisoning), accommodation disorders, heat build-up through decline in sweat secretion, micturition disorders and constipation can occur as side effects, particularly with overdoses.

OVERDOSAGE

Because of the high content of scopolamine in the drug, poisonings lead at first to somnolence, but then also, after the intake of very high dosages, to central excitation (restlessness, hallucinations, delirium and manic episodes), followed by exhaustion and sleep. Lethal dosages (for adults starting at 100 mg atropine, considerably less for children) carry with them the danger of respiratory failure. Severe poisonings are particularly conceivable in connection with the misuse of the drug as an intoxicant.

The treatment for poisonings include stomach emptying; temperature-lowering measures with wet cloths (no antipyretics!); oxygen respiration for respiratory distress; intubation; parenteral physostigmine salts as antidote; diazepam for spasms while monitoring respiratory function; catheter for cystoparalysis.

DOSAGE

Mode of Administration: The drug is now obsolete and is only rarely used in medicinal preparations. In homeopathy, dilutions from the fresh herb are used.

LITERATURE

Al-Khali S, Alkofahi A, The chemical constituents of Mandragora autumnalis. In: PM 62, Abstracts of the 44th Ann Congress of GA, 149. 1996.

Frohne D, Pfänder HJ, Giftpflanzen - Ein Handbuch für Apotheker, Toxikologen und Biologen, 4. Aufl., Wiss. Verlags-Ges. Stuttgart 1997.

Hänsel R, Keller K, Rimpler H, Schneider G (Hrsg.), Hagers Handbuch der Pharmazeutischen Praxis, 5. Aufl., Bde 4-6 (Drogen), Springer Verlag Berlin, Heidelberg, New York, 1992-1994.

Jackson BP, Berry MI, Hydroxytropane tigliates in the roots of Mandragora species. In: PH 12(5): 1165-1166. 1973.

Kraft K, Europäische Rauschdrogen. In: ZPT 17(6):343-355. 1996.

Lewin L, Gifte und Vergiftungen, 6. Aufl., Nachdruck, Haug Verlag, Heidelberg 1992.

Madaus G, Lehrbuch der Biologischen Arzneimittel, Bde 1-3, Nachdruck, Georg Olms Verlag Hildesheim 1979.

Roth L, Daunderer M, Kormann K, Giftpflanzen, Pflanzengifte, 4. Aufl., Ecomed Fachverlag Landsberg Lech 1993.

Scholz E, Alraunenfrüchte - ein biblisches Aphrodisiakum. In: ZPT 16(2):109-110. 1995.

Teuscher E, Lindequist U, Biogene Gifte - Biologie, Chemie, Pharmakologie, 2. Aufl., Fischer Verlag Stuttgart 1994.

Wagner H, Wiesenauer M, Phytotherapie. Phytopharmaka und pflanzliche Homöopathika, Fischer-Verlag, Stuttgart, Jena, New York 1995.

Manna

Fraxinus ornus

DESCRIPTION

Medicinal Parts: The medicinal part is the juice extracted from the bark starting from the 8th to the 10th year. This tree yields from its bark a sugary sap known in pharmacy as Manna.

Flower and Fruit: The inflorescence is in upright, later hanging, feathery panicles. The sepals are very short. The petals are fused at the base in pairs. They are linear to narrowly linguiform and white. The 2 stamens have very long filaments. The fruit is a nutlet. It is hanging, linguiform, 3 to 4 mm long and 7 to 10 mm wide. It is rounded at the base or narrowed wedge-shaped, glossy dark brown, flat and longitudinally striped. The seeds are ovate, 15 to 20 mm by 4 to 5 mm, broad, flat, longitudinally striped and brown.

Leaves, Stem and Root: Fraxinus ornus is a tree growing up to 8 m tall with gray, crust-embossed bark. The new-year's branchlets are olive-green or browny gray-green, somewhat glossy, with numerous, light-brown lenticels. The long shoots are downy to the tip; the short shoots are awned at the base. The terminal and lateral buds are orbicular and 4-scaled. The leaflets are elliptical-ovate-lanceolate or ovate, tapering to a tip and crenate-serrate. The upper surface is rich green and the underside lighter green with pink veins. The nerves are pink-tomentose.

Habitat: The tree is indigenous to southern Europe, extending to the southern borders of the Alps and as far as European Turkey. The tree is cultivated in Italy.

Production: Manna consists of the dried sap generated from the slit bark of trunk and branches of Fraxinus ornus, as well as its preparations in effective dosage. The eight to ten year-old trees are incised. The manna flows out of the bark and is collected.

Other Names: Flowering Ash, Manna Ash, Flake Manna

ACTIONS AND PHARMACOLOGY

COMPOUNDS

Alditols: Mannitol (70-90%)

Oligosaccharides: Stachyose, Mannotriose, Glucose, Fructose

EFFECTS

Manna acts as a laxative.

INDICATIONS AND USAGE

Approved by Commission E:

■ Constipation

Unproven Uses: Manna is also used for ailments where an easier elimination and a soft stool is desirable, such as anal fissures, hemorrhoids, and post-rectal/anal surgery.

CONTRAINDICATIONS

The drug is not to be used in the presence of ileus.

PRECAUTIONS AND ADVERSE REACTIONS

No health hazards or side effects are known in conjunction with the proper administration of designated therapeutic dosages. Susceptible persons could experience flatulence and nausea.

DOSAGE

Mode of Administration: Comminuted herb and other galenic preparations for internal use.

Daily Dosage: For adults, 20 to 30 gm of drug; For children, 2 to 16 gm of drug. Manna, like other laxatives, should not be used for an extended period of time.

LITERATURE

Hänsel R, Keller K, Rimpler H, Schneider G (Hrsg.), Hagers Handbuch der Pharmazeutischen Praxis, 5. Aufl., Bde 4-6 (Drogen), Springer Verlag Berlin, Heidelberg, New York, 1992-1994 (unter Fraxinus ornus).

Maranta arundinacea

See Arrowroot

Marigold

Calendula officinalis

TRADE NAMES

Califlora Calndula Gel, Calendula Gel, Calendula Ointment

DESCRIPTION

Flower and Fruit: On the tip of each stem there is a 5 to 7 cm composite flower head consisting of an epicalyx of numerous narrow-lanceolate sepals, which are densely covered on both sides with glandular hairs. The inner section of the flower head is made up of orange-yellow tubular florets. The disc florets are pseudohermaphrodites; the female sterile. The zygomorphic ray florets at the edge are female, their stamens are completely absent, and their inferior ovaries are much more developed than those of the tubular florets. Fruit forms only in the female ray flowers. The heterocarp achenes are sickle-shaped, curved and ringed.

Leaves, Stem and Root: The plant is usually an annual, seldom biennial. It grows to between 30 and 50 cm high and has a 20 cm long tap root and numerous thin, secondary roots. The stem is erect, angular, downy and branched from the base up or higher. The alternate leaves are almost spatulate at the base, oblong to lanceolate above and are all tomentose.

Characteristics: The plant has a strong, unpleasant smell.

Habitat: Central and southern Europe, western Asia and the U.S.

Production: Marigold flowers are the ray florets of the completely unfolded, collected and dried capitula of Calendula officinalis. Harvest begins in July. Drying takes place in the shade at a maximum of 45° C. Calendula herb consists of the fresh or dried above-ground parts of Calendula officinalis harvested during flowering season.

Not to be Confused With: Other Asteraceae; arnica and saffron are often adulterated with Marigold.

Other Names: Calendula, Holligold, Goldbloom, Golds, Mary Bud, Ruddes, Mary Gowles, Holigold, Marybud

ACTIONS AND PHARMACOLOGY

COMPOUNDS: MARIGOLD FLOWERS

Triterpene saponins (2 to 10%): glycosides A to F (mono- or bisdemosidic oleanolic acid glycosides)

Triterpene alcohols: tirterpene monooles (0.8%), triterpene dioles (4%) and triterpene trioles, including lupeol, taraxasterol, psi-taraxasterol, faradiol, arnidiol, their mono- and diesters (chiefly acetic acid, lauric, myristic and palmitic acid as acid components)

Flavonoids (0.3 to 0.8%): including isorhamnetin and quercetin glycosides

Hydroxycoumarins: including scopoletin, umbelliferone, esculetin

Carotinoids: chief components lutein, zeaxanthine

Volatile oil (0.2%): chief components alpha-cadinol, T-cadinol, fatty acids

Water-soluble polysaccharides (15%): rhamnoarabinogalactans, arabinogalactans

Polyynes

EFFECTS: MARIGOLD FLOWERS

The results of numerous studies on the mode of action are available. The flowers are antimicrobial due to the terpene alkaloids, lactone and flavones contained in the essential oil. Flavonoids isolated from flowers of Calendula officinalis demonstrated positive antimicrobial activity against *Staphylococcus aureus* (at a concentration of 1 milligram/milliliter (Dumenil et al., 1980). Other studies have demonstrated the flavones to be effective against *Klebsiella pneumoniae, Sarcina lutea* and *Candida monosa.*

Organic extracts of the dried flowers of Calendula officinalis exhibited potent anti-HIV activity in an in-vitro MTT/ tetrazolium-based assay. It was also found that the organic extract caused a significant dose- and time-dependent reduction of HIV-1 reverse transcription activity (Kalvatchev et al, 1997).

Antiviral tests performed using the oleanolic acid glycosides from the aerial parts of the plant demonstrated an inhibitory effect against *Vesicular stomatitis virus* (VSV). Only one compound (3.MH) significantly affected replication in *Rhinovirus* (HRV) cultures (De Tommasi et al., 1991).

Topical application of Calendula has been shown to enhance the granulation and epithelialization of damaged skin (Klouchek-Popova et al., 1982).

CLINICAL STUDIES

Wound Treatment/Tissue Repair

In one study, surgically induced skin wounds in rats were treated with a 5% Calendula ointment in combination with allantoin. Histological studies of the damaged tissue at 8 hours, 24 hours and 48 hours after inflicting the wounds were performed. The drug combination was found to markedly stimulate physiological regeneration and epithelialization. This effect was attributed to more extensive metabolism of glycoproteins, nucleoproteins and collagen protein during the regenerative period in the tissues (Klouchek-Popova et al., 1982).

In another in-vitro study, an extract of Calendula was shown to induce formation of new blood vessels, which is important in the process of granulation (Patrick et al., 1996).

Anti-Inflammatory Action

The anti-inflammatory activity of the 3 main triterpendiol esters of Marigold were tested against croton oil-induced edema of the ears in mice. Faradiol-3-myristic acid ester and faradiol-3-palmitic acid ester were found to have the same dose-dependent anti-inflammatory activity. The non-esterified faradiol was more active than the esters and had an equivalent effect on inflammation as an equimolar dose of indomethacin (Zitterl-Eglseer, et al., 1997).

In another study, the faradiol monoester was proven to be the most relevent anti-inflammatory principle due to its quantitative prevalence in the flowers. The unesterified faradiol was found to be the most active of all tested compounds, equal to indomethacin in effect (Della Loggia et al., 1994).

COMPOUNDS: MARIGOLD HERB

Triterpene saponins

Flavonoids

Carotinoids

Volatile oil

EFFECTS: MARIGOLD HERB

The astringent and granulation-promoting effect may be attributable to the essential oil, saponin and the amaroid loliolid. Efficacy has not been documented with valid data.

INDICATIONS AND USAGE

MARIGOLD FLOWERS

Approved by Commission E:

- Inflammation of the mouth and pharynx
- Wounds and burns

Externally, Marigold is used for inflammation of the oral and pharyngeal mucosa, poorly healing wounds, leg ulcers, to clean wounds, and for acute and chronic skin inflammation.

Unproven Uses: Marigold has been used extensively as a folk medicine. Externally it is used for varicosis, vascular disease wounds, inflammatory skin disease, anal eczema, proctitis, conjunctivitis. It is a constituent in treatments for sore, dry skin, bee stings and frostbite.

Marigold is used internally for inflammatory conditions of internal organs, gastrointestinal ulcers, constipation, worm infestation and dysmenorrhea. It is also used as a diuretic and diaphoretic. In the past (19th century), Marigold was used as a cancer therapy but is no longer in use today for this purpose.

Homeopathic Uses: Calendula officinalis is used for frostbite, burns to the skin and poorly healing wounds. The efficacy of the homeopathic uses has not been proven.

MARIGOLD HERB

Unproven Uses: Preparations are used for circulation, ulcers, spasms, swelling of the glands, jaundice, and for wounds and eczema. The herb is used in Russia for strep throat, on the Canaries for coughs and cramps and in China for irregular menstruation.

PRECAUTIONS AND ADVERSE REACTIONS

MARIGOLD FLOWERS AND HERB

No health hazards or side effects are known in conjunction with the proper administration of designated therapeutic dosages. There is a low potential for sensitization after frequent skin contact with the drug. A low rate of contact dermatitis (less than 1%) occurred in patients patch-tested with a tincture of 10% Calendula. Only 2 of 1032 patients had a positive skin reaction to Calendula (Bruynzeel et al, 1992).

DOSAGE

MARIGOLD FLOWERS

Mode of Administration: Comminuted drug for decoctions, and other preparations to be applied topically. It is available as tinctures, liquid extracts and infusions.

How Supplied: Powder, gel ointment, ophthalmic solution, tincture (10%), tea (infusion), shampoo and hand cream.

Cream

Gel — 7%, 10%

Ointment — 4%

Ophthalmic solution

Tea

Tincture

Shampoo

Preparation:

Tea — 150 ml of hot water are poured over 1 to 2 teaspoons drug and strained after approximately 10 minutes.

Diaphoretic — 2 to 4 ml tincture to 250 to 500 ml water or 0.5 to 1 ml liquid extract 1:1 ethanol 40%.

Ointment (10 to 20%) — 2 to 5 g drug in 100 g ointment with a fatty base.

Marigold oil — olive oil extraction 1:10 peanut oil; this 1:1 in 40% ethanol or 1:5 in 90% ethanol.

Daily Dosage:

Sore Throat and Inflammation, powder — 1 to 2 grams of Calendula powder to 150 milliliters of water (Bisset, 1994).

Sore Throat and Inflammation, tea — 1 to 2 grams in one cup of water, steep 10 to 15 minutes.

Peptic Ulcer, tea — 1 to 4 grams in one cup of water, steep 10 to 15 minutes. Take three times daily (Mills, 1991).

Wound Treatment, ointment 2% to 5% — Apply topically to the affected area (Bisset, 1994).

Wound Treatment, compress — Steep one tablespoon herb in 500 milliliters water for 10 to 15 minutes and apply as a moist compress (Weiss, 1985).

Homeopathic Dosage: 5 to 10 drops, 1 tablet or 5 to 10 globules 1 to 3 times daily or 1 ml injection solution sc twice weekly (HAB1).

Storage: Protect from light and moisture. May be stored a maximum of 3 years.

MARIGOLD HERB

Mode of Administration: Since efficacy has not been proven the therapeutic value is uncertain.

Preparation: Contained in Kneipp's Calendula Ointment.

LITERATURE

MARIGOLD FLOWERS

Ahmed AA et al., Sesquiterpene glycosides from Calendula officinalis. In: JNP 56(10):1821. 1993.

Antibiotika und Immunabwehr. In: Symbiose 4(2):20. 1992.

Bisset NG, Calendulae floss - marigold, in Herbal Drugsand Phytopharmaceuticals; a Handbook for Practice on a Scientific Basis. Medpharm Scientific Publishers, Stuttgart and CRC Press, Boca Raton, FL, USA, 1994.

Bruynzeel DP, Van Ketel WG, Young E et al., Contact sensitization by alternative topical medicaments containing plant extracts. Contact Dermatitis 1992; 27:278-279.

Della Loggia R et al., The role of triterpenoids in the topical antiinflammatory activity of Calendula officinalis flowers. In: PM 60(6):516-520. 1994.

De Tommasi N, Conti C, Stein ML, Pizza C, Structure and in vitro antiviral activity of triterpenoid saponins from Calendula arvensis. Planta Med (1991 Jun) 57(3):250-3.

Dumenil G, Chemli R & Balansard G et al., Evaluation of antibacterial properties of marigold glowers (Calendula officinalis L.) and mother homeopathic tinctures of C. officinalis L. and C. arvensis L. Ann Pharm Fr 1980; 38(6):493-499.

Hänsel R, Keller K, Rimpler H, Schneider G (Hrsg.), Hagers Handbuch der Pharmazeutischen Praxis, 5. Aufl., Bde 4-6 (Drogen), Springer Verlag Berlin, Heidelberg, New York, 1992-1994.

Hausen B, Allergiepflanzen, Pflanzenallergene, ecomed Verlagsgesellsch. mbH, Landsberg 1988.

Isaac O, Calendula officinalis L.- Die Ringelblume, Portrait einer Arzneipflanze. In: ZPT 15(6):357-370. 1994.

Isaac O, Die Ringelblume. Botanik, Chemie, Pharmakologie, Toxikologie, Pharmazie und therapeutsche Verwendung, Wissenschaftl. Verlagsges. mbH Stuttgart, 1992.

Kalvatchev Z, Walder R & Garzaro D, Anti-HIV activity of extracts from Calendula officinalis flowers. Biomed Pharmacother 1997; 51:176-180.

Kasprzyk Z, Pyrek J, (1968) Phytochemistry 7:1631.

Kasprzyk Z, Wilkomyrski B, (1973) Phytochemistry 13:2299.

Kloucek-Popova E, Popov A, Pavlova N et al., Influence of the physiological regeneration and epithelization using fractions isolated from Calendula officinalis. Acta Physiol Pharmacol Bulg 1982; 8(4):63-67.

Madaus G, Lehrbuch der Biologischen Arzneimittel, Bde 1-3, Nachdruck, Georg Olms Verlag Hildesheim 1979.

Mennet-von Eiff M, Meier B, Phytotherapie in der Dermatologie. In: ZPT 16(4):201-210. 1995.

Mills SY, Out of the Earth: The Essential Book of Herbal Medicine. Viking Arkana, London, 1991.

Patrick KFM, Kumar S, Edwardson PAD et al., Induction of vascularisation by an aqueous extract of the flowers of Calendula officinalis L the European marigold. Phytomedicine 1996; 3(1):11-18.

Pyrek J, (1977) Roczniki Chemii 51:1141, 2331, 2493.

Samochowiec E et al., (1979) Wiad Parazytol 25(1):77.

Steinegger E, Hänsel R, Pharmakognosie, 5. Aufl., Springer Verlag Heidelberg 1992.

Teuscher E, Biogene Arzneimittel, 5. Aufl., Wiss. Verlagsges. Stuttgart 1997.

Vecherko LP et al., (1975) Khim Prir Soed 11(3):366.

Weiss RF, Herbal Medicine. Ab Arcanum, Gothernburg, Sweden, 1985.

Wichtl M (Hrsg.), Teedrogen, 4. Aufl., Wiss. Verlagsges. Stuttgart 1997.

Wilkomirski B, (1985) Phytochemistry 24(12):3067.

Wagner H, Wiesenauer M, Phytotherapie. Phytopharmaka und pflanzliche Homöopathika, Fischer-Verlag, Stuttgart, Jena, New York 1995.

Willuhn G, Ringenblumenblüten (Calendulablüten). In: Tägl Praxis 33(3):685. 1992.

Zitterl-Eglseer K, Sosa S, Jurenitsch J et al., Anti-oedematous activities of the main triterpendiol esters of Marigold (Calendula officinalis L.). J Ethnopharmacol 1997; 57:139-144.

Marijuana

Cannabis sativa

DESCRIPTION

Medicinal Parts: The medicinal parts are the twig tips of the female flowers, with either flowers or fruit attached, the flower-bearing twigs that have been dried; the ripe hemp fruit and various homeopathic preparations of the fresh dried plant-parts.

Flower and Fruit: Hemp is dioecious. The female flowers are reduced to the perigone with one bract. The complete inflorescences form a leafy, false spike. The male flowers form panicles rich in pollen. Pollination is by wind. The fruit is a gray-green, glossy achene, 3.5 to 5 mm long and 2.5 to 4 mm wide. The seeds have little endosperm, are white, oily-fleshy and hooked.

Leaves, Stem and Root: Cannabis is an annual or biennial plant, which is usually branched and grows up to 5 m. The plant has erect, rough-haired and compressed bristles. The leaves are long-petioled and 3 to 7 pinnate. The leaflets are lanceolate and serrate.

Habitat: The plant probably originated in the Middle East. Today it is grown worldwide in temperate and tropical regions.

Production: Indian hemp is the dried flowering or fruiting branch tips of Cannabis sativa var. indica. Production depends on the origin. One method is by striping the leaves. Another method is stripping the resin exuded from the flowers and multiple fruit, which is shaped into balls or sheet forms. The final method involves cutting 5 cm to 10 cm long branch tips, which have just borne fruit, removing the leaves, pressing the shooting tips and gathering them into bundles.

Not to be Confused With: Prior to being used as a narcotic, marijuana was often combined with Nicotiana tabacum, Lavandula officinalis, Nepeta catarina or Origanum vulgare. It is possible to confuse Marijuana with varieties of Urtica, Moraceae, Ulmaceae and Boraginaceae.

Other Names: Cannabis, Pot, Bhang, Grass, Indian Hemp, Weed, Ganja, Kif

ACTIONS AND PHARMACOLOGY

COMPOUNDS

Cannabinoids: chief active agent 9-tetrahydrocannabinol (9-THC = 1-THC), in addition to 60 additional cannabinoids

Volatile oil: of a very complex composition, with, among other things beta-caryophyllenes, humules, caryophyllene oxide, alpha-pinenes, beta-pinenes, limonene, myrcene, beta-ocimene

Flavonoids: including canniflavone-1, canniflavone-2

EFFECTS

Psychotropic action: In most subjects the effect is registered following an oral dose of 20 mg d-9-tetrahydrocannabinol or after inhaling a cigarette with 2% d-9-tetrahydrocannabinol. The symptoms are mood swings, reduction in drive, inability to think clearly, confusion, lack of concentration, impairment of short term memory and perception of time. Sensory impressions become heightened or experienced differently.

Complex tasks become more difficult, the capacity to understand or empathize is impaired. Negative reactions such as anxiety, panic and psychosis can occur.

It is only possible to describe this effect in animal tests, on the basis of free behavioral and controlled behavioral tests. A stimulating effect has also been observed with lower doses. Not all cannaboids cause the same effect. CBC, CBD and CBG have no psychomimetic effect. Various interactions occur in combination with d-9-tetrahydrocannabinol.

Antiemetic action: has been reported in clinical studies involving cancer patients receiving chemotherapy.

Anticonvulsive action: d-9-tetrahydrocannabinol reduces the clinical and electrographic convulsion intensity in cats.

Analgesic characteristics: d-9-tetrahydrocannabinol displays analgesic characteristics, while at the same time partially increasing sensitivity to pain.

Body temperature: In animal tests, d-9-tetrahydrocannabinol and other cannaboids reduced body temperature. The maximum reduction was relatively small. A stronger hypothermic effect was observed in higher doses, which affected behavior.

Respiratory tract: The inhalation of marihuana smoke caused bronchial dilation in healthy subjects. Methacholine-induced asthma attacks can be terminated by inhaling marihuana, in this case only psychomimetic cannaboids are active.

Eyes: The ability of cannabis products to reduce intraocular pressure was discovered accidentally during trials on the effect of inhaling high doses. During the tests, intraocular pressure dropped by 45%. Eye drops applied locally had the same effect as standard medication but the effect lasted longer.

Immune system: In vitro and in animal testing, depending on the tissue, the immune system was significantly suppressed after cannaboid administration.

Antimicrobial action: CBC, CBDA, CBG and d-9-tetrahydrocannabinol displayed antibacterial effects. CBC and d-9-tetrahydrocannabinol are bacteriostatic and bactericidal against *streptococci* and *staphylococci.*

Tumor inhibiting effect: The in-vitro inhibiting effect of d-9-tetrahydrocannabinol, d-8-tetrahydrocannabinol and CBN on the growth of transplanted lung tumors has been documented.

Heart, circulation: Cannaboids increase heart frequency, peripheral vasodilatation causes an increase in systolic blood pressure in the prone position and a decrease in the supine position.

Other effects: d-9-tetrahydrocannabinol is said to be an appetite stimulant. Long term usage leads to a clear increase in tolerance for most of the pharmacological effects.

Mode of action: Most cannaboids act on the CNS. The multiplicity of effects does not point to just one receptor. Possible interaction with cell-wall lipids or effects on prostoglandin biosynthesis is under discussion at present.

When administered orally, the first psychotropic reactions take effect 30 to 60 minutes later. The effect is at its optimum between 2 to 3 hours later and lasts for a total of 8 hours. When inhaled the effect sets in within a few minutes, reaches its climax or maximum after 30 minutes and lasts for 3 hours.

INDICATIONS AND USAGE

Unproven Uses: Cannabis was first mentioned in the pharmacopoeia of the Chinese Emperor about 3,000 years ago. Cannabis resin was used for beriberi, constipation, female conditions, gout, malaria, rheumatism and absentmindedness. In medieval herbals, it was mostly used externally. There are recipes for balms for healing contractures and for cooling poultices for the head and joints and for podagra.

In 1845, the herb tips were mentioned for internal administration for gonorrhea, angina pectoris and choking fits. It was not until the nineteenth century that Indian hemp was described as having a euphoric effect; it was used for insomnia, neuralgia, painful rheumatism, painful gastrointestinal disorders, cholera, tetanus, epilepsy, strychnine poisoning, acute bronchitis, whooping cough, asthma, impending abortion and weak contractions. The extract was used as a sedative and mild soporific.

Current literature on phytotherapeutic drugs cite as indications for Indian hemp: painful disorders of the alimentary canal such as ulcers or cancer; respiratory disorders such as asthma, emphysema or chronic bronchitis; neuralgia, migraine; urinary tract disorders; mental disorders such as anxiety, neurasthenia or hysteria.

Dronabinol (delta-9-tetrahydrocannabinol, Marinol®) is marketed as an appetite stimulant in the treatment of AIDS-related anorexia and as an antiemetic for chemotherapy-induced emeses.

Indian and Chinese Medicine: In early Indian and Chinese medicine, it was used for nervous depressive states, insomnia, vomiting, tetanus and coughs.

PRECAUTIONS AND ADVERSE REACTIONS

No health hazards or side effects are known in conjunction with the proper administration of designated therapeutic dosages. The intake of toxic dosages, as is common with the smoking of cannabis, leads almost at once to euphoric states (pronounced gaiety, laughing fits) with exaggerated apprehension of sensual impressions. Alterations in the perception of time and space, as well as acoustical, visual and sensory hallucinations, lasting for 2 to 3 hours are common in higher dosages.

Driving ability can be disturbed for as long as 8 hours. Although only rarely reported, acute poisoning symptoms include nausea, vomiting, tear flow, hacking cough, disturbance of cardiac function and numbness of the limbs. Despite its widespread use as a recreational drug, instances of death are very rare. The results of chronic abuse are laryngitis, bronchitis, apathy, psychic decline and disturbances of genital functions.

DOSAGE

Mode of Administration: Marijuana is widely used as an illegal recreational drug. It is usually either smoked or eaten to produce mind-altering effects. The extracted or synthetically produced delta-9-tetrahydrocannabinol component is used legally in capsule form for oral administration.

How Supplied:

Capsules — (Marinol®) 2.5 mg, 5 mg, 10 mg

Dried Herb

Daily Dosage: The former average oral single dose of the drug was 0.1 gm.

Appetite stimulation — (Marinol®) 2.5 mg to 10 mg twice daily

Antiemetic — (Marinol®) 5 mg/m² to 15 mg/m² four to six times daily

Narcotic — hash and tobacco are mixed. 1 cigarette contains 0.5 gm to 1 gm of the drug with at least 5 mg to 10 mg d-9-tetrahydrocannabinol for the psychotropic effect. More exact dosages are almost impossible to stipulate due to the varieties of action of the different cannaboids and because of varying breathing techniques.

Storage: Store with care, protected from light. Studies have shown that 9-tetrahydrocannabinol has a strong affinity with synthetics and rubber and is easily absorbed by them.

LITERATURE

Anonym, Cannabis: Hanf als Nutzpflanze. In: DAZ 135(27):2538-2541. 1995.

Anonym, Rezeptorforschung: Körpereigener Ligand des Cannabis-Rezeptors isoliert. In: DAZ 133(24):2214. 1993.

Bayewitch M, Rhee MH, Avidor-Reiss T, Breuer A, Mechoulam R, Vogel Z Cannabis sativa - deceptive weed? S Afr Med J, 271:1269-70, 1995 Dec

Bonnin A et al Effects of perinatal exposure to delta 9-tetrahydrocannabinol on the fetal and early postnatal development of tyrosine hydroxylase-containing neurons in rat brain. J Mol Neurosci, 7:291-308, 1996 Winter

Castle DJ, Ames FR Cannabis and the brain. Aust N Z J Psychiatry, 30:179-83, 1996 Apr

Clarke CC, Marijuana botany. In: And/Or Press, Berkeley, California. 1981.

Drogenmiβbrauch: Drogen im Straβenverkehr. In: DAZ 134(27):2575. 1994.

Evans AT et al., (1985) J Pharm Pharmacol.

Evans AT et al., (1987) FEBS 211:119.

Evans AT et al., (1987) Biochem Pharmacol 36:2035.

Evans FJ, Cannabinoids - The separation of central from peripheral effects on a structural basis. In: PM 57:60. 1991.

Fairbairn JW et al., J Pharm Pharmacol 28:130.

Fairbairn JW, Pickens JT (1981) Br. J Pharmacol 72:401.

Gil EW et al., (1970) Nature 228:135.

Goedecke H, Karkos J, Die arzneiliche Verwendung von Cannabisprodukten. In: DAZ 136(34):2859-2862. 1996.

Jungmayr P, Rauschmittel: Macht Marihuana dumm? In: DAZ 136(34):2867-2868. 1996.

Kovar KA, Cannabis - was ist das? In: DAZ 132(43):2302. 1992.

Nahas, B, In: Marihuana in Science and Medicine. Nahas G (Ed.) Raven Press New York. 1984.

Paris RR et al., (1976) Plant Med Phytother 10:144.

Ross SA, ElSohly MA, The volatile oil composition of fresh and air-dried buds of Cannabis. In: JNP 59(1):49-51. 1996.

Ruh MF, Taylor JA, Howlett AC, Welshons WV Failure of cannabinoid compounds to stimulate estrogen receptors. Biochem Pharmacol, 53:35-41, 1997 Jan 10

Ruh MF, Taylor JA, Howlett AC, Welshons WV The volatile oil composition of fresh and air-dried buds of Cannabis sativa. J Nat Prod, 53:49-51, 1996 Jan

Segelman A et al., (1977) J Pharm Sci 66:1358.

Täschner KL, Drogen und Straβenverkehr. In: DAZ 134(35):3299. 1994.

Taura F, Morimoto S, Shoyama Y Three acyclic bis-phenylpropane lignanamides from fruits of Cannabis sativa. Phytochemistry, 271:1003-7, 1995 Mar

Turner CE et al., (1980) J Nat Prod 43:169.

Vidal C, Fuente R, Iglesias A, Saez A Bronchial asthma due to Cannabis sativa seed. Allergy, 40:647-9, 1991 Nov

Yamamoto I, Matsunaga T, Kobayashi H, Watanabe K, Yoshimura H Analysis and pharmacotoxicity of feruloyltyramine as a new constituent and p-coumaroyltyramine in Cannabis sativa L. Pharmacol Biochem Behav, 40:465-9, 1991 Nov

Yamaudi T, (1975) Phytochemistry 14:2189.

Further information in:

Barrett ML et al Biochem Pharmacol 34 (1985), 2019

Burstein S, Ozman K Biochem Pharmacol 34 (1982), 2019

Frohne D, Pfänder HJ, Giftpflanzen - Ein Handbuch für Apotheker, Toxikologen und Biologen, 4. Aufl., Wiss. Verlags-Ges. Stuttgart 1997.

Gruenwald J, Brendler T, Jaenicke C (Eds) Physicians Desk Reference for Herbal Medicines. Medical Economics Company Inc., Montvale, 1998

Hänsel R, Keller K, Rimpler H, Schneider G (Hrsg.), Hagers Handbuch der Pharmazeutischen Praxis, 5. Aufl., Bde 4-6 (Drogen), Springer Verlag Berlin, Heidelberg, New York, 1992-1994.

Hernandez ML, Garcia-Gil L, Berrendero F, Ramos JA, Fernandez-Ruiz JJ delta 9-Tetrahydrocannabinol increases activity of tyrosine hydroxylase in cultured fetal mesencephalic neurons. J Mol Neurosci, 8:83-91, 1997 Apr

Lercker G, Bocci F, Frega N, Bortolomeazzi R Cannabinoid acids analysis. Farmaco, 40:367-78, 1992 Mar

Lewin L, Gifte und Vergiftungen, 6. Aufl., Nachdruck, Haug Verlag, Heidelberg 1992.

Mackie K, Hille B Cannabinoids inhibit N-type calcium channels in neuroblastoma-glioma cells. Proc Natl Acad Sci U S A, 89:3825-9, 1992 May 1

Mackie K, Hille B Passive consumption of mariJuana through milk: a low level chronic exposure to delta-9-tetrahydrocannabinol(THC). J Toxicol Clin Toxicol, 89:255-60, 1990

Madaus G, Lehrbuch der Biologischen Arzneimittel, Bde 1-3, Nachdruck, Georg Olms Verlag Hildesheim 1979.

Navarro M, Rubio P, de Fonseca FR Behavioural consequences of maternal exposure to natural cannabinoids in rats. Psychopharmacology (Berl), 122:1-14, 1995 Nov

Romero J, Garcia-Palomero E, Lin SY, Ramos JA, Makriyannis A, Fernandez-Ruiz JJ Cannabis sativa—a plea for decriminalisation. S Afr Med J, 58:1268-9, 1995 Dec

Roth L, Daunderer M, Kormann K, Giftpflanzen, Pflanzengifte, 4. Aufl., Ecomed Fachverlag Landsberg Lech 1993.

Teuscher E, Lindequist U, Biogene Gifte - Biologie, Chemie, Pharmakologie, 2. Aufl., Fischer Verlag Stuttgart 1994.

Teuscher E, Biogene Arzneimittel, 5. Aufl., Wiss. Verlagsges. Stuttgart 1997.

Thomas BF, Adams IB, Mascarella SW, Martin BR, Razdan RK Structure-activity analysis of anandamide analogs: relationship to a cannabinoid pharmacophore. J Med Chem, 58:471-9, 1996 Jan 19

Marrubium vulgare

See Horehound

Marsdenia condurango

See Condurango

Marsh Blazing Star

Liatris spicata

DESCRIPTION

Medicinal Parts: The medicinal parts are the roots.

Flower and Fruit: The inflorescence is compound spikes of carmine red flowers, 4 to 8 mm in diameter.

Leaves, Stem and Root: The plant is a perennial and has an erect, leafy stem up 2 m. The leaves are opposite, up to 30 cm long and 1 cm wide. The rhizome is 1 cm or more in diameter. It is gnarled with several cup-shaped scars. The rhizome is brownish and slightly wrinkled on the outside. Inside it is whitish with dark gray spots.

Characteristics: The root is very solid. The taste is bitter, and the odor is faintly aromatic, resembling cedar.

Habitat: U.S., cultivated in parts of Europe.

Production: Marsh Blazing Star is the rhizome of Liatris spicata.

Other Names: Button Snakeroot, Gay-Feather, Backache Root, Colic Root, Devil's Bite

ACTIONS AND PHARMACOLOGY

COMPOUNDS

Coumarin

Flavonoids: including rutin, quercetin-3-O-glucoside

EFFECTS

Main active principle: Coumarin. There is no reliable information available.

INDICATIONS AND USAGE

Unproven Uses: Marsh Blazing Star has been used for disorders of the kidney, dysmenorrhea, as a diuretic and for gonorrhea treatment.

PRECAUTIONS AND ADVERSE REACTIONS

No health hazards or side effects are known in conjunction with the proper administration of designated therapeutic dosages.

DOSAGE

Mode of Administration: Ground drug as an infusion.

LITERATURE

Kern W, List PH, Hörhammer L (Hrsg.), Hagers Handbuch der Pharmazeutischen Praxis, 4. Aufl., Bde. 1-8, Springer Verlag Berlin, Heidelberg, New York, 1969.

Lowry JB, (1973) Nature 241:61.

Madaus G, Lehrbuch der Biologischen Arzneimittel, Bde 1-3, Nachdruck, Georg Olms Verlag Hildesheim 1979.

Seshadri TF, (1972) Phytochemistry 11:881.

Marsh Marigold

Caltha palustris

DESCRIPTION

Medicinal Parts: The medicinal part is the dried aerial part of the flowering plant.

Flower and Fruit: The flowers are about 4 cm in diameter. The involucre is simple and has 5 or more yolk-yellow, 12 to 18 mm long ovate bracts, that are glossy greenish on the outside. There are numerous stamens and 5 to 8 ovaries. The fruit is a star-shaped follicle with a short beak. The seeds are dark brown to black, measuring about 2.5 cm long by 1.3 cm wide.

Leaves, Stem and Root: Caltha palustris is a 15 to 30 cm high perennial marsh plant with a sturdy, many-headed rhizome. The glabrous, hollow stem is ascending or decumbent. The leaves are dark green and have an oily-glossy, cordate to reniform, crenate or serrate-margined leaf blade. The petioles are grooved. The cauline leaves have shorter petioles and are smaller, clasping, and often have a membranous leaf sheath.

Characteristics: The plant is highly poisonous.

Habitat: Caltha palustris is found in all temperate regions of the Northern Hemisphere.

Other Names: Cowslip, Kingcups, Water Blobs, Horse Blobs, Bull's Eyes, Leopard's Foot, Meadow Routs, Verrucaria, Solsequia, Sponsa Solis, Palsy Root, Water Dragon

ACTIONS AND PHARMACOLOGY

COMPOUNDS

Protoanemonine-forming agents: In the freshly harvested plant, it is presumably the glycoside ranunculin that changes enzymatically when the plant is cut into small pieces, and probably also when it is dried. It then changes into the pungent, volatile protoanemonine that is severely irritating to skin and mucous membranes but quickly dimerizes to anemonine; when dried, the plant is not capable of protoanemonine formation

Triterpene saponins: including hederagenin glycosides

Triterpene lactones: caltholid, palustrolid

Isoquinoline alkaloids (aporphine type, very small quantities): including corytuberine, magnoflorine, protopine

EFFECTS

The drug lowers cholesterol levels and raises blood sugar levels in rats subsequent to oral administration (according to unavailable Russian research). There are also reports of anti-inflammatory effects on formaldehyde-induced inflammation.

The drug contains alkaloids of the benzylisoquinoline type (magnoflorine, triterpene saponins, triterpene lactones). In animal tests magnoflorine temporally lowers blood pressure and induces hypothermia in mice. An effect on the nicotine receptor in the parasympathetic nervous system is under discussion.

Insufficient information is available for an authoritative assessment of these effects.

INDICATIONS AND USAGE

Unproven Uses: Marsh Marigold was formerly used for jaundice, liver and bilious complaints. Some Native American tribes and those practicing Russian folk medicine used the plant for dressing and cleansing skin lesions and sores. When administered internally, it is meant to have a laxative and diuretic effect. Since this has not been sufficiently proven, and the side effects of Marsh Marigold are so dangerous, its internal use is not recommended.

Homeopathic Uses: The drug is used externally for skin rashes.

PRECAUTIONS AND ADVERSE REACTIONS

No health hazards or side effects are known in conjunction with the proper administration of designated therapeutic dosages of the dehydrated drug.

Extended skin contact with the freshly harvested, bruised plant can lead to treatment-resistant blisters and cauterizations due to the release of protoanemonine, which is severely irritating to skin and mucous membranes.

If taken internally, large quantities could lead to severe irritation of the gastrointestinal tract, combined with colic and diarrhea, as well as with irritation of the urinary drainage passages.

OVERDOSAGE

Symptomatic treatment for external contact should consist of irrigation with diluted potassium permanganate solution followed by mucilage. Ingestion of the drug should be treated with gastric lavage followed by activated charcoal. The toxicity of this plant is less than that of many other Ranunculaceae (Anemones nemorosae) due to the relatively low levels of protoanemonine-forming agents.

DOSAGE

Mode of Administration: Because of the herb's toxicity, its use is not recommended other than topically and as an extract.

LITERATURE

Bhandari P et al., Triterpenoid saponins from Caltha palsutris. In: PM 53(1):98-100. 1987.

Bhandari P et al., Two nortriterpene lactones from Caltha palustris. In: PH 23(8):1699-1702. 1984.

Bonora A et al., PH 26:2277. 1987.

Bruni A et al., Protoanemonin detection in Caltha palustris. In: JNP 49(6): 1172-1173. 1986.

Frohne D, Pfänder HJ, Giftpflanzen - Ein Handbuch für Apotheker, Toxikologen und Biologen, 4. Aufl., Wiss. Verlags-Ges Stuttgart 1997.

Hänsel R, Keller K, Rimpler H, Schneider G (Hrsg.), Hagers Handbuch der Pharmazeutischen Praxis, 5. Aufl., Bde 4-6 (Drogen): Springer Verlag Berlin, Heidelberg, New York, 1992-1994.

Lewin L, Gifte und Vergiftungen, 6. Aufl., Nachdruck, Haug Verlag, Heidelberg 1992.

Madaus G, Lehrbuch der Biologischen Arzneimittel, Bde 1-3, Nachdruck, Georg Olms Verlag Hildesheim 1979.

Roth L, Daunderer M, Kormann K, Giftpflanzen, Pflanzengifte, 4. Aufl., Ecomed Fachverlag Landsberg Lech 1993.

Teuscher E, Lindequist U, Biogene Gifte - Biologie, Chemie, Pharmakologie, 2. Aufl., Fischer Verlag Stuttgart 1994.

Marshmallow

Althaea officinalis

TRADE NAMES

Marshmallow is available from a number of manufacturers, often as Marshmallow Root.

DESCRIPTION

Medicinal Parts: The medicinal parts are the mallow flowers, leaves, syrup and roots.

Flower and Fruit: The reddish-white flowers are usually in axillary or terminal clusters. The 6 to 9 sepals of the epicalyx are fused at the base, pointed and 8 to 10 mm long. There are 5 sepals, 5 heart-shaped petals and numerous stamens fused together with the anthers to a column. The ovaries are in a ring. There are numerous styles. The mericarps are smooth and downy. The 5 to 8 mm fruit is disc-like and breaks up into the mericarps, which are downy on the outside and often have fine, branched and radiating ribs. The seeds are dark-brown, glabrous, kidney-shaped and somewhat compressed.

Leaves, Stem and Root: The 60 to 120 cm high, hardy, velvety plant has a thick erect root up to 50 cm long by a few cm with secondary roots. The erect, succulent stem is usually woody at the base but unbranched. The leaves are short-petioled with an ovate, acute leaf-blade. The secondary leaves are narrow and drooping. The lower leaves are 5-lobed, and the upper cauline leaves are often triangular, wider than they are long, and irregularly and roughly dentate.

Habitat: The plant was originally indigenous to Asia and then spread westward to southeast Europe and eastward to China. In temperate latitudes, Marshmallow is established as a garden plant.

Production: Marshmallow root consists of the dried root, unpeeled or peeled, of Althaea officinalis. The root cultures are harvested from October to November, and after cleaning, are carefully dried at a maximum temperature of 35°C. Marshmallow leaves consist of the dried leaves of Althaea officinalis. After harvest, the leaves are dried at a temperature of 40°C.

Not to be Confused With: May be confused with other Althea species.

Other Names: Moorish Mallow, Cheeses, White Maoow, Althea, Mortification Root, Sweet Weed, Wymote, Mallards, Schloss Tea

ACTIONS AND PHARMACOLOGY

COMPOUNDS

Mucilages: mixture of colloidally soluble polysaccharides, particularly galacturonic rhamnans, arabinogalactans, arabans and glucans

Pectins

Starch

EFFECTS

The drug alleviates local irritation, inhibits mucociliary activity, stimulates phagocytosis, and functions as an anti-inflammatory and anticomplementary agent, immune stimulant and hypoglycemic. Efficacy has been demonstrated when used as a gargle for inflammation of the mucous membrane of the mouth and throat.

INDICATIONS AND USAGE

Approved by Commission E:

■ Cough/bronchitis

Unproven Uses: Uses of the drug include irritation of the oral and pharyngeal mucosa and associated dry cough; mild inflammation of the gastric mucosa; as cataplasm for light inflammations and skin burns; and for insect bites. In folk medicine, marshmallow is employed for catarrh of the mouth, throat, gastrointestinal tract and urinary tract, as well as for inflammation, ulcers, abscesses, burns, constipation and diarrhea.

PRECAUTIONS AND ADVERSE REACTIONS

General: No health hazards or side effects are known in conjunction with the proper administration of designated therapeutic dosages.

Drug Interactions: The absorption of other drugs taken simultaneously may be delayed.

DOSAGE

Mode of Administration: Cut leaves for aqueous extracts as well as other galenic preparations for internal use. Cut or ground root for aqueous extracts as well as other galenic preparations for internal use. Marshmallow syrup is to be used only for treatment of dry coughs.

Note: Diabetics need to consider sugar concentration of marshmallow syrup.

How Supplied:
Capsules — 460 mg

Cough mixture

Drops

Liquid — Generally in syrup form, which is also called ‘‘snail juice’’: (1:1)

Powder

Tablets (coated and uncoated)

Preparation: To prepare a tea, use 10 to 15 g with 150 ml of cold water and allow to stand for 90 minutes, then warm to drink.

Daily Dosage: The average daily dose is 6 gm of the root and 5 gm of the leaf. The tea dosage is several cups of the slightly warmed tea taken during the course of the day. A single dose of the syrup is 10 gm.

Storage: The drug should be protected from light sources and insects.

LITERATURE

Blaschek W, Franz G, (1986) Planta Med 6:76P.

Capek P, et al., Carbohydr Res 164:443. 1987.

Franz G, Madaus A, Stabilität von Polysacchariden. Untersuchungen am Beispiel des Eibischschleims. In: DAZ 130(40):2194. 1990.

Franz G, PM 14:90. 1966.

Franz G, PM 55:493. 1989.

Gudej J, (1981) Acta Pol Pharm 38:385.

Gudej J, Bieganowska HL, Chromatographia 30:333. 1990.

Gudej J, PM 57:284. 1991.

Hahn-Deinstrop E, Eibischwurzel Identifizierung von Eibischwurzel-Extrakt und Gehaltsbestimmung in einem Instant-Tee. In: DAZ 135(13):1147-1149. 1995.

Kardosova A, et al., (1983) Coll Czech Commun 45:2082.

Kochich P, et al., (1983) Sov J Bioorg Chem 9(2):121.

Nosál'ova G, Strapková A, Kardosova A, Capek P, Zatureck'y L, Bukovska E, Antitussive Wirkung des Extraktes und der Polysaccharide aus Eibisch (Althaea officinalis L. var. robusta). In: PA 47(3):224-226. 1992.

Nosolova G, et al., PA 47:224. 1993.

Shimizu N, Tomoda T, Chem Pharm Bull 33:5539. 1985.

Tomoda M et al., (1977) Chem Pharm Bull 25:1357.

Tomoda M et al., (1980) Chem Pharm Bull 28:824.

Tomoda M et al., (1987) Planta Med 53(1):8.

Wunderer H, Zentral und peripher wirksame Antitussiva: eine kritische Übersicht. In: PZ 142(11):847-852. 1997.

Further information in:

Hänsel R, Keller K, Rimpler H, Schneider G (Hrsg.), Hagers Handbuch der Pharmazeutischen Praxis, 5. Aufl., Bde 4-6 (Drogen), Springer Verlag Berlin, Heidelberg, New York, 1992-1994.

Madaus G, Lehrbuch der Biologischen Arzneimittel, Bde 1-3, Nachdruck, Georg Olms Verlag Hildesheim 1979.

Schulz R, Hänsel R, Rationale Phytotherapie, Springer Verlag Heidelberg 1996.

Steinegger E, Hänsel R, Pharmakognosie, 5. Aufl., Springer Verlag Heidelberg 1992.

Teuscher E, Biogene Arzneimittel, 5. Aufl., Wiss. Verlagsges. Stuttgart 1997.

Wagner H, Wiesenauer M, Phytotherapie. Phytopharmaka und pflanzliche Homöopathika, Fischer-Verlag, Stuttgart, Jena, New York 1995.

Wichtl M (Hrsg.), Teedrogen, 4. Aufl., Wiss. Verlagsges. Stuttgart 1997.

Martagon

Lilium martagon

DESCRIPTION

Medicinal Parts: The medicinal parts are the leaves, stem and flowers, which are collected when the plant is completely mature.

Flower and Fruit: The inflorescence is terminal and racemous with 3 to 10 inclined flowers. The flower buds are globose or oblong-ovate. The tepal petals are 3 to 3.5 cm long, involute and orange with dark spots. They contain a ciliate mauve honey gland. The anthers are red. The fruit is a 2-winged capsule with an erect fruit stem. The seeds are flat, light brown and 6 to 8 mm long. Since the seeds do not ripen in northern regions, propagation takes place by means of bulbils, which occur at the leaf axils. Flowers are produced during the third year of growth.

Leaves, Stem and Root: The plant is a perennial, 30 to 60 cm high or higher. The bulb is golden yellow, ovate and about 5 cm long. The stem is erect, round, glabrous or with short rough hairs on the upper section. The stem is green or spotted red and leafy in the middle. The leaves are 7 to 11 ribbed, oblong-spatulate, shortly ciliated and up to 15 cm long.

Habitat: The plant comes from China and Japan, but is also cultivated in central and southern Europe.

Production: Martagon is the tuber of Lilium martagon.

Other Names: Purple Turk's Cap Lily, Turk's Cap

ACTIONS AND PHARMACOLOGY

COMPOUNDS

Soluble polysaccharides

Starch

Gamma-methylene glutamic acid

Tuliposide

The constituents of the drug have not been fully investigated.

EFFECTS

No information is available.

INDICATIONS AND USAGE

Unproven Uses: The drug is used as a diuretic and in the treatment of dysmenorrhea. It is used externally for ulcers.

Homeopathic Uses: All the above uses are also employed in homeopathic medicine.

PRECAUTIONS AND ADVERSE REACTIONS

No health hazards or side effects are known in conjunction with the proper administration of designated therapeutic dosages.

DOSAGE

Mode of Administration: Martagon is available as cut drug for internal use in infusions and external use in poultices. Homeopathic dilutions are also available.

LITERATURE

Satou T, Mimaki Y, Kuroda M, Sashida Y, Hatakeyama Y, A pyrroline glucoside ester and steroidal saponins from Lilium martagon. Phytochemistry, 41:1225-30, 1996 Mar.

Masterwort

Peucedanum ostruthium

DESCRIPTION

Medicinal Parts: The medicinal part is the dried root.

Flower and Fruit: The white flowers form many-blossomed compound umbels. There is no involucre. The epicalyx has only a few leaves. The calyx is indistinct. The petals have indented, pointed tips.

Leaves, Stem and Root: The plant grows from 50 to 100 cm high. The rhizome is gray-brown and produces runners. The stem is round, slightly grooved and glabrous. The basal leaves are doubly trifoliate. The leaflets are ovate to oblong, about 4 cm wide, roughly serrate and pale green beneath. The lateral leaflets are dipinnate. The terminal leaflet is tripinnate. The cauline leaves are small with a bulbous, membranous sheath.

Characteristics: Masterwort has an aromatic-bitter taste.

Habitat: The plant grows in central Europe.

Production: Masterwort rootstock is the rhizome of Peucedanum ostruthium. The thickened rhizomes are harvested. These are dug up in autumn or spring, then cleaned, freed from any root or green residue, cut and dried at a temperature of 35° C.

ACTIONS AND PHARMACOLOGY

COMPOUNDS

Volatile oil: chief components alpha-pinene, (+)-phellandrene, (+)-limonene, esters of isobutyric and isovaleric acid

Furocoumarins: in particular imperatorin, oxypeucedanin, osthrutol gamma-chromones: peucenine

Phthalides

Polyynes

EFFECTS

Masterwort is said to be stomachic and to have a mild sedative effect. Its main action is as a diuretic.

INDICATIONS AND USAGE

Unproven Uses: Masterwort is used for bloating, flatulence, Roemheld syndrome, digestive disorders, weak stomach and intestinal catarrh.

PRECAUTIONS AND ADVERSE REACTIONS

General: No health hazards or side effects are known in conjunction with the proper administration of designated therapeutic dosages. Light-skinned individuals may experience an increase in UV-sensitivity, due to the phototoxic effect of the furocoumarins.

DOSAGE

Mode of Administration: Masterwort is obsolete as a drug in German-speaking countries. It is occasionally used as a constituent in medicinal preparations in combination with other bitters. It is administered as a powder or as an infusion.

Preparation: To prepare an infusion, use a cold extraction of 1 teaspoonful of the drug over a period of 8 hours.

Daily Dosage:

Infusion — Can be drunk throughout the day.

Powder — 0.5 gm to 2 gm can be taken 2 to 3 times daily.

Storage: Store in a dry place, in closed containers.

LITERATURE

Gijbels MJM et al., (1985) Fitoterapia 61(1):17.

Hegnauer R, Chemotaxonomie der Pflanzen, Bde 1-11, Birkhäuser Verlag Basel, Boston, Berlin 1962-1997.

Kern W, List PH, Hörhammer L (Hrsg.), Hagers Handbuch der Pharmazeutischen Praxis, 4. Aufl., Bde. 1-8, Springer Verlag Berlin, Heidelberg, New York, 1969.

Madaus G, Lehrbuch der Biologischen Arzneimittel, Bde 1-3, Nachdruck, Georg Olms Verlag Hildesheim 1979.

Schimmer O et al., (1980) Planta Med 40(1):68.

Teuscher E, Lindequist U, Biogene Gifte - Biologie, Chemie, Pharmakologie, 2. Aufl., Fischer Verlag Stuttgart 1994.

Mastic Tree

Pistacia lentiscus

DESCRIPTION

Medicinal Parts: The medicinal part is the resin.

Flower and Fruit: The inflorescence is compact and spike-like. The flowers are yellowish or purplish. The drupe is approximately 4 mm, globose, apiculate and is red, but later turns black.

Leaves, Stem and Root: The plant is a small evergreen tree or shrub 1 to 8 m high. The trees are said to be exclusively male. The leaves are bipinnate. The 8 to 12 leaflets measure 1 to 5 cm by 0.5 to 1.5 cm. They are lanceolate to ovate-lanceolate, mucronate and coriaceous. The rhachis is broadly winged. The petioles are glabrous.

Habitat: The tree thrives in the Mediterranean region, Portugal, Turkey, on the Canaries and in tropical Africa.

Production: Mastic resin is the resin from the trunk of Pistacia lentiscus.

Other Names: Lentisk

ACTIONS AND PHARMACOLOGY

COMPOUNDS

Resins (90%): chief components are the triterpenes mastic acid, isomastic acid, oleanolic acid and tirucallol

Volatile oil (1-3%): including alpha-pinene, myrcene, linalool, beta-pinene, beta-caryophyllene (constituents vary a great deal)

EFFECTS

In animal experiments Mastic is ulcer protective. The amaroids and essential oil are astringent and aromatic.

INDICATIONS AND USAGE

Unproven Uses: Mastic Tree resin was formerly used in dentistry, as a material for fillings. The masticated resin releases substances that freshen the breath and tighten the gums.

PRECAUTIONS AND ADVERSE REACTIONS

General: No health hazards or side effects are known in conjunction with the proper administration of designated therapeutic dosages.

Pediatric Use: There is an occasional risk of diarrhea in small children.

DOSAGE

Mode of Administration: The resin is used for the production of chewing gum and is used in the food and drink industries.

LITERATURE

Al-Said MS et al., Evaluation of Mastic, a crude drug obtained from Pistacia lentiscus for gastric and duodenal anti-ulcer activity. In: ETH 15:271. 1986.

Marner FJ, Freyer A, Lex J, Triterpenoids from gum Mastic, the resin of Pistacia lentiscus. In: PH 30(11):3709-3712. 1991.

Further information in:

Kern W, List PH, Hörhammer L (Hrsg.), Hagers Handbuch der Pharmazeutischen Praxis, 4. Aufl., Bde. 1-8, Springer Verlag Berlin, Heidelberg, New York, 1969.

Teuscher E, Biogene Arzneimittel, 5. Aufl., Wiss. Verlagsges. Stuttgart 1997.

Maté

Ilex paraguariensis

DESCRIPTION

Medicinal Parts: The medicinal parts are the dried or roasted leaves.

Flower and Fruit: The white flowers are axillary and are in clusters of 40 to 50. They have a 4 to 5 sepaled calyx and 4 to 5 petalled corolla, are unisexual and dioecious. The fruit is a globoid reddish drupe with 5 to 8 seeds.

Leaves, Stem and Root: The plant is an evergreen shrub or tree up to 20 m tall with pale bark and an oblong-oval crown. The leaves are alternate, obovate, acuminate with a crenate or serrate margin. They are dark green above and pale green beneath and are tough, coriaceous and 6 to 20 cm long and 3 to 9 cm wide.

Characteristics: The taste is astringent and bitter. The odor is characteristic and aromatic.

Habitat: The plant is only found in South America between the 20th and 30th parallel.

Production: Maté consists of the dried leaf and leaf stem of Ilex paraguariensis. It is harvested every 2 years from May to September, then dried and cut.

Other Names: Yerba Maté, Jesuit's Tea, Paraguay Tea

ACTIONS AND PHARMACOLOGY

COMPOUNDS

Purine alkaloids: chief alkaloids caffeine (0.4-2.4%) and theobromine (0.3-0.5%)

Caffeic acid derivatives: including among others chlorogenic acid, neochlorogenic acid, cryptochlorogenic acid

Flavonoids: including among others rutin, isoquercitrin, kaempferol glycosides

Triterpene saponins (mate saponins)

Nitrile glycosides: menisdaurin, not cyanogenic

Volatile oil

EFFECTS

The main active principles are caffeine in varying amounts, tannins and small amounts of essential oil. Depending on the caffeine content the drug can display analeptic, diuretic, positively inotropic and positively chronotropic, glycogenolytic and lipolytic effects.

The centrally stimulating effect of the drug is due to the chlorogenic acids.

INDICATIONS AND USAGE

Approved by Commission E:

■ Lack of stamina

Maté is used for mental and physical fatigue.

Unproven Uses: In folk medicine Maté is used internally for ulcers, rheumatism, anemia, neurasthenia, depression, as a diuretic for oliguria and as a prophylaxis against fever and infections. Externally Maté is used as a poultice for ulcers and inflammation.

Homeopathic Uses: Ilex paraguariensis is used to treat poor digestion.

PRECAUTIONS AND ADVERSE REACTIONS

No health hazards or side effects are known in conjunction with the proper administration of designated therapeutic dosages.

DOSAGE

Mode of Administration: Maté is available as comminuted herb for infusions, herb powder and as galenic preparations for internal use. The drug is available as filter teas in mono tea form and in various tea combinations such as bladder and kidney teas.

Preparation: To prepare an infusion, pour water that has just been brought to boil over 1 teaspoonful drug (2 gm) and leave to draw for 5 to 10 minutes, then strain. The briefly infused drink is more stimulating, less astringent and tastes better (caffeine dissolves more quickly than the tannins).

Roasted leaves: The dried leaves are heated for 20 minutes to 100° C and then rinsed with water. The leaves are stored for 3 to 4 days to allow the taste and aroma to develop (DAC86).

Daily Dosage: 3 gm of drug.

Tea: as required (1 teaspoon corresponds to 2 gm drug).

Homeopathic Dosage: 5 drops, 1 tablet or 10 globules every 30 to 60 minutes (acute) or 1 to 3 times daily (chronic); parenterally: 1 to 2 ml sc acute, 3 times daily; chronic: once a day (HAB34).

LITERATURE

Baltassat F et al., (1985) Plant Med Phytother 18(4):194.

Gosmann G et al., Triterpenoid saponins from Ilex paraguariensis. In: JNP 58(3):438-441. 1995.

Fenaroli's Handbook of Flavor Ingredients, Vol. 1, 2nd Ed., CRC Press Boca Raton 1975.

Hänsel R, Keller K, Rimpler H, Schneider G (Hrsg.), Hagers Handbuch der Pharmazeutischen Praxis, 5. Aufl., Bde 4-6 (Drogen), Springer Verlag Berlin, Heidelberg, New York, 1992-1994 (unter Ilex paraguariensis).

Kraemer KH et al., A new polar saponin from Ilex paraguariensis. In: PM 61 (Abstracts of 43rd Ann Congr):62. 1995.

Roth L, Daunderer M, Kormann K, Giftpflanzen, Pflanzengifte, 4. Aufl., Ecomed Fachverlag Landsberg Lech 1993.

Teuscher E, Lindequist U, Biogene Gifte - Biologie, Chemie, Pharmakologie, 2. Aufl., Fischer Verlag Stuttgart 1994.

Teuscher E, Biogene Arzneimittel, 5. Aufl., Wiss. Verlagsges. Stuttgart 1997.

Wichtl M (Hrsg.),Teedrogen, 4. Aufl., Wiss. Verlagsges. Stuttgart 1997.

Matico

Piper elongatum

DESCRIPTION

Medicinal Parts: The medicinal part of the plant is the leaf.

Flower and Fruit: The inflorescence is a long spike of up to 20 cm, opposite the leaf. The flowers have no tepals and are very small with 4 stamens and an obovoid ovary with a very short 3-stigmaed style. The fruit is a very narrow, black, 1-seeded drupe.

Leaves, Stem and Root: Piper elongatum is a shrub that typically grows to over 2 m high. The leaves are alternate, entire, up to 20 cm long and 4 cm wide, short petiolate and coriaceous. The lamina is elongate-lanceolate, long acuminate and punctate with oil glands. The leaf base is unevenly cordate; the petiole is winged and clasps the stem. The stem is round, conspicuously jointed and pubescent toward the top.

Characteristics: The leaves have an aromatic smell when rubbed and a bitter, mildly astringent taste.

Habitat: The plant is indigenous to Argentina, Columbia and Tanzania.

Production: Piper elongatum is cultivated as a medicinal plant in the countries of origin. Matico leaves are the dried leaves of Piper elongatum. The fresh leaves are also used medicinally.

Not to be Confused With: Confusion can occur with Piper aduncum.

ACTIONS AND PHARMACOLOGY

COMPOUNDS

Volatile oil (0.3 to 6.0%): chief component dill apiol, as well as asarone, parsley apiol

Tannins

Sesquiterpene: maticin

EFFECTS

Use as a hemostyptic could possibly be a result of the tannin content.

INDICATIONS AND USAGE

Unproven Uses: The hemostyptic effect of the leaves is used externally for bleeding wounds and in the treatment of ulcers. Internally, it is used for urogenital complaints (primarily bacterial infections), atonic diarrhea and dysentery. In Peru, Matico is considered to be an aphrodisiac. It has also been used for minor wounds such as leech bites and after tooth extraction.

PRECAUTIONS AND ADVERSE REACTIONS

No health hazards are known in conjunction with the proper administration of designated therapeutic dosages.

DOSAGE

Mode of Administration: The leaves are administered as whole, cut and powdered forms for internal and external use.

Preparation: There is no information in the literature.

Daily Dosage:

Powder — 0.5 to 2 g drug, 3 to 4 times daily

Infusion — single dose: 1 g drug per cup; or 10% infusion: taken 3 or 4 times daily.

LITERATURE

Hänsel R, Keller K, Rimpler H, Schneider G (Ed), Hagers Handbuch der Pharmazeutischen Praxis, 5. Aufl., Bde 4 - 6 (Drogen), Springer Verlag Berlin, Heidelberg, New York, 1992-1994.

Matricaria Recutita

See German Chamomile

Mayapple

Podophyllum peltatum

DESCRIPTION

Medicinal Parts: The medicinal parts are the dried rhizome and the resin extracted from it.

Flower and Fruit: The solitary white flowers are located in the stem bifurcation between 2 leaves. When the flower drops, the developing fruit swells to the size and shape of a 2.5 to 5 cm long rosehip. It is yellow and fleshy.

Leaves, Stem and Root: The plant is a perennial reaching a height of 40 cm. It has a bifurcated, 45 cm high stem and deeply indented, umbrella-like, hand-sized leaves. The rhizome is reddish-brown and is 0.5 cm in diameter. Depending on the time of harvesting, the surface of the rhizome may be smooth or wrinkled. Nodes occur at intervals of 3 to 5 cm, and the fracture is whitish.

Characteristics: The odor is unpleasant and acrid.

Habitat: The plant is indigenous to northeast North America.

Production: Mayapple rhizome consists of the dried rhizome and connected roots of Podophyllum peltatum. Mayapple resin consists of the resin of the dried and aged rhizome of Podophyllum peltatum.

Not to be Confused With: Mayapple should not be confused with English Mandrake or Bryonia dioica.

Other Names: Duck's Foot, Ground Lemon, Hog Apple, Indian Apple, Mandrake, Raccoon Berry, Wild Lemon

ACTIONS AND PHARMACOLOGY

COMPOUNDS: IN THE ROOT

Podophyllin: mixture of ethanol-soluble extractive material from the root

Lignans: chief components podophyllotoxin (20%), including as well, alpha-peltatin (5%), beta-peltatin (10%), 4′-dimethyl podophyllotoxin, dioxypodophyllotoxin

EFFECTS

The drug is antimitotic.

INDICATIONS AND USAGE

Approved by Commission E:

■ Warts

Preparations of Mayapple are used externally for removal of pointed condyloma. The treated skin surface must not be larger than 25 sq. cm. Be sure to protect skin adjacent to the treated area.

CONTRAINDICATIONS

The drug is contraindicated in pregnancy.

PRECAUTIONS AND ADVERSE REACTIONS

General: The drug is severely irritating to skin and mucous membranes. External administration of the drug over large skin areas can also bring about resorptive poisonings. The drug should not be taken internally in allophathic medicine. With external use, the skin area to be treated should not exceed 25 sq. cm. The drug serves as an industrial drug for the extraction of podophyllotoxin and its semi-synthetic derivatives that are used in tumor therapy.

Use in Pregnancy: The drug is contraindicated in pregnancy.

OVERDOSAGE

In dosages over 0.2 gm, it causes severe abdominal pain, bloody-watery diarrhea, vomiting of liquid bile, dizziness, headache, coordination disorders, spasms, nephritis, later collapse and death in coma through respiratory failure.

Following gastrointestinal emptying (inducement of vomiting, gastric lavage with burgundy-colored potassium permanganate solution, sodium sulfate) and instillation of activated charcoal, the therapy for poisonings consists of treating spasms with diazepam (i.v.), electrolyte substitution and treating possible cases of acidosis with sodium bicarbonate infusions. In case of shock, plasma volume expanders should be used. Monitoring of kidney function is essential. Intubation and oxygen respiration may also be necessary.

DOSAGE

Mode of Administration: The dried rhizome is used for production of resin exclusively for external application.

Daily Dosage: The daily dosage is 1.5 to 3.0 gm root, 1.5 to 3.0 gm liquid extract or 2.5 to 7.5 gm tincture.

LITERATURE

Anonym, Dermatologie: Gemeine Warze, Flachwarze und spitze Feigwarze. In: DAZ 134(22):2059. 1994.

Auterhoff H, May O, (1958) Planta Med 6:240.

Chatterjee R, (1952) Econ Bot 6:342.

Dewick P et al., (1982) Phytochemistry 20:2277.

Enzell CR, Wahlberg I, Aaasen AI, Fortschr Chem Org Naturstoffe 34:1. 1977.

Franz G, Biogene Cytostatica. In: DAZ 130(35):2003. 1990.

Hartwell JL, Detly WE, (1950) J Am. Chem Soc 72:246.

Jardine I, In: Anticancer Agents Based on Natural Product Models, Ed. Cassady JM, Douros JD., Academic Press 1980.

MacRae WD, Towers GHN, Biological activities of lignans. In: PH 23(6):1207-1220. 1984.

Stoll A et al., (1954) J Am Chem Soc 76:5004, 6431.

Stoll A et al., (1955) J Am. Chem Soc 77:1710.

Wartburg A et al., (1957) Helv Chim. Acta 40:1331.

Further information in:

Frohne D, Pfänder HJ, Giftpflanzen - Ein Handbuch für Apotheker, Toxikologen und Biologen, 4. Aufl., Wiss. Verlags-Ges. Stuttgart 1997.

Lewin L, Gifte und Vergiftungen, 6. Aufl., Nachdruck, Haug Verlag, Heidelberg 1992.

Madaus G, Lehrbuch der Biologischen Arzneimittel, Bde. 1-3, Nachdruck, Georg Olms Verlag Hildesheim 1979.

Roth L, Daunderer M, Kormann K, Giftpflanzen, Pflanzengifte, 4. Aufl., Ecomed Fachverlag Landsberg Lech 1993.

Schulz R, Hänsel R, Rationale Phytotherapie, Springer Verlag Heidelberg 1996.

Steinegger E, Hänsel R, Pharmakognosie, 5. Aufl., Springer Verlag Heidelberg 1992.

Teuscher E, Lindequist U, Biogene Gifte - Biologie, Chemie, Pharmakologie, 2. Aufl., Fischer Verlag Stuttgart 1994.

Teuscher E, Biogene Arzneimittel, 5. Aufl., Wiss. Verlagsges. Stuttgart 1997.

Maytenus ilicifolia

See Congorosa

Meadowsweet

Filipendula ulmaria

DESCRIPTION

Medicinal Parts: The medicinal parts are the dried flowers, the dried aerial parts of the flowering plant, and the fresh underground and aerial parts of the flowering plant.

Flower and Fruit: The radial flowers are in terminal compound, loose cymes arranged with erect, very irregular branches. The 5 to 6 free sepals are triangular, pointed, 1 mm long, downy on the outside and fused to the flat receptacle at the base. The 5 to 6 petals are obviate, narrowed to a short stem, yellowish white and 2 to 5 mm long. The ovaries are glabrous or downy and have a flattened-stigma-bearing style under 1 mm. The one-seeded indehiscent fruit twine in a spiral.

Leaves, Stem and Root: The plant is perennial and grows to about 50 to 200 cm high. The stem is erect, simple or branched above, woody below, angular, usually glabrous or occasionally tomentose. The leaves are alternate, long-petioled to almost sessile, irregularly odd-pinnate with paired opposite pinna. These are ovate, rounded at the base or short-wedge-shaped, double serrate to dentate. The pinna is dark green and usually glabrous above and gray to white tomentose beneath and only pubescent on the ribs.

Characteristics: The leaves smell very different from the flowers, having a pleasant, almond-like fragrance.

Habitat: The plant is found in northern and southern Europe, North America and northern Asia.

Production: Meadowsweet flower consists of the dried flower of Filipendula ulmaria (syn. Spiraea ulmaria), as well as its preparations. Meadowsweet herb consists of the dried above-ground parts of Filipendula ulmaria, harvested during flowering season, as well as its preparations. The plant is combed off during the flowering season and air-dried in a dark place.

Not to be Confused With: May be confused with elder flowers and Filipendula hexapetala.

Other Names: Bridewort, Dolloff, Meadsweet, Meadow Queen, Meadow-Wort, Queen of the Meadow, Lady of the Meadow, Spireaea ulmaria

ACTIONS AND PHARMACOLOGY

COMPOUNDS: MEADOWSWEET FLOWER

Flavonoids: chief components - spiraeoside (quercetin-4′-O-glucosides, 3-4%), further including among others kaempferol-4′-O-glucosides, hyperoside, rutin

Volatile oil (0.2%): chief components salicylaldehyde and methyl salicylate (yielded through dehydration from monotropitin - salicylaldehyde primveroside - and spiraeine - salicylic acid ester primveroside), further, a little vanillin and heliotropine

Tannins: ellagic tannins

EFFECTS: MEADOWSWEET FLOWER

Meadowsweet has antiphlogistic and astringent effects. The drug, which contains salicylate, has an antimicrobial, antipyretic and diuretic effect. In animal tests the flavonoid fraction had a positive effect on the healing of stomach ulcers and a tone-increasing effect on smooth muscle was observed.

COMPOUNDS: MEADOWSWEET HERB

Etheric oil (traces): including salicylic acid ester

Flavonoids: including rutin, hyperoside, quercetin-3-O-glucuronide, quercetin-3-O-arabinoside

Tannins: ellagic tannins

EFFECTS: MEADOWSWEET HERB

The drug, which contains salicylate, has an antimicrobial, antipyretic and diuretic effect. In animal tests the flavonoid fraction had a positive effect on the healing of stomach ulcers and a tone-increasing effect on smooth muscle was observed.

INDICATIONS AND USAGE

Approved by Commission E:

- Cough
- Bronchitis
- Fever and cold

Meadowsweet is used as supportive therapy for colds, for febrile colds, and as a diuretic.

Unproven Uses: In folk medicine Meadowsweet is used as a diuretic, for rheumatism of the joints and muscles, for gout, for bladder and kidney disease and for headaches. Meadowsweet herb is used for stomach complaints with hyperacidity, prophylaxis and therapy of stomach ulcers and for diarrhea in children.

Homeopathic Uses: Filipendula ulmaria is used for rheumatism and inflammation of mucous membrane.

CONTRAINDICATIONS

Preparations are contraindicated when sensitivity to salicylate exists.

PRECAUTIONS AND ADVERSE REACTIONS

No health hazards or side effects are known in conjunction with the proper administration of designated therapeutic dosages.

OVERDOSAGE

Overdosage can lead to queasiness and stomach complaints.

DOSAGE

Mode of Administration: Comminuted drug and other galenic preparations for infusions. Meadowsweet flower is contained in various tea mixtures which are used for the flu, rheumatism, kidney and bladder inflammations.

Preparation: To prepare an infusion, pour boiling water over 3 to 6 gm cut drug, steam for 10 minutes and then strain. Fluid extract (herb): 1:1 in 25% ethanol (BHP83). Tincture (herb): 1:5 in 45% ethanol (BHP83)

Daily Dosage: 2.5 to 3.5 gm of Meadowsweet flower or 4 to 5 gm Meadowsweet herb. Infusion dosage is 1 cup several times a day (1 tsp. = 1.4 gm drug). Liquid extract (herb) daily dose: 1.5 to 6 ml; Tincture (herb) daily dose: 2 to 4 ml

Homeopathic Dosage: 5 drops, 1 tablet or 10 globules every 30 to 60 minutes (acute) or 1 to 3 times daily (chronic); from D6: parenterally: 1 to 2 ml sc acute: 3 times daily; chronic: once a day (HAB1)

Storage: Should be protected from light and moisture.

LITERATURE

Barnaulov OD, (1978) Rastit Resur 14(4):573.

Barnaulov OD et al., (1977) Rastit Resur 13(4):661.

Barnaulov OD, Denisenko P, (19809 Farmakol Toksicol 43(6):700.

Csedö K et al., The antibiotic activity of Filipendula ulmaria. 1988. In: PM 59(7)75. 1993.

Genig AY et al., (1977) Mater S'ezola Farm B SSR 3:162.

Gräfe AK, Besonderheiten der Arzneimitteltherapie im Säuglings- und Kindesalter. In: PZ 140(30):2659-2667. 1995.

Haslam E et al., (1985) Ann Proc Phytochemistry Soc Eur 25: 252.

Hörhammer L et al., Arch Pharm 61:133. 1956.

Kasarnovski LS, (1962) Tr Khar'kovsk Farmats Inst 2:23.

Lindeman A et al., (1982) Lebensm Wiss Technol. 15(5):286.

Thieme H, (1965) Pharmazie 20:113.

Valle MG et al., PM 54:181.

Further information in:

Hänsel R, Keller K, Rimpler H, Schneider G (Hrsg.), Hagers Handbuch der Pharmazeutischen Praxis, 5. Aufl., Bde 4-6 (Drogen): Springer Verlag Berlin, Heidelberg, New York, 1992-1994.

Madaus G, Lehrbuch der Biologischen Arzneimittel, Bde 1-3, Nachdruck, Georg Olms Verlag Hildesheim 1979.

Steinegger E, Hänsel R, Pharmakognosie, 5. Aufl., Springer Verlag Heidelberg 1992.

Wichtl M (Hrsg.), Teedrogen, 4. Aufl., Wiss. Verlagsges. Stuttgart 1997.

Medicago sativa

See Alfalfa

Melaleuca alternifolia

See Tea Tree

Melaleuca leucadendra

See Cajuput

Melaleucaea viridiflora

See Niauli

Melilotus officinalis

See Sweet Clover

Melissa officinalis

See Lemon Balm

Mentha aquatica

See Wild Mint

Mentha arvensis var. piperascens

See Japanese Mint

Mentha longifolia

See English Horsemint

Mentha piperita

See Peppermint

Mentha pulegium

See Pennyroyal

Mentha spicata

See Spearmint

Menyanthes trifoliata

See Bog Bean

Mercurialis annua

See Mercury Herb

Mercury Herb

Mercurialis annua

DESCRIPTION

Medicinal Parts: The drug is the flowering plant.

Flower and Fruit: The plant has yellow-green flowers. The male flowers are in tightly packed, interrupted ears, on thin, hair-like pedicles. They have 12 stamens. The female flowers are short-petioled in twos or threes in the leaf axils. The style is short or non-existent. There are 2 stigmas. The fruit is a 2-headed capsule.

Leaves, Stem and Root: The plant is an annual that grows 20 to 50 cm high. The stem is erect, cross-branched, obtuse, quadrangular, glabrous and segmented. The leaves are opposite, petiolate, ovate to lanceolate, light green and have a ciliate margin.

Characteristics: The plant has an unpleasant smell when rubbed. The whole plant has no latex.

Habitat: The plant grows in Europe and is naturalized in the eastern U.S.

Production: Mercury Herb is the flowering herb of Mercurialis annua.

ACTIONS AND PHARMACOLOGY

COMPOUNDS

Cyanogenic glycosides (small amounts)

Pyridone derivatives (that color the urine red): including among others hermidin

Saponins (1%)

Amines: including among others, methyl amine (mercurialine), ethyl amine, propyl amine, isobutyl amine, isoamyl amine

Flavonoids: including among others, rutin, narcissine, isorhamnetin.

Nothing is known regarding the type of the toxins. The cyanogenic glycosides are probably not responsible for the toxicity.

EFFECTS

The drug is slightly poisonous, and it can lead to diarrhea and an overactive bladder. The root and stock act as strong laxatives.

INDICATIONS AND USAGE

Unproven Uses: The drug is used for suppurating inflammation, as a laxative and diuretic, and as an adjuvant in the treatment of gastrointestinal and urinary tract diseases.

Homeopathic Uses: Mercury Herb is used for rheumatism and colds.

PRECAUTIONS AND ADVERSE REACTIONS

The fresh plant, in particular the root and the rhizome, are considered poisonous. Symptoms of poisoning include diarrhea, nerve paralysis, and liver and kidney damage. Poisonings, including fatal ones, are only known among animals. There are no reports available on the drug's toxicity in humans. The intake of small doses would likely lead to nothing more than diarrhea.

DOSAGE

Mode of Administration: The drug is administered ground, as an extract, in juice and in homeopathic dilutions.

LITERATURE

Frohne D, Pfänder HJ, Giftpflanzen - Ein Handbuch für Apotheker, Toxikologen und Biologen, 4. Aufl., Wiss. Verlags-Ges. Stuttgart 1997.

Kern W, List PH, Hörhammer L (Hrsg.), Hagers Handbuch der Pharmazeutischen Praxis, 4. Aufl., Bde. 1-8, Springer Verlag Berlin, Heidelberg, New York, 1969.

Lewin L, Gifte und Vergiftungen, 6. Aufl., Nachdruck, Haug Verlag, Heidelberg 1992.

Madaus G, Lehrbuch der Biologischen Arzneimittel, Bde 1-3, Nachdruck, Georg Olms Verlag Hildesheim 1979.

Roth L, Daunderer M, Kormann K, Giftpflanzen, Pflanzengifte, 4. Aufl., Ecomed Fachverlag Landsberg Lech 1993.

Teuscher E, Lindequist U, Biogene Gifte - Biologie, Chemie, Pharmakologie, 2. Aufl., Fischer Verlag Stuttgart 1994.

Mexican Scammony Root

Ipomoea orizabensis

DESCRIPTION

Medicinal Parts: The medicinal parts are the dried roots and the steamed ethanol extract from the roots.

Flower and Fruit: The plant has reddish-purple, campanulate flowers.

Leaves, Stem and Root: Mexican Scammony Root is a twining plant with large cordate leaves. The root tuber is about 18 to 25 cm long, 9 to 10 cm wide and cylindrical-fusiform. It is grayish-brown to brownish-black and wrinkled externally. Inside the section shows irregular concentric rings and scattered resin glands, resembling jalap.

Characteristics: The taste is acrid and resinous. The odor is slight.

Habitat: Mexico

Production: Mexican Scammony Root is the root extracted from Ipomoea orizabensis. Both the root and the yielded resin are effective as drugs.

Other Names: Ipomoea, Jalap, Mexican Jalap

ACTIONS AND PHARMACOLOGY

COMPOUNDS

Glycoretines (12-15%, resinous): polymeric ester glycosides made up of hydroxy- and dihydroxy fatty acids bonded in ester-like fashion (including 11-hydroxy palmitic acid = jalapinolic acid), on the hydroxyl groups of which oligosaccharide remnants are bonded as glycosides. These bear in turn short-chained acyl remnants (acetyl, isobutyryl, isovaleryl, and tigoyl remnants).

EFFECTS

The drug has a strong laxative effect on the small and large intestines caused by resin (Resina Scammoniae) combined with ester glycoside mixtures (glycoretine).

INDICATIONS AND USAGE

Unproven Uses: Preparations have been used as a very drastic purgative for constipation.

CONTRAINDICATIONS

The drug is contraindicated in pregnancy.

PRECAUTIONS AND ADVERSE REACTIONS

General: No health hazards are known in conjunction with the proper administration of designated therapeutic dosages. Intestinal colic occurs frequently as a side effect.

Pregnancy: Mexican Scammony Root is contraindicated in pregnancy.

OVERDOSAGE

Overdosages cause vomiting.

DOSAGE

Mode of Administration: The herb is obsolete as a drug in many countries. Used on rare occasions in combination preparations. The same applies to other Ipomoea varieties e.g., I. turpethum, I. operculata.

Daily Dosage: The average single dose is 1 gm of drug.

LITERATURE

Hänsel R, Keller K, Rimpler H, Schneider G (Hrsg.), Hagers Handbuch der Pharmazeutischen Praxis, 5. Aufl., Bde 4-6 (Drogen): Springer Verlag Berlin, Heidelberg, New York, 1992-1994.

Lewin L, Gifte und Vergiftungen, 6. Aufl., Nachdruck, Haug Verlag, Heidelberg 1992.

Madaus G, Lehrbuch der Biologischen Arzneimittel, Bde 1-3, Nachdruck, Georg Olms Verlag Hildesheim 1979.

Noda N et al., Tetrahedron 43:3889. 1987.

Roth L, Daunderer M, Kormann K, Giftpflanzen, Pflanzengifte, 4. Aufl., Ecomed Fachverlag Landsberg Lech 1993.

Shellard EJ, PM 9:146-152. 1961.

Singh S, Stacey BE, (1973) Phytochemistry 12:1701.

Steinegger E, Hänsel R, Pharmakognosie, 5. Aufl., Springer Verlag Heidelberg 1992.

Wagner H, (1973) In "Chemistry in Biochemical Classification", Nobel Symposium (1973).

Mezereon

Daphne mezereum

DESCRIPTION

Medicinal Parts: The medicinal part is the bark, which is collected before the flowering season.

Flower and Fruit: The flowers are dark pink. They appear before the leaves in irregular, sessile clusters usually in threes. There is a 4-tipped calyx with an external silky-haired tube. There are 8 stamens in 2 rows and 1 free ovary. The fruit consists of a bright red, pea-sized, juicy, ovoid, 1-seeded berry.

Leaves, Stem and Root: The plant is a 50 to 150 cm high perennial. It is a deciduous, sparsely branched shrub with reed-like, grayish or yellow-brown branches that are very tough. The leaves are short-petioled, lanceolate, narrowing toward the petiole and entire-margined.

Characteristics: Mezereon has a strong, pleasant fragrance. The plant is poisonous and can be fatal if ingested. It is a protected species.

Habitat: The plant is indigenous to Europe as far as Siberia. It is cultivated in the U.S., Canada and elsewhere.

Production: Mezereon root, root bark and bark are from Daphne mezereum. The bark of the trunk and the root are gathered before flowering, dried and rolled up but with the phloem facing outward. Care should be taken not to destroy the plant during the harvest.

Other Names: Spurge Olive, Spurge Laurel, Daphne, Spurge Flax, Wild Pepper, Dwarf Bay, Camolea

ACTIONS AND PHARMACOLOGY

COMPOUNDS

Diterpenes: diterpene esters, daphnane derivatives, including mezerein, daphnetoxin

Hydroxycoumarins: including umbelliferone, daphnetin, daphnoretin (dimerous), triumbellin (trimerous) and hydroxycoumarin glycosides, for example daphnin, daphnorin

Flavonoids

EFFECTS

The drug acts as a powerful skin stimulant, hallucinogenic and a rubifacient. A possible immunostimulating effect has been observed in vitro. Antitumoral, anticoagulant and abortifacient effects have been observed in animal tests.

INDICATIONS AND USAGE

Unproven Uses: Use of Mezeron is no longer recommended due to its toxicity.

In the past, Mezeron root was used to relieve headache, toothache, gout, whooping cough, syphilis, constipation and worm infestation. It was used externally for joint pains and to increase circulation in the case of rheumatic complaints, skin conditions and conjunctivitis. The drug is known in old drug manuals as 'Spanish fly plaster' or Drouotic plaster and recommended for various pain symptoms.

Homeopathic Uses: In homeopathic medicine, Daphne mezereon is used for skin conditions such as cradle cap, shingles, weeping eczema and encrusted, weeping blisters, as well as for neuralgia and pains in the bones.

PRECAUTIONS AND ADVERSE REACTIONS

External contact with the severely irritating toxic diterpenes of Daphne mezereon causes erysipeloid reddening of the skin, swelling, blister formation and shedding of the epidermis. Extended exposure leads to the formation of necroses. Contact with the eyes causes severe conjunctivitis. If taken internally, reddening and swelling of the oral mucous membranes, feeling of thirst, salivation, stomach pains, vomiting and severe diarrhea occur.

Resorption of the drug may cause headache, dizziness, stupor, tachycardia, spasms and possibly death through circulatory collapse. Cool wrappings and anesthetic salves are recommended for treatment of the skin injuries.

OVERDOSAGE

Poisoning resulting from ingestion of the drug should be treated with gastric lavage and calcium gluconate, IV. Administration of corticosteroids may also be indicated.

DOSAGE

Mode of Administration: The drug is seldom used today. Used in homeopathic dilutions, topically and internally.

Homeopathic Dosage: 5 drops, 1 tablet or 10 globules every 30 to 60 minutes (acute) or 1 to 3 times daily (chronic); parenterally: 1 to 2 ml sc acute, 3 times daily; chronic: once a day (HAB1).

Storage: The effect fades if it is stored for too long. Therefore, do not store for a period of more than 2 years.

LITERATURE

Evans B, In: Evans FJ:Naturally Occuring Phorbolesters, CRC Press Inc., Boca Raton, Florida. 1986.

Kupchan SM, Baxter RL, (1974) Science 187:652.

Nyborg J, La Cour, T, (1975) Nature 257:824.

Ronlan A, Wickberg B, Tetrahedron Lett 4261. 1970.

Schildknecht H et al., (1970) Chem Ztg 94:347.

Schindler H, PM 10:232. 1962.

Stout GH et al., (1970) J Am Chem Soc 92:1070.

Further information in:

Frohne D, Pfänder HJ, Giftpflanzen - Ein Handbuch für Apotheker, Toxikologen und Biologen, 4. Aufl., Wiss. Verlagsges. mbH Stuttgart 1997.

Kern W, List PH, Hörhammer L (Hrsg.), Hagers Handbuch der Pharmazeutischen Praxis, 4. Aufl., Bde 1-8, Springer Verlag Berlin, Heidelberg, New York, 1969.

Lewin L, Gifte und Vergiftungen, 6. Aufl., Nachdruck, Haug Verlag, Heidelberg 1992.

Madaus G, Lehrbuch der Biologischen Arzneimittel, Bde 1-3, Nachdruck, Georg Olms Verlag Hildesheim 1979.

Roth L, Daunderer M, Kormann K: Giftpflanzen, Pflanzengifte, 4. Aufl., Ecomed Fachverlag Landsberg Lech 1993.

Teuscher E, Lindequist U, Biogene Gifte - Biologie, Chemie, Pharmakologie, 2. Aufl., Fischer Verlag Stuttgart 1994.

Wagner H, Wiesenauer M, Phytotherapie. Phytopharmaka und pflanzliche Homöopathika, Fischer-Verlag, Stuttgart, Jena, New York 1995.

Milk Thistle

Silybum marianum

TRADE NAMES

Milk Thistle (available from numerous manafacturers), Silymarin, Milk Thistle Extract, Milk Thistle Super Complex, Milk Thistle Phytosome, Alcohol Free Milk Thistle Seed, Milk Thistle Extract, Milk Thistle Plus, Silymarin Milk Thistle, Milk Thistle Power, Time Release Milk Thistle Power, Thisilyn Standardized Milk Thistle Extract

DESCRIPTION

Medicinal Parts: The medicinal parts of the plant are the ripe seeds.

Flower and Fruit: The inflorescences are large, solitary and purple. They consist of somewhat nodding, composite flower heads. The perigone is globular. The inner tepals taper to a slender point, and the outer tepals are tough at the base, then spread and terminate at a horny tip. There are only tubular florets. The fruit is brown, spotted and glossy, with a white tuft of hair.

Leaves, Stem and Root: The plant grows from 70 to 150 cm high with an erect stem. The leaves are arranged in different levels with the lower leaves indented-pinnatisect, and the upper ones lanceolate and clasping. There are white spots along the ribs of the leaf and yellow thorns at the margin.

Habitat: The plant is indigenous to Europe.

Other Names: Marian Thistle, Mediterranean Milk Thistle, Mary Thistle

ACTIONS AND PHARMACOLOGY

COMPOUNDS: MILK THISTLE HERB

Flavonoids: in particular, apigenin-, luteolin- and kaempferol-7-0-glycosides, apigenin-4,7′-di-0-glucoside, kaempferol-7-0-glucoside-3-sulfate

Steroids: sterols, including beta-sitosterol, beta-sitosterol glucoside

Polyynes

Organic Acids: fumaric acid (3.3%)

(Silymarin is absent; it is localized only in the seed case)

EFFECTS: MILK THISTLE HERB

The cholagogue effect of the drug has not been documented.

COMPOUNDS: MILK THISTLE SEED

Silymarin (flavonolignan mixture, 1.5-3%): chief components silybin A, silybin B (mixture known as silibinin), isosilybin A, isosilybin B, silychristin, silydianin

Flavonoids: apigenin, chrysoeriol, eriodictyol, naringenin, quercetin, taxifolin

Fatty oil (20-30%)

EFFECTS: MILK THISTLE SEED

Hepatoprotective Effects

The hepatoprotective activity of the seed is from silymarin, in particular, silychristin and silydianin. The compounds seem to inhibit the entrance of toxins and block toxin-binding sites through alteration of the liver cell's outer membrane. (Hikino, 1994; Leng-Peschlow, 1996). The hepatoprotective effect of silibinin also involves different functions of the Kupffer cells. Silibinin decreases production of superoxide anion radicals and nitric oxide (free-radical scavenger or antioxidant) by the Kupffer cells. Silibinin also inhibits leukotriene formation by the Kupffer cells (Dehmlow, 1996). Silymarin increases glutathione production by the liver, intestines and stomach. Glutathione is used for detoxification cells in the liver (Valenzuela, 1989). Silibinin decreases hepatic and mitochondrial glutathione oxidation induced by iron overload and is a mild chelator of iron (Pietrangelo, 1995).

Protective Effects

The seed exerts an anti-inflammatory effect through inhibition of leukotriene production by silymarin (Leng-Peschlow, 1996). A renoprotective effect of the herb on kidney cells damaged by acetaminophen, cisplatin and vincristin was demonstrated in a recent study. Silibinin and silychristin demonstrated remarkable stimulatory effects on proliferation rate, biosynthesis of protein and DNA, and activity of the enzyme lactate dehydrogenase in kidney cells (Sonnenbichler, 1999). Silibinin reduces intracellular and secreted forms of prostate-specific antigen (PSA) levels and inhibits cell growth via a G1 arrest in cell cycle progression in hormone-refractory prostate carcinomas. Silibinin-induced G1 arrest decreases the kinase activity of cyclin-dependent kinases (CDKs) and associated cyclins for an anticarcinogenic effect (Zi, 1999; Zi, 1998)

Liver Regenerative Effects

Silymarin stimulates RNA polymerase I in the cell nucleus of the hepatocytes, resulting in an increase of ribosomal protein synthesis and the regenerative ability of the liver. This mechanism is of particular importance in the antidote effect against death-cap mushroom poisoning since the poison which it contains, alpha-Amanitin, inhibits this enzyme in the cell nucleus. The drug also has a cholagogic effect.

CLINICAL TRIALS

Hepatoprotection

A double-blind, randomized, placebo-controlled trial was conducted to determine the hepatoprotective effect of silymarin in 170 cirrhosis patients. The patients were given either 140 mg silymarin three times daily or a placebo. After treatment for two years, biochemical markers did not change significantly. After a four-year analysis, treatment was seen most effective in patients with alcoholic cirrhosis and Child's A group classification of portal hypertension. The drug was ineffective in patients with Child's B and C group hypertension (Ferenci, 1989).

The effect of silymarin in 200 alcoholic patients with cirrhosis of the liver was demonstrated in a controlled, double-blind, randomized and multicenter trial. The study was comparing 450 mg of silymarin (150 mg/ three times per day) with placebo. Patient survival was similar in the silymarin and placebo treatment group after 2 years of therapy. No relevant side effects were observed in either group, and the results indicated that silymarin has no effect on survival and the clinical course in alcoholics with liver cirrhosis (Pares, 1998).

Silymarin 420 mg per day was compared to placebo in a double-blind, controlled study to determine the effect on chemical, functional and morphological alterations of the liver. The study involved 106 patients with relatively slight and subacute liver disease induced by alcohol abuse. The patients were selected on the basis of elevated serum transaminase levels. After 4 weeks, there was a highly significant decrease of S-SGPT and S-SGOT in the silymarin treatment group. There was also a decrease in the serum total and conjugated bilirubin with the silymarin treatment group, although the decrease was not significant. Histological changes normalized significantly more in the silymarin treatment group (Salmi, 1982).

INDICATIONS AND USAGE

MILK THISTLE HERB

Unproven Uses: Preparations of Milk Thistle herb are used as a stimulant, for functional disorders of liver and gallbladder including jaundice, gallbladder colic and diseases of the spleen. The herb was formerly used as a malaria treatment, emmenagogue and for uterine complaints.

MILK THISTLE SEED

Approved by Commission E:

- Dyspeptic complaints
- Liver and gallbladder complaints

The drug is used for toxic liver damage, adjunctive treatment in chronic inflammatory liver disease and hepatic cirrhosis.

Unproven Uses: The drug is also used as an antidote to death-cap mushroom poisoning.

PRECAUTIONS AND ADVERSE REACTIONS

MILK THISTLE HERB AND SEED

No health hazards or side effects are known in conjunction with the proper administration of designated therapeutic dosages. Episodes of severe sweating, abdominal cramping, nausea, vomiting, diarrhea and weakness were recently reported in Australia, but the reaction was found to be due to a substance in the Milk Thistle product other than silybin (Adverse Drug Reaction Advisory Committee, 1999).

Drug Interactions: The concomitant use of silymarin and butyrophenones or phenothiazines results in a reduction of lipid peroxidation (Palasciano, 1994). Silymarin has an atagonistic effect with yohimbine and phentolamine when given simutaneously (Di Carlo, 1993).

DOSAGE

MILK THISTLE HERB

Preparation: An infusion is prepared by pouring boiling water over 1/2 teaspoonful of the drug and then straining after 5 to 10 minutes.

Daily Dosage: The average dose of the infusion is 2 to 3 cups daily.

MILK THISTLE SEED

Mode of Administration: Comminuted drug for infusions and extracts; tinctures for liquids and solid forms.

How Supplied:

Capsules—70 mg, 100 mg, 140 mg, 150 mg, 175 mg, 180 mg, 500 mg, 540 mg, 1000 mg, 1050 mg

Liquid—1:1, 1:2

Tablet—50 mg, 500 mg

Preparation: To prepare an infusion, add 3 gm of the drug to cold water and bring to a boil. Drain after 10 to 20 minutes.

Daily Dosage: For liver dysfunction or ailments, the daily dosage has been effective and well tolerated at 140 to 420 mg divided in 2 to 3 doses (Ferenci, 1989; Frerick, 1990; Pares, 1998; Schuppan, 1998). The average dose of silymarin was approximately 33 milligrams/kilogram/day for cyclopeptide mushroom poisoning. Silymarin administered up to 48 hours after mushroom ingestion appears to be effective in preventing severe liver damage in Amanita phalloides poisoning (Hruby, 1983).

Although products are usually standardized to 70% to 80% (not milligrams) of silymarin, the silymarin concentrations may vary without government regulation (Flora et al, 1998).

Storage: Store away from direct light, heat and moisture; keep at room temperature.

LITERATURE

MILK THISTLE HERB

Ahmed AA et al., PH 28:1751. 1989.

DAZ 25:1427. 1990.

Khafagy SM et al., Sci Pharm 49:157. 1981.

Kern W, List PH, Hörhammer L (Hrsg.), Hagers Handbuch der Pharmazeutischen Praxis, 4. Aufl., Bde. 1-8, Springer Verlag Berlin, Heidelberg, New York, 1969.

Madaus G, Lehrbuch der Biologischen Arzneimittel, Bde 1-3, Nachdruck, Georg Olms Verlag Hildesheim 1979.

Mericli AH, PM 54:44. 1988.

Wichtl M (Hrsg.), Teedrogen, 4. Aufl., Wiss. Verlagsges. Stuttgart 1997.

MILK THISTLE SEED

Baumann J, (1975) Über die Wirkung von Chelidonium, Curcuma, Absinth und Carduus marianus auf die Gálle- und Pankreassekretion bei Hepatopathien. Med Mschr 29:173.

Benda I, Zenz W, (1973) Wien Med Wschr 123:512.

Desplaces A et al., (1975) Arzneim Forsch 25, 89.

Dehmlow C, Erhard J, de Groot H, Inhibition of Kupffer cell functions as an explanation for the hepatoprotective properties of silibinin. Hepatology 1996 Apr;23(4):749-54.

Devault RL, Rosenbrook W, (1973) J Antibiotic 26:532.

Hruby K et al., (1983) Hum Toxicol 2(2):183.

Neu R, (1960) Arch Pharm 293:269.

Pelter A, Hänsel R, (1968) Tetrahedron Letters 19:2911.

Poser G, (1971) Arzneim Forsch 21:1209.

Qiu SJ et al., (1981) Chin J Cardiol 9:61.

Tuchweber B et al., (1973) J Med 4:327.

Vogel G et al., (1984) Toxicol Appl Pharmacol 51:265.

Wagner H et al., (1971) Tetrahedron Letters 22:1985.

An adverse reaction to the herbal medication milk thistle (Silybum marianum). Adverse Drug Reactions Advisory Committee. Med J Aust 1999 Mar 1;170(5):218-9.

Arnone A, Merlini L, Zanarotti A, (1979) Constituents of Silybum marianum. Structure of isosilybin and stereochemistry of isosilybin. J Chem Soc (Chem Commun):696-697.

Benda L, Dittrich H, Ferenzi P, Frank H, Wewalka F, (1980) The influence of therapy with silymarin on the survial rate of patients with liver cirrhosis. Wien Klin Wschr 92(19):678-683.

Bode JCh, (1986) Arzneimittel für die Indikation "Lebererkrankungen". In: Dölle W, Müller-Oerlingshausen B, Schwabe U (Hrsg.), Grundlagen der Arzneimitteltherapie. Entwicklung, Beurteilung und Anwendung von Arzneimitteln. B.I.- Wissenschaftsverlag, Mannheim Wien Zürich, S 202-211.

Bode JCh, (1981) Die alkoholische Hepatitis, ein Krankheitsspektrum. Internist 220:536-545.

Di Carlo G, Autore G, Izzo AA et al., Inhibition of intestinal motility and secretion by flavonoids in mice and rats: structure-activity relationships. J Pharm Pharmacol 1993; 45:1054-1059.

Dölle W, Schwabe U, (1988) Leber- und Gallenwegstherapeutika. In: Schwabe U, Paffrath D (Hrsg.), Arzneiverordnungsreport 88, Gustav Fischer, Stuttgart New York, S 242-253.

Feher J, Deak G, Muezes G, Lang I, Niederland V, Nekam K, Karteszi M, (1989) Hepatoprotective activity of silymarin legalon therapy in patients with chronic alcoholic liver disease. Orv Hetil 130(51):2723-2727.

Frerick H, Kuhn U, Strenge-Hesse A et al. Silymarin - ein Phytopharmakon zur Behandlung von toxischen Leberschäden.Der Kassenarzt 1990;33/34:36-41.

Ferenci P, Dragosics B, Dittrich H, Frank H, Benda L, Lochs H, Meryn S, Base W, Schneider B, (1989) Randomized controlled trial of silymarin treatment in patients with cirrhosis of the liver. J Hepatol 9(1):105-113.

Fintelmann V, Albert A, (1980) Nachweis der therapeutischen Wirksamkeit von Legalon bei toxischen Lebererkrankungen im Doppelblindversuch. Therapiewoche 30(35):5589-5594.

Flora K, Hahn M, Rosen H et al., Milk Thistle (Silybum marianum) for the therapy of liver disease. Am JGastroenterol 1998; 93:139-143.

Hahn G, Lehmann HD, Kürten M et al., (1968) Zur Pharmakologie und Toxikologie von Silymarin, des antihepatotocischen Wirkprinzips aus Silybum marianum (L.) Gaertn. Arzneim Forsch/Drug Res 18:698-704.

Hruby K, Fuhrmann M, Csomos G, Thaler H, (1983) Pharmakotherapie der Knollenblätterpilzvergiftung mit Silibinin. Wien Klein Wschr 95(7):225-231.

Hruby K, Csomos G, Fuhrmann M, Thaler H, Chemotherapy of Amanita phalloides poisoning with intravenous silibinin. Hum Toxicol 1983 Apr;2(2):183-95.

Kalmar L, Kadar J, Somogyi A et al., Silibinin (Legalon-70) enhances the motility of human neutrophils immobilized by formyl-tripeptide, calcium ionophore, lymphokine and by normal human serum. Agents Actions 1990; 29:239-246.

Koch H, (1980) Leberschutz-Therapeutika. Pharmazie in unserer Zeit 9:33-44:65-74.

Leng-Peschlow E, Properties and medical use of flavonolignans (silymarin) from Silybum marianum. Phytother Res1996; 10(suppl): S25-S26.

Leng-Peschlow E, Strenge-Hesse A, (1991) Die Mariendistel (Silybum marianum) und Silymarin als Lebertherapeutikum. Z Phytother 12:162-174.

Lorenz D, Mennicke WH, Behrendt W, (1992) Untersuchungen zur Elimination von Silymarin bei cholecystektomierten Patienten. Planta Med 45:216-233.

Martines G, Copponi V, Cagnetta G, (1980) Aspetti del danno epatico dopo somministrazione sperimentale di alcuni farmaci. Arch Sci Med 137:367-386.

Martini GA, (1988) Hepatozelluläre Erkrankungen, Leberkrankheiten. In: Riecker G (Hrsg.), Therapie innerer Krankheiten, Springer, Berlin Heidelberg New York, S 638-652.

Marugg D, Reutter FW, (1985) Die Amanita-phalloides-Intoxikation. Moderne therapeutische Maβnahmen und klinischer Verlauf. Schweiz Rundschau Med (Praxis) 14(37):972-982.

Mennicke WH, (1975) Zur biologischen Verfügbarkeit und Verstoffwechselung von Silybin. Dtsch Apoth Ztg 115(33):1205-1206.

Palasciano G, Portinacasa P, Palmieri V et al., The effect of silymarin on plasma levels of malondialdehyde in patients receiving long-term treatment with psychotropic drugs. Curr Ther Res 1994; 55:537-545.

Pares A, Planas R, Torres M et al., Effects of silymarin in alcoholic patients with cirrhosis of the liver: results of a controlled, double-blind, randomized and multicenter trial. J Hepatol 1998 Apr;28(4):615-21.

Peeters H (Ed.), (1976) Phosphatidylcholine. Biochemical and Clinical Aspects of Essential Phospholipids. Springer Verlag, Berlin Heidelberg New York.

Rauen HM, Schriewer H, (1971) Die antihepatotoxische Wirkung von Silymarin bei experimentellen Leberschäden der Ratte durch Tetrachlorkohlenstoff, D-Galaktosamin und Allylalkohol. Arzneim Forsch/Drug Res 21:1194-1201.

Reuter HD, (1992) Spektrum Mariendistel und andere leber- und gallewirksame Phytopharmaka. In: Bundesverband Dtschr Ärzte für Naturheilverfahren (Hrsg.) Arzneimitteltherapie heute. Aesopus Verlag, Basel.

Salmi HA, Sarna S, (1982) Effect of silymarin on chemical, functional and morphological alterations of the liver. A double-blind controlled study. Scand J Gastroenterol 17(4):517-521.

Schulz HU, Schürer M, Krumbiegel G, Wächter W, Weyhenmeyer R, Seidel G, (1995) Untersuchungen zum Freisetzungsverhalten und zur Bioäquivalenz von Silymarin-Präparaten. Arzneim Forsch/Drug Res 45:61-64.

Schuppan D, Strösser W, Burkard G, Walosek G et al., Verminderung der Fibrosierungsaktivität durch Legalon bei chronischen Lebererkrankungen

Z Allgemeinmed 1998;11/12:577-584.

Sonnebichler J, Zetl I, (1984) Untersuchungen zum Wirkungsmechanismus von Silibinin, Einfluβ von Silibinin auf die Synthese ribosomaler RNA, mRNA und tRNA in Rattenlebern in vivo. Hoppe-Seyler's Physiol Chem 365:555-556.

Sonnenbichler J, Zetl I, (1986) Biochemical effects of the flavonolignane silibinin in RNA, protein and DANN synthesis of rat livers. Prog Clin Biol Res 213:319-331.

Sonnenbichler J, Zetl I, (1987) Stimulating influence of a flavonolignane on proliferation, RNA synthesis and protein Synthesis in liver cells. In, Okoliczányi L, Csomós G, Crepaldi G (Eds.), Assessment and management of hepatobiliary disease. Springer, Berlin Heidelberg New York, S 265-272.

Sonnenbichler J, Zetl I, (1988) Specific binding of a flavonolignane to an estradiol receptor. In: Plant flavonoids in Biology and Medicine II, Biochemical, cellular, and medicinal properties. Alan R Liss, New York, S 369-374.

Sonnenbichler J, Scalera F, Sonnenbichler I et al., Stimulatory effects of silibinin and silicristin from the Milk Thistle Silybum marianum on kidney cells. J Pharmacol Exp Ther 1999 Sep;290(3):1375-83.

Varis K, Salmi HA, Siurala M, (1978) Die Therapie der Lebererkrankung mit Legalon; eine kontrollierte Doppelblindstudie. In: Aktuelle Hepatologie, III. Internationales Symposium Köln 15.-17. November 1978. Hanseatisches Verlagskontor. Lübeck, S 42-43.

Valenzuela A, Aspillaga M, Vial S, Guerra, Selectivity of silymarin on the increase of the glutathione content in different tissues of the rat. Planta Med 1989 Oct;55(5):420-2.

Vogel G, (1980) The anti-amanita effect of silymarin. In: Faulstich et al., (Eds.), Amanita toxins and poisoning. Witzstrock, Baden-Baden Köln New York, S 180-187.

Wagner H, Seligmann O, Seilz M, Abraham D, Sonnenbichler J, (1976) Silydianin und Silychristin, zwei isomere Silymarine aus Silybum marianum L. Gaertn. (Mariendistel). Z Naturforsch 31b:876-884.

Zi X, Agarwal R, Silibinin decreases prostate-specific antigen with cell growth inhibition via G1 arrest, leading to differentiation of prostate carcinoma cells: implications for prostate cancer intervention. Proc Natl Acad Sci U S A 1999 Jun 22;96(13):7490-5.

Zi X, Feyes DK, Agarwal R, Anticarcinogenic effect of a flavonoid antioxidant, silymarin, in human breast cancer cells MDA-MB 468: induction of G1 arrest through an increase in Cip1/p21 concomitant with a decrease in kinase activity of cyclin-dependent kinases and associated cyclins. Clin Cancer Res 1998 Apr;4(4):1055-64.

Further information in:

Kern W, List PH, Hörhammer L (Hrsg.), Hagers Handbuch der Pharmazeutischen Praxis, 4. Aufl., Bde 1-8, Springer Verlag Berlin, Heidelberg, New York, 1969.

Madaus G, Lehrbuch der Biologischen Arzneimittel, Bde 1-3, Nachdruck, Georg Olms Verlag Hildesheim 1979.

Roth L, Daunderer M, Kormann K, Giftpflanzen, Pflanzengifte, 4. Aufl., Ecomed Fachverlag Landsberg Lech 1993.

Schulz R, Hänsel R, Rationale Phytotherapie, Springer Verlag Heidelberg 1996.

Steinegger E, Hänsel R, Pharmakognosie, 5. Aufl., Springer Verlag Heidelberg 1992.

Teuscher E, Biogene Arzneimittel, 5. Aufl., Wiss. Verlagsges. mbH Stuttgart 1997.

Wagner H, Wiesenauer M, Phytotherapie. Phytopharmaka und pflanzliche Homöopathika, Fischer-Verlag, Stuttgart, Jena, New York 1995.

Wichtl M (Hrsg.), Teedrogen, 4. Aufl., Wiss. Verlagsges. Stuttgart 1997.

Monarda didyma

See Oswego Tea

Monarda Punctata

See Horsemint

Moneywort

Lysimachia nummularia

DESCRIPTION

Medicinal Parts: The medicinal parts are the fresh or dried whole flowering plant.

Fruit and Flower: The flowers are solitary or in pairs. The leaf axils have 5 free, almost cordate sepals. The corolla is rotate, divided into 5 and fused at the base. It is rich yellow and spotted with dark red glands on the inside. There are 5 glandular-haired stamens fused at the base and 1 ovary. The fruit is a 4- to 5-mm long globular capsule. The seeds are triangular, blackish-brown, warty and 1.5 mm long.

Leaves, Stem and Root: The plant is a perennial. The stem is a runner-like creeper, lightly branched, quadrangular, glabrous to slightly pubescent with roots at the nodes. It grows from 10 to 45 cm. The leaves are entire-margined, crossed-opposite, short-petioled, red-glandular punctate and orbicular elliptical.

Habitat: The plant is indigenous to all of Europe and the Caucasus and has been introduced into America and Japan.

Production: Moneywort is the complete plant of Lysimachia nummularia. The whole flowering plant, including the root, is collected, cleaned and dried in the shade.

Other Names: Creeping Jenny, Creeping Joan, Herb Two-pence, Meadow Runagates, Running Jenny, Serpentaria, String of Sovereigns, Twopenny Grass, Wandering Jenny, Wandering Tailor

ACTIONS AND PHARMACOLOGY

COMPOUNDS

Flavonoids: including among others glycosides of myricetins, kempferols and quercetins, including rutin, hyperosides

Tannins

Triterpene saponins

The constituents of the drug have not been fully investigated.

EFFECTS

Moneywort is mildly astringent and expectorant. Extracts of the aerial plant parts are said to be antibacterial in vitro; however, scientific results are not available.

INDICATIONS AND USAGE

Unproven Uses: Moneywort is used externally as a vulnerary and for acute and chronic eczema. It is used internally for diarrhea and excessive salivation, and as an expectorant for coughs.

PRECAUTIONS AND ADVERSE REACTIONS

No health hazards or side effects are known in conjunction with the proper administration of designated therapeutic dosages.

DOSAGE

Preparation: To make a tea, pour 250 ml boiling water over 2 heaping teaspoonfuls drug and leave to draw for 5 minutes. For a wound poultice, dilute the tea preparation with the same amount of chamomile tea.

Daily Dosage: For the treatment of coughs, drink 1 cup of tea, 2 to 3 times daily with honey if desired.

LITERATURE

Hänsel R, Keller K, Rimpler H, Schneider G (Hrsg.), Hagers Handbuch der Pharmazeutischen Praxis, 5. Aufl., Bde 4-6 (Drogen), Springer Verlag Berlin, Heidelberg, New York, 1992-1994.

Madaus G, Lehrbuch der Biologischen Arzneimittel, Bde 1-3, Nachdruck, Georg Olms Verlag Hildesheim 1979.

Prum N et al., PA 38:494. 1083.

Monkshood

Aconitum napellus

DESCRIPTION

Medicinal Parts: Deadly poison.

Flower and Fruit: The flowers are 50 to 160 cm long and form violet, bluish or reddish upright racemes. The calyx has 5 petal-like sepals. The upper sepal is convex and helmet-shaped. There are 2 petals with nectar-releasing spurs under the upper sepal. There are numerous glabrous or ciliate stamens. There are 3 glabrous ovaries with 10 to 14 ovules. The fruit is a 16 to 20 mm long by 5 mm thick follicle. The seeds are glossy black and triangular with narrow wings on the edges.

Leaves, Stem and Root: Aconitum napellus is a 0.5 to 1.5 m high shrub with a tuberous, thickened, fleshy root and an erect, rigid, undivided stem. The racem axis and petioles are glabrous or hairy. The leaves are dark green, glossy above and lighter beneath. They are palmate and 5 to 7-pinnatasect. The sections of the leaf are rhomboid in outline and deeply indented with oblong tips.

Characteristics: The plant is extremely poisonous.

Habitat: Aconitum napellus is common to the Alps and the Carpathians and is to be found in all the mountainous regions of Europe. The plant is found as far as Sweden in the north, as far as England and Portugal in the west, as far as the Pyrenees in the south and as far as the Carpathians in the east.

Production: Monkshood tuber consists of the fresh or dried tubers and roots of Aconitum napellus harvested in autumn after flowering. Monkshood herb consists of the dried herb of Aconitum napellus collected at the beginning of the flowering season. The collected roots are quickly dried at 40° C.

Not to be Confused With: Other blue-flowering Aconitum species.

Other names: Aconite, Wolfsbane, Blue Rocket, Friar's Cap, Mousebane

ACTIONS AND PHARMACOLOGY

COMPOUNDS

Nor-diterpene alkaloids: including aconitine, mesaconitine, hypaconitine, N-desethyl aconitine, oxoaconitine

EFFECTS

The efficacy of the drug is based on the di-ester alkaloids aconitin, mesaconitin and hypaconitin. Aconitin raises membrane permeability for sodium ions and retards repolarization. Aconitin is initially stimulating, and then causes paralysis in the motor and sensitive nerve ends, and in the

CNS. The other di-ester alkaloids function in a similar fashion. Hypaconitin works more intensely. Aconitin applied in small doses triggers bradycardia and hypotension; in higher doses it has at first, a positive inotropic effect, followed by tachycardia, cardiac arrhythmia and cardiac arrest. Di-ester alkaloids were shown to be analgesic in animal experiments. Applied topically in humans, the drug is initially stimulating, in the form of itchiness or burning, and then anesthetizing. The drug has an anti-febrile effect. Therapeutic doses influence the heart minimally; the heart rate may increase slightly. Given orally, the drug is active after a few minutes.

INDICATIONS AND USAGE

Unproven Uses: The drug is used to reduce pain from neuralgia, particularly with trigeminus and intercostal neuralgia. It is also used for myalgia, muscular and articular rheumatism, serous skin inflammation and migraine. Preparations of blue monkshood are used for pain, facial paralyses, ailments of the joints, arthritis, gout, rheumatic complaints, inflammation, pleurisy, pericarditis sicca, fever, and skin and mucosal diseases, as well as for disinfecting and wound treatment. In experimental pharmacology, Aconitin is used due to its ability to trigger cardiac arrhythmia.

Chinese Medicine: Monkshood is used for analgesia, as an anti-inflammatory and a cardiac tonic.

Homeopathic Uses: Aconitum napellus is used for acute inflammatory illnesses, cardiac palpitations with anxiety states and painful peripheral nerve disease.

PRECAUTIONS AND ADVERSE REACTIONS

The drug is highly toxic. Signs of poisoning can appear even with the administration of therapeutic dosages. The first sign of poisoning is a tingling of the mouth, fingers and toes, which then spreads over the entire body surface and changes into a furry sensation. Body temperature decreases quickly and queasiness, vomiting, diarrhea and urination follow.

OVERDOSAGE

With fatal doses, breathing becomes irregular and the heartbeat slows down and becomes arrythmic. Intense pains are characteristic. Death usually follows within 6 hours due to heart failure or asphyxiation. For adults, the estimated fatal dosage lies between 1 to 2 g. Countermeasures include gastrointestinal emptying, keeping the patient warm, cardiovascular and pulmonary support, magnesium and calcium infusions, administration of atropine to fight bradycardia, lidocaine for relieving the arrythmias, possibly artificial respiration, pain relief (no opiates).

DOSAGE

Mode of Administration:

The use of the drug is risky and not recommended.

Preparation: Aconiti tinctura: 1:1

Daily Dosage:

Aconiti tinctura: Average dose 0.1 gm; maximum dose 0.2 gm; maximum daily dose 0.6 gm. Only standardized preparations should be used.

Externally: Aconiti tinctura is applied with a brush.

Homeopathic Dosage: 5 drops, 1 tablet or 10 globules every 30 to 60 minutes (acute) and 1 to 3 times per day (chronic); Parenterally: 1 to 2 ml 3 times daily sc; Ointment 1 to 2 times daily (HAB1).

Storage: The herb must be kept in a dry place protected from light and insects.

LITERATURE

Bugatti C, Colombo ML, Tomé F, Extraction and purification of lipoalkaloids from Aconitum napellus roots and leaves. In: PM 58(7)95. 1992.

Hikino H et al., J Pharm Dyn 2:78-83. 1979.

Honerjäger P, Meissner A, Naunyn-Schmiedeberg's Arch Pharmacol 322:49-58. 1983.

Katz A, Rudin HP, Staehlin E, Pharm Acta Helv 62: 216-220. 1987.

Katz A, Staehlin E, Pharm Acta Helv 54:253-265. 1979.

Kimura M et al., Japan J Pharmacol 48:290-299. 1988.

Liu H, Katz A, Norditerpenoid alkaloids from Aconitum napellus ssp. neomontanum. In: PM 62(2):190-191. 1997.

Rao MR, (1966) Acta Pharm Sinica 3, 195.

Further information in:

Chan H, But P (Eds.), Pharmacology and Applications of Chinese Materia Medica, Vol 1, Ed. World Scientific Singapore 1986.

Frohne D, Pfänder HJ, Giftpflanzen - Ein Handbuch für Apotheker, Toxikologen und Biologen, 4. Aufl., Wiss. Verlags-Ges Stuttgart 1997.

Hänsel R, Keller K, Rimpler H, Schneider G (Hrsg.), Hagers Handbuch der Pharmazeutischen Praxis, 5. Aufl., Bde 4-6 (Drogen), Springer Verlag Berlin, Heidelberg, New York, 1992-1994.

Lewin L, Gifte und Vergiftungen, 6. Aufl., Nachdruck, Haug Verlag, Heidelberg 1992.

Madaus G, Lehrbuch der Biologischen Arzneimittel, Bde 1-3, Nachdruck, Georg Olms Verlag Hildesheim 1979.

Roth L, Daunderer M, Kormann K, Giftpflanzen, Pflanzengifte, 4. Aufl., Ecomed Fachverlag Landsberg Lech 1993.

Steinegger E, Hänsel R, Pharmakognosie, 5. Aufl., Springer Verlag Heidelberg 1992.

Teuscher E, Biogene Arzneimittel, 5. Aufl., Wiss. Verlagsges. Stuttgart 1997.

Teuscher E, Lindequist U, Biogene Gifte - Biologie, Chemie, Pharmakologie, 2. Aufl., Fischer Verlag Stuttgart 1994.

Wagner H, Wiesenauer M, Phytotherapie. Phytopharmaka und pflanzliche Homöopathika, Fischer-Verlag, Stuttgart, Jena, New York 1995.

Morinda citrifolia

See Noni

Moringa oleifera

See Behen

Morning Glory

Impomoea hederacea

DESCRIPTION

Medicinal Parts: The medicinal parts are the seeds and root.

Flower and Fruit: The flowering branches bear 1 to 5 radial flowers with structures in fives. The 5 sepals are 1.3 to 2.5 cm long, narrow-lanceolate, acuminate and rough-haired at the base. The 5 petals are 3.8 to 5 cm long, funnel-shaped, spotted blue-pink or are fused at the base of the orange corolla. The plant has 5 stamens and a superior 3-chambered ovary. The fruit is a capsule with a diameter of approximately 8 mm containing 4 to 6 smooth seeds.

Leaves, Stem and Root: This winding herb grows 1 to 3 m high. The leaves are alternate, ovate-cordate and entire, with a diameter of 5 to 12.5 cm. The stem is slightly pubescent.

Habitat: The plant is indigenous to China, India, and Central and South America.

Production: Morning Glory seeds are the dried, ripe seeds of Ipomoea hederacea. The plants are harvested in autumn before the seeds open, then dried in the sun. The seeds are then removed and cleaned.

Not to be Confused With: Morning Glory seeds are similar to and sometimes confused with the seeds of other Ipomoea species.

ACTIONS AND PHARMACOLOGY

COMPOUNDS

Indole alkaloids of the ergoline type (0.5%): chief alkaloids lysergol (50%) and chanoclavine (35%). Smaller amounts of penniclavine and elymoclavine

Fatty oil (12 to 14%): chief fatty acids oleic acid, palmitic acid, stearic acid

Resins (15%): glycoretines (macromolecular, resinous glycosides of hydroxy-fatty acids [C12 to C16]) with oligosaccharides, the so-called pharbitinic acids; the latter's hydroxyl groups are estered with (among others) alpha-methylbutyric acid, tiglic acida and valeric acid to the fatty acid remnant

EFFECTS

The drug has a drastic laxative effect due to the glycoretines it contains, which presumably explains its usefulness against ascarid and tapeworm infestations.

INDICATIONS AND USAGE

Unproven Uses: Morning Glory has been used for worm infestation and constipation.

Indian Medicine: Morning Glory is used for constipation, flatulence, parasite infestation, scabies and dyspepsia. According to the Tschirch manual, the roots of Ipomoea species have long been in use in India, and the drug also was used extensively by the Persians and Arabs.

Chinese Medicine: Uses of Morning Glory include edema, constipation, parasite infestation and feelings of fullness.

PRECAUTIONS AND ADVERSE REACTIONS

The drug's laxative effect is frequently accompanied by cramp-like pains.

CONTRAINDICATIONS

Because of the possible teratogenic effect, the drug should not be used during pregnancy.

DOSAGE

Mode of Administration: Whole, cut and powdered drug.

Preparation: Resin is made by heating the powdered drug until it melts, then cooling it to form a pale translucent mass.

Daily dosage:

Drug — 0.5 to 3 g drug

Resin — daily dose: 0.3 g; maximum single dose: 0.1 g

Chinese Dosage:

Powder — 1.5 to 5 g drug, can be raised to 12 to 15 g

Tea — 24 to 30 g drug

Storage: Store in dry place.

LITERATURE

Hänsel R, Keller K, Rimpler H, Schneider G (Ed), Hagers Handbuch der Pharmazeutischen Praxis, 5. Aufl., Bde 4 - 6 (Drogen), Springer Verlag Berlin, Heidelberg, New York, 1992-1994.

Morus nigra

See Black Mulberry

Motherwort

Leonurus cardiaca

DESCRIPTION

Medicinal Parts: The medicinal parts are the fresh aerial parts collected during the flowering season.

Flower and Fruit: Small, bright red, bilabiate flowers are in dense false whorls in the upper leaf axils. The calyx is funnel-shaped with 5 rigid, awned tips, which are bent outward. The corolla is densely villous on the outside and longer than the calyx. The stamens stretch out longer than the flower. The fruit is a brown, triangular, 2.5 to 3 mm long nutlet with a tuft of hair at the tip.

Leaves, Stem and Root: The plant is perennial and has a short woody rhizome. It grows to about 120 cm. The stem is erect, quadrangular, grooved, hollow, often red-violet and usually hairy. The leaves are long-petioled, pubescent or glabrous. The lower leaves are palmate and cordate at the base. The upper leaves are 3-lobed. The upper surface is dark green, the lower surface light green.

Characteristics: Motherwort has an unpleasant smell.

Habitat: The plant is indigenous to central Europe and Scandinavia through temperate Russia to central Asia. It was introduced to North America and has become established in the wild there.

Production: Motherwort herb consists of the above-ground parts of Leonurus cardiaca, gathered during flowering season, as well as their preparations. They are collected in the wild and dried at 35° C.

Other Names: Lion's Tail, Lion's Ear, Throw-Wort

ACTIONS AND PHARMACOLOGY

COMPOUNDS

Diterpene bitter principles: leocardin

Iridoide monoterpenes: ajugoside (leonuride), ajugol, galiridoside, reptoside

Flavonoids: including, among others, rutin, quercitrin, isoquercitrin, hyperoside, genkwanin

Leonurin: (syringa acid esters of 4-guanidino-butane-1-ols)

Betaine: stachydrine (N-dimethyl-L-proline)

Caffeic acid derivatives: caffeic acid-4-O-rutinoside

Tannins

Volatile oil (traces)

EFFECTS

Mildly negatively chronotropic, hypotonic, sedative.

INDICATIONS AND USAGE

Approved by Commission E:

■ Nervous heart complaints

Unproven Uses: Hyperthyroidism and flatulence. In folk medicine it is used for bronchial asthma, climacteric symptoms and amenorrhea.

Homeopathic Uses: Homeopathic treatments include use for cardiac complaints, flatulence and hyperthyroidism.

PRECAUTIONS AND ADVERSE REACTIONS

General: No health hazards or side effects are known in conjunction with the proper administration of designated therapeutic dosages.

Pregnancy: Not to be used during pregnancy.

DOSAGE

Mode of Administration: Comminuted herb for infusions and other galenic preparations for internal use.

Daily Dosage: 4.5 gm herb; infusion: 2 to 4 gm drug 3 times daily; liquid extract (1:1): 2 to 4 ml 3 times daily; tincture: daily dose: 2 to 6 ml.

Homeopathic Dosage: Acute states: 5 drops, 1 tablet or 10 globules every 30 to 60 minutes. Chronic states: 5 drops, 1 tablet, 10 pellets or a knife tip 1 to 3 times daily. Parenterally: Acute: 1 to 2 ml sc., 3 times daily; chronic: 1 to 2 ml once a day (HAB1).

LITERATURE

Buzogany K, Cucu V, Accumulation, distribution and conservation dynamics of iridoids in Leonurus cardiaca L. and L. villosus Desf. In: Farmacia (Bukarest): 34(3):173-176. 1986.

Chang CF, Li CZ, (1986) Chung I Chieh Ho Tsa Chih 6(1):39.

Kartnig T et al., (1985) J Nat Prod 48(3):494.

Kooiman P, (1972) Acta Bot Neerl. 21(4):417.

Malakov P et al., (1985) Phytochemistry 24(10):2341.

Peng Y, (1983) Bull Chin. Mat Med 8:41.

Reuter G, Diehl HJ, (1970) Pharmazie 25:586.

Schilling G et al., (1975) Liebigs Ann Chem:230.

Tschesche R et al., (1980) Phytochemistry 19:2783.

Weischer ML, Okpanyi SN, Pharmakologie eines pflanzlichen Schlafmittels. In: ZPT 15(5):257-262. 1994.

Xia XX, (1983) J Trad Chin Med 3:185.

Further information in:

Hänsel R, Keller K, Rimpler H, Schneider G (Hrsg.), Hagers Handbuch der Pharmazeutischen Praxis, 5. Aufl., Bde 4-6 (Drogen), Springer Verlag Berlin, Heidelberg, New York, 1992-1994.

Madaus G, Lehrbuch der Biologischen Arzneimittel, Bde 1-3, Nachdruck, Georg Olms Verlag Hildesheim 1979.

Steinegger E, Hänsel R, Pharmakognosie, 5. Aufl., Springer Verlag Heidelberg 1992.

Teuscher E, Biogene Arzneimittel, 5. Aufl., Wiss. Verlagsges. Stuttgart 1997.

Wagner H, Wiesenauer M, Phytotherapie. Phytopharmaka und pflanzliche Homöopathika, Fischer-Verlag, Stuttgart, Jena, New York 1995.

Wichtl M (Hrsg.), Teedrogen, 4. Aufl., Wiss. Verlagsges. Stuttgart 1997.

Mountain Ash Berry

Sorbus aucuparia

DESCRIPTION

Medicinal Parts: The medicinal parts are the ripe, dried fruit or the dried and then boiled fruit.

Flower and Fruit: The inflorescence is broadly umbelliferous-paniculate, erect, floriferous, loosely tomentose, occasionally completely or almost completely glabrous. The calyx has 5 segments. There are 5 white petals and numerous stamens. The ovary is inferior and has 2 to 4 free styles, which are pubescent in the lower portion. The false fruit is almost globular with a diameter of 9 to 10 mm and is scarlet. There are usually 3 seeds which are narrow-oblong, acute and reddish.

Leaves, Stem and Root: The plant is usually a medium-sized tree up to 16 m high with a round, rather loose crown. The bark is smooth and pale gray, later becoming vertically fissured and blackish. The leaves are odd-pinnate with 5 to 11 almost sessile leaflets. These are oblong-lanceolate, irregularly thorny-tipped and serrate, pubescent or almost glabrous.

Characteristics: The flowers have an unpleasant smell and the berries are sharp-tasting and sour. Sorbus moravica tastes sweet in contrast.

Habitat: The plant is indigenous to almost all of Europe, to Western Siberia and Asia Minor, and is found in North America.

Production: Mountain Ash Berry consists of the fresh or dried fruit, or fruit cooked and dried thereafter, of Sorbus aucuparia as well as its preparations. The ripe, shiny red fruit is harvested from August to October

Other Names: Quick-Beam, Rowan Tree, Witchen, European Mountain Ash, Sorb Apple

ACTIONS AND PHARMACOLOGY

COMPOUNDS

Cyanogenic glycosides (0.06%; in the seeds 0.2 to 0.5%; traces in the fruit pulp): in the seeds amygdalin, in the fruit pulp prunasin

Fruit acids: malic acid (3 to 5%), tartaric acid

Monosaccharides/oligosaccharides: saccharose, glucose, fructose, sorbose

Parasorboside (bitter substance): parasorbic acid is formed from it through cell destruction (lactone of the (5S)-Hydroxyhex-2-en-acid-1, pungent in odor, mucus-membrane-irritating, 0.1 to 0.3% of the fresh weight). Parasorbic acid is destroyed through dehydration or volatilized during cooking. It is present only in traces (less than 0.01%) in the cultivated variety, that contains few bitter substances.

Sugar alcohols: sorbitol

Tannins

Vitamins: ascorbic acid (vitamin C, 0.03 to 0.13%, higher content in the non-bitter fruits)

EFFECTS

The parascorbic acid is weakly laxative and irritating to the mucous membrane. Ascorbic acid is a vitamin C supplement.

INDICATIONS AND USAGE

Unproven uses: Mountain Ash is used in folk medicine for kidney diseases, diabetes, rheumatism, disorders of the uric acid metabolism, for dissolution of uric acid deposits, menstruation disturbances, the alkalization of the blood, to improve the metabolism and for vitamin C deficiency.

PRECAUTIONS AND ADVERSE REACTIONS

No health hazards or side effects are known in conjunction with the proper administration of designated therapeutic dosages of the dehydrated drug or with the consumption of fruit sauces, juices, jellies, jams, etc. produced through cooking.

OVERDOSAGE

Because of the formation of the mucus-membrane-irritating parasorboside that results from cutting up the fruit, the intake of very large quantities ofthe fresh fruit leads to gastroenteritis, vomiting, queasiness, gastric pain, diarrhea, kidney damage (albuminuria, glycosuria) and to polymorphic exanthemas.

DOSAGE

Mode of Administration: Mountain Ash is available as whole and crude drug forms.

Daily Dosage: A purée is used for diarrhea. Freshly pressed juice (or juice with sugar) is taken by the dessertspoonful for conditions of the lungs and pleura with fever.

LITERATURE

Fikenscher LH et al., PM 41:313. 1981.

Letzig E et al., Nahrung 7:591. 1963.

Sicher O, Salama O, PM 39:269. 1980.

Further information in:

Frohne D, Pfänder HJ, Giftpflanzen - Ein Handbuch für Apotheker, Toxikologen und Biologen, 4. Aufl., Wiss. Verlags-Ges. Stuttgart 1997.

Hänsel R, Keller K, Rimpler H, Schneider G (Hrsg.), Hagers Handbuch der Pharmazeutischen Praxis, 5. Aufl., Bde 4-6 (Drogen): Springer Verlag Berlin, Heidelberg, New York, 1992-1994.

Lewin L, Gifte und Vergiftungen, 6. Aufl., Nachdruck, Haug Verlag, Heidelberg 1992.

Madaus G, Lehrbuch der Biologischen Arzneimittel, Bde 1-3, Nachdruck, Georg Olms Verlag Hildesheim 1979.

Roth L, Daunderer M, Kormann K, Giftpflanzen, Pflanzengifte, 4. Aufl., Ecomed Fachverlag Landsberg Lech 1993.

Teuscher E, Lindequist U, Biogene Gifte - Biologie, Chemie, Pharmakologie, 2. Aufl., Fischer Verlag Stuttgart 1994.

Mountain Avens

Dryas octopetala

DESCRIPTION

Medicinal Parts: Mountain Avens or Silverweed Herb is the whole dried plant of Dryas octopetala.

Flower and Fruit: The flower stalk is upright, 2 to 8 cm long. The diameter of the flowers is 2 to 4 cm; there are 6 to 9 sepals, which are glabrous on the inside and brown, felt-like and glandular on the outside. There are 6 to 9 white petals and numerous stamens. The carpels are numerous, free and densely haired, with apical styles twisted like screws. The fruit is like a nut.

Leaves, Stem and Root: This evergreen dwarf shrub grows up to 0.5 m high. The leaves are 0.5 to 4 cm long, up to 2.5 cm wide, coriaceous, crenate, short-petiolate; the lamina is spatulate, obovate or elongate-elliptical, with a cordate base, wrinkled and glabrous above, tomentose beneath; the stipules are dry-membranous and sharply acuminate. The small stem is heavily branched, the leaves on the horizontal branches are double-rowed, the upright stem has leaves all around. The plant has a primary taproot.

Habitat: The shrub grows in the Arctic, subarctic and high mountainous regions.

Production: The plant is collected in the wild, cut and powdered.

Other Names: Silverweed Herb

ACTIONS AND PHARMACOLOGY

COMPOUNDS

Tannins (2.5 to 5.5% in the root; 7.5 to 14% in the leaves)

Catechin tannins (7 to 14%)

Flavonoids (0.7 to 1.6%): glycosides of quercetin, kaempferol, isorhamnetin, limocitrin, gossypetin, corniculatusin and sexangularetin

Triterpenes: including tormentoside

EFFECTS

Due to its tannin and flavonoid glycoside content, the drug is astringent in effect.

INDICATIONS AND USAGE

Unproven Uses: Folk medicine uses include stomach pains and diarrhea.

The effect appears to be plausible because of the flavonoid glycoside content, but is unproven.

PRECAUTIONS AND ADVERSE REACTIONS

No health hazards are known in conjunction with the proper administration of designated therapeutic dosages. The ingestion of larger dosages can lead to digestive complaints and constipation, due to the high tannin content. Available data are insufficient to classify the drug's safety.

LITERATURE

Hänsel R, Keller K, Rimpler H, Schneider G (Ed.), Hagers Handbuch der Pharmazeutischen Praxis, 5. Aufl., Bde 4 - 6 (Drogen), Springer Verlag Berlin, Heidelberg, New York, 1992-1994.

Schulthess H, Dissertation Zurich; 1945.

Mountain Flax

Linum catharticum

DESCRIPTION

Medicinal Parts: The medicinal parts are the herb, the fresh flowering plant and the whole plant.

Flower and Fruit: The flowers are on loose, panicled, branched, sparsely leafed twining stems on long peduncles in the leaf axils. They hang before flowering. The sepals are elliptically acuminate, 2 to 2.5 mm long with ciliate glands. The 5 white petals are up to 5 mm long, and yellow at the base. There are 5 stamens fused at the base and 1 ovary with 5 headed stigma on long thin styles. The fruit is erect, globular, 2 to 3 cm long and incomplete 10-valved with long, pubescent, dividing membranes. The seeds are elliptical, 1 to 1.5 mm long, flat, smooth and light brown.

Leaves, Stem and Root: The plant is an inconspicuous annual (occasionally perennial) that grows up to 30 cm. It has a long erect or ascending stem, which is undivided or dividing into the flowering branches. The leaves are opposite or alternate, entire-margined, sessile and have a partly ciliate margin.

Habitat: Found in central Europe as far as the British Isles and southward as far as the Mediterranean countries, the Caucasus, Iran and northern Africa.

Production: Mountain Flax is the flowering plant (aerial part) of Linum catharticum, collected in the uncultivated regions.

Other Names: Purging Flax, Dwarf Flax, Fairy Flax, Mill Mountain

ACTIONS AND PHARMACOLOGY

COMPOUNDS

Lignans: achromatin (bitter), presumably present in the fresh plant as a glycoside

Tannins

Volatile oil

The constituents of the drug have not been extensively investigated.

EFFECTS

Mountain Flax has a laxative effect in therapeutic doses of up to 0.5 gm. High doses cause vomiting and gastroenteritis.

Although the amaroid linin is not laxative, it is probably present in the form of a glycoside, which has a stronger laxative effect.

INDICATIONS AND USAGE

Unproven Uses: Its use as a laxative is obsolete. In folk medicine Mountain Flax is used for constipation, oliguria, edema, worm infestation, catarrhal and rheumatic conditions.

Homeopathic Uses: Used homeopathically for coughs, hemorrhoids, diarrhea, catarrh and rheumatic disorders, dropsy and worm infestation. Also used as a purgative and emetic.

PRECAUTIONS AND ADVERSE REACTIONS

No health hazards or side effects are known in conjunction with the proper administration of designated therapeutic dosages. The drug can lead to vomiting, inflammations of the gastrointestinal tract and diarrhea. The emetic and laxative effects are used therapeutically.

DOSAGE

Mode of Administration: Ground and as an extract.

Preparation: To prepare an infusion, add 2.5 gm to 1 cup of hot water.

Dosage: 2.0 gm powder as a single dose.

LITERATURE

Hänsel R, Keller K, Rimpler H, Schneider G (Hrsg.), Hagers Handbuch der Pharmazeutischen Praxis, 5. Aufl., Bde 4-6 (Drogen), Springer Verlag Berlin, Heidelberg, New York, 1992-1994.

Madaus G, Lehrbuch der Biologischen Arzneimittel, Bde 1-3, Nachdruck, Georg Olms Verlag Hildesheim 1979.

Mountain Grape

Mahonia aquifolium

TRADE NAMES

Oregon Grape (Berberis aquifolium variety available from numerous manufacturers) Oregon Grape Root

DESCRIPTION

Medicinal Parts: The medicinal parts are the dried rhizome and the roots, the dried branch and twig bark, as well as the root bark.

Flower and Fruit: The heavily scented flowers are either in dense 5 to 10 cm panicles or in groups of 3 to 6 in erect 5 to 8 cm racemes in the leaf axils. The flowers are yellow and have 9 sepals, 6 petals and 6 stamens, which are about 8 cm long. The pedicles are 5 to 10 mm long. The fruit is a globose, purple-black, frosted berry with red juice. The 2 to 5 seeds are glossy brown.

Leaves, Stem and Root: The plant is a fast-growing, evergreen, stoloniferous shrub about 50 to 150 cm high with stout stems, sparingly branched. The leaves are odd-pinnate, 10 to 20 cm long with 3 to 6 pairs of leaflets. The leaflets are 4 to 8 cm by 2 to 4 cm, ovate, distally spinose dentate, coriaceous, dark and shining green.

Habitat: Indigenous to the Pacific U.S.; ornamental or cultivated in Europe.

Production: Mountain Grape bark consists of the branch and twig bark as well as the twig tips of Mahonia aquifolium.

Other Names: Holly-Leaved Berberis, Oregon Grape

ACTIONS AND PHARMACOLOGY

COMPOUNDS

Isoquinoline alkaloids (in the root bark, 7 to 16%, in the stem bark, 2.4-4.5%):

benzyl isoquinoline type: including among others berberine

bisbenzyl isoquinoline type: including among others berbamine, oxyacanthine

aporphine type: including among others isocorydine

EFFECTS

The use of the drug as a tonic for loss of appetite is plausible in view of the alkaloid and amaroid content. The berberine has a mild mutagenic effect. It is an antipsoriatic when used externally.

INDICATIONS AND USAGE

Unproven Uses: The drug is used internally for scaly skin, psoriasis, eczema, bronchitis, gastritis, cholecystitis and digestion problems.

Homeopathic Uses: Mountain Grape is used for dry skin rashes (e.g., for psoriasis between the acute phases) and for liver and gallbladder conditions.

PRECAUTIONS AND ADVERSE REACTIONS

General: No health hazards or side effects are known in conjunction with the proper administration of designated therapeutic dosages.

Pregnancy: The drug should not be used during pregnancy.

DOSAGE

Mode of Administration: The drug is available in commercial ointments for external use.

Storage: Protect from light.

LITERATURE

Anonym, Ein Lichtblick in der Psoriasistherapie. In: DAZ 134(8):646. 1994.

Augustin M, Mahonia aquifolium bei Psoriasis. In: ZPT 17(1):44. 1996.

Galle K, Bladt S, Wagner H, Mahonia. In: DAZ 134(49):4883. 1994.

Mennet-von Eiff M, Meier B, Phytotherapie in der Dermatologie. In: ZPT 16(4):201-210. 1995.

Misik V et al., Lipoxygenase inhibition and antioxidant properties of protoberberine and aporphine alkaloids isolated from Mahonia aquifolium. In: PM 61(4):372-373. 1995.

Müller K, Ziereis K, Gawlik I, The antipsoriatic Mahonia aquifolium and its active constituents II: Antiproliferative activity against cell growth of human keratinocytes. In: PM 61(1):74-75. 1995.

Müller K, Ziereis K, The antisporiatic Mahonia aquifolium and its active constitutents; Pro- and antioxidant properties and inhibition of 5-lipoxygenase. In: PM 60(5):421. 1994.

Niedner R, Wiesnauer M, Dermatologie: Mahonia aquifolium - ein Phytopharmakon in der Psoriasistherapie. In: DAZ 132(37):1890. 1992.

Petersen-Lehmann J, Homöopathische Salbe gegen Schuppenflechte. In: PZ 137(38):2892. 1992.

Willaman JJ, Hui-Li L, (1970) Lloydia 33(3A):1.

Further information in:

Frohne D, Pfänder HJ: Giftpflanzen - Ein Handbuch für Apotheker, Toxikologen und Biologen, 4. Aufl., Wiss. Verlags-Ges. Stuttgart 1997.

Hänsel R, Keller K, Rimpler H, Schneider G (Hrsg.), Hagers Handbuch der Pharmazeutischen Praxis, 5. Aufl., Bde 4-6 (Drogen), Springer Verlag Berlin, Heidelberg, New York, 1992-1994.

Madaus G, Lehrbuch der Biologischen Arzneimittel, Bde 1-3, Nachdruck, Georg Olms Verlag Hildesheim 1979 (unter Berberis aquifolium).

Roth L, Daunderer M, Kormann K, Giftpflanzen, Pflanzengifte, 4. Aufl., Ecomed Fachverlag Landsberg Lech 1993.

Teuscher E, Lindequist U, Biogene Gifte - Biologie, Chemie, Pharmakologie, 2. Aufl., Fischer Verlag Stuttgart 1994.

Wagner H, Wiesenauer M, Phytotherapie. Phytopharmaka und pflanzliche Homöopathika, Fischer-Verlag, Stuttgart, Jena, New York 1995.

Mountain Laurel

Kalmia latifolia

DESCRIPTION

Medicinal Parts: The medicinal parts are the fresh or dried leaves.

Flower and Fruit: The inflorescence is a compound umbelled-raceme with numerous flowers. The flowers are red, whitish or purple-brown to chocolate brown; solitary on long glandular-hairy pedicles in the axils of the bracts and 2 lateral, brown bracteoles. The bud has 10 folds and spreads out in a bowl shape. There are 10 stamens, red anthers without appendages that burst open at irregular holes. The fruit is an erect, orbicular, 5-to-7-valvular capsule. The numerous seeds are flat, oblong, 1 mm long and fly easily.

Leaves, Stem and Root: The plant is a heavily branched shrub or tree about 4 m high with reddish-brown or gray branches. The evergreen, laurel-like, ovate-lanceolate acuminate, glabrous leaves are alternate, 4 to 12 cm long and have a 1 to 3 cm long petiole. They are red-brown on the lower surface, have numerous glandular hairs and a distinct midrib. The upper surface is dark green.

Habitat: Eastern U.S.

Production: Mountain Laurel leaves are the leaves (fresh or dried) of Kalmia latifolia.

Other Names: Broad-Leafed Laurel, Calico Bush, Spoonwood, Sheep Laurel, Rose Laurel, Laurel, Lambkill, Mountain Ivy

ACTIONS AND PHARMACOLOGY

COMPOUNDS

Diterpenes (andromedan- derivatives): including among others grayanotoxin I (andromedotoxin, asebotoxin, acetylandromedol, rhodotoxin), grayanotoxin II, III, XVIII, lyonol A, leucothol A, kalmiatoxine

Acylphloroglucinols: including among others 2',6'-dihydroxy-4'-methoxy-acetophenone, phloretin

Flavonoids: including among others asebotin, hyperoside

EFFECTS

Use of Mountain Laurel is no longer recommended because of the formation of grayanotoxins, which are highly toxic. Efficacy for the recorded indications has not been proven.

According to earlier sources (which are questionable), the drug is antiphlogistic and mildly diuretic.

INDICATIONS AND USAGE

Unproven Uses: Today, the drug is only used in homeopathic dilutions. In the past it was used as a decoction in the treatment of tinea capitis and to treat psoriasis, herpes and secondary syphilis.

Homeopathic Uses: Uses include rheumatism, shingles, nerve pain, rheumatic and cardiac pain.

PRECAUTIONS AND ADVERSE REACTIONS

The andromedan derivatives of the drug prevent the closure of the excitable cells of the sodium channels and thereby prevent conduction. Painful mucous membranes in the mouth and in the stomach, increased salivation, cold sweat, nausea, vomiting, diarrhea and paresthesias are experienced following intake of the drug. Dizziness, headache, fever attacks, as well as intoxicated states with temporary loss of vision, follow later. Muscle weakness, coordination disorders and spasms can also occur. Bradycardia, cardiac arrhythmias, drops in blood pressure, eventual cardiac arrest and respiratory failure can lead to death.

OVERDOSAGE

Following gastrointestinal emptying, (inducement of vomiting, gastric lavage with burgundy-colored potassium permanganate solution, sodium sulfate) and instillation of activated charcoal, the treatment of poisoning consists of electrolyte replacement, countering of acidosis with sodium bicarbonate, plasma volume expanders if required, diazepam (I.V.) in case of spasms and oxygen in case of respiratory failure.

DOSAGE

Mode of Administration: Available in homeopathic preparations.

Homeopathic Dosage: 5 drops, 1 tablet or 10 globules every 30 to 60 minutes (acute) or 1 to 3 times daily (chronic); parenterally: 1 to 2 ml sc acute, 3 times daily; chronic: once a day (HAB1).

LITERATURE

Frohne D, Pfänder HJ, Giftpflanzen - Ein Handbuch für Apotheker, Toxikologen und Biologen, 4. Aufl., Wiss. Verlags-Ges Stuttgart 1997.

Hänsel R, Keller K, Rimpler H, Schneider G (Hrsg.), Hagers Handbuch der Pharmazeutischen Praxis, 5. Aufl., Bde 4-6 (Drogen), Springer Verlag Berlin, Heidelberg, New York, 1992-1994.

Lewin L, Gifte und Vergiftungen, 6. Aufl., Nachdruck, Haug Verlag, Heidelberg 1992.

Madaus G, Lehrbuch der Biologischen Arzneimittel, Bde 1-3, Nachdruck, Georg Olms Verlag Hildesheim 1979.

Roth L, Daunderer M, Kormann K, Giftpflanzen, Pflanzengifte, 4. Aufl., Ecomed Fachverlag Landsberg Lech 1993.

Teuscher E, Lindequist U, Biogene Gifte - Biologie, Chemie, Pharmakologie, 2. Aufl., Fischer Verlag Stuttgart 1994.

Wagner H, Wiesenauer M, Phytotherapie. Phytopharmaka und pflanzliche Homöopathika, Fischer-Verlag, Stuttgart, Jena, New York 1995.

Wolters B, Zierpflanzen aus Nordamerika. In: DAZ 137(26):2253-2261. 1997.

Mouse Ear

Pilosella officinarum

DESCRIPTION

Medicinal Parts: The medicinal parts are the flowering aerial parts.

Flower and Fruit: The yellow, composite flowers are solitary at the end of long pedicles. There are bright yellow, lingual florets. The lateral ones are usually striped reddish underneath. The bracts are linear and acute, have a membranous margin and are covered in star-hairs. They have black glandular hairs at the base. The fruit is cylindrical and has a simple, brittle tuft of hair.

Leaves, Stem and Root: The plant is a perennial herb, which grows up to 30 cm. Erect, leafless stems grow from the rosette of basal leaves. The plant produces long, leafy runners. The leaves are oblong or obovate to lanceolate. They bear long bristles, which are thickened at the base and are star-haired to tomentose beneath.

Habitat: The plant grows in large areas of Europe and temperate Asia. It is also found in North America.

Production: Mouse Ear is the aerial part of Pilosella officinarum.

ACTIONS AND PHARMACOLOGY

COMPOUNDS

Flavonoids: including among others luteolin-7-glucoside, isoetin

Hydroxycoumarins: umbelliferone, skimmine

Tannins

EFFECTS

The plant has been shown to have diuretic, spasmolytic and diaphoretic effects.

INDICATIONS AND USAGE

Unproven Uses: Mouse Ear is used internally in the treatment of asthma, bronchitis, coughs and whooping cough and externally in the treatment of wounds.

PRECAUTIONS AND ADVERSE REACTIONS

No health hazards or side effects are known in conjunction with the proper administration of designated therapeutic dosages.

DOSAGE

Mode of Administration: The drug is used internally and externally as a liquid extract.

LITERATURE

Bate-Smith EC et al., Phytochemistry 7:1165.

Duquenois P, (1965) Mem Soc Bot Franc 41.

Guerin JC, Reveillere HP, (1985) Ann Farm Franc 43(1):77.

Hegnauer R, Chemotaxonomie der Pflanzen, Bde 1-11, Birkhäuser Verlag Basel, Boston, Berlin 1962-1997.

Kern W, List PH, Hörhammer L (Hrsg.), Hagers Handbuch der Pharmazeutischen Praxis, 4. Aufl., Bde. 1-8, Springer Verlag Berlin, Heidelberg, New York, 1969.

Madaus G, Lehrbuch der Biologischen Arzneimittel, Bde 1-3, Nachdruck, Georg Olms Verlag Hildesheim 1979.

Mucuna pruriens

See Cowhage

Mugwort

Artemisia vulgaris

DESCRIPTION

Medicinal Parts: The medicinal parts are the root and the above-ground parts of the plant, particularly the dried branch tips.

Flower and Fruit: The flower heads are ovoid, 3 to 4 mm long by 2 mm wide. The numerous flowers are short-stemmed, erect or slightly drooping. They are in dense, heavily branched panicles with numerous lanceolate bracts. The bracts are downy white with a green midrib. The inner bracts are lanceolate and acuminate. The outside ones are oblong and obtuse with broad membranous margin. The flowers are yellowish or red-brown and almost glabrous. The inner flowers are androgynous and those on the outside are female. The receptacle is glabrous. The fruit has an indistinct margin.

Leaves, Stem and Root: The plant is a long-stemmed, 70 to 150 cm high shrub with a branched, many-headed and creeping rhizome without runners or rosette. The shoots are slightly pubescent, often red-tinged and have a weak unpleasant smell. The erect or ascending, edged, coriaceous stems die off each year. They are in branched panicles and downy. The leaves are 5 to 10 cm long, coriaceous, and the margins are often rolled back. The upper surface is usually dark green and glabrous, occasionally pubescent, and the lower surface is tomentose. The basal leaves are short-petioled and lobed with an end section and 1 to 2 pairs of small side leaflets. The rest of the leaves are sessile or almost sessile with a slit base. The lower leaves are double-pinnate, the middle and upper ones are pinnatifid and lanceolate, acuminate, entire-margined or slightly serrated.

Characteristics: Mugwort has a pleasant tangy taste. The root is sweet and pungent, the herb is aromatic and bitter.

Habitat: The plant is indigenous to Asia and North America, and is also distributed all over Europe except in the south.

Production: Mugwort herb consists of the above-ground parts of Artemisia vulgaris. The branch tips are gathered during the flowering season and carefully dried. Other fresh above- and underground parts of the plant are harvested at the beginning of winter, primarily from the wild. Mugwort root consists of the below-ground parts of Artemisia vulgaris.

Not to be Confused With: Some confusion can arise with Asinthii herba.

Other Names: Felon Herb, St. John's Plant, Wormwood

ACTIONS AND PHARMACOLOGY

COMPOUNDS

Volatile oil (complex composition): chief constituents, according to plant variety, 1,8- cineol, camphor, linalool or thujone

Sesquiterpene lactones: including vulgarin, pilostachyin, pilostachyin C

Lipophilic flavonoids

Polyynes

Hydroxycoumarins: for example, umbelliferone, aesculetin

EFFECTS

The aqueous extract and essential oil show antimicrobial activity in laboratory tests.

CONTRAINDICATIONS

Mugwort is not to be used during pregnancy.

INDICATIONS AND USAGE

Unproven Uses: Mugwort is used in complaints and problems involving the gastrointestinal tract such as stomach ulcers and indigestion. The plant is also used for worm infestations, epilepsy, persistent vomiting, to promote circulation, as a sedative, and for delayed or irregular menstuation. The root is used for asthenic states as a tonic, and in combination with other remedies also for psychoneuroses, neurasthenia, depression, hypochondria, autonomic neuroses, general irritability and restlessness, insomnia and anxiety states. The efficacy of Mugwort for the listed indications has not been substantiated.

Chinese Medicine: Mugwort is used in China for female complaints as well as for ulcers and burns.

Homeopathic Uses: Homeopathic uses of the root include convulsions and worm infestations.

PRECAUTIONS AND ADVERSE REACTIONS

General: No health hazards or side effects are known in conjunction with the proper administration of designated therapeutic dosages. Sensitization through skin contact has been observed, although very rarely.

Pregnancy: Mugwort is not to be used during pregnancy.

DOSAGE

Mode of Administration: Since the efficacy for the claimed applications is not verified, therapeutic administration is not recommended.

Preparation: ''Moxibustion'' (China, Japan) leaves are ground with water in a mortar and, after removal of the larger remnants, small cones are formed and dried to be later burnt onto the skin of the patient. Tea is prepared by allowing 1 tsp. to draw in 150 to 200 ml boiling water for 10 minutes. A liquid extract is prepared in a 1:1 proportion from a mixture of the drug in 25% ethanol.

Daily Dosage: An infusion (drug 0.5 to 2 g) is given 3 times daily. Usual dosage of tea is one cup 2 or 3 times daily.

Homeopathic Dosage: 5 drops, 1 tablet, 10 globules every 30 to 60 minutes (acute) or 1 to 3 times daily (chronic); Parenterally: 1 to 2 ml 3 times daily sc (HAB1).

LITERATURE

Hoffmann B, Herrmann K, (1982) Z Lebensm Unters Forsch 174 (3):211.

Jork H, Juel S, (1979) Arch Pharm 312:540.

Juel S et al., (1976) Arch Pharm 309:458.

Kaul VK et al., (1976) Ind J Pharm 38 (1):21.

Marco JA et al., Sesquiterpenes lactones from Artemisia species. In: PH 32:460. 1993.

Marco JA, Sanz JF, Hierro P, Two eudesmane acids from Artemisia vulgaris. In: PH 30:2403-2404. 1991.

Michaelis K et al., On the essential oil components from blossoms of Artemisia vulgaris L. In: Z Naturfosch 37(3/4):152. 1982.

Nano GM et al., (1976) Planta Med 30:211.

Nano GM et al., Composition of some oils from Artemisia vulgaris. In: PM 30(3):211. 1976.

Stefanovic M et al., (1982) Glas Khem Drush Beogr 47 (3):7.

Wallnöfer B, Hofer O, Greger H, Polyacetylenes from Artemsia ''Vulgares'' Group. In: PH 28(10):2687. 1989.

Further information in:

Hänsel R, Keller K, Rimpler H, Schneider G (Hrsg.), Hagers Handbuch der Pharmazeutischen Praxis, 5. Aufl., Bde 4-6 (Drogen): Springer Verlag Berlin, Heidelberg, New York, 1992-1994.

Hausen B, Allergiepflanzen, Pflanzenallergene, ecomed Verlagsgesellsch. mbH, Landsberg 1988.

Madaus G, Lehrbuch der Biologischen Arzneimittel, Bde 1-3, Nachdruck, Georg Olms Verlag Hildesheim 1979.

Wichtl M (Hrsg.), Teedrogen, 4. Aufl., Wiss. Verlagsges. Stuttgart 1997.

Muira-Puama

Ptychopetalum olacoides

DESCRIPTION

Medicinal Parts: The medicinal parts are the dried roots and the dried trunk with bark.

Flower and Fruit: The inflorescences are racemous; there are 1 or 2 per axil. They have 5 to 8 flowers and are about 2 cm long. The calyx is narrow and has 5 tips. The corolla is white, oblong and about 1.3 to 2 mm long. The outside is smooth, and the inside is white pubescent. There are usually 10 stamens with long anthers. The ovary is clavate. The fruit is a long elliptical drupe that is initially green and changes to pink and finally to lilac-black when ripening. The pericarp is thin, and the endocarp is crusty.

Leaves, Stem and Root: The plant is a 5 to 15 m high tree with a trunk 25 cm in diameter, which is vertically grooved. The leaves are oblong-lanceolate, very tapered and narrow toward the base. They are sometimes acute, coriaceous, smooth and gray or frosted to blue-green beneath. The dried leaves are matte with a dark green to black upper surface and a dark gray undersurface. The ribs are pinnatifid, curved, becoming distinct at the margin and protruding on the undersurface. The petioles are deeply grooved and do not thicken.

Habitat: The plant is indigenous to Guyana and the Amazon region of Brazil.

Production: Muira-Puama consists of the wood from the trunk and/or roots of Ptychopetalum olacoides and/or Ptychopetalum unicatum.

ACTIONS AND PHARMACOLOGY

COMPOUNDS

Triterpene acid esters (0.4-0.5%): chief components are behenolic acid esters of lupeol (60%), including, among others, fatty acid esters of beta-sitosterol

Sterols: beta-sitosterol, campesterol, lupeol

Volatile oil: chief components are alpha-pinene (25%), alpha-humulene (10%), beta-pinene (8%), beta-caryophyllene (8%) camphene (7%), camphor (6%),

EFFECTS

No information is available.

INDICATIONS AND USAGE

Unproven Uses: Muira-Puama is used internally for diarrhea, loss of appetite and for the prevention of sexual disorders. The herb is also used externally for the prevention of sexual disorders.

PRECAUTIONS AND ADVERSE REACTIONS

No health hazards or side effects are known in conjunction with the proper administration of designated therapeutic dosages.

DOSAGE

Mode of Administration: Muira-Puama is administered whole, ground, as a powder and as an extract.

Preparation: To prepare a liquid extract, mix the powdered herb in a ratio of 10:2:1 with spirit of wine and glycerine. Then percolate the mixture with spirit of wine, yielding 10 parts liquid extract.

Daily Dosage: When used internally, a single dose is 0.5 gm drug. The daily dosage for the liquid extract and the decoction is 0.5 to 2 ml 3 times daily. For external use, the herb can be added to baths.

LITERATURE

Auterhoff H, Momberger B, Arch Pharm 304:223-228. 1971.

Hänsel R, Keller K, Rimpler H, Schneider G (Hrsg.), Hagers Handbuch der Pharmazeutischen Praxis, 5. Aufl., Bde 4-6 (Drogen), Springer Verlag Berlin, Heidelberg, New York, 1992-1994.

Steinegger E, Hänsel R, Pharmakognosie, 5. Aufl., Springer Verlag Heidelberg 1992.

Mullein

Verbascum densiflorum

TRADE NAMES

Mullein Leaf, Alcohol-Free Mullein Leaves, Mullein Leaves

DESCRIPTION

Medicinal Parts: The medicinal parts are the herb at the beginning of the flowering season, the flowers and the root.

Flower and Fruit: The large, yellow flowers with a diameter of 30 to 35 mm are in apical spike-like racemes. The calyx is divided deeply into five. The corolla is rotate, has a short tube and a 5-lobed, uneven margin. There are 5 stamens of uneven length. The 3 upper ones are lanate and have long anthers. There is 1 superior ovary. The fruit is a 2-lobed capsule.

Leaves, Stem and Root: The plant is biennial. It has petiolate basal leaves and is up to 2 m high. The stem is erect, undivided or lightly branched above. It is tomentose like the leaves and calyx. The leaves are alternate, turned downward and finely crenate. The lower ones are lanceolate or oblong lanceolate; the upper ones, ovate.

Characteristics: The flowers have a honey-like fragrance and an almond-like taste. The leaves are slimy and bitter.

Habitat: The plant is widespread in Europe, temperate Asia and North America.

Production: Mullein flower consists of the dried petals of Verbascum densiflorum and/or of Verbascum phlomoides.

Not to be Confused With: Other Verbascum species.

Other Names: Torch Weed, Aaron's Rod, Blanket-Leaf, Candlewick Plant, Flannelflower, Feltwort, Hedge-Taper, Jacob's Staff, Shepherd's Club, Velvet Plant, Shepherd's Staff, Torches, Our Lady's Flannel, Blanket Herb, Woollen, Rag Paper, Wild Ice Leaf, Clown's Lungwort, Golden Rod, Adam's Flannel, Beggar's Blanket, Clot-Bur, Cuddy's lungs, Duffle, Fluffweed, Hare's Beard, Hag's Taper

ACTIONS AND PHARMACOLOGY

COMPOUNDS

Mucilage (3%): including among others, arabino galactans, xyloglucans

Triterpene saponins: chief components verbascosaponine (0.007%)

Iridoide monoterpenes: including among others, aucubin, 6beta-xylosylaucubin, catalpol, isocatalpol, methyl catalpol

Caffeic acid derivatives: verbascoside (acteoside)

Flavonoids (0.5-4.0%): including among others, rutin, diosmin, quercetin-7-O-glucoside, hesperidine, apigenin-7-O-glucoside, kempferol-7-O-glucoside

Invert sugar (11%)

EFFECTS

Mullein alleviates irritation and has an expectorant effect due to its mucin and saponin content.

INDICATIONS AND USAGE

Approved by Commission E:

■ Cough/bronchitis

Unproven Uses: Mullein is used internally for catarrh of the respiratory tract, bladder and kidney conditions, enteritis, rheumatism, coughs, flu, intestinal pain caused by colic, asthma, cystitis, hemorrhoids, dermatoses, and painful diarrhea. The plant is used externally for earache, ear furuncles, eczema of the auditory canal, middle ear infection, inflammatory skin diseases with itch, burns, eczema, weeping eczema, nappy dermatitis, insect bites, and itching in the anal and genital regions.

PRECAUTIONS AND ADVERSE REACTIONS

No health hazards or side effects are known in conjunction with the proper administration of designated therapeutic dosages.

DOSAGE

Mode of Administration: Whole, cut, and powdered drug is available in the form of teas and other galenic preparations for internal and external use.

How Supplied:

Liquid — 250 mg/ml, 285 mg/ml

Liquid Extract — 1:1

Preparation: To prepare tea, pour boiling water over 1.5 to 2 gm finely cut drug and strain after 10 to 15 minutes (1 teaspoonful is equivalent to 0.5 gm drug).

To make an oil preparation, pour 100 gm of olive oil over a handful of fresh flowers. Leave the mixture outdoors in the sun, stirring several times a day, then filter after 3 to 4 weeks.

To prepare a tincture, add 20 gm cut drug to 80 gm of 70% ethanol and leave to draw for 10 days.

Daily Dose: The daily dose is 3 to 4 gm of drug. The tincture dose is 20 to 30 drops taken several times a day.

Storage: Mullein must be protected from light and particularly from moisture to prevent the drug from changing color to brown or dark brown due to the iridoid content.

LITERATURE

Grzybek J, Szewczyk A, Verbascum-Arten - Königskerze oder Wollblume Portrait einer Arzneipflanze. In: ZPT 17(6):389-398. 1996.

Haslinger E, Schröder H, Sci Pharm 60:202. 1992.

Klimek B, PA 48:51. 1991.

Kraus K, Franz G, DAZ 127:665. 1987.

Seifert K et al., PM 51:409. 1985.

Swiatek L et al., PM 45:153. 1982.

Swiatek L et al., Pharm Weekbl (Sci Ed) 9:246. 1987.

Further information in:

Kern W, List PH, Hörhammer L (Hrsg.), Hagers Handbuch der Pharmazeutischen Praxis, 4. Aufl., Bde. 1-8: Springer Verlag Berlin, Heidelberg, New York, 1969.

Madaus G, Lehrbuch der Biologischen Arzneimittel, Bde 1-3, Nachdruck, Georg Olms Verlag Hildesheim 1979.

Roth L, Daunderer M, Kormann K, Giftpflanzen, Pflanzengifte, 4. Aufl., Ecomed Fachverlag Landsberg Lech 1993.

Steinegger E, Hänsel R, Pharmakognosie, 5. Aufl., Springer Verlag Heidelberg 1992.

Teuscher E, Biogene Arzneimittel, 5. Aufl., Wiss. Verlagsges. Stuttgart 1997.

Wichtl M (Hrsg.), Teedrogen, 4. Aufl., Wiss. Verlagsges. Stuttgart 1997.

Musa paradisiaca

See Plantain

Muskmallow

Abelmoschus moschatus

DESCRIPTION

Medicinal Parts: The medicinal parts are the seeds of the plant and the oil extracted from them.

Flower and Fruit: The flowers are solitary and axillary. They have 5 to 7 pubescent, linear, 1.5 cm long epicalyx leaves. The sepals are about 3 cm long. The corolla has a diameter of 7.5 cm. The petals are sulfur yellow with a crimson spot at the base. The petals are ovate and lightly pubescent. The fruit is a 5 to 8 cm long capsule, which is shaped like a pentagonal pyramid and filled with numerous large seeds. The seeds are kidney-shaped, compressed and about 3 mm in diameter. They are grayish-brown, with numerous striations that are concentric around the hilum.

Leaves, Stem and Root: The plant is an annual erect herb about 1 to 2 m high with star-shaped, pubescent stem, stalks and leaves. The leaves are 15 to 25 cm long, cordate to round with 3 to 7 lobes, which taper to a point. The petioles are as long or longer than the leaves. The stipules are oblong and pubescent.

Characteristics: The seeds have a strong, musky smell, and the taste is oily. The seed pods have an aromatic flavor and are used in some parts of the Middle East to mix with and flavor coffee.

Habitat: The plant is indigenous to Africa, India, Java and South America and is cultivated in all tropical regions.

Production: Muskmallow seeds are the dried seeds of Hibiscus abelmoschus. The seeds are dried in the open air.

Not to be Confused With: Foenugraeci semen.

Other Names: Muskseed, Ambrette Seed, Abelmosk, Ambretta, Egyptian Alcée, Target-Leaved Hibiscus, Okra

ACTIONS AND PHARMACOLOGY

COMPOUNDS

Fatty oil and chief fatty acids: palmitic acid, linoleic acid, stearic acid

Volatile oil: ambrette oil, chief components farnesylacetate, macrocyclic lactones as carriers of the musk smell such as hexadec-7-en-16-olide (ambrettolide), tetradec-5-en-14-olide

Sterols: including beta-sitosterin, beta-sitosterin-beta-D-glucoside

EFFECTS

Muskmallow is said to be an aromatic, a stimulant and carminative.

INDICATIONS AND USAGE

Unproven Uses: The various preparations are used internally and externally for snake bite, cramps, stomach and intestinal disorders with cramps, loss of appetite and headache.

Homeopathic Uses: Muskmallow is used for feelings of tightness in the rib cage area.

PRECAUTIONS AND ADVERSE REACTIONS

Health risks or side effects following the proper administration of designated therapeutic dosages are not recorded.

DOSAGE

Mode of Administration: Muskmallow is used as a tea or tincture, and is administered both internally and externally.

Homeopathic Dosage: 5 to 10 drops, 1 tablet, 5 to 10 globules, 1 to 3 times a day (HAB34).

LITERATURE

Maurer B, Greider A, (1977) Helv Chim Acta 60:1155.

Srivastava KC, Rastogi SC, (1969) Planta Med 17:189.

Further information in:

Hänsel R, Keller K, Rimpler H, Schneider G (Hrsg.), Hagers Handbuch der Pharmazeutischen Praxis, 5. Aufl., Bde 4-6 (Drogen), Springer Verlag Berlin, Heidelberg, New York, 1992-1994 (unter Abelmoschus moschatus).

Myosotis arvensis

See Forget-Me-Not

Myrica cerifera

See Southern Bayberry

Myrica gale

See Sweet Gale

Myristica fragrans

See Nutmeg

Myroxylon balsamum

See Tolu Balsam

Myrrh

Commiphora molmol

TRADE NAMES

Myrrh is sold as Myrrh Commiphora, Myrrh Gum, Guggal Resin, Wild Countryside Myrrh Gum (available from numerous manufacturers).

DESCRIPTION

Medicinal Parts: The resin, which has exuded from the bark and dried in the air, is the medicinal part. Myrrh is the pale yellow granular secretion that is discharged into cavities in the bark when it is wounded. The exudate hardens to a red-brown mass about the size of a walnut.

Flower and Fruit: The yellowish-red inflorescences are panicled. The fruit is brown, about 7 mm long, ovate and acuminate.

Leaves, Stem and Root: Commiphora molmol is a thorny shrub or small tree up 3 m high. It has a thick trunk and numerous irregular knotted branches and smaller clustered branchlets. A few trifoliate leaves grow at the end of short branches, with very small lateral leaflets dentate only at the tip. The terminal leaflet is 1 cm long, obovate and glabrous. The oleo-gum resin exudes from fissures or incisions in the bark and is collected as irregular masses or tears, varying in color from yellowish to reddish-brown, often with white patches.

Characteristics: The surface may be oily or covered with fine dust. The taste is bitter and acrid. The odor is aromatic.

Habitat: The plant is indigenous to eastern Mediterranean countries, Somalia, Ethiopia, Eritrea, Yemen and South Arabia.

Production: Myrrh is collected in the wild from June to August and consists of oleo-gum resin exuded from the stems of Commiphora molmol after incisions have been made in the bark. It is then air-dried. Myrrh can also originate from other Commiphora species if the chemical composition is comparable to the official drug.

Not to be Confused With: Some confusion can arise with ''False myrrh'' or Commiphora mukul.

Other Names: Guggal Gum, Guggal Resin, Didin, Didthin

ACTIONS AND PHARMACOLOGY

COMPOUNDS

Volatile oil (2-10%): chief components are sesquiterpenes including, among others, delta-elemene, beta-eudesmol, alpha-copaene and furosesquiterpenes, especially 5-acetoxy-2-methoxy-4,5-dienone (aroma-bearer), furanoeudesma-1,3-dien, isofuranogermacren (curzeren), curzenenone, 2-methoxy-furanoguaia-9-ene

Triterpenes (30-50%): including 3-epi-alpha-amyrin, alpha-amyrenone

Mucilages (30-60%): chiefly methyl-glucurono-galactans)

EFFECTS

Myrrh has a local astringent, disinfectant and granulation-promoting effect because of its essential oil (consisting mainly of sesquiterpenes) and amaroids.

INDICATIONS AND USAGE

Approved by Commission E:

- Inflammation of the mouth and pharynx

Unproven Uses: Myrrh is used for the topical treatment of mild inflammations of the oral and pharyngeal mucosa. In folk medicine, Myrrh is occasionally used internally as a carminative for non-specific intestinal infections and also as an expectorant for coughs. Folk medicine uses have also included stimulating the appetite and the flow of digestive juices.

Chinese Medicine: Uses include carbuncles, furuncles, wounds (as a styptic), amenorrhea and abdominal tumors.

Indian Medicine: Among uses in Indian medicine are menstrual disorders, stomach complaints, wounds, ulcers and inflammations of the skin and mouth.

CONTRAINDICATIONS

Use of myrrh is contraindicated during pregnancy.

PRECAUTIONS AND ADVERSE REACTIONS

No health hazards or side effects are known in conjunction with the proper administration of designated therapeutic dosages.

DOSAGE

Mode of Administration: Powdered resin, myrrh tincture and other galenic preparations for topical use.

How Supplied:

Capsules — 657 mg

Dental powders — 10% powdered resin

Liquid — 1:1 (Myrrh gum)

Oil — 100% (Myrrh commiphora)

Preparation: Prepare 1:5 tincture using 90% ethanol (V/V) in accordance with DAB10.

Daily Dosage: Myrrh tincture: Paint an undiluted tincture (1:5) on 2 to 3 times daily for external applications. As a rinse, use 5 to 10 drops in a glass of water; as a gargle, 30 to 60 drops in a glass of water. In dental powders: 10% of powdered resin.

Storage: The herb and its preparations should be stored in sealed containers that protect them from light and moisture. A desiccant should be present because the carbohydrate component of the drug readily absorbs water. For this reason, powdered forms should not be stored.

LITERATURE

Arora RB et al., (1972) Ind J Med Res 60(6):929.

Bajaj AC, Dev S, (1982) Tetrahedron 38(19):2949.

Brieskorn CH, (1980) Tetrahedron Lett 21(6):1511.

Brieskorn CH et al., (1983) Phytochemistry 22:187 et 1207.

Delaveau P et al., (1980) Planta Med 40:49.

Kodama M et al., (1975) Tetrahedron Lett 35:3065.

Malhotra SC, Ahuja MMS, (1971) Ind J Med Res 59(10):1621.

Mester L et al., (1979) Planta Med 37(4):367.

Mincione E, Iavarone C, (1972) Chim Ind 54:424 and 525.

Pernet R, (1972) Lloydia 35:280.

Ruecker G, (1972) Arch Pharm 305(7):486.

Srivastava M et al., (1984) J Biosci 6(3):277.

Tripathi SN et al., (1975) Ind. J Exp Biol 13(1):15.

Wiendl RM, Franz G, Myrrhe. Neue Chemie einer alten Droge. In: DAZ 134(1):25. 1994.

Wylegalla R, Biblische Botanik: Pflanzen und Früchte aus dem gelobten Land. In: DAZ 137(11):867-869. 1997.

Further information in:

Hänsel R, Keller K, Rimpler H, Schneider G (Hrsg.), Hagers Handbuch der Pharmazeutischen Praxis, 5. Aufl., Bde 4-6 (Drogen), Springer Verlag Berlin, Heidelberg, New York, 1992-1994.

Leung AY, Encyclopedia of Common Natural Ingredients Used in Food, Drugs and Cosmetics, John Wiley & Sons Inc., New York 1980.

Madaus G, Lehrbuch der Biologischen Arzneimittel, Bde 1-3, Nachdruck, Georg Olms Verlag Hildesheim 1979.

Steinegger E, Hänsel R, Pharmakognosie, 5. Aufl., Springer Verlag Heidelberg 1992.

Teuscher E, Biogene Arzneimittel, 5. Aufl., Wiss. Verlagsges. Stuttgart 1997.

Wichtl M (Hrsg.), Teedrogen, 4. Aufl., Wiss. Verlagsges. Stuttgart 1997.

Myrrhis odorata

See Sweet Cicely

Myrtle

Myrtus communis

DESCRIPTION

Medicinal Parts: The medicinal parts are the leaves (dried and as a source of oil), twigs and the fresh, flowering branches.

Flower and Fruit: The flowers are medium-sized and stiff. They are short, glandular-haired pedicles, which are covered in bracteoles. They grow solitary in the leaf axils. The petals are white with fine glands and a somewhat tomentose margin covered with fine hairs. The anthers are yellow. The berries are pea-sized, orbicular or ovoid-ellipsoid, blue-black or white. They are crowned by the calyx.

Leaves, Stem and Root: Myrtle is an evergreen, bushy shrub or a small tree growing up to 5 m high with opposite branches and quadrangular cane-shaped, initially delicately glandular, downy branches. The dark green leaves are glossy, glabrous, coriaceous, opposite-paired or whorled, ovate to lanceolate, entire-margined, acuminate and 1-3 cm long.

Characteristics: The berries have a sweet-spicy taste.

Habitat: Myrtle grows from the Mediterranean region to the northwestern Himalayas.

Production: Myrtle leaves are the dried leaves of Myrtus communis. Myrtle oil is the essential oil of Myrtus communis, which is extracted from the leaves and branches through steam distillation. (The percentage extracted ranges from 0.1 to 0.5%.) May and June are the best months for harvesting, since the plant has the highest concentration of essential oil during this period.

Not to be Confused With: Confusion can arise with the leaves of Bux semper-virens and Vaccinium vitisidaea, which resemble Myrtle.

ACTIONS AND PHARMACOLOGY

COMPOUNDS: MYRTLE OIL

Chief components: 1,8-cineol (15-45%), alpha-pinene (15-38%), myrtenol (1-5%), myrtenylacetate (4-20%), limonene (4-10%), alpha-terpineol (2-12%), geraniol (0.5-1.5%), geranylacetate (1-5%), myrtol (a myrtle oil fraction that boils between 160-180°C, chief components 1.8-cineole and alpha-pinene)

EFFECTS: MYRTLE OIL

The oil's mono- and sesquiterterpenes display antibacterial, fungicidal and disinfectant activity.

COMPOUNDS: MYRTLE LEAVES

Volatile oil (0.1-0.5%): (see Myrtle Oil compounds listing above for composition)

Tannins (gallotannins, condensed tannins)

Acylphloroglucinols: myrtocommulon A and B

EFFECTS: MYRTLE LEAVES

The leaves, which contain essential oil and tannins, display antimicrobial activity. An antiademic and hypoglycemic effect was demonstrated in animal experiments. An effect on the central nervous system (an increase in the duration of sleep) was also proven. The efficacy in cold infections may be attributable to the deodorizing and bronchosecretolytic effect of the essential oil.

INDICATIONS AND USAGE

MYRTLE OIL

Unproven Uses: Myrtle oil is used internally in folk medicine for acute and chronic infections of the respiratory tract such as bronchitis, whooping cough, tuberculosis of the lung, as well as for bladder conditions, diarrhea, hemorrhoids, prostatitis and worm infestation. It is sometimes used as a substitute for Buchu.

MYRTLE LEAVES

Unproven Uses: Folk medicine internal uses include diarrhea, hemorrhoids, prostatitis, bronchitis, sinusitis, tuberculosis and colds. Among external uses are ear infections, tired limbs, fatigue and leukorrhea. External applications include ear infections, tired limbs, and leukorrhea.

CONTRAINDICATIONS

No internal administration of the drug should take place in the presence of inflammatory illnesses of the gastrointestinal area or of the biliary ducts, or in the case of severe liver diseases.

PRECAUTIONS AND ADVERSE REACTIONS

General: No health hazards or side effects are known in conjunction with the proper administration of designated therapeutic dosages. In rare cases, the internal administration of Myrtle oil as a drug leads to nausea, vomiting and diarrhea.

Pediatric Use: Preparations containing the oil should not be applied to the faces of infants or small children because of the possibility of triggering glottal spasm, bronchial spasm, asthma-like attacks or even respiratory failure.

OVERDOSAGE

Overdoses of Myrtle oil (more than 10 g) can lead to life-threatening poisoning, due to the high cineole content. Symptoms include, among others, a decrease in or loss of blood pressure, circulatory disorders, collapse and respiratory failure. Do not induce vomiting if poisoning occurs, because of the danger of aspiration. Following administration of activated charcoal, the therapy for poisonings consists of treating spasms with diazepam (i.v.); treating colic with atropine; and providing electrolyte substitution. Treat possible cases of acidosis with sodium bicarbonate infusions. Intubation and oxygen respiration may also be necessary.

DOSAGE

MYRTLE OIL

Mode of Administration: Myrtle is available in various medicinal/pharmaceutical preparations for internal use.

Preparation: Prepare an infusion by mixing 15 to 30 g of the drug with 1 L water and leave to draw for 15 minutes.

Daily Dosage: Single dose: 0.2 g of drug to be taken internally.

Storage: Protect from light and keep tightly sealed.

MYRTLE LEAVES

Preparation: Prepare an infusion by mixing 15 to 30 g of the drug with 1 L water and leave to draw for 15 minutes. A wash is prepared by adding 30 g of leaves to 1 L of water and letting it stand.

Daily Dosage: The average daily dosage of powder from the leaves is 5 g taken before meals. 3 cups of an infusion may be taken each day. Washes may be used several times daily.

Storage: Store the leaves in a tightly sealed container that blocks exposure to light.

LITERATURE

Hänsel R, Keller K, Rimpler H, Schneider G (Hrsg.), Hagers Handbuch der Pharmazeutischen Praxis, 5. Aufl., Bde 4-6 (Drogen), Springer Verlag Berlin, Heidelberg, New York, 1992-1994.

Joseph MI et al., (1987) Pharmazie 42 (2):142.

Lawrence BM, Perfumer Flavorist 15:65-66. 1990.

Madaus G, Lehrbuch der Biologischen Arzneimittel, Bde 1-3, Nachdruck, Georg Olms Verlag Hildesheim 1979.

Morton JF, An Atlas of Medicinal Plants of Middle America, Charles C Thomas USA 1981.

Peyron L, Plantes Méd Phytothér 4:279-285. 1970.

Roth L, Daunderer M, Kormann K, Giftpflanzen, Pflanzengifte, 4. Aufl., Ecomed Fachverlag Landsberg Lech 1993.

Steinegger E, Hänsel R, Pharmakognosie, 5. Aufl., Springer Verlag Heidelberg 1992.

Wagner H, Wiesenauer M, Phytotherapie. Phytopharmaka und pflanzliche Homöopathika, Fischer-Verlag, Stuttgart, Jena, New York 1995.

Myrtus communis

See Myrtle

Narcissus pseudonarcissus

See Daffodil

Nardostachys jatamansi

See Jatamansi

Nasturtium

Tropaeolum majus

DESCRIPTION

Medicinal Parts: The medicinal parts are the fresh herb, the whole fresh flowering plant and the seeds.

Flower and Fruit: The handsome campanulate flowers are orange with flame-red to fiery red stripes. The calyx is bilabiate, colored and has a spurred upper lip. There are 5 uneven petals. The 2 upper petals are unstemmed, the 3 lower ones are stemmed and fringed at the base. There are 8 stamens and a superior ovary with a 3-stigmaed style. The fruit is a 3-valved pericarp. It is orbicular-reniform, fleshy, wrinkled when ripe and dirty yellow.

Leaves, Stem and Root: The plant is an annual, sometimes perennial and often creeping or climbing plant, 0.3 to 5 m long. The main root is thin and forms an underground runner. The stem is round, branched, fleshy and glabrous, like the whole plant. The leaves are alternate, long-petioled, hastate and almost circular. The leaves are 3 to 5 cm and deeply lobed at the petiole.

Characteristics: The flowers are fragrant and the leafy parts smell and taste like cress.

Habitat: The plant is indigenous to warmer regions of South America and is becoming naturalized in the Mediterranean region, otherwise found as a garden or ornamental plant.

Production: Garden Nasturtium consists of the aerial parts, the seeds or leaves of Tropaeolum majus.

Other Names: Indian Cress

ACTIONS AND PHARMACOLOGY

COMPOUNDS

Glucosinolates (0.1%): in the fresh, unbruised plant: chief components are glucotropaeolin, yielding benzyl isothiocyanate after cell destruction

Ascorbic acid (vitamin C, 300 mg/100 gm fresh weight)

Cucurbitacins (in the fruits): including cucurbitacins B and E

Fatty oil (in the seeds, 7.5%): chief fatty acids erucic acid (50%), 11-cis-eiconsenic acid (25%), oleic acid (12%)

Oxalates

Flavonoids: including among others, isoquercetin and quercetin glycosides

Carotinoids (as blossom pigments): lutein, zeaxanthine

EFFECTS

Benzyl mustard oil extracted from Nasturtium is bacteriostatic, virostatic, and antimycotic in vitro. Mustard oils are eliminated mainly via the breath or are collected and eliminated in the urine; used externally, Nasturtium is a rubefacient.

INDICATIONS AND USAGE

Approved by Commission E:

- Infections of the urinary tract
- Cough
- Bronchitis

Unproven Uses: Nastertium is used internally for infections of the urinary tract and catarrh of the upper respiratory tract. It is also used internally for mild muscular pain, skin diseases, scurvy, tuberculosis, conditions of the respiratory and urinary tracts, and menstrual disorders. The herb is used externally for hair loss and for infected and poorly healing wounds.

CONTRAINDICATIONS

Do not administer to patients with gastrointestinal ulcers or kidney diseases.

Do not administer to infants or small children.

PRECAUTIONS AND ADVERSE REACTIONS

General: No health hazards or side effects are known in conjunction with the proper administration of designated therapeutic dosages. Administration of higher dosages of the fresh plant or of its volatile oil can lead to mucous membrane irritation of the gastrointestinal tract. External administration involving long-term intensive contact with the fresh plant can lead to skin irritations. The plant possesses a low potential for sensitization.

Pediatric Use: Not to be administered to infants or small children.

DOSAGE

Mode of Administration: The cut drug is available in the form of coated and filmed tablets and compound preparations.

Preparation: To make an infusion, add 30 gm of leaves to 1 liter of water.

Daily Dosage: The dose for the extract is 14.4 mg of benzylisothiocyanate taken 3 times daily. The dose for the infusion is 2 to 3 cups per day; for the pressed juice, 30 gm per day.

LITERATURE

Franz G, Kapuzinerkresse (Tropaeolum majus L.) Portrait einer Arzneipflanze. In: ZPT 17(4):255-622. 1996.

Frohne D, Pfänder HJ, Giftpflanzen - Ein Handbuch für Apotheker, Toxikologen und Biologen, 4. Aufl., Wiss. Verlags-Ges. Stuttgart 1997.

Hänsel R, Keller K, Rimpler H, Schneider G (Hrsg.), Hagers Handbuch der Pharmazeutischen Praxis, 5. Aufl., Bde 4-6 (Drogen): Springer Verlag Berlin, Heidelberg, New York, 1992-1994.

Madaus G, Lehrbuch der Biologischen Arzneimittel, Bde 1-3, Nachdruck, Georg Olms Verlag Hildesheim 1979.

Pintao AM et al., In vitro and in vivo antitumor activity of benzyl isothiocyanate: a natural product from Tropaeolum majus. In: PH 61(3):233-236. 1995.

Roth L, Daunderer M, Kormann K, Giftpflanzen, Pflanzengifte, 4. Aufl., Ecomed Fachverlag Landsberg Lech 1993.

Steinegger E, Hänsel R, Pharmakognosie, 5. Aufl., Springer Verlag Heidelberg 1992.

Teuscher E, Lindequist U, Biogene Gifte - Biologie, Chemie, Pharmakologie, 2. Aufl., Fischer Verlag Stuttgart 1994.

Wagner H, Wiesenauer M, Phytotherapie. Phytopharmaka und pflanzliche Homöopathika, Fischer-Verlag, Stuttgart, Jena, New York 1995.

Wichtl M (Hrsg.), Teedrogen, 4. Aufl., Wiss. Verlagsges. Stuttgart 1997.

Nasturtium officinale

See Watercress

Neem

Antelaea azadirachta

TRADE NAMES

Neem (available from numerous manufacturers)

DESCRIPTION

Medicinal Parts: The medicinal parts of the plant are the bark, the leaves, the branches, the seeds and the latex.

Flower and Fruit: The plant has small white flowers.

Leaves, Stem and Root: Antelaea azadirachta is a deciduous tree up to 16 m high with leaves that are compound, alternate, oblong, ovate-lanceolate and pointed. The bark is grayish-brown, externally fissured, and has a buff inner surface and fibrous fracture.

Characteristics: The plant has no odor; the taste is bitter.

Habitat: Indigenous to the woods of India and Sri Lanka. Found today in other tropical regions such as Indonesia, Australia and western Africa.

Production: Neem tree bark, leaves and seeds are the trunk and branch bark, leaves and seeds of Azadirachta indica or of the closely related variety (in the literature often given as a synonym) of Melia azedarach.

Other Names: Azedarach, Holy Tree, Nim

ACTIONS AND PHARMACOLOGY

COMPOUNDS: NEEM SEED OIL

Triterpenes and tetranortriterpenes (limonoids and protolimonoids of the gedunin-group): for example nimbolin A and B, nimbin, gedunin

COMPOUNDS: NEEM BARK AND LEAVES

Tannin

Volatile oil

EFFECTS

Azadirachta indica has anti-inflammatory and antipyretic properties. Melia azedarach has an anthelmintic effect.

INDICATIONS AND USAGE

Unproven Uses: Azadirachta indica is used in inflammatory and febrile diseases (including malaria, although unconfirmed). Melia azedarach is used for worm infestation.

Indian Medicine: Antelaea azadirachta is used for inflammatory and febrile diseases (including malaria and leprosy, although unconfirmed), dyspeptic complaints and worm infestation.

PRECAUTIONS AND ADVERSE REACTIONS

No health hazards or side effects are known in conjunction with the proper administration of designated therapeutic dosages.

DOSAGE

Mode of Administration: The drug is available as a tincture. A slightly narcotic decoction can be prepared (said to lower a fever). An ointment for killing lice is administered topically.

How Supplied:
Capsules — 475 mg

LITERATURE

Adnrei GM et al., (1986) Experientia 42 (7):843.

Anon Pat. Appl 83/234, 294 Japan 1983.

Bray DH et al., (1985) Trans Royal Soc Trop Med Hyg 79: 426.

Ekong DEU, (1967) Chem Comm 808.

Ekong DEU, Ibiyemi SA, (1971) Chem Comm: 1177.

El Said et al., (1968), Study of certain Nigerian plants used in Fever. Communication at the Inter-Africa Symposium Dakar.

Garg GP, Nigam SK, Ogle CW, The gastric antiulcer effects of the leaves of Neem tree. In: PM 59(3):215. 1993.

Godvindachari T et al., JNP 55:596-601. 1992.

Kraus W, Bokel M, (1981) Chemische Berichte 114:267.

Lavie D, Levy EC, (1969) Tetrahedron Letters 3525.

Okpanyi SN, Ezenkwu GC, (1981) Planta Med 41:34.

Pat. Appl 83/234, 294 Japan (1983).

Rojatkar SR et al., 1-Tigloyl-3-acteyl-11-hydroxy-4β-methylmeliacarpin from Azadirachta indica. In: PH 32:213. 1993.

Rücker G, Malariawirksame Verbindungen aus Pflanzen, insbesondere Peroxide. In: PUZ 24(4):189-195. 1995.

Siidiqui S et al., JNP 55:303-310. 1992.

Further information in:

Hänsel R, Keller K, Rimpler H, Schneider G (Hrsg.), Hagers Handbuch der Pharmazeutischen Praxis, 5. Aufl., Bde 4-6 (Drogen), Springer Verlag Berlin, Heidelberg, New York, 1992-1994.

Kern W, List PH, Hörhammer L (Hrsg.), Hagers Handbuch der Pharmazeutischen Praxis, 4. Aufl., Bde. 1-8, Springer Verlag Berlin, Heidelberg, New York, 1969.

Lewin L, Gifte und Vergiftungen, 6. Aufl., Nachdruck, Haug Verlag, Heidelberg 1992.

Madaus G, Lehrbuch der Biologischen Arzneimittel, Bde 1-3, Nachdruck, Georg Olms Verlag Hildesheim 1979.

Oliver-Bever B (Ed.), Medicinal Plants of Tropical West Africa, Cambridge University Press Cambridge, London 1986.

Nelumbo nucifera

See Lotus

Nepalese Cardamom

Amomum aromaticum

DESCRIPTION

Medicinal Parts: The medicinal parts of the plant are the bark and fruit.

Flower and Fruit: The flowers are arranged in globose, 4 cm long spikes with single flowers in the axils of the scale-like, stem-clasping bracts. The inner flower bracts are elongate, ribbed and thorn-tipped. The flowers are pale yellow with a tubular, 3-toothed calyx. The corolla petals are tubular. The flower tube is approximately 2.5 cm long. The petals are 2.5 cm long, lanceolate, blunt and somewhat cap-shaped. The lip is twice as long as the petals. The lip is round with a cuneiform base and single stamen. The fruit is 3-chambered and narrow ovoid in shape. It is approximately 3 cm long and has numerous 3 mm long seeds in each chamber.

Leaves, Stem and Root: Amomum aromaticum is a herbaceous perennial, which grows up to 1 m high. The leaves are lanceolate, up to 25 cm long and 6 cm wide. They are pubescent beneath, with a 2 mm long ligule. The rhizome is up to 5 m long with shoots growing in clusters from it.

Habitat: India

Production: The ripe fruit is harvested in autumn and dried in the sun at low temperatures. Nepalese cardamoms are the dried, ripe fruit of Amomum aromaticum.

Not to be Confused With: Amomum aromaticum may be confused with Amomum subulatum.

ACTIONS AND PHARMACOLOGY

COMPOUNDS

Volatile oil (1%): chief constituent 1.8-cineole, including as well, alpha- and beta-pinene, limonene, myrcene, terpinene, p-cymol, terpineol, nerolidol, 1H-indene-2,3-dihydro-5-carboxyl aldehyde

EFFECTS

The efficacy of the drug in the context of folk medicine is believed to be traceable to the cineole contained in the essential oil, although scientific data regarding this are not available.

INDICATIONS AND USAGE

Chinese Medicine: Nepalese cardamom is used for malaria, diarrhea, vomiting and digestive disturbances.

PRECAUTIONS AND ADVERSE REACTIONS

No health hazards are known in conjunction with the proper administration of designated therapeutic dosages.

OVERDOSAGE

Overdoses of the essential oil can lead to life-threatening poisoning, due to the high levels of cineole. Symptoms include reduced blood pressure, circulatory disorders, circulary collapse and asphyxiation. Vomiting is not to be induced in the case of poisoning, due to the danger of aspiration.

Following instillation of activated charcoal, the therapy for poisoning consists of the treatment of spasms with diazepam, of colic with atropine, electrolyte substitution and the countering of any acidosis that may appear with sodium bicarbonate infusions. Intubation and oxygen respiration may also be required.

DOSAGE

Mode of Administration: Whole herb, cut drug and liquid preparations for internal use.

Daily Dosage: As decoction 3-6 gm.

Storage: Should be protected from light and moisture.

LITERATURE

Hänsel R, Keller K, Rimpler H, Schneider G (Ed), Hagers Handbuch der Pharmazeutischen Praxis, 5. Aufl., Bde 4 - 6 (Drogen), Springer Verlag Berlin, Heidelberg, New York, 1992-1994.

Nepeta cataria

See Catnip

Nerium oleander

See Oleander

Nerve Root

Cypripedium calceolus

DESCRIPTION

Medicinal Parts: The medicinal parts are the dried rhizome with the roots, the fresh underground parts harvested in autumn and the fresh roots. The roots of several varieties are used as a sedative and antispasmodic.

Flower and Fruit: The plant develops terminal inflorescences with 1 to 2 flowers that have leaf-like bracts. The flowers are 4 to 9 cm long by 0.5 to 1 cm wide. They are linear-lanceolate and twisted. The petals are green, green-brown or yellow. The petals, including the protruding lip or shoe, are splayed. The shoe is 3 to 4 cm long in the shape of an inflated sack. It is lemon yellow to gold with purple spots and veins. The pollen is powdery. The pollen seeds are in 4 groups. The ovary is single-valved and pubescent.

Leaves, Stem and Root: Nerve Root is a perennial, 15 to 70 cm high. The plant has a horizontal rootstock with scales and thick root fibers. The stem is round with short hairs, and is covered at the base with scaly brown leaves. There are 3 to 4 leaves above these, which are broad, elliptical, sheath-like, folded and acute. The upper surface is bright green, the underside is paler.

Characteristics: The plant has a faintly gentian-like smell and has an irritating effect on the skin.

Habitat: Indigenous to the U.S. and Canada, cultivated in Europe.

Production: Lady's Slipper rhizome is the rhizome of Cypripedium calceolus.

Not to be Confused With: Other Cypripedium varieties

Other Names: Lady's Slipper, American Valerian, Bleeding Heart, Moccasin Flower, Monkey Flower, Noah's Ark, Slipper Root, Venus Shoe, Yellows

ACTIONS AND PHARMACOLOGY

COMPOUNDS

Volatile oil

Phenanthrene quinones: including cypripedine (2,8-dimethoxy-7-hydroxy-1,4-phenanthrene quinone

Tannins

EFFECTS

The constituents of the drug have not been investigated. Some species of Cypripedium contain allergens and skin-irritating phenanthrene quinones. Nerve Root is astringent and hemostyptic. No additional information is available.

INDICATIONS AND USAGE

Unproven Uses: In folk medicine, the drug is used for insomnia, emotional tension, states of agitation, nervousness and hysteria. It is also used internally in the treatment of menorrhagia and diarrhea, as well as externally in the treatment of pruritus vulvae.

PRECAUTIONS AND ADVERSE REACTIONS

Health risks or side effects following the proper administration of designated therapeutic dosages are not recorded. The plant possesses a medium potential for sensitization through skin contact.

DOSAGE

Mode of Administration: The drug is administered in its dry form or as liquid extract. The supply of higher (concentrated) doses should be avoided.

Preparation: Liquid extract: 1:1 in 45% alcohol.

Daily Dosage: To be taken internally, 2 teaspoonfuls (2 to 4 gm) of the dried drug as an infusion.

LITERATURE

Hänsel R, Keller K, Rimpler H, Schneider G (Hrsg.), Hagers Handbuch der Pharmazeutischen Praxis, 5. Aufl., Bde 4-6 (Drogen), Springer Verlag Berlin, Heidelberg, New York, 1992-1994.

Hausen B, Allergiepflanzen, Pflanzenallergene, ecomed Verlagsgesellsch. mbH, Landsberg 1988.

Madaus G, Lehrbuch der Biologischen Arzneimittel, Bde 1-3, Nachdruck, Georg Olms Verlag Hildesheim 1979.

Schmalle HW, Hausen BM, Naturwissenschaften: 66:527. 1979.

New Jersey Tea

Ceanothus americanus

DESCRIPTION

Medicinal Parts: The medicinal parts are the dried leaves, the dried root bark and the fresh leaves.

Flower and Fruit: The inflorescences grow in the axils of the upper leaves and have long peduncles. They are 5 to 15 cm long, panicled, and have numerous cyme-like partial inflorescences. The flowers are white, the petals are 2 to 3 mm long and twice as long as the sepals. The fruit is a globose capsule with a diameter of about 7 mm.

Leaves, Stem and Root: Ceanothus americanus is a low deciduous shrub 40 to 100 cm high with greenish-purple branches. The petioled leaves are alternate, 3 to 10 cm long by 1.5 to 5 cm wide, ovate or oblong-ovate, rounded at the base, lightly pointed at the tip, and with pinnatifid nerves. The upper surface is glabrous or has finely compressed silky hairs. The lower surface is densely gray and pubescent. The leaf blade is finely and irregularly serrated. The root is tough, woody, dark brown, and striated or finely wrinkled longitudinally. The bark is thin, brittle and dark brown.

Characteristics: The taste is astringent; odorless.

Habitat: Indigenous to eastern and central North America. It is also used for breeding garden hybrids.

Production: Red Root is the root of Ceanothus americanus. The shrub is cultivated.

Other Names: Red Root, Wild Snowball, Jersey Tea, Mountain-Sweet, Walpole Tea, Redroot

ACTIONS AND PHARMACOLOGY

COMPOUNDS

Cyclic peptide alkaloids (0.16% in the root cortex): including ceanothines A to E, americine, adouetines X and Y cyclic peptines

Triterpenes: including ceanothusic acid, ceanothenic acid, and betulic acid

EFFECTS

The tannins have an astringent effect. In blood taken from young rats, an aqueous-ethanol extract of the drug reduced blood-clotting time by 25%. However, the results are difficult to assess. The hemostyptic effect is attributed to the acid fraction of the drug. The drug is still useful as an astringent, expectorant and antispasmodic. There is no valid data on the expectorant and antispasmodic effect.

INDICATIONS AND USAGE

Unproven Uses: Formerly, New Jersey Tea was used as an astringent, in the clotting of the blood, for fever, gonorrhea, syphilis, and for colds and chills, especially of the respiratory organs.

Homeopathic Uses: In homeopathy, Ceanothus americanus is used to treat enlarged spleen.

PRECAUTIONS AND ADVERSE REACTIONS

No health hazards or side effects are known in conjunction with the proper administration of designated therapeutic dosages.

DOSAGE

Mode of Administration: Orally as a liquid extract.

Homeopathic Dosage: 5 drops, 1 tablet or 10 globules every 30 to 60 minutes (acute) or 1 to 3 times daily (chronic); parenterally: 1 to 2 ml sc 3 times daily (HAB1).

LITERATURE

Hänsel R, Keller K, Rimpler H, Schneider G (Hrsg.), Hagers Handbuch der Pharmazeutischen Praxis, 5. Aufl., Bde 4-6 (Drogen), Springer Verlag Berlin, Heidelberg, New York, 1992-1994.

Lagarias JC et al., (1979) J Nat Prod 42:220 et 663

Mayo de P, Starratt AN, Canad J Chem 40:1632-1641. 1962.

Servis RE et al., J Am Chem Soc 91:5619-5624. 1969.

Niauli

Melaleucaea viridiflora

DESCRIPTION

Medicinal Parts: The medicinal parts are the young or shrubby plants and the oil, which is distilled from the fresh leaves and twigs.

Flower and Fruit: The plant grows up to 15 m.

Characteristics: The presence of traces of copper in the Niauli oil make it slightly greenish. The aromatic odor is reminiscent of camphor.

Habitat: The plant grows in tropical parts of southeast Asia and Australia.

Production: Niauli oil consists of the essential oil from the leaves of Melaleucaea viridiflora, obtained by water distillation.

ACTIONS AND PHARMACOLOGY

COMPOUNDS

Chief components: 1,8-cineole (up to 40%), viridiflorol (up to 25%), nerolidol (up to 95%), linalool (up to 30%), (+)-alpha-terpineol and (-)-alpha-terpineol as well as their valeric acid esters, alpha-pinene, limonene

EFFECTS

The drug is antibacterial and stimulates circulation.

INDICATIONS AND USAGE

Approved by Commission E:

■ Cough/bronchitis

Unproven Uses: Niauli is used for catarrhs of the upper respiratory tract, rheumatism, neuralgia, cystitis.

CONTRAINDICATIONS

Contraindications to internal use include inflammatory illnesses of the gastrointestinal area or of the biliary ducts, and severe liver diseases.

PRECAUTIONS AND ADVERSE REACTIONS

General: No health hazards or side effects are known in conjunction with the proper administration of designated therapeutic dosages. The internal administration of Niauli oil as a drug leads, in rare cases, to nausea, vomiting and diarrhea.

Drug Interactions: Niauli oil contains 35-60% cineole. Cineole causes the induction of the enzymes involved in the detoxification of the liver. The effect of other drugs can therefore be reduced and/or shortened.

Pediatric Use: Preparations containing the oil should not be applied to the faces of infants or small children, since glottal spasm, bronchial spasm and asthma-like attacks are possible, as is respiratory failure.

OVERDOSAGE

Overdosages of Niauli oil (more than 10 gm), can lead to life-threatening poisonings due to the high cineole content. Symptoms include, among others, fall in blood pressure, circulatory disorders, collapse and respiratory failure. In case of poisoning, vomiting should not be induced because of the danger of aspiration. Following administration of activated charcoal, the therapy for poisonings consists of treating spasms with diazepam (i.v.), treating colics with atropine, electrolyte substitution and treating possible cases of acidosis with sodium bicarbonate infusions. Intubation and oxygen respiration may also be necessary.

DOSAGE

Mode of Administration: The oil and other galenic preparations are for internal and external application.

Preparation: Oily nose drops are prepared in a 2 to 5% concentration in vegetable oil. For external use, preparations contain 10 to 30% active ingredient in oil.

Daily Dosage: For internal use, the single dose is 0.2 gm, with the daily dosage ranging from 0.2 to 2.0 gm.

LITERATURE

Kern W, List PH, Hörhammer L (Hrsg.), Hagers Handbuch der Pharmazeutischen Praxis, 4. Aufl., Bde. 1-8, Springer Verlag Berlin, Heidelberg, New York, 1969.

Steinegger E, Hänsel R, Pharmakognosie, 5. Aufl., Springer Verlag Heidelberg 1992.

Teuscher E, Biogene Arzneimittel, 5. Aufl., Wiss. Verlagsges. Stuttgart 1997.

Nicotiana tabacum

See Tobacco

Night-Blooming Cereus

Selenicereus grandiflorus

DESCRIPTION

Medicinal Parts: The medicinal parts are the fresh or dried flowers, the fresh young stems and flowers, and the fresh young shoots and sprouts.

Flower and Fruit: The flowers are 18 to 25 cm long and have a diameter of 15 to 27 cm. They have numerous, long-acute, lanceolate tepals that are arranged in a spiral. The outer tepals are brown; the middle ones are light yellow and the inner ones are spatulate to acute, lanceolate and snow white. The numerous stamens are white and have yellow anthers. The styles with the 4-rayed stigmas become yellow toward the top. The ovary is globular and bumpy, with triangular scales and many brownish-gray hairs and thorns, which are approximately 10 mm long, dark brown and bristly.

Leaves, Stem and Root: The plant has a succulent trunk as well as a 1 to 4 cm thick snake-like, creeping or climbing, branched stem, which can grow to 10 m long or longer. The stem is 4- to 8-sided, green to bluish, has no bumps and is covered in adventitious roots. It has white tomentose axis buds on the protruding vertical ribs with 6 to 11 needle-like thorns that are 4 to 6 mm long.

Characteristics: The plant has sweet-smelling flowers, which only bloom for about 6 hours before dying.

Habitat: The plant is indigenous to Central America and is cultivated in Mexico and also in Europe.

Production: The young shoots and flowers are harvested in June or July and then preserved in alcohol. Some cultivated production is done in greenhouse settings, particularly in Europe.

Not to be Confused With: Confusion can arise with the flowers of Opuntia maxima, Selenicereus hamatus, and Selenicereus pteranthus. The drug is adulterated commercially with the flowers of Opuntia vulgaris and Opuntia ficus-indica.

Other Names: Sweet-Scented Cactus

ACTIONS AND PHARMACOLOGY

COMPOUNDS

Flavonoids (1.5%): including among others, narcissin, rutin, cacticine, kaempferitine, grandiflorin, hyperoside

Amines: (found only in the shoots) chief components are hordenine (cactine), tyramine, N-methyltyramine, N,N-dimethyl tyramine

Betacyans: (in the blossoms, yellow pigments)

EFFECTS

The drug has an effect similar to digitalis, which includes cardiac stimulation as well as coronary and peripheral vessel dilation. The drug is also said to stimulate the motor neurons of the spinal cord. In addition, the drug may act topically as an antiphlogistic, but this is unproven.

INDICATIONS AND USAGE

Unproven Uses: Preparations of Selenicereus grandiflorus are used for nervous cardiac disorders, angina pectoris, stenocardia, and urinary ailments. In Mexico and Central America, folk medicine internal uses include hemoptysis, menorrhagia, dysmenorrhea, hemorrhage, cardiac complaints, cystitis, shortness of breath and dropsy. Externally, it also is used in these countries as a skin stimulant for rheumatism.

Homeopathic Uses: Night-Blooming Cereus is used to treat heart disease in homeopathy.

PRECAUTIONS AND ADVERSE REACTIONS

No health hazards or side effects are known in conjunction with the proper administration of designated therapeutic dosages. Intake of the fresh juice is said to cause itching and pustules on the skin, burning of the mouth, queasiness, vomiting and diarrhea.

DOSAGE

Mode of Administration: Fluid extracts and tinctures are used internally and externally.

Preparations: Fluid extract (Extractum Cerei liquidum 1:1); Tinctura Cerei (1:4) BPC 34; Tincture in sweetened water (1:10).

Daily Dosage: For the folk medicine dosages, a liquid extract is used in doses up to 0.6 ml, one to 10 times daily. The Tincture Cerei dosage is 0.12 to 2 ml taken 2 to 3 times daily. Dosage for the tincture in sweetened water is 10 drops, 3 to 5 times daily.

LITERATURE

Hänsel R, Keller K, Rimpler H, Schneider G (Hrsg.), Hagers Handbuch der Pharmazeutischen Praxis, 5. Aufl., Bde 4-6 (Drogen): Springer Verlag Berlin, Heidelberg, New York, 1992-1994.

Madaus G: Lehrbuch der Biologischen Arzneimittel, Bde 1-3, Nachdruck, Georg Olms Verlag Hildesheim 1979 (unter Cactus grandiflorus).

Roth L, Daunderer M, Kormann K, Giftpflanzen, Pflanzengifte, 4. Aufl., Ecomed Fachverlag Landsberg Lech 1993.

Wagner H, Wiesenauer M, Phytotherapie. Phytopharmaka und pflanzliche Homöopathika, Fischer-Verlag, Stuttgart, Jena, New York 1995.

Willaman JJ, Schubert BG (1961) Tech. Bull 1234: USDA Washington DC.

Noni

Morinda citrifolia

DESCRIPTION

Medicinal Parts: The medicinal parts of the plant are the leaf, fruit and root.

Flower and Fruit: The inflorescence is globose. The flowers are radial, their structures in fives with fused yellowish-white tepals. The ovary is inferior with 1 stigma. The fruit is a many-seeded, glassy-white berry the size of a chicken egg.

Leaves, Branches: Morinda citrifolia is a tree that is occasionally shrub-like. It grows up to 10 m high. The leaves are opposite, 10 to 30 cm long. The petiole is approximately 12 mm long. The lamina is coriaceous, glossy, elliptical to elliptical-ovate, acuminate, somewhat crenate and cuneiform at the base with stipules. The branches are square, divided jointed and contain nodes.

Characteristics: The fruit is inedible.

Habitat: Malaysia

Production: Noni fruit and leaves are the fresh ripe fruit and dried leaves of Morinda citrifolia.

Other Names: Mengkudu

ACTIONS AND PHARMACOLOGY

COMPOUNDS

Volatile oil

Iridoids: asperulosid, deacetylasperuloside

EFFECTS

No definitive data available.

INDICATIONS AND USAGE

Unproven Uses: Noni is used for diabetes, as a blood purifier (for women), for fever and stomachache (Malaysia).

PRECAUTIONS AND ADVERSE REACTIONS

No health hazards are known in conjunction with the proper administration of designated therapeutic dosages.

DOSAGE

Preparation: The dried leaves are used as hot compresses on the chest and stomach (for fever and stomachache).

LITERATURE

Hirazumi A, Furusawa E, Chou SC, Hokama Y, Immunomodulation contributes to the anticancer activity of morinda citrifolia (noni) fruit juice. Planta Med, 39:7-9, 1996.

Younos C, Rolland A, Fleurentin J, Lanhers MC, Misslin R, Mortier F, Analgesic and behavioral effects of Morinda citrifolia. Planta Med, 56:430-4, 1990 Oct.

Northern Prickly Ash

Zanthoxylum americanum

TRADE NAMES

Prickly Ash Autumn-Harvested

DESCRIPTION

Medicinal Parts: The medicinal parts are the root bark and the berries.

Flower and Fruit: The greenish-yellow flowers are in terminal umbels. The fruit is black or deep blue and enclosed in a gray shell.

Leaves, Stem and Root: The plant is an aromatic shrub or small tree up to 3 m tall. The branches are alternate and the leaves pinnatifid. The bark and the petioles are covered in sharp spines about 5 mm long. The bark is brownish-gray on the outside and faintly furrowed with whitish patches and flattened spines that are about 5 mm long.

Characteristics: The leaves and berries have an aromatic lemon-like fragrance, and the bark has a pungent, acrid taste.

Habitat: The plant grows in North America.

Other Names: Prickly Ash, Toothache Tree, Yellow Wood, Suterberry

ACTIONS AND PHARMACOLOGY

COMPOUNDS

Pyranocoumarins: xanthoxyletin (xanthoxyloin), xanthyletin, alloxanthyletin

Isoquinoline alkaloids: chelerythrine, berberine, N-methylisocorydine, laurifoline, magnoflorine, nitidine

Volatile oil

Resins

EFFECTS

No information is available.

INDICATIONS AND USAGE

Unproven Uses: Northern Prickly Ash is used for low blood pressure, rheumatic disorders, fever and inflammation.

Indian Medicine: The drug is used for toothache, headache, eye and ear conditions, dyspeptic symptoms, colic, flatulence, worm infestation, diarrhea, fever, coughs, asthma, paralyses and leprosy.

PRECAUTIONS AND ADVERSE REACTIONS

No health hazards or side effects are known in conjunction with the proper administration of designated therapeutic dosages.

OVERDOSAGE

Overdosage is said to lead to salivation, increased cardiac function and elevated blood pressure. Severe poisonings resulting from intake of the drug have not been recorded.

DOSAGE

Mode of Administration: Liquid extract, in preparations and in combinations.

How Supplied: Liquid extract—1:4

LITERATURE

Fish F et al., (1975) Lloydia 38:268.

Fish F, Waterman PG, (1973) J Pharm Pharmac. 25S, 115.

Kern W, List PH, Hörhammer L (Hrsg.), Hagers Handbuch der Pharmazeutischen Praxis, 4. Aufl., Bde 1-8: Springer Verlag Berlin, Heidelberg, New York, 1969.

Leung AY, Encyclopedia of Common Natural Ingredients Used in Food, Drugs, Cosmetics, John Wiley & Sons Inc., New York 1980.

Madaus G, Lehrbuch der Biologischen Arzneimittel, Bde 1-3, Nachdruck, Georg Olms Verlag Hildesheim 1979.

Oliver-Bever B (Ed.), Medicinal Plants of Tropical West Africa, Cambridge University Press, Cambrigde 1986.

Roth L, Daunderer M, Kormann K, Giftpflanzen, Pflanzengifte, 4. Aufl., Ecomed Fachverlag Landsberg Lech 1993.

Nutmeg

Myristica fragrans

DESCRIPTION

Medicinal Parts: The medicinal parts are the nutmeg seeds, which through various processes yield several therapeutic components. They include the essential oil of the seed; the compressed, dried aril; the mixture of fat, oil and color pigment from the pressed seeds; the dried seed kernels freed from the aril and shell of the nut; calcified seed kernels; and the dried seed kernels.

Flower and Fruit: Myristica fragans is either male or female, although there are male trees with female flowers and fruit. The flowers are unisexual. The male flowers are in sparsely flowered inflorescence; the female ones are solitary and inconspicuous. The flowers have a simple 3-lobed involucre; the filaments are fused to a tube. The fruit ripens 7 to 10 months after flowering. The fruit is fleshy, almost round, acuminate at the stem end, 3 to 6 cm long and 2.5 to 5 cm thick. The fruit is light yellow and about the size of a peach. The fruit flesh bursts open when ripe and exposes the bright red seed's aril that surrounds the dark brown seed. Within the aril, the seed kernel is covered in a hard brown testis that shows the marks of the aril.

Leaves, Stem and Root: Nutmeg is an evergreen tree up to 15 m in height. The smooth bark is green on the young branches, then turns grayish-brown. The alternate leaves are dark green, entire-margined, sharp edged, short-petioled, ovate-elliptical and up to 8 cm long.

Habitat: The plant is indigenous to the Molucca Islands and New Guinea and has spread to Indonesia, the West Indies and other tropical areas, where it also is cultivated.

Production: Nutmeg is the seed of Myristica fragrans. After harvesting, the nut is shelled and dried (maximum 45° C), and the seed is opened after 4 to 8 weeks. The lacy, fleshy covering of the nut, which is scarlet when fresh and dark orange when dried, yields Nutmeg and Mace. After being separated, both parts are dried slowly. The nut is ground and then distilled. Nutmeg butter is made by pressing and steaming the nuts to extract the fatty and essential oils from the seeds.

Not to be Confused With: Several other nuts are often given the name nutmeg. Confusion may occur with calabash nutmeg (Monodora myristica), Papua nutmeg (Myristica succedanea) and Myristica malabarica, Laurelia sempervirens, Atherosperma moschatum, Ravensara aromatica, Cryptocarya moschata, Torreya californica. Nutmeg oil is sometimes confused with the oil from the green leaves of Myristica fragrans.

Other Names: Mace

ACTIONS AND PHARMACOLOGY

COMPOUNDS: NUTMEG

Volatile oil (7-16%)

Fatty oil (30-40%): fatty acids including among others lauric, myristic, pentadecanoic, palmitic, heptadecanoic, stearic, oleic acid

Triterpene saponins

Sterols: including among others beta-sitosterol, campesterol

COMPOUNDS: NUTMEG OIL

Monoterpene hydrocarbons 80%): including sabinene (39%), alpha-pinene (13%), beta-pinene (9%)

monoterpene alcohols (5%): including 1,8-cineole (3.5%)

phenyl propane derivatives (10 to 18%): including myristicin (2 to 5%), elemicin (1 to 2.5%)

Fatty oil (30 to 40%) in the nutmeg oil rendered through pressing

EFFECTS

In animal experiments, the eugenol in the essential oil inhibits, dose-dependently, medicinally induced diarrhea and slows down the transport of active carbon in the gastrointestinal tract. An effect on prostaglandin synthesis and an antimicrobial effect have also been demonstrated. The use of the drug for dysentery and rheumatic complaints seems plausible.

INDICATIONS AND USAGE

Unproven Uses: Internal folk medicine uses of nutmeg include diarrhea and dysentery, inflammation of the stomach membranes, cramps, flatulence and vomiting. Externally, the oil is used for rheumatism, sciatica, neuralgia and disorders of the upper respiratory tract.

Chinese Medicine: Indications include diarrhea, vomiting and digestive problems.

Indian Medicine: Indications in Indian medicine include headaches, poor vision, insomnia, fever and malaria, cholera, impotence and general debility.

Homeopathic Uses: Among uses in homeopathy are nervous physical symptoms, digestive problems with flatulence and disturbed perception.

CONTRAINDICATIONS

The drug is not to be used during pregnancy.

PRECAUTIONS AND ADVERSE REACTIONS

No health hazards or side effects are known in conjunction with the proper administration of designated therapeutic dosages. However, the drug can trigger allergic contact dermatitis.

OVERDOSAGE: NUTMEG SEED AND OIL

Ingestion of 1 to 3 "nuts" (or even fewer) can produce amphetamine derivatives through bioconversion of the phenylpropane derivatives in the human body. This eventually leads to intense thirst, nausea, reddening and swelling of the face, and alterations of consciousness from mild changes, such as anxiety or lethargy, to intensive hallucinations. The stupor can last from 2 to 3 days. The therapy for poisonings consists of gastrointestinal emptying (inducement of vomiting, gastric lavage with burgundy-colored potassium permanganate solution, sodium sulfate), and installation of activated charcoal. That is followed by treating spasms intravenously with diazepam; treating colic with atropine; electrolyte substitution; and treating possible cases of acidosis with sodium bicarbonate infusions. In case of shock, plasma volume expanders should be infused. Monitoring of kidney function is essential. Intubation and oxygen respiration may also be necessary.

DOSAGE

Mode of Administration: Nutmeg oils, extracts, powders, syrups and butters are used internally. The oil also is used externally as a liniment 10%

Preparation: There is no information in the literature.

Daily Dosage:

Infusion/decoction: 1%, 50 to 200 ml daily.

Liquid extract: 1 to 2 times daily.

Oil: 1 to 3 drops internally 2 to 3 times a day.

Powder: 0.3 to 1 g; not to exceed 3 times daily.

Syrup: 10 to 40 ml daily.

Tincture: 2 to 10 ml daily.

Homeopathic Dosage: 5 drops, 1 tablet or 10 globules every 30 to 60 minutes (acute) or 1 to 3 times daily (chronic); parenterally: 1 to 2 sc acute, 3 times daily; chronic: once a day (HAB1).

Storage: Nutmeg should be stored in tightly sealed containers and kept cool and dry. The oil should be protected from light in containers that are tightly sealed, completely filled and kept at a temperature not to exceed 25° C.

LITERATURE: NUTMEG SEED AND OIL

Baldry J et al., (1976) Int Flav Food Add 7:28.

Bennett A et al., New Eng J Med 290:110.

Effertz B et al., (1979) Z Pflanzenphysiol 92:319.

Forrest JE et al., (1974) J Chem Soc Perkin Trans 1(2):205.

Forrest JE, Heacock RA, (1972) Lloydia 35:440.

Forrest TP et al., (1973) Naturwissenschaften 60:257.

Gottlieb OR, (1979) J Ethnopharmacol 1:309.

Isogai A et al., (1973) Agric Biol Chem 37:198 et 1479.

Kim et al., (1978) Biochim. Biophys Acta 537:22.

Miller EC et al., (1983) Cancer Res 43:1124.

Misra V et al., (1978) Ind J Med Res 67:482.

Pecevski J et al., (1980) Toxicol Lett 7:739.

Rasheed A et al., (1984) Planta Med 50(2):222.

Sanford KJ, Heinz DE, (1971) Pharm Acta Helv 59(9/10):242.

Sanford KJ, Heinz DE, (1971) Phytochemistry 10:1245.

Sarath-Kumara SJ et al., (1985) J Sci Food Agric 36(2):93.

Shafkan I et al., (1977) New Eng J Med 296:694.

Further information in:

Frohne D, Pfänder HJ, Giftpflanzen - Ein Handbuch für Apotheker, Toxikologen und Biologen, 4. Aufl., Wiss. Verlags-Ges. Stuttgart 1997.

Hänsel R, Keller K, Rimpler H, Schneider G (Hrsg.), Hagers Handbuch der Pharmazeutischen Praxis, 5. Aufl., Bde 4-6 (Drogen), Springer Verlag Berlin, Heidelberg, New York, 1992-1994.

Leung AY, Encyclopedia of Common Natural Ingredients Used in Food, Drugs and Cosmetics, John Wiley & Sons Inc., New York 1980.

Lewin L, Gifte und Vergiftungen, 6. Aufl., Nachdruck, Haug Verlag, Heidelberg 1992.

Roth L, Daunderer M, Kormann K, Giftpflanzen, Pflanzengifte, 4. Aufl., Ecomed Fachverlag Landsberg Lech 1993.

Steinegger E, Hänsel R, Pharmakognosie, 5. Aufl., Springer Verlag Heidelberg 1992.

Teuscher E, Lindequist U, Biogene Gifte - Biologie, Chemie, Pharmakologie, 2. Aufl., Fischer Verlag Stuttgart 1994.

Teuscher E, Biogene Arzneimittel, 5. Aufl., Wiss. Verlagsges. Stuttgart 1997.

Nux Vomica

Strychnos nux vomica

DESCRIPTION

Medicinal Parts: The medicinal parts are the ripe, dried seeds and the dried bark.

Flower and Fruit: The inflorescences are terminal and cyme-like. The flowers have a 5-tipped calyx and a white to greenish-white plate-shaped corolla with a long tube. There are 5 sessile stamens in the mouth of the corolla tube. The ovary is superior, 2-valved and has a long style and a 2-lobed stigma. The fruit, when ripe, is an orange-red, globular berry with a diameter of 4 to 6 cm. The pulp is white, bitter and surrounded by a tough, brittle exocarp about 1.5 mm thick. There are usually 1 to 9 seeds in the pulp, of which 2 to 4 are erect. The seeds are disc-like, orbicular, 12 to 25 mm wide, radially striped, appressed pubescent and exceptionally bitter.

Leaves, Stem and Root: The plant is a tree up to 25 m high with a trunk circumference of up to 3 m. The branches are obtuse-quadrangular, close together and repeatedly bifurcated. They are glabrous and they have 1 to 2 leaf pairs, which are thickened at the nodes. The trunk bark is blackish-ash-gray and the branch bark is gray. The twigs are green and glossy. The leaves are petiolate and crossed-opposite. The leaf blade is glabrous, broadly ovate, entire-margined and has a curved main rib. The broad stipules dry later.

Habitat: The plant grows all over southeast Asia from Pakistan to Vietnam.

Production: Nux Vomica consists of the seeds of Strychnos nux-vomica. The berries are picked when ripe. The hard exocarp is removed and the seeds are taken out and washed to remove any pulp residue. They are subsequently dried in the sun.

Not to be Confused With: The seeds of Strychnos nux-blanda, Strychnos potatorum and Strychnos wallichiana. Nux vomica powder may be confused with the powder of date nuts or olive stones and with by-products of stone-nut processing.

Other Names: Poison Nut, Quaker Button's

ACTIONS AND PHARMACOLOGY

COMPOUNDS

Indole alkaloids (2.0-5.0%): chief alkaloids strychnine and brucine (approximately in a 1:1 ratio), including among others, 12-hydroxystrychnine, 15-hydroxystrychnine, alpha-colubrine, beta-colubrine, icajine

Fatty oil

Polysaccharides as insoluble reserve substances

Iridoide monoterpenes: including among others, loganin

EFFECTS

Nux Vomica increases reflex excitability. Endogenic and exogenic stimuli reach the targeted organ without hindrance and, as a result, possess a strengthened effect that can be attributed to the alkaloid strychnine. The toxic principle strychnine deadens the inhibitory synapse of the CNS and results in overextended musculature reactions.

The strychnine and brucine components act as competitive antagonists of the neurotransmitter glycine. The drug is psychoanaleptic due to an increase in reflex action, i.e., endogenic and exogenic stimuli reach the targeted organ without hindrance and as a result have a strengthened effect. In addition, strychnine is cholinolytic in animal experiments.

In lower doses, the drug causes a reflexive increase of glandular secretion in the gastrointestinal tract through the amaroids.

INDICATIONS AND USAGE

Unproven Uses: Nux Vomica and its preparations are used in combinations for diseases and conditions of the gastrointestinal tract, organic and functional disorders of the heart and circulatory system, diseases of the eye, nervous conditions, depression, migraine, and climacteric complaints. In addition, the herb is used as a tonic, an appetite stimulant, for respiratory complaints, for secondary anemia and for unspecific geriatric complaints.

Chinese Medicine: The drug is used for general pain, febrile illnesses, sore throat and abdominal tumors.

Indian Medicine: The drug is used for loss of appetite, anemia, lumbago, asthma, bronchitis, constipation, diabetes, intermittent and malarial fever, skin diseases, paralyses, and muscle weakness; a special procedure is supposed to detoxify the seeds.

Homeopathic Uses: The drug is used for inflammations of the respiratory and gastrointestinal tracts, disorders of the urinary tract, febrile illnesses, hepatocystic disorders, hemorrhoids, dizziness, headache, neuralgia, rheumatic pain, cramps, paralyses, insomnia and nervous irritability.

PRECAUTIONS AND ADVERSE REACTIONS

The drug is severely toxic due to the strychnine content and is not recommended for use.

OVERDOSAGE

Symptoms of poisoning can occur after ingestion of one bean. Strychnine doses of as little as 1.5 mg (30-50 mg of the drug) initially cause restlessness, feelings of anxiety, heightening of sense perception, enhanced reflexes, equilibrium disorders, and painful stiffness of the neck and back musculature. Later, twitching, tonic spasms of the masseter and neck musculature, and finally painful convulsions of the entire body that are triggered by visual or tactile stimulation occur. Dyspnea comes following spasm of the breathing musculature. Death occurs through suffocation or exhaustion. The lethal dosage for an adult is approximately 50 mg strychnine (1-2 gm of the drug). Chronic intake of subconvulsive dosages can also lead to death under similar conditions after a period of weeks. This is due to an accumulation of drug in the body, particularly in those who have liver damage.

Following the administration of a watery suspension of activated charcoal, the therapy for poisoning consists of keeping external stimulation to a minimum through placement in a quiet, warm, darkened room. Convulsions should be treated with dosages of diazepam or barbital (i.v.). High-calorie glucose infusions should also be given. Intubation and oxygen respiration may also be required. Gastric lavage should be avoided, due to the danger of triggering convulsions. Analeptics or phenothiazines should not be administered. Because of the possibility of unwanted effects occurring in conjunction with the administration of therapeutic dosages, one should forgo any administration of the drug.

DOSAGE

Mode of Administration: Nux Vomica is used almost exclusively in homeopathy. Radioactively tagged strychnine is used in medicine to detect glycinergic receptors. In industry, the drug is used as an active agent for pest control.

Daily Dosage: The average single dose is 0.02-0.05 gm.

The daily dosages for various preparations are as follows: liquid (0.05 to 2 ml), extract (0.005 gm, with a maximun dose of 0.1 gm), tincture (0.5 to 2 ml (BP80), or Strychninum nitricum (maximum single dose of 0.005 gm).

Homeopathic Dosage: 5 drops, 1 tablet or 10 globules every 30 to 60 minutes (acute) or 1 to 3 times daily (chronic); parenterally: 1 to 2 ml sc, acute: 3 times daily; chronic: once a day (HAB1).

Storage: Mark the container as ''poisonous'' and keep tightly sealed; protect the drug from cool air and light.

LITERATURE

Bisset NG, Phillipson JD, JNP 39:263. 1976.

Galeffi C, ETH:2:129-134. 1980.

Hänsel R, Keller K, Rimpler H, Schneider G (Hrsg.), Hagers Handbuch der Pharmazeutischen Praxis, 5. Aufl., Bde 4-6 (Drogen): Springer Verlag Berlin, Heidelberg, New York, 1992-1994.

Lewin L, Gifte und Vergiftungen, 6. Aufl., Nachdruck, Haug Verlag, Heidelberg 1992.

Madaus G, Lehrbuch der Biologischen Arzneimittel, Bde 1-3, Nachdruck, Georg Olms Verlag Hildesheim 1979.

Maier W, Gröger D, Pharm Zentralhalle 107:883. 1968.

Marini-Bettolo GB, Advances in the research of curare and Strychnos. In: Rend Accad Naz 40:1975-1976, 1-2, 61-76. 1977. Roth L, Daunderer M, Kormann K, Giftpflanzen, Pflanzengifte, 4. Aufl., Ecomed Fachverlag Landsberg Lech 1993.

Rodriguez F et al. PH 18:2065. 1980.

Steinegger E, Hänsel R, Pharmakognosie, 5. Aufl., Springer Verlag Heidelberg 1992.

Teuscher E, Biogene Arzneimittel, 5. Aufl., Wiss. Verlagsges. Stuttgart 1997.

Teuscher E, Lindequist U, Biogene Gifte - Biologie, Chemie, Pharmakologie, 2. Aufl., Fischer Verlag Stuttgart 1994.

Wagner H, Wiesenauer M, Phytotherapie. Phytopharmaka und pflanzliche Homöopathika, Fischer-Verlag, Stuttgart, Jena, New York 1995.

Nymphaea odorata

See American White Pond Lily

Oak

Quercus robur

DESCRIPTION

Medicinal Parts: The medicinal parts are the dried bark of the young branches and the lateral shoots, the dried bark of the trunk and branches, the dried leaves of various oak species and the seed kernels without the seed coats.

Flower and Fruit: The flowers are reddish brown and monoecious. The male flowers consist of a 5-part perigone with 6 to 10 stamens that appear in small groups in limp, hanging catkins. The female flowers, solitary or in groups of up to 5, appear in a involucre which clasps the base of the fruit and which later becomes bowl-shaped. The fruit is solitary or in groups of up to 5 on 1 shared, glabrous or occasionally sparsely pubescent stem. They are oblong-ovate, acuminate and enclosed in the cupule.

Leaves, Stem and Root: The tree is about 50 m high with a broad, irregular, heavily branched crown and a trunk which divides into gnarled, strong, bent branches. The bark is deeply fissured, thick and grey-brown. The leaves are short-petioled, almost sessile, oblong-obovate, almost lobed, usually cordate or polled at the base.

Habitat: The tree is widespread in Europe, Asia Minor and the Caucasus region.

Production: Oak bark consists of the dried bark of young branches and saplings of Quercus robur and/or Quercus petraea, harvested in the spring, as well as their preparations. Oak bark is harvested from March to April. The trees fall every 10 years. The bark is dried rapidly.

Other Names: Common Oak, Pedunculate Oak, English Oak, Tanner's Bark

ACTIONS AND PHARMACOLOGY

COMPOUNDS

Catechin tannins: oligomeric proanthocyanidins

Ellagitannins: (including castalagin, pedunculagin, vesvalagin, 2,3-(S)-hexahydroxy diphenoyl glucose), flavano-ellagitannins (acutissimins A and B, eugenigrandin, guajavacin B, stenophyllanin C)

Gallo tannins

Monomeric and dimeric catechins and leucocyanidins

Tannins (12 to 16%)

EFFECTS

The drug, which contains tannins, is astringent, antiphlogistic, antiviral and anthelmintic.

INDICATIONS AND USAGE

Approved by Commission E:

- Cough/bronchitis
- Diarrhea
- Inflammation of the mouth and pharynx
- Inflammation of the skin

Unproven Uses: Oak is used internally for non-specific diarrhea. In smaller doses it is used as a stomach tonic. The drug is used externally for inflammatory skin diseases, inflammation of the mouth and throat as well as the genital and anal area, suppurating eczema, hyperhydrosis, intertrigo and as an adjuvant treatment of chilblains.

Oak is also used in folk medicine internally for hemorrhagic stool, non-menstrual uterine bleeding, hemoptysis and chronic inflammation of the gastrointestinal tract. External uses include hemorrhoid bleeding, varicose veins, uterine bleeding, vaginal discharge (washes/douches), rashes, chronic, itching, scaley and suppurating eczema and eye inflammations.

CONTRAINDICATIONS

Whole-body baths are contraindicated with large-area weeping eczemas and skin injuries, with feverish and infectious illnesses, with cardiac insufficiency in stages III and IV (NYHA) and with hypertonia in stage IV (WHO).

PRECAUTIONS AND ADVERSE REACTIONS

General: No health hazards or side effects are known in conjunction with the proper administration of designated therapeutic dosages. Internal administration could lead to digestive complaints because of the secretion-inhibiting effect of the tannins.

Drug-Interactions: The absorption of alkaloids and other alkaline drugs may be reduced or inhibited.

DOSAGE

Mode of Administration: Oak is available as whole, crude and powdered drug form, as a bath additive and in compounded preparations. It is also available in solid pharmaceutical form for oral intake.

Preparation:

Tea — 1 gm finely cut or coarse powdered drug is put in cold water, rapidly boiled and strained after some time (1 teaspoon corresponds to 3 gm drug).

Bath additive — 5 gm drug is boiled with 1 Liter water and added to the full or hip bath.

Daily Dosage:

Internally — 3 gm of drug; Tea: 1 cup 3 times a day.

Externally — Rinses/gargles: boil 2 dessertspoons finely cut drug with 3 cups water.

Bath additive — duration: 20 minutes at 32 to 37° C.

Storage: Should be tightly sealed and protected from light

LITERATURE

Ahn BZ et al., Arch Pharm 304:666. 1971.

Glasl H, DAZ 123:1979. 1983.

König M et al., Ellegitannins and complex tannins from Quercus petraea bark. In: JNP 57(10):1411-1415. 1994.

Pallenbach E, Scholz E, König M, Rimpler H, Proanthocyanidins from Quercus petraea bark. In: PM 59(3):264. 1993.

Scalbert A et al., PH 27:3483. 1988.

Willuhn G, Pflanzliche Dermatika. Eine kritische Übersicht. In: DAZ 132(37):1873. 1992.

Further information in:

Hänsel R, Keller K, Rimpler H, Schneider G (Hrsg.), Hagers Handbuch der Pharmazeutischen Praxis, 5. Aufl., Bde 4-6 (Drogen): Springer Verlag Berlin, Heidelberg, New York, 1992-1994.

Madaus G, Lehrbuch der Biologischen Arzneimittel, Bde. 1-3, Nachdruck, Georg Olms Verlag Hildesheim 1979.

Roth L, Daunderer M, Kormann K, Giftpflanzen, Pflanzengifte, 4. Aufl., Ecomed Fachverlag Landsberg Lech 1993.

Schulz R, Hänsel R, Rationale Phytotherapie, Springer Verlag Heidelberg 1996.

Steinegger E, Hänsel R, Pharmakognosie, 5. Aufl., Springer Verlag Heidelberg 1992.

Teuscher E, Biogene Arzneimittel, 5. Aufl., Wiss. Verlagsges. Stuttgart 1997.

Wagner H, Wiesenauer M, Phytotherapie. Phytopharmaka und pflanzliche Homöopathika, Fischer-Verlag, Stuttgart, Jena, New York 1995.

Wichtl M (Hrsg.), Teedrogen, 4. Aufl., Wiss. Verlagsges. Stuttgart 1997.

Oak Gall

Quercus infectoria

DESCRIPTION

Medicinal Parts: The medicinal part of the plant is the leaf.

Flower and Fruit: The male flowers are tangled into hanging, axillary catkins, with a 6- to 8-tepaled perigone and 6 to 10 stamens. The female sessile flowers are single or in small groups in the leaf axils of dropping stipules. The perigone is 6-tipped with an inferior 3-chambered ovary surrounded by an initially inconspicuous and then later cup-shaped cupula. The fruit is up to 4 cm long, cylindrical, shiny brown and is 3 times longer than the cupula, which is covered with narrow scales.

Leaves, Stem and Root: The plant grows as a shrub or small tree, diclinous and monoecious. The leaves are alternate, approximately 5 cm long, short-petiolate, elongate, sinuate, roughly thorny-tipped serrate.

Characteristics: Apical galls are formed by the laying of eggs by the gall wasp (Andricus gallae-tinctoriae) in the young leaf buds.

Habitat: The various Quercus species originated in Iran, Iraq and Turkey, but are now widespread and particularly common in Asia Minor, Europe and North Africa.

Production: Oak Gall is the gall of Quercus infectoria produced by gall wasps (Andricus gallae-tinktoriae) laying their eggs in the leaf buds. The development of the larva probably stimulates the bud as an infection would and produces the gall as a reaction.

Other Names: Gallinaccia Oak

ACTIONS AND PHARMACOLOGY

COMPOUNDS

Tannins (60 to 70%): gallotannins, particularly hexa- and heptagalloyl-glucoses

Phenol carboxylic acids: gallic acid (3%), ellagic acid (2%)

EFFECTS

The astringent quality of the drug can be explained by the tannins it contains. The dry extract exhibits analgetic, hypoglycemic and sedative-hypnotic efficacy.

INDICATIONS AND USAGE

Unproven Uses: External uses include treatment of inflammation of the skin and frostbite and as an adjuvant in the treatment of infectious skin conditions. Oak gall is used externally for chilblains and gingivitis, for which efficacy appears plausible but has not yet been sufficiently documented.

Indian Medicine: Uses include intestinal hemorrhaging, coughing blood, diarrhea, dysentery, ulcerative stomatitis, coughs, bronchitis, dyspepsia, fever, gonorrhea, leucorrhea, menorrhagia, impetigo, eczema, hemorrhoids, pharyngodynia, diabetes, hyperhidrosis and tonsillitis.

Chinese Medicine: Dysentery, hyperhidrosis, oral ulceration, leucorrhea, hemorrhoids, wounds and rectal prolapse are considered to be indications. Efficacy for these indications has not yet been proven.

PRECAUTIONS AND ADVERSE REACTIONS

No health hazards are known in conjunction with the proper external administration of designated therapeutic dosages.

DOSAGE

Mode of Administration: Preparations of the whole, cut and powdered drug have internal and external applications.

Preparation:

Tincture — Powdered gall apples are mixed roughly 1:5 with spirit of wine.

Storage: The drug should be stored in a tightly sealed container.

LITERATURE

Dar MS, Ikram M, Fakouhi T, Constituents of Quercus infectoria. Planta Med, 65:286-7, 1977 May.

Dar MS, Ikram M, Fakouhi T, Pharmacology of Quercus infectoria. J Pharm Sci, 65:1791-4, 1976 Dec.

Dar MS, Ikram M, Fakouhi T, Studies on Quercus infectoria; isolation of syringic acid and determination of its central depressive activity. Planta Med, 65:156-61, 1979 Feb.

Hänsel R, Keller K, Rimpler H, Schneider G (Ed), Hagers Handbuch der Pharmazeutischen Praxis, 5. Aufl., Bde 4 - 6 (Drogen), Springer Verlag Berlin, Heidelberg, New York, 1992-1994.

Oats

Avena sativa

TRADE NAMES

Wild Oats, Oat Bran, Oatstraw

DESCRIPTION

Medicinal Parts: The medicinal parts are the fresh or dried above-ground plant, the ripe, dried fruits, and the dried, threshed leaf and stem.

Flower and Fruit: The spikelet has 2 to 3 flowers. The outer glume has no awn, is 18 to 30 mm long and has 7 to 11 ribs. The top glumes grow from 12 to 24 mm long, have 2 divisions and a dentate tip. They have 7 ribs and can either be awned or unawned. The awn is 15 to 40 mm long, upright and rough. The double ribbed husks are 10 to 20 mm long and are thickly ciliate on the short ridge. The 3 stamens are 2.5 to 4 mm long. The ovary has a pinnatifid stigma. The fruit is 7 to 12 mm long, narrowly elliptoid and pubescent.

Leaves, Stem and Root: Oat is a light-green annual grass with a bushy root. The stalks are 60 to 100 cm high, smooth and glabrous. The linear-lanceolate tapering, flat leaves are in double rows, and the leaf sheath is clasping. The ligula is short and ovate with triangular pointed teeth. The leaf blade is linear-lanceolate and is 45 cm long by 5 to 15 mm wide.

Habitat: Oats originated in England, France, Poland, Germany and Russia, and are now cultivated worldwide.

Production: Wild oat herb consists of the fresh above-ground parts of Avena sativa, which are harvested shortly before the height of the flowering season and then quickly dried. Oats consist of the ripe, dried fruits of Avena sativa. Oat bran is taken from the outer layer of the husked fruit. To make rolled oats, the husked fruit is treated with steam, then crushed. Oat straw consists of the dried, threshed leaves and stems of Avena sativa, also harvested shortly before the height of the flowering season.

Other Names: Grain, Groats, Oatmeal, Straw

ACTIONS AND PHARMACOLOGY

COMPOUNDS: OAT HERB

Soluble oligo- and polysaccharides: including saccharose, kestose, neokestose, bifurcose, beta- glucans, galactoarabinoxylans

Silicic acid (partially water-soluble)

Steroid saponins: avenacoside A and B

Unusual amino acids: avenic acid A and B

Flavonoids: including vitexin-, isovitexin-, apigenin-, isoorientin-, tricinglycosides

EFFECTS: OAT HERB

In one poorly constructed experimental investigation, the drug was said to lower the uric acid level and to display an antihepatoxin effect in animal experiments. The mode of action was not explained.

COMPOUNDS: OAT FRUIT

Starch

Soluble polysaccharides: in particular beta-glucans and arabinoxylans

Proteic substances: including gliadin, avenin, avenalin

Peptides: alpha-avenothionine, beta-avenothionine

Steroid saponins: avenacoside A and B

Sterols: including beta-sitosterol, delta-5-avenasterol

Fatty oil

Vitamins of the B-group

Amines: including gramine

EFFECTS: OAT FRUIT

Dehusked oats are, according to various studies, able to lower serum cholesterol and to hinder prostaglandin biosynthesis. The latest research attributes the cholesterol-lowering effect to the water-soluble polysaccharides, in particular beta-glucans.

COMPOUNDS: OAT STRAW

Soluble oligo- and polysaccharides: including saccharose, kestose, neokestose, bifurcose, beta-glucans, galactoarabinoxylans

Silicic acid (partially water-soluble)

Steroid saponins: avenacoside A and B

Unusual amino acids: avenic acid A and B

Flavonoids: including vitexin-, isovitexin-, apigenin-, isoorientin-, tricinglycosides

EFFECTS: OAT STRAW

There is no information available concerning the efficacy of oat straw.

INDICATIONS AND USAGE

OAT HERB

Unproven Uses: Wild oat herb preparations are used for many purposes, including acute and chronic anxiety, atonia of the bladder and connective tissue, connective tissue deficiencies, excitation, gout, kidney ailments in Kneipp therapy, neurasthenic and pseudoneurasthenic syndromes, old age symptoms, opium and tobacco withdrawal treatment, rheumatism, skin diseases, sleeplessness, stress, weakness of the bladder, and as a tonic and roborant. The efficacy for the claimed applications is not documented.

Homeopathic Uses: Oats are used in homeopathy for exhaustion and insomnia.

OAT FRUIT

Unproven Uses: Oat preparations are used for diseases and complaints of the gastrointestinal tract, gallbladder and kidneys, for cardiovascular disorders, constipation, diabetes, diarrhea, physical fatigue, rheumatism, and as a gruel for chest and throat complaints. The claimed efficacy has not been fully substantiated.

OAT STRAW

Approved by Commission E:

- Inflammation of the skin
- Warts

Unproven Uses: The drug is employed externally for seborrheic skin disorders, especially those accompanied by itch. Oat straw is used for abdominal fatigue, bladder and rheumatic disorders, eye ailments, frostbite, gout, impetigo and metabolic diseases. It is used in foot baths for chronically cold or tired feet. It is also used as a tea for flu and coughs.

PRECAUTIONS AND ADVERSE REACTIONS

OAT HERB, FRUIT AND STRAW

No health hazards or side effects are known in conjunction with the proper administration of designated therapeutic dosages.

DOSAGE

AVENA HERB

Mode of Administration: The herb is used in combination therapy, as a tea for internal use, and in homeopathic mother tinctures and dilutions.

How Supplied:

Liquid — 1000 mg/ml

Preparation: To make a tea, 3 gm drug is boiled in 250 ml water, which is strained after cooling.

Daily Dosage: The tea is taken repeatedly throughout the day and shortly before going to bed.

Homeopathic Dosage: 5 to 10 drops, 1 tablet or 5 to 10 globules 1 to 3 times daily or 1 ml injection solution twice weekly sc (HAB1).

Storage: The herb should be protected from light and moisture.

OAT FRUIT

Mode of Administration: The fruit is used in homeopathy and in combination preparations.

OAT STRAW

Mode of Administration: As a comminuted herb for decoctions and other galenic preparations as teas and bath additives.

Preparation: To make oat straw bath, 100 g chopped drug is boiled with 3 liters water for 20 minutes and the decoction is added to the bath.

Daily Dosage: 100 g of herb is used for one full bath.

LITERATURE

OAT HERB

Anand CL, (1971) Nature 233:496.

Connor J et al., (1975) J Pharm Pharmacol 27:92.

Effertz B et al., (1979) Z Pflanzenphysiol 92:319.

Gabrinowicz JW, (1974) Med J Aust Ii:306.

Kim et al., (1978) Biochim Biophys Acta 537:22.

Schneider E, Lösliche Silikate im grünen Hafer. In: ZPT 11(4):129. 1990.

Willuhn G, Pflanzliche Dermatika. Eine kritische Übersicht.. In: DAZ 132(37):1873. 1992.

Further information in:

Hänsel R, Keller K, Rimpler H, Schneider G (Hrsg.), Hagers Handbuch der Pharmazeutischen Praxis, 5. Aufl., Bde 4-6 (Drogen), Springer Verlag Berlin, Heidelberg, New York, 1992-1994.

Madaus G, Lehrbuch der Biologischen Arzneimittel, Bde 1-3, Nachdruck, Georg Olms Verlag Hildesheim 1979.

Teuscher E, Lindequist U, Biogene Gifte - Biologie, Chemie, Pharmakologie, 2. Aufl., Fischer Verlag Stuttgart 1994.

Wichtl M (Hrsg.), Teedrogen, 4. Aufl., Wiss. Verlagsges. Stuttgart 1997.

OAT FRUIT

Connor J et al., (1975) J Pharm Pharmacol 27:92.

Effertz B et al., (1979) Z Pflanzenphysiol 92: 319Anand CL (1971) Nature 233:496.

Gabrinowicz JW, (1974) Med J Aust Ii: 306.

Kim et al., (1978) Biochim Biophys Acta 537:22.

Schneider E, Lösliche Silikate im grünen Hafer. In: ZPT 11(4):129. 1990.

Willuhn G, Pflanzliche Dermatika. Eine kritische Übersicht.. In: DAZ 132(37):1873. 1992.

Further information in:

Hänsel R, Keller K, Rimpler H, Schneider G (Hrsg.), Hagers Handbuch der Pharmazeutischen Praxis, 5. Aufl., Bde 4-6 (Drogen), Springer Verlag Berlin, Heidelberg, New York, 1992-1994.

Madaus G, Lehrbuch der Biologischen Arzneimittel, Bde 1-3, Nachdruck, Georg Olms Verlag Hildesheim 1979.

Wagner H, Wiesenauer M, Phytotherapie. Phytopharmaka und pflanzliche Homöopathika, Fischer-Verlag, Stuttgart, Jena, New York 1995.

OAT STRAW

Kim et al., (1978) Biochim Biophys Acta 537:22.

Anand CL, (1971) Nature 233:496.

Connr J et al., (1975) J Pharm Pharmacol 27:92.

Effertz B et al., (1979) Z Pflanzenphysiol 92:319.

Gabrinowicz JW, (1974) Med J Aust Ii: 306.

Jaspersen-Schib R, Ballaststoffe als Lipidsenker. In: DAZ 132(39):1991. 1992.

Schneider E, Lösliche Silikate im grünen Hafer. In: ZPT 11(4):129. 1990.

Willuhn G, Pflanzliche Dermatika. Eine kritische Übersicht.. In: DAZ 132(37):1873. 1992.

Further information in:

Hänsel R, Keller K, Rimpler H, Schneider G (Hrsg.), Hagers Handbuch der Pharmazeutischen Praxis, 5. Aufl., Bde 4-6 (Drogen), Springer Verlag Berlin, Heidelberg, New York, 1992-1994.

Madaus G, Lehrbuch der Biologischen Arzneimittel, Bde 1-3, Nachdruck, Georg Olms Verlag Hildesheim 1979.

Teuscher E, Lindequist U, Biogene Gifte - Biologie, Chemie, Pharmakologie, 2. Aufl., Fischer Verlag Stuttgart 1994.

Wichtl M (Hrsg.), Teedrogen, 4. Aufl., Wiss. Verlagsges. Stuttgart 1997.

Ocimum basilicum

See Basil

Oenanthe aquatica

See Water Fennel

Oenanthe crocata

See Water Dropwort

Oenothera biennis

See Evening Primrose

Oilseed Rape

Brassica napus

DESCRIPTION

Medicinal Parts: The medicinal parts of the plant are the roots and seeds.

Flower and Fruit: The flowers are in racemes with 4 upright, splayed sepals. The 4 petals are yellow, 11 to 14 mm long, almost twice as long as the calyx, with an orbicular-elliptical surface. There are 2 short and 4 long stamens. The ovary is superior, with 4 fused carpels. The fruit is 4.5 to 11 cm long and is a dehiscent pod opening on 2 sides with a septum and 20 to 40 seeds. The seeds are globose and approximately 1.5 to 3 mm in diameter.

Leaves, Stem and Root: Oilseed Rape is an annual or biennial herb that grows up to 1.4 m high. The leaves are alternate with a bluish bloom; the lower ones are petiolate and pinnatisect, with relatively large terminal lobes and are slightly pubescent. The middle and upper leaves are sessile, partly clasping, simple, glabrous, dentate or entire. The stem of larger plants is branched. The root is thin and spindle-shaped.

Habitat: Europe, North Africa, U.S.

Production: The seeds are cold-pressed and then refined. Rapeseed oil is the cold-pressed and refined oil from the ripe seeds of Brassica napus.

Not to be Confused With: Rapeseed oil may be adulterated with resins and mineral oil. Sinapis arvensis is a permitted substitute.

Other Names: Colza, Cole, Rape, Rape Seed

ACTIONS AND PHARMACOLOGY

COMPOUNDS

Fatty oil: chief fatty acids: oleic acid (60%), linoleic acid (20%), linolenic acid (10%), as well as palmitic acid, stearic acid, eicosanoic acid, behenic acid. Varieties with high erucic acid content (40 to 50%) are no longer cultivated (reduction of the erucic acid content in the Common Market countries to below 5%)

Sterols: beta-sitosterol, campesterol, brassicasterol, estered to some extent

EFFECTS

Rapeseed oil, when ingested in high dosages over an extended period of time, is cardiotoxic. The drug is chiefly used as a substitute for olive oil and in the manufacture of salves and liniments.

INDICATIONS AND USAGE

No medicinal indications

PRECAUTIONS AND ADVERSE REACTIONS

No health hazards are known in conjunction with the proper administration of designated therapeutic dosages of the oil, which is low on erucic acid.

DOSAGE

Storage: Store in the dark, in well-filled containers.

LITERATURE

Butcher RD, Goodman BA, Deighton N, Smith WH, Evaluation of the allergic/irritant potential of air pollutants: detection of proteins modified by volatile organic compounds from oilseed rape (Brassica napus ssp. oleifera) using electrospray ionization-mass spectrometry. Clin Exp Allergy, 25 (1995).

Hänsel R, Keller K, Rimpler H, Schneider G (Ed), Hagers Handbuch der Pharmazeutischen Praxis, 5. Aufl., Bde 4 - 6 (Drogen), Springer Verlag Berlin, Heidelberg, New York, 1992-1994.

Slabas AR, Cottingham IR, Austin A, Hellyer A, Safford R, Smith CG, Immunological detection of NADH-specific enoyl-ACP reductase from rape seed (Brassica napus) - induction, relationship of alpha and beta polypeptides, mRNA translation and interaction with ACP. Biochim Biophys Acta, 1039:181-8, 1990 Jun 19.

Olea europaea

See Olive

Oleander

Nerium oleander

DESCRIPTION

Medicinal Parts: The leaves are the medicinal part of the plant.

Flower and Fruit: The corolla is 4 to 7 mm in diameter, usually pink to red but sometimes white. The petals are thickly covered in glands. The tube is 2 cm long as are the obtuse and patent lobes. The anther appendages are long, pubescent and twisted. The follicles are 8 to 16 cm by 0.5 to 1 cm, erect and reddish-brown.

Leaves, Stem and Root: The evergreen plant can be tree or shrub-like. The trunks are up to 4 m high. The leaves are 6 to 12 by 1.2 to 2 cm, linear-lanceolate, sharp-edged, coriaceous, dark green.

Habitat: Nerium oleander grows mainly in the Mediterranean region but also in parts of Asia. It is cultivated in Europe.

Production: Oleander leaf is the leaf of Nerium oleander, collected shortly before flowering and then dried in the shade.

Other Names: Rose Laurel

ACTIONS AND PHARMACOLOGY

COMPOUNDS

Cardiac steroids (cardenolide): chief components are 16-acetyl neogistonin, adynerin, 5alpha-adynerin, gentiobiosyl-adynerin, delta16-dehydroadynerin, digitoxigenin oleandroside, gentibioosyl-odoroside A, gentiobiosyl-oleandrin, glucosyl-oleandrin, oleandrigenin glucoside, kaneroside, neriaside, nerigoside, neriumoside

Pregnanes and pregnane glycosides: including 12beta-hydroxy-16alpha-methoxy-pregna-4,6-dien-3,20-dione

EFFECTS

Oleander is positively inotropic and negatively chronotropic. The cardenolide glycosides of the drug are qualitatively digitoxin-like in their action, but generally weaker, probably due to the lower rate of absorption.

INDICATIONS AND USAGE

Unproven Uses: Folk medicine uses of Oleander leaf include diseases and functional disorders of the heart, as well as skin diseases. Previous internal application for myocardial insufficiency, decompensated hypertonia and cardiac insufficiency is no longer common.

Indian Medicine: Among uses in Indian medicine are scabies, eye diseases (using only the juice of the leaves) and hemorrhoids.

PRECAUTIONS AND ADVERSE REACTIONS

General: No health hazards are known in conjunction with the proper administration of designated therapeutic dosages. Side effects can include, particularly in the case of overdosages, nausea, vomiting, diarrhea, headache, stupor and cardiac arrhythmias.

Drug Interactions: The simultaneous administration of the drug with quinidine, calcium salts, saluretics, laxatives or glucocorticoids increases both efficacy and side effects. For symptoms of an acute poisoning and therapy see Digitalis. The scientific literature (Lewin) contains numerous descriptions of fatalities.

OVERDOSAGE

See PRECAUTIONS and ADVERSE REACTIONS.

DOSAGE

How Supplied: Forms of commercial pharmaceutical preparations include solutions, coated tablets and compound preparations.

Dosage: No information is available.

Storage: Oleander should be stored where it is protected from dampness and light.

LITERATURE

Loew D, Phytotherapie bei Herzinsuffizienz. In: ZPT 18(2):92-96. 1997.

Loew DA, Loew AD, Pharmakokinetik von herzglykosidhaltigen Pflanzenextrakten. In: ZPT 15(4):197-202. 1994.

Siddiqui S et al., Isolation and structure of two cardiac glycosides from the leaves of Nerium oleander. In: PH 26(1):237-241. 1985.

Yamauchi T et al., Quantitative variations in the cardiac glycosides of oleander. In: PH 22:2211-2214. 1983.

Further information in:

Frohne D, Pfänder HJ, Giftpflanzen - Ein Handbuch für Apotheker, Toxikologen und Biologen, 4. Aufl., Wiss. Verlags-Ges. Stuttgart 1997.

Kern W, List PH, Hörhammer L (Hrsg.), Hagers Handbuch der Pharmazeutischen Praxis, 4. Aufl., Bde. 1-8, Springer Verlag Berlin, Heidelberg, New York, 1969.

Lewin L, Gifte und Vergiftungen, 6. Aufl., Nachdruck, Haug Verlag, Heidelberg 1992.

Madaus G, Lehrbuch der Biologischen Arzneimittel, Bde 1-3, Nachdruck, Georg Olms Verlag Hildesheim 1979.

Roth L, Daunderer M, Kormann K: Giftpflanzen, Pflanzengifte, 4. Aufl., Ecomed Fachverlag Landsberg Lech 1993.

Schulz R, Hänsel R, Rationale Phytotherapie, Springer Verlag Heidelberg 1996.

Steinegger E, Hänsel R, Pharmakognosie, 5. Aufl., Springer Verlag Heidelberg 1992.

Teuscher E, Lindequist U, Biogene Gifte - Biologie, Chemie, Pharmakologie, 2. Aufl., Fischer Verlag Stuttgart 1994.

Teuscher E, Biogene Arzneimittel, 5. Aufl., Wiss. Verlagsges. Stuttgart 1997.

Wagner H, Wiesenauer M, Phytotherapie. Phytopharmaka und pflanzliche Homöopathika, Fischer-Verlag, Stuttgart, Jena, New York 1995.

Olive

Olea europaea

TRADE NAMES

Olive oil and Olive leaves are available from numerous manufacturers. The leaves are sometimes marketed as Olive Leaf-Powder.

DESCRIPTION

Medicinal Parts: The medicinal parts are the dried leaves, the oil extracted from the ripe drupes, and the fresh branches containing leaves and clusters of flowers.

Flower and Fruit: The flowers are in small axillary clustered inflorescence. The calyx has 4 tips. The white corolla has a short tube and 4 lobes. The superior ovary is bilocular, with each side having 2 hanging anatropal ovules. The drupe has 1 to 2 seeds, is fleshy, plum-like or round. The smooth drupe is initially green, then red and finally blue-black when ripe. The very hard stone contains oblong compact seeds with many endosperm.

Leaves, Stem and Root: Olive grows as a medium high shrub or a tree up to 10 m high. The plant has pale bark and cane-like, quadrangular to round, initially downy, thorny or thornless branches. The leaves are opposite, entire, stiff, coriaceous, narrow-elliptical to lanceolate or cordate with thorny tips. The upper surface is dark green, glabrous or covered with scattered scutiform hairs; the underside shimmers silver with scuitform hairs.

Habitat: The plant grows in almost all of the southern European countries and throughout the entire Mediterranean region as far as Iran and beyond the Caucasus. Olive trees are cultivated in many regions of the world.

Production: Olive leaves consist of the fresh or dried leaves of Olea europaea. The leaves are harvested from cultivated trees and dried in the shade. Olive oil is the fatty oil extracted from the drupes of Olea europaea, using the cold-press method.

Not to be Confused With: Confusion can arise between Olive leaves and the leaves of Nerium oleander. The oils of Camellia sasanqua and other Camellia species can be mistaken for Olive oil.

Other Names: Olivier

ACTIONS AND PHARMACOLOGY

COMPOUNDS: OLIVE LEAVES

Iridoide monoterpenes: including among others, oleoropine (6-9%), additionally 6-O-oleoropinesaccharose, ligstroside, oleoroside, oleoside-7,11-dimeth-ylether

Triterpenes: including oleanolic acid, maslinic acid

Flavonoids: luteolin-7-O-glucoside, apigenine-7-O-glucoside

Chalcones: olivin, olivin-4'-O-diglucoside

EFFECTS: OLIVE LEAVES

Animal tests demonstrated hypotensive, antiarrhythmic and spasmolytic effects on the smooth muscle of the intestine, caused by the terpenes and phenols of the drug.

COMPOUNDS: OLIVE OIL

Chief fatty acids: oleic acid (56-83%), palmitic acid (8-20%), linoleic acid (4-20%)

Steroids (0.125 to 0.25%): beta-sitosterol, delta7-stigmasterol, delta5-avenasterol, campesterol, stigmasterol

Tocopherols (0.02%)

EFFECTS: OLIVE OIL

Through the presence of polyunsaturated fatty acids, the drug has an antisclerotic effect by positively influencing the serum lipids. A reduction of plasma glucose was also observed. Contraction of the gallbladder was observed with the increase of cholecystokinin in the plasma.

(Use for gallstones is not advised because efficacy has not been proven and use may cause colic.)

INDICATIONS AND USAGE

OLIVE LEAVES

Unproven Uses: Folk medicine uses include hypertonia, arteriosclerosis, rheumatism and gout, diabetes mellitus and fever.

OLIVE OIL

Unproven Uses: Internal uses of the oil in folk medicine include cholangitis, inflammation of the gallbladder, flatulence, constipation, icterus, Roemhel syndrome, gastrointestinal ulcers and kidney stones. Externally, it has been used for psoriasis, eczema, sunburn, mild burns and rheumatism. Its use as a lubricant for constipation and dry skin conditions appears plausible because of the oily characteristics.

CONTRAINDICATIONS

The internal administration of the drug can trigger colic among gallstone sufferers, so its use is contraindicated.

PRECAUTIONS AND ADVERSE REACTIONS

No health hazards or side effects are known in conjunction with the proper administration of designated therapeutic dosages.

DOSAGE

OLIVE LEAVES

Mode of Administration: The drug is available for oral use in mono and combination tea mixture preparations.

How Supplied:

Capsules — 580 mg

Drops

Preparation: An infusion is prepared by pouring 150 ml of hot water over 7 to 8 g of the dried leaves. Prepare a tea by pouring hot water over 2 teaspoonfuls of the drug and allowing it to steep for 30 minutes.

Daily Dosage: Tea: 3 to 4 cups throughout the day.

OLIVE OIL

Daily Dosage:

Constipation — 100 to 500 ml Olive oil at body temperature applied rectally.

Gastrointestinal ulcers — 15 to 30 ml 3 taken times daily at mealtimes.

LITERATURE

OLIVE LEAVES

Bianchi G, Pozzi N, 3,4-Dihydroxyphenylglycol, a major C6-C2 phenolic in Olea europaea. In: PH 35(5):1335. 1994.

Bianco A et al., Partial synthesis of oleuropein. In: JNP 55(6):760-766. 1992.

Duarte J et al., Effects of oleuropeosid in isolated guinea-pig atria. In: PM 59(4):318. 1993.

Hänsel R, Keller K, Rimpler H, Schneider G (Hrsg.), Hagers Handbuch der Pharmazeutischen Praxis, 5. Aufl., Bde 4-6 (Drogen), Springer Verlag Berlin, Heidelberg, New York, 1992-1994.

Kuwajima H et al., A secoiridoid glucoside from Olea europaea. In: PH 27(6):1757. 1988.

Lasser B et al., (1983) Naturwissenschaften 70:95.

OLIVE OIL

Anonym, Positive Auswirkungen von Olivenöl auf den Blutdruck. In: ZPT 12(1):13. 1991.

Flemming S, Ist Olivenöl erlaubt? In: DAZ 131(29):1525. 1991.

Hänsel R, Keller K, Rimpler H, Schneider G (Hrsg.), Hagers Handbuch der Pharmazeutischen Praxis, 5. Aufl., Bde 4-6 (Drogen), Springer Verlag Berlin, Heidelberg, New York, 1992-1994.

Lasser B et al., (1983) Naturwissensch. 70:95.

Steinegger E, Hänsel R, Pharmakognosie, 5. Aufl., Springer Verlag Heidelberg 1992.

Teuscher E, Biogene Arzneimittel, 5. Aufl., Wiss. Verlagsges. Stuttgart 1997.

Onion

Allium cepa

DESCRIPTION

Medicinal Parts: The medicinal part is the bulb.

Flower and Fruit: The peduncles are up to 3 cm long. The flowers are greenish-white, in orbicular umbels, with 6 free flower bracts that are shorter than the 6 stamens. The pedicles are eight times as long as the flowers. The fruit is a thin-skinned capsule. The seeds are black and angular. The flowers are in globular umbels, before blooming in membranous sheaths.

Leaves, Stem and Root: The plant is perennial or biennial. There are many varieties and can be compressed-globose, ovate or oblong. Most varieties have secondary bulbs. Leaves are shorter than the peduncle, tubular or swollen, and blue-green. There is a hollow scape, which is gray-blue, expanded and bloated below the middle.

Habitat: Central Asia is considered to be the region of origin. Onion was introduced to the Mediterranean and is cultivated worldwide.

Production: Onion consists of the fresh or dried, thick and fleshy leaf sheaths and stipules of Allium cepa.

ACTIONS AND PHARMACOLOGY

COMPOUNDS

Alliins (alkylcysteine sulphoxides): in particular allylalliin (allyl-L-(+)-cysteine sulphoxide) and its gamma-glutamyl conjugates, that in the course of cutting up either the freshly harvested bulbs or those that have been already dried and then re-moistened, are transformed into the so-called alliaceous oils.

Fructosans (polysaccharides, 10-40%)

Saccharose and other sugars

Flavonoids: including quercetin-4′-O-beta-D-glucoside (spiraeoside)

Steroid Saponins

EFFECTS

The thiosulphinate exhibits an antimicrobial effect, and is effective against *Bacillus subtilis*, *Salmonella typhi*, *Pseudomonas aeroginosa* and *Escherichia coli.*

Lipid and blood pressure lowering effect: Certain constituents function similarly to those in garlic, although this is not yet clinically proven.

Inhibits thrombocyte aggregation: Dimethyl and diphenylthiosulphinateboth retard thrombocyte biosynthesis using thrombase stimulation.

Antiasthmatic and antiallergic effect: Guinea pigs sensitized using ovalbumin were protected from asthma attack through the oral administration of onion juice. Administration of an ethanol onion extract significantly reduced allergy-induced bronchial constriction in asthma patients.

INDICATIONS AND USAGE

Approved by Commission E:

- Loss of appetite
- Arteriosclerosis
- Dyspeptic complaints
- Fevers and colds
- Cough/bronchitis
- Hypertension
- Tendency to infection
- Inflammation of the mouth and pharynx
- Common cold

Unproven Uses: In folk medicine, the drug is administered internally for cough, whooping cough, bronchitis, asthma and angina. Onion has been used to stimulate gallbladder functions, for digestive disorders with bloating and colic pain, for dehydration, as an aid at the introduction of menstruation. Onion is also used for ascariasis, high blood pressure, arteriosclerosis and in the treatment of diabetes. Externally the drug is used for insect bites, wounds, light burns, furuncles, warts, and in the after-care of bruises.

Indian Medicine: Onion preparations are used for dyspeptic conditions, respiratory conditions, wounds, pain and for malarial fever.

Chinese Medicine: Preparations are used for worm infestation, fungal and bacterial infections.

Homeopathic Uses: Allium cepa is used for acute inflammatory illnesses, pain syndrome, flatulent colic.

PRECAUTIONS AND ADVERSE REACTIONS

No health hazards or side effects are known in conjunction with the proper administration of designated therapeutic dosages. The intake of large quantities can lead to stomach complaints. Frequent contact with the drug leads on rare occasion to allergic reactions (hand eczema).

DOSAGE

Mode of Administration: Cut onions, pressed juice from fresh onions and other oral galenic preparations.

Preparation: Onion oil maceration: same as garlic maceration drug extract 1:1.

Old recipe: Siripus Cepae: freshly grated onions 15 g; water 60 ml; ethanol 90% (V/V) 15 ml; saccharose 150 g; the ethanolic extract is boiled with the saccharose.

Popular: pressed juice and onion syrup: made of 500 g onions, 500 g water, 100 g honey and 350 g sugar.

Onion tincture: 100 g minced onions in 300 g ethanol 70% macerated for 10 days.

Daily Dosage: Raw drug is used therapeutically.

Externally the juice is spread or laid on as a poultice or in slices.

Internally: onion tincture 4 to 5 teaspoonfuls daily; onion syrup 4 to 5 tablespoons daily.

Average daily dose: 50 g of fresh onions or 20 g of dried drug.

Homeopathic Dosage: 5 drops, 1 tablet, 10 globules every 30 to 60 minutes (acute) or 1 to 3 times daily (chronic); Parenterally: 1 to 2 ml 3 times daily sc; Ointment 1 to 2 times daily (HAB1)

LITERATURE

Agarwal RH, Controlled trial of the effect of cycloalliin on the fibrinolytic activity of venous blood. In: Atherosclerosis 27:347-351. 1977.

Augusti KT, Benaim ME, (1974) Clin Chim Acta 60:121.

Augusti KT, (1976) Curr Sci 45:863.

Dorsch W, et al., (1984) Eur J Pharmacol 107(1):17.

Jain RC, Vyas CR, (1974) Brit Med J 2:730.

Kabelik J, (1970) Pharmazie 25:266.

Koch HP, Hormonwirkungen bei Allium-Arten. In: ZPT 13(6):177. 1992.

Kumari K, Augusti KT, Antidiabetic effects of S-methylcystein sulphoxide on alloxan diabetes. In: PM 61(1):72-74. 1995.

Liakopoulou-Kyriakides M, et al., (1985) Phytochemistry 24: 600 and 1593.

Maugh TH, (1979) Science 204:293.

Spare CG, Virtanen AI, (1963) Acta Chem Scand 17:641.

Tverskoy L, Dmetriev A, Kozlovsky A, Grodzinsky D, Two phytoalexins from Allium-cepa bulbs. In: PH 30:799. 1991.

Vollhardt BR, Zwiebelölmazerat (z.B. Alligerol). In: Intern Praxis 32(1):201. 1992.

Wagner H, Bayer Th, Dorsch W, Das antiasthmatische Wirkprinzip der Zwiebel (Allium cepa L.). In: ZPT 9(6):165. 1988.

Whitaker JR, (1976) Adv Food Res 22:73.

Zwiebeln gegen Durchfall. In: Medical Tribune 14:26. 1993.

Further information in:

Hänsel R, Keller K, Rimpler H, Schneider G (Hrsg.), Hagers Handbuch der Pharmazeutischen Praxis, 5. Aufl., Bde 4 - 6 (Drogen), Springer Verlag Berlin, Heidelberg, New York, 1992-1994.

Madaus G, Lehrbuch der Biologischen Arzneimittel, Bde 1-3, Nachdruck, Georg Olms Verlag Hildesheim. 1979.

Wagner H, Wiesenauer M, Phytotherapie. Phytopharmaka und pflanzliche Homöopathika, Fischer-Verlag, Stuttgart, Jena, New York. 1995.

Ononis spinosa

See Spiny Rest Harrow

Onopordum acanthium

See Scotch Thistle

Ophioglossum vulgatum

See English Adder's Tongue

Opium Antidote

Combretum micranthum

DESCRIPTION

Medicinal Parts: The dry leaves and stems are the medicinal parts of the plant.

Leaves, Stem and Root: The leaves are 10 to 13 cm long and about 6 cm wide, with 8 to 10 lateral spreading veins, transparent in the axils. The surface of the young leaves has small scales.

Characteristics: The taste is astringent and strong.

Habitat: The plant is indigenous to China, Malaysia and Indonesia.

Production: Combretum leaves are the dried leaves of Combretum micramthum.

Other Names: Combretum, Jungle Weed

ACTIONS AND PHARMACOLOGY

COMPOUNDS

Pyrrolidine alkaloid betaines: stachydrines, 4-hydroxystachydrines, combretin-A (betaines drawn from the proline)

Catechin tannins

Flavonoids: including vitexin, saponaretin, orietin

EFFECTS

The drug has mild choleric and astringent effects.

INDICATIONS AND USAGE

Unproven Uses: The drug has been used for cholecystopathy, dyspepsia and liver disease. It is obsolete as a drug and now found only in combination preparations.

PRECAUTIONS AND ADVERSE REACTIONS

Health risks or side effects following the proper administration of designated therapeutic dosages are not recorded.

LITERATURE

Bassène E, Plantes Med Phytotherapie 21:173. 1987.

Bassène E et al., Ann Pharm Franc 44:491. 1986.

Further information in:

Hegnauer R, Chemotaxonomie der Pflanzen, Bde 1-11, Birkhäuser Verlag Basel, Boston, Berlin 1962-1997.

Kern W, List PH, Hörhammer L (Hrsg.), Hagers Handbuch der Pharmazeutischen Praxis, 4. Aufl., Bde 1-8, Springer Verlag Berlin, Heidelberg, New York, 1969.

Orchis species

See Salep

Oregano

Origanum vulgare

DESCRIPTION

Medicinal Parts: The medicinal parts are the oil extracted from the fresh or dried leaves through a process of steam distillation, the herb picked during the flowering season and freed from the thicker stems and dried, as well as the fresh flowering herb.

Flower and Fruit: The bright purple labiate flowers are in cyme-like panicles with elliptical, pointed and usually dark purple bracts, which are longer than the calyx. The calyx is tubular and has 5 even tips. The upper lip of the corolla is flat. The lower lip has 3 lobes; the middle lobe is the widest. There are 4 stamens, the longer ones extending beyond the lower lip.

Leaves, Stem and Root: Origanum vulgare is a woody perennial plant, which grows up to 90 cm high. The upper part is branched. The plant has rhizome-like runners and is downy, bristly or velvet-like. The leaves are 10 to 40 cm long and 4 to 25 mm wide, ovate, entire-margined or slightly crenate, glabrous or pubescent, translucent-punctate and petiolate.

Characteristics: The plant has an aromatic scent, similar to Origanum majorana.

Habitat: The plant is common throughout Asia, Europe and northern Africa.

Production: Oregano consists of the above-ground parts of Origanum vulgare. It is harvested 5 cm above the ground during the flowering season and dried carefully on the field or under a roofed loft.

Other Names: Mountain Mint, Origano, Wild Marjoram, Winter Marjoram, Wintersweet

ACTIONS AND PHARMACOLOGY

COMPOUNDS

Volatile oil (0.15-1.0%): chief components carvacrol (share 40-70%), gamma-terpinene (8-10%), p-cymene (5-10%), additionally alpha-pinene, myrcene, thymol. There are also strains with thymol, linalool + terpinene-4-ol, linalool, caryophyllene +germacren D, or germacren D as chief components

Flavonoids: including naringin

Caffeic acid derivatives: in particular, rosmaric acid (5%)

EFFECTS

The essential oil, which contains carvacrol, is antimicrobial *in vitro*.

INDICATIONS AND USAGE

Unproven Uses: Oregano herb is used for respiratory disorders such as coughs, inflammation of the bronchial mucous membranes and as an expectorant. In folk medicine, it is used for coughs, dyspepsia, painful menstruation, rheumatoid arthritis, scrofulosis, urinary tract disorders and as a diaphoretic.

Chinese Medicine: In China, Oregano is used for colds, fever, vomiting, dysentery, jaundice and malnutrition for children.

Homeopathy Uses: Oregano is used to increase sexual excitability.

PRECAUTIONS AND ADVERSE REACTIONS

No health hazards or side effects are known in conjunction with the proper administration of designated therapeutic dosages.

DOSAGE

Mode of Administration: Oregano infusions and powders are used as teas, gargles and bath additives.

Preparation: For internal use, pour 250 ml boiling water over 1 heaped teaspoonful and strain after 10 minutes; the tea can be sweetened with honey. The unsweetened infusion is used as gargle and mouthwash. To use as a bath additive, pour 1 l of water over 100 g drug, strain after 10 minutes and add to a full bath.

Daily Dosage: Tea: 1 cup several times a day. Powder: 0.5 to 1 dessertspoon 2 to 3 times daily with food.

Homeopathic Dosage: 5 to 10 drops, 1 tablet or 5 to 10 globules 1 to 3 times daily or 1 ml injection solution sc twice weekly (HAB34).

Storage: Store Oregano where it is protected from moisture and light.

LITERATURE

Afshaypuor S et al., Volatile constituents of Origanum vulgare ssp. viride (syn. O. heracleoticum) from Iran. In: PM 63(2):179-180. 1997.

Afshaypuor S, Essential oil constituents of wild marjoram from Iran. In: PM 62, Abstracts of the 44th Ann Congress of GA, 133. 1996.

Hänsel R, Keller K, Rimpler H, Schneider G (Hrsg.), Hagers Handbuch der Pharmazeutischen Praxis, 5. Aufl., Bde 4-6 (Drogen), Springer Verlag Berlin, Heidelberg, New York, 1992-1994.

Madaus G, Lehrbuch der Biologischen Arzneimittel, Bde 1-3, Nachdruck, Georg Olms Verlag Hildesheim 1979.

Steinegger E, Hänsel R, Pharmakognosie, 5. Aufl., Springer Verlag Heidelberg 1992.

Oriental Arborvitae

Thuja orientalis

DESCRIPTION

Medicinal Parts: The medicinal parts are the dried leaves and leafy branches.

Flower and Fruit: The inflorescence forms cones with horned cone scales. The male cones are apical and globose with 3 to 6 stamens. The female cones are small, ovoid to globose with 3 pairs of scales, the upper one sterile, the middle one with 1 ovule and the lower one with three. The seeds are ovoid to elliptical and have no wings.

Leaves, Stem and Root: Oriental arborvitae is a diclinous, monoecious, evergreen tree, which grows up to 10 m high. The leaves are decussately arranged, scale-like, imbricate, appressed to the branches, thick and acute. The edge leaves are pressed together and keeled. The surface leaves are ovate-rhomboid, grooved on the back, needle-like when young and acutely splayed. The branches are vertical, flattened and vertically branched. The smaller branches are the same color on both sides.

Habitat: China, Korea, Afghanistan, Iran

Production: Oriental Aborvitae tops are the dried leaves and leafy branches of Thuja orientalis. They are harvested from cultivated stock in late summer or early autumn, followed by drying in the shade.

Not to be Confused With: May be confused with other Thujae species.

Other Names: Chinese Arborvitae

ACTIONS AND PHARMACOLOGY

COMPOUNDS

Volatile oil (0.4%): containing alpha-pinene, alpha-thujone (6%)

Flavonoids: including tricetin-3-glucoside

Wax (0.5%, estolides): chief acid juniperic acid

EFFECTS

The terpene-containing drug is severely toxic. The hemostyptic and hair growth-promoting effects with which it is credited have not yet been documented in experimental data.

INDICATIONS AND USAGE

Chinese Medicine: Oriental Arborvitae is used for coughing blood, nose bleeds, dysentery, hematuria and hair loss.

PRECAUTIONS AND ADVERSE REACTIONS

No health hazards are known in conjunction with the proper administration of designated therapeutic dosages.

DOSAGE

Mode of Administration: Whole herb preparations, cut and powdered drug for internal and external use.

Preparation: to prepare Biotae Cacumen. The rubbed branches are roasted in an iron pan until the surface blackens.

Daily Dosage: 3 to 18 gm of drug

Storage: Should be stored in a dry place and protected from light.

LITERATURE

Hänsel R, Keller K, Rimpler H, Schneider G (Ed), Hagers Handbuch der Pharmazeutischen Praxis, 5. Aufl., Bde 4 - 6 (Drogen), Springer Verlag Berlin, Heidelberg, New York, 1992-1994.

Origanum majorana

See Sweet Marjoram

Origanum vulgare

See Oregano

Orris

Iris species

DESCRIPTION

Medicinal Parts: The medicinal part is the rhizome with the roots.

Flower and Fruit: The flowers are long-pedicled and perfumed. The tepals are white or slightly blue. The outer ones are darker with a yellow beard. The anthers are as big as the filaments. The upper lip of the stigma branch is inclined forward. The fruit is a large capsule with a number of sections in which the brown seeds are lined up like rolls of coins.

Leaves, Stem and Root: The plants are perennial, 30 to 100 cm high. The rhizome is thick and short. The strong flower-bearing stem is branched from the middle. The leaves are broad, sword-shaped, usually curved and gray-green.

Habitat: Indigenous to southern Europe.

Production: Orris root is the root of Iris germanica, Iris versicolor and other varieties.

Other Names: Iris, Florentine Orris, White Flag Root, Blue Flag, Flag Lily, Liver Lily, Poison Flag, Snake Lily, Water Flag, Wild Iris, Yellow Flag, Yellow Iris, Dragon Flower, Myrtle Flower, Fliggers, Flaggon, Sheggs, Segg, Daggers, Jacob's Sword, Gladyne

ACTIONS AND PHARMACOLOGY

COMPOUNDS

Volatile oil: chief constituent's irone, in particular alpha-, beta- and gamma-irone (odor resembling violets)

Triterpenes: Iridale (mono-, bi- and spirocyclic compounds, precursors of the irones), including among others irigermanal

Isoflavonoids: including, among others, irilon, irisolone, irigenine, tectorigenin and their glycosides including iridine

Flavonoids

Xanthones: C-glucosylxanthones, for example iris xanthone, magniferin

Starch

EFFECTS

Orris root is mildly expectorant. Some of the flavonoids (in particular the isoflavon irigenin) have an inhibitory effect on c-AMP phosphodiesterase. Root extracts are said to have an ulcer-protective, spasmolytic and serotonin-antagonistic effect.

INDICATIONS AND USAGE

Unproven Uses: Orris has been used for disorders of the respiratory system.

Homeopathic Uses: This species has been used to treat disorders of the respiratory tract or thyroid gland, for digestion complaints and headaches.

PRECAUTIONS AND ADVERSE REACTIONS

General: No health hazards or side effects are known in conjunction with the proper administration of designated therapeutic dosages. The juice of the fresh plant has a severely irritating effect upon skin and mucous membranes. If taken internally, it can lead to vomiting, abdominal pain and bloody diarrhea. Severe inflammation occurs following mucous membrane contact.

Pregnancy: Not to be used during pregnancy.

DOSAGE

Mode of Administration: Iris is available in homeopathic dilutions, as a constituent of various combination preparations and in various tea mixtures.

LITERATURE

Bambhole VD, Jiddewar GG, (1985) Sach Ayurveda 37(9):557.

Duke JA, A Handbook of Medicinal Herbs, Pub. CRC Press Boca Raton 1985.

El Moghazy AM et al., (1980) Fitoterapia 5:237.

Frohne D, Pfänder HJ, Giftpflanzen - Ein Handbuch für Apotheker, Toxikologen und Biologen, 4. Aufl., Wiss. Verlags-Ges Stuttgart 1997.

Kern W, List PH, Hörhammer L (Hrsg.), Hagers Handbuch der Pharmazeutischen Praxis, 4. Aufl., Bde. 1-8, Springer Verlag Berlin, Heidelberg, New York, 1969.

Krick W et al., (1983) Z Naturforsch Sect C Biosci 38 (9/10): 689.

Lewin L, Gifte und Vergiftungen, 6. Aufl., Nachdruck, Haug Verlag, Heidelberg 1992.

Madaus G, Lehrbuch der Biologischen Arzneimittel, Bde 1-3, Nachdruck, Georg Olms Verlag Hildesheim 1979.

Morita N et al., (1973) Chem Pharm Bull 21, 600.

Poisonous Plants in Britain and Their Effects on Animals and Man, Ministry of Agriculture Fisheries and Food, Pub; HMSO UK 1984.

Steinegger E, Hänsel R, Pharmakognosie, 5. Aufl., Springer Verlag Heidelberg 1992.

Teuscher E, Lindequist U, Biogene Gifte - Biologie, Chemie, Pharmakologie, 2. Aufl., Fischer Verlag Stuttgart 1994.

Tsukida K et al., (1973) Phytochemistry 12:2318.

Wagner H, Wiesenauer M, Phytotherapie. Phytopharmaka und pflanzliche Homöopathika, Fischer-Verlag, Stuttgart, Jena, New York 1995.

Wichtl M (Hrsg.), Teedrogen, 4. Aufl., Wiss. Verlagsges. Stuttgart 1997.

Orthosiphon spicatus

See Java Tea

Oryza sativa

See Rice

Oswego Tea

Monarda didyma

DESCRIPTION

Medicinal Parts: The medicinal part of the plant is the herb.

Flower and Fruit: The terminal flowers are in 1 to 3 richly blossomed false whorls supported by bracts. The bracts bear leaflets that are pale green with a reddish tinge. The calyx tips are awl-shaped. The corolla is scarlet and 3.5 to 6 cm in length. The plant is propagated using root cuttings.

Leaves, Stem and Root: The plant is a bristly haired to glabrous 50 to 90 cm high herbaceous perennial with runners. The stems are erect, acutely quadrangular, grooved and hard. The leaves are in pairs, ovate-lanceolate, clearly petiolate, crenate and often rough on both sides.

Characteristics: Monarda didyma has a scent similar to that of the bergamot orange.

Habitat: The plant is indigenous to swampy regions from Georgia and Michigan in the U.S. and to wet areas extending northward to Ontario, Canada.

Other Names: Scarlet Monarda, Bee Balm, Blue Balm, High Balm, Low Balm, Mountain Balm, Mountain Mint, Bergamot

ACTIONS AND PHARMACOLOGY

COMPOUNDS

Volatile oil (0.1-0.3%): including among others carvacrol, thymol, p-cymene, linalool, linalyl acetate, limonene, ocimene, alpha-pinene, camphene, Delta3-carene

Flavonoids: including linarin, didymin (isosakurenatin-7-O-beta-D), isosakuranin, genkwanin

Anthocyans: monardein (triacyliertes pelargonidine-3, 5-di-O-glucoside, 2 malonyl- and 1 p-cumaroyl- residue)

EFFECTS

The drug has antispasmodic, digestive, carminative and diuretic effects; it is also used to regulate menstruation.

CONTRAINDICATIONS

Oswego Tea is not to be used during pregnancy.

INDICATIONS AND USAGE

Unproven Uses: The drug is used for flatulence and other digestive disorders and also menstrual complaints including premenstrual syndrome (PMS). In Europe, the herb is sometimes used as an aromatic, carminative and antipryreticum. Former use of the drug as an alternative to quinine is no longer common.

PRECAUTIONS AND ADVERSE REACTIONS

No health hazards or side effects are known in conjunction with the proper administration of designated therapeutic dosages.

DOSAGE

Mode of Administration: Ground drug (powder) prepared as an infusion or tea.

LITERATURE

Hegnauer R, Chemotaxonomie der Pflanzen, Bde 1-11, Birkhäuser Verlag Basel, Boston, Berlin 1962-1997.

Kern W, List PH, Hörhammer L (Hrsg.), Hagers Handbuch der Pharmazeutischen Praxis, 4. Aufl., Bde. 1-8, Springer Verlag Berlin, Heidelberg, New York, 1969.

Nikolaevski VV, Kononova NS, Pertsovski i AI, Shinkarchuk IF, Effect of essential oils on the course of experimental atherosclerosis. Patol Fiziol Eksp Ter:52-3, Sep-Oct, 1990.

Shubina LP, Siurin SA, Savchenko VM, Inhalations of essential oils in the combined treatment of patients with chronic bronchitis. Vrach Delo:66-7, May 1990.

Ox-Eye Daisy

Chrysanthemum leucanthemum

DESCRIPTION

Flower and Fruit: Long pedicled flowers with a semi-globular calyx. Sepals are imbricate, green and wide, the corolla golden-yellow and orbicular. The young flowers are white and 1 to 2 cm long. The fruit is 2.5 to 3 mm long and top-shaped.

Leaves, Stem and Root: Ox-Eye Daisy is a perennial growing 10 to 100 cm high. It is somewhat hairy or glabrous with cylindrical knotted root. The stem is erect, glabrous, simple or divided into numerous oblong 1-headed branches. The leaves are tough, compound and glabrous or slightly pubescent. The cauline leaves are petiolate, linear to ovate-oblong, roughly dentate to almost pinnatisect.

Habitat: The plant is found in Britain, Europe, Russia, Asia and numerous other parts of the world.

Production: Ox-Eye Daisy is the above-ground part of Chrysanthemum leucanthemum.

Other Names: White Weed, Golden Daisy, Herb Margaret, Maudlinwort, White Daisy, Great Ox-Eye, Goldenseal, Marguerite, Moon Daisy, Horse Gowan, Maudlin Daisy, Dun Daisy, Butter Daisy, Horse Daisy, Moon Flower, Moon Penny, Poverty Weed

ACTIONS AND PHARMACOLOGY

COMPOUNDS

Cyclitols: including meso-inositol, L(-)-quercitol, meso-inositol, L(-)-quercitol

Polyynes: among them the strongly sensitizing trideca-3,5,7,9,11-pentain-1-ol and its acetate

Flavonoids: including niviaside (a C-glycosyl flavone, containing a cyclitol instead of a sugar), apigenein-7-0-glucuronide

EFFECTS

Ox-Eye Daisy herb and flowers are used similarly to Chamomile as a tonic, although they have a much weaker effect. They are also considered to have an antispasmodic and diuretic effect.

INDICATIONS AND USAGE

Unproven Uses: Internal folk medicine uses include asthma, whooping cough and nervous agitation. Among external applications are skin ulcers, wounds and nose bleeds. (Also see Chamomile.)

PRECAUTIONS AND ADVERSE REACTIONS

No health hazards or side effects are known in conjunction with the proper administration of designated therapeutic dosages. There is, however, a strong potential for sensitization resulting from skin contact with the drug.

DOSAGE

Mode of Administration: See Chamomile.

Daily Dosage: Decoction: 1 cup 3 times daily.

LITERATURE

Hausen B, Allergiepflanzen, Pflanzenallergene, ecomed Verlagsgesellsch. mbH, Landsberg 1988.

Hegnauer R, Chemotaxonomie der Pflanzen, Bde 1-11, Birkhäuser Verlag Basel, Boston, Berlin 1962-1997.

Kern W, List PH, Hörhammer L (Hrsg.), Hagers Handbuch der Pharmazeutischen Praxis, 4. Aufl., Bde 1-8, Springer Verlag Berlin, Heidelberg, New York, 1969.

Teuscher E, Lindequist U, Biogene Gifte - Biologie, Chemie, Pharmakologie, 2. Aufl., Fischer Verlag Stuttgart 1994.

Oxalis acetosella

See Wood Sorrel

Paeonia officinalis

See European Peony

Pagoda Tree

Sophora japonica

DESCRIPTION

Medicinal Parts: The medicinal parts are the ripe seeds.

Flower and Fruit: The white flowers are in large, broad, sweeping terminal panicles made up of racemes. The flowers are papilionaceous with a patent standard. The lower edge of the lateral wing petals are bent over so that one surrounds the others. The fruit is a round pod tied in around the seeds like a string of pearls.

Leaves, Stem and Trunk: The tree is reminiscent of the robinia, with a densely branched crown. It grows 12 to 15 m high. It has smooth, green branches. The leaves are odd-pinnate with 11 to 15 leaflets. The leaflets are ovate, acute, dark green above and glaucous beneath. The main leaf petiole is very thick at the base.

Habitat: The plant is indigenous to China and Japan, and is found in Europe as an ornamental and roadside tree.

Production: Pagoda Tree seeds are the ripe seeds of Sophora japonica.

ACTIONS AND PHARMACOLOGY

COMPOUNDS

Quinolizidine alkaloids (0-0.04%): including among others cytisine, N-methyl cytisine, matrine, sophocarpine

Flavonoids: including rutin, sophorine

Toxic lectins

Polysaccharides: galactomannans

Fatty oil

Proteins

EFFECTS

The active agent, rutin, increases the permeability of the capillaries.

INDICATIONS AND USAGE

Homeopathic Uses: Pagoda Tree is used in homeopathy for dysentery.

PRECAUTIONS AND ADVERSE REACTIONS

No health hazards, side effects, or cases of poisoning are known in conjunction with the proper administration of designated therapeutic dosages. Nevertheless, according to older reports, regular consumption of the seed meal can cause facial edema and even death. Cystine poisonings are possible through the intake of very high dosages.

DOSAGE

Mode of Administration: As a mother tincture in homeopathic dilutions. Sophora is used by the pharmaceutical industry in the production of rutin (a substance that influences the resolution and porousness of the dilation of the capillaries). The drug is contained in medicinal preparations, which are used to stabilize blood circulation and as a cure for nervous disorders and inflammation.

LITERATURE

Izaddoost M, PH 14:203. 1975.

Kern W, List PH, Hörhammer L (Hrsg.), Hagers Handbuch der Pharmazeutischen Praxis, 4. Aufl., Bde. 1-8: Springer Verlag Berlin, Heidelberg, New York, 1969.

Roth L, Daunderer M, Kormann K, Giftpflanzen, Pflanzengifte, 4. Aufl., Ecomed Fachverlag Landsberg Lech 1993.

Tang W, Eisenbrand G, Chinese Drugs of Plant Origin, Springer Verlag Heidelberg 1992.

Teuscher E, Lindequist U, Biogene Gifte - Biologie, Chemie, Pharmakologie, 2. Aufl., Fischer Verlag Stuttgart 1994.

Panax ginseng

See Ginseng

Papaver rhoeas

See Corn Poppy

Papaver somniferum

See Poppyseed

Papaya

Carica papaya

TRADE NAMES

Papaya (available from numerous manufacturers), Papaya Digestive Enzyme, Papaya Enzyme Double Strength, Papaya with Papain

DESCRIPTION

Medicinal Parts: The medicinal parts are the leaves and fruits.

Flower and Fruit: The plant has varying yellow to yellowish-white flowers of both sexes. The male flowers form many-branched, hanging panicles with small flowers. The female flowers are almost sessile in the leaf axils on the trunk. In addition there are androgynous, fertile flowers. The yellow to yellow-green berry fruit is up to 30 cm long, 15 cm thick and weighs 2 to 5 kg. The fruit is clavate and lightly grooved. It contains numerous peppercorn-sized seeds surrounded by orange-yellow and melon-flavored flesh.

Leaves, Stem and Root: Carica papaya is a 4 to 8 m high bushy tree with an unbranched fleshy-woody trunk that is hollow in the middle. The leaves are long-petioled, very large and segmented into 5 to 7 palmate lobes, which terminate in sharp tips.

Habitat: Indigenous to tropical America. Cultivated in all tropical regions today.

Production: Papaya leaves consist of the fresh or dried leaves of Carica papaya harvested before the fruit appears. Raw papain is the latex from Carica papaya, which has been dried using various methods; where necessary the latex is decontaminated mechanically or by filtration.

Other Names: Melon Tree, Papaw, Mamaeire

ACTIONS AND PHARMACOLOGY

COMPOUNDS: RAW PAPAIN

Proteolytic enzymes (proteinases): papain, chymopapain A and B, proteinase A and B, papaya peptidase A

Other enzymes: lysozyme, chitotransferase, glycosidases, callase, pectinesterases, lipases, phosphatases, cycloligases

EFFECTS: RAW PAPAIN

The proteolytic activity of the raw papain enzymes can be used within the parameters of enzyme substitution for digestive complaints, particularly pancreatic conditions. Papain has an antimicrobial, anthelmintic and anti-ulcerative effect.

The results of the analgesic and anti-inflammatory effects are contradictory. Experiments have shown that papain has an edema-reducing effect. The fibrinogenous effect has not been sufficiently proven.

COMPOUNDS: PAPAYA LEAVES

Polyketide alkaloids: carpaine, pseudocarpaine

Glucosinolates

Cyanogenic glycosides (traces): including prunasin

Saponins

Proteolytic ferments (ficin)

EFFECTS: PAPAYA LEAVES

No information is available.

INDICATIONS AND USAGE

RAW PAPAIN

Unproven Uses: Papaya is used for gastrointestinal digestion complaints, inflammations and ulcers in the gastro-duodenal area, and pancreas excretion insufficiency.

PAPAYA LEAVES

Unproven Uses: Papaya leaf preparations are used singly or in combinations for prophylaxis and therapy of diseases and disorders of the gastrointestinal tract and for infections with intestinal parasites.

Indian Medicine: Worm infestation, damage to the urinary tract and stones, hemorrhoids, coughs and bronchitis have been treated with Papaya leaves.

CONTRAINDICATIONS

RAW PAPAIN AND PAPAYA LEAVES

Papaya is contraindicated in pregnancy.

PRECAUTIONS AND ADVERSE REACTIONS

RAW PAPAIN

General: No health hazards or side effects are known in conjunction with the proper administration of designated therapeutic dosages. Because of the fibrinolytic effect, a tendency to bleed is possible when there is a predisposition to clotting delay and during treatment with anticoagulants. Allergic reactions, including asthma attacks, are also possible.

Drug Interactions: There has been some documented interactions with warfarin. Papaya extract has been shown to increase the international normalized ratio (INR) levels when used in conjunction with warfarin.

Pregnancy: Because of the experimentally proven embryotoxic and teratogenic effects, as well as its known abortifacient effect in humans, unripe papain fruit should not be used during pregnancy.

PAPAYA LEAVES

No health hazards or side effects are known in conjunction with the proper administration of designated therapeutic dosages.

DOSAGE

RAW PAPAIN

Daily Dosage: The dosage depends on the composition of the enzyme substitute preparation.

How Supplied:

Chewable Tablets

Tablets

PAPAYA LEAVES

Daily Dosage: No information is available.

LITERATURE

RAW PAPAIN

Buttle DJ et al., Affinity purification of the novel cysteine proteinase papaya proteinase IV, and papain from papaya latex. In: Biochem J 261(2):469-476.

Lohiya NK et al., Antifertility effects of aqueous extract of Carica papaya seeds in male rats. In: PM 60(5):400. 1994.

McKee RA, Smith H, Purification of proteinases from Carica papaya. In: PH 25:2283. 1986.

Zoch E, Über die Inhaltsstoffe des Handelspapains. In: Arzneim Forsch 19:1593. 1969.

Further information in:

Kern W, List PH, Hörhammer L (Hrsg.), Hagers Handbuch der Pharmazeutischen Praxis, 4. Aufl., Bde. 1-8, Springer Verlag Berlin, Heidelberg, New York, 1969.

Madaus G, Lehrbuch der Biologischen Arzneimittel, Bde 1-3, Nachdruck, Georg Olms Verlag Hildesheim 1979.

Shaw D, Leon C, Kolex S, Traditional remedies and food supplements: a 5-year toxicological study (1991-1995). Drug Saf 1997 Nov; 17(5):342-56.

Steinegger E, Hänsel R, Pharmakognosie, 5. Aufl., Springer Verlag Heidelberg 1992.

Teuscher E, Biogene Arzneimittel, 5. Aufl., Wiss. Verlagsges. Stuttgart 1997.

PAPAYA LEAVES

Hegnauer R, Chemotaxonomie der Pflanzen, Bde 1-11, Birkhäuser Verlag Basel, Boston, Berlin 1962-1997.

Kern W, List PH, Hörhammer L (Hrsg.), Hagers Handbuch der Pharmazeutischen Praxis, 4. Aufl., Bde. 1-8, Springer Verlag Berlin, Heidelberg, New York, 1969.

Madaus G, Lehrbuch der Biologischen Arzneimittel, Bde 1-3, Nachdruck, Georg Olms Verlag Hildesheim 1979.

Oliver-Bever B (Ed.), Medicinal Plants of Tropical West Africa, Cambridge University Press Cambridge, London 1986.

Roth L, Daunderer M, Kormann K, Giftpflanzen, Pflanzengifte, 4. Aufl., Ecomed Fachverlag Landsberg Lech 1993.

Pareira

Chondrodendron tomentosum

DESCRIPTION

Medicinal Parts: The medicinal parts are the curare, which is the extract from the fresh or dried trunk, along with the bark and the dried roots.

Flower and Fruit: The flowers grow in axillary clusters 10 to 15 cm long on stems that are often unbranched. There are 9 outer pubescent sepals about 1 mm long. The inner 6 sepals are about 3.5 mm long and glabrous. The petals are 0.4 mm long. The fruit is a drupe about 12 mm long and 9 mm wide on a stem 4 mm long.

Leaves, Stem and Root: The plant is a climber that grows up to 30 m in height. The stems are velvety. The petioles are short-haired at the base, have long erect hairs near the leaf blade and are about 8 to 12 cm long. The leaves are somewhat coriaceous, entire-margined, sparse above and tomentose beneath. They are mildly cordate, triangular-ovate or roundish and obtuse, 10 to 15 cm in length and width. The root is about 2 to 5 cm in diameter, tortuous, black, longitudinally furrowed with transverse ridges and some constrictions. Internally the root is grayish-brown, and the transverse section shows three or four concentric rings traversed by wide medullary rays. The stem pieces are similar but the external surface is grayish and marked with numerous round, warty lenticels.

Characteristics: The taste is at first bitter, then slightly sweet. The plant is odorless.

Habitat: The plant is found in western Bolivia, Peru, Ecuador, central Columbia and Panama.

Production: Pareira root is the root of Chondrodendron tomentosum. Tubocurare is extracted from the fresh or dried trunk with bark of the same plant.

Other Names: Pereira Brava, Velvet Leaf, Ice Vine

ACTIONS AND PHARMACOLOGY

COMPOUNDS

Bibenzyl isoquinoline alkaloids: including, among others, D-tubocurarine, chondrocurarine, (-)-curine, (+)-chondrofoline, chondrocurine, isochondrodendrine

EFFECTS

Tubocurare contains tubocurarine and acts as an emmenagogic and diuretic.

INDICATIONS AND USAGE

Unproven Uses: Only the tubocurarine extracted from the bark and twigs is in use. It is a peripheral muscle relaxant, which inhibits the stimulation of transference in the neuromuscular, hence causing a paralysis of the skeletal muscles. Tubocurare is used in modern anesthetics as tubocurarine. In Brazil, an infusion of the root is taken internally and the crushed leaves applied externally as treatments for poisonous snake bites.

Homeopathic Uses: Uses in homeopathy include inflammations of the urinary tract and enlarged prostate.

PRECAUTIONS AND ADVERSE REACTIONS

No health hazards or side effects are known in conjunction with the oral administration of designated therapeutic dosages of the drug. The alkaloids with curare-like effect, such as tubocurarine, are not resorbed with oral administration of the drug.

OVERDOSAGE

Nausea and heavy urine flow have been observed in individuals poisoned with tubocurare.

DOSAGE

Mode of Administration: Use of drug is no longer common.

Storage: The plant is considered poisonous and should be stored in clearly marked containers that are impervious to insects.

LITERATURE

Guha et al., (1979) J Nat Prod 42:1.

Further information in:

Hänsel R, Keller K, Rimpler H, Schneider G (Hrsg.), Hagers Handbuch der Pharmazeutischen Praxis, 5. Aufl., Bde 4-6 (Drogen), Springer Verlag Berlin, Heidelberg, New York, 1992-1994.

Madaus G, Lehrbuch der Biologischen Arzneimittel, Bde 1-3, Nachdruck, Georg Olms Verlag Hildesheim 1979.

Teuscher E, Lindequist U, Biogene Gifte - Biologie, Chemie, Pharmakologie, 2. Aufl., Fischer Verlag Stuttgart 1994.

Parietaria officinalis

See Pellitory-of-the-Wall

Paris quadrifolia

See Herb Paris

Parsley

Petroselinum crispum

TRADE NAME

Parsley Leaf, Parsley Herb (available from numerous manufacturers)

DESCRIPTION

Medicinal Parts: The medicinal parts are the oil extracted from the parsley fruit, the dried, separated schizocarp, the fresh or dried aerial parts, the dried underground parts and the whole fresh plant at the beginning of the flowering season.

Flower and Fruit: The inflorescences are long pedicled, terminal, occasionally apical, 10 to 20 rayed yellowish umbels. The involucre has 1 to 2 bracts, and the epicalyx has 6 to 8 leaves. The petals are splayed with a curved tip. The style thickening is very developed. The fruit is orbicular-ovate, 2.5 mm long and greenish-gray.

Leaves, Stem and Root: The plant is a biennial. It is glabrous, has a characteristic odor and grows from 60 to 100 cm high. The usually numerous stems grow from 1 root and are erect, round, finely grooved, glabrous and branched. The root is thin or thick fusiform to tuberous, vertical and almost fiberless. The leaves are ovate and tripinnate. The upper ones are shorter stemmed and less compound. The leaflets are tripinnate.

Characteristics: Parsley has a spicy smell.

Habitat: The plant originated in the Mediterranean region and is cultivated worldwide today.

Production: Parsley consists of the fresh or dried plant section of Petroselinum. Parsley root is the dried root of Petroselinum crispum. The fresh herb is harvested from cultivations. Parsley seed consists of the dried ripe fruits of Petroselinum crispum.

Not to be Confused With: The leaves of Aethusa cynapium.

Other Names: Hamburg Parsley, Persely, Petersylinge, Rock Parsley

ACTIONS AND PHARMACOLOGY

COMPOUNDS: PARSLEY HERB

Volatile oil (0.02-0.3%): chief components, according to breed, up to 90%

Apiole

Myristicin

1-allyl-2,3,4,5-tetramethoxybenzole: additionally including among others mentha-1,3,8-triene (up to 50%, aroma-bearer). alpha- and beta-pinene, alpha- and beta-phellandrene, hybrid strains also exist

Furocoumarins: including among others, bergapten, oxypeucedanin, isopimpinellin, psoralen, xanthotoxin, imperatorin

Flavonoids (1.9-5.6%): chief components apiin

Vitamins: in particular ascorbic acid (up to 165 mg per 100 gm)

COMPOUNDS: PARSLEY ROOT

Volatile oil (0.05-0.12%): chief components of Petroselinum crispum ssp. crispum apiole, myristicin, terpinolene, tuberosum apiole, beta-pinene, additionally including among others, alpha- and beta-pinene, (+)-limonene, beta-bisabolene

Phthalides: including among others, ligustilide, senkyunolide

Furocoumarins: including among others, bergaptene, oxypeucedanin, isopimpinellin, psoralen, xanthotoxin and imperatorin

Flavonoids (0.2-1.3%): chief components apiin

Polyynes: including among others, falcarinol, falcarindiol

EFFECTS: PARSLEY HERB AND ROOT

Although its mode of action has not been clearly explained, its use for urinary tract complaints seems plausible.

COMPOUNDS: PARSLEY FRUIT

Volatile oil (2-6%): chief components, according to breed

Apiole (58-80%)

Myristicin (49-77%)

1-allyl-2,3,4,5-tetramethoxybenzole (50-60%)

Alpha- and beta-pinene, beta-phellandrene: among others

Furocoumarins: including among others bergapten, oxypeucedanin, isopimpinellin, psoralen, xanthotoxin and imperatorin

Fatty oil: chief fatty acid petroselic acid (60-80%)

EFFECTS: PARSLEY FRUIT

In animal experiments, a diuretic effect is said to have been demonstrated with low doses as well as a moderate increase in uterine tone. Higher doses increase contractility of the smooth muscle of the intestine, bladder and especially the uterus and therefore may be abortifacient; this explains its use for menstruation complaints.

INDICATIONS AND USAGE

PARSLEY HERB AND ROOT

Approved by Commission E:

- Infections of the urinary tract
- Kidney and bladder stones

Unproven Uses: The herb is used for flushing the efferent urinary tract and for the prevention and treatment of kidney gravel. In folk medicine, it is used for gastrointestinal disorders, jaundice, kidney and bladder inflammation, as a diuretic and as an emmenagogue.

Homeopathic Uses: Inflammation of the urinary tract and irritable bladder.

PARSLEY FRUIT

Unproven Uses: In folk medicine, the fruit has been used for menstrual disturbances, disorders of the gastrointestinal tract, the kidneys and lower urinary tract, and as a digestive.

CONTRAINDICATIONS

PARSLEY HERB, ROOT AND FRUIT

The herb is contraindicated in patients allergic to parsley or apiole, those with kidney inflammations and in pregnant women. Irrigation therapy should not be carried out in the presence of edema resulting from reduced cardiac and kidney function.

PRECAUTIONS AND ADVERSE REACTIONS

PARSLEY HERB AND ROOT

General: No health hazards or side effects are known in conjunction with the proper administration of designated therapeutic dosages. The drug leads rarely to contact allergies; photodermatosis is also conceivable following intensive skin contact between freshly harvested plant parts and light-skinned individuals.

Pregnancy: Therapeutic doses are contraindicated in pregnancy.

PARSLEY FRUIT

General: No health hazards or side effects are known in conjunction with the proper administration of designated therapeutic dosages. The drug leads rarely to contact allergies; photodermatoses occur somewhat more frequently following skin contact.

Pregnancy: Parsley fruit preparations are contraindicated in pregnancy; an abortive effect has been observed.

OVERDOSAGE

PARSLEY HERB, ROOT AND FRUIT

The administration of higher dosages of the volatile oil or of preparations with high concentrations of the volatile oil can lead to poisonings. Symptoms include elevated contractility of the smooth musculature, in particular of the urinary bladder, of the intestines and of the uterus. Other symptoms may include anuria, bloody stools, emaciation, fatty liver, hemolysis, methemoglobinuria and mucous membrane bleeding.

DOSAGE

PARSLEY HERB AND ROOT

Mode of Administration: Comminuted drug for infusions as well as other galenic preparations with a comparably small proportion of essential oil to be taken orally. Dry extracts are used in pharmaceutical products, such as tablets.

How Supplied:

Capsules — 450 mg, 455 mg

Liquid — 1:1

Preparation: Infusion: Pour boiling water over 2 gm finely cut drug and strain after 10 to 15 minutes.

Daily Dosage: A total of 6 gm in the appropriate preparations.

Infusion: 2 to 3 cups over the course of the day.

Adequate intake of liquid is essential for flushing out treatment.

Homeopathic Dosage: 5 drops, 1 tablet or 10 globules every 30 to 60 minutes (acute) or 1 to 3 times a day (chronic); parenterally: 1 to 2 ml sc, acute: 3 times daily; chronic: once a day (HAB1). The daily dosage is 6 gm drug. Adequate intake of liquid is essential for flushing out treatment.

Storage: Protect from light and moisture and tightly sealed.

PARSLEY FRUIT

Mode of Administration: Preparations of the fruit are for internal use.

Preparation: To make an infusion, pour boiling water over 1gm freshly pressed drug and strain after 10 minutes.

Daily Dosage: The average single dose is 1 gm.

Tea — Two to 3 cups of the infusion can be taken daily.

Storage: Protect from light and moisture.

LITERATURE

PARSLEY HERB AND ROOT

Ashraf M et al., (1980) Pak J Sci Ind Res 23(3/4):128.

Bjeldanes LF, Kim I, (1977) J Org Chem 42:2333.

Busse WW et al., (1984) J All Clin. Immunol. 73:801.

Chaudhary SK et al., (1986) Planta Med (6):462.

Gijbels MJM et al., (1985) Fitoterapia 61(1):17.

Hänsel R, Keller K, Rimpler H, Schneider G (Eds.), Hagers Handbuch der Pharmazeutischen Praxis, 5. Aufl., Bde 4-6 (Drogen), Springer Verlag Berlin, Heidelberg, New York, 1992-1994.

Harborne Jr. B, Williams CE, (1972) Phytochemistry 11:1741.

Hausen B, Allergiepflanzen, Pflanzenallergene, ecomed Verlagsgesellsch. mbH, Landsberg 1988.

Innocenti G et al., (1976) Planta Med 29:165.

Leung AY, Encyclopedia of Common Natural Ingredients Used in Food Drugs and Cosmetics, John Wiley & Sons Inc., New York 1980.

MacLeod AJ et al., (1985) Phytochemistry 24(11):2623.

MacLeod AJ, Snyder CH, Subramanian G, Volatile aroma constituents from parsley leafs. In: PH 24(11):2623-2627. 1985.

Madaus G, Lehrbuch der Biologischen Arzneimittel, Bde 1-3, Nachdruck, Georg Olms Verlag Hildesheim 1979.

Middleton E, Drzewiecki G, (1984) Biochem Pharmacol 33:3333.

Neuhaus-Carlisle K et al., Calcium-antagonistic activity of extracts and constituents of Petroselinum crispum and other phenylpropane derivatives. In: PM 59(7):A582. 1992.

Roth L, Daunderer M, Jormann K, Giftpflanzen, Pflanzengifle. 4. Aufl., Ecomed Fachverlag Landsberg/ Lech 1993.

Sökeland J, Phytotherapie in der Urologie. In: ZPT 10(1):8. 1989.

Stahl E, Jork H, Chemische Rssen bei Arzneipflanzen. I. Mitt. Untersuchung der Kulturvarietäten europäischer Petersilienhrkünfte. In: Arch Pharmaz 297:273-281. 1964.

Steinegger E, Hänsel R, Pharmakognosie, 5. Aufl., Springer Verlag Heidelberg 1992.

Teuscher E, Lindequist U, Biogene Gifte - Biologie, Chemie, Pharmakologie, 2. Aufl., Fischer Verlag Stuttgart 1994.

Teuscher E, Biogene Arzneimittel, 5. Aufl., Wiss. Verlagsges. Stuttgart 1997.

Wagner H, Wiesenauer M, Phytotherapie. Phytopharmaka und pflanzliche Homöopathika, Fischer-Verlag, Stuttgart, Jena, New York, 1995.

Warncke D, Petroselinum crispum - Die Gartenpetersilie. In: ZPT 15(1):50-58. 1994.

Wichtl M (Ed.), Teedrogen, 4. Aufl., Wiss. Verlagsges. Stuttgart 1997.

Zheng GQ, Kenney PM, Lam LKT, Myristicin - a potential cancer chemopreventive agent from parsley leaf oil. In: J Agric Food Chem 40(1):107. 1992.

PARSLEY FRUIT

Ashraf M et al., (1980) Pak J Sci Ind Res 23(3/4):128.

Bjeldanes LF, Kim I, (1977) J Org Chem 42:2333.

Busse WW et al., (1984) J All Clin. Immunol. 73:801.

Chaudhary SK et al., (1986) Planta Med (6):462.

Gijbels MJM et al., (1985) Fitoterapia 61(1):17.

Hänsel R, Keller K, Rimpler H, Schneider G (Eds.), Hagers Handbuch der Pharmazeutischen Praxis, 5. Aufl., Bde 4-6 (Drogen), Springer Verlag Berlin, Heidelberg, New York, 1992-1994.

Harborne Jr. B, Williams CE, (1972) Phytochemistry 11:1741.

Hausen B, Allergiepflanzen, Pflanzenallergene, ecomed Verlagsgesellsch. mbH, Landsberg 1988.

Innocenti G et al., (1976) Planta Med 29:165.

Leung AY, Encyclopedia of Common Natural Ingredients Used in Food Drugs and Cosmetics, John Wiley & Sons Inc., New York 1980.

MacLeod AJ et al., (1985) Phytochemistry 24(11):2623.

Madaus G, Lehrbuch der Biologischen Arzneimittel, Bde 1-3, Nachdruck, Georg Olms Verlag Hildesheim 1979.

Middleton E, Drzewiecki G, (1984) Biochem Pharmacol 33:3333.

Neuhaus-Carlisle K et al., Calcium-antagonistic activity of extracts and constituents of Petroselinum crispum and other phenylpropane derivatives. In: PM 59(7):A582. 1992.

Roth L, Daunderer M, Jormann K, Giftpflanzen, Pflanzengifle. 4. Aufl., Ecomed Fachverlag Landsberg/ Lech 1993.

Sökeland J, Phytotherapie in der Urologie. In: ZPT 10(1):8. 1989.

Stahl E, Jork H, Chemische Rssen bei Arzneipflanzen. I. Mitt. Untersuchung der Kulturvarietäten europäischer Petersilienhrkünfte. In: Arch Pharmaz 297:273-281. 1964.

Steinegger E, Hänsel R, Pharmakognosie, 5. Aufl., Springer Verlag Heidelberg 1992.

Teuscher E, Lindequist U, Biogene Gifte - Biologie, Chemie, Pharmakologie, 2. Aufl., Fischer Verlag Stuttgart 1994.

Teuscher E, Biogene Arzneimittel, 5. Aufl., Wiss. Verlagsges. Stuttgart 1997.

Wagner H, Wiesenauer M, Phytotherapie. Phytopharmaka und pflanzliche Homöopathika, Fischer-Verlag, Stuttgart, Jena, New York, 1995.

Warncke D, Petroselinum crispum - Die Gartenpetersilie. In: ZPT 15(1):50-58. 1994.

Wichtl M (Ed.), Teedrogen, 4. Aufl., Wiss. Verlagsges. Stuttgart 1997.

Zheng GQ, Kenney PM, Lam LKT, Myristicin - a potential cancer chemopreventive agent from parsley leaf oil. In: J Agric Food Chem 40(1):107. 1992.

Parsley Piert

Aphanes arvensis

DESCRIPTION

Medicinal Parts: The medicinal part of the plant is the above-ground section.

Flower and Fruit: The flowers are in axillary clusters of 10 to 20. They are encircled by stipules. The sepals are erect, acuminate-ovate and pubescent on the outside and on the margins. They are glabrous on the inside and draw together when the fruit ripens. The fruit is 1 mm long, ovate, keeled, flat and jug-shaped. The calyx is vertically wrinkled and pubescent.

Leaves, Stem and Root: The plant is an annual or hardy annual 2 to 30 cm long and dull green in color. The root is thin, branched and fusiform. The stem is generally branched and decumbent, with short internodes. The leaves are 3 to 5 lobed fan- or diamond-shaped. The upper ones are short-petioled. The lower leaves are sessile and usually rough-haired, occasionally only ciliate. The stipules are semi-ovate, indentate-serrate, leafy and pubescent.

Habitat: Parsley Piert grows in Britain, Europe, northern Africa, and the U.S.

Production: Parsley Piert herb is the above-ground part of Aphanes arvensis.

Not to be Confused With: The plants name is a reference to the serrated shape of the leaves; it is not related to the parsley herb.

Other Names: Parsley Breakstone, Field Lady's Mantle, Parsley Piercestone

ACTIONS AND PHARMACOLOGY

COMPOUNDS

Tannin

EFFECTS

The herb is claimed to be effective as a diuretic and a psychostimulant.

INDICATIONS AND USAGE

Unproven Uses: Parsley Piert is used in folk remedies in the treatment of urinary tract disorders, especially kidney and bladder stones, and as a diuretic.

PRECAUTIONS AND ADVERSE REACTIONS

No health hazards or side effects are known in conjunction with the proper administration of designated therapeutic dosages.

DOSAGE

Mode of Administration: The fresh or dried drug and the liquid extract are used.

LITERATURE

Kern W, List PH, Hörhammer L (Hrsg.), Hagers Handbuch der Pharmazeutischen Praxis, 4. Aufl., Bde 1-8, Springer Verlag Berlin, Heidelberg, New York, 1969.

Parsnip

Pastinaca sativa

DESCRIPTION

Medicinal Parts: The medicinal parts are the dried fruit, the dried herb, the dried root and the fresh, 2-year-old root of cultivated plants.

Flower and Fruit: The golden yellow flowers are in 8- to 12-rayed umbels, which are quite flat and contain androgynous blooms. There is usually no involucre or epicalyx, or they consist of 1 or 2 dropping bracts. The petals are even-sized, golden yellow, 0.5 mm long when rolled up and 1 mm wide. The fruit is broad-elliptical, compressed, similar to a lentil, 5 to 7 mm long and 4 to 5.5 mm wide. It is yellow-brownish when ripe. The fruit is marked with oil marks and hollows.

Leaves, Stem and Root: The plant is a biennial, which grows from 30 to 100 cm. The root is fusiform or tuberous like a carrot or turnip. It is whitish and usually bears only 1 stem. The stem is erect, angular, grooved, short-haired to glabrous and branched above. The leaves are simple pinnate, glossy above, paler and soft-haired beneath. The cauline leaves are on a long sheath, which is rolled at the edge. The basal leaves are petiolate; the leaflets are ovate-oblong and deeply lobed at the base. The terminal leaflet is 3 lobed and roughly crenate to serrate.

Characteristics: The turnip-like root tastes like carrot.

Habitat: Parsnip grows wild in most parts of Europe and Asia Minor as far as western Siberia. It is naturalized in the U.S. It is cultivated in Europe, America, Australia, India, China and southern Africa.

Production: Parsnip root or herb are the dried parts of Pastinaca sativa.

Not to be Confused With: Other types of root such as Corium, Parsley Roots and the root of Bear's Breech (also known as Hogweed).

ACTIONS AND PHARMACOLOGY

COMPOUNDS: PARSNIP HERB

Furocoumarins: in particular angelicin, bergaptene, xanthotoxin, imperatorin, psoralen

Volatile oil: chief components cis- and trans-beta-ocimene, trans-beta-farnesene, terpineols, palmitolactone

Flavonoids: including rutin

COMPOUNDS: PARSNIP ROOT

Furocoumarins: in particular angelicin, bergaptene, xanthotoxin, imperatorin, psoralen

Volatile oil (1.9-3.1%): chief components including aliphatic ester, in particular octylbutyrate (29-85%), in certain strains also octylacetate, additionally other esters and some myristicin (depending on strain, 5-65%)

Fatty oil: chief fatty acid petroselic acid (46%)

EFFECTS

No information is available.

INDICATIONS AND USAGE

PARSNIP HERB

Unproven Uses: The herb is used in kidney and gastrointestinal complaints and for digestion problems.

Homeopathic Uses: The herb is used for delirium.

PARSNIP ROOT

Unproven Uses: The root is used for kidney stones, sprains and fever.

Homeopathic Uses: The root is used for delirium.

PRECAUTIONS AND ADVERSE REACTIONS

No health hazards or side effects are known in conjunction with the proper administration of designated therapeutic dosages. An increase in UV-sensitivity is possible among light-skinned persons (due to phototoxic effect of the furocoumarins).

DOSAGE

PARSNIP HERB

Mode of Administration: Available ground, as a decoction of the dried herb.

Preparation: 1 handful of Parsnip herb cooked in 1 liter of water for 10 minutes.

Daily Dosage: For the first 8 days, drink one wine-glassful 3 times daily; during the second week drink one water glassful. The daily intake can be increased up to 2 liters. The cure takes 4 to 6 weeks.

Homeopathic Dosage: 5 drops, 1 tablet or 10 globules every 30 to 60 minutes (acute) or 1 to 3 times daily (chronic); parenterally: 1 to 2 ml sc, acute, 3 times daily; chronic: once daily (HAB34).

PARSNIP ROOT

Daily Dosage: Take 1 teaspoon of freshly grated root, containing 50% plant material, 3 times daily.

Homeopathic Dosage: 5 drops, 1 tablet or 10 globules every 30 to 60 minutes (acute) or 1 to 3 times daily (chronic); parenterally: 1 to 2 ml sc, acute, 3 times daily; chronic: once daily (HAB34).

LITERATURE

Ivie GW, Holt DL, Ivey MC, Natural toxicants in human foods: psoralen an raw and cooked parsnip roots. In: Science 213:909. 1981.

Kubeczka KH et al., Über das ätherische Öl der Apiaceae (Umbeliiferae). II. Das ätherische Öl der oberirdischen Teile von Pastinaca sativa. In: PM 31(2):173-184. 1977.

Stahl E et al., Über das ätherische Öl der Apiaceae (Umbeliiferae). VI.Untersuchungen zum Vorkommen von Chemotypen bei Pastinaca sativa. In: PM 371(12):49-56. 1979.

Further information in:

Hänsel R, Keller K, Rimpler H, Schneider G (Hrsg.), Hagers Handbuch der Pharmazeutischen Praxis, 5. Aufl., Bde 4-6 (Drogen), Springer Verlag Berlin, Heidelberg, New York, 1992-1994.

Madaus G, Lehrbuch der Biologischen Arzneimittel, Bde 1-3, Nachdruck, Georg Olms Verlag Hildesheim 1979.

Teuscher E, Lindequist U, Biogene Gifte - Biologie, Chemie, Pharmakologie, 2. Aufl., Fischer Verlag Stuttgart 1994.

Parthenocissus quinquefolia

See American Ivy

Pasque Flower

Pulsatilla pratensis

DESCRIPTION

Medicinal Parts: The medicinal part is the whole fresh plant collected during the flowering season.

Flower and Fruit: The flowers are solitary and almost always nodding. They have 6 campanulate, close, bright-violet tepals. These are usually thickly silky-haired on the outside with revolute tips, and are 1.5 to 3 cm long. The stamens are yellow and numerous; the longer ones are at least two-thirds the length of the tepals. The carpels with the style are as long as the tepals. The ripe fruit is oblong and densely pubescent. The protruding style is up to 6 cm long.

Leaves, Stem and Root: The plant is a perennial, 7 to 50 cm high with a strong, dark, usually divided, rhizome. The basal leaves usually appear after the flowers and are not hardy. They are 3 to 4 pinnate with narrow linear acuminate end sections that, along with the petioles, are thickly white villous. The stems are erect and densely pubescent with 3 whorled high leaves, divided into linear, pubescent tips.

Characteristics: The plant is poisonous.

Habitat: The plant originated in southwestern Europe and now also grows in central and eastern Europe.

Production: Pasque Flower herb consists of the dried, above-ground parts of Pulsatilla vulgaris and/or Pulsatilla pratensis.

Other Names: Easter Flower, Meadow Anemone, Passe Flower, Pulsatilla, Wind Flower

ACTIONS AND PHARMACOLOGY

COMPOUNDS

Protoanemonine-forming agents: In the freshly harvested plant, presumably the glycoside ranunculin changes enzymatically when the plant is cut into small pieces, and probably also when it is dried, into the pungent, volatile protoanemonine that quickly dimerizes to anemonin. When dried, the plant is not capable of protoanemonine-formation.

Triterpene saponins

EFFECTS

In animal experiments, the protoanemonin and anemonin had an antipyretic and motility-inhibiting effect. In the inhibition test, an antibiotic effect was shown. Protoanemonin is a strong local irritant to the mucous membranes and skin.

INDICATIONS AND USAGE

Unproven Uses: Pasque Flower is used for diseases and functional disorders of genital organs; inflammatory and infectious diseases of skin and mucosa; diseases and functional disorders of the gastrointestinal tract and the urinary tract; neuralgia; migraine; and general restlessness. It has also been used to treat iritis, scleritis, gray cataract and glaucoma.

Homeopathic Uses: Homeopathic uses include inflammation of the respiratory tract, digestive organs, female genital organs, bladder, eyes, middle ear, menstruation complaints, problems during pregnancy and nursing, rheumatism, problems with voiding urine, headaches, insomnia, measles, mumps and depressive states.

CONTRAINDICATIONS

The drug is contraindicated during pregnancy.

PRECAUTIONS AND ADVERSE REACTIONS

General: No health hazards or side effects are known in conjunction with the proper administration of designated therapeutic dosages of the dehydrated drug. Extended skin contact with the freshly harvested, bruised plant (which releases protoanemonine that is severely irritating to skin and mucous membranes) can lead to blister formation and cauterizations that are difficult to heal. If taken internally, severe irritation to the gastrointestinal tract, combined with colic and diarrhea, as well as irritation of the urinary drainage passages, are possible.

Pregnancy: Administration of the drug during pregnancy is absolutely contraindicated.

OVERDOSAGE

Death by asphyxiation following the intake of large quantities of protoanemonine-forming plants has been observed in animal experiments.

Symptomatic treatment for external contact should consist of mucilaginosa, after irrigation with diluted potassium permanganate solution; in case of internal contact, activated charcoal should follow gastric lavage.

DOSAGE

Mode of Administration: Whole, cut and powdered forms of the drug are used, as are homeopathic forms for internal use.

Daily Dosage: A single dose of a decoction/liquid extract/infusion is 0.12 to 0.3 g taken 3 times daily. The usual single dose of the drug is 0.2 g; Powder 0.1 to 0.4 g; Tincture: single dose: 0.3 to 1 ml.

Conditions of the inner eye: 1 to 3 pills 3 times daily (from powder and extract at 50 g /75 pills).

Homeopathic Dosage: From D2: 5 to 10 drops, 1 tablet or 5 to 10 globules 1 to 3 times a day; from D3: 1 suppository 2 to 3 times a day; from D4: 1 ml injection solution sc twice weekly and 3 to 4 nose drops 3 to 5 times a day (HAB1).

LITERATURE

Pourrat A et al., (1980) Planta Med 38:289.

Ruijgrok HWL, PM 11:338-347. 1963.

Siess M, Seybold G, Untersuchungen über die Wirkung von Pulsatilla pratensis, Cimicifuga racemosa und Aristolochia clematis auf den Östrus infantiler und kastrierter weißer Mäuse. In: Arzneim Forsch 10:514. 1960.

Further information in:

Chan H, But P (Eds.), Pharmacology and Applications of Chinese Materia Medica, Vol 1, World Scientific Singapore 1986.

Frohne D, Pfänder HJ, Giftpflanzen - Ein Handbuch für Apotheker, Toxikologen und Biologen, 4. Aufl., Wiss. Verlags-Ges. Stuttgart 1997.

Hänsel R, Keller K, Rimpler H, Schneider G (Hrsg.), Hagers Handbuch der Pharmazeutischen Praxis, 5. Aufl., Bde 4-6 (Drogen), Springer Verlag Berlin, Heidelberg, New York, 1992-1994.

Madaus G, Lehrbuch der Biologischen Arzneimittel, Bde 1-3, Nachdruck, Georg Olms Verlag Hildesheim 1979.

Roth L, Daunderer M, Kormann K, Giftpflanzen, Pflanzengifte, 4. Aufl., Ecomed Fachverlag Landsberg Lech 1993.

Teuscher E, Lindequist U, Biogene Gifte - Biologie, Chemie, Pharmakologie, 2. Aufl., Fischer Verlag Stuttgart 1994.

Wagner H, Wiesenauer M, Phytotherapie. Phytopharmaka und pflanzliche Homöopathika, Fischer-Verlag, Stuttgart, Jena, New York 1995.

Passiflora incarnata

See Passion Flower

Passion Flower

Passiflora incarnata

TRADE NAME

Passion Flower (available from numerous manufacturers), Alcohol Free Passion Flower Liquid

DESCRIPTION

Medicinal Parts: The medicinal parts are the whole or cut dried herb and the fresh aerial parts. The yellow pulp from the berry is edible. Several other related species also have edible fruits or healing properties.

Flower and Fruit: The axillary pedicle grows up to 8 cm and bears 1 flower. The flowers are androgynous and rayed with a diameter of 5 to 9 cm and have an involucre. The 5 sepals are green on the outside, white on the inside and tough. The 5 petals are white to pale red. There is a secondary corolla inside the petals made up of 4 thread wreaths arranged in rays around the axis of the flower, which are white on the inside and purple on the outside. The ovary has 3 carpels and 3 style branches, which end in a thickened stigma. The 5 stamens are joined at the base and fused to the androgynophor.

Leaves, Stem and Root: The Passion Flower is a perennial vine on a strong, woody stem reaching up to about 10 m in length. The vine is initially angular, later gray and rounded with longitudinally striated bark. The leaves are alternate, petiolate, serrate and very finely pubescent. The under surface is hairier than the upper surface. There are bumpy extra-floral nectaries on the leaf blades. Stipules and tendrils grow from the leaf axils.

Habitat: The plant is indigenous to an area from the southeast U.S. to Argentina and Brazil. It is cultivated in Europe as a garden plant.

Production: Passion Flower herb consists of the fresh or dried aerial parts of Passiflora incarnata. The flowering shoots are cut 10 to 15 cm above the ground, usually after the formation of the first apple-sized fruit. The harvest is dried in a hay drier or in the air. For a maximum flavonoid content in the flowering shoot, twice yearly harvest is recommended; opinions are not, however, unanimous.

Not to be Confused With: Passiflora caeulea, Passiflora foetida or Passiflora edulis

Other Names: Granadilla, Maypop, Passion Vine

ACTIONS AND PHARMACOLOGY

COMPOUNDS

Flavonoids (up to 2.5%): in particular C-glycosyl-flavones, including among others isovitexin-2''-o-glucoside, schaftoside, isoschaftoside, isoorientin, isoorientin-2''-o-glucoside, vicenin-2, lucenin-2

Cyanogenic glycosides: gynocardine (less than 0.1%)

Volatile oil (trace)

The frequently postulated presence of harmaline alkaloids could not be confirmed.

EFFECTS

Passion Flower contains glycosides and in animal tests is hypotensive and stimulates respiration. Sedative or spasmolytic effects could not be definitively proven. The use of the herb for nervous agitation, difficulty falling asleep or nervous gastrointestinal symptoms needs further investigation. A motility-inhibiting effect has been observed in animal tests.

INDICATIONS AND USAGE

Approved by Commission E:

■ Nervousness and insomnia

Unproven Uses: Passion Flower is used internally for depressive states such as hysteria, general nervous agitation, insomnia and nervous gastrointestinal complaints. The herb is used externally for hemorrhoids and as a bath additive for nervous agitation.

Homeopathic Uses: Passifloraincarnata is used for insomnia, convulsions and agitation.

PRECAUTIONS AND ADVERSE REACTIONS

No health hazards or side effects are known in conjunction with the proper administration of designated therapeutic dosages.

DOSAGE

Mode of Administration: As a comminuted herb for tea and other galenic preparations for internal use or as sedative bath additives.

How Supplied:

Capsules — 400 mg

Liquid (alcohol free) — 1:1

Preparation: To make an infusion, pour 150 ml of hot water over 1 teaspoon drug and strain after 10 minutes. To make a rinse for the external treatment of hemorrhoids, put 20 gm drug into 200 ml simmering water, strain and use when cooled.

Daily Dosage:

Tea — Pour 150 ml of hot water over 1 teaspoon of the herb and strain after 10 minutes. Drink 2 to 3 times throughout the day and one-half hour before bedtime.

Tincture — 0.5 to 2 ml, 3 times daily.

External use — 20 gm of the herb in 200 ml simmering water. Strain and use when cool as a wash or rinse.

Homeopathic Dosage: 5 drops, 1 tablet, 10 globules every 30 to 60 minutes (acute) or 1 to 3 times daily (chronic); parenterally: 1 to 2 ml SC, acute: 3 times daily; chronic: once a day; ointment: 1 to 2 times daily; 1 suppository 2 to 3 times daily (acute and chronic) (HAB1).

LITERATURE

Anon, Phytotherapeutika: Nachgewiesene Wirkung, aber wirksame Stoffe meist nicht bekannt. In: DAZ 137(15):1221-1222. 1997.

Aoyagi N et al., (1974) Chem Pharm Bull 22:1008.

Bennati E, (1968), Boll Chim Farm 110:664.

Bennati E, Fedeli E, (1968) Boll Chim Farm 107:716.

Busse WW et al., (1984) J All Clin. Immunol. 73:801.

Caesar W, Passionsblume Kulturhistorische Aspekte einer Arzneipflanze. In: DAZ 137(8): 587-93. 1997.

Hänsel R, Pflanzliche Beruhigungsmittel Möglichkeiten und Grenzen der Selbstmedikation. In: DAZ 135(32), 2935-2943. 1995.

Hänsel R, Keller K, Rimpler H, Schneider G (Ed.), Hagers Handbuch der Pharmazeutischen Praxis, 5. Aufl., Bde 4 - 6 (Drogen), Springer Verlag Berlin, Heidelberg, New York, 1992-1994.

Leung AY, Encyclopedia of Common Natural Ingredients Used in Food Drugs and Cosmetics. John Wiley & Sons Inc. New York 1980.

Loehdefink J, Kating H, (1974) Planta Med 25:101.

Lutomski J, Malek B, (1975) Planta Med 27:381.

Lutomski J, Wrocinski T, (1960) Bui Inst Ros Lec 6:176.

Madaus G, Lehrbuch der Biologischen Arzneimittel, Bde 1-3, Nachdruck, Georg Olms Verlag Hildesheim 1979.

Maluf E, Barros HMT, Frochtengarten ML et al., (1991) Assessment of the Hypnotic/Sedative Effects and Toxicity of Passiflora edulis Aqueous Extract in Rodents and Humans. Phytother Res 5:262-266.

Meier B, (1995) Passiflora incarnata - Portrait einer Arzneipflanze. Z Phytother 16:115-126.

Meier B, (1995) Passiflorae herba - pharmazeutische Qualität. Z Phytother 16:90-99.

Middleton E, Drzewiecki G, (1984) Biochem Pharmacol 33:3333.

Poethke W, et al., (1970) Planta Med 18:303.

Proliac A, Raynaud J, (1986) Pharmazie 41:673.

Roth L, Daunderer M, Kormann K, Giftpflanzen, Pflanzengifte. 4. Aufl., Ecomed Fachverlag Landsberg / Lech 1993.

Schilcher H, (1995) Pflanzliche Psychopharmaka. Eine neue Klassifizierung nach Indikationsgruppen. Deutsche Apotheker Ztg 135:1811-1822.

Schilcher H Z, (1968) Naturforsch 23B:1393.

Schulz R, Hänsel R, Rationale Phytotherapie. Springer Verlag Heidelberg 1996.

Speroni E, Minghetti A, (1988) Neuropharmacological activity of extracts from Passiflora incarnata. Planta Med:488-491.

Steinegger E, Hänsel R, Pharmakognosie. 5. Aufl., Springer Verlag Heidelberg 1992.

Teuscher E, Biogene Arzneimittel. 5. Aufl., Wiss. Verlagsgesellschaft Stuttgart 1997.

Wagner H, Wiesenauer M, Phytotherapie. Phytopharmaka und pflanzliche Homöopathika. Fischer-Verlag, Stuttgart, Jena, New York 1995.

Wichtl M, (Ed) Teedrogen. 4. Aufl., Wiss. Verlagsges. Stuttgart 1997.

Pastinaca sativa

See Parsnip

Patchouli

Pogostemon cablin

DESCRIPTION

Medicinal Parts: The medicinal parts are the young leaves and shoots and the oil extracted from them.

Flower and Fruit: The flowers, which are whitish and often have reddish marks, grow in terminal and axillary spikes.

Leaves, Stem and Root: The plant is a pubescent, perennial herb, which grows from 60 to 90 cm high. The stem is erect and quandrangular, and the leaves are ovate, opposite and soft.

Characteristics: The ovate leaves have a strong characteristic odor when rubbed. The extracted oil is used in perfumery. The desired characteristics improve with age.

Habitat: The plant is cultivated in tropical and subtropical regions worldwide.

Production: Patchouli oil is extracted from the leaves of Pogostemon cablin.

Other Names: Putcha-Pat, Patchouly

ACTIONS AND PHARMACOLOGY

COMPOUNDS

Volatile oil (1.5-4%): chief components are sesquiterpenes, including among others patchouli alcohol (35%), alpha-guaiene (20%), alpha-bulnesen (20%), beta-patchoulen (2%) as well as nordehydropatchoulol (aroma-bearer); Sesquiterpene pyridine alkaloids were isolated from the volatile oil, including among others patchouli pyridine, epiguai pyridine

EFFECTS

No information is available.

INDICATIONS AND USAGE

There is no known medicinal use. The herb is used in perfumes and cosmetics.

PRECAUTIONS AND ADVERSE REACTIONS

No health hazards or side effects are known in conjunction with the proper administration of designated therapeutic dosages.

DOSAGE

Mode of Administration: It is used only in the perfume and cosmetic industry.

LITERATURE

Kern W, List PH, Hörhammer L (Hrsg.), Hagers Handbuch der Pharmazeutischen Praxis, 4. Aufl., Bde. 1-8, Springer Verlag Berlin, Heidelberg, New York, 1969.

Leung AY, Encyclopedia of Common Natural Ingredients Used in Food Drugs and Cosmetics, John Wiley & Sons Inc., New York 1980.

Paullinia cupana

See Guarana

Pausinystalia yohimbe

See Yohimbe Bark

Peanut

Arachis hypogaea

DESCRIPTION

Medicinal Parts: The oil has medicinal applications.

Flower and Fruit: The flowers are 5 to 7 cm long, monosymmetrical and have a large golden-yellow standard. The flowers have lemon-yellow wings and a pure white carina. They are arranged singularly or in pairs in the leaf axils. They blossom at sunrise and wilt in the same morning, during which time they stretch from 5 to 20 cm and act negatively phototropically downward. After pollination, a meristem develops at the base of the ovary, from which the fruit axis grows. The fruit only starts to grow when the stem is 5 to 10 cm underground, where it grows horizontally. The fruit is a 4 cm long by 1.5 cm thick closed pod with a fibrous, reticulate-wrinkled wall and 1 to 4 large seeds with no endosperm and a thin, red shell.

Leaves, Stem and Root: The peanut plant is an annual herbaceous 30 to 70 cm high legume, with glabrous, double pinnate leaves and a decumbent to upright stem.

Habitat: Peanuts were originally indigenous to tropical and sub-tropical South America. Today, Arachis hypogaea is cultivated in all tropical and sub-tropical regions worldwide except in the rain forests.

Production: Peanut oil is the fatty oil extracted from the husked seeds of Arachis hypogaea by means of a ''cold press'' method or by hexane extraction and refining.

Other Names: Arachis, Groundnuts, Monkey Nuts

ACTIONS AND PHARMACOLOGY

COMPOUNDS

Fatty oil: chief fatty acids include oleic acid, linolic acid and palmitin acid. Also present in small quantities are longer-chained fatty acids such as eicosanoic acid and tetracosanoic acid.

EFFECTS

The effect obtained when used as an enema for constipation and in dermatology for dry skin, eczema and dandruff is achieved primarily from the drug's oiliness, although it has been shown to contain lectines.

INDICATIONS AND USAGE

Unproven Uses: Peanut oil is added to ointments and medicinal oils, and applied rectally in rectal constipation. It is also used in dermatology for crusting and scaling of the scalp (with hair), baby care and dry skin. Other applications include use as a bath additive for subacute and chronic eczema and for atrophic eczema and ichthyosis.

The pharmaceutical and medical industries use peanut oil as a vehicle for medication in external, enteral or parenteral preparations; the cosmetics industry uses it in skin, sun and massage oil. Domestically, it is used as a salad or cooking oil that is said to lower blood cholesterol levels.

Indian Medicine: Peanut oil is used for constipation, neuralgia and dislocated joints.

PRECAUTIONS AND ADVERSE REACTIONS

No health hazards or side effects are known in conjunction with the proper administration of designated therapeutic dosages.

DOSAGE

Mode of Administration: As an enema, oil, bath additive and medicinal base component.

Daily Dosage: As a rectal enema, use 130 ml of oil at body temperature. For use in a bath, the recommended concentration is 4 ml per 10 liters of water. Adults should bathe for 15 to 20 minutes 2 to 3 times weekly. Children and babies should bathe for a few minutes 2 to 3 times weekly.

Storage: Protect from light in well-sealed and, if possible, fully filled containers. Oils from different deliveries should not be stored together. Oils with a tocopherol content less than 50 mg/100 mg do not store well.

LITERATURE

Adrian J, Jacquot R, Valeur Alimentaire de l'Arachide et ses Derives, Maisonneuve et Larose, Paris 1968.

Avichezer D, Arnon R, Differential reactivities of the Arachis hypogaea (peanut) and Vicia villosa B4 lectins with human ovarian carcinoma cells grown either in vitro or in vivo xenograft model. FEBS Lett, 395:103-8, 1996 Oct 21.

Boudreaux HB, Frampton VL, (1960) Nature 185:469.

Codex Alimentarius Commission, Alinorm 79/17, Report 10th Session. Codex Committee on Fats and Oils, London 1987.

Eghafona NO, Immune responses following cocktails of inactivated measles vaccine and Arachis hypogaea L. (groundnut) or Cocos nucifera L. (coconut) oils adjuvant. Vaccine, 14:1703-6, 1996 Dec.

Garcia GM, Stalker HT, Shroeder E, Kochert G, Identification of RAPD SCAR and RFLP markers tightly linked to nematode resistance genes introgressed from Arachis cardenasii into Arachis hypogaea. Genome, 39:836-45, 1996 Oct.

Hänsel R, Keller K, Rimpler H, Schneider G (Hrsg.), Hagers Handbuch der Pharmazeutischen Praxis, 5. Aufl., Bde 4-6 (Drogen): Springer Verlag Berlin, Heidelberg, New York, 1992-1994.

Further information in:

Bhagya S, Prakash V, Srinivasan KS, Effect of different proteolytic enzymes on the nature of subunit composition of arachins from groundnut (Arachis hypogaea L.). Indian J Biochem Biophys, 12:154-9, 1992 Apr.

Boudreaux HB, Frampton VL, Nature 185 (1960), 469.

Burks AW, et al., Identification and characterization of a second major peanut allergen Ara h II with use of the sera of patients with atopic dermatitis and positive peanut challenge. J Allergy Clin Immunol, 90:962-9, 1992 Dec.

Calori-Domingues MA, Fonseca H, Laboratory evaluation of chemical control of aflatoxin production in unshelled peanuts

(Arachis hypogaea L.). Food Addit Contam, 12:347-50, 1995 May-Jun.

Codex Alimentarius Commission Alinorm 79/17, Report 10th Session. Codex Committee on Fats and Oils, London 1987. 1987.

Hänsel R, Keller K, Rimpler H, Schneider G (Ed), Hagers Handbuch der Pharmazeutischen Praxis, 5. Aufl., Bde 4 - 6 (Drogen), Springer Verlag Berlin, Heidelberg, New York, 1992-1994.

Langkilde NC et al., Human urinary bladder carcinoma glycoconjugates expressing T-(Gal beta(1-3)GalNAc alpha 1-O-R) and T-like antigens: a comparative study using peanut agglutinin, poly- and monoclonal antibodies. Cancer Res, 52:5030-6, 1992 Sep 15.

Roth L, Daunderer M, Kormann K, Giftpflanzen, Pflanzengifte, 4. Aufl., Ecomed Fachverlag Landsberg Lech 1993.

Sanford GL, Harris-Hooker S, Stimulation of vascular cell proliferation by beta-galactoside specific lectins. FASEB J, 52:2912-8, 1990 Aug.

Sreenivas A, Sastry PS, A soluble preparation from developing groundnut seeds (Arachis hypogaea) catalyzes de novo synthesis of long chain fatty acids. Indian J Biochem Biophys, 14:213-7, 1995 Aug.

Srivastava R, Rajput YS, Khare SK, Tyagi R, Gupta MN, Purification and characterization of an acid phosphatase from Arachis hypogaea. Biochem Mol Biol Int, 224:949-56, 1995 Apr.

Steinegger E, Hänsel R, Pharmakognosie, 5. Aufl., Springer Verlag Heidelberg 1992.

Swamy MJ, Gupta D, Mahanta SK, Surolia A, Further characterization of the saccharide specificity of peanut (Arachis hypogaea) agglutinin. Carbohydr Res, 137:59-67, 1991 Jun 25.

Teuscher E, Biogene Arzneimittel, 5. Aufl., Wiss. Verlagsges. Stuttgart 1997.

Urtz BE, Elkan GH, Purification and partial characterization of acyl carrier proteins from developing oil seeds of pisa (Actinodaphne hookeri) and ground nut (Arachis hypogaea). Indian J Biochem Biophys, 224:137-46, 1995 Jun.

Zhang X, Ling L, Dai R, Constituents of the seed coat of Arachis hypogaea L. Chung Kuo Chung Yao Tsa Chih, 137:356-8 384, 1990 Jun.

Pear

Pyrus communis

DESCRIPTION

Medicinal Parts: The medicinal part is the fruit.

Flower and Fruit: The fleshy fruit is typically smaller near the stem and larger at the apical end, with a relatively tough skin. The core has a number of carpels, which are large and edible. The seeds are pointed at one end and rounded at the other. When ripe, they are dark brown to black, glabrous and about 0.5 cm long.

Leaves, Stem and Root: The pear is a tree, up to 20 m tall, with a long-clavate crown. The bark is dark brown to black and broken into square plates. The glabrous or slightly pubescent branches are glossy brown or thorny. The leaves are 2 to 8 cm long, ovate-round, acuminate, tough and serrate. The ribs are protruding.

Habitat: The Pear Tree grows mainly in the temperate regions of the Northern Hemisphere.

Production: Pears are the fruit of Pyrus communis.

ACTIONS AND PHARMACOLOGY

COMPOUNDS

Fruit acids: malic acid (0.06-0.1%), additionally citric acid, quinic acid

Cyanogenic glycosides: amygdalin (only in the seeds)

Aromatic substances: including (E,Z)-2,4-deca-dien-(E)-2-octen and -(Z)-4-decenacylethylester, acetic acid hexylester

Caffeic acid derivatives: in particular 5-caffeoyl quinic acid

Pectin

EFFECTS

In folk remedies, Pear is said to be astringent and cooling.

INDICATIONS AND USAGE

Unproven Uses: Pear is used in the treatment of mild digestive disorders, while its syrup is used as a diuretic and laxative.

PRECAUTIONS AND ADVERSE REACTIONS

No health hazards or side effects are known in conjunction with the proper administration of designated therapeutic dosages.

DOSAGE

Mode of Administration: Fresh fruit (as food)

LITERATURE

Belitz HD, Grosch W, Lehrbuch der Lebensmittelchemie, 4. Aufl., Springer Verlag Berlin, Heidelberg, New York 1992.

Kern W, List PH, Hörhammer L (Hrsg.), Hagers Handbuch der Pharmazeutischen Praxis, 4. Aufl., Bde 1-8, Springer Verlag Berlin, Heidelberg, New York, 1969.

Pellitory

Anacyclus pyrethrum

DESCRIPTION

Medicinal Parts: The medicinal part of the plant is the root.

Flower and Fruit: Each stem bears a 1 cm wide flower. The bracts are fused. The ray florets are white and tinged purple beneath. The disc florets are pointed. The fruit has transparent wings.

Leaves, Stem and Root: Pellitory is a perennial grass plant whose thickened, hollow stems grow a short distance along the ground before turning upward. The plant grows to about 45 cm high and has double-pinnate, tough leaves. The root is almost cylindrical, easily twisted, tapered and crowned with a tuft of gray hair. The outside is brown and fissured with shiny black markings.

Habitat: The plant grows in North Africa and is cultivated in the Mediterranean.

Production: Pellitory root is the root of Anacyclus pyrethrum.

Other Names: Pellitory of Spain, Pyrethre, Pyrethrum, Roman Pellitory, Spanish Camomile

ACTIONS AND PHARMACOLOGY

COMPOUNDS

Alkamides: including deca-2, 4-dien acid-isobutylamide, anacycline, dehydroanacycline

Lignans: including sesamine

Inulin (fructosan)

Tannins

EFFECTS

Application to the skin stimulates the nerve ends, resulting in redness and irritation (hot, burning sensation). Pellitorin (rather than anacycline) is the local irritant. The drug, which contains alkamides (pellitorin) and tannins, had an inhibitory effect in vitro on cyclo-oxygenase and 5-lipoxygenase (affecting prostaglandin metabolism), and also an antimicrobial, insecticidal and molluscicidal effect. In tests on animals and humans, a local anesthetic effect was observed indicating ptery mandibular block with infiltration of the long buccal nerves after extraction of mandibular molars.

INDICATIONS AND USAGE

Unproven Uses: Pellitory is used externally for rheumatic conditions, the treatment of toothache. Pellitory is used internally as a tonic to aid digestion and as an insecticide.

Indian Medicine: Used as a gargle for toothache and as a powder mixed with honey for epilepsy.

PRECAUTIONS AND ADVERSE REACTIONS

No health hazards or side effects are known in conjunction with the proper administration of designated therapeutic dosages.

OVERDOSAGE

Signs of irritation are possible in connection with overdoses due to the mucous-membrane-stimulating character of the alkamides.

DOSAGE

Mode of Administration: There is mention of use as a gargle and as a powder, but no precise information is available.

LITERATURE

Kern W, List PH, Hörhammer L (Hrsg.), Hagers Handbuch der Pharmazeutischen Praxis, 4. Aufl., Bde 1-8, Springer Verlag Berlin, Heidelberg, New York, 1969.

Pellitory-of-the-Wall

Parietaria officinalis

DESCRIPTION

Medicinal Parts: The medicinal part is the herb.

Flower and Fruit: The small, green, sessile flowers grow in axillary racemes and bloom throughout the summer. The bracteoles are free and shorter than the calyx. The filaments of the stamens are strangely jointed and so elastic that when they are touched before the flower has opened, they uncoil from their rolled-up position and distribute the pollen. The achaenes are black.

Leaves, Stem and Root: The plant is a perennial, heavily branched, bushy and leafy. It grows to 70 cm high. It has a reddish hard stem and narrow petiolate, ovate-lanceolate or elliptical, long-acuminate leaves 2.5 to 5 cm long. The leaf stalk is shorter than the leaf blade. The stem and the undersurface of the leaf ribs are pubescent with short, soft hairs. The uppersurface of the leaves is almost glabrous and the ribs sunken.

Habitat: The herb is indigenous to Europe.

Production: Pellitory-of-the-Wall is the aerial part of Parietaria officinalis.

Other Names: Lichwort

ACTIONS AND PHARMACOLOGY

COMPOUNDS

Flavonoids: including among others kaempferol-, quercetin- and isorhamnetin-3-glucosides, -3-sophoroside, -3-rutinosides, -3-neohesperidosides

Caffeic acid derivatives: including caffeoyl malic acid

Bitter principles

EFFECTS

The drug is a mild diuretic.

INDICATIONS AND USAGE

The herb is used to treat diseases of the urinary tract.

PRECAUTIONS AND ADVERSE REACTIONS

No health hazards or side effects are known in conjunction with the proper administration of designated therapeutic dosages.

DOSAGE

Mode of Administration: The herb is obsolete as a drug, but is occasionally used in commercial medicinal preparations.

LITERATURE

Budzianowski J et al., (1985) J Nat Prod 48(2):336.

Geraci D et al., (1978) Immunochemistry 15:491.

Hegnauer R, Chemotaxonomie der Pflanzen, Bde 1-11, Birkhäuser Verlag Basel, Boston, Berlin 1962-1997.

Kern W, List PH, Hörhammer L (Hrsg.), Hagers Handbuch der Pharmazeutischen Praxis, 4. Aufl., Bde. 1-8, Springer Verlag Berlin, Heidelberg, New York, 1969.

Madaus G, Lehrbuch der Biologischen Arzneimittel, Bde 1-3, Nachdruck, Georg Olms Verlag Hildesheim 1979.

Pennyroyal

Mentha pulegium

DESCRIPTION

Medicinal Parts: The medicinal parts are the essential oil extracted from the fresh plant, the dried aerial parts and the whole plant.

Flower and Fruit: The flowers are in axillary, loose and globular false whorls. The calyx is cylindrical-funnel-shaped, grooved and is awned in the tube. The lower tips are awl-shaped, the upper ones shorter and wider. The upper lip has 3 tips and is curved slightly upward. The lower lip is divided in two and is straight. The corolla is violet, glabrous or downy. It has a tube, which suddenly widens in a sack-like manner and has a slightly developed ring of hair as well as lobes. These extend well beyond the calyx. The nutlets are glossy brown.

Leaves, Stem and Root: Pennyroyal is a glabrous to downy perennial, which grows from 10 to 40 cm high. The stem is ascendent or decumbent, branched and slightly downy. The leaves are elliptical to narrow ovate-elliptical, short-petioled, entire-margined, translucently glandular punctate with 1 to 3 pairs of shallow teeth and curved pinnate ribs.

Characteristics: Strongly aromatic.

Habitat: The plant thrives in western, southern and central Europe, in Asia as far as Turkmenistan, Iran, in the Arab countries and Ethiopia. It is naturalized in America.

Production: Pennyroyal is the flowering herb of Mentha pulegium. The plants are harvested during the flowering season and dried.

Other Names: Pulegium, Run-by-the-Ground, Lurk-in-the-Ditch, Pudding Grass, Piliolerial, Mosquito Plant, Squaw Balm, Squawmint Tickweed

ACTIONS AND PHARMACOLOGY

COMPOUNDS

Volatile oil (1-2%): chief constituents D-pulegone (60-90%), menthone (10-20%), isomenthone (2-10%), additionally including among others piperitone, neoisomenthylacetate

Tannins: presumably rosmaric acid

Flavonoids: including among others diosmin, hesperidin

EFFECTS

Pennyroyal oil (main component pulegone) has an antimicrobial and insecticidal effect. There is no scientific proof of the described effects.

INDICATIONS AND USAGE

Unproven Uses: The drug is used for digestive disorders, liver and gallbladder disorders, amenorrhea, gout, colds and increased micturation; externally, it is used for skin diseases.

PRECAUTIONS AND ADVERSE REACTIONS

General: European Pennyroyal oil is hepatotoxic in effect.

Acute poisonings are not to be feared in conjunction with the proper administration of designated therapeutic dosages of the foliage drug. Still, because of its hepatotoxicity, it is recommended that the drug not be used.

Pregnancy: In high doses, Pennyroyal has been reported to cause abortion. Use in pregnancy is not recommended.

OVERDOSAGE

Severely acute poisonings have been observed following administration of 5 gm of the volatile oil. Vomiting, blood-pressure elevation, anesthetic-like paralysis and death through respiratory failure have been reported following larger dosages. Cases of death have been described following misuse of the volatile oil to induce abortion.

DOSAGE

See: PRECAUTIONS AND ADVERSE REACTIONS.

Mode of Administration: Internally as a ground drug, an extract and a tea. The oil is applied topically.

Daily Dosage: The average daily internal dose of the dried drug is 1 to 4 gm, taken 3 times daily. Pennyroyal is prepared as an infusion. Drink one cupful at a time during the course of the day. Extract: 1 to 4 ml, 3 times daily.

LITERATURE

Frohne D, Pfänder HJ, Giftpflanzen - Ein Handbuch für Apotheker, Toxikologen und Biologen, 4. Aufl., Wiss. Verlags-Ges. Stuttgart 1997.

Hänsel R, Keller K, Rimpler H, Schneider G (Hrsg.), Hagers Handbuch der Pharmazeutischen Praxis, 5. Aufl., Bde 4-6 (Drogen), Springer Verlag Berlin, Heidelberg, New York, 1992-1994.

Lewin L, Gifte und Vergiftungen, 6. Aufl., Nachdruck, Haug Verlag, Heidelberg 1992.

Madaus G, Lehrbuch der Biologischen Arzneimittel, Bde 1-3, Nachdruck, Georg Olms Verlag Hildesheim 1979.

Miller EC et al., (1983) Cancer Res 43: 1124.

Roth L, Daunderer M, Kormann K, Giftpflanzen, Pflanzengifte, 4. Aufl., Ecomed Fachverlag Landsberg Lech 1993.

Steinegger E, Hänsel R, Pharmakognosie, 5. Aufl., Springer Verlag Heidelberg 1992.

Peppermint

Mentha piperita

DESCRIPTION

Medicinal Parts: The medicinal parts are the oil extracted from the aerial parts of the flowering plant, the dried leaves and flowering branch tips, the fresh flowering plant and the whole plant.

Flower and Fruit: The flowers are false spikes with numerous inconspicuous bracts. The calyx is tubular with a ring of hair. The corolla is violet, glabrous inside and has an almost even margin divided into four parts.

Leaves, Stem and Root: The plant is a perennial, 50 to 90 cm high. The usually branched stems are normally glabrous, but sometimes they are gray-tomentose and are often tinged violet. The leaves are short-petioled, oblong-ovate and serrate. The plant has over- and underground runners.

Habitat: Common in Europe and the U.S., usually cultivated.

Production: Peppermint oil consists of the essential oil of Mentha piperita obtained by aqueous steam distillation from freshly harvested, flowering springs and preparations of same. Peppermint leaves consist of the fresh or dried leaf of Peppermint as well as its preparations.

Peppermint leaf is harvested several times a year. The maximum leaf harvest and highest oil content is shortly before the flowering season. The harvest is dried mechanically on drying belts at a temperature of 42° C. Peppermint is harvested mechanically shortly after flowering and dried in the field.

Not to be Confused With: Peppermint should not be confused with rectified mint oil. Sometimes adulterated by increasing the ester content with racemic menthol acetate.

Other Names: Brandy Mint, Lamb Mint

ACTIONS AND PHARMACOLOGY

COMPOUNDS: PEPPERMINT LEAVES

Volatile oil: chief components: menthol (35-45%), menthone (15-20%), menthyl acetate (3-5%), neomenthol (2.5-3.5%), isomenthone (2-3%), menthofurane (2-7%), additionally including among others limonene, pulegone, alpha- and beta-pinene, trans-sabinene hydrate

Caffeic acid: including among others, rosmaric acid

Flavonoids: apigenine-, diosmetin- and luteolin glycosides, free lipophile methoxylized flavone including among others, xanthomicrol, gardenine D

EFFECTS: PEPPERMINT LEAVES

The drug has a spasmolytic effect on the smooth muscle of the digestive tract. It also has antiviral, antimicrobial, diuretic, cholagogic, carminative and mild sedative effect.

COMPOUNDS: PEPPERMINT OIL

Chief components: menthol (35-45%), menthone (15-20%), menthyl acetate (3-5%), neomenthol (2.5-3.5%), isomenthone (2-3%), menthofurane (2-7%), additionally including among others limonene, pulegone, alpha- and beta-pinene, trans-sabinene hydrate

Labiatentannins: including, among others rosmaric acid

Flavonoids: apigenine-, diosmetin- and luteolin glycosides, free lipophile methoxylized flavone including, among others xanthomicrol, gardenine D

EFFECTS: PEPPERMINT OIL

The drug has a spasmolytic effect on smooth muscle of the gastrointestinal tract. It is a carminative, cholagogue, antibacterial, insecticidal and secretolytic agent; it also has a cooling effect on the skin.

INDICATIONS AND USAGE

PEPPERMINT LEAVES

Approved by Commission E:

- Liver and gallbladder complaints
- Dyspeptic complaints

The drug is used for convulsive complaints of the gastrointestinal tract as well as gallbladder and bile ducts.

Unproven Uses: In folk use, peppermint is utilized for nausea, vomiting, morning sickness, respiratory infections, dysmenorrhea and colds.

Homeopathic Uses: The drug is used for colds.

PEPPERMINT OIL

Approved by Commission E:

- Common cold
- Cough/bronchitis
- Fevers and colds
- Inflammation of the mouth and pharynx
- Liver and gallbladder complaints
- Dyspeptic complaints
- Tendency to infection

The drug is used internally for cramps of the upper gastrointestinal tract and bile ducts, irritable colon, catarrhs of the respiratory tract, and inflammation of the oral and pharyngeal mucosa.

Unproven Uses: Externally, Peppermint oil is used for myalgia and neuralgia.

CONTRAINDICATIONS

PEPPERMINT LEAVES

Contraindicated in cases of gallstones.

PEPPERMINT OIL

Contraindications for the internal administration of the drug include occlusion of the biliary ducts, gallbladder inflammation and severe liver damage. Gallstone carriers could experience colic due to the cholagogic effect.

PRECAUTIONS AND ADVERSE REACTIONS

PEPPERMINT LEAVES

No health hazards are known in conjunction with the proper administration of designated therapeutic dosages. Gallstone carriers could experience colic due to the cholagogic effect.

PEPPERMINT OIL

General: No health hazards are known in conjunction with the proper administration of designated therapeutic dosages. The intake can lead to gastric complaints in susceptible persons. The volatile oil possesses a weak potential for sensitization due to its menthol content. One is advised against administration of the drug in the presence of a tendency to gastroesophageal reflux.

Pediatric Use: Preparations containing the oil should not be applied to the faces of infants or small children, particularly not in the nasal area (glottal spasm or bronchial spasm up to asthma-like attacks or even possible respiratory failure).

OVERDOSAGE

Cases of poisoning are not recorded. The minimal lethal dosage of menthol is estimated to be 2 gm, although individuals have survived higher dosages (8 to 9 gm).

DOSAGE

PEPPERMINT LEAVES

Mode of Administration: Comminuted herb for infusions, extracts of peppermint leaves for internal use.

Preparation: To prepare an infusion, pour 150 ml of hot water over 1 dessertspoonful of the drug, strain after 10 minutes (one study has shown that the maximum level of menthol and methon is present after this time).

Tincture: leave 200 parts leaves in spirit of wine for 10 days (shaken at intervals), which is filtered after this time (EB6).

Daily Dosage: The average daily dose of the drug is 3 to 6 gm. The average daily dose of the tincture (1:10) is 5 to 15 gm. Tea: 1 cup to be consumed 3 to 4 times a day between meals. Infusion: 2 to 4 gm drug, drink slowly in sips while warm.

Homeopathic Dosage: 5 drops, 1 tablet or 10 globules every 30 to 60 minutes (acute) or 1 to 3 times a day (chronic); parenterally: 1 to 2 ml sc acute, 3 times daily; chronic: once a day (HAB34).

Storage: Peppermint should be stored cool and dry and protected from light in non-plastic containers.

PEPPERMINT OIL

Mode of Administration: The essential oil and the galenic preparations are for internal and external use.

Daily Dosage: The average daily internal dose is 6 to 12 drops; inhalation, 3 to 4 drops in hot water; for irritable colon, daily dose: 0.6 ml; single dose: 0.2 ml in enteric coated form.

Externally, a few drops rubbed into the affected skin areas several times a day (2 to 4 times). For young children: Rub 5 to 15 drops on the chest and back. The drug is available as semi-solid and oily preparations (5 to 20%); aqueous-ethanol preparations (5 to 10%); nasal ointments with 1 to 5% essential oil.

Storage: Peppermint should be stored cool and dry and protected from light in non-plastic containers.

LITERATURE

Bowen ICH, Cubbin IJ, (1993) Mentha piperita and Mentha spicata. In: De Smet PAGM

Bromm B, Scharein E, Darsow U, Ring J, (1995) Effects of menthol and cold on histamine-induced itch and skin reactions in man. Neuroscience Lett 187:157-160.

Burrow A, Eccles R, Jones AS, (1983) The effects of camphor, eucalyptus and menthol vapor on nasal resistance to airflow and nasal sensation. Acta Otolaryng (Stockholm) 96: 157-161.

Clark M, (1981) Econ Bot 35:59.

Dew MJ, Evans BK, Rhodes J, (1984) Peppermint oil for the irritable bowel syndrome: a multicentre trial. Br J Clin Pract 38:394-395.

Eccles R, Jones AS, (1982) The effects of menthol on nasal resistance to airflow. J Laryngology Otology 97:705-709.

Eccles R, Lancashire B, Tolley NS, (1987) Experimental studies on nasal sensation of airflow. Acta Otolaryngol (Stockholm) 103:303-306.

Eccles R, Morris S, Tolley NS, (1988) The effects of nasal anaesthesia upon nasal sensation of airflow. Acta Otolaryngol (Stockholm) 106:152-155.

Fintelmann V, Möglichkeiten und Grenzen der Phytotherapie bei Magen-Darm- Krankheiten. In: ZPT 10(1):29. 1989.

Fintelmann V, Phytopharmaka in der Gastroenterologie. In: ZPT 15(3):137. 1994.

Friederich HC, Vogelsberg, H, Neiss A, (1978) Ein Beitrag zur Bewertung von intern wirksamen Venenpharmaka. Z Hautkrankheiten 53 (11):369-374.

Göbel H, Schmidt G, (1995a) Effekt von Pfefferminz- und Eukalyptusölpräparationen in experimentellen Kopfschmerzmodellen. Z Phytother 16:23-33.

Göbel H, Schmidt G, Dworschak M, Stolze H, Heuss D, (1995) Essential plant oils and headache mechanisms. Phytomedicine 2:93-102.

Göbel H, Schmidt G, Dworschak M, Stolze H, Heuss D, (1995b) Essential plant oils and headache mechanisms. Phytomedicine 2:93-103.

Göbel H, Schmidt G, Effekt von Pfefferminz- und Eukalyptusölpräparationen in experimentellen Kopfschmerzmodellen. In: ZPT 16(1):23-33. 1995.

Göbel H, Schmidt G, Soyka D, (1994) Effect of peppermint and eucalyptus oil preparations on neurophysiological and experimental algesimetric headache parameters. Cephalalgia 14:228-234.

Gräfe AK, Besonderheiten der Arzneimitteltherapie im Säuglings- und Kindesalter. In: PZ 140(30):2659-2667. 1995.

Hamann KF, Bonkowsky V, (1987) Minzölwirkung auf die Nasenschleimhaut von Gesunden. Dtsch Apoth Z 125:429-436.

Harries N et al., (1978) J Clin Pharm 2:171.

Hawthorn M, Ferranthe J, Luchowski E, Rutledge A, Wie XY, Triggle DJ, (1988) The actions of peppermint oil and menthol on calcium channel dependent processes in intestinal, neuronal and cardiac preparations. Aliment Pharmacol Therap 2:101-118.

Hefendehl FW, Murray MJ, (1973) Planta Med 23:101.

Heinze A, (1995c) Oleum menthae piperitae: Wirkmechanismen und klinische Effektivität bei Kopfschmerz vom Spannungstyp. In: Loew D, Rietbrock N (Hrsg) Phytopharmaka in Forschung und klinischer Anwendung. Steinkopff Verlag, Darmstadt, S 177-184.

Herrmann EC Jr., Kucera LS, Antiviral substances in plants of the mint family (Labiatae). III. Peppermint (Mentha piperita) and other mint plants. In: Proc Soc Exp Biol Med 124:874-878. 1995.

Hills JM, Aaronson PI, (1991) The mechanisms of action of peppermint oil on gastrointestinal smooth muscle. Gastroenterol 101:55-65.

Kantarev N, Peicev P, (1977) Folia Med 19(1):41.

Keller K, Hänsel R, Chandler RF, (eds) Adverse Effects of Herbal Drugs 1. Springer Verlag, Berlin Heidelberg New York, S 171-178.

Kucera LS, Hermann EC Jr, (1967) Proc Soc Exp Biol Med 124:865 et 874.

Leiber B, (1967) Dieskussionsbemerkung. In: Dost FH, Leiber B (Hrsg) Menthol and menthol-containing external remedies. Thieme Stuttgart 1967, S. 22.

Leicester RJ, Hunt RH, (1982) Peppermint oil to reduce solonic spasm during endoscopy. Lancet: 989.

Nash P, Gould SR, Barnardo DE, (1986) Peppermint oil does not relieve the pain of irritable bowel syndrome. Br J Clin Pract 40:292-293.

Nöller HG, (1967) Elektronische Messungen an der Nasenschleimhaut unter Mentholwirkung. In: Menthol and menthol-containung external remedies. Thieme, Stuttgart, S 146-153, 179.

Rees WDW, Evans BK, Rhoes J, (1979) Treating irritable bowel syndrome with peppermint oil. Brit med J II:835-838.

Reuter HD, Pflanzliche Gallentherapeutika (Teil I) und (Teil II). In: ZPT 16(1):13-20 u. 77-89. 1995.

Rohmeder J, Menthol: Verum statt Racemicum. In: PZ 139(4):300. 1994.

Sommerville KW, Richmond CR, Bell GD, (1984) Delayed release peppermint oil capsules (Colpermin) for the spastic colon syndrome: a pharmacokinetic study. Br J Clin Pharmac 18:638-640.

Taylor BA, Luscombe DK, Duthie HL, (1983) Inhibitory effect of peppermint on gastrointestinal smooth muscle. Gut 24: A 992 (Abstract).

Weizel A, (1980) Colon irritabile. Therapiewoche 30:3898-3900.

White DA, Thompson SP, Wilson CG, Bel JD, (1987) A pharmacokinetic comparison of two delayed release peppermint oil preparations, Colpermin and Mintec for treatment of the irritable bowel syndrome. Int J Pharmaceutics 40:151-155.

Wildgrube HJ, (1988) Untersuchung zur Wirksamkeit von Pfefferminzöl auf Beschwerdebild und funktionelle Parameter bei Patienten mit Reizdarmsyndrom (Studie). NaturHeilpraxis 41:2-5.

Further information in:

Fenarolis Handbook of Flavor Ingredients, Vol. 1, 2nd Ed., CRC Press Boca Raton 1975.

Hänsel R, Keller K, Rimpler H, Schneider G (Hrsg.), Hagers Handbuch der Pharmazeutischen Praxis, 5. Aufl., Bde 4-6 (Drogen), Springer Verlag Berlin, Heidelberg, New York, 1992-1994.

Hausen B, Allergiepflanzen, Pflanzenallergene, ecomed Verlagsgesellsch. mbH, Landsberg 1988.

Leung AY, Encyclopedia of Common Natural Ingredients Used in Food Drugs and Cosmetics, John Wiley & Sons Inc., New York 1980.

Madaus G, Lehrbuch der Biologischen Arzneimittel, Bde 1-3, Nachdruck, Georg Olms Verlag Hildesheim 1979.

Schulz R, Hänsel R, Rationale Phytotherapie, Springer Verlag Heidelberg 1996.

Steinegger E, Hänsel R, Pharmakognosie, 5. Aufl., Springer Verlag Heidelberg 1992.

Teuscher E, Biogene Arzneimittel, 5. Aufl., Wiss. Verlagsges. Stuttgart 1997.

Wagner H, Wiesenauer M, Phytotherapie. Phytopharmaka und pflanzliche Homöopathika, Fischer-Verlag, Stuttgart, Jena, New York 1995.

Wichtl M (Hrsg.), Teedrogen, 4. Aufl., Wiss. Verlagsges. Stuttgart 1997.

Perilla

Perilla fructescens

DESCRIPTION

Medicinal Parts: The medicinal parts of the plants are the leaf-bearing branches and leaves.

Flower and Fruit: The flowers are in 2-blossomed false whorls in the axils of the triangular bracts in 5 to 15 cm long, spike-like, downy-haired inflorescences. The calyx is campanulate, bilabiate, 3 to 10 mm long, with a triple-toothed upper lip and a lower lip divided in two. The corolla is 4 to 5 mm long, almost radial, with a short tube and a broadened, almost circular section having a whitish, 5-lobed margin. There are 4 stamens of almost equal length and a superior, 2-carpeled, 4-chambered ovary. The fruit is globose, gray-brown, with purple reticulate stripes and a diameter of approximately 1.5 mm. The pericarp is thin and brittle; the seeds yellowish-white.

Leaves, Stem and Root: The herb, stands up to 1 m high. The leaves are long-petiolate. The lamina is wide-ovate, acuminate, rounded at the base, crenate, curly, dull green with brown-red spots to blackish-purple. The leaves are glossy and downy-haired along the veins. The stem is square, branched and downy.

Habitat: The species is found in India, Burma, Japan and China.

Production: Perilla leaves are the dried leaves and leaf-bearing branches of Perilla fructescens. Harvesting is from July to August, after which the leaves and branches are dried in the sun or shade.

Other Names: Beefsteak Plant

ACTIONS AND PHARMACOLOGY

COMPOUNDS

Volatile oil: constituents vary greatly according to chemotype, with perillaldehyde, L-limonene + perillaldehyde, perilla ketone, myristicin, dill apiole or elsholtzia ketone predominating

Caffeic acid derivatives: rosmarinic acid (0.4 to 1.7%)

Monoterpene glucosides: including perillosides A to D, citrusine C

Flavonoids: apigenin glucoside and luteolin glucoside, estered to some extent with caffeic acid

EFFECTS

Perilla aldehyde (chemotype PA) is sedative and antibacterial in effect; perilla ketone (chemotype PK) acts as a propulsive in the gastrointestinal tract. In addition, a cytotoxic and antitumorous effect was able to be demonstrated. Perilla leaves may trigger allergic skin reactions (Kanzaki & Kimura, 1992.) In at least one study, serum cholesterol and triglyceride levels in rats that were fed Perilla oil were lowered (Sakono et al, 1993.)

INDICATIONS AND USAGE

Unproven Uses: The herb is used pharmaceutically as an antiseptic and for diseases of the mouth. The oil may also have positive antilipidemic effects.

Chinese Medicine: Perilla is used in traditional Chinese medicine for colds with fever, coughs, shortness of breath, chills, swelling of the nasal mucous membrane, headache and to treat poisoning from ingestion of fish or crab. Efficacy for these indications has not yet been proven.

CONTRAINDICATIONS

Use during pregnancy is contraindicated because perillaldehyde was demonstrated to have a mutagenic effect in some in vitro studies.

PRECAUTIONS AND ADVERSE REACTIONS

No health hazards are known in conjunction with the proper administration of designated therapeutic dosages. The plant possesses potential for sensitization. In tests with sheep using 15 to 20 mg/kg body weight administration per infusion, Perilla ketone triggered pulmonary edema. Perillaldehyde had mutagenic effect in some in vitro studies.

DOSAGE

Mode of Administration: Whole, cut, powdered drug preparations and oil for internal use.

Daily Dosage: Extract (aqueous): 3 to 10 g

LITERATURE

Blaschek W, Hänsel R, Keller K, Reichling J, Rimpler G, Schneider G (Eds), Hagers Handbuch der Pharmazeutischen

Praxis. Folgebände 1 und 2. Drogen A-Z. Springer. Berlin, Heidelberg 1998.

Kanzaki T, Kimura S, Occupational allergic contact dermatitis from Perilla frutescens (shiso). Contact Dermatitis (1992 Jan) 26(1):55-6.

Sakono M, Yoshida K, Yahiro M, Combined effects of dietary protein and fat on lipid metabolism in rats. J Nutr Sci Vitaminol (Tokyo) (1993 Aug) 39(4):335-43.

Perilla fructescens

See Perilla

Periwinkle

Vinca minor

DESCRIPTION

Medicinal Parts: The medicinal parts are the dried leaves, the fresh aerial parts of the flowering plant and the whole fresh flowering plant.

Flower and Fruit: The flowers are solitary, long-pedicled, 40 to 50 mm in diameter and grow in the axils of the upper leaves. The calyx is funnel-shaped with long, narrow-linear, pointed-ciliated tips. The corolla is light blue or violet with a funnel-shaped tube and 5 irregularly terminated tips. The fruit is a follicle. It is oblong, acuminate, 15 to 2 mm long and has 2 to 3 seeds.

Leaves, Stem and Root: The plant is a perennial subshrub, 10 to 60 cm high. The non-flowering shoots are prostrate root at the nodes. The flowering shoots are ascending, up to 20 cm high and woody at the base. The leaves are evergreen, ovate, tapering at the front and distinctly pinnate-ribbed. They are 5 cm by 2 cm, petiolate with finely ciliated margins, which become glabrous later.

Habitat: The plant is indigenous to northern Spain, through western France, eastward via central and southern Europe as far as the Caucasus; it has been naturalized in many regions.

Production: Periwinkle herb consists of the above-ground parts of Vinca minor.

ACTIONS AND PHARMACOLOGY

COMPOUNDS

Indole alkaloids (0.15-1.4%): chief alkaloid vincamine (eburnamine-type, 25-65%), including as well vincine, apovincamine, vincadifformin

Flavonoids: including kempferol-3-O-rhamnoside-7-O-glucoside, kempferol-3-O-rhamnoglucoside-3-O-galactoside, kempferol-3-O-rhamnoglucoside-3-O-glucoside, quercetin-3-O-rhamnoglucoside-7-O-glucoside

EFFECTS

The alkaloid vincamine is hypotensive, negatively chronotropic, spasmolytic, hypoglycemic and sympatholytic. Scientifically validated studies on the hypotensive effect on humans have not yet been carried out. Its use as an amaroid seems plausible.

INDICATIONS AND USAGE

Unproven Uses: Periwinkle is used internally for circulatory disorders, cerebral circulatory impairment and support for the metabolism of the brain. It is also used internally for loss of memory, hypertension, cystitis, gastritis and enteritis, diarrhea, raised blood sugar levels and to help weaning. Periwinkle is used externally for sore throats, nose bleeds, bruising, abscesses, eczema and to stop bleeding.

Homeopathic Uses: Periwinkle is used for weeping eczema and bleeding mucous membranes.

PRECAUTIONS AND ADVERSE REACTIONS

No health hazards are known in conjunction with the proper administration of designated therapeutic dosages. Gastrointestinal complaints and skin flushing have been observed as side effects.

OVERDOSAGE

Overdosage will bring about a severe drop in blood pressure. Cases of poisonings have not yet been recorded.

Treatment includes gastrointestinal emptying (inducement of vomiting, gastric lavage with burgundy-coloured potassium permanganate solution, sodium sulphate), instillation of activated charcoal and shock prophylaxis (appropriate body position, quiet, warmth). The therapy for poisonings consists of treating bradycardia with atropine or Alupent, cardiac arrhythmias with lidocaine or phenytoin and treating possible cases of acidosis with sodium bicarbonate infusions. In case of shock, plasma volume expanders should be infused.

DOSAGE

Mode of Administration: Whole, cut and powdered drug is available in the form of capsules, ampules, coated and filmed tablets, and compound preparations.

Preparation: To make a tea, pour 200 ml boiling water over 1 teaspoonful of drug, steep for 10 minutes, then strain. To make a decoction, boil 60 gm of drug in 1 liter of water for 2 minutes, steep for 10 minutes, then strain.

To make an infusion, boil 15 gm of drug in 1/4 liter of water. To make wine, macerate 100 gm of drug in 1 liter of wine for 10 days, decant, then press. To make a liquid for gargling, boil 2 dessertspoonfuls of drug for a few minutes in 1/2 liter water.

Daily Dosage: The usual drug dosage is as follows: Tea—2 to 3 cups daily; Decoction—2 to 4 cups between meals; Infusion—drink after meals for diarrhea; Wine—1 dessertspoonful after meals; a gargle or wash can be used externally as needed.

Homeopathic Dosage: 5 drops, 1 tablet or 10 globules every 30 to 60 minutes (acute) or 1 to 3 times daily (chronic); parenterally: 1 to 2 ml sc, acute: 3 times daily; chronic: once a day (HAB1).

LITERATURE

Behninger C, Abel G, Schneider E, Vinca minor zeigt keine antimitotische Eigenschaften. In: ZPT 13(2):35. 1992.

Gosset-Garnier J et al., (1965) Bull Soc Chim Franc 676.

Janot MM et al., (1962) Bull Soc Chim Franc 1079.

Kaul JL, Trojanek (1966) Lloydia 29:25.

Neczypor W, PA 24:273. 1969.

Taylor, B, In: Taylor WI, Farnsworth N (Ed.): The Vinca Alkaloids, Marcel Dekker Inc., New York. 1973.

Trunzler G, Phytotherapeutische Möglichkeiten bei Herz- und arteriellen Gefäßerkrankungen. In: ZPT 10(5):147. 1989.

Vinpocetin. In: ZPT 14(1):11. 1993.

Further information in:

Hänsel R, Keller K, Rimpler H, Schneider G (Hrsg.), Hagers Handbuch der Pharmazeutischen Praxis, 5. Aufl., Bde 4-6 (Drogen): Springer Verlag Berlin, Heidelberg, New York, 1992-1994.

Madaus G, Lehrbuch der Biologischen Arzneimittel, Bde 1-3, Nachdruck, Georg Olms Verlag Hildesheim 1979.

Roth L, Daunderer M, Kormann K, Giftpflanzen, Pflanzengifte, 4. Aufl., Ecomed Fachverlag Landsberg Lech 1993.

Steinegger E, Hänsel R, Pharmakognosie, 5. Aufl., Springer Verlag Heidelberg 1992.

Teuscher E, Lindequist U, Biogene Gifte - Biologie, Chemie, Pharmakologie, 2. Aufl., Fischer Verlag Stuttgart 1994.

Teuscher E, Biogene Arzneimittel, 5. Aufl., Wiss. Verlagsges. Stuttgart 1997.

Wagner H, Wiesenauer M, Phytotherapie. Phytopharmaka und pflanzliche Homöopathika, Fischer-Verlag, Stuttgart, Jena, New York 1995.

Persea americana

See Avocado

Persicaria bistorta

See Bistort

Persicaria hydropiper

See Smartweed

Petasites

Petasites hybridus

DESCRIPTION

Medicinal Parts: The medicinal parts are the dried or fresh leaves, the underground parts collected in autumn and dried, the aerial parts collected toward the end of the flowering season and the whole fresh plant.

Flower and Fruit: The reddish flowers appear before the leaves, immediately after the snow has melted. They grow on flowering shafts from the base of the plant. The shaft is erect, thick and has purplish scales. The ones bearing the male flowers are 15 to 20 cm high and those bearing the female flowers are 40 cm high. The capitula of the mainly male flowers are initially in ovate, compact racemes. The flowers are tubular campanulate. The female flowers have a thread-like, tight tube and a bilabiate margin. The involucre is in 1 to 2 rows and is reddish. A prismatic fruit with a yellowish-whitish pappus develops from the flower.

Leaves, Stem and Root: The short and gnarled rhizome lies vertically or somewhat slanted in the ground. It is about 4 cm thick, brownish and thickened at the nodes. The root creeps and branches under the surface. The leaves are large, basal, long-petioled and roundish with a deeply cordate base. It is gray underneath and irregularly dentate.

Characteristics: Petasite has the largest leaves of all indigenous flora and has an unpleasant smell.

Habitat: The species is found in northern Asia, Europe and some areas of North America.

Production: Petasite consists of the whole plant of Petasites hybridus. Petasite leaf consists of the leaves of Petasites hybridis. The leaves are harvested before the end of the flowering season and quickly dried. Only leaves that are the size of the palm of the hand are picked, as these are said to have a higher level of active principles than the larger leaves. Petasite root consists of the dried underground parts of Petasites hybridus. A distinction is made between androdynamic and gynodynamic varieties. The roots of the former are dug up in autumn and of the latter in spring. After being dug up they are washed and dried. If drugs containing petasin are to be extracted, then cultivation must be carried out under laboratory conditions.

Not to be Confused With: Other Petasite varieties and the leaves of Adenostyles alliariae or Tussilago farfara.

Other Names: Blatterdock, Bog Rhubarb, Bogshorns, Butterbur, Butter-Dock, Butterfly Dock, Capdockin, Flapperdock, Langwort, P. Vulgaris, Umbrella Leaves

ACTIONS AND PHARMACOLOGY

COMPOUNDS: PETASITES LEAF

Sesquiterpene alcohol esters: chief components including among others according to chemotype - petasitine, neopetasitine and isopetasitine, or furanopetasin and 9-hydroxyfuranoeremophilone

Pyrrolizidine alkaloids: senecionine, integerrimine, senkirkine, presumably only in traces

Volatile oil: including, among others, dodecanal (aroma-bearer)

Flavonoids: including among others, isoquercitrin, astragaline

Mucilages

Tannins

EFFECTS: PETASITES LEAF

A spasmolytic effect has been demonstrated in animals.

COMPOUNDS: PETASITES ROOT

Sesquiterpene alcohol esters: including among others, chief components according to chemotype - petasitine, neopetasitine and isopetasitine or furanopetasine and 9-hydroxyfuranoeremophilone

Volatile oil (0.1-0.4%): including among others, 1-nonen, eremophilone, furanoeremophilone

Pyrrolizidine alkaloids: senecionine, integerrimine

EFFECTS: PETASITES ROOT

In animals, the pyrrolizidine alkaloids inhibit leukotriene synthesis and are spasmolytic and spasmoanalgesic as well as cytoprotective. In humans, it provides analgesia for nervous headaches. Its application for psychasthenic symptoms seems plausible.

In higher doses and with chronic use, a hepatotoxic, mutagenic, teratogenic and carcinogenic effect may be expected.

INDICATIONS AND USAGE

PETASITES LEAF

Unproven Uses: Petasite leaves are used to stimulate the appetite and to treat nervous cramp-like states and states associated with pain, colic and headaches. In folk medicine, the leaves are used internally for respiratory disorders, liver, gallbladder or pancreas disorders, as a prophylaxis for agitation and to induce sleep. Externally, the leaves are used to heal wounds and as a poultice for malignant ulcers.

PETASITES ROOT

Approved by Commission E:

■ Kidney and bladder stones

Unproven Uses: The underground stem is used as an adjunct in the treatment of acute spastic pain in the efferent urinary tract, particularly if stones are present. It is also used for respiratory disorders, particularly for coughs, whooping cough and bronchial asthma. Other uses include gastrointestinal disorders, migraine and tension headaches.

Homeopathic Uses: Smooth muscle cramps.

CONTRAINDICATIONS

All forms of the drug should not be used during pregnancy or by nursing mothers.

PRECAUTIONS AND ADVERSE REACTIONS

PETASITES LEAF

General: One should entirely forgo any administration of the drug, due to the presence of pyrrolizidine alkaloids with hepatotoxic and carcinogenic effects in the parts of the plant above ground, as even mere traces of the alkaloids present a danger. The industrial manufacture of extracts virtually free of pyrrolizidine alkaloids is possible. The drug should not be used without knowledge of the pyrrolizidine alkaloids content.

Note: Alkaloid-free varieties are cultivated.

Pregnancy: The administration of the drug during pregnancy is to be completely ruled out.

Nursing Mothers: The drug should not be consumed by nursing mothers.

PETASITES ROOT

One should unconditionally forgo any administration of the drug, due to the presence of pyrrolizidine alkaloids with hepatotoxic and carcinogenic effect. The industrial manufacture of extracts virtually free of pyrrolizidine alkaloids is possible.

DOSAGE

PETASITES LEAF

Preparation: To make an infusion, pour boiling water over 1.2 to 2 gm comminuted drug and strain after 10 minutes.

Daily Dosage: Drink 2 to 3 cups of the infusion per day.

Note: The herb should not be used unless the pyrrolizidine content is known. The maximum daily dose of pyrrolizidine alkaloids is 0.1 micrograms.

PETASITES ROOT

Mode of Administration: Extracts obtained with ethanol or lipophilic solvents and other galenic preparations for internal use.

Daily Dosage: Dosing of herbal preparations is highly dependent on a variety of factors, such as growing and harvesting conditions, plant parts, extraction methods used and the dosage form chosen by the manufacturer. Standardization to single constituent makers has proven unreliable. Since no official standards have been established to date to regulate production of herbal medicines in the United States, dosage ranges must be employed as guidelines.

Preparations equivalent to 4.5 to 7 gm drug may be used. When used internally, the daily dosage must not exceed 0.1 micrograms of pyrrolizidine alkaloids with 1.2 unsaturated necine structure including their N-oxides. When used externally, the maximum daily dosage should not exceed 10 micrograms of pyrrolizidine alkaloids with 1.2 unsaturated necine structure including their N-oxides. Teas should not be used.

Homeopathic Uses: 5 drops, 1 tablet or 10 globules every 30 to 60 minutes (acute) or 1 to 3 times daily (chronic); parenterally: 1 to 2 ml sc, acute: 3 times daily; chronic: once a day (HAB1).

LITERATURE

PETASITES LEAF

Bicket D et al., Identification and characterization of inhibitors of peptide-leukotriene-synthesis from Petasites hybridus. In: PM 60(4):318. 1994.

Brune K, Analgetische Wirkung von Pestwurz. In: DAZ 133(37):3296. 1993.

Brune K, Bickel D, Peskar BA, Gastro-Protective Effects by Extracts of Petasites hybridus: The Role of Inhibition of Peptido-leukotriene Synthesis. In: PM 59(6):494. 1993.

Bucher K, (1951) Über ein antispastisches Prinzip in Petasites officinalis Moench. Arch Exp Path Pharmacol 213:69.

Carle R, Pflanzliche Antiphlogistika und Spasmolytika. In: ZPT 9(3):67. 1988.

Chizzola R, Distribution of the pyrrolizidine alkaloids senecionine and intergerrimine within the Petasites hybridus. In: PM 58(7)93. 1992.

Dorsch W, Neues über antientzündliche Drogen. In: ZPT 14(1):26. 1993.

Frohne D, Pfänder HJ, Giftpflanzen - Ein Handbuch für Apotheker, Toxikologen und Biologen, 4. Aufl., Wiss. Verlags-Ges. Stuttgart 1997.

Hänsel R, Keller K, Rimpler H, Schneider G (Hrsg.), Hagers Handbuch der Pharmazeutischen Praxis, 5. Aufl., Bde 4-6 (Drogen), Springer Verlag Berlin, Heidelberg, New York, 1992-1994.

Hasler A et al., Trace analysis of pyrrolizidine alkaloids by GC-NPD of extracts from the roots of Petasites hybridus. In: PM 62, Abstracts of the 44th Ann Congress of GA, 147. 1996.

Madaus G, Lehrbuch der Biologischen Arzneimittel, Bde 1-3, Nachdruck, Georg Olms Verlag Hildesheim 1979.

Mauz Ch et al., (1985) Pharm Acta Helv 60:4.

Meier B, Die Pestwurz - Stand der Forschung. In: ZPT 15(5):268-284. 1994.

Röder E, Pyrrolizidinhaltige Arzneipflanzen. In: DAZ 132(45):2427-2435. 1992.

Roth L, Daunderer M, Kormann K, Giftpflanzen, Pflanzengifte, 4. Aufl., Ecomed Fachverlag Landsberg Lech 1993.

Teuscher E, Lindequist U, Biogene Gifte - Biologie, Chemie, Pharmakologie, 2. Aufl., Fischer Verlag Stuttgart 1994.

Wichtl M (Hrsg.), Teedrogen, 4. Aufl., Wiss. Verlagsges. Stuttgart 1997.

PETASITES ROOT

Bicket D et al., Identification and characterization of inhibitors of peptide-leukotriene-synthesis from Petasites hybridus. In: PM 60(4):318. 1994.

Brune K, Analgetische Wirkung von Pestwurz. In: DAZ 133(37):3296. 1993.

Brune K, Bickel D, Peskar BA, Gastro-Protective Effects by Extracts of Petasites hybridus: The Role of Inhibition of Peptido-leukotriene Synthesis. In: PM 59(6):494. 1993.

Bucher K, (1951) Über ein antispastisches Prinzip in Petasites officinalis Moench. Arch Exp Path Pharmacol 213:69.

Carle R, Pflanzliche Antiphlogistika und Spasmolytika. In: ZPT 9(3):67. 1988.

Chizzola R, Distribution of the pyrrolizidine alkaloids senecionine and intergerrimine within the Petasites hybridus. In: PM 58(7)93. 1992.

Dorsch W, Neues über antientzündliche Drogen. In: ZPT 14(1):26. 1993.

Frohne D, Pfänder HJ, Giftpflanzen - Ein Handbuch für Apotheker, Toxikologen und Biologen, 4. Aufl., Wiss. Verlags-Ges. Stuttgart 1997.

Gruenwald J, Brendler T, Jaenicke C (Eds.), Physicians' Desk Reference for Herbal Medicines. Medical Economics Company Inc., Montvale, 1998.

Hänsel R, Keller K, Rimpler H, Schneider G (Hrsg.), Hagers Handbuch der Pharmazeutischen Praxis, 5. Aufl., Bde 4-6 (Drogen), Springer Verlag Berlin, Heidelberg, New York, 1992-1994.

Hasler A et al., Trace analysis of pyrrolizidine alkaloids by GC-NPD of extracts from the roots of Petasites hybridus. In: PM 62, Abstracts of the 44th Ann Congress of GA, 147. 1996.

Madaus G, Lehrbuch der Biologischen Arzneimittel, Bde 1-3, Nachdruck, Georg Olms Verlag Hildesheim 1979.

Mauz Ch et al., (1985) Pharm Acta Helv 60:4.

Meier B, Die Pestwurz - Stand der Forschung. In: ZPT 15(5):268-284. 1994.

Röder E, Pyrrolizidinhaltige Arzneipflanzen. In: DAZ 132(45):2427-2435. 1992.

Roth L, Daunderer M, Kormann K, Giftpflanzen, Pflanzengifte, 4. Aufl., Ecomed Fachverlag Landsberg Lech 1993.

Teuscher E, Lindequist U, Biogene Gifte - Biologie, Chemie, Pharmakologie, 2. Aufl., Fischer Verlag Stuttgart 1994.

Wichtl M (Hrsg.), Teedrogen, 4. Aufl., Wiss. Verlagsges. Stuttgart 1997.

Petasites hybridus

See Petasites

Petroselinum crispum

See Parsley

Peucedanum ostruthium

See Masterwort

Peumus boldo

See Boldo

Peyote

Lophophora williamsii

DESCRIPTION

Medicinal Parts: The medicinal parts are the pincushion-like, aerial, transversely cut and dried, tough-corky shoot, and the fresh plant.

Flower and Fruit: The flowers grow from the center of the cactus head. They are 1 to 2.5 cm long and 1 to 2.2 cm across. The outer petals are green with a darker middle stripe and have green-pink or white margins. The filaments are white with yellow anthers. The ovary is glabrous. The fruit is a 15 to 20 mm long berry, which is 2 to 3.5 mm across, sturdy, clavate, initially fleshy, glabrous and red. It turns brown-white and dries out when ripe. The seeds are black, rough, 1 to 1.5 mm long and 1 mm wide.

Leaves, Stem and Root: The plant is a succulent, spineless, globular or top-shaped, bluish-green cactus with up to 13 distinct vertical ribs. It grows to 20 cm. From one rhizome side shoots are produced to create a cactus formation of 1.5 m across. The roots are tuberous and 8 to 11 cm long. The aerial part has a diameter of 4 to 12 cm, and the pressed-in top is filled with gray, woolly bushels of hair. The head is divided into irregular flat warts by horizontal grooves. Roundish aueroles of paintbrush-like yellowish or whitish tufts of hair grow from the tip of the warts.

Habitat: The plant grows in northern Mexico and bordering southern Texas.

Production: Mescal Button stem consists of the pincushion-like cactus Lophophora willamsii, cut into slices and dried. The root and hair tuft of the Peyote plant are cut off. Particularly mescaline and chlorophyll-rich center is dried as a slice. This slice is referred to as the Mescal Button.

Other Names: Pellote, Mescal Buttons, Devil's Root, Dumpling Cactus, Sacred Mushroom

ACTIONS AND PHARMACOLOGY

COMPOUNDS

Alkaloids phenylethylamine type: chief among them mescaline (up to 7%), hordenine; tetrahydroisoquinoline type: including among others pellotin, anhalonidine, anhalamine

EFFECTS

Peyote has an emetic and a hallucinogenic effect. The psychotropic effects of Peyote consumption are mainly due to the mescaline content. Controlled pharmacological studies on the Peyote cactus are unknown. Mescal beans cause visual, auditory, taste and kinesthetic hallucinations.

INDICATIONS AND USAGE

Unproven Uses: Peyote is rarely used as a medicinal preparation. In folk medicine, Peyote is one of the oldest hallucinogens.

PRECAUTIONS AND ADVERSE REACTIONS

Due to its mescaline content, the drug causes chiefly visual, but also aural, kinesthetic and synesthetic hallucinations when taken in dosages of between 4 and 12 dried slices of the sprout (so-called Mescal Buttons: diameter 3 to 4.5 cm, thickness 0.5 cm).

DOSAGE

Mode of Administration: Peyote is obsolete as a drug; it is often ingested illegally for its hallucinogenic effect.

LITERATURE

Hänsel R, Keller K, Rimpler H, Schneider G (Hrsg.), Hagers Handbuch der Pharmazeutischen Praxis, 5. Aufl., Bde 4-6 (Drogen), Springer Verlag Berlin, Heidelberg, New York, 1992-1994.

Kapadia GJ, Fayez MB, (1970) J Pharm Sci 59:1699.

Madaus G, Lehrbuch der Biologischen Arzneimittel, Bde 1-3, Nachdruck, Georg Olms Verlag Hildesheim 1979 (unter Anhalonium).

Roth L, Daunderer M, Kormann K, Giftpflanzen, Pflanzengifte, 4. Aufl., Ecomed Fachverlag Landsberg Lech 1993.

Seeger R, Mescalin. In: DAZ 133(2):24. 1993.

Steinegger E, Hänsel R, Pharmakognosie, 5. Aufl., Springer Verlag Heidelberg 1992.

Teuscher E, Lindequist U, Biogene Gifte - Biologie, Chemie, Pharmakologie, 2. Aufl., Fischer Verlag Stuttgart 1994.

Willaman JJ, Hui-Li L, (1970) Lloydia 33(3A):1.

Phaseolus vulgaris

See Bean Pod

Phoenix dactylifera

See Date Palm

Phragmites communis

See Reed Herb

Phyllanthus amarus

See Black Catnip

Physalis alkekengi

See Winter Cherry

Physostigma venenosum

See Calabar Bean

Phytolacca americana

See Poke

Picea species

See Spruce

Picrasma excelsa

See Quassia

Picrorhiza

Picrorhiza kurroa

DESCRIPTION

Medicinal Parts: The medicinal part of the plant is the rhizome, which is cut and dried.

Flower and Fruit: The inflorescence is a terminal, dense spike, 5 to 10 cm long, on an upright peduncle over a rosette of dentate leaves (may be absent). The sepals are fused, approximately 6 mm long. The calyx is 5-lobed and pubescent, the corolla 5-lobed, radial, pale blue or reddish-blue. There are 4 stamens, and the ovary is 2-chambered with numerous ovules. The flowers are dimorphic, having either 6 to 8 mm long corollas and 8 mm long filaments or a single 6 mm long corolla and 2 cm long filaments. The fruit is an approximately 1.3 cm long, ovoid, 4-sided capsule. The seeds are ellipsoid with a translucent, thick, blistery aril.

Leaves, Stem and Roots: The leaves on this herbaceous creeping perennial are alternate, 5 to 15 cm long and 2 to 6 cm wide. The lamina is coriaceous, spatulate to narrow-elliptical with a rounded tip. The margin is dentate and the petiole winged. The rhizome is woody, up to 25 cm long, and covered in the remains of dried leaf bases.

Habitat: The plant is native to the mountains of India, Nepal, Tibet and Pakistan.

Production: Kharbagehindi (Arabic name) roots are the cut and dried rhizome of Picrorhiza kurroa, which are collected in the wild.

Not to be Confused With: Mistaken identity can occur with Lagotis cashmiriana.

Other Names: Kharbagehindi

ACTIONS AND PHARMACOLOGY

COMPOUNDS

Iridoids: catalpol derivatives, including picroside I (0.6 to 7.4%, extremely bitter), kutkoside (10-O-vanilloyl catalpol, with picroside I present in a stable state as a mixed crystal: kutkin), picroside II (3 to 5%), minecoside (0.5%), veronicoside and picroside III

Acetophenone derivatives: androsine (0.1 to 0.7%), apocynin (0.1%), picein

Cucurbitacins: chief component 25-acetoxy-2beta-D-glucosyloxy-3,16,20-trihydroxy-9-methyl-19-norlanosta-5,23-dien-22-one (1.0 to 1.5%. extremely bitter)

Glycoproteins

EFFECTS

The acetophenone derivatives androsine and apocynine are bronchospasmolytic and antiasthmatic in effect. In addition, antiphlogistic, immunostimulating, antibacterial and antiviral, hepatoprotective, choleretic, spasmolytic and insecticidal action mechanisms were able to be demonstrated. The positive influence of Picrorhiza kurroa in the treatment of vitiligo is traceable to the immunomodulating and hepatoprotective characteristics of the drug.

INDICATIONS AND USAGE

Unproven Uses: Folk medicine uses have included menstrual complaints, enteritis, gall bladder complaints, for stomach conditions as an emetic, fever, constipation, chronic dysentery, scabies, leucoderma, joint pain, chronic asthma, infections, inflammations, coughs, hepatitis and snakebite.

Chinese Medicine: Picrorhiza is used for fever induced by strain, hyperemia, dysentery, jaundice, carbuncles, hemorrhoids, epilepsy and malnutrition in children.

PRECAUTIONS AND ADVERSE REACTIONS

No health hazards are known in conjunction with the proper administration of designated therapeutic dosages.

DOSAGE

Mode of Administration: Preparations for internal use.

Preparation: To prepare a tincture, 100 g finely cut and crushed Kharbagehindi root with 37.5 g dried and crushed orange peels, 12.5 g crushed cardamom to 1000 ml 45% ethanol.

Daily Dosage: Powder: 0.6 to 1.2 g drug; as an antiperiodic 3 to 4 g. Tincture: 2 to 4 ml.

LITERATURE

Blaschek W, Hänsel R, Keller K, Reichling J, Rimpler G, Schneider G (Eds), Hagers Handbuch der Pharmazeutischen Praxis. Folgeb nde 1 und 2. Drogen A-Z. Springer. Berlin, Heidelberg 1998.

Chander R, Dwivedi Y, Rastogi R, Sharma SK, Garg NK, Kapoor NK, Dhawan BN, Effect of different extracts of kutaki (Picrorhiza kurroa) on experimentally induced abnormalities in the liver. Indian J Med Res, 95:34-7, 1990 Feb.

Chander R, Dwivedi Y, Rastogi R, Sharma SK, Garg NK, Kapoor NK, Dhawan BN, Evaluation of hepatoprotective activity of picroliv (from Picrorhiza kurroa) in Mastomys natalensis infected with Plasmodium berghei. Indian J Med Res, 95:34-7, 1990 Feb.

Dorsch W, Stuppner H, Wagner H, Gropp M, Demoulin S, Ring J, Antiasthmatic effects of Picrorhiza kurroa: androsin prevents allergen- and PAF-induced bronchial obstruction in guinea pigs. Int Arch Allergy Appl Immunol, 95:128-33, 1991.

Mahajani SS, Kulkarni RD, Effect of disodium cromoglycate and Picrorhiza kurroa root powder on sensitivity of guinea pigs to histamine and sympathomimetic amines. Int Arch Allergy Appl Immunol, 42:137-44, 1977.

Pandey BL, Das PK, Immunopharmacological studies on Picrorhiza kurroa Royle-ex-Benth. Part III: Adrenergic mechanisms of anti-inflammatory action. Indian J Physiol Pharmacol, 42:120-5, 1988 Apr-Jun.

Pandey BL, Das PK, Immunopharmacological studies on Picrorhiza kurroa Royle-ex-Benth. Part IV: Cellular mechanisms of anti-inflammatory action. Indian J Physiol Pharmacol, 42:28-30, 1989 Jan-Mar.

Shukla B, Visen PK, Patnaik GK, Dhawan BN, Choleretic effect of picroliv, the hepatoprotective principle of Picrorhiza kurroa. Planta Med, 95:29-33, 1991 Feb.

Vaidya AB, Antarkar DS, Doshi JC, Bhatt AD, Ramesh V, Vora PV, Perissond D, Baxi AJ, Kale PM, Picrorhiza kurroa (Kutaki) Royle ex Benth as a hepatoprotective agent - experimental & clinical studies. J Postgrad Med, 42:105-8, 1996 Oct-Dec.

Picrorhiza kurroa

See Picrorhiza

Pilocarpus microphyllus

See Jaborandi

Pilosella officinarum

See Mouse Ear

Pimenta racemosa

See Pimento

Pimento

Pimenta racemosa

DESCRIPTION

Medicinal Parts: The medicinal parts are the berries and the oil extracted from them.

Flower and Fruit: The inflorescences are racemes of white or lilac flowers, which develop very quickly into the infructescence. The fruit is a brown, globular berry, which is about 0.75 cm in diameter. The fruit has a rough surface and the remains of the calyx are present as a toothed ring at the apex. It contains 2 reniform seeds.

Leaves, Stem and Root: The tree is an evergreen up to 12 m in height. The leaves are oblong and coriaceous.

Characteristics: The odor is aromatic and reminiscent of cloves.

Habitat: The plant is indigenous to the West Indies and is cultivated in South America, Central America and Jamaica.

Production: Pimento leaves are the foliage leaves of Pimenta racemosa. Pimentae fructus is obsolete as a drug.

Other Names: Allspice, Clove Pepper, Jamaica Pepper, Pimenta

ACTIONS AND PHARMACOLOGY

COMPOUNDS

Volatile oil (bay oil, 0.7-1.2%): chief components- eugenol (50-60%), chavicol (20%), additionally including among others eugenol methyl ether, methyl chavicol, myrcene, limonene, (-)-phellandrene, 3- octanon, 1-octen-3-ole, citral

EFFECTS

Pimento is antiseptic and analgesic, and is a skin irritant.

INDICATIONS AND USAGE

Unproven Uses: Pimento is used externally in rubefacient lotions or liniments.

PRECAUTIONS AND ADVERSE REACTIONS

General: No health hazards or side effects are known in conjunction with the proper administration of designated therapeutic dosages. Allergic reactions to eugenol occur rarely.

DOSAGE

Mode of Administration: Pimento preparations are administered externally as lotions or liniments.

LITERATURE

Hogg JW et al., (1971) Am Perf Cosmet 86:33.

Kato Y, (1975) Koryo 113:17 et 24.

Kern W, List PH, Hörhammer L (Eds.), Hagers Handbuch der Pharmazeutischen Praxis, 4. Aufl., Bde. 1-8, Springer Verlag Berlin, Heidelberg, New York, 1969.

Leung AY, Encyclopedia of Common Natural Ingredients Used in Food Drugs and Cosmetics, John Wiley & Sons Inc., New York 1980.

Oishi K et al., (1974) Nippon Suisan Gakaishi 40:1241.

Saito Y et al., (1976) Eiyo To Shokuryo 29:505.

Steinegger E, Hänsel R, Pharmakognosie, 5. Aufl., Springer Verlag Heidelberg 1992.

Pimpinella

Pimpinella major

DESCRIPTION

Medicinal Parts: The medicinal parts are the dried rhizome, the dried roots and the fresh roots collected in May.

Flower and Fruit: The white flowers are in compound 5- to 15-rayed umbels. There is no involucre or epicalyx. The flowers are small. The petals are uneven with curved lobes. The style is longer than the ovary during the flowering season. The fruit is dark brown to black, oblong-ovate, compressed at the sides, 2 to 3.5 mm long, heavily grooved and has no beak.

Leaves, Stem and Root: The 50 to 100 cm high plant is a perennial. During the flowering season, it develops lateral rosettes of leaves for the following year. These are usually glabrous, occasionally finely downy to short-bristly. The root is fusiform or carrot-shaped. The root is 10 to 20 cm long and 1 to 1.5 cm thick, gray-yellow and somewhat ringed. The stem is erect, angular, grooved, hollow, glabrous, somewhat leafy and branched from the ground up. The leaves are simple pinnate and glossy. The leaflets of the lower leaves are petiolate. They are ovate or oblong-indented or serrate acuminate.

Characteristics: The fresh root smells rancid, suet or carrot-like. The taste is tangy at first then burning-hot.

Habitat: The plant grows all over Europe with the exception of Scandinavia and the southern Balkans. It has been introduced to North America.

Production: Pimpinella herb consists of the above-ground parts of Pimpinella saxifrage and/or Pimpinella major. Pimpinella root consists of the dried rhizomes and roots of Pimpinella saxifrage and/or Pimpinella major. The root is dug up in spring and autumn. The uncut root is dried at temperatures of 40° C to prevent loss of essential oils. The drying process is completed when the roots can be broken.

Not to be Confused With: Pimpinellae radix should not be confused with other Apiaca roots. It is often adulterated with the roots of Heracleum sphondylium, Heracleum mantegazzianum and Pastinaca sativa.

Other Names: Pimpernell, Saxifrage, Burnet Saxifrage

ACTIONS AND PHARMACOLOGY

COMPOUNDS: PIMPINELLA HERB

Flavonoids

The foliage of the plant has not been fully investigated.

EFFECTS: PIMPINELLA HERB

No information is available.

COMPOUNDS: PIMPINELLA ROOT

Volatile oil (0.05 to 0.7%): chief components- trans-epoxy-pseudo-isoeugenol (20-57%), additionally pregeijeren (10%), geijerene (3%), beta-bisabolene, germacrenes A to D, 1,4-dimethyl azulene

Furocoumarins (1.2-2.3%): including among others bergaptene, isopimpinellin, pimpinellin, isobergapten, sphondine

Hydroxycoumarins: umbelliferone, scopoletin

Caffeic acid esters: including among others, chlorogenic acid

Polyynes: including trideca-2,8,10-trien-4,6-diine; trideca-2,8-dien-4,6-diin-10-ole

EFFECTS: PIMPINELLA ROOT

The drug contains essential oil. The efficacy of the drug as a flushing-out therapy in bacterial infections of the urinary tract seems plausible. The expectorant effect has not been proven.

INDICATIONS AND USAGE

PIMPINELLA HERB

Preparations of Pimpinella herb are used internally for lung ailments and to stimulate gastrointestinal activity. The herb is used externally for varicose veins.

PIMPINELLA ROOT

Approved by Commission E:

- Cough/bronchitis

Preparations of the root are also used for colds, chills and catarrh of the upper respiratory tract.

Unproven Uses: In folk medicine, it is used internally for disorders of the urinary organs, inflammation of the bladder and kidney, bladder and kidney stones, and edema. It is also used as flushing-out therapy in bacterial inflammation of the efferent urinary tract. Externally, it is used for inflammation of the oral and pharyngeal mucous membrane and as a bath additive for poorly healing wounds.

Homeopathic Uses: Homeopathic uses include febrile states and spinal pain. Efficacy of the flushing-out therapy seems plausible, efficacy for the other indications has not been sufficiently proven.

PRECAUTIONS AND ADVERSE REACTIONS

PIMPINELLA HERB

No health hazards or side effects are known in conjunction with the proper administration of designated therapeutic dosages.

PIMPINELLA ROOT

No health hazards or side effects are known in conjunction with the proper administration of designated therapeutic dosages. Photosensitivity may occur in light-skinned individuals.

DOSAGE

PIMPINELLA ROOT

Mode of Administration: Pimpinella root is administered as a tincture (Tinctura Pimpinellae) and as a comminuted herb for teas and other galenic preparations for internal use.

Daily Dosage: 6 to 12 g drug for infusions or 6 to 15 ml pimpernel tincture (1:5).

Folk medicine — Add freshly cut drug to cold water and bring to the boil, use as a gargle and as a bath additive.

Infusion — 3 to 10 g; 1 cup 3 to 4 times daily (sweetened with honey).

Gargle tincture — 30 drops in a glass of water.

For coughs — 5 to 10 drops on a sugar lump.

Homeopathic Dosage: 5 drops, 1 tablet or 10 globules every 30 to 60 minutes (acute) or 1 to 3 times daily (chronic); parenterally: 1 to 2 ml sc, acute: 3 times daily; chronic: once a day (HAB1).

LITERATURE

PIMPINELLA HERB

Bohn IU, Pimpinella saxifraga und Pimpinella major-Kleine und Große Bibernelle. In: ZPT 12(3):98. 1991.

Kubeczka KH, Formacek V, New Constituents from the Essential Oils of Pimpinella. In: Brunke EJ (Ed.) Progress in Essential Oil Research, Walter de Gruyter & Co, Berlin 1986. 1986.

Martin R et al., (1985) Planta Med 51(3):198.

Reichling J, Martin R, Pseudoisoeugenole - eine Gruppe seltener Phenylpropanoide im Genus Pimpinella: Biosynthese unfd biologische Wirkung. In: PZW 136(5/6)225. 1991.

Further information in:

Hänsel R, Keller K, Rimpler H, Schneider G (Hrsg.), Hagers Handbuch der Pharmazeutischen Praxis, 5. Aufl., Bde 4-6 (Drogen), Springer Verlag Berlin, Heidelberg, New York, 1992-1994.

Madaus G, Lehrbuch der Biologischen Arzneimittel, Bde 1-3, Nachdruck, Georg Olms Verlag Hildesheim 1979.

PIMPINELLA ROOT

Bohn IU, Pimpinella saxifraga und Pimpinella major-Kleine und Große Bibernelle. In: ZPT 12(3):98. 1991.

Kubeczka KH, Formacek V, New Constituents from the Essential Oils of Pimpinella. In: Brunke EJ (Ed.) Progress in Essential Oil Research, Walter de Gruyter & Co, Berlin 1986.

Martin R et al., (1985) Planta Med 51(3):198.

Reichling J, Martin R, Pseudoisoeugenole - eine Gruppe seltener Phenylpropanoide im Genus Pimpinella: Biosynthese unfd biologische Wirkung. In: PZW 136(5/6)225. 1991.

Further information in:

Hänsel R, Keller K, Rimpler H, Schneider G (Hrsg.), Hagers Handbuch der Pharmazeutischen Praxis, 5. Aufl., Bde 4-6 (Drogen), Springer Verlag Berlin, Heidelberg, New York, 1992-1994.

Madaus G, Lehrbuch der Biologischen Arzneimittel, Bde 1-3, Nachdruck, Georg Olms Verlag Hildesheim 1979.

Steinegger E, Hänsel R, Pharmakognosie, 5. Aufl., Springer Verlag Heidelberg 1992.

Teuscher E, Lindequist U, Biogene Gifte - Biologie, Chemie, Pharmakologie, 2. Aufl., Fischer Verlag Stuttgart 1994.

Teuscher E, Biogene Arzneimittel, 5. Aufl., Wiss. Verlagsges. Stuttgart 1997.

Wichtl M (Hrsg.), Teedrogen, 4. Aufl., Wiss. Verlagsges. Stuttgart 1997.

Pimpinella anisum

See Anise

Pimpinella major

See Pimpinella

Pineapple

Ananas comosus

DESCRIPTION

Medicinal Parts: The medicinal part of the plant is the fruit.

Flower and Fruit: The white, blue or purple flowers are arranged in approximately 30 cm long spikes. The flowers are in the axils of reddish, thorny bracts. The 3 sepals are free or fused at the base, and the 3 petals form a tube. There are 6 stamens and a 3-chambered ovary. The fruit is fused with the thickening receptacle to an oval to cylindrical, cone-like pseudocarp. The pseudocarp is 10 to 25 cm thick, 15 to 25 cm high, 0.5 to 5 kg in weight, yellow to orange-red with large warts and a hexagonal area bearing a leaf cluster at the tip.

Leaves, Stem and Root: Ananas comosus is a leafy rosette perennial plant, which grows up to 1.2 m high. The leaves are narrow-linear, thorny-tipped, up to 0.9 m long and 6 cm wide. They are usually thorny dentate and arranged in rosette. The stem is short.

Characteristics: The fruit is usually parthenocarpic. The cultivated fruits are seedless. The fruit pulp is white to yellow with a sourish-sweet, aromatic smell and taste.

Habitat: Hawaii, Japan, Taiwan

Production: Bromelain is a mixture of proteolytic enzymes from the main stump of Ananas comosus. Bromelain is produced from the main pineapple stumps harvested after 4 years. The main stumps are pressed and put through an extraction process with water. The juice is then precipitated with acetone to produce raw bromelain. The resulting waste product is a soft wax, which is used in the cosmetic industry.

ACTIONS AND PHARMACOLOGY

COMPOUNDS

Proteases: mixture of at least 5 chemically very similar cysteine proteinases, including EC 3.4.22.4 and EC 3.4.22.5, that can be deactivated with oxidizing substances or activated with thiols such as cysteine, as well as small amounts of a phosphatase, a peroxidase or protease inhibitors.

EFFECTS

Pineapple is antiphlogistic, fibrinolytic and proteolytic. The proteolytic enzymes promote the healing of wounds. In addition, an inhibition of thrombocyte aggregation and an antineoplastic effect have been observed, as well as an elevation of the serum level of antibiotics when administered concurrently.

INDICATIONS AND USAGE

Approved by Commission E:

- Wounds and burns

Unproven Uses: Internal application: For post traumatic and postoperative swelling to stimulate healing and as an enzyme substitution for digestive symptoms after pancreatic disease. The drug can also be used for edema, digestive complaints, for inflammation and febrile conditions (Hawaiian Islands, Philippines and South America), for asthmatic conditions in children (Zaire) and as a vermifuge (Brazil). Pineapple bran is used in weight reduction.

Indian Medicine: The fruit is used for dyspeptic symptoms, constipation, amenorrhea and dysmenorrhea, as well as for black vomiting and fever.

PRECAUTIONS AND ADVERSE REACTIONS

No health hazards are known in conjunction with the proper administration of designated therapeutic dosages. Gastric complaints and diarrhea may occur as side effects of internal administration. Allergic reactions following repeated administration have been observed.

DOSAGE

Mode of Administration: Available as tablets, granules and galenic preparations for internal use; compounded preparations for external use.

Daily Dosage: Internal application: 80 to 240 mg of raw bromelain in galenic preparations, corresponding to 200 to 600 FIP units.

Storage: Seal tightly and air dry.

LITERATURE

Hänsel R, Keller K, Rimpler H, Schneider G (Ed), Hagers Handbuch der Pharmazeutischen Praxis, 5. Aufl., Bde 4 - 6 (Drogen), Springer Verlag Berlin, Heidelberg, New York, 1992-1994.

Harrach T, Eckert K, Schulze-Forster K, Nuck R, Grunow D, Maurer HR, Isolation and partial characterization of basic proteinases from stem bromelain. J Protein Chem, 57:41-52, 1995 Jan.

Holtum JA, Summons R, Roeske CA, Comins HN, O'Leary MH, Allergic reactions, including asthma, to the pineapple protease bromelain following occupational exposure. Clin Allergy, 57:443-50, 1979 Sep.

Hotz G, Frank T, Zöller J, Wiebelt H, Antiphlogistic effect of bromelaine following third molar removal. Dtsch Zahnarztl Z, 57:830-2, 1989 Nov.

Taussig SJ, Batkin S, Abortifacient effect of steroids from Ananas comosus and their analogues on mice. J Reprod Fertil, 22:461-2, 1976 Mar.

Taussig SJ, Batkin S, Bromelain, the enzyme complex of pineapple (Ananas comosus) and its clinical application. An update. J Ethnopharmacol, 22:191-203, 1988 Feb-Mar.

Taussig SJ, Batkin S, Modulation of pulmonary metastasis (Lewis lung carcinoma) by bromelain, an extract of the pineapple stem (Ananas comosus). Letter Cancer Invest, 22:241-2, 1988.

Pink Root

Spigelia marilandica

DESCRIPTION

Medicinal Parts: The medicinal parts are the dried rhizomes and roots.

Fruit and Flower: The inflorescences are terminal, sometimes branched spikes inclined to one side. The flowers are erect. The high leaves are tiny or awl-shaped in fives, and they are narrow. The 5-petaled corolla is red or yellow. The fruit is a 2-valved capsule. The seeds are angular and packed tightly in the fruit.

Leaves, Stem and Root: The plant is a perennial that grows up to 45 cm high and has fibrous, twisted roots. The stem is quadrangular and glabrous. The foliage leaves are opposite, membranous, ovate to ovate-lanceolate, acuminate, rounded at the base, entire-margined and sessile. The stipules are small.

Habitat: The plant is indigenous to the U.S.

Production: Pink Root and herb are the rhizome and aerial parts of Spigelia marilandica.

Other Names: American Wormgrass, Indian Pink, Maryland Pink, Pinkroot, Starbloom, Wormgrass

ACTIONS AND PHARMACOLOGY

COMPOUNDS

The drug has not been investigated in recent times. Older sources include, among others, references to the presence of acidic resins, volatile oil, tannins, waxes and a volatile base (presumably identical with isoquinoline).

EFFECTS

Pink Root has anthelmintic actions.

INDICATIONS AND USAGE

Unproven Uses: The herb is used for worm infestation, as a febrifuge and for malaria.

Homeopathic Uses: Spigelia marilandica is used as a calmative during states of excitement.

PRECAUTIONS AND ADVERSE REACTIONS

According to older sources, the drug allegedly contains a toxin that paralyzes the spinal marrow and leads to death through asphyxiation.

DOSAGE

Mode of Administration: As a powdered root or herb or as a liquid extract.

LITERATURE

Hänsel R, Keller K, Rimpler H, Schneider G (Hrsg.), Hagers Handbuch der Pharmazeutischen Praxis, 5. Aufl., Bde 4-6 (Drogen): Springer Verlag Berlin, Heidelberg, New York, 1992-1994.

Lewin L, Gifte und Vergiftungen, 6. Aufl., Nachdruck, Haug Verlag, Heidelberg 1992.

Pinus Bark

Tsuga canadensis

DESCRIPTION

Medicinal Parts: The medicinal parts are the latex, which exudes from the plant and the essential oil.

Flower and Fruit: The pedicle of the male flower is shorter than the scale sheath. The cones are small (1.5 to 2.5 cm long) and light brown. The wood contains no resin.

Leaves, Stem and Root: The young shoots are villous, becoming pubescent. The leaves have a leaf cushion and are flat, short (1 to 1.5 cm long) and obtuse. The upper surface is dark green and the under surface has 2 blue-white long stripes.

Habitat: The plant is indigenous to North America.

Other Names: Hemlock Bark, Canada Pitch, Hemlock Gum

ACTIONS AND PHARMACOLOGY

COMPOUNDS

Tannins (8-15%)

Flavonoids: hemlock tannin

Stilbene derivatives (8-10%): picea tannols

EFFECTS

The active agents are the tannin, hemlock tannin, and picea tannols. The drug has astringent, anti-inflammatory, diaphoretic, and diuretic properties.

INDICATIONS AND USAGE

Unproven Uses: Pinus Bark is used for digestive disorders, diarrhea, and diseases of the mouth and throat. It was formerly used to treat scurvy.

PRECAUTIONS AND ADVERSE REACTIONS

No health hazards or side effects are known in conjunction with the proper administration of designated therapeutic dosages. Administration in allopathic medicine is not common.

DOSAGE

Mode of Administration: The drug is available as a liquid extract, in medicinal preparations and combinations.

LITERATURE

Hoppe HA, (1975-1987) Drogenkunde, 8. Aufl., Bde 1-3: W de Gruyter Verlag, Berlin, New York.

Kern W, List PH, Hörhammer L (Hrsg.), Hagers Handbuch der Pharmazeutischen Praxis, 4. Aufl., Bde 1-8: Springer Verlag Berlin, Heidelberg, New York, 1969.

Pinus species

See Scotch Pine

Piper betle

See Betel Nut

Piper cubeba

See Cubeb

Piper elongatum

See Matico

Piper methysticum

See Kava Kava

Piper nigrum

See Black Pepper

Pipsissewa

Chimaphila umbellata

DESCRIPTION

Medicinal Parts: The medicinal parts are the dried leaves (occasionally mixed with twigs and flowers), the fresh aerial parts of the flowering plant and the complete dried plant.

Flower and Fruit: The plant has terminal inflorescences 10 cm long with umbels of 2 to 7 flowers. The flowers, which are initially bright pink and then white, are nodding and mildly campanulate. The 5 sepals are obovate, dentate and about a third as long as the 5 petals. The petals are broadly ovate, domed, pink and 5 to 6 mm long. The 10 stamens are thickened at the base, the edges are winged and ciliate. The anthers are short, thick and red. The style is very short and the stigma broad and shorter than the anthers. The fruit is a 5-grooved capsule with erect stems.

Leaves, Stem and Root: The plant is a perennial semi-shrub growing up to 25 cm high with an upright, angular stem and a creeping white rhizome. The evergreen, alternate leaves are short-petioled, coriaceous, ovate-spatulate to linear and wedge-shaped. The leaf margin is sharply serrate.

Habitat: The plant grows extensively in Europe, Asia, Siberia, and North and South America. It is a protected species in Germany.

Production: Pipsissewa is the aerial part of Chimaphila umbellata, which is collected in the wild.

Not to be Confused With: Confusion sometimes arises with Chimaphila maculata.

Other Names: Prince's Pine, Ground Holly, Umbellate Wintergreen, Butter Winter, King's Cureall, Love in Winter, Rheumatism Weed, King's Cure

ACTIONS AND PHARMACOLOGY

COMPOUNDS

Hydroquinone glycosides: chief component isohomoarbutin, additionally homoarbutin

Naphthacene derivatives (naphthoquinone): chimaphilin (2,7-dimethyl-1,4-naphthoquinone)

Flavonoids: including among others hyperoside, avicularin

Tannins: (4-5%)

EFFECTS

The drug contains quinine, which is said to be a urinary antiseptic. (See Uva Ursi) Alcoholic and aqueous extracts of the plant are said to have antimicrobial properties in vitro.

INDICATIONS AND USAGE

Unproven Uses: Internal applications include acute and chronic cystitis and edema.

Indian Medicine: Pipsissewa is used internally by American Indians for complaints of the kidneys and bladder, and to regulate menstruation, both before and after giving birth. It is also used for rheumatism and cancerous conditions. It is used externally for skin diseases and smallpox.

Homeopathic Uses: Among uses in homeopathy are chronic inflammation of the efferent urinary tracts, prostate gland and mammary glands.

PRECAUTIONS AND ADVERSE REACTIONS

No health hazards or side effects are known in conjunction with the proper administration of designated therapeutic dosages. The drug possesses a weak sensitizing effect, due to its chimaphilin content. The drug is not suitable for long-term use because of its hydroquinone glycoside content. (See Uva-Ursi leaf.)

DOSAGE

Mode of Administration: Constituent of homeopathic preparations in dilutions or as a mother tincture.

Preparation: A liquid extract is prepared 1:1 with ethanol.

Daily Dosage: The usual single dose is 2 g drug, 1 to 3 g drug in a tea, or 1 to 4 ml of extract.

Homeopathic Dosage: 5 to 10 drops, 1 tablet, 5 to 10 globules 1 to 3 times daily, or 1 ml injection solution sc twice weekly (HAB1).

LITERATURE

Bolkart KH et al., (1968) Naturwissenschaften 55:445.

Hänsel R, Keller K, Rimpler H, Schneider G (Hrsg.), Hagers Handbuch der Pharmazeutischen Praxis, 5. Aufl., Bde 4-6 (Drogen), Springer Verlag Berlin, Heidelberg, New York, 1992-1994.

Madaus G, Lehrbuch der Biologischen Arzneimittel, Bde 1-3, Nachdruck, Georg Olms Verlag Hildesheim 1979.

Thomson RH, Naturally Occuring Quinones, 2nd Ed., Academic Press New York 1971.

Walewska E, Thieme H, (1969) Pharmazie 24:423.

Piscidia piscipula

See Jamaica Dogwood

Pistacia lentiscus

See Mastic Tree

Pitcher Plant

Sarracenia purpurea

DESCRIPTION

Medicinal Parts: The medicinal parts are the leaves and roots.

Flower and Fruit: The androgynous flowers usually have numerous stamens and a large 3- to 5-valved superior ovary. The style spreads into a wide, stemmed umbrella, which spreads over the stamens. The 5 stigma sit as small cone-like structures on the underside of the roof of the tips. The numerous marginal ovules are on individual axillary shafts. The fruit is a valved capsule. The small, membranous, thin-skinned seeds contain an abundance of endosperm.

Leaves, Stem and Root: Sarracenia purpurea is a strange, perennial plant with leaves that are in a basal rosette and change into a tube or beaker-like formation. The beaker bears a long wing-like strip on the side turned towards the stem. These beakers are often very colorful and fill up with rainwater and insects. During hot weather they are closed because of a concentration of fibers. The enclosed rainwater and insects form a mass, which probably acts as a fertilizer and has a strong odor.

Habitat: The plant is indigenous to the U.S.

Production: Pitcher Plant root and leaves are the root and leaves of Sarracenia purpurea.

Other Names: Eve's Cups, Fly-Catcher, Fly-Trap, Huntsman's Cup, Purple Side-Saddle Flower, Side-Saddle Plant, Water-Cup, Smallpox Plant

ACTIONS AND PHARMACOLOGY

COMPOUNDS

Piperidine alkaloids: coniine, gamma-conicein (particularly in the trapping fluid of the pitcher leaves)

EFFECTS

The drug has stomachic, diuretic, and laxative effects due to its active agents, which include sarracenia acid, tannin, resin, and the alkaloid sarracenin, which is similar to veratrin.

INDICATIONS AND USAGE

Unproven Uses: Pitcher Plant was formerly used for digestive disorders, particularly constipation, also for urinary tract diseases, and as a cure for smallpox. Indigenous North American Indians believe the drug not only saved lives of smallpox victims, but they also administered it to prevent scar formation.

PRECAUTIONS AND ADVERSE REACTIONS

No health hazards or side effects are known in conjunction with the proper administration of designated therapeutic dosages.

DOSAGE

Mode of Administration: Both the root and leaf preparations are considered completely obsolete.

LITERATURE

Foder GB, Colasenko B, In: Alkaloids, Vol. 3, Ed. SW Pelletier, Pub. John Wiley 1985.

Kern W, List PH, Hörhammer L (Hrsg.), Hagers Handbuch der Pharmazeutischen Praxis, 4. Aufl., Bde. 1-8: Springer Verlag Berlin, Heidelberg, New York, 1969.

Teuscher E, Lindequist U, Biogene Gifte - Biologie, Chemie, Pharmakologie, 2. Aufl., Fischer Verlag Stuttgart 1994.

Plantago afra

See Psyllium Seed

Plantago lanceolata

See English Plantain

Plantago ovata

See Psyllium

Plantain

Musa paradisiaca

DESCRIPTION

Medicinal Parts: The medicinal part of the plant is the fruit.

Flower and Fruit: The inflorescence, growing through the false trunk and curving downward, bears groups of male flowers in the axils of the bracts at the tip, groups of androgynous flowers beneath and finally female flowers. The flowers are zygomorphic with 5 fused and 1 free tepal. There are 5 stamens and a superior ovary. The fruit is a berry. The 10 to 16 single fruits that develop from the flowers of a bract are called a hand.

Leaves, Stem and Root: The herbaceous perennial grows up to 6 m high. The leaves are very large, entire and simple. They are often pinnatifid and grow from an underground rhizome. The leaf sheaths form a hollow false trunk. There are adventitious roots.

Characteristics: A seedless berry fruit develops from the female flowers without pollination.

Habitat: The plant grows in tropical areas.

Production: Plantain banana pulp is the unripened pulp of Musa paradisiaca. Plantains are harvested when still green and ripened in special rooms for 3 to 10 days.

Other Names: Banana, Banana Tree

ACTIONS AND PHARMACOLOGY

COMPOUNDS

Polysaccharides: starch (20% of fresh weight)

Protein (1% of fresh weight)

Ascorbic acid (vitamin C): 10 to 20 mg/100 g fresh weight

Amines: serotonin (28 g/g fresh weight), tyramine (7 g/g fresh weight), dopamine (8 g/g fresh weight), noradrenaline (2 g/g fresh weight)

Fruit acids: including malic and citric acid

Aromatic substances: 180 components, including isopentenyl acetate (chief aroma-bearer)

EFFECTS

The starchy fruit has antiulcerogenic and cholesterol-reducing effects, and is a source of potassium. In East Africa and elsewhere, Plantain is used to prepare a narcotic drink.

INDICATIONS AND USAGE

Unproven Uses: The drug is used for dyspepsia, gastrointestinal complaints, diabetes, scurvy, diarrhea, hypertension and gout. The roots of the tree have been used as an anthelmintic and considered useful in alleviating bronchocele. The juice was used as a snakebite antidote.

Indian Medicine: Uses include worm disease, scabies, severe thirst, bronchitis, itching, kidney disease, pharyngalgia and dysuria. Efficacy for these indications has not yet been proven.

PRECAUTIONS AND ADVERSE REACTIONS

No health hazards are known in conjunction with the proper administration of designated therapeutic dosages. It is conceivable that the amine content could trigger attacks of migraine headache. The freqency of myocardial fibrosis in tropical countries is said to be caused by chronic ingestion of the plant. (Plantain should never be eaten raw; it must be cooked or fried.)

DOSAGE

Mode of Administration: Preparations of the whole, cut and powdered drug are administered orally.

Preparation: Plantain starch is extracted through the elutriation of the ground fruit pulp. Plantain powder is produced by dividing the fruit into slices and air- or chamber-drying them to a water content of only 15%, and then grinding. Plantain powder (or the unripened mashed fruit) is added to milk and drunk or made into bread called Chapatis.

LITERATURE

Chattopadhyay S, Chaudhuri S, Ghosal S, Activation of peritoneal macrophages by sitoindoside-IV, an anti-ulcerogenic acylsterylglycoside from Musa paradisiaca. Planta Med, 94:16-8, 1987 Feb.

Englyst HN, Cummings JH, Digestion of the carbohydrates of banana (Musa paradisiaca sapientum) in the human small intestine. Am J Clin Nutr, 44:42-50, 1986 Jul.

Goel RK, Gupta S, Shankar R, Sanyal AK, Anti-ulcerogenic effect of banana powder (Musa sapientum var. paradisiaca) and its effect on mucosal resistance. J Ethnopharmacol, 18:33-44, 1986 Oct.

Lyte M, Induction of gram-negative bacterial growth by neurochemical containing banana (Musa x paradisiaca) extracts. FEMS Microbiol Lett, 44:245-50, 1997 Sep 15.

Mukhopadhyaya K, Bhattacharya D, Chakraborty A, Goel RK, Sanyal AK, Effect of banana powder (Musa sapientum var. paradisiaca) on gastric mucosal shedding. J Ethnopharmacol, 21:11-9, 1987 Sep-Oct.

Srivastava A, Raj SK, Haq QM, Srivastava KM, Singh BP, Sane PV, Association of a cucumber mosaic virus strain with mosaic disease of banana, Musa paradisiaca - an evidence using immuno/nucleic acid probe. Indian J Exp Biol, 94:986-8, 1995 Dec.

Usha V, Vijayammal PL, Kurup PA, Aortic/glycosaminoglycans alterations in antiatherogenic action of dietary fiber from unripe banana (Musa paradisiaca). Indian J Med Res, 94:143-6, 1991 Apr.

Usha V, Vijayammal PL, Kurup PA, Effect of dietary fiber from banana (Musa paradisiaca) on cholesterol metabolism. Indian J Exp Biol, 44:550-4, 1984 Oct.

Usha V, Vijayammal PL, Kurup PA, Effect of dietary fiber from banana (Musa paradisiaca) on metabolism of carbohydrates in rats fed cholesterol free diet. Indian J Exp Biol, 44:445-9, 1989 May.

Platycodon grandiflorum

See Balloon-Flower (Jie-Geng)

Pleurisy Root

Asclepias tuberosa

DESCRIPTION

Medicinal Parts: The medicinal part of the plant is the root.

Flower and Fruit: The plant bears panicles of deep yellow and orange petalous flowers on the apex of the stem.

Leaves, Stem and Root: The plant is perennial, erect, 50 to 100 cm high with a fleshy tuberous root stock bearing a few stout, hairy stems. The leaves are alternate, oblong, glabrous, narrowly lanceolate and dark green. The under surface of the leaves is somewhat lighter than the upper surface. The rootstock is mildly ring-shaped with a branched crown. The roots are grooved lengthwise, grayish brown on the outside and whitish on the inside. The tissue is made up of concentric rings, which divide easily. The root is tough, short and starchy. Asclepias tuberosa is devoid of the latex typical of the genus (see Asclepias incarnata).

Characteristics: Pleurisy Root has a nutty and bitter taste. The odor is faint.

Habitat: Indigenous to America and Canada.

Production: Pleurisy Root is the root of Asclepias tuberosa.

Other Names: Butterfly Weed, Canada Root, Flux Root, Orange Swallow-Wort, Swallow-Wort, Tuber Root, White Root, Wind Root, Orange Milkweed

ACTIONS AND PHARMACOLOGY

COMPOUNDS

Cardioactive steroids (cardenolids) : including frugoside, glucofrugoside, coriglaucigenin (aglycone)

EFFECTS

Pleurisy Root is said to act as an expectorant, tonic, diaphoretic and antispasmodic.

INDICATIONS AND USAGE

Unproven Uses: Pleurisy Root is used for coughs, pleurisy, disorders of the uterus, as an analgesic and to ease breathing.

The plant plays a particularly important role in the medicine of American Indians as a remedy for pleurisy. It is also used as a diaphoretic in treating pneumonia, inflammation of the mucous membranes, local or general atrophy, diarrhea, dysentery, rheumatism and stomach ache. Pleurisy Root is also used as a diaphoretic and expectorant.

CONTRAINDICATIONS

Pleurisy Root is not to be used during pregnancy.

PRECAUTIONS AND ADVERSE REACTIONS

No health hazards or side effects are known in conjunction with the proper administration of designated therapeutic dosages.

OVERDOSAGE

The drug has an emetic effect in higher dosages, and digitalis-like poisonings are possible due to the cardioactive steroid content. For possible symptoms and treatments for poisonings, see Digitalis purpurea.

DOSAGE

Mode of Administration: The drug is used internally as a liquid extract and is also available in combination preparations.

LITERATURE

Costello CH, Butler CL, (1950) J Am Pharm Ass Sci Ed 39:233.

Pagani F, (1975) Boll Chim Farm 114(8):450.

Petricic J, (1966) Arch Pharm Ber Dtsch. Pharm Ges 299(12):1007.

Further information in:

Kern W, List PH, Hörhammer L (Hrsg.), Hagers Handbuch der Pharmazeutischen Praxis, 4. Aufl., Bde. 1-8, Springer Verlag Berlin, Heidelberg, New York, 1969.

Madaus G, Lehrbuch der Biologischen Arzneimittel, Bde. 1-3, Nachdruck, Georg Olms Verlag Hildesheim 1979.

Roth L, Daunderer M, Kormann K, Giftpflanzen, Pflanzengifte, 4. Aufl., Ecomed Fachverlag Landsberg Lech 1993.

Plumbago

Plumbago zeylanica

DESCRIPTION

Medicinal Parts: The medicinal parts of the plant are the leaf and root.

Flower and Fruit: The flowers are radial, their structures are arranged in fives with white petals and a superior ovary. The fruit is a 1-seeded nut.

Leaves, Stem and Root: Plumbago is a semi-shrub. The leaves are simple and entire.

Habitat: The plant is indigenous to Malaysia and China.

Production: Plumbago herb is the dried aerial part of Plumbago zeylandica.

ACTIONS AND PHARMACOLOGY

COMPOUNDS

Naphthalene derivatives: chief component plumbagin (0.04%), including as well 3-chlorplumbagin, isoshinanolone, 3,3′-biplumbagin, elliptinone (6,6′-biplumbagin), droserone, 3,6′-biplumbagin (chitranone), zeylanone, isozeylanone, maritinone, 2-methyl naphthazarine

EFFECTS

No definitive data available.

INDICATIONS AND USAGE

Chinese Medicine: The herb has been used for rheumatism, intestinal parasites, joint pain, anemia, scabies and furuncles.

PRECAUTIONS AND ADVERSE REACTIONS

No health hazards are known in conjunction with the proper administration of designated therapeutic dosages.

DOSAGE

Daily Dosage: 9 to 15 gm of drug

LITERATURE

No data available.

Plumbago zeylanica

See Plumbago

Podophyllum peltatum

See Mayapple

Pogostemon cablin

See Patchouli

Poison Ivy

Rhus toxicodendron

DESCRIPTION

Medicinal Parts: The medicinal parts are the leaves collected after flowering and dried, the fresh young shoots, the young flowering branches and the fresh leaves.

Flower and Fruit: The pedicled flowers are in axillary, pubescent panicles. They are dioecious, sometimes androgynous. The stemmed petals are whitish-green with red hearts. The fruit is an almost globular, glabrous, yellow or yellowish-white, 10-grooved drupe. The fruit varies in size and contains a viscous latex in resin channels, which turns black in the air.

Leaves, Stem and Root: The plant is a dioecious shrub up to 1 m high with ascending, procumbent or climbing rooting branches and underground runners. The branches are initially green and softly pubescent, later brown and glabrous. There are numerous lenticels on the two-year old shoots. The leaves are trifoliate with 8 to 14 cm long petioles. The leaflets are oblong, acute or obtuse, entire-margined or roughly serrate in the middle. They have a dark-green upper surface and slightly pubescent lower surface, which is a lighter green.

Habitat: The plant is indigenous to North America; it is also found in east Asia and is cultivated in Germany in botanical and apothecary gardens.

Production: Poison Ivy leaves are the leaves of Rhus toxicodendron. Subsequent to the flowering period, the leaves of R. toxicodendron are gathered and then well-dried. Gloves should be worn to protect hands while gathering the leaves, as they can cause unpleasant inflammation of the skin.

Not to be Confused With: Although it is sometimes called ''Ampelopsis hoggii,'' Rhus toxicodendron actually has nothing in common with the Ampelopsis group of vines.

Other Names: Poison Oak, Poison Vine, Epright Sumach

ACTIONS AND PHARMACOLOGY

COMPOUNDS

Alkyl phenols: urushiol, chiefly cis,cis-3-(n-heptadeca-8',11'-dienyl)catechol, cis,cis, cis-3-(n-heptadeca-8',11',14'-trienyl)catechol, cis-3-(n-heptadec-8'-enyl)catechol

Tannins

Flavonoids

EFFECTS

''Rhus poison,'' even in very small amounts, causes severe irritation to the skin. Following contact it can result in reddening, swelling and herpes simplex-like blisters. It also has a strong toxic effect if taken internally. The mother tincture (main constituents: gallic acid and urushiol) inhibits in vitro prostaglandin biosynthesis.

INDICATIONS AND USAGE

Homeopathic uses: The drug is used to treat rheumatism in the joints and muscles; overexertion (stress and strain); febrile infections with giddiness; inflammation of the respiratory tract, gastrointestinal tract and the eyes; menstrual disturbances; anxiety and depressive states; and itching skin diseases.

PRECAUTIONS AND ADVERSE REACTIONS

Contact with larger quantities of the allergen can bring about resorption and generalized erythema; in severe cases also fever and unconsciousness. Severe conjunctivitis and corneal inflammations, with possible loss of sight, may result after contact with the eyes. External application of the drug should be avoided. Skin affected by accidental contact should be intensively rinsed with a soapy solution and then cleaned with ether or ethanol. The points of inflammation should be covered with bicarbonate of soda paste (mixed with water). Internal treatment is carried out with systematically effective corticosteroids. Cooling bandages give relief in mild cases.

OVERDOSAGE

Overdoses of homeopathic preparations lead to severe mucous membrane irritation, accompanied by queasiness, vomiting, intestinal colic and diarrhea, as well as signs of resorption, e.g., vertigo, stupor, kidney damage (nephritis, hematuria).

Following gastrointestinal emptying (gastric lavage with burgundy-colored potassium permanganate solution, sodium sulfate), installation of activated charcoal and shock prophylaxis (quiet, warmth), the therapy for these sorts of poisonings consists of treating spasms with diazepam (i.v.), electrolyte substitution and treating possible cases of acidosis with sodium bicarbonate infusions. In case of shock, plasma volume expanders should be infused. Monitoring of kidney function is essential. Intubation and oxygen respiration may also be necessary. Furthermore, the leaves possess a very severe potential for sensitization, due to their urushiol content. Following sensitization (which can also occur through contact with decorative art from the Far East, such as wooden chairs that have been treated with toxicodendron lacquers), renewed contact leads within a few hours to itching eczemas and eventual blister formation.

DOSAGE

Mode of Administration: Homeopathic dilutions of the mother tincture.

Homeopathic Dosage: 5 drops, 1 tablet or 10 globules every 30 to 60 minutes (acute) or 1 to 3 times daily (chronic);

parenterally: 1 to 2 ml sc; acute: 3 times daily; chronic: once a day (HAB34); children are given different doses.

Storage: In tightly sealed containers, not to be kept for more than a year.

LITERATURE

Gross M et al., PH 14:2263. 1975.

Millet S et al., PH 15:553. 1976.

Randall RC, Phillips GO, Williams PA, Food Hydrocolloids 3:65-75. 1989.

Shobha SV et al., Inhibition of soybean lipoxygenase-1 by anacardic acids, cardols, and cardanols. In: JNP 57(12):1755-1757. 1994.

Symes WF, Dawson CR, Nature 171:841. 1953.

Further information in:

Frohne D, Pfänder HJ, Giftpflanzen - Ein Handbuch für Apotheker, Toxikologen und Biologen, 4. Aufl., Wiss. Verlags-Ges. Stuttgart 1997.

Hausen B, Allergiepflanzen, Pflanzenallergene, ecomed Verlagsgesellsch. mbH, Landsberg 1988.

Lewin L, Gifte und Vergiftungen, 6. Aufl., Nachdruck, Haug Verlag, Heidelberg 1992.

Madaus G, Lehrbuch der Biologischen Arzneimittel, Bde 1-3, Nachdruck, Georg Olms Verlag Hildesheim 1979.

Roth L, Daunderer M, Kormann K: Giftpflanzen, Pflanzengifte, 4. Aufl., Ecomed Fachverlag Landsberg Lech 1993 (unter Toxicodendron).

Steinegger E, Hänsel R, Pharmakognosie, 5. Aufl., Springer Verlag Heidelberg 1992.

Teuscher E, Lindequist U, Biogene Gifte - Biologie, Chemie, Pharmakologie, 2. Aufl., Fischer Verlag Stuttgart 1994.

Wagner H, Wiesenauer M, Phytotherapie. Phytopharmaka und pflanzliche Homöopathika, Fischer-Verlag, Stuttgart, Jena, New York 1995.

Poisonous Buttercup

Ranunculus sceleratus

DESCRIPTION

Medicinal Parts: The medicinal part is the fresh herb.

Flower and Fruit: The plant produces numerous flowers. They are small, pale yellow and 4 to 10 mm in size. The petals are as long as the calyx. The sepals are revolute, ovate and downy. There are many stamens and numerous ovaries. The fruit consists of an oblong, ear-like capitula. The calyx and corolla drop easily.

Leaves, Stem and Root: The plant grows from 20 to 60 cm high with an annual root. The plant is pale, glossy, yellowish-green, fleshy and glabrous. The upper part of the stem is occasionally pubescent. The stem is erect, tubular, glabrous and branched. The leaves are palmate: The lower ones are long-petioled with 2- to 3-lobed segments, and the upper ones are sessile and usually trifoliate.

Characteristics: A bruised leaf coming into contact with the skin creates a blister that heals very slowly.

Habitat: The plant is indigenous to central and northern Europe.

Production: Poisonous Buttercup is the fresh herb of R. sceleratus, which is gathered in October.

Other Names: Celery-Leaved Crowfoot, Cursed Crowfoot

ACTIONS AND PHARMACOLOGY

COMPOUNDS

Glycoside ranunculin: as protoanemonine-forming agent in the freshly harvested plant (1.4% of the fresh weight) that changes enzymatically when the plant is cut into small pieces, and probably also while it is drying, into the pungent, volatile protoanemonine that quickly dimerizes to non-mucous-membrane-irritating anemonine. When dried, the plant may not be capable of protoanemonine formation.

Saponins

EFFECTS

The active agents are ranunculin, protoanemonin and anemonin and flavoid in the leaves. The plant is highly toxic. The juice contains protoanemonin, which causes pain and burning sensations, increases saliva secretion and causes severe inflammation of the tongue.

INDICATIONS AND USAGE

Unproven Uses: Poisonous Buttercup is used as a skin stimulant for skin diseases (such as scabies) and leukoderma.

Homeopathic Uses: Poisonous Buttercup is used for skin complaints, swollen muscles and joints, and influenza.

PRECAUTIONS AND ADVERSE REACTIONS

No health hazards or side effects are known in conjunction with the proper administration of designated therapeutic dosages of the dehydrated drug. Extended skin contact with the freshly harvested, bruised plant can lead to blister formation and cauterizations that are difficult to heal due to the resulting protoanemonine, which is severely irritating to skin and mucous membranes. If taken internally, severe irritation to the gastrointestinal tract, combined with colic and diarrhea, as well as irritation of the urinary drainage passages, may occur. Symptomatic treatment for external contact consists of mucilaginosa after irrigation with diluted potassium permanganate solution. In case of internal contact, administration of activated charcoal should follow gastric lavage.

OVERDOSAGE

Death by asphyxiation following the intake of large quantities of protoanemonine-forming plants has been observed in animal experiments.

DOSAGE

Mode of Administration: The herb is available as a mother tincture and extract in homeopathic dilutions.

LITERATURE

Bonora A et al., PH 26:2277. 1987.

Frohne D, Pfänder HJ, Giftpflanzen - Ein Handbuch für Apotheker, Toxikologen und Biologen, 4. Aufl., Wiss. Verlags-Ges. Stuttgart 1997.

Hegnauer R, Chemotaxonomie der Pflanzen, Bde 1-11: Birkhäuser Verlag Basel, Boston, Berlin 1962-1997.

Kern W, List PH, Hörhammer L (Hrsg.), Hagers Handbuch der Pharmazeutischen Praxis, 4. Aufl., Bde. 1-8: Springer Verlag Berlin, Heidelberg, New York, 1969.

Madaus G, Lehrbuch der Biologischen Arzneimittel, Bde 1-3, Nachdruck, Georg Olms Verlag Hildesheim 1979.

Roth L, Daunderer M, Kormann K, Giftpflanzen, Pflanzengifte, 4. Aufl., Ecomed Fachverlag Landsberg Lech 1993.

Ruijgrok HWL, PM 11:338-347. 1963.

Teuscher E, Lindequist U, Biogene Gifte - Biologie, Chemie, Pharmakologie, 2. Aufl., Fischer Verlag Stuttgart 1994.

Poke

Phytolacca americana

DESCRIPTION

Medicinal Parts: The medicinal parts are the dried root and the berries.

Flower and Fruit: The racemes are about 10 cm long and more or less erect. The flowers are androgynous. There is a calyx without a corolla. The involucre segments are 2.5 cm, broadly ovate, greenish-white and turn reddish at the fruit. There are 10 stamens and 10 carpels, which are fused. The fruits are 10 mm depressed-globose, purplish-black berries, which cover the stem like a raceme. They are similar to blueberries.

Leaves, Stem and Root: The plant is a glabrous, perennial herb, somewhat woody at the base. The root is long and fleshy. The stems are 1 to 3 m high, hollow, bifurcated and often marked with grooves. The leaves are alternate, entire-margined, unpleasantly scented, 12 to 25 cm by 5 to 10 cm, ovate-lanceolate and petiolate.

Habitat: The plant is indigenous to the U.S. and has also become common in Mediterranean countries.

Production: Poke Root and berries are the root and fruit of Phytolacca americana.

Other Names: American Nightshade, American Spinach, Bear's Grape, Branching Phytolacca, Cancer-Root, Coakum-Chongras, Cokan, Crowberry, Inkberry, Jalap, Phytolacca Berry, Phytolacca Root, Pigeon Berry, Pocan, Poke Root, Poke Berry, Pokeweed, Red Weed, Red-Ink Plant, Scoke, Skoke, Virginian Poke

ACTIONS AND PHARMACOLOGY

COMPOUNDS: POKE FRUIT

Triterpene saponins (mixture termed phytolaccatoxin): phytolaccoside A-G, phytolaccasaponin B, aglycones 28,30-dicarboxy-oleans, including jaligonic acid, esculentic acid, phytolaccagenic acid, pokeberrygenin

Triterpenes: including alpha-amyrin, beta-amyrin, taraxasterol, psi-taraxasterol, tirucallol

Lectins (pokeweed-mitogens)

Ribosome: inactivating proteins (1-RIP), in the seeds

Betacyans (red pigments): including among others phytolaccanin (betanin), particularly in the fruits

Lignans: caffeic acid aldehyde-oligomerics; including among others americanine A, B and D

Histamine: gamma-aminobutyric acid (in the rhizomes)

Saccharose: cyclitols

EFFECTS: POKE FRUIT

An antihepatotoxic and antiviral effect has been demonstrated for the fruit. The saponins have an emetic effect.

COMPOUNDS: POKE ROOT

Triterpene saponins (mixture termed phytolaccatoxin): phytolaccosides A, B, D, D2, E (chief component, aglycone phytolaccagenin), F, G, phytollaccasaponin B, aglycone 28,30-dicarboxy-oleans, including jaligonic acid, jaligonic acid-30-methyl ester, esculentic acid, phytolaccagenic acid

Amines: histamine (0.13 to 0.16%), in the roots

Starch

EFFECTS: POKE ROOT

An anti-edemic and immune-stimulating effect has been demonstrated for the root. The saponins have an emetic effect.

INDICATIONS AND USAGE

POKE FRUIT

Unproven Uses: Rheumatism and skin ulcers

POKE ROOT

Unproven Uses: Poke has been used to treat dysmenorrhoea, dyspepsia, catarrh, rheumatism, tonsillitis, pharyngitis, syphilis, mumps, conjunctivitis, scabies, ring worm infestation, ulcers, constipation and as an emetic.

Homeopathic Uses: Uses in homeopathic medicine include inflammation of the mucous membranes (particularly of the respiratory tract), feverish infections, inflammation of conditions of the mammary glands and rheumatic conditions.

PRECAUTIONS AND ADVERSE REACTIONS

General: All parts of the plants are poisonous, due to the presence of mucous membrane-irritating saponins and of the toxic, perorally effective lectins. The toxicity is reduced through cooking, since this destroys the lectins.

Pediatric Use: Emergency poison treatment procedures should be instituted in small children who consume even one berry.

OVERDOSAGE

Symptoms of poisoning include diarrhea (sometimes bloody), dizziness, hypotension, severe thirst, somnolence, tachycardia, vomiting, and in severe cases, spasm and death through respiratory failure. Up to 10 berries are considered harmless for an adult, but could be dangerous for a small child. Adults who consume more than 10 berries and small children who consume any berries should be treated for poisoning. This includes stomach and intestinal emptying (inducement of vomiting, gastric lavage with burgundy-colored potassium permanganate solution, sodium sulphate) and instillation of activated charcoal. Electrolyte substitution and the use of sodium bicarbonate to treat possible acidosis may be necessary.

DOSAGE

Mode of Administration: Administered as a powder, liquid extract and tincture.

Daily Dosage: Usual dosage is 60 to 100 mg

Homeopathic Dosage: 5 drops, 1 tablet or 10 globules every 30 to 60 minutes (acute) or 1 to 3 times daily (chronic); parenterally: 1 to 2 ml SC, IV., IM, acute: 3 times daily; chronic: once a day (HAB1).

Storage: The drug should be stored in paper or sacks made from cloth.

LITERATURE

Aron GM, Irvin JD, (1980) Antimicrob Agents Chem 17:1032.

Kang SS, Woo WS, Triterpenes from the berries of Phytolacca americana. In: JNP 43(4):510-513. 1980.

Kern W, List PH, Hörhammer L (Hrsg.), Hagers Handbuch der Pharmazeutischen Praxis, 4. Aufl., Bde. 1-8, Springer Verlag Berlin, Heidelberg, New York, 1969.

Lewin L, Gifte und Vergiftungen, 6. Aufl., Nachdruck, Haug Verlag, Heidelberg 1992.

Lewis WH, JAMA. 1979 Dec. 21; 242(25):2759-60.

Madaus G, Lehrbuch der Biologischen Arzneimittel, Bde 1-3, Nachdruck, Georg Olms Verlag Hildesheim 1979.

MecPherson A, In: Toxic Plants, Ed. AD Kinghorn, Columbia Press 1979.

Roth L, Daunderer M, Kormann K, Giftpflanzen, Pflanzengifte, 4. Aufl., Ecomed Fachverlag Landsberg Lech 1993.

Shin KH et al., (1979) Soul Taehakkyo Saengyak Opjukjip 18: 90.

Sick WW, Shin KH, (1976) Yakhak Hoe Chi 20(3):149.

Sick WW et al., (1976) Soul Taehakkyo Saengyak Opjukjip 15: 103.

Steinegger E, Hänsel R, Pharmakognosie, 5. Aufl., Springer Verlag Heidelberg 1992.

Tang W, Eisenbrand G, Chinese Drugs of Plant Origin, Springer Verlag Heidelberg 1992.

Teuscher E, Lindequist U, Biogene Gifte - Biologie, Chemie, Pharmakologie, 2. Aufl., Fischer Verlag Stuttgart 1994.

Tomlinson JA et al., (1974) J Gen Virol 22:225.

Ussberg MA et al., (1977) Ann N Y Acad Sci 284:431.

Wagner H, Wiesenauer M, Phytotherapie. Phytopharmaka und pflanzliche Homöopathika, Fischer-Verlag, Stuttgart, Jena, New York 1995.

Woo WS, Kang SS, (1978), 88:4750.

Polemonium caeruleum

See Jacob's Ladder

Polemonium reptans

See Abscess Root

Poley

Teucrium polium

DESCRIPTION

Medicinal Parts: The medicinal part is the whole herb.

Flower and Fruit: The flowers are axillary forming a capitula. They are fused and sessile, and their structures are in fives. The calyx is turned slightly upward with 5 acuminate tips and is white-gray pubescent. The corolla is reddish-white or yellowish. The upper lip is deeply divided into two and fused to half of the lower lip so that it appears 5-tipped. There are 4 stamens, which are much longer than the corolla, and a 2-carpeled ovary, divided, but not to the base. The fruit is a nutlet.

Leaves, Stem and Root: Poley is a dwarf shrub that grows up to 45 cm high. The leaves are decussate, obovate to elongate, crenate, involute and pubescent. The stem is densely covered with white, greenish or golden hairs.

Habitat: Mediterranean region

Production: Poley herb is the dried aerial part of Teucrium polium collected during the flowering season.

ACTIONS AND PHARMACOLOGY

COMPOUNDS

Diterpenes: including picropolin, picropolinol, picropolinon, teucrin A, teucrin P1 , teucrin H3 , montanines B and C, teupolins I to V, gnaphalidin, the diterpene spectrum varies a great deal according to both the subspecies being investigated and its source

Volatile oil (0.1 to 1%): the following have been demonstrated to be chief components, varying according to chemical race, alpha-pinene and beta-pinene, alpha-cadinol, alpha-humulene, beta-caryophyllene, caryophyllene oxide, cedrol, gamma-cadinene, delta-cadinene, limonene, linalool, menthofurane, myrcene, ocimene, T-cadinol, terpine-4-ol

Iridoids: iridoid glycosides, including 8-O-acetyl harpagide, harpagide, teucardoside

Flavonoids: including apigenin-7-O-glucoside, luteolin-7-O-glucoside, acacetine, apigenin, cirsiliol, cirsimaritin, eupatorin, luteolin, salvigenin

EFFECTS

The antidiabetic and anti-ulcer efficacy with which the drug has been credited has not yet been documented in definitive clinical studies. A reduction of the ulcer index was described in connection with animal experiments; furthermore, a definite reduction of the blood sugar levels was exhibited following the I.V. administration of a 4% decoction of the dried herb. The drug is additionally antibacterial, antipyretic and possibly anti-edematic and antiexudative in effect.

INDICATIONS AND USAGE

Unproven Uses: Poley is used for diabetes (Israel), gastric complaints (North Africa), fever (Italy) and as a vulnerary (Spain).

PRECAUTIONS AND ADVERSE REACTIONS

No health hazards are known in conjunction with the proper administration of designated therapeutic dosages.

DOSAGE

Mode of Administration: Cut drug and liquid extract for internal use.

Daily Dosage: Single dose for infusion: 1.5 gm drug per cup

Storage: Should be tightly sealed and protected from light.

LITERATURE

Autore G, Capasso F, De Fusco R, Fasulo MP, Lembo M, Mascolo N, Menghini A, Antipyretic and antibacterial actions of Teucrium polium (L.). Pharmacol Res Commun, 16:21-9, 1984 Jan.

Capasso F, Cerri R, Morrica P, Senatore F, Chemical composition and anti-inflammatory activity of an alcoholic extract of Teucrium polium L. Boll Soc Ital Biol Sper, 59:1639-43, 1983 Nov 30.

Gharaibeh MN, Elayan HH, Salhab AS, Hypoglycemic effects of Teucrium polium. J Ethnopharmacol, 24:93-9, 1988 Sep.

Hänsel R, Keller K, Rimpler H, Schneider G (Ed), Hagers Handbuch der Pharmazeutischen Praxis, 5. Aufl., Bde 4 - 6 (Drogen), Springer Verlag Berlin, Heidelberg, New York, 1992-1994.

Mattéi A, Rucay P, Samuel D, Feray C, Reynes M, Bismuth H, Liver transplantation for severe acute liver failure after herbal medicine (Teucrium polium) administration. letter J Hepatol, 22:597, 1995 May.

Rizk AM, Hammouda FM, Rimpler H, Kamel A, Chemical composition of the wild Egyptian plant Teucrium polium L. Pharmazie, 22:540-1, 1974 Aug.

Rizk AM, Hammouda FM, Rimpler H, Kamel A, Iridoids and flavonoids of Teucrium polium herb. Planta Med, 22:87-8, 1986 Apr.

Rizk AM, Hammouda FM, Rimpler H, Kamel A, On the essential oil of Teucrium polium L. Pharmazie, 22:351-2, 1974 May.

Suleiman MS, Abdul-Ghani AS, Al-Khalil S, Amin R, Effect of Teucrium polium boiled leaf extract on intestinal motility and blood pressure. J Ethnopharmacol, 22:111-6, 1988 Jan.

Polygala amara

See Bitter Milkwort

Polygala senega

See Seneca Snakeroot

Polygonatum multiflorum

See Solomon's Seal

Polygonum aviculare

See Knotweed

Pomegranate

Punica granatum

DESCRIPTION

Medicinal Parts: The medicinal parts are the root, the bark, the fruits, the peel of the fruit and the flowers.

Flower and Fruit: The flowers are infundibulate or rotate, usually solitary or in pairs of threes at the tips of the branches. The calyx and receptacle are bright coral-red and have a tough margin. There are 5 to 8 bright-red campanulate nodding petals and numerous stamens. The filaments are orange-red and the anthers yellow-gold. The ovary consists of 2 or 3 layers lying on top of one another. The fruit is an apple-sized, round, 1.6 to 12 cm wide false berry whose skin turns from bright red to leather-brown. The seeds are roughly square and purple, later acquiring a soft red outer skin.

Leaves, Stem and Root: The plant is an erect, roughly branched shrub up to 1.5 m high or a small, tree 3 to 5 m tall with a curved trunk and glabrous 4- to 6-edged, sometimes spiny-tipped branches. The branches are narrowly winged when young. The trunk later becomes fissured and twisted. The leaves are generally opposite or in clusters on the short shoots. They are deciduous, simple, pinnate-veined, short-petioled, glabrous, hard, oval-lanceolate with a tough middle rib.

Habitat: The plant probably originated in Asia. Today it is widespread in the Mediterranean region as far as South Tyrol, the Near East, South Africa, South Asia, China, Australia, U.S., and South America.

Production: Pomegranate bark is the dried bark of the trunk roots and branches of Punica granatum. The roots, trunk and older branches are collected at the beginning of autumn. Their bark is peeled off and air-dried.

Other Names: Delima, Grenadier

ACTIONS AND PHARMACOLOGY

COMPOUNDS: POMEGRANATE FRUIT PEEL

Tannins (25 to 28%; gallo tannins): including punicalin (granatine D), punicalagin (granatine C), granatine A, granatine B

COMPOUNDS: POMEGRANATE STEMS AND ROOT

Tannins (20 to 25% gallo tannins): including punicalagin, punicacortein C, casuarin

Piperidine alkaloids (0.4% in the rind of the stem, up to 0.8% in the rind of the root): chief alkaloids isopelletierine, N-methylisopelletierine, pseudopelletierine

EFFECTS

The drug, which contains tannins and alkaloids, is anthelmintic and amoeboid.

Pelletierin triggers, like strychnine, a raised stimulant reflex, which can escalate to tetanus and is effective against diverse tapeworms, ring worms and nematodes.

The tannins in the drug makes it useful as an astringent for sore throats, diarrhea and dysentery.

INDICATIONS AND USAGE

Unproven Uses: In folk medicine Pomegranate is used for infestation with tapeworm and other worms, for diarrhea and dysentery, as an abortifacient and astringent; externally used for hemorrhoids and as a gargle in cases of sore throat.

Homeopathic Uses: Punica granatum is used for gastrointestinal disturbances.

Chinese Medicine: In China, Pomegranate is used to treat chronic diarrhea and dysentery, blood in the stool, worm infestation and anal prolapses.

Indian Medicine: In India, uses include diarrhea, dysentery, vomiting and eye pain.

PRECAUTIONS AND ADVERSE REACTIONS

No health hazards are known in conjunction with the proper administration of designated therapeutic dosages. The high levels of tannin content in the drug could lead to gastric irritation.

OVERDOSAGE

Due to the alkaloid content, overdoses with the rind of the stem or the root (above 80 gm) lead to vomiting, including the vomiting of blood, later to dizziness, chills, vision disorders, collapse and possible death through respiratory failure. Total blindness (amaurosis) could occur within a few hours or a few days.

Following gastrointestinal emptying, (inducement of vomiting, gastric lavage with burgundy-colored potassium permanganate solution, sodium sulfate), installation of medicinal charcoal and shock prophylaxis (quiet, warmth), the therapy for poisonings consists of treating spasms with diazepam (i.v.), electrolyte substitution and treating possible cases of acidosis with sodium bicarbonate infusions. In case of shock, plasma volume expanders should be infused. Monitoring of kidney function is essential. Intubation and oxygen respiration may also be necessary.

DOSAGE

Mode of Administration: Pomegranate is available as whole, crude and powder forms for internal and external use. It is also available in parenteral form for homeopathic use.

Preparation:

Decoction — 1 part drug and 5 parts water.

Macerations — 60 parts drug and 400 parts water macerated for 12 hours to half the initial volume.

Liquid extract — percolation of 1000 parts coarse powder and 59% ethanol (V/V). The percolate is evaporated to the initial amount of the drug (EB6).

Decoction — 250 parts bark powder and 1500 parts water boiled for 30 minutes (Belg IV).

Daily Dosage:

Tapeworm treatment 1 (decoction) — 4 doses of 60 ml with 2 hour intervals between doses accompanied before treatment and after treatment by a laxative.

Tapeworm treatment 2 (maceration) — administration of 3 doses of 65 ml with a duodenal probe at 30 minute intervals; a laxative is administered after an hour.

As pomegranate bark juice extract — single dose: for tapeworm 20 gm.

Homeopathic Dosage: 5 drops, 1 tablet or 10 globules every 30 to 60 minutes (acute) or 1 to 3 times daily (chronic); parenterally: 1 to 2 ml sc acute: 3 times daily; chronic: once a day (HAB1).

Storage: Pomegranate should be sealed in containers and protected from moisture.

LITERATURE

Beckham N, Phyto-oestrogens and compounds that affect oestrogen metabolism. In: Aust Herbalism 7:11-16. 1995.

Foder GB, Colasenko B, In: Alkaloids, Vol. 3, Ed. SW. Pelletier, John Wiley 1985.

Neuhöfer H et al., The occurence of pelletierine derivatives in Punica granatum. In: 37. Annual Congr Med Plant Res Braunschweig 1989 P1-13. 1989.

Schilling G, Schick H, On the structure of punicalagin and punicalin. In: Liebigs Ann Chem (11):2240. 1985.

Tanake T et al., (1986) Chem Pharm Bull 34(2):656.

Wylegalla R, Biblische Botanik: Pflanzen und Früchte aus dem gelobten Land. In: DAZ 137(11):867-869. 1997.

Further information in:

Hänsel R, Keller K, Rimpler H, Schneider G (Hrsg.), Hagers Handbuch der Pharmazeutischen Praxis, 5. Aufl., Bde 4-6 (Drogen), Springer Verlag Berlin, Heidelberg, New York, 1992-1994.

Lewin L, Gifte und Vergiftungen, 6. Aufl., Nachdruck, Haug Verlag, Heidelberg 1992.

Madaus G, Lehrbuch der Biologischen Arzneimittel, Bde 1-3, Nachdruck, Georg Olms Verlag Hildesheim 1979.

Roth L, Daunderer M, Kormann K, Giftpflanzen, Pflanzengifte, 4. Aufl., Ecomed Fachverlag Landsberg Lech 1993.

Pontian Rhododendron

Rhododendron ponticum

DESCRIPTION

Medicinal Parts: The medicinal part of the plant is its leafy branches.

Flower and Fruit: The inflorescence is an umbelliferous raceme with 8 to 15 single flowers on 3 pubescent pedicles that are up to 3.5 cm long. The flower structures are in fives and fused. The calyx is inconspicuous, up to 3 mm long, and 5-toothed. The corolla is campanulate, 5-lobed, 4 to 5 cm in diameter, violet to pink-violet with green-yellow spots on the upper lobes. There are 10 stamens and a multi-chambered ovary on sessile disc. The fruit is an elongate-cylindrical capsule. The seeds are small and can fly.

Leaves, Stem and Root: Rhododendron ponticum is an evergreen shrub typically growing up to 5 m high, occasionally up to a tree height of 8 m. The leaves are 8 to 15 cm long, 3 to 5 cm wide with a 1 to 2 cm long petiole. The lamina is elliptical-elongate, acute at both ends, entire, coriaceous, dark green, smooth and glabrous above, pale green and glabrous beneath. The plant is heavily branched. The branches are glabrous.

Habitat: The plant is indigenous to the Balkan states, the Commonwealth of Independent States, Spain, Portugal and England.

Production: Pontian rhododendron herb is the dried leafy branches of Rhododendron ponticum.

ACTIONS AND PHARMACOLOGY

COMPOUNDS

Diterpenes of the andromedan type: grayanotoxin I (andromedotoxin, acetylandromedol, asebotoxin, rhodotoxin, 0.001 to 0.02%), grayanotoxin II (andromedol), grayanotoxin III (andromedenol)

Flavonoids: myricetin, gossypetin, azaleatin, malvin

Steroids: sterols, including beta-sitosterol, alpha-amyrin, ursolic acid

EFFECTS

The drug has the effect of reducing blood pressure in animal experiments, due to the diterpenes it contains of the andromedan type (grayanotoxins). Historically, effects also have been described as stimulating, narcotic, diaphoretic and diuretic.

INDICATIONS AND USAGE

Therapeutic use is no longer recommended because of the drug's possibly dangerous side-effects due to its toxic content.

Unproven Uses: Folk medicine uses have focused on primary hypertension and arthritis. Various species of Rhododendron have been used for rheumatic and gouty conditions and for stones.

PRECAUTIONS AND ADVERSE REACTIONS

All medicinal administration of the drug is discouraged. The observed effect (lowered blood pressure resulting from bradycardia) is the first sign of a toxic reaction.

The plant is toxic because of its andromedan derivative content. The grayanotoxins it contains prevent the closure of the sodium channels and thus inhibit conduction.

OVERDOSAGE

Symptoms of poisoning in case of overdosage could include salivation, cold sweats, paresthesia, vomiting, diarrhea, severe stupor, coordination disorders, spasm, bradycardia, cardiac arrhythmias, hypotension, and eventually death through cardiac failure or apnea. While poisonings among humans have not been documented, poisonings (including fatal ones such as ''goat death'') occur frequently among animals. The presumed explanation is that the leathery leaves are not tempting to humans to eat, and because of the low levels of andromendan derivatives present in medicinal preparations.

Toxic and/or lethal dosage levels cannot be determined with any precision because the plant's andromendan derivative content can vary so wildly. The LD50 for mice amounts to 5.1 mg grayonotoxin I/kg body weight, p.o.

Following gastrointestinal emptying (inducement of vomiting, gastric lavage with burgundy-colored potassium permanganate solution, sodium sulfate), installation of medicinal charcoal and shock prophylaxis (quiet, warmth), the therapy for poisonings consists of treating spasms with diazepam (IV), bradycardia with atropine and electrolyte substitution, and treating possible cases of acidosis with sodium bicarbonate infusions. In case of shock, plasma volume expanders should be infused. It is crucial that no opiates are administered. Monitoring of kidney function is essential. Intubation and oxygen respiration may also be necessary.

DOSAGE

Mode of Administration: Whole drug. Folk medicine modes also include administration as a tea or cigarette.

How Supplied: Forms of commercial pharmaceutical preparations include coated tablets and compound preparations.

Daily Dosage: There are no more exact details available.

LITERATURE

Hänsel R, Keller K, Rimpler H, Schneider G (Ed), Hagers Handbuch der Pharmazeutischen Praxis, 5. Aufl., Bde 4 - 6 (Drogen), Springer Verlag Berlin, Heidelberg, New York, 1992-1994.

Keller S, von Kürten S, Pachaly P, Zymalkowski F, Sterines and triterpenes from Rhododendron ponticum. Pharmazie, 25:621-5, 1970 Oct.

Thieme H, Walewska E, Winkler HJ, Isolation of salidroside from leaves of Rhododendron ponticum x catawbiense. Pharmazie, 24:783, 1969 Dec 12.

Poplar

Populus species

DESCRIPTION

Medicinal Parts: The medicinal parts are the bark, leaves, and leaf buds.

Flower and Fruit: The plant is dioecious. The carmine red flowers are in large, cylindrical hanging, thick catkins with carmine anthers. The male flowers have carmine red anthers; the female flowers have carmine stigmas. The flowers appear before the leaves. The seeds, which ripen in May/June, are very small and have a white lanate tuft of hair.

Leaves, Stem and Root: The tree may grow up to 30 m. The bark is initially yellow brown and later black-gray and fissured. The leaf buds are viscid. The leaves are almost circular with a dark green upper surface and a light grey-green under surface. They are dentate or lobed with obtuse teeth, initially silky-haired, later glabrous. The petioles are long, thin and laterally compressed.

Habitat: There are both European and North American species within the genus that have spread to other temperate zones.

Other Names: White Poplar, Canadian Poplar, Black Poplar, Trembling Poplar, European Aspen, Quaking Aspen

Production: Poplar bark consists of the fresh or dried bark of salicin-rich Poplar species as well as their preparations. Poplar leaves consist of the leaves of salicin-rich Poplar species as well as their preparations. Poplar buds consist of the dried, unopened leaf buds of Populus species, as well as their preparations.

ACTIONS AND PHARMACOLOGY

COMPOUNDS: POPLAR BARK AND LEAVES

Glycosides and esters yielding salicylic acid:

In Populus alba (leaf 6%, bark 2%) chief components: salicortin, tremulacin, salicin

In Populus nigra (leaf 2%, bark 1.5%) chief components: salicortin, salicin

In Populus tremula (leaf 3%, bark 2%) chief components: salicin, tremulacin, salicortin including as well as salireposide, populin, tremuloidin

EFFECTS

Poplar bark and leaves have antiphlogistic, analgesic, antibacterial and spasmolytic effects.

The salicylate acid derivatives and flavonoids are responsible for the antiphlogistic, analgesic, spasmolytic and antibacterial characteristics of the drug. The beneficial effect in micturition complaints due to prostate hypertrophy may be due to the content of zinc lignans in the drug.

COMPOUNDS: POPLAR LEAF BUDS

Flavonoids: (particularly in the glutinous coating of the buds, also yielding propolis) including chrysin, tectochrysin, galengine, izalpinine, galangin-3-methyl ether, kaempferol-3-methyl ether, pinocembrin, pinocembrin-7-methyl ether, apigenin

Glycosides and esters yielding salicylic acid: including salicin, populin

Volatile oil: chief components alpha- and beta-caryophyllene

EFFECTS: POPLAR LEAF BUDS

Poplar buds have antiphlogistic, antibacterial and wound healing effects.

INDICATIONS

POPLAR BARK AND LEAVES

Unproven Uses: Poplar bark and leaves are used for pain and rheumatism therapy; and in micturition complaints due to prostate hypertrophy.

POPLAR LEAF BUDS

Approved by Commission E:

- Hemorrhoids
- Wounds and burns

Unproven Uses: Poplar buds are used for superficial skin injuries, external hemorrhoids, frostbite and sunburn.

CONTRAINDICATIONS

POPLAR BARK AND LEAVES

Contraindicated in cases of hypersensitivity to salicylates.

POPLAR LEAF BUDS

Contraindicated in cases of hypersensitivity to salicylates, propolis and balsam of Peru, which may be a componant in commercially available ointments.

PRECAUTIONS

POPLAR BARK AND LEAVES

No health hazards or side effects are known in conjunction with the proper administration of designated therapeutic dosages.

POPLAR LEAF BUDS

No health hazards are known in conjunction with the proper administration of designated therapeutic dosages. External administration of the drug occasionally leads to allergic skin reactions.

DOSAGE

POPLAR BARK AND LEAVES

Mode of Administration: Poplar leaves are available in crude form as well as galenic preparations for internal use. Poplar bark is only available in compounded preparations.

Daily Dosage: 10 gm of drug

POPLAR LEAF BUDS

Mode of Administration: Poplar buds are available in semi-solid preparations for application to the skin.

How Supplied : Semi-solid preparations equivalent to 20% to 30% of drug.

Daily Dosage: Externally, 5 gm drug.

LITERATURE

POPLAR BARK AND LEAVES

Anonym, Phytotherapie: Pflanzliche Antirheumatika - was bringen sie? In: DAZ 136(45):4012-4015. 1996.

Jossang A et al., Cinnamrutinoses A and B, glycosides from Populus tremula. In: PH 35(2):547. 1994.

Picard S et al., Isolation of a new phenolic compound from leaves of Populus deltoides. In: JNP 57(6):808-810. 1994.

Thieme H, Benecke R, (1969) Pharmazie 24:567.

Vonkruedener S et al., Effects of extracts from Populus tremula L., Solidago virgaurea L. and Fraxinus excelsior L. on various myeloperoxidase systems. In: Arzneim Forsch 46(8):809-814. 1996.

Further information in:

Fenaroli's Handbook of Flavor Ingredients, Vol. 1. 2nd Ed. Pub. CRC Press Boca Raton 1975.

Hegnauer R, Chemotaxonomie der Pflanzen, Bde 1-11, Birkhäuser Verlag Basel, Boston, Berlin 1962-1997.

Kern W, List PH, Hörhammer L (Hrsg.), Hagers Handbuch der Pharmazeutischen Praxis, 4. Aufl., Bde. 1-8, Springer Verlag Berlin, Heidelberg, New York, 1969.

Leung AY, Encyclopedia of Common Natural Ingredients Used in Food, Drugs and Cosmetics, John Wiley & Sons Inc., New York 1980.

Madaus G, Lehrbuch der Biologischen Arzneimittel, Bde 1-3, Nachdruck, Georg Olms Verlag Hildesheim 1979.

Wagner H, Wiesenauer M, Phytotherapie. Phytopharmaka und pflanzliche Homöopathika, Fischer-Verlag, Stuttgart, Jena, New York 1995.

POPLAR LEAF BUDS

Anonym, Phytotherapie: Pflanzliche Antirheumatika - was bringen sie? In: DAZ 136(45):4012-4015. 1996.

Jossang A et al., Cinnamrutinoses A and B, glycosides from Populus tremula. In: PH 35(2):547. 1994.

Picard S et al., Isolation of a new phenolic compound from leaves of Populus deltoides. In: JNP 57(6):808-810. 1994.

Thieme H, Benecke R, (1969) Pharmazie 24:567.

Vonkruedener S et al., Effects of extracts from Populus tremula L., Solidago virgaurea L. and Fraxinus excelsior L. on various myeloperoxidase systems. In: Arzneim Forsch 46(8):809-814. 1996.

Further information in:

Fenaroli's Handbook of Flavor Ingredients, Vol. 1. 2nd Ed. Pub. CRC Press Boca Raton 1975.

Hegnauer R, Chemotaxonomie der Pflanzen, Bde 1-11, Birkhäuser Verlag Basel, Boston, Berlin 1962-1997.

Kern W, List PH, Hörhammer L (Hrsg.), Hagers Handbuch der Pharmazeutischen Praxis, 4. Aufl., Bde. 1-8, Springer Verlag Berlin, Heidelberg, New York, 1969.

Leung AY, Encyclopedia of Common Natural Ingredients Used in Food Drugs and Cosmetics, John Wiley & Sons Inc., New York 1980.

Madaus G, Lehrbuch der Biologischen Arzneimittel, Bde. 1-3, Nachdruck, Georg Olms Verlag Hildesheim 1979.

Wagner H, Wiesenauer M, Phytotherapie. Phytopharmaka und pflanzliche Homöopathika, Fischer-Verlag, Stuttgart, Jena, New York 1995.

Poppyseed

Papaver somniferum

DESCRIPTION

Medicinal Parts: The medicinal part is the latex extracted from the seed capsule.

Flower and Fruit: A solitary flower grows on a long, glabrous or pubescent pedicle. The flowers are erect with a diameter of 10 cm. There are 2 green, glabrous, falling sepals and 4 violet-white or red petals with a darker mark at the base. The fruit is round or ellipsoid and often has a very large capsule. The numerous seeds are reniform, pitted, black, and blue-frosted or whitish.

Leaves, Stem and Root: The opium Poppy is an annual that grows 30 to 150 cm high. It is a 1-stemmed blue-gray frosted plant. The stem is erect, straight or branched and produces, as does the whole plant, white milky latex. The leaves are entire, glabrous, serrated or crenate at the margin and clasping.

Characteristics: The cultivation of the plant and the extraction and sale of opium is banned in many countries.

Habitat: The plant originated in western Asia. It is cultivated worldwide commercially.

Production: Opium is the thickened latex collected from the outside of immature Poppy capsules that have had incisions made in the fruit capsules. The unripe seed capsules suitable for the production of opium are trimmed. Subsequent to drying, the processed latex is scraped off and formed into pieces of varying size. The obtained material is referred to as raw opium (Rohopium) and is also the basic substance used for the production of heroin.

Other Names: Garden-Poppy, Mawseed, Opium Poppy

ACTIONS AND PHARMACOLOGY

COMPOUNDS

Isoquinoline alkaloids (20-30%): chief alkaloids morphine (3-23%), narcotine (2-10%), codeine (0.2-3.5%), papaverine (0.5-3%), thebaine (0.2-1%).] The alkaloids are present as salts of meconic acid, lactic acid or fumaric acid.

Benzyl isoquinoline type: papaverine (0.5 to 3%)

Phthalide isochinoline type: narcotine (noscapine, 2 to 10%)

Rubber (5-10%)

Resins

Mucilages

EFFECTS

The main alkaloid is morphine, which is a strong analgesic that, even in small doses, causes euphoria, sedation then narcotic sleep. It depresses breathing and slows down evacuation of the stomach, causing constipation and urine retention. Codeine has an antitussive effect and papaverine is spasmolytic and vasodilatory.

INDICATIONS AND USAGE

Unproven Uses: Opium is used most frequently as a sedative and/or analgesic. Uses in folk medicine include as a sedative in cases of typhus, intestinal tuberculosis and intestinal ulcers; for spasms of smooth muscle, bile ducts and urinary tract; for peritonitis; for gallstones, kidney stones and bladder colic; as well as for coughs and certain types of depression.

Chinese Medicine: Uses in Chinese medicine include chronic coughs, diarrhea, dysentery, anal prolapse and abdominal symptoms.

Indian Medicine: Irritable cough, ear and eye inflammation, proctologic symptoms, diarrhea and dysentery are considered indications for use in Indian medicine.

CONTRAINDICATIONS

Contraindications include pregnancy (alkaloids pass through the placenta barrier), nursing (alkaloids entering the mother's milk), illnesses connected with reduced respiratory function, pancreatitis, colon ulcers, elevated internal cranial pressure, acute hepatitis propheria and biliary colic. Caution is to be observed when administering in the presence of Addison's disease and hypothyroidism because of opium's centrally depressive effect.

PRECAUTIONS AND ADVERSE REACTIONS

No health hazards are known in conjunction with the proper administration of designated therapeutic dosages. However, the following can occur as side effects: clonic twitching, constipation, dizziness, general weakness, headache, hyperthermia, itchy skin, rashes and trembling of the hands. Sensitization has been reported, with papaverin the presumed allergen.

OVERDOSAGE

Overdosage leads initially to reduction of mental capacity, reactive euphoria, analgesia, miosis, bradycardia, slowed respiration. That can progress to respiratory failure, cyanosis, tonic-clonic spasms, pylorospasm and sphincterism, intestinal atonia, nausea, vomiting, pulmonary and brain edemas. Following gastrointestinal emptying (inducement of vomiting, gastric lavage with burgundy-colored potassium permanganate solution, sodium sulfate) and instillation of activated charcoal, the therapy for poisoning consists of electrolyte substitution, treating possible cases of acidosis with sodium bicarbonate infusions and administration of plasma volume expanders in the event of shock. Intubation and oxygen respiration may also be necessary. Naloxone (i.v.) is suitable as an antidote.

DOSAGE

Mode of Administration: Opium is obsolete as a drug. Morphine is administered as a pure substance and in combination with other active substances, although it has been extensively replaced by synthetic analgesia. Codeine is used by itself and in combination with other agents. Numerous cases of death due to opium use are known.

LITERATURE

Amann T, Zenk MH, Endogenes Morphin. In: DAZ 136(7):519-527. 1996.

Bethke T, Codein. In: DAZ 133(6):433. 1993.

Buch, In: Handbook of Experimental Pharmacology. Volume 104/I und 104/II: Opioids I und II. Springer-Verlag Berlin, Heidelberg, New York, 1993.

Buchbauer G et al., Headspace constituents of opium. In: PM 60(2):181. 1994.

Czygan FC, Hellas und Phytopharmaka. In: DAZ 135(51/52):4707-4711. 1995.

Freye E, Leopold C, Opiate und Opiatantagonisten. I. Theoretischen Grundlagen der Opioidwirkung. In: DAZ 131(29):1517. 1991.

Pfeifer S, Mohn - eine Arzneipflanze seit mehr als zweitausend Jahren, Teil 1 und 2. In: PA 17:467-479 et 536-554. 1962.

Répási J, Hosztafi S, Szabó Z, 5'-O-Demethylnarcotin: A New Alkaloide from Papaver somniferum. In: PM 59(5):477. 1993.

Znek MH, Über das Opium, das den Schmerz besiegt und die Sucht weckt. In: PZ 139(48):4185. 1994.

Further information in:

Frohne D, Pfänder HJ, Giftpflanzen - Ein Handbuch für Apotheker, Toxikologen und Biologen, 4. Aufl., Wiss. Verlags-Ges. Stuttgart 1997.

Kern W, List PH, Hörhammer L (Hrsg.), Hagers Handbuch der Pharmazeutischen Praxis, 4. Aufl., Bde. 1-8, Springer Verlag Berlin, Heidelberg, New York, 1969.

Lewin L, Gifte und Vergiftungen, 6. Aufl., Nachdruck, Haug Verlag, Heidelberg 1992.

Roth L, Daunderer M, Kormann K, Giftpflanzen, Pflanzengifte, 4. Aufl., Ecomed Fachverlag Landsberg Lech 1993.

Schulz R, Hänsel R, Rationale Phytotherapie, Springer Verlag Heidelberg 1996.

Steinegger E, Hänsel R, Pharmakognosie, 5. Aufl., Springer Verlag Heidelberg 1992.

Teuscher E, Biogene Arzneimittel, 5. Aufl., Wiss. Verlagsges. Stuttgart 1997.

Teuscher E, Lindequist U, Biogene Gifte - Biologie, Chemie, Pharmakologie, 2. Aufl., Fischer Verlag Stuttgart 1994.

Wagner H, Wiesenauer M, Phytotherapie. Phytopharmaka und pflanzliche Homöopathika, Fischer-Verlag, Stuttgart, Jena, New York 1995.

Populus species

See Poplar

Potentilla

Potentilla anserina

DESCRIPTION

Medicinal Parts: The medicinal parts are leaves and flowers, whole or macerated, collected during or shortly before the flowering season and dried.

Flower and Fruit: The flowers are solitary on long pedicles of lateral shoots growing from the stem nodes. They are 1.5 to 3 cm wide. There are 5 epicalyx bracts, 5 sepals and 5 petals. The last are twice as long as the sepals and are golden yellow, ovate and without a distinct margin. The 20 stamens have ovate anthers. The styles occur laterally, are thread-like and only thickened at the stigmas. The ripe fruit is glabrous, ovate to almost globular and grooved on the back.

Leaves, Stem and Root: The plant is a two-axis herbacious perennial with a short, thick, branched rhizome and rosettes of basal leaves. The stems are 80 cm long, creeping, rooting at the nodes, softly pubescent eventually becoming glabrous. The leaves are unevenly paired, pinnate and glossy with silky white hairs beneath, tomentose and fresh green above.

Characteristics: The plant has an almond-like fragrance and dry taste.

Habitat: The plant is found in temperate and colder regions of the entire Northern Hemisphere.

Production: Potentilla herb consists of the fresh or dried leaf and flowers of Potentilla anserina harvested shortly before or during flowering, as well as its preparations.

Other Names: Cinquefoil, Crampweed, Goosegrass, Goose Tansy, Moor Grass, Silver Cinquefoil, Goosewort, Prince's Feathers, Trailing Tansy, Wild Agrimony

ACTIONS AND PHARMACOLOGY

COMPOUNDS

Tannins (5 to 10%): chiefly ellagitannins

Flavonoids: including quercitrin

Hydroxycoumarins: umbelliferone, scopoletin

EFFECTS

The drug is astringent because of the tannin concentration.

On isolated rat uterus a paralyzing effect was proven which is due to the presence of ammonium salts. The empirical evidence of a spasmolytic effect in dysmenorrhea could not be definitively proven.

INDICATIONS

Approved by Commission E:

- Diarrhea
- Inflammation of the mouth and pharynx
- Premenstrual syndrome (PMS)

Internal application for topical treatment of inflammation of the oral and pharyngeal mucosa, adjuvant treatment of non-specific, acute diarrhea, and dysmenorrhea symptoms.

Unproven Uses: In folk medicine, Potentilla is used externally as a wash for poorly healing wounds.

PRECAUTIONS

No health hazards or side effects are known in conjunction with the proper administration of designated therapeutic dosages. There have been complaints of stomach irritation associated with Potentilla.

DOSAGE

Mode of Administration: Potentilla is available in commercial forms for oral intake. It is also available in crude and powder forms.

Preparation: To prepare a tea, pour boiling water over 2 gm finely cut drug, strain after 10 minutes (1 teaspoon corresponds to approximately 0.7 gm drug).

Daily Dosage: 4 to 6 gm of drug; Tea: 1 cup freshly prepared several times a day between meals.

Storage: Protect from light and moisture.

LITERATURE

Eisenreichova E et al., Cesk Farm 23:82-84. 1974.

Kombal R, Glasl H, Flavan-3-ols and flavonoids from Potentilla anserina. In: PM 61(5):484-485. 1995.

Schimmer O, Lindenbaum M, Tannins with antimutagenic properties in the herb of Alchemilla species and Potentilla anserina. In: PM 61(2):141-145. 1995.

Further information in:

Hänsel R, Keller K, Rimpler H, Schneider G (Hrsg.), Hagers Handbuch der Pharmazeutischen Praxis, 5. Aufl., Bde 4-6 (Drogen), Springer Verlag Berlin, Heidelberg, New York, 1992-1994.

Madaus G, Lehrbuch der Biologischen Arzneimittel, Bde 1-3, Nachdruck, Georg Olms Verlag Hildesheim 1979.

Schulz R, Hänsel R, Rationale Phytotherapie, Springer Verlag Heidelberg 1996.

Steinegger E, Hänsel R, Pharmakognosie, 5. Aufl., Springer Verlag Heidelberg 1992.

Teuscher E, Biogene Arzneimittel, 5. Aufl., Wiss. Verlagsges. Stuttgart 1997.

Potentilla anserina

See Potentilla

Potentilla erecta

See Cinquefoil

Potentilla reptans

See European Five-Finger Grass

Premorse

Scabiosa succisa

DESCRIPTION

Medicinal Parts: The medicinal part is the dried herb.

Flower and Fruit: The flowers are purple-blue, globular and long pedicled composite blooms, with a 2 to 3 rowed involucre. The florets are all the same size. The epicalyx has thorn-tipped teeth and the calyx has 5 bristles. The corolla is fused and has 4 tips. There are 4 stamens and 1 inferior ovary. The fruit is a nutlet.

Leaves, Stem and Root: The plant grows from 15 to 80 cm high. It has a short, finger-thick rhizome, which looks bitten off. In the first year of growth, the root resembles a carrot. Later it becomes woody and dies off except for the upper part, which accounts for its appearance. The remaining upper part then develops lateral roots. The stem is erect, sparsely branched, pubescent and has few leaves. The basal leaves are petiolate, oblong and obtuse. The cauline leaves are narrow and acute.

Habitat: Scabiosae succisae is indigenous to all of Europe.

Production: Premorse is the aerial part of Scabiosa succisa.

Other Names: Devil's Bit, Ofbit, Premorse scaboius

ACTIONS AND PHARMACOLOGY

COMPOUNDS

Iridoide monoterpenes: including among others, dipsacan, cephalaroside (structures unknown)

Saponins

Tannins

Flavonoids: including among others, saponarine (C-glycosyl-flavone)

Triterpenes: including among others, ursolic acid

EFFECTS

Premorse is a febrifuge and a diaphoretic.

INDICATIONS AND USAGE

Unproven Uses: The herb is used for febrile colds and coughs.

PRECAUTIONS AND ADVERSE REACTIONS

No health hazards or side effects are known in conjunction with the proper administration of designated therapeutic dosages.

DOSAGE

Mode of Administration: The herb is ground as a drug for infusion.

LITERATURE

Hegnauer R, Chemotaxonomie der Pflanzen, Bde 1-11: Birkhäuser Verlag Basel, Boston, Berlin 1962-1997.

Kern W, List PH, Hörhammer L (Hrsg.), Hagers Handbuch der Pharmazeutischen Praxis, 4. Aufl., Bde 1-8: Springer Verlag Berlin, Heidelberg, New York, 1969 (unter Succisa pratensis).

Madaus G, Lehrbuch der Biologischen Arzneimittel, Bde 1-3, Nachdruck, Georg Olms Verlag Hildesheim 1979.

Primula veris

See Cowslip

Prunella vulgaris

See Self-Heal

Prunus laurocerasus

See Cherry Laurel

Prunus serotina

See Wild Cherry

Prunus species

See Almond

Prunus spinosa

See Sloe

Psyllium

Plantago ovata

TRADE NAMES

Psyllium Husk, Psyllium Husk Bulk-Forming Laxative, Psyllium Husks, Konsyl Easy Mix, Konsyl for Kids, Konsyl Powder Sugar Free Unflavored, Metamucil

DESCRIPTION

Medicinal Parts: The medicinal parts are the ripe and dried seeds, the epidermis, the adjacent, broken-down layers of the Indian variety and the fresh plant.

Flower and Fruit: The flowers are on cylindrical, glabrous or finely pubescent scapes, which are only slightly longer than the leaves. They form 0.5 to 3.5 cm long spikes. The bracts are about 3 mm, suborbicular to ovate and sometimes shortly pubescent. The sepals are about 2.5 mm, similarly shaped, almost free, keeled at the apex with wide scarious margins. The anterior ones are usually pubescent. The corolla-tube is 1.5 to 2 mm long and glabrous. The lobes are 2.5 mm, ovate-orbicular, subobtuse to very shortly acuminate. The stamens are exserted up to 1 mm and the capsule is about 3 mm. The seeds are 2.2 to 2.5 mm and cymbiform.

Leaves, Stem and Root: The plant is an annual almost stemless, softly pubescent plant. The plant may have one or several rosettes. The leaves are 2.5 to 12 cm by 0.1 to 0.8 cm, linear to linear-lanceolate. The leaves are entire-margined or slightly denticulate and sparsely to densely villous-lanate.

Habitat: The plant grows in India, Afghanistan, Iran, Israel, northern Africa, Spain and the Canary Islands. The plant is cultivated in India and neighboring countries, Arizona and southern Brazil.

Production: Psyllium consists of the ripe seeds or epidermis of Plantago ovata (synonym: Plantago isphagula).

Other Names: Blood Plantago, Indian Plantago, Ispaghula, Sand Plantain, Spogel, Blond Psyllium, Black Psyllium

ACTIONS AND PHARMACOLOGY

COMPOUNDS: PSYLLIUM SEED

Mucilages (20-30%): chiefly arabinoxylans and glacturonosidorhamnoses

Fatty oil

Iridoids: aucubin

Proteic Substances

COMPOUNDS: PSYLLIUM SEED EPIDERMIS

Mucilages (parent substances arabinoxylans)

EFFECTS

The drug is rich in mucins with swelling properties that exert laxative and anti-diarrheal effects. Psyllium also lowers serum cholesterol levels, reduces postprandial blood glucose, decreases gallstone formation, and decreases the feeling of fullness.

Antidiarrheal: When used for diarrhea, psyllium absorbs water to increase the bowel content viscosity and delay gastric emptying (Washington, 1998).

Decreases Hypercholesterolemia: Psyllium increases cholesterol and bile acid fecal excretion but does not affect cholesterol synthesis (Miettinen, 1989). Psyllium may lower serum cholesterol levels by replacing dietary fats, thereby reducing the amount available for absorption, and not directly affecting cholesterol (Swain, 1990). A decrease in low-density lipoprotein (LDL) cholesterol levels and total cholesterol with the herb have been seen in many studies (Davidson, 1998; MacMahon, 1998; Rodriguez-Moran, 1998; Romero, 1998). Although one study indicated an increase in high-density lipoprotein (HDL) cholesterol and a decrease in serum triglycerides (TG) with Psyllium, other studies have reported no change in these parameters (Anderson, 1988; Bell, 1989; Davidson, 1998; Rodriguez-Moran, 1998).

Glucose Control: Postprandial glucose and fasting plasma glucose significantly improved in type 2 diabetic patients taking psyllium (Anderson, 1999; Rodriguez-Moran, 1998).

Inhibition of Gallstones: Psyllium hydrocolloid exerts bile acid sequestrant properties determined by a rise in the cholic/chenodeoxycholic acid ratio. This activity protects against cholesterol gallstone formation (Berman, 1975). Psyllium also protects against cholesterol gallstone formation by reducing biliary cholesterol saturation index. The protective effect is associated with a selective decrease in biliary cholesterol and chenodeoxycholic acid (Schwesinger, 1999).

Irritable Bowel Syndrome/Ulcerative Colitis: Stool frequency and consistency, abdominal pain and abdominal distention have shown improvement in irritable bowel syndrome patients taking psyllium (Hotz, 1994; Prior, 1987). A decrease in transit time of bowel content may also be seen with the herb (Prior, 1987).

Laxative Effects: Psyllium decreases the passage time of the bowel content by increasing the volume of the stool, thus exerting a laxative effect. The herb acts as stool softener by increasing stool water content. Psyllium was superior to docusate sodium in subjects with chronic idiopathic constipation (McRorie, 1998).

Weight Reduction: Psyllium may be a useful supplement in weight control diets as it decreases fat intake, and increases the subjective feeling of fullness (Turnbull, 1995). The herb exerts these actions by increasing the time for intestinal absorption by inhibition of pancreatic enzymes such as amylase (Hansen, 1982; Hansen, 1987; Rigaud, 1998).

CLINICAL TRIALS

Hypercholesterolemia/Hyperglycemia

A randomized, double-blind, placebo-controlled study was conducted to determine the lipid and glucose lowering effects of Psyllium in type 2 diabetic patients. One hundred twenty-five subjects were included in the study and received either placebo or Psyllium (5 gm three times daily) over a 6-week period. Prior to the treatment period, all patients participated in a 6-week period of diet counseling. Fasting plasma glucose, total cholesterol, LDL cholesterol and triglyceride levels were significantly reduced in the Psyllium treatment group compared to placebo. HDL significantly increased in the Psyllium treatment group compared to the placebo group, suggesting Psyllium as a useful adjunct to diet in Type 2 diabetes (Rodriguez-Moran, 1998).

Hypercholesterolemia/Hyperglycemia

The safety and effectiveness of Psyllium husk fiber as an adjunct to diet was evaluated in patients with type 2 diabetes and mild- to-moderate hypercholesterolemia. After a 2-week dietary stabilization phase, 34 patients were randomly assigned to receive 5.1 gm psyllium or placebo twice daily for an 8 week period. The Psyllium group had significant improvements in glucose and lipid values compared with the placebo group. Serum total and LDL-cholesterol concentrations were 8.9% ($P < 0.05$) and 13.0% ($P = 0.07$) lower, respectively, in the Psyllium treatment group compared to the placebo group. All day and postprandial glucose concentrations were 11.0% ($P < 0.05$) and 19.2% ($P < 0.01$) lower in the Psyllium treatment group than in the placebo group (Anderson, 1999).

Ulcerative Colitis

The objective of an open label, parallel-group, randomized clinical trial was to assess the efficacy and safety of Plantago ovata seeds compared to mesalamine in maintaining remission in ulcerative colitis patients. One hundred and five ulcerative colitis patients who were in remission received oral treatment with Plantago ovata seeds (10 gm twice daily), mesalamine (500 mg three times daily), or Plantago ovata seeds plus mesalamine at the same doses. After 12 months, treatment failure rate was 40% in the Plantago ovata seed group, 35% in the mesalamine group, and 30% in the Plantago ovata plus mesalamine group. The probability of continued remission was similar between all treatment groups (Mantel-Cox test, $p = 0.67$; intent-to-treat analysis), thus implicating the herb might be as effective as mesalamine to maintain remission in ulcerative colitis (Fernandez-Banares F, 1999).

INDICATIONS AND USAGE

Approved by Commission E:

- Constipation
- Diarrhea
- Raised levels of cholesterol
- Hemorrhoids

Psyllium is used for disorders where easy bowel movements with a loose stool is desirable (e.g., in patients with anal fissures and hemorrhoids; following anal/rectal surgery; and during pregnancy).

Unproven Uses: In Folk medicine, the herb is used internally for inflammation of the mucous membrane of the urogenital tract and gastrointestinal tract, and dysentery. Externally, Psyllium is used for gout, rheumatism, furuncles and as an analgesic.

Indian Medicine: Psyllium is used for gastritis, chronic diarrhea, constipation, dysentery, dry cough, gout, gonorrhea, nephropathy, dysuria, duodenal ulcers and hemorrhoids.

CONTRAINDICATIONS

The drug is contraindicated in patients who have pathological narrowing in the gastrointestinal tract, obstruction or threatening obstruction of the bowel (ileus), or difficulties in regulating diabetes mellitus.

PRECAUTIONS AND ADVERSE REACTIONS

General: Incorrect administration procedures (with too little fluid) can cause the product to swell and lead to obstruction of the esophagus or of the intestine, particularly with older people. Patients with exocrine pancreatic insufficiency should avoid use of Psyllium due to inhibitory actions on pancreatic lipase (Hansen, 1987).

Allergic Reactions/Anaphylaxis: Allergic reactions ranging from sneezing to chest congestion and wheezing were reported in three nurses after Psyllium use (Ford, 1992). One patient reported anaphylaxis after Psyllium ingestion, and had experienced recurrent rhinitis and asthma related to Psyllium exposure for the past 15 years (Vaswani, 1996). IgE mediated anaphylaxis was reported after the ingestion of Psyllium seed laxative (Seggav, 1984). Occupational allergic rhinitis reaction was confirmed by elevation of antipsyllium IgE after exposure to a Psyllium-based powdered laxative (Schwartz, 1989).

Flatulence Symptoms: Psyllium did not cause greater gaseous symptoms compared to placebo reported in one study (Zumarraga, 1997). One study decreased flatulence symptoms by adding psyllium to half the usual dose of bile acid sequestrant resins to maintain efficacy and tolerability of resins (Spence, 1995).

Drug Interactions: The absorption of other drugs taken simultaneously may be delayed. There is a possibility that insulin dosage adjustment (downward) will be necessary when diabetics use psyllium products.

DOSAGE

Mode of Administration: The whole or coarsely-chopped drug as well as other galenic preparations are used internally.

Sufficient fluid must be taken with the drug (150 ml water per 5 gm drug). One study did show a greater effect of Psyllium on cholesterol after mixing with food (Wolever, 1994). The dose should be taken one-half hour to one hour after taking other medication.

How Supplied:
Capsule — 525 mg, 567 mg, 610 mg, 625 mg

Powder — 2.0 gm Psyllium per dose, 3.4 gm Psyllium per dose, 6.0 gm Psyllium per dose (available in a variety of package sizes)

Daily Dosage: The daily dosage ranges from 12 to 40 gm of the drug. The powder products should be administered as 1 teaspoonful (3.4 gm to 6.0 gm drug) in 8 oz. of fruit juice or cool water. Either stir briskly or shake for 3-5 seconds, depending on the specific product. Psyllium may be taken up to 3 times daily (Prod. Info. Konsyl®, 1999; Prod. Info. Metamucil®, 1999).

Children: For children 6 to 12 years of age administer 1 teaspoonful (2.0 gm of the drug) in an empty glass and add 8 oz. of cool water. Stir briskly for 3-5 seconds. The dose may be taken up to 3 times daily (Prod Info Konsyl for Kids®, 1999)

LITERATURE

Anderson JW, Zettwoch N, Tietyen-Clark et al. Cholesterol lowering effects of PSYLLIUM hydrophilic mucilloid for hypercholesterolemic men. Arch Intern Med 1988; 148:292-296.

Anderson JW; Allgood LD; Turner J et al. Effects of psyllium on glucose and serum lipid responses in men with type 2 diabetes and hypercholesterolemia. Am J Clin Nutr 1999 Oct;70(4):466-73.

Anonym, Pharmaceutical Care: ''Den Mißbrauch von Laxanzien vermeiden helfen.'' In: DAZ 135(20):1867-1868. 1995.

Bell LP; Hectorne K; Reynolds H et al. Cholesterol-lowering effects of psyllium hydrophilic mucilloid. Adjunct therapy to a prudent diet for patients with mild to moderate hypercholesterolemia. JAMA 1989 Jun 16;261(23):3419-23.

Bergman F; van der Linden W. Effect of dietary fibre on gallstone formation in hamsters. Z Ernahrungswiss 1975 Sep;14(3):217-24.

Curry CE, (1982) Laxative products. In: Handbook of Nonprescription Drugs, Am Pharmac Assoc, Washington, S 69-92.

Davidson MH; Maki KC; Kong JC et al. Long-term effects of consuming foods containing psyllium seed husk on serum lipids in subjects with hypercholesterolemia. Am J Clin Nutr 1998 Mar;67(3):367-76.

Ershoff BH, (1976) J Food Sci 41:949.

Fernandez-Banares F; Hinojosa J; Sanchez-Lombrana JL. Randomized clinical trial of Plantago ovata seeds (dietary fiber) as compared with mesalamine in maintaining remission in ulcerative colitis. Spanish Group for the Study of Crohn's Disease and Ulcerative Colitis (GETECCU). Am J Gastroenterol 1999 Feb;94(2):427-33.

Fintelmann V, Phytopharmaka in der Gastroenterologie. In: ZPT 15(3):137. 1994.

Ford MA; Cristea G Jr; Robbins WD et al. Delayed psyllium allergy in three nurses. Hosp Pharm 1992 Dec;27(12):1061-2.

Gelpi E et al., PH 8:2077-2081. 1969.

Hansen WE. Effect of dietary fiber on pancreatic lipase activity in vitro. Pancreas 1987;2(2):195-8.

Hansen WE; Schulz G. The effect of dietary fiber on pancreatic amylase activity in vitro. Hepatogastroenterology 1982 Aug;29(4):157-60.

Hotz J; Plein K. Effectiveness of plantago seed husks in comparison with wheat bran on stool frequency and manifestations of irritable colon syndrome with constipation. Med Klin 1994 Dec 15;89(12):645-51.

Kasper H, (1985) Ernährungsmedizin und Diätetik. 5. Aufl. Urban & Schwarzenberg, München Wien. Leng-Peschlow E.

Jaspersen-Schib R, Ballaststoffe als Lipidsenker. In: DAZ 132(39):1991. 1992.

Kasper H, (1985) Ernährungsmedizin und Diätetik. 5. Aufl. Urban & Schwarzenberg, München Wien. Leng-Peschlow E.

Kennedy JF et al., Carbohydr Res 75:265-274. 1979.

Khorana ML et al., (1958) Ind J Pharm 20:3.

Koedam A, Plantago - history and use. In: Pharm Weekbl 112(10):246-252. 1977.

McRorie JW; Daggy BP; Morel JG et al. Psyllium is superior to docusate sodium for treatment of chronic constipation. Aliment Pharmacol Ther 1998 May;12(5):491-7.

Maciejko JJ; Brazg R; Shah A et al. Psyllium for the reduction of cholestyramine-associated gastrointestinal symptoms in the treatment of primary hypercholesterolemia. Arch Fam Med 1994 Nov;3(11):955-60.

MacMahon M; Carless J. Ispaghula husk in the treatment of hypercholesterolaemia: a double- blind controlled study. J Cardiovasc Risk 1998 Jun;5(3):167-72.

Mengs U, (1990) No renal pigmentation by plantago ovata seeds or husks. Med Sci Res 18:37-38.

Miettinen TA; Tarpila S. Serum lipids and cholesterol metabolism during guar gum, plantago ovata and high fibre treatments. Clin Chim Acta 1989 Aug 31;183(3):253-62.

Miller JN, In: Industrial Gums, Ed. R. L. Whistler, Academic Press 1973.

Oshio H, Inouye H, (1982) Planta Med 44:204.

Popov S, (1978) IUPAC Int Symp Chem Nat Prod 11(2):61 (via CA 92:59170).

Prior A & Whorwell PJ. Double-blind study of ispaghula in irritable bowel syndrome. Gut 1987; 28:1510-1513.

Product Information: Metamucil®, Proctor & Gamble, Cincinnati, OH, 1999.

Product Information: Konsyl for Kids®, Konsyl Pharmaceuticals, Inc., Fort Worth, Texas, 1999.

Product Information: Konsyl®, Konsyl Pharmaceuticals, Inc., Fort Worth, Texas, 1999.

Rigaud D; Paycha F; Meulemans A et al. Effect of psyllium on gastric emptying, hunger feeling and food intake in normal volunteers: a double blind study. Eur J Clin Nutr 1998 Apr;52(4):239-45.

Rodriguez-Moran M; Guerrero-Romero F; Lazcano-Burciaga G. Lipid- and glucose-lowering efficacy of Plantago Psyllium in type II diabetes. J Diabetes Complications 1998 Sep-Oct;12(5):273-8.

Romero AL; Romero JE; Galaviz S; Fernandez ML. Cookies enriched with psyllium or oat bran lower plasma LDL cholesterol in normal and hypercholesterolemic men from Northern Mexico. J Am Coll Nutr 1998 Dec;17(6):601-8.

Sandhu JS et al., Carbohdr Res 93:247-259. 1981.

Schwartz HJ; Arnold JL; Strohl KP. Occupational allergic rhinitis reaction to psyllium. J Occup Med 1989 Jul;31(7):624-6.

Schwesinger WH; Kurtin WE; Page CP et al. Soluble dietary fiber protects against cholesterol gallstone formation. Am J Surg 1999 Apr;177(4):307-10.

Seggev JS; Ohta K; Tipton WR. IgE mediated anaphylaxis due to a psyllium-containing drug. Ann Allergy 1984 Oct;53(4):325-6.

Spence JD; Huff MW; Heidenheim P et al. Combination therapy with colestipol and psyllium mucilloid in patients with hyperlipidemia. Ann Intern Med 1995 Oct 1;123(7):493-9.

Swain JF; Rouse IL; Curley CB; Sacks FM. Comparison of the effects of oat bran and low-fiber wheat on serum lipoprotein levels and blood pressure. N Engl J Med 1990 Jan 18;322(3):147-52.

Tomoda M et al., (1987) Planta Med 53(1):8.

Turnbull WH; Thomas HG. The effect of a Plantago ovata seed containing preparation on appetite variables, nutrient and energy intake. Int J Obes Relat Metab Disord 1995 May;19(5):338-42.

Washington N; Harris M; Mussellwhite A; Spiller RC. Moderation of lactulose-induced diarrhea by psyllium: effects on motility and fermentation. Am J Clin Nutr 1998 Feb;67(2):317-21.

Wolever TM; Jenkins DJ; Mueller S et al. Method of administration influences the serum cholesterol-lowering effect of psyllium. Am J Clin Nutr 1994 May;59(5):1055-9.

Zumarraga L; Levitt MD; Suarez F. Absence of gaseous symptoms during ingestion of commercial fibre preparations. Aliment Pharmacol Ther 1997 Dec;11(6):1067-72.

Further information in:

Chan EH et al. (Ed.), Advances in Chinese Medicinal Materials Research, World Scientific Pub. Co. Singapore 1985.

Hänsel R, Keller K, Rimpler H, Schneider G (Hrsg.), Hagers Handbuch der Pharmazeutischen Praxis, 5. Aufl., Bde 4-6 (Drogen): Springer Verlag Berlin, Heidelberg, New York, 1992-1994.

Leung AY, Encyclopedia of Common Natural Ingredients Used in Food, Drugs and Cosmetics, John Wiley & Sons Inc., New York 1980.

Steinegger E, Hänsel R, Pharmakognosie, 5. Aufl., Springer Verlag Heidelberg 1992.

Teuscher E, Biogene Arzneimittel, 5. Aufl., Wiss. Verlagsges. Stuttgart 1997.

Wagner H, Wiesenauer M, Phytotherapie. Phytopharmaka und pflanzliche Homöopathika, Fischer-Verlag, Stuttgart, Jena, New York 1995.

Wichtl M (Hrsg.), Teedrogen, 4. Aufl., Wiss. Verlagsges. Stuttgart 1997.

Psyllium Seed

Plantago afra

DESCRIPTION

Medicinal Parts: The medicinal parts are the ripe seeds.

Flower and Fruit: The inflorescence is a 12-mm long spike with glandular hairs and ovate-lanceolate bracts with a midrib and translucent lateral lamina. The corolla is disc-shaped with 4 translucent petals. The edge of the calyx has 4 acute lobes. The sepals are 3 to 4.5 cm and lanceolate. The ovary is superior, and the fruit is a 2-sectioned, membranous pyxidium. The seeds are dark brown, glossy and narrowly oblong in outline.

Leaves, Stem and Root: The plant is an annual that is erect with stems up to 60 cm high. The stems have ascending, pubescent branches with patent or ascending hairs and are more or less minutely glandular above. The leaves are 3 to 8 by 0.1 to 0.3 cm, linear or linear-lanceolate and are not fleshy. The bracts are 3.5 to 8 mm and all have a similar shape. They are ovate-lanceolate to lanceolate, sharp-edged or acuminate with a broad dry membranous margin without lateral ribs.

Habitat: The plant is indigenous to the Mediterranean region and western Asia. Psyllium Seeds are cultivated in Spain, central Europe, Israel, Russia, India, Pakistan, Japan, Cuba and southern Brazil.

Production: Psyllium Seed (blonde) consists of the dried, ripe seed of Plantago psyllium (syn. Plantago afra) and of Plantago indica (syn. Plantago arenaria), with a swell index of at least 10, and its formulations.

Not to be Confused With: The seeds of other Plantago seeds.

Other Names: Plantain, Fleaseed, Flea Wort, Psyllion, Psyllios

ACTIONS AND PHARMACOLOGY

COMPOUNDS

Mucilages (only in the epidermis of the seed coat, 10-12%): chiefly arabinoxylans

Iridoids: aucubin (0.14%)

Pyrridine alkaloids: boschniakines, including plantagonine, indicaine, indicainine

Proteic substances

Fatty oil

EFFECTS

The mucins are laxative and antidiarrheal; they regulate intestinal peristalsis through the swelling effect.

INDICATIONS AND USAGE

Approved by Commission E:

- Diarrhea
- Constipation

Unproven Uses: Psyllium Seed is used internally for constipation, diarrhea, cystitis and all conditions in which a soft stool is desirable, such as anal fissures, hemorrhoids, anal-rectal surgery and pregnancy. It is also used externally for furunculosis.

CONTRAINDICATIONS

Psyllium Seed is contraindicated in pathologic constriction of the gastrointestinal tract, inflammatory illnesses of the gastrointestinal tract, the threat or presence of ileus and in severely variable diabetes mellitus.

PRECAUTIONS AND ADVERSE REACTIONS

General: No health hazards or side effects are known in conjunction with the proper administration of designated therapeutic dosages. Allergic reactions could, however, arise in isolated cases (rhinitis, conjunctivitis, asthma and urticaria). Incorrect administration procedures (with too little fluid) can lead to obstruction (blockage) of the esophagus or the intestine, particularly with older people.

Drug Interactions: Absorption of other drugs taken simultaneously could be delayed.

DOSAGE

Mode of Administration: Internally as whole, cut or powdered drug, and externally as a poultice.

Preparation: The ratio for the liquid extract is 1:1 (25% ethanol).

Daily Dosage: The recommended daily dose is 12 to 40 g drug. The dose for the liquid extract is 2 to 5 ml.

Storage: The cut drug should be protected from light and moisture and used within 24 hours.

LITERATURE

Anonym, Pharmaceutical Care: ''Den Miβbrauch von Laxanzien vermeiden helfen''. In: DAZ 135(20):1867-1868. 1995.

Curry CE, (1982) Laxative products. In: Handbook of Nonprescription Drugs, Am Pharmac Assoc, Washington, S 69-92.

Fintelmann V, Phytopharmaka in der Gastroenterologie. In: ZPT 15(3):137. 1994.

Hänsel R, Keller K, Rimpler H, Schneider G (Hrsg.), Hagers Handbuch der Pharmazeutischen Praxis, 5. Aufl., Bde 4-6 (Drogen), Springer Verlag Berlin, Heidelberg, New York, 1992-1994.

Jaspersen-Schib R, Ballaststoffe als Lipidsenker. In: DAZ 132(39):1991. 1992.

Karawya MS et al., PM 20:14-35. 1971.

Kennedy JF et al., Carbohydr Res 75:265-274. 1979.

Schulz R, Hänsel R, Rationale Phytotherapie, Springer Verlag Heidelberg 1996.

Steinegger E, Hänsel R, Pharmakognosie, 5. Aufl., Springer Verlag Heidelberg 1992.

Teuscher E, Biogene Arzneimittel, 5. Aufl., Wiss. Verlagsges. Stuttgart 1997.

Wagner H, Wiesenauer M, Phytotherapie. Phytopharmaka und pflanzliche Homöopathika, Fischer-Verlag, Stuttgart, Jena, New York 1995.

Wichtl M (Hrsg.), Teedrogen, 4. Aufl., Wiss. Verlagsges. Stuttgart 1997.

Ptelea trifoliata

See Wafer Ash

Pterocarpus santalinus

See Red Sandalwood

Ptychopetalum olacoides

See Muira-Puama

Puff Ball

Lycoperdon species

DESCRIPTION

Medicinal Parts: The medicinal parts are the aerial parts and the mature spores of the fungus.

Flower and Fruit: The giant form of this fungus attains a diameter of 20 to 50 cm and a weight of 9 kg. The outer covering is at first whitish, smooth and downy. It later turns gray-yellow or ochre, develops grooves and patches, and starts to break off from above. The now-visible inner section bursts at the vertex and disintegrates. The content is composed of a whitish mass, which turns yellow and mushy and finally breaks down into greenish-brown spore dust. A cup-shaped receptacle with torn edges remains.

Habitat: Lycoperdon species are indigenous to Europe.

Production: Puff Ball is the aerial part and the mature spores of Lycoperdon species.

Other Names: Bovista, Hart's Truffle, Deer Balls

ACTIONS AND PHARMACOLOGY

COMPOUNDS

Calvacin (mucoprotein)

Steroids: mycosterols

Urea

EFFECTS

The main active agents are various amino acids, glucosamine, sterol, enzymes and approximately 3% urea.

INDICATIONS AND USAGE

Unproven Uses: The drug is used for dysmenorrhea, nose bleeds and skin disorders.

Homeopathic Uses: Lycoperdon is used for anemia, skin complaints and chronic catarrh.

PRECAUTIONS AND ADVERSE REACTIONS

No health hazards or side effects are known in conjunction with the proper administration of designated therapeutic dosages. The young mushroom is edible.

DOSAGE

Mode of Administration: Puff Ball is available ground or in alcoholic extracts.

LITERATURE

Gasco A et al., (1974) Tetrahedron Lett 38:3431.

Kern W, List PH, Hörhammer L (Hrsg.), Hagers Handbuch der Pharmazeutischen Praxis, 4. Aufl., Bde. 1-8, Springer Verlag Berlin, Heidelberg, New York, 1969.

Madaus G, Lehrbuch der Biologischen Arzneimittel, Bde 1-3, Nachdruck, Georg Olms Verlag Hildesheim 1979.

Pulmonaria officinalis

See Lungwort

Pulsatilla pratensis

See Pasque Flower

Pumpkin

Cucurbita pepo

DESCRIPTION

Medicinal Parts: The medicinal parts are the fresh and dried seeds.

Flower and Fruit: The flower is yellow, monoecious, very large and solitary in the leaf axils. The male flower has a longer pedicle. The calyx is fused to the corolla except for the 5 awl-shaped tips. The corolla is 5-tipped and funnel-shaped. The interior is pubescent. There are 3 stamens fused to the anther. The ovary is inferior and 3-locular. The fruit is very large with many seeds. The flesh is fibrous, yellow-orange to white, and has a viscous placenta. The seeds are 7 to 15 mm long, narrow, broad or narrow-ovate with a shallow groove and flat ridge around the margin.

Leaves, Stem and Root: Annual plant 3 to 8 m long. The stem is sharply-angular with longitudinal grooves and hairy spines. The leaves are alternate, very large and bristly, petiolate with 5 to 7 lobes from a cordate base.

Characteristics: The seeds taste somewhat like almonds.

Habitat: Pumpkin is indigenous to America and widely cultivated, especially in temperate climates.

Production: Pumpkin seed consists of the ripe, dried seed of Cucurbita pepo and cultivated varieties of Cucurbita pepo.

Other Names: Field Pumpkin

ACTIONS AND PHARMACOLOGY

COMPOUNDS

Steroids: Delta5-, Delta7- and Delta8-phytosterols (24- alkyl sterols), including clerosterol, isofucosterol, sitosterol, stigmasterol, cholesterol, isoavenasterol, spinasterol

Fatty oil: chief fatty acids are oleic acid and linoleic acid

Proteic substances (25 to 42%)

Unusual amino acids: including cucurbitin (vermifuge)

Gamma-tocopherol

EFFECTS

As well as amaroids (cucurbitacin), the drug contains delta-7-sterols, which are similar in conformation to the dihydrostesterone. Cucurbitacin has anthelmintic properties.

There are no pharmacological studies that substantiate the empirically documented clinical efficacy; the empirical evidence indicates efficacy for prostate hyperplasia. Pumpkin is also antiphlogistic and antioxidative.

INDICATIONS AND USAGE

Approved by Commission E:

- Irritable bladder
- Prostate complaints

Unproven Uses: Pumpkin is used for irritable bladder, micturition problems accompanying prostate adenoma stages I to II. This medication relieves only the difficulties associated with an enlarged prostate without reducing the enlargement. Medical supervision is essential.

In folk medicine, it is also used for kidney inflammation, intestinal parasites, particularly tape worm, and vulnary.

PRECAUTIONS AND ADVERSE REACTIONS

Health risks or side effects following the proper administration of designated therapeutic dosages are not recorded.

DOSAGE

Mode of Administration: Whole and coarsely ground seed and other galenic preparations are for internal use.

Daily Dosage: The average daily dose is 10 gm of ground seeds; 1 to 2 heaping dessert spoons with liquid in the mornings and evenings.

Storage: It should be protected from light and moisture.

LITERATURE

Anonym, Welche Bedeutung haben pflanzliche Prostatamittel. In: DAZ 133(9):720. 1993.

Koch E, (1995) Pharmakologie und Wirkmechanismen von Extrakten aus Sabalfrüchten (Sabal fructus), Brennesselwurzeln (Urticae radix) und Kürbissamen (Cucurbitae peponis semen) bei der Behandlung der benignen Prostatahyperplasie. In: Loew D, Rietbrock N (Hrsg.) Phytopharmaka in Forschung und klinischer Anwendung. Steinkopff Verlag, Darmstadt, S 57-79.

Miersch WDE, Benigne Prostatahyperplasie. In: DAZ 133(29):2653. 1993.

Nahrstedt A, (1993) Pflanzliche Urologica - eine kritische Übersicht. Pharm Z 138:1439-1450.

Schabort JC, (1978) Phytochemistry 17:1062.

Schiebel-Schlosser G., Kürbiskerne stärken die Blasenfunktion. In: PTA 4(11):552. 1990.

Schilcher H, Möglichkeiten und Grenzen der Phytotherapie am Beispiel pflanzlicher Urologika. Urologe [B] 27 (1987), 316-319

Schilcher H, (1987a) Pflanzliche Diuretika. Urologe [B] 27:215-222; (1987b)n Möglichkeiten und Grenzen der Phytotherapie am Beispiel pflanzlicher Urologika. Urologe [B] 27:316-319.

Schilcher H, Boesel R, Effenberger ST Segebrecht S, Neuere Untersuchungsergebnisse mit aquaretisch, antibakteriell und prostatotrop wirksamen Arzneipflanzen. In: ZPT 10(3):77. 1989.

Schilcher H, Dunzendorfer U, Ascali F, Dekta-7-Sterole, das prostatatrope Wirkprinzip des Kürbis? In: Urologe (B) 27:316-319. 1987.

Tewary JP, Srivasta MC, (1968) J Pharm Sci 57:328.

Further information in:

Hänsel R, Keller K, Rimpler H, Schneider G (Hrsg.), Hagers Handbuch der Pharmazeutischen Praxis, 5. Aufl., Bde 4-6 (Drogen), Springer Verlag Berlin, Heidelberg, New York, 1992-1994.

Madaus G, Lehrbuch der Biologischen Arzneimittel, Bde 1-3, Nachdruck, Georg Olms Verlag Hildesheim 1979.

Oliver-Bever B (Ed.), Medicinal Plants of Tropical West Africa, Cambridge University Press, Cambridge, London 1986.

Steinegger E, Hänsel R, Pharmakognosie, 5. Aufl., Springer Verlag Heidelberg 1992.

Teuscher E, Biogene Arzneimittel, 5. Aufl., Wiss. Verlagsges. mbH Stuttgart 1997.

Wagner H, Wiesenauer M, Phytotherapie. Phytopharmaka und pflanzliche Homöopathika, Fischer-Verlag, Stuttgart, Jena, New York 1995.

Wichtl M (Hrsg.), Teedrogen, 4. Aufl., Wiss. Verlagsges. Stuttgart 1997.

Punica granatum

See Pomegranate

Purple Gromwell (Ying Zicao)

Lithospermum erytrorhizon

DESCRIPTION

Medicinal Parts: The medicinal part of the plant is the root, which is dried.

Flower and Fruit: The radial flowers are in axillary or apical racemes. The calyx has up to 5 tips, and the sepals are fused. The petals are white and also fused. The corolla tube is approximately 4 mm long. The diameter of the corolla is approximately 4 mm. There are 5 stamens and one superior, 2-carpeled, 4-chambered ovary. The fruit is a glossy nutlet, approximately 3 mm long, ovoid and gray-white.

Leaves, Stem and Root: This herbaceous perennial grows up to 80 cm high. The leaves are alternate, sessile, simple, lanceolate to elongate-lanceolate with acute tips and parallel veins. It has a few upright, roughly pubescent stems and a thick root.

Characteristics: The root becomes purple when dried.

Habitat: This herb is indigenous to Korea, China and Japan.

Production: Purple Gromwell root or Ying Zicao (Chinese) is the dried root of Lithospermum erythrorhizon. The 3-year-old roots are collected in spring or autumn, cleaned, cut in slices and then dried.

Other Names: Ying Zicao

ACTION AND PHARMACOLOGY

COMPOUNDS

Naphthalene derivatives (0.5 to 3%): isohexenylnaphthazarines, particularly esters of the (R)-(+)-shikonins with short-chained fatty acids, including acetic acid, isobutyric acid, isovaleric acid

Water-soluble polysaccharides: lithospermans A to C

Pyrrolizidine alkaloids: chief alkaloid intermedine, as well as myoscorpine, hydroxymyoscorpine

Hydroquinone derivatives (0.3%): furylhydroquinones and furylquinones, including shikonofurane A to E

Caffeic acid derivatives: rosmarinic acid, lithospermic acid, caffeic acid esters of higher alcohols, for example docosanylcaffeat

EFFECTS

The naphthoquinone derivatives contained in the drug are antimicrobial, antiphlogistic, analgetic, antipyretic tumor-inhibiting and immunomodulating in their activity. In addition, a hypoglycemic effect from the glycane fraction has been described.

INDICATIONS AND USAGE

Unproven Uses: Uses in folk medicine include fever, constipation, smallpox, strangury, bacterial skin conditions and insect bites (Korea).

Chinese Medicine: Uses include constipation, swellings, tumors and eczema of the skin. Efficacy for these indications has not yet been proven.

PRECAUTIONS AND ADVERSE REACTIONS

The drug is no longer considered safe for internal use. Hepatotoxicity and carcinogenicity are to be assumed for the drug, due to the pyrrolizidine alkaloid content with 1,2-unsaturated necic parent substances.

DOSAGE

Mode of Administration: Whole drug.

Preparation: There is no exact information in the literature.

Daily Dosage: Drug/tea: 3 to 10 g. The traditional daily dose for smallpox is 5 to 8 g drug to taken internally. (The drug is no longer considered safe for internal use.)

LITERATURE

Bechthold A, Berger U, Heide L, Partial purification, properties, and kinetic studies of UDP-glucose:p-hydroxybenzoate glucosyltransferase from cell cultures of Lithospermum erythrorhizon. Arch Biochem Biophys, 288:39-47, 1991 Jul.

Blaschek W, Hänsel R, Keller K, Reichling J, Rimpler G, Schneider G, (Eds) Hagers Handbuch der Pharmazeutischen Praxis. Folgeb nde 1 und 2. Drogen A-Z. Springer. Berlin, Heidelberg 1998.

Hisa T, Kimura Y, Takada K, Suzuki F, Takigawa M, Isolation and hypoglycemic activity of lithospermans A, B and C, glycans of Lithospermum erythrorhizon roots. Planta Med, 18:157-8, 1998 Mar-Apr.

Hisa T, Kimura Y, Takada K, Suzuki F, Takigawa M, Shikonin, an ingredient of Lithospermum erythrorhizon, inhibits angiogenesis in vivo and in vitro. Anticancer Res, 18:783-90, 1998 Mar-Apr.

Purple Loosestrife

Lythrum salicaria

DESCRIPTION

Medicinal Parts: The medicinal parts are the flowering plant without the roots and flowering branch tips.

Flower and Fruit: The purple flowers are in axillary whorls and form terminal spikes. There are 6 small sepals, 6 long thin tips, 6 free petals, 12 stamens and 1 half-superior ovary. There are flowers with long, short or medium-long styles and similar stamens.

Leaves, Stem and Root: The plant is an annual and grows from 60 to 120 cm high. It has a creeping rhizome with 4 to 6 unbranched, erect, 6-sided, reddish-brown, pubescent stems. The leaves are simple lanceolate, 7.5 to 15 cm long, sometimes opposite and sometimes clasping whorls.

Habitat: The plant is indigenous to Europe including Russia, central Asia, Australia and North America.

Production: Purple Loosestrife is the plant in flower, excluding the root, of Lythrum salicaria. Before the seeds form, the plants are cut and gathered during the blossoming period, which occurs from June to August. The material is bound into small bundles. It is hung in an open-air, shaded area to dry.

Other Names: Loosestrife, Lythrum, Purple Willow-Herb, Long Purples, Milk Willow-Herb, Rainbow Weed, Soldiers,

Spiked Loosestrife, Spiked, Willow Sage, Salicaire, Flowering Sally, Blooming Sally

ACTIONS AND PHARMACOLOGY

COMPOUNDS

Tannins (ellagitannins = lythrartannin, condensed tannins)

Flavonoids: including among others vitexin, orientin

Phthalides: diisobutyl-, butyl-, isobutyl-, dibutylphthalides

Steroids: beta-sitosterol

EFFECTS

The active agents are tannin, pectin, resins, cholin and salicarin.

The drug has an anti-inflammatory, astringent, and antibiotic effect. The astringent properties of the Purple Loosestrife is attributed not just to the tannin content, but also to the glycoside salcarin, which has a special antimicrobial effect on various bacteria in the intestinal tract.

INDICATIONS AND USAGE

Unproven Uses: The drug is used internally for diarrhea, chronic intestinal catarrh and menstrual complaints; externally, in the treatment of varicose veins, bleeding of the gums, hemorrhoids and eczema.

PRECAUTIONS AND ADVERSE REACTIONS

No health hazards or side effects are known in conjunction with the proper administration of designated therapeutic dosages.

DOSAGE

Mode of Administration: The drug is used internally as well as externally.

Preparation: For internal use, an infusion is made from 3 gm of the drug added to 100 ml of water. To prepare a tincture, add 20 gm of the drug to 100 ml of 20% alcohol (leave to set for 5 days).

Daily Dosage: Two to 3 cups of an infusion are to be taken per day. Two to 3 teaspoons of the tincture should be taken per day.

Storage: Keep wrapped in paper or in cloth sacks.

LITERATURE

Kern W, List PH, Hörhammer L (Hrsg.), Hagers Handbuch der Pharmazeutischen Praxis, 4. Aufl., Bde. 1-8, Springer Verlag Berlin, Heidelberg, New York, 1969.

Madaus G, Lehrbuch der Biologischen Arzneimittel, Bde 1-3, Nachdruck, Georg Olms Verlag Hildesheim 1979.

Pyrethrum

Chrysanthemum cinerariifolium

DESCRIPTION

Medicinal Parts: The part of the plant used for medicinal purposes (primary as an insecticide) is the flower.

Flower and Fruit: Solitary flower heads are at the end of long slender peduncles, consisting of white lingual florets and yellow tubular florets. The fruit is an achene.

Leaves, Stem and Root: Pyrethrum is a perennial, 20 to 60 cm high plant with an erect stem covered in alternating, pinnate, roughly serrated leaves. The underside of the leaves is downy.

Characteristics: The entire plant gives off a heavy perfume.

Habitat: Pyrethrum is indigenous to Kenya and the Mediterranean region and is widely cultivated in other parts of the world.

Production: Pyrethrum flowers are the just-opening compound flower heads of 2-to-8-year-old Chrysanthemum cinerariifolium and/or Chrysanthemum coccineum. The heads are left to wilt and then dried in special drying plants.

Other Names: Dalmatian Pellitory, Dalmation Insect Flowers

ACTIONS AND PHARMACOLOGY

COMPOUNDS

Pyrethrine (ester of monoterpene acid with alkylcyclopentenolone, 1%): chief components pyrethrines I and II, cinerines I and II, jasmoline I and II

Flavonoids: including apigenin-, luteolin- and quercetin-7-O-glucosides and —glucuronides

Sesquiterpenes: sesquiterpene lactones, including pyrethrosine, cyclopyrethrosine

Lignans: sesamine

Polyynes: thiophenes, including 5-(4-hydroxy-1-butenyl)-2,2′-bithienyl

EFFECTS

Pyrethrum exhibits a neurotoxic effect on the sodium canal of insects with no development of habitual immunity. Pyrethrine and cinerine are contact insecticides that paralyze the nerve center of lower animals.

INDICATIONS AND USAGE

Unproven Uses: Pyrethrum is used as an insecticide for scabies, head lice, crab lice and their nits.

PRECAUTIONS AND ADVERSE REACTIONS

No health hazards or side effects are known in conjunction with the proper administration of designated therapeutic dosages. The pyrethrines possess only limited toxicity in humans, with dosages up to 2 g of the drug are considered non-toxic.

OVERDOSAGE

Dosages exceeding 2 g of the drug have been observed to produce poisoning symptoms including headache, ringing in the ears, nausea, paresthesias, respiratory disturbances and other neurotoxic complaints.

Following gastric lavage with burgundy-colored potassium permanganate solution and installation of activated charcoal, the therapy for poisonings consists of treating possible cases of acidosis with sodium bicarbonate infusions. In case of shock, plasma volume expanders should be infused. Monitoring of kidney function is essential. Intubation and oxygen respiration may also be necessary.

DOSAGE

Mode of Administration: Externally as a liquid extract. (Area must be rinsed after use.) Some homeopathic remedies contain Pyrethrum mother tincture and dilutions.

How Supplied: Solutions, sprays and shampoos.

LITERATURE

Anonym, Bio-Insektensprays: Wirken Pyrethroide als Nervengifte? In: DAZ 132(31):1632. 1992.

Kern W, List PH, Hörhammer L (Hrsg.), Hagers Handbuch der Pharmazeutischen Praxis, 4. Aufl., Bde. 1-8, Springer Verlag Berlin, Heidelberg, New York, 1969.

Lewin L, Gifte und Vergiftungen, 6. Aufl., Nachdruck, Haug Verlag, Heidelberg 1992.

Pachaly P, Pflanzenschutzmittel in der Apotheke - Pyrethrum. In: DAZ 132(19):1032. 1992.

Roth L, Daunderer M, Kormann K, Giftpflanzen, Pflanzengifte, 4. Aufl., Ecomed Fachverlag Landsberg Lech 1993 (unter Chrysanthemum cinerariifolium).

Stüttgen G, Skabies und Läuse heute. In: DAZ 132(34):1745. 1992.

Teuscher E, Lindequist U, Biogene Gifte - Biologie, Chemie, Pharmakologie, 2. Aufl., Fischer Verlag Stuttgart 1994.

Teuscher E, Biogene Arzneimittel, 5. Aufl., Wiss. Verlagsges. Stuttgart 1997.

Pyrola rotundifolia

See Round-Leafed Wintergreen

Pyrus communis

See Pear

Quassia

Picrasma excelsa

DESCRIPTION

Medicinal Parts: The medicinal part of the plant is the dried trunk wood.

Flower and Fruit: The flowers are in leaf-axillary, richly blossomed cymose panicles. The flower structures are in fours or fives. There are 5, 0.6 to 0.9 mm long, pubescent sepals, 5 yellow-green (in male flowers approximately 2 mm long, in androgynous flowers 3 mm long) petals, 10 stamens and 5 carpels surrounded by a disc. The fruit is a 1-seeded, orbicular to oval, blue-black drupe.

Leaves, Stem and Root: An evergreen, this tree is usually dioecious and grows to a height of up to 25 m. The leaves are alternate, 15 to 35 cm long, odd pinnate, with 9 to 13 leaflets. The leaflets are 5 to 13 cm long, 20 to 45 cm wide, blunt-acuminate and glossy. The trunk has gray grooved bark.

Habitat: The tree is indigenous to the Caribbean and northern Venezuela.

Production: Bitterwood is the dried trunk wood of Picrasma excelsa, collected in the wild.

Not to be Confused With: Mistaken identity can occur with Rhus metopium.

Other Names: Ash, Bitter Ash, Bitterwood

ACTIONS AND PHARMACOLOGY

COMPOUNDS

Triterpenes: decanor-triterpenes (picrasan derivatives, quassinoids, simaroubolides, 0.15 to 0.3%), chief components quassin (nigaki lactone D) and neoquassin (both extremely bitter), and also including isoquassin (picrasmine) and 18-hydroxyquassin

Indole alkaloids: beta-carboline types, including N-methoxy-2-vinyl-beta-carboline and canthinone types, including canthine-6-one, 4-methoxy-5-hydroxycanthine-6-one

EFFECTS

The bitter substances contained in the drug (quassinoids and canthinones) exhibit antimicrobial, antiviral, anthelminthic and insecticidal effects. Quassia extract is positively inotropic and negatively chronotropic in animal experiment models. An antitumorous activity was able to be demonstrated for various quassionoids. The drug's use to stimulate appetite and promote digestion is traceable to the bitter substances it contains.

INDICATIONS AND USAGE

Unproven Uses: Folk medicine uses include dyspepsia (Mexico and Brazil), loss of appetite, and stimulation of gastric juice and saliva production. These effects are attributed to the amaroid content. Quassia is also used for fever (Costa Rica and Surinam), malaria, dysentery, gonorrhea (Brazil), lice and worm infestations, as an antiseptic wound treatment, for diarrhea (Costa Rica and Brazil), for snake bites (Guyana), for liver disease, edema and menstrual complaints.

Homeopathic Uses: Uses in homeopathy include poor digestion and liver disease.

CONTRAINDICATIONS

Not to be used during pregnancy.

PRECAUTIONS AND ADVERSE REACTIONS

No health hazards are known in conjunction with the proper administration of designated therapeutic dosages. Internal administration has occasionally led to dizziness and headache, as well as uterine pain.

OVERDOSAGE

Gastric mucous membrane irritation has been observed with cases of overdosage, followed by vomiting. It is said that prolonged use can lead to weakened vision and total blindness.

DOSAGE

Mode of Administration: Preparations are available for internal and external use.

Daily Dosage:

Drug — single dose, 0.3 to 0.6 g, 3 times daily; Tincture: daily dose; 2 to 4 ml; Lice: apply tincture twice weekly to the scalp.

Homeopathic Dosage: 5 drops, 1 tablet, 10 globules, every 30 to 60 minutes (acute), and 1 to 3 times daily (chronic); Parenterally: 1 to 2 ml sc, IV, IF; Acute: 3 times daily; Chronic: 1 to 3 times daily (HA).

Storage: Store protected from light and moisture.

LITERATURE

Hänsel R, Keller K, Rimpler H, Schneider G (Ed), Hagers Handbuch der Pharmazeutischen Praxis, 5. Aufl., Bde 4 - 6 (Drogen), Springer Verlag Berlin, Heidelberg, New York, 1992-1994.

Wagner H, Nestler T, Neszmelyi A, New constituents of Picrasma excelsa. Planta Med, 36:113-8, 1979 Jun.

Quassia amara

See Amargo

Quebracho

Aspidosperma quebracho-blanco

DESCRIPTION

Medicinal Parts: The medicinal part of the plant is the bark.

Flower and Fruit: The inflorescences, which grow from the upper leaf axils, are opposite or in threes. They are shaped like a thyrsus and are warty to almost glabrous with numerous flowers. The flowers are 1 to 3 cm long. The bracts, which fall off, are very small and have a 2 to 3 mm stem. The sepals are ovate, obtuse, 1 to 2 mm long and uneven. The corolla is white, yellow or yellowish-green, smooth or uneven on the outside. The tube is 3 to 5 mm long and has long, narrow, lanceolate petals. The stamens are in the middle of the corolla tube. The anthers are 1 mm long. The follicles are cylindrical to ovoid, 4 to 10 cm long and 1 to 7 cm wide. They are very woody, slightly warty, with or without a midrib, uneven and stemless.

Leaves, Stem and Root: The tree grows to a height of 20 m and has slim branches. The young branches are warty; the older branches are smooth with thin orange-brown bark. The leaves are opposite or trifoliate, oblong-elliptoid, ovate-lanceolate to lanceolate, acuminate and gradually narrow at the base. They are 3 to 5 cm long by 0.5 to 1.5 cm wide, coriaceous, often yellow-green and smooth. The leaves have 20 to 30 pairs of steeply ascending secondary ribs, which are very close to each other and sunk into a thick mesophyll. The exterior of the bark is grayish and deeply fissured. The inner surface is yellowish-brown, often with a reddish tint, and is grooved. The transverse fracture shows a coarsely granular outer layer and a fibrous or splintery, darker inner layer.

Characteristics: The bark has a bitter taste and is odorless.

Habitat: The plant grows in Chile, Argentina, southeast Bolivia and southeast Brazil.

Production: Quebracho bark is the bark of Aspidosperma quebracho-blanco.

Not to be Confused With: Confusion can arise with Aspidosperma horco kebracho.

ACTIONS AND PHARMACOLOGY

COMPOUNDS

Indole alkaloids (0.5-1.5%): chief alkaloids aspidospermine (30%), yohimbine (quebrachine, 10%), further including, among others, (-)-quebrachamine, akuammidine

Tannins

EFFECTS

Quebracho bark works as an expectorant and stimulates the respiratory center. A respiratory-stimulating effect has been proven for the main alkaloid aspidospermin in animal tests, but there are no studies available on the effect of the whole drug.

INDICATIONS AND USAGE

Unproven Uses: Internal folk medicine uses of Quebracho include bronchial asthma, breathing difficulties, bronchitis, fever, cramps and loss of appetite.

Homeopathic Uses: Uses in homeopathy are primarily chronic respiratory tract conditions with accompanying breathing difficulties.

PRECAUTIONS AND ADVERSE REACTIONS

No health hazards are known in conjunction with the proper administration of designated therapeutic dosages. Side effects can include, among others, salivation, headache, outbreaks of sweating, vertigo, stupor and sleepiness.

OVERDOSAGE

Intakes of larger-than-recommended therapeutic dosages lead to queasiness and vomiting.

DOSAGE

Mode of Administration: The drug is available in extract and powder form, and is often used in combination bronchial preparations. However, it is rarely used as a drug in asthma remedies.

How Supplied: Commercial pharmaceutical preparations include powder, tablets, coated tablets, drops and elixir.

Preparation: Quebracho tincture is a 1:5 (ethanol 70%) combination.

Daily Dosage: A single dose of the drug is 1 to 2 g. (Recommended daily amount not specified.)

Homeopathic Dosage: 5 to 10 drops, 1 tablet, 5 to 10 globules, 1 to 3 times daily or 1 ml injection solution sc twice weekly (HAB1).

Storage: Keep the drug in tightly sealed containers.

LITERATURE

Biemann K et al., J Am Chem Soc 85:631. 1963.

Jemec GB, Hausen BM, Contact dermatitis from Brazilian box tree wood (Aspidosperma sp.). Contact Dermatitis, 25:58-60, 1991.

Hänsel R, Keller K, Rimpler H, Schneider G (Ed), Hagers Handbuch der Pharmazeutischen Praxis, 5. Aufl., Bde 4 - 6 (Drogen), Springer Verlag Berlin, Heidelberg, New York, 1992-1994.

Lyon RL et al., (1973) J Pharm Sci 62: 218.

Markey S et al., Tetrahedron Lett 157. 1967.

Willaman JJ, Hui-Li L, (1970) Lloydia 33 (3A): 1.

Wilson E et al., Rev farm (Buenos Aires) 125:9, 1983.

Further information in:

Hänsel R, Keller K, Rimpler H, Schneider G (Hrsg.), Hagers Handbuch der Pharmazeutischen Praxis, 5. Aufl., Bde 4-6 (Drogen): Springer Verlag Berlin, Heidelberg, New York, 1992-1994.

Leung AY, Encyclopedia of Common Natural Ingredients Used in Food Drugs, Cosmetics, John Wiley & Sons Inc., New York 1980.

Lewin L, Gifte und Vergiftungen, 6. Aufl., Nachdruck, Haug Verlag, Heidelberg 1992.

Madaus G, Lehrbuch der Biologischen Arzneimittel, Bde 1-3, Nachdruck, Georg Olms Verlag Hildesheim 1979.

Makkar HP, Blümmel M, Becker K, Formation of complexes between polyvinyl pyrrolidones or polyethylene glycols and tannins and their implication in gas production and true digestibility in in vitro techniques. Br J Nutr, 73:897-913, 1995.

Roth L, Daunderer M, Kormann K: Giftpflanzen, Pflanzengifte, 4. Aufl., Ecomed Fachverlag Landsberg Lech 1993.

Steinegger E, Hänsel R, Pharmakognosie, 5. Aufl., Springer Verlag Heidelberg 1992.

Teuscher E, Biogene Arzneimittel, 5. Aufl., Wiss. Verlagsges. Stuttgart 1997.

Wichtl M (Hrsg.), Teedrogen, 4. Aufl., Wiss. Verlagsges. Stuttgart 1997.

Quercus infectoria

See Oak Gall

Quercus robur

See Oak

Quillaja

Quillaja saponaria

DESCRIPTION

Medicinal Parts: The medicinal part is the inner bark.

Flower and Fruit: The terminal inflorescence consists of white androgynous flowers with a calyx and corolla but no epicalyx. They are arranged in groups of 3 to 5 on the peduncle. The flower head is 5-lobed, splayed flat and formed into a disc on the upper surface. The many-seeded carpels spread into a star shape in the ripe fruit. The seeds are winged with little or no endosperm.

Leaves, Stem and Root: The tree is up to 18 m tall. The leaves are smooth, glossy, short petioled, and oval. The bark is thick, dark and very hard. It is odorless, very bitter and astringent.

Habitat: The plant is indigenous to Chile, Peru and is cultivated in India and California.

Production: Quillaja Bark is the bark of Quillaja saponaria.

Other Names: Quillai, Quillaja Bark, Soap Tree, Panama Bark, and Cullay

ACTIONS AND PHARMACOLOGY

COMPOUNDS

Tannins (10 to 15%)

Triterpene saponins (8.5 to 17%): chief saponins quillajasaponins 17 (QS 17, QS III), 18 (QS 18), 21 (QS 21), chief saponin quillaic acid

EFFECTS

Because of its saponin content the drug is lipid-lowering, anti-exudative and immune-stimulating in animal experiments. The expectorant and purgative effect is also attributed to the saponin content.

INDICATIONS AND USAGE

Unproven Uses: Quillaja is used internally for coughs, chronic bronchitis, and conditions of the respiratory tract. It is used externally for dandruff.

PRECAUTIONS AND ADVERSE REACTIONS

No health hazards or side effects are known in conjunction with the proper administration of designated therapeutic dosages.

OVERDOSAGE

Mucus membrane irritation could occur in the event of overdosage. Overdosage complaints include gastroenteritis, combined with vertigo, stomach pain and diarrhea. The drug possesses a low potential for sensitization.

DOSAGE

Mode of Administration: Quillaja is available as liquid extract and tincture for internal and external use.

LITERATURE

Higuchi R et al., (1987) Phytochemistry 26 (1):229.

Higuchi R et al., PH 27:1165. 1988.

Higuchi R, Komori T, PH 26:2357. 1987.

Labriola RA, Denlofeu, V, (1969) Experientia 25:124.

Lallouette P et al., (1967) C R A S Paris D 265:582.

Topping DL et al., (1980) Proc Nutr Soc Aust 5:195.

Wolters B, Arzneipflanzen und Volksmedizin Chiles. In: DAZ 134(39):3693. 1994.

Further information in:

Kern W, List PH, Hörhammer L (Hrsg.), Hagers Handbuch der Pharmazeutischen Praxis, 4. Aufl., Bde 1-8: Springer Verlag Berlin, Heidelberg, New York, 1969.

Leung AY, Encyclopedia of Common Natural Ingredients Used in Food Drugs, Cosmetics, John Wiley & Sons Inc., New York 1980.

Madaus G, Lehrbuch der Biologischen Arzneimittel, Bde 1-3, Nachdruck, Georg Olms Verlag Hildesheim 1979.

Steinegger E, Hänsel R, Pharmakognosie, 5. Aufl., Springer Verlag Heidelberg 1992.

Teuscher E, Biogene Arzneimittel, 5. Aufl., Wiss. Verlagsges. Stuttgart 1997.

Wichtl M (Hrsg.), Teedrogen, 4. Aufl., Wiss. Verlagsges. Stuttgart 1997.

Quillaja saponaria

See Quillaja

Quince

Cydonia oblongata

DESCRIPTION

Medicinal Parts: The medicinal parts are the fruit and seeds.

Flower and Fruit: The flowers are pink, relatively large, solitary and perfumed. The fruit is yellow, downy and apple or pear-shaped.

Leaves, Stem and Root: Qunice is a 3 to 6 m high tree or shrub with tomentose branches covered in alternate, ovate leaves. The undersurface of the leaves is grass-green and tomentose.

Habitat: Quince is indigenous to southwest and central Asia, but it has also spread to Europe and in particularly the Mediterranean.

Production: Quince seeds are the seeds of Cydonia oblongata. The ripe quinces are picked, stored for a period, then cut and finally dried at temperatures not exceeding 50°C. The seeds are gathered up and used in whole or ground form.

ACTIONS AND PHARMACOLOGY

COMPOUNDS

Cyanogenic glycosides: amygdalin (corresponding to 0.4 - 1.5%, 27 to 75 mg HCN/100 g)

Mucilages

Fatty oil

EFFECTS

The main active principles are mucilage, some tannins and vitamin C. There is no information is available on the mode of action.

INDICATIONS AND USAGE

Unproven Uses: Quince is used as a demulcent in digestive disorders and diarrhea. As a lotion, it is used to soothe the eyes. The seeds are also used to treat coughs and gastrointestinal catarrh. Additionally, the herb is used as compresses or poultices for injuries, inflammation of the joints, injuries of the nipples and gashed or deeply cut fingers.

PRECAUTIONS AND ADVERSE REACTIONS

Health risks or side effects following the proper administration of designated therapeutic dosages are not recorded. Because quince mucilage is prepared from the whole seeds, and/or the whole seeds are taken internally, the cyanogenic glycosides are credited with a slight toxicological relevance.

DOSAGE

Mode of Administration: The drug is used as a powder, a lotion, a decoction and an extract.

Preparation: Extract/decoction: 1 tsp. of whole seeds per cup of water. A viscous poultice is prepared from the ground seeds.

LITERATURE

De Tommasi N et al., New tetracyclic sesterterpenes from Cydonia vulgaris. In: JNP 59(3):267-270. 1996.

Huber P, Landw Versuchst 75:462. 1911.

Sommer W, Dissertation Universität Kiel. 1984.

Further information in:

Kern W, List PH, Hörhammer L (Hrsg.), Hagers Handbuch der Pharmazeutischen Praxis, 4. Aufl., Bde. 1-8, Springer Verlag Berlin, Heidelberg, New York, 1969.

Reis D, Vian B, Chanzy H, Roland JC, Liquid crystal-type assembly of native cellulose-glucuronoxylans extracted from plant cell wall. Biol Cell, 30:173-8, 1991

Steinegger E, Hänsel R, Pharmakognosie, 5. Aufl., Springer Verlag Heidelberg 1992

Teuscher E, Lindequist U, Biogene Gifte - Biologie, Chemie, Pharmakologie, 2. Aufl., Fischer Verlag Stuttgart 1994.

Quinine

Cinchona pubescens

DESCRIPTION

Medicinal Parts: The medicinal part is the dried bark of 6- to 8-year-old trees.

Flower and Fruit: The 35 cm long inflorescence is panicled, opposite, often leafy and densely blossomed. The flowers are almost sessile, and the tube is thickly covered in silky hairs. The calyx has appressed hairs, and the tips are short and widely acuminate. The corolla is red or pink and 10 to 12 mm long. The fruit is an oblong, glabrous and longitudinally grooved capsule.

Leaves, Stem and Root: The plant is an evergreen tree, sometimes a bush, which grows from 5 to 15 m high, with a dense crown. The branches are at right angles to the trunk. The young branches are usually pubescent. The stipules are large, ovate, obtuse or acuminate, silky-haired or glabrous. The leaves have an up to 8 cm long petiole. The leaf blade is 15 to 40 cm long and 7 to 25 cm wide, oblong-elliptoid to roundish with curved side ribs. The bark occurs in quills or flat pieces up to 30 cm long and 3 to 6 mm thick. The external surface is brownish-gray, usually fissured with an exfoliating cork. Lichens and mosses may be seen as grayish-white or greenish patches. The inner surface is yellowish to reddish-brown. The fracture is fibrous.

Characteristics: The bark has an astringent, bitter taste and the odor is slight.

Habitat: The herb is indigenous to mountainous regions of the tropical U.S. and is cultivated elsewhere.

Production: Cinchona bark consists of the dried bark of Cinchona pubescens or other varieties. Trees are felled at between 6 and 12 years. They are dried slowly in the sun initially and then artificially dried at maximum temperatures of 70° C.

Not to be Confused With: Yellow factory bark

Other Names: Peruvian Bark, Jesuit's Bark, Cinchona

ACTIONS AND PHARMACOLOGY

COMPOUNDS

Quinoline alkaloids (5-15%): main alkaloids are quinine (0.8-4%), quinidine (0.02-0.4%), cinchonine (1.5-3%), cinchonidine (1.5-5%)

Triterpenes: bitter acid monoglycosides, in particular chinovic acid-3-O-chinovoside, chinovic acid-3-O-glucoside

Catechin tannins (3-5%)

EFFECTS

Quinine promotes stimulation of the secretion of saliva and gastric juices.

INDICATIONS AND USAGE

Approved by Commission E:

- Loss of appetite
- Dyspeptic complaints

Unproven Uses: Quinine is used internally to correct loss of appetite, dyspepsia and flatulence with a sense of fullness. The bark is used for malaria, flu, enlarged spleen, muscle cramps, muscle pain, cancer and gastric disorders. Externally, it is used for scrapes and skin ulcers.

Chinese Medicine: Quinine is used for malaria, fever and alcohol intoxication.

Indian Medicine: The drug is used to treat intermittent fever, malaria, intercostal neuralgia, sciatica and neuritis (especially of the arm).

Homeopathic Uses: Quinine is used to treat general poisoning, attacks of fever, inflammation of the respiratory tract, acute diarrhea, anemia, general debility, skin rashes and neuralgia.

CONTRAINDICATIONS

Quinine should not be used during pregnancy.

PRECAUTIONS AND ADVERSE REACTIONS

General: Sensitization to Quinine and Quinidine have been observed (eczema, itching). Even at therapeutic dosages, an enhanced pseudohemophiliac effect can occur through the triggering of thrombocytopenia.

Drug Interactions: Because of the possibility of thrombocytopenia, care must be taken when Quinine preparations are administered along with other drugs that are known to precipitate thrombocytopenia.

OVERDOSAGE

In cases of overdose (more than 3 gm Quinine) or of long-term administration of the drug or its alkaloids, nausea, summer cholera, headache, fall of body temperature, intravascular hemolysis, cardiac arrhythmias, buzzing in the ears, hearing and visual disorders (all the way to complete deafness and blindness) may occur. Death comes with dosages of 10 to 15 gm of Quinine through heart failure and asphyxiation. Following gastric lavage, the symptomatic therapy for acute poisonings includes atropine for bradycardia and phenytoin in the presence of tachycardic heart rhythm disorders. Forced diuresis and hemodialysis are not suitable as therapeutic measures.

DOSAGE

Mode of Administration: Whole, cut and powdered drug are used in various galenic preparations, including tonics, drops, tablets, compresses, ampules, coated tablets, suppositories and compound preparations.

Preparation: A tea is prepared by pouring 150 ml of boiling water over 1/2 teaspoonful of the drug and allowing it to draw for 10 minutes. A decoction is prepared by adding 0.5 g to 1 teacup of water. A tincture in the proportion of 1:5 in 75% ethanol is also used.

Daily Dosage: Total daily dose is 1 to 3 gm of drug. The liquid extract daily dose is 0.6 to 3 gm of cinchona liquid extract, which contains 4 to 5% total alkaloids. A daily dose of 0.15 to 0.6 g cinchona extract with 15 to 20% total alkaloids may also be used.

The standard single dose of the extract is 0.2 gm. The liquid extract single dose is 0.5 to 1 gm.

Homeopathic Dosage: 5 drops, 1 tablet or 10 globules, every 30 to 60 minutes (acute) or 1 to 3 times a day (chronic); parenterally: 1 to 2 ml sc, acute: 3 times daily; chronic: once a day (HAB1).

Storage: Keep protected from light and moisture.

LITERATURE

Chinidin: Photoallergische Reaktion. In: DAZ 133(30):2765. 1993.

Hämorrhoidenbehandlung: Ambulant oder stationär. In: DAZ 133(40):3616. 1993.

Risdale CE, Hasskarls cinchona barks. 1. Historical review. In: Reinwardtia 10, Teil 2: 245-264. 1985.

Schönfeld, Fleischer K, Eichenlaub D, Die Malariavorbeugung. Mückenschutz und Arzneimittel zur Kurzzeitprophylaxe und Notfallbehandlung. In: DAZ 133(21):1981. 1993.

Further information in:

Chan, EH et al. (Eds.), Advances in Chinese Medicinal Materials Research, World Scientific Pub. Co. Singapore 1985.

Hänsel R, Keller K, Rimpler H, Schneider G (Hrsg.), Hagers Handbuch der Pharmazeutischen Praxis, 5. Aufl., Bde 4-6 (Drogen): Springer Verlag Berlin, Heidelberg, New York, 1992-1994.

Leung AY, Encyclopedia of Common Natural Ingredients Used in Food Drugs and Cosmetics, John Wiley & Sons Inc., New York 1980.

Lewin L, Gifte und Vergiftungen, 6. Aufl., Nachdruck, Haug Verlag, Heidelberg 1992.

Madaus G, Lehrbuch der Biologischen Arzneimittel, Bde 1-3, Nachdruck, Georg Olms Verlag Hildesheim 1979.

Manske RHF, Holmes HL, fortgeführt von Rodrigo RGA, Brossi A): The Alkaloids - Chemistry and Physiology, III:1, XIV:181, XXXIV:331, Academic Press New York 1950-1997.

Roth L, Daunderer M, Kormann K, Giftpflanzen, Pflanzengifte, 4. Aufl., Ecomed Fachverlag Landsberg Lech 1993.

Steinegger E, Hänsel R, Pharmakognosie, 5. Aufl., Springer Verlag Heidelberg 1992.

Teuscher E, Lindequist U, Biogene Gifte - Biologie, Chemie, Pharmakologie, 2. Aufl., Fischer Verlag Stuttgart 1994.

Teuscher E, Biogene Arzneimittel, 5. Aufl., Wiss. Verlagsges. mbH Stuttgart 1997.

Wagner H, Wiesenauer M, Phytotherapie. Phytopharmaka und pflanzliche Homöopathika, Fischer-Verlag, Stuttgart, Jena, New York 1995.

Wichtl M (Hrsg.), Teedrogen, 4. Aufl., Wiss. Verlagsges. Stuttgart 1997.

Radish

Raphanus sativus

DESCRIPTION

Medicinal Parts: The medicinal part is the fresh root. The plant is an important drug in homeopathic medicine.

Flower and Fruit: The raceme is loose and has about 30 flowers. The pedicles are 1 to 2 cm long and are covered in scattered bristles. The sepals are 6.5 to 10 mm long, oblong, acute, glabrous or with scattered bristles and red or green. The petals are 17 to 22 mm long, obovate, slightly margined, violet or white with dark veins. The fruit is on upright, patent stems. They are upright, cylindrical and conically acuminate. The upper segment is up to 9 cm long and even or slightly constricted between the seeds, and straw-like on the outside. The seeds are ovate, 4 mm long and 3 mm wide, light brown with a black hilum.

Leaves, Stem and Root: The root is annual or biennial and thin. The stem is up to 1 m high, bent, cane-like, branched, glabrous or covered with bristles and often violet, particularly in the axils of the lateral branches. The lower leaves are lyrate-pinnatisect with large sweeping crenate end segments and smaller, oblong-ovate, obtuse, dentate lateral lobes. They are light green, often red-veined and covered with scattered, appressed bristles.

Characteristics: The large, thick, tuberous, fleshy root, is hot to the taste.

Habitat: The plant is probably indigenous to China and Japan and today is cultivated in most temperate regions of the world.

Production: Radish consists of the fresh roots of Raphanus sativus and/or of Raphanus sativus, as well as their preparations. It is a cultivated plant.

Other Names: Common Radish, Garden Radish

ACTIONS AND PHARMACOLOGY

COMPOUNDS

Glucosinolates in the fresh, unbruised rhizome: chief component 4-methylthio-3-butenyl-glucosinolate, glucobrassin, sinigrin, glucoraphanine

EFFECTS

The drug is said to be choleretic, antimicrobial and to increase motility in the upper gastrointestinal tract, an effect caused by the mustard oils.

A choleretic effect and an antiviral effect were proven in animal experiments.

Radish has a secretolytic effect in patients suffering from chronic bronchitis.

INDICATIONS AND USAGE

Approved by Commission E:

- Cough/Bronchitis
- Dyspeptic complaints

Radish is used internally for respiratory catarrh and dyspeptic disorders, especially those related to dyskinesia of the bile ducts.

Unproven Uses: In folk medicine Radish is used for whooping cough and gallstones.

Chinese Medicine: In China, Radish is used to treat coughs, diarrhea and abdominal pain.

Indian Medicine: Uses in India include dyspeptic complaints, nausea, flatulence, gallbladder disturbances, headache, neuralgias, and urological conditions.

Homeopathic Uses: Raphanus sativus is used for poor digestion and oily skin.

PRECAUTIONS AND ADVERSE REACTIONS

No health hazards or side effects are known in conjunction with the proper administration of designated therapeutic dosages.

OVERDOSAGE

Administration of higher dosages of the fresh root could lead to mucus membrane irritation of the gastrointestinal tract. Due to the cholagogic effect of the drug, biliary colic could be triggered in patients with gallstones.

DOSAGE

Preparation:

Radish-honey juice — 1 radish is grated and the resulting juice is mixed with honey, then allowed to stand for 10 hours.

Radish plant juice — The Radish is washed, cut and grated and up to 17% of the liquid is pressed out. 1-liter of juice is extracted from 1.3 kg of fresh drug.

Daily Dosage:

Pressed juice — 50 to 100 ml; ½ tablespoon several times daily over a 3-day period.

Radish-honey juice — spoonfuls taken over the course of the day for whooping cough.

Homeopathic Dosage: 5 drops, 1 tablet or 10 globules every 30 to 60 minutes (acute) or 1 to 3 times daily (chronic); parenterally: 1 to 2 ml sc acute: 3 times daily; chronic: once a day (HAB1)

LITERATURE

Hänsel R, Keller K, Rimpler H, Schneider G (Hrsg.), Hagers Handbuch der Pharmazeutischen Praxis, 5. Aufl., Bde 4-6 (Drogen): Springer Verlag Berlin, Heidelberg, New York, 1992-1994.

Teuscher E, Lindequist U, Biogene Gifte - Biologie, Chemie, Pharmakologie, 2. Aufl., Fischer Verlag Stuttgart 1994.

Ragwort

Senecio jacoboea

DESCRIPTION

Medicinal Parts: The medicinal parts are the dried aerial parts of the flowering plant and the entire fresh plant gathered during the flowering season.

Flower and Fruit: The golden yellow composite flowers grow in dense, terminal, erect, branched cymes. The linguiform ray florets are female. The disc florets are tubular and androgynous. The capitula has a diameter of 15 to 20 mm. The involucre is cylindrical. The bracts are in 1 row and are oblong-lanceolate, acuminate and black at the tip, with a short 1- to 4-leafed epicalyx. The lateral fruit is glabrous and has drooping tufts of hair. The other fruit is covered in thick tufts of loosely attached hair.

Leaves, Stem and Root: The plant is biennial to perennial and grows 30 to 90 cm high. The stem is erect, branched above and cobweb-pubescent. The basal leaves are lyrate-pinnatifid. The cauline leaves are pinnatifid with indented pinna. The lateral tips are almost at right angles and have small, 4-sectioned, slit ears that clasp the stem.

Habitat: The plant is indigenous to all of Europe, Asia Minor and northern Africa, and is naturalized in North America.

Production: Ragwort is the flowering plant of Senecio jacoboea. The plant is gathered in the wild, usually during the flowering season. The cut drug is dried away from direct sunlight.

Other Names: Ragweed, St. James Wort, Stinking Nanny, Staggerwort, Dog Standard, Cankerwort, Stammerwort

ACTIONS AND PHARMACOLOGY

COMPOUNDS

Pyrrolizidine alkaloids (0.1-0.9%): the alkaloid spectrum depends upon the chemotype. Jacobine chemotype: chief alkaloid jacobine; erucifoline chemotype: chief alkaloids erucifoline and O-acetylerucifoline

Volatile oil (traces)

EFFECTS

The toxic principles of the drug are the pyrrolizidine alkaloids, which should be assumed to be hepatotoxic and carcinogenic. Countless experiments have shown the plant to be acutely and chronically poisonous in animals.

INDICATIONS AND USAGE

Because of its potential carcinogenic effect, Ragwort should not be used. Traditional folk medicine uses have included painful menstruation, urinary tract inflammation, chronic cough, rheumatism, anemia and anemic headaches.

PRECAUTIONS AND ADVERSE REACTIONS

Ragwort should not be taken internally since hepatotoxicity and carcinogenicity are possible due to the pyrrolizidine alkaloids with 1,2-unsaturated necic parent substances in its makeup.

DOSAGE

Mode of Administration: The drug is used externally as a component of lotions, but should not be taken internally.

Preparation: The lotion is made using 1 part of the drug and 5 parts of 10% ethanol.

Daily Dosage: The lotion is applied topically for the treatment of rheumatic arthritis.

LITERATURE

Bradbury RB, Culvenor CCJ, (1954) Austr J Chem 7. 378.

Deinzer ML et al., Science 195:497. 1977.

Schoental R, (1968) Cancer Res 28:2237.

Van Dooren, Bos R et al., (1981) Planta Med 42:385.

Van Dorren B et al., PM 42:385. 1981.

Witte L et al., PH 31:559. 1985.

Further information in:

Frohne D, Pfänder HJ: Giftpflanzen - Ein Handbuch für Apotheker, Toxikologen und Biologen, 4. Aufl., Wiss. Verlags-Ges. Stuttgart 1997.

Hänsel R, Keller K, Rimpler H, Schneider G (Hrsg.), Hagers Handbuch der Pharmazeutischen Praxis, 5. Aufl., Bde 4-6 (Drogen): Springer Verlag Berlin, Heidelberg, New York, 1992-1994.

Madaus G: Lehrbuch der Biologischen Arzneimittel, Bde 1-3, Nachdruck, Georg Olms Verlag Hildesheim 1979.

Roth L, Daunderer M, Kormann K, Giftpflanzen, Pflanzengifte, 4. Aufl., Ecomed Fachverlag Landsberg Lech 1993.

Teuscher E, Lindequist U, Biogene Gifte - Biologie, Chemie, Pharmakologie, 2. Aufl., Fischer Verlag Stuttgart 1994.

Ranunculus acris

See Buttercup

Ranunculus bulbosus

See Bulbous Buttercup

Ranunculus ficaria

See Lesser Celandine

Ranunculus sceleratus

See Poisonous Buttercup

Raphanus raphanistrum

See Wild Radish

Raphanus sativus

See Radish

Raspberry

Rubus idaeus

TRADE NAMES

Alcohol Free Red Raspberry Leaf, Certified Organic Red Raspberry, Red Raspberry Leaves, Red Raspberry Leaves Glycerine, Wild Countryside Red Raspberry Leafs

DESCRIPTION

Medicinal Parts: The medicinal parts are the leaves and fruit.

Flower and Fruit: The white flowers are in cymes. The calyx has 5 sepals and the corolla is 5-petalled. There are numerous stamens and ovaries. Similar to the blackberry, the small fruit forms a red aggregate fruit, the raspberry.

Leaves, Stem and Root: Raspberry is a 2 m high deciduous bush with erect, woody stems, which are densely covered in tough thorns. The aerial part is usually biennial while the creeping root is perennial. The leaves are pale green. There are 3 leaves that sit atop 7 leaflets.

Habitat: The plant is indigenous to Europe and Asia and is cultivated in temperate climates.

Production: Raspberry leaf consists of the leaf of Rubus idaeus.

Not to be Confused With: Blackberry leaves.

Other Names: Red Raspberry

ACTIONS AND PHARMACOLOGY

COMPOUNDS

Tannins: gallo tannins, ellagic tannins

Flavonoids

EFFECTS

The main active agents are tannin, flavonoids, and vitamin C. The tannins give the fruit an astringent effect.

INDICATIONS AND USAGE

Unproven Uses: Raspberry leaf is used for disorders of the gastrointestinal tract, the respiratory tract, the cardiovascular system, and the mouth and throat. In folk medicine, Raspberry preparations were used to facilitate childbirth.

PRECAUTIONS AND ADVERSE REACTIONS

No health hazards or side effects are known in conjunction with the proper administration of designated therapeutic dosages.

DOSAGE

Mode of Administration: As a component of purgative and ''blood purifying'' teas, and in fruit tea mixtures.

Preparation: To prepare an infusion, scald 1.5 gm finely cut drug, steep for 5 minutes and then strain. (1 teaspoonful = 0.8 gm drug).

LITERATURE

Bamford DS et al., (1970) Brit J Pharmacol 40(1):161P.

Beckett A et al., (1954) J Pharm Pharmacol 6:785.

Czygan FC, Die Himbeere - Rubus idaeus L. In: ZPT 16(6):366-74. 1995.

Henning W, (1981) Lebensm Unters Forsch 173:1.

Henning W, (1981) Lebensm Unters Forsch 173:180.

Marczal G, (1963) Herba Hung 2:343.

Further information in:

Kern W, List PH, Hörhammer L (Hrsg.), Hagers Handbuch der Pharmazeutischen Praxis, 4. Aufl., Bde. 1-8: Springer Verlag Berlin, Heidelberg, New York, 1969.

Wichtl M (Hrsg.), Teedrogen, 4. Aufl., Wiss. Verlagsges. Stuttgart 1997.

Rauwolfia

Rauwolfia serpentina

DESCRIPTION

Medicinal Parts: The medicinal part is the dried root.

Flower and Fruit: The white to pink flowers are in terminal or axillary cymes which have a diameter of 2.5 to 5 cm and are 5 to 13 cm long in main axis. The corolla tube is 11 to 19 cm long and therefore much longer than the tips, which form a plate-like margin. The fruit is a bilabiate drupe, which is purple-black when ripe.

Leaves, Stem and Root: The plant is an erect, glabrous evergreen semishrub 0.5 to 1 m in height. The trunk is pale and unbranched. The leaves are concentrated toward the top of the trunk and are entire-margined. They are in whorls of 3 to 5 and occasionally opposite. The leaves are 7 to 18 cm long, 2.5 to 5 cm wide, oblong-ovate or lanceolate and taper to an irregular base. The petiole is 5 to 15 cm long.

The rhizome is vertical and woody, the root is gray-brown with a wrinkled surface and is 3 to 22 mm in diameter.

Characteristics: The fresh root has a very bitter, unpleasant taste.

Habitat: The plant is indigenous to India, Indochina, Borneo, Sri Lanka and Sumatra.

The drug is derived from wild collections in India, Pakistan, Thailand and Indonesia.

Production: Rauwolfia root consists of the dried root of Rauwolfia serpentina as well as its preparations. It is collected in the uncultivated regions, mostly from 4-year-old plants. When cultivated, 2-year-old plants are harvested. Roots are air-dried at 60° C.

Not to be Confused With: The roots of other Rauwolfia species and Withania sonnifera.

ACTIONS AND PHARMACOLOGY

COMPOUNDS

Ajmalane-type: including ajmaline

Heteroyohimbane-type: including serpentinine, serpentine, raubasine, ajmalicine

Indole alkaloids (1 to 2.5%)

Sarpagan-type: including raupine, sarpagine

Starch

Yohimbine-type: including reserpine, isorauhimbine, rescinnamine, reserpinine

EFFECTS

The drug contains alkaloids of the rauwolfia type. Reserpine and other alkaloids in the root have a sympatholytic effect by releasing noradrenaline and inhibiting its resorption in the vesicles of the noradrenergic nerve ends. This results in a lowering of catecholamine, which causes a hypotensive effect. The ajmalin in the root has an antiarrhythmic effect brought about by membrane stabilization. In animal experiments a centrally generated sedative effect was demonstrated.

INDICATIONS AND USAGE

Approved by Commission E:

- Hypertension
- Nervousness and insomnia

Rauwolfia is used internally for hypertension due to vascular hypertonia. It is also useful for anxiety and tension states and other psychomotoric disorders.

Unproven Uses: Rauwolfia is also used in folk medicine for flatulence, vomiting, insomnia, eclampsia, hypertension and liver disease. It is used to encourage uterine contraction during birth, and is used locally in the treatment of wounds.

Indian Medicine: The drug is used as an antidote for snakebites and the poisonous bites of other reptiles; also for high blood pressure, dysuria, fever, colic and in the treatment of wounds.

CONTRAINDICATIONS

Rauwolfia is contraindicated in depression, ulceration, pheochromocytoma, pregnancy, and lactation.

PRECAUTIONS AND ADVERSE REACTIONS

General: No health hazards are known in conjunction with the proper administration of designated therapeutic dosages. Side effects could include nasal congestion, states of depression, tiredness erectile dysfunction. The drug may cause drowsiness and care must be taken when operating an automobile or machinery.

Drug-Interactions:

Alcohol: — Combination with alcohol considerably increases the impairment of reactions.

Neuroleptics and Barbiturates — An increase of drug effect occurs with these medications.

Digitalis-Glycosides — Severe bradycardia occurs in combination with digitalis glycosides.

Levodopa — Drug effect is reduced in combination with levodopa along with an increase in the undesired extra-pyramidal motor symptoms in combination with sympathomimetics. Cough or 'flu' remedies and appetite suppressants may cause a significant increase in blood pressure in combination with Rawolfia.

DOSAGE

Mode of Administration: Rauwolfia is available in whole, crude and powder form for internal and external use. It is also available in solid pharmaceutical form and in compounded preparations.

Preparation: Rauwolfia serpentina dry extract contains 7% total alkaloids (DAB10). Various processes are used to isolate reserpine.

Daily Dosage: 600 mg drug/6 mg total alkaloids

Storage: The drug should be protected from light.

LITERATURE

Beim HJ, Pharmacol Rev 8:281. 1978.

Cornett GBR, World Crops 17:33. 1965.

Lounasmaa M et al., On the structure of the indole alkaloid ajmalicidine. In: PM 60(5):480. 1994.

Nattkämper G, PA 22:281. 1967.

Further information in:

Hänsel R, Keller K, Rimpler H, Schneider G (Hrsg.), Hagers Handbuch der Pharmazeutischen Praxis, 5. Aufl., Bde 4-6 (Drogen): Springer Verlag Berlin, Heidelberg, New York, 1992-1994.

Roth L, Daunderer M, Kormann K, Giftpflanzen, Pflanzengifte, 4. Aufl., Ecomed Fachverlag Landsberg Lech 1993.

Schulz R, Hänsel R, Rationale Phytotherapie, Springer Verlag Heidelberg 1996.

Steinegger E, Hänsel R, Pharmakognosie, 5. Aufl., Springer Verlag Heidelberg 1992.

Teuscher E, Biogene Arzneimittel, 5. Aufl., Wiss. Verlagsges. Stuttgart 1997.

Wagner H, Wiesenauer M, Phytotherapie. Phytopharmaka und pflanzliche Homöopathika, Fischer-Verlag, Stuttgart, Jena, New York 1995.

Wichtl M (Hrsg.), Teedrogen, 4. Aufl., Wiss. Verlagsges. Stuttgart 1997.

Rauwolfia serpentina

See Rauwolfia

Red Bryony

Bryonia cretica

DESCRIPTION

Medicinal Parts: The medicinal part of the plant is the root.

Flower and Fruit: The female flowers are in short-pedicled clusters; the male flowers are in long-pedicled racemes. The flowers are radial and their structures are arranged in fives. The corolla of the female flowers are up to 10 mm wide. The sepals are half as a long as the petals. The ovary is inferior and 3-chambered. The corolla of the male flowers is up to 20 mm wide, yellowish and green-veined; the 5 stamens are fused in groups (2+2+1). The fruit is a 1 to 2 seeded, globose berry, 6 to 10 mm thick. They are scarlet when ripe.

Leaves, Stem and Root: Bryonia cretica is a herbaceous perennial. The stem is dioecious and 2 to 4 m long. It climbs with the aid of simple tendrils. The leaves are alternate, short petiolate, broad-cordate to palmate-5-lobed. The lobes are entire or have blunt teeth. Both surfaces of the leaf are covered in short bristly hairs. Each leaf is positioned opposite a tendril. The root is tuberous, up to 2.5 kg, light yellow and white slimy inside.

Habitat: Central and southern Europe

Production: Bryonia cretica root is the dried root of Bryonia cretica. The plant is cultivated.

Other Names: White Bryony, Devil's Turnip, English Mandrake

ACTIONS AND PHARMACOLOGY

COMPOUNDS

Cucurbitacins: cucurbitacins B, D, E, I, J, K, L and S (present in the fresh root as aglycones of the glycosides, presumably the result of decomposition after dehydration), small quantities of intact glycosides, for example bryoamarid, bryoside, bryodiosides A to C

Triterpenes: triterpene acids, including bryonolic acid, bryocoumaric acid, 3alpha-hydroxymultiflora-8-ene-29alpha-acid

Fatty acids (polyhydroxyderivatives, resembling the eicosanoids): for example 9,12,13-trihydroxy-octadeca-10 (E)-15(Z)-dienic acid

Ribosome-inactivating proteins: bryodine-L and bryodine-R

EFFECTS

The protein bryodine has cytotoxic effect in vitro. The drug is used as a laxative and an emetic. The chief active ingredients are the cucurbitacins, which even in low dosages lead to irritation of the mucous membrane of the gastrointestinal tract with subsequent increase of peristalsis. The drug is severely toxic in higher dosages.

INDICATIONS AND USAGE

Unproven Uses: The drug can be used for respiratory tract and rheumatic conditions, gastrointestinal tract, metabolic disorders, liver disease, and acute and chronic infectious conditions.

Homeopathic Uses: Bryonia cretica is used for acute and chronic rheumatism, peritonitis, and inflammation of the respiratory organs and the pleura.

PRECAUTIONS AND ADVERSE REACTIONS

No health hazards are known in conjunction with the proper administration of designated homeopathic therapeutic dosages. Side effects connected with the ingestion of the base tincture and D1 include signs of irritation in the gastrointestinal tract. All parts of the plant are strongly toxic, due to the cucurbitacins content, which is irritating to mucous membranes.

OVERDOSAGE

Symptoms of poisoning include vomiting, bloody diarrhea, colic, kidney irritation, anuria, spasms, palsies and aborted pregnancy. Death occurs through asphyxiation. Forty berries are considered lethal for an adult, 15 for a child. 3.5 gm of the drug is considered poisonous; one death has been documented following the ingestion of an infusion made from 30 gm of the root.

Following gastrointestinal emptying (in case vomiting has not occurred, gastric lavage with burgundy-colored potassium permanganate solution, sodium sulfate) and installation of activated charcoal, the therapy for poisoning consists of treating spasms with diazepam (i.v.), electrolyte substitution and treating possible cases of acidosis with sodium bicarbonate infusions. In the event of shock, plasma volume expanders should be infused. Monitoring of kidney function is imperative. Intubation and oxygen respiration may also be necessary.

DOSAGE

Mode of Administration: Liquid and solid preparations for internal use; semi-solid preparations for external use.

Preparation:

Wine — 40 gm drug to 1 L white wine, leave to draw for 1 day.

Tincture — 10 gm to 90 gm ethyl alcohol (60%), leave to draw for 8 days.

Honey decoction — 20 gm drug to 250 gm honey and 350 gm wine vinegar, simmer for 30 minutes at a low temperature, strain when cool and store in a well-sealed bottle.

Ointment — Mix 30 gm cut drug with the same amount of Vaseline or wax.

Daily Dosage:

Powder — 0.3 to 0.5 gm as a laxative and emetic.

Decoction — 0.5 gm to 1 gm per cup.

Wine — 1 to 2 dessertspoons daily.

Tincture — 1 to 10 drops per day; maximum 20 drops.

Homeopathic Dosage: 5 to 10 drops, 1 tablet, 5 to 10 globules, 1 to 3 times daily or 1 ml injection solution sc. twice weekly; ointment 1 to 2 times daily; mother tincture D1 diluted to be taken with liquid (HAB1)

Storage: Should be sealed tightly.

LITERATURE

Hänsel R, Keller K, Rimpler H, Schneider G (Ed), Hagers Handbuch der Pharmazeutischen Praxis, 5. Aufl., Bde 4 - 6 (Drogen), Springer Verlag Berlin, Heidelberg, New York, 1992-1994.

Red Clover

Trifolium pratense

TRADE NAMES

Red Clover liquid, Red Clover Blossom, Red Clover Herb, Promensil, EuroQuality Red Clover Blossoms, NuVeg Red Clover Concentrate

DESCRIPTION

Medicinal Parts: The medicinal parts are the dried and the fresh flower heads.

Flower and Fruit: One to 4 globular, ovate flower heads form on the tip of the stem. The calyx is tubular-campanulate. The petals are light carmine to fleshy red, occasionally yellowish-white or pure white. The fruit is a pod, which is ovate, 1-seeded and thin-skinned. The seed is oblong-ovate, yellow to brownish or violet.

Leaves, Stem and Root: The plant is a perennial herb, 15 to 40 cm high with a bushy rhizome and a basal leaf rosette. An erect, angular stem grows from the rhizome. The rhizome is covered in alternate, trifoliate, elliptical or ovate leaves, which have a characteristic arrow-shaped white spot on the upper surface. The leaflets are short-petioled, almost entire-margined, appressed, softly pubescent on both surfaces or only on the upper surface.

Habitat: The plant is indigenous to Europe, central Asia, northern Africa and is naturalized in many other parts of the world.

Production: Red Clover flowers are the flowers of Trifolium pratense. The dried flower buds are used to produce the drug.

Other Names: Purple Clover, Trefoil, Wild Clover

ACTIONS AND PHARMACOLOGY

COMPOUNDS

Volatile oil: including among others, benzyl alcohol, 2-phenyl ethanol, their formates and acetates, methyl salicylate, methyl anthranilate (likely only in the fresh blossoms)

Isoflavonoids: including among others, biochanin A

Coumarin derivatives

Cyanogenic glycosides: presumably lotaustralin, linamarin

EFFECTS

Red Clover has antispasmodic and expectorant effects and also promotes the skin's healing process.

INDICATIONS AND USAGE

Unproven Uses: Internally, Red Clover is used for coughs and respiratory conditions, particularly whooping cough. Externally, it is used in the treatment of chronic skin conditions such as psoriasis and eczema.

PRECAUTIONS AND ADVERSE REACTIONS

No health hazards or side effects are known in conjunction with the proper administration of designated therapeutic dosages.

DOSAGE

Mode of Administration: The drug is used internally and externally as a liquid extract and in medicinal preparations.

Preparation: Liquid extract 1:1 can be prepared in 25% ethanol.

Daily Dosage: The daily dosage is 4 gm of drug, taken as an infusion, up to 3 times a day. Alternately, 1.5 to 3 ml of the liquid extract can be taken 3 times daily.

LITERATURE

Dewick P, (1977) Phytochemistry 16:93.

Fenaroli's Handbook of Flavor Ingredients, Vol. 1, 2nd Ed., CRC Press 1975.

Guggolz J et al., (1961) Agric Food Chem 9(4):331.

Hänsel R, Keller K, Rimpler H, Schneider G (Hrsg.), Hagers Handbuch der Pharmazeutischen Praxis, 5. Aufl., Bde 4-6 (Drogen): Springer Verlag Berlin, Heidelberg, New York, 1992-1994.

Kattaev NS et al., (1972) Khim Prir Soed 6:806.

Madaus G, Lehrbuch der Biologischen Arzneimittel, Bde 1-3, Nachdruck, Georg Olms Verlag Hildesheim 1979.

Sachse J, (1974) J Chrom 96(1):123.

Wagner H, Wiesenauer M, Phytotherapie. Phytopharmaka und pflanzliche Homöopathika, Fischer-Verlag, Stuttgart, Jena, New York 1995.

Yoshihara T et al., (1977) Agric Biol Chem 41(9):1679.

Red Currant

Ribes rubrum

DESCRIPTION

Medicinal Parts: The medicinal parts are the fruit and leaves.

Flower and Fruit: The flowers are in hanging, many-blossomed racemes. The green flowers are inconspicuous and their structures are in fives. The sepals and petals are fused with the hollowed receptacle. The calyx tips are wide obovate and longer than the petals. The corolla tube is flat with a pentagonal ring swelling. There are 2 carpels fused with the corolla tube to an inferior, single-chambered ovary. The ovary has a concave tip and a disc ring. The fruit is multi-seeded red berry. The cultivated forms are pink or white.

Leaves, Stem and Root: Ribes rubrum grows as a shrub, reaching up to 2 m high. The leaves are alternate, over 10 cm wide with a petiole half as long as the lamina, which is 3- to 5-lobed. The lobes are blunt to acute, double crenate and cordate at the base with an acute indentation.

Habitat: The plant is indigenous to Western Europe.

Production: Red Currants are the fresh ripe berries of Ribes rubrum.

ACTIONS AND PHARMACOLOGY

COMPOUNDS

Fruit acids: chief fruit acid is citric acid; other acids include malic acid, isocitric acid and tartartic acid

Monosaccharides/polysaccharides (7%): D-glucose, D-fructose

Pectins (15%)

Fatty oil (in the seeds 20%) with gamma-linolenic acid (6%)

Ascorbic acid (vitamin C, 0.005 to 0.015%)

Caffeic acid derivatives: including caffeoyl glucose, p-cumaric acid-O-glucoside

EFFECTS

Red Currant is a source of vitamin C and exhibits in vitro radical scavenger qualities. The fruit and juice are considered cooling and antiscorbutic and have often been used as a febrifuge. The jelly prepared from the berries has an antiseptic effect and was often used to treat burns to prevent the formation of blisters. The leaves are said to have emmenagogic properties.

INDICATIONS AND USAGE

Unproven Uses: Red currant has been used in folk medicine to treat febrile conditions.

PRECAUTIONS AND CONTRAINDICATIONS

No health hazards are known in conjunction with the proper administration of designated therapeutic dosages.

DOSAGE

No data are available in the literature.

LITERATURE

Hänsel R, Keller K, Rimpler H, Schneider G (Ed), Hagers Handbuch der Pharmazeutischen Praxis, 5. Aufl., Bde 4 - 6 (Drogen), Springer Verlag Berlin, Heidelberg, New York, 1992-1994.

Red Maple

Acer rubrum

DESCRIPTION

Medicinal Parts: The medicinal part is the bark.

Flower and Fruit: The flowers are red and aromatic, forming round bunches. The ovary is formed from 2 simple carpels pressed together at the sides, which are also present in the male flowers in rudimentary form. Each section contains 2 ovules. The fruit is a schizocarp with 2 one-sided or many-sided, often heavily veined wings. There is usually only one seed in each section.

Leaves, Stem and Root: The Red Maple tree grows to a height of up to 36 m. The leaves are crossed-opposite, petiolate and partially 3-lobed.

Habitat: Canada and the U.S., introduced into England and Europe around 1650.

Production: Red Acorn bark is the trunk bark of Acer rubrum.

Other Names: Swamp Maple, Bird's Eye Maple, Sugar Maple

ACTIONS AND PHARMACOLOGY

COMPOUNDS

Tannins

Triterpenoid saponins

Allantoins

EFFECTS

Red maple has an astringent effect.

INDICATIONS AND USAGE

Unproven Uses: Red Maple is used for eye conditions (folk medicine of the North American Indians).

This product should not be used otherwise.

PRECAUTIONS AND ADVERSE REACTIONS

No health hazards or side effects are known in conjunction with the proper administration of designated therapeutic dosages.

DOSAGE

Mode of Administration: Comminuted drug.

LITERATURE

No literature references are available.

Red Sandalwood

Pterocarpus santalinus

DESCRIPTION

Medicinal Parts: The medicinal part is the wood.

Flower and Fruit: The tree bears spikes of yellow flowers.

Leaves, Stem and Root: The plant is a 6 to 8 m high tree with red bark.

Habitat: The plant grows in South India, Sri Lanka and the Philippines.

Production: Red Sandalwood consists of the heartwood of the trunk of Pterocarpus santalinus separated from the sapwood, in some regions also obtained from other Pterocarpus species. It is collected in uncultivated regions.

Other Names: Real Sandalwood, Rubywood, Red Saunders, Sappan, and Sanderswood Red

ACTIONS AND PHARMACOLOGY

COMPOUNDS

Benzxanthenone derivatives (red pigments): chief components santalins A and B (red), additionally santalin AC and santalin Y (yellow)

Isoflavonoids: santal, pterocarpine, and homopterocarpine

Stilbene derivatives: pterostilbene

Volatile oil (traces): chief components cedrol (cedar camphor, up to 50%), including as well pterocarpol, isopterocarpol, eudesmol

EFFECTS

In animal experiments, extracts of the wood are hypoglycemic. Insecticidal and antidiabetic effects are attributed to the pterostilbene constituent. In addition CNS-suppressive, spasmolytic and anti-exudative affects have been described, although detailed information is unavailable.

INDICATIONS AND USAGE

Indian Medicine: Red Sandalwood is used for headaches, toothaches, vomiting, black vomit, diarrhea, fever and conditions of the eye. It is also used to treat stomach ulcers, gallbladder complaints, diabetes, and snakebite poisoning.

PRECAUTIONS AND ADVERSE REACTIONS

No health hazards or side effects are known in conjunction with the proper administration of designated therapeutic dosages.

DOSAGE

Mode of Administration: Red Sandalwood is available as whole, crude and powdered drug forms for internal and external use.

Preparation: To prepare a tincture, 200 parts coarsely powdered drug are mixed with 1000 parts ethanol (EB6).

Daily Dosage: As a tincture, 5 gm.

Storage: Red Sandalwood should be tightly sealed, powdered and protected from light.

LITERATURE

Kumar N et al., PH 13:633. 1974.

Kumar N et al., PH 14:521. 1974.

Kumar N et al., PH 15:1417. 1976.

Seshadri TR, (1972) Phytochemistry 11:881.

Seshadri TR, PH 11:881. 1972.

Singh S et al., Fitoterapia 63:555. 1992.

Singh S et al., Fitoterapia 64:84. 1993.

Further information in:

Kern W, List PH, Hörhammer L (Hrsg.), Hagers Handbuch der Pharmazeutischen Praxis, 4. Aufl., Bde. 1-8: Springer Verlag Berlin, Heidelberg, New York, 1969.

Wichtl M (Hrsg.), Teedrogen, 4. Aufl., Wiss. Verlagsges. Stuttgart 1997.

Red-Rooted Sage (Dan-Shen)

Salvia miltiorrhiza

DESCRIPTION

Medicinal Parts: The medicinal parts of the plant are the dried rhizome and root.

Flower and Fruit: The inflorescences are false whorls with 6 to 8 flowers arranged very close together in glandularly haired racemes with a few lanceolate bracts. The calyx is campanulate, dark purple and glandularly pubescent. The upper lip is simple, the lower lip is longer than the upper lip and thorny-double-dentate with an inner dense ring of white hairs. The petals are violet and glandularly pubescent on the outside. The corolla tube is approximately 1.9 cm long; the upper lip slightly enlarged and turned out. There are 2 long and 2 short stamens and a superior, 2-carpeled, 4-chambered ovary. The fruit breaks up into 4, 1-seeded mericarps.

Leaves, Stem and Root: Salvia miltiorrhiza is a herbaceous perennial growing upright to a height of up to 80 cm. The lower leaves are cordate to ovate. The upper leaves are trifoliolate, crenate-dentate, pubescent above and along the ribs of the lower surface. The rhizome is thick and short.

Habitat: The plant is found in China and Japan.

Production: Red sage (red ginseng) root is the dried rhizome and root of Salvia miltiorrhiza. The plant is dug up in spring or autumn, cleaned, cut and dried.

Not to be Confused With: Mistaken identity can occur with Salvia przewalskii or Salvia trijuga.

Other Names: Red Ginseng, Red-Rooted Salvia, Dan-Shen

ACTIONS AND PHARMACOLOGY

COMPOUNDS

Diterpenes: the so-called tanshinones, including cryptotanshinone, isocryptotanshinone, isotanshinones I and II, tanshinones I and II, miltiron, ferruginol, salviol

Caffeic acid derivatives: including rosmarinic acid, lithospermic acid ethyl ester, salvianolic acids A to E

EFFECTS

Patients with coronary heart disease experienced an improvement in various hemodynamic parameters. At the same time, a significant increase in coronary blood flow due to a reduction of vascular resistance was demonstrated. The drug is antithrombotic, antihypertonic, antimicrobial, antipyretic/anti-inflammatory and hepatoprotective in its effect; it is also said to possess sedative characteristics.

INDICATIONS AND USAGE

Chinese Medicine: Preparations of the root are used for metrorrhagia, pain following menstruation, amenorrhea, post partum bleeding and pain, angina pectoris, furuncles, carbuncles, painful swellings, swelling of the liver and spleen, and joint pain. Efficacy for these indications has not yet been proven.

PRECAUTIONS AND ADVERSE REACTIONS

No health hazards are known in conjunction with the proper administration of designated therapeutic dosages.

DOSAGE

Mode of Administration: Whole and cut drug and their preparations are for internal use.

Preparation: Jiudanshen - Slices of the root, to which wine has been added in accordance with the Jiuzhi method, are roasted until dry.

Daily Dosage: The daily dosage of the drug is 9 to 15 g. The daily dosage of tea is an amount prepared from 3 to 15 g of the drug.

Storage: The drug should be stored in a dry place.

LITERATURE

Chang HM, Chui KY, Tan FW, Yang Y, Zhong ZP, Lee CM, Sham HL, Wong HN, Effect of abietane-type pigments from Salvia miltiorrhiza on post-hypoxic recovery of cardiac contractile force in rats. letter Planta Med, 56:288-9, 1991 Jun.

Chang HM, Chui KY, Tan FW, Yang Y, Zhong ZP, Lee CM, Sham HL, Wong HN, Effect of Liqustrazini and Salvia miltiorrhiza on extracorporeal fibroblast culture. Chung Hsi I Chieh Ho Tsa Chih, 56:547-8, 518, 1987 Sep.

Chang HM, Chui KY, Tan FW, Yang Y, Zhong ZP, Lee CM, Sham HL, Wong HN, Structure-activity relationship of miltirone, an active central benzodiazepine receptor ligand isolated from Salvia miltiorrhiza Bunge (Danshen). J Med Chem, 56:1675-92, 1991 May.

Chang HM, Chui KY, Tan FW, Yang Y, Zhong ZP, Lee CM, Sham HL, Wong HN, Studies on the chemical components of Dan-shen (Salvia miltiorrhiza Bunge) (author's transl). Yao Hsueh Hsueh Pao, 56:489-94, 1980 Aug.

Chen KY, Wen SF, Zhi ZJ, Shao JS, Preliminary observation of 131Cs distribution in experimental acute myocardial infarction and coronary insufficiency treated with root of Salvia miltiorrhiza, flower of Chrysanthemum morifolium and Chrysanthemum indicum. J Tradit Chin Med, 56:265-70, 1983.

Chen WZ, Pharmacology of Salvia miltiorrhiza Yao Hsueh Hsueh Pao, 56:876-80, 1984 Nov.

Cheng YY, Fong SM, Chang HM, Protective action of Salvia miltiorrhiza aqueous extract on chemically induced acute myocardial ischemia in rats. Chung Hsi I Chieh Ho Tsa Chih, 56:609-11, 582, 1990 Oct.

Cheng YY, Fong SM, Hon PM, Effect of Salvia miltiorrhiza on the cardial ischemia in rats induced by ligation. Chung Kuo Chung Hsi I Chieh Ho Tsa Chih, 26:424-6, 390, 1992 Jul.

Cheng YY, Fong SM, Hon PM, Li CM, Chang HM, Prevention and treatment of isoproterenol induced ventricular fibrillation in rats by aqueous extract of Salvia miltiorrhiza. Chung Hsi I Chieh Ho Tsa Chih, 18:543-6, 518, 1991 Sep.

Ding Y, Soma S, Takano-Yamamoto T, Matsumoto S, Sakuda M, Effects of Salvia miltiorrhiza bunge (SMB) on MC3T3-E1 cells. J Osaka Univ Dent Sch, 26:21-7, 1995 Dec.

Dong JC, Xu LN, Beneficial effects of acetylsalvianolic acid A on focal cerebral ischemic rats subjected to middle cerebral artery thrombosis. Yao Hsueh Hsueh Pao, 56:6-9, 1996.

Du H, Qian Z, Wang Z, Prevention of radiation injury of the lungs by Salvia miltiorrhiza in mice. Chung Hsi I Chieh Ho Tsa Chih, 26:230-1, 198, 1990 Apr.

Fu X, Tian H, Sheng Z, Wang D, Multiple organ injuries after abdominal high energy wounding in animals and the protective effect of antioxidants. Chin Med Sci J, 56:86-91, 1992 Jun.

H nsel R, Keller K, Rimpler H, Schneider G (Ed), Hagers Handbuch der Pharmazeutischen Praxis, 5. Aufl., Bde 4 - 6 (Drogen), Springer Verlag Berlin, Heidelberg, New York, 1992-1994.

Hu L, Yu T, Jia Z, Experimental study of the protective effects of astragalus and Salvia miltiorrhiza bunge on glycerol induced acute renal failure in rabbits. Chung Hua Wai Ko Tsa Chih, 26:311-4, 1996 May.

Huang YS, Zhang JT, Antioxidative effect of three water-soluble components isolated from Salvia miltiorrhiza in vitro. Yao Hsueh Hsueh Pao, 18:96-100, 1992.

Li W, Zhou CH, Lu QL, Effects of Chinese materia medica in activating blood and stimulating menstrual flow on the endocrine function of ovary-uterus and its mechanisms. Chung Kuo Chung Hsi I Chieh Ho Tsa Chih, 56:165-8, 134, 1992 Mar.

Liu GT, Zhang TM, Wang BE, Wang YW, Isolation and bioactivity of new tanshinones. J Nat Prod, 43:157-60, 1987 Mar-Apr.

Liu GT, Zhang TM, Wang BE, Wang YW, Prediction and prevention of hypertension syndrome of pregnancy. Chung Hsi I Chieh Ho Tsa Chih, 43:530-2, 516, 1992 Jan 22.

Liu GT, Zhang TM, Wang BE, Wang YW, Prognostic factors and treatment of severe acute pancreatitis. Chung Hua Nei Ko Tsa Chih, 43:82-5, 125, 1991 Feb.

Liu GT, Zhang TM, Wang BE, Wang YW, Protective action of seven natural phenolic compounds against peroxidative damage to biomembranes. Biochem Pharmacol, 43:147-52, 1992 Jan 22.

Lo AC, Chan K, Yeung JH, Woo KS, The effects of Danshen (Salvia miltiorrhiza) on pharmacokinetics and pharmacodynamics of warfarin in rats. Eur J Drug Metab Pharmacokinet, 56:257-62, 1992 Oct-Dec.

Luo HW, Hu XJ, Wang N, Ji J, Platelet aggregation inhibitors from Salvia miltiorrhiza. Bunge Yao Hsueh Hsueh Pao, 56:830-4, 1988 Nov.

Ma XH, Effect of Salvia miltiorrhiza on experimental hepatic regeneration. Chung Hsi I Chieh Ho Tsa Chih, 56:180-1, 1983 May.

Murakami S, Kijima H, Isobe Y, Muramatsu M, Aihara H, Otomo S, Li LN, Ai CB, Effect of salvianolic acid A, a depside from roots of Salvia miltiorrhiza, on gastric H+,K(+)-ATPase. Planta Med, 56:360-3, 1990 Aug.

Qi XG, Protective mechanism of Salvia miltiorrhiza and Paeonia lactiflora for experimental liver damage. Chung Hsi I Chieh Ho Tsa Chih, 18:102-4, 69, 1991 Feb.

Sato M, Sato T, Ose Y, Nagase H, Kito H, Sakai Y, Modulating effect of tanshinones on mutagenic activity of Trp-P-1 and benzoapyrene in Salmonella typhimurium. Mutat Res, 56:149-54, 1992 Feb.

Shen YC, The protective effects of Salvia miltiorrhiza on the warm ischemic kidney: experimental study in animals. Chung Hua Wai Ko Tsa Chih, 56:759-61, 783, 1988 Dec.

Sun RY, Dilative effect of injection of radix Angelicae, Salvia miltiorrhiza and ligustrazin on the pulmonary vessels in rats. Chung Kuo I Hsueh Ko Hsueh Yuan Hsueh Pao, 56:40-4, 1988 Feb.

Wang JZ, Chen ME, Xu YQ, Effect of Salvia miltiorrhiza co. on angiotensin II and atrial natriuretic polypeptide in rabbits. Chung Hsi I Chieh Ho Tsa Chih, 18:420-1, 390, 1991 Jul.

Wang L, Huang X, Ding Z, Chen H, Peng R, Yuan G, Zhou D, The effects of Salvia miltiorrhiza and polysaccharide sulphate on the adhesion of erythrocytes of the patients with cerebral thrombosis to cultured endothelial cells. Hua Hsi I Ko Ta Hsueh Hsueh Pao, 26:381-5, 1995 Dec.

Wu BQ, Cerebral infarction in 141 cases treated by traditional Chinese medicine and Western medicine. Chung Hsi I Chieh Ho Tsa Chih, 56:656-7, 644, 1989 Nov.

Wu YJ, Hong CY, Lin SJ, Wu P, Shiao MS, Cardiovascular pharmacology of Panax notoginseng (Burk). F.H. Chen and Salvia miltiorrhiza. Am J Chin Med, 18:145-52, 1986.

Wu YJ, Hong CY, Lin SJ, Wu P, Shiao MS, Effect of Salvia miltiorrhiza on serum lipid peroxide, superoxide dismutase of the patients with coronary heart disease. Chung Kuo Chung Hsi I Chieh Ho Tsa Chih, 18:287-8, 1996 May.

Wu YJ, Hong CY, Lin SJ, Wu P, Shiao MS, Effects of Salvia miltiorrhiza Bunge on isolated perfused liver and portal vein of rats. Chung Kuo Chung Yao Tsa Chih, 18:749-51, 764, 1992 Dec.

Wu YJ, Hong CY, Lin SJ, Wu P, Shiao MS, Experimental study of Salvia miltiorrhiza on prevention of restenosis after angioplasty. Chung Kuo Chung Hsi I Chieh Ho Tsa Chih, 18:480-2, 1996 Aug.

Wu YJ, Hong CY, Lin SJ, Wu P, Shiao MS, Hypotensive action of Salvia miltiorrhiza cell culture extract. Am J.Chin Med, 18:157-66, 1990.

Wu YJ, Hong CY, Lin SJ, Wu P, Shiao MS, In vitro cytotoxicity of tanshinones from Salvia miltiorrhiza. Planta Med, 18:339-42, 1997 Aug.

Wu YJ, Hong CY, Lin SJ, Wu P, Shiao MS, Increase of vitamin E content in LDL and reduction of atherosclerosis in cholesterol-fed rabbits by a water-soluble antioxidant-rich fraction of Salvia miltiorrhiza. Arterioscler Thromb Vasc Biol, 18:481-6, 1998 Mar.

Wu YJ, Hong CY, Lin SJ, Wu P, Shiao MS, Possible active components of tan-shen (Salvia miltiorrhiza) for protection of the myocardium against ischemia-induced derangements. Planta Med, 18:51-4, 1989 Feb.

Wu YJ, Hong CY, Lin SJ, Wu P, Shiao MS, Prevention of reperfusion injury of an ischemic flap: an experimental study Chung Hua Cheng Hsing Shao Shang Wai Ko Tsa Chih, 18:216-7, 249, 1992 Sep.

Wu YJ, Hong CY, Lin SJ, Wu P, Shiao MS, Studies on cardiovascular actions of Salvia miltiorrhiza. Am J Chin Med, 18:26-32, 1986.

Wu YJ, Hong CY, Lin SJ, Wu P, Shiao MS, The effects of Danshen (Salvia miltiorrhiza) on warfarin pharmacodynamics and pharmacokinetics of warfarin enantiomers in rats. J Pharm Pharmacol, 18:402-6, 1995 May.

Xie M, Jin ZY, Ye GH, Clinical research of compound salviae miltiorrhizae injection for severe pancreatitis. Chung Kuo Chung Hsi I Chieh Ho Tsa Chih, 43:269-70, 1995 May.

Xu HT, Chen SL, Li LS, Effect of Salvia miltiorrhiza on the left ventricular diastolic function in coronary artery stenosis. Chung Hsi I Chieh Ho Tsa Chih, 26:737-9, 710, 1990 Dec.

Xue QF, Effect of ligustrazine and Salvia miltiorrhiza on microcirculation in the hamster cheek pouch. Chung Hua I Hsueh Tsa Chih, 56:334-7, 382, 1986 Jun.

Yu GR, Clinical and experimental study on the effect of Salvia miltiorrhiza on microcirculation and 2,3 diphosphoglyceric acid in patients with coronary heart disease. Chung Hsi I Chieh Ho Tsa Chih, 56:596-8, 581, 1988 Oct.

Yu GR, Effect of Salvia miltiorrhiza on mesenteric microcirculatory blood flow in the dog measured by the Doppler effect of laser light. Chung Hsi I Chieh Ho Tsa Chih, 56:546-7, 516, 1984 Sep.

Yu NC, Zhu YL, Cai LJ, Changes in plasma 6-keto-PGF1 alpha, TXB2 lipid peroxides in acute cerebral infarction patients and the effects of Salvia miltiorrhiza on these three indices. Chung Hua Nei Ko Tsa Chih, 56:596-9, 651, 1988 Oct.

Yu NC, Zhu YL, Cai LJ, New platelet aggregation inhibitors from Tan-Shen; radix of Salvia miltiorrhiza Bunge. Chem Pharm Bull (Tokyo), 56:1670-5, 1983 May.

Yu NC, Zhu YL, Cai LJ, The effect of Salvia miltiorrhiza on the ischemic injury of the intercalated disc of heart in rabbits. (author's transl) Yao Hsueh Hsueh Pao, 56:416-20, 1979 Jul.

Zhang FC, Zheng LJ, Effects of different administration of Salvia miltiorrhiza and heparin on antithrombin IIIAg, antithrombin III: A and alpha 2-macroglobulin in patients with cor pulmonale. Chung Hsi I Chieh Ho Tsa Chih, 18:589-91, 579, 1991 Oct.

Zhang JQ, Zhou YP, Inhibition of aldose reductase from rat lens by some Chinese herbs and their components. Chung Kuo Chung Yao Tsa Chih, 56:557-9, 576, 1989 Sep.

Zhang JY, Effect of Salvia miltiorrhiza root on calcium deposition in experimental fracture healing. Chung Hsi I Chieh Ho Tsa Chih, 56:536-9, 515, 1984 Sep.

Zhang XL, Preliminary study of rose shu-xin oral liquid in the treatment of angina pectoris in coronary heart disease. Chung Kuo Chung Hsi I Chieh Ho Tsa Chih, 56:414-6, 389, 1992 Jul.

Zhang YW, Xue Y, Zhang BQ, Effect of Salvia miltiorrhiza on hyperfibrinogen in patients with malignant lymphoma. Chung Hsi I Chieh Ho Tsa Chih, 56:607-8, 582, 1988 Oct.

Zhao BL, Jiang W, Zhao Y, Hou JW, Xin WJ, Scavenging effects of Salvia miltiorrhiza on free radicals and its protection for myocardial mitochondrial membranes from ischemia-reperfusion injury. Biochem Mol Biol Int, 38:1171-82, 1996 May.

Zhou Y, Pan LM, Zhan S, Studies and preparations of fufang danshen granules. Chung Kuo Chung Yao Tsa Chih, 56:540-3, 575-6, 1992 Sep.

Zhu P, Experimental study on myocardial protection with verapamil and Salvia miltiorrhiza Bunge cardioplegia. Chung Hua Wai Ko Tsa Chih, 26:9-12, 60, 1990 Jan.

Zhuang HM, Zhu HY, Qin ZL, Effect of Salvia miltiorrhiza on the survival time of a heart allograft in experimental animals. Chung Hsi I Chieh Ho Tsa Chih, 56:29-30, 6, 1988 Jan.

Red-Spur Valerian

Centranthus ruber

DESCRIPTION

Medicinal Parts: The medicinal part is the root of the plant.

Flower and Fruit: The numerous flowers are in dense cymes, red, pink or seldom white. The corolla is tubular and spurred at the base. Each flower contains 1 stamen. The fruit is small and dry. The margin of the surrounding calyx forms a pinnatifid rosette or a papus.

Leaves, Stem and Root: The plant grows from about 30 to 80 cm high. The rhizome is perennial and very branched. The stems are tough, bushy at the base, hollow and smooth. The leaves are 5 to 10 cm long in opposite pairs, somewhat fleshy and entire-margined.

Habitat: The plant is probably indigenous to the Mediterranean region, although it is found in Europe.

Other Names: Pretty Betsy, Bouncing Bess, Delicate Bess, Drunken Sailor, Bovisand Soldier

ACTIONS AND PHARMACOLOGY

COMPOUNDS

Iridoids (iridoid epoxy compounds, 1-3%): valepotriates, including valtrate, acevaltrate, didrovaltrate

EFFECTS

The drug has sedative and equilibratory effects.

INDICATIONS AND USAGE

Unproven Uses: The drug is not in current use. It was previously used as a sedative.

PRECAUTIONS AND ADVERSE REACTIONS

No health hazards or side effects are known in conjunction with the proper administration of designated therapeutic dosages.

DOSAGE

No information is available.

LITERATURE

Handjieva N et al., PM 34:203. 1978.

Hegnauer R: Chemotaxonomie der Pflanzen, Bde 1-11, Birkhäuser Verlag Basel, Boston, Berlin 1962-1997.

Kern W, List PH, Hörhammer L (Hrsg.), Hagers Handbuch der Pharmazeutischen Praxis, 4. Aufl., Bde 1-8, Springer Verlag Berlin, Heidelberg, New York, 1969.

Marekow NL, PM 23A:48. 1977.

Schneider G, Valepotriat-Artefakte aus Centrantus ruber. In: Arch Pharmaz 318(6):515- 519. 1985.

Reed Herb

Phragmites communis

DESCRIPTION

Medicinal Parts: The medicinal parts are the stem and the rhizome.

Flower and Fruit: The grassy flowers appear in long panicles of up to 30 cm with a thick crown of hair.

Leaves, Stem and Root: The plant is a sturdy grass with a long, creeping rhizome. It grows up to 3 m and has gray-green leaves.

Habitat: Reed Herb is common worldwide.

Production: Reed Herb and rhizome are the stem (base) and rhizome of Phragmites communis.

Other Names: Common Reed

ACTIONS AND PHARMACOLOGY

COMPOUNDS

Flavonoids: including tricine, luteolin, chrysoeriol, rutin, isoquercitrin

Vitamin A (5 mg/100 gm in the fresh foliage)

Ascorbic acid (vitamin C, 100 mg/100 gm in the fresh foliage)

B vitamins

Sugar: in particular saccharose, inverted sugar (relatively high content in the rhizome)

Triterpenes: including beta-amyrin, taraxerol, taraxerone

EFFECTS

The plant has diuretic and diaphoretic effects.

INDICATIONS AND USAGE

Unproven Uses: Reed Herb is used as a diuretic and diaphoretic to treat digestive disorders. The juice is used to soothe insect bites.

Chinese Medicine: Reed Herb is used for diabetes, leukemia and breast cancer.

PRECAUTIONS AND ADVERSE REACTIONS

No health hazards or side effects are known in conjunction with the proper administration of designated therapeutic dosages.

DOSAGE

Mode of Administration: Preparations are used internally and externally. The fresh and dried forms are used as infusions.

LITERATURE

Hegnauer R, Chemotaxonomie der Pflanzen, Bde 1-11, Birkhäuser Verlag Basel, Boston, Berlin 1962-1997.

Kern W, List PH, Hörhammer L (Hrsg.), Hagers Handbuch der Pharmazeutischen Praxis, 4. Aufl., Bde. 1-8, Springer Verlag Berlin, Heidelberg, New York, 1969.

Tsitsa-Tzardi E, Skaltsa-Diamantidis H, Philianos S, Delitheos A, Chemical and pharmacological study of Phragmites communis Trin. Ann Pharm Fr, 48:185-91, 1990.

Van Ree R, Driessen MN, Van Leeuwen WA, Stapel SO, Aalberse RC, Variability of crossreactivity of IgE antibodies to group I and V allergens in eight grass pollen species. Clin Exp Allergy, 22:611-7, 1992 Jun.

Rehmannia (Di-Huang)

Rehmannia glutinosa

DESCRIPTION

Medicinal Parts: The medicinal part of the plant is the root tuber.

Flower and Fruit: The inflorescences are racemes with approximately 10 flowers. The flower structures are in fives; the calyx is approximately 1.5 cm long, 5-tipped and campanulate. The corolla is a tube that broadens higher up, is 3 to 4 cm long and red-violet. There are 4 stamens and a superior, 2-chambered ovary. The fruit is a loculicidal capsule.

Leaves, Stem and Root: This herbaceous perennial grows up to 40 cm high. The leaves are alternate, 3 to 10 cm long and 1.5 to 4 cm wide. The lamina is obovate to lanceolate and undulating with a crenate margin; the leaves and stem are velvet-pubescent. The roots are partly thickened to tubers.

Habitat: Rehmannia glutinosa is indigenous to China, Japan and Korea.

Production: Rehmannia glutinosa is harvested in autumn; the root tuber is either cleaned and used as it is (called Shoudihuang or Xiandihuang) or is moistened with steam, cut into slices and dried over a fire until the water is reduced by 80% (Shengdihuang).

ACTIONS AND PHARMACOLOGY

COMPOUNDS

Iridoids: chief component catalpol (0.3 to 0.5%), including ajugol, aucubin, melittoside, rehmaniosides A to D

Monoterpene: rehmapicroside

Ionone glucosides: rehmaionones A and B

Monosaccharides/oligosaccharides: stachyose (10%, based upon the fresh weight), saccharose, raffinose, D-fructose, D-glucose, D-galactose

Steroids: sterols, including beta-sitosterol, campesterol, stigmasterol

EFFECTS

The phenolic glycosides of the drug are antibacterial, immunosuppressive and antihepatotoxic in effect. Verbascoside inhibits the thromboxane synthetase system; its efficacy with rheumatic diseases, among others, is thus plausible.

INDICATIONS AND USAGE

Chinese Medicine: The drug is used in traditional Chinese medicine as a diuretic and for its nourishing and strengthening effect on the liver, kidney and heart. The fresh and dried forms are used differently.

Shoudihuang (fresh root tuber) is used in the liver and kidney meridians for paralysis of the larynx, irregular menstruation, allergic lowered immunity, insomnia, vertigo, tinnitus, impaired hearing, hyperhidrosis, diabetes and increased frequency of urination.

Shengdihuang (dried root tuber) is used mainly in the heart, kidney and liver meridians for febrile conditions, dry mouth, nose bleeds, internal bleeding, rheumatism, constipation, hepatitis, diabetes and metrorrhagia.

Efficacy for the indications rheumatism, eczema and viral hepatitis (IV) has been proven in clinical trials with decoctions of the fresh root. Efficacy for the other indications has not yet been proven.

PRECAUTIONS AND ADVERSE REACTIONS

No health hazards are known in conjunction with the proper administration of designated therapeutic dosages.

DOSAGE

Mode of Administration: Whole and powdered drug. Preparations are for internal use.

Preparation: Shoudihuang can be prepared in two ways:

Jiushoudihuang (jiudun method): The drug is simmered in yellow rice wine over a low flame until all of the wine has been absorbed (30 to 50 kg for 100 kg drug). It is then dried in the sun until the outer skin (initially slimy) is dry, and is then cut into 2 to 4 mm thick slices, which are dried.

Zhengshoudihuang (zheng method): Using this method, the drug is steamed until it is smooth and black (80% loss of moisture). It is then cut into 2 to 4 mm thick slices and dried.

Daily Dosage: Decoction — 9 to 15 g drug

Storage: The fresh root is stored in sandy earth, protected from frost. The dried drug is stored dry in areas having good air circulation.

LITERATURE

Feng GP, Zhang SD, Yi NY, Effects of Rehmannia glutinosa, Plastrum testudinis, Aconitum carmichaeli and Cinnamomum cassia on the beta-adrenergic receptors of hyperthyroid rat kidneys. Chung Hsi I Chieh Ho Tsa Chih, 116:606-8, 582, 1986 Oct.

Hänsel R, Keller K, Rimpler H, Schneider G (Ed), Hagers Handbuch der Pharmazeutischen Praxis, 5. Aufl., Bde 4 - 6 (Drogen), Springer Verlag Berlin, Heidelberg, New York, 1992-1994.

Kubo M, Asano T, Matsuda H, Yutani S, Honda S, Studies on Rehmanniae radix. III. The relation between changes of constituents and improvable effects on hemorheology with the processing of roots of Rehmannia glutinosa. Yakugaku Zasshi, 116:158-68, 1996 Feb.

Lu CS, Effects of Rehmannia glutinosa in the treatment of Sheehan's syndrome. Chung Hsi I Chieh Ho Tsa Chih, 116:476-8, 451, 1985 Aug.

Ni M, Bian B, Wang H, Constituents of the dry roots of Rehmannia glutinosa. Libosch Chung Kuo Chung Yao Tsa Chih, 116:297-8, inside backcover, 1992 May.

Ni M, Bian B, Wang H, On the constituents of rhizome of Rehmannia glutinosa Libosch. forma hueichingensis. Hsiao Yakugaku Zasshi, 116:593-6, 1971 May.

Yuan Y, Hou S, Lian T, Han Y, Studies of Rehmannia glutinosa Libosch. f. hueichingensis as a blood tonic. Chung Kuo Chung Yao Tsa Chih, 17:366-8, inside backcover, 1992 Jun.

Zha LL, Experimental effect of Rehmannia glutinosa on the pituitary and adrenal cortex in a glucocorticoid inhibition model using rabbits. Chung Hsi I Chieh Ho Tsa Chih, 116:95-7, 70, 1988 Feb.

Rehmannia glutinosa

See Rehmannia (Di-Huang)

Rhamnus catharticus

See Buckthorn

Rhamnus frangula

See Frangula

Rhamnus purshiana

See Cascara Sagrada

Rhatany

Krameria triandra

DESCRIPTION

Medicinal Parts: The medicinal part is the air-dried root, separated from the rhizome.

Flower and Fruit: The 7 to 12 mm long flowers are spare terminal racemes. The calyx is petaloid. The sepals are splayed, lanceolate, dark red, silky-haired on the outside. The petals are irregular, with 2 glands, wedge-shaped, 3 to 5 mm wide, crimson and spatulate. The flower has 3 stamens. The ovary is ovate, covered in bristly hairs with a thick glabrous style. The fruit is solitary angular and bristled. It is ovate and has numerous red-black bristly thorns.

Leaves, Stem and Root: The plant is a 0.3 to 1 m high subshrub whose long, 3 cm thick root is covered in a brown-red, smooth, peeling bark. The younger branches are dark green, silky to bristly haired, the older ones are black and often gnarled. The leaves are entire-margined, ovate, silver-gray pubescent, 6 to 15 mm long and 2 to 6 mm wide.

Habitat: Rhatany is mostly found in Peru, but there are a few areas in countries bordering Peru and in the central Andes where it is also found.

Production: Rhatany root consists of the dried root of Krameria triandra Ruiz et Pavon as well as its preparations collected in the wild, washed and air-dried in the shade.

Not to be Confused With: roots of other Krameria species

Other Names: Rhatania, Krameria Root, Mapato

ACTIONS AND PHARMACOLOGY

COMPOUNDS

Tannins (10-15%): oligomeric proanthocyanidins

Tanner's reds (phlobaphenes): polymeric, insoluble oxydation products of the tannins

Neolignans: including among others rhatany phenols I-III (0.3%)

EFFECTS

In vitro the drug is antimicrobial, fungitoxic and astringent. Because of the tannin and lignan content, local treatment of oral and pharyngeal mucous membrane inflammation seems reasonable.

INDICATIONS AND USAGE

Approved by Commission E:

■ Inflammation of the mouth and pharynx

Unproven Uses: In folk medicine used internally as an antidiarrheal agent for enteritis, inflammation of female genital organs and urinary tract. It is used externally to strengthen gums and clean teeth.

Homeopathic Uses: Krameria triandra is used for bleeding mucous membranes and painful conditions of the rectum.

PRECAUTIONS AND ADVERSE REACTIONS

No health hazards or side effects are known in conjunction with the proper administration of designated therapeutic dosages. Internal administration can lead to digestive complaints because of the secretion-inhibiting efficacy. Allergic mucus membrane reactions have been observed in rare cases.

DOSAGE

Mode of Administration: Comminuted herb for decoctions and other galenic preparations for topical application, especially in oral and pharyngeal areas.

The drug is a component of various standardized preparations of pharyngeal remedies.

Preparation: 1.5 to 2 gm coarsely powdered drug in boiling water, strain after 10 to 15 minutes (1 teaspoonful = approx. 3 g drug).

Daily Dosage: About 1 gm comminuted drug in 1 cup of water as decoction or 5 to 10 drops of Rhatany tincture in 1 glass of water, 2 to 3 times daily. Undiluted Rhatany tincture painted on the affected surface 2 to 3 times daily. Tea: freshly prepared as a rinse or gargle 2 to 3 times a day.

Storage: Rhatany should be protected from light.

LITERATURE

Hänsel R, Keller K, Rimpler H, Schneider G (Hrsg.), Hagers Handbuch der Pharmazeutischen Praxis, 5. Aufl., Bde 4-6 (Drogen): Springer Verlag Berlin, Heidelberg, New York, 1992-1994.

Madaus G, Lehrbuch der Biologischen Arzneimittel, Bde 1-3, Nachdruck, Georg Olms Verlag Hildesheim 1979.

Scholz E, Rimpler H, Österr Apoth Ztg 48:138. 1994.

Scholz E, Rimpler H, PM 55:379. 1098.

Scholz R, Rimpler H, (1986) Planta Med (6):58P.

Steinegger E, Hänsel R, Pharmakognosie, 5. Aufl., Springer Verlag Heidelberg 1992.

Teuscher E, Biogene Arzneimittel, 5. Aufl., Wiss. Verlagsges. Stuttgart 1997.

Wichtl M (Hrsg.), Teedrogen, 4. Aufl., Wiss. Verlagsges. Stuttgart 1997.

Williams V et al., (1983) Phytochemistry 22:569.

Rheum palmatum

See Chinese Rhubarb (Da-Huang)

Rhododendron ferrugineum

See Rust-Red Rhododendron

Rhododendron ponticum

See Pontian Rhododendron

Rhus aromatica

See Sweet Sumach

Rhus toxicodendron

See Poison Ivy

Ribes nigrum

See Black Currant

Ribes rubrum

See Red Currant

Rice

Oryza sativa

DESCRIPTION

Medicinal Parts: The medicinal parts of the plant are the seeds.

Flower and Fruit: The panicle is up to 30 cm long. The husk is 7 to 9 mm long with 5 clearly protruding veins. They have 8 cm long, light or dark red awns, or no awns at all. The seed is tightly covered by the layers of the husk and is compressed from the side.

Leaves, Stem and Root: Rice is an annual. The stem is hollow, leafy and erect. The leaves are clasping and sheath-like at the base and grow up to 1 m in length. The leaf surface is up to 60 cm long and 1.5 cm wide. The leaves have bristly ciliate spikelets at the base.

Habitat: Rice is probably native to China and India. Today it is cultivated widely in wet areas in the tropics and sub-tropics.

Production: Rice is the seed of Oryza sativa.

Other Names: Nivara

ACTIONS AND PHARMACOLOGY

COMPOUNDS

Starch (70%)

Proteins: including prolamines, glutelins, globulins, albumins

Fatty oil (1.0-1.8% in the entire fruit, 7—12 % in the germ): chief fatty acid linoleic acid (45%)

Polysaccharides, soluble: galactoarabinoxylan

Monosaccharides, oligosaccharides: glucose, fructose, saccharose

Flavonoids: including tricine, tricine-7-O-glucoside, tricinine

Steroids: sterols, including beta-sitosterol, gamma-sitosterol, campesterol

Diterpenes: momilactone A, momilactone B

Trigonelline

Trypsin inhibitors

Lectins

Vitamins of the B-group

EFFECTS

Rice has been shown to be effective for pain relief and sedation of the digestive tract.

INDICATIONS AND USAGE

Unproven Uses: Rice is used during recovery from disorders of the gastrointestinal tract, illnesses of the gastrointestinal tract and diarrhea.

Chinese Medicine: Among uses in Chinese medicine are diabetes, spontaneous perspiration, diarrhea and debility.

Indian Medicine: Rice is used for pneumonia, diarrhea and diseases of the colon.

PRECAUTIONS AND ADVERSE REACTIONS

No health hazards or side effects are known in conjunction with the proper administration of designated therapeutic dosages.

DOSAGE

Preparation: Rice seeds are boiled in water before ingestion.

LITERATURE

Belitz HD, Grosch W, Lehrbuch der Lebensmittelchemie, 4. Aufl., Springer Verlag Berlin, Heidelberg, New York 1992.

Huesing JE, Murdock LL, Shade RE, Rice and stinging nettle lectins - insecticidal activity similar to wheat germ agglutinin. In: PH 30:3565. 1991.

Kern W, List PH, Hörhammer L (Hrsg.), Hagers Handbuch der Pharmazeutischen Praxis, 4. Aufl., Bde. 1-8, Springer Verlag Berlin, Heidelberg, New York, 1969.

Swaminathan S, Rice, This member of the grass family is one of three on which the human species largely subsists. In: Scientific American 250(1):80. 1984.

Vignols F, Wigger M, Garcia-Garrido JM, Grellet F, Kader JC, Delseny M, Rice lipid transfer protein (LTP) genes belong to a complex multigene family and are differentially regulated. Gene, 195:177-86, Aug 22, 1997.

Ricinus communis

See Castor Oil

Rosa canina

See Dog Rose

Rosa gallica & Rosa centifolia

See Rose

Rose

Rosa gallica & Rosa centifolia

DESCRIPTION

Medicinal Parts: The medicinal parts are the petals and the oil extracted from them. Rose is also used in homeopathic medicine.

Flower and Fruit: The flowers are usually solitary, more rarely in twos and threes, on 2 to 3 cm long, thickly-glandular pedicles. The calyx is round to pear-shaped and is usually thickly covered with stem glands and gland bristles. The velvety petals are pink to purple, 2 to 3 cm long and wide. The style and stigma form the ovary that is surrounded by carpels enclosed in the calyx, forming woolly capitula. The ripe, red-brown false fruit is 1 to 1.5 cm long.

Leaves, Stem and Root: The plant, a descendant of Rosa gallica is a low shrub with extensive runners and above ground reed-like shoots, which are erect and branched. They usually grow to between 0.5 to 1 m and are covered with long, revolute or erect thorns and stem glands of different length. The leaves, which are usually penfoliate, less frequently trifoliate, have long glanular, dark green above, lighter and bluer below, leaflets. They grow together at the leaf stem that terminate in free tips.

Habitat: Rose is probably indigenous to Iran and is cultivated worldwide.

Production: Rose flowers consist of the dried petals of Rosa gallica and Rosa centifolia that are gathered prior to fully unfolding. The petals are harvested by hand and dried in the shade.

Other Names: Cabbage Rose, Hundred-Leafed Rose, French Rose, Damask Rose

ACTIONS AND PHARMACOLOGY

COMPOUNDS

Tannins: oligomeric proanthocyanidins

Volatile oil (in the fresh blossoms): chief components (-)-citronellol, geraniol, nerol, phenyl ethanol, Including as well (-)-linalool, and citral

EFFECTS

The astringent effect attributed to the drug is due to the tannin content.

INDICATIONS AND USAGE

Approved by Commission E:

■ Inflammation of the mouth and pharynx

Unproven Uses: Rose flowers are used in folk medicine internally for diarrhea, tuberculosis of the lungs, pulmonary catarrh and asthma, hemorrhage and leucorrhea. Externally, it is used for inflammations of the oral and pharyngeal mucosa, suppurating wounds and lid inflammation.

Indian Medicine: In India, Rose is used for coughs, bronchitis, asthma, fever and general debility. It is also used for wounds and hyperhydrosis.

PRECAUTIONS AND ADVERSE REACTIONS

No health hazards or side effects are known in conjunction with the proper administration of designated therapeutic dosages.

DOSAGE

Mode of Administration: Rose flowers are available as whole, crude and powdered drug forms for internal and external use.

Preparation:

Tea — 1 to 2 gm drug added to 1 cup (200 ml) water.

Rose vinegar — 60 gm petals added to 750 ml red wine vinegar.

Daily Dosage:

Tea infusion — up to 3 cups per day. It is also used for rinses and washes.

Powder — 5 to 10 gm with honey or liquid.

The leaves can be applied directly to the eyes.

Storage: Should be tightly sealed and stored in dry and cool place.

LITERATURE

Kern W, List PH, Hörhammer L (Hrsg.), Hagers Handbuch der Pharmazeutischen Praxis, 4. Aufl., Bde. 1-8: Springer Verlag Berlin, Heidelberg, New York, 1969.

Leung AY, Encyclopedia of Common Natural Ingredients Used in Food Drugs, Cosmetics, John Wiley & Sons Inc., New York 1980.

Madaus G, Lehrbuch der Biologischen Arzneimittel, Bde 1-3, Nachdruck, Georg Olms Verlag Hildesheim 1979.

Rosemary

Rosmarinus officinalis

TRADE NAMES

Rosemary Leaf (available from numerous manufacturers and as combination product)

DESCRIPTION

Medicinal Parts: The medicinal parts are the oil extracted from the leaves and the leafy stems, the flowering, dried twig tips, the dried leaves, the fresh leaves, the fresh aerial parts collected during flowering and the flowering branches.

Flower and Fruit: Labiate flowers grow on tometose inflorescences in the leaf axils of the upper part of the branches. The calyx is 3 to 4 mm, green or reddish, initially tomentose, later 5 to 7 mm and glabrous. The venation is conspicuous. The corolla is 10 to 12 mm long, bluish, occasionally pink or white. The nutlet is brown.

Leaves, Stem and Root: The plant is an evergreen, branched subshrub, 50 to 150 cm high with erect, climbing or occasionally decumbent brown branches. The leaves are linear, coriaceous, entire-margined, light green and somewhat rugose above. They are tomentose, 15 to 40 mm by 1.2 to 3.5 mm.

Characteristics: The plant has a very pungent aroma.

Habitat: The plant is indigenous to the Mediterranean region and Portugal and is cultivated there as well as on the Crimea, in the Transcaucasus, Central Asia, India, Southeast Asia, South Africa, Australia and the U.S.

Production: Rosemary leaves consist of the fresh or dried leaves of Rosmarinus officinalis collected after flowering as well as their preparations. The leaves are harvested after flowering on sunny, warm days and dried.

Not to be Confused With: May be confused with Ledum palustre, Andromeda polifolia, Teucrium montanum, Taxus baccata, Santolina rosmarinfolia, and S. chamaecyparissus.

Other Names: Polar Plant, Compass-Weed, Compass Plant

ACTIONS AND PHARMACOLOGY

COMPOUNDS

Caffeic acid derivatives: chief component rosmarinic acid

Diterpenes (bitter): including carnosolic acid (picrosalvin), isorosmanol, rosmadial, rosmaridiphenol, rosmariquinone

Flavonoids: including cirsimarin, diosmin, hesperidin, homoplantiginin, phegopolin

Triterpenes: chief components oleanolic acid, ursolic acid and their 3-acetyl esters

Volatile oil (1.0 to 2.5%): chief components 1,8-cineole (20 to 50%), alpha-pinene (15 to 25%), camphor (10 to 25%), including as well camphene, borneol, bornyl acetate, beta-caryophyllene, p-cymene, limonene, linalool, myrcene, alpha-terpineol, verbenone

EFFECTS

The drug is mildly antimicrobial and antiviral (probably because of the diterpenes).

Animal tests have demonstrated spasmolytic effects on the gallbladder ducts and on the upper intestine. The tests have confirmed choleretic, liver-protective, anti-convulsive, anti-mutagenic and tumor-inhibiting effects. The metabolism of the drug is accelerated by the presence of 1,8 cineol. In humans Rosemary oil improves circulation when applied externally because of a certain skin irritating effect.

INDICATIONS AND USAGE

Approved by Commission E:

- Blood pressure problems
- Dyspeptic complaints
- Loss of appetite
- Rheumatism

Rosemary is used internally for dyspeptic disorders and externally for hypotonic circulatory disorders and rheumatic conditions.

Unproven Uses: Rosemary is used in folk medicine for digestive symptoms, headaches and migraine, dysmenorrhea, amenorrhea and oligomenorrhea, states of exhaustion, dizziness and poor memory. It is used externally as a poultice for poorly healing wounds, for eczema, as an analgesic for injuries of the mouth and throat, topically for myalgias, intercostal neuralgia and sciatica.

Homeopathic Uses: Rosmarinus officinalis is used for gastrointestinal disorders.

CONTRAINDICATIONS

Rosemary preparations should not be used during pregnancy.

PRECAUTIONS AND ADVERSE REACTIONS

General: No health hazards or side effects are known in conjunction with the proper administration of designated therapeutic dosages. Contact allergies have been observed on occasion.

Pregnancy: Not to be used during pregnancy.

OVERDOSAGE

Very large quantities of rosemary leaves misused for the purpose of abortion, can lead to deep coma, spasm, vomiting, gastroenteritis, uterine bleeding, kidney irritation, and to death in humans.

DOSAGE

Mode of Administration: Rosemary is available as whole, crude and powdered drug forms for internal and external use. It is also available in compounded preparations.

How Supplied:
Liquid — 1:1

Preparation:
Tea — pour boiling water over 2 gm finely cut drug and strain after 15 minutes (1 teaspoon corresponds to approximately 2 gm drug).

Rosemary wine — Add 20 gm drug in 1 Liter wine, let stand for 5 days, shake occasionally.

Tincture — 1:5 with 70% ethanol (V/V)

Liquid extract — 1:1 45% ethanol (V/V)

Daily Dosage: The daily dose is 4 to 6 gm drug.
Tea — 1 cup several times a day

Tincture (1:5) — single dose: 20 to 40 drops

Liquid extract — single dose: 2 to 4 ml

Externally — semi-solid and liquid forms with 6 to 10% essential oil

Bath additive — 50 gm drug to 1 Liter hot water added to full or hip bath

Washes — use 1% infusion

Homeopathic Dosage: 5 drops, 1 tablet or 10 globules every 30 to 60 minutes (acute) or 1 to 3 times daily (chronic); parenterally: 1 to 2 ml sc acute: 3 times daily; chronic: once a day (HAB1)

Storage: Rosemary should be protected from light and moisture.

LITERATURE

Anonym, Phytotherapie:Pflanzliche Antirheumatika - was bringen sie? In: DAZ 136(45):4012-4015. 1996.

Boehlens MH, Perfum Flav 10:21-24, 26 et 28-37. 1985.

Brieskorn CH, Zweyrohn G, (1970) Pharmazie 25:488.

Brieskorn CH, Domling HJ, (1969) Z Lebensm Unters Forsch 14:10.

Brieskorn CH, Michel H, (1968) Tetrahedron Letters 30:3447.

Czygan I, Czygan FC, Rosmarin - Rosmarinus officinalis L. In: ZPZ 18(3):182-186. 1997.

Haraguchi H et al., Inhibition of lipid peroxidation and superoxide generation by diterpenoids from Rosmarinus officinalis. In: PM 61(4):333-336. 1995.

Houlihan CM et al., (1985) J Am Oil Chem Soc 62(1):96.

Koedan A, Gijbels MJM, (1978) Z Natur Forsch 33C, 144.

Kreis P, Juchelka D, Motz C, Mosandl A, Chirale Inhaltstoffe ätherischer Öle. In: DAZ 131(39):1984. 1991.

Litvinenko VI et al., (1970) Planta Med 18:243.

Mascolo N et al., (1987) Phytother Res 1(1):28.

Tattje DHE, (1970) Pharm Weekbl 105:1241.

Further information in:

Fenaroli's Handbook of Flavor Ingredients, Vol. 1, 2nd Ed., CRC Press 1975.

Hänsel R, Keller K, Rimpler H, Schneider G (Hrsg.), Hagers Handbuch der Pharmazeutischen Praxis, 5. Aufl., Bde 4-6 (Drogen): Springer Verlag Berlin, Heidelberg, New York, 1992-1994.

Leung AY, Encyclopedia of Common Natural Ingredients Used in Food, Drugs, Cosmetics, John Wiley & Sons Inc., New York 1980.

Madaus G, Lehrbuch der Biologischen Arzneimittel, Bde 1-3, Nachdruck, Georg Olms Verlag Hildesheim 1979.

Roth L, Daunderer M, Kormann K, Giftpflanzen, Pflanzengifte, 4. Aufl., Ecomed Fachverlag Landsberg Lech 1993.

Steinegger E, Hänsel R, Pharmakognosie, 5. Aufl., Springer Verlag Heidelberg 1992.

Teuscher E, Biogene Arzneimittel, 5. Aufl., Wiss. Verlagsges. Stuttgart 1997.

Wagner H, Wiesenauer M, Phytotherapie. Phytopharmaka und pflanzliche Homöopathika, Fischer-Verlag, Stuttgart, Jena, New York 1995.

Wichtl M (Hrsg.), Teedrogen, 4. Aufl., Wiss. Verlagsges. Stuttgart 1997.

Rosinweed

Silphium laciniatum

DESCRIPTION

Medicinal Parts: The medicinal part is the root.

Leaves, Stem and Root: The plant is a stately 1 to 4 m high herbaceous perennial, with an almost leafless, round shaft. The leaves are 30 to 60 cm long. They are long-petioled, simple or double pinnate leaves. The leaves are alternate, with their edges turned upward and downward and their surfaces facing north and south.

Characteristics: The taste of the root is bitter and then acrid. The roots are odorless.

Habitat: The plant grows in the midwestern U.S., especially Ohio.

Other Names: Compass Weed, Polar Plant, Pilot Weed

ACTIONS AND PHARMACOLOGY

COMPOUNDS

Resins (smelling terpene-like, mastic-like)

Volatile oil

Inulin (in the root)

EFFECTS

The active agents are resin, with 19% terpene and 37% of a resin acid, and inulin in the root. The drug has antispasmodic, diuretic and diaphoretic effects.

INDICATIONS AND USAGE

Homeopathic Uses: In homeopathy, the drug is used for the treatment of digestive disorders.

PRECAUTIONS AND ADVERSE REACTIONS

No health hazards or side effects are known in conjunction with the proper administration of designated therapeutic dosages.

DOSAGE

Mode of Administration: Rosinweed is available as a tincture or liquid extract.

LITERATURE

Kern W, List PH, Hörhammer L (Hrsg.), Hagers Handbuch der Pharmazeutischen Praxis, 4. Aufl., Bde. 1-8: Springer Verlag Berlin, Heidelberg, New York, 1969.

Madaus G, Lehrbuch der Biologischen Arzneimittel, Bde 1-3, Nachdruck, Georg Olms Verlag Hildesheim 1979.

Rosmarinus officinalis

See Rosemary

Round-Leafed Wintergreen

Pyrola rotundifolia

DESCRIPTION

Medicinal Parts: The medicinal parts are the leaves.

Flower and Fruit: The white, sometimes reddish flowers are in many-blossomed, nodding racemes turning to all sides. The calyx is divided in 5 almost to the base and has lanceolate, revolute, splayed tips. The corolla has 5 petals and is flatly campanulate. The 10 stamens are curved upward. The ovary is superior with 5 sections and a downward curving style. The fruit is a 5-sectioned capsule.

Leaves, Stem and Root: The plant grows from 15 to 30 cm high. The stem is erect, obtusely angular and glabrous; it has 2 sheath-like bracts. The leaves in the basal rosette are petiolate, orbicular and glabrous. They are grass-green, glossy, somewhat cordate at the base, shallowly crenate, coriaceous and evergreen.

Characteristics: The flowers have a slight, pleasant fragrance, and the leaves are astringent.

Habitat: The plant originated in the South Sea islands but is now naturalized in other climates.

Production: Wintergreen leaves are the leaves of Pyrola rotundifolia.

Other Names: Wintergreen

ACTIONS AND PHARMACOLOGY

COMPOUNDS

Hydroquinone derivatives (4-8%): chief components isohomoarbutin, additionally homoarbutin (arbutin)

Naphthacene derivatives (naphthoquinone): chimaphilin (2,7-dimethyl-1,4-naphthoquinone)

Tannins (up to 18%)

EFFECTS

No information is available.

INDICATIONS AND USAGE

Unproven Uses: Wintergreen is used for bladder inflammation and urinary tract diseases, diseases of the prostate and kidney disorders.

PRECAUTIONS AND ADVERSE REACTIONS

No health hazards or side effects are known in conjunction with the proper administration of designated therapeutic dosages. The drug possesses a weak sensitizing effect due to its chimaphilin content. The drug is not suitable for long-term use because of its hydroquinone glycoside content.

DOSAGE

Mode of Administration: The drug is administered ground and as an extract.

LITERATURE

Hegnauer R, Chemotaxonomie der Pflanzen, Bde 1-11, Birkhäuser Verlag Basel, Boston, Berlin 1962-1997.

Kern W, List PH, Hörhammer L (Hrsg.), Hagers Handbuch der Pharmazeutischen Praxis, 4. Aufl., Bde. 1-8, Springer Verlag Berlin, Heidelberg, New York, 1969 (unter Pirola rotundifolia).

Madaus G, Lehrbuch der Biologischen Arzneimittel, Bde 1-3, Nachdruck, Georg Olms Verlag Hildesheim 1979 (unter Pirola rotundifolia).

Rubia tinctorum

See Madder

Rubus fruticosus

See Blackberry

Rubus idaeus

See Raspberry

Rue

Ruta graveolens

DESCRIPTION

Medicinal Parts: The medicinal parts are oil extracted from the herb, the herbal parts of the plant harvested after flowering, the fresh aerial parts of the plant collected at the beginning of the flowering season and the whole plant.

Flower and Fruit: The yellow flowers are in cymes, which are on twining branches with entire or 3-lobed bracts. The calyx has 4 or 5 segments. The 4 to 5 petals are spoon-like concave, ovate and end suddenly in the stem. The 8 to 10 stamens are in 2 circles. The single short, broadly ovate ovary has 4 to 5 grooves and is covered with hemispherical glands. The fruit is a globular, 4 to 5 valvular, many-seeded capsule. The seeds are angular and have a bumpy brown skin.

Leaves, Stem and Root: The plant is a sturdy shrub 30 to 80 cm high with a woody root and a crooked, branched rhizome. The shoots are glabrous, pale green and more or less covered in oil glands. The stems are erect, rigid, round, lightly branched and woody from below. The leaves are 4 to 11 cm long and 3 to 7 cm wide, odd-pinate, with 1 to 3 pinnatesect pinna. The terminal segments are spatulate to lanceolate. The front leaves are very finely crenate or serrate, somewhat fleshy, pale yellowish or bluish green.

Characteristics: The odor is tangy and the taste is hot, somewhat bitter and can cause skin irritation.

Habitat: The plant grows in the Balkans as far as Siebengebirge, upper Italy and central Italy and is cultivated elsewhere. Rue is completely naturalized in the southern Alps, southern France and Spain.

Production: Rue leaves consist of the dried leaves of Ruta graveolens. Rue herb consists of the dried above-ground parts of Ruta graveolens. Both are dried in the shade at a maximum of 35° C.

Not to be Confused With: Confusion can arise with other Ruta species.

Other Names: Herb-of-Grace, Herbygrass

ACTIONS AND PHARMACOLOGY

COMPOUNDS

Alkaloids (0.4-0.4%): furoquinoline alkaloids including among others, skimmianin, gamma-fagarine, dictamnin, kokusaginine, ptelein

Acridine alkaloids: including arborinine- 2-arylquinoline

Quinazoline alkaloids: including among others, arborine

Quinoline alkaloids: including graveoline, graveolineine

Volatile oil (0.2-0.4%): chief components are nonan-2-one (50%), nonan-2-ylacetate, undecan-2-one, undec-2-ylacetate further including, among others, linalyl acetate, 1,8-cineole, menthol

Flavonoids: chief component is rutin (2-5%)

Hydroxycoumarins: umbelliferone, herniarin, gravelliferon, rutacultin

Furocoumarins: bergapten, psoralen, xanthotoxin, chalepensin, isopimpinellin, isoimperatorin, rutarin, rutaretine

Pyranocoumarins: including among others, xanthyletine

Lignans: savinin, helioxanthine

EFFECTS

The alkaloids in the drug are anti-exudative. Chalepensin inhibits fertility, and the coumarin derivatives and alkaloids are spasmolytic. In addition, the drug is antimicrobial, abortifacient and photosensitizing.

INDICATIONS AND USAGE

Unproven Uses: Preparations of rue herb and/or leaves are used for menstrual disorders, as an effective uterine remedy and as an abortive agent. In folk medicine, Rue is used for menstrual complaints, as a contraceptive and as an abortive agent. The herb is also used for inflammation of the skin, oral and pharyngeal cavities, earache, toothache, for feverish infectious diseases, for cramps, as an obstetric remedy, hepatitis, dyspepsia, diarrhea and intestinal worm infestations.

Homeopathic Uses: Among uses in homeopathy are contusions, sprains, bruising, varicose veins and rheumatism (especially of the spine).

CONTRAINDICATIONS

Rue is not to be used during pregnancy.

PRECAUTIONS AND ADVERSE REACTIONS

General: No health hazards are known in conjunction with the proper administration of designated therapeutic dosages. The drug can lead to photosensitization, due to its furocoumarine and furoquinoline content; photodermatoses have been observed following skin contact with the fresh leaves. Sensitization is possible following skin contact.

Pregnancy: Vomiting, epigastric pain, liver damage, kidney damage, depression, sleep disorders, feelings of vertigo, delirium, fainting, tremor, and spasm, occasionally with fatal outcome, have occurred after misuse of extracts of the plant as an abortive agent.

OVERDOSAGE

Vomiting, epigastric pain, liver damage, kidney damage, depression, sleep disorders, feelings of vertigo, delirium, fainting, tremor, and spasm, occasionally with fatal outcome, have occurred in cases of overdose.

DOSAGE

Mode of Administration: Preparations of the leaves and root are used internally as a tea and also externally.

Preparation: Tea or a cold decoction is prepared by adding 1 heaping teaspoonful to 1/4 liter of water. (1 teaspoonful is roughly equivalent to 2.8 g drug).

Daily Dosage: 0.5 g of the drug is considered a medium single dose; 1.0 g the maximum daily dose. The tea may be taken several times a day.

Delayed menstruation—2 cups per day of the infusion

For topical use, leaves are used to fill hollow teeth for toothache and juice from the leaves is used as an ear drop for earaches.

Homeopathic Dosage: 5 to 10 drops, 1 tablet or 5 to 10 globules 1 to 3 times a day or 1 ml injection solution sc twice a week (HAB1)

LITERATURE

Amling R, Phytotherapeutika in der Neurologie. In: ZPT 12(1):9. 1991.

Becela-Deller C, Die Weinraute. Heilpflanze zwischen Magie und Wissenschaft. In: DAZ 131(51/52):2705. 1991.

Becela-Deller C, Ruta graveolens L. - Weinraute. In: ZPT 16(5):275-281. 1995.

Grundon, MF, In "The Alkaloids Vol. 11", Pub. Royal Soc Chem (1981).

Hellwig B, Phytochemie, Hauterkrankungen und zentrales Nervensystem, 21. Seminarkongreβ der Bundesapothekerkammer in Erfurt. In: DAZ 135(38):3492 ff. 1995.

Mascolo N et al., (1987) Phytother Res 1(1):28.

Novak I et al., (1967) Planta Med 15:132.

Opdyke DLJ, (1975) Food Cosmet Toxicol 13: Suppl 713.

Paulini H, Waibel R, Kiefer J, Schimmer O, Gravacridondiolacetat, a new dihydrofuroacridone alkaloid from Ruta graveolens. In: PM 57:82. 1991.

Reisch J et al., (1967) Pharmazie 22: 220 et (1970) 25:435.

Reisch J et al., (1976) Phytochemistry 15:240.

Robbins RC, (1967) J Atheroscler Res 7:3.

Rozsa Z et al., (1980) Planta Med 39:218.

Schimmer O, Furochinolinalkaloide als biologisch aktive Naturstoffe. In: ZPT 12(5):151. 1991.

Van Duuren BL et al., (1971) J Natl Cancer Inst 46:1039.

Varga E et al., (1976) Fitoterapia 47:107.

Further information in:

Frohne D, Pfänder HJ, Giftpflanzen - Ein Handbuch für Apotheker, Toxikologen und Biologen, 4. Aufl., Wiss. Verlags-Ges. Stuttgart 1997.

Hänsel R, Keller K, Rimpler H, Schneider G (Hrsg.), Hagers Handbuch der Pharmazeutischen Praxis, 5. Aufl., Bde 4-6 (Drogen): Springer Verlag Berlin, Heidelberg, New York, 1992-1994.

Leung AY, Encyclopedia of Common Natural Ingredients Used in Food Drugs, Cosmetics, John Wiley & Sons Inc., New York 1980.

Lewin L, Gifte und Vergiftungen, 6. Aufl., Nachdruck, Haug Verlag, Heidelberg 1992.

Madaus G, Lehrbuch der Biologischen Arzneimittel, Bde 1-3, Nachdruck, Georg Olms Verlag Hildesheim 1979.

Roth L, Daunderer M, Kormann K, Giftpflanzen, Pflanzengifte, 4. Aufl., Ecomed Fachverlag Landsberg Lech 1993.

Steinegger E, Hänsel R, Pharmakognosie, 5. Aufl., Springer Verlag Heidelberg 1992.

Teuscher E, Lindequist U, Biogene Gifte - Biologie, Chemie, Pharmakologie, 2. Aufl., Fischer Verlag Stuttgart 1994.

Teuscher E, Biogene Arzneimittel, 5. Aufl., Wiss. Verlagsges. Stuttgart 1997.

Wagner H, Wiesenauer M, Phytotherapie. Phytopharmaka und pflanzliche Homöopathika, Fischer-Verlag, Stuttgart, Jena, New York 1995.

Rumex acetosa

See Sorrel

Rumex aquaticus

See Water Dock

Rumex crispus

See Yellow Dock

Rupturewort

Herniaria glabra

DESCRIPTION

Medicinal Parts: The medicinal part is the fresh flowering plant.

Flower and Fruit: The flowers are in flat clusters of 7 to 10 in the leaf axils or opposite the leaves along the stem. They are yellow-white and very small. The fruit is a membranous capsule covered by the calyx and contains 1 seed.

Leaves, Stem and Root: The plant is an annual small shrub of about 15 cm. The stem tends to be decumbent. It is round and branched. The leaves are sessile, entire-margined, elliptical and opposite. The leaves are alternate.

Characteristics: The plant is yellow-green and glabrous; it creates suds when rubbed under water.

Habitat: The plant is found in the temperate and southern regions of Europe and in Asian Russia.

Production: Rupturewort is the complete aerial part of Herniaria glabra or Herniaria hirsuta.

Other Names: Flax Weed, Herniary

ACTIONS AND PHARMACOLOGY

COMPOUNDS

Triterpene saponins: herniaria saponins I-VII (aglycones medicagen, gypsogen, 16-hydroxy-medicagen)

Flavonoids: including hyperoside

Hydroxycoumarins: umbelliferone, herniarin

EFFECTS

The main active principles (saponins, flavonoids, coumarins and small amounts of tannins) are reported to have mild spasmolytic and diuretic effects, which have not been scientifically proven.

INDICATIONS AND USAGE

Unproven Uses: Herniaria glabra is used for disorders of the efferent urinary tract, inflammatory disorders of the kidneys and bladder, respiratory disorders, nerve inflammation, gout and rheumatism, and as a blood purifier.

PRECAUTIONS AND ADVERSE REACTIONS

Health risks or side effects following the proper administration of designated therapeutic dosages are not recorded.

DOSAGE

Mode of Administration: The drug is administered as an infusion and in tea mixtures, as an extract in drops and in urological pharmaceutical preparations.

Preparation: Put 1.5 gm comminuted drug (1 teaspoonful is equal to 1.4 gm) in cold water and bring briefly to a boil. Strain after 5 minutes.

Daily Dosage: Drink 1 cup 2 to 3 times daily as a diuretic.

LITERATURE

Cart J, Reznicek G, Korhammer S, Haslinger E, Jurenitsch J, Kubelka W, The first spectroscopically confirmed saponin from Herniaria glabra. In: PM 58(7)09. 1992.

Franck HP, (1975) Dtsch. Apoth Ztg 115:1206.

Freiler M et al., A new triterpenesaponin from Herniaria glabra. In: PM 61(Abstracts of 43rd Ann Congr):66. 1995.

Freiler M et al., Sci Pharm 64:359. 1996. f Krolikowska M, Wolbis M, (1979) Acta Pol Pharm 36:469.

Reznicek G et al., PA 48:450. 1993.

Tama M et al., (1981) Clujul Med 54(1):73.

Zoz et al., (1976) Rastit Resur 12(3):411 (via CA 85:174257). f Kern W, List PH, Hörhammer L (Hrsg.), Hagers Handbuch der Pharmazeutischen Praxis, 4. Aufl., Bde. 1-8, Springer

Verlag Berlin, Heidelberg, New York, 1969.

Madaus G, Lehrbuch der Biologischen Arzneimittel, Bde 1-3, Nachdruck, Georg Olms Verlag Hildesheim 1979.

Steinegger E, Hänsel R, Pharmakognosie, 5. Aufl., Springer Verlag Heidelberg 1992.

Teuscher E, Biogene Arzneimittel, 5. Aufl., Wiss. Verlagsges. mbH Stuttgart 1997.

Wichtl M (Hrsg.), Teedrogen, 4. Aufl., Wiss. Verlagsges. Stuttgart 1997.

Ruscus aculeatus

See Butcher's Broom

Rust-Red Rhododendron

Rhododendron ferrugineum

DESCRIPTION

Medicinal Parts: The medicinal parts are the dried foliage leaves, the dried leafy branches and the fresh leafy branches.

Flower and Fruit: The pink flowers are in umbel-like racemes. The calyx has 5 short ovate tips. The corolla is fused and funnel-shaped with an edge divided into 5 segments. It is covered on the outside with white or golden-yellow resin spots. There are 10 stamens and 1 superior ovary. The fruit is a 5-valved capsule. The seeds are fusiform, about 1 mm long and light brown.

Leaves, Stem and Root: The plant is an evergreen shrub up to 1 m high and is richly branched from the base upward. The branches are sturdy and elastic with gray-brown bark. The leaves are oblong-lanceolate, tough and glabrous. The margin is entire, involuted. The leaves are dark green above, densely scaled underneath and sometimes rust-colored.

Characteristics: The leaves are not ciliate at the edge.

Habitat: The plant grows in the Alpine chain from the Pyrenees to the southern Croatian mountains, but not in the Carpathians.

Production: Rust-Red Rhododendron consists of the dried leaves of Rhododendron ferrugineum.

Not to be Confused With: The leaves of R. hirsutum. The plant product may be altered through the addition of cranberry leaves.

Other Names: Rosebay, Snow Rose

ACTIONS AND PHARMACOLOGY

COMPOUNDS: RHODODENDRON AUREUM

Diterpenes of the andromedan type (presence questionable)

Hydroquinone glycosides: arbutin (ericolin)

Flavonoids: including polystachoside, avicularin, myricetin, gossypetin, azaleatin

Phenol glycosides (bitter substances): rhododendrine (betuloside, 4-(3'-glucosyloxybutyl)-phenol)

COMPOUNDS: RHODODENDRON FERRUGINEUM

Diterpenes of the andromedan type (presence questionable, but probable)

Flavonoids: including myricetin, gossypetin, azaleatin

Phenol glycosides (bitter substances): rhododendrine (betuloside, 4-(3'-glucosyloxybutyl)-phenol)

COMPOUNDS: RHODODENDRON PONTICUM

Diterpenes of the andromedan type: grayanotoxin I (andromedotoxin, acetyl andromedol, asebotoxin, rhodotoxin), grayanotoxin II (andromedol), grayanotoxin III (andromedenol).

Flavonoids: including myricetin, gossypetin, azaleatin

Phenol glycosides (bitter substances): rhododendrine (betuloside, 4-(3'-glucosyloxybutyl)-phenol)

EFFECTS

No information is available.

INDICATIONS AND USAGE

Because the drug's composition is not fully known, its use cannot be recommended.

Unproven Uses: Rust-Red Rhododendron is used to treat rheumatic symptoms, calculosis, geriatric complaints, gout, high blood pressure, meteorosensitiveness, migraine, muscular pain and neuralgia.

Homeopathic Uses: The drug is used for neuralgia, rheumatism, and inflammation of the testicles.

PRECAUTIONS AND ADVERSE REACTIONS

The Rhododendron species mentioned are considered poisonous. The grayanotoxins prevent the closure of the sodium channels and thus paralyze conduction.

OVERDOSAGE

Signs of poisoning could include cardiac arrhythmias, coordination disorders, diarrhea, hypotension, cold sweats, paresthesia, salivation, severe stupor, spasm bradycardia, vomiting and eventually death through cardiac failure or apnea. Unambiguous proof of toxicity is available only for the foliage, blossoms and sap of Rhododendron ponticum.

Following gastrointestinal emptying (inducement of vomiting, gastric lavage with burgundy-colored potassium permanganate solution, sodium sulphate), administration of activated charcoal and shock prophylaxis (quiet, warmth), therapy for poisonings consists of treating spasms with diazepam (i.v.), bradycardia with atropine, electrolyte substitution and treating possible cases of acidosis with sodium bicarbonate infusions. In case of shock, plasma volume expanders should be infused. Opiates should not be given. Monitoring of kidney function is essential. Intubation and oxygen respiration may also be necessary.

DOSAGE

Daily Dosage: The daily dosage is 5 to 6 gm of drug as an infusion.

LITERATURE

Bewuβtlos nach Verzehr eines Honigbrötchens. In: DAZ 132(27):1440. 1992.

Frohne D, Pfänder HJ, Giftpflanzen - Ein Handbuch für Apotheker, Toxikologen und Biologen, 4. Aufl., Wiss. Verlags-Ges. Stuttgart 1997.

Hänsel R, Keller K, Rimpler H, Schneider G (Hrsg.), Hagers Handbuch der Pharmazeutischen Praxis, 5. Aufl., Bde 4-6 (Drogen): Springer Verlag Berlin, Heidelberg, New York, 1992-1994.

Keller S auf dem et al., PA 25:621-625. 1970.

Lewin L, Gifte und Vergiftungen, 6. Aufl., Nachdruck, Haug Verlag, Heidelberg 1992.

Madaus G, Lehrbuch der Biologischen Arzneimittel, Bde 1-3, Nachdruck, Georg Olms Verlag Hildesheim 1979.

Roth L, Daunderer M, Kormann K: Giftpflanzen, Pflanzengifte, 4. Aufl., Ecomed Fachverlag Landsberg Lech 1993.

Schulz R, Hänsel R, Rationale Phytotherapie, Springer Verlag Heidelberg 1996.

Tang W, Eisenbrand G, Chinese Drugs of Plant Origin, Springer Verlag Heidelberg 1992.

Teuscher E, Lindequist U, Biogene Gifte - Biologie, Chemie, Pharmakologie, 2. Aufl., Fischer Verlag Stuttgart 1994.

Wagner H, Wiesenauer M, Phytotherapie. Phytopharmaka und pflanzliche Homöopathika, Fischer-Verlag, Stuttgart, Jena, New York 1995.

Wichtl M (Hrsg.), Teedrogen, 4. Aufl., Wiss. Verlagsges. Stuttgart 1997.

Ruta graveolens

See Rue

Saccharomyces cerevisiae

See Brewer's Yeast

Safflower

Carthamus tinctorius

DESCRIPTION

Medicinal Parts: The medicinal parts are the flowers, seeds and the oil extracted from its embryos.

Flower and Fruit: Axillary flowers grow in the leaf axils. They are initially red-yellow, later bright orange. The heads are up to 4 by 3 cm and are encircled by upper leaves. The bracts are light green and have thorny tips with a thorny appendage. The fruit is 6 to 8 cm long, obovate or pear-shaped and bluntly wedge-shaped at the base with protruding long ribs. The pappus consists of scales.

Leaves, Stem and Root: Carthamus tinctorius is an annual plant, that grows up to 90 cm high. It has a thin fusiform root. The stem is erect, simple or branched at the top into stiff, glabrous, whitish-yellow and glossy branches. The leaves are long, fairly soft, and glabrous with a thorny-serrate margin and tip.

Habitat: The plant is said to be indigenous to Iran, northwest India and possibly parts of Africa. It is also found in the Far East and North America, and can be cultivated.

Production: Safflower blooms are the dried flowers of Carthamus tinctorius. The flowers are gathered as they begin to wilt, the calyx and inferior ovary are removed, the remainder is put in the shade where it is mildly warm, and left to dry. Direct sunlight destroys the coloring pigment. Safflower or thistle oil is the oil extracted from the embryos of the fruits of Carthamus tinctorius.

Other Names: Dyer's Saffron, American Saffron, Fake Saffron, Bastard Saffron, Zaffer

ACTIONS AND PHARMACOLOGY

COMPOUNDS: SAFFLOWER FLOWERS

Chalcones and their p-quinones: carthamin (yellow), carthamone (red-orange)

Flavonoids

EFFECTS: SAFFLOWER FLOWERS

No information is available.

COMPOUNDS: SAFFLOWER OIL

Fatty oil: chief fatty acids linoleic acid (55-88%), linolenic acid

Carotinoids

EFFECTS: SAFFLOWER OIL

Safflower oil lowers the serum cholesterol levels.

INDICATIONS AND USAGE

SAFFLOWER FLOWERS

Unproven Uses: In folk medicine, it is mainly used as a stimulant, purgative, antihydrotic, emmenagogue, abortifacient, expectorant, pneumonic and for tumors. It is also added to teas for soothing which soothe coughs and bronchial conditions.

Chinese Medicine: In China, Safflower flowers treat amenorrhoea and stomach tumors, as well as for external and internal wounds.

Indian Medicine: The flowers are used for scabies, arthritis, and chest pains.

SAFFLOWER OIL

Unproven Uses: Safflower oil is used for the prophylaxis of arteriosclerosis.

PRECAUTIONS AND ADVERSE REACTIONS

SAFFLOWER FLOWERS AND OIL

General: No health hazards or side effects are known in conjunction with the proper administration of designated therapeutic dosages.

SAFFLOWER FLOWERS

Pregnancy: Not to be used during pregnancy.

DOSAGE

SAFFLOWER FLOWERS

Daily Dosage: The average daily dose is 3 gm of decoction; single dose is 1 gm.

LITERATURE

SAFFLOWER FLOWERS

Akihisa T, Yasukawa K, Oinuma H, Kasahara Y, Yamanouchi S, Takido M, Kumaki K, Tamura T, Triterpene alcohols from the flowers of compositae and their anti-inflammatory effects. Phytochemistry, 12:1255-60, 1996 Dec.

Amling R, Phytotherapeutika in der Neurologie. In: ZPT 12(1):9. 1991.

Caldes G et al., (1981) J Gen Appl Microbiol 27, 157.

Chan, EH et al., (Eds.), Advances in Chinese Medicinal Materials Research, World Scientific Pub. Co. Singapore 1985.

Kern W, List PH, Hörhammer L (Hrsg.), Hagers Handbuch der Pharmazeutischen Praxis, 4. Aufl., Bde. 1-8, Springer Verlag Berlin, Heidelberg, New York, 1969.

Liu F, Wei Y, Yang XZ, Li FG, Hu J, Cheng RF, Hypotensive effects of safflower yellow in spontaneously hypertensive rats and influence on plasma renin activity and angiotensin II level. Yao Hsueh Hsueh Pao, 27:785-7, 1992.

Lu ZW, Liu F, Hu J, Bian D, Li FG, Suppressive effects of safflower yellow on immune functions. Chung Kuo Yao Li Hsueh Pao, 12:537-42, 1991 Nov.

Martinez Flores H, Cruz Mondragon C, Larios Saldana A Reduction of crude fiber content in safflower meal (Carthamus tinctorius L) and its potential use in human food. Arch Latinoam Nutr, 284:295-8, 1996 Dec.

Nose M, FuJimoto T, Takeda T, Nishibe S, Ogihara Y, Structural transformation of lignan compounds in rat gastrointestinal tract. Planta Med, 53:520-3, 1992 Dec.

Shi M, Chang L, He G, Stimulating action of Carthamus tinctorius L. Angelica sinensis (Oliv.) Diels and Leonurus sibiricus L. on the uterus. Chung Kuo Chung Yao Tsa Chih, 20:173-5 192, 1995 Mar.

Thomson RH, Naturally Occurring Quinones, 2nd Ed., Academic Press New York 1971.

Yasukawa K et al., Inhibitory effect of alkane-68-diols the components of safflower on tumor promotion by 12-O-tetradecanoylphorbol-13-acetate in two-stage carcinogenesis in mouse skin. Oncology, 53:133-6, 1996 Mar-Apr.

Zhang HL, Nagatsu A, Watanabe T, Sakakibara J, Okuyama H, Antioxidative compounds isolated from safflower (Carthamus tinctorius L.) oil cake. Chem Pharm Bull (Tokyo), 45:1910-4, 1997 Dec.

Zhang HL, Nagatsu A, Watanabe T, Sakakibara J, Okuyama H, Tinctormine a novel Ca2+ antagonist N-containing quinochalcone C-glycoside from Carthamus tinctorius L. Chem Pharm Bull (Tokyo), 45:3355-7, 1992 Dec.

SAFFLOWER OIL

Caldes, G et al., (1981) J Gen Appl Microbiol 27, 157.

Chan, EH et al., (Eds.), Advances in Chinese Medicinal Materials Research, World Scientific Pub. Co. Singapore 1985.

Kern W, List PH, Hörhammer L (Hrsg.), Hagers Handbuch der Pharmazeutischen Praxis, 4. Aufl., Bde. 1-8, Springer Verlag Berlin, Heidelberg, New York, 1969.

Steinegger E, Hänsel R, Pharmakognosie, 5. Aufl., Springer Verlag Heidelberg 1992.

Teuscher E, Biogene Arzneimittel, 5. Aufl., Wiss. Verlagsges. mbH Stuttgart 1997.

Xu SX, (1986) Chung Yao Tung Pao 11(2):42.

Saffron

Crocus sativus

DESCRIPTION

Medicinal Parts: The medicinal parts are the stigma and style.

Flower and Fruit: The lily-like flowers have two 2 bracts at the base. There is a pale violet-veined calyx, yellow anthers and a white filament. The thread-like style is 10 mm long. The stigma is bright orange. The plant is non-fruit-bearing.

Leaves, Stem and Root: The grass-like plant is a perennial that grows 8 to 30 cm high. There is a large squat tuber, surrounded by reticulate and fibrous sheaths. The leaves are erect or splayed, narrow, and have a ciliate margin and keel.

Habitat: The plant is indigenous to India, the Balkans and the eastern Mediterranean region. It is cultivated in India, Spain, France, Italy and the Middle East.

Production: Saffron is produced by drying the brown-red stigma over fire.

Not to be Confused With: The powdered drug is more or less always adulterated; Calsendula officinalis, Carthamus tinctorius are usually used.

Other Names: Spanish Saffron

ACTIONS AND PHARMACOLOGY

COMPOUNDS

Apocarotinoid glycosides: in particular crocin (crocetin-beta-digentiobioside), colored intensive yellow orange

Picrocrocin (glycosidic bitter principle, up to 4%): the apocarotinoids and picrocrocin are presumably breakdown products of a carotinoid-digentiobioside-diglucoside (protocrocin)

Volatile oil (0.4 to 1.3%): components 4,5-dehydro-beta-cyclocitral (safranal), 4-hydroxy-beta-cyclocitral (breakdown products of the picrocrocin)

Carotinoids: lycopene, alpha-, beta-, gamma-carotene

Fatty oil

Starch

EFFECTS

Small doses of Saffron stimulate the secretion of the gastric juices. Large doses stimulate the smooth muscle of the uterus.

INDICATIONS AND USAGE

Unproven Uses: Saffron is no longer of interest medicinally. It is sometimes used in folk medicine to stimulate digestion.

Chinese Medicine: Chinese uses include menorrhagia, amenorrhea, high-risk deliveries and postpartum lochiostasis.

Indian Medicine: In India, Saffron is used for bronchitis, sore throat, headache, vomiting and fever.

PRECAUTIONS AND ADVERSE REACTIONS

General: Health risks or side effects following the proper administration of designated therapeutic dosages are not recorded.

Pregnancy: The herb is not to be used during pregnancy.

OVERDOSAGE

Lethal poisonings can occur with overdoses or through the abuse of larger doses as an abortient (abortive dosage approximately 10 gm, lethal dosage approximately 12 to 20 gm).

Symptoms of poisoning include vomiting, uterine bleeding, intestinal colic, bloody diarrhea, hematuria, severe schwere purpuras, hemorrhaging of skin of the nose, lips and eyelids, attacks of dizziness, stupor, yellowing of the skin and the mucous membranes (through inclusion of the apocarotinodermas) and central paralysis.

The treatment consists of stomach and intestinal emptying (gastric lavage, sodium sulfate) and the administration of activated charcoal; convulsions to be treated with diazepam, colics with atropine, and any eventual acidosis with sodium bicarbonate infusions. Intubation and oxygen respiration may also be necessary.

DOSAGE

Storage: It is stored in air-tight, non-synthetic containers and protected from light.

LITERATURE

Dhingra VK et al., (1975) Ind J Chem 13:339.

Dufresne C, Cormier F, Dorion S, In vitro formation of crocetin glucosyl esters by Crocus sativus callus extract. Planta Med, 16:150-3, 1997 Apr.

Duquenois P, (1972) Bull Soc Pharm Strasbourg 15:149.

Escribano J, Alonso GL, Coca-Prados M, Fernandez JA, Crocin safranal and picrocrocin from saffron (Crocus sativus L.) inhibit the growth of human cancer cells in vitro. Cancer Lett, 100:23-30, 1996 Feb 27.

Morimoto S et al., Post-harvest degradation of carotenoid glucose esters in saffron. In: PM 60(5):438. 1994.

Thesen R, Phytotherapeutika - nicht immer harmlos. In: ZPT 9(49):105. 1988.

Wagner K, Dissertation Universität Saarbrücken. 1969.

Further information in:

Fenaroli's Handbook of Flavor Ingredients, Vol. 1, 2nd Ed., CRC Press 1975.

Frohne D, Pfänder HJ: Giftpflanzen - Ein Handbuch für Apotheker, Toxikologen und Biologen, 4. Aufl., Wiss. Verlagsges. mbH Stuttgart 1997.

Kern W, List PH, Hörhammer L (Hrsg.), Hagers Handbuch der Pharmazeutischen Praxis, 4. Aufl., Bde 1-8, Springer Verlag Berlin, Heidelberg, New York, 1969.

Leung AY, Encyclopedia of Common Natural Ingredients Used in Food Drugs and Cosmetics, John Wiley & Sons Inc., New York 1980.

Lewin L, Gifte und Vergiftungen, 6. Aufl., Nachdruck, Haug Verlag, Heidelberg 1992.

Liakopoulou-Kyriakides M, Skubas AI, Characterization of the platelet aggregation inducer and inhibitor isolated from Crocus sativus. Biochem Int, 22:103-10, 1990 Oct.

Madaus G, Lehrbuch der Biologischen Arzneimittel, Bde 1-3, Nachdruck, Georg Olms Verlag Hildesheim 1979.

Nair SC, Kurumboor SK, Hasegawa JH, Saffron chemoprevention in biology and medicine: a review. Cancer Biother, 5:257-64, 1995 Winter.

Nair SC, Pannikar B, Panikkar KR, Antitumor activity of saffron (Crocus sativus). Cancer Lett, 57:109-14, 1991 May 1.

Nair SC, Salomi MJ, Panikkar B, Panikkar KR, Modulatory effects of Crocus sativus and Nigella sativa extracts on cisplatin-induced toxicity in mice. J Ethnopharmacol, 16:75-83, 1991 Jan.

Roth L, Daunderer M, Kormann K, Giftpflanzen, Pflanzengifte, 4. Aufl., Ecomed Fachverlag Landsberg Lech 1993.

Salomi MJ, Nair SC, Panikkar KR, Inhibitory effects of Nigella sativa and saffron (Crocus sativus) on chemical carcinogenesis in mice. Nutr Cancer, 16:67-72, 1991.

Steinegger E, Hänsel R, Pharmakognosie, 5. Aufl., Springer Verlag Heidelberg 1992.

Tang W, Eisenbrand G, Chinese Drugs of Plant Origin, Springer Verlag Heidelberg 1992.

Teuscher E, Lindequist U, Biogene Gifte - Biologie, Chemie, Pharmakologie, 2. Aufl., Fischer Verlag Stuttgart 1994.

Teuscher E, Biogene Arzneimittel, 5. Aufl., Wiss. Verlagsges. mbH Stuttgart 1997.

Wichtl M (Hrsg.), Teedrogen, 4. Aufl., Wiss. Verlagsges. Stuttgart 1997.

Sage

Salvia officinalis

TRADE NAMES

Sage (available from a number of manufacturers), Alcohol-Free Sage.

DESCRIPTION

Medicinal Parts: The medicinal parts are the fresh leaves and the fresh flowering aerial parts, the dried leaves, and the oils extracted from the flowers and stems.

Flower and Fruit: The medium-sized, pale violet, white or pink labiate flowers are in 6- to 12- blossomed false whorls, which are arranged above each other in 4 to 8 rows. The surrounding leaves fall early. The calyx is 10 to 14 mm long, funnel-shaped-campanulate, downy, glandular punctate and bilabiate. The upper lip has 3 throrny-awned teeth; the lower lip has 2. The corolla tube has a ring of hair inside. The upper lip is almost straight and the lower lip has 3 segments. There are 2 stamens with almost semicircular bent filaments.

Leaves, Stem and Root: Sage grows as a bush up to 60 cm high. The stem is erect and woody at the base with leafy, quadrangular, white-gray tomentose branches. The leaves are simple, oblong or oblong-lanceolate and narrowed at the base. They are petiolate, densely and finely crenate, ribbed-wrinkled, and white-gray tomentose initially, tough, and evergreen.

Characteristics: The leaves are aromatic, tangy, and bitterly astringent.

Habitat: The plant is indigenous to the Mediterranean region and has naturalized in all of Europe. It is cultivated in North America.

Production: Sage leaf consists of the fresh or dried leaf of Salvia officinalis. In the wild, sage is collected from the former Yugoslavia, the Adriatic coast and those areas that are farther from the coast but are still under Mediterranean influence. The harvest lasts from mid-July until December, depending on the area. October is recommended as the most favorable time to harvest Dalmatian sage.

When Sage is cultivated, it is recommended that the harvest take place beginning in the second vegetation year at the beginning of the flowering period and in the afternoon.

Sage can be dried in direct sunlight, but up to 25% of the oil can be lost. Drying in shade reduces oil loss to 2 to 10%. Optimum drying conditions for preventing oil loss use a drying chamber with vertical incoming air currents at 50° C with 0.9% absolute humidity.

Not to be Confused With: Confusion can arise with the leaves of Salvia triloba and also with Salvia or Phlomis species.

ACTIONS AND PHARMACOLOGY

COMPOUNDS

Volatile oil (1.5-3.5%): chief constituents alpha-thujone and beta-thujone(20-60%), 1,8-cineole (6-16%), camphor (14-37%), borneol, isobutyl acetate, camphene, linalool, alpha- and beta-pinene, viridiflorol, alpha- and beta-caryophyllene (humulene)

Caffeic acid derivatives (3-6%): rosmarinic acid, chlorogenic acid

Diterpenes: chief components carnosolic acid (picrosalvin, 0.2-0.4%), rosmanol, safficinolide

Flavonoids: including, among others, apigenin- and luteolin-7-glucosides, numerous methoxylated aglycones, including among others, genkwanin, genkwanin-6-methylether

Triterpenes: chief components ursolic acid (5%)

EFFECTS

Sage has antibacterial, fungistatic, virostatic, astringent, secretolytic, and perspiration-inhibiting effects. In animal experiments, the herb was found to be antihypertensive and choleretic. It acts on the CNS and is a spasmolytic agent. Proof of an antidiabetic effect found in one study has not yet been confirmed. The essential oil has bactericidal, fungistatic, and virostatic.

INDICATIONS AND USAGE

Approved by Commission E:

- Loss of appetite
- Inflammation of the mouth and pharynx
- Excessive perspiration

Sage is used externally for inflammation of the mucous membranes of the nose and throat and internally for dyspeptic symptoms and as a diaphoretic.

Unproven Uses: In folk medicine, the drug is used internally for gastric disorders such as loss of appetite, bloating, flatulence, diarrhea, enteritis, and excessive perspiration. Externally, Sage is used as a rinse and gargle for light injuries and skin inflammation, bleeding gums, stomatitis, laryngitis, pharyngitis, and for firming the gums.

Homeopathic Uses: The most common application in homeopathy is for excessive perspiration.

CONTRAINDICATIONS

Sage preparations are contraindicated during pregnancy.

PRECAUTIONS AND ADVERSE REACTIONS

General: No health hazards or side effects are known in conjunction with the proper administration of designated therapeutic dosages.

Pregnancy: Sage preparations should not be taken during pregnancy.

OVERDOSAGE

A sense of heat, tachycardia, feelings of vertigo and epileptiform convulsions can occur following extended intake of ethanolic extracts of the drug or volatile oil, or through overdosage (corresponding to more than 15 g of the sage leaves).

DOSAGE

Mode of Administration: Cut herb for infusions, alcoholic extracts, and distillates for gargles, rinses, and other topical applications such as compresses or poultices. The pressed juice of fresh plants is also used. In folk medicine, Sage is used internally as an antihidrotic infusion and ''medicinal cigarettes'' are used for asthma.

How Supplied: Sage is available as an alcohol-free 1:1 liquid.

Preparation:
Tincture — prepared 1:10 with 70% ethanol.

Liquid extract — 1:1 with 45% ethanol.

The formulas for several ''generic'' folk medicine decoctions and infusions follows.

Decoction No. 1 — One spoonful of powdered drug scalded with 1 cup of water, quickly strained, and sweetened.

Decoction No. 2 — 15 g of the fresh leaves with 200 ml of water heated for 3 minutes.

Infusion No.1 — Scald 20 g dried leaves with 1 liter water, steep for 15 minutes, strain, press, and sweeten if required.

Infusion No. 2 — Pour 1 liter boiling water over 50 g drug, strain after 15 minutes and sweeten with honey.

Antihidrotic infusion — Scald 20 g of the dried leaves with 1 liter water, steep 15 minutes, strain, compress and sweeten if required.

Cardiac insufficiency — A tonic infusion is prepared by pouring 1 liter boiling water over 50 g of the drug, strain after 15 minutes, sweeten with sugar or honey.

Diabetes — Prepare a fortified wine made by boiling 100 g of the leaves with one liter wine for 2 minutes.

Inflammation of the bronchial mucous membranes — An expectorant honey is made by mixing 50 g of the powdered drug with 80 g of honey.

Nervous exhaustion — A fortified wine is manufactured using an 8-day maceration of 100 g of the leaves with one liter of wine.

Tumors — The drug is worked into an ointment base or pounded into a paste together with salt and vinegar to make an adhesive paste.

Wounds — The drug is prepared as a cleanser or rinse to heal wounds using a wine made by heating 100 g of the leaves with 0.5 liter white wine for 1 minute.

Daily Dosage: The average daily internal dose is 4 to 6 g of the drug; 0.1 to 0.3 g of the essential oil; 2.5 to 7.5 g of the tincture; 1.5 to 3 g of the liquid extract.

Antihidrotic — 0.25 g of the powdered drug (spoonful or capsules) taken before meals for excessive perspiration and nervous complaints.

Cardiac insufficiency — 1 glass of the tonic infusion can be taken 4 times daily. The decoction dosage (using No. 1 or No. 2) is 1 glass at hourly intervals.

Diabetes — 1 glass of the wine preparation after meals.

Halitosis — The leaves may be chewed occasionally.

Inflammation of the bronchial mucous membranes — 1 spoonful of the expectorant in the morning and at bedtime.

Nervous complaints — 0.25 g of the powdered drug (spoonful or capsules) before meals.

Externally, the following dosages/applications are often used:

Antihidrotic infusion — 200 ml of infusion 1 to three times daily.

Gargles and rinses — 2.5 g of the drug or 2 to 3 drops of essential oil in 100 ml of water as infusion or 5 g of the alcoholic extract in 1 glass of water.

Inflamed mucous membranes — Undiluted alcohol extract is applied repeatedly.

Homeopathic Dosage: 5 drops, 1 tablet or 10 globules every 30 to 60 minutes (acute) or 1 to 3 times daily (chronic); parenterally: 1 to 2 ml sc acute: 3 times daily; chronic: once a day (HAB1), Special doses must be prepared for children.

Storage: Sage leaves are to be protected from light and humidity in sealed containers. Storage duration of coarsely cut drug is 18 months; powder, maximum 24 hours. The tincture is stored in tightly sealed containers away from light. The liquid extract may be kept for up to 2 years.

LITERATURE

Brieskorn CH, Bichele W, (1971) Dtsch Apoth Ztg 111:141.

Brieskorn CH, Salbei - seine Inhaltstoffe und sein therapeutischer Wert. In: ZPT 12(2):91. 1991.

Ferguson G et al., (1973) J Chem Soc Chem Comm 281.

Länger R, Mechtler C, Tanzler HO, Jurenitsch J, Differences of the composition of the essential oil within an individium of Salva officinalis. In: PM 59(7)35. 1993.

Murko D et al., (1974) Planta Med 25:295.

Paris A, Strukelj B, Renko M, Turk V, Puki M, Umek A, Korant BD, Inhibitory effect of carnosolic acid on HIV-1 protease in cell free assays. In: JNP 56(8):1426-1430. 1993.

Raic D, Novina R, Petricic J, Acta Pharm Jugosl 35:121. 1985.

Tada M et al., Antiviral diterpenes from Salvia officinalis. In: PH 35(2):539. 1994.

Telekova D et al., PA 49:299. 1994.

Further information in:

Fenaroli's Handbook of Flavor Ingredients, Vol. 1, 2nd Ed., CRC Press 1975.

Frohne D, Pfänder HJ, Giftpflanzen - Ein Handbuch für Apotheker, Toxikologen und Biologen, 4. Aufl., Wiss. Verlags-Ges. Stuttgart 1997.

Hänsel R, Keller K, Rimpler H, Schneider G (Hrsg.), Hagers Handbuch der Pharmazeutischen Praxis, 5. Aufl., Bde 4-6 (Drogen): Springer Verlag Berlin, Heidelberg, New York, 1992-1994.

Leung AY, Encyclopedia of Common Natural Ingredients Used in Food, Drugs, Cosmetics, John Wiley & Sons Inc., New York 1980.

Lewin L, Gifte und Vergiftungen, 6. Aufl., Nachdruck, Haug Verlag, Heidelberg 1992.

Madaus G, Lehrbuch der Biologischen Arzneimittel, Bde 1-3, Nachdruck, Georg Olms Verlag Hildesheim 1979.

Roth L, Daunderer M, Kormann K, Giftpflanzen, Pflanzengifte, 4. Aufl., Ecomed Fachverlag Landsberg Lech 1993.

Steinegger E, Hänsel R, Pharmakognosie, 5. Aufl., Springer Verlag Heidelberg 1992.

Teuscher E, Lindequist U, Biogene Gifte - Biologie, Chemie, Pharmakologie, 2. Aufl., Fischer Verlag Stuttgart 1994.

Teuscher E, Biogene Arzneimittel, 5. Aufl., Wiss. Verlagsges. Stuttgart 1997.

Wagner H, Wiesenauer M, Phytotherapie. Phytopharmaka und pflanzliche Homöopathika, Fischer-Verlag, Stuttgart, Jena, New York 1995.

Wichtl M (Hrsg.), Teedrogen, 4. Aufl., Wiss. Verlagsges. Stuttgart 1997.

Salep

Orchis species

DESCRIPTION

Medicinal Parts: The medicinal parts of the plant are the tubers of Orchis morio and other varieties.

Flower and Fruit: The flowers form erect spikes. The surrounding leaves are sometimes large and longer than the flowers; they are often colored. The pollen mass is enclosed in 1 to 2 sectioned anthers. The ovary is almost always twisted. The seed skins can be with or without a reticulate thickening.

Leaves, Stem and Root: The species are perennial, medium-sized, glabrous plants with a round, ovate or variously palmate tuber. The leaves are green, sheath-like and tapering.

Habitat: The plant comes from central and southern Europe.

Production: Salep tubers are the subterranean parts of Orchis morio and other varieties of Orchis. They are gathered during flowering season, dried and processed into Salep powder.

Other Names: Cuckoo Flower, Levant Salep, Orchid, Sahlep, Saloop, Satyrion

ACTIONS AND PHARMACOLOGY

COMPOUNDS

Mucilage (Salep mannan, up to 50%): glucans, glucomannans (partially acetylized)

Starch (25%)

Proteins (5-15%)

EFFECTS

The mucilage is rich in mucine and polysaccharides, which act as a demulcent and have protective and sequestering effects on mucous membranes. In animal tests, a lowering of the plasma cholesterol effect was proven. In addition, the drug is said to be analgesic, cholagogic and hypoglycemic, but no further details are available.

INDICATIONS AND USAGE

Unproven Uses: The drug is used for unspecified diarrhea, particularly in children, and for heartburn, flatulence and indigestion.

Indian Medicine: Uses in Indian medicine include diabetes, hemiplegia, chronic diarrhea, neurasthenia and general debility.

PRECAUTIONS AND ADVERSE REACTIONS

No health hazards or side effects are known in conjunction with the proper administration of designated therapeutic dosages.

DOSAGE

Mode of Administration: As a powdered formulation in medicinal preparations.

Daily Dosage: Dosage for commercial pharmaceutical preparations for heartburn, flatulence and indigestion is often 1 teaspoon of powder stirred into a glass of warm water and drunk before or after meals.

LITERATURE

Kern W, List PH, Hörhammer L (Hrsg.), Hagers Handbuch der Pharmazeutischen Praxis, 4. Aufl., Bde 1-8: Springer Verlag Berlin, Heidelberg, New York, 1969.

Steinegger E, Hänsel R, Pharmakognosie, 5. Aufl., Springer Verlag Heidelberg 1992.

Salix Species

See White Willow

Salvia miltiorrhiza

See Red-Rooted Sage (Dan-Shen)

Salvia officinalis

See Sage

Salvia triloba

See Greek Sage

Sambucus ebulus

See Dwarf Elder

Sambucus nigra

See European Alder

Samphire

Crithmum maritimum

DESCRIPTION

Medicinal Parts: The aerial parts of the plant are the medicinal parts.

Flower and Fruit: The 10 to 20 radiating umbels are medium-sized, sturdy and domed. The barely 1 mm long petals are yellow or greenish-white. The style is very short and barely visible. The fruit is ovate-oblong. The fruit wall is thick and filled with a spongy, air-retaining tissue.

Leaves, Stem and Root: The plant is a perennial, glabrous shrub with woody base. The root is long, cylindrical, thick, hard, knotty, ringed, gray, branching upward and polycephalous. The stem is erect, 20 to 50 cm high, round, tender, grooved, hollowed, woody and with fewer branches higher up. The leaves are sea green, fleshy and glossy.

Habitat: The plant grows on the Atlantic, Mediterranean and Baltic coasts.

Production: Samphire herb is the above-ground part of Crithmum maritimum.

Other Names: Sea Fennel, Sampier, Crest Marine, Pierce-Stone, Peter's Cress.

ACTIONS AND PHARMACOLOGY

COMPOUNDS

Volatile oil

Polyynes: including falcarindiol

Furanocoumarins

Ascorbic acid (high content)

EFFECTS

Samphire is a diuretic and also a source of vitamin C.

INDICATIONS AND USAGE

Unproven Uses: The herb is used for scurvy and states of general resistance.

PRECAUTIONS AND ADVERSE REACTIONS

Health risks or side effects following the proper administration of designated therapeutic dosages are not recorded.

DOSAGE

Mode of Administration: Samphire is used internally and is available as an extract and a food additive.

LITERATURE

Francke W, (1982) Econ Bot 36 (2):163.

Hegnauer R, Chemotaxonomie der Pflanzen, Bde 1-11, Birkhäuser Verlag Basel, Boston, Berlin 1962-1997.

Sandalwood

Santalum album

DESCRIPTION

Medicinal Parts: The medicinal parts are the oil extracted from the trunk wood, the heartwood freed from the sapwood and the bark, and the dried wood.

Flower and Fruit: The flowers are in numerous, small, short pedicled, odorless and erect paniculate inflorescences. There is no calyx. The perianth is 4 to 5 mm long, campanulate and changes from yellow to deep red. There are 4 stamens at the mouth of the tube, which have simple hairs at their base. The semi-inferior ovary with 3 ovules is free in the bud and later enclosed in the disc. The fruit is a round, black, pea-sized drupe with a crown made up of the perianth remains.

Leaves, Stem and Root: The plant is a small evergreen tree up to 10 m high that flowers the whole year round. It has smooth bark and pendulous branches. The leaves are opposite, 4 to 6 cm long and 2 cm wide, lanceolate, entire-margined, and matte underneath. The petiole is approximately 1 cm long.

Characteristics: The wood has a characteristic odor.

Habitat: The tree grows wild in India and also is cultivated there and on Timor and the Sunda Islands.

Production: Sandalwood consists of the heartwood, the trunk and branches of Santalum album or Pterocarpus santalinius, which has been freed from the bark and sapwood.

Not to be Confused With: Confusion can arise with other sandalwoods, i.e. the heartwood of Pterocarpus santalinus. The white sapwood, which contains almost no essential oil, is occasionally marketed as Lignum santali albi. The brownish-yellow to brown-red root wood is, in contrast, rich in essential oil, but is disallowed as a drug in EB6.

Other Names: Sanderswood, White Saunders, Yellow Saunders

ACTIONS AND PHARMACOLOGY

COMPOUNDS

Volatile oil (3-5%): chief components santalols (50% cis-alpha-santalol, 20% cis-beta-santalol, 4% epi-beta-santalol), further including among others, alpha-bergamotol, alpha-bergamotal

Tannins

Resins

EFFECTS

The essential oil of Sandalwood has disinfecting effect on the urinary tract. However, if used in high doses and for long periods, it can be toxic to the kidneys.

INDICATIONS AND USAGE

Approved by Commission E:

- Infections of the urinary tract

Sandalwood is used for inflammatory conditions of the efferent urinary tract. It is generally used in combination with other diuretic or urinary disinfecting drugs.

Chinese Medicine: The Chinese use Sandalwood primarily for epigastric pain, chest pain and vomiting.

Homeopathic Uses: Uses of the drug in homeopathy include urethral inflammation. It is advisable to use Sandalwood in combination with other diuretic or urinary disinfecting drugs.

Indian Medicine: Internal uses include heat stroke, sunstroke and resulting fever. It is used as an infusion mixed with honey (in Kerala); with water cooked in rice (in Nepal); in the treatment of gonorrhea and as an anti-aphrodisiac in ayurvedic medicine.

CONTRAINDICATIONS

Sandalwood is contraindicated in diseases of the kidney.

PRECAUTIONS AND ADVERSE REACTIONS

No health hazards are known in conjunction with the proper administration of designated therapeutic dosages. Intake can occasionally lead to skin itching, queasiness, gastrointestinal complaints and hematuria. The drug possesses minimal potential for sensitization.

DOSAGE

Mode of Administration: Sandalwood is used internally in preparations derived from comminuted drug.

Preparation: Sandalwood oil should only be taken in an enteric-coated form.

Daily Dosage: The average daily dose is 10 g of the drug; 1 to 1.5 g of the essential oil.

Homeopathic Dosage: 5 drops, 1 tablet or 10 globules every 30 to 60 minutes (acute) or 1 to 3 times daily (chronic); parenterally: 1 to 2 ml sc acute: 3 times daily; chronic: once a day (HAB34).

LITERATURE

Adams DR et al., (1975) Phytochemistry 14:1459.

Brunke EJ, Dragoco Rep 35:102-109. 1980.

Demole DR et al., (1976) Helv Chim Acta 59:737.

Hänsel R, Keller K, Rimpler H, Schneider G (Hrsg.), Hagers Handbuch der Pharmazeutischen Praxis, 5. Aufl., Bde 4-6 (Drogen), Springer Verlag Berlin, Heidelberg, New York, 1992-1994.

Lewin L, Gifte und Vergiftungen, 6. Aufl., Nachdruck, Haug Verlag, Heidelberg 1992.

Madaus G, Lehrbuch der Biologischen Arzneimittel, Bde 1-3, Nachdruck, Georg Olms Verlag Hildesheim 1979.

Patnikar SK, Naik CG, (1975) Tetrahedron Letters 15:1293.

Roth L, Daunderer M, Kormann K, Giftpflanzen, Pflanzengifte, 4. Aufl., Ecomed Fachverlag Landsberg Lech 1993.

Steinegger E, Hänsel R, Pharmakognosie, 5. Aufl., Springer Verlag Heidelberg 1992.

Wagner H, Wiesenauer M, Phytotherapie. Phytopharmaka und pflanzliche Homöopathika, Fischer-Verlag, Stuttgart, Jena, New York 1995.

Sandarac

Tetraclinis articulata

DESCRIPTION

Medicinal Parts: The medicinal parts of the plant are the naturally flowing resin and the bark.

Flowers and Fruit: The inflorescences are apical on the lateral branches and conical. The male flowers are 4 to 5 mm wide. There are 4 stamens with very short filaments and scale-like anthers. The female flowers are very small, with 4 scales in 2 pairs arranged like whorls. The upper surface of the flower is fleshy, with a swelling at the base almost completely covering the ovules, which are on woody, dark-brown, approximately 12 mm long cone scales. The seeds are narrow ovoid with large, membranous wings on both sides.

Leaves, Stem and Root: Tetraclinis articulata grows as a monoclinous, monoecious evergreen shrub or tree, reaching a height of up to 12 m. The leaves are opposite, scaly, long and down-turned. They grow close together in groups of 2 pairs on young branches in whorls. The branches are jointed and somewhat pressed together.

Habitat: North Africa, particularly Morocco and Algeria

Production: Sandarac gum is the resin that flows naturally from the branches and bark of Tetraclines articulata.

Other Names: Arartree, Alerce, Sandarac Gum Tree, Gharghar

ACTIONS AND PHARMACOLOGY

COMPOUNDS

Diterpenes (95%): diterpene acids: including pimaric acid, callitrolic acid, sandaracinic acid, sandaracinolic acid, sandaracolic acid, callitrisinic acid

Bitter substances

Volatile oil (1.3%): including alpha- and beta-pinene, limonene, thymoquinone

EFFECTS

The resin is said to be antibacterial and bacteriostatic in effect. Experimental data supporting these effects is not available.

INDICATIONS AND USAGE

Unproven Uses: The plant's use as a fumigant for rheumatic and gouty complaints and edematous swellings has been known since the 19th century. Other folk medicine uses include fever and diarrhea.

PRECAUTIONS AND ADVERSE REACTIONS

No health hazards are known in conjunction with the proper administration of designated therapeutic dosages.

DOSAGE

Mode of Administration: Whole and cut drug is either inhaled or used in the form of compresses.

LITERATURE

Blaschek W, Hänsel R, Keller K, Reichling J, Rimpler G, Schneider G (Eds), Hagers Handbuch der Pharmazeutischen Praxis. Folgebände 1 und 2. Drogen A-Z. Springer. Berlin, Heidelberg 1998.

Sanguinaria canadensis

See Bloodroot

Sanguisorba officinalis

See Great Burnet

Sanicula europaea

See European Sanicle

Santalum album

See Sandalwood

Santolina chamaecyparissias

See Lavender Cotton

Saponaria officinalis

See Soapwort

Sarracenia purpurea

See Pitcher Plant

Sarsaparilla

Smilax species

TRADE NAMES

Sarsaparilla (available from numerous manufacturers) Sarsaparilla Root

DESCRIPTION

Medicinal Parts: The medicinal parts are the dried roots, the entire underground part and the tuberous swellings produced by the runners.

Flower and Fruit: The flowers are white to pale green, yellow or brown. They are dioecious, usually in axillary cymes or racemes, and contain 6 petals in 2 circles. The ovate to lanceolate tepals are curved outward. The male flowers have 6 stamens with thick filaments and anthers, which are fused at the base of the petals. The female flowers have 6, sometimes only 3, staminoids. The ovate ovary has 3 carpels, each with 1 to 2 atropic ovules and with an almost sessile, bent-back, 3-lobed stigma. The fruit is a globular, red, blue or black berry with 1 to 6 seeds.

Leaves, Stem and Root: The species are evergreen shrubs or semishrubs with climbing branches and stipular tendrils. They have a short, gnarled, perennial, creeping or ascending rhizome with numerous long roots stretching over many meters. The branched, thorny, nodular stem has the thickness of an arm and is yellowish-green. The leaves are in 2 rows. They are alternate, simple and often hardy, with 3, occasionally 5, reticulately joined main ribs. The leaf sheaths are ovate and cordate, sagittate and petiolate, or often stipule-like. They turn into climbing tendrils above and break off at this point when they die.

Habitat: The species is indigenous to tropical and subtropical regions of America, eastern Asia and India. In Europe, only the variety S. aspera is found in the Mediterranean region.

Production: Sarsaparilla consists of the dried root of Smilax species, such as Smilax aristolochiaefolii, Smilax regelii and Smilax febrifuga. The plant is collected in the wild from January to May. The roots are cut up and air-dried.

Not to be Confused With: Adulterations and mistaken identity often occurs among the Smilax species.

ACTIONS AND PHARMACOLOGY

COMPOUNDS

Steroid saponins (0.5-3%): chief components are sarsaparilloside, along with parillin, as a breakdown product; also including among others desglucoparillin, desglucorhamnoparillin, aglycones sarsapogenin

EFFECTS

The steroid saponins in the drug are responsible for its irritating effect on the skin and the strong diuretic and diaphoretic effect in high doses, as well as its effect as an emulsifier and foam stabilizer.

INDICATIONS AND USAGE

Unproven Uses: Preparations of Sarsaparilla root are used for skin diseases, psoriasis, rheumatic complaints, kidney diseases, and as a diuretic and diaphoretic.

Homeopathic Uses: In homeopathy Smilax is used for itching skin rashes, rheumatism and inflammation of the urinary organs.

PRECAUTIONS AND ADVERSE REACTIONS

No health hazards are known in conjunction with the proper administration of designated therapeutic dosages. Stomach complaints and queasiness may occur in rare cases, as could kidney irritation.

DOSAGE

Daily Dosage:

Powder — 0.3 to 1.5 g drug

Tea — 3 cups daily with meals

Cold water extract — 500 ml mornings and evenings

Decoction — 1 to 5 g 3 times daily

Tincture — 5 to 15 g per day

Liquid extract — 8 to 15 ml

Homeopathic Dosage: 5 drops, 1 tablet or 10 globules every 30 to 60 minutes (acute) or 1 to 3 times daily (chronic); parenterally: 1 to 2 ml sc, acute: 3 times daily; chronic: once a day (HAB34)

LITERATURE

Elmunajied DT et al., (1965) Phytochemistry 4(4):587.

Thurmon FM, (1942) New Eng. J Med 227(4):128.

Tschesche R et al., (1969) Chem Ber 102:1253.

Tschesche R et al., Chem Ber 102:53-61. 1969.

Tschesche R et al., Liebigs Ann Chem 699:212. 1966.

Tschesche R, In: Pharmacognosy, Phytochemistry, Ed. H Wagner, L Hörhammer, Pub. Springer-Verlag (1971).

Further information in:

Hänsel R, Keller K, Rimpler H, Schneider G (Hrsg.), Hagers Handbuch der Pharmazeutischen Praxis, 5. Aufl., Bde 4-6 (Drogen): Springer Verlag Berlin, Heidelberg, New York, 1992-1994.

Leung AY, Encyclopedia of Common Natural Ingredients Used in Food Drugs, Cosmetics, John Wiley & Sons Inc., New York 1980.

Madaus G, Lehrbuch der Biologischen Arzneimittel, Bde 1-3, Nachdruck, Georg Olmserlag Hildesheim 1979.

Roth L, Daunderer M, Kormann K, Giftpflanzen, Pflanzengifte, 4. Aufl., Ecomed Fachverlag Landsberg Lech 1993.

Teuscher E, Biogene Arzneimittel, 5. Aufl., Wiss. Verlagsges. Stuttgart 1997.

Wagner H, Wiesenauer M, Phytotherapie. Phytopharmaka und pflanzliche Homöopathika, Fischer-Verlag, Stuttgart, Jena, New York, 1995.

Sassafras

Sassafras albidum

DESCRIPTION

Medicinal Parts: The medicinal parts are the essential oil of the root wood, the peeled and dried root bark, and the root wood.

Flower and Fruit: The flowers appear before the leaves. They are dioecious, small and yellowish, and form loose cymes. The perigone has 6 tepals. The male flower has 6 filaments and the female has 1 ovate ovary and 6 bent stamens. The fruit is a pea-sized, oval drupe that, when ripe, is dark blue and appears in the beaker-shaped receptacle.

Leaves, Stem and Root: Sassafras albidum is a deciduous tree up to 30 m tall with numerous branches. The bark of the trunk and of the thicker branches is rough, deeply grooved and grayish. The bark of the outer branches is green. The alternate leaves are petiolate and 7 to 12 cm long. Some are simple ovate, others deeply 2- or 3-lobed. The root bark is a bright, rusty-brown and its irregular pieces are soft, brittle and corky. They grow in distinct layers and show numerous oil glands. The root itself is brownish-white with clear concentric rings traversed by narrow medullary rays.

Characteristics: The taste is sweet and slightly astringent and the odor is pleasantly aromatic. Sassafras' carcinogenic effect, however, has made its use inadvisable.

Habitat: The plant is common to eastern North America, Mexico, and Taiwan.

Production: Sassafras wood is the root wood of Sassafras albidium. The woody roots (up to 20 cm thick) are dug up in autumn, then shredded, cut or sawn into cubes. The wood must not be moistened when being cut because moisture will cause a deterioration of smell and taste in the later drying process.

Not to be Confused With: Sassafras root wood is sometimes confused with the wood of the tree's trunk, which has distinctive annual ring growth and marrow, or with the bark, which has calculus and primary fibers. Another difference is that the trunk wood and bark have little smell or taste.

Other Names: Ague Tree, Cinnamon Wood, Saxifrax, Sassafrax

ACTIONS AND PHARMACOLOGY

COMPOUNDS

Volatile oil (6-9%): chief components safrole (up to 90%), 5-methoxyeugenol (up to 30%), asarone (up to 18%), camphor (up to 5%)

Isoquinoline alkaloids: representatives of the aporphine and reticuline type (less than 0.1%)

EFFECTS

The drug is said to have a mild diuretic effect, which is undocumented. The toxic characteristics are determined by the essential oil, which contains safrole (sassafras aetheroleum that is renal toxic and carcinogenic).

INDICATIONS AND USAGE

Unproven Uses: Sassafras is considered obsolete, but previously was used for disorders of the urinary tract. The drug, which was formerly an ingredient of ''blood-cleaning tea,'' has also been used for skin disorders, inflammation of the mucous membranes, rheumatism and syphilis.

PRECAUTIONS AND ADVERSE REACTIONS

Because of the carcinogenic effect of the safrole, neither the drug nor its volatile oil should be administered.

DOSAGE

Mode of Administration: The drug is a constituent of tea mixtures.

Preparation: To prepare an infusion, add 50 g of the drug to 1 liter of water. To prepare a tea, add 1 teaspoonful (3 g) of the drug to boiling water and strain after 10 minutes. A tincture is prepared using 200 parts coarse powder mixed with 100 parts diluted wine spirit.

Daily Dosage: A single dose of tincture consists of 5 g.

Storage: Keep Sassafras in a tightly sealed tin container.

LITERATURE

Albert K, Sassafrasöl zum Abtanzen? In: PZ 142(11):878. 1997.

Borchet P et al., (1973) Cancer Res 33:575.

Brophy JJ, Goldsack RJ, House APN, Lassak EV, J Ess Oil Res 5:117-122. 1993.

Chowdhury BK et al., (1976) Phytochemistry 15:1803.

Kamdem DP et al., Chemical composition of essential oil from the root bark of Sassafras albidum. In: PM 61(6):574-575. 1995.

Kampen KR van, Sudan grass and sorghum poisoning of horse: a possible lathyrogenic disease. In: J Am Vet Medic Assoc 156, 629-630. 1970.

Miller EC et al., (1983) Cancer Res 43:1124.

Segelman AB et al., (1976) J Am Med Ass 236:477.

Sethi ML et al., (1976) Phytochemistry 15:1773.

Further information in:

Frohne D, Pfänder HJ, Giftpflanzen - Ein Handbuch für Apotheker, Toxikologen und Biologen, 4. Aufl., Wiss. Verlags-Ges. Stuttgart 1997.

Hänsel R, Keller K, Rimpler H, Schneider G (Hrsg.), Hagers Handbuch der Pharmazeutischen Praxis, 5. Aufl., Bde 4-6 (Drogen), Springer Verlag Berlin, Heidelberg, New York, 1992-1994.

Lewin L, Gifte und Vergiftungen, 6. Aufl., Nachdruck, Haug Verlag, Heidelberg 1992.

Madaus G, Lehrbuch der Biologischen Arzneimittel, Bde 1-3, Nachdruck, Georg Olms Verlag Hildesheim 1979.

Roth L, Daunderer M, Kormann K, Giftpflanzen, Pflanzengifte, 4. Aufl., Ecomed Fachverlag Landsberg Lech 1993.

Steinegger E, Hänsel R, Pharmakognosie, 5. Aufl., Springer Verlag Heidelberg 1992.

Teuscher E, Lindequist U, Biogene Gifte - Biologie, Chemie, Pharmakologie, 2. Aufl., Fischer Verlag Stuttgart 1994.

Wichtl M (Hrsg.), Teedrogen, 4. Aufl., Wiss. Verlagsges. Stuttgart 1997.

Sassafras albidum

See Sassafras

Satureja hortensis

See Summer Savory

Saussurea costus

See Costus

Savin Tops

Juniperus sabina

DESCRIPTION

Medicinal Parts: The medicinal parts are the essential oil of the leaves and branch tips; the dried leafy branch tips; the fresh, youngest non-woody branch tips with leaves; and the branches and leaves.

Flower and Fruit: The male and female flowers are at the end of the twigs, which are covered in leaf-scales. The male flowers are up to 2 mm wide and oblong to ovate. The female flowering branch bears the flowers erect when in bloom, later curved inward. The flowers have 4 carpels, which develop into pea-sized berry-cones with 4 ovate seeds. The seeds are ovate and striped with numerous edges.

Leaves, Stem and Root: It is generally a 4.5 m high, dioecious, evergreen shrub with either an erect trunk, an irregular crown or numerous low-lying branches with erect tips. The bark of the young branches are light brown, of more mature branches red-brown and peeling. The young plants up to 10 years have only needle-like 4 mm long, blue-green leaves whose tips stand out. Mature plants have triangular, scale-like, imbricate leaves.

Habitat: Found in southern and central Europe, the Caucasus and the southern mountains of Asian Russia, as well as in the northern U.S.

Production: Savin Tops is the young shoots and twig tips of Juniperus sabina.

Other Names: Savin, Savine

ACTIONS AND PHARMACOLOGY

COMPOUNDS

Volatile oil (3-5%): chief components sabinyl acetate, sabinene, further including among others beta-myrcene, terpin-4-ol, gamma-terpinene, alpha-pinene, limonene

Lignans: including among others deoxypodorhizone, deoxypodophyllotoxin, junaphtoinsäure, deoxypicropodophyllotoxin, and dehydropodophyllotoxin

Hydroxycoumarins: including among others cumarsabine, 8-methoxycumarsabine, siderin, 4-methoxy-5-methylcoumarin- propiophenone

Propiophenone derivatives: including among others 2-hydroxy-3,4-dimethoxy-6-methyl-propiophenone

EFFECTS

The drug is hyperemic both internally and externally, and is a strong irritant to the skin and mucous membrane.

Lignans are also said to have antineoplastic and antiviral properties: The main substance is 3 to 5% essential oil with thujon acting as the principal ingredient, along with containing podophyllotoxin and other lignans.

A diuretic effect has been described for the essential oil and the drug is also said to be emmenagogic and hemostyptic.

The use of the drug on viral warts seems justified because of the podophyllotoxin content.

INDICATIONS AND USAGE

Unproven Uses: For external use only, in the treatment of fig warts.

Homeopathic Uses: Juniperus sabina is used for metrorrhagia, gout, inflammation of the urogenital tract, rheumatism and warts.

PRECAUTIONS AND ADVERSE REACTIONS

The drug is severely toxic. External administration, in particular of the volatile oil, can lead to severe skin irritation, blister formation, necroses and resorbent poisonings.

OVERDOSAGE

One is cautioned against internal administration of the drug and of the volatile oil. Fatal poisonings have occurred repeatedly following administration of the drug in either powder form or infusion as an abortient. Symptoms include, among others, queasiness, cardiac rhythm disorders, spasm, kidney damage and hematuria. Death finds the patient in a state of central paralysis and deep unconsciousness. The internal administration of 6 drops of the volatile oil is life-threatening for humans.

Following gastrointestinal emptying, (inducement of vomiting, gastric lavage, sodium sulfate) and instillation of activated charcoal, the therapy for poisonings consists of treating spasms with diazepam (I.V.), colic with atropine, electrolyte substitution and treating possible cases of acidosis with sodium bicarbonate infusions. Monitoring of kidney function, blood coagulation and liver values is essential. Intubation and oxygen respiration may also be necessary. The level of danger depends upon the age of the drug of the volatile oil, as the toxicity probably develops chiefly through the formation of terpene peroxides during storage. The fresh tips of the branches contain presumably very little toxicity.

DOSAGE

Mode of Administration: For external use, as a powdered drug. Internal application is obsolete because of the danger of intoxication.

Daily Dosage: maximum 1 gm externally.

Savin Tops powder - Powder twice daily, put bandages into the folds of skin.

Skin ointment - Average content: 50% drug.

Homeopathic Dosage: 5 drops, 1 tablet or 10 globules every 30 to 60 minutes (acute) or 1 to 3 times daily (chronic); parenterally: 1 to 2 ml sc acute, 3 times daily; chronic: once a day (HAB1).

LITERATURE

Feliciano AS, Del Corral JMM, Gordaliza M, Castro A, Acid and phenolic lignans from Juniperus sabina. In: PH 30: 3483-3485. 1991.

Fournier G et al., PM 57:392-393. 1991.

Fournier G et al., Pharm Belg 45:293. 1990.

Frohne D, Pfänder HJ, Giftpflanzen - Ein Handbuch für Apotheker, Toxikologen und Biologen, 4. Aufl., Wiss. Verlags-Ges. Stuttgart 1997.

Hänsel R, Keller K, Rimpler H, Schneider G (Hrsg.), Hagers Handbuch der Pharmazeutischen Praxis, 5. Aufl., Bde 4-6 (Drogen): Springer Verlag Berlin, Heidelberg, New York, 1992-1994.

Hartwell, JL et al., (1953) J Chem Soc 75: 235.

Lewin L, Gifte und Vergiftungen, 6. Aufl., Nachdruck, Haug Verlag, Heidelberg 1992.

Madaus G, Lehrbuch der Biologischen Arzneimittel, Bde 1-3, Nachdruck, Georg Olms Verlag Hildesheim 1979.

Roth L, Daunderer M, Kormann K, Giftpflanzen, Pflanzengifte, 4. Aufl., Ecomed Fachverlag Landsberg Lech 1993.

Steinegger E, Hänsel R, Pharmakognosie, 5. Aufl., Springer Verlag Heidelberg 1992.

Teuscher E, Lindequist U, Biogene Gifte - Biologie, Chemie, Pharmakologie, 2. Aufl., Fischer Verlag Stuttgart 1994.

Saw Palmetto

Serenoa repens

TRADE NAMES

Saw Palmetto (available from numerous manafacturers), Saw Palmetto Berries, Saw Palmetto Standardized, Centrum Saw Palmetto, Proactive Saw Palmetto, Standardized Saw Palmetto ExtractCap, Saw Palmetto Extract, Saw Palmetto Power, Premium Blend Saw Palmetto, Herbal Sure Saw Palmetto, Quanterra Prostate, Super Saw Palmetto Plus

DESCRIPTION

Medicinal Parts: The medicinal parts are the partially dried ripe fruit, the ripe fresh fruit and the ripe dried fruit.

Flower and Fruit: The inconspicuous cream flowers are in short, densely pubescent, paniculately branched inflorescences. The fruit is deep purple to almost black. It is an ovate, 3 cm long, 1-seeded berry. It has a hard but fragile pericarp that covers a pale brown, spongy pulp. The endocarp is thin and papery. The fruit is slightly wrinkled,

1.25 to 2.5 cm long and 1.25 cm in diameter. The hard seed is pale brown, oval or globular, and has a hilum near the base. The whole panicle can weigh up to 4 kg.

Leaves, Stem and Root: The plant is a bushy palm with a maximum height of 6 m. The large, yellow-green leaves have up to 20 segments and form a crown.

Characteristics: The taste of the seeds is soapy and unpleasant.

Habitat: The plant is indigenous to the coastal regions of the southern states of the U.S., from South Carolina to Florida and southern California.

Other Names: Sabal, Shrub Palmetto

ACTIONS AND PHARMACOLOGY

COMPOUNDS

Steroids: Sterols, including beta-sitosterol, beta-sitosterol-3-O-glucosides, beta-sitosterol-3-O-diglucoside, beta-sitosterol-fatty acid esters and their glucosides, for example beta-sitosterol-3-O-myristate, beta-sitosterol-3-O-(6-O-myristyl-beta-glucosides)

Flavonoids: including isoquercitrin, kaempferol-3-O-glucosides, rhoifolin

Water-soluble polysaccharides (galactoarabane with uronic acid)

Fatty oil: free fatty acids

The lipophilic components (fatty oil with phytosterines) can be found in ethanolic and hexane-extracts. The anti-exudative components (polysaccharides) are found in aqueous extracts. Ethanolic extracts contain both component groups.

EFFECTS

Anti-Androgenic Effects

The lipophilic extract of the herb inhibits binding of dihydrotestosterone (DHT) to the cytosolic androgenic receptor and alpha1-adrenoceptor in the prostate, thus preventing accumulation of the steroid, which may lead to prostate hyperplasia (Carilla, 1984; Goepel, 1999). Anti-androgenic effects of the lipophilic extract also consist of 5-alpha-reductase and 3- ketosteroid reductase inhibition. These enzymes are responsible for the conversion of testosterone to DHT and for conversion of DHT to an androgen compound, respectively (Sultan, 1984).

Anti-Estrogenic Effects

The herb lowers cytosol and nuclear receptor values for estrogen which result in an anti-estrogen effect since progesterone receptor content is linked to estrogenic activity. Anti-estrogenic agents inhibit stromatic prostate mass growth in patients with benign prostate hypertrophy (DiSilverio, 1992). There is also some evidence with inhibition of several steps involved in prolactin receptor signal transduction in ovary cells (Vacher, 1995).

Anti-Inflammatory Effects

The hexane extracts of the herb have demonstrated anti-inflammatory activity (Champault, 1984). Inhibition of the synthesis of arachidonic acid inflammatory metabolites, through a double blocking of cyclooxygenas and 5-lipoxygenase pathways results in anti-inflammatory properties. (Breu, 1992). The drug also contains anti-spasmodic properties by inhibiting calcium influx and activation of the sodium/calcium ion exchanger. Induction of protein synthesis plays a role in the antispasmotic effect with cyclic AMP as a possible mediator. Extracts of the drug may also antagonize the contracting effect of acetylcholine on urinary bladders. (Gutierrez, 1996).

CLINICAL TRIALS

Benign Prostatic Hyperplasia

The effect of Saw Palmetto on voiding symptoms and urodynamic parameters was determined in men with lower urinary tract symptoms (LUTS) presumed secondary to benign prostatic hyperplasia (BPH). The study was conducted over a 6-month period with Saw Palmetto 160 mg given twice daily. Parameters evaluated included peak urinary flow rate, postvoid residual urine volume, pressure-flow study and serum prostate-specific antigen. The herb was well-tolerated and significantly improved urinary tract symptoms. There was no significant improvement in objective measures of bladder outlet obstruction (Gerber, 1998).

A 6-month, double-blind, randomized equivalence study was conducted to compare the effects of a Saw Palmetto extract (320 mg Permixon) with those of a 5 alpha-reductase inhibitor (5 mg finasteride). The study included 1098 men with moderate benign prostate hypertrophy (BPH) using the International Prostate Symptom Score (IPSS) as the primary end-point. The finasteride and Permixon treatment groups relieved the symptoms of BPH including a decrease in IPSS, improved quality of life and increased peak urinary flow rate. There was no statistical difference in improvement between the two treatment groups. Finasteride markedly decreased serum PSA levels and prostate volume while Permixon had little effect on androgen-dependent parameters. This conclusion suggests that other pathways might also be involved in the symptomatology of BPH (Carraro, 1996).

Serenoa repens given 160 mg twice daily was compared to alfuzosin 2.5 mg three times daily to determine the effect on 63 benign prostatic hyperplasia. The double-blind, comparative, parallel-groups study determined efficacy by assessment of clinical symptoms (Boyarsky's nscale, visual analogue scale, clinical global impression), urinary flow rates (uroflowmetry) and residual urinary volume (transabdominal ultrasound). The Serenoa repens treatment group had similar improvement to that of the alfuzosin treatment group, but significant effects were in favor of the alfuzosin treatment group with overall clinical impression and visual analogue scale (Grasso, 1995).

INDICATIONS AND USAGE

Approved by Commission E:

- Prostate complaints
- Irritable bladder

Saw Palmetto is used for urination problems in benign prostate hyperplasia stages I and II. This medication relieves only the difficulties associated with an enlarged prostate without reducing the enlargement.

Unproven Uses: In folk medicine, Saw Palmetto is used for inflammation of the urinary tract, bladder, testicles and mammary glands. It has been used for nocturnal enuresis, persistant cough, eczema and improvement of libido.

Homeopathic Uses: The herb is used for micturation problems and inflammation of the urinary tract.

PRECAUTIONS AND ADVERSE REACTIONS

No health hazards or side effects are known in conjunction with the proper administration of designated therapeutic dosages. Stomach complaints following intake have been observed in rare cases. Patients with hormone-dependent cancers should observe caution and speak to a physician regarding the use of Saw Palmetto because of its anti-estrogenic, estrogenic and anti-androgenic effects. The use of Saw Palmetto with pregnancy and breast feeding is not recommended due to its potential hormonal effects.

Drug Interactions: Saw Palmetto is believed to exert estrogen, androgen and alpha-adrenergic blocking effects. Because of this, the use of hormones, hormone-like drugs or adrenergic drugs concomitantly may need to be adjusted.

DOSAGE

Mode of Administration: Comminuted herb and other galenic preparations for oral use.

How Supplied:

Capsule—80 mg, 125 mg,160 mg, 227 mg, 250 mg, 320 mg 450 mg, 500 mg, 565 mg, 570 mg, 585 mg, 600 mg, 1000 mg

Liquid—1:1

Daily Dosage: The average daily dose is 1 to 2 gm of the drug or 320 mg of the lipophilic extract (hexane or ethanol 90% v/v). Dosages used in studies demonstrated efficacy at 160 mg given twice daily or 320 mg given once daily (Carraro, 1996; Gerber, 1998; Grasso, 1995).

LITERATURE

Anonym, Welche Bedeutung haben pflanzliche Prostatamittel. In: DAZ 133(9):720. 1993.

Aso Y, Boccon-Gibob L, Brendler CB et al., (1993) Clinical research criteria. In: Cockett AT, Aso Y, Chatelain C, Denis L, Griffith K, Murphy G (eds.), Proceedings of the second international consultation on benign prostatic hyperplasia (BPH). Paris, SCI S. 345-355.

Bach D, (1995) Medikamentöse Langheitbehandlung der BPH Ergebnisse einer prospektiven 3-Jahres-Studie mit dem Sabalextrakt IDS 89. Urologe [B]35:178-183.

Bach D, Behandlung der benignen Prostatahypertrophie. In: ZPT 17(4):209-218. 1996.

Bach D, Ebeling L, Long-term drug treatment of benign prostatic hyperplasia - Results of a prospective 3-year multicenter study using Sabal extract IDS 89. In: Phytomedicine 3(2):105-111. 1996.

Bauer R, Neues von ''immunmodulierenden Drogen'' und ''Drogen mit antiallergischer und antiinflammatorischer Wirkung''. In: ZPT 14(1):23-24. 1993.

Bazan NG, Authie D, Braquet P, Effect of Serenoa repens extract (Permixon (r)) on estradiol/testosteron-induced experimental prostate enlargement in the rat. In: Pharmacol Res 34(3/4):171-179. 1996.

Becker H, Ebeling L, (1988) Konservative Therapie der benignen Prostata-Hyperplasie (BPH) mit Cernilton (N) - Ergebnisse einer placebokontrollierten Doppelblindstudie. Urologe [B]28:301.

Becker H, Ebeling L, (1991) Phytotherapie der BPH mit Cernilton(N) - Ergebnisse einer kontrollierten Verlaufsstudie. Urologe [B]31:113.

Berges RR, Windeler J, Trampisch HJ, Senge TH, (1995) Randomised, placebo-controlled, double-blind clinical trial of β-sitosterol in patients with benign prostatic hyperplasia. Lancet 345:1529-1532.

Breu W, Hagenlocher M, Redl K et al., Antiphlogistische Wirkung eines mit hyperkritischem Kohlendioxid gewonnenen Sabalfrucht-Extraktes. In vitro Hemmung des Cyclooxygenase- und 5-Lipoxygenase-Metabolismus. Arzneimittelforschung 1992; 42:547.

Breu W, Stadler F, Hagenlocher M et al., Der Sabalfrucht-Extrakt SG 291. Ein Phytotherapeutikum zur Behandlung der benignen Prostatahyperplasie. Z Phytother 1992; 13:107-115.

Carraro JC et al., Comparision of phytotherapy (Permixon (R)) with finasteride in the treatment of benign prostate hyperplasia: a randomized international study of 1,098 patients. In: Prostate 29(4):231-240. 1996.

Carilla E, Briley M, Fauran F et al., Binding of Permixon(R), a new treatment for prostatic benign hyperplasia, to the cytosolic androgen receptor in rat prostate. J Steroid Biochem 1984; 20:521-523.

Carraro J, Raynaud J, Koch G et al., Comparison of phytotherapy (Permixon) with finasteride in the treatment of benign prostate hyperplasia: a randomized international study of 1,098 patients. Prostate 1996 Oct;29(4):231-40.

Casarosa C, Cosci M, o di Coscio, Fratta M, (1988) Lack of effects of a lyposterolic extract of Serenoa repens on plasma levels of testosterone, follicle-stimulating hormone, luteinizing hormone. Clin Ther 10:5.

DiSilverio F, D'Eramo GD, Lubrano C et al., Evidence that Serenoa repens extract displays an anti-estrogenic activity in prostatic tissue of benign prostatic hypertrophy patients. Eur Urol 1992: 21:309.

DiSilverio F, D'Eramo G, Flammia GP et al., Pharmacological combinations in the treatment of benign prostatic hypertrophy. J Urol (Paris) 1993a; 99:316-320.

Engelmann U, Phytopharmaka und Synthetika bei der Behandlung der benignen Prostatahypertrophie. In: ZPT 18(1):13-19. 1997.

Gerber GS, Zagaja GP, Bales GT, et al., Saw Palmetto (Seronoa repens) in men with lower urinary tract symptoms: effects on urodynamic parameters and voiding symptoms. Urology 1998 Jun;51(6):1003-7.

Goepel M, Hecker U, Krege S et al., Saw Palmetto extracts potently and noncompetitively inhibit human alpha1-adrenoceptors in vitro. Prostate 1999 Feb 15;38(3):208-15.

Gutierrez M, Garcia De Boto MJ, Cantabrana B et al., Mechanisms involved in the spasmolytic effect of extracts from Sabal serrulata fruit on smooth muscle. Gen Pharmacol 1996; 27:171-176.

Grasso M, Montesano A, Buonaguidi A et al., Comparative effects of alfuzosin versus Serenoa repens in the treatment of symptomatic benign prostatic hyperplasia. Arch Esp Urol 1995 Jan-Feb;48(1):97-103.

Gutierrez M, Hidalgo A & Cantabrana B, Spasmolytic activity of a lipidic extract from Sabal serrulata fruits further study of the mechanism underlying this activity. Planta Med 1996; 62:507-511.

Hänsel R et al., (1964) Planta Med 12:169.

Harnischfeger G, Stolze H, (1989) Serenoa repens - Die Sägezahnpalme. Z Phytother 10:71-76.

Koch E, (1995) Pharmakologie und Wirkmechanismen von Extrakten aus Sabalfrüchten (Sabal fructus): Brennesselwurzeln (Urticae radix) und Kürbissamen (Cucurbitae peponis semen) bei der Behandlung der benignen Prostatahyperplasie. In: Loew D, Rietbrock N (Hrsg) Phytopharmaka in Forschung und klinischer Anwendung. Steinkopff Verlag, Darmstadt, S 57-79.

Mattei FM, Capone M, Acconia A, Medikamentöse Therapie der benignen Prostatahyperplasie mit einem Exktrakt der Sägepalme. In: Therapiewoche Urologie, Nephrologie 2:346-350. 1990.

Miersch WDE, Benigne Prostatahyperplasie. In: DAZ 133(29):2653. 1993.

Nahrstedt A, (1993) Pflanzliche Urologica - eine kritische Übersicht. Pharm Z 138:1439-1450.

Niederprüm HJ, Schweikert HU, Zänker KS, (1994) Testosteron 5D-reductase inhibition by free fatty acids from Sabal serrulata fruits. Phytomedicine 1:127-133.

Plosker GL, Brogden RN, Serenoa repens (Permixon (R)): A review of its pharmacological and therapeutic efficacy in benign prostatic hyperplasia. In: Drugs & Aging 9(5):379-395. 1996.

Ravenna L et al., Effects of the lipidosterolic extract of Serenoa repens (Permixon (R)) on human prostatic cell lines. In: Prostate 29(4):219-230. 1996.

Rhodes L, Primka RL, Berman CH, Vergult F, Gabriel M, Pierre-Malice M, Gibelin B, Comparision of Finasteride (Proscar(R)), a 5alpha-reductase inhibitor, and various commercial plant extracts in in vitro and in vivo 5alpha reductase inhibition. In: Prostate.

Schilcher H, (1987) Möglichkeiten und Grenzen der Phytotherapie am Beispiel pflanzlicher Urologika. Urologe [B] 27:316-319.

Schilcher H, (1987) Pflanzliche Diuretika. Urologe [B]27:215-222.

Schilcher B, In: Schilcher H: Phytotherapie in der Urologie. Hippokrates Verlag Stuttgart. 1992.

Shimada H et al., Biological active acylglycerides from the berries of Saw Palmetto (Serenoa repens). In: JNP 60(4):417-418. 1997.

Sultan C, Terraza A, Devillier C et al., Inhibition of androgen metabolism and binding by a liposterolic extract of 'Serenoa repens B' in human foreskin fibroblasts. J Steroid Biochem 1984; 20:515-519.

Vacher P, Prevarskaya N, Skryma R et al., The lipidosterolic extract from Serenoa repens interferes with prolactin receptor signal transduction. J Biomed Sci 1995; 2:357-365.

Wagner H, Flachsbarth H, (1981) Planta Med 41:244.

Wichtl M, Pflanzliche Geriatrika. In: DAZ 132(30):1576. 1992.

Further information in:

Hänsel R, Keller K, Rimpler H, Schneider G (Hrsg.), Hagers Handbuch der Pharmazeutischen Praxis, 5. Aufl., Bde 4-6 (Drogen): Springer Verlag Berlin, Heidelberg, New York, 1992-1994.

Madaus G, Lehrbuch der Biologischen Arzneimittel, Bde 1-3, Nachdruck, Georg Olms Verlag Hildesheim 1979.

Schulz R, Hänsel R, Rationale Phytotherapie, Springer Verlag Heidelberg 1996.

Teuscher E, Biogene Arzneimittel, 5. Aufl., Wiss. Verlagsges. Stuttgart 1997.

Wagner H, Wiesenauer M, Phytotherapie. Phytopharmaka und pflanzliche Homöopathika, Fischer-Verlag, Stuttgart, Jena, New York 1995.

Scabiosa succisa

See Premorse

Scarlet Pimpernel

Anagallis arvensis

DESCRIPTION

Medicinal Parts: The medicinal part of the plant is the dried flowering herb, usually with the roots removed.

Flower and Fruit: The plant has 6 to 10 brick-red flowers in the leaf axils, which are up to 2.5 times as long as the bracts. The symmetrically radiating flower has a double perianth. It has 5 sepals that are 4 to 5 mm long, entire-margined, narrow-lanceolate and acute. The wheel-shaped corolla is usually vermilion, but occasionally blue-flesh colored, lilac or white. The tip of the corolla is obovate to oval, about 7 mm long by 6 mm wide, overlapping at the base, entire-margined or slightly crenate with 50 to 70 glandular hairs. Its 5 stamens have a distinct awn and are fused to a funnel at the tube. The anthers are short, ellipsoid and cordate at the base. The superior ovary is globose and one-valved with an oblong style and head-like stigma. The fruit is a globose pyxidum, 4 to 5 mm in diameter, that contains 20 to 22 rough wart-like, brown seeds 1.3 mm long by 1 mm wide.

Leaves, Stem and Root: Anagallis arvensis is an annual herb with prostrate, creeping, square stems up to 30 cm long. Its thinner, branched, ascending stems grow to a length of 6 to 30 cm. The square shoots, like the leaves, are thickly covered with short hairs when young; they later become glabrous. The leaves are opposite, occasionally in whorls of 3, ovate to lanceolate, up to 20 mm long by 10 mm wide, sessile, entire-margined, acute and spotted black on the underside.

Characteristics: The flowers, which are poisonous, close at night and open at about 9:00 each morning. They also close at the first sign of rain.

Habitat: The plant is widely distributed throughout Europe, Asia, the U.S. and non-tropical South America.

Production: Scarlet Pimpernel herb is the dried herb in flower of Anagallis arvensis, generally without the root but occasionally including the whole plant. It is collected in the wild and also cultivated.

Not to be Confused With: The blue flowering form of Scarlet Pimpernel is often confused with Anagallis foemina, and occasionally with Stellaria media.

Other Names: Adder's Eyes, Poor Man's Weatherglass, Red Chickweed, Red Pimpernel, Shepherd's Barometer

ACTIONS AND PHARMACOLOGY

COMPOUNDS

Triterpene saponins: including anagalline, chief sapogenine 13, 28-epoxy-16- oxooleanan

Cucurbitacins: including cucurbitacins E, B, D, I and L

Flavonoids

Caffeic acid derivatives

EFFECTS

In vitro and animal tests showed the drug (main constituents saponins and amaroids of the cucurbitacin group) to have fungitoxic, antiviral, taecidal, spermicidal, estrogenic, oxytocic and hemolytic effects. The aqueous extract of the dried leaves is fungitoxic. Triterpenglycoside, anagalloside and aglycon anagalligenones, when isolated from the drug, displayed inhibitory results against numerous micro-organisms. Aqueous extracts showed uterine contracting activity in rats, guinea pigs, rabbits, and on strips of human uterine material. The triterpene saponins isolated from the drug demonstrated action against human sperm. The methanol extract of the drug demonstrated estrogen activity in the Allen-Doisy test. The saponins isolated from the powder drug with ethanol demonstrated hemolytic activity in human blood. The methanol extract of the dried powdered drug is antiviral against *Herpes simplex Type I, Adenovirus Type II* and *Polio Type II*, among others. The saponins are the active constituents. The acetyl-saponin isolated from the drug acts as a teniacide.

INDICATIONS AND USAGE

Unproven Uses: The drug is used to treat depression, disorders of the mucous membranes, hemorrhoids, herpes, painful kidney and liver disorders (in particular, to increase urination), poorly healing wounds and pruritus. The herb is used as a supporting treatment in various carcinomas. It is used both internally and externally (as a poultice) to treat pains in the joints.

Chinese Medicine: The herb is used for snake bites, dog bites, fish poisoning, joint ailments and edema.

Indian Medicine: Employed as a treatment for menstruation disorders.

Homeopathic Uses: Used in the treatment of skin rashes, warts and urinary tract infections.

Efficacy has not been proven.

PRECAUTIONS AND ADVERSE REACTIONS

No health hazards or side effects are known in conjunction with the proper administration of designated therapeutic dosages. Large doses or long-term administration could lead to gastroenteritis and nephritis, due to the cucurbitacins content of the drug.

OVERDOSAGE

Higher dosages (no amounts specified) are said to have a strong diuretic, diarrheic and mildly narcotic effect.

DOSAGE

Mode of Administration: Scarlet Pimpernel topically as a poultice and internally as an infusion.

Preparation: For the treatment of liver and kidney disorders as well as dropsy, add one teaspoonful of the drug to a glass of hot water and let it steep for 10 minutes. Drink throughout the day.

Daily Dosage: The usual dosage is 1.8 g of the powder 4 times a day.

Homeopathic Dosage: The oral dosage is 5 to 10 drops, 1 tablet or 10 globules daily. The parenteral dosage is 1 ml twice a week sc. Topically, ointment can be applied 1 to 2 times daily.

LITERATURE

Alimbaeva PK, Mukhamedziev MM, Rast Resur 5:380-385. 1969.

Aliotta G, De Napoli L, Giordano F, Piccialli G, Piccialli V, Santacroce C, An oleanen triterpene from Anagallis arvensis. In: PH 31(3):929-933. 1992.

Amoros M and Girre RL, (1977) Phytochemistry 26(3):787.

Amoros M et al., (1979) PlantMed Phytother 13:122.

Amoros M, Fauconnier B, Girre RL, In vitro antiviral activity of a saponin from Anagallis arvensis, Primulaceae, against herpes simplex virus and poliovirus. In: Antiviral Res 8:13-25. 1987.

Banerji R et al., (1981) Indian Drugs 19:121.

Büechi S, Antivirale Saponine, pharmakologische und klinische Untersuchungen. In: DAZ 136(2):89-98. 1996.

Yamada Y et al., (1978) Phytochemistry 17:1798.

Yamada Y et al., Chem Pharm Bull 26:3107-3112. 1978.

Further information in:

Hänsel R, Keller K, Rimpler H, Schneider G (Hrsg.), Hagers Handbuch der Pharmazeutischen Praxis, 5. Aufl., Bde 4-6 (Drogen), Springer Verlag Berlin, Heidelberg, New York, 1992-1994.

Hausen B, Allergiepflanzen, Pflanzenallergene, ecomed Verlagsgesellsch. mbH, Landsberg 1988.

Madaus G, Lehrbuch der Biologischen Arzneimittel, Bde 1-3, Nachdruck, Georg Olms Verlag Hildesheim 1979.

Roth L, Daunderer M, Kormann K, Giftpflanzen, Pflanzengifte, 4. Aufl., Ecomed Fachverlag Landsberg Lech 1993.

Schinus molle

See California Peppertree

Schinus terebinthifolius

See Brazilian Pepper Tree

Schisandra chinensis

See Schisandra (Wu-Wei-Zi)

Schisandra sphenanthera

See Lemon-Wood

Schisandra (Wu-Wei-Zi)

Schisandra chinensis

DESCRIPTION

Medicinal Parts: The medicinal part of the plant is the fruit.

Flower and Fruit: The flowers are in clusters with a few blossoms in the axils of the bracts. There are 6 to 8 tepals. The perigone of the male flowers has 6 to 8 tepals that are 6 to 11 mm long and 5 mm wide, and 5 to 15 stamens. The female flowers have a similar perigone and 17 to 40 elongated, elliptical ovaries. The round, fleshy, berry-like fruit grows as a slim, hanging aggregate or as bloomed individual fruits. The fruit is deep red to black-brown and appears partly white-powdered. The fruit has a diameter of 5 to 8 mm and contains 1 to 2 reniform seeds.

Leaves, Stem and Root: This liana plant can be monoecious or dioecious. The leaves are alternate. They are arranged like whorls on short shoots. The petiole is 1 to 4 cm long. The lamina is 5 to 11 cm long, 3 to 9 cm wide, elongate to ovate-elliptical, serrate to dentate with up to 3 teeth per cm. The upper surface is green or brown. The lower surface is partly pubescent. The young branches are brown to purple.

Characteristics: The crushed seeds taste hot and are aromatic.

Habitat: The plant is indigenous to northeastern China and Korea.

Production: Northern schisandra fruit is the dried, ripe fruit of Schisandra chinensis. The fruit is harvested in autumn, then steamed before being dried in the sun.

Other Names: Chinese Mock-Barberry, Lemonwood

ACTIONS AND PHARMACOLOGY

COMPOUNDS

Volatile oil: containing among others, alpha- and beta-chamigrene, chamigrenal, sesquicarene, (+)-ylangene

Ascorbic acid (vitamin C)

Lignans (in the seeds 5 to 20%): dibenzo[a,c]cyclooctene derivatives, including schizandrine A to C, schizandrol A and B, schizantherine A and B, gomisins D to J, K1 to K3, L1 and L2, M1 and M2, N and O, P to T, the gomisins present to some extent as esters, among them those of angelic acid, benzoic acid and acetic acid; additional lignans with other parent substances, including pregomisin

Fatty oil (in the seeds): chief fatty acids oleic acid and linoleic acid

EFFECTS

The lignans isolated from the drug (schizandrin, schizandrol) are liver-protective in effect, acting as radical scavengers and promoting liver regeneration. Anti-inflammatory and tumor-inhibiting characteristics have also been demonstrated. Schizandrol A is said to be neuroleptic, anticonvulsive and sedative in effect. Schisandra fruits and seeds are believed to bring about a non-specific increase in physical performance ability and to be antithelminthic in effect.

INDICATIONS AND USAGE

Chinese Medicine: The plant is used mainly for conditions of the digestive tract such as intestinal inflammation, and also for insomnia, enuresis, pollakisuria, nightly ejaculation, coughs, chronic diarrhea, dyspnea, insomnia, spontaneous outbreaks of sweating, hepatitis, neurasthenia and anxiety states. Efficacy for these indications has not yet been proven.

PRECAUTIONS AND ADVERSE REACTIONS

No health hazards are known in conjunction with the proper administration of designated therapeutic dosages.

DOSAGE

Mode of Administration: Whole and powdered drug and their preparations for internal use.

Preparation: To prepare Cuwuweizi powder, the drug is evaporated in the ratio of 1:5 with vinegar in closed containers until the surface turns black. This substance is then ground to a powder.

Daily Dosage: Powder/tincture/extract: 1.5 to 6 g daily

Storage: Store in dry area with good air circulation to avoid fungal formation.

LITERATURE

Hänsel R, Keller K, Rimpler H, Schneider G (Ed), Hagers Handbuch der Pharmazeutischen Praxis, 5. Aufl., Bde 4 - 6 (Drogen), Springer Verlag Berlin, Heidelberg, New York, 1992-1994.

Ip SP, Mak DH, Li PC, Poon MK, Ko KM, Determination and study of lignan distribution in the fruits of Schisandra chinensis (Turcz.). Baill Farmatsiia, 78:34-7, 1972 May-Jun.

Ip SP, Mak DH, Li PC, Poon MK, Ko KM, Determination of lignans in the fruits of Schisandra chinensis (Trucz.) Baill. and S. Sphenanthern Rehd. et Wils. using HPLC and their chromatograms. Chung Kuo Chung Yao Tsa Chih, 78:611-4, 639-40, 1989 Oct.

Ip SP, Mak DH, Li PC, Poon MK, Ko KM, Determination of the active ingredients in Chinese drug wuweizi (Schisandra chinensis) by TLC-densitometry. Yao Hsueh Hsueh Pao, 78:49-53, 1990.

Ip SP, Mak DH, Li PC, Poon MK, Ko KM, Ecological investigation on Schisandra chinensis (Turcz.) Baill. of the Changbai Mountain. Chung Kuo Chung Yao Tsa Chih, 78:204-5, 255, 1992 Apr.

Ip SP, Mak DH, Li PC, Poon MK, Ko KM, Effect of a lignan-enriched extract of Schisandra chinensis on aflatoxin B1 and cadmium chloride-induced hepatotoxicity in rats. Pharmacol Toxicol, 78:413-6, 1996 Jun.

Ip SP, Mak DH, Li PC, Poon MK, Ko KM, Pharmacological studies on an oil emulsion of Schisandra chinensis. Chung Yao Tung Pao, 78:185-6, 1984 Jul.

Ip SP, Mak DH, Li PC, Poon MK, Ko KM, Preliminary studies on the processing of Schisandra chinensis. Chung Yao Tung Pao, 78:26-7, 1986 Mar.

Ip SP, Mak DH, Li PC, Poon MK, Ko KM, Schisandra chinensis-dependent myocardial protective action of sheng-mai-san in rats. Am J Chin Med, 78:255-62, 1996.

Ip SP, Mak DH, Li PC, Poon MK, Ko KM, The occurrence of some important lignans in Wu Wei Zi (Schisandra chinensis) and its allied species. Yao Hsueh Hsueh Pao, 78:138-43, 1983 Feb.

Ip SP, Poon MK, Che CT, Ng KH, Kong YC, Ko KM, Anti-oxidant activity of dibenzocyclooctene lignans isolated from Schisandraceae. Planta Med, 21:311-3, 1992 Aug.

Ip SP, Poon MK, Che CT, Ng KH, Kong YC, Ko KM, Schisandrin B protects against carbon tetrachloride toxicity by enhancing the mitochondrial glutathione redox status in mouse liver. Free Radic Biol Med, 21:709-12, 1996.

Ko KM, Ip SP, Poon MK, Wu SS, Che CT, Ng KH, Kong YC, Effect of a lignan-enriched fructus schisandrae extract on hepatic glutathione status in rats: protection against carbon tetrachloride toxicity. Planta Med, 21:134-7, 1995 Apr.

Liu CS, Fang SD, Huang MF, Kao YL, Hsu JS, Studies on the active principles of Schisandra sphenanthera Rehd. et Wils. The structures of schisantherin A, B, C, D, E and the related compounds. Sci Sin, 21:483-502, 1978 Jul-Aug.

Nishiyama N, Wang YL, Saito H, Beneficial effects of S-113m, a novel herbal prescription, on learning impairment model in mice. Biol Pharm Bull, 21:1498-503, 1995 Nov.

Tong Q, Deuteration of dimethyl 4,4′-dimethoxy-5,6,5′,6′-dimethylenedioxybiphenyl-2,2′-dicarboxylate (BDD): a remedy for chronic hepatitis. Chung Kuo I Hsueh Ko Hsueh Yuan Hsueh Pao, 21:42-5, 1990 Feb.

Yasukawa K, Ikeya Y, Mitsuhashi H, Iwasaki M, Aburada M, Nakagawa S, Takeuchi M, Takido M, Gomisin A inhibits tumor promotion by 12-O-tetradecanoylphorbol-13-acetate in two-stage carcinogenesis in mouse skin. Oncology, 21:68-71, 1992.

Scolopendrium vulgare

See Hartstongue

Scopolia

Scopolia carniolica

DESCRIPTION

Medicinal Parts: The medicinal part is the dried rhizome.

Flower and Fruit: The nodding flowers are solitary and axillary on long bending pedicles. The calyx is campanulate with obtuse tips. The corolla is tubular-campanulate, glossy brown outside, and matte olive-green inside. The anthers are large and yellowish. The fruit is a 2-valved pixidium. The seeds are 3 to 4 mm long, brownish-yellow and bumpy.

Leaves, Stem and Root: The erect perennial plant grows from 30 to 60 cm high. The rhizome is horizontal, slightly bent and almost cylindrical. The rhizome grows up to 12 cm long and 5 cm thick, and is covered in tough, loose-skinned fibers. The color varies between yellowish-brown to dark brownish-gray. The stems bear scale-like stipules at the base that are bifurcated, fleshy and also glabrous or with scattered hairs. The 12 cm by 4 to 9 cm foliage leaves are petiolate, obovate, entire-margined or lightly sinuate and dull green.

Characteristics: Scopolia is considered to be a narcotic. The taste is initially somewhat sweet, then bitter and biting. The plant is odorless.

Habitat: The plant is indigenous to southern Germany, Austria, Hungary, and southwest Russia.

Production: Scopolia root consists of the dried rhizome of Scopolia carniolica.

Other Names: Scopola, Japanese Belladonna, Belladonna Scopola, Russian Belladonna

ACTIONS AND PHARMACOLOGY

COMPOUNDS

Tropane alkaloids (0.2-0.5%): chief alkaloid (-)-hyoscyamine, which changes (to some extent) under drying conditions into atropine; also including scopolamine

Hydroxycoumarins: including among others, scopoletins, scopoline

Caffeic acid derivatives: chlorogenic acids

EFFECTS

The drug acts as a parasympatholytic/anticholinergic via competitive antagonism of the neuromuscular transmitter acetylcholine. Because of its parasympatholytic properties, Scopolia root relaxes the smooth muscle organs and eliminates spastic conditions, especially of the gastrointestinal tract and the bile ducts.

Conditions of muscular tremors and muscular rigidity caused by central nervous impulses, are alleviated. The action on the heart is positively chronotropic and positively dromotropic.

INDICATIONS AND USAGE

Approved by Commission E:

■ Liver and gallbladder complaints

The drug is used for spasms and colic-like pain of the gastrointestinal tract, bile ducts, and urinary tract for adults and for children over 6 years of age.

CONTRAINDICATIONS

The drug is contraindicated in angle-closure glaucoma, prostatic adenoma with residual urine, tachycardia, mechanical stenosis in the area of the gastrointestinal tract, and megacolon.

PRECAUTIONS AND ADVERSE REACTIONS

General: No health hazards are known in conjunction with the proper administration of designated therapeutic dosages. However, accommodation disorders, heat build-up due to a decline in sweat secretion, micturition disorders, and obstipation can occur as side effects, particularly with overdosages. Scopolia should be used only under the supervision of an expert qualified in its appropriate use.

Drug Interactions: Scopolia increases the effectiveness of simultaneously administered tricyclic antidepressants, amantadine, and quinidine.

OVERDOSAGE

The four early warning symptoms of atropine poisoning are skin reddening, dryness of the mouth, and tachycardiac arrhythmias and mydriasis. In addition, other side effects, particularly with overdosages, can include accommodation disorders, heat build-up through decline in sweat secretion, micturition disorders, and obstipation.

The intake of very high dosages leads to central excitation (restlessness, compulsive speech, hallucinations, delirium, manic episodes, followed by exhaustion and sleep). Potentially lethal dosages for adults start at 100 mg of atropine, depending upon alkaloid content, and may result from use of between 20 to 50 g of the drug; considerably less can prove lethal for children.

The treatment for poisonings includes gastric lavage; temperature-lowering measures with wet cloths (no antipyretics!); oxygen respiration for respiratory distress; intubation; parenteral physostigmine salts as antidote; diazepam for spasms and chlorpromazine for severe excitation.

DOSAGE

Mode of Administration: Comminuted root, powder and other galenic preparations for oral application.

Daily Dosage: The average daily dose is equivalent to 0.25 mg of total alkaloids, calculated as hyoscyamine. The maximum daily dose should not exceed the equivalent of 3.0 mg of total alkaloids, calculated as hyoscyamine. The maximum recommended single dose is equivalent to 1.0 mg of total alkaloids, calculated as hyoscyamine.

LITERATURE

Frohne D, Pfänder HJ, Giftpflanzen - Ein Handbuch für Apotheker, Toxikologen und Biologen, 4. Aufl., Wiss. Verlags-Ges. Stuttgart 1997.

Kern W, List PH, Hörhammer L (Hrsg.), Hagers Handbuch der Pharmazeutischen Praxis, 4. Aufl., Bde. 1-8: Springer Verlag Berlin, Heidelberg, New York, 1969.

Lewin L, Gifte und Vergiftungen, 6. Aufl., Nachdruck, Haug Verlag, Heidelberg 1992.

Nicolic R et al., Acta Pharm Jugosl 26:257. 1976.

Roth L, Daunderer M, Kormann K, Giftpflanzen, Pflanzengifte, 4. Aufl., Ecomed Fachverlag Landsberg Lech 1993.

Smart RG et al., J Forens Sci 32:303. 1987.

Teuscher E, Lindequist U, Biogene Gifte - Biologie, Chemie, Pharmakologie, 2. Aufl., Fischer Verlag Stuttgart 1994.

Scopolia carniolica

See Scopolia

Scotch Broom

Cytisus scoparius

DESCRIPTION

Medicinal Parts: The medicinal parts are the dried and stripped broom flowers, the dried aerial parts (broom herb) and freshly picked flowers.

Flower and Fruit: The bilabiate flowers are bright yellow, 20 to 25 mm long, large, solitary or in pairs. The flowers are on 2 or 3 obovate bracts on short stems, or singly in the leaf axils. They seem to form long racemes. The corolla is bright yellow, sometimes white. The standard is revolute, the wings obtuse. The ovary is short-stemmed and villous with a glabrous, strongly hooked style. The pod is oblong, compressed, glabrous on the surfaces, villous on the seams and is a matte black. There are numerous brown-black seeds.

Leaves, Stem and Root: Scotch Broom is a shrub that grows from 0.5 to 2 m high. The tap root is very sturdy and woody. The bark of the root is brown. The branches are thick, usually crooked, and the bark is also brown. Young shoots are glabrous, later pubescent. The branchlets are cane-like, erect and pentagular. The leaves are small, short-petioled, with 3 obovate to lanceolate, 1 to 2 cm long and 1.5 to 9 mm wide, pointed leaflets. The leaflets, particularly on the undersurface, are silky pubescent. After flowering, sessile and entire leaves form on the upper shoot.

Habitat: The herb is found in Europe, northern Africa, Canary Islands, North America, Chile, South Africa and Japan.

Production: Scotch Broom herb consists of the aerial parts of Cytisus scoparius. Broom flowers consist of the flowers of Cytisus scoparius.

Not to be Confused With: The herb should not be confused with other Cytisus or Genista varieties. The flowers should not be confused with Spanish Broom.

Other Names: Broom, Broomtops, Besom, Scoparium, Irish Tops, Basam, Bizzom, Browme, Brum, Breeam

ACTIONS AND PHARMACOLOGY

COMPOUNDS: SCOTCH BROOM HERB

Quinolizidine alkaloids (0.5 to 1.6%): main alkaloid (-)-sparteine, including among others 11, 12-dehydrosparteine, 17-oxosparteine, lupanine, alpha-isosparteine

Biogenic amines: including tyramine, epinine, dopamine

Flavonoids: including spirasoside, isoquercitrin, scoparin

Isoflavonoids: including genistein, sarothamnoside

EFFECTS: SCOTCH BROOM HERB

No specific studies are available. Tyramine acts indirectly on the sympathetic nervous system as a vasoconstrictor and hypertensive.

COMPOUNDS: SCOTCH BROOM FLOWERS

Quinolizidine alkaloids (0.004%) (very small quantities): main alkaloid (-)-sparteine

Biogenic amines: including tyramine (0.13 to 2%)

Flavonoids: including scoparin (C-glycosylflavone)

EFFECTS: SCOTCH BROOM FLOWERS

The drug can contain over 2% tyramine. It contains small amounts of alkaloids. The main alkaloid is sparteine. Tyramine acts as an indirect sympathicomimetic, vasoconstrictoral and hypotensive. Sparteine acts negatively inotropic and negatively chronotropic; because of the very minimal amounts of sparteine no intense effect can be expected.

INDICATIONS AND USAGE

SCOTCH BROOM HERB

Approved by Commission E:

- Circulatory disorders
- Hypertension

Unproven Uses: The herb is used for functional heart and circulatory disorders, as an adjunct in the stabilization of circulation and to raise blood pressure. Folk medicine uses include pathological edema, cardiac arrhythmia, nervous cardiac complaints, low blood pressure, heavy menstruation, hemorrhaging after birth, as a contraction stimulant, for bleeding gums, hemophilia, gout, rheumatism, sciatica, gall and kidney stones, enlarged spleen, jaundice, bronchial conditions and snake bites.

SCOTCH BROOM FLOWERS

Unproven Uses: The use of the pure drug cannot be recommended except as an inactive ingredient in teas. In folk medicine, the flowers are used for edema, rheumatism, gout, kidney stones, jaundice, liver disorders, enlarged spleen and as a blood purifier.

CONTRAINDICATIONS

SCOTCH BROOM HERB AND FLOWERS

The drug is contraindicated in high blood pressure, A-V block, pregnancy and with MAO inhibitor drugs.

PRECAUTIONS AND ADVERSE REACTIONS

SCOTCH BROOM HERB

General: Health risks or side effects following the proper administration of designated therapeutic dosages are not recorded. Scotch Broom preparations should not be used in cases of high blood pressure or with atrioventricular block.

Drug Interactions: Use of Scotch Broom herb with monoamine oxidase inhibitors (amine content) may cause a hypertensive crisis.

Pregnancy: The herb should not be used during pregnancy (abortive effect).

SCOTCH BROOM FLOWERS

Health risks or side effects following the proper administration of designated therapeutic dosages are not recorded. The drug should not be used in cases of high blood pressure or when the patient is being treated with monoamine oxidase inhibitors (amine content).

OVERDOSAGE

SCOTCH BROOM HERB

Doses corresponding to more than 300 mg sparteine (approximately 30 gm of the drug), lead to dizziness, headache, palpitations, prickling in the extremities, feeling of weakness in the legs, outbreaks of sweat, sleepiness, pupil dilation and ocular palsy. If no vomiting has occurred, poisonings are treated with gastric lavage and administration of activated charcoal. Spasms are to be treated with chlorpromazine or diazepam. In cases of asphyxiation, intubation and oxygen respiration are to be carried out. No deaths through poisonings with this drug have been proven beyond a doubt (though they certainly have been with sparteine).

DOSAGE

SCOTCH BROOM HERB

Mode of Administration: The herb is available in aqueous essential oil extracts for internal administration.

Preparation: Tea: Pour 150 ml boiling water over 1 to 2 gm drug and strain after 10 minutes

Decoction — from 1 to 2 gm drug.

Liquid extract — 1:1 25% ethanol (V/V) (BHP83).

Tincture — 1:5 45% ethanol (V/V) (BHP83).

Daily Dosage: The daily dose of the infusion is 1 cup fresh infusion 3 times daily. The liquid extract dosage is 1 to 2 ml daily. The tincture internal use dosage is 0.5 to 2 ml. Aqueous-ethanol extracts corresponding to 1:1.5 drug are also used.

Storage: Carefully protect from light and moisture.

SCOTCH BROOM FLOWERS

Mode of Administration: Since the efficacy for the claimed uses has not been documented, and considering the risks, a therapeutic application cannot be justified. To be used only under the supervision of an expert qualified in the appropriate use of this substance.

Preparation: To prepare an infusion, Pour 200 ml boiling water over 1 teaspoon of flowers and strain after 10 minutes.

Daily Dosage: Infusion dosage is 1 cup daily. For pathological edema, 1 liter infusion per day is administered in 4 portions during meals for 1 month.

LITERATURE

SCOTCH BROOM HERB

Brum-Bousquet M, Delaveau P, (1981) Plant Med Phytother 15(4):201.

Brum-Bousquet M et al., (1981) Planta Med 43(4):367.

Kurihara T, Kikuchi M, (1980) Yakugaku Zasshi 100(10):1054.

Murakoshi I et al., (1986) Phytochemistry 25(2):521.

Seeger R, Neumann HG, Spartein. In: DAZ 132(30):1577. 1992.

Vixcardi P et al., (1984) Pharmazie 39(11):781.

Wink M, Heinen HJ, Vogt H, Schiebel HM, Plant Cell Rep 3:230-233. 1984.

Wink M et al., (1981) Planta Med 43(4):342.

Young N et al., (1984) Biochem J 222(1):41.

Further information in:

Chan EH et al., (Eds.), Advances in Chinese Medicinal Materials Research, World Scientific Pub. Co. Singapore 1985.

Gresser G, Der Besenginster - Cytisus scoparius (L.) LINK. Z Phytother 17 (1996), 320-330.

Hänsel R, Keller K, Rimpler H, Schneider G (Hrsg.), Hagers Handbuch der Pharmazeutischen Praxis, 5. Aufl., Bde 4-6 (Drogen): Springer Verlag Berlin, Heidelberg, New York, 1992-1994.

Konami Y, Yamamoto K, Osawa T, Irimura T, The primary structure of the Cytisus scoparius seed lectin and a carbohydrate-binding peptide. J Biochem (Tokyo), 112:366-75, 1992 Sep.

Leung AY, Encyclopedia of Common Natural Ingredients Used in Food, Drugs and Cosmetics, John Wiley & Sons Inc., New York 1980.

Lewin L, Gifte und Vergiftungen, 6. Aufl., Nachdruck, Haug Verlag, Heidelberg 1992.

Madaus G, Lehrbuch der Biologischen Arzneimittel, Bde 1-3, Nachdruck, Georg Olms Verlag Hildesheim 1979.

Roth L, Daunderer M, Kormann K Giftpflanzen, Pflanzengifte. 4. Aufl., Ecomed Fachverlag Landsberg / Lech 1993.

Steinegger E, Hänsel R, Pharmakognosie, 5. Aufl., Springer Verlag Heidelberg 1992.

Teuscher E, Lindequist U, Biogene Gifte - Biologie, Chemie, Pharmakologie, 2. Aufl., Fischer Verlag Stuttgart 1994.

Teuscher E, Biogene Arzneimittel, 5. Aufl., Wiss. Verlagsges. mbH Stuttgart 1997.

Wagner H, Wiesenauer M, Phytotherapie. Phytopharmaka und pflanzliche Homöopathika, Fischer-Verlag, Stuttgart, Jena, New York 1995.

SCOTCH BROOM FLOWERS

Brum-Bousquet M, Delaveau P, (1981) Plant Med Phytother 15(4):201.

Brum-Bousquet M et al., (1981) Planta Med 43(4):367.

Kurihara T, Kikuchi M, (1980) Yakugaku Zasshi 100(10):1054.

Murakoshi I et al., (1986) Phytochemistry 25(2):521-524.

Seeger R, Neumann HG, Spartein. In: DAZ 132(30):1577. 1992.

Vixcardi P et al., (1984) Pharmazie 39(11):781.

Wink M, Heinen HJ, Vogt H, Schiebel HM, Plant Cell Rep 3:230-233. 1984.

Wink M et al., (1981) Planta Med 43(4):342-352.

Young N et al., (1984) Biochem J 222(1):41.

Further information in:

Chan EH et al., (Eds.), Advances in Chinese Medicinal Materials Research, World Scientific Pub. Co. Singapore 1985.

Hänsel R, Keller K, Rimpler H, Schneider G (Hrsg.), Hagers Handbuch der Pharmazeutischen Praxis, 5. Aufl., Bde 4-6 (Drogen): Springer Verlag Berlin, Heidelberg, New York, 1992-1994.

Leung AY, Encyclopedia of Common Natural Ingredients Used in Food Drugs and Cosmetics, John Wiley & Sons Inc., New York 1980.

Lewin L, Gifte und Vergiftungen, 6. Aufl., Nachdruck, Haug Verlag, Heidelberg 1992.

Madaus G, Lehrbuch der Biologischen Arzneimittel, Bde 1-3, Nachdruck, Georg Olms Verlag Hildesheim 1979.

Roth L, Daunderer M, Kormann K, Giftpflanzen, Pflanzengifte, 4. Aufl., Ecomed Fachverlag Landsberg Lech 1993.

Steinegger E, Hänsel R, Pharmakognosie, 5. Aufl., Springer Verlag Heidelberg 1992.

Teuscher E, Lindequist U, Biogene Gifte - Biologie, Chemie, Pharmakologie, 2. Aufl., Fischer Verlag Stuttgart 1994.

Teuscher E, Biogene Arzneimittel, 5. Aufl., Wiss. Verlagsges. mbH Stuttgart 1997.

Wagner H, Wiesenauer M, Phytotherapie. Phytopharmaka und pflanzliche Homöopathika, Fischer-Verlag, Stuttgart, Jena, New York 1995.

Scotch Pine

Pinus species

DESCRIPTION

Medicinal Parts: The medicinal parts are the tar extracted from the trunks, branches and roots. The oil extracted from the fresh needles, branch tips or fresh twigs is also used medicinally, as are the pine tips from fresh and dried shoots. The purified oil from the resin balsam, the tar extracted from the wood, the young shoots and the flowering branches of male and female flowers with pollen are also used.

Flower and Fruit: The male flowers are sulfur-yellow in the form of ovate catkins. The female flowers are purple and long-pedicled in erect, 5 to 6 mm long cones that hang down after flowering. The ripe cones are ovate-clavate, matte brown and have rhomboid scales. The hilum is small, smooth and light brown. The seeds are 3 to 4 mm long, oblong with wings, which are 3 times as long as the seed.

Leaves, Stem and Root: The tree is 10 to 30 m high with a straight, slim, cylindrical trunk or a gnarled twisted one. It has a girth of 1.8 to 3.6 m. The crown is umbrella-shaped. The bark of the older trees is gray-brown on the outside and rust red on the inside. Bark of older trees is deeply fissured below and peeling. The bark of the young trees is fox-red and thinly peeling. The buds are reddish, 6 to 12 mm long, oblong-oval and somewhat resinous. The needles are in pairs and remain on the trees for 3 years. They are various lengths, rigid, twisted, bluish-green with interrupted rows on the outside and minimally dentate.

Habitat: Pinus sylvestris is found in Europe, Siberia, the Crimea, the Caucasus and Iran.

Production: Pine shoots (Pini turiones) consist of the fresh or dried, 3 to 5 cm long shoots of Pinus sylvestris. Pine shoots are collected at the beginning of spring. The essential oil (Pini aetheroleum) is obtained from fresh needles, tips of the branches or fresh branches with needles and tips of Pinus sylvestris, Pinus mugo ssp. pumilio, Pinus nigra or Pinus pinaster. The oil is recovered form the fresh needles and branch tips using steam distillation with a successful yield of 0.15-0.6%. Purified turpentine oil (Terebinthinae aetheroleum rectificatum) is the essential oil obtained from the turpentine of Pinus species, especially Pinus palustries (syn. Pinus australis), and Pinus pinaster.

Not to be Confused With: Pine shoots should not be confused with the shoots of Picea abies and Abies alba. Pine oil should not be confused with "pine oils" that are synthetically produced.

Other Names: Dwarf-Pine, Pine Oils, Pix Liquida, Pumilio Pine, Scotch Fir, Stockholm Tar, Swiss Mountain Pine

ACTIONS AND PHARMACOLOGY

COMPOUNDS: PINE SHOOTS

Volatile oil (0.2-0.5%): including among others bornyl acetate, cadinene, Delta3 -carene, limonene, phellandrene, alpha-pinene

Resins

Bitter principles: pinicrin

Ascorbic acid (vitamin C)

EFFECTS: PINE SHOOTS

Pine shoots have secretolytic and mildly antiseptic effects and stimulate the peripheral circulation.

COMPOUNDS: PINE NEEDLE OIL

From Pinus mugo: chief components include Delta3-carene (up to 35%), alpha- and beta-pinene (20%), beta-phellandrene (15%)

From Pinus nigra: chief components include alpha-pinene (48-65%), beta-pinene (up to 32%), germacren D (up to 19%)

From Pinus palustris: chief components include alpha-and beta-pinene (95%)

From Pinus silvestris: chief components include alpha-pinene (10-50%), Delta3-carene (up to 20%), camphene (up to 12%), beta-pinene (10-25%), limonene (up to 10%), additionally including among others myrcene, terpinolene, bornyl acetate

EFFECTS: PINE NEEDLE OIL

The essential oil is secretolytic, hyperemic and weakly antiseptic.

COMPOUNDS: TURPENTINE OIL, PURIFIED

Chief components of the raw turpentine oil yielded from turpentine from Pinus silvestris include: (-)-alpha-pinene (ca. 39-87%), Delta3-carene (ca. 14-33%), (-)-beta-pinene (share up to 27%), limonene (6%), camphene (ca. 5%), from out of which and from out of the volatile oils of other pine species purified turpentine oil. Therebinthinae aetheroleum rectici-factum is realized through fractional distillation. It must contain at least 90% pinenes, but no more than 0.5 % Delta3-carene.

EFFECTS: TURPENTINE OIL, PURIFIED

The essential oil is hyperaemic, antiseptic and increases bronchial secretion in animal tests.

INDICATIONS AND USAGE

PINE SHOOTS

Approved by Commission E:

- Blood pressure problems
- Common cold
- Cough/bronchitis
- Fevers and colds
- Inflammation of the mouth and pharynx
- Neuralgias
- Tendency to infection

Pine shoots are used internally for catarrhal conditions of the upper and lower respiratory tract. Externally, it is used for mild muscular pain and neuralgia.

Unproven Uses: In folk medicine, preparations of pine shoot are used internally for uncomplicated coughs and acute bronchial diseases and topically for nasal congestion and hoarseness.

Homeopathic Uses: Homeopathic uses include weak ligaments of the upper ankle joint, inflammation of the respiratory tract, chronic rheumatism, eczema and urticaria.

PINE NEEDLE OIL
Approved by Commission E:

- Common cold
- Cough/bronchitis
- Fevers and colds
- Inflammation of the mouth and pharynx
- Neuralgias
- Rheumatism
- Tendency to infection

The essential oil is used internally and externally for congestive diseases of the upper and lower respiratory tract. Externally, it is used for rheumatic and neuralgic ailments.

TURPENTINE OIL, PURIFIED
Approved by Commission E:

- Cough/bronchitis
- Inflammation of the mouth and pharynx
- Rheumatism

Purified turpentine oil is used internally and externally for chronic diseases of the bronchi with profuse secretion. It is used externally for rheumatic and neuralgic ailments.

Unproven Uses: Folk medicine uses include bladder catarrh, gallstones and phosphorous poisoning. Externally, the oil is used for scabies, burns, frostbite and skin injuries.

CONTRAINDICATIONS

PINE SHOOTS AND PINE NEEDLE OIL
Contraindications include bronchial asthma and whooping cough.

PRECAUTIONS AND ADVERSE REACTIONS

PINE SHOOTS
No health hazards or side effects are known in conjunction with the proper administration of designated therapeutic dosages. Patients with extensive skin injuries, acute skin diseases, feverish or infectious diseases, cardiac insufficiency or hypertonia should not use the drug as a bath additive.

PINE NEEDLE OIL
No health hazards are known in conjunction with the proper administration of designated therapeutic dosages. Signs of irritation could appear on skin and mucous membranes. Bronchial spasms could worsen. Patients with extensive skin injuries, acute skin diseases, feverish or infectious diseases, cardiac insufficiency or hypertonia should not use the drug as a bath additive.

TURPENTINE OIL, PURIFIED
General: No health hazards or side effects are known in conjunction with the proper external administration of designated therapeutic dosages. However, resorptive poisonings, such as kidney and central nervous system damage, are possible with large-area administration. Where large skin injuries, severe feverish or infectious diseases, cardiac insufficiency or hypertonia are present, entire-body baths with the volatile oil added should be carried out only following consultation with a physician.

Kidney damage is conceivable with internal administration of therapeutic dosages. Inhalation should be avoided with acute inflammation of the breathing passages.

Pediatric Use: Cases of death, in particular among children, following intake of the oil have been reported in the scientific literature.

OVERDOSAGE

TURPENTINE OIL, PURIFIED
Severe poisonings are possible with the intake of large dosages. Symptoms include albuminuria, diarrhea, dyspnea, dysuria, feelings of vertigo, hematuria, intestinal colic, queasiness, reddening of the face, salivation, skin efflorescences, sore throat, staggering walk, strangury, thirst, twitching and vomiting. Poisonings can also occur through inhalation of the vapors or through skin contact. Fifty grams is the approximate lethal dosage for an adult. Cases of death, in particular among children, following intake of the oil are known from the scientific literature. Gastric lavage with bicarbonate of soda solution, intestinal emptying through administration of sodium sulphate, the administration of paraffin oil, activated charcoal and shock prophylaxis (suitable body position, quiet, warmth) should be instituted. Thereafter, therapy for poisonings consists of treating spasms with diazepam (i.v.), electrolyte substitution, and treating possible cases of acidosis with sodium bicarbonate infusions. In case of shock, plasma volume expanders should be infused. Monitoring of kidney function is essential. Intubation and oxygen respiration may also be necessary.

DOSAGE

PINE SHOOTS
Mode of Administration: Pine shoot is available as a comminuted herb for internal use in teas, syrups and tinctures. Alcoholic solutions, oils or ointments are used externally.

Daily Dosage:
Internal — daily dose: 2 to 3 g drug several times a day.

External — as a bath additive: 100 g alcoholic extract in a full bath.

Semi-solid preparations — 20 to 50% ointment to be rubbed in several times a day.

Homeopathic Dosage: 5 drops, 1 tablet or 10 globules every 30 to 60 minutes (acute) or 1 to 3 times daily (chronic); parenterally: 1 to 2 ml sc, acute: 3 times daily; chronic: once a day (HAB1). The dose is different for children.

PINE NEEDLE OIL

Mode of Administration: The essential oil is administered in alcoholic solutions, ointments, gels, emulsions, oils or as an inhalant. It is used externally as bubble baths and bath salts.

Daily Dosage: For internal use, the daily dose is 5 gm drug. For inhalation therapy, add 2 g oil to 2 cups hot water and breathe in the vapors several times daily. When used externally, several drops of a liquid or semi-solid preparation containing 10 to 50% drug may be rubbed onto the affected area. To use as a bath additive, use 0.025 gm drug per liter water and bathe for 10 to 20 minutes at a temperature 35 to 38° C.

Storage: Keep protected from light in tightly sealed containers.

TURPENTINE OIL, PURIFIED

Mode of Administration: Purified turpentine oil is administered externally in the form of ointments, gels, emulsions, oils, as a plaster and as an inhalant.

Daily Dosage:

External Dose — Varies according to the type and severity of the condition as well as the instructions of manufacturer.

As a bath additive and plaster — Use as directed by manufacturer.

Ointment/gel — 20% ointment/gel to be applied to the affected area several times a day.

Inhalation — 5 drops oil in hot water 3 times a day, inhale.

LITERATURE

PINE SHOOTS

Glasl H et al., Gaschromatographische Untersuchung von Arzneibuchdrogen 7. Mitt.: GC-Untersuchung von Pinaceen-Ölen des Handels und Versuche zu ihrer Standardisierung. In: DAZ 120(2):64-67. 1980.

Ikeda RM, (1962) J Food Sci 27:455.

Roschin VI et al., (1985) Khim Prir Soedin 1:122.

Zinkel DF, (1975) Chemtech 5(4):235.

Further information in:

Hänsel R, Keller K, Rimpler H, Schneider G (Hrsg.), Hagers Handbuch der Pharmazeutischen Praxis, 5. Aufl., Bde 4-6 (Drogen), Springer Verlag Berlin, Heidelberg, New York, 1992-1994.

Leung AY, Encyclopedia of Common Natural Ingredients Used in Food Drugs and Cosmetics, John Wiley & Sons Inc., New York, 1980.

Madaus G, Lehrbuch der Biologischen Arzneimittel, Bde 1-3, Nachdruck, Georg Olms Verlag Hildesheim 1979.

PINE NEEDLE OIL

Glasl H et al., Gaschromatographische Untersuchung von Arzneibuchdrogen 7. Mitt.: GC-Untersuchung von Pinaceen-Ölen des Handels und Versuche zu ihrer Standardisierung. In: DAZ 120(2):64-67. 1980.

Ikeda RM, (1962) J Food Sci 27:455.

Roschin VI et al., (1985) Khim Prir Soedin 1:122.

Zinkel DF, (1975) Chemtech 5(4):235.

Further information in:

Hänsel R, Keller K, Rimpler H, Schneider G (Hrsg.), Hagers Handbuch der Pharmazeutischen Praxis, 5. Aufl., Bde 4-6 (Drogen), Springer Verlag Berlin, Heidelberg, New York, 1992-1994.

Leung AY, Encyclopedia of Common Natural Ingredients Used in Food Drugs and Cosmetics, John Wiley & Sons Inc., New York, 1980.

Madaus G, Lehrbuch der Biologischen Arzneimittel, Bde 1-3, Nachdruck, Georg Olms Verlag Hildesheim 1979.

Steinegger E, Hänsel R, Pharmakognosie, 5. Aufl., Springer Verlag Heidelberg 1992.

Teuscher E, Biogene Arzneimittel, 5. Aufl., Wiss. Verlagsges. Stuttgart 1997.

Wagner H, Wiesenauer M, Phytotherapie. Phytopharmaka und pflanzliche Homöopathika, Fischer-Verlag, Stuttgart, Jena, New York, 1995.

TURPENTINE OIL, PURIFIED

Bauer L, (1973) Die Feinstruktur der menschlichen Bronchialschleimhaut nach Behandlung mit Ozothin. Klin Wochenschr 51:450-453.

Glasl H, Wagner H, DAZ 120:64-67. 1980.

Iconomou N et al., J Chromatogr 16:29. 1964.

Ikeda RM, (1962) J Food Sci 27:455.

Iravani J, (1972) Wirkung eines Broncholytikums auf die tracheobronchiale Reinigung. Arzneim Forsch (Drug Res) 22:1744-1746.

Roschin VI et al., (1985) Khim Prir Soedin 1:122.

Zänker KS, Blümel G, Probst J, Reiterer W, (1984) Theoretical, experimental evidence for the action of terpens as modulators in lung function. Prog Resp Res 18:302-304.

Zinkel DF, (1975) Chemtech 5(4):235.

Further information in:

Hänsel R, Keller K, Rimpler H, Schneider G (Hrsg.), Hagers Handbuch der Pharmazeutischen Praxis, 5. Aufl., Bde 4-6 (Drogen): Springer Verlag Berlin, Heidelberg, New York, 1992-1994.

Steinegger E, Hänsel R, Pharmakognosie, 5. Aufl., Springer Verlag Heidelberg 1992.

Teuscher E, Biogene Arzneimittel, 5. Aufl., Wiss. Verlagsges. Stuttgart 1997.

Wagner H, Wiesenauer M, Phytotherapie. Phytopharmaka und pflanzliche Homöopathika, Fischer-Verlag, Stuttgart, Jena, New York, 1995.

Scotch Thistle

Onopordum acanthium

DESCRIPTION

Medicinal Parts: The medicinal parts are the herb and the root.

Flower and Fruit: The large, light-red composite flowers are terminal on the branches. The bracts are linear-lanceolate, thorny-tipped, splayed at the bottom and like cobwebs. The plant has only tubular androgynous flowers. The bristles of the hair calyx are reddish, short pinnate and almost twice as long as the fruit. The flower heads fall after the fruit ripens and the seeds fall out.

Leaves, Stem and Root: The plant is biennial and grows from 30 to 150 cm. The stem is erect and branched. It appears to be winged because of the downward leaves, which are broader than the stem. The leaves are rough, irregularly thorny and dentate to pinnatisect. When young they appear almost white.

Habitat: The plant is indigenous to almost all of Europe, with the exception of the far north; it was introduced to North America.

Production: Scotch Thistle is the aerial part of Onopordum acanthium.

Other Names: Woolly Thistle

ACTIONS AND PHARMACOLOGY

COMPOUNDS

Sesquiterpene lactones (bitter principles): including, among others onopordopicrin

Flavonoids: including luteolin-7-O-glucoside

Hydroxycoumarins: esculin

Caffeic acid derivatives

Betaine: stachydrine

Polyynes

EFFECTS

A cardiotonic effect is questionable.

INDICATIONS AND USAGE

Unproven Uses: The drug is considered obsolete. In the religious system of anthroposophy, Scotch Thistle is used as a cardiac stimulant.

PRECAUTIONS AND ADVERSE REACTIONS

No health hazards or side effects are known in conjunction with the proper administration of designated therapeutic dosages.

DOSAGE

Mode of Administration: Scotch Thistle is available in the form of drops, ampules and tablets. In anthroposophic medicine, a preparation of the fresh leaves is used internally.

LITERATURE

Kern W, List PH, Hörhammer L (Hrsg.), Hagers Handbuch der Pharmazeutischen Praxis, 4. Aufl., Bde 1-8, Springer Verlag Berlin, Heidelberg, New York, 1969.

Madaus G, Lehrbuch der Biologischen Arzneimittel, Bde 1-3, Nachdruck, Georg Olms Verlag Hildesheim 1979.

Scrophularia nodosa

See Figwort

Scullcap

Scutellaria lateriflora

TRADE NAMES

Scullcap (available from numerous manufacturers), Wild American Scullcap, Wild Countryside Scullcap

DESCRIPTION

Medicinal Parts: The medicinal part of the plant is the herb.

Flower and Fruit: The pink or blue flowers are in short, chiefly lateral false spikes. The calyx is fluffy, dorsiventral and flattened, with 2 rounded, entire-margined lips. The lower lip has a helmet-shaped, concave appendage. The 4 ascending stamens have pairs of ciliated anthers. The fruit is a globular to flattened-ovoid warty nutlet.

Leaves, Stem and Root: The perennial herb grows to 60 cm in height and is thickly covered with simple and glandular hairs. The stem is erect and heavily branched. The foliage leaves are usually ovate to lanceolate or linear, petioled, entire-margined or crenate.

Characteristics: The herb has a bitter, slightly astringent taste.

Habitat: The plant is indigenous to North America and is cultivated in Europe.

Production: Scullcap is the aerial part of 3- to 4-year-old Scutellaria lateriflora and related species, which is harvested in June and then pulverized.

Other Names: Blue Pimpernel, Helmet Flower, Hoodwort, Mad-Dog Weed, Madweed, Quaker Bonnet

ACTIONS AND PHARMACOLOGY

COMPOUNDS

Iridoids

Flavonoids: including among others, scutellarin

Volatile oil

Tannins

EFFECTS

Scullcap has sedative, antispasmodic (little research), anti-inflammatory, and also lipid peroxidation inhibitor effects.

INDICATIONS AND USAGE

Unproven Uses: The drug was formerly used for hysteria and nervous tension, epilepsy, chorea, and other nervous disorders. It has also been used as a bitter tonic and febrifuge.

PRECAUTIONS AND ADVERSE REACTIONS

No health hazards or side effects are known in conjunction with the proper administration of designated therapeutic dosages.

DOSAGE

Mode of Administration: The herb is available as a powder and liquid extract for internal use.

How Supplied:

Capsules — 425 mg, 429 mg, 430 mg

LITERATURE

Barberan FAT, (1986) Fitoterapia 57(2):67.

Kimura Y et al., (1984) Planta Med 50:290.

Kimura Y et al., (1985) Planta Med 51:132.

Kimura Y et al., (1987) Phytother Res 1(1):48.

Kooiman P, (1972) Acta Bot Neerl. 21(4):417.

Kubo M et al., (1984) Chem Pharm Bull 32(7):2724.

Nicollier GF et al., (1981) J Agric Food Chem 29:1179.

Takido M et al., (1979) Yakugaku Zasshi 99(4):443-444.

Yagma, MS, Benson GG, (1979) J Nat Prod 42(2):229.

Further information in:

Chan, EH et al. (Eds.), Advances in Chinese Medicinal Materials Research, World Scientific Pub. Co. Singapore 1985.

Kern W, List PH, Hörhammer L (Hrsg.), Hagers Handbuch der Pharmazeutischen Praxis, 4. Aufl., Bde 1-8: Springer Verlag Berlin, Heidelberg, New York, 1969.

Madaus G, Lehrbuch der Biologischen Arzneimittel, Bde 1-3, Nachdruck, Georg Olms Verlag Hildesheim 1979.

Scurvy Grass

Cochlearia officinalis

DESCRIPTION

Medicinal Parts: The medicinal parts of the plant are the harvested and dried basal leaves of the first or second year; the aerial parts harvested shortly before or during flowering in the second year; or the fresh aerial parts of the plant collected at the onset of flowering.

Flower and Fruit: The flowers are arranged in racemes that are initially tight and somewhat hanging, which then grow longer. The flower is large, white and fragrant. The sepals are about 1.5 to 2 mm long, narrowly elliptoid, with a white membranous edge. The petals are about 4 to 5 mm long, oblong-obovate. The stamens are yellow. The fruit is a 4 to 7 mm long, globular or ovate pod, crowned by the short style. The 2 to 4 seeds in each loculus are roundish-elliptoid, a little compressed and 1 to 3 mm long. The seed shell is usually red-brown and finely warty.

Leaves, Stem and Root: The glabrous biennial or perennial plant is a 15 to 35 cm high evergreen. It has a fusiform, fibrous rhizome from which grows one or more stemmed shoots that are sterile and fertile. The leafy stems are ascending or almost erect, simple or branched, angular and grooved. The long-petioled basal leaves are in loose whorls. The fleshy, juicy cauline leaves are petiolate, ovate, angular-dentate, and the upper ones are stem-clasping.

Characteristics: The flowers have a strong taste and, when rubbed, a strong fragrance.

Habitat: The plant is found in central and northern Europe, Asia and North America.

Production: True Scurvy Grass consists of the dried basal leaves of Cochlearia officinalis harvested in the first year, or the aerial parts harvested during the flowering season in the second year. The cultivated plant is dried rapidly with artificial heat at temperatures below 35°C.

Not to be Confused With: Scurvy Grass is occasionally confused with Ranunculus ficaria.

Other Names: Scrubby Grass, Spoonwort

ACTIONS AND PHARMACOLOGY

COMPOUNDS

Glucosinolates: chief components in the freshly harvested, unbruised plant include glucocochlearin; with the destruction of the cells, the plants yield secretions of butyl mustard oil, and among others, glucotropaeolin (yielding butyl mustard oil) and sinigrin (yielding allyl mustard oil).

Flavonoids

Tropane alkaloids: tropine, m-hydroxybenzoyl-tropine (cochlearin)

Vitamin C

EFFECTS

The mustard oil glycosides in the drug, in ethereal oil and in an ethanol solution are strong external skin and mucous membrane irritants.

INDICATIONS AND USAGE

Unproven Uses: Scurvy Grass is used internally for vitamin C deficiency, and was used in folk medicine primarily as an agent for scurvy and scrofula. However, it was also valued for nose bleeds, rheumatism, gonorrhea, ''blood-cleansing or purification'' cures, gout, rheumatism, stomachache and as a diuretic. External applications include use as a mouthwash for gum disease and as a poultice for ulcers.

Homeopathic Uses: Among uses in homeopathy are eye inflammation and stomach disorders.

Efficacy has not been proven.

PRECAUTIONS AND ADVERSE REACTIONS

Health risks or side effects following the proper administration of designated therapeutic dosages are not recorded. The administration of higher dosages can lead to irritation of the mucous membrane of the gastrointestinal tract.

DOSAGE

Mode of Administration: Alcoholic extracts of Scurvy Grass are used topically. Freshly pressed juice is for internal use.

Homeopathic Dosage: 5 to 10 drops, 1 tablet, 5 to 10 globules 1 to 3 times a day; or 1 ml injection solution sc twice weekly; as an eye drop: 1 drop 1 to 3 times daily (HAB1)

LITERATURE

Cole RA, PH 15:759-762. 1976.

Hänsel R, Keller K, Rimpler H, Schneider G (Hrsg.), Hagers Handbuch der Pharmazeutischen Praxis, 5. Aufl., Bde 4-6 (Drogen): Springer Verlag Berlin, Heidelberg, New York, 1992-1994.

Madaus G, Lehrbuch der Biologischen Arzneimittel, Bde 1-3, Nachdruck, Georg Olms Verlag Hildesheim 1979.

Scutellaria lateriflora

See Scullcap

Sea Buckthorn

Hippophaë rhamnoides

DESCRIPTION

Medicinal Parts: The medicinal parts are the ripe, yellow-red berries.

Flower and Fruit: The plant is dioecious and has greenish-yellow, insignificant flowers in numerous, sturdy clusters in the axils of scales. There are 2 bracts and a simple calyx. The male calyx is divided in 2 down to the base, with brown-spotted ovate sepals; it has 4 stamens attached to the base. The female calyx is a tight tube clasping the ovary with erect, inward-inclined tips. The fruit is a bright orange, globular, ellipsoid, false berry.

Leaves, Stem and Root: The plant is an angular, thorny 1.5 to 4.5 m high shrub with numerous thorn-tipped and thorny branches. The leaves are 5 to 8 cm long, linear-lanceolate, short petioled, glabrous above, tomentose beneath. The plant spreads by underground runners.

Habitat: Hippophaë rhamnoides is indigenous to Europe and some northern regions of Asia.

Production: Sea Buckthorn berries are the false fruit of Hippophaë rhamnoides. The fatty oil is extracted from both the seeds and the fruit flesh. The harvest is from August to December, until the first snow. As soon as the fruit has been picked, it is immediately processed. The juice is produced without any contact with metal substances.

Other Names: Sallow Thorn

ACTIONS AND PHARMACOLOGY

COMPOUNDS

Fruit acids: chiefly malic acid, additionally acetic acid, quinic acid

Ascorbic acid (Vitamin C): 0.2-1.4%

Flavonoids: in particular kaempferol, isorhamnetin-as well as quercetin tri- and tetra-glycosides

Carotinoids: beta-carotine, gamma-carotine, lycopene

Fatty oil (in the seeds 12%): chief fatty acids oleic acid, isolinol acid, linolenic acid, stearic acid

Sugar alcohols: mannitol, quebrachit

EFFECTS

The drug is used as a vitamin C supplement. The vitamin C constituent encourages the healing of wounds and epithelization. It strengthens sight and inhibits sclerosis and the aging process.

The oil has a liver-protective, ulcer-protective, tumor-protective, anti-oxidative and wound-healing effect. The oil is said to be anticoagulative. The flavones are said to improve the contractility and pumping ability of cardiac muscle, reduce peripheral resistance and promote vascular elasticity.

INDICATIONS AND USAGE

Unproven Uses: The drug is used as an infection prophylaxis, in particular during the time just before spring and during periods of convalescence. It is used externally as a treatment for radiation damage, such as x-ray damage and sunburn, and as fatty oil for the treatment of wounds.

PRECAUTIONS AND ADVERSE REACTIONS

No health hazards or side effects are known in conjunction with the proper administration of designated therapeutic dosages.

DOSAGE

Mode of Administration: Buckthorn is an extract constituent in various vitamin C concentrates and juices.

Daily Dosage: The recommended daily dose is 5 to 10 gm of one of the Buckthorn products.

LITERATURE

Kern W, List PH, Hörhammer L (Hrsg.), Hagers Handbuch der Pharmazeutischen Praxis, 4. Aufl., Bde. 1-8, Springer Verlag Berlin, Heidelberg, New York, 1969.

Sedum acre

See Common Stonecrop

Selenicereus grandiflorus

See Night-Blooming Cereus

Self-Heal

Prunella vulgaris

DESCRIPTION

Medicinal Parts: The medicinal part is the whole flowering plant.

Flower and Fruit: The blue-violet or brownish-blue labiate flowers are clustered in semi-whorls at the end of stems and lateral branches. The accompanying leaves are red-brown. The upper lip of the calyx has 3 tips and the lower lip has 2 tips. The corolla is about 1 cm longer than the domed upper lip. The lower lip has 3 lobes. There are 4 stamens, the longer ones have a straight awl-shaped tip. The style is divided into two. The small fruit is flung out of the calyx.

Leaves, Stem and Root: The plant grows from 10 to 30 cm high. The stems are usually ascendant, sometimes creeping. The leaves are petiolate, ovate to lanceolate, dentate or entire-margined and crossed opposite.

Habitat: Prunella vulgaris is indigenous to Europe and Asia and practically all temperate regions of the world.

Production: Self-Heal is the complete plant in flower of Prunella vulgaris.

Other Names: Woundwort, Prunella, Hook-Heal, Slough-Heal, Brunella, Heart of the Earth, Blue Curls, Heal-All, Brownwort, Carpenter's Herb, Carpenter's Weed, Sicklewort

ACTIONS AND PHARMACOLOGY

COMPOUNDS

Bitter principles

Flavonoids: including rutin, hyperoside.

Tannins

Triterpene saponins

Triterpenes, ursolic acid, oleanolic acid

EFFECTS

There is no information available.

INDICATIONS AND USAGE

Unproven Uses: Self-Heal is used for inflammatory diseases and ulcers in the mouth and throat, gastrointestinal catarrh, as a remedy for diarrhea, hemorrhage and gynecological disorders.

PRECAUTIONS AND ADVERSE REACTIONS

No health hazards or side effects are known in conjunction with the proper administration of designated therapeutic dosages.

DOSAGE

Mode of Administration: Self-Heal is available as crude drug, as an extract and as a gargle solution.

Preparation: To prepare a tea, use 1 dessertspoon of the drug per cup of water.

LITERATURE

Kojima H. et al., (1987) Phytochemistry 26(4):1107.

Tabba HD, Chang RSh, Smith KM, Isolation, purification and partial characterization of prunellin, an anti-HIV component from aqueous extracts of Prunella vulgaris. In: Antiviral Res 11:263-274. 1989.

Further information in:

Hegnauer R, Chemotaxonomie der Pflanzen, Bde 1-11, Birkhäuser Verlag Basel, Boston, Berlin 1962-1997.

Kern W, List PH, Hörhammer L (Hrsg.), Hagers Handbuch der Pharmazeutischen Praxis, 4. Aufl., Bde. 1-8, Springer Verlag Berlin, Heidelberg, New York, 1969.

Sempervivum tectorum

See Houseleek

Senburi

Swertia japonica

DESCRIPTION

Medicinal Parts: The medicinal parts of the plant are the leaves and stems, which are used as an amaroid and tonic.

Flower and Fruit: The flowers are in dense apical panicles. The flowers are radial and fused, and their structures are in fives. The 5 calyx tips are up to 5 mm long and linear to lanceolate. The petals are 12 to 17 mm long, fused to a tube, with 5 broadened, elongate elliptical tips. The petals are white with reddish veins at the margin. Pairs of villous glandular scales are ciliate and twisted in the bud. There are 5 stamens and a superior, single-chambered ovary. The style is very short and the stigma 2-lobed. The fruit is a capsule; the seeds are ovate to clavate.

Leaves, Stem and Root: The herbaceous plant grows to approximately 20 cm high. The leaves are opposite and simple. The lower leaves are small and lanceolate. The cauline leaves are 1.5 to 3.5 cm long and 1 to 3 mm wide, linear to elongate-lanceolate, and acuminate with an involute margin. The stem is square in cross-section, 2 mm thick, dark green to dark red. The root is woody.

Characteristics: All parts of the plant taste very bitter.

Habitat: Swertia japonica is found in Korea, China and Japan.

Production: Japanese chirata is the dried herb of Swertia japonica harvested during its flowering season.

ACTIONS AND PHARMACOLOGY

COMPOUNDS

Iridoids (bitter substances): secoiridoid glycosides, including amarogentin (0.01 to 0.05%) and amaroswerin (0.05 to 0.3%), the representatives that are chiefly responsible for the bitter taste, as well as the less bitter representatives swertiamarin (1.0 to 2.5%), gentiopicroside (0.5%) and sweroside (0.2%)

Flavonoids: including swertisin, isoswertisin, swertiajaponin, isovitexin

Xanthone derivatives (yellow): including swertianin, norswertianin, methyl swertianin, swertianol (bellidifolin)

Monoterpene alkaloids

EFFECTS

The use of the drug as an amarum is traceable to the bitter substances it contains (secoiridoid glucoside). The allergenic effect connected with topical application should be taken into consideration.

INDICATIONS AND USAGE

Unproven Uses: Uses in folk medicine include poor digestion and loss of appetite.

Chinese Medicine: Insomnia and poor digestion are considered indications for use in Chinese medicine. Efficacy for these indications has not yet been proven.

PRECAUTIONS AND ADVERSE REACTIONS

No health hazards are known in conjunction with the proper administration of designated therapeutic dosages.

DOSAGE

Mode of Administration: Whole, cut and powdered drug.

How Supplied: Forms of commercial pharmaceutical preparations: Drops.

Daily Dosage: 30 to 50 mg of the powder.

LITERATURE

Basnet P, Kadota S, Shimizu M, Takata Y, Kobayashi M, Namba T, Bellidifolin stimulates glucose uptake in rat 1 fibroblasts and ameliorates hyperglycemia in streptozotocin (STZ)-induced diabetic rats. Planta Med, 61:402-5, 1995 Oct.

Blaschek W, Hänsel R, Keller K, Reichling J, Rimpler G, Schneider G, (Eds) Hagers Handbuch der Pharmazeutischen Praxis. Folgebä nde 1 und 2. Drogen A-Z. Springer. Berlin, Heidelberg 1998.

el-Sedawy AI, Shu YZ, Hattori M, Kobashi K, Namba T, Metabolism of swertiamarin from Swertia japonica by human intestinal bacteria. Planta Med, 33:147-50, 1989 Apr.

Hase K, Li J, Basnet P, Xiong Q, Takamura S, Namba T, Kadota S, Artificial bases from Swertia japonica. Makino Yakugaku Zasshi, 45:1202-4, 1966 Dec.

Hase K, Li J, Basnet P, Xiong Q, Takamura S, Namba T, Kadota S, Biologically active principles of crude drugs: pharmacological actions of Swertia japonica extracts, swertiamarin and gentianine (author's transl.). Yakugaku Zasshi, 45:1446-51, 1978 Nov.

Hase K, Li J, Basnet P, Xiong Q, Takamura S, Namba T, Kadota S, Biosynthesis of C-glucosylflavones in Swertia japonica (author's transl.). Yakugaku Zasshi, 45:165-71, 1979 Feb.

Hase K, Li J, Basnet P, Xiong Q, Takamura S, Namba T, Kadota S, Hepatoprotective principles of Swertia japonica Makino on D-galactosamine/lipopolysaccharide-induced liver injury in mice. Chem Pharm Bull (Tokyo), 45:1823-7, 1997 Nov.

Hase K, Li J, Basnet P, Xiong Q, Takamura S, Namba T, Kadota S, Studies on the constituents of Swertia japonica. I. On the structures of swertisin and isoswertisin. Chem Pharm Bull (Tokyo), 45:263-9, 1967 Mar.

Hase K, Li J, Basnet P, Xiong Q, Takamura S, Namba T, Kadota S, Studies on the constituents of Swertia japonica. II. Isolation and structure of new flavonoid, swertiajaponin. Chem Pharm Bull (Tokyo), 45:1567-72, 1967 Oct.

Hase K, Li J, Basnet P, Xiong Q, Takamura S, Namba T, Kadota S, Studies on the constituents of Swertia japonica. III. On the flavonoid constituents of the plants of Swertia. Yakugaku Zasshi, 45:832-7, 1968 Jul.

Hase K, Li J, Basnet P, Xiong Q, Takamura S, Namba T, Kadota S, Studies on the constituents of Swertia japonica. IV. Isolation and structure of xanthones. Chem Pharm Bull (Tokyo), 45:155-62, 1969 Jan.

Hase K, Li J, Basnet P, Xiong Q, Takamura S, Namba T, Kadota S, Studies on the constituents of Swertia japonica. V. On the xanthone constituents of the plants of Swertia. Yakugaku Zasshi, 45:410-7, 1969 Mar.

Hase K, Li J, Basnet P, Xiong Q, Takamura S, Namba T, Kadota S, Studies on the constituents of Swertia japonica. VI. On the flavonoid and xanthone constituents of Swertia randaiensis. Hayata and S. swertopsis Makino Yakugaku Zasshi, 45:1276-82, 1969 Sep.

Yamahara J, Kobayashi M, Matsuda H, Aoki S, Anticholinergic action of Swertia japonica and an active constituent. J Ethnopharmacol, 33:31-5, 1991 May-Jun.

Seneca Snakeroot

Polygala senega

DESCRIPTION

Medicinal Parts: The medicinal part is the dried root.

Flower and Fruit: The raceme is 8 cm long and is smaller than the bracts. The petals are pale red, the wings are yellowish-white with green veins.

Leaves, Stem and Root: The plant is a perennial herb with up to 40 cm high stems, which sprout in the axils of the scale-like bracts of the previous year's growth. The leaves are 8 cm long and 3 cm wide, alternate, ovate-lanceolate to lanceolate, acuminate and denticulate. The upper surface is rich green; the under surface somewhat paler. The root varies in color from pale yellowish-gray to brownish-gray. It is usually twisted or almost spiral and has a thick, irregular, gnarled crown.

Habitat: Polygala senega is indigenous to the central and western U.S.

Production: Seneca Snakeroot consists of the dried root with remains of aerial stems of Polygala senega and/or other closely related species or a mixture of Polygala species.

Not to be Confused With: The roots of other Polygala species.

Other Names: Milkwort, Mountain Flax, Rattlesnake Root, Seneca, Senega Snake Root, Senega, Seneka, Snake Root

ACTIONS AND PHARMACOLOGY

COMPOUNDS: SNAKEROOT (SENEGA SPECIES)

Triterpene saponins (6-12%): chief components senegins II to IV, chief aglycone presenegin

Oligosaccharide esters: senegosene A-I

Xanthone derivatives

Methyl salicylate (traces) and its glucoside

COMPOUNDS: SNAKEROOT (TENUIFOLIA SPECIES)

Triterpene saponins (6-12%): chief components onjisapo-nine aglycone presenegenin

Oligosaccharide esters: tenuifolosen A-P

Polygalite (acerite, 1.5-anhydrosorbite) and its glycosides, for example polygalite-2-alpha-galactoside

EFFECTS

The rhizome is secretolytic and works as an expectorant.

INDICATIONS AND USAGE

Approved by Commission E:

■ Cough/bronchitis

Unproven Uses: The drug is used for congestion of the respiratory tract, as an expectorant in cases of bronchitis with minor sputum output and tracheitis.

PRECAUTIONS AND ADVERSE REACTIONS

General: No health hazards or side effects are known in conjunction with the proper administration of designated therapeutic dosages. With prolonged use, gastrointestinal irritation can occur.

Pregnancy: Not to be used during pregnancy.

OVERDOSAGE

Overdosage leads to nausea, diarrhea, gastric complaints and queasiness.

DOSAGE

Mode of Administration: As a comminuted root for decoctions and other galenic preparations for internal use or as an extract. It is a component of various standardized antitussive preparations.

Preparation: To make an infusion, place 0.5 gm comminuted drug in cold water, heat to a simmer and strain after 10 minutes (1 teaspoonful = 2.5 gm drug).

Daily Dosage: The daily dosage is 1.5 to 3.0 gm root or liquid extract (1:2) or 2.5 to 7.5 gm tincture (1:10). To use the infusion as an expectorant, drink 1 cup of tea 2 to 3 times daily. In serious cases, the tea can be taken every two hours if the patient is observed for side effects.

LITERATURE

Corner JJ et al., (1962) Phytochemistry 1:73.

Kako M et al., Hypoglycemic effect of the rhizomes of Polygala senega in normal and diabetic mice and its main component, the triterpenoid glycoside senegin-II. In: PM 62(5)440-443. 1996.

Shibata S, In: Progress in Phytochemistry, Vol. 6, Ed. Reinhold et al., Pergamon Press 1980.

Shoji J et al., (1971) Yakugaku Zasshi 91:198.

Further information in:

Kern W, List PH, Hörhammer L (Hrsg.), Hagers Handbuch der Pharmazeutischen Praxis, 4. Aufl., Bde 1-8, Springer Verlag Berlin, Heidelberg, New York, 1969.

Madaus G, Lehrbuch der Biologischen Arzneimittel, Bde 1-3, Nachdruck, Georg Olms Verlag Hildesheim 1979.

Steinegger E, Hänsel R, Pharmakognosie, 5. Aufl., Springer Verlag Heidelberg 1992.

Teuscher E, Biogene Arzneimittel, 5. Aufl., Wiss. Verlagsges. Stuttgart 1997.

Wichtl M (Hrsg.), Teedrogen, 4. Aufl., Wiss. Verlagsges. Stuttgart 1997.

Senecio aureus

See Golden Ragwort

Senecio bicolor

See Dusty Miller

Senecio jacoboea

See Ragwort

Senecio nemorensis

See Alpine Ragwort

Senecio vulgaris

See Groundsel

Senna

Cassia species

TRADE NAMES

Senna Extract, Senna Leaf, Ex-Lax Regular Strength, Ex-Lax Maximum Strength, X-Prep Bowel Evacuant Liquid, SenokotXTRA, Senokot, Senokot Children's Syrup

DESCRIPTION

Medicinal Parts: The medicinal parts are the leaves, fruit and flowers.

Flower and Fruit: The flowers are yellow, occasionally white or pink. They are located in axillary or terminal positions on erect racemes. The calyx is deeply divided with a short tube and 5 regular, imbricate sepals. There are 5 layered petals. The 4 to 10 stamens are often irregular and partially sterile. The ovary is sessile or short-stemmed with a short or oblong style. The pod can be cylindrical or flat, angular or winged and often with horizontal walls between the seeds. The seeds are numerous and either horizontally or vertically compressed.

Leaves, Stem and Root: The genus Cassia comprises shrubs, subshrubs, and herbaceous perennials with paired-pinnate leaves. There are axes with stem glands either between the leaflets or on the petiole. The stipules have varying shapes.

Habitat: Cassia species is found in the tropical and subtropical regions of all continents except Europe. Most varieties are indigenous to North, Central, and South America.

Other Names: Tinnevelly Senna, India Senna, Alexandrian Senna, Khartoum Senna

ACTIONS AND PHARMACOLOGY

COMPOUNDS

Anthracene derivatives (2.5-3.5%): chief components sennosides A, A1 and B, as well as sennosides C and D

Naphthacene derivatives: including 6-hydroxymusizin glucoside (0.85% in Cassia senna), tinnevellin-6-glucosides (0.3% in Cassia angustifolia)

EFFECTS

Laxative Effects

Senna is an anthranoid-type stimulating laxative. The laxative effect is due to the action of sennosides and their active metabolite, rhein anthrone, in the colon. The laxative effect is realized by inhibition of water and electrolyte absorption from the large intestine, which increases the volume and pressure of the intestinal contents. This will stimulate colon motility resulting in propulsive contractions.

In addition, stimulation of active chloride secretion increases water and electrolyte content of the intestine. These changes in active electrolyte transport are dependent on calcium in the serosal surface (Donowitz, 1984; Yamauchi, 1993). The laxative action of Senna is partially via stimulation of colonic fluid and electrolyte secretion, and this secretion is mediated by stimulation of endogenous prostaglandin E2 formation (Beubler, 1988; Yamauchi, 1993).

CLINICAL TRIALS

Laxative Effects

A randomized, single-blind study evaluated the efficacy of Senna compared to polyethylene glycol (PEG) for mechanical preparation for elective colorectal resection. Five hundred twenty-three patients included in the study were undergoing resection, followed by anastomosis. All patients received 5% providone iodine antiseptic enema before surgery, and ceftriaxone sodium and metronidazole were given at anesthesia induction. Senna was significantly better than PEG with regard to colonic cleanliness and less fecal matter in the colonic lumen. The risk for moderate or large intraoperative fecal soiling was lower with senna and overall clinical tolerance did not differ significantly between the treatment groups. Senna was better tolerated in patients with stenosis. There was no statistical difference between the treatment groups with postoperative infective complications or anastomotic leakage (Valverde, 1999).

A prospective randomized trial evaluated the efficacy of the addition of senna to a polethylene glycol electrolyte lavage solution (PEG-ELS). One hundred and twenty patients received either a Senna extract with PEG-ELS or placebo with PEG-ELS before a total colonoscopy. Superiority by physician assessment was seen in the group with Senna. The colon was free of solid debris in 66.7% of patients after PEG-ELS and in 90% after Senna/PEG-ELS administration, which was a significant difference. Patient tolerance was similar in both groups, and significantly less lavage fluid was needed in the Senna/PEG-ELS treatment group (Ziegenhagen, 1991).

A randomized, open, parallel group study was conducted to determine the efficacy of senna compared to lactulose in terminal cancer patients treated with opioids. Ninety-one terminal cancer patients were treated with either senna (starting with 0.4 mL daily) or lactulose (starting with 15 mL daily) for a 27-day period. The main outcome measures were defecation-free intervals of 72 hr, days with defecation, general health status, and treatment cost. Both treatment groups had similar scores for defecation-free intervals and in days with defecation. The final scores for general health status were similar in both groups (Agra, 1998).

INDICATIONS AND USAGE

- Constipation

Senna is used for constipation and for evacuation of the bowel prior to diagnostic tests of the gastrointestinal and colorectal area.

Indian Medicine: The herb is used for constipation, liver disease, jaundice, splenomegaly, anemia, and typhoid fever.

Note: Stimulating laxatives must not be used over a period of more than 1 to 2 weeks without medical advice.

CONTRAINDICATIONS

The herb is not to be administered in the presence of intestinal obstruction, acute inflammatory intestinal diseases or appendicitis.

PRECAUTIONS AND ADVERSE REACTIONS

General: Spasmodic gastrointestinal complaints can occur as a side effect to the drug's purgative effect or from overdosage. In rare cases, prolonged use may lead to cardiac arrhythmias, nephropathies, edema and accelerated bone deterioration. Senna abuse has also resulted in tetany, aspartylglucosamine excretion, and hypogammaglobulinemia (Levine, 1981; Malmquist, 1980; Prior, 1978).

Electrolyte Abnormalies: Long-term use leads to loss of electrolytes, in particular potassium ions. As a result of hypokalemia, hyperaldosteronism, albuminuria, hematuria, inhibition of intestinal motility, and muscle weakness may occur. Enhancement of cardioactive glycosides and antiarrythics may also occur with hypokalemia.

Finger Clubbing: Senna abuse has resulted in finger clubbing, which was reversible upon discontinuation of the drug (Levine, 1981; Malmquist, 1980; Prior, 1978; Silk, 1975).

Cathartic Colon: Anatomic alteration of the colon is seen secondary to chronic use with Senna (more than three times weekly for 1 year or longer). The result is a loss of haustral folds, a finding that suggests neuronal injury or damage to colonic longitudinal musculature (Joo, 1998).

Carcinogenesis: Carcinogenic activity in the colon following long-term administration of anthracene drugs has not yet been fully clarified. Study findings are controversial regarding the correlation between the administration of anthracene drugs and the frequency of carcinomas in the colon (al-Dakan, 1995; Mereto, 1996).

Melanosis Coli: Prolonged use of Senna may lead to melanosis coli. Precursors of the melanic substance in melanosis coli may be derived from anthranoid laxatives (Benavides, 1997).

Occupational Sensitization: IgE-mediated allergy, asthma, and rhinoconjunctivitis have been reported after occupational exposure to senna products (Helin, 1996, Marks, 1991).

Tissue Damage: Chronic treatment with anthranoids in high doses reduces vasoactive intestinal polypeptide and somatostatin levels in the colon, which may represent damage to the enteric nervous tissue (Tzavella, 1985).

Drug Interactions:

Digitalis Glycosides — With prolonged use or abuse of Senna, loss of potassium may potentiate digitalis toxicity.

Antiarrythmics — Loss of potassium associated with prolonged use of Senna may potentiate arrhythmias when given concomitantly with antiarrhythmic medications.

Estrogen — The serum level of estrogen is decreased when given concomitantly with Senna due to the effect of intestinal transit on the absorption of estrogens (Lewis, 1998).

Indomethacin (NSAIDS) — Indomethacin given concomitantly with Senna pod extract had a dose-dependent inhibition of net fluid transport due to the inhibition of prostaglandin E2 (SEE EFFECTS), which decreases the therapeutic effect of the Senna (Beubler, 1985).

Nifedipine (calcium channel blocker) — Therapeutic effects induced by rhein anthrone also involve the calcium channel which can be blocked by nifedipine, but not verapamil (SEE EFFECTS) (Yamauchi, 1993).

Pregnancy: The drug should not be used during pregnancy or while nursing.

Pediatric Use: Not to be used by children under 2 years of age. Children between the ages of 2-12 years should follow proper dosage recommendations.

Elderly: Elderly patients should initially take half of the normal prescribing dose.

DOSAGE

Mode of Administration: Comminuted herb, powder or dried extracts for teas, decoctions, cold macerates, or elixirs. Liquid or solid forms of medication exclusively for oral use.

How Supplied:

Capsule — 25 mg, 450 mg

Chewable tablet — 15 mg sennosides

Granules — 15 mg sennosides per teaspoon

Liquid — 2.5 oz. (alcohol 7% by volume), 8.8 mg sennosides per teaspoon

Tablet — 8.6 mg sennosides, 15 mg sennosides, 17 mg sennosides, 25 mg sennosides

Preparation: To prepare an infusion, pour hot water (not boiling) over 0.5 to 2 gm of comminuted drug, steep for 10 minutes, then strain; or steep in cold water for 10 to 12 hours, then strain. The cold water method, according to various authors, should result in a solution containing less resin, which is responsible for abdominal pain. The drug takes effect after a latency period of 10 to 12 hours.

Daily Dosage:

Constipation — The average dose is 20 to 60 mg sennosides.

Chewable Tab — Adults and children 12 years of age and over, chew 2 tabs once or twice daily. Children 6 to under 12 years of age, chew 1 tab once or twice daily (Prod Info Ex-Lax®, 1998).

Granules (15 mg sennosides per teaspoon) — Adults and children 12 years of age, administer 1 teaspoon once daily with a maximum of 2 teaspoons twice daily. Children 6 to 12 years of age, administer 1/2 teaspoon once daily with a maximum of 1 teaspoon twice a day. Children 2 to 6 years of age, administer 1/4 teaspoon daily with a maximum of 1/2 teaspoon twice daily (Prod Info Senokot®, 1993).

Liquid (8.8 mg sennoside per teaspoon) — Children 6 to 12 years of age, administer 1 to 1 1/2 teaspoon once daily with a maximum of 1 1/2 teaspoon twice daily. Children 2 to 6 years of age, administer 1/2 to 3/4 teaspoon once daily with a maximum of 3/4 teaspoon twice daily (Prod Info Senokot®, 1991).

Pills — Adults and children 12 years of age and over should take 2 pills once or twice daily with a glass of water. Children 6 to under 12 years of age: take 1 pill once or twice daily with a glass of water. Children under 6 years of age: consult a doctor (Prod Info Ex-Lax®, 1998).

Tablets (8.6 mg sennosides) — Adults and children 12 years of age, administer 2 tablets once daily with a maximum of 4 tablets twice daily. Children 6 to 12 years of age, administer 1 tablet once daily, with a maximum of 2 tablets twice daily. Children 2 to 6 years of age, adminster 1/2 tablet once daily with a maximum of 1 tablet twice daily (Prod Info Senokot®, 1993).

Tablets (17 mg sennosides) — Adults and children 12 years of age, administer 1 tablet once daily with a maximum of 2 tablets twice daily. Children 6 to 12 years of age, administer 1/2 tablet once daily with a maximum of 1 tablet twice daily (Prod Info SenokotXTRA®, 1993).

Bowel Evacuation:

Liquid (alcohol 7% by volume) — Adults and children 12 years of age and older should take one bottle between 2 and 4 p.m. on day prior to x-ray or other diagnostic procedures. Drink entire contents of bottle. A strong bowel action can be expected approximately 6 hours after drinking the preparation (Prod Info X-Prep®,1998).

Storage: Senna should be protected from light (DAB10 EUR), and stored for a maximum of 3 years (2.AB-DDR).

LITERATURE

Agra Y; Sacristan A; Gonzalez M et al. Efficacy of senna versus lactulose in terminal cancer patients treated with opioids. J Pain Symptom Manage 1998 Jan;15(1):1-7.

al-Dakan AA; al-Tuffail M; Hannan MA. Cassia senna inhibits mutagenic activities of benzo[a]-pyrene, aflatoxin B1, shamma and methyl methanesulfonate. Pharmacol Toxicol 1995 Oct;77(4):288-92.

Anonym, Sennahaltige Laxanzien: Alte Arzneipflanze in neuem Licht? In: DAZ 133(28):2594. 1993.

BGA, Arzneimittelrisiken: Anthranoide. In: DAZ 132(21):1164. 1992.

Benavides SH; Morgante PE; Monserrat AJ et al. The pigment of melanosis coli: a lectin histochemical study. Gastrointest Endosc 1997 Aug;46(2):131-8.

Beubler E, Kollar G. Stimulation of PGE2 synthesis and water and electrolyte secretion by senna anthraquinones is inhibited by indomethacin. J Pharm Pharmacol 1985 Apr;37(4):248-51.

Beubler E; Kollar G. Prostaglandin-mediated action of sennosides. Pharmacology 1988;36 Suppl 1:85-91.

Choi JS et al., In vitro antimutagenic effects of anthraquinone aglycones and naphthoquinones. In: PM 63(1):11-14. 1997.

Christ B et al., (1978) Arzneim Forsch 28:225.

Donowitz M; Wicks J; Battisti L et al. Effect of Senokot on rat intestinal electrolyte transport. Evidence of Ca+ dependence. Gastroenterology 1984 Sep;87(3):503-12.

Dufour P, Gendre P, (1988) Long-Termin mucosal alterations by sennosides, related compounds. Pharmacology 36(Suppl 1):194-202.

Fairbairn JW (1964) Lloydia 27:79.

Fairbairn JW (1976) Pharmacol 14(Suppl 1):48.

Fairbairn JW, Shrestha AB, (1967) Lloydia 30:67.

Helin T; Makinen-Kiljunen. Occupational asthma and rhinoconjunctivitis caused by senna. Allergy 1996 Mar;51(3):181-4.

Jahn K et al., Toxicology of Cassia fikifiki Aubréville 6 Pellegrin in relation to other species of the genus Cassia (s.l.). In: PM 62, Abstracts of the 44th Ann Congress of GA, 57. 1996.

Joo JS; Ehrenpreis ED; Gonzalez L et al. Alterations in colonic anatomy induced by chronic stimulant laxatives: the cathartic colon revisited. J Clin Gastroenterol 1998 Jun;26(4):283-6.

Klimpel BE et al., Anthranoidhaltige Laxantien - ein Risiko für die Entwicklung von Tumoren der ableitenden Harnwege. In: PUZ 26(1):33, Jahrestagung der DPhG, Berlin, 1996. 1997.

Lemli J, Cuveele J, (1975) Phytochemistry 14:1397.

Lemli, J et al., (1981) Planta Med 43:11.

Leng-Peschlow E, Mengs U, Sennalaxantien: Sicher und wirksam. In: PZ 140(8):668-676. 1995.

Levine D; Goode AW; Wingate DL. Purgative abuse associated with reversible cachexia, hypogammaglobulinaemia, and finger clubbing. Lancet 1981 Apr 25;1(8226):919-20.

Lewis SJ, Oakey RE, Heaton KW. Intestinal absorption of estrogen: the effect of altering transit-time. Eur J Gastroenterol Hepatol 1998 Jan;10(1):33-9.

Malmquist J; Ericsson B; Hulten-Nosslin MB et al. Finger clubbing and aspartylglucosamine excretion in a laxative-abusing patient. Postgrad Med J 1980 Dec;56(662):862-4.

Marks GB; Salome CM; Woolcock AJ. Asthma and allergy associated with occupational exposure to ispaghula and senna products in a pharmaceutical work force. Am Rev Respir Dis 1991 Nov;144(5):1065-9.

Mereto E; Ghia M; Brambilla G. Evaluation of the potential carcinogenic activity of Senna and Cascara glycosides for the rat colon. Cancer Lett 1996 Mar 19;101(1):79-83.

Prior J, White I. Tetany and clubbing in patient who ingested large quantities of senna. Lancet 1978 Oct 28;2(8096):947.

Product Information: Ex-Lax®, chocolated laxative pieces. Novartis, Summit, NJ, USA, 1998.

Product Information: Ex-Lax®, regular and maximum strength laxative pills. Novartis, Summit, NJ, USA, 1998.

Product Information: SenokotXTRA®, standardized senna concentrate. Purdue Frederick, Norwalk, CT, USA, 1993.

Product Information: Senokot®, extract of standardized senna. Purdue Frederick, Norwalk, CT, USA, 1991.

Product Information: Senokot®, standardized senna concentrate. Purdue Frederick, Norwalk, CT, USA, 1993.

Product Information X-Prep®, extract of standardized senna. Gray Pharmaceuticals, Norwalk, CT, USA, 1998.

Schultze W, Jahn K, Richter R, Volatile constituents of the dried leaves of Cassia angustifolia and C. acutifolia (Sennae folium). In: PM 61(6):540-543. 1996.

Silber W, Sprühgetrockneter Senna-Extrakt. In: DAZ 131(9):349. 1991.

Silk DB; Gibson JA; Murray CR. Reversible finger clubbing in a case of purgative abuse. Gastroenterology 1975 Apr;68(4 Pt 1):790-4.

Sprecher E, Über die Qualität von Phytopharmaka. In: ZPT 12(4):105. 1991.

Sydiskis RJ, Owen DG, Lohr JL, Rosler KHA, Blosmster RN, Inactivation of enveloped viruses by anthraquinones extracted from plants. In: Antimicrob Agents Chemother 35:2463-2466. 1991.

Tzavella K; Schenkirsch G; Riepl RL et al. Effects of long-term treatment with anthranoids and sodium picosulphate on the contents of vasoactive intestinal polypeptide, somatostatin and substance P in the rat colon. Eur J Gastroenterol Hepatol 1995 Jan;7(1):13-20.

Valverde A; Hay JM; Fingerhut A et al. Senna vs polyethylene glycol for mechanical preparation the evening before elective colonic or rectal resection: a multicenter controlled trial. French Association for Surgical Research. Arch Surg 1999 May;134(5):514-9.

Van Os FHL (1976) Pharmacol 14(Suppl 1):7.

Yamauchi K; Yagi T; Kuwano S. Suppression of the purgative action of rhein anthrone, the active metabolite of sennosides A and B, by calcium channel blockers, calmodulin antagonists and indomethacin. Pharmacology 1993 Oct;47 Suppl 1:22-31.

Ziegenhagen DJ; Zehnter E; Tacke W et al. Addition of senna improves colonoscopy preparation with lavage: a prospective randomized trial. Gastrointest Endosc 1991 Sep-Oct;37(5):547-9.

Further information in:

Hänsel R, Keller K, Rimpler H, Schneider G (Hrsg.), Hagers Handbuch der Pharmazeutischen Praxis, 5. Aufl., Bde 4-6 (Drogen): Springer Verlag Berlin, Heidelberg, New York, 1992-1994.

Leung AY, Encyclopedia of Common Natural Ingredients Used in Food Drugs, Cosmetics, John Wiley & Sons Inc., New York 1980.

Lewin L, Gifte und Vergiftungen, 6. Aufl., Nachdruck, Haug Verlag, Heidelberg 1992.

Madaus G, Lehrbuch der Biologischen Arzneimittel, Bde 1-3, Nachdruck, Georg Olms Verlag Hildesheim 1979.

Roth L, Daunderer M, Kormann K, Giftpflanzen, Pflanzengifte, 4. Aufl., Ecomed Fachverlag Landsberg Lech 1993.

Schulz R, Hänsel R, Rationale Phytotherapie, Springer Verlag Heidelberg 1996.

Steinegger E, Hänsel R, Pharmakognosie, 5. Aufl., Springer Verlag Heidelberg 1992.

Teuscher E, Lindequist U, Biogene Gifte - Biologie, Chemie, Pharmakologie, 2. Aufl., Fischer Verlag Stuttgart 1994.

Teuscher E, Biogene Arzneimittel, 5. Aufl., Wiss. Verlagsges. Stuttgart 1997.

Wagner H, Wiesenauer M, Phytotherapie. Phytopharmaka und pflanzliche Homöopathika, Fischer-Verlag, Stuttgart, Jena, New York 1995.

Wichtl M (Hrsg.), Teedrogen, 4. Aufl., Wiss. Verlagsges. Stuttgart 1997.

Serenoa repens

See Saw Palmetto

Sesame

Sesamum orientale

DESCRIPTION

Medicinal Parts: The medicinal part of the plant is the seed.

Flower and Fruit: The flowers are short-pedicled, single or in groups of 2 or 3 in the leaf axils. The flowers are zygomorphic; the calyx 5-tipped, 2 to 5 mm long, pubescent and does not drop. The corolla is campanulate, 5-lobed and distinctly bilabiate. It is 1.5 to 3.5 cm long, white or reddish. The lower lobes are the longest. There are 4 stamens. The ovary is usually 2-chambered (but can be up to 10-chambered) with a false septum, 1 to 1.5 mm long and pubescent. The fruit is a square, brownish, 2 to 3 cm long and up to 1 cm wide, multi-seeded capsule. The seeds are yellowish-white, brownish, reddish or black, 1.5 to 4 mm long, 1 to 2 mm wide, 0.5 to 1 mm thick, and smooth or finely ribbed.

Leaves, Stem and Root: The herb grows upright to a height of 1.2 m. The lower leaves are opposite and the petiole is 3 to 11 cm long. The lamina 4 to 20 cm long and 2 to 10 cm wide. It is elongate-ovate, entire or 3-lobed, then dentate. The upper leaves are opposite or alternate. The petiole is up to 3 cm long. The lamina is 0.5 to 2.5 cm wide, lanceolate and usually entire. Young leaves are pubescent and sticky. The stem is square to hexagonal, either completely pubescent or only on the upper section. The taproot grows down to a depth of almost 1 m. The stem is branched or unbranched.

Characteristics: The plant's oily seeds are odorless with a sweet taste.

Habitat: Sesame orientale is cultivated worldwide in tropical and subtropical temperate zones, but the main sesame oil-producing countries are India, Sudan, Burma and China.

Production: Sesame oil is the oil of Sesamum orientale, which is pressed or extracted from the ripe seeds and refined.

Other Names: Beniseed, Gingelly, Oriental Sesame

ACTIONS AND PHARMACOLOGY

COMPOUNDS

Fatty oil (97 to 98%): chief fatty acids are oleic acid (35 to 50%), linoleic acid (35 to 50%), palmitic acid (7 to 12%), stearic acid (3 to 6%)

Lignans (0.8 to 1.7%): including sesamine sesamolin

Steroids: sterols, including beta-sitosterol (0.4%), campesterol

EFFECTS

The lignan sesamine contained in the drug is immunosuppressive in vitro. In view of its oily nature, use as a clysma for softening the stool and topically on dry skin diseases is plausible. Its effect as a purgative seems logical but has not been clinically proven. Sesame oil treated with lipase is cytotoxic in vitro. Because of its high levels of linoleic acid, sesame oil is a valuable dietetic.

INDICATIONS AND USAGE

Unproven Uses: Folk medicine internal uses include treating constipation, especially dyschezia; external uses include removal of scabs and crust formations, for swellings, rheumatism and as a massage oil. Its use as a laxative is considered obsolete.

PRECAUTIONS AND ADVERSE REACTIONS

No health hazards are known in conjunction with the proper administration of designated therapeutic dosages. The drug possesses a limited potential for sensitization.

DOSAGE

Mode of Administration: Preparations are available for internal and external use.

Preparation: Sesame oil for parenteral application is produced from Sesamum orientale by heating in a drying chamber to 140°C or by means of germ filtration with the addition of 5% benzyl alcohol followed by heating at 120° C for 1 hour in the drying chamber.

Storage: Store in tightly sealed containers and protect from light.

LITERATURE

Aregheore EM, A review of implications of antiquality and toxic components in unconventional feedstuffs advocated for use in intensive animal production in Nigeria. Vet Hum Toxicol, 40:35-9, 1998 Feb.

Badifu GI, Akpagher EM, Effects of debittering methods on the proximate composition, organoleptic and functional properties of sesame (Sesamum indicum L.) seed flour. Plant Foods Hum Nutr, 51:119-26, 1996 Feb.

Bhatnagar A, Gupta A, Chlorpyriphos, quinalphos and lindane residues in sesame seed and oil (Sesamum indicum L.). J Sci Food Agric, 60:596-600, 1998 Apr.

Bhatnagar A, Gupta A, Dissociation and denaturation behaviour of sesame alpha-globulin in sodium dodecyl sulphate solution. Int J Pept Protein Res, 60:385-92, 1998 Apr.

Chambers SJ, Carr HJ, Lambert N, An investigation of the dissociation and denaturation of legumin by salts using laser light scattering and circular dichroism spectroscopy. Biochim Biophys Acta, 1037:66-72, 1990 Jan 19.

Egbekun MK, Ehieze MU, Proximate composition and functional properties of fullfat and defatted beniseed (Sesamum indicum L.) flour. Plant Foods Hum Nutr, 51:35-41, 1997.

Guerra MJ, Jaffe WG, Sangronis E, Obtaining protein fractions from commercial sesame cakes (Sesamum indicum). Arch Latinoam Nutr, 34:477-87, 1984 Sep.

Guerra MJ, Jaffe WG, Sangronis E, Os sesamum genus proximale tibiale. Cesk Radiol, 34:477-87, 1984 Sep.

Hansel R, Keller K, Rimpler H, Schneider G (Ed), Hagers Handbuch der Pharmazeutischen Praxis, 5. Aufl., Bde 4 - 6 (Drogen), Springer Verlag Berlin, Heidelberg, New York, 1992-1994.

Kadirvel R, Studies on sesame oil cake meal (Sesamum indicum) in chick mash. Indian Vet J, 45:529-36, 1968 Jun.

Kumar KS, Murthy SK, Studies on lipolytic enzymes of oil seeds. Part I. Sesamum indicum (gingelly). Enzymologia, 33:243-9, 1967 Nov 30.

Lakshmi TS, Nandi PK, Prakash V, Interactions of sugars with alpha-globulin from Sesamum indicum L. Indian J Biochem Biophys, 51:135-41, 1985 Jun.

Marston A, Potterat O, Hostettmann K, Isolation of biologically active plant constituents by liquid chromatography. J Chromatogr, 60:3-11, 1988 Oct 19.

Mehrotra RS, Tiwari DP, Organic amendments and control of foot rot of Piper betle caused by Phytophthora parasitica var. piperina. Ann Microbiol (Paris), 35:415-21, 1976 Apr.

Otaiza ER, Valeri H, Cumare V, Selenium content in the blood of cattle from Venezuela. I. Central and Portuguese zones. Arch Latinoam Nutr, 60:233-46, 1977 Jun.

Perez C, Saad R, Enzymatic modification of proteins of commercial sesame meals (Sesamum indicum, L.). Arch Latinoam Nutr, 34:735-48, 1984 Dec.

Plietz P, Damaschun G, Zirwer D, Gast K, Schwenke KD, Prakash V, Shape and quaternary structure of alpha-globulin from sesame (Sesamum indicum L.) seed as revealed by small angle x-ray scattering and quasi-elastic light scattering. J Biol Chem, 1986 Sep 25; 261(27):12686-91.

Prakash V, Nandi PK, Association-dissociation behavior of sesame alpha-globulin in electrolyte solutions. J Biol Chem, 60:240-3, 1977 Jan 10.

Prakash V, Nandi PK, Dissociation, aggregation and denaturation of sesame alpha-globulin in urea and guanidine hydrochloride solutions. Int J Pept Protein Res, 60:97-106, 1977.

Prakash V, Nandi PK, Jirgensons B, Effect of sodium dodecyl sulfate, acid, alkali, urea and guanidine hydrochloride on the circular dichroism of alpha-globulin of Sesamum indicum L. Int J Pept Protein Res, 51:305-13, 1980 Apr.

Rajamohan T, Kurup PA, Histopathologic studies on sesamoid bones of the hoof in cattle with purulent podotrochlitis. Berl Munch Tierarztl Wochenschr, 35:289-93 concl, 1976 Aug 1.

Rajamohan T, Kurup PA, Lysine: arginine ratio of a protein influences cholesterol metabolism. Part 1 - Studies on sesame protein having low lysine: arginine ratio. Indian J Exp Biol, 35:1218-23, 1997 Nov.

Saad R, Perez C, Functional and nutritional properties of modified proteins of sesame (Sesamum indicum, L.). Arch Latinoam Nutr, 34:749-62, 1984 Dec.

Saad R, Perez C, Persistance of antibiotics in leaves of sesamum (Sesamum indicum L.). Hindustan Antibiot Bull, 34:107-8, 1984 Aug-Nov.

Salgado JM, Goncalves CM, Sesame seed (Sesamum indicum, L.). I. Methods for preparing an edible white flour. Arch Latinoam Nutr, 38:306-11, 1988 Jun.

Sheela P, Amuthan G, Mahadevan A, Cloning of extracellular lipase gene from Xanthomonas campestris pathovar sesami on to Escherichia coli. Indian J Exp Biol, 60:27-31, 1996 Jan.

Tasneem R, Prakash V, Aggregation, dissociation and denaturation of sesame (Sesamum indicum L.) alpha-globulin in cetyl trimethyl ammonium bromide solution. Int J Pept Protein Res, 8:120-8, 1977.

Tasneem R, Prakash V, Association-dissociation and denaturation behaviour of an oligomeric seed protein alpha-globulin of Sesamum indicum L. in acid and alkaline solutions. Int J Pept Protein Res, 8:319-28, 1977.

Tasneem R, Prakash V, Resistance of alpha-globulin from Sesamum indicum L. to proteases in relationship to its structure. J Protein Chem, 8:251-61, 1989 Apr.

Tasneem R, Prakash V, The nature of the unhydrolysed fraction of alpha-globulin, the major protein component of Sesamum indicum L. hydrolysed by alpha-chymotrypsin. Indian J Biochem Biophys, 29:160-7, 1992 Apr.

Thompson EW, Richardson M, Boulter D, The amino acid sequence of sesame (Sesamum indicum L.) and castor (Ricinus communis L.) cytochrome c. Biochem J, 51:439-46, 1971 Feb.

Wankhede DB, Tharanathan RN, Sesame (Sesamum indicum) carbohydrates. J Agric Food Chem, 51:655-9, 1976 May-Jun.

Yukawa Y, Takaiwa F, Shoji K, Masuda K, Yamada K, Structure and expression of two seed-specific cDNA clones encoding stearoyl-acyl carrier protein desaturase from sesame, Sesamum indicum L. Plant Cell Physiol, 37:201-5, 1996 Mar.

Yun TK, Kim SH, Lee YS, Trial of a new medium-term model using benzo(a)pyrene induced lung tumor in newborn mice. Anticancer Res, 15:839-45, 1995 May-Jun.

Sesamum orientale

See Sesame

Shepherd's Purse

Capsella bursa-pastoris

DESCRIPTION

Medicinal Parts: The medicinal part is the aerial portion of the plant.

Flower and Fruit: The plant stays in bloom for almost the whole year. The flowers are white and about 4 to 6 mm long. The 4 sepals are 1 to 2 mm long and the 4 petals are 2 to 3 mm long. There are 6 stamens. The inflorescence is extended after flowering. The many-seeded pod is 4 to 9 mm long and almost as wide. It is glabrous, flattened, long-stemmed, triangular and obcordate. The seeds are 0.8 to 1 mm long and red-brown with a short style.

Leaves, Stem and Root: Shepard's purse is a 2 to 40 cm high plant with a simple fusiform root and a simple upright stem. The stem is glabrous or has scattered hairs on the lower section. The basal leaves form a rosette and are petioled, entire-margined or pinnatifid. The few cauline leaves are alternate, smaller, sessile, entire, very wrinkled and involute.

Habitat: Worldwide, except tropical regions.

Production: Shepherd's Purse herb consists of the fresh or dried aboveground parts of Capsella bursa, collected in the wild during the summer and dried rapidly.

Other Names: Shepherd's Scrip, Shepherd's Sprout, Lady's Purse, Witches' Pouches, Rattle Pouches, Case-Weed, Pick-Pocket, Blindweed, Pepper-and-Salt, Poor Man's Parmacettie, Sanguinary, Mother's Heart, Cocowort, St. James' Weed, Shepherd's Heart, Toywort

ACTIONS AND PHARMACOLOGY

COMPOUNDS

Cardioactive steroids: presumably only in the seeds

Glucosinolates, sinigrin: 9-methyl sulfinyl nonyl glucosinolate, 9-methyl sulfinyl decyl glucosinolate

Flavonoids: including rutin, luteolin-7-rutinoside

Caffeic acid derivatives: including chlorogenic acid.

The plant very often acts as a host to endophytic fungi (*Albugo candida, Peronospora parasitica*), so the presence of mytotoxins is a possibility.

EFFECTS

A number of different studies have shown both a lowering and elevation of blood pressure, positive inotropic and chronotropic cardiac effects, and increased uterine contraction. Despite numerous studies a clear therapeutic use could not be identified.

INDICATIONS AND USAGE

Approved by Commission E:

- Nosebleeds
- Premenstrual syndrome (PMS)
- Wounds and burns

Unproven Uses: Internally, the plant is used for mild menstrual irregularities such as menorrhagia and metrorrhagia. Externally, it is used for nosebleeds and superficially bleeding skin injuries. Shepherd's Purse is seldom used in folk medicine today. In America it is used for headaches. In Spain a decoction of the fresh plant is used for bladder inflammation.

Homeopathic Uses: Capsella bursa-pastoris is used for uterine and mucous membrane bleeding as well as for calculosis.

PRECAUTIONS AND ADVERSE REACTIONS

General: No health hazards or side effects are known in conjunction with the proper administration of designated therapeutic dosages.

Pregnancy: Not to be used during pregnancy.

DOSAGE

Mode of Administration: Comminuted drug for tea and other galenic preparations for internal use and external administration.

Daily Dosage: Internally, the average daily dose is 10 to 15 gm of drug. The liquid extract daily dose is 5 to 8 gm drug. The infusion may be drunk throughout the day. Externally an infusion is prepared by adding 3 to 5 gm drug to 150 ml water.

Homeopathic Dosage: 5 drops or 1 tablet or 10 globules every 30 to 60 minutes (acute) or 1 to 3 times a day (chronic); parenterally: 1 to 2 ml 3 times a day sc (HAB1)

Storage: Shepard's Purse should be protected from light and moisture.

LITERATURE

Farkas L, In "Pharmacognosy and Phytochemistry 1st Int Cong. Munich 1971", Springer-Verlag 1971.

Hänsel R, Keller K, Rimpler H, Schneider G (Hrsg.), Hagers Handbuch der Pharmazeutischen Praxis, 5. Aufl., Bde 4-6 (Drogen), Springer Verlag Berlin, Heidelberg, New York, 1992-1994.

Hill RK, in "The Alkaloids Vol. 2", Ed. SW Pelletier, John Wiley 1984.

Kuroda K, Tagaki K, (1968) Nature 220:707.

Kuroda K et al., (1976) Cancer Res 36:1900.

Kuroda K, Kaku T, (1969) Life Sci 8(1):151.

Kuroda K, Tagaki K, (1969) Arch Int Pharmacodyn 178(2): 382, 392.

Madaus G, Lehrbuch der Biologischen Arzneimittel, Bde 1-3, Nachdruck, Georg Olms Verlag Hildesheim 1979.

Teuscher E, Lindequist U, Giftstoffe mikrobieller Endo- und Epiphyten. Gefahren für Mensch und Tier? In: DAZ 132(42):2231. 1992.

Teuscher E, Lindequist U, Biogene Gifte - Biologie, Chemie, Pharmakologie, 2. Aufl., Fischer Verlag Stuttgart 1994.

Vermathen M, Glasl H, Effect of the herb extract of Capsella bursa pastoris on blood coagulation. In: PM 59(7)70. 1993.

Wichtl M (Hrsg.), Teedrogen, 4. Aufl., Wiss. Verlagsges. Stuttgart 1997.

Short Buchu

Barosma species

DESCRIPTION

Medicinal Parts: The medicinal parts are the leaves of Barosma betulina, Barosma crenulata and Barosma serratifolia gathered during the flowering season, as well as the ethereal oil extracted from the dried leaves of Barosma betulina.

Flower and Fruit: The pentamerous flowers of Barosma betulina form a white or pink corolla 12 mm in diameter with lanceolate petals. The fruit is a 7 mm long capsule with 5 chambers and one seed per chamber. The upper surface is greenish-brown and rough. The fruit springs open at the 5 valves. The seeds are ovoid, oblong, about 5 mm long and 2 mm wide, glossy black and hard with no endosperm. The flowers of Barosma crenulata are pink or white and attached to short leafy side branches.

Leaves, Stem and Root: Barosma betulina is a small shrub with light green to yellowish leaves. The leaves are 12 to 20 mm in length, opposite, rigid and coriaceous. They are rhomboid or obovate, short-petioled and slightly pubescent, blunt and revolute at the apex. Each indentation has an oil gland. The oil glands form small raised structures on the leaf surface. The stem is about 2 to 3 mm in diameter, reddish-brown and rough (due to the oil glands) with 4 long grooves. The internodes are 8 to 20 mm long.

Barosma crenulata is a slender glabrous bush 2 to 3 m high. It is branched somewhat angularly. The bark is violet-brown. The leaves of Barosma crenulata vary in form, and are opposite and pubescent on both surfaces. They reach up to 3 cm in length with an obtuse, but not a revolute, tip.

Barosma serratifolia bush is very similar to the above, although the leaves are longer, obtuse at the tip and narrowed on both edges. The leaves are lanceolate, have a long, serrated, saw-shaped margin and a blunt apex. They are yellowish green and up to 4 cm long with an oil gland at the apex and indentations on the margin. There are smaller oil glands spread over the leaf blade.

Characteristics: The leaves have a peppermint odor.

Habitat: The plant is indigenous to the Cape region of South Africa.

Production: Short Buchu leaf consists of the dried leaves of Barosma betulina harvested when in flower and in fruit. In South Africa, collection of the leaves is strictly controlled by the government to prevent destruction of the plant in the wild.

Not to be Confused With: Other Barosma and Diosma species.

Other Names: Buchu

ACTIONS AND PHARMACOLOGY

COMPOUNDS

Volatile oil: chief components diosphenol and psi-diosphenol (as a mixture known as buccocamphor), limonene, (+)-menthone, 8-9-isomenthone, pulegone, furthermore (-)- cis- and (+)-trans-8-mercapto-p-menth-3-one (odor-determining, so-called cassis aroma)

Flavonoids: including rutin and diosmetin

EFFECTS

No studies of the drug are currently available.

INDICATIONS AND USAGE

Unproven Uses: Short Buchu leaf is used for inflammation and infection of the kidneys and urinary tract, for bladder irritation, as a disinfectant of the urinary tract and as a diuretic. In Europe the drug has been in use since the 16th century for the treatment of gout, various bladder disorders and rheumatism, and for the prostate gland. In South Africa it is still widely used, typically as a brandy made from the plant and used to treat stomach complaints.

CONTRAINDICATIONS

Short Buchu is not to be used during pregnancy.

PRECAUTIONS AND ADVERSE REACTIONS

No health hazards or side effects are known in conjunction with the proper administration of designated therapeutic dosages, but it is noted that the volatile oil could lead to signs of irritation.

DOSAGE

Mode of Administration: Since the claimed efficacy has not been documented, the application of Buchu leaf cannot be recommended. Buchu is used in various preparations and combinations.

How Supplied: Short Buchu is available as an extract, tincture and infusion.

Preparation: A fluid extract is prepared using 1000 parts powdered Buchu leaves plus 400 parts 90% ethanol (V/V) 7:3 water produce 1000 parts fluid extract (EB6).

Infusion — fluid extract 1:1 90% ethanol (V/V) (BHP83).

Buchu leaf tincture — 1:5 60% ethanol (V/V) (BHP83).

Daily Dose: The daily dose of the drug is 1 g to 2 g. Fluid extracts of 0.3 to 1.2 ml are taken 3 times daily. Dosage for the tincture is 2 to 4 ml up to 3 times daily. Infusion usage is typically 1 g per cup.

Homeopathic Dosage: 5 drops, 1 tablet, 10 globules every 30 to 60 minutes (acute) or 1 to 3 times daily (chronic); parenterally: 1 to 2 ml 3 times daily sc (HAB34).

Storage: The drug must be kept cool, dry and away from the light in sealed containers.

LITERATURE

Didry N, Pinkas M, (1982) Plant Med Phytother 16 (4): 249.

Hänsel R, Keller K, Rimpler H, Schneider G (Hrsg.), Hagers Handbuch der Pharmazeutischen Praxis, 5. Aufl., Bde 4-6 (Drogen), Springer Verlag Berlin, Heidelberg, New York, 1992-1994.

Kaiser R et al., (1975) J Agric Food Chem 23: 943-950.

Leung AY, Encyclopedia of Common Natural Ingredients Used in Food Drugs and Cosmetics, John Wiley & Sons Inc., New York 1980.

Madaus G, Lehrbuch der Biologischen Arzneimittel, Bde 1-3, Nachdruck, Georg Olms Verlag Hildesheim 1979.

Steinegger E, Hänsel R, Pharmakognosie, 5. Aufl., Springer Verlag Heidelberg 1992.

Wichtl M (Hrsg.), Teedrogen, 4. Aufl., Wiss. Verlagsges. Stuttgart 1997.

Siam Benzoin

Styrax tonkinensis

DESCRIPTION

Medicinal Parts: The medicinal part of the plant is the resin obtained from the trunk.

Flower and Fruit: Styrax tonkinensis is a tree that grows up to 20 m high. It is very similar to Styrax benzoin, but the flowers are smaller, the calyx is 3 to 4 mm long, the corolla is white and up to 9 mm long. The fruit is up to 12 mm long.

Leaves, Stem and Root: The leaves are oval, 4.5 to 10 cm long and 2 to 6 cm wide.

Habitat: Laos

Production: Siam Benzoin is the balsam of Styrax tonkinensis, or other related species, obtained by making cuts in the trunk. The optimal age of tree to be harvested is 7 years. The tree is cut, which stimulates it to exude resin to heal the cuts. The resin is then collected in a vessel, and left to melt to a homogenous mass in the sun.

ACTIONS AND PHARMACOLOGY

COMPOUNDS

Ester mixture (90%): bestehend aus coniferyl benzoate (60 to 70%), p-cumaryl benzoate (10 to 15%), as well as cinnamyl benzoate, cinnamyl cinnamate

Benzoic acid (10 to 20%)

Vanillin (0.5%)

Triterpenes: alpha-siaresinolic acid (5%)

EFFECTS

The expectorant effect with which the drug is credited could not be proven experimentally (it possibly originated in connection with an ''aroma therapy,'' due to its vanilla content).

INDICATIONS AND USAGE

Unproven Uses: Siam Benzoin is used for respiratory catarrh.

Chinese Medicine: In China, preparations are used for stroke, syncope, post partal syncope due to heavy loss of blood, chest and stomach pain.

PRECAUTIONS AND ADVERSE REACTIONS

No health hazards are known in conjunction with the proper administration of designated therapeutic dosages.

DOSAGE

Mode of Administration: Whole herb, powdered drug and other galenic preparations for internal use.

Preparation: To prepare a tincture, use powder in 90% ethanol (V/V) 1:5 macerate (DAB9).

Daily Dosage: 0.5 gm; single dose: 0.05 gm

Storage: Should be tightly sealed, and protected from light.

LITERATURE

Hänsel R, Keller K, Rimpler H, Schneider G (Ed), Hagers Handbuch der Pharmazeutischen Praxis, 5. Aufl., Bde 4 - 6 (Drogen), Springer Verlag Berlin, Heidelberg, New York, 1992-1994.

James WD, White SW, Yanklowitz B, Allergic contact dermatitis to compound tincture of benzoin. J Am Acad Dermatol, 11:847-50, 1984 Nov.

Siberian Ginseng

Eleutherococcus senticosus

DESCRIPTION

Medicinal Parts: The medicinal parts are the pulverized root rind, the pulverized root and an alcoholic fluid extract of the rhizome and the roots.

Flower and Fruit: The flowers are in umbels. The central umbel is on a long, thick peduncle. The style is fused into a column to the tip and has 5 small stigma lobes.

Leaves, Stem and Root: Siberian Ginseng is a 1 to 3 m high shrub whose branches are thickly covered with pale, thorny bristles pointing downward at an angle. The leaves are in groups of 5 and are thorny-serrate. The petiole is covered in fine bristles.

Habitat: Siberian Ginseng grows in Siberia, northern China, Korea and Japan.

Production: Siberian Ginseng consists of the dried roots and/or rhizome of Eleutherococcus senticosus as well as their preparations in effective dosage.

ACTIONS AND PHARMACOLOGY

COMPOUNDS

Caffeic acid derivatives: including chlorogenic acid

Hydroxycoumarins: isofraxidin

Lignans: sesamine, eleutheroside D (epimeric diglucosides of syringaresinols)

Steroids: including beta-sitosterol-3-O-beta-D-glucoside (daucosterol, eleutheroside A, 0.1%)

Phenylacrylic acid derivatives: eleutheroside B (syringin)

Polysaccharides: immunostimulatingly effective polysaccharides (eleutherane A-G)

Steroid glycosides: eleutheroside A (daucosterol, beta-stigmasterol-3-O-beta-D-glucoside)

Triterpene saponins: eleutheroside I, eleutheroside K (beta-hederin), eleutheroside L, eleutheroside M (hederasaponin B), for all of these aglycone oleanolic acid

EFFECTS

The liquid extract of the drug has an immune-stimulating/immune-modulating and antiviral effect. In various stress models, e.g., immobilization test and coldness test, the endurance of rodents was enhanced. With healthy volunteers, the lymphocyte count, especially that of T-lymphocytes, increased following intake of liquid extracts.

Hypoglycemic effects have also been demonstrated with the herb along with enhancement of platelet aggregation-inhibiting effects (Hikino, 1986; Yun-Coi, 1987).

INDICATIONS AND USAGE

Approved By Commission E:

- Lack of stamina
- Tendency to infection

Unproven Uses: Siberian Ginseng is used as a tonic for invigoration and fortification in times of fatigue and debility or declining capacity for work and concentration, and during convalescence.

Chinese Medicine: Siberian Ginseng is used for kidney pain, retention of urine, impotence, sleep disturbance, loss of appetite, pain and weakness in the hip and knee joints, rheumatoid arthritis and as a stimulant for the immune system.

CONTRAINDICATIONS

The drug should not be administered to patients with hypertension.

PRECAUTIONS AND ADVERSE REACTIONS

Health risks or side effects following the proper administration of designated therapeutic dosages are not recorded.

Drug Interactions:

Digoxin — elevated serum levels (McRae, 1996)

Antidiabetic Agents/Insulin — may potentiate effects (Hikino, 1986)

Anticoagulants/Antiplatelets/Antithrombotics — may enhance effects (Yun-Choi, 1987)

DOSAGE

Mode of Administration: Powdered or cut root for teas, as well as aqueous-alcoholic extracts for internal use.

Preparation:

Extract (Siberian Ginseng) — root powder 1:7 75% ethanol extracted with back flow to which is added a 10% alpha-naphthol solution until there is no reaction. It is then evaporated to a paste (ChinP IX).

Liquid extract — medium fine root powder can be produced using a through flow procedure with 40% ethanol (V/V) (1000 gm drug to 1 Liter extract), (Ross XI).

Daily Dosage: 9 to 15 gm root bark; 9 to 27 gm root; 0.3 to 0.5 gm drug extract 3 times daily. The average daily dosage is 2 to 3 gm of root.

Storage: Should be stored in well-aired, dry place, protected from light

LITERATURE

Bauer R, Neues von ''immunmodulierenden Drogen'' und ''Drogen mit antiallergischer und antiinflammatorischer Wirkung.'' In: ZPT 14(1):23-24. 1993.

Bladt S, Wagner H, Woo WS, (1990) Taiga-Wurzel. Dtsch Apoth Ztg 27:1499-1508.

Bohn B, Nebe Cr, Birr C, (1987) Flow-cytometric studies with Eleutherococcus senticosus extract as an immunomodulatory agent. Arzneim Forsch (Drug Res) 37:1193-1196.

Hikino H, Takahashi M, Otake K, Konno C, Isolation and hypoglycemic activity of A, B, C, D, E, F, and G: glycans of Eleutherococcus senticosus roots. J Nat Prod 1986 Mar-Apr; 49(2):293-7.

Kaemmerer K, Fink J, (1980) Untersuchungen von Eleutherococcus-Extrakt auf trophanabole Wirkungen bei Ratten. Der Praktische Tierarzt 61:748-753.

Koch HP, Eidler S, (1988) Eleutherococcus Senticosus. Sibirischer Ginseng. Wissenschaftlicher Bericht. Kooperation Phytopharmaka, Köln Bonn Frankfurt Bad Homburg.

McRae S, Elevated serum digoxin levels in a patient taking digoxin and Siberian ginseng. CMAJ 1996 Aug 1;155(3):293-5.

Obermeier A, (1980) Zur Analytik der Ginseng-und Eteutherococcusdroge. Dissertation Ludwig-Maximilians-Universität München.

Sprecher E, Pflanzliche Geriatrika. In: ZPT 9(2):40. 1988.

Wagner H, Nörr H, Winterhoff H, Drogen mit ''Adaptogenwirkung'' zur Stärkung der Widerstandskräfte. In: ZPT 13(2):42. 1992.

Wagner H, Pflanzliche Immunstimulanzien. In: DAZ 131(4):117. 1991.

Weber R, Eleutherococcus senticosus. In: PTA 4(11):558. 1990.

Wichtl M, Pflanzliche Geriatrika. In: DAZ 132(30):1576. 1992.

Yun-Choi HS, Kim JH, Lee, Potential inhibitors of platelet aggregation from plant sources, III. J Nat Prod 1987 Nov-Dec;50(6):1059

Zorikov PS, Lyapustina TA, (1974) Change in a concentration of protein and nitrogen in the reproductive organs of hens under the effect of Eleutherococcus extract. Deposited DOC VIN1:732-774, 58-63: ref Chem Abstracts 86 (1977).

Further information in:

Schulz R, Hänsel R, Rationale Phytotherapie, Springer Verlag Heidelberg 1996.

Steinegger E, Hänsel R, Pharmakognosie, 5. Aufl., Springer Verlag Heidelberg 1992.

Tang W, Eisenbrand G, Chinese Drugs of Plant Origin, Springer Verlag Heidelberg 1992.

Teuscher E, Biogene Arzneimittel, 5. Aufl., Wiss. Verlagsges. mbH Stuttgart 1997.

Wagner H, Wiesenauer M, Phytotherapie. Phytopharmaka und pflanzliche Homöopathika, Fischer-Verlag, Stuttgart, Jena, New York 1995.

Silphium laciniatum

See Rosinweed

Silphium perfoliatum

See Cup Plant

Silybum marianum

See Milk Thistle

Simaruba

Simaruba amara

DESCRIPTION

Medicinal Parts: The medicinal part is the dried root bark.

Flower and Fruit: The flowers grow in small racemes with dense matte-white petals.

Leaves, Stem and Root: Simaruba amara is a tree that grows over 18 m high. The roots are long and spread horizontally. The leaves are 22 to 27 cm long. The tree has numerous long, bent branches covered in smooth, grayish bark. The bark that is used commercially is thin and flat with a yellowish or grayish-yellow color. The bark is tough, fibrous and almost impossible to break.

Characteristics: The taste is very bitter and odorless.

Habitat: The plant grows on the Caribbean islands and the northern parts of South America.

Other Names: Dysentery Bark, Mountain Damson, Bitter Damson, Slave Wood, Stave Wood, Sumaruba

ACTIONS AND PHARMACOLOGY

COMPOUNDS

Bitter substances: quassinoids (breakdown products of triterpenes), including among others simarubin (1%), simarubidin, simarolide, 13,18-dehydro-glaucarubinone

Tannins (20-27%)

Volatile oil (0.1-0.2%)

5-hydroxy-canthin-6-one

Alkaloids

EFFECTS

The active agents are tannin, simarubin, essential oil and fat. The drug has a sedative effect on the smooth muscle of the intestine. It constricts the vessels of the intestinal tract. Simaruba is a tonic and febrifuge.

INDICATIONS AND USAGE

Unproven Uses: Simaruba was formerly used in the treatment of febrile illnesses and dysentery. Recent research indicates that it may be effective in treating malaria. The drug is used for unspecified enteritis, diarrhea and as a bitter. It may cause vomiting, and is also used as an abortive.

PRECAUTIONS AND ADVERSE REACTIONS

No health hazards or side effects are known in conjunction with the proper administration of designated therapeutic dosages. The drug triggers vomiting in high dosages.

DOSAGE

Mode of Administration: The drug is available as a liquid extract for internal use.

Daily Dosage: The average dose is 1 gm of the drug to be taken internally.

Storage: Protect against dampness.

LITERATURE

Bray DH et al., (1987) Phytother Res 1 (1):22.

Geissmann T, (1964) Ann Rev Pharmacol 4:305.

Kuroda K et al., (1976) Cancer Res 36:1900.

Polonsky J et al., (1978) Experientia 34 (9):1122.

Further information in:

Hegnauer R, Chemotaxonomie der Pflanzen, Bde 1-11: Birkhäuser Verlag Basel, Boston, Berlin 1962-1997.

Kern W, List PH, Hörhammer L (Hrsg.), Hagers Handbuch der Pharmazeutischen Praxis, 4. Aufl., Bde 1-8: Springer Verlag Berlin, Heidelberg, New York, 1969.

Simaruba amara

See Simaruba

Simmondsia chinesis

See Jojoba

Sinapis alba

See White Mustard

Sisymbrium officinale

See Hedge Mustard

Sium sisarum

See Skirret

Skirret

Sium sisarum

DESCRIPTION

Medicinal Parts: The medicinal part is the root.

Flower and Fruit: The inflorescence has 10 to 30 rayed-umbels with 1 to 5 lanceolate-narrow involucral bracts. The petals are white, about 1 mm long and broad orbicular-elliptical. The fruit is broad-ovate, about 3.5 by 2 to 2.5 mm in diameter and brownish with light ribs. The fruit segments in cross-section are obtuse pentagons with thin walls.

Leaves, Stem and Root: Sium sisarum is a perennial glabrous plant on a stubby rhizome with clustered, often tuberous roots. The stem is about 30 to 80 cm high, round and branched. The lower leaves are simple pinnate, oblong and serrate. The upper leaves are narrower and more acuminate, and are usually lanceolate.

Habitat: The plant is indigenous to China; it is cultivated in Europe.

Production: Skirret root is the root of Sium sisarum.

ACTIONS AND PHARMACOLOGY

COMPOUNDS

Oligosaccharides: saccharose (4-8%)

Starch (4-18%)

Mucilage

EFFECTS

No information is available.

INDICATIONS AND USAGE

Unproven Uses: The drug is used for digestive disorders and loss of appetite.

PRECAUTIONS AND ADVERSE REACTIONS

No health hazards or side effects are known in conjunction with the proper administration of designated therapeutic dosages.

DOSAGE

Mode of Administration: Skirret root is available as cut drug for internal use.

LITERATURE

Kern W, List PH, Hörhammer L (Hrsg.), Hagers Handbuch der Pharmazeutischen Praxis, 4. Aufl., Bde. 1-8: Springer Verlag Berlin, Heidelberg, New York, 1969.

Skunk Cabbage

Symplocarpus foetidus

DESCRIPTION

Medicinal Parts: The medicinal parts are the seeds, the rhizome and the roots.

Flower and Fruit: The plant has numerous small purple flowers in a red-brown, oval, high, spadix-like inflorescence.

Leaves, Stem and Root: The plant is a perennial and grows up to 75 cm high. It has a thick tuberous rhizome, which is truncate at both ends, dark brown and up to 4 cm in diameter. The rhizome is gnarled and woody and bears numerous roots and root scars. The roots are up to 8 cm long, 0.5 cm in diameter and transversely wrinkled. The leaves are similar to cabbage leaves and they surround the inflorescence.

Characteristics: The taste is hot and the odor is unpleasant.

Habitat: The plant is indigenous to the northern U.S.

Production: Skunk Cabbage root and rootstock are the rhizome and roots of Symplocarpus foetidus.

Other Names: Dracontium, Meadow Cabbage, Polecatweed, Skunkweed

ACTIONS AND PHARMACOLOGY

COMPOUNDS

Volatile oil (bad-smelling)

Resins

The constituents of the drug have not been fully investigated.

EFFECTS

Skunk Cabbage is an antispasmodic, a diaphoretic, an expectorant and a sedative.

INDICATIONS AND USAGE

Unproven Uses: The plant is used for bronchitis and asthma.

PRECAUTIONS AND ADVERSE REACTIONS

No health hazards or side effects are known in conjunction with the proper administration of designated therapeutic dosages.

OVERDOSAGE

Overdosage results in queasiness and vomiting.

DOSAGE

Mode of Administration: Skunk Cabbage is administered as a liquid extract in various medicinal preparations.

LITERATURE

Adolf A, Hecker E (1980) Tetrahedron Letters 21:2887

Hegnauer R, Chemotaxonomie der Pflanzen, Bde 1-11: Birkhäuser Verlag Basel, Boston, Berlin 1962-1997.

Kern W, List PH, Hörhammer L (Hrsg.), Hagers Handbuch der Pharmazeutischen Praxis, 4. Aufl., Bde 1-8: Springer Verlag Berlin, Heidelberg, New York, 1969.

Slippery Elm

Ulmus rubra

TRADE NAMES

Slippery Elm Bark

DESCRIPTION

Medicinal Parts: The medicinal part is the dried inner rind separated from the outer bark.

Flower and Fruit: The flowers are in dense, almost sessile clusters. There are 5 to 9 tepals and the same number of stamens. The stigmas are bright red. The fruit is almost top-shaped to broad-elliptical, 1 to 2 cm long, wide and glabrous, except for the rust-red downy center. The seeds are inserted in the center.

Leaves, Stem and Root: The tree is medium-sized and grows up to 20 m tall with spread branches forming an open crown. The younger branches are red-brown or orange and more or less downy. The bark is deeply fissured. The buds are large, rust-red and downy. The leaves are obovate to oblong, 10 to 20 cm long and have a double-serrate margin. The lamina is long acuminate and sharply asymmetrical at the base. The leaves, are dark green above and very rough, densely downy beneath. They darken in autumn.

Characteristics: The texture is mucilaginous and the odor slight but characteristic. The powdered inner bark is used for its mucilaginous quality. Taken as a drink, it relieves irritation of the mucous membrane. The same water-retaining properties allow the powder to be used as an emollient poultice.

Habitat: The plant is indigenous to North America.

Production: Slippery Elm bark is the inner bark and wood of Ulmus fulva.

Other Names: Red Elm, Sweet Elm

ACTIONS AND PHARMACOLOGY

COMPOUNDS

Steroids: sterols, including cholesterol, campesterol, beta-sitosterol

Sesquiterpenes: including 5-isopropyl-3,8-dimethyl-2-naphthol, 2-hydroxy-5-isopropyl-8-methyl-5,6,7,8-tetrahydro-3-naphthyl aldehyde

Tannins (very little)

EFFECTS

Slippery Elm is demulcent, emollient and soothing to the alimentary canal.

INDICATIONS AND USAGE

Unproven Uses: Internally, the drug is used in the treatment of gastritis and gastric or duodenal ulcers. Externally, it is used in the treatment of wounds, burns, skin conditions, swollen glands, gout, and rheumatism.

PRECAUTIONS AND ADVERSE REACTIONS

No health hazards or side effects are known in conjunction with the proper administration of designated therapeutic dosages.

DOSAGE

Mode of Administration: Whole and cut drug is available in the form of a decoction for internal use and poultices for external use.

How Supplied: Capsules — 370 mg

Preparation: A decoction is made in a ratio of 1:8 with ethanol.

Daily Dosage: The dose for the decoction is 4 to 16 ml per day. Externally, the coarsely ground drug is used as a poultice.

LITERATURE

Hänsel R, Keller K, Rimpler H, Schneider G (Hrsg.), Hagers Handbuch der Pharmazeutischen Praxis, 5. Aufl., Bde 4-6 (Drogen): Springer Verlag Berlin, Heidelberg, New York, 1992-1994.

Kim JP, Kim WG, Koshino H, Jung J, Yoo ID Sesquiterpene O-naphthoquinones from the root bark of Ulmus davidiana. Phytochemistry, 43:425-30, 1996 Sep.

Sloe

Prunus spinosa

DESCRIPTION

Medicinal Parts: The medicinal parts are the flowers.

Flower and Fruit: The white, pedicled flowers are solitary but appear close to each other on the branches. The bush finishes flowering before the leaves unfold. The calyx is campanulate with long tips, which are twice as long as the tips of the 5 petals. The fruit is dark blue, frosted, globular, diameter approximately 10 mm.

Leaves, Stem and Root: Sloe is a bulky bush about 3 m high. The branches are velvet-haired when young. The numerous lateral branches are almost horizontal and end in sharp thorns. The bark is black-brown.

Characteristics: The fruit tastes exceptionally sour and is only really edible after several frosts.

Habitat: The plant grows in Europe and parts of Asia.

Production: Sloe fruit consists of the fresh or dried ripe fruit of Prunus spinosa as well as its preparations. Sloe flower consists of the dried flowers of Prunus spinosa as well as its preparations.

Not to be Confused With: May be confused with the flowers of Prunus padus syn. Padus avium.

Other Names: Blackthorn, Wild Plum

ACTIONS AND PHARMACOLOGY

COMPOUNDS: SLOE FRUIT

Cyanogenic glycosides: amygdalin, only in the seeds

Fruit acids

Monosaccharides/oligosaccharides

Tannins

EFFECTS: SLOE FRUIT

Sloe fruit has an astringent effect.

COMPOUNDS: SLOE FLOWER

Cyanogenic glycosides: amygdalin (traces, likely only in the fresh blossoms)

Flavonoids: including quercitrin, rutin, and hyperoside

EFFECTS: SLOE FLOWER

There is no reliable information available.

INDICATIONS AND USAGE

SLOE FRUIT

Approved by Commission E:

■ Inflammation of the mouth and pharynx

Sloe fruit is used externally for inflammation of the oral and pharyngeal mucosa (as a gargle).

Unproven Uses: In folk medicine the fruit juice is used as a gargle for mouth, throat, and gum inflammation. Syrup and wine are employed as a purgative or diuretic and as jam for a weak stomach.

SLOE FLOWER

Unproven Uses: Preparations of Sloe flower are used for common colds, diseases and ailments of the respiratory tract, as a laxative, for diarrhea, for prophylaxis and treatment of gastric spasms, flatulence, intestinal diseases and gastric insufficiency.

Homeopathic Uses: Prunus spinosa is used for cardiac insufficiency and 'nervous headaches'.

PRECAUTIONS AND ADVERSE REACTIONS

SLOE FRUIT AND FLOWER

No health hazards or side effects are known in conjunction with the proper administration of designated therapeutic dosages.

DOSAGE

SLOE FRUIT

Mode of Administration: Sloe fruit is available as crude drug for infusions and other galenic preparations for mouth rinses.

Daily Dosage: External use — 2 to 4 gm drug

SLOE FLOWER

Mode of Administration: Sloe flower preparations are available in various commercial compounded preparations.

Preparation: Tea: pour boiling water over 1 to 2 heaped teaspoons, stir occasionally for 5 to 10 minutes and strain.

Daily Dosage: Drink 1 to 2 cups during the day or 2 cups in the evening. (1 teaspoon corresponds approximately to 1 gm drug)

Storage: Should be protected from light and moisture, at best not longer than 1 year.

LITERATURE

SLOE FLOWER

Irizar AC, Fernandez MF, Constituents of Prunus spinosa. In: JNP 55:450-454. 1992.

Kern W, List PH, Hörhammer L (Hrsg.), Hagers Handbuch der Pharmazeutischen Praxis, 4. Aufl., Bde. 1-8, Springer Verlag Berlin, Heidelberg, New York, 1969.

Madaus G, Lehrbuch der Biologischen Arzneimittel, Bde 1-3, Nachdruck, Georg Olms Verlag Hildesheim 1979.

Steinegger E, Hänsel R, Pharmakognosie, 5. Aufl., Springer Verlag Heidelberg 1992.

Teuscher E, Biogene Arzneimittel, 5. Aufl., Wiss. Verlagsges. Stuttgart 1997.

Wichtl M (Hrsg.), Teedrogen, 4. Aufl., Wiss. Verlagsges. Stuttgart 1997.

SLOE FRUIT

Irizar AC, Fernandez MF, Constituents of Prunus spinosa. In: JNP 55:450-454. 1992.

Further information in:

Kern W, List PH, Hörhammer L (Hrsg.), Hagers Handbuch der Pharmazeutischen Praxis, 4. Aufl., Bde. 1-8, Springer Verlag Berlin, Heidelberg, New York, 1969.

Madaus G, Lehrbuch der Biologischen Arzneimittel, Bde 1-3, Nachdruck, Georg Olms Verlag Hildesheim 1979.

Smartweed

Persicaria hydropiper

DESCRIPTION

Medicinal Parts: The medicinal parts are the leaves and the whole plant harvested during the flowering season.

Flower and Fruit: The greenish pink flowers are in sparse, thin, hanging false ears. The 4-bract involucre is inconspicuous with a reddish tip and is glandular-punctate. The flowers are androgynous. There are 6 to 8 stamens, 2 of which have no function. The fruit has a flat and a domed side. It is black, punctate, nut-like, roughly bumpy and surrounded by a remaining epicalyx.

Leaves, Stem and Root: The plant grows from 30 to 50 cm high. The branched stems, which are from 60 to 90 cm long, are first creeping and later semi-erect and often tinged red. The leaves are oblong-lanceolate, short petioled, narrowed at both ends and alternate; they are glandular and ciliate on the under surface. The leaf sheaths at the base of the leaves are loose, glabrous and ciliated at the margin.

Characteristics: Smartweed has an extraordinarily hot, pepper-like taste and is often used as a pepper substitute. The plant has characteristic long, thinly curved, hanging, flowering branches.

Habitat: The plant is indigenous to large parts of Europe, Asian Russia and Arctic regions.

Production: Smartweed is the fresh plant, in flower, of Polygonum hydropiper. The flowering herb is cut and washed, the roots are removed and discarded and the herb is dried in the shade.

Not to be Confused With: Polygonum hydropiper is sometimes adultered with polygonum persicaria, P. mite and P. minus.

Other Names: Water Pepper, Arsesmart

ACTIONS AND PHARMACOLOGY

COMPOUNDS

Flavonoids: including rhamnazin, rhamnazin bisulfate, persicarin (isorhamnetine sulfate) quercitrin, and hyperoside

P-cumaroyl glycosides: hydropiperoside

Sesquiterpenes: sesquiterpene aldehydes (pungent substances), polygoidal (tadeonal), and warburganal

Tannins

EFFECTS

Smartweed is a hemostyptic.

INDICATIONS

Unproven Uses: In folk medicine Smartweed is used internally for uterine bleeding, menstrual bleeding, bleeding of hemorrhoids (piles), gastrointestinal bleeding, rheumatic pain, as a diuretic, for bladder and kidney disease and gout; and used externally for poorly healing wounds, sprains, contusions, rheumatism and gout.

Chinese Medicine: Smartweed is used for severe digestive problems, vomiting, diarrhea, dysentery, scabies and external wounds in China.

Homeopathic Uses: Polygonum hydropiper is used to treat varicose veins.

PRECAUTIONS

No health hazards or side effects are known in conjunction with the proper administration of designated therapeutic dosages. The consumption of larger quantities of the fresh kraut can lead to gastroenteritis. External use is not advisable because of the drugs irritant effect on the skin.

DOSAGE

Mode of Administration: Smartweed is available in crude powder form for oral intake and in parenteral form for homeopathic use.

Preparation: Tea — Pour 1/4 Liter hot water over 1 heaped teaspoon drug and strain after 10 minutes.

Daily Dosage: Tea — 3 times a day.

Homeopathic Dosage: 5 drops, 1 tablet or 10 globules every 30 to 60 minutes (acute) or 1 to 3 times daily (chronic); parenterally: 1 to 2 ml sc acute: 3 times daily; chronic: once a day (HAB34)

LITERATURE

Asakawa Y, Takemoto T, (1979) Experientia 35:1429.

Barnes CS, Loder JW, (1962) Aust J Chem 15:322.

Furuta, T. et al., (1986) Phytochemistry 25(2):517.

Fukujama Y et al., Hydropiperoside, a novel coumaroly glycoside from the root of Polygonum hydropiper. In: PH 22:549-552. 1983.

Kifakh SY, Blinova KF, (1984) Khim Prir Soedin 5:658.

Further information in:

Kern W, List PH, Hörhammer L (Hrsg.), Hagers Handbuch der Pharmazeutischen Praxis, 4. Aufl., Bde. 1-8, Springer Verlag Berlin, Heidelberg, New York, 1969.

Madaus G, Lehrbuch der Biologischen Arzneimittel, Bde. 1-3, Nachdruck, Georg Olms Verlag Hildesheim 1979.

Steinegger E, Hänsel R, Pharmakognosie, 5. Aufl., Springer Verlag Heidelberg 1992.

Teuscher E, Lindequist U, Biogene Gifte - Biologie, Chemie, Pharmakologie, 2. Aufl., Fischer Verlag Stuttgart 1994.

Wagner H, Wiesenauer M, Phytotherapie. Phytopharmaka und pflanzliche Homöopathika, Fischer-Verlag, Stuttgart, Jena, New York 1995.

Smilax species

See Sarsaparilla

Sneezewort

Achillea ptarmica

DESCRIPTION

Medicinal Parts: The medicinal part is the dried root.

Flower and Fruit: The flowers are white, composite and in cymes at the tip of the stem. The bracts are lanceolate and short-haired. The ray florets are linguiform and female. The disc florets are tubular and androgynous. The chaff scales are lanceolate and hairy-tipped. The fruit is hairless.

Leaves, Stem and Root: The plant grows from 30 to 80 cm high. The rhizome is creeping, and the stem is upright and glabrous. The leaves are glabrous, alternate, simple, lanceolate, acute, sessile and finely serrated. They are slightly glossy and dark green.

Habitat: The plant is indigenous to northern and central Europe.

Production: The rhizome is dug up in the autumn of its second year of bearing fruit, washed, freed of any green areas and dried in the shade at a temperature of 35° C.

ACTIONS AND PHARMACOLOGY

COMPOUNDS

Volatile oil

Polyynes: including pontica expoxide, tridecatrien-(1,3,5)-triin-(7,9,11)-cis-dehydromatricaria ester

Alkamides: including trans-dehydromatricaria acid isobutylamide

EFFECTS

No information is available.

INDICATIONS AND USAGE

Unproven Uses: In the past, Sneezewort was used as a remedy for tiredness, loss of appetite, urinary tract complaints, nausea, vomiting, diarrhea, rheumatism and other painful disorders. Today it is considered a remedy for toothache, flatulence and problems with elimination; the herb also helps to regulate bowel movements.

PRECAUTIONS AND ADVERSE REACTIONS

No health hazards or side effects are known in conjunction with the proper administration of designated therapeutic dosages, although persons with compound allergies should avoid salves prepared from the drug.

DOSAGE

Mode of Administration: Sneezewort is available as a topical preparation and in alcoholic extracts.

Preparation: To prepare an infusion, use 2 teaspoonfuls of the comminuted drug to 2 cups of water.

Daily Dosage: A daily infusion can be drunk, or the fresh root can be chewed.

LITERATURE

Kuropka G, Neugebauer M, Glombitza KW, Essential oils of Achillea ptarmica. In: PM 57:492. 1991.

Rücker G et al., trans-Pinocarveylhydroxid aus Achillea ptarmica. In: PM 60(2):194. 1994.

Snowdrop

Galanthus nivalis

DESCRIPTION

Medicinal Parts: Although disputed, some attribute medicinal properties to the bulb.

Flower and Fruit: The flowers are single on approximately 10 cm long peduncles, are campanulate, drooping and shorter than the hood-like bract. The perigone has 6 tepals, the outer 3 oval, white, 14 to 18 mm long and free. The inner 3 tepals are shorter, with an indentate tip, a green longitudinal stripe on the inside and a green half-moon- shaped spot on the outside. The 6 stamens are short and inclined toward each other. The ovary is barrel-shaped and has 1 style. The fruit is a yellowish-green, 3-chambered capsule with up to 12 seeds in each chamber. It is initially fleshy, and later springs open in folds. The seeds are elliptical, 3 to 4 mm long, with a thin membranous skin and a small and narrow horn-like appendage.

Leaves, Stem and Root: This bulb plant is hardy and grows to 10 to 25 cm high. There are only 2 basal leaves, up to 0.8 cm wide and up to 10 cm long, with a blue-green bloom.

They are linear and slightly keeled on the underside. The outer leaf has an open sheath, the inner leaf a closed sheath. The bulb is globose to ovoid and approximately 1.5 cm wide.

Habitat: The plant is native to Switzerland and Austria as well as other sections of southern Europe, but also has spread to other parts of Europe including Bulgaria and the Commonwealth of Independent States.

Production: The Snowdrop bulb is the fresh bulb of Galanthus nivalis, which is harvested in the flowering season.

ACTION AND PHARMACOLOGY

COMPOUNDS

Amaryllidaceae alkaloids (0.2 to 1.6%): including galanthamine, hemanthamin, narwedine, nivalidine, hippeastrine, lycorine, nivaline, narciclasine, pretazettine. The alkaloid spectrum depends greatly upon the variety.

Lectins

EFFECTS

The drug is now considered toxic. Previous use was based on the effect of the alkaloid galanthamine contained in the drug as a competitive inhibitor of true cholinesterase. The administration of this isolated alkaloid for decurarization in connection with anesthetics thus appeared plausible, as did use for postoperative atonia of the gastrointestinal tract and of the bladder, myasthenia and other conditions. The effects of other alkaloids contained in the drug are virostatic, tumor-inhibiting, positively inotropic and negatively chronotropic, as well as being respiratory analeptics.

INDICATIONS AND USAGE

Unproven Uses: Internal application: Snowdrop has been used for myasthenia, myopathy, symptoms resulting from polyneuropathy, neuritis, myelitis and injuries to the spine, as well as postoperative intestinal, gastric and bladder atonia. It has also been used in anesthetics, for thrombosis and thrombo-embolism, Glaucoma (rare) and Alzheimer's disease.

DOSAGE

The drug is no longer used therapeutically. The literature includes mention of previous use of an aqueous solution of Galanthamine hydrobromide 0.15 to 0.35 mg per kg of body weight IV, IM, sc.

PRECAUTIONS AND ADVERSE REACTIONS

The drug is toxic. Oral ingestion leads to symptoms resembling those of physostigmine poisoning: diarrhea, colic and vomiting (acetylcholine esterase inhibition through galanthamine). Fatal poisonings have not been recorded.

LITERATURE

Amin K, Beillevaire D, Mahmoud E, Hammar L, Mardh PA, Frman G, Binding of Galanthus nivalis lectin to Chlamydia trachomatis and inhibition of in vitro infection. APMIS, 103:714-20, 1995 Oct.

Hänsel R, Keller K, Rimpler H, Schneider G (Ed.), Hagers Handbuch der Pharmazeutischen Praxis, 5. Aufl., Bde 4 - 6 (Drogen), Springer Verlag Berlin, Heidelberg, New York, 1992-1994.

Kalashnikov ID, Isolation of alkaloids from Galanthus nivalis L Farm Zh, 103:40-4, 1970

Plaitakis A, Duvoisin RC, Homer's moly identified as Galanthus nivalis L.: physiologic antidote to stramonium poisoning. Clin Neuropharmacol, 6:1-5, 1983 Mar.

Venturi VM, Piccinin GL, Taddei I, Pharmacognostic study of self-sown Galanthus nivalis (var. gracilis) in Italy Boll Soc Ital Biol Sper, 103:593-7, 1965 Jun 15.

Soapwort

Saponaria officinalis

DESCRIPTION

Medicinal Parts: The medicinal parts are the fresh or dried roots, and the leaves harvested in summer before or during the flowering season of the first and second year of growth.

Flower and Fruit: The flowers generally are flesh-colored, sometimes white, grow in racemes and have a 5-tipped fused calyx. The petals have long stems. The ovary is superior and has 1 style. The fruit is a capsule with 4 teeth at the tip and bursts open when ripe. The seeds are reniform-globular and black-brown.

Leaves, Stem and Root: The perennial plant is leafy and grows about 100 cm high. The stems are round, erect, and finely downy. The leaves are crossed opposite, oblong to lanceolate, acute, entire-margined, 3-veined and taper to a short petiole.

Characteristics: The plant has a weak fragrance. The leaves and root contain bitter tasting saponine and produce suds when rubbed under water.

Habitat: The plant is indigenous to the temperate regions of North America, Asia, and Europe.

Production: Soapwort herb consists of the dried, above ground parts of Saponaria officinalis. The herb is harvested in the summer before flowering in the first and second years of the plant's growth.

Soapwort root consists of the dried roots, rhizomes and runners of Saponaria officinalis. The roots are plowed up in autumn, after the herb has been mown. The root is cleaned and then dried artificially at 50° C.

White Soapwort root consists of the dried, underground parts of Gypsophila species, particularly Gypsophila paniculata. The roots of Gypsophilae radix are dried quickly under high temperatures or in direct sunlight. The roots are cut into 5 mm thick slices to avoid a separation of the sugars from the saponines.

Not to be Confused With: Saponaria officinalis should not be confused with Gypsophilae species and Solanum dulcamara.

Other Names: Soapwood, Soap Root, Latherwort, Bouncing Bet, Fuller's Herb, Bruisewort, Crow Soap, Sweet Betty, Wild Sweet William, Dog Cloves, Old Maids' Pink

ACTIONS AND PHARMACOLOGY

COMPOUNDS: SOAPWORT HERB

Triterpene saponins: chiefly aglycone quillaic acid

Flavonoids: including among others, saponarine (C-glycosyl-flavone)

Ribosome-inactivating proteins (in the seeds)

EFFECTS: SOAPWORT HERB

Because of the high saponin content, the drug is antibiotic, expectorant, antiphlogistic, cholesterol-lowering and spermicidal. In high doses, it becomes irritating to the mucous membrane, cytotoxic and emetic.

COMPOUNDS: SOAPWORT ROOT

Triterpene saponins (2 to 8%): aglycones quillaic acid, gypsogenic acid

EFFECTS: SOAPWORT ROOT

Because of the high saponin content, the Soapwort root is antibiotic, expectorant, antiphlogistic, cholesterol-lowering and spermicidal. The drug is expectorant because of its effect on the gastric mucosa. In high concentrations, it has been shown to be irritating to the mucous membranes, cytotoxic and emetic.

INDICATIONS AND USAGE

SOAPWORT HERB

Unproven Uses: In addition to uses as an expectorant for cough and other diseases of the respiratory tract, folk medicine internal uses also encompass constipation, gastrointestinal disorders, liver and kidney disorders, rheumatic gout, neurasthenia and oxyuriasis. External folk medicine indications include skin rashes, eczema and as a gargle for tonsillitis.

SOAPWORT ROOT

Approved by Commission E:

- Cough/bronchitis

The drug is used for inflammation of the mucous membranes of the upper respiratory tract.

Unproven Uses: In addition to respiratory applications, internal folk medicine uses occasionally include diseases of the liver, gallbladder and kidney, constipation, gout and as an emmenagogue. Among external uses are skin disorders, lingual mycoses and rheumatic complaints.

PRECAUTIONS AND ADVERSE REACTIONS

SOAPWORT HERB AND ROOT

No health hazards are known in conjunction with the proper administration of designated therapeutic dosages. Localized skin and mucus membrane irritations are possible with the administration of larger dosages.

DOSAGE

SOAPWORT HERB

Daily Dosage: As an aqueous extract, take 1 to 2 g daily.

Constipation—2 glasses daily of a decoction, (Preparation instructions are not given.)

Storage: The herb should be stored in a container that protects it from light and moisture.

SOAPWORT ROOT

Mode of Administration: Comminuted herb for teas and other galenic preparations for internal use. Drug extracts are contained in a few standardized preparations of antitussives.

Preparation: To prepare tea, use 0.4 g of medium fine cut (1 teaspoonful is approximately equal to 2.6 g of the drug).

Decoction—10 g/180 g drug with the addition of 1 g sodium carbonate and simple syrup to 200 g.

Daily Dosage: The average daily dose is 30 to 150 mg of the drug corresponding to 3 to 15 mg of gypsophilia saponin. As an expectorant, 1 dessertspoonful of the decoction is taken every 2 hours.

Storage: The root should be stored tightly sealed and protected from light.

LITERATURE

SOAPWORT HERB

Kern W, List PH, Hörhammer L (Hrsg.), Hagers Handbuch der Pharmazeutischen Praxis, 4. Aufl., Bde 1-8: Springer Verlag Berlin, Heidelberg, New York, 1969.

Madaus G, Lehrbuch der Biologischen Arzneimittel, Bde 1-3, Nachdruck, Georg Olms Verlag Hildesheim 1979.

SOAPWORT ROOT

Carzaniga R et al., Planta 194:461. 1994.

Henry M et al., Plantes Med Phytothér 15:192. 1981.

Kern W, List PH, Hörhammer L (Hrsg.), Hagers Handbuch der Pharmazeutischen Praxis, 4. Aufl., Bde. 1-8: Springer Verlag Berlin, Heidelberg, New York, 1969.

Lewin L, Gifte und Vergiftungen, 6. Aufl., Nachdruck, Haug Verlag, Heidelberg 1992.

Madaus G, Lehrbuch der Biologischen Arzneimittel, Bde 1-3, Nachdruck, Georg Olms Verlag Hildesheim 1979.

Roth L, Daunderer M, Kormann K: Giftpflanzen, Pflanzengifte, 4. Aufl., Ecomed Fachverlag Landsberg Lech 1993.

Teuscher E, Biogene Arzneimittel, 5. Aufl., Wiss. Verlagsges. Stuttgart 1997.

Wichtl M (Hrsg.), Teedrogen, 4. Aufl., Wiss. Verlagsges. Stuttgart 1997.

Solanum dulcamara

See Bittersweet Nightshade

Solanum nigrum

See Black Nightshade

Solidago canadensis

See Canadian Golden Rod

Solidago virgaurea

See European Golden Rod

Solomon's Seal

Polygonatum multiflorum

DESCRIPTION

Medicinal Parts: The medicinal parts of the plant are the dried rhizome and roots.

Flower and Fruit: The odorless, greenish-white campanulate flowers are in 2 to 6 blossomed racemes, usually without an accompanying leaf. The perigone tube is tightly cylindrical, 9 to 20 mm long and 2 to 4 mm wide. It is drawn together over the ovary and opens out like a funnel at the top. The tepals at the tip are pubescent on the inside, and the filaments are softly pubescent. The fruit is a blue-black, frosted berry, 8 to 9 mm in diameter with a disgusting, sweet taste.

Leaves, Stem and Root: The plant is a perennial 30 to 80 cm high herb. The stems are sturdy, round and glabrous. The leaves are ovate to elliptical, 5 to 15 cm long and 3 to 7.5 cm wide, narrowing suddenly at the base. They are glabrous, dark green above and gray-green frosted beneath.

Habitat: The plant is indigenous to Europe, the Near East, eastern Asia, the Himalayas, Siberia and North America.

Production: Solomon's Seal rhizome is the rhizome of Polygonatum multiflorum. The root-stocks should be dug up during the dormant seasons, autumn and spring. Earth and roots are removed and the rhizomes cut into pieces of a few centimeters in length.

Other Names: Dropberry, Lady's Seals, Sealroot, Sealwort, St. Mary's Seal

ACTIONS AND PHARMACOLOGY

COMPOUNDS

Steroid saponins (2.5%): 2 unnamed saponins, aglycones diosgenin, or else (25R)-furost-5-en-3beta,22alpha,26-triole

Mucilages

Acetidin-2-carboxylic acid

EFFECTS

The steroid saponins may be responsible for the anti-inflammatory effect of the drug. It works as a tonic, and relieves and soothes upset stomach.

INDICATIONS AND USAGE

Unproven Uses: The plant was formerly used in the treatment of respiratory and lung disorders. It was used externally in the treatment of bruises, furuncles, ulcers or boils on the fingers, hemorrhoids, redness of the skin, and for edema and hematoma.

PRECAUTIONS AND ADVERSE REACTIONS

No health hazards or side effects are known in conjunction with the proper administration of designated therapeutic dosages. Extended administration of the drug in therapeutic dosages can lead to gastrointestinal irritation.

OVERDOSAGE

Overdosage leads to nausea, diarrhea, gastric complaints and queasiness.

DOSAGE

Mode of Administration: The drug has been used internally as an infusion and externally as a poultice, but is now obsolete.

Storage: Store in paper and cloth sacks.

LITERATURE

Janeczko Z, (1980) Acta Polon. Pharm 37:559.

Kato A, Miura T, Hypoglycemic action of the rhizomes of Polygonatum officinale in normal and diabetic mice. In: PM 60(3):201. 1994.

Sugiyama M et al., Chem Pharm Bull 32:1365-1372. 1984.

Tomoda M et al., Chem Pharm Bull 21:2511-2516. 1973.

Further information in:

Frohne D, Pfänder HJ, Giftpflanzen - Ein Handbuch für Apotheker, Toxikologen und Biologen, 4. Aufl., Wiss. Verlags-Ges. Stuttgart 1997.

Hänsel R, Keller K, Rimpler H, Schneider G (Hrsg.), Hagers Handbuch der Pharmazeutischen Praxis, 5. Aufl., Bde 4-6 (Drogen), Springer Verlag Berlin, Heidelberg, New York, 1992-1994.

Madaus G, Lehrbuch der Biologischen Arzneimittel, Bde 1-3, Nachdruck, Georg Olms Verlag Hildesheim 1979.

Roth L, Daunderer M, Kormann K, Giftpflanzen, Pflanzengifte, 4. Aufl., Ecomed Fachverlag Landsberg Lech 1993.

Teuscher E, Lindequist U, Biogene Gifte - Biologie, Chemie, Pharmakologie, 2. Aufl., Fischer Verlag Stuttgart 1994.

Sophora japonica

See Pagoda Tree

Sorb Apple

Sorbus domestica

DESCRIPTION

Medicinal Parts: The medicinal part is the ripe fruit.

Flower and Fruit: The inflorescence is umbelliferous-racemous and tomentose. The sepals and petals are also tomentose. The petals are white to light red, and the carpels are pubescent. The dividing membranes are not split. There are 2 ovules in each ovary chamber. The fruit is false pear-shaped-globular, yellow, speckled red on the sun side. The seed is flat, brown and sharp-edged.

Leaves, Stem and Root: Sorbus domestica is a bush or tree up to 13 m high, with branches that are initially gray-tomentose, later glabrous. The winter buds are glabrous or have hairy tips, and are sticky. The leaves are pinnatifid with 13 to 21 sessile, serrate and acuminate leaflets. The serrate teeth are long and finely acuminate. The lower surface is bluish-green and initially villous-cobweb pubescent, later glabrous.

Habitat: The plant is cultivated in Europe and elsewhere.

Production: Sorb Apple berries are the fruit of Sorbus domestica.

Other Names: Sorvice Tree, Cheque Tree, Ash

ACTIONS AND PHARMACOLOGY

COMPOUNDS

Sugar alcohols: sorbitol

The fruits do not contain parasorboside, in contrast to those of Sorbus aucuparia.

The drug has not been fully researched.

EFFECTS

The active agents are pectin, tannin, organic acids (sorbic acid) and sorbitol. The fruit has astringent, anti-inflammatory and pain-relieving properties.

INDICATIONS AND USAGE

Unproven Uses: Internally, the berries act as an astringent for the intestinal tract. Externally, preparations are used for skin cleansing.

PRECAUTIONS AND ADVERSE REACTIONS

No health hazards or side effects are known in conjunction with the proper administration of designated therapeutic dosages.

DOSAGE

Mode of Administration: Fresh juice from the berries and a decoction made from the dried fruit are used internally. The decoction is also applied externally as a wash to the affected areas. See also Mountain Ash Berry (Sorbus aucuparia).

Daily Dosage: Fresh juice: 50 to 80 gm; decoction: add 5 gm of drug to 100 ml of water and drink 1 to 2 cups.

LITERATURE

No literature is available.

Sorbus aucuparia

See Mountain Ash Berry

Sorbus domestica

See Sorb Apple

Sorbus torminalis

See Wild Service Tree

Sorghum vulgare

See Broom Corn

Sorrel

Rumex acetosa

TRADE NAMES

Sorrel (available from a number of manufacturers), Sheep Sorrel

DESCRIPTION

Medicinal Parts: The medicinal parts are the fresh leaves and the whole herb.

Flower and Fruit: The plant has small greenish unisexual, dioecious flowers growing in narrow, loose panicles. There are 6 tepals. The 3 inner ones are longer, closer together, and turn red when the fruit ripens. When mature they are often red-tinged, membranous, entire-margined and have a scale-like downwardly curved welt at the base. The three outermost tips are revolute. There are 6 stamens and 3 styles with a paintbrush-like stigma. The fruit is a triangular, brown-black nut enclosed in the wing-like enlarged inner tepal.

Leaves, Stem and Root: The plant can grow up to 100 cm high. The leaves alternate on the erect, grooved stems, which are unbranched up to the panicles. The leaves are fleshy, grass green, hastate or spit-shaped. The lower leaves are long-petioled; the upper ones are short-petioled, sessile and clasping. There is a membranous, dentate or fringed cone at the base of the leaves.

Characteristics: The stem is red-tinged, and the herb has a sour taste. It gets its acidity from the same salt that is present in Rhubarb.

Habitat: The plant is common in Europe.

Production: Sorrel is the aerial part of Rumex acetosa.

ACTIONS AND PHARMACOLOGY

COMPOUNDS

Oxalates: oxalic acid, calcium oxalate

Tannins (7-10%)

Flavonoids

Anthracene derivatives: anthranoids, aglycones, physcion, chryosphanol, emodin, aloe-emodin, rhein, and their glucosides, as well as aloe-emodin acetate

EFFECTS

Sorrel acts as a diuretic. It stimulates secretion, and improves resistance to infections (antibacterial), although some of these effects are questionable.

INDICATIONS AND USAGE

Unproven Uses: The herb is used for acute and chronic inflammation of the nasal passages and respiratory tract. It is also used as an adjuvant in antibacterial therapy. Folk medicine uses include stomach ailments, liver and biliary ailments and purification of the blood.

PRECAUTIONS AND ADVERSE REACTIONS

No health hazards or side effects are known in conjunction with the proper administration of designated therapeutic dosages.

OVERDOSAGE

Oxalate poisonings are conceivable only with the consumption of very large quantities of the leaves as a salad.

DOSAGE

Mode of Administration: The drug is described as obsolete.

How Supplied:

Tablets

Liquid — 1:4

Daily Dosage: The dosage for adults is 2 coated tablets or 50 drops (drops with 19% Ethanol) taken 3 times daily.

LITERATURE

Ito H. Effects of the antitumor agents from various natural sources on drug-metabolizing system, phagocytic activity and complement system in sarcoma 180-bearing mice. Jpn J Pharmacol, 40:435-43, Mar 1986.

Southern Bayberry

Myrica cerifera

TRADE NAMES

Southern Bayberry is available from a number of manufacturers, sometimes labeled Bayberry Bark or Bayberry Root Bark.

DESCRIPTION

Medicinal Parts: The medicinal parts are the dried root bark and the wax extracted from the berries.

Flower and Fruit: The flowers are unisexual and have no calyx or corolla. They are small and yellowish in scaly catkins. The fruit is small groups of round, gray-white berries containing numerous black seeds, which have a crust of usable greenish-white wax. The wax helps keep the berries in a suitable state for germination for a period of 2 to 3 years.

Leaves, Stem and Root: Southern Bayberry is an evergreen shrub or small tree that grows up to 10 m high. The bark has a white, peeling outer layer, which covers a red-brown inner layer. The leaves are lanceolate to oblong-lanceolate, glossy or resinous, and punctate on both sides.

Characteristics: The taste is astringent and bitter. The leaves have an aromatic odor.

Habitat: The plant is found in the eastern and southern regions of the U.S. and around Lake Erie.

Production: Bayberry bark is the bark from the trunk and branches of Myrica cerifera.

Other Names: Bayberry, Candleberry, Tallow Shrub, Vegetable Tallow, Waxberry, Wax Myrtle, Myrica

ACTIONS AND PHARMACOLOGY

COMPOUNDS

Volatile oil (traces)

Tannins

Resins

The constituents of the drug have not been extensively investigated.

EFFECTS

The active compounds have diaphoretic, stimulant and astringent effects.

INDICATIONS AND USAGE

Unproven Uses: The drug is used internally for coughs and colds, and externally for skin diseases and ulcers.

PRECAUTIONS AND ADVERSE REACTIONS

No health hazards or side effects are known in conjunction with the proper administration of designated therapeutic dosages. Higher dosages of the drug are said to trigger vomiting, and are used as an emetic.

DOSAGE

Mode of Administration: The drug is available as a liquid extract for internal use, and in powder form.

How Supplied:

Capsules — 450 mg, 475 mg

Liquid Extract — 1:1

LITERATURE

Kern W, List PH, Hörhammer L (Hrsg.), Hagers Handbuch der Pharmazeutischen Praxis, 4. Aufl., Bde. 1-8, Springer Verlag Berlin, Heidelberg, New York, 1969.

Leung AY, Encyclopedia of Common Natural Ingredients Used in Food Drugs and Cosmetics, John Wiley & Sons Inc., New York 1980.

Madaus G, Lehrbuch der Biologischen Arzneimittel, Bde 1-3, Nachdruck, Georg Olms Verlag Hildesheim 1979.

Paul BD et al., (1974) J Pharm Sci 63:958.

Yoshizawa S et al., (1987) Phytother Res 1(1):44.

Southern Tsangshu (Cang-Zhu)

Atractylodes lancea

DESCRIPTION

Medicinal Parts: The medicinal parts of the plant are the whole plant and roots.

Flower and Fruit: The composite flowers are surrounded by bracts. The capitulas are apical and upright, with a diameter of 1.5 to 2 cm. The calyx is double-rowed and double-pinnate. The lingual florets are in 7 or 8 rows, whitish and 1 to 1.2 cm long. The fruit is an achaene. The pappus is brownish and 8 to 9 mm long.

Leaves, Stem and Root: Southern Tsangshu is an upright, herbaceous perennial with a rhizome that extends up to 1 m high. The basal leaves wilt rapidly, the upper cauline leaves are alternate, small, usually simple and sessile. The lower leaves are long-petiolate and 8 to 10 cm long. The lamina is pergament-like, single pinnate with 3 to 5 elongate-elliptical leaflets. The apical leaflet is larger with short thorns on the margin. The rhizome is elongate, gnarled, 2 to 3 cm thick and up to 8 cm long.

Habitat: Cang-Zhu is indigenous to Japan and China.

Production: Southern Tsangshu rhizome is the dried rhizome of Atractylodes lancea. The rhizome is dug up in spring or autumn and dried. In order to obtain the cut drug, the rhizome is soaked after being cleaned and cut into slices.

ACTIONS AND PHARMACOLOGY

COMPOUNDS

Volatile oil (1.5%): components including p-cymol, beta-selinene, alpha curcumene, elemol, hinesol, beta-eudesmol

Sesquiterpenes: 3 beta-hydroxyatractylon, 3beta-acetoxy-atractylon

Polyynes: including atractylodin, atractylodinol, acetylatratylodinol

EFFECTS

The sesquiterpenes and furanosesquiterpenes contained in the essential oil of the drug have hepatoprotective, immunostimulating and intestinal motility-enhancing effects, while also inhibiting the secretion of gastric juices. The smoke of the drug is said to have antiseptic characteristics, while the essential oil is additionally credited with a sedative effect, derived from its beta-eudesmol and hinesol content.

INDICATIONS AND USAGE

Unproven Uses: Southern Tsangshu is used for diarrhea, feelings of fullness in the lower abdomen, lack of strength including atrophy, rheumatic pain, colds and night blindness.

Chinese Medicine: The herb is used for gastroenteritis, edema, disturbances of renal function and generalized pain.

PRECAUTIONS AND ADVERSE REACTIONS

No health hazards are known in conjunction with the proper administration of designated therapeutic dosages.

DOSAGE

Mode of Administration: Whole herb, cut and powdered drug for internal use.

Preparation: The powder is prepared in accordance with Jap XI or ChinP IX. It is roasted using the Fuchao method.

Dosage: 3 to 9 of gm of drug

Storage: Should be stored in a dry and cool place and in tightly sealed containers.

LITERATURE

Blaschek W, Hänsel R, Keller K, Reichling J, Rimpler G, Schneider G (Eds), Hagers Handbuch der Pharmazeutischen Praxis. Folgebände 1 und 2. Drogen A-Z. Springer. Berlin, Heidelberg 1998.

Gong QM, Wang SL, Gan C, A clinical study on the treatment of acute upper digestive tract hemorrhage with wen-she decoction. Chung Hsi I Chieh Ho Tsa Chih, 29:272-3, 260, 1989 May.

Hiraoka N, Atractylodes lancea autotetraploids induced by colchicine treatment of shoot cultures. Biol Pharm Bull, 16:479-83, 1998 May.

Hwang JM, Tseng TH, Hsieh YS, Chou FP, Wang CJ, Chu CY, Inhibitory effect of atractylon on tert-butyl hydroperoxide induced DNA damage and hepatic toxicity in rat hepatocytes. Arch Toxicol, 70:640-4, 1996.

Kimura M, Diwan PV, Yanagi S, Kon-no Y, Nojima H, Kimura I, Potentiating effects of beta-eudesmol-related cyclohexylidene derivatives on succinylcholine-induced neuromuscular block in isolated phrenic nerve-diaphragm muscles of normal and alloxan-diabetic mice. Biol Pharm Bull, 18:407-10, 1995 Mar.

Kimura M, Nojima H, Muroi M, Kimura I, Mechanism of the blocking action of beta-eudesmol on the nicotinic acetylcholine receptor channel in mouse skeletal muscles. Neuropharmacology, 30:835-41, 1991 Aug.

Kiso Y, Tohkin M, Hikino H, Antihepatotoxic principles of Atractylodes rhizomes. J Nat Prod, 46:651-4, 1983 Sep-Oct.

Muroi M, Tanaka K, Kimura I, Kimura M, Anti-inflammatory principles of Atractylodes rhizomes. Chem Pharm Bull (Tokyo), 50:2954-8, 1979 Dec.

Muroi M, Tanaka K, Kimura I, Kimura M, Beta-eudesmol (a main component of Atractylodes lancea)-induced potentiation of depolarizing neuromuscular blockade in diaphragm muscles of normal and diabetic mice. Jpn J Pharmacol, 50:69-71, 1989 May.

Nojima H, Kimura I, Kimura M Blocking action of succinylcholine with beta-eudesmol on acetylcholine-activated channel activity at endplates of single muscle cells of adult mice. Brain Res, 575:337-40, 1992 Mar 20.

Resch M, Steigel A, Chen ZL, Bauer R 5-Lipoxygenase and cyclooxygenase-1 inhibitory active compounds from Atractylodes lancea. J Nat Prod, 61:347-50, 1998 Mar.

Sakamoto S, Kudo H, Suzuki S, Sassa S, Yoshimura S, Nakayama T, Maemura M, Mitamura T, Qi Z, Liu XD, Yagishita Y, Asai A Pharmacotherapeutic effects of toki-shakuyaku-san on leukorrhagia in young women. Am J Chin Med, 24:165-8, 1996.

Satoh K, Nagai F, Ushiyama K, Kano I Specific inhibition of Na+,K(+)-ATPase activity by atractylon, a major component of byaku-jutsu, by interaction with enzyme in the E2 state. Biochem Pharmacol, 51:339-43, 1996 Feb 9.

Usuki S Blended effects of herbal components of tokishakuyakusan on rat corpus luteum function in vivo. Am J Chin Med, 16:107-16, 1988.

Wang GT Antianoxic action and active constituents of atractylodis lanceae rhizoma. Chem Pharm Bull (Tokyo), 10:2033-4, 1990 Jul.

Wang GT Treatment of operated late gastric carcinoma with prescription of strengthening the patient's resistance and dispelling the invading evil in combination with chemotherapy: follow-up study of 158 patients and experimental study in animals Chung Hsi I Chieh.

Yamahara J, Matsuda H, Huang Q, Li Y, Fujimura H Intestinal motility enhancing effect of Atractylodes lancea rhizome. J Ethnopharmacol, 29:341-4, 1990 Jul.

Soybean

Glycine soja

DESCRIPTION

Medicinal Parts: The medicinal parts are the soya lecithin extracted from the soya bean, the soya oil and the soya seed.

Flower and Fruit: The flowers are small, inconspicuous, short pedicled, upright, axillary and in 3 to 8 blossomed clusters. The sepals are campanulate or tubular-campanulate and somewhat bilabiate. The corolla is usually purple, exceeding the calyx only slightly or not at all. The stamens are diadelphous or monodelphous. The style is glabrous. The pod is linear or oblong and constricted between the seeds. The pod is septate and dehiscent. There are 2 to 4 seeds, which are oblong-ovate, white, yellow or black-brown.

Leaves, Stem and Root: The soya plant is an erect or twining annual bushy plant. The stem and leaves are thickly villous. The leaves are trifoliate, the leaflets are large, ovate, entire-margined and, particularly on the margins and on the ribs of the lower surface, pubescent.

Habitat: The soya plant is indigenous to east Asia but has never been found in the wild. Glycine soja is found in the Amur-Ussuri area, northern China, Taiwan, Korea and Japan.

Production: Lecithin consists of the phospholipid mixture from Glycine soja seeds and its preparations. Virgin Soybean oil is mixed with 2% water at 60° to 80° C. After the swelling times it is separated by centrifugation and the lecithin paste is evaporated at 100° C in a vacuum until the remaining water content is 0.2 to 0.8%.

ACTIONS AND PHARMACOLOGY

COMPOUNDS

Phospholipids (45-60%): in particular phosphatidylcholine, phosphatidylethanolamine, phosphatidylinositol

Fatty oil (30-35%)

Steroids: Phytosterols (2-5%)

EFFECTS

The phospholipids extracted from soya lecithin was shown to have lipid-reducing properties in animal experiments and clinical trials.

INDICATIONS AND USAGE

Approved by Commission E:

- Raised levels of cholesterol

Unproven Uses: Soybean is used for less severe forms of hypercholesterolemia when dietary measures are required. Soybean is also used for liver and gallbladder complaints, anemia, poor concentration, cerebral and nerve conditions, and general debility.

Chinese Medicine: Soybean is used for hyperhidrosis, night sweats, confusion and joint pain.

PRECAUTIONS AND ADVERSE REACTIONS

No health hazards or major side effects are known in conjunction with the proper administration of designated therapeutic dosages. Minor side effects include occasional gastrointestinal effects, such as stomach pain, loose stool and diarrhea.

DOSAGE

Mode of Administration: Preparations for oral administration.

Daily Dosage: The average dose is 3.5 gm of phospholipids (phosphatidylcholine).

Storage: Soybean preparations must be protected from light and tightly sealed.

LITERATURE

Hänsel R, Keller K, Rimpler H, Schneider G (Hrsg.), Hagers Handbuch der Pharmazeutischen Praxis, 5. Aufl., Bde 4-6 (Drogen): Springer Verlag Berlin, Heidelberg, New York, 1992-1994 (unter Glycine).

Steinegger E, Hänsel R: Pharmakognosie, 5. Aufl., Springer Verlag Heidelberg 1992.

Teuscher E, Biogene Arzneimittel, 5. Aufl., Wiss. Verlagsges. Stuttgart 1997.

Spanish Chestnut

Castanea sativa

DESCRIPTION

Medicinal Parts: The medicinal parts are the leaves collected and dried in autumn, and preparations of the fresh leaves.

Flower and Fruit: The male, monoecious, yellowish-white flowers are in 12 to 20 cm long, erect catkins consisting of numerous, 7-flowered clusters. These are located in the leaf axils of the upper branches. There are 3 to 6 female flowers at the base of unopened male catkins. When the fruit ripens in October, the outer soft thorny husk bursts into 4 lobes, revealing a brown-skinned sweet chestnut that needs "wine weather" to ripen.

Leaves, Stem and Root: The tree grows from 15 to 30 m high. The bark is smooth at first, olive green, later dark brown, and vertically reticulate. The leaves are 8 to 25 cm long, coriaceous, oblong-lanceolate with long, pointed, serrated teeth.

Habitat: Northern temperate hemispheres; prefers maritime climate.

Production: Spanish Chestnut leaves consist of the leaves of Castanea sativa collected from September to October. The leaves are collected and air-dried.

Other Names: Sweet Chestnut, Husked Nut, Jupiter's Nut, Sardian Nut, Chestnut

ACTIONS AND PHARMACOLOGY

COMPOUNDS

Tannins (6 to 8%): ellagitannins, including pedunculagin, tellimagrandin I and II, casuarictin, potentillin, castalagin, vescalagin

Flavonoids: including rutin, quercitrin, myricetin

EFFECTS

No information is available.

INDICATIONS AND USAGE

Unproven Uses: Spanish Chestnut leaves are used for complaints affecting the respiratory tract, such as bronchitis and whooping cough, leg pain, circulation and diarrhea, and as a gargle for sore throats.

PRECAUTIONS AND ADVERSE REACTIONS

No health hazards or side effects are known in conjunction with the proper administration of designated therapeutic dosages.

DOSAGE

Preparation: An infusion is prepared by pouring boiling water over 5 gm of comminuted drug and then straining it.

Daily Dosage: The average single dose is 5 gm of drug or 5 gm of liquid extract.

LITERATURE

Haddock EA et al., PH 21:1049-1062. 1982.

Hänsel R, Keller K, Rimpler H, Schneider G (Hrsg.), Hagers Handbuch der Pharmazeutischen Praxis, 5. Aufl., Bde 4-6 (Drogen), Springer Verlag Berlin, Heidelberg, New York, 1992-1994.

Leung AY, Encyclopedia of Common Natural Ingredients Used in Food Drugs and Cosmetics, John Wiley & Sons Inc., New York 1980.

Madaus G, Lehrbuch der Biologischen Arzneimittel, Bde 1-3, Nachdruck, Georg Olms Verlag Hildesheim 1979.

Wichtl M (Hrsg.), Teedrogen, 4. Aufl., Wiss. Verlagsges. Stuttgart 1997.

Spearmint

Mentha spicata

DESCRIPTION

Medicinal Parts: The medicinal parts are the steamed distillation of the fresh, flowering, aerial parts, and the leaves collected during the flowering season and dried.

Flower and Fruit: The spike-like inflorescence consists of false whorls in the axils of the bracts. The 5-tipped calyx is campanulate, glabrous or pubescent and is surrounded by a 5-tipped, pale lilac, pink or white corolla, which is almost half as long again as the calyx. The nutlet is reticulate in pubescent plants and smooth in glabrous plants.

Leaves, Stem and Root: The plant is 30 to 60 cm during the flowering season. Runners grow from the buds at the base of the stem. The quadrangular stem is ascendent or erect and usually thickly pubescent. The leaves are oblong-ovate or lanceolate, decussate, smooth or wrinkled, regularly serrate, and glabrous to thickly pubescent. The upper leaves are sessile, the lower ones short petiolate.

Habitat: The plant probably originates from the Mediterranean region and is now naturalized in large parts of Europe and North America.

Production: Spearmint is the aerial part of Mentha spicata. Spearmint oil is the essential oil extracted from the plant.

Other Names: Curled Mint, Garden Mint, Mackerel Mint, Our Lady's Mint, Green Mint, Spire Mint, Sage of Bethlehem, Fish Mint, Lamb Mint

ACTIONS AND PHARMACOLOGY

COMPOUNDS: IN THE FOLIAGE

Volatile oil (0.8-2.5%)

Flavonoids: thymonin

Caffeic acid derivatives: including among others rosmaric acid in the volatile oil

Chief components: L-carvone (40-80%, aroma-carrier), (-)-limonene (5-15%), additionally including among others beta-bourbonene, cis- and transcarvylacetate, caryophyllene, 1,8-cineole, dihydrocarveol, trans-sabinene hydrate

EFFECTS

The oil produced contains a high proportion of carvon, which produces the spearmint smell. It has antispasmodic, carminative and stimulant effects.

In vitro, an antimicrobial effect was observed. The drug is insecticidal and shows a neurodepressive effect in animal experiments (increased duration of sleep).

INDICATIONS AND USAGE

Unproven Uses: Spearmint is used for digestive disorders and as a remedy for flatulence. The essential oil is used as an aromatic preparation. Spearmint leaves are used as carminative.

PRECAUTIONS AND ADVERSE REACTIONS

No health hazards or side effects are known in conjunction with the proper administration of designated therapeutic dosages. The volatile oil possesses a weak potential for sensitization due to its menthol and L-carvone content.

DOSAGE

Mode of Administration: Spearmint is mainly used internally in the form of an oil or concentrate.

LITERATURE

Hänsel R, Keller K, Rimpler H, Schneider G (Hrsg.), Hagers Handbuch der Pharmazeutischen Praxis, 5. Aufl., Bde 4-6 (Drogen), Springer Verlag Berlin, Heidelberg, New York, 1992-1994.

Hausen B, Allergiepflanzen, Pflanzenallergene, ecomed Verlagsgesellsch. mbH, Landsberg 1988.

Hefendehl FW, Murray MJ, (1973) Planta Med 23:101.

Leung AY, Encyclopedia of Common Natural Ingredients Used in Food Drugs and Cosmetics, John Wiley & Sons Inc., New York 1980.

Murray MJ et al., (1972) Crop Sci 12:723.

Steinegger E, Hänsel R, Pharmakognosie, 5. Aufl., Springer Verlag Heidelberg 1992.

Subramanian SS, Nair AGR, (1972) Phytochemistry 11:452.

Teuscher E, Biogene Arzneimittel, 5. Aufl., Wiss. Verlagsges. Stuttgart 1997.

Wichtl M (Hrsg.), Teedrogen, 4. Aufl., Wiss. Verlagsges. Stuttgart 1997.

Speedwell

Veronica officinalis

DESCRIPTION

Medicinal Parts: The medicinal parts are the dried herb collected during the flowering season, the fresh aerial parts of the flowering plant and the dried aerial parts collected during the flowering season.

Flower and Fruit: The erect bright blue or lilac flowers are in axillary, peduncled, spike-like racemes. The flowers are small, pedicled and have 4 slightly fused sepals. The corolla has a very short tube, is flatly splayed and has 4 uneven tips. There are 2 stamens and 1 superior ovary. The fruit is a triangular capsule narrowed at the base. The fruit chambers each have 5 to 10 seeds. The seeds are about 1 mm long, oval and flat; the back of the seed is smooth.

Leaves, Stem and Root: The plant is a 10 to 20 cm high herbaceous perennial with runners that tend to form grass. The root system consists mainly of shoot-producing roots. The stem is creeping, and the flower-bearing branches are erect. The whole plant is roughly pubescent. The leaves are obovate-ovate, elliptical or oblong, short-petioled and serrate.

Habitat: The plant is indigenous to almost all of Europe, parts of Asia and North America. The sources of the drug are Bulgaria, the former Yugoslavia and Hungary.

Production: Speedwell consists of the above-ground parts of Veronica officinalis imported from Bulgaria, the former Yugoslavia and Hungary. Only the flowering herb is harvested (without roots or lower parts) and subsequently dried fully in the shade before it is cut.

Not to be Confused With: Veronica chamaedrys or Veronica allionii.

ACTIONS AND PHARMACOLOGY

COMPOUNDS

Iridoide monoterpenes (0.5-1.0%): including among others aucubin, catalpol, catalpol esters (including among others minecoside, verminoside, veronicoside), mussaenoside, ladroside

Flavonoids (0.7%): including among others luteolin-7-O-glucosides (cinaroside), 6-hydroxyluteolin-7-monoglucoside

Triterpene saponins (10%)

Caffeic acid derivatives: chlorogenic acid (0.5%)

EFFECTS

Speedwell exhibits a protective effect against ulcers and accelerates ulcer healing. Its use as an astringent in the treatment of wounds and as a gargle for inflammations of the mouth and throat is plausible because of the amaroid-like properties of the drug.

INDICATIONS AND USAGE

Unproven Uses: Speedwell preparations are used for diseases and discomfort of the respiratory, gastrointestinal and lower urinary tracts. It is also used for the liver and kidneys, and to treat gout, rheumatoid arthritis and rheumatic complaints.

In addition, Speedwell is used internally to improve metabolism (''blood-purifying'') and for nervous agitation. Externally, the herb is used as a gargle for inflammation of the oral and pharyngeal mucosa, promotion of wound healing, chronic skin complaints, itching and sweating of the feet.

PRECAUTIONS AND ADVERSE REACTIONS

No health hazards or side effects are known in conjunction with the proper administration of designated therapeutic dosages.

DOSAGE

Mode of Administration: The herb is available as a whole, cut and powdered drug for internal and external use in compound preparations.

Preparation: To prepare a tea, pour 1 cup of boiling water over 1.5 gm of drug (1 gm is approximately 1 teaspoonful). For the preparation of external lavages and compresses for ulcers, wounds and eczema, add 1 handful of drug to1 liter of water and boil for 10 minutes.

Daily Dosage: The average single dose is 1.5 gm of drug. The dose of the tea (used as an expectorant) is 1 cup taken 2 to 3 times daily.

Storage: Speedwell must be protected from light sources.

LITERATURE

Afifi-Yazar F, Sticher O, (1980) Helv Chim Acta 63:1905.

Afifi-Yazar FÜ et al., Helv Chim Acta 64:16. 1981.

Sticher O et al., (1982) Planta Med 45:159.

Sticher O et al., Helv Chim Acta 62:530 et 535. 1979.

Tamas M et al., Clujul Med 57:169. 1985.

Wojcik E, Acta Polon, Pharm 38:621.

Further information in:

Hänsel R, Keller K, Rimpler H, Schneider G (Hrsg.), Hagers Handbuch der Pharmazeutischen Praxis, 5. Aufl., Bde 4-6 (Drogen): Springer Verlag Berlin, Heidelberg, New York, 1992-1994.

Madaus G, Lehrbuch der Biologischen Arzneimittel, Bde 1-3, Nachdruck, Georg Olms Verlag Hildesheim 1979.

Steinegger E, Hänsel R, Pharmakognosie, 5. Aufl., Springer Verlag Heidelberg 1992.

Wichtl M (Hrsg.), Teedrogen, 4. Aufl., Wiss. Verlagsges. Stuttgart 1997.

Spergularia rubra

See Arenaria Rubra

Spigelia anthelmia

See Wormwood Grass

Spigelia marilandica

See Pink Root

Spikenard

Aralia racemosa

DESCRIPTION

Medicinal Parts: The medicinal parts are the fresh and dried rhizome and roots.

Flower and Fruit: The inflorescence is a large panicle, each branch of which carries a simple, round, 10 to 15 flower umbel. The flowers are small and have greenish-white petals. The drupes are dark red to crimson, roundish and 5-ribbed. The seeds are compressed and have a similarly formed endosperm.

Leaves, Stem and Root: Aralia racemosa is a herbaceous, bushy, stiffly branched perennial with a woody base. The stem extends up to 2 m high and is glabrous and grooved. The leaflets are thin and oval. The leaflets can grow up to 20 cm long and 16 cm wide, but are usually much smaller and cordate at the base. The rhizome is up to 15 cm long and has a diameter of roughly 2.5 cm with prominent concave scars. The roots are about 2 cm thick at the base, pale brown, and wrinkled. The root fracture is short and whitish.

Characteristics: Spikenard has an aromatic odor and taste.

Habitat: The plant grows in North America from central Canada southward to Virginia.

Production: The root and rhizome of Aralia racemosa are gathered from the wild in summer and autumn and chopped while fresh. The freshly chopped roots and rhizomes are either dried or processed immediately to form a thick paste.

Not to be Confused With: It is possible to confuse Spikenard with the Aralia nudicaulis root. However, Spikenard can be distinguished by its lack of spotted hypodermis cells, which are a feature of the Aralia nudicaulis root.

Other Names: Indian Root, Life of Man, Old Man's Root, Petty Morell, Spignet

ACTIONS AND PHARMACOLOGY

COMPOUNDS

Polyynes: including falcarinole, falcarindiole

Triterpene saponins

Volatile oil (very little)

EFFECTS

Due to its saponin content, the drug's effectiveness as a reflex expectorant for colds seems plausible. It is also diaphoretic and stimulates tissue renewal. Its efficacy has not been proven.

INDICATIONS AND USAGE

Unproven Uses: Preparations are used internally for colds, chronic coughs and asthma. It is used as an alternative to sarsaparilla in the treatment of skin diseases and for rheumatic conditions. North American Indians use Spikenard internally to treat backache and externally for bruises, wounds, swellings and inflammations.

Homeopathic Uses: Spikenard is used for colds, hay fever and asthma. Efficacy for colds appears plausible; efficacy for other uses has not been documented.

PRECAUTIONS AND ADVERSE REACTIONS

General: No health hazards or side effects are known in conjunction with the proper administration of designated therapeutic dosages. Because of the polyyne spectrum, sensitization and dermatoses connected with the plant are also possible through skin contact.

Pregnancy: The drug is not to be used during pregnancy.

DOSAGE

Mode of Administration: The drug is administered internally as a fluid extract.

Preparation: It is prepared as a liquid extract (1:1); information on the ethanol content is unavailable.

Daily Dosage: When the drug is prepared as an infusion, the recommended daily dosage is approximately 15 g per 500 ml, to be drunk, one cup at a time, during the course of the day. The recommended dosage of the liquid extract is 0.9 g to 1.8 g.

Homeopathic Dosage: 5 to 10 drops, 1 tablet, 5 to 10 globules, 1 to 3 times daily or 1 ml injection solution twice a week sc (HAB1).

LITERATURE

Ahn Y-J, Kim M-J, Yamamoto T, Fujiwawa T, Mitsouka T, (1990) Selective growth responses of human intestinal bacteria to Araliaceae extracts. Microbial Ecol Health Disease 3:223-229.

Hansen L and Boll PM, (1986) Phytochemistry 25 (2):285.

Further information in:

Hänsel R, Keller K, Rimpler H, Schneider G (Hrsg.), Hagers Handbuch der Pharmazeutischen Praxis, 5. Aufl., Bde 4-6 (Drogen): Springer Verlag Berlin, Heidelberg, New York, 1992-1994.

Hoppe HA (1975-1987) Drogenkunde, 8. Aufl., Bde 1-3, W. de Gruyter Verlag, Berlin, New York.

Madaus G, Lehrbuch der Biologischen Arzneimittel, Bde 1-3, Nachdruck, Georg Olms Verlag Hildesheim 1979.

Roth L, Daunderer M, Kormann K, Giftpflanzen, Pflanzengifte, 4. Aufl., Ecomed Fachverlag Landsberg Lech 1993.

Teuscher E, Lindequist U, Biogene Gifte - Biologie, Chemie, Pharmakologie, 2. Aufl., Fischer Verlag Stuttgart 1994.

Wagner H, Wiesenauer M, Phytotherapie. Phytopharmaka und pflanzliche Homöopathika, Fischer-Verlag, Stuttgart, Jena, New York 1995.

Spinach

Spinacia oleracea

DESCRIPTION

Medicinal Parts: The medicinal parts are the leaves.

Leaves, Stem and Root: Spinach is an annual plant that can be planted at various times during the vegetation period to guarantee a year-round supply. The stems may grow up to 1 m or more and are erect. The leaves are ovate to deltoid-hastate, entire or dentate. When the plant ripens, the bracteoles are almost orbicular-obovate, usually wider than long. They often have a divergent spine at the apex.

Habitat: The plant probably originated in Iran and is cultivated worldwide today.

Production: Spinach consists of the fresh or dried leaf of Spinacia oleracea.

ACTIONS AND PHARMACOLOGY

COMPOUNDS

Triterpene saponins: including among others spinach saponins A and B

Oxalic acid (in young leaves 6-8%, in older leaves up to 16%)

Histamine (up to 140 mg/100 gm fresh weight)

Flavonoids: including among others patuletin, spinacetin, spinatoside

Chlorophyll (0.3-1.0%)

Vitamins: including among others ascorbic acid (vitamin C, 40-155 mg/100 g)

Nitrates (depending on the fertilizer, 0.3-0.6%)

EFFECTS

No information is available.

INDICATIONS AND USAGE

Unproven Uses: Spinach preparations are used for ailments and complaints of the gastrointestinal tract, as a blood-generating remedy, to stimulate growth in children, as an appetite stimulant, for fatigue and for supporting convalescence.

PRECAUTIONS AND ADVERSE REACTIONS

General: No health hazards or side effects are known in conjunction with the proper administration of designated therapeutic dosages. The relatively high nitrate content makes it advisable to forgo consuming spinach as a foodstuff too often. Circumstances that lead to reduction (e.g., leaving spinach standing at room temperature) should also be avoided to prevent nitrite formation. In addition, the oxalate content of spinach could reduce calcium resorption.

Pediatric Use: Infants should not receive spinach as a foodstuff until after their fourth month (danger of methemoglobin formation through nitrites).

DOSAGE

No information is available.

LITERATURE

Hegnauer R, Chemotaxonomie der Pflanzen, Bde 1-11: Birkhäuser Verlag Basel, Boston, Berlin 1962-1997.

Kern W, List PH, Hörhammer L (Hrsg.), Hagers Handbuch der Pharmazeutischen Praxis, 4. Aufl., Bde. 1-8: Springer Verlag Berlin, Heidelberg, New York, 1969.

Teuscher E, Lindequist U, Biogene Gifte - Biologie, Chemie, Pharmakologie, 2. Aufl., Fischer Verlag Stuttgart 1994.

Spinacia oleracea

See Spinach

Spiny Rest Harrow

Ononis spinosa

DESCRIPTION

Medicinal Parts: The medicinal parts are the roots and flowering branches.

Flower and Fruit: The pink flowers are solitary or in pairs in the leaf axils. The calyx is campanulate with 5 segments. The standard is large and has dark stripes. The ovoid, erect fruit is a pod as long as or longer than the calyx.

Leaves, Stem and Root: The plant is a low subshrub of about 30 to 60 cm with a long taproot. The branches are erect, spreading, villous and more or less densely covered in short shoots, which terminate in straight thorns. The leaves are trifoliate with 3 small, dentate, oblong leaflets. The upper leaves are entire.

Characteristics: The plant has an unpleasant smell.

Habitat: Spiny Rest Harrow is common in almost all of Europe, as well as in North Africa and western Asia.

Production: Spiny Rest Harrow root consists of the dried roots and rhizomes of Ononis spinosa. The plant is harvested in autumn.

Other Names: Cammock, Petty Whin, Stayplough, Rest-Harrow, Wild Liquorice, Stinking Tommy, Ground Furze, Land Whin

ACTIONS AND PHARMACOLOGY

COMPOUNDS

Isoflavonoids: glycosides, including among others, trifolirhizin (maackiain-7-0-glucoside), ononin (formononetin-7-0-glucoside), ononin-6-malonylester, homopterocarpin-7-0-glucoside

Free isoflavonoids: including among others, formononetin, genistein, biochanin

Volatile oil (0.02-0.2%): chief components anethole, carvone, menthol

Triterpenes: including among others, alpha-onocerin (alpha-onoceradiendiol)

Lectins

EFFECTS

In combination with sufficient liquid intake, the drug is said to be diuretic. The diuretic effect is disputed because it is not sufficiently documented and can be attributed neither to the essential oil nor to the flavonoids. In animal tests, an anti-edemic effect was proven. The genistein is mildly estrogenic.

INDICATIONS AND USAGE

Approved by Commission E:

- Infections of the urinary tract
- Kidney and bladder stones

Preparations of the drug are used for flushing-out therapy for inflammatory diseases of the lower urinary tract and also for prevention and treatment of kidney gravel.

Unproven Uses: Spiny Rest Harrow is popularly used for gout, rheumatic complaints, as a flushing-out therapy for inflammatory diseases of the lower urinary tract, and for prevention and treatment of kidney gravel.

CONTRAINDICATIONS

The drug should not be used in the presence of edema resulting from reduced cardiac or renal activity.

PRECAUTIONS AND ADVERSE REACTIONS

No health hazards or side effects are known in conjunction with the proper administration of designated therapeutic dosages.

DOSAGE

Mode of Administration: The drug is ground for teas and other galenic preparations for internal use. Ample liquid intake (at least 2 liters per day) should accompany use of the drug.

Preparation: To prepare an infusion (tea), pour boiling water over 2 to 2.5 g finely cut or coarsely powdered drug and strain after 20 to 30 minutes (1 teaspoonful equals approximately 3 g).

Daily Dosage: 6 to 12 gm of drug.

LITERATURE

Dedio I, Kozlowski J, (1977) Acta Pol Pharm 34:97.

Fujise Y et al., (1965) Chem Pharm Bull 13:93.

Haznagy A, Thot G, Tamas J, Constituents of the aqueous extracts from Ononis spinosa L. In: Arch Pharm 311(4):318-323. 1978.

Hilp K et al., (1975) Arch Pharm 308:429.

Horejsi V, Kocourek J, (1978) Biochim Biophys Acta 538.

Kartnig T et al., (1985) Pharm Acta Helv 60(9/19):253.

Kern W, List PH, Hörhammer L (Hrsg.), Hagers Handbuch der Pharmazeutischen Praxis, 4. Aufl., Bde 1-8, Springer Verlag Berlin, Heidelberg, New York, 1969.

Kirmizigül S et al., Spinonin, a novel glycoside from Ononis spinosa subsp. leiosperma. In: JNP 60(4):378-381. 1997.

Koster J et al., (1983) Planta Med 48:131.

Madaus G, Lehrbuch der Biologischen Arzneimittel, Bde 1-3, Nachdruck, Georg Olms Verlag Hildesheim 1979.

Steinegger E, Hänsel R, Pharmakognosie, 5. Aufl., Springer Verlag Heidelberg 1992.

Teuscher E, Biogene Arzneimittel, 5. Aufl., Wiss. Verlagsges. Stuttgart 1997.

Wagner H, Wiesenauer M, Phytotherapie. Phytopharmaka und pflanzliche Homöopathika, Fischer-Verlag, Stuttgart, Jena, New York 1995.

Wichtl M (Hrsg.), Teedrogen, 4. Aufl., Wiss. Verlagsges. Stuttgart 1997.

Spruce

Picea species

DESCRIPTION

Medicinal Parts: The medicinal parts are the oil extracted from the needles, branch tips or branches and the fresh Spruce shoots.

Flower and Fruit: The male flowers are strawberry colored, the female are crimson or green. The male flowers are in short-stemmed, cylindrical catkins scattered over the crown. The female flowers are in elliptical-cylindrical cones at the top of the crown. The ripe cones are sessile, hanging, globular-clavate and covered in rhomboid scales, which are thin, undulating at the tip and dentate. The wings of the small seeds are 3 times as long as the seeds themselves.

Leaves, Stem and Root: Picea excelsa is a tree that grows from 30 to 60 m high and has a column-like trunk with brown-red bark and a girth of about 2 m. The trunk is usually branched. The branches are horizontal and flat. The young shoots are reddish-brown or orange-red. The crossed-opposite leaves are scaly and imbricate. The needles remain on the tree for a number of years. On the upper surface of the shoots they are pointed forward, on the lower surface they are pointed toward the sides. They are 1.3 to 2.5 cm long, rigid or curved, rich green and have a blunt horn-like tip.

Habitat: The tree is found in northern and central Europe.

Production: The essential oil is obtained from the fresh needles and twig tops or branches of Picea abies (Syn: Picea excelsa), Abies alba, Abies sachalinensis or Abies sibirica. The essential oil is recovered from the needles by a 5 to 6 hour continuous process of aqueous steam distillation on a sieve base of layered and crushed fresh twigs. Preparations from the fresh 10 to 15 cm long shoots of Picea abies and/or Abies alba (Syn.: Abies pectinata) are collected in the spring.

Other Names: Balm of Gilead Fir, Balsam Fir, Canada Balsam, Fir Tree, Hemlock Spruce, Norway Pine, Norway Spruce, Spruce Fir

ACTIONS AND PHARMACOLOGY

COMPOUNDS: SPRUCE NEEDLE OIL

From Picea abies:

Bornyl acetate (5-25%)

Limonene (10-30%)

Camphene (10-25%)

Alpha-pinene (10-25%): additionally, including among others santene, beta-pinene, Delta3-carene, myrcene

From Picea mariana:

Bornyl acetate (37-49%)

Camphene (10-17%)

Alpha-pinene (10%): additionally, including among others beta-pinene, limonene, Delta3-carene, myrcene, santene

From Abies alba:

Bornyl acetate (2-10%)

Limonene (25-55%)

Camphene (9-20%)

Alpha-pinene (6-35%): additionally, including among others beta-pinene, beta-phellandrene, Delta-carene, myrcene, santene

EFFECTS: SPRUCE NEEDLE OIL

The plants are secretolytic, antibacterial and hyperemic.

COMPOUNDS: SPRUCE SHOOTS (FRESH)

Volatile oil (0.2-0.5%): chief components limonene, alpha-pinene, borneol, bornyl acetate

Ascorbic acid (vitamin C)

EFFECTS: SPRUCE SHOOTS (FRESH)

The essential oil has a secretory, mild antiseptic and hyperemic effect.

INDICATIONS AND USAGE

SPRUCE NEEDLE OIL

Approved by Commission E:

- Common cold
- Cough/bronchitis
- Fevers and colds

- Inflammation of the mouth and pharynx
- Neuralgias
- Rheumatism
- Tendency to infection

Unproven Uses: The essential oil is used internally for catarrhal conditions of the respiratory tract. Externally, it is used for catarrhal conditions of the respiratory tract, rheumatic and neuralgic pain, and tension states.

SPRUCE SHOOTS (FRESH)

Approved by Commission E:

- Common cold
- Cough/bronchitis
- Fevers and colds
- Inflammation of the mouth and pharynx
- Muscular and nerve pains
- Tendency to infection

Unproven Uses: The drug is used internally as a respiratory-tract catarrh and externally for muscle pains and neuralgia. In folk medicine, it is used internally for tuberculosis and externally as a bath additive for patients with neurological illnesses.

CONTRAINDICATIONS

Contraindications include bronchial asthma and whooping cough. Patients with extensive skin injuries, acute skin diseases, feverish or infectious diseases, cardiac insufficiency or hypertonia should not use the drug as a bath additive.

PRECAUTIONS AND ADVERSE REACTIONS

No health hazards or side effects are known in conjunction with the proper administration of designated therapeutic dosages, although bronchial spasms could be worsened.

DOSAGE

SPRUCE NEEDLE OIL

Mode of Administration: Embrocations of alcohol solutions, ointments, gels, emulsions and oils are available, as well as bath additives and inhalants.

Daily Dosage:

Infusion — Place 4 drops of oil on a lump of sugar or in a little water and take 3 times a day.

Inhalation — Add 2 gm of oil to hot water and inhale several times a day.

External application — A 20 to 30% ointment is rubbed onto the affected area several times a day.

Bath additive — Add 5 gm oil to a full bath at a temperature of 35 to 38° C.

Storage: Store in a cool place, in a tightly sealed container, protected from light.

SPRUCE SHOOTS (FRESH)

Mode of Administration: In galenic preparations for internal and external application.

Preparation: For inhalation therapy, place 2 gm of oil in hot water and inhale the vapors. To make a bath additive, boil 200 to 300 gm drug in 1 liter water and strain after 5 minutes; add to a full bath. Make sure it is possible to relax after the bath.

Daily Dosage: For internal use: 5 to 6 gm of drug is administered per day.

Four drops of the essential oil may be placed in a little water or on a lump of sugar and taken 3 times a day.

The inhalation therapy mentioned in the *Preparation* section can be used several times a day.

LITERATURE

SPRUCE NEEDLE OIL

Glasl H, Wagner H, DAZ 120:64-67. 1980.

Hänsel R, Keller K, Rimpler H, Schneider G (Eds.), Hagers Handbuch der Pharmazeutischen Praxis, 5. Aufl., Bde 4-6 (Drogen), Springer Verlag Berlin, Heidelberg, New York, 1992-1994.

Kubeczka KH, Schultze W, Flavour Fragrance J:2.137-148. 1987.

Madaus G, Lehrbuch der Biologischen Arzneimittel, Bde 1-3, Nachdruck, Georg Olms Verlag Hildesheim 1979.

Schantz von M, Juvonen S, Acta Bot Fenn 73:5-51. 1966.

Schantz von M, Juvonen S, PM 15:337-341. 1967.

Steinegger E, Hänsel R, Pharmakognosie, 5. Aufl., Springer Verlag Heidelberg 1992.

Teuscher E, Biogene Arzneimittel, 5. Aufl., Wiss. Verlagsges. Stuttgart 1997.

Wagner H, Wiesenauer M, Phytotherapie. Phytopharmaka und pflanzliche Homöopathika, Fischer-Verlag, Stuttgart, Jena, New York 1995.

SPRUCE SHOOTS (FRESH)

Glasl H, Wagner H, DAZ 120:64-67. 1980.

Hänsel R, Keller K, Rimpler H, Schneider G (Hrsg.), Hagers Handbuch der Pharmazeutischen Praxis, 5. Aufl., Bde 4-6 (Drogen), Springer Verlag Berlin, Heidelberg, New York, 1992-1994.

Kubeczka KH, Schultze W, Flavour Fragrance J:2.137-148. 1987.

Madaus G, Lehrbuch der Biologischen Arzneimittel, Bde 1-3, Nachdruck, Georg Olms Verlag Hildesheim 1979.

Schantz M von, Juvonen S, Acta Bot Fenn 73:5-51. 1966.

Schantz M von, Juvonen S, PM 15:337-341. 1967.

Spurge

Euphorbia resinifera

DESCRIPTION

Medicinal Parts: The medicinal part of the plant is the milky resin that is exuded when cuts are made into this plant.

Flower and Fruit: The inflorescence is arranged in a dichasium above the thorn-bearing scales. They are typical cyathia of the Euphorbia species, which have one female and a number of male flowers surrounded by 5 greenish-yellowish, tubularly fused bracts. The female flower has a 3-carpeled ovary with 3 styles; the male flower consists of only 1 stamen. The fruit separates into 3 mericarps.

Leaves, Stem and Root: This diclinous, monoecious leafless shrub has the appearance of cactus and grows to a height of up to 2.5 m. The trunk is thick at the base, and only slightly branched higher up. The diameter of the 3- or 4-edged, fleshy branches is approximately 2 cm. There are scales at intervals of 1 cm at the edges, each with 2 short thorns, which are splayed and approximately 5 mm long.

Characteristics: The plant produces a milk latex when the surface is scored.

Habitat: The shrub grows in the folds of the Great Atlas Mountains in Morocco and also in North America and the Canary Islands.

Production: Gum euphorbium or Spurge is the air-dried latex of Euphorbia resinifera. The plant is cut in late summer to produce the latex.

Other Names: Poisonous Gum-Thistle, Dergmuse, Darkmous, Gum Euphorbium

ACTIONS AND PHARMACOLOGY

COMPOUNDS

Diterpenes: diterpene esters of the ingenan-, tiglic- and daphnan-types (0.1 to 2%): resinifera factors RL 1 to RL 23, among them resiniferatoxin, 12-desoxyphorbol-13-isobutyrate-20-acetate, 12-Desoxyphorbol-13-phenylacetate-20-acetate

Triterpenes: particularly alpha- and beta-euphorbol, beta-amyrin, resiniferol

Fruit acids: including malic acid, succinic acid, citric acid

Resins (40%)

Polyterpenes

EFFECTS

The diterpene esters contained in the drug have laxative and non-specific immunostimulating effects. Severe skin and mucous membrane irritation arises in conjunction with topical administration.

INDICATIONS AND USAGE

Use of the medication has been discontinued because of the related dangers. Because of its harsh effects, the plant's resin is no longer administered internally despite its properties as a strong emetic and laxative.

Unproven Uses: External uses in folk medicine have included application to remove proliferating flesh, warts and malignant ulcers, as well as for chronic inflammatory conditions. It was also used as a plaster for gout. Internal uses included the treatment of dropsy, chronic headaches, and ear or eye complaints.

Homeopathic Uses: The drug is used homeopathically for acute inflammation of the respiratory tract and skin.

Indian Medicine: Uses include constipation and menstrual complaints and also as an abortifacient. Because of the danger of rapid intoxication, the drug's use is not advised. Efficacy for these indications has not been proven.

PRECAUTIONS AND ADVERSE REACTIONS

The drug is severely irritating to mucous membranes and skin. Ingestion leads to salivation, burning pains in the stomach, colic, diarrhea and nephritis. One case of death has been reported. Chronic application of the drug promotes tumor formation, so its administration in human medicine is no longer advised.

DOSAGE

Mode of Administration: Administration of preparations of Spurge are no longer recommended.

How Supplied: Skin stimulating ointment: 5% drug content

Homeopathic Dosage: 5 drops, 1 tablet, 10 globules every 30 to 60 minutes (acute from D4) and 1 to 3 times daily (chronic); parenterally: 1 to 2 ml sc; IV; IM acute: 3 times daily; chronic once a day (HAB1); children are given special doses.

Storage: Due to the plant's poisonous nature, store securely.

LITERATURE

Blaschek W, Hänsel R, Keller K, Reichling J, Rimpler G, Schneider G (Eds), Hagers Handbuch der Pharmazeutischen Praxis. Folgebände 1 und 2. Drogen A-Z. Springer. Berlin, Heidelberg 1998.

Hergenhahn M, Kusumoto S, Hecker E, New constituents of Euphorbia resinifera Berg. Acta Chem Scand, 108:3609, 1984.

Hergenhahn M, Kusumoto S, Hecker E, On the active principles of the spurge family (Euphorbiaceae). V. Extremely skin-irritant and moderately tumor-promoting diterpene esters from Euphorbia resinifera Berg. J Cancer Res Clin Oncol, 108:98-109, 1984.

Squill

Urginea maritima

DESCRIPTION

Medicinal Parts: The medicinal parts come from the bulbs of the white latex variety collected after flowering and the fresh, fleshy bulb scales of the white variety and of the red variety.

Flower and Fruit: The flowering stem is erect and 50 to 150 cm high. It is often a washed purple color and glabrous. The flowers, which often number 100, are arranged in richly flowered, dense racemes up to 60 cm long. The bracts are membranous and pointed. They are shorter than the pedicles and drop early. The pedicles are up to 3 cm long, thin and smooth. The flowers are white, radial and star-shaped. The ovary is ovate to oblong triangular. The capsule is ovate to oblong, 3-valved, obtuse or almost pointed. Each chamber has 1 to 4 seeds, which are elongate, flattened, smooth, glossy and winged.

Leaves, Stem and Root: The plant is a perennial bulb plant. The bulbs are pear-shaped, about 15 to 30 cm in diameter. They are rarely sold whole commercially, as they tend to start growing. The fracture is short, tough and flexible.

Characteristics: The taste is bitter and acrid.

Habitat: Indigenous to the Mediterranean and is cultivated there too.

Production: Squill consists of the sliced, dried, fleshy middle scales of the onion of the white variety of Urginea maritima, harvested during the flowering season. It is collected mostly from uncultivated regions.

Other Names: Scilla

ACTIONS AND PHARMACOLOGY

COMPOUNDS

Cardioactive steroid glycosides (bufadienolides, 1-3%): chief components glucoscillarene A, proscillaridin A, scillarene A; including among others, scillicyanoside, scilliglaucoside

Mucilage

EFFECTS

The drug is inotropic on myocardial work capacity and negatively chronotropic. The overall effect is economy of heart action. There is a lowering of increased, left ventricular diastolic pressure and pathologically elevated venous pressure.

INDICATIONS AND USAGE

Approved by Commission E:

- Cardiac insufficiency NYHA I and II
- Arrhythmia
- Nervous heart complaints
- Venous conditions

Unproven Uses: Squill is used for reduced kidney capacity. In folk medicine it is used for catarrhal conditions of the upper respiratory tract, bronchitis, asthma and whooping cough, also for wounds and fractures, back pain and hemorrhoids and for the disinfection of septic wounds.

CONTRAINDICATIONS

The drug and pure glycosides, among others, should not be administered in the presence of second or third degree atrioventricular block, hypercalcemia, hypokalemia, hypertrophic cardiomyopathy, carotid sinus syndrome, ventricular tachycardia, thoracic aortic aneurysm or WPW-syndrome.

PRECAUTIONS AND ADVERSE REACTIONS

General: No health hazards are known in conjunction with the proper administration of designated therapeutic dosages. Because of the narrow therapeutic range of cardioactive steroid glycosides, side effects could appear even with therapeutic dosages. Side effects include tonus elevation of the gastrointestinal area, loss of appetite, vomiting, diarrhea, headache and irregular pulse.

Contact with the juice of the fresh bulb can lead to skin inflammation (squill dermatitis). The administration of pure glycoside is preferable due to the difficulties of standardizing the drug (proscillaridin A).

Drug Interactions: Increase of effectiveness and thus also of side effects is possible with concomitant administration of quinidine, calcium, saluretics, laxatives and extended therapy with glucocorticoids.

Squill potentiates the positive inotropic and negative chronotropic effects of digoxin.

The simultaneous administration of arrhythmogenic substances (sympathomimetics, methylxanthines, phosphodiesterase inhibitors, and quinidine) increases the risk of cardiac arrhythmias.

OVERDOSAGE

Besides the already-mentioned symptoms, overdosage can lead to cardiac rhythm disorders, life-threatening ventricular tachycardia, atrial tachycardia with atrioventricular block, stupor, vision disorders, depression, confused states, hallucinations and psychosis. Fatal dosages lead to cardiac arrest or asphyxiation.

Treatment of poisoning includes gastric lavage and instillation of activated charcoal. All other measures are to be carried out according to the symptoms. In case of potassium loss, careful replenishment; for ectopic impulse formation in the ventricle, administration of phenytoin as antiarrhythmic drug; lidocaine for ventricular extrasystole; for pronounced bradycardia, atropine or orciprenaline. The prophylactic use of a pacemaker is recommended. Hemoperfusion for eliminating the glycosides or the administration of cholestyramine for interrupting the enterohepatic circulation are possible.

DOSAGE

Mode of Administration: Comminuted drug and other galenic preparations for internal use.

Preparation: Stabilized powder is standardized according to content, there are no more exact specifications in the literature, standardization according to DAB10.

Squill Extract — Evaporated extract 1:4; drug: diluted spirit of wine (EB6)

Acetum Scillae — drug: spirit of wine 1:1 (EB6)

Oxymel Scillae — 5 parts Acetum Scillae: 10 parts purified honey evaporated in a water bath to 10 parts

Daily Dosage: Single dose: 60 to 200 mg; Daily dose: 180 to 200 mg; Average daily dosage: 0.1 to 0.5 gm of standardized sea onion powder.

Squill Extract: 1.0 gm; Liquid extract: 0.03 to 2.0 ml; Tincture: 0.3 to 2.0 ml; Acetum Scillae: 1.0 gm; Acetic acid maceration: 0.6 to 2.0 ml

Oxymel Scillae: 2.5 gm

Storage: Squill should be protected from light and moisture at temperatures below 25°C.

LITERATURE

Brisse B, Anwendung pflanzlicher Wirkstoffe bei kardialen Erkrankungen. In: ZPT 10(4):107. 1989.

Eichstädt H, Hansen G, Danne O, Koch HP, Minge C, Richter W, Schröder R, Die positiv inotrope Wirkung eines Scilla-Extraktes nach Einmal-Applikation. In: ZPT 12(2):46. 1991.

Garcia-Casado P et al., (1977) Pharm Acta Helv 52:218.

Hakim FS, Evans FJ, (1976) Pharm Acta Helv 52:117.

Kamano Y, Satoh N, Nakayoshi H, Pettit GR, Smith CR, Rhinovirus inhibition by bufadienolides. In: Chem Pharm Bull 36:326-332. 1988.

Karawya MS et al., (1973) Planta Med 23:213.

Kopp B, Krenn L, Jurenitsch J, Bufadienolide in Meerzwiebeln. In: DAZ 130(40):2175. 1990.

Krenn L, Ferth R, Robien W, Kopp B, Bufadienolide aus Urginea-maritima-sensu-strictu. In: PM 57:560. 1991.

Krenn L, Kopp B, 9-Hydroxyscilliphaeosid, a new bufadienolide from Urginea maritima. In: JNP 59(6):612-613. 1996.

Loew D, Phytotherapie bei Herzinsuffizienz. In: ZPT 18(2):92-96. 1997.

Loew DA, Loew AD, Pharmakokinetik von herzglykosidhaltigen Pflanzenextrakten. In: ZPT 15(4):197-202. 1994.

Majinda RRT et al., Bufadienolides and other constituents of Urginea sanguinea. In: PM 63(2):188-190. 1997.

Mathic C, Ourrison G, (1964) Phytochemistry 3:115, 133, 377 et 379.

Sato, Muro T, Antiviral activity of scillarenin, a plant bufadienolide. In: Jap J Microbiol 18:441-448. 1974.

Vega FA, (1976) An Rev Acad Farm. 42(1):81.

Further information in:

Frohne D, Pfänder HJ, Giftpflanzen - Ein Handbuch für Apotheker, Toxikologen und Biologen, 4. Aufl., Wiss. Verlags-Ges. Stuttgart 1997.

Hänsel R, Keller K, Rimpler H, Schneider G (Hrsg.), Hagers Handbuch der Pharmazeutischen Praxis, 5. Aufl., Bde 4-6 (Drogen): Springer Verlag Berlin, Heidelberg, New York, 1992-1994.

Joubert JP, Schultz RA Detection of scilliroside in the preparation of maritime Scille. (Urginea maritima Baker) Ann Pharm Fr, 42:17-21, 1967 Jan.

Leung AY, Encyclopedia of Common Natural Ingredients Used in Food, Drugs, Cosmetics, John Wiley & Sons Inc., New York 1980.

Lewin L, Gifte und Vergiftungen, 6. Aufl., Nachdruck, Haug Verlag, Heidelberg 1992.

Madaus G, Lehrbuch der Biologischen Arzneimittel, Bde 1-3, Nachdruck, Georg Olms Verlag Hildesheim 1979.

Roth L, Daunderer M, Kormann K, Giftpflanzen, Pflanzengifte, 4. Aufl., Ecomed Fachverlag Landsberg Lech 1993.

Schulz R, Hänsel R, Rationale Phytotherapie, Springer Verlag Heidelberg 1996.

Spies T, Praznik W, Hofinger A, Altmann F, Nitsch E, Wutka R A new bufadienolide from Urginea pancration Planta Med, 235:284-5, Jun, 1992.

Spies T, Praznik W, Hofinger A, Altmann F, Nitsch E, Wutka R The structure of the fructan sinistrin from Urginea maritima. Carbohydr Res, 235:221-30, Nov 4, 1992.

Steinegger E, Hänsel R, Pharmakognosie, 5. Aufl., Springer Verlag Heidelberg 1992.

Teuscher E, Lindequist U, Biogene Gifte - Biologie, Chemie, Pharmakologie, 2. Aufl., Fischer Verlag Stuttgart 1994.

Teuscher E, Biogene Arzneimittel, 5. Aufl., Wiss. Verlagsges. Stuttgart 1997.

Tuncok Y, Kozan O, Cavdar C, Guven H, Fowler J Estimation of scilladienolides of Urginea maritima as well as in galenicals and formulations. Planta Med, 33:213-20, May, 1973.

Tuncok Y, Kozan O, Cavdar C, Guven H, Fowler J Preparation of the naturally occurring complex of the initial scilladienolides of Urginea maritima. Planta Med, 33:290-7, May, 1973.

Tuncok Y, Kozan O, Cavdar C, Guven H, Fowler J Separation of cardiotonic from flavonoid compounds of the squill, Urginea maritima Baker. Experientia, 33:447-8, Apr 15, 1969.

Tuncok Y, Kozan O, Cavdar C, Guven H, Fowler J Urginea maritima (squill) toxicity. J Toxicol Clin Toxicol, 33:83-6, 1995.

Wagner H, Wiesenauer M, Phytotherapie. Phytopharmaka und pflanzliche Homöopathika, Fischer-Verlag, Stuttgart, Jena, New York 1995.

Wälli F, Grob PJ, Müller-Schoop J Antineoplastic constituents of some Southern African plants. J Ethnopharmacol, 111:323-35, Dec, 1980.

Wälli F, Grob PJ, Müller-Schoop J Pseudo-(venocuran-)lupus - a minor episode in the history of medicine Schweiz Med Wochenschr, 111:1398-405, Sep 19, 1981.

Wälli F, Grob PJ, Müller-Schoop J Traditional medicine in health care. J Ethnopharmacol, 111:19-22, Mar, 1980.

St. John's Wort

Hypericum perforatum

TRADE NAMES

St. John's Wort (available from numerous manufacturers and as combination product), St. John's Wort Extract, Alterra, Advanced St. John's Wort, St. John's Wort Herb, St. John's Wort High Potency, St. John's Wort Preferred, St. John's Wort Standardized Extract, St. John's Power Time Release, Mood Support, KIRA, Centrum St. John's Wort, Hypericalm, St. John's Powder 0.3%, Tension Tamer, Hypercalm, St. John's Powder, St. John's Extra Strength

DESCRIPTION

Medicinal Parts: The medicinal parts include the fresh buds and flowers separated from the inflorescences, the aerial parts collected during the flowering season and dried, and the entire fresh flowering plant.

Flower and Fruit: The golden yellow flowers are in sparsely blossomed terminal cymes. The 5 sepals are ovate-lanceolate to lanceolate and very pointed. The sepals are also smooth, serrate at the tip, and marked by many light and dark glands. The 5 petals and numerous stamens are fused into 3 bundles. The ovary has a broad or narrow oval shape. The fruit is a 3-valvular capsule, which is triangular and oval. The seeds are cylindrical and shortly pointed at both ends. The seeds are 1 to 3 mm long, either black or dark brown, and covered in small warts.

Leaves, Stem and Root: The perennial plant is 30 to 60 cm and contains a long-living branched root and rhizome, which tapers toward each end. The reddish stem is erect, includes 2 raised edges and can reach 100 cm in height. The oval-shaped, translucent, punctate leaves are attached directly at the base and often covered in black glands.

Characteristics: The flowers release an odorless red juice when squeezed, which tastes weakly bitter and irritating.

Habitat: The plant is indigenous to all of Europe, western Asia and northern Africa. It has been introduced to eastern Asia, Australia and New Zealand, and it is cultivated in Poland and Siberia.

Production: St. John's Wort consists of the dried above-ground parts of Hypericum perforatum gathered during flowering season. The herb is cut at the start of the flowering season and dried quickly in bunches in order to preserve the oil and secreted contents.

Not to be Confused With: The plant may be mistaken for other Hypericum species, such as Hypericum barbatum, Hypericum hirsutum, Hypericum maculatum, Hypericum montanum and Hypericum tetrapterum.

Other Names: Hardhay, Amber, Goatweed, Klamath Weed, Tipton Weed, Saint John's Word, St. Johnswort

ACTIONS AND PHARMACOLOGY

COMPOUNDS

Anthracene derivatives (0.1-0.15%): favoring naphthodianthrones, especially hypericin, pseudohypericin

Flavonoids (2-4%): in particular hyperoside, quercitrin, rutin, isoquercitrin, and also biflavonolids including amentoflavone

Xanthones (0.15-0.72%): 1,3,6,7-tetrahydroxy-xanthone

Acylphloroglucinols: hyperforin with small quantities of adhhyperforin

Volatile oil: chief components aliphatic hydrocarbons, including, among others, 2- methyloctane, undecane, furthermore dodecanol, mono- and sesquiterpenes: including, among others, alpha-pinene, caryophyllene, additionally also 2-methyl-3-but-3-en-2-ol

Oligomers

Procyanidines and other catechin tannins (6.5-15%)

Caffeic acid derivatives: including chlorogenic acid

EFFECTS

The main active principles of the herb are the flavone and flavonol derivatives, xanthones and naphthodianthrone (hypericins). A mild antidepressant, sedative and anxiolytic action of the herb and its preparations has been documented in clinical studies. Historically, hypericin was thought to have a weak MAO inhibitor effect. However, recent literature suggests hypericin is devoid of MAO inhibitory activity (Bladt, 1994).

More recent studies have indicated that the antidepressive effect may be largely due to the ability of the herb to inhibit the reuptake of serotonin and other neurotransmitters. The activity of the herb could be attributable to the combined contribution of several mechanisms, each one too weak by itself to account for the overall effect (Bennett, 1998). A study concluded that hydroalcoholic hypericum extract inhibits the reuptake of serotonin, norepinephrine and dopamine with similar affinities, which leads to a significant down-regulation of cortical beta- adrenoceptors and serotonin (5HT-2) receptors. This data suggested hyperforin is the active principle of hypericum extracts in biochemical models of antidepressant activity (Muller, 1998). The antidepressive action not only results from the effect on adrenergic transmitter systems (norepinephrine, dopamine, serotonin), but also from an endocrine effect (melatonin).

Oily Hypericum preparations demonstrate an anti-inflammatory action due to their high flavonoid content. Antiviral (retroviruses) properties of the herb have not been proven. No antiretroviral activity determined by virologic markers and CD4 cell count of hypericin was seen in a study of HIV-infected patients (Gulick, 1999).

The antibacterial effect of hyperforin was demonstrated in a recent study. Hyperforin inhibited the growth of gram positive bacteria, such as *Streptococcus pyogenes* and *Streptococcus agalactiae*. Hyperforin also demonstrated efficacy against penicillin-resistant *Staphylococcus aureus* (PRSA) and methicillin-resistant *Staphylococcus aureus* (MRSA). These data indicate the possible use of the herb for local treatment of infected wounds and eczematous skin lesions (Schempp, 1999).

CLINICAL TRIALS

A meta-analysis of 23 randomized trials consisting of 1757 outpatients with mild to moderately severe depressive disorders was conducted to determine the effectiveness of Hypericum perforatum. Although Hypericum was significantly superior to placebo with fewer adverse effects (19.9% with Hypericum compared to 52.8% with standard antidepressants), there was little standardization and a lack of information with regard to the diagnostic criteria, compliance control, and dosage regimen of Hypericum and standard antidepressants (Linde K, 1996).

The equivalence between St. John's Wort and fluoxetine was demonstrated in a randomized, double-blind, comparative trial involving 149 outpatients with mild or moderate depressive episodes (according to International Statistical Classification of Diseases and Related Health Problems). Patients were treated for 6 weeks. A daily dose of 800 mg St. John's Wort extract LoHyp-57 (dry extract of St. John's Wort, drug extract ratio 5-7:1, solvent, ethanol 60% [w/w]) was found to be equivilent in efficacy to 20 mg fluoxetine (Harrer, 1999).

The effectiveness and tolerance of Hypericum extract LI 160 with a dosage of 300 mg three times daily was compared to imipramine 25 mg three times daily in a double-blind, clinical study. The study involved 135 depressed patients (according to DSM-III-R criteria) treated over a 6-week period. The analysis demonstrated comparable results between the treatment groups, with fewer and milder side effects in the Hypericum group (Vorbach, 1994).

INDICATIONS AND USAGE

Approved by Commission E:

- Anxiety
- Depressive moods
- Inflammation of the skin
- Blunt injuries
- Wounds and burns

Internally, the drug is used for psychovegetative disturbances, depressive moods, anxiety and nervous unrest. Externally, the oily Hypericum preparations are used for treatment and post-therapy of acute and contused injuries and for first-degree burns.

Unproven uses: The herb has been used for worm infestation, bronchitis and asthma, gallbladder disease, gastritis (also diarrhea), nocturnal enuresis, gout and rheumatism. Oily Hypericum preparations are used internally for dyspeptic complaints, and externally for the treatment of myalgia.

Chinese Medicine: In a gargle solution, the herb is used externally for tonsillitis. The herb is also administered externally as a lotion for dermatoses.

Homeopathic Uses: The herb has been used for treatment of peripheral and central nervous system injuries, depressive moods, asthma and cerebral-vascular calcification.

CONTRAINDICATIONS

Simultaneous use of a MAO inhibitor: St. John's Wort contains some weak monoamine oxidase inhibitor (MAOI) properties that may add to the effects of other MAOI drugs, therefore theoretically increasing the risk for hypertensive crisis (Hoelzl & Ostrowski, 1986; Muller & Schaefer, 1996; Suzuki, 1984).

PRECAUTIONS AND ADVERSE REACTIONS

General: No health hazards are known in conjunction with the proper administration of designated therapeutic dosages. The tannin content of the drug can lead to digestive complaints, such as feeling of fullness or constipation. Patients with a previous history of photosensitization to various chemicals should be cautious of direct sun exposure (Wheatley, 1998).

Central Nervous System Effects: Restlessness (0.3%) and fatigue (0.4%) occurred in 3250 patients in one study of depressed patients (Woelk, 1994). In another study, fatigue/tiredness was reported in 5% of subjects, and restlessness in 6% (Vorbach, 1997). Symptoms are difficult to evaluate since the herb is being used to treat depression, which may have similar symptoms. Headache was noted in 7% of studies reviewed (Wheatley, 1998).

Fertility Effects: High concentrations of St. John's Wort *in vitro,* was mutagenic to sperm cells and adversely effected oocytes. The data suggests St. John's Wort given at high concentrations damages reproductive cells (Ondrizek, 1999).

Gastrointestinal Effects: Gastrointestinal effects were noted in 0.6% of patients in one study. Anorexia occurred in 0.55% (n=18), diarrhea occurred in 0.55% (n=18), nausea occurred in 0.55% (n=18), and gastrointestinal pain or stomachache occurred in 0.55% (n=18) of 3250 patients taking Hypericum extract 300 milligrams 3 times daily (Woelk, 1994). Three percent of patients in one study developed dry mouth and 5% had gastrointestinal complaints Vorbach, 1997). Constipation was reported in 5% of cases reviewed (Wheatley, 1998).

Dermatologic Effects: Photosensitization has been observed in animals following intakes of large quantities of the drug (starting at 3 g per kg body weight, which would be 150 g for a person weighing 50 kg). St. John's Wort photosensitization is dose-related, and has occurred with plasma concentrations of 50 mcg of hypericin per ml, according to Schulz' Rational Phytotherapy—six orders of magnitude above that of patients taking an extract of 300 mg of 0.6% hypericin three times a day. Hypericism is defined as a sensitivity to light seen in animals who have ingested certain Hypericum species. The Hypericum pigments are carried to the skin, and in the unpigmented, unhaired portions of the skin of sheep, cattle, horses, goats and swine may produce sunlight induced rash and blisters (Giese, 1980; Southwell & Campbell, 1991). However, such a reaction is unlikely with administration of therapeutic dosages in humans.

1. Hypericum extract, especially at higher doses or with long-term use, may cause photosensitivity with sunburn-like lesions and inflammation of the mucous membranes, at least in animals (Duran & Song, 1986). Photosensitization has been demonstrated in a controlled clinical trial using metered doses of hypericin and subsequent exposure to UVA/UVB radiation (Roots, 1996).

2. Significant phototoxicity did occur in HIV-infected persons administered intravenous hypericim, 0.25-0.5 mg/kg twice weekly, or 0.25 mg three times weekly, or oral hypericin 0.25 mg/kg daily (Gulick, 1999).

3. Pruritus and exanthema occurred in 17 of 3250 patients (0.52%) taking Hypericum extract 300 milligrams three times a day (Woelk, 1994). Pruritus was found in 2% of patients taking Hypericum for depression (Wheatley, 1998).

4. A case report involved one patient taking St. John's Wort who developed subacute polyneuropathy after sun exposure (Bove, 1998).

Drug Interactions:

MAOI—Although there is poor documentation, concomitant administration of St. John's Wort and a MAOI , such as tranylcypromine, phenelzine, may lead to increased effects and possible toxicity (hypertensive crisis)-See Contraindications (Hoelzl & Ostrowski, 1986; Mueller & Schaefer, 1996; Suzuki, 1984). It is prudent to avoid concomitant use with beta-sympathomimetic amines, e.g., ma huang or pseudoephedrine (Miller, 1998).

SSRI's—St. John's Wort taken concomitantly with an SSRI, such as fluoxetine, paroxetine, sertraline, fluvoxamine or citalopram, may lead to an increased effect and possible toxicity "serotonin syndrome", e.g., sweating, tremor, flushing, confusion and agitation. St. John's Wort has slight serotonin reuptake properties. A case report suggests that co-administration of St. John's Wort with paroxetine has resulted in a clinical syndrome resembling a sedative/hypnotic intoxication (Gordon, 1998).

Tannic acids present in St. John's Wort may inhibit the absorption of iron (Miller, 1998).

Concomitant use with other photosensitizers, such as tetracyclines, sulfonamides, thiazides, quinolones, piroxicam and others should be avoided (Miller, 1998).

Hypericum extract has been reported to significantly prolong narcotic-induced sleeping times and to antagonize the effects of reserpine (Okpanyi, 1987).

Cyclosporine — Decreased serum concentrations have occurred with use of St. John's Wort (Bon, 1999). Acute cellular transplant rejection in heart transplant patients due to an interaction between St. John's Wort and Cyclosporine has been reported. St. John's Wort has been proven to induce the cytochrome P450 enzyme system, the major pathway for cyclosporine metabolism. Heart transplant rejection has been reported as soon as 3 weeks after St. John's Wort is added to the drug regimen of heart transplant patients maintained on cyclosporine therapy (Ruschitzka, et al., 2000).

Indinavir — An open label study was conducted involving healthy volunteers that were administered 800 mg indinavir every 8 hours along with 300 mg St. John's Wort standardized to 0.3% hypericin 3 times daily. Results showed a 57% reduction in the area under the curve for the protease inhibitor and an 81% decrease of the extrapolated 8-hour indinavir trough value. The authors concluded that a reduction of this magnitude could lead to development of drug resistance and treatment failure (Piscitelli, et al., 2000). Clinicians are warned that St. John's Wort may significantly affect plasma concentrations of any drug that is metabolized by the cytochrome P450 system.

Ethinyloestradiol and desogestrel (combined oral contraceptive) — Breakthrough bleeding has occurred with concomitant use of St. John's Wort (Bon, 1999).

Hypericin causes a reduction in barbiturate-induced sleeping times (Ozturk, 1992).

Theophylline — The herb has decreased theophylline levels on a patient stabilized on theophylline therapy (Nebel, 1999).

Co-administration of St. John's Wort extract (LI160) with digoxin resulted in a significant decrease in digoxin C_{trough}, AUC (0-24), and C_{max} values compared to placebo. Therefore, St. John's Wort may reduce efficacy of digoxin and make a patient a nonresponder, whereas increased toxicity may be anticipated after withdrawal of the herb (Andreas, 1999).

St. John's Wort (600-900 mg/day) taken concomitantly with sertraline (50-75 mg/day) after 2 to 4 days, resulted in a presumed serotonin syndrome consisting of dizziness, nausea, vomiting, headache, epigastric pain, anxiety, confusion, and/or feelings of restlessness and irritability. Cyproheptadine was used to reverse the symptoms and after discontinuation of the herb-drug therapy, all symptoms resolved (Lantz, 1999).

Nefazadine (100 mg BID) and St. John's Wort (300 mg TID) taken simutaneously resulted in nausea, vomiting and restlessness after 3 days of therapy. The symptoms improved after stopping the nefazadine and continuing with St. John's Wort (Lantz, 1999).

DOSAGE

Mode of Administration: Comminuted drug, herb powder, liquid and solid preparations for internal use; liquid and semi-solid preparations for external use; preparations made with fatty oils for external and internal use.

How Supplied:

Capsules—(standardized at 0.3% hypericin) 125mg, 150mg, 250mg, 300mg, 350mg, 370mg, 375mg, 400mg, 424mg, 434mg, 450mg, 500mg, 510mg

Capsules, Extended Release—(standardized at 0.3% hypericin) 450mg, 900mg, 1000mg

Dried Herb

Extract—1:1

Injection—1%

Liquid—300 mg/5ml, 250 mg/ml

Liquid Dilutions—3x, 6x, 30x,12c, 30c

Pellets—3x, 6x, 12x, 12c, 30c

Tablets—(standardized at 0.3% hypericin) 100mg, 150mg, 300mg, 450mg

Tincture—1:10

Transdermal—900mg/24hr

Preparation: To prepare an infusion, use 2 teaspoonfuls of drug in 150 ml boiling water and steep for 10 minutes.

Daily Dosage: In general, a range of 200 to 1000 micrograms/day of hypericin is recommended for treatment of depression (Anon, 1996). Total hypericin concentrations of Hypericum extracts may vary widely, therefore caution should be taken in determining dosage (Fachinfo Helarium Hypericum, 1996; Fachinfo Remotiv, 1996; Hansgen, 1993; Schmidt & Sommer, 1993; Vorbach, 1994; Woelk, 1994).

For depressive moods, it is recommended the herb be administered for the duration of 4 to 6 weeks; if no improvement is apparent, a different therapy should be initiated.

Depression:

Capsules/tablets — 300 mg of the standardized extract should be administered three times daily (Clausson & Muller, 1997; Fachinfo Helarium Hypericum, 1996).

Dried herb — 2 to 4 grams taken 3 times daily (Fachinfo Helarium Hypericum, 1996; Fachinfo Remotiv, 1996; Hansgen, 1993; Schmidt & Sommer, 1993; Vorbach, 1994; Woelk, 1994).

Tea — St. John's Wort as a tea is the traditional method of administration, with a single dose of 2-3 grams dried herb placed in boiling water. If dried herb of 2 grams is used, and the dried herb to extract ratio is 6, a usual dose of the extract would be 300 milligrams (Schultz, 1997).

Liquid extract 1:1 in 25% ethanol — 2 to 4 milliliters taken 3 times daily (Fachinfo Helarium Hypericum, 1996; Fachinfo Remotiv, 1996; Haensgen, 1993; Schmidt & Sommer, 1993; Vorbach, 1994; Woelk, 1994).

Tincture: (1:10) in 45% ethanol — 2 to 4 milliliters, 3 times a day (Fachinfo Helarium Hypericum, 1996; Fachinfo Remotiv, 1996; Hansgen, 1993; Schmidt & Sommer, 1993; Vorbach, 1994; Woelk, 1994).

Wounds, bruising and swelling: The herb is applied topically and locally for treatment. The activity of the topical preparations is based on the hyperforin content, which is highly variable depending on the method of oil preparation. The preparation may be stable for a few weeks up to 6 months. (Maisenbacher & Kovar, 1992)

Homeopathic Dosage: The daily dosage for homeopathic indications is 5 drops, 1 tablet or 10 globules every 30 to 60 minutes for acute therapy, and 1 to 3 times daily for chronic use. Parenterally, 1 to 2 ml subcutaneously administered three times daily for acute therapy and once daily for chronic therapy. The ointment is applied 1 to 2 times daily for acute and chronic use (HAB1).

Storage: Store at room temperature, away from heat, moisture and direct light. Hyperici oleum has a limited shelf life. One study showed that a sample containing 62 milligrams of hyperforin (the active ingredient in the oil) contained no hypericin in 14 days. If sunlight is not used to prepare the oil, then the breakdown is slower, but still less than 30 days. Various oil preparation methods have been described, including one with eutanol G, which showed stability for 6 months. Researchers evaluated 6 commercial samples of oil of Hypericum containing 2.2 to 20.8 milligrams/deciliter. All hyperforin was gone by the end of five weeks (Maisenbacher, 1992).

LITERATURE

Andreas J, J. Brockmoller et al., Pharmacokientic interaction of digoxin with an herbal extract from St. John's wort. Clinical Pharmacology & Therapeutics. 1999;66:338-345.

Araya OS, Ford EJH, (1981) An investigation of the type of photosensitization caused by the ingestion of St. John's Wort (hypericum perforatum) by calves. J Comp Pathol 91:135-141.

Baldt S, Wagner H, (1994) Inhibition of MAO by Fractions and Constiuents of Hypericum Extract. J Geriatr Psychiatry Neurol 7(Suppl 1):57-59.

Bennett DA, Phun L, Polk JF, Neuropharmacology of St. John's Wort (Hypericum). Ann Pharmacother 1998 Nov;32(11):1201-8.

Bon D, Hartmann K, Kuhn M. Schweitzer Apothekerzeitung 1999; 16:535-36.

Borsini F, Meli A, (1988) Is the forced swimming test a suitable model for revealing antidepressant activity? Psychopharmacology 94:147-160.

Bove GM, Acute neuropathy after exposure to sun in a patient treated with St. John's Wort, The Lancet 1998;352:1121-1122.

Butterweck V et al., Isolation by MLCCC and NMR spectroscopy of hypericin, pseudohypericin and I3,II8-biapigenin from Hypericum perforatum. In: PM 62, Abstracts of the 44th Ann Congress of GA, 119. 1996.

Butterweck V, Winterhoff H, Schulz V, Nahrstedt A, Pharmacological in vivo testing of fractions obtained from Hypericum perforatum L. In: PM 62, Abstracts of the 44th Ann Congress of GA, 65. 1996.

Carpenter S, Kraus GA, Photosensitization required for inactivation of equine infectious anaemia virus by hypericin. In: Photochem Photobiol 53:169-174. 1991.

Czygan FC, (1993) Kulturgeschichte und Mystik des Johanniskrautes. Z Phytother 14:276-281.

Danie K, (1939) Inhaltsstoffe und Prüfmethoden homöopathisch verwendeter Arzneipflanzen. Hippokrates 10:5-6.

Decoaterd LA, Hoffmann E, Kyburz D, Bray D, Hostettmann K, A new phloroglucinol derivative from Hypericum-calycinum with antifungal and in vitro antimalarial activity. In: PM 57:548. 1991.

Dingermann T, Phytopharmaka im Alter: Crataegus, Ginkgo, Hypericum und Kava-Kava. In: PZ 140(23):2017-2024. 1995.

Engelhardt A, (1962) Justinus Kerner und das Johanniskraut. Apotheker-Dienst Roche 3:51-55.

Ernst E, (1959) St. John's Wort, an anti-depressant? A systematic, criteria-based overview. Phytomedicine 2:67-71.

Fachinformation: Helarium (R) Hypericum, hypericum extract. Bionorica GmbH, Neumarkt, 1996.

Fachinformation: Remotiv (R), hypericum extract. Bayer AG, Pharma Deutschland, Leverkusen, 1996.

Freytag WE, (1984) Dtsch Apoth Ztg 124(46):2383.

Giese AC, (1980) Hypericism. Photochem Photobiol Rev 5:229-255.

Gulick RM, McAuliffe V, Holden-Wiltse J et al., Phase I studies of hypericum, the active compound in St. John's Wort, as an antiretroviral agent in HIV-infected adults. AIDS clinical trials group protocols 150 and 258. Ann Intern Med 1999 Mar 16;130(6):510-4.

Hänsel R, Keller K, Rimpler H, Schneider G, (Hrsg.), (1993) Hagers Handbuch der Pharmazeutischen Praxis, 5. Auflage, Drogen E-O. Springer Verlag, Berlin Heidelberg New York, S 268-292.

Hansgen KD, Vesper J, Plock M, Multicenter double-blind study examining the antidepressant effectiveness of the hypericum extract LI 160. J Geriatr Psychiatry Neurol 1994 Oct;7 Suppl 1:S15-8.

Hänsgen KD, Vesper J, (1996) Antidepressive Wirksamkeit eines hochdosierten Hypericum-Extraktes. Münch Med Wschr 138:29-33.

Harrer G, Payk TR, Schulz V, (Hrsg) Hypericum als pflanzliches Antidepressivum. Nervenheilkunde 12:268-366.

Harrer G, Schulz V, (1993) Zur Prüfung der antidepressiven Wirksamkeit von Hypericum. Nervenheilkunde 12:271-273.

Harrer G, Sommer H, Treatment of mild/moderate depressions with Hypericum. Phytomedicine 1:3-8. 1994.

Harrer G, Schmidt U, Kuhn U, Biller A., Comparison of equivalence between the St. John's Wort extract LoHyp-57 and fluoxetine. Arzneimittelforschung 1999 Apr;(4):289-96.

Hiller KO, Rahlfs V, Therapeutische Äquivalenz eines hochdosierten Phytopharmakons mit Amytriptylin bei ängstlich-depressiven Versimmungen - Reanalyse einer randomisierten Studie unter besonderer Beachtung biometrischer und klinischer Aspekte. In: Forsch.

Hölzl J, Inhaltsstoffe und Wirkungsmechanismen des Johanniskrautes. In: ZPT 14(5):255. 1993.

Hölzl J, Ostrowski E, (1986) Planta Med 6:62P.

Hölzl J, Sattler S, Schütt H, Johanniskraut: eine Alternative zu synthetischen Antidepressiva. In: PZ 139(46):3959. 1994.

Jenike MA (Ed), (1994) Hypericum: A Novel Antidepressant. J Geriatr Psychiatry Neurol 7: S1-S68.

Kil KS, Yum YN, Seo SH, Antitumor activities of hypericin as a protein tyrosine kinase blocker. In: Arch Pharmacal Res 19(6):490-496. 1996.

Kitanov G et al., (1984) Khim Prir Soedin 2:269.

Koren H, Schenk GM, Jindra RH, Alth G, Ebermann R, Kubin A, Koderhold G, Kreitner M, Hypericin in phototherapy. In: J Photochem Photobiol B - Biology 36(2): 113-119. 1996.

Lantz MS, Buchalter E, Giambanco V, St. John's Wort and antidepressant drug interactions in the elderly. J Geriatr Psychiatry Neurol 1999 Spring;2(1):7-10.

Laux G, (1995) Kontrollierte Vergleichsstudien mit Moclobemid in der Depressionsbehandlung. Münch Med Wschr 137:296-300.

Leuschner J, (1995) Gutachten zur experimentellen Toxikologie von Hypericum-Extrakt LI 160. Lichtwer Pharma GmbH, Berlin.

Linde K et al., St John's Wort for depression - An overview and meta-analysis of randomized clinical trials. BMJ 1996 Aug 3;313(7052):253-8.

Lopez-Bazzocchi I, Hudson JB, Towers GHN, Antiviral activity of the photoactive plant pigment hypericin. In: Photochem Photobiol 54:95-98. 1991.

Maisenbacher P, Johanniskrautöl. In: DAZ 132(6):281. 1992.

Maisenbacher P, Kovar KA, Analysis and stability of Hyperici oleum. Planta Med 1992 Aug;58(4):351-4.

Mathic C, Ourrison G, (1964) Phytochemistry 3: 115, 133, 377, 379.

Maurer A, Johne A, Bauer S et al. Interaction of St. John's wort extract with phenprocoumon. Eur J Clin Pharmacol 1999;55: A22.

Miller LG, Selected clinical considerations focusing on known or potential drug-herb interactions. Arch Intern Med vol 158, Nov 9, 1998: 2200-2211.

Muller WE, Singer A, Wonnemann M et al., Hyperforin represents the neurotransmitter reuptake inhibiting constituent of Hypericum extract. Pharmacopsychiatry 1998 Jun;31 Suppl 1:16-21.

Müller WE, Schäfer C, Johanniskraut In-vitro-Studie über Hypericum-Extrakt, Hypericin und Kämpferol. In: DAZ 136(13):1015-1022. 1996.

Müller WEG, Rossol R, (1994) Effects of Hypericum Extract on the Expression of Serotonin Receptors. J Geriatr Psychiatry Neurol 7(Suppl 1):63-64.

Muldner H, Zoller M, (1984) Arzneim Forsch. 34II(8):918.

Nebel A, Schneider BJ, Baker R et al: Potential metabolic interaction between St. John's Wort and theophylline. Ann Pharmacother 1999; 33(4):502.

Niesel S, (1992) Untersuchungen zum Freisetzungsverhalten und zur Stabilität ausgewählter wertbestimmender Pflanzeninhaltsstoffe unter besonderer Berücksichtigung moderner phytochemischer Analysenverfahren. Inaugural-Dissertation. Freie Universität Berlin.

Okpanvi SN, Weischer ML, (1987) Arzneim-Forsch, 37:10-13.

Ozturk Y et al., (1992) op cit.

Piscitelli, S et al., Indinavir concentrations and St. John's Wort. In: Lancet 2000; 355: 547-548.

Popovic M et al., Biochemical and pharmacodynamic study of Hypericum perforatum. In: PM 62, Abstracts of the 44th Ann Congress of GA, 67. 1996.

Rammert K, Phytopharmaka: Johanniskraut als Antidepressivum. In: DAZ 136(46):4131-4132. 1996.

Reuter HD, Hypericum als pflanzliches Antidepressivum. In: ZPT 14(5):239. 1993.

Roth L, Hypericum - Hypericin: Botanik, Inhaltsstoffe, Wirkung. In: ZPT 13(5):174. 1992.

Roth L, Hypericum. In: Roth L: Hypericum Hypericin, Botanik, Inhaltsstoffe, Wirkung. 1990.

Ruschitzka, F, et al., Acute heart transplant rejection due to Saint John's Wort. In: Lancet 2000; 355: 548-549.

Saller R, Hellenbrecht D, Johanniskraut (Hypericum perforatum). In: Tägl Praxis 33(3):689. 1992.

Schempp CM, Pelz K, Wittmer A, et al., Antibacterial activity of hyperforin from St John's Wort, against multiresistant Staphylococcus aureus and gram-positive bacteria. Lancet 1999 Jun 19;353(9170):2129.

Schmidt U, Sommer H, St. John's Wort extract in the ambulatory therapy of depression. Attention and reaction ability are preserved. Fortschr Med 1993 Jul 10;111(19):339-42.

Southwell IA, Campbell MH, Hypericin content variation in Hypericum perforatum in Australia. In: Phytochemistry 30:475-478. 1991.

Sparenberg B, Demisch L, Hölzl J, Untersuchungen über antidepressive Wirkstoffe von Johanniskraut. In: PZW 138(2)50. 1993.

Suzuki O et al., (1984) Planta Med 3:272.

Thiele, B, Brink I, Ploch M, (1993) Modulation der Zytkokin-Expression durch Hypericum-Extrakt. Mervemjeoölimde 12:353-356.

Volz HP, Hänsel R, (1995) Hypericum (Johanniskraut) als pflanzliches Antidepressivum. Psychopharmakotherapie 2:1-9.

Vorbach EU, Arnold KH, Hubner WD, Efficacy and tolerability of St. John's Wort extract Hypericum extract LI 160 in patients with severe depressive incidents according to ICD-10. Pharmacopsychiatry 1997; 30 (suppl 1): S81-S85.

Vorbach EU, Hubner WD, Arnoldt KH, Effectiveness and tolerance of the Hypericum extract LI 160 in comparison with imipramine: randomized double-blind study with 135 outpatients. J Geriatr Psychiatry Neurol 1994 Oct;7 Suppl 1: S19-23.

Wagner H, Bladt S, (1993) Pharmazeutische Qualität der Hypericum-Extrakte. Nervenheilkunde 12:362-366.

Wheatley D, Hypericum extract. Potential in the treatment of depression. CNS Drugs 1998; 9:431-440.

Wheatley D, LI 160, and extract of St. John's Wort, versus amitriptyline in mildly to moderately depressed outpatients - a controlled 6-week clinical trial. Pharmacopsychiatry 1997; 30(suppl II): S77-S80.

Willner P, (1984) The validity of animal models of depression. Psychopharmacology 83:1-16.

Winterhoff H, Butterweck V, Nahrstedt A, Gumbinger HG, Schulz V, Erping S, Boßhammer F, Wieligmann A, (1995) Pharmakologische Untersuchungen zur antidepressiven Wirkung von Hypericum perforatum L. In: Loew D, Rietbrock N (Hrsg.) Phytopharmaka in Forschung und klinischer Anwendung. Steinkopff Verlag, Darmstadt, S 39-56.

Winterhoff H, Hambrügge M, Vahlensieck W, (1993) Testung von Hypericum perforatum L. im Tierexperiment. Nervenheilkunde 12:341-345.

Woelk H, Burkard G, Grunwald J, Benefits and risks of the hypericum extract LI 160: drug monitoring study with 3250 patients. J Geriatric Psychiatry Neurol 1994; 7(suppl 1):3438.

Further information in:

Frohne D, Pfänder HJ, Giftpflanzen - Ein Handbuch für Apotheker, Toxikologen und Biologen, 4. Aufl., Wiss. Verlags-Ges. Stuttgart 1997.

Hänsel R, Keller K, Rimpler H, Schneider G (Hrsg.), Hagers Handbuch der Pharmazeutischen Praxis, 5. Aufl., Bde 4-6 (Drogen), Springer Verlag Berlin, Heidelberg, New York, 1992-1994.

Lewin L, Gifte und Vergiftungen, 6. Aufl., Nachdruck, Haug Verlag, Heidelberg 1992.

Madaus G, Lehrbuch der Biologischen Arzneimittel, Bde 1-3, Nachdruck, Georg Olms Verlag Hildesheim 1979.

Roth L, Daunderer M, Kormann K, Giftpflanzen, Pflanzengifte, 4. Aufl., Ecomed Fachverlag Landsberg Lech 1993.

Schulz R, Hänsel R, Rationale Phytotherapie, Springer Verlag Heidelberg 1996.

Steinegger E, Hänsel R, Pharmakognosie, 5. Aufl., Springer Verlag Heidelberg 1992.

Teuscher E, Lindequist U, Biogene Gifte - Biologie, Chemie, Pharmakologie, 2. Aufl., Fischer Verlag Stuttgart 1994.

Teuscher E, Biogene Arzneimittel, 5. Aufl., Wiss. Verlagsges. Stuttgart 1997.

Wagner H, Wiesenauer M, Phytotherapie. Phytopharmaka und pflanzliche Homöopathika, Fischer-Verlag, Stuttgart, Jena, New York 1995.

Wichtl M (Hrsg.), Teedrogen, 4. Aufl., Wiss. Verlagsges. Stuttgart 1997.

Stachys palustris

See Woundwort

Star Anise

Illicium verum

DESCRIPTION

Medicinal Parts: The medicinal parts are the oil extracted from the ripe fruit, the whole dried fruit and the seeds.

Flower and Fruit: The flowers are yellowish or reddish-white. The follicles have a diameter of about 2 cm. They are star-like and formed from eight cybiform carpels. The follicles open when ripe, each containing one smooth, polished, brown seed. The pericarp of the seed is brown and wrinkled below.

Leaves, Stem and Root: The plant is an evergreen tree up to 10 m tall with white, birch-like bark. The leaves are 7.5 cm long, entire-margined, glossy, elliptic-lanceolate and acuminate.

Habitat: The plant is only known in its cultivated form. It is cultivated in China and Vietnam.

Production: Star anise consists of the ripe syncarp of Illicium verum, as well as its preparations in effective dosage. The fruit is harvested shortly before it is fully ripe (August to October).

Not to be Confused With: Should not be confused with the smaller Japanese star anise (I. lanceolatum or I. religiosum), which is poisonous.

Other Names: Aniseed Stars, Badiana

ACTIONS AND PHARMACOLOGY

COMPOUNDS

Volatile oil: chief constituent trans-anethol, chavicol methyl ether (estragole), d-limonene, l-limonene, d-fenchone, d-pinene, dl-limonene, anisaldehyde

Fatty oil

Flavonoids: including rutin, kaempferol-3-O-rutinoside

Tannins

EFFECTS

Star Anise is a bronchial expectorant and antispasmodic for the gastrointestinal tract. The essential oils (star anise oil) and flavonoids act on the smooth muscle of the gastrointestinal tract and the mucous membrane of the respiratory tract.

INDICATIONS AND USAGE

Approved by Commission E:

- Loss of appetite
- Cough/bronchitis

Unproven Uses: Star Anise is used for catarrh of the respiratory tract and peptic discomfort.

Indian Medicine: Star Anise is used for dyspeptic complaints, flatulence, spasmodic colon pain, dysentery, facial paralysis, hemiparesis and rheumatoid arthritis.

PRECAUTIONS AND ADVERSE REACTIONS

No health hazards or side effects are known in conjunction with the proper administration of designated therapeutic dosages. Sensitization has occurred very rarely in cases of repeated administration. Berries of Illicium anisatum are similar, but contain spasmogenic sesquiterpene lactones; confusions with Star Anise have been observed.

DOSAGE

Mode of Administration: Herb, ground fresh just prior to use, and other galenic preparations for internal use.

Daily Dosage: 3 gm of drug or 0.3 gm of essential oil. Single dose: 0.5 to 1 gm prepared as tea.

Storage: Keep Star Anise protected from light.

LITERATURE

Frohne D, Pfänder HJ, Giftpflanzen - Ein Handbuch für Apotheker, Toxikologen und Biologen, 4. Aufl., Wiss. Verlags-Ges Stuttgart 1997.

Hänsel R, Keller K, Rimpler H, Schneider G (Hrsg.), Hagers Handbuch der Pharmazeutischen Praxis, 5. Aufl., Bde 4-6 (Drogen), Springer Verlag Berlin, Heidelberg, New York, 1992-1994.

Kubeczka KH, DAZ 122:2309. 1982.

Leung AY, Encyclopedia of Common Natural Ingredients Used in Food Drugs and Cosmetics, John Wiley & Sons Inc., New York 1980.

Schulz R, Hänsel R, Rationale Phytotherapie, Springer Verlag Heidelberg 1996.

Steinegger E, Hänsel R, Pharmakognosie, 5. Aufl., Springer Verlag Heidelberg 1992.

Teuscher E, Lindequist U, Biogene Gifte - Biologie, Chemie, Pharmakologie, 2. Aufl., Fischer Verlag Stuttgart 1994.

Teuscher E, Biogene Arzneimittel, 5. Aufl., Wiss. Verlagsges. Stuttgart 1997.

Wichtl M (Hrsg.), Teedrogen, 4. Aufl., Wiss. Verlagsges. Stuttgart 1997.

Zänglein A, Schultze W, Illicium verum - Sternanis. In: ZPT 10(6):191. 1989.

Stavesacre

Delphinium staphisagria

DESCRIPTION

Medicinal Parts: The medicinal parts are the ripe, dried seeds.

Flower and Fruit: The flowers are deep blue. The sections of the involucres are 13 to 20 mm long. The limb of the lateral honey-leaves gradually narrows to a claw. The follicles are 8 to 11 mm wide and swollen. The seeds are grayish-black, wrinkled and pitted. They are triangular or square and convex at the back. The seeds are about 2 cm long.

Leaves, Stem and Root: The plant is annual and has a 30 to 100 cm high stem that is stout and sparsely pubescent. The leaves are are palmatiform digitate with 5 to 7 lobes, pubescent on both surfaces with a mixture of very short and longer hairs. The segments are entire-margined or are made up of ovate-lanceolate or oblong, sharp-edged lobes.

Characteristics: The seeds are poisonous. They taste bitter and tingling, and are odorless.

Habitat: The plant is found in Asia Minor and Europe, and is cultivated in Italy and France.

Production: Stavesacre seeds are the seeds of *Delphinium staphisagria.*

Other Names: Lousewort

ACTIONS AND PHARMACOLOGY

COMPOUNDS

Diterpene alkaloids: main alkaloid delphinine, including among others the bi-diterpene alkaloids staphisine, staphisagroine

EFFECTS

Stavesacre is arrythmogenic and has an effect similar to aconitine.

INDICATIONS AND USAGE

Unproven Uses: The herb is used in washes and ointments to kill lice.

Homeopathic Uses: Stavesacre is used for the treatment of anxiety, urinary tract diseases, acute or acutely recurring hordeolum or chalazion, seborrheal skin with a tendency to inflammation, odorous perspiration, nervous exhaustion, neurasthenia with poor memory and hypochondria, sexual neurasthenia, gonorrhea, melancholia, hysteria, leukorrhea, headaches, general debility and delicate health, weak bladder, scrofulous and swollen glands, hair loss, rheumatism, nervous diarrhea, habitual obstipation, gastric ulcer, gastritis, trigeminal neuralgia and conditions of the eyelids.

PRECAUTIONS AND ADVERSE REACTIONS

External administration of extracts of the drug leads to reddening, inflammation and eczema. Internal administration could lead to inflammation of the throat, salivation, nausea, ructus, skin itching, and urinary and stool urgency.

OVERDOSAGE

The intake of 2 teaspoonfuls of seeds leads to weakened pulse, stomach pain, labored breathing and collapse.

Treatment of poisoning consists of stomach and intestinal emptying (gastric lavage, sodium sulphate), and the administration of activated charcoal. Further treatment should proceed symptomatically (i.e. diazepam for spasms, sodium bicarbonate for acidoses, intubation and oxygen respiration may also be required).

DOSAGE

Mode of Administration: An extract from the seeds is used in homeopathic dilutions.

Storage: The drug should be stored cautiously, as it is poisonous.

LITERATURE

Kern W, List PH, Hörhammer L (Hrsg.), Hagers Handbuch der Pharmazeutischen Praxis, 4. Aufl., Bde. 1-8, Springer Verlag Berlin, Heidelberg, New York, 1969.

Lewin L, Gifte und Vergiftungen, 6. Aufl., Nachdruck, Haug Verlag, Heidelberg 1992.

Madaus G, Lehrbuch der Biologischen Arzneimittel, Bde 1-3, Nachdruck, Georg Olms Verlag Hildesheim 1979.

Micovic IV, J Serb Chem Soc 51:355. 1986.

Roth L, Daunderer M, Kormann K, Giftpflanzen, Pflanzengifte, 4. Aufl., Ecomed Fachverlag Landsberg Lech 1993.

Teuscher E, Lindequist U, Biogene Gifte - Biologie, Chemie, Pharmakologie, 2. Aufl., Fischer Verlag Stuttgart 1994.

Wagner H, Wiesenauer M, Phytotherapie. Phytopharmaka und pflanzliche Homöopathika, Fischer-Verlag, Stuttgart, Jena, New York 1995.

Stellaria media

See Chickweed

Stevia

Stevia rebaudiana

DESCRIPTION

Medicinal Parts: The medicinal part of the plant is the dried leaves.

Flower and Fruit: The composite flowers are surrounded by an involucre. The capitula are in loose, irregular, sympodial cymes. There are 5 overlapping epicalyx sepals, with 5 tubular florets per composite flower. The flowers have light purple rhacis, white tips and 5 stamens. The fruit is a 5-ribbed, spindle-shaped achene with 15 to 17 awns.

Leaves, Stem and Root: Stevia rebaudiana is a semi-shrub that grows up to 30 cm high. The leaves are sessile, 3 to 4 cm long with an elongate-lanceolate or spatulate, blunt-tipped lamina. The leaves are serrate from the middle to the tip and entire below. The upper surface of the leaf is slightly glandular pubescent. The stem is weakly downy-pubescent at the bottom and woody. The tough rhizome has slightly branching roots.

Characteristics: All plant parts taste intensively sweet.

Habitat: The plant is indigenous to Paraguay.

Production: Stevia leaves are the dried leaves of Stevia rebaudiana.

Other Names: Sweet Herb, Sweetleaf

ACTIONS AND PHARMACOLOGY

COMPOUNDS

Diterpenes: diterpene glycosides, particularly stevioside (5 to 10%), rebaudoside A (2 to 4%), including as well rebaudoside C and dulcoside A

Volatile oil (0.1%): chief components nerolidol and caryophyllene oxide

Flavonoids: including apigenin-4′-O-glucoside, luteolin-7-O-glucoside

EFFECTS

The use of the drug as a sweetener is based upon the glycosidal diterpenes present (stevioside's sweetening power is 300 times that of saccharose). In animal experiments, stevioside significantly elevated the glucose clearance while at the same time increasing both salt excretion and urine flow (measured in percentage of glomerular filtration rate), which led to a significant lowering of blood pressure.

INDICATIONS AND USAGE

Unproven Uses: Folk medicine uses include hypertension, diabetes and as a contraceptive.

PRECAUTIONS AND ADVERSE REACTIONS

No health hazards are known in conjunction with the proper use of the drug as a sweetener.

DOSAGE

Mode of Administration: Stevia is available as cut drug for oral administration.

LITERATURE

Constantin J, Ishii-Iwamoto EL, Ferraresi-Filho O, Kelmer-Bracht AM, Bracht A, Sensitivity of ketogenesis and citric acid cycle to stevioside inhibition of palmitate transport across the cell membrane. Braz J Med Biol Res, 11:767-71, 1991.

Das S, Das AK, Murphy RA, Punwani IC, Nasution MP, Kinghorn AD, Evaluation of the cariogenic potential of the intense natural sweeteners stevioside and rebaudioside A. Caries Res, 26:363-6, 1992.

Hänsel R, Keller K, Rimpler H, Schneider G (Ed), Hagers Handbuch der Pharmazeutischen Praxis, 5. Aufl., Bde 4 - 6 (Drogen), Springer Verlag Berlin, Heidelberg, New York, 1992-1994.

Ishii EL, Bracht A, Stevioside, the sweet glycoside of Stevia rebaudiana, inhibits the action of atractyloside in the isolated perfused rat liver. Res Commun Chem Pathol Pharmacol, 34:79-91, 1986 Jul.

Ishii-Iwamoto EL, Bracht A, Stevioside is not metabolized in the isolated perfused rat liver. Res Commun Mol Pathol Pharmacol, 82:167-75, 1995 Feb.

Ishikawa H, Kitahata S, Ohtani K, Tanaka O, Transfructosylation of rebaudioside A (a sweet glycoside of Stevia leaves) with Microbacterium beta-fructofuranosidase. Chem Pharm Bull (Tokyo), 6:2043-5, 1991 Aug.

Jakinovich W Jr, Moon C, Choi YH, Kinghorn AD, Evaluation of plant extracts for sweetness using the Mongolian gerbil. J Nat Prod, 82:190-5, 1990 Jan-Feb.

Kawano T, Simoes LC, Effect of Stevia rebaudiana in Biomphalaria glabrata. Rev Bras Biol, 34:555-62, 1986 Aug.

Kelmer Bracht A, Alvarez M, Bracht A, Effect of Stevia rebaudiana on glucose tolerance in normal adult humans. Braz J Med Biol Res, 34:771-4, 1986.

Kelmer Bracht A, Alvarez M, Bracht A, Effects of Stevia rebaudiana natural products on rat liver mitochondria. Biochem Pharmacol, 34:873-82, 1985 Mar 15.

Kelmer Bracht A, Alvarez M, Bracht A, Sterols in Stevia rebaudiana Bertoni. Boll Soc Ital Biol Sper, 34:2237-40, 1984 Dec 30.

Kim KK, Sawa Y, Shibata H, Hydroxylation of ent-kaurenoic acid to steviol in Stevia rebaudiana Bertoni - purification and partial characterization of the enzyme. Arch Biochem Biophys, 34:223-30, 1996 Aug 15.

Klongpanichpak S, Temcharoen P, Toskulkao C, Apibal S, Glinsukon T, Lack of mutagenicity of stevioside and steviol in Salmonella typhimurium TA 98 and TA 100. J Med Assoc Thai, 82:S121-8, 1997 Sep.

Matsui M, Matsui K, Kawasaki Y, Oda Y, Noguchi T, Kitagawa Y, Sawada M, Hayashi M, Nohmi T, Yoshihira K, Ishidate M Jr, Sofuni T, Evaluation of the genotoxicity of stevioside and steviol using six in vitro and one in vivo mutagenicity assays. Mutagenesis, 11:573-9, 1996 Nov.

Melis MS, A crude extract of Stevia rebaudiana increases the renal plasma flow of normal and hypertensive rats. Braz J Med Biol Res, 29:669-75, 1996 May.

Melis MS, Chronic administration of aqueous extract of Stevia rebaudiana in rats: renal effects. J Ethnopharmacol, 47:129-34, 1995 Jul 28.

Melis MS, Renal excretion of stevioside in rats. J Nat Prod, 26:688-90, 1992 May.

Melis MS, Stevioside effect on renal function of normal and hypertensive rats. J Ethnopharmacol, 26:213-7, 1992 Jun.

Melis MS, Sainati AR, Effect of calcium and verapamil on renal function of rats during treatment with stevioside. J Ethnopharmacol, 11:257-62, 1991 Jul.

Oliveira-Filho RM, Uehara OA, Minetti CA, Valle LB, Chronic administration of aqueous extract of Stevia rebaudiana (Bert.) Bertoni in rats: endocrine effects. Gen Pharmacol, 34:187-91, 1989.

Pezzuto JM, Compadre CM, Swanson SM, Nanayakkara D, Kinghorn AD, Metabolically activated steviol, the aglycone of stevioside, is mutagenic. Proc Natl Acad Sci U S A, 82:2478-82, 1985 Apr.

Pezzuto JM, Nanayakkara NP, Compadre CM, Swanson SM, Kinghorn AD, Guenthner TM, Sparnins VL, Lam LK, Characterization of bacterial mutagenicity mediated by 13-hydroxy-ent-kaurenoic acid (steviol) and several structurally related derivatives and evaluation of potential to induce glutathione S-transferase in mice. Mutat Res, 169:93-103, 1986 Mar.

Shibata H, Sawa Y, Oka T, Sonoke S, Kim KK, Yoshioka M, Steviol and steviol-glycoside: glucosyltransferase activities in Stevia rebaudiana Bertoni - purification and partial characterization. Arch Biochem Biophys, 34:390-6, 1995 Aug 20.

Smoliar VI, Karpilovskaia ED, Salii NS, Tsapko EV, Lavrushenko LF, Gulich MP, Kryshevich LP, Grigorenko SN, Effect of a new sweetening agent from Stevia rebaudiana on animals. Planta Med, 32:60-3, 1992 Jan-Feb.

Tomita T, Sato N, Arai T, Shiraishi H, Sato M, Takeuchi M, Kamio Y, Bactericidal activity of a fermented hot-water extract from Stevia rebaudiana Bertoni towards enterohemorrhagic Escherichia coli O157:H7 and other food-borne pathogenic bacteria. Microbiol Immunol, 34:1005-9, 1997.

Yodyingyuad V, Bunyawong S, Analysis of Stevia glycosides by capillary electrophoresis. Electrophoresis, 6:367-71, 1996 Feb.

Yodyingyuad V, Bunyawong S, Effect of stevioside on growth and reproduction. Hum Reprod, 6:158-65, 1991 Jan.

Yodyingyuad V, Bunyawong S, Potential sweetening agents of plant origin. III. Organoleptic evaluation of Stevia leaf herbarium samples for sweetness. J Nat Prod, 6:590-99, 1982 Sep-Oct.

Stevia rebaudiana

See Stevia

Stillingia

Stillingia sylvatica

DESCRIPTION

Medicinal Parts: The medicinal part is the fresh or dried root.

Flower and Fruit: The yellow flowers are in terminal spikes and are apetalous. The fruit is a 3-seeded capsule.

Leaves, Stem and Root: The plant is a perennial herb up to 100 cm tall. It has an angular, smooth stem, which contains a milky latex. The leaves are sessile, coriaceous and narrow at the base. They are variable in form and color and are 3 to 11 cm long. The root is usually reddish-white on the outside and has numerous resin glands.

Characteristics: The taste is bitter and acrid, the smell is characteristic and unpleasant.

Habitat: The plant is indigenous to the southern U.S.

Production: Stillingia root is the root of Stillingia sylvatica.

Other Names: Cockup Hat, Marcory, Silver Leaf, Queen's Delight, Yaw Root

ACTIONS AND PHARMACOLOGY

COMPOUNDS

Diterpenes: diterpene esters of the tiglic or daphnan type, including diesters of 12-deoxyphorbol, of 12-deoxy-5β-hydroxyphorbol, of 5β, 12β-dihydroxyresiniferonol-6α,7α-oxide, referred to as stillingia factors S1 to S9 (S6 = gniditilactin, yuanhuacin, S7 = prostratin)

Volatile oil

Tannins (10 to 12%)

EFFECTS

The juice of the green root causes inflammation of the skin and swelling. The drug has laxative, tonic and diuretic properties.

INDICATIONS AND USAGE

Unproven Uses: The herb is used as a 'blood purifier', for digestive disorders, and for the treatment of liver, billiary and skin diseases.

Homeopathic Uses: Stillingia sylvatica is used for secondary and tertiary syphilis.

PRECAUTIONS AND ADVERSE REACTIONS

General: The drug is strongly irritating to skin and mucous membranes. Taken internally, it triggers vomiting (it is used as an emetic) and diarrhea (it is used as a laxative). Skin contact leads to inflammation and swelling. The diterpenes cause inflammation and are likely to be carcinogenic and virus-activating.

Nursing Mothers: Stillingia should not be administered to nursing mothers.

DOSAGE

Mode of Administration: As a liquid extract or tincture.

Storage: The drug should not be kept longer than 2 years.

LITERATURE

Adolf A, Hecker E, (1980) Tetrahedron Letters 21:2887.

British Herbal Pharmacopoeia, British Herbal Medicine Association, UK 1983.

Hegnauer R, Chemotaxonomie der Pflanzen, Bde 1-11: Birkhäuser Verlag Basel, Boston, Berlin 1962-1997.

Kern W, List PH, Hörhammer L (Hrsg.), Hagers Handbuch der Pharmazeutischen Praxis, 4. Aufl., Bde. 1-8: Springer Verlag Berlin, Heidelberg, New York, 1969.

Lewin L, Gifte und Vergiftungen, 6. Aufl., Nachdruck, Haug Verlag, Heidelberg 1992.

Madaus G, Lehrbuch der Biologischen Arzneimittel, Bde 1-3, Nachdruck, Georg Olms Verlag Hildesheim 1979.

Teuscher E, Lindequist U, Biogene Gifte - Biologie, Chemie, Pharmakologie, 2. Aufl., Fischer Verlag Stuttgart 1994.

Zahn P et al., Investigations of homeopathic drugs derived from Hippomane mancinella and Stillingia sylvatica: A potential iatrogenic risk of cancer? In: PM 59(7)84. 1993.

Stillingia sylvatica

See Stillingia

Stinging Nettle

Urtica dioica

TRADE NAMES

Alcohol Free Nettles Leaf, Basics Stinging Nettle, Certified Organic Nettles Leaf, Nettle Leaf, Nettle Herb, Nettle Power

DESCRIPTION

Medicinal Parts: The medicinal parts are the fresh and dried flowering plant and the roots.

Flower and Fruit: The flowers are greenish-white in axillary, clustered, hanging panicles. The perigone has 4 tepals. There are 4 stamens and 1 ovary with a brush-like stigma. The flowers are dioecious. The male flowers have only stamens and the female flowers only a style or a seed-producing organ. The male flower consists of a perianth of 4 segments, which enclose an even number of stamens. The stamens curve inward in the bud stage and spring back at the end of flowering for the anthers to fling out the pollen. The fruit is a small 1-seeded nutlet.

Leaves, Stem and Root: The plant grows from 60 to 150 cm high and has a winter hard rhizome. The leaves are opposite, oblong-cordate and roughly serrate. The whole plant is covered in stinging hairs.

Habitat: The plant is common in most temperate regions of the world.

Production: Stinging Nettle herb consists of the fresh or dried above-ground parts of Urtica dioica, Urtica urens and/or hybrids of these species, collected during flowering season. Stinging nettle leaf consists of fresh or dried leaves of Urtica dioica, Urtica urens and/or hybrids of these species, gathered during flowering season.

Not to be Confused With: The leaves of Laminum album.

Other Names: Nettle

ACTIONS AND PHARMACOLOGY

COMPOUNDS: STINGING NETTLE FLOWERING PLANT

In the stings of the fresh plant: histamine, serotonin, acetylcholine, formic acid, leukotriens (LTB4, LTC4, LTD4)

Flavonoids (0.7-1.8%): including rutin, isoquercitrin (0.02%), astragalin, kaempferol-3-O-rutinoside

Silicic acid (1-4%): partially water-soluble

Volatile oil: chief components are ketones, including, among others, 2-methylhept-2-en-6-on

Potassium-ions (0.6% in the fresh foliage)

Nitrates (1.5 to 3%)

EFFECTS: STINGING NETTLE FLOWERING PLANT

The fresh leaves contain acetylcholine, serotin and histamine. The pressed juice (main active principles scopoletine, beta-sitosterol and caffeoyl malic acid) is diuretic in combination with sufficient fluid intake. In animal experiments, a local anaesthetic and analgesic effect has been observed. Caffeoyl acid in vitro, inhibits 5-lipoxygenase-dependent leukotriene synthesis. In various studies, an antirheumatic and anti-arthritic effect was demonstrated.

Anti-inflammatory Effect - In one study, an extract from Stinging Nettle leaves (IDS 23) was tested for the ability to inhibit the biosynthesis of arachidonic acid metabolites in vitro. IDS 23 showed a strong concentration dependent inhibition of cyclooxygenase derived reactions. A phenolic acid isolate from the extract inhibited the synthesis of leukotriene B4 in a concentration dependent manner. The authors concluded that the combination of these effects may account for the antiphlogistic effects of this extract of Stinging Nettle (Obertreis, 1996.)

COMPOUNDS: STINGING NETTLE ROOT

Steroids: sterols, including beta-sitosterol (0.03 to 0.06%), beta-sitosterol-3-O-beta-glucoside (0.03 to 0.5%), (6′-Palmitoyl)-sitosterol-3-O-beta-D-glucoside (0.003%), 7alpha-hydroxysitosterol (0.001%), 7eta-Hydroxysitosterol (0.001%), stigmasterol, campesterol, stigmast-4-en-3-one

Lectins (0.1%): UDA (Urtica dioica Agglutinin, isolectine mixture)

Polysaccharides: glucans, glucogalacturonans, acidic arabinogalactans water-soluble with immunostimulating effect)

Hydroxycoumarins: scopoletin

Lignans: including secoisolariciresinol-9-O-glucoside (0.004%), neo-olivil (0.003%), neo-olivil-4-O-glucoside (0.004%)

Ceramides

EFFECTS: STINGING NETTLE ROOT

Effects on Prostate Tissue - The root has been show to cause an increase in the volume of urine, increase of maximum urinary flow and reduction of residual urine. One study found that an aqueous extract of the root was the most effective in treating benign prostatic hyperplasia. The extract inhibited the binding of sex hormone-binding globulin (SHBG) to its receptor on human prostatic membranes in a dose related manner. Inhibition was noted at 0.6 mg/ml and complete inhibition was achieved at 10 mg/ml (Hryb et al, 1995.) In a second study, most ligans that were tested were found to have an affinity for SHBG. The affinity of (-)-3,4-divanillyltetrahydrofuran was found to be extremely high (Schottner, 1997.)

Viral Inhibition - The (N-acetylglucosamine) n-specific lectin fron Stinging Nettle was found to be inhibitory to HIV-1, HIV-2, CMV, RSV and influenza A virus in-vitro at an EC-50 (50% inhibitory concentration) ranging from 0.3 to 0.9 micrograms/ml (Balzarini, 1992.)

Effects on Systemic Lupus Erythematosus-like Pathology - Urtica dioica agglutinin (UDA) treated MRL lpr/lpr mice were shown to be protected from developing clinical signs of lupus and nephritis (Musette, 1996.)

CLINICAL TRIALS

One randomized, reference-controlled, multicenter double blind clinical trial compared therapeutic efficacy of a Sabal and Urtica extract (PRO 160/120) with finasteride in benign prostatic hyperplasia (Aiken stages I to II). The study involved 543 patients that were treated for 48 weeks with either the PRO 160/120 extract or finasteride in a double blind design. The primary marker was the change of maximum urinary flow after 24 weeks of therapy. Secondary markers included average urinary flow, miction volume and miction time. Urinary symptoms were recorded by the International-Prostate-Symptom-Score (I-PSS). There was also a quality of life questionnaire that was developed by the American Urological Associacion Ameasurement Committee (1991). Results were similar for both groups. There was an increase in urinary flow rate (1.9 ml with PRO 160/120; 2.4 ml with finasteride). Urinary flow increase and miction time decreases were comparable for both groups. The I-PSS decreased from 11.3 at the start to 8.2 at 24 weeks and 6.5 by week 48 for the PRO 16/120 group, and went from 11.8 to 8.0 and 6.2 respectively for the finasteride group. The life quality scores went from 7.5 at the start of treatment, to 4.2 in the PRO 160/120 group, and from 7.7 to 4.1 in the finasteride group. The most notable differences between the groups were in the lower adverse events categories where the PRO 160/120 group reported less events, in particular in the areas of diminished ejaculation volume, erectile dysfunction and headache (Sokeland & Albrecht, 1997.)

INDICATIONS AND USAGE

STINGING NETTLE FLOWERING PLANT

- Infections of the urinary tract
- Kidney and bladder stones
- Rheumatism

The drug is used internally and externally as supportive therapy for rheumatic ailments. It is used internally as flushing-out therapy for inflammatory diseases of the lower urinary tract. Also used as irrigation therapy for prevention and treatment of kidney stones.

Unproven Uses: In folk medicine, the plant is used internally as a hematogenic remedy, diuretic for arthritis, rheumatism of the joints and muscles, and as a component of diabetic teas (this indication is not recommended). Externally, the drug is used as a hair and scalp remedy against oily hair and dandruff.

STINGING NETTLE ROOT

- Prostate complaints, irritable bladder

Preparations of the root are used for micturition disorders in prostate adenoma stages I to II. This drug only relieves the symptoms of an enlarged prostate without eliminating the enlargement itself.

Unproven Uses: In folk medicine, the root is used for edema, rheumatism, gout and prostatitis.

CONTRAINDICATIONS

STINGING NETTLE FLOWERING PLANT

The drug is contraindicated when there is fluid retention resulting from reduced cardiac or renal function.

PRECAUTIONS AND ADVERSE REACTIONS

STINGING NETTLE FLOWERING PLANT

General: No health hazards or side effects are known in conjunction with the proper administration of designated therapeutic dosages. Possible allergic reactions (skin afflictions, edema) have been observed in rare cases following intake of the drug. Contact urticaria frequently occurs when skin is exposed to the plant. The urticaria is accompanied by a stinging sensation that may last as long as 12 hours post exposure (Oliver, 1991.)

Drug Interactions: Studies have demonstrated that leaf extracts of Stinging Nettle when used along with diclofenac, enhance the anti-inflammatory effect of diclofenac.

STINGING NETTLE ROOT

No health hazards are known in conjunction with the proper administration of designated therapeutic dosages. Occasional, mild gastrointestinal complaints may occur as side effects of drug intake.

DOSAGE

STINGING NETTLE FLOWERING PLANT

Mode of Administration: Comminuted herb for infusions and other galenic preparations for internal use; as stinging nettle spirit for external application. Drug extracts are contained in diuretic tea mixtures and in blood-purifying teas.

Preparation: To prepare an infusion, use 1.5 g finely cut herb in cold water, briefly bring to a boil and steep for 10 minutes, then strain.

Daily Dose: The average daily dose is 8 to 12 g of drug. Observe ample intake of liquid (minimum 2 liters/day). One cup several times daily as a diuretic (1 teaspoonful = 0.8 g drug). For external application, a tincture/spiritus (1:10) may be administered.

STINGING NETTLE ROOT

Mode of Administration: Comminuted drug from the root for infusions as well as other galenic preparations for oral use.

Preparation: To prepare an infusion use 1.5 g coarse powdered drug in cold water, heat to boiling point for 1 minute, then steep, covered, for 10 minutes, and strain. (1 teaspoonful = 1.3 g drug)

Daily Dose: 4 to 6 g drug.

Tea — 1.5 g coarse powderd drug to water

Dry Extract — 120 mg twice daily

LITERATURE

STINGING NETTLE FLOWERING PLANT

Anonym (1982) Vet Hum Toxicol 24:247.

Chaurasia N, Wichtl M, PM 53:432. 1987.

Hughes RE et al., (1980) J Sci Food Agric 31:1279.

Obertreis B, Giller K et al., Anti-inflammatory effect of Urtica dioica folia extract in comparison to caffeic malic acid. In: Arzneimittelforschung 46(1): 52-6, Jan, 1996.

Oliver F, Amon EU, Breathnach A et al., Contact urticaria due to the common stinging nettle (Urtica dioica)—histological, ultrastructural and pharmacological studies. Clin Exp Dermatol 16:1-7. 1991.

Schiebel-Schlosser G, Die Brennessel. In: PTA 8(1):53. 1994.

Schilcher H, Urtica-Arten - Die Brennessel. In: ZPT 9(5):160. 1988.

Schomakers J, Bollbach FD Hagels H, Brennesselkraut - Phytochemische und anatomische Unterscheidung der Herba-Drogen von Urtica dioica und U. urens. In: DAZ 135(7):578-584. 1995.

Further information in:

Frohne D, Pfänder HJ, Giftpflanzen - Ein Handbuch für Apotheker, Toxikologen und Biologen, 4. Aufl., Wiss. Verlags-Ges. Stuttgart 1997.

Kern W, List PH, Hörhammer L (Hrsg.), Hagers Handbuch der Pharmazeutischen Praxis, 4. Aufl., Bde 1-8: Springer Verlag Berlin, Heidelberg, New York, 1969.

Lewin L, Gifte und Vergiftungen, 6. Aufl., Nachdruck, Haug Verlag, Heidelberg 1992.

Madaus G, Lehrbuch der Biologischen Arzneimittel, Bde 1-3, Nachdruck, Georg Olms Verlag Hildesheim 1979.

Roth L, Daunderer M, Kormann K, Giftpflanzen, Pflanzengifte, 4. Aufl., Ecomed Fachverlag Landsberg Lech 1993.

Steinegger E, Hänsel R, Pharmakognosie, 5. Aufl., Springer Verlag Heidelberg 1992.

Teuscher E, Lindequist U, Biogene Gifte - Biologie, Chemie, Pharmakologie, 2. Aufl., Fischer Verlag Stuttgart 1994.

Teuscher E, Biogene Arzneimittel, 5. Aufl., Wiss. Verlagsges. Stuttgart 1997.

Wagner H, Wiesenauer M, Phytotherapie. Phytopharmaka und pflanzliche Homöopathika, Fischer-Verlag, Stuttgart, Jena, New York 1995.

Wichtl M (Hrsg.), Teedrogen, 4. Aufl., Wiss. Verlagsges. Stuttgart 1997.

STINGING NETTLE ROOT

Anonym (1982) Vet Hum Toxicol 24:247.

Anonym, Extrakt aus Brennesselwurzel wirksam bei benigner Prostatahyperplasie. In: ZPT 12(5):8. 1991.

Anonym, Phytotherapie: Pflanzliche Antirheumatika - was bringen sie? In: DAZ 136(45):4012-4015. 1996.

Anonym, Welche Bedeutung haben pflanzliche Prostatamittel. In: DAZ 133(9):720. 1993.

Balzarini J, Neyts J, Schols D et al., The mannose-specific plant lectins from Cymbidium hybrid and Epipactishelleborine and the (N-acetylglucosamine)(n)-specific plant lectin from Urtica dioica are potent and selective inhibitors of human immunodeficiency virus and cytomegalovirus replication in vitro. In: Antivir Res 18(12):191-207, 1992.

Dathe G, Schmid H, (1987) Phytotherapie der benignen Prostatahyperplasie (BPH). Doppelblindstudie mit Extraktum Radicis Uricae (ERU). Urologe [B]27:223-226.

Fessler B, Brennesselwurzel bei Prostataadenom. In: Med Mo Pharm 16(9):287. 1993.

Ganβer D, Spiteller G, Aromatase inhibitors from Urtica dioica. In: PM 61(2):138-140. 1995.

Goetz P, Die Behandlung der benignen Prostatahyperplasie mit Brennesselwurzeln. In: ZPT 10(6):175. 1990.

Hirano T et al., Effect of stinging nettle root extract and their steroidal components on the Na+,K+-ATPase of the benign prostic hyperplasia. In: PM 60:30. 1994.

Hryb DJ, Khan MS, Romas NA, Rosner W, (1995) The Effect of Extracts of the Roots of the Stinging Nettle (Urtica dioica) on the Interaction of SHBG with 1st Receptor on Human Prostatic Membranes. Planta Med 61:31-32.

Huesing JE, Murdock LL, Shade RE, Rice and stinging nettle lectins - insecticidal activity similar to wheat germ agglutinin. In: PH 30:3565. 1991.

Hughes RE et al., (1980) J Sci Food Agric 31:1279.

Koch E, (1995) Pharmakologie und Wirkmechanismen von Extrakten aus Sabalfrüchten (Sabal fructus): Brennesselwurzeln (Urticae radix) und Kürbissamen (Cucurbitae peponis semen) bei der Behandlung der benignen Prostatahyperplasie. In: Loew D, Rietbrock N (Hrsg.) Phytopharmaka in Forschung und klinischer Anwendung. Steinkopff Verlag, Darmstadt, S 57-79.

Lauel H, Extrakt aus Radix Urticae normalisiert Hormonhaushalt. In: DAZ 130(51/52):2789. 1990.

Lichius JJ et al., Inhibition of experimentally induced mouse prostatic hyperplasia by methanolic extracts of Urtica dioica roots. In: PM 61(Abstracts of 43rd Ann Congr):89. 1995.

Lichius JJ, Muth C, A new biological evaluation of Urtica dioica root-extracts. In: PM 62, Abstracts of the 44th Ann Congress of GA, 20. 1996.

Miersch WDE, Benigne Prostatahyperplasie. In: DAZ 133(29):2653. 1993.

Musette P, Galelli A, Chabre H et al., Urtica dioica agglutinin, a V beta 8.3-specific superantigen, prevents the development of the systemic lupus erythematosus-like pathology of MRL lpr/lpr mice. In: Eur J Immunol 26:1707-1711, 1996.

Nahrstedt A (1993) Pflanzliche Urologica - eine kritische Übersicht. Pharm Z 138: 1439-1450.

Nöske HD (1994) Die Effektivität pflanzlicher Prostatamittel am Beispiel von Brennesselwurzelextrakt. ÄrzteZ Naturheilverfahren 35 (1):18-27.

Sabo A et al., Radix Urticae (Urtica dioica): Influence on erythrocyte deformability and enzymes. In: PM 62, Abstracts of the 44th Ann Congress of GA, 60. 1996.

Schiebel-Schlosser G, Die Brennessel. In: PTA 8(1):53. 1994.

Schilcher H (1987a) Pflanzliche Diuretika. Urologe [B]27:215-222; (1987b) Möglichkeiten und Grenzen der Phytotherapie am Beispiel pflanzlicher Urologika. Urologe [B]27:316-319.

Schilcher H, Boesel R, Effenberger ST Segebrecht S, Neuere Untersuchungsergebnisse mit aquaretisch, antibakteriell und prostatotrop wirksamen Arzneipflanzen. In: ZPT 10(3):77. 1989.

Schilcher H, Urtica-Arten - Die Brennessel. In: ZPT 9(5):160. 1988.

Schmidt K (1983) Die Wirkung eines Radix Urticae-Extrakts und einzelner Nebenextrakte auf das SHBG des Blutplasmas bei der benignen Prostatahyperplasie. Fortschr Med 101:713-716.

Schmidt K (1983) Die Wirkung eines Radix Urticae-Extrakts und einzelner Nebenextrakte auf das SHGB des Blutplasmas bei der benignen Prostatahyperplasie. Fortschr Med 101:713-716.

Schoettner M, Gansser D & Spiteller G: Lignans from the roots of Urtica dioica and their metabolites bind to human sex hormone binding globlin (SHBG). In: Planta Med 63:529-532, 1997.

Sokeland J, Albrecht J, Combination of Sabal and Urtica extract vs. finasteride in benign prostatic hyperplasia (Aiken stages I to II). Comparison of therapeutic effectiveness in a one year double-blind study. In: Urologe A 36(4):327-33, July, 1997.

Sonnenschein R (1987) Untersuchung der Wirksamkeit eines prostatotropen Phytotherapeutikums (Urtica plus) bei benigner Prostatahyperplasie und Prostatitis - eine prospektive multizentrische Studie. Urologe [B]27:232-237.

Wagner H et al., Studies on the binding of Urtica dioica agglutinin (UDA) and other lectins in an in vitro epidermal growth factor receptor test. In: Phytomedicine 1:287-290. 1994.

Wagner H, Willer F, Samtleben R, Boos G (1994) Search for the antiprostatic principle of stinging nettle (Urtica dioica) roots. Phytomedicine 1:213-224.

Willer F, Wagner H, Schecklies E, Urtica-Wurzelextrakte. In: DAZ 131(24):1217. 1991.

Further information in:

Madaus G, Lehrbuch der Biologischen Arzneimittel, Bde 1-3, Nachdruck, Georg Olms Verlag Hildesheim 1979.

Schulz R, Hänsel R, Rationale Phytotherapie, Springer Verlag Heidelberg 1996.

Steinegger E, Hänsel R, Pharmakognosie, 5. Aufl., Springer Verlag Heidelberg 1992.

Teuscher E, Biogene Arzneimittel, 5. Aufl., Wiss. Verlagsges. Stuttgart 1997.

Wichtl M (Hrsg.), Teedrogen, 4. Aufl., Wiss. Verlagsges. Stuttgart 1997.

Stone Root

Collinsonia canadensis

DESCRIPTION

Medicinal Parts: The medicinal parts of the plant are the fresh or dried roots and rhizomes.

Flower and Fruit: The flowers are dirty yellow, labiate, with red venation on the inside in richly blossomed panicles. The upper lip has an obtuse tip. The side tips of the lower lip are small and rounded; the middle tips are larger and fringed. The calyx is acuminate and has 2 stamens. The fruit is a small globose nutlet.

Leaves, Stem and Root: The plant is a perennial that grows 90 to 120 cm high. The rhizome is grayish-brown, very hard, fibrous and up to 8 cm long. The shoots are glabrous, often tinged red, with few side shoots. The bark is very thin. The leaves are light green above and pale green, glabrous, broad, cordate or ovate below, becoming narrower and shorter above.

Characteristics: The smell is strongly aromatic, unpleasant, and numbing in large amounts. The taste is unpleasantly bitter.

Habitat: The plant is indigenous to North America from Canada to the Carolinas in the U.S. It is also found in central Europe.

Production: Stone Root, the rhizome and root of Collinsonia canadensis, is gathered and dried in autumn.

Other Names: Hardhack, Horseweed, Heal-All, Knob Grass, Knob Root, Richweed, Richleaf, Knobweed, Hardback

ACTIONS AND PHARMACOLOGY

COMPOUNDS

Volatile oil: chief components are caryophyllene, germacrene D, limonene, alpha- and beta-pinenes

Caffeic acid derivatives: including rosmaric acid

EFFECTS

Stone Root has stomachic, tonic and diuretic effects, probably due to the presence of the essential oil and rosmaric acid.

INDICATIONS AND USAGE

Unproven Uses: Stone Root is used for calculi, kidney stones, urea (bladder semolina), bladder inflammation, dropsy and gastrointestinal disorders.

Homeopathic Uses: Preparations of Collinsonia canadensis are used for hemorrhoids and constipation.

DOSAGE

Mode of Administration: The drug is used internally as an extract, infusion or tincture.

Preparation: Liquid extract (1:1) 1 ml to 4 ml; tincture (1:5) 2 ml to 8 ml.

Daily Dosage: The drug is generally used as a single dose, 1 to 4 g, internally as an infusion.

Homeopathic Dosage: 5 to 10 drops, 1 tablet or 5 to 10 globules 1 to 3 times daily; or 1 ml injection solution sc twice weekly (HAB1).

LITERATURE

Joshi BS, Moore KM, Pelletier SW, Saponins from Collinsonia canadensis. In: JNP 55(10):1468-1476. 1992.

Lawrence BM et al., PH 11:2636-2638. 1972.

Wolters B, Zierpflanzen aus Nordamerika. In: DAZ 137(26):2253-2261. 1997.

Further information in:

Hänsel R, Keller K, Rimpler H, Schneider G (Hrsg.), Hagers Handbuch der Pharmazeutischen Praxis, 5. Aufl., Bde 4-6 (Drogen), Springer Verlag Berlin, Heidelberg, New York, 1992-1994.

Madaus G, Lehrbuch der Biologischen Arzneimittel, Bde 1-3, Nachdruck, Georg Olms Verlag Hildesheim 1979.

Storax

Liquidambar orientalis

DESCRIPTION

Medicinal Parts: The medicinal part is the balsam from the trunk and the inner bark.

Flower and Fruit: The flowers and inflorescences are unisexual, monoecious and arranged in small, round solitary capitula. The flowers are yellow. The male flowers show no signs of a calyx or corolla. The female flowers have tiny scaly sepals, and the floret tubes are fused. There are numerous stamens, and the ovary is semi-inferior. The fruit is a hard globular schizocarp.

Leaves, Stem and Root: Liquidambar orientalis is a deciduous tree about 12 m tall with many branches and a thick reddish-gray bark. It has alternate, usually 5-lobed leaves. The leaf blades are usually roughly toothed.

Characteristics: Raw Storax is a thick, viscous, sticky, aromatic and somewhat bitter-tasting gray-brown mass. When stored, the drug becomes clearer, an effect caused by a reduction in the water content.

Habitat: The tree is indigenous from Asia Minor to Syria.

Production: Storax (amber tree balm) is extracted from Liquidambar orientalis. To extract the balsam, the trunk is beaten, causing the bark to soak up the exuding resin. The bark is then boiled and the resulting decoction further refined.

Not to be Confused With: Fir resin, turpentine, colophony, olive oil

Other Names: Balsam Styracis, Sweet Gum, Copalm, Gum Tree, Liquid Amber, Opossum Tree, Red Gum, White Gum

ACTIONS AND PHARMACOLOGY

COMPOUNDS

Aromatic alcohols: phenylpropyl-, cinnamic-, benzyl alcohol

Cinnamic acid (up to 30%): cinnamic acid esters, including among others cinnamylcinnamate (styracine), cinnamic acid ethyl esters

Styrene

Triterpenes: oleanolic acid, 3-epioleanolic acid (resin fraction)

Vanillin (up to 2%)

Volatile oil (depending upon source, 1 to 20%): with styrol, benzyl alcohol, cinnamic alcohol

EFFECTS

Storax has anti-inflammatory, diaphoretic and stimulant effects.

INDICATIONS AND USAGE

Unproven Uses: Storax is used for coughs and bronchitis as an inhalation, externally for wounds and ulcers.

Chinese Medicine: In China, Storax is used in the treatment of syncope, epilepsy and lactose intolerance in young children.

Indian Medicine: In India, Storax is used for itching, suppurating wounds, leprosy, chronic coughs and fever.

PRECAUTIONS AND ADVERSE REACTIONS

No health hazards are known in conjunction with the proper administration of designated therapeutic dosages. Internal administration of the drug occasionally leads to diarrhea. Storax can also trigger contact allergies.

OVERDOSAGE

External administration over large areas can lead to absorptive poisonings that are characterized by kidney damage (albuminuria, hemorrhagic nephritis).

DOSAGE

Mode of Administration: Storax is used in combination preparations for coughs and bronchitis as an inhalation, externally for wounds and ulcers.

LITERATURE

Hänsel R, Keller K, Rimpler H, Schneider G (Hrsg.), Hagers Handbuch der Pharmazeutischen Praxis, 5. Aufl., Bde 4-6 (Drogen), Springer Verlag Berlin, Heidelberg, New York, 1992-1994.

Huneck S, (1968) Tetrahedron 19: 479.

Leung AY, Encyclopedia of Common Natural Ingredients Used in Food Drugs and Cosmetics, John Wiley & Sons Inc., New York 1980.

Lewin L, Gifte und Vergiftungen, 6. Aufl., Nachdruck, Haug Verlag, Heidelberg 1992.

Strawberry

Fragaria vesca

DESCRIPTION

Medicinal Parts: The medicinal parts are dried leaves collected during the flowering season, the dried rhizome and ripe fruit.

Flower and Fruit: The small white flowers are arranged on a repeatedly bifurcated pedicle. They are usually androgynous. There are 5 sepals and 5 petals. The sepals are triangular, pointed or briefly acuminate appressed pubescent. The petals are oribicular or ovate, glabrous and pure white. There are 20 stamens and numerous ovate, glabrous carpels and a style at the side. After flowering the receptacle turns into a fleshy false fruit. The receptacle is 2 cm long, ovate, globular or clavate, carmine red when ripe. The nutlets are ovate, 0.8 to 1.5 mm long, brown and matte.

Leaves, Stem and Root: The perennial, herbaceous plant grows from 20 to 30 cm high. The rhizome is cylindrical, horizontal or crooked and thickly covered with the residual died off leaves and stipules. Long runners grow from the axils of the basal leaves. The stem is erect and is slightly longer than the basal leaves. The cauline leaves are trifoliate and roughly serrate from the first quarter upward. The petioles are very long and, like the stem have patent hairs. The stipules are lanceolate, long-acuminate, entire-margined, reddish brown, glabrous above and hairy beneath.

Habitat: Found in almost all of the temperate zones of Europe and Asia.

Production: Strawberry leaf consists of the dried leaf of Fragaria species, mainly Fragaria vesca. The leaves are collected in the wild and air-dried in a shady place.

Not to be Confused With: Other Fragaria species, although they have the same value.

Other Names: Wild Strawberry, Mountain Strawberry, Wood Strawberry, Alpine Strawberry

ACTIONS AND PHARMACOLOGY

COMPOUNDS

Caffeic acid derivatives: including chlorogenic acid

Flavonoids: including rutin, quercetin

Tannins: ellagic acid tannins, oligomeric proanthocyanidins

EFFECTS

Strawberry leaf has astringent and diuretic properties; but no studies are available.

INDICATIONS AND USAGE

Unproven Uses: Preparations of strawberry leaf are used externally as compresses for rashes, and internally for catarrh of the gastrointestinal tract, diarrhea, intestinal sluggishness, liver disease, jaundice, catarrh of the respiratory tract, gout, rheumatoid arthritis, nervous tension, kidney ailments involving gravel and stones and as a diuretic. Because of the tannin content, its efficacy in treating mouth and throat inflammation and diarrhea is plausible.

PRECAUTIONS AND ADVERSE REACTIONS

Health risks or side effects following the proper administration of designated therapeutic dosages are not recorded. The drug should not be taken in presence of strawberry allergy.

DOSAGE

Mode of Administration: Strawberry leaves are only used occasionally in folk medicine, the berries are used more commonly.

Preparation: Pour boiling water over 1 gm of comminuted drug and strain after 5 to 10 minutes.

Decoction — boil 375 gm green leaves with 1.15 Liter water until only 550 ml remain.

Infusion — add 4 gm drug to 150 ml boiling water.

Extract — boil 20 gm drug with 500 ml water until only half remains.

Daily Dosage: Tea: As an antidiarrheal agent, several cups per day.

Decoction — for diarrhea, 1 teaspoon every 3 to 4 hours.

Extract — for diarrhea, a spoonful before bed and on rising.

Infusion — one dose only for children with diarrhea. The decoction is used as a gargle.

LITERATURE

Haddock EA et al., PH 21:1049. 1982.

Hänsel R, Keller K, Rimpler H, Schneider G (Hrsg.), Hagers Handbuch der Pharmazeutischen Praxis, 5. Aufl., Bde 4-6 (Drogen), Springer Verlag Berlin, Heidelberg, New York, 1992-1994.

Henning W (1981) Z Lebensm Unters Forsch 173:180.

Lund K, Dissertation Universität Freiburg i. Br. 1986.

Teuscher E, Biogene Arzneimittel, 5. Aufl., Wiss. Verlagsges. mbH Stuttgart 1997.

Wichtl M (Hrsg.), Teedrogen, 4. Aufl., Wiss. Verlagsges. Stuttgart 1997.

Strophanthus

Strophanthus species

DESCRIPTION

Medicinal Parts: The medicinal parts are the ripe seeds, which have been freed from their appendages and dried. Most of the species are poisonous.

Flower and Fruit: The flowers are in terminal or lateral panicles with few flowers or in richly blossomed, umbelliferous panicles. Their parts are in fives. They are white or yellowish, radially symmetrical and sometimes fragrant. The calyx has 5 elliptical-lanceolate to obovate sepals and a short tube with a campanulately splayed upper part, which has 10 scales on the margin. The anthers are acute with a partly tailed middle section. The ovary is 2-valved, semi-inferior and has numerous ovules. The fruit has 1 to 2 follicles, which are oblong, 8 to 58 cm long, splayed or horizontal on one level. The greenish-brown seeds are 8 to 25 mm long, fusiform and often flattened. The seeds have an awn-like appendage and a long tuft of hair at the base, which eventually drops off.

Leaves, Stem and Root: The plants are climbing lianes, occasionally erect shrubs, subshrubs or trees. They contain milky latex. The leaves are opposite, ovate to elliptical, short-petioled, simple, entire-margined and usually coriaceous.

Habitat: Strophanthus is indigenous to tropical Africa.

Production: Strophanthus seeds are the seeds of Strophanthus gratus. Kombe-Strophanthus seeds are the seeds of Strophanthus kombé. The plant is harvested mostly by African tribes in the wilderness or in protected areas in the vicinity of African settlements.

Not to be Confused With: Strophanthi semen should not be confused with African Strophantus species.

Other Names: Kombé

ACTIONS AND PHARMACOLOGY

COMPOUNDS: STROPHANTHUS GRATUS SEEDS

Cardioactive steroid glycosides (cardenolides, 3-8%): chief glycoside strophanthin-G (ouabain, over 80%), further including acolongifloroside K, strogoside, among others

Saponins (0.2%)

Fatty oil (35%)

EFFECTS: STROPHANTHUS GRATUS SEEDS

The active agent, Strophanthin-G, is a cardioactive glycoside that has actions similar to digitalis, but is milder. No clinical test results are available. The drug is poorly absorbed by the gastrointestinal tract.

COMPOUNDS: STROPHANTHUS KOMBE SEEDS

Cardioactive steroid glycosides: (cardenolides, 4.0-4.5%, the mixture known as Strophanthin-K) chief glycoside K-strophanthoside (60-80%), erysimoside (15-25%), strophoside, (10-15%)

Saponins (0.2%)

Fatty oil (35%)

EFFECTS: STROPHANTHUS KOMBE SEEDS

The effects are similar to Strophanthus gratus, but milder.

INDICATIONS AND USAGE

STROPHANTHUS GRATUS SEEDS

Unproven Uses: Strophanthus is used for arteriosclerosis, cardiac insufficiency, gastrocardial symptoms, hypertension and neurodystonia.

Homeopathic Uses: Strophanthus gratus is used for cardiac insufficiency and anxiety.

PRECAUTIONS AND ADVERSE REACTIONS

General: No health hazards are known in conjunction with the proper administration of designated therapeutic dosages. Queasiness, vomiting, headache, stupor, disturbance of color vision and cardiac arrhythmias could occur as side effects, in particular through overdosages connected with parenteral administration of strophanthin-G or glycoside mixtures.

Drug Interactions: Simultaneous administration of quinidine, calcium salts, saluretics, laxatives and glucocorticoids enhance both effects and side effects.

OVERDOSAGE

Queasiness, vomiting, headache, stupor, disturbance of color vision and cardiac arrhythmias are the most likely consequence of overdosage. Overdosage is more likely to occur with parenteral administration of strophanthin-G or glycoside mixtures.

For a review of symptoms of an acute poisoning and therapy, see Digitalis folium. The danger of poisoning after oral administration is relatively low, due to the poor absorption of the glycosides.

DOSAGE

STROPHANTHUS GRATUS SEEDS

Mode of Administration: The drug is available as injection solutions and capsules and in combination preparations.

Preparation: A tincture is prepared by using 1 part coarsely ground powder (previously specially treated) stabilized for content with 10 parts 70% ethanol (V/V) (DAB6)

Daily Dosage: Tincture daily dose is 1.5 g. The single dose is 0.5 g.

Homeopathic Dosage: From D4: 5 drops, 1 tablet or 10 globules (from D2); Tincture: single dose: 0.5 g and daily dose: 1.5 g.

STROPHANTHUS KOMBE SEEDS

Mode of Administration: The drug is available in monopreparations, and is rarely used in combinations.

Homeopathic Dosage: From D4: 5 drops, 1 tablet or 10 globules (from D2) every 30 to 60 minutes (acute) or 1 to 3 times daily (chronic); parenterally: 1 to 2 ml sc, acute: 3 times daily; chronic: once a day (HAB1).

LITERATURE

STROPHANTHUS GRATUS SEEDS

Brisse B, Anwendung pflanzlicher Wirkstoffe bei kardialen Erkrankungen. In: ZPT 10(4):107. 1989.

Geiger UP et al., Helv Cheim Acta 50:179. 1967.

Jäger HH et al., Helv Chim Acta 48:202. 1965.

Tittel G et al., PM 45:207. 1982.

Tittel G et al., Pharm Ind 48:822. 1986.

Further information in:

Hänsel R, Keller K, Rimpler H, Schneider G (Hrsg.), Hagers Handbuch der Pharmazeutischen Praxis, 5. Aufl., Bde 4-6 (Drogen): Springer Verlag Berlin, Heidelberg, New York, 1992-1994.

Lewin L, Gifte und Vergiftungen, 6. Aufl., Nachdruck, Haug Verlag, Heidelberg 1992.

Madaus G, Lehrbuch der Biologischen Arzneimittel, Bde 1-3, Nachdruck, Georg Olms Verlag Hildesheim 1979.

Roth L, Daunderer M, Kormann K, Giftpflanzen, Pflanzengifte, 4. Aufl., Ecomed Fachverlag Landsberg Lech 1993.

Steinegger E, Hänsel R, Pharmakognosie, 5. Aufl., Springer Verlag Heidelberg 1992.

Teuscher E, Biogene Arzneimittel, 5. Aufl., Wiss. Verlagsges. Stuttgart 1997.

Teuscher E, Lindequist U, Biogene Gifte - Biologie, Chemie, Pharmakologie, 2. Aufl., Fischer Verlag Stuttgart 1994.

Wagner H, Wiesenauer M, Phytotherapie. Phytopharmaka und pflanzliche Homöopathika, Fischer-Verlag, Stuttgart, Jena, New York 1995.

STROPHANTHUS KOMBE SEEDS

Kaiser F et al., Liebigs Ann Chem 643:192. 1961.

Kaiser F et al., Naturwissenschaften 46:670. 1959.

Kartnig T et al., J Chromatogr 52:313. 1970.

Makarevich IF, Khim Prir Soedin 180. 1972.

Puchkova EI et al., Rastit Resu 11:268. 1975.

Further information in:

Hänsel R, Keller K, Rimpler H, Schneider G (Hrsg.), Hagers Handbuch der Pharmazeutischen Praxis, 5. Aufl., Bde 4-6 (Drogen): Springer Verlag Berlin, Heidelberg, New York, 1992-1994.

Lewin L, Gifte und Vergiftungen, 6. Aufl., Nachdruck, Haug Verlag, Heidelberg 1992.

Roth L, Daunderer M, Kormann K, Giftpflanzen, Pflanzengifte, 4. Aufl., Ecomed Fachverlag Landsberg Lech 1993.

Steinegger E, Hänsel R, Pharmakognosie, 5. Aufl., Springer Verlag Heidelberg 1992.

Teuscher E, Lindequist U, Biogene Gifte - Biologie, Chemie, Pharmakologie, 2. Aufl., Fischer Verlag Stuttgart 1994.

Teuscher E, Biogene Arzneimittel, 5. Aufl., Wiss. Verlagsges. Stuttgart 1997.

Strophanthus hispidus

See Kombe Seed

Strophanthus species

See Strophanthus

Strychnos ignatii

See Ignatius Beans

Strychnos nux vomica

See Nux Vomica

Styrax benzoin

See Benzoin

Styrax paralleloneurum

See Sumatra Benzoin

Styrax tonkinensis

See Siam Benzoin

Sumatra Benzoin

Styrax paralleloneurum

DESCRIPTION

Medicinal Parts: The medicinal part of the plant is the balsamic resin obtained from the damaged trunk.

Flower and Fruit: Styrax paralleloneurum is a tree that grows up to 35 m high. The flowers are small, the corolla is violet, and the calyx is 3 to 4.5 mm high. The fruit is 5 to 9 mm in diameter.

Leaves, Stem and Root: The leaves are ovate or lanceolate and 6 to 16 cm long.

Habitat: Sumatra

Production: Sumatra Benzoin (Gum Benzoin) is the balsamic resin from the damaged trunk of Styrax benzoin and Styrax paralleloneurum. The optimal age of a tree to be harvested is 7 years. The tree is cut which causes it to exude resin to heal the cuts. The resin is then collected in a vessel and left to melt to a homogenous mass in the sun.

ACTIONS AND PHARMACOLOGY

COMPOUNDS

Ester mixture (70 to 80%): composed of coniferyl benzoate and cinnamyl benzoate, as well as cinnamyl cinnamoate (styracine), propyl cinnamoate

Phenylacrylic acids: cinnamic acid (10 to 20%)

Vanillin (0.4 to 0.6%)

Triterpenes: including sumaresinolic acid

EFFECTS

Sumatra Benzoin has a mild expectorant effect possibly due to its vanilla content.

INDICATIONS AND USAGE

Unproven Uses: Preparations of the resin have been used for respiratory catarrh.

Chinese Medicine: Sumatra Benzoin preparations are used for stroke, syncopes, postpartum syncope due to heavy loss of blood, chest and stomach pain.

PRECAUTIONS AND ADVERSE REACTIONS

No health hazards are known in conjunction with the proper administration of designated therapeutic dosages.

DOSAGE

Mode of Administration: Whole herb preparations for internal use.

Storage: Should be tightly sealed and stored below 25° C.

LITERATURE

Hänsel R, Keller K, Rimpler H, Schneider G (Ed), Hagers Handbuch der Pharmazeutischen Praxis, 5. Aufl., Bde 4 - 6 (Drogen), Springer Verlag Berlin, Heidelberg, New York, 1992-1994.

James WD, White SW, Yanklowitz B, Allergic contact dermatitis to compound tincture of benzoin. J Am Acad Dermatol, 11:847-50, 1984 Nov.

Sumbul

Ferula sumbul

DESCRIPTION

Medicinal Parts: The medicinal part is the rhizome with the roots.

Leaves, Stem and Root: The plant is a 2.5 m tall shrub. It has a solid, cylindrical, thin stem, which produces about 12 branches. The fern-like leaflets are blue-gray. The basal leaves are about 50 cm long and triangular while the cauline leaves reduce gradually in size until they are little more than sheath leaves. The roots are 2.5 to 7.5 cm thick. They are covered on the outside with a blackish-brown, paper-like, horizontally folded cork, which is sometimes fibrous. The fracture is spongy and roughly fibrous with white spots and resin drops.

Characteristics: The odor is strong and musk-like; the taste is bitter and aromatic.

Habitat: The plant is found in some parts of Russia, Turkestan, and northern India.

Production: Sumbul or Musk root is the root of Ferula moschata (Reinsch, Kozo) or Ferula sumbul.

Other Names: Ferula, Musk Root

ACTIONS AND PHARMACOLOGY

COMPOUNDS

Volatile oil (0.3-0.5%)

Resins (17%)

Bitter substances

Hydroxycoumarins: including among others, umbelliferone

Short-chained acids: butyric acid, angelic acid, methylcrotonic acid, and valeric acid

EFFECTS

The active agents include essential oil, resin, angelic acid, umbelliferon.

The effects are unclear; and sedative effect has not been proven

INDICATIONS AND USAGE

Indian Medicine: Sumbul root is used for states of debility, asthma, bronchitis, pneumonia, dysmenorrhea, diarrhea, hypertension and excessive excitability

Homeopathic Uses: Ferula sumbul is used to treat nervous cardiac symptoms.

PRECAUTIONS AND ADVERSE REACTIONS

No health hazards or side effects are known in conjunction with the proper administration of designated therapeutic dosages.

DOSAGE

Mode of Administration: Sumbul is used as liquid extract or tincture.

LITERATURE

Kern W, List PH, Hörhammer L (Hrsg.), Hagers Handbuch der Pharmazeutischen Praxis, 4. Aufl., Bde. 1-8: Springer Verlag Berlin, Heidelberg, New York, 1969.

Madaus G, Lehrbuch der Biologischen Arzneimittel, Bde 1-3, Nachdruck, Georg Olms Verlag Hildesheim 1979.

Summer Savory

Satureja hortensis

DESCRIPTION

Medicinal Parts: The medicinal part is the fresh or dried plant harvested during the flowering stage.

Flower and Fruit: The lilac or whitish labiate flowers are in axillary, 5-blossomed, false whorls. The calyx is tubular-campanulate, regular, and has 5 tips. The corolla does not have a ring of hair. The upper lip is straight and margined. The lower lip has 3 divisions and is red-spotted at the mouth of the tube.

Leaves, Stem and Root: The herb grows 30 to 45 cm in height with erect, heavily branched, and shortly pubescent stems. The leaves are crossed opposite, up to 3 cm long, short-petioled, lanceolate to linear-lanceolate and entire-margined. They are rather thick with a ciliate margin and are glandular punctate on both surfaces.

Characteristics: Summer Savory has a spicy scent and a taste that is spicy and peppery.

Habitat: The plant is indigenous to southern Europe and northern Africa, and is extensively cultivated elsewhere.

Production: Summer Savory is the aerial part of Satureja hortensis.

Other Names: Bean Herb, Savory

ACTIONS AND PHARMACOLOGY

COMPOUNDS

Volatile oil (0.2-3.0%): chief components carvacrol (30%), p-cymene (20-30%), alpha-thujene, alpha-pinene, beta-myrcene, alpha- and beta-terpinene, beta-caryophyllene, thymol

Caffeic acid derivatives: rosmarinic acid (0.2 to 1.3%), chlorogenic acid

EFFECTS

The tannin content of the drug provides astringent qualities. Summer Savory also has a mild antiseptic effect due to the presence of cymol and carvacrol in the essential oil. An aqueous extract of the herb has antiviral properties.

INDICATIONS AND USAGE

Unproven Uses: Savory is used for acute gastrointestinal enteritis.

PRECAUTIONS AND ADVERSE REACTIONS

No health hazards or side effects are known in conjunction with the proper administration of designated therapeutic dosages.

DOSAGE

Mode of Administration: The drug is used internally as an infusion that is prepared from ground plant.

Daily Dosage: Three teaspoonfuls of the drug can be taken daily in the form of a hot tea. To prepare the tea, do not boil but leave the drug to steep in scalding hot water.

LITERATURE

Herisset A et al., (1974) Plant Med Phytother 8(4):306, 287.

Kern W, List PH, Hörhammer L (Hrsg.), Hagers Handbuch der Pharmazeutischen Praxis, 4. Aufl., Bde 1-8: Springer Verlag Berlin, Heidelberg, New York, 1969.

Leung AY: Encyclopedia of Common Natural Ingredients Used in Food, Drugs, Cosmetics, John Wiley & Sons Inc., New York 1980.

Madaus G: Lehrbuch der Biologischen Arzneimittel, Bde 1-3, Nachdruck, Georg Olms Verlag Hildesheim 1979.

Opdyke DLJ (1976) Food Cosmet Toxicol: 14.

Zani F et al., Studies on the genotoxic properties of essential oils with Bacillus subtilis rec-assay and Salmonella/microsome reversion assay. Planta Med, 57:237-41, 1991 Jun

Sundew

Drosera ramentacea

DESCRIPTION

Medicinal Parts: The medicinal part is the whole herb.

Flower and Fruit: Size: The plant is from 7 to 20 cm tall. The flowers are white and arranged in racemes turned to one side. There are 5 sepals, 5 petals and 1 ovary with 3 to 5 styles. The fruit is capsular.

Leaves, Stem and Root: The leaves are basal rosette, long-petioled and thickly covered in red glandular hairs. The thickened ends have a drop of viscid juice to trap insects.

Characteristics: The herb has a sour, bitter, hot taste.

Habitat: Europe, India, China, North and South America, on wet and peat ground.

Production: Sundew consists of the dried, above- and below-ground parts of Drosera ramentacea.

Not to be Confused With: Asian varieties.

Other Names: Dew Plant, Lustwort, Youthwort, Red Rot

ACTIONS AND PHARMACOLOGY

COMPOUNDS

Naphthaquinone derivatives:

If the source is Drosera rotundifolia: plumbagin, ramentaceone

If the source is Drosera ramentacea: ramentone, ramentaceone, biramentaceone, plumbagin

If the source is Drosera madagascariensis: 7-methyl juglone, plumbagin

If the source is Drosera peltata: plumbagin, droserone, 8-hydroxydroserone

EFFECTS

The drug has secretolytic, broncho-spasmolytic, and antitussive effects.

The pharmacological mode of action can be traced to 1, 4 naphtoquinone and plumbagin. Plumbagin showed an antiphlogistic effect in vitro through the inhibition of prostaglandin synthesis and an antimicrobial and cytostatic effect in animal experiments.

A possible immune-stimulant effect is the subject of recent studies, the results of which are not yet available.

INDICATIONS AND USAGE

Approved By Commission E:

■ Cough/Bronchitis

Sundew is used for respiratory problems, particularly for coughing fits and dry coughs.

Unproven Uses: In folk medicine, Sundew is used for asthma and warts.

PRECAUTIONS AND ADVERSE REACTIONS

Health risks or side effects following the proper administration of designated therapeutic dosages are not recorded.

DOSAGE

Mode of Administration: Liquid and solid preparations for external and internal application. The plant is a protected species and is in danger of extinction.

Preparation: To prepare an infusion, pour boiling water over 1 to 2 gm drug and strain after 10 minutes.

Daily Dosage: The average daily dose is 3 gm drug. The dosage of the infusion when used as a broncholytic is 1 cup, 3 to 4 times daily.

LITERATURE

Ayuga C et al., (1985) An R Acad Farm 51(2):321.

Budzianowski J et al., Ellagic acid derivatives and further naphthoquinones from Dionea muscipula and four species of the genus Drosera in vitro cultures. In: PM 59(7)54. 1993.

Croft S et al., (1985) Ann Trop Med Parasitol 79(6):651.

Franz G, Workshop über Sonnentaukraut. In: DAZ 135(47):4431-4433. 1995.

Krenn L, Länger R, Kopp B, DAZ 135:867. 1995.

Langer R, Kopp B, Qualitätsprüfung von Sonnentaukraut. In: DAZ 135(8):657-664. 1995.

Schilcher H, Elzer M, Drosera - der Sonnentau, ein bewährtes Antitussivum. In: ZPT 14(1):50. 1993.

Vichnanova SA et al., (1973) Planta Med (Suppl):185.

Wunderer H, Zentral und peripher wirksame Antitussiva: eine kritische Übersicht. In: PZ 142(11):847-852. 1997.

Zenk MH, Fürbringer M, Steglich W, PH 8:2199. 1969.

Further information in:

Kern W, List PH, Hörhammer L (Hrsg.), Hagers Handbuch der Pharmazeutischen Praxis, 4. Aufl., Bde 1-8, Springer Verlag Berlin, Heidelberg, New York, 1969.

Madaus G, Lehrbuch der Biologischen Arzneimittel, Bde 1-3, Nachdruck, Georg Olms Verlag Hildesheim 1979.

Teuscher E, Biogene Arzneimittel, 5. Aufl., Wiss. Verlagsges. mbH Stuttgart 1997.

Thomson RH, Naturally Occurring Quinones, 2nd Ed., Academic Press New York 1971.

Wichtl M (Hrsg.), Teedrogen, 4. Aufl., Wiss. Verlagsges. Stuttgart 1997.

Sunflower

Helianthus annuus

DESCRIPTION

Medicinal Parts: The medicinal parts of the plant are the ray florets, the leaves, the ripe fruit, the oil extracted from the seeds and the mature flower heads.

Flower and Fruit: The very large, composite flowers are solitary or in small clusters, usually nodding, and 10 to 40 cm wide on the stems. The bracts in a number of rows are leaf-like, ovate, acute and sparsely bristly. The 20 to 70 asexual, linguiform golden-yellow ray florets are 3 to 10 cm long and 1 to 3 cm wide. The numerous tubular disc florets are androgynous. They may be brown, purple or yellow, with black or purple anthers. There are small 3-pointed paleas on the base of the capitula. The fruit is compressed at the sides, obovate to almost wedge-shaped; it is an achaene. It is densely appressed, downy and whitish, straw yellow or gray to black.

Leaves, Stem and Root: The sunflower is a 1 to 3 m high annual plant with a long primary root and numerous lateral roots. The stem is erect, branchless or branched higher up, densely covered in hairs, and filled with thin white pith. The leaves are alternate, cordate-triangular, long-petioled, irregularly crenately serrate and covered with short bristles on both sides.

Habitat: Helianthus annuus is indigenous to central and eastern North America and is cultivated worldwide.

Production: Sunflower oil is the fatty oil of the achenes of Helianthus annuus, which is recovered from the fruits, excluding the shell, by cold pressing. The ray florets and leaves are collected at the beginning of the flowering season.

Other Names: Corona Solis, Marigold of Peru

ACTIONS AND PHARMACOLOGY

COMPOUNDS: SUNFLOWER OIL

Triglycerides: chief fatty acids linoleic acid (35-62%), oleic acid (25-42%), palmitic acid (4-7%)

Steroids: Sterols including campesterol, cholesterol, beta-sitosterol

EFFECTS: SUNFLOWER OIL

Useful as a dietary supplement.

INDICATIONS AND USAGE

SUNFLOWER OIL

Sunflower oil is used internally to alleviate constipation (as a lubricant). It is used externally as massage oil, for poorly healing wounds (as an oil dressing) and in the treatment of skin lesions, psoriasis and rheumatism. Sufficient information on the efficacy of the drug is not available.

PRECAUTIONS AND ADVERSE REACTIONS

SUNFLOWER OIL

Health risks or side effects following the proper administration of designated therapeutic dosages are not recorded.

DOSAGE

SUNFLOWER OIL

Mode of Administration: In folk medicine, the drug is mainly for external use. In other areas, it is used as an inactive ingredient in pharmaceutical preparations.

Storage: Keep protected from light, in tightly sealed containers. Oils from different deliveries should not be mixed.

LITERATURE

Bader G, Streich S, Gründemann E, Flatau S, Hiller K, Enzymatic degradation of the triterpenoid saponin helianthoside 2. Pharmazie, 52:836-8, 1997 Nov.

Grotjohann N, Janning A, Eising R, In vitro photoinactivation of catalase isoforms from cotyledons of sunflower (Helianthus annuus L.). Arch Biochem Biophys, 346:208-18, 1997 Oct 15.

Hänsel R, Keller K, Rimpler H, Schneider G (Hrsg.), Hagers Handbuch der Pharmazeutischen Praxis, 5. Aufl., Bde 4-6 (Drogen), Springer Verlag Berlin, Heidelberg, New York, 1992-1994.

Huesa Lope J et al., Grasas Aceites 25:350-353, 1974.

Madaus G, Lehrbuch der Biologischen Arzneimittel, Bde 1-3, Nachdruck, Georg Olms Verlag Hildesheim 1979.

Matsumoto T, Nagakawa M, Itoh T, PH 23:921-923. 1984.

Plohmann B, Bader G, Hiller K, Franz G, Immunomodulatory and antitumoral effects of triterpenoid saponins. Pharmazie, 52:953-7, 1997 Dec.

Teuscher E, Biogene Arzneimittel, 5. Aufl., Wiss. Verlagsges. mbH Stuttgart 1997.

Surinam Cherry

Eugenia uniflora

DESCRIPTION

Medicinal Parts: The medicinal parts are the bark of the plant's main stem, the leaves and its fruit.

Flower and Fruit: The flowers are radial, in clusters of 1 to 8. The sepals are fused; the calyx has 4 or 5 points and a tube approximately 1.5 mm long. The sepals are ovate-elliptical, revolute and up to 4 mm long. The 4 or 5 petals are white, elongate-ovate and 8 to 12 mm long. There are numerous very conspicuous stamens. The ovary is an inferior coenocarp. The fruit is a red, juicy berry with 8 vertical grooves and a diameter of 1 to 3 cm; it is usually 1-seeded.

Leaves, Stem and Root: The plant grows as a shrub or low evergreen tree, which reaches a height of 3 to 10 m. The leaves are opposite, 2.5 to 7 cm long and 1.5 to 4.5 cm wide, short-petiolate, elliptical-ovate, blunt-tipped, slightly cordate at the base, entire, densely and translucently punctate. The trunk is slim (about the thickness of an arm), the bark is smooth and light brown.

Characteristics: The plant produces a shiny red, cherry-sized vitamin-rich fruit, whose strongly acidic taste is like that of a nectarine.

Habitat: The plant grows abundantly in the tropics, especially in Brazil, Uruguay and Paraguay.

Production: Surinam Cherries are the fresh fruit of Eugenia uniflora, and Surinam Cherry leaves are the dried leaves of the same plant.

ACTIONS AND PHARMACOLOGY

COMPOUNDS: SURINAM CHERRY LEAVES

Volatile oil (0.2 to 1%): composition very dependent on the variety.

Components of an African variety include: furanodien (20%), selina-1,3,7(11)-trien-8-one (17%), oxidoselina-1,3,7(11)-trien-8-one (14%), in addition to caryophyllene, germacrene B, germacrene D, cis- and trans-ocimene, beta-selinene, spathulenol and viridiflorol

In a South American variety, the chief components include carvone, pulegone, nerolidol, limonene and verbenone, flavonoids: including quercitrin, myricitrin, and tannins.

EFFECTS: SURINAM CHERRY LEAVES

The flavonoids quercitrin and myricitrin contained in the drug have an inhibiting effect on the xanthine oxidase; the essential oil exhibits antimicrobial and antimycotic effect. A possible protective effect in relation to hyperlipidemia has been proposed. The drug may also exhibit astringent effects due to tannins and flavonoids whose identities have not yet been determined.

COMPOUNDS: SURINAM CHERRY FRUIT

Volatile oil: components including isofuranodiene, germacrene B, selina-4(14),7(11)-diene

Monosaccharides/oligosaccharides (6%): L-fructose, D-glucose, saccharose

Carotinoids: including lycopine, gamma-carotine, beta-cryptoxanthine

Fatty oil (in the seeds and the pulp)

Fruit acids: citric acid (2%)

EFFECTS: SURINAM CHERRY FRUIT

The fruit contains vitamin C, tannins and citric acid, which explain its use as a dietetic. The essential oil of the fruit is said to have an antimicrobial effect.

INDICATIONS AND USAGE

SURINAM CHERRY LEAVES

Unproven uses: Folk medicine practices include use of the bark as an astringent in the treatment of diarrhea, gout, fever, hypertension, gastrointestinal complaint, edema and eye infections. The leaves have been made into a tea and as a component of a distilled oil, used for treating chronic inflammation of the mucous membranes of the respiratory organs, primarily rhinitis.

SURINAM CHERRY FRUIT

Unproven Uses: Folk medicine includes use as a dietetic, but efficacy for that use has not yet been proven.

PRECAUTIONS AND ADVERSE REACTIONS

No health hazards are known in conjunction with the proper administration of designated therapeutic dosages of either drug.

DOSAGE

There is no information in the literature.

LITERATURE

Hänsel R, Keller K, Rimpler H, Schneider G (Ed.), Hagers Handbuch der Pharmazeutischen Praxis, 5. Aufl., Bde 4 - 6 (Drogen), Springer Verlag Berlin, Heidelberg, New York, 1992-1994.

Wazlawik E, Da Silva MA, Peters RR, Correia JF, Farias MR, Calixto JB, Ribeiro-Do-Valle RM, Analysis of the role of nitric oxide in the relaxant effect of the crude extract and fractions from Eugenia uniflora in the rat thoracic aorta. J Pharm Pharmacol, 49:433-7, 1997 Apr.

Swamp Milkweed

Asclepias incarnata

DESCRIPTION

Medicinal Parts: The medicinal parts are the rhizome with roots.

Flower and Fruit: The flowers are reddish-purple. They are located on terminal umbels in clusters of 2 to 6 on a 5 cm long peduncle. The umbels consist of 10 to 20 small florets. The fruit is a long pod.

Leaves, Stem and Root: The herbaceous plant is up to 80 cm high. The stem is erect and smooth. The upper part of the stem is branched and very leafy. The leaves are opposite, petiolate, oblong, lanceolate, hairy, acute and cordate at the base. They are 10 to 18 cm long, 2.5 to 5 cm wide and sharp-edged. The rhizome is about 2 to 3 cm in diameter, yellowish-brown, irregularly globular or oblong, hard and knotty. The rhizome is covered with a thin, tough bark and is surrounded by light brown rootlets that are about 10 cm long.

Characteristics: The taste is sweetish, acrid and bitter. The plant's roots exude latex that is typical of the genus (and giving rise to the name Milkweed,) which is slightly acrid and has a strong odor that decreases on drying.

Habitat: Swamp Milkweed is indigenous to America, Canada and Asia.

Other Names: Swamp Silkweed, Rose-Colored Silkweed

ACTIONS AND PHARMACOLOGY

COMPOUNDS

Cardioactive steroids (cardenolids): including asclepiadin

EFFECTS

The root is said to contain asclepiadin (cardiac glycoside), which is positively inotropic and emetic.

INDICATIONS AND USAGE

Unproven Uses: Similar to other Asclepiadaceae, Swamp Milkweed is mainly used for digestive disorders.

Homeopathic Uses: The main importance of medicinal use of the American varieties is in homeopathy, but further details are not available.

PRECAUTIONS AND ADVERSE REACTIONS

No health hazards or side effects are known in conjunction with the proper administration of designated therapeutic dosages. The drug has an emetic effect in higher dosages, and digitalis-like poisonings are possible due to the cardioactive steroid content. For possible symptoms and treatments for poisonings, see Digitalis folium.

LITERATURE

Kern W, List PH, Hörhammer L (Hrsg.), Hagers Handbuch der Pharmazeutischen Praxis, 4. Aufl., Bde. 1-8, Springer Verlag Berlin, Heidelberg, New York, 1969.

Sweet Cicely

Myrrhis odorata

DESCRIPTION

Medicinal Parts: The medicinal parts of the plant are the entire herb and the seeds.

Flower and Fruit: The white flowers appear in early summer. The complex umbels are flattened on top, many-rayed and more cyme-like at the end of the branches. The rays of the androgynous flowers are covered in thick down. The pedicles of the male flowers are hollow. In the flowering season, the umbels are erect and closed. The fruit is elongate-pyramid-shaped, 2 to 2.5 cm long, compressed at the sides and brown to glossy black.

Leaves, Stem and Root: The plant is a perennial with a thick, gnarled, brown, branched and polycephalous rhizome. The stem is erect, 50 to 120 cm high, cane-like and, higher up, is glabrous or villous and branched. The nodes are covered in long, fine hairs. The 2- to 4-pinnatisect leaves are large, soft, triangular and covered underneath with short, soft bristles.

Characteristics: The leaves smell like garden lovage and taste like anise.

Habitat: The herb is found in mountainous regions from the Pyrenees to the Caucasus and is cultivated elsewhere.

Production: Sweet Cicely root and herb are the whole plant of Myrrhis odorata.

Other Names: Sweet Chervil, Sweet Bracken, Sweet-Fern, Sweet-Cus, Sweet-Humlock, Sweets, The Roman Plant, Shepherd's Needle, British Myrrh

ACTIONS AND PHARMACOLOGY

COMPOUNDS

Volatile oil: chief components are trans-anethole, additionally germacrene-D, anisaldehyde, limonene, chavicolmethyl ether, beta-caryophyllene, alpha-pinene, alpha-farnesene, myrcene. Also, in the roots, trans-isoosmorhizol.

Flavonoids: apigenine-7-O-glucoside, luteolin-7-O-glucoside

EFFECTS

The drug is said to be a carminative, digestive and expectorant.

INDICATIONS AND USAGE

Unproven Uses: The herb is used as a blood purifier and an expectorant, as well as for asthma and other breathing difficulties. Balms and salves made from it are used to treat fresh wounds and sores and relieve the pains of gout.

The roots are used to treat chest and throat complaints and also urinary complaints. The fresh herb is used externally for gout swelling and indurations. Previous folk medicine uses also included use of a decoction from the roots for snake and dog bites.

PRECAUTIONS AND ADVERSE REACTIONS

No health hazards or side effects are known in conjunction with the proper administration of designated therapeutic dosages.

DOSAGE

Mode of Administration: Ground root is used to make tonics and infusions for internal and external use. Salves are used externally.

LITERATURE

Hegnauer R, Chemotaxonomie der Pflanzen, Bde 1-11, Birkhäuser Verlag Basel, Boston, Berlin 1962-1997.

Kern W, List PH, Hörhammer L (Hrsg.), Hagers Handbuch der Pharmazeutischen Praxis, 4. Aufl., Bde. 1-8, Springer Verlag Berlin, Heidelberg, New York, 1969.

Sweet Clover

Melilotus officinalis

DESCRIPTION

Medicinal Parts: The medicinal part is the flowering herb.

Flower and Fruit: The small yellow flowers are in many-blossomed, long-peduncled racemes. The standard and wings are the same length, but longer than the carina. Of the 10 stamens, 9 are fused. The fruit is an obtuse, glabrous, light brown to black, thorny-tipped, horizontally wrinkled and usually one-seeded pod.

Leaves, Stem and Root: The plant is perennial and 60 to 120 cm high. The smooth ascending or decumbent stems are heavily branched. The leaves are alternate, glabrous, trifoliate and long petioled. The leaflets are obovate and dentate. The stipules are awl-like bristly.

Characteristics: The plant has a fragrance similar to woodruff or hay.

Habitat: The plant is found all over Europe, Australia and North America, as well as in temperate regions of Asia.

Production: Sweet Clover consists of the dried or fresh leaf and flowering branches of Melilotus officinalis, and/or Melilotus altissimus.

Other Names: Melilot, King's Clover, Yellow Sweet Clover, Hay Flowers, Sweet Lucerne, Wild Laburnum, Hart's Tree

ACTIONS AND PHARMACOLOGY

COMPOUNDS: IN THE FRESH PLANT

Coumarinic acids glycosides: including melilotoside

COMPOUNDS: IN THE DEHYDRATED DRUG

Free coumarin (0.4-0.9%): formed from the coumarinic acids during dehydration, furthermore 3,4-dihydrocoumarin, melilotol, melilotin

Hydroxycoumarins: including among others umbelliferone, scopoletin, herniarin, fraxidin

Flavonoids: including, among others, kampferol- and quercetin glycosides

Triterpene saponins: including azuki saponin-V-carboxylate, azuki saponin II, aglycones soya sapogenols B and E, melilotigenin

Volatile oil: traces of very complex composition

COMPOUNDS: IN THE SEEDS

Canavanin

Trigonelline

EFFECTS

The drug has an antiphlogistic, antiexudative and anti-edematous effect, which explain its use for inflammatory and congestive edema. It increases venous reflux and improves lymphatic kinetics.

Animal experiments showed an increase in healing wounds.

INDICATIONS AND USAGE

Approved by Commission E:

- Blunt injuries
- Hemorrhoids
- Venous conditions

The drug is used internally for problems arising from chronic venous insufficiency, such as pain and heaviness in legs, night cramps in the legs, itching and swelling; for the supportive treatment of thrombophlebitis, postthrombotic syndromes, hemorrhoids and lymphatic congestion. Externally, the drug is used for contusions, sprains and superficial effusions of blood.

Unproven Uses: In folk medicine, Sweet Clover is used as a diuretic.

PRECAUTIONS AND ADVERSE REACTIONS

No health hazards or side effects are known in conjunction with the proper administration of designated therapeutic dosages. Administration of the drug in higher dosages can lead to headache and stupor, transitory liver damage is possible for a very small number of particularly susceptible patients. Elevation of liver enzyme values usually disappears following discontinuance of the drug. (Monitoring of the liver enzyme values is recommended.)

DOSAGE

Mode of Administration: Comminuted drug for infusions and other galenic preparations for oral use; liquid forms of medication for parenteral application; ointments, liniments, cataplasms and herbal sachets for external use; ointments and suppositories for rectal use.

Preparation: To prepare an infusion, pour boiling water over 1 to 2 teaspoonfuls of comminuted, cut drug, then strain after 5 to 10 minutes.

Daily Dosage: The average daily dose of the herb or preparation in amounts corresponding to 3 to 30 mg of coumarin; parenteral application corresponding to 1.0 to 7.5 mg of coumarin.

Infusion — As a therapy for varicose veins, 2 to 3 cups daily.

External — As a poultice for hemorrhoids.

Storage - The drug must be stored away from light in sealed containers to prevent loss of coumarin.

LITERATURE

Abou-Donia AHA, (1976) Ph. D. Thesis, Faculty of Pharmacy, University of Alexandria, Egypt.

Bos R et al., Analysis of coumarin in Melilotus officinalis. In: PM 61(Abstracts of 43rd Ann Congr):68. 1995.

Földi M, Kovach AGB, Varga L, Zoltan ÖT, Die Wirkung des Melilotus-Präparates Esberiven R auf die Lymphströmung. In: Ärztl Forsch 16:99. 1962.

Földi M, Zoltán ÖT, Obál F, Experimentelle lymphostatische Encephalopathie als Folgeerscheinung einer cervikalen . Lymphangiothrombophlebitis und deren Therapie mit Cumarin aus Melilotus officinalis. In: Arzneim Forsch 20:1626-1628. 1970.

Földi-Börcsök E, Bedall FK, Rahlfs VW, Die antiphlogistische und ödemhemmende Wirkung von Cumarin aus Melilotus officinalis. In: Arzneim Forsch 21:2025-2030. 1971.

Hammouda FM, Rizk AM, Seif EL-Nazar MM, Abou-Youssef AA, Ghaleb HA, Madkour MK, Pholand AE, Wood G, Flavonoids and coumarins from elilotus. In: Fitotherapia 54(6):249-255. 1983.

Hong ND et al., (1983) Korean J Pharmacognosy 14(2):51.

Johne HO, Experimentelle und klinische Untersuchung mit dem Melilotuspräparat Esberiven. In: Ärztl Forsch 14:473-474. 1960.

Marshall M, Wüstenberg P, Klinik und Therapie der chronischen enösen Insuffizienz. In: Klinik und Therapie der chronischen venösen Insuffizienz, Braun Fachverlage, Karlsruhe 1994.

Mislin H, Die Wirkung von Cumarin aus Melilotus officinalis auf die Funktion des Lymphangioms. In: Arzneim Forsch 21:852-853. 1971.

Plouvier V, (1963) Compt Rend 257:4061.

Wüstenberg, P, Baumann G, Verdacht der Toxizität von Cumarin nicht bestätigt. In: PZ 139(13):1058. 1994.

Further information in:

Kern W, List PH, Hörhammer L (Hrsg.), Hagers Handbuch der Pharmazeutischen Praxis, 4. Aufl., Bde 1-8, Springer Verlag Berlin, Heidelberg, New York, 1969.

Madaus G, Lehrbuch der Biologischen Arzneimittel, Bde 1-3, Nachdruck, Georg Olms Verlag Hildesheim 1979.

Roth L, Daunderer M, Kormann K, Giftpflanzen, Pflanzengifte, 4. Aufl., Ecomed Fachverlag Landsberg Lech 1993.

Steinegger E, Hänsel R, Pharmakognosie, 5. Aufl., Springer Verlag Heidelberg 1992.

Teuscher E, Lindequist U, Biogene Gifte - Biologie, Chemie, Pharmakologie, 2. Aufl., Fischer Verlag Stuttgart 1994.

Teuscher E, Biogene Arzneimittel, 5. Aufl., Wiss. Verlagsges. Stuttgart 1997.

Wagner H, Wiesenauer M, Phytotherapie. Phytopharmaka und pflanzliche Homöopathika, Fischer-Verlag, Stuttgart, Jena, New York 1995.

Wichtl M (Hrsg.), Teedrogen, 4. Aufl., Wiss. Verlagsges. Stuttgart 1997.

Sweet Gale

Myrica gale

DESCRIPTION

Medicinal Parts: The medicinal parts are the leaves and branches as well as the wax extracted from the catkins.

Flower and Fruit: Sweet Gale plants are either male or female. The male plants produce groups of stemless catkins on the leafless branches of the previous year's growth. The fruit catkins are about the same size but somewhat thicker and grow in closely packed resinous nutlets. They are dry and compressed.

Leaves, Stem and Root: The plant is usually dioecious, but plants may change sex from year to year. Sweet Gale is a deciduous shrub up to 2.5 m high. The branches have scattered yellowish glands. The leaves are 2 to 6 cm long, almost lanceolate, cuneate at the base and more or less serrate near the apex. They are pubescent beneath with shiny yellow, fragrant glands on both surfaces.

Characteristics: The branches and leaves are fragrant when bruised.

Habitat: Sweet Gale is indigenous to the higher latitudes of the northern hemisphere.

Production: Sweet Gale is the aerial part of Myrica gale.

Other Names: Bog Myrtle, Dutch Myrtle, Bayberry

ACTIONS AND PHARMACOLOGY

COMPOUNDS

Volatile oil (0.4-0.7%): including among others alpha-pinene, delta-cadinene, gamma-cadinene, limonene, beta-myrcene, alpha-phellandrene, beta-phellandrene, 1,8-cineole, nerolidol, p-cymene, alpha-copaene, beta-caryophyllene

Flavonoids: including myricitrin

Triterpenes: including ursolic acid, oleanolic acid

EFFECTS

Sweet Gale has an astringent and aromatic effect.

INDICATIONS AND USAGE

Unproven Uses: Sweet Gale has been used in digestive disorders. A strong brew of dried bark is also used in Sweden as a vermifuge and to cure itching.

PRECAUTIONS AND ADVERSE REACTIONS

The volatile oil of the drug is considered toxic. Mixing plant extracts with beer, as practiced in the Middle Ages, is said to have led to manic episodes.

DOSAGE

Mode of Administration: The drug is ground. Information on preparations is not available.

LITERATURE

Hegnauer R, Chemotaxonomie der Pflanzen, Bde 1-11, Birkhäuser Verlag Basel, Boston, Berlin 1962-1997.

Kern W, List PH, Hörhammer L (Hrsg.), Hagers Handbuch der Pharmazeutischen Praxis, 4. Aufl., Bde. 1-8, Springer Verlag Berlin, Heidelberg, New York, 1969.

Malteru KE, Faegri A, (1982) Acta Pharm Suec 19: 43

Roth L, Daunderer M, Kormann K, Giftpflanzen, Pflanzengifte, 4. Aufl., Ecomed Fachverlag Landsberg Lech 1993.

Von Schantz M, Kapétanidis I, Qualitative und qunatitative Untersuchung des ätherischen Öls von Myrica gale L. (Myricaceae). In: Pharm Acta Helv 46(10/11):649. 1071.

Sweet Marjoram

Origanum majorana

DESCRIPTION

Medicinal Parts: The medicinal parts of the plant are the leaves and flowers, the fresh aerial parts of the flowering plant and the whole of the fresh, flowering plant.

Flower and Fruit: The inconspicuous, sessile flowers barely extend above the gray tomentose bracts surrounding them. The calyx appears to have only 1 sepal because the 2 lower sepals are almost non-existent and the upper 3 are completely fused. The calyx is 2.5 cm long and otherwise resembles the bracts. The corolla is white to pale lilac or pink, 4 mm long, with a few uneven, pointed tips. The 2 upper tips are fused together to form a lip. The stamens are enclosed in the corolla or extend above it. The fruit is a smooth, light brown nutlet, 0.75 to 1 mm long.

Leaves, Stem and Root: The plant is biennial with a main shoot that is heavily branched. It grows 20 to 25 cm high. The downy to tomentose shoots are gray-green to whitish, and sometimes tinged with red. The leaves are spatulate, short-petioled, 0.5 to 2 cm long and 0.5 to 1 cm wide, entire-margined and rounded. They are gray-tomentose on both surfaces, somewhat thick and usually without distinct ribs. The false whorls are mostly covered by the 3 to 4 wide, circular, gray-green bracts, which are fused to globular, racemous or panicled capitula.

Characteristics: The plant has a distinctive tangy odor and a bitter taste.

Habitat: The plant is indigenous to the southeastern Mediterranean region and is cultivated in Germany.

Production: Marjoram herb consists of the dried leaf and flower of Origanum majorana (synonymous with Majorana hortensis), gathered during the flowering season and stripped off the stems. Drying must be fast to avoid blackening of the leaves. Marjoram oil consists of the essential oil of Origanum majorana obtained by aqueous steam distillation of the fresh or dried leaves and flowers stripped from the stems and harvested during flowering season. Depending on the area of cultivation, there may be two crops of the aerial plant parts per year.

ACTIONS AND PHARMACOLOGY

COMPOUNDS: MARJORAM HERB

Chief components in the volatile oil of the foliage: cis-sabinene hydrate (40 to 50%), cis-sabinene hydrate acetate (20 to 30%), sabinene (10%) and trans-sabinene hydrate (2%); cis-sabinene hydrate acetate transforms itself with steam distillation into (among others) terpinene-4-ol (in volatile oil yielded through steam distillation, 15 to 40%), gamma-terpinene (in volatile oil yielded through steam distillation, 2 to 12%), alpha-terpinene, limonene and terpinols, that leads to change of aroma

COMPOUNDS: MARJORAM OIL

Volatile oil (1 to 3%)

Flavonoids: including diosmetin, luteolin, apigenin and their C- and O-glycosides, including vitexin, orientin, thymonine

Hhydroquinone glycosides: including arbutin (0.15 to 0.45%), methyl arbutin

Caffeic acid derivatives: rosmarinic acid, chlorogenic acid

Water soluble polysaccharides (13%)

Triterpenes: including ursolic acid (0.5%), oleanolic acid (0.2%)

EFFECTS: MARJORAM HERB AND OIL

In vitro, Marjoram is antimicrobial, antiviral and insecticidal.

INDICATIONS AND USAGE

Unproven Uses: The herb is used for rhinitis and colds in infants, rhinitis in small children and gastritis. In folk medicine, Majoram herb and oil are used for cramps, depression, dizziness, gastrointestinal disorders, migraine, nervous headaches, neurasthenia, paralysis, paroxysmal coughs, rhinitis and as a diuretic.

Homeopathic Uses: Homeopathy sometimes uses Marjoram to increase sexual excitability.

PRECAUTIONS AND ADVERSE REACTIONS

General: No health hazards or side effects are known in conjunction with the proper administration of designated therapeutic dosages. The drug is not suitable for longer-term use because of its arbutin content.

Pediatric Use: Marjoram salve should not be administered to infants or small children.

DOSAGE

Mode of Administration: Marjoram herb is used as an infusion for teas, mouthwashes and poultices (5% infusion). The oil is used in ointments and a few compound preparations.

Preparation: To prepare a tea, pour 250 ml boiling water over 1 to 2 teaspoonfuls of Marjoram herb and strain after 5 minutes. An ointment is prepared by leaving 20 parts Marjoram herb to stand with 1 part ammonia and 10 parts spirit of wine for a few hours. It is then heated with 100 parts Vaseline in a water bath until the spirit of wine and ammonia have evaporated. Then the ointment is filtered (EB6).

Daily Dosage: Sip 1 to 2 cups of tea throughout the day.

Homeopathic Dosage: 5 to 10 drops, 1 tablet or 5 to 10 globules 1 to 3 times a day or 1 ml injection solution sc twice weekly (HAB1).

Storage: Dried Marjoram herb may be stored for up to 2 years in air-tight containers.

LITERATURE

Brosche T, Vostrowsky O, Über die Komponenten des ätherischen Öls aus Majorana hortensis

Hänsel R, Keller K, Rimpler H, Schneider G (Hrsg.), Hagers Handbuch der Pharmazeutischen Praxis, 5. Aufl., Bde 4-6 (Drogen), Springer Verlag Berlin, Heidelberg, New York, 1992-1994 (unter Orignum majorana).

Herrmann K, (1962) Lebensm Unters Forsch. 116:224.

Kucera LS, Hermann Jr EC, (1967) Proc Soc Exp Biol Med 124: 865-874.

Leung AY, Encyclopedia of Common Natural Ingredients Used in Food Drugs and Cosmetics, John Wiley & Sons Inc., New York 1980.

Lossner G, (1968) Planta Med 16:54.

Madaus G, Lehrbuch der Biologischen Arzneimittel, Bde 1-3, Nachdruck, Georg Olms Verlag Hildesheim 1979.

Moench, In: Z Naturforsch 36C:23-29. 1981.

Steinegger E, Hänsel R, Pharmakognosie, 5. Aufl., Springer Verlag Heidelberg 1992.

Teuscher E, Biogene Arzneimittel, 5. Aufl., Wiss. Verlagsges. Stuttgart 1997.

Sweet Orange

Citrus sinensis

DESCRIPTION

Medicinal Parts: The medicinal parts are the fresh and dried peel as well as the oil extracted from the peel.

Flower and Fruit: The fragrant flowers are arranged singly or in short, limp racemes. The fruit is depressed-globose to shortly ovoid, 10- to 13-locular. The peel is thin to rather thick, nearly smooth, orange to orange-yellow when ripe. The pulp is sweet. The core remains solid when ripe.

Leaves, Stem and Root: Citrus sinensis is an evergreen tree with rounded crown. The branches are angular when young, then become terete, with a few slender, rather flexible axillary spines. The leaves are acute, rounded below; the petioles are narrowly winged.

Habitat: Like other Citrus varieties, the plant is indigenous to Asia and is cultivated in the Mediterranean and other subtropical regions in many parts of the world.

Production: Orange peel consists of the fresh or dried outer peel of ripe fruits of Citrus sinensis, separated from the white pith layer, as well as its preparations in effective dosage.

Other Names: Orange, China Orange, Citrus dulcis

ACTIONS AND PHARMACOLOGY

COMPOUNDS

Volatile oil: chief components in the fresh pericarp include (+)-limonene, furthermore citral (as an odor-bearer), citronellal, nootkatone, sinesal, n-nonanal, n-decanal, n-dodecanal, linalyl acetate, geranyl acetat, citronellyl acetat, methyl anthranilate. Pressed oils also contain lipophilic flavonoids and furocoumarins.

Flavonoids

EFFECTS

Sweet Orange promotes gastric juice secretion.

INDICATIONS AND USAGE

- Dyspeptic complaints
- Loss of appetite

PRECAUTIONS AND ADVERSE REACTIONS

No health hazards or side effects are known in conjunction with the proper administration of designated therapeutic dosages. There is a low potential for sensitization through skin contact with the volatile oil.

DOSAGE

Mode of Administration: Comminuted herb for teas and other bitter-tasting galenic preparations for oral administration.

Daily Dosage: 10 to 15 gm of drug.

LITERATURE

Ihrig M, Qualitätskontrolle von süβem Orangenschalenöl. In: PZ 140(26):2350-2353. 1995.

Further information in:

Hausen B, Allergiepflanzen, Pflanzenallergene, ecomed Verlagsgesellsch. mbH, Landsberg 1988.

Kern W, List PH, Hörhammer L (Hrsg.), Hagers Handbuch der Pharmazeutischen Praxis, 4. Aufl., Bde. 1-8, Springer Verlag Berlin, Heidelberg, New York, 1969.

Sweet Sumach

Rhus aromatica

DESCRIPTION

Medicinal Parts: The medicinal parts are the dried and fresh root bark.

Flower and Fruit: The flowers are in 1 to 1.5 cm long, false spikes. They are yellow-green and often appear before the leaves are fully developed. The fruit is a globular, yellow-red, pubescent drupe.

Leaves, Stem and Root: The plant is a fragrant 1 to 2.4 m high shrub with glabrous red-brown annual growth and small to 10 cm-long trifoliate leaves. The leaflets are oval and the middle one is cuneate at the base. The leaflets are irregularly dentate and initially pubescent on both sides. Later the leaflets turn glabrous on the upper surface and eventually pubescent only on the ribs of the lower surface.

Habitat: The plant is indigenous to Atlantic North America.

Production: Sweet Sumach root-bark is the root-bark of Rhus aromatica.

Other Names: Polecat-Bush, Smooth, Sumach, Sweet Fragrant Sumach, Sumac

ACTIONS AND PHARMACOLOGY

COMPOUNDS

Phenol glycosides: orcin-O-beta-D-glucoside

Steroids: sterols, including beta-sitosterol, stigmast-7-en-3beta-ole

Tannins

Triterpenes: including oleanolic aldehyde

Volatile oil (0.01 to 0.07%); very complex in mixture, with constituents including delta-cadinene, camphene, delta3-carene, beta-elemene, farnesyl acetone, alpha- and beta-pinene, fatty acids

EFFECTS

The drug has an antimicrobial and antiviral effect due to the tannins (gallic acid). In animal experiments it increased contraction of the smooth muscles of ileum. Two older studies describe an improvement in the symptoms of urinary incontinence.

INDICATIONS AND USAGE

Unproven Uses: In folk medicine Sweet Sumach is used for irritable bladder, urinary incontinence, enuresis nocturna and uterine bleeding.

Homeopathic Uses: Rhus aromatica is used for weak bladder conditions.

PRECAUTIONS AND ADVERSE REACTIONS

No health hazards or side effects are known in conjunction with the proper administration of designated therapeutic dosages.

DOSAGE

Mode of Administration: Sweet Sumach is available in crude powder form and in compounded preparations for oral intake. It is also available in parenteral form for homeopathic use.

Daily Dosage: Single dose is 1 gm.

Bed-wetting—5 to 20 drops depending on age, to be taken 2 to 3 times daily, over an extended period.

Homeopathic Dosage: 5 drops, 1 tablet or 10 globules every 30 to 60 minutes (acute) or 1 to 3 times daily (chronic); parenterally: 1 to 2 ml sc acute: 3 times daily; chronic: once a day (HAB34)

Storage: Should be stored in dry place, protected from direct light.

LITERATURE

Baer H, In: Toxic Plants, Ed. AD Kinghorn, Columbia Press 1979.

Effenberger S, Schilcher H, Gewürzsumachrinde. In: ZPT 11(4):113. 1990.

Schilcher H, Boesel R, Effenberger ST Segebrecht S, Neuere Untersuchungsergebnisse mit aquaretisch, antibakteriell und prostatotrop wirksamen Arzneipflanzen. In: ZPT 10(3):77. 1989.

Further information in:

Hänsel R, Keller K, Rimpler H, Schneider G (Hrsg.), Hagers Handbuch der Pharmazeutischen Praxis, 5. Aufl., Bde 4-6 (Drogen): Springer Verlag Berlin, Heidelberg, New York, 1992-1994.

Madaus G, Lehrbuch der Biologischen Arzneimittel, Bde 1-3, Nachdruck, Georg Olms Verlag Hildesheim 1979.

Sweet Vernal Grass

Anthoxanthum odoratum

DESCRIPTION

Medicinal Parts: The whole plant is considered to have medicinal properties.

Flower and Fruit: The green, solitary, flowered spikelet has 4 spelts, the lower half of which are as large as the upper and taller than the flowers. Both of the upper spelts are awned, with 2 stamens. The style is long, the stigma pinnate, and spikelets form an oblong false ear.

Leaves, Stem and Root: The plant size ranges from 15 to 50 cm. The plant grows as thick grass. The leaves are ciliate at the base of the lamina. The leaf sheath is deeply grooved and hairy.

Characteristics: Sweet Vernal Grass has a scent of dried woodruff or new-mown hay and a tangy taste.

Habitat: The plant is indigenous to Britain, Europe and temperate Asia.

Production: Sweet Vernal Grass is the whole Anthoxanthum odoratum plant in flower.

ACTIONS AND PHARMACOLOGY

COMPOUNDS

Hydroxy cinnamic acid glycosides: in the fresh plant

Melilotoside and coumarin: triggered by a beta-glucosidase during dehydration of the plant

Iridoids: asperuloside, monotropein, scandoside

EFFECTS

No information is available.

INDICATIONS AND USAGE

Unproven Uses: The drug is used for headache, nausea, sleeplessness and conditions of the urinary tract.

PRECAUTIONS AND ADVERSE REACTIONS

The freshly harvested plant contains glycosidic precursors of coumarin, which release coumarin in the process of dehydration (the drug contains up to 1.5% coumarin). No health hazards or side effects are known in conjunction with the proper administration of designated therapeutic dosages.

OVERDOSAGE

The administration of higher levels of the drug can lead to headache and dizziness. Liver injuries are possible among susceptible patients during long-term treatment. The abnormal liver values disappear when the drug is discontinued, but on going observation of liver enzyme values of the blood is recommended.

DOSAGE

Mode of Administration: The drug is used externally as an extract.

LITERATURE

Brown SA, C and J Biochem Physiol 38:143. 1960.

Fentem JH, Fry JR, Thomas NW, Species differences in the hepatotoxicity of coumarin-a comparision of rat and Mongolian gerbil. In: Toxicology 71(1-2):129. 1992.

Further information in:

Kern W, List PH, Hörhammer L (Hrsg.), Hagers Handbuch der Pharmazeutischen Praxis, 4. Aufl., Bde. 1-8, Springer Verlag Berlin, Heidelberg, New York, 1969.

Lewin L, Gifte und Vergiftungen, 6. Aufl., Nachdruck, Haug Verlag, Heidelberg 1992.

Poisonous Plants in Britain and their effects on Animals and Man, Ministry of Agriculture Fisheries and Food, Pub; HMSO (1984) UK.

Roth L, Daunderer M, Kormann K, Giftpflanzen, Pflanzengifte, 4. Aufl., Ecomed Fachverlag Landsberg Lech 1993.

Teuscher E, Lindequist U, Biogene Gifte - Biologie, Chemie, Pharmakologie, 2. Aufl., Fischer Verlag Stuttgart 1994.

Sweet Violet

Viola odorata

DESCRIPTION

Medicinal Parts: The medicinal parts are the essential oil from the leaves, the dried flowers, the air-dried leaves collected during the flowering season, the flowering herb, the dried rhizome, the fresh aerial parts collected during the flowering season and the whole plant.

Flower and Fruit: The dark violet flowers are solitary on 3 to 7 cm long pedicles. The flowers are 1.5 to 2 cm long and fragrant. The 5 sepals are obtuse, glabrous and have an appendage. There are 5 uneven petals, which are unevenly spurred and which have a broad margin. The 5 stamens have an appendage at the tip. The flower has 3 fused ovaries. The fruit is a globular capsule, approximately 7.5 mm. It is 3 to 6 sided, clearly and densely short-pubescent and often violet. It can be found pressed to the receptacle.

Leaves, Stem and Root: The Violet is 5 to 10 cm high. It is a rosette plant with a short, thick but soft ground axis. The rooting runners are 10 to 20 cm long and 1.5 mm thick. They produce flowers in the second year. The shoots are a strong dark green with scattered appressed hairs or almost glabrous. The leaves are petiolate, broadly cordate, obtuse or short-acuminate and crenate. The leaves, which appear first, are reniform-cordate and the younger ones are rolled up. There are lanceolate stipules at the base of the leaves.

Characteristics: The plant is strongly scented.

Habitat: The plant is indigenous to or naturalized in large parts of Europe and the Middle East as far as central Asia; it is also found in North America.

Production: Sweet Violet root consists of the dried root of Viola odorata. Sweet Violet herb is the dried plant section of Viola odorata. The rhizome is imported from the former Czechoslovakia and Romania. The rootstock is dug up, pounded to remove any soil residue, washed and air-dried.

Other Names: Garden Violet

ACTIONS AND PHARMACOLOGY

COMPOUNDS: SWEET VIOLET RHIZOME AND HERB

Volatile oil (0.04%): salicylic acid methyl ester (formed out of glycosidic precursors during plant drying), beta-nitropropionic acid

Saponins

Alkaloids

EFFECTS: SWEET VIOLET RHIZOME AND HERB

The drug acts as an expectorant due to its saponin content. The alkaloid violin has an emetine-like effect.

COMPOUNDS: SWEET VIOLET FLOWER

Volatile oil (0.003%): aroma-carrier trans-alpha-ionone (parmone), chief constituents (-)-zingiberene, (+)-curcumene, dihydro-beta-ionone, 2,6-nonadien-1-al, undecan-2-one, isoborneol

EFFECTS: SWEET VIOLET FLOWER

The drug has antimicrobial and broncho-secretolytic effects due to the saponin content.

INDICATIONS AND USAGE

SWEET VIOLET RHIZOME AND HERB

Unproven Uses: The rhizome is used for conditions of the respiratory organs, particularly for dry catarrh and rheumatism of the minor joints; it is additionally used for fever, skin diseases, inflammation of the oral mucosa, nervous strain, headache and insomnia.

The herb is used internally for coughs, hoarseness, pneumonia, throat inflammations, bronchitis accompanied by fixed mucous, nervous strain, insomnia and hysteria. It is also used to induce sweating. Externally, the herb is used to treat various skin diseases.

SWEET VIOLET FLOWER

Unproven Uses: The flowers are used to prepare an infusion tea, which is used as an expectorant for bronchial catarrh; as an antitussive for chronic bronchitis; and for whooping cough, asthma and migraine. Sweet Violet syrup is used as an expectorant and to lessen irritation for bronchial catarrh (children's remedy).

Homeopathic Uses: The flowers are used for inflammation of the respiratory tract and rheumatism of the wrist.

PRECAUTIONS AND ADVERSE REACTIONS

SWEET VIOLET RHIZOME, HERB, AND FLOWER

No health hazards or side effects are known in conjunction with the proper administration of designated therapeutic dosages.

DOSAGE

SWEET VIOLET RHIZOME AND HERB

Preparation: An herbal tea is prepared by adding 2 teaspoonfuls Sweet Violet herb with 1/4 liter water.

Daily Dosage: The average single dose of the rhizome is 1 gm orally. The 5% rhizome decoction dosage is 20 gm. The 5% rhizome infusion dosage is 1 dessertspoonful 5 to 6 times daily. The herbal tea dosage is 1 cup 2 to 3 times daily.

SWEET VIOLET FLOWER

Preparation: To prepare an infusion, decoction or tea, use 1 heaping teaspoonful of drug with 1 cup of water.

Daily Dosage: The dosage for the infusion, decoction or tea is 1 cup twice daily, or taken in sips 1 to 2 times per hour.

The dosage of Sweet Violet syrup is 1 to 2 dessertspoonfuls every 2 hours.

Homeopathic Dosage: 5 drops, 1 tablet or 10 globules every 30 to 60 minutes (acute) or 1 to 3 times daily (chronic); parenterally: 1 to 2 ml sc, acute: 3 times daily; chronic: once a day (HAB34).

LITERATURE

SWEET VIOLET RHIZOME AND HERB

Farnsworth NR, (1968) Lloydia 246.

Hänsel R, Keller K, Rimpler H, Schneider G (Hrsg.), Hagers Handbuch der Pharmazeutischen Praxis, 5. Aufl., Bde 4-6 (Drogen): Springer Verlag Berlin, Heidelberg, New York, 1992-1994.

Madaus G, Lehrbuch der Biologischen Arzneimittel, Bde 1-3, Nachdruck, Georg Olms Verlag Hildesheim 1979.

Watt JM, Breyer-Brandwijk MG, The Medicinal, Poisonous Plants of Southern, Eastern Africa, 2nd Ed, Livingstone 1962.

Willaman JJ, Hui-Li L, (1970) Lloydia 33 (3A):1.

SWEET VIOLET FLOWER

Farnsworth NR, (1968) Lloydia 246.

Roberg M, Arch Pharm 275,145. 1937.

Ruzicka L, Schinz H, Helv Chim Acta 25:760. 1942.

Uhde G et al., Helv Chim Acta 55:2621. 1972.

Willaman JJ, Hui-Li L, (1970) Lloydia 33 (3A):1.

Further information in:

Hänsel R, Keller K, Rimpler H, Schneider G (Hrsg.), Hagers Handbuch der Pharmazeutischen Praxis, 5. Aufl., Bde 4-6 (Drogen): Springer Verlag Berlin, Heidelberg, New York, 1992-1994.

Madaus G, Lehrbuch der Biologischen Arzneimittel, Bde 1-3, Nachdruck, Georg Olms Verlag Hildesheim 1979.

Watt JM, Breyer-Brandwijk MG, The Medicinal, Poisonous Plants of Southern, Eastern Africa, 2nd Ed, Livingstone 1962.

Sweet Woodruff

Galium odoratum

DESCRIPTION

Medicinal Parts: The medicinal parts are the dried or fresh aerial parts collected during or shortly before the flowering season.

Flower and Fruit: The flowers are in loose terminal cymes. The petals are fused to a funnel-shaped, white, 1.5 mm long tube. The border of the tube is divided in 4 and is 2 to 3.5 mm long. The 4 stamens are fused with the corolla. The involucre bracts are small, lanceolate or almost bristle-like. The 2-seeded indehiscent fruit is globular, 2 to 3 mm long and thickly covered with white barbed bristles.

Leaves, Stem and Root: Sweet Woodruff is a 10 to 35 cm herbaceous perennial with a thin cylindrical circular rhizome. The stem is erect, quadrangular, smooth and, apart from the bristly nodes, glabrous and glossy. The leaves are in false whorls of 6 to 9, the lower ones are obovate-oblong, the middle and upper ones are lanceolate to oblong-lanceolate. They are entire-margined, thorny tipped, glabrous and rough-edged.

Characteristics: Sweet Woodruff is aromatic when dried; the taste is bitter and tangy.

Habitat: The plant grows in northern and central Europe, Siberian and northern Africa.

Production: Sweet Woodruff herb is the fresh or dried aerial part of Galium odoratum. It is gathered during or shortly before flowering. The herb must be turned regularly while being dried.

Not to be Confused With: Gallium mollugo or Gallium sylvaticum

Other Names: Master of the Wood, Woodwrad, Woodruff

ACTIONS AND PHARMACOLOGY

COMPOUNDS: IN THE FRESH PLANT

O-hydroxycinnamic acid glucoside: melilotoside

COMPOUNDS: IN THE DRIED PLANT

Coumarin (0.4-1%)

Iridoids: asperuloside (0.05-0.3%), monotropein (0.04%), scandoside

EFFECTS

The coumarin content may impart antiphlogistic, antiedematic, spasmolytic and lymphokinetic properties. However, due to the low level of coumarin, the therapeutic effect is doubtful.

INDICATIONS AND USAGE

Unproven Uses: Sweet Woodruff is used as a treatment for nervous agitation, sleeplessness, nervous menstrual disorders, congested liver, jaundice, hemorrhoids, circulation disorders and venous conditions.

PRECAUTIONS AND ADVERSE REACTIONS

The freshly harvested plant contains melilotoside as glycosidic precursor of coumarins. In the process of dehydration, coumarin is released (content up to 1% coumarin in freshly dried drug). Health risks or side effects following the proper administration of designated therapeutic dosages are not recorded. Headache and stupor can occur with the administration of higher dosages of the drug. Susceptible patients could experience liver damage following long-term administration. This effect is reversible following discontinuation of the drug. Liver enzyme values should be monitored.

DOSAGE

Mode of Administration: The herb is obsolete as a drug in many countries, and since 1981 is not allowed to be used in the manufacture of aroma or flavoring in German-speaking countries.

Preparation: To make a tea, place 2 teaspoonfuls (1.8 gm drug) in one glass water. An infusion of 5% drug is used for insomnia, and a forehead poultice made of crushed herb is used for headache.

Daily Dosage: The average single dose is 1.0 gm drug. The preparations can be taken during the day or shortly before going to bed.

Storage: The drug should be protected from light sources to avoid brown coloring.

LITERATURE

Anonym, Cumarin (1,2-b-Benzopyron) - Neue Erkenntnisse zur Tumortherapie. In: Med Welt 45(5):62-63. 1994.

Anonym, Leberschäden durch Cumarin? In: DAZ 134(15):1372. 1994.

Berkowitz WF et al., (1982) J Org Chem 47:824.

Böjthe-Horvath K et al., PH 21:2917-2919. 1982.

Burnett AR, Thomsom RH, (1968) J Clin Soc (6):854.

Casley-Smith JR, Casley-Smith JR, Effects of varying doses of 7-hydroxy-coumarin and coumarin in acute lymphoedema and other high-protein oedemas. In: Progress in Lymphology, X, Adelaide, 1985: 194-196. 1985.

Cox D, O'Kennedy R, Thornes RD, The rarity of liver toxicity in patients treated with coumarine (1,2-Benzopyrone). In: Human Toxikol 8:501-506. 1989.

Egan D, O'Kennedy R, Moran E, Cox D, Prosser E, Thornes RD, The pharmacology, metabolism, analysis, and applications of coumarin and coumarin-related compounds. In: Drug Metabolism Reviews 22(5):503-529. 1990.

Ellinger A, Zur pharmako-dynamischen Charakterisierung des Cumarins. In: Schmiedebergs Arch exp Pathol Pharmakol Suppl. Festschrift, S.150-163. 1908.

Fentem JH, Fry JR, Thomas NW, Species differences in the hepatotoxicity of coumarin - a comparision of rat and Mongolian gerbil. In: Toxicology 71(1-2):129. 1992.

Hardt TJ, Ritschel WA, The effect of coumarin and 7-hydroxycoumarin on in vitro macrophage phagocytosis of latex particles. In: Methods Find Exp Clin Pharmacol 5(1):39-43. 1983.

Hausen BM, Schmieder M, The sensitizing capacity of coumarins. In: Contact Dermatitis 15(3):157-163. 1986.

Hazleton LW, Tusing TW, Zeitlin BR, Thiesen R, Murer HK, Toxicity of coumarin. In: J Pharmacol Exp Ther 116:348-358. 1956.

Inouye H et al., (1974) Planta Med 25:285.

Kooiman P, Acta Bot Neerl 18:124-137. 1966.

Laub E, Olszowski W, Woller R, Waldmeister und Maibowle. Pharmazeutisch und lebensmittelchemische Aspekte. In: Dtsch Apoth Ztg 125:848-850. 1985.

Mascolo N et al., (1987) Phytother Res 1 (1):28.

Rosskopf F, Kraus J, Franz G, Immunological and antitumor effects of coumarin and some derivatives. In: PA 47(2):139-142. 1992.

Sporn A, Toxicity of coumarin as a flavoring agent. In: Igenia (Bucharest)9:121-126. 1960.

Sticher O et al., (1971) Dtsch Apoth Ztg 111:1795.

Wüstenberg, P, Baumann G, Verdacht der Toxizität von Cumarin nicht bestätigt. In: PZ 139(13):1058. 1994.

Further information in:

Frohne D, Pfänder HJ: Giftpflanzen - Ein Handbuch für Apotheker, Toxikologen und Biologen, 4. Aufl., Wiss. Verlagsges. mbH Stuttgart 1997.

Hänsel R, Keller K, Rimpler H, Schneider G (Hrsg.), Hagers Handbuch der Pharmazeutischen Praxis, 5. Aufl., Bde 4-6 (Drogen), Springer Verlag Berlin, Heidelberg, New York, 1992-1994.

Leung AY, Encyclopedia of Common Natural Ingredients Used in Food Drugs and Cosmetics, John Wiley & Sons Inc., New York 1980.

Madaus G, Lehrbuch der Biologischen Arzneimittel, Bde 1-3, Nachdruck, Georg Olms Verlag Hildesheim 1979.

Roth L, Daunderer M, Kormann K, Giftpflanzen, Pflanzengifte, 4. Aufl., Ecomed Fachverlag Landsberg Lech 1993.

Steinegger E, Hänsel R, Pharmakognosie, 5. Aufl., Springer Verlag Heidelberg 1992.

Teuscher E, Lindequist U, Biogene Gifte - Biologie, Chemie, Pharmakologie, 2. Aufl., Fischer Verlag Stuttgart 1994.

Teuscher E, Biogene Arzneimittel, 5. Aufl., Wiss. Verlagsges. mbH Stuttgart 1997.

Swertia chirata

See Chiretta

Swertia japonica

See Senburi

Symphytum officinale

See Comfrey

Symplocarpus foetidus

See Skunk Cabbage

Syzygium aromaticum

See Clove

Syzygium cumini

See Jambolan

Tamarind

Tamarindus indica

DESCRIPTION

Medicinal Parts: The medicinal parts are the fruit pulp and the dried seeds.

Flower and Fruit: The flowers form a terminal raceme and have three, 1 cm long petals which are initially whitish, then yellowish with light-red stripes. They have a calyx with a narrow, top-shaped base and 4 thickly covered segments. The stamens are fused in a sheath, which is open at the top. The fruit is a 20 cm long and 3 cm wide, matt-brown, slightly compressed, indehiscent, bean-like pod. The fruit has 3 to 12 seeds that are very hard and glossy brown. The seeds are 14 mm long and have an irregular, roundish-quadrangular shape. The mesocarp is odorless, mushy and sweet-tasting.

Habitat: The plant is indigenous to tropical Africa and is naturalized in North and South America from Florida to Brazil. It is cultivated in subtropical China, India, Pakistan, Indochina, on the Phillippines and in Java and Spain.

Production: Tamarind paste is derived from the fruit of Tamarindus indica. The fruit is fermented for a long time in the sun. The initially red-brown fruit attains a black or black-brown hue and becomes more aromatic and sour. The paste is boiled to a glutinous mass, which is the finished product.

Other Names: Imlee

ACTIONS AND PHARMACOLOGY

COMPOUNDS

Fruit acids: tartaric acid (3-10%); including among others, malic acid, citric acid, lactic acid

Invert sugar (25-30%)

Pectin

Pyrazines and thiazols (aromatic substances)

EFFECTS

The drug, which contains organic acids and pectine, is said to be laxative; however, the mode of action has not been documented.

INDICATIONS AND USAGE

Unproven Uses: The drug is used for chronic or acute constipation and liver and gallbladder ailments.

Indian Medicine: The drug is used for bilious vomiting, alcohol intoxication, fever, pharyngitis, stomatitis, constipation and hemorrhoids.

Homeopathic Uses: Tamarindus indica is used for stomachaches.

PRECAUTIONS AND ADVERSE REACTIONS

No health hazards or side effects are known in conjunction with the proper administration of designated therapeutic dosages.

DOSAGE

Mode of Administration: Tamarind is taken orally and is usually used in combination with other laxatives, such as figs.

Preparation: To make a clean paste, soften the raw tamarind paste in hot water, strain through a sieve, and steam to a soft consistency in a water bath; mix the paste with sugar.

Daily Dosage: 10 to 50 gm of cleaned tamarind paste, pure or with other purgatives, is taken in fruit cubes.

Homeopathic Dosage: 5 drops, 1 tablet or 10 globules, every 30 to 60 minutes (acute) or 1 to 3 times daily (chronic); parenterally: 1 to 2 ml sc, acute: 3 times daily; chronic: once a day (HAB34).

Storage: Store in a tightly sealed container.

LITERATURE

Hänsel R, Keller K, Rimpler H, Schneider G (Hrsg.), Hagers Handbuch der Pharmazeutischen Praxis, 5. Aufl., Bde 4-6 (Drogen): Springer Verlag Berlin, Heidelberg, New York, 1992-1994.

Ishola MM et al., J Sci Food Agric 51:141. 1990.

Khurana AL, Ho CT, J Liq Chromatogr 12:419-430. 1989.

Lee PL et al., (1975) J Agric Food Chem 23:1195.

Leung AY, Encyclopedia of Common Natural Ingredients Used in Food Drugs, Cosmetics, John Wiley & Sons Inc., New York 1980.

Madaus G, Lehrbuch der Biologischen Arzneimittel, Bde 1-3, Nachdruck, Georg Olms Verlag Hildesheim 1979.

Steinegger E, Hänsel R, Pharmakognosie, 5. Aufl., Springer Verlag Heidelberg 1992.

Teuscher E, Biogene Arzneimittel, 5. Aufl., Wiss. Verlagsges. Stuttgart 1997.

Tamarindus indica

See Tamarind

Tamus communis

See Black Bryony

Tanacetum parthenium

See Feverfew

Tanacetum vulgare

See Tansy

Tansy

Tanacetum vulgare

DESCRIPTION

Medicinal Parts: The medicinal part consists of the dried flowering herb.

Flower and Fruit: The inflorescences are flat, round and button-like composite flowers in cymes. The bright golden yellow flowers consist only of tubular flowers. The fruit has 5 ribs without tufts of hair.

Leaves, Stem and Root: The plants grow from 60 to 120 cm high. The stem is erect, glabrous, angular, red-tinged and leafy. The leaves are alternate, simple or double pinnatifid, 15 cm long and 12 cm wide and have a long emarginate tip.

Characteristics: The herb has a strong aromatic smell. The taste is bitter and camphor-like. The plant is poisonous.

Habitat: The plant is indigenous to Europe.

Production: Tansy flower consists of the inflorescence of Chrysanthemum vulgare (syn. Tanacetum vulgare). Tansy herb consists of the above-ground parts of Chrysanthemum vulgare (syn. Tanacetum vulgare). Tansy oil is the oil extracted from Tanacetum vulgare.

Other Names: Buttons, Daisy, Hindheal, Parsley Fern

ACTIONS AND PHARMACOLOGY

COMPOUNDS: TANSY FLOWER AND HERB

Volatile oil (0.5 to 0.9% in the foliage, 0.8 to 1.8% in the blossoms): constituents of the volatile oil vary greatly according to variety. The following could appear as main constituents: artemisia ketone, (-)-thujone, (+)-isothujone, 1,8-cineole, alpha-pinene, alpha-terpinyl acetate, borneol, bornyl acetate, davanone, germacrene D, L-camphor (+) umbellulone, camphor, lyratol (+) lyratol acetate, piperitone, sabinene, thuj-4-en-2-ylacetate (+) trans-Carveyl acetate, trans-chrysanthenol (+) trans-chrysanthenyl acetate, umbellulone, as well as (+)-vulgarol A (8%), vulgaron B (up to 12%). Hybrid varieties exist.

Sesquiterpenes: sesquiterpene lactones, including crispolid, deacetyl crispolid, tatridins A and B, tavulin, artemorin, parthenolide (in some varieties), reynosine, armefoline, dentatin A, santamarin, chrysanthemine

Flavonoids: including cosmosiin, apigenin-7-O-glycoside, cynaroside, luteolin-7-O-glucoside, quercimetrin, eupatilin, acacetin-7-glucobioside

Hydroxycoumarins: including scopoletin

Polyynes: including diterthiophene, triterthiophene (phototoxic)

EFFECTS: TANSY FLOWER AND HERB

The oil, which contains thujone, is an insect repellent. The sesquiterpenes in the leaves are antimicrobial. A leaf extract has displayed an anti-edemic effect, and the polysaccharide fraction is said to have an ulcer-protective effect in rats.

COMPOUNDS: TANSY OIL

Constituents of the volatile oil vary greatly according to variety. The following could appear as chief constituents: artemisia ketone, (-)-thujone, (+)-isothujone, 1,8-cineole, alpha-pinene, alpha-terpinyl acetate, borneol, bornyl acetate, davanone, germacrene D, L-camphor (+) umbellulone, L-camphor, lyratol (+) lyratol acetate, piperitone, sabinene, thuj-4-en-2-ylacetate (+) trans-carvyl acetate, trans-chrysanthenol (+) trans-chrysanthenyl acetate, umbellulone, among others. Hybrid varieties exist.

EFFECTS: TANSY OIL

The thujone-type oil is antimicrobial, anthelmintic, and repellent to various insects.

INDICATIONS AND USAGE

TANSY FLOWER AND HERB

Unproven Uses: Tansy preparations are used as an anthelmintic, for migraine, neuralgia, rheumatism, bloating and loss of appetite.

TANSY OIL

Unproven Uses: Tansy oil is used internally for gout, rheumatic complaints, joint pains, stomach cramps, gastrointestinal infections, intermittent fever, dizziness and dysmenorrhea. It is used externally for rheumatism, gout, contusions, sprains and wounds.

CONTRAINDICATIONS

The drug should not be used during pregnancy.

PRECAUTIONS AND ADVERSE REACTIONS

TANSY FLOWER AND HERB

The administration of therapeutic dosages of drugs that have a high thujone content (see Tanaceti aetheroleum) can lead to poisoning. Beyond that, there is a medium potential for sensitization via skin contact with the drug. Internal administration of the drug in allopathic dosages is to be avoided.

TANSY OIL

Particularly toxic are volatile oils with high thujone content. Poisonings occur chiefly through the misuse of the drug as an abortifacient. Administration in allopathic dosages is to be avoided.

OVERDOSAGE

TANSY OIL

Symptoms of poisoning include vomiting, abdominal pain, gastroenteritis, severe reddening of the face, mydriasis, fixed pupil, tonic-clonic spasms, cardiac arrhythmias, uterine bleeding, kidney damage and liver damage. Death occurs after 1 to 3.5 hours. The lethal dosage is approximately 15-30 gm. The treatment for poisonings can only proceed symptomatically.

DOSAGE

TANSY FLOWER AND HERB

Daily Dosage: Administration in allopathic dosages is to be avoided.

TANSY OIL

Mode of Administration: The drug is found in extract form in a small number of combination preparations.

Daily Dosage: Administration in allopathic dosages is to be avoided. The documented single dose is 0.1 gm.

LITERATURE

TANSY FLOWER AND HERB

Banthorpe DV et al., (1973) Planta Med 23:64.

Brown AMG et al., Tissue culture, biochemistry and pharmacology of Tanacetum ssp. In: PM 62, Abstracts of the 44th Ann Congress of GA, 33. 1996.

Hendriks H, Bos R, Woerdenbag, Der Rainfarn - eine potentielle Arzneipflanze? In: ZPT 14(6):333. 1993.

Holopainen M, (1968) Planta Med (6):20P.

Nano GM et al., (1983) Fitoterapia (4):135.

Ognyanov I, Tochorova M, (1983) Planta Med 48:181.

Schearer WR, (1984) J Nat Prod 47(6):964.

Frohne D, Pfänder HJ, Giftpflanzen - Ein Handbuch für Apotheker, Toxikologen und Biologen, 4. Aufl., Wiss. Verlagsges. mbH Stuttgart 1997.

Hausen B, Allergiepflanzen, Pflanzenallergene, ecomed Verlagsgesellsch. mbH, Landsberg 1988.

Kern W, List PH, Hörhammer L (Hrsg.), Hagers Handbuch der Pharmazeutischen Praxis, 4. Aufl., Bde. 1-8, Springer Verlag Berlin, Heidelberg, New York, 1969.

Lewin L, Gifte und Vergiftungen, 6. Aufl., Nachdruck, Haug Verlag, Heidelberg 1992.

Madaus G, Lehrbuch der Biologischen Arzneimittel, Bde 1-3, Nachdruck, Georg Olms Verlag Hildesheim 1979.

Roth L, Daunderer M, Kormann K, Giftpflanzen, Pflanzengifte, 4. Aufl., Ecomed Fachverlag Landsberg Lech 1993.

Teuscher E, Lindequist U, Biogene Gifte - Biologie, Chemie, Pharmakologie, 2. Aufl., Fischer Verlag Stuttgart 1994.

TANSY OIL

Banthorpe DV et al., (1973) Planta Med 23:64.

Brown AMG et al., Tissue culture, biochemistry and pharmacology of Tanacetum ssp. In: PM 62, Abstracts of the 44th Ann Congress of GA, 33. 1996.

Hendriks H, Bos R, Woerdenbag, Der Rainfarn - eine potentielle Arzneipflanze? In: ZPT 14(6):333. 1993.

Holopainen M, (1968) Planta Med (6):20P.

Nano GM et al., (1983) Fitoterapia (4):135.

Ognyanov I, Tochorova M, (1983) Planta Med 48:181.

Schearer WR, (1984) J Nat Prod 47(6):964.

Further information in:

Frohne D, Pfänder HJ, Giftpflanzen - Ein Handbuch für Apotheker, Toxikologen und Biologen, 4. Aufl., Wiss. Verlagsges. mbH Stuttgart 1997.

Hausen B, Allergiepflanzen, Pflanzenallergene, ecomed Verlagsgesellsch. mbH, Landsberg 1988.

Kern W, List PH, Hörhammer L (Hrsg.), Hagers Handbuch der Pharmazeutischen Praxis, 4. Aufl., Bde. 1-8, Springer Verlag Berlin, Heidelberg, New York, 1969.

Lewin L, Gifte und Vergiftungen, 6. Aufl., Nachdruck, Haug Verlag, Heidelberg 1992.

Madaus G, Lehrbuch der Biologischen Arzneimittel, Bde 1-3, Nachdruck, Georg Olms Verlag Hildesheim 1979.

Roth L, Daunderer M, Kormann K, Giftpflanzen, Pflanzengifte, 4. Aufl., Ecomed Fachverlag Landsberg Lech 1993.

Teuscher E, Lindequist U, Biogene Gifte - Biologie, Chemie, Pharmakologie, 2. Aufl., Fischer Verlag Stuttgart 1994.

Taraxacum officinale

See Dandelion

Taumelloolch

Lolium temulentum

DESCRIPTION

Medicinal Parts: The medicinal parts are the ripe seeds.

Flower and Fruit: The spikes are uninterrupted, 30 cm long and green. The 5 to 7 spikelets form the ear. The glume is longer than the spikelet, which has 7 ribs and no awn. The husk is cartilaginous, with 5 ribs and a stiff, straight awn.

Leaves, Stem and Root: The stalk is rigid and erect. The leaf sheaths are rough and weakly bulbous on the upper leaves.

Characteristics: The spikelets have their narrow sides turned toward the main axis (in contrast to the couch grass). A parasitic fungus, which is often present on the plant, forms an alkaloid, making the plant poisonous.

Habitat: The plant grows in Europe and Mediterranean regions.

Production: Taumelloolch seeds are the ripe seeds of Lolium temulentum.

Other Names: Bearded Darnel, Cheat, Drake, Ray-Grass, Tare

ACTIONS AND PHARMACOLOGY

COMPOUNDS

The active ingredients are not known. However, the toxicity of Lolium rigidum is caused by bacterial toxins, the so-called kidney toxins, which are unusual nucleosides with uracil as the base.

EFFECTS

The active agents are temulentin, temulentic acid, free fatty acids, tannin and glycosides. The fruit has been suspected of poisoning for some time; however, the toxic principle generally remains unexplained. The drug's ability to relieve gastroenteritis can possibly be attributed to the free fatty acids.

INDICATIONS AND USAGE

Unproven Uses: Taumelloolch is used for dizziness, nerve pain, nose bleeds, sleeplessness, stomach cramps and urinary incontinence.

PRECAUTIONS AND ADVERSE REACTIONS

The drug can be toxic. In earlier times, poisonings were frequently caused by the presence of the plant's berries in grain. No cases of poisoning are known in recent times. The plant has now become extremely rare through intensive seed-corn purification.

OVERDOSAGE

Symptoms of poisoning include dizziness, headache, colic, confusion, staggering, vision and speech disorders, somnolence, and, in rare cases, death through respiratory failure. The treatment of poisoning consists of gastrointestinal emptying (inducement of vomiting, gastric lavage with burgundy-colored potassium permanganate solution, sodium sulphate), administration of activated charcoal and shock prophylaxis (quiet, warmth). Further management consists of treating spasms with careful administration of diazepam (i.v.) and icepacks for fever. Phenothiazines and analeptics should not be administered. Intubation and oxygen therapy may be required.

DOSAGE

Mode of Administration: The plant is administered ground and as a liquid extract.

LITERATURE

Frohne D, Pfänder HJ, Giftpflanzen - Ein Handbuch für Apotheker, Toxikologen und Biologen, 4. Aufl., Wiss. Verlags-Ges Stuttgart 1997.

Kern W, List PH, Hörhammer L, (Hrsg.), Hagers Handbuch der Pharmazeutischen Praxis, 4. Aufl., Bde 1-8, Springer Verlag Berlin, Heidelberg, New York, 1969.

Lewin L, Gifte und Vergiftungen, 6. Aufl., Nachdruck, Haug Verlag, Heidelberg 1992.

Madaus G, Lehrbuch der Biologischen Arzneimittel, Bde 1-3, Nachdruck, Georg Olms Verlag Hildesheim 1979.

Roth L, Daunderer M, Kormann K, Giftpflanzen, Pflanzengifte, 4. Aufl., Ecomed Fachverlag Landsberg Lech 1993.

Teuscher E, Lindequist U, Biogene Gifte - Biologie, Chemie, Pharmakologie, 2. Aufl., Fischer Verlag Stuttgart 1994.

Taxus baccata

See Yew

Tea Tree

Melaleuca alternifolia

DESCRIPTION

Medicinal Parts: The medicinal parts of the plant are the leaves and branch tips from which an oil is extracted by steam distillation.

Flower and Fruit: The inflorescence is a 3 to 5 cm long spike. The flowers are sessile with a campanulate epicalyx on which the sepals sit like tips. The tips are 3 to 4 mm long. The petals are free, approximately twice as large as the calyx tips. There are numerous conspicuous stamens, in 5 bundles approximately 2 cm long. The ovary is inferior and partially fused with the hollow receptacle. It is in 3 parts with a thick pistil and a capitular stigma. The fruit is a woody, cylindrical capsule with a diameter of 3 to 4 mm.

Leaves, Stem and Root: This tree reaches heights up to 7 m. The leaves are simple, coriaceous, 1 to 2.5 cm long, acute-lanceolate, and sometimes slightly sickle-shaped with oil glands. The young shoots are tomentose, the older branches glabrous. The trunk has a paper-like, whitish bark.

Habitat: Melaleuca alternifolia is indigenous to Australia.

Production: Tea tree oil is the essential oil extracted from the leaves and branch tips of Melaleuca alternifolia, Melaleuca dissitifolia and other Melaleuca species by aqueous steam distillation. Ideally, the leaves and shoots have first been stored for six weeks.

ACTIONS AND PHARMACOLOGY

COMPOUNDS

Terpinenes: Primarily terpinene-4-ol (45%), gamma-terpinene (18%), alpha-terpinene (8%), 1.8-cineole (6%), alpha-terpineol (5%), as well as alpha-pinene, limonene, p-cymol, terpinolene, viridiflorene

EFFECTS

The terpenes present in the essential oil exhibit efficacy that is antimicrobial, possibly antiviral and weakly antimycotic.

INDICATIONS AND USAGE

Tea Tree Oil is used for conditions of the respiratory tract and for skin conditions. It is also used as a disinfectant. The oil's administration against acne has been demonstrated in at least one clinical test.

Unproven Uses: Folk medicine internal uses have included tonsillitis, pharyngitis, colitis and sinusitis. Externally, Tea Tree Oil is used for ulcers of the oral mucous membrane, gingivitis, root canal treatment, mycosis of the nail, skin infections, ulcers, burns and insect bites.

PRECAUTIONS AND ADVERSE REACTIONS

No health hazards are known in conjunction with the proper administration of designated therapeutic dosages.

OVERDOSAGE

In several cases involving children, overdosage (10 ml for a child) led to coordination weakness and a state of confusion. A very high dosage (70 ml) led to coma.

DOSAGE

Mode of Administration: Preparations of the oil are used internally and externally.

Storage: Store tightly sealed and protected from light.

LITERATURE

Blaschek W, Hänsel R, Keller K, Reichling J, Rimpler G, Schneider G (Eds), Hagers Handbuch der Pharmazeutischen Praxis. Folgebände 1 und 2. Drogen A-Z. Springer. Berlin, Heidelberg 1998.

Carson CF, Cookson BD, Farrelly HD, Riley TV, Susceptibility of methicillin-resistant Staphylococcus aureus to the essential oil of Melaleuca alternifolia. J Antimicrob Chemother, 35:421-4, 1995 Mar.

Carson CF, Hammer KA, Riley TV, Broth micro-dilution method for determining the susceptibility of Escherichia coli and Staphylococcus aureus to the essential oil of Melaleuca alternifolia (tea tree oil). Microbios, 82:181-5, 1995.

Carson CF, Riley TV, Antimicrobial activity of the major components of the essential oil of Melaleuca alternifolia. J Appl Bacteriol, 78:264-9, 1995 Mar.

Carson CF, Riley TV, In-vitro activity of the essential oil of Melaleuca alternifolia against Streptococcus. spp letter J Antimicrob Chemother, 78:1177-8, 1996 Jun.

Carson CF, Riley TV, Toxicity of the essential oil of Melaleuca alternifolia or tea tree oil. letter; comment. J Toxicol Clin Toxicol, 33:193-4, 1995.

Hammer KA, Carson CF, Riley TV, Susceptibility of transient and commensal skin flora to the essential oil of Melaleuca alternifolia (tea tree oil). Am J Infect Control, 24:186-9, 1996 Jun.

Nenoff P, Haustein UF, Brandt W, Antifungal activity of the essential oil of Melaleuca alternifolia (tea tree oil) against pathogenic fungi in vitro. Skin Pharmacol, 9:388-94, 1996.

Teazle

Dipsacus silvestris

DESCRIPTION

Medicinal Parts: The medicinal part is the whole flowering plant with root.

Flower and Fruit: The flowers are lilac with 8 cm long, cylindrical capitula. The bracts are lanceolate-awl-shaped, curved upward, thorny and longer than the capitulum. The outer bracts with their straight, flexible, thorny tips are longer than the flowers. The calyx is basin-shaped, and the corolla is fused with 4 tips. There are 4 stamens and 1 inferior ovary. The fruit is a nutlet.

Leaves, Stem and Root: The plant is a biennial that grows 80 to 150 cm high. The stem is erect, angular and thorny. The basal leaves are rosette-like, crenate-serrate. The cauline leaves are oblong with a thorny midrib underneath.

Habitat: With the exception of northern Norway, Sweden and Finland, wild Teazle is grown throughout all of Europe, North Africa and Asia Minor.

Production: Common Teazle root is the underground part of Dipsacus silvestris.

Other Names: Barber's Brush, Brushes and Combs, Card Thistle, Church Broom, Venus' Basin

ACTIONS AND PHARMACOLOGY

COMPOUNDS

Iridoide monoterpenes: including cantleyoside, loganin, sweroside, sylvestroside III and IV

Caffeic acid derivatives: including chlorogenic acid

EFFECTS

No information is available.

INDICATIONS AND USAGE

Unproven Uses: Teazle is used externally for small wounds, fistulae, eczema and as a rub in the treatment of rheumatism.

PRECAUTIONS AND ADVERSE REACTIONS

Health risks or side effects following the proper administration of designated therapeutic dosages are not recorded.

DOSAGE

Mode of Administration: Teazle is used externally in alcoholic extracts.

LITERATURE

Hegnauer R, Chemotaxonomie der Pflanzen, Bde 1-11, Birkhäuser Verlag Basel, Boston, Berlin 1962-1997.

Kern W, List PH, Hörhammer L (Hrsg.), Hagers Handbuch der Pharmazeutischen Praxis, 4. Aufl., Bde. 1-8, Springer Verlag Berlin, Heidelberg, New York, 1969.

Madaus G, Lehrbuch der Biologischen Arzneimittel, Bde 1-3, Nachdruck, Georg Olms Verlag Hildesheim, 1979.

Suh HW, Song DK, Son KH, Wie MB, Lee KH, Jung KY, Do JC, Kim YH, An iridoid glucoside from dipsacus asperoides. Phytochemistry, 27:239-40, 1996 May.

Suh HW, Song DK, Son KH, Wie MB, Lee KH, Jung KY, Do JC, Kim YH, Studies on the chemical constituents of Dipsacus asper Wall. Yao Hsueh Hsueh Pao, 27:1167-72, 1996 Oct.

Zhang Y, Kiyohara H, Matsumoto T, Yamada H, Fractionation and chemical properties of immunomodulating polysaccharides from roots of Dipsacus asperoides. Planta Med, 27:393-9, 1997 Oct.

Terminalia arjuna

See Arjun Tree

Terminalia chebula

See Tropical Almond

Tetraclinis articulata

See Sandarac

Teucrium chamaedrys

See Germander

Teucrium polium

See Poley

Teucrium scordium

See Water Germander

Teucrium scorodonia

See Wood Sage

Theobroma cacao

See Cocoa

Thuja

Thuja occidentalis

DESCRIPTION

Medicinal Parts: The medicinal parts are the oil extracted from the leaves and branch tips, the young dried branches, the fresh, leafy annual branches and the fresh, leafy branches collected in spring.

Flower and Fruit: The male flowers are dark brown, the female flowers are yellow-green. They are monoecious. The male flowers are arranged in small, terminal catkins and the female flowers are almost star-shaped. The ripe cones are brown-yellow, 6 to 8 mm long, ovate and covered in coriaceous, obtuse scales. The lower ones are patent at the tips. The seeds are brown-yellow, 3 to 5 mm long and approximately 1 mm wide. They are narrowly winged the whole way around.

Leaves, Stem and Root: The plant is a narrowly clavate, 12 to 21 m high tree with short horizontally spread branches and red-brown, striped peeling trunk. The trunk is usually branched from the base up. The leaves are scale-like, crossed opposite, imbricate, flattened on the branch side and folded at the margins. They are dark green above and matte-green beneath. The scales on the upper part of the branches have a globular glandular swelling.

Habitat: The plant originated from eastern North America and is found in Europe mainly as an ornamental plant and is partly naturalized.

Production: Thuja herb is the young branch tips and young shoots of Thuja occidentalis. The harvest should take place in spring when the content of the active agents is optimal. The herb should be dried in the shade and handled with care.

Not to be Confused With: Other forms of Thuja.

Other Names: Arborvitae, Hackmatack, Swamp Cedar, Tree of Life, White Cedar

ACTIONS AND PHARMACOLOGY

COMPOUNDS

Water-soluble immunostimulating polysaccharides and glycoproteins

Water-soluble immunostimulating glycoproteins

Volatile oil (1.4-4%): chief components (-)-thujone (alpha-thujone, 59%), (+)-isothujone (beta-thujone, 7-10%), fenchone (10-15%)

Flavonoids: including among others, quercitrin, mearusitrin, the biflavonoids hinoki flavone, amentoflavone, bilobetin-procyanidins

Lignans

Tannins

EFFECTS

The antiviral effect of the drug is attributed to many reasons. The topical use for viral wart growth is plausible. Proliferation of T cells caused by polysaccharides (esp. CD-4 and T-helper/inducer-cells) and an increase in the production of interleukin-2 has been demonstrated.

The essential oil, because of its thujone content, causes spasm and leads in high doses to clonic-tonic convulsions, severe metabolism disturbances through fatty degeneration of the liver, and damage of the renal parenchyma.

INDICATIONS AND USAGE

Unproven Uses: Thuja is used for respiratory tract infections and in conjunction with antibiotics in the treatment of bacterial skin infections and *herpes simplex*. Other possible uses include the treatment of rheumatism, trigeminal neuralgia, strep throat, gout, pruritus, blepharitis, conjunctivitis, otitis media, pertussis, tracheitis, kidney and bladder complaints, enuresis, psoriasis, amenorrhea, and cardiac insufficiency. The drug is used externally as an ointment for treating pains in the joints, arthritis, and muscle rheumatism, as well as infected wounds and burns.

Homeopathic Uses: Thuja occidentalis is used for rheumatism, depressive states, poor digestion, and skin and mucous membrane conditions.

CONTRAINDICATIONS

The drug should not be used during pregnancy.

PRECAUTIONS AND ADVERSE REACTIONS

General: The drug's toxic effect is due to the thujone content. The doses should be strictly followed because of the toxicity of the drug. Allopathic preparations do not contain any thujone.

The toxicological limit, up to which thujone can be administered orally without risk to health, has been established at 1.25 mg/kg body weight. Only poisonings connected with the consumption of the leaves and shoots of fresh plants have been recorded since 1980. In therapeutic dosages of medications, the thujone content is far below the toxicological limit.

Use in Pregnancy: The drug is misused as an abortifacient. Thuja should not be taken during pregnancy.

OVERDOSAGE

Symptoms of poisoning, often seen after misuse of the drug as an abortifacient, include queasiness, vomiting, painful diarrhea, and mucous membrane hemorrhaging. Instances of death have been reported.

Following gastrointestinal emptying (inducement of vomiting, gastric lavage with burgundy-colored potassium permanganate solution, sodium sulphate), administration of activated charcoal, and shock prophylaxis (appropriate body position, quiet, warmth), the treatment for poisoning consists of treating spasms with diazepam (i.v.), colic with atropine, administering electrolytes and treating possible cases of acidosis with sodium bicarbonate infusions. Monitoring of kidney function is essential. Intubation and oxygen respiration may also be necessary.

DOSAGE

Mode of Administration: Whole, cut, and powdered drug is found in compound preparations.

Preparation: To make an extract of 1:1, use 50% ethanol; for an extract of 1:10, use 60% ethanol. To make a tincture, mix 100 parts Thuja powder and 1,000 parts diluted spirit of wine (EB6).

Daily Dosage: The daily dose for the extract is 1 to 2 ml 3 times daily.

Homeopathic Dosage: 5 drops, 1 tablet or 10 globules every 30 to 60 minutes (acute) or 1 to 3 times daily (chronic); parenterally: 1 to 2 ml sc, acute: 3 times daily; chronic: once a day (HAB1).

Storage: Mark the container as ''poisonous'' and protect from light and excessive heat.

LITERATURE

Anonym, Behandlung mit pflanzlichen Immunmodulatoren. In: Symbiose 5(2):9. 1993.

Anonym, Echinacea-Präparate. In: DAZ 136(22):1814-1820. 1996.

Baumann J, Flamme D, Harnischfeger G, DAZ 127:2518-2522. 1987.

Baumann J, Vergleichende pharmakognostisch-phytochemische Untersuchungen an Drogen der Familie der Cupressaceae. In: Diplomarbeit Göttingen. 1987.

Beuscher N, Kopanski L, Purification and biological characterization of antiviral substances from Thuja occidentalis. In: PM 52:555-556. 1986.

Beuscher N, Kopanski L, Reinigung und biologische Charakterisierung von antiviralen Substanzen aus Thuja occidentalis. In: PM 52(6):555-556. 1086.

Beuscher N, Über die medikamentöse Beeinflussung zellulärer Resistenzmechanismen im Tierversuch. Aktivierung von Peritonealmakrophagen der Maus durch pflanzliche Reizkörper. In: Arzneim Forsch 32(I):134-138. 1977.

Beuscher N, Über die medikamentöse Beeinflussung zellulärer Resistenzmechanismen im Tierversuch. III. Steigerung der Leukozytenmobilisation bei der Maus durch pflanzliche Reizkörper. In: Arzneim Forsch 30(I):821-825. 1977.

Gohla S, Dissertation Universität Hamburg. 1988.

Gross G, Papillomvirus-Infektionen der Haut. In: Med Welt 36:437-440. 1985.

Khurana SMP, Effect of homoeopathic drugs on plant viruses. In: PM 20:142-146. 1971.

Sait MA, Garg BR, Indian J Dermatol Vernerol Leprol 51:96-98. 1985.

Schubert W, Die Inhaltsstoffe von Thuja occidentalis. In: Dissertation Technische Universität Braunschweig. 1987.

Tachibana Y et al., Mitogenic activities in african traditional herbal medicines. In: PM 59(4):354. 1993.

Von R, (1961) Can J Chem 39:1200.

Wagner H, Antivirales Prinzip von Thuja aufgeklärt. In: Phytoformum (Medisculab) 1/93:4. 1993.

Zellner J, Arch Pharm 262:381-397. 1924.

Further information in:

Frohne D, Pfänder HJ, Giftpflanzen - Ein Handbuch für Apotheker, Toxikologen und Biologen, 4. Aufl., Wiss. Verlags-Ges. Stuttgart 1997.

Hänsel R, Keller K, Rimpler H, Schneider G (Hrsg.), Hagers Handbuch der Pharmazeutischen Praxis, 5. Aufl., Bde 4-6 (Drogen): Springer Verlag Berlin, Heidelberg, New York, 1992-1994.

Leung AY, Encyclopedia of Common Natural Ingredients Used in Food Drugs, Cosmetics, John Wiley & Sons Inc., New York 1980.

Lewin L, Gifte und Vergiftungen, 6. Aufl., Nachdruck, Haug Verlag, Heidelberg 1992.

Madaus G, Lehrbuch der Biologischen Arzneimittel, Bde 1-3, Nachdruck, Georg Olms Verlag Hildesheim 1979.

Roth L, Daunderer M, Kormann K, Giftpflanzen, Pflanzengifte, 4. Aufl., Ecomed Fachverlag Landsberg Lech 1993.

Steinegger E, Hänsel R, Pharmakognosie, 5. Aufl., Springer Verlag Heidelberg 1992.

Teuscher E, Lindequist U, Biogene Gifte - Biologie, Chemie, Pharmakologie, 2. Aufl., Fischer Verlag Stuttgart 1994.

Teuscher E, Biogene Arzneimittel, 5. Aufl., Wiss. Verlagsges. Stuttgart 1997.

Wagner H, Wiesenauer M, Phytotherapie. Phytopharmaka und pflanzliche Homöopathika, Fischer-Verlag, Stuttgart, Jena, New York 1995.

Thuja occidentalis

See Thuja

Thuja orientalis

See Oriental Arborvitae

Thyme

Thymus vulgaris

TRADE NAMES

Red Thyme and White Thyme, Thyme Herb, Thyme Leaf and Flower

DESCRIPTION

Medicinal Parts: The medicinal parts are the oil extracted from the fresh, flowering herb; the dried leaves; the striped and dried leaves; and the fresh aerial part of the flowering plant.

Flower and Fruit: The blue-violet to bright red labiate flowers are arranged in 3 to 6 blossomed axillary clusters. The calyx is bilabiate with a 3-tipped upper lip and a 2-tipped lower lip. The upper lip of the corolla is straight and the lower lip is divided in 3. The stamens are splayed from the base.

Leaves, Stem and Root: The plant is a dwarf shrub that grows up to 50 cm high with an erect, woody and very branched-bushy and downy stem, which never roots. The leaves are short-petioled, linear or oblong-round, acute, glandular-punctate with an involute margin and a tomentose under surface.

Characteristics: The odor is aromatic and the taste tangy, somewhat bitter and camphor-like.

Habitat: The plant is indigenous to the Mediterranean region and neighboring countries, northern Africa and parts of Asia. It is extensively cultivated.

Production: Thyme consists of the stripped and dried leaves and flowers of Thymus vulgaris, Thymus zygis, or both species.

ACTIONS AND PHARMACOLOGY

COMPOUNDS

Volatile oil (1.0-2.5%): chief components thymol (20-55%), p-cymene (14-45%), carvacrol (1-10%), gamma-terpinene (5-10%), borneol (up to 8%), linalool (up to 8%)

Caffeic acid derivatives: rosmarinic acid (0.15-1.35%)

Flavonoids: including among others, luteolin, apigenin, naringenin, eriodictyol, cirsilineol, salvigenin, cirsimaritin, thymonine, thymusine, partially present as glycosides

Triterpenes: including among others, ursolic acid (1.9%), oleanolic acid (0.6%)

EFFECTS

Thyme is a bronchial antispasmodic, an expectorant, and an antibacterial agent. In animal experiments, a spasmolytic effect was demonstrated for the flavone fraction and an expectorant effect on ciliary activity for the terpenes.

INDICATIONS AND USAGE

Approved by Commission E:

- Cough
- Bronchitis

Unproven Uses: The herb is used internally for catarrh of the upper respiratory tract, dyspeptic complaints, asthma, laryngitis, chronic gastritis and whooping cough. Externally, it is used as a mouthwash and gargle for inflammations of the mouth and throat, pruritus, and dermatoses. It is also used externally for tonsillitis and poorly healing wounds.

PRECAUTIONS AND ADVERSE REACTIONS

No health hazards or side effects are known in conjunction with the proper administration of designated therapeutic dosages. The drug possesses a low potential for sensitization.

DOSAGE

Mode of Administration: Thyme is available as a comminuted drug, powder, liquid extract or dry extract for infusions and other galenic preparations. Liquid and solid medicinal forms for internal and external application are available. Combinations with other herbs, which have expectorant action, are also available. Extracts of the drug are components of standardized preparations of antitussive and cough remedy teas.

How Supplied:

Oil — 100%

Liquid — 1:1, 1:5

Preparation: To prepare a tea, use 1.5 to 2 gm drug with boiling water, steep for 10 minutes, then strain. (1 teaspoonful is equivalent to 1.4 gm drug.) To prepare an infusion, add 1 to 2 gm drug to 150 ml of water. For a bath, add a minimum of 0.004 gm thyme oil to 1 liter of water, filter, then add to bath water drawn at a temperature of 35-38° C. Alternatively, add 500 gm of drug to 4 liters of boiling water, filter, then add to bath water.

Daily Dosage: The recommended daily dosage is 10 gm drug with 0.03% phenol, calculated as thymol. When using a liquid extract, 1 to 2 gm is taken 1 to 3 times daily. The single dose for the infusion is 1.5 gm drug, or 1 to 2 gm drug per cup of water taken several times a day. The dose for the powder is 1 to 4 gm drug twice daily.

The tea can be taken several times a day as needed. A 5% infusion can be used for compresses. Baths should be taken for 10 to 20 minutes.

Storage: Keep the herb in a tightly sealed container, and protect from light and moisture.

LITERATURE

Czygan FC, Hänsel R, Thymian und Quendel - Arznei und Gewürzpflanzen. In: ZPT 14(2):104. 1992.

Haraguchi H et al., Antiperoxidative components in Thymus vulgaris. In: PM 62(3):217-221. 1996.

Hiller K, Pharmazeutische Bewertung ausgewählter Teedrogen. In: DAZ 135(16):1425-1440. 1995.

Kreis P, Juchelka D, Motz C, Mosandl A, Chirale Inhaltstoffe ätherischer Öle. In: DAZ 131(39):1984. 1991.

Messerschmidt W, PM 13:56-72. 1965.

Miguel JD, (1976) J Agric Food Chem 24:833.

Montes GM et al., (1981) An Real Acad Farm 47(3):285.

Schratz E, Hörster H, PM 19:160. 1970.

Sourgens H et al., (1982) Planta Med 45:78.

Svendsen AB, Karlsen J, (1966) Planta Med 14:376.

Vampa G et al., Plantes Med Phytothér 22:195. 1988.

Van den Broucke CO et al., (1983) Pharm Weekbl 5(1):9.

Weiss B, Flück H, Pharm Acta Helv 45:169. 1970.

Further information in:

Hänsel R, Keller K, Rimpler H, Schneider G (Hrsg.), Hagers Handbuch der Pharmazeutischen Praxis, 5. Aufl., Bde 4-6 (Drogen): Springer Verlag Berlin, Heidelberg, New York, 1992-1994.

Leung AY, Encyclopedia of Common Natural Ingredients Used in Food Drugs, Cosmetics, John Wiley & Sons Inc., New York 1980.

Madaus G, Lehrbuch der Biologischen Arzneimittel, Bde 1-3, Nachdruck, Georg Olms Verlag Hildesheim 1979.

Steinegger E, Hänsel R, Pharmakognosie, 5. Aufl., Springer Verlag Heidelberg 1992.

Teuscher E, Biogene Arzneimittel, 5. Aufl., Wiss. Verlagsges. Stuttgart 1997.

Teuscher E, Lindequist U, Biogene Gifte - Biologie, Chemie, Pharmakologie, 2. Aufl., Fischer Verlag Stuttgart 1994.

Wichtl M (Hrsg.), Teedrogen, 4. Aufl., Wiss. Verlagsges. Stuttgart 1997.

Thymus serpyllum

See Wild Thyme

Thymus vulgaris

See Thyme

Tiarella cordifolia

See Coolwort

Tilia species

See Linden

Tobacco

Nicotiana tabacum

DESCRIPTION

Medicinal Parts: The medicinal parts are the dried leaves.

Flower and Fruit: The numerous flowers are in many-branched panicles. The sepals are 12 to 25 mm long and tubular to tubular-campanulate. The tips are triangular, pointed and unequal. The corolla is 30 to 55 mm long, funnel-shaped, pale greenish-cream and often pinkish distally. The limb is 10 to 15 mm with pointed lobes, which are sometimes subentire. The four stamens are unequal and sometimes slightly exerted. The capsule is 15 to 20 mm long, ellipsoid to globose.

Leaves, Stem and Root: Tobacco is an annual or biennial plant, 1 to 3 m in height. The plant has a long fibrous root and an upright, round, pubescent and stick stem, which is heavily branched at the top. The leaves are up to 50 cm in length. They are ovate to elliptical or lanceolate, pointed, alternate and sessile. They sometimes have a short, winged petiole.

Habitat: The plant originates from tropical America and is cultivated worldwide, in particular in the U.S., China, Turkey, Greece, Holland, France, Germany and most subtropical countries.

Production: Tobacco leaves are the cultivated, unfermented leaves of Nicotiana tabacum.

ACTIONS AND PHARMACOLOGY

COMPOUNDS

Pyridine alkaloids (0.5-8.0%, among select cultivars 1.5%): chief alkaloid nicotine (30-60% share of the alkaloid mixture) including among others N-formyl nor-nicotine, cotinine, myosmine, nicotyrine, anabasine, nicotelline

EFFECTS

In small doses, Tobacco increases blood pressure and the activity of the gastric mucous membrane. In larger doses, it reduces blood pressure and lowers muscle tone of the gastrointestinal tract. Tobacco is a stimulant to the respiratory and central nervous system.

INDICATIONS AND USAGE

Unproven Uses: Nicotine is used to help break the smoking habit.

Apache Indians use the drug to treat toothache, mosquito bites and bee stings. In Brazil and Guyana, Tobacco is used for worm infestation, skin parasites and biliary flow disturbances. The drug's use in these conditions is not advised because of the risk of toxicity.

Indian Medicine: Tobacco is used for toothache, dental caries, earache, suppurating rhinitis, hernias, and painful swellings.

Homeopathic Uses: Tobacco is used for angina pectoris, low blood pressure and vomiting with diarrhea.

PRECAUTIONS AND ADVERSE REACTIONS

Tobacco leaves are severely poisonous. The chief toxin is nicotine, a liquid alkaloid, that can be resorbed through the skin.

OVERDOSAGE

The lethal dosage for nicotine for an adult is 40 to 100 mg, although this can be considerably elevated through habituation (with smoking Tobacco, 2 to 7 g of the drug; one cigarette contains 10 mg nicotine, of which 1 to 2 mg are inhaled during smoking). Symptoms of an acute poisoning include dizziness, salivation, vomiting, diarrhea, trembling of the hands and feelings of weakness in the legs; very high dosages can lead rapidly to spasms, unconsciousness, cardiac arrest and respiratory failure. Poisonings occur in particular through the ingestion of cigarettes by children, the handling of insecticides containing nicotine (through skin contact) and in connection with the harvesting of Tobacco (also through cutaneous resorption). Nicotine patches also represent a danger for children.

Following gastric lavage with burgundy-colored potassium permanganate solution, instillation of activated charcoal and sodium sulphate solution, the therapy for poisonings consists of treating spasms with diazepam (i.v.), chloral hydrate for children (rectal); cardiac massage; administration of orciprenaline; and atropine for severe sympathetic excitation. Intubation and oxygen respiration may also be necessary. No centrally effective analeptics are to be given.

DOSAGE

Mode of Administration: The nicotine alkaloid is used internally as a gum and externally as a transdermal patch.

Preparation: Nicorette (chewing gum); also as transdermal patches.

Daily Dosage: Nicotine as a pure alkaloid in smoker's remedies; nicotine (2 to 4 mg) bound by polacrilin (8 to 16 mg). Nicorette is an ion exchanger and therefore causes the slow release of nicotine, which is absorbed in the saliva over and over again. Eventually, the doses are reduced as the breaking of the habit progresses.

Homeopathic Dosage: 5 drops, 1 tablet or 10 globules every 30 to 60 minutes (acute) or 1 to 3 times daily (chronic); parenterally: 1 to 2 ml sc, acute: 3 times daily; chronic: once a day (HAB1).

LITERATURE

Anonym, Harvard-Studie: Herzkrank durch Passivrauchen. In: DAZ 137(22):1860. 1997.

Anonym, Passivrauchen:Risiko für vorzeitigen Herztod. In: DAZ 137(14):1097. 1997.

Anonym, Rauchen und Gesundheit. In: DAZ 131(25):1313. 1991.

Anonym, Rauchen während der Schwangerschaft - Lungenfunktion von Säuglingen gestört. In: DAZ 137(8):554. 1997.

Anonym, Raucherinnen schaden ihren Knochen. In: DAZ 137(26):2226. 1997.

Anonym, Risiken des Rauchens in der Schwangerschaft. In: DAZ 131(20):1010. 1991.

Anonym, Risikofaktoren: Primäre Prävention des Schlaganfalls. In: DAZ 136(24):1999-2003. 1996.

Anonym, Zigaretten: Raucher haben ein doppeltes Alzheimer-Risiko. In: DAZ 137(17):1423. 1997.

Bakoula C et al., Obective passive smoking indicators and respiratory morbidity in young children. In: DAZ 135(46):4330-4331 et 4334. 1995.

Bhide SV et al., Beitrag Tabakforsch Int 14:29. 1987.

Borisjuk NV, Davidjuk YM, Kostishin SS, Miroshnichenco GP, Velasco R, Hemleben V, Volkov RA, Structural analysis of rDNA in the genus Nicotiana. Plant Mol Biol, 35:655-60. 1997 Nov.

Devarenne TP, Shin DH, Back K, Yin S, Chappell J, Characterization of cucumber mosaic virus. IV. Movement protein and coat protein are both essential for cell-to-cell movement of cucumber mosaic virus. Virology, 349:237-48. 1997 Oct 27.

Duncker S, Atemwegserkrankungen: Passivrauchen verschlimmert Bronchialasthma bei Kindern. In: DAZ 136(3):184. 1996.

Enzell CR, Wahlberg I, Aaasen AI, Fortschr Chem Org Naturstoffe 34:1. 1977.

Frohne D, Pfänder HJ: Giftpflanzen - Ein Handbuch für Apotheker, Toxikologen und Biologen, 4. Aufl., Wiss. Verlags-Ges. Stuttgart 1997.

Jungmayr P, Schlaganfall: Wie hoch ist das Risiko für Exraucher? In: DAZ 136(2):28. 1996.

Kammerer S, Nichtraucherschutz. Passivrauchen erhöht Lungenkrebsrisiko. In: DAZ 135(14):1264-1266. 1995.

Kern W, List PH, Hörhammer L (Hrsg.), Hagers Handbuch der Pharmazeutischen Praxis, 4. Aufl., Bde. 1-8, Springer Verlag Berlin, Heidelberg, New York, 1969.

Klotz KL, Liu TT, Liu L, Lagrimini LM, Expression of the Tobacco anionic peroxidase gene is tissue-specific and developmentally regulated. Plant Mol Biol, 36:509-20. 1998 Mar.

Langheimer P, Rauchen und freie Radikale. In: DAZ 134(10):836. 1994.

Lewin L, Gifte und Vergiftungen, 6. Aufl., Nachdruck, Haug Verlag, Heidelberg 1992.

Lippiello, Buch. In: The Biology of Nicotine. Current Research Issue. Lippiello PM, Collins AC, Gray JA, Robinson JH (Eds.). Raven Press New York. 1992.

Matsushima S, Ohsumi T, Sugawara S, Agric Biol Chem (Tokyo) 47:507. 1983.

Müller CE, Nicotin - Genuβmittel oder Arzneistoff. In: DAZ 135(36):3253-3268. 1995.

Olbrich A, Das Lungenemphysem - Neuere Apsekte zu Pathogenese und Therapie. In: DAZ 135(47):4393-4405. 1995.

Piotrowski M, Oecking C, Five new 14-3-3 isoforms from Nicotiana tabacum L.: implications for the phylogeny of plant 14-3-3 proteins. Planta, 204:127-30. 1998 Jan.

Roth L, Daunderer M, Kormann K, Giftpflanzen, Pflanzengifte, 4. Aufl., Ecomed Fachverlag Landsberg Lech 1993.

Seigel R, Collings PR, Diaz JL, Econ Botany 32:16. 1977.

Teuscher E, Lindequist U, Biogene Gifte - Biologie, Chemie, Pharmakologie, 2. Aufl., Fischer Verlag Stuttgart 1994.

Wasielewski S, Neuropharmakologie:MAO-B-Hemmung: Psychoaktiver Zigarettenrauch. In: DAZ 136(30):2529-2530. 1996.

Wasielewski S, Zigarettenrauch: Wie Passivrauchen Herz und Kreislauf schädigt. In: DAZ 135(28):2605-2606, siehe auch S. 2606 rechts. 1995.

Willaman JJ, Hui-Li L, Lloydia 33(3A):1. 1970.

Tolu Balsam

Myroxylon balsamum

DESCRIPTION

Medicinal Parts: The medicinal parts are the balsam from the sweltered trunks, the hardened resin balsam that has been extracted from damaged trunks, softened and purified through a process of melting and sweltering.

Flower and Fruit: The androgynous flowers grow on pedicles approximately 12 cm long on simple, richly blossomed racemes. The calyx is inferior, broadly tubular or oblong-campanulate, dark green with short, rough hairs. The 5 petals are white and stemmed. The standard is almost circular. The stamens are bright red and the 1-valve ovary is on a long stem. The fruit is a 1-seeded, indehiscent, winged pod. The seeds are distinctly curved, brow-red and reniform.

Leaves, Stem and Root: These balsam trees grow to 25 m tall with a round, spreading crown that only starts to branch at a height of 13 to 19 m. The bark is smooth, yellow-gray or brown with numerous lenticles. The leaves are usually odd-pinnate and have 4 to 7 obovate, acuminate, coreacious, short-petioled leaflets. The upper surface is dark green and the lower surface pale green.

Characteristics: Before drying, the resin smells strongly of vanilla or benzoin.

Habitat: Myroxylon balsamum is indigenous to South and Central America, Sri Lanka and Jamaica.

Production: Peruvian balsam consists of the balsam generated from scorched tree trunks of Myroxylon balsamum. The bark of 10-year-old trees is removed just above ground level and this area is scorched with a flame, after which the balsam is collected in cloths placed on the scorched area.

Tolu Balsam consists of the balsam generated from the incised tree trunks of Myroxylon balsamum. The balsam is purified by melting, straining and solidifying. A V-shaped incision is made in the tree trunk, and a vessel is secured under the incision to collect the resin, which is then cleaned.

Other Names: Balsam Tree, Peruvian Balsam, Tolu Opobalsam

ACTIONS AND PHARMACOLOGY

COMPOUNDS: PERUVIAN BALSAM

Ester mixture, so-called cinnamein (50-70%): made up of benzyl benzoate and benzyl cinnamoate

Resins (20-30%): chief constituent cinnamic acid ester of the so-called peruresitannols (polymer)

Volatile oils: including some with nerolidol

EFFECTS: PERUVIAN BALSAM

The drug has an antibacterial/antiseptic effect, promotes the granulation process and is antiparasitic (especially for scabies). The main active constituent is an ester mixture that mainly contains benzyl benzoate.

COMPOUNDS: TOLU BALSAM

Ester mixture (10-20%): made up of benzyl benzoate and benzyl cinnamoate

Free benzoic acid/free cinnamic acid (10 to 30%)

Resins (up to 80%)

Volatile oil

EFFECTS: TOLU BALSAM

The undiluted oil showed antibacterial and fungicidal effects in the diffusion test. The drug also acts as an expectorant. The effect on the respiratory tract appears to work in the field of aromatherapy.

INDICATIONS AND USAGE

PERUVIAN BALSUM

Approved by Commission E:

- Wounds and burns
- Hemorrhoids

External Use: for infected and poorly healing wounds, for burns, decubitus ulcers, frostbite, leg ulcers, bruises caused by prostheses and hemorrhoids.

Unproven Uses: Although no longer used internally, it was used previously for fevers, colds, coughs, bronchitis, inflammation of the mouth and pharynx, and a tendency to infection. External folk medicine uses are the treatment of eczema and itching. Outdated uses include treatment of scabies; as a liniment for headaches, toothache and rheumatic symptoms; and use of the resin for uterine and umbilical venous bleeding.

Homeopathic Uses: Indications in homeopathy include chronic mucous membrane inflammation of the respiratory and urinary organs.

TOLU BALSAM

Approved by Commission E:

- Cough
- Bronchitis

Tolu Balsam is used to treat inflammation of the mucous membranes of the respiratory tract.

Unproven Uses: Folk medicine external uses include the approved indications above, as well as the treatment of wounds.

PRECAUTIONS AND ADVERSE REACTIONS

PERUVIAN BALSAM

Peruvian balsam often causes contact allergies. Urticaria, recurring aphthoid oral ulcers, Quincke's disease and diffuse purpura can all occur, among other ailments (possibly also following internal administration, for example, of foods containing Peruvian Balsam). Photodermatoses and phototoxic reactions are possible without ingestion. Kidney damage has been observed following internal as well as external use of large dosages (such as albuminuria, pyelitis and necroses of the canaliculus epithelia).

TOLU BALSAM

No health hazards or side effects are known in conjunction with the proper administration of designated therapeutic dosages. However, just as is the case with Peruvian Balsam, allergic reactions are possible.

DOSAGE

PERUVIAN BALSAM

Mode of Administration: Galenic preparations for external use.

How Supplied: Commercial pharmaceutical preparations include ointments and suppositories.

Homeopathic Dosage: 5 drops, 1 tablet or 10 globules every 30 to 60 minutes (acute) or 1 to 3 times daily (chronic); parenterally: 1 to 2 ml sc acute, 3 times daily; chronic: once a day (HAB34).

Daily Dosage: Galenic preparations containing 5 to 20% Peruvian Balsam, for extensive surface application not more than 10% Peruvian Balsam. Duration of application should not exceed 1 week.

Storage: Store Peruvian Balsam in a container that seals tightly and prevents exposure to light.

TOLU BALSAM

Mode of Administration: Various preparations of Tolu Balsam are used internally.

Preparation: To prepare Tolu Balsam syrup, dissolve the drug in 96% alcohol in a water bath with reflux; add 85% glycerol and water, then warm the mixture. Let stand for a week before adding saccharose. Prepare a 1000 ml tincture with 200 g Tolu Balsam and 92.3% ethanol.

Daily Dosage: Average daily dosage is 0.6 g of drug, depending on the preparation.

Storage: Store protected from light in tightly sealed containers with a suitable drying agent. Do not store Tolu Balsam in powder form.

LITERATURE

PERUVIAN BALSAM

Friedel HD, Dissertation Marburg. 1986.

Gharbo SA, Hussein FT, Nassra AA, UAR J Pharm Sci 11:170-173. 1970.

Glasl H, Wagner H, DAZ 114:45-47. 1974.

Lund K, Rimpler H, (1985) Dtsch Apoth Ztg 125(3):105.

Rudski E, Grzywaz Z, (1977) Dermatologia 155(2):115.

Further information in:

Hänsel R, Keller K, Rimpler H, Schneider G (Hrsg.), Hagers Handbuch der Pharmazeutischen Praxis, 5. Aufl., Bde 4-6 (Drogen), Springer Verlag Berlin, Heidelberg, New York, 1992-1994.

Leung AY, Encyclopedia of Common Natural Ingredients Used in Food Drugs and Cosmetics, John Wiley & Sons Inc., New York 1980.

Lewin L, Gifte und Vergiftungen, 6. Aufl., Nachdruck, Haug Verlag, Heidelberg 1992.

Madaus G, Lehrbuch der Biologischen Arzneimittel, Bde 1-3, Nachdruck, Georg Olms Verlag Hildesheim 1979.

Morton JF, An Atlas of Medicinal Plants of Middle America, Charles C. Thomas, USA 1981.

Roth L, Daunderer M, Kormann K, Giftpflanzen, Pflanzengifte, 4. Aufl., Ecomed Fachverlag Landsberg Lech 1993.

Steinegger E, Hänsel R, Pharmakognosie, 5. Aufl., Springer Verlag Heidelberg 1992.

Teuscher E, Biogene Arzneimittel, 5. Aufl., Wiss. Verlagsges. Stuttgart 1997.

Wagner H, Wiesenauer M, Phytotherapie. Phytopharmaka und pflanzliche Homöopathika, Fischer-Verlag, Stuttgart, Jena, New York 1995.

TOLU BALSAM

Harkiss KJ, Linley PA, PM 35:61-65. 1979.

Lund K, Rimpler H, (1985) Dtsch Apoth Ztg 125(3):105.

Morton JF, An Atlas of Medicinal Plants of Middle America, Charles C. Thomas, USA 1981.

Rudski E, Grzywaz Z, (1977) Dermatologia 155(2):115.

Wahlberg I, Enzell CR, Acta Chem Scand 25:352-354. 1971.

Further information in:

Hänsel R, Keller K, Rimpler H, Schneider G (Hrsg.), Hagers Handbuch der Pharmazeutischen Praxis, 5. Aufl., Bde 4-6 (Drogen), Springer Verlag Berlin, Heidelberg, New York, 1992-1994.

Leung AY, Encyclopedia of Common Natural Ingredients Used in Food Drugs and Cosmetics, John Wiley & Sons Inc., New York 1980.

Madaus G, Lehrbuch der Biologischen Arzneimittel, Bde 1-3, Nachdruck, Georg Olms Verlag Hildesheim 1979.

Steinegger E, Hänsel R, Pharmakognosie, 5. Aufl., Springer Verlag Heidelberg 1992.

Teuscher E, Biogene Arzneimittel, 5. Aufl., Wiss. Verlagsges. Stuttgart 1997.

Tomato

Lycopersicon esculentum

DESCRIPTION

Medicinal Parts: The medicinal parts are the fresh leaves, the fresh herb collected during the flowering season or the whole plant.

Flower and Fruit: The flowers are in lateral, cyme-like coils. The tips of the calyx are linear-lanceolate. The corolla is yellow, as long as the calyx and has a very short tube. It is divided into pointed, lanceolate lobes. The stamens are fused to the tube. The stigma is greenish and capitular. The fruit is a large, juicy, smooth, round to ovoid berry with a short, obtuse tip. It is scarlet, occasionally yellow or whitish with a diameter of 2 to 10 cm. The seeds are reniform, flattened, whitish-gray-yellow and villous-tomentose.

Leaves, Stem and Root: The tomato plant is an annual with a fusiform, fibrous root. The stem grows to 120 cm, and is leafy, heavily branched and glandular-haired. The leaves are broad-petiolate, odd-pinnate, petiolate, ovate-lanceolate, pinnatifid, dentate and slightly involute leaflets. The leaves have a gray-green underside.

Habitat: The plant probably originated in southern or Central America; today it is only cultivated.

Production: Tomato tincture is the homeopathic mother tincture of the whole plant Lycopersicon esculentum.

Other Names: Love Apple

ACTIONS AND PHARMACOLOGY

COMPOUNDS

Steroid alkaloid glycosides: chief alkaloid alpha-tomatine

EFFECTS

The tomatin content has been shown to be antibacterial. In animal experiments, a lowering of blood pressure was observed after IV administration of tomatin hydrochloride. Lectin isolated from the fruit is said to have an effect on cell division and DANN synthesis in human leukocyte cultures.

INDICATIONS AND USAGE

Unproven Uses: In folk medicine, Tomato is used externally for sore eyes (extract) and inflammations of the mouth and throat (decoction).

Indian Medicine: Tomato is used for 'flu' infections (tea), also for flatulence, atonic dyspepsia and anorexia.

Homeopathic Uses: Lycopersicon esculentum is used to treat rheumatic conditions, colds, chills and digestive disorders.

PRECAUTIONS AND ADVERSE REACTIONS

No health hazards or side effects are known in conjunction with the proper administration of designated therapeutic dosages.

OVERDOSAGE

Signs of poisoning are not to be expected with less than 100 gm of the fresh leaves (or green tomatoes) and for that reason is unlikely. Symptoms would be severe mucous membrane irritation (vomiting, diarrhea, and colic). Following absorption, dizziness, stupor, headache, bradycardia, respiratory disturbances, mild spasms and, in very severe cases, death through respiratory failure could occur.

Case studies are not known.

DOSAGE

Mode of Administration: The drug is commonly used in homeopathic dilutions.

Preparation: The mother tincture is produced by maceration or percolation of the fresh or dried drug, with an ethanol content of 45%.

Homeopathic Dosage: 5 drops, 1 tablet or 10 globules every 30 to 60 minutes (acute) or 1 to 3 times daily (chronic); parenterally: 1 to 2 ml sc acute, 3 times daily; chronic: once a day (HAB1).

LITERATURE

Hänsel R, Keller K, Rimpler H, Schneider G (Hrsg.), Hagers Handbuch der Pharmazeutischen Praxis, 5. Aufl., Bde 4-6 (Drogen), Springer Verlag Berlin, Heidelberg, New York, 1992-1994.

Tomaten als Krebsschutz. In: DAZ 134(6):485. 1994.

Tonka Beans

Dipteryx odorata

DESCRIPTION

Medicinal Parts: The medicinal part is the seeds.

Flower and Fruit: The beans are usually 2 to 5 cm long and 1 cm in diameter. They have a grayish or black color.

Characteristics: The bean has a characteristic odor, like new-mown hay of coumarin.

Habitat: South America

Production: Tonka Beans are the seeds of Dipteryx odorata.

Other Names: Tonquin Bean

ACTIONS AND PHARMACOLOGY

COMPOUNDS

Coumarin (1-3% to 10%)

Fatty oil

EFFECTS

Tonka Beans have a tonic and aromatic effect.

INDICATIONS AND USAGE

Unproven Uses: Whooping cough (no longer used).

PRECAUTIONS AND ADVERSE REACTIONS

Health risks or side effects following the proper administration of designated therapeutic dosages are not recorded. The therapeutic administration of drugs containing coumarin can lead to slight liver damage (elevated liver enzyme values in the blood) in a very small number of patients, that is, however, reversible following discontinuance of the drug.

OVERDOSAGE

The intake of very high dosages (4 gm coumarin, equivalent to 150 gm of the drug) could bring about stupor, headache, nausea and vomiting.

DOSAGE

Mode of Administration: Tonka Beans are obsolete as a drug.

LITERATURE

Kalume DE, Sousa MV, Morhy L, Purification characterization sequence determination and mass spectrometric analysis of a trypsin inhibitor from seeds of the Brazilian tree Dipteryx alata (Leguminosae). J Protein Chem, 14:685-93, Nov, 1995.

Lewin L, Gifte und Vergiftungen, 6. Aufl., Nachdruck, Haug Verlag, Heidelberg 1992.

Roth L, Daunderer M, Kormann K, Giftpflanzen, Pflanzengifte, 4. Aufl., Ecomed Fachverlag Landsberg Lech 1993.

Steinegger E, Hänsel R, Pharmakognosie, 5. Aufl., Springer Verlag Heidelberg 1992.

Sullivan G, (1968) J Agric Food Chem 30(3):609.

Teuscher E, Lindequist U, Biogene Gifte - Biologie, Chemie, Pharmakologie, 2. Aufl., Fischer Verlag Stuttgart 1994.

Tragacanth

Astragalus gummifer

DESCRIPTION

Medicinal Parts: The medicinal product of the plant is the gum-like exudation from the trunk and branches.

Flower and Fruit: The axillary flowers are solitary or in groups of 2 or 3 and are sessile. The calyx is 6 to 7 mm long and densely pubescent. The corolla is yellowish to white and sometimes has bluish or reddish veins. The standard, wings and carina are each 9 to 10 mm long. The fruit is ovoid, 4 mm long with dense, silky hairs. The seed is oval, smooth and about 3 mm long.

Leaves, Stem and Root: Astralagus gummifer is a low shrub that grows up to 30 cm high and has gray branches that become glabrous. The older branches have scale-like remains of the stipules from the previous year, which disappear later, and a 1 to 4 cm long perennial, thorny leaf column. The 8 to 14 leaflets are folded, oblong-ovate, 2.5 to 6 mm long and 0.7 to 2.5 mm wide, blue-gray and glabrous or sparsely pubescent beneath.

Habitat: The plant grows in Turkey, Syria, Lebanon, northwest Iraq and the border area between Iran and Iraq.

Production: Tragacanth is the latex that exudes primarily from immediately under the bark of Astralagus gummifer and other varieties. It is extracted by making an incision in the trunk and branches of shrubs growing in the wild. When dried, it forms flakes that swell in water to form a gelatinous mass.

Other Names: Gum Dragon

ACTIONS AND PHARMACOLOGY

COMPOUNDS

Polysaccharides (water-soluble part, approximately 40%): tragacanthine, which can decompose into tragacanthic acid (galacturonane with side chains consisting of D-xylose, L-fucose, D-galactose)

Arabino-galactane-protein complex (non-water soluable part, approximately 60%): containing bassorin, a composition similar to that of tragacanthine

EFFECTS

Tragacanth has a laxative effect, primarily due to stimulating stretching of the intestinal wall, which results in increased peristalis.

INDICATIONS AND USAGE

Unproven Uses: Tragacanth is used as a laxative. Folk medicine uses in Europe and the Arab world have included treatment for tumors of the eyes, liver and throat. Efficacy has not been proven.

PRECAUTIONS AND ADVERSE REACTIONS

No health hazards or side effects are known in conjunction with the proper administration of designated therapeutic dosages. Allergic reactions have been observed in rare cases. Insufficient fluid supply following intake of large quantities of tragacanth can lead to obstruction ileus, as well as to esophageal closure.

DOSAGE

Mode of Administration: Tragacanth is used in various combinations and preparations.

Daily Dosage: Recommended daily dosage is not specified. A typical single dose is 1 tsp. granulated drug (approximately 3g) added to 250 to 300 ml liquid for oral administration.

Storage: Tragacanth cannot be stored for any significant length of time because of its instability.

LITERATURE

Anderson DMW, Bridgeman MME, PH 24:2301-2304. 1985.

Aspinall GO, Baillie J, J Chem Soc: 1702-1714. 1963.

Fang S et al., (1982): You Ji Hua Xue 2: 26.

Gralen N, Kärrholm M, J Colloid Sci 5:21-36. 1950.

Osswald H, (1968) Arzneim Forsch 18: 1495.

Srimal RC, Dhawan CN, (1973) J Pharm Pharmacol 25: 447.

Whistler RL et al., (1976) Adv Carbohydr Chem Biochem 32: 235.

Further information in:

Hänsel R, Keller K, Rimpler H, Schneider G (Hrsg.), Hagers Handbuch der Pharmazeutischen Praxis, 5. Aufl., Bde 4-6 (Drogen): Springer Verlag Berlin, Heidelberg, New York, 1992-1994.

Leung AY, Encyclopedia of Common Natural Ingredients Used in Food Drugs, Cosmetics, John Wiley & Sons Inc., New York 1980.

Steinegger E, Hänsel R, Pharmakognosie, 5. Aufl., Springer Verlag Heidelberg 1992.

Teuscher E, Biogene Arzneimittel, 5. Aufl., Wiss. Verlagsges. Stuttgart 1997.

Trailing Arbutus

Epigae repens

DESCRIPTION

Medicinal Parts: The medicinal parts are the fresh or dried leaves.

Flower and Fruit: The flowers are in apical dense racemes. They are white with a reddish tinge and are very fragrant. They are divided at the tip into 5 segments which open in a star shape.

Leaves, Stem and Root: The plant is a fragrant evergreen branching shrub with rust-colored, pubescent, round stems. Roots develop at the stem nodes, which spread quickly. The leaves are petioled, broadly ovate, 2.5 to 4 cm long and about 2 cm wide, coriaceous, entire-margined, reticulate, with a cordate base and short pointed apex and short hairs on the undersurface. The branches, petioles and leaf nerves are very pubescent.

Characteristics: The plant has a similar action to Buchu on the urinary system.

Habitat: Indigenous to North America, established as an ornamental plant in Europe.

Production: Trailing Arbutus is the aerial part of Epigae repens.

Other Names: Eleuthero, Gravel Plant, Ground Laurel, Mountain Pink, Water Pink, Winter Pink

ACTIONS AND PHARMACOLOGY

COMPOUNDS

Arbutin (hydroquinone glucoside)

Tannins

EFFECTS

Eleuthero has astringent and diuretic properties.

INDICATIONS AND USAGE

Unproven Uses: Trailing Arbutus is used for urinary tract conditions.

PRECAUTIONS AND ADVERSE REACTIONS

Health risks or side effects following the proper administration of designated therapeutic dosages are not recorded. Nausea and vomiting can also occur with stomach sensitivity in children. Liver damage, cachexia, hemolytic anemia and depigmentation of the hair is possible with long-term use of the drug.

OVERDOSAGE

Overdosages could lead to inflammatory reactions of the mucous membranes of the bladder and urinary passages, accompanied by strangury and possible blood in the urine.

DOSAGE

Mode of Administration: Trailing Arbutus is available as an infusion or extract for internal use.

LITERATURE

Kern W, List PH, Hörhammer L (Hrsg.), Hagers Handbuch der Pharmazeutischen Praxis, 4. Aufl., Bde. 1-8, Springer Verlag Berlin, Heidelberg, New York, 1969.

Traveller's Joy

Clematis vitalba

DESCRIPTION

Medicinal Parts: The medicinal parts of the plant are the fresh leaves.

Flower and Fruit: The flowers are arranged in leafy cymes. The blossoms are small and white with 4 downy, revolute or splayed bracts. The stamens and ovaries are numerous. The fruit is a red-brown, long-tailed nut.

Leaves, Stem and Root: The plant grows to about 1.5 to 5 m high. The leaves are petiolate and 5-pinnate. The leaflets are ovate or slightly cordate, acute and lobed. The petioles are clinging and the stems climbing, grooved, at first leafy then woody.

Characteristics: The flowers have a slight scent resembling white thorn. The plant is poisonous if ingested in large amounts.

Habitat: The plant is indigenous to Europe.

ACTIONS AND PHARMACOLOGY

COMPOUNDS

Protoanemonine-forming agents: In the freshly harvested plant, it is presumably the glycoside ranunculin that changes enzymatically when the plant is cut into small pieces, and probably also when it is dried. It then changes into the pungent, volatile protoanemonine that is severely irritating to skin and mucous membranes but quickly dimerizes to anemonine; when dried, the plant is not capable of protoanemonine formation.

Saponins

EFFECTS

No information is available.

INDICATIONS AND USAGE

Unproven Uses: The drug causes blistering and was formerly used to treat diseases of the male genitals, as well as for poorly healing wounds. Today, it is used in small doses, both internally and externally, for migraine.

PRECAUTIONS AND ADVERSE REACTIONS

No health hazards or side effects are known in conjunction with the proper administration of designated therapeutic dosages of the dehydrated drug.

Extended skin contact with the freshly harvested, bruised plant can lead to treatment-resistant blisters and cauterizations due to the release of protoanemonine, which is severely irritating to skin and mucous membranes. If taken internally, severe irritation to the gastrointestinal tract, combined with colic, diarrhea and irritation of the urinary drainage passages, are possible. Symptomatic treatment for external contact should consist of irrigation with diluted potassium permanganate solution followed by mucilage.

OVERDOSAGE

Ingestion of the drug should be treated with gastric lavage followed by activated charcoal. Death by asphyxiation following the intake of large quantities of protoanemonine-forming plants has been observed in animal experiments. The toxicity of this plant is less than that of many other Ranunculaceae (Anemones nemorosae) due to the relatively low levels of protoanemonine-forming agents.

DOSAGE

Mode of Administration: The drug is used topically and is also available in alcoholic extracts.

LITERATURE

Bonora A et al., PH 26:2277. 1987.

Frohne D, Pfänder HJ: Giftpflanzen - Ein Handbuch für Apotheker, Toxikologen und Biologen, 4. Aufl., Wiss. Verlagsges. mbH Stuttgart 1997.

Kern W, List PH, Hörhammer L (Hrsg.), Hagers Handbuch der Pharmazeutischen Praxis, 4. Aufl., Bde 1-8, Springer Verlag Berlin, Heidelberg, New York, 1969.

Lewin L, Gifte und Vergiftungen, 6. Aufl., Nachdruck, Haug Verlag, Heidelberg 1992.

Madaus G, Lehrbuch der Biologischen Arzneimittel, Bde 1-3, Nachdruck, Georg Olms Verlag Hildesheim 1979.

Roth L, Daunderer M, Kormann K: Giftpflanzen, Pflanzengifte, 4. Aufl., Ecomed Fachverlag Landsberg Lech 1993.

Ruijgrok HWL, PM 11:338-347. 1963.

Southwell IA et al., Protoanemonin in australian Clematis. In: PH 33:1099. 1993.

Teuscher E, Lindequist U, Biogene Gifte - Biologie, Chemie, Pharmakologie, 2. Aufl., Fischer Verlag Stuttgart 1994.

Tree of Heaven

Ailanthus altissima

DESCRIPTION

Medicinal Parts: The medicinal parts are the dried trunk and root bark.

Flower and Fruit: The small, greenish-yellow flower is in branched, axillary or terminal panicles. Some of the flowers are male, some female and some androgynous. The calyx is short and has 5 glandular, fused sepals. The sepals are much longer than the corolla and have 5 hollow, splayed petals. There are 10 stamens, often only 5 in the androgynous and rudimentary remains in the female flowers. There are 5 obovate, compressed ovaries with 5 splayed stigmas. There is a narrow, oblong-lanceolate schizocarp, 4 to 5 cm by 1 cm. It is winged above and below, first green then brown-red and finally brown. The seed is orbicular and found in the middle of the fruit section. It is thin-skinned, without any recognizable endosperm and has an ovate, flat cotyledon.

Leaves, Stem and Root: Ailanthus altissima is a beautiful, fast-growing tree, up to 30 m high. The bark is smooth, pale and vertically striated. The branches are initially fine-haired, yellow or red-brown. The leaves are up to 1 m long and odd-pinnate. The upper surface of the leaves is dark green and the under-surface is light gray-green. Both sides of the leaf are glandular-haired. The leaflets are ovate to oblong-lanceolate. The shallow, cordate base of the leaflets has 1 to 3 small lobes at either side, each with 1 gland. The wood surface is satin-like and white.

Characteristics: The flowers have a strong elder flower scent. The fresh bark and leaves give off an unpleasant, nauseating smell.

Habitat: The tree was originally indigenous to China. Today it grows in the wild and is cultivated in tropical and subtropical eastern Asia, northern Europe and North America.

Production: Tree of Heaven bark is the trunk and branch bark of Ailanthus altissima. The bark is gathered year-round. The outer bark is removed and dried in the sun. After drying, there is a process of sorting and removing foreign bodies, washing, macerating and a second drying.

Other Names: Ailanto, Chinese Sumach, Vernis de Japon

ACTIONS AND PHARMACOLOGY

COMPOUNDS

Quassinoids: including ailanthone, quassin

Indole alkaloids of the beta-carbolic type

Tannins

EFFECTS

An antimalarial action is being tested in an in-vitro trial. The active agents also have astringent, antipyretic, and antispasmodic properties.

INDICATIONS AND USAGE

Unproven Uses: In Africa, Tree of Heaven is used for cramps, asthma, fast heart rate, gonorrhea, epilepsy and tapeworm infestation. It is increasingly used in the treatment of malaria.

Chinese Medicine: The drug is used for pathological leukorrhea, diarrhea, chronic diarrhea, chronic dysentery and dysmenorrhea.

PRECAUTIONS AND ADVERSE REACTIONS

Large doses of the drug are said to lead to queasiness, dizziness, headache, tingling in the limbs and diarrhea.

OVERDOSAGE

Fatal poisonings have been observed in animal experiments. Treatment of poisonings should be conducted symptomatically, following stomach and intestinal emptying.

DOSAGE

Mode of Administration: Tree of Heaven is still being researched as a drug; up until now it has only been used in folk medicine.

Daily Dosage: 6 to 9 gm of drug

Storage: Keep in a dry, well-ventilated area away from moths.

LITERATURE

Bray DH, et al., (1987) Phytother Res 1(1):22.

Casinovi CG, et al., (1964) Tetrahedron Lett: 3991.

Casinovi CG, et al., (1965) Tetrahedron Lett: 2273.

Furuno T, et al., (1984) Bull Chem Soc Jpn 57:2484-2489.

Geissmann T, (1964) Ann Rev Pharmacol 4:305.

Ghosh P et al, (1977) Lloydia 40(4):636.

Ishibashi M, et al., (1983) Bull Chem Soc Jpn 56:3683-3693.

Ishibashi M, et al., (1984) Bull Chem Soc Jpn 57:2013-2014.

Ishibashi M, et al., (1985) Bull Chem Soc Jpn 58:2723-2724.

Ishibashi M, et al., (1983) Chem Pharm Bull 31:2179-2182.

Ishibashi M, et al., (1985) Tetrahedron Lett:1205-1206.

Naora H, et al., (1983) Bull Chem Soc Jpn 56:3694-3698.

Niimi Y, et al., (1987) Chem Pharm Bull 35:4302-4306.

Ohmoto T, et al., (1981) Chem Pharm Bull 29:390-395.

Ohmoto T, et al., (1984) Chem Pharm Bull 32:170-173.

Polonski J, (1985) Prog Chem Org Nat Prod 47:221.

Polonsky J, (1973) Fortschr Chem Org Naturst 30:101.

Rücker G, (1995) Malariawirksame Verbindungen aus Pflanzen, insbesondere Peroxide. In: PUZ 24(4):189-195.

Varga E, et al., (1980) Planta Med 40:337-339.

Varga E, et al., (1981) Fitoterapia 52:183-186.

Further information in:

Hänsel R, Keller K, Rimpler H, Schneider G (Hrsg.), Hagers Handbuch der Pharmazeutischen Praxis, 5. Aufl., Bde 4 - 6 (Drogen), Springer Verlag Berlin, Heidelberg, New York, 1992-1994.

Lewin L, (1992) Gifte und Vergiftungen, 6. Aufl., Nachdruck, Haug Verlag, Heidelberg.

Madaus G, (1979) Lehrbuch der Biologischen Arzneimittel, Bde 1-3, Nachdruck, Georg Olms Verlag Hildesheim.

Roth L, Daunderer M, Kormann K, (1993) Giftpflanzen, Pflanzengifte, 4. Aufl., Ecomed Fachverlag Landsberg Lech.

Trifolium pratense

See Red Clover

Trigonella foenum-graecum

See Fenugreek

Trillium erectum

See Beth Root

Triticum

Agropyron repens

DESCRIPTION

Medicinal Parts: The medicinal part is the rhizome collected in spring or autumn.

Flower and Fruit: Five to 7 flowered spikelets in groups of 20 form a 10 cm-long ear. The ears are usually short, upright and usually dense green and inconspicuous grass with 5 veined, lanceolate, sharply keeled glume. The spike stem is glabrous. The glume is 8 to 11 mm long, acuminate or awned. The anthers are 5 to 6 mm. The fruit is 6 to 7 mm long, flat to the front with 1 groove.

Leaves, Stem and Root: Triticum is a 0.2 to 1.5 m perennial plant with a hardy creeping rhizome. The rhizome has long white runners, is segmented and hollow. The leaves are thin, flat, grass-green or gray-green. The upper surface is rough and often covered in solitary, long hairs.

Characteristics: The spikelets have their broad side turned toward the wave-like curved main axis. The plant is odorless; the taste sweetish.

Habitat: Indigenous to the temperate regions of the Northern Hemisphere. Introduced to Greenland, South America, Australia and New Zealand.

Production: Triticum rhizome consists of the rhizome, roots and short stems of Agropyron repens, harvested in spring before the blade develops, as well as its preparations. The rhizomes are collected after the fields are harrowed. They are cleaned, washed and dried at approximately 35° C.

Not to be Confused With: The rhizomes of Cynodon dactylon, Poaceae and Carex species (a frequent occurrence).

Other Names: Couch Grass Quitch Grass, Witch Grass, Twitch-Grass, Scotch Quelch, Dog-Grass, Quickgrass, Cutch, Durfa Grass, Quack Grass, Elytrigia repens

ACTIONS AND PHARMACOLOGY

COMPOUNDS

Mucilages

Triticin (polyfructosan)

Sugar alcohols

Soluble silicic acid

Volatile oil: including carvacrol and carvone-containing P-hydroxyalkyl cinnamic acid alkyl ester

EFFECTS

The essential oil has an antimicrobial effect.

INDICATIONS AND USAGE

Approved by Commission E:

- Infections of the urinary tract
- Kidney and bladder stones

Unproven Uses: Triticum is used as a flushing-out therapy, for inflammatory diseases of the urinary tract and the prevention of kidney gravel. The drug is also used for cystitis, kidney stones, gout, rheumatic pain and chronic skin disorders. Due to the high mucilage content, the drug is used as a soothing cough remedy. The infusion is used for constipation. It is also used as fructose-containing additive for diabetics.

Homeopathic Uses: Agropyron repens is used to treat urinary tract infections.

CONTRAINDICATIONS

No flushing-out therapy if edema is present due to cardiac or renal insufficiency.

PRECAUTIONS AND ADVERSE REACTIONS

No health hazards or side effects are known in conjunction with the proper administration of designated therapeutic dosages. For flushing-out therapy, ensure copious fluid intake.

DOSAGE

Mode of Administration: Comminuted herb decoctions and other galenic preparations for internal use.

Preparation: Liquid extract: 1:1; Tincture: 1:5; Tea: Pour boiling water over the drug and strain after 10 minutes.

Daily Dosage: The average single dose is 3 to 10 gm of drug in 1 cup of boiling water; average daily dose is 6 to 9 gm of drug.

Tea: 12 to 24 gm drunk fresh several times a day; Liquid extract: 4 to 8 ml 3 times daily; Tincture: 5 to 15 ml 3 times daily.

Homeopathic Dosage: 5 drops, 1 tablet, 10 globules every 30 to 60 minutes (acute) or 1 to 3 times a day (chronic); Parenterally: 1 to 2 ml sc acute, 3 times daily; Chronic: once a day (HAB1).

Storage: The drug must be kept in sealed containers, protected from light and moisture.

LITERATURE

Bell EA, Jansen DH, (1971) Nature 229:136.

Boesel R, Schilcher H, PM 55:399-400. 1989.

Kiesewetter R, Müller M, (1958) Pharmazie 13:777.

Koetter U, et al., Isolierung und Strukturaufklärung von p-Hydroxyzimtsäurealkylesterverbindungen aus dem Rhizom von Agropyron repens, 2. Mitt. In: PM 60(5):488. 1994.

Koetter U, Kaloga M, Schilcher H, Isolierung und Strukturaufklärung von p-Hydroxyzimtsäurealkylester-Verbindungen aus dem Rhizom von Agropyron repens; 1. Mitt. In: PM 59(3):279. 1993.

Paslawska S, Piekos R, (1976) Planta Med 30:216.

Racz-Kotilla E and Mozes E, (1971) Rev Med 17:82.

Schilcher H, Boesel R, Effenberger ST, Segebrecht S, Neuere Untersuchungsergebnisse mit aquaretisch, antibakteriell und prostatotrop wirksamen Arzneipflanzen. In: ZPT 10(3):77. 1989.

Further information in:

Hänsel R, Keller K, Rimpler H, Schneider G (Hrsg.), Hagers Handbuch der Pharmazeutischen Praxis, 5. Aufl., Bde 4 - 6 (Drogen), Springer Verlag Berlin, Heidelberg, New York, 1992-1994.

Wagner H, Wiesenauer M, Phytotherapie. Phytopharmaka und pflanzliche Homöopathika, Fischer-Verlag, Stuttgart, Jena, New York 1995.

Wichtl M (Hrsg.), Teedrogen, 4. Aufl., Wiss. Verlagsges. Stuttgart 1997.

Triticum aestivum

See Wheat

Trollius europaeus

See Globe Flower

Tropaeolum majus

See Nasturtium

Tropical Almond

Terminalia chebula

DESCRIPTION

Medicinal Parts: The medicinal part of the tree is the fruit.

Flower and Fruit: The flowers are arranged in 5 to 7 cm long, axillary spikes. The flowers are small and fused. Their structures are arranged in fives. The sepals are almost glabrous and yellowish-white; the calyx tube is 5-tipped. There are no petals, but there are 10 stamens and a single-chambered, inferior ovary. The style is long and projects out of the bud. The fruit is a glabrous, ovoid drupe, yellow to orange-brown when ripe and 2 to 4 cm long.

Leaves, Stem and Root: Tropical Almond is a tree that grows up to 25 m high. The leaves are alternate or opposite, 7 to 18 cm long, 4 to 6 cm wide and coriaceous. The petiole is approximately 2.5 cm long, with 2 glands at the upper end. The lamina is ovate or elliptical, blunt and orbicular at the base. It is finely crenate and woolly pubescent beneath. The branches are rust colored, woolly or glabrous, and the trunk has a brown, longitudinally fissured bark.

Habitat: India

Production: Tropical Almond fruit is the dried ripe fruit of Terminalia chebula.

Not to be Confused With: Can be confused with emblica and Terminalia bellirica.

Other Names: Black Myrobalan, Chebulic Myrobalan, Myrobalan

ACTIONS AND PHARMACOLOGY

COMPOUNDS

Tannins (20 to 45%): gallotannins, including terchebulin, terflavin A, punicalagin, corilagin, chebulic acid, and chebulinic acid

Monosaccharides/oligosaccharides (9%): including D-glucose, D-fructose, saccharose

Fruit acids: including quinic acid (1.5%), shikimic acid (2%)

Fatty oil (in the seeds, to 40%)

EFFECTS

Its high tannin content explains the use of the drug as an astringent. A variety of experiments have demonstrated antibacterial, cardiotonic and antiarteriosclerotic (lowering of cholesterol levels) effects for the drug.

INDICATIONS AND USAGE

Chinese Medicine: Tropical Almond is used for chronic diarrhea, chronic dysentery, rectal prolapse, loss of voice because of chronic coughs, blood in the stool, leucorrhea, night sweats and undesired discharges.

Indian Medicine: The drug is used in the treatment of wounds, ulcers, gingivitis, excitation, gastric complaints, anorexia, worm infestation, flatulence, hemorrhoids, jaundice, for liver and spleen disease, pharyngodynia, hiccups, coughs, epilepsy, eye disease, skin changes, leprosy, intermittent fever, cardiac dysfunction, gastritis and neuropathy.

PRECAUTIONS AND ADVERSE REACTIONS

No health hazards are known in conjunction with the proper administration of designated therapeutic dosages, although even therapeutic dosages could lead to constipation, due to the high tannin content (administration as an antidiarrheal).

OVERDOSAGE

The administration of extremely high doses (25% of the fodder) over a period of 4 weeks to rats led to kidney and liver damage; mice developed liver tumors in a related experiment (750 mg/kg body weight of the tannin fraction over a period of 12 weeks).

DOSAGE

Mode of Administration: Whole herb preparations for internal and external use.

Daily Dosage: 3 to 9 gm

Storage: Should be stored in a dry and cool place.

LITERATURE

el-Mekkawy S, Meselhy MR, Kusumoto IT, Kadota S, Hattori M, Namba T, Inhibitory effects of Egyptian folk medicines on human immunodeficiency virus (HIV) reverse transcriptase. Chem Pharm Bull (Tokyo), 20:641-8, 1995 Apr.

Grover IS, Bala S, Antimutagenic activity of Terminalia chebula (myroblan) in Salmonella typhimurium. Indian J Exp Biol, 30:339-41, 1992 Apr.

Hamada S, Kataoka T, Woo JT, Yamada A, Yoshida T, Nishimura T, Otake N, Nagai K, Immunosuppressive effects of gallic acid and chebulagic acid on CTL-mediated cytotoxicity. Biol Pharm Bull, 20:1017-9, 1997 Sep.

Hänsel R, Keller K, Rimpler H, Schneider G (Ed), Hagers Handbuch der Pharmazeutischen Praxis, 5. Aufl., Bde 4 - 6 (Drogen), Springer Verlag Berlin, Heidelberg, New York, 1992-1994.

Jiang JY, Influence of processing methods on the quality of Terminalia chebula. Chung Yao Tung Pao, 20:24-6, 1986 Sep.

Kurokawa M, Nagasaka K, Hirabayashi T, Uyama S, Sato H, Kageyama T, Kadota S, Ohyama H, Hozumi T, Namba T, et al Efficacy of traditional herbal medicines in combination with acyclovir against herpes simplex virus type 1 infection in vitro and in vivo. Antiviral Res, 45:19-37, 1995 May.

Miglani BD, Sen P, Sanyal RK, Purgative action of an oil obtained from Terminalia chebula. Indian J Med Res, 20:281-3, 1971 Feb.

Phadke SA, Kulkarni SD, Screening of in vitro antibacterial activity of Terminalia chebula, Eclapta alba and Ocimum sanctum. Indian J Med Sci, 43:113-7, 1989 May.

Sato Y, Oketani H, Singyouchi K, Ohtsubo T, Kihara M, Shibata H, Higuti T, Extraction and purification of effective antimicrobial constituents of Terminalia chebula Retz. against methicillin-resistant Staphylococcus aureus. Biol Pharm Bull, 20:401-4, 1997 Apr.

Shiraki K, Yukawa T, Kurokawa M, Kageyama S, Cytomegalovirus infection and its possible treatment with herbal medicines. Nippon Rinsho, 56:156-60, 1998 Jan.

Shiraki K, Yukawa T, Kurokawa M, Kageyama S, Influence of processing methods on the quality of Terminalia chebula. Chung Yao Tung Pao, 56:24-6, 1986 Sep.

Sohni YR, Bhatt RM, Activity of a crude extract formulation in experimental hepatic amoebiasis and in immunomodulation studies. J Ethnopharmacol, 45:119-24, 1996 Nov.

Sohni YR, Kaimal P, Bhatt RM, The antiamoebic effect of a crude drug formulation of herbal extracts against Entamoeba histolytica in vitro and in vivo. J Ethnopharmacol, 45:43-52, 1995 Jan.

Thakur CP, Thakur B, Singh S, Sinha PK, Sinha SK, The Ayurvedic medicines Haritaki, Amala and Bahira reduce cholesterol-induced atherosclerosis in rabbits. Int J Cardiol, 21:167-75, 1988 Nov.

Yukawa TA, Kurokawa M, Sato H, Yoshida Y, Kageyama S, Hasegawa T, Namba T, Imakita M, Hozumi T, Shiraki K, Effect of tannins from Terminalia chebula Retz. on the infectivity of potato virus X. Acta Microbiol Pol B, 32:127-32, 1970.

Yukawa TA, Kurokawa M, Sato H, Yoshida Y, Kageyama S, Hasegawa T, Namba T, Imakita M, Hozumi T, Shiraki K, Prophylactic treatment of cytomegalovirus infection with traditional herbs. Antiviral Res, 32:63-70, 1996 Oct.

Tsuga canadensis

See Pinus Bark

Tulip Tree

Liriodendron tulipifera

DESCRIPTION

Medicinal Parts: The bark is said to have medicinal properties.

Flower and Fruit: The flowers are apical, single with 3 revolute, greenish-white sepals. There are 6 petals, 4 to 5 cm long, greenish-yellow with orange bands near the base on the inside similar to the tepals of the tulip. The flower has numerous stamens and numerous apocarpic ovaries on a spindle-shaped column. The small, 1-seeded nut with pointed wings is in a 6 to 8 cm long, cone-like, aggregate fruit that is light green when ripe.

Leaves, Stem and Root: Liriodendron tulipifera is a tree, up to 60 m high. The leaves are alternate with saddle-shaped middle lobes and 2 large lateral lobes, almost square in outline, 8 to 15 cm long and wide, and usually rounded at the base. The upper leaf surface is fresh green, the lower surface a weak blue. The petioles are 5 to 10 cm long. The young branches are yellow-green in summer and reddish-brown in winter and spotted with lenticles. The young trunks are dark green to gray and spotted white with lenticles. The trunks (up to 3 m thick) of older trees have a brown, deeply grooved bark.

Characteristics: The leaves are bright golden-yellow in autumn.

Habitat: Indigenous to North America, Europe and China.

Production: The Tulip Tree bark is the peeled and dried branch bark of Liriodendron tulipifera.

Other Names: Yellow Poplar

ACTIONS AND PHARMACOLOGY

COMPOUNDS

Isoquinoline alkaloids (0.1%), particularly of the aporphine type: including remerine, lysicamine, liriodenine, lanugosine

Lignans (0.1%): including liriodendrin

Volatile oil (0.1%): chief components cis-beta-ocimene, beta-pinene, bornyl acetate

Hydroxycumarins: esculetin methyl and dimethyl esters

EFFECTS

The alkaloids contained in the drug are antimicrobial in effect, and a positively inotropic effect has been described. Its usefulness as a tonic and a stimulant appears to be plausible, based upon its qualities as a bitter substance.

INDICATIONS AND USAGE

Unproven Uses: According to Hoppe's 1958 work on drugs, Linodendron tulipifera is used as a febrifuge and antiperiodic. Folk medicine indications have included fever, menstrual complaints, insomnia and malaria.

PRECAUTIONS AND ADVERSE REACTIONS

The drug is considered toxic, due to its alkaloid content. Administration in animal experiments led to coma (exact details unavailable). No case of poisoning among humans has been recorded.

DOSAGE

Preparation: There is no information in the literature.

Daily dosage: Powder: 4 to 8 g daily; decoction (30:500) 60 g daily.

LITERATURE

Doskotch RW, el-Feraly FS, Antitumor agents. II. Tulipinolide, a new germacranolide sesquiterpene, and constunolide. Two cytotoxic substances from Liriodendron tulipifera L. J Pharm Sci, 28:877-80, 1969 Jul.

Hufford CD, Funderburk MJ, Morgan JM, Robertson LW, Two antimicrobial alkaloids from heartwood of Liriodendron tulipifera L. J Pharm Sci, 64:789-92, 1975 May.

Rzedowski M, Furmanowa M, Molak W, Liriodenine in tissue culture of Liriodendron tulipifera L. II. Quantitative analysis and antifungal effect. Acta Pol Pharm, 42:300-4, 1985.

Schulz HK, Hausen BM, White wood allergy (author's transl) Derm Beruf Umwelt, 28:158-60, 1980.

Turkey Corn

Dicentra cucullaria

DESCRIPTION

Medicinal Parts: The medicinal part is the dried tuber.

Flower and Fruit: The inflorescence is racemous. The 4 to 10 flowers are odorless, white and often tinged pink. The flowers are hanging, with yellow to yellow-orange tips and widely splayed spurs. The fruit is oval and 9 to 13 mm long. The seeds are reniform, 2 mm long, black and glossy.

Leaves, Stem and Root: Turkey Corn is a delicate, glabrous, 15 to 40 cm high plant on a tawny yellow, tuberous rhizome. The rhizome has subglobular, pink, smaller tubers about 0.5 cm in diameter, with a scar on both depressed sides. All the leaves are basal and almost triangular in outline. They are 3-pinnate and bluish-green on the underside.

Characteristics: The taste of the tuber is bitter.

Habitat: Canada and U.S.

Production: Turkey Corn root is the root of Dicentra cucullaria.

Other Names: Squirrel Corn, Staggerweed, Bleeding Heart, Corydalis, Dutchman's Breeches

ACTIONS AND PHARMACOLOGY

COMPOUNDS

Isoquinoline alkaloids: including bicuculline, corlumine, protopine, cryptopine, cularine

EFFECTS

Diuretic and tonic

INDICATIONS AND USAGE

Unproven Uses: Turkey corn is used for digestive disorders, urinary tract diseases, menstrual disorders and skin rashes. Formerly it was used for syphilis.

PRECAUTIONS AND ADVERSE REACTIONS

Health risks or side effects following the proper administration of designated therapeutic dosages are not recorded. Bicuculline is a centrally acting, spasmogenic antagonist of gamma-aminobutyric acid (GABA). Due to the bicuculline componant, poisonings are possible if higher dosages are consumed, but none have been reported to date.

DOSAGE

Mode of Administration: The drug is available as a liquid extract.

LITERATURE

Kanamori H, Sakamoto I, Mizuta M, Chem Pharm Bull 34:1826. 1986.

Manske RHF, Canad J Res 7:265-269. 1932.

Manske RHF, Canad J Res Sect B 16:81-90. 1938.

Tusboi NS, J Labelled compd Radiopharm 13:353. 1977.

Further information in:

Hänsel R, Keller K, Rimpler H, Schneider G (Hrsg.), Hagers Handbuch der Pharmazeutischen Praxis, 5. Aufl., Bde 4-6 (Drogen): Springer Verlag Berlin, Heidelberg, New York, 1992-1994.

Madaus G, Lehrbuch der Biologischen Arzneimittel, Bde 1-3, Nachdruck, Georg Olms Verlag Hildesheim 1979.

Roth L, Daunderer M, Kormann K, Giftpflanzen, Pflanzengifte, 4. Aufl., Ecomed Fachverlag Landsberg Lech 1993.

Steinegger E, Hänsel R, Pharmakognosie, 5. Aufl., Springer Verlag Heidelberg 1992.

Teuscher E, Lindequist U, Biogene Gifte - Biologie, Chemie, Pharmakologie, 2. Aufl., Fischer Verlag Stuttgart 1994.

Turmeric

Curcuma domestica

DESCRIPTION

Medicinal Parts: The medicinal parts are the stewed and dried rhizome.

Flower and Fruit: The inflorescence is cone-like, 10 to 15 cm long, and is attached to a stem enclosed in a sheathing petiole. The flower has 2 pale green bracts, which are 5 to 6 cm long. The covering bracts are whitish, often red-tinged. The individual flowers are yellowish-white or yellow. The flowers have a tubular, 3-lobed calyx and funnel-shaped, 3-tipped corolla. The fruit is a gobular capsule.

Leaves, Stem and Root: Curcuma domestica is a perennial, erect and leafy plant with very large, lily-like leaves up to 1.2 m long. The leaf blade is ovate-lanceolate, thin, entire-margined and narrows to a long sheath-like petiole. The main rhizome is thickened to a tuber and has numerous roots. The roots in turn terminate in partially elliptical tubers. The secondary rhizomes are digit-shaped with no roots. All rhizomes are yellowish-brown with stipules and appear transversely ringed when they die.

Habitat: Turmeric is probably indigenous to India; it is cultivated today in India and other tropical regions of southeast Asia.

Production: Turmeric root consists of the finger-like, often tuber-like, scalded and dried rhizomes of Curcuma longa. It is harvested from February to April. The rhizomes are boiled in water for 5 to 10 minutes and then dried in the sun.

Adulterations: The synthetic color pigments azo and anilin are sometimes added to the herb.

Not to be Confused With: Curcuma xanthorrhiza, Curcuma aromatica and Curcuma zedoaria

ACTIONS AND PHARMACOLOGY

COMPOUNDS

Volatile oil (3-5%): alpha- and beta-tumerone (aroma source), artumerone, alpha- and gamma-atlantone, curlone, zingiberene, curcumol

Curcuminoids (3-5%): including curcumin, demethoxy curcumin, bidemethoxy curcumin

1,5-diaryl-penta-1,4-dien-3-one derivatives

Starch (30-40%)

EFFECTS

Turmeric has antihepatotoxic, antihyperlipidemic and anti-inflammatory effects. It is also antioxidative (inhibits lipid peroxide formation in the liver), antitumoral and antimicrobial (in particular, the sesquiterpene derivatives). It has insect repellent and antifertile effects. It also inhibits prostaglandin formation, *in vitro*.

INDICATIONS AND USAGE

Approved by Commission E:

- Dyspeptic complaints
- Loss of appetite

Unproven Uses: Turmeric is used for dyspeptic disorders, particularly feelings of fullness after meals and regular abdominal distention due to gas. The drug is also used for diarrhea, intermittent fever, edema, bronchitis, colds, worms, leprosy, kidney inflammation and cystitis. Other uses include headaches, flatulence, upper abdominal pain, chest infections, colic, amenorrhea and blood rushes. It is used externally for bruising, leech bites, festering eye infections, inflammation of the oral mucosa, inflammatory skin conditions and infected wounds.

Chinese Medicine: Turmeric is used for pains in the chest, ribs, abdomen, liver and stomach; nose bleeds; vomiting with bleeding; and heat stroke.

Indian Medicine: Turmeric is used for inflammation, wounds and skin ulcers, itching, stomach complaints, flatulence, conjunctivitis, constipation, ringworm infestation and colic.

CONTRAINDICATIONS

General: The drug should not be used by people with obstructed biliary ducts; those with gallstones should take it only under the supervision of a physician.

Pregnancy: Turmeric should not be used during pregnancy.

PRECAUTIONS AND ADVERSE REACTIONS

Health risks or side effects following the proper administration of designated therapeutic dosages are not recorded. Stomach complaints can occur following extended use or in the case of overdose.

DOSAGE

Mode of Administration: Whole, cut and powdered drug available as capsules, solution, coated tablets and compound preparations.

Preparation: To prepare a tea, scald 0.5 to 1 gm drug in boiling water, cover, draw for 5 minutes and then strain. The tincture strength is 1:10.

Daily Dosage: The average dose is 1.5 to 3 gm of drug. The powder should be taken 2 to 3 times daily after meals; the tea (2 to 3 cups) should be taken between meals. The tincture dose is 10 to 15 drops 2 to 3 times daily.

Storage: Turmeric should be protected from light.

LITERATURE

Ammon HP, Wahl MA, Pharmacology of Curcuma longa. Planta Med, 57:1-7, 1991.

Ammon HPT, Anazodo MI, Safayhi H et al., Planta Med 58:226, 1992.

Ammon HPT, Wahl MA, Pharmacology of Curcuma longa. Planta Med 57:1-7, 1991.

Anto RJ, George J, Babu KV, RaJasekharan KN, Kuttan R, Antimutagenic and anticarcinogenic activity of natural and synthetic curcuminoids. Mutat Res, 42:127-31, 1996.

Apisariyakul A, Vanittanakom N, Buddhasukh D, Antifungal activity of Turmeric oil extracted from Curcuma longa (Zingiberaceae). J Ethnopharmacol, 30:163-9, 1995.

Babu PS, Srinivasan K, Hypolipidemic action of curcumin the active principle of Turmeric (Curcuma longa) in streptozotocin induced diabetic rats. Mol Cell Biochem, 30:169-75, 1997.

Basu AB, Ind J Pharm 33:131, 1971.

Bonte F, Noel-Hudson MS, Wepierre J, Meybeck A, Protective effect of curcuminoids on epidermal skin cells under free oxygen radical stress. Planta Med, 8:265-6, 1997.

Chan MM, Inhibition of tumor necrosis factor by curcumin a phytochemical. Biochem Pharmacol, 42:1551-6, 1995.

Charles V, Charles SX, The use and efficacy of Azadirachta indica ADR ('Neem') and Curcuma longa ('Turmeric') in scabies. A pilot study. Trop Geogr Med, 30:178-81, 1992.

Dhar ML, et al Indian J Exp Biol 6:232, 1968.

Donatus IA, SardJoko, Vermeulen NP, Cytotoxic and cytoprotective activities of curcumin. Effects on paracetamol-induced cytotoxicity lipid peroxidation and glutathione depletion in rat hepatocytes. Biochem Pharmacol, 39:1869-75, 1990.

Ferreira LA, Henriques OB, Andreoni AA, Vital GR, Campos MM, Habermehl GG, de Moraes VL, Antivenom and biological effects of ar-turmerone isolated from Curcuma longa (Zingiberaceae). Toxicon, 30:1211-8, 1992.

Ferreira LA, Henriques OB, Andreoni AA, Vital GR, Campos MM, Habermehl GG, de Moraes VL, Toxicity studies on Alpinia galanga and Curcuma longa. Planta Med, 30:124-7, 1992.

Garg SK, Planta Med 26:225, 1974.

Hanif R, Qiao L, Shiff SJ, Rigas B, Curcumin a natural plant phenolic food additive inhibits cell proliferation and induces cell cycle changes in colon adenocarcinoma cell lines by a prostaglandin-independent pathway. J Lab Clin Med, 42:576-84, 1997.

Hänsel R, Keller K, Rimpler H, Schneider G (Ed.), Hagers Handbuch der Pharmazeutischen Praxis, 5. Aufl., Bde 4 - 6 (Drogen), Springer Verlag Berlin, Heidelberg, New York, 1992-1994.

Hasmeda M, Polya GM, Inhibition of cyclic AMP-dependent protein kinase by curcumin. Phytochemistry, 42:599-605, 1996.

Huang HC, Jan TR, Yeh SF, Inhibitory effect of curcumin an anti-inflammatory agent on vascular smooth muscle cell proliferation. Eur J Pharmacol, 54:381-4, 1992.

Inagawa H et al., Homeostasis as regulated by activated macrophage. II. LPS of plant origin other than wheat flour and their concomitant bacteria. Chem Pharm Bull (Tokyo), 54:994-7, 1992.

Kiso Y et al., Planta Med 49:185, 1983.

Krishnamurthy N et al., Trop Sci 18:37, 1976.

Leung AY, Encyclopedia of Common Natural Ingredients Used in Food Drugs and Cosmetics. John Wiley & Sons Inc. New York 1980.

Limtrakul P, Lipigorngoson S, Namwong O, Apisariyakul A, Dunn FW, Inhibitory effect of dietary curcumin on skin carcinogenesis in mice. Cancer Lett, 8:197-203, 1997.

Masuda T et al., Anti-oxidative and anti-inflammatory curcumin-related phenolics from rhizomes of Curcuma domestica. Phytochemistry 32:1557, 1986.

Mehta K, Pantazis P, McQueen T, Aggarwal BB, Antiproliferative effect of curcumin (diferuloylmethane) against human breast tumor cell lines. Anticancer Drugs, 8:470-81, 1997.

Nagarajan K, Arya VP, J Sci Ind Res 41:232, 1982.

Nakayama R et al., Two curcuminoid pigments from Curcuma domestica. Phytochemistry 33:501, 1993.

Polasa K, Sesikaran B, Krishna TP, Krishnaswamy K, Turmeric (Curcuma longa)-induced reduction in urinary mutagens. Food Chem Toxicol, 47:699-706, 1991.

Priyadarsini KI, Free radical reactions of curcumin in membrane models. Free Radic Biol Med, 54:838-43, 1997.

Rafatullah S, Tariq M, Al-Yahya MA, Mossa JS, Ageel AM, Evaluation of Turmeric (Curcuma longa) for gastric and duodenal antiulcer activity in rats. J Ethnopharmacol, 47:25-34, 1990.

Ravindranath V, Satyanarayana MN, Phytochemistry 19:2031, 1980.

Ruby AJ, Kuttan G, Babu KD, RaJasekharan KN, Kuttan R, Anti-tumour and antioxidant activity of natural curcuminoids. Cancer Lett, 42:79-83, 1995.

Selvam R, Subramanian L, Gayathri R, Angayarkanni N, The anti-oxidant activity of Turmeric (Curcuma longa). J Ethnopharmacol, 47:59-67, 1995.

Sikora E, Bielak-ZmiJewska A, Piwocka K, Skierski J, Radziszewska E, Inhibition of proliferation and apoptosis of human and rat T lymphocytes by curcumin a curry pigment. Biochem Pharmacol, 54:899-907, 1997.

Soni KB, RaJan A, Kuttan R, Reversal of aflatoxin induced liver damage by Turmeric and curcumin. Cancer Lett, 66:115-21, 1992.

Srimal RC, Dhawan CN, J Pharm Pharmacol 25:447, 1973.

Srinivas L, Shalini VK, ShylaJa M, Turmerin: a water soluble antioxidant peptide from Turmeric Curcuma longa. Arch Biochem Biophys, 30:617-23, 1992.

Srivastava KC, Bordia A, Verma SK, Curcumin a major component of food spice Turmeric (Curcuma longa) inhibits aggregation and alters eicosanoid metabolism in human blood platelets. Prostaglandins Leukot Essent Fatty Acids, 52:223-7, 1995.

Steinegger E, Hänsel R, Pharmakognosie. 5. Aufl., Springer Verlag Heidelberg 1992.

Tang W, Eisenbrand G, Chinese Drugs of Plant Origin. Springer Verlag Heidelberg 1992.

Teuscher E, Biogene Arzneimittel. 5. Aufl., Wiss. Verlagsgesellschaft Stuttgart 1997.

Veit M, Beeinflussung der Leukotrien-Biosynthese durch Curcumin. Z Phytother 14:46, 1993.

Verma SP, Salamone E, Goldin B, Curcumin and genistein plant natural products show synergistic inhibitory effects on the growth of human breast cancer MCF-7 cells induced by estrogenic pesticides. Biochem Biophys Res Commun, 233:692-6, 1997.

Wagner H et al., 6th Int Conf. Prostaglandins and Related Compounds. Florence, Italy. Pub. Fondzione Giovanni Lorenzini. June 3-6, 1986.

Wichtl M (Ed.), Teedrogen, 4. Aufl., Wiss. Verlagsges. Stuttgart 1997.

Turnera diffusa

See Damiana

Tussilago farfara

See Colt's Foot

Ulmus minor

See Elm Bark

Ulmus rubra

See Slippery Elm

Uncaria species

See Gambir

Uncaria tomentosa

See Cat's Claw

Urginea indica

See Indian Squill

Urginea maritima

See Squill

Urtica dioica

See Stinging Nettle

Usnea

Usnea species

DESCRIPTION

Medicinal Parts: Research into this species is not yet complete, making it difficult to establish which lichens are used for the extraction of which drug, and which lichens have been described by earlier botanists.

Flower and Fruit: Mycelia flourishes on a variety of trees (on the trunk, branches branchlets) as a whitish, reddish, or black lichen.

Habitat: Usnea is found worldwide in cool, damp places.

Production: Usnea consists of the dried thallus of Usnea species, primarily of Usnea barbata, Usnea florida, Usnea hirta and Usnea plicata.

Other Names: Tree Moss, Old Man's Beard, Beard Moss

ACTIONS AND PHARMACOLOGY

COMPOUNDS

Lichen acids (polyketides): including among others (+)-usnic acid, thamnolic acid (hirtellic acid), usnaric acid (salazinic acid), lobaric acid, stictinic acid, protocetraric acid, everninic acid, barbatinic acid (rhizonic acid), diffractaic acid (dirhizonic acid), barbatolic acid. The lichen acid spectrums of the different species vary from one another, with usnic acid the chief constituent.

Mucilage

EFFECTS

The drug is antimicrobial.

INDICATIONS AND USAGE

Approved by Commission E:

- Inflammation of the mouth and pharynx

Unproven Uses: The species are used for mild inflammation of the oral and pharyngeal mucosa.

PRECAUTIONS AND ADVERSE REACTIONS

No health hazards or side effects are known in conjunction with the proper administration of designated therapeutic dosages. Following overdosage, signs of poisoning could appear. These signs have yet to be described.

DOSAGE

Mode of Administration: The drug is available as lozenges and equivalent solid forms of medication.

Daily Dose: The daily dose is 600 mg. For lozenge preparations, use the equivalent of 100 mg of herb; take 1 lozenge 3 to 6 times daily.

LITERATURE

Kern W, List PH, Hörhammer L (Hrsg.), Hagers Handbuch der Pharmazeutischen Praxis, 4. Aufl., Bde 1-8: Springer Verlag Berlin, Heidelberg, New York, 1969.

Okuyama E et al., Usnic acid and diffractic acid as analgesic and antipyretic components of Usnea diffracta. In: PM 61(2):113-115. 1995.

Roth L, Daunderer M, Kormann K, Giftpflanzen, Pflanzengifte, 4. Aufl., Ecomed Fachverlag Landsberg Lech 1993.

Steinegger E, Hänsel R, Pharmakognosie, 5. Aufl., Springer Verlag Heidelberg 1992.

Usnea species

See Usnea

Utricularia vulgaris

See Bladderwort

Uva-Ursi

Arctostaphylos uva-ursi

TRADE NAMES

Uva-Ursi (available from numerous manufacturers), Uva-Ursi Leaf, Uva Ursi Leaves, Standardized Uva-Ursi Extract

DESCRIPTION

Medicinal Parts: The medicinal parts of the plant are the dried leaves and preparations of the fresh leaves.

Flower and Fruit: The flowers are on 3 to 12 short, hanging stalks, where they are in clusters at equal length and distance on the terminal end of the stalks. The pedicle has 2 small, ciliate, oval-shaped leaves at the base with the subtending flower clusters. The calyx is 1 mm long, palmate and has 5 membranous tips. The corolla (fused petals of the inner whorl) is ovoid to jug-shaped, white or reddish with a red border, 5 to 6 mm long with 5 short tips rolled backward. The 10 stamens are half in length as the corolla tube. The filaments are heavily thickened at the base. The crimson anthers have porous openings and a long whip-like, curling appendage. The ovaries are 5- to 7-valved, and the style is longer than the stamens. The fruit is a globular, pea-sized, scarlet, floury drupe. The fruit has 5 to 7 stone seeds, 4 mm in length, which are kidney-shaped and also compressed at the sides.

Leaves, Stem and Root: The plant is a decumbent (reclining on the ground with ascending extremities), up to 1.5 m long, creeping espalier with elastic, red-brown branches. The leaves are alternate, coriaceous, short-petioled, spatulate-obovate or wedge-shaped, entire-margined and slightly revolute. They are 12 to 30 mm long by 4 to 15 mm wide, glabrous, glossy and evergreen. The underside is distinctly reticulate, and the midrib and the margins are often downy.

Characteristics: The leaves have a bitter, astringent taste. They are distinguished from the cranberry by the reticulate vein structure and non-glandular spots beneath.

Habitat: The plant has spread from the Iberian Peninsula across Central Europe north to Scandinavia and east to Siberia. The plant is also found in the Altai mountains, the Himalayas and North America.

Production: Uva-Ursi (Bearberry) leaves consist of the fresh or dried leaves of Arctostaphylos uva-ursi, which are gathered in the wild. The arbutin content is highest in December and January and also when the leaves are dried rapidly. The main sources are Spain, Italy, Austria, Switzerland, Scandinavia, Poland, Russia and Bulgaria.

Not to be Confused With: The leaves are sometimes confused with the leaves of other Ericaceae, such as Buxus sempervirens.

Other Names: Arberry, Bearberry, Bear's Grape, Kinnikinnick, Mealberry, Mountain Box, Mountain Cranberry, Red-Berried Trailing Arbutus, Redberry Leaves, Rockbeery, Sagackhomi, Sandberry, Upland Cranberry, Red-Beery, Upland Cranbeery, Common Bearberry, Arbutus Uva-Ursi, Red Bearberry, Kinnickinick

ACTIONS AND PHARMACOLOGY

COMPOUNDS

Hydroquinone glycosides: arbutin (arbutoside, hydroquinone-O-beta-D-glucoside, 5-16%), methyl arbutin (O-methyl hydroquinone-O-beta-D-glycoside, up to 4%), galloyl derivatives of arbutin (0.05%): O-galloyl hydroquinone-O-beta-D-glucoside (p-galloyl oxyphenyl-O-beta-D-glucoside), 2′-O- galloyl arbutin, 6′-O-galloyl arbutin, free hydroquinone (usually under 0.3%) as decomposition product of arbutin, emerging as the leaves age or during dehydration

Piceoside: (4-hydroxyacetophenone-O-beta-D-glucopyranoside)

Phenol carboxylic acids: including gallic acid (free 180 mg/100 g), p-coumaric acid (18.0 mg/100 g), syringic acid (16.8 mg/100 g), salicylic acid (12.0 mg/100 g), p-hydroxybenzoic acid (9.6 mg/100 g), ferulic acid (6.0 mg/100 g), caffeic acid (6.0 mg/100 g), lithospermic acid (dimeric caffeic acid)

Tannins (15-20%): gallo tannins including penta-O-galloyl-beta-D-Glucose and hexa-O-galloyl-beta-D-glucose; ellagitannins, including corilagin (1-0-galloyl-3, 6-di-O-hexahydroxydophenol-beta-D-gulcoside); condensed tannins, chiefly proanthocyanidins and their monomerics, including cyanidin, delphinidin

Iridoide: monotropein (0.025%)

Flavonoids: flavonol glycosides, including hyperoside (0.8-1.5%) which is the chief flavonol glycoside, quercitrin-3-

beta-D-O-6′-galloyl galactoside, quercitrin, isoquercitrin, myricitrin, myricetin-3-O-beta-D-galactoside, 2 isomeric quercetin arabinosides, aglycones of these compounds

Enzymes: including a beta-glucosidase (arbutase), that is rendered inactive with dehydration and processing of the drug, due to the high tannin content

Triterpenes: including among others ursolic acid (0.4-0.8%), alcohol uvaol, beta-amyrin

EFFECTS

The tannins in Uva-Ursi act as an astringent, and the phenol glucocsides and their aglyca have an antibacterial effect. The antimicrobial effect is associated with the aglycon hydroquinone released from arbutin (transport form) or arbutin waste products in the alkaline urine. The drug has urine-sterilizing properties that are attributed to bacteriostatic hydroquinones, conjugates of glucuronic acid and sulfuric acid. The maximum antibacterial effect is expected 3 to 4 hours after administration. There are no clinical studies available that have been definitively evaluated.

CLINICAL TRIALS

Nephrolithiasis

The effects of Uva-Ursi with prevention and treatment of kidney stone formation was studied in rats. It concluded that beneficial effects from Uva-Ursi on urolithiasis can be attributed to some disinfectant action (Grases, 1994).

Diuresis

The aqueous extract of Arctostaphylos uva-ursi was studied in rats involoving diuresis. The pharmacological evaluation revealed an increase in urine flow without an increase in urinary sodium excretion (Beaux, 1999).

Antibacterial Properties

The effect of aqueous extracts of Uva-Ursi leaves to decrease surface hydrophobicity of 155 Escherichia coli strains was determined in cattle. The adhesion of microbes on host cells is important for development of Gram-negative microbe-induced infections and is influenced by the surface hydrophobicity of the microbial cell. Bactericidal action of Uva-Ursi was low, but the decrease in cell surface hydrophobicity may influence the bacteria's virulent properties (Turi, 1997). The aqueous extract of Uva-Ursi leaves was also studied in Helicobacter pylori (H. pylori) strains to determine possible changes in cell surface hydrophobicity. The tannic acid in the Uva-Ursi was determined to have the highest activity of decreasing cell surface hydrophobicity as well as antibacterial activity against H. Pylori (Annuck, 1999)

INDICATIONS AND USAGE

Approved by Commission E:

■ Infections of the urinary tract

Uva-Ursi is used for inflammatory disorders of the efferent urinary tract.

Unproven Uses: In folk medicine, the herb is used for all forms of urogenital and biliary tract disease.

Homeopathic Uses: The herb is used for inflammations of the efferent urinary tract.

CONTRAINDICATIONS

The drug is contraindicated in pregnant women, nursing mothers and children under 12 years of age.

PRECAUTIONS AND ADVERSE REACTIONS

General: No health hazards are known in conjunction with the proper administration of designated therapeutic dosages. Individuals with gastric sensitivity may experience nausea and vomiting following intake of preparations made from the drug due to its high tannin content.

Pregnancy: The drug is contraindicated during pregnancy.

Nursing Mothers: The drug is contraindicated in nursing mothers.

Pediatric Use: Liver damage is conceivable in connection with administration of the drug over extended periods, particularly with children, due to the possible hepatotoxicity of the hydroquinones released. The drug is contraindicated in children under 12 years of age.

Drug Interactions: Uva-Ursi preparations should not be administered with any substance that causes acidic urine since this reduces the antibacterial effect. Because the urine-disinfecting effect of the hydroquinones released in the urinary tract only occurs in an alkali environment, the simultaneous administration of medication or food that increase uric acid levels in the bladder is to be avoided.

The sodium sparing effect of Uva-Ursi may offset the diuretic effect of thiazide and loop diuretics.

Uva-Ursi may add to the gastrointestinal irritation that occurs with NSAID use.

OVERDOSAGE

Overdosage can lead to inflammation and irritation of the bladder and urinary tract mucous membranes. Liver damage is conceivable in connection with administration of the drug over extended periods, particularly with children, due to the possible hepatotoxicity of the hydroquinones released.

DOSAGE

Mode of Administration: Uva-Ursi is available as comminuted drug, drug powder or dried extract for infusions or cold macerations, and also as extracts and solid forms for oral administration. It is also a component of urologic combination and single-component preparations.

How Supplied:

Capsules—150 mg, 455 mg, 505 mg

Teas

Solutions

Preparation: To make a tea, pour boiling water over 2.5 gm finely cut or coarse powdered drug (1 teaspoonful is equivalent to 2.5 g drug.), or place the drug in cold water that is rapidly brought to a boil. The tea should draw (to extract the essence) for 15 minutes and then be strained. Teas may contain up to 30% Uva-Ursi in combination with other drugs. For higher Uva-Ursi content, prepare cold macerate (over 6 to 12 hours) to lower the tannin content.

Daily Dosage: The daily dosage of finely cut or powdered drug is 10 g (corresponding to arbutin content of 400 to 840 mg) or 0.4 g dry extract in a single dose. A single dose of liquid extract is 2 g. Daily dosages of an infusion or cold maceration are 3 g drug to 150 ml water as an infusion or cold maceration up to 4 times a day or 400 to 840 mg hydroquinone derivatives calculated as water-free arbutin. The urine should be alkaline.

Homeopathic Dosage: 5 to 10 drops, 1 tablet or 5 to 10 globules 1 to 3 times daily or 1 ml injection solution twice weekly sc (HAB1).

Storage: Store in well-sealed containers protected from light.

LITERATURE

Annuk H, Hirmo S, Turi E et al., Effect on cell surface hydrophobicity and susceptibility of Helicobacter pylori to medicinal plant extracts. FEMS Microbiol Lett 1999 Mar 1;172(1):41-5.

Beaux D, Fleurentin J, Mortier F, Effect of extracts of Orthosiphon stamineus Benth, Hieracium pilosella L., Sambucus nigra L. and Arctostaphylos uva-ursi (L.) Spreng. in rats. Phytother Res 1999 May;13(3):222-5.

Britton G, Haslam E, J Chem Soc (London): 7312. 1965.

Denford KE, (1973) Experientia 29:939.

Frohne D, (1970) Planta Med 18:1.

Frohne D, (1986) Arctostaphylos uva-ursi: Die Bärentraube. Z Phytother 7:45-47.

Hiller K, Pharmazeutische Bewertung ausgewählter Teedrogen. In: DAZ 135(16):1425-1440. 1995.

Ihring M, Blume H, Zur pharmazeutischen Qualität von Phytopharmaka 2. Mitt.: Vergleichende Bewertung von Arbutin enthaltenden Urologika. In: PZW 135(6)267. 1990.

Jahodar L et al., (1978) Pharmazie 33(8):536.

Jahodar L et al., (1981) Pharmazie 36(2):294.

Jahodar L et al., (1985) Cesk Farm. 34(5):174.

Kraus L, DAZ 111:1225. 1974.

Kubo M et al., Pharmacological studies on leaf of Arctostaphylos uva-ursi: Combined effect of 50% methanolic extract from Arctostaphylos uva-ursi and prednisolone on immuno-inflammation.

Matsuda H et al., Pharmacological studies on leaf of Arctostaphylos uva-ursi: Effect of 50% methanolic extract from Arctostaphylos uva-ursi on melanin synthesis. Yakugaku Zasshi, 112:276-82, 1992 Apr

Matsuda H et al., Pharmacological studies on leaf of Arctostaphylos uva-ursi: Effect of water extract from Arctostaphylos uva-ursi on the antiallergic and anti-inflammatory activities of dexamethasone ointment. Yakugaku Zasshi, 112:673-7, 1992 Sep.

Matsuda H, Nakata H, Tanaka T, Kubo M, Phenolic acids in leaves of Arctostaphylos uva ursi L. Vaccinium vitis idaea L. and Vaccinium myrtillus L. Pharmazie, 110:680-1, 1991 Sep.

Matsuda H, Tanaka T, Kubo M, Pharmacological studies on leaf of Arctostaphylos uva-ursi (L.) Spreng. III. Combined effect of arbutin and indomethacin on immuno-inflammation. Yakugaku Zasshi, 111:253-8, 1991 Apr-May.

Matsuda H, Nakata H, Tanaka T, Kubo M, Pharmacological study on Arctostaphylos uva-ursi (L.) Spreng. II. Combined effects of arbutin and prednisolone or dexamethazone on immuno-inflammation. Yakugaku Zasshi, 110:68-76, 1990 Jan.

Matsuo K, Kobayashi M, Takuno Y, Kuwajima H, Ito H, Yoshida T, Anti-tyrosinase activity constituents of Arctostaphylos uva-ursi. Yakugaku Zasshi, 117:1028-32, 1997 Dec.

Ng TB et al., Examination of coumarins, flavonoids and polysaccharopeptides for antibacterial activity. In: General Pharmacology 27(7):1237-1240. 1996.

Paper DH, Koehler J, Franz G, Bioavailalibilty of drug preparations containing a leaf extract of Arctostaphylos uva-ursi (Uvae Ursi Folium). In: PM 59(7)

Thesen R, Phytotherapeutika-nicht immer harmlos. In: ZPT 9(49):105. 1988.

Thieme H, Winkler HJ, PA 26:235 et 419. 1971.

Turi M, Turi E, Koljalg S et al., Influence of aqueous extracts of medicinal plants on surface hydrophobicity of Escherichia coli strains of different origin. APMIS 1997 Dec; 105(12):956-62.

Grases F, Melero G, Costa-Bauza A et al., Urolithiasis and phytotherapy. Int Urol Nephrol 1994;26(5):507-11.

Further information in:

Hänsel R, Keller K, Rimpler H, Schneider G (Hrsg.), Hagers Handbuch der Pharmazeutischen Praxis, 5. Aufl., Bde 4-6 (Drogen): Springer Verlag Berlin, Heidelberg, New York, 1992-1994.

Madaus G, Lehrbuch der Biologischen Arzneimittel, Bde 1-3, Nachdruck, Georg Olms Verlag Hildesheim 1979.

Ritch-Krc EM, Thomas S, Turner NJ, Towers GH, Carrier herbal medicine: traditional and contemporary plant use. J Ethnopharmacol, 117:85-94, 1996 Jun.

Roth L, Daunderer M, Kormann K, Giftpflanzen, Pflanzengifte, 4. Aufl., Ecomed Fachverlag Landsberg Lech 1993.

Schulz R, Hänsel R, Rationale Phytotherapie, Springer Verlag Heidelberg 1996.

Stammwitz U, Pflanzliche Harnwegsdesinfizienzien - heute noch aktuell? Z Phytother 19(1998), 90-95.

Steinegger E, Hänsel R, Pharmakognosie, 5. Aufl., Springer Verlag Heidelberg 1992.

Teuscher E, Biogene Arzneimittel, 5. Aufl., Wiss. Verlagsges. Stuttgart 1997.

Wagner H, Wiesenauer M, Phytotherapie. Phytopharmaka und pflanzliche Homöopathika, Fischer-Verlag, Stuttgart, Jena, New York 1995.

Wichtl M (Hrsg.), Teedrogen, 4. Aufl., Wiss. Verlagsges. Stuttgart 1997.

Uzara

Xysmalobium undulatum

DESCRIPTION

Medicinal Parts: Different varieties are used for drug extraction depending on the area. The drug is therefore easier to categorize according to its definitive active substances (bitters) than to its particular varieties.

Flower and Fruit: The root has a weak and unusual odor. The taste is bitter with a burning effect after it has been chewed for a long time.

Habitat: South Africa

Production: Uzara root consists of the dried, underground parts of 2- to 3-year-old plants of Xysmalobium undulatum.

ACTIONS AND PHARMACOLOGY

COMPOUNDS

Cardioactive steroid glycosides (cardenolides, mixture referred to as uzarone or xysmalobin): including among others uzarin (5.5%), xysmalorin (1.5%), allo-uzarine, allo-xysmalobin, urezin, uzaroside, ascleposide, glucoascleposide

Pregnane derivatives: delta5-pregnene-3beta-ol-20-one glucoside, 5alpha-pregnane-3beta-ol-20-one glucoside

EFFECTS

Uzara inhibits intestinal motility. In high dosages, it has digitalis-like effects on the heart.

INDICATIONS AND USAGE

Approved by Commission E:

■ Diarrhea

Unproven Uses: Uzara is used as a treatment for dysentery.

CONTRAINDICATIONS

Uzara should not be administered concomitantly with other cardioactive glycosides.

PRECAUTIONS AND ADVERSE REACTIONS

General: No health hazards or side effects are known in conjunction with the proper administration of designated therapeutic dosages.

Drug Interactions: Because Uzara contains cardioactive glycosides, there is a potential for interaction with digoxin and other cardiac glycosides. This interaction has not been reported in the literature for orally administered Uzara. The lack of reports may be due to the fact that the glycocides are not well absorbed from the gut.

OVERDOSAGE

Because the glycosides are absorbed only with difficulty and because their cardiac effect is minimal, poisonings following oral intake are unlikely, although conceivable. There have been cases of fatalities following parenteral application of Uzara drugs.

DOSAGE

Mode of Administration: The drug is available as ethanol-water extracts in liquid form or as dry extracts for internal use. Pharmaceutical forms include coated tablets, drops and compound preparations.

Daily Dose: The daily dose should be equivalent to 45 to 90 mg of total glycosides, calculated as uzarin. Follow the manufacturer's dosing instructions.

LITERATURE

Kern W, List PH, Hörhammer L (Hrsg.), Hagers Handbuch der Pharmazeutischen Praxis, 4. Aufl., Bde. 1-8: Springer Verlag Berlin, Heidelberg, New York, 1969.

Madaus G, Lehrbuch der Biologischen Arzneimittel, Bde 1-3, Nachdruck, Georg Olms Verlag Hildesheim 1979 (unter Gomphocarpus).

Pauli G, Schiller H, Asymmetric key position in Uzara steroids. In: PM 62, Abstracts of the 44th Ann Congress of GA, 113. 1996.

Roth L, Daunderer M, Kormann K, Giftpflanzen, Pflanzengifte, 4. Aufl., Ecomed Fachverlag Landsberg Lech 1993.

Schmidt M, Uzarawurzel. In: PTA 8(6):498. 1994.

Steinegger E, Hänsel R, Pharmakognosie, 5. Aufl., Springer Verlag Heidelberg 1992.

Wagner H, Wiesenauer M, Phytotherapie. Phytopharmaka und pflanzliche Homöopathika, Fischer-Verlag, Stuttgart, Jena, New York 1995.

Vaccinium myrtillus

See Bilberry

Vaccinium uliginosum

See Bog Bilberry

Vaccinium vitis-ideae

See Alpine Cranberry

Valerian

Valeriana officinalis

TRADE NAMES

Valerian Root (available from numerous manufacturers,) Herbal Sure Valerian Root, NuVeg Valerian Root, Valerian Root Alcohol Free, Valerian Power Time Release, Valerian Root Power, Standardized Valerian, Natural Herbal Valerian Root, Nature's Root Nighttime, Quanterra Sleep

DESCRIPTION

Medicinal Parts: The medicinal parts are the carefully dried underground parts and the dried roots.

Flower and Fruit: The androgynous, bright, pink-to-white flowers are in panicled cymes. The calyx consists of 10 revolute tips. The corolla is funnel-shaped with a 5-sectioned margin. The tube has a bump at the base. There are 3 stamens. The ovary is inferior and has 3 chambers. The fruit is ovate-oblong, yellow, indehiscent and has a 10-rayed tuft of white hair.

Leaves, Stem and Root: The plant is 50 to 100 cm high and has a short, cylindrical rhizome with finger-length, bushy round roots. The stem is erect and unbranched. The leaves are odd-pinnate with 11 to 23 lanceolate, indented-dentate leaflets. The lower ones are petiolate and the upper ones sessile and clasping with a white sheath.

Characteristics: The flowers are fragrant and the rhizome smells strongly when dried. The odor is not present in the fresh plant. Hydrolysis of componants in the root form isovaleric acid which is responsible for the offensive smell.

Habitat: The plant is found in Europe and in the temperate regions of Asia. It is cultivated mainly in central Europe, England, France, eastern Europe, Japan and the U.S.

Production: Valerian root, consisting of fresh underground plant parts, or parts carefully dried below 40° C of the species Valeriana officinalis. Cultivation is possible in low-lying, sandy, humus soil that is well supplied with lime and situated in a damp area. The root is harvested in September. The fresh roots are washed, chopped, and carefully dried in circulating air under 40° C.

Not to be Confused With: Confusion with other species seldom occurs since the plant is primarily supplied via cultivation. The most dangerous adulteration of the plant occurs by the addition of the roots of Veratrum album.

Other Names: All-Heal, Amantilla, Setwall, Setewale, Capon's Tail, Heliotrope, Vandal Root

ACTIONS AND PHARMACOLOGY

COMPOUNDS

Iridoids: valepotriates (valeriana-epoxy-triacylates, iridoide monoterpenes, 0.5-2.0%) chief components (50-80%), isovaltrate (up to 46%), isovaleroxyhydroxy didrovaltrate (IVDH-valtrate, 10-20%), including among others, didrovaltrate, acevaltrate

Volatile oil (0.2-1.0%): chief components (-)-bornyl isovalerenate and isovalerenic acid (both aroma-carriers), including among others, (-)-bornyl acetate, isoeugenyl valerenate, isoeugenyl isovalerenate, also with some strains valerenal, valeranone, cryptofaurinol

Sesquiterpenes: valerenic acid (0.1-0.9%), 2-hydroxyvalerenic acid, 2-acetoxy-valerenic acid

Pyridine alkaloids (traces, cat pheromone): actinidine, valerianine, alpha-methylpyrrylketone

Caffeic acid derivatives: chlorogenic acid.

The subspecies within the collective species differ in their constituent substances spectra.

EFFECTS

In animal experiments, the interaction of the various constituents are centrally depressive, sedative, anxiolytic, spasmolytic, muscle relaxing and anti-ulcerogenic. The pharmacological efficacy is heavily dependent on the quality of the extract used.The main effect in humans is to reduce sleep induction time. In vitro the valerenic acid componants have been shown to decrease the degradation of gamma—aminobutyric acid (GABA.) Animal experiments have demonstrated an increase of GABA at the synaptic cleft via inhibition of re-uptake and an increase in secretion of the neurotransmitter. The increase of available GABA is one factor that may be responsible for the sedative properties of

Valerian root (Houghton, 1998; Santos et al, 1994.) One other mechanism that may contribute to the sedative properties of Valerian could be the high levels of glutamine present in the extract Unlike GABA, glutamine more effectively crosses the blood-brain barrier where it can be taken up by the nerve terminals and converted to GABA (Santos, Fero, 1994.)

CLINICAL TRIALS

Improvements in sleep quality ratings were demonstrated in a well constructed, randomized, placebo-controlled, multi-center study involving 121 patients. Subjects were given either 600 mg of a 70% ethanol extract (5:1, n = 61) of Valerian root that was standardized to 0.4 - 0.6% valerenic acid or placebo (n = 60) one hour before bedtime for 28 consecutive nights. Patients were given two standardized sleep questionaires; one that measured the depression/mood scale and another global clinical impression scale. Sixty-six percent of the Valerian treatment arm rated the therapeutic effect as either good or very good at the end of the 28 day trial. This compared to only a 29% equally positive rating by the placebo participants. (Vorbach, 1996).

INDICATIONS AND USAGE

Approved by Commission E:

■ Nervousness and insomnia

Unproven Uses: Valerian is used for restlessness, sleeping disorders based on nervous conditions, mental strain, lack of concentration, excitability, stress, headache, neurasthenia, epilepsy, hysteria, nervous cardiopathy, menstrual states of agitation, pregnancy, menopause, neuralgia, fainting, nervous stomach cramps, colic, uterine spasticity and states of anxiety.

PRECAUTIONS AND ADVERSE REACTIONS

General: No health hazards are known in conjunction with the proper administration of designated therapeutic dosages. Gastrointestinal complaints can occur in rare cases, contact allergies in very rare ones.

With long-term administration, the following can occasionally appear: headache, restless states, sleeplessness, mydriasis, disorders of cardiac function.

When large skin injuries or acute skin illnesses, severe feverish or infectious diseases, cardiac insufficiency or hypertonia are present, entire-body baths with the addition of the volatile oil or of extracts from the drug should be avoided.

Drug Interactions: Valerian may potentiate the effect of other CNS depressants. Animal studies have shown that Valerian has an additive effect when used in combination with barbiturates and benzodiazepines (Leuschner, 1993; Hiller, 1996.) Though there has been no evidence of potentiation of the CNS depressive effect when combined with alcohol, it is not recommended that Valerian be used in conjunction with alcohol. Because of the sedative effect of Valerian, operation of machinery or motor vehicles should be avoided for several hours after injesting Valerian products.

Pregnancy: Use of Valerian during pregnancy or in nursing mothers is not recommended.

DOSAGE

Mode of Administration: Valerian is used internally as expressed juice from fresh plants, tincture, extracts, and other galenic preparations. Externally, it is used as a bath additive, though efficacy is unproven for this indication.

How Supplied:

Capsules — 100 mg, 250 mg, 380 mg, 400 mg, 445 mg, 450 g, 475 mg, 493 mg, 495 mg, 500 mg, 530 mg, 550 mg, 1000 mg

Liquid — 1:1

Tablets — 160 mg, 550 mg

Tea Bags

Preparation: To prepare an infusion, use 2 to 3 g of drug per cup. A tea is prepared by adding 1 teaspoonful (3 to 5 g) of drug to 150 ml of hot water and strain after 10 to 15 minutes. An extract is prepared by mixing 2 parts root powder to 6 parts spirit of wine and 9 parts water. For external use, 100 g of comminuted drug is mixed with 2 liters hot water; this is then added to the bath.

Daily Dosage: The daily dose of Valerian extract is 100 mg to 1800 mg. Total internal daily dose is 15 g of root powder.

Infusion — One cup one to several times per day

Tea — One cup (150 ml) 2 to 3 times daily and before bedtime.

Tincture — 1/2 to 1 teaspoonful (1 to 3 ml) one to several times per day.

Tincture (1:5) — several times daily 15 to 20 drops in water.

Extract — equivalent 2 to 3 g drug, one to several times per day.

Plant juice — Adults take 1 tablespoonful 3 times daily. Children take 1 teaspoonful 3 times daily.

External use — As a bath according to preparation instructions above.

Sleep Aid — 400 mg to 900 mg of the extract 30 minutes before bedtime

Restlessness — 220 mg extract three times daily

Storage: Must be kept from sources of light; tinctures and extracts should be stored at room temperature in tightly closed, non-plastic containers.

LITERATURE

Anonym, Phytotherapeutika: Nachgewiesene Wirkung, aber wirksame Stoffe meist nicht bekannt. In: DAZ 137(15):1221-1222. 1997.

Becker H et al., (1983) Planta Med 49(1):64.

Bodesheim U, Hölzl J, Isolation and receptor binding properties of alkaloids and lignans from Valeriana officinalis L. In: PA 52(5):386-391. 1997.

Bos R et al., (1983) Phytochemistry 22 (6):1505.

Bos R et al., Seasonal variation of the essential oil, valerenic acid derivatives, and valepotriates in Valeriana officinalis roots. In: PM 59(7)98. 1993.

Bounthanh C et al., (1981) Planta Med 41:21.

Bounthanh C et al., (1983) Planta Med 49:138.

Bounthanh C, Bergmann C, Beck JP, Haag-Berrurier M, Anton R (1981) Valepotriates, a new class of cytotoxic, antitumor agents. Planta Med 41:21-28.

Braun R et al., (1982) Dtsch Apoth Ztg 122:1109.

Braun R et al., (1984) Planta Med 1.

Braun R, Dittmar W, Machut M, Weickmann S, (1982) Valepotriate mit Epoxidstruktur - beachtliche Alkylantien. Dtsch Apoth Z 122:1109-1113.

Braun R, Dittmar W, von der Hude W, Scheutwinkel-Reich M, (1985) Bacterial mutagenicity of the tranquilizing constituents of valerianaceae roots. Naunyn- Schmiedeberg's Arch Pharmacol Suppl 329:R28.

Donath F, Roots I, (1995) Untersuchung zur Erfassung der Wirkung von Baldrianextrakt (LI 156) auf das Pharmako-EEG bei 16 Probanden. Z Phytother Abstractband, S. 10.

Eickstedt KW von, (1969) Arzneim Forsch 19:995.

Eickstedt KW von, Rahmann R, (1969) Psychopharmakologische Wirkungen von Valepotriaten. Arzneim-Forsch 19:316-319.

Funk ED, Friedrich H, (1975) Planta Med 28:215.

Gross D et al., (1971) Arch Pharm 304:19.

Grusla D, (1987) Nachweis der Wirkung eines Baldrianextraktes im Rattenhirn mit der 14C-2-Desoxyglucose-Technik. Dissertation, Phillipps-Universität, Marburg.

Hänsel R, (1984) Bewertung von Baldrian-Präparaten: Differenzierung wesentlich: Dtsch Apoth Z 124:2085.

Hänsel R, Pflanzliche Beruhigungsmittel Möglichkeiten und Grenzen der Selbstmedikation. In: DAZ 135(32):2935-2943. 1995.

Hänsel R, Pflanzliche Sedativa. In: ZPT 11(1):14. 1990.

Hänsel R, Schultz J, (1982) Dtsch Apoth Ztg 122(5):215.

Hänsel R, Schulz J, (1982) Valerensäuren und Valerenal als Leitstoffe des offizinellen Baldrians. Dtsch Apoth Z 122:215-219.

Hänsel R, Schulz J, (1985) Beitrag zur Qulaitätssicherung von Baldrianextrakten. Pharm Industrie 47:531-533.

Hardy M, Kirk-Smith MD, Stretch DD (1995) Replacement of drug treatment for insomnia by ambient odour. Lancet 346:701.

Hazelhoff B, (1984) Phytochemical, Pharmacological Aspects of Valeriana compounds. Dissertation, Universität Groningen.

Hazelhoff B et al., (1979) Pharm Weekbl Sci Ed. 1:71.

Hendricks H, Bruins AB, (1980) J Chromatogr 190:321.

Hendricks R et al., (1977) Phytochemistry 16:1853.

Hendriks H et al., (1981) Planta Med 42(1):62.

Hendriks H et al., (1985) Planta Med (3):28.

Hendriks H, Bos R, Woerdenbag HJ, Koster AS, (1985) Central Nervous Depressant Activity of Valerenic Acid in the Mouse. Planta Med 51:28-31.

Hiller KO, Zetler G, (1996) Neuropharmacological Studies on Ethanol Extracts of Valeriana officinalis: Behavioural, Anticonvulsant Properties. Phytotherapy Res 10:145-151.

Hiller KO, Kato G, Anxiolytic activity of psychotropic plant extracts. I. Test of ethanolic Valeriana extract STEI Val. In: PM 62, Abstracts of the 44th Ann Congress of GA, 65. 1996.

Hiller KO, Rahlfs V, Therapeutische Äquivalenz eines hochdosierten Phytopharmakons mit Amytriptylin bei ängstlich-depressiven Versimmungen - Reanalyse einer randomisierten Studie unter besonderer Beachtung biometrischer und klinischer Aspekte. In: Forsch.

Hölzl J, Baldrian ein Mittel gegen Schlafstörungen. In: DAZ 136(10):751-759. 1996.

Jansen W, (1977) Doppelblindstudie mit Baldrisedon. Therapiewoche 27:2779-2786.

Kamm-Kohl AV, Jansen W Brockmann P, (1984) Moderne Baldriantherapie gegen nervöse Störungen im Senium. Med Welt 35:1450-1454.

Krieglstein J, Grusla D, (1988) Zentraldämpfende Inhaltsstoffe im Baldrian. Dtsch Apoth Z 128:2041-2046.

Kubitschek J, Baldrian beeinflußt die Melatoninwirkung. In: PZ 142(6):433 1997.

Leathwood PD et al., (1982) Pharmacol Biochem Behav 17:65.

Leathwood PD, Chauffard F (1983) J Psychiatr. Res 17(2):115.

Leathwood PD, Chauffard F, (1983) Quantifying the effects of mild sedatives. J Psychiat Res 17:115-122.

Leathwood PD, Chauffard F, (1984) Aqueous extract of valerian reduces latency to fall asleep in man. Planta Med 50:144-148.

Meier B, Linnenbrink N, Status und Vergleichbarkeit pflanzlicher Arzneimittel. In: DAZ 136(47):4205-4220. 1996.

Müller-Bohn T, Pflanzliche Sedativa und Antidepressiva. In: DAZ 136(24):2032-2033. 1996.

Orth-Wagner S, Ressin WJ, Friedrich I, Phytosedativum gegen Schlafstörungen. In: ZPT 16(3):147-156. 1995.

Popov S et al., (1974) Phytochemistry 13:2815.

Reidel E et al., (1982) Planta Med 46:219.

Riedel E, Hänsel R, Ehrke G, (1982) Hemmung des Gamma-Aminobuttersäureabbaus durch Valerensäurederivate. Planta Med 46:219-220.

Rücker G, Tautges J, Sieek A, Wenzel H, Frag E, (1978) Untersuchungen zur Isolierung und pharmakodynamischen Aktivität des Sesquiterpens Valeranon aus Nardostrachys jatamansi DC Arzneim-Forsch/Drug Res 28:7.

Santos MS, Ferreira F, Cunha AP et al., (1994) An Aqueous Extract of Valerian Influences the Transport of GABA in Synaptosomes. Planta Med 60:278-279.

Schilcher H, Pflanzliche Psychopharmaka. Eine neue Klassifizierung nach Indikationsgruppen. In: DAZ 135(20):1811-1822. 1995.

Schimmer O, Röder A, Valerensäuren in Fertigarzneimitteln und selbst bereiteten Auszügen aus der Wurzel von Valeriana officinalis L.s.l. In: PZW 137(1):31-36. 1992.

Schulz H, Jobert M, (1995) Die Darstellung sedierender/ Tranquilisierender Wirkungen von Phytopharmaka im quantifizierten EEG Z Phytother Abstractband, S. 10.

Schulz H, Stolz C, Müller J, (1994) The effect of a valerian extract on sleep polygraphy in poor sleepers. A pilot study. Pharmacopsychiat 27:147-151.

Schulz V, Hübner WD, Ploch M, Klinische Studien mit Psycho-Phytopharmaka. In: ZPT 18(3):141-154. 1997.

Sprecher E, Pflanzliche Geriatrika. In: ZPT 9(2):40. 1988.

Sprecher E, Über die Qualität von Phytopharmaka. In: ZPT 12(4):105. 1991.

Thies PW, Funke S, (1966) Tetrahedron Letters 11:1155.

Torii S, Fukuda H, Kanemoto H, Miyanchi R, Hamauzu Y, Kawasaki M, (1988) Contingent negative variation (CNV), the psychological effects of odour. In: Van Toller St, Dodd GH (eds) Perfumery, The psychology, biology of fragrance. Chapman, Hall, London New York, S 107-146.

Trossell K, Wahlberg K, (1966) Tetrahedron Letters 4:445.

Tyler VE, (1987) The new honest herbal. A sensible guide to herbs, related remedies. 2nd ed Stickley Co., Philadelphia, S 125-126.

Van Meer JH, Labadine RP, (1981) J Chromatogr. 205(1):206.

Veith J et al., (1986) Planta Med (3):179.

Vorbach EU, Arnold KH, (1995) Wirksamkeit und Verträglichkeit von Baldrianextrakt (LI 156) versus Placebo bei behandlungsbedürftigen Insomnien. Z Phytother Abstractband, S 11.

Vorbach EU, Gortelmeyer R & Bruning J: Therapie von Insomnien. Wirksamkeit und Vertraeglichkeit eine Baldrianpraeparats. Psychopharmakotherapie 1996; 3:109-115.

Werner, Arzneipflanzen in der Volksmedizin. In: DAZ 130(45):2510. 1990.

Wichtl M, Volksmedizinisch verwendete pflanzliche Arzneimittel. In: ZPT 11(3):71. 1990.

Further information in:

Hänsel R, Keller K, Rimpler H, Schneider G (Hrsg.), Hagers Handbuch der Pharmazeutischen Praxis, 5. Aufl., Bde 4-6 (Drogen): Springer Verlag Berlin, Heidelberg, New York, 1992-1994.

Leung AY, Encyclopedia of Common Natural Ingredients Used in Food Drugs, Cosmetics, John Wiley & Sons Inc., New York 1980.

Madaus G, Lehrbuch der Biologischen Arzneimittel, Bde 1-3, Nachdruck, Georg Olms Verlag Hildesheim 1979.

Roth L, Daunderer M, Kormann K, Giftpflanzen, Pflanzengifte, 4. Aufl., Ecomed Fachverlag Landsberg Lech 1993.

Schulz R, Hänsel R, Rationale Phytotherapie, Springer Verlag Heidelberg 1996.

Steinegger E, Hänsel R, Pharmakognosie, 5. Aufl., Springer Verlag Heidelberg 1992.

Teuscher E, Lindequist U, Biogene Gifte - Biologie, Chemie, Pharmakologie, 2. Aufl., Fischer Verlag Stuttgart 1994.

Teuscher E, Biogene Arzneimittel, 5. Aufl., Wiss. Verlagsges. Stuttgart 1997.

Wagner H, Wiesenauer M, Phytotherapie. Phytopharmaka und pflanzliche Homöopathika, Fischer-Verlag, Stuttgart, Jena, New York 1995.

Wichtl M (Hrsg.), Teedrogen, 4. Aufl., Wiss. Verlagsges. Stuttgart 1997.

Valeriana officinalis

See Valerian

Venus Flytrap

Dionaea muscipula

DESCRIPTION

Medicinal Parts: The entire fresh plant is used medicinally.

Flower and Fruit: The peduncles are leafless, up to 45 cm long with 3 to 10 radial flowers arranged in an umbelliferous raceme. The sepals are fused, and the 5 petals are free and white. There are 15 to 20 stamens and 5 superior carpels. The styles are fused to a column with 5 stigmas on the tip. The fruit is an ovoid capsule, which splits when ripe. The numerous seeds are ovoid, black and smooth.

Leaves, Stem and Root: This herbaceous perennial grows up to 45 cm high with leaves that are arranged in a basal rosette. The leaves are 6.5 to 13 cm long, have a cuneiform broadened petiole and an orbicular lamina with 2 sides forming a trap. The leaf sides have 15 to 20 stiff bristles on the edge and 3 sensitive bristles on the surface. The nectar glands are on the periphery and the digestive glands toward the center. When the sensitive bristles are stimulated, the lamina halves snap shut and the bristles on the edge lock together. Digestion of the trapped insect takes approximately 6 days after which the trap slowly opens again. There are only adventitious roots on the fully grown plant.

Characteristics: The plant is carnivorous.

Habitat: Dionaea muscipula is native to North America.

Production: Venus flytrap herb is the whole fresh, aerial plant of Dionaea muscipula, which is harvested shortly before the flowering season and processed immediately.

ACTIONS AND PHARMACOLOGY

COMPOUNDS

Naphthalene derivatives: napthoquinones, including hydroplumbagin-4-O-beta-glucoside, (0.6%), plumbagin (0.2%)

Flavonoids: including quercetin-3-O-galactoside, quercetin-3-O-glucoside, kaempferol-3-O-galactoside, kaempferol-3-O-glucoside

Phenol carboxylic acids: glucosides of gallic acid, ellagic acid, 3-O-methyl-ellagic acid and 3,3-dimethyl ellagic acid

Enzymes (in the secretions of the digestive glands): proteases, phosphatases, nucleases

EFFECTS

The pressed fresh plant (chief active ingredient plumbagin) is immunostimulating, antineoplastic and spasmogenic due to the lysophosphatidinic acid component.

INDICATIONS AND USAGE

Unproven Uses: The drug extracted from the plant is used chiefly in the treatment of malignant conditions such as tumors in advanced stages (mammary carcinoma, bladder carcinoma, prostate carcinoma and osteosarcoma) and also for hematological systemic conditions (such as Hodgkin and non-Hodgkin lymphoma) as well as solid tumors.

PRECAUTIONS AND ADVERSE REACTIONS

Parenteral administration of medicinal preparations made from the fresh plant led to elevated body temperature, chills and circulatory damage. Circulatory collapse, possibly as a result of contamination with endotoxins is possible. Skin contact with the fresh plant may cause irritation.

DOSAGE

Mode of Administration: Preparations of the pressed juice have been administered orally, by inhalation and parenterally.

How Supplied: Availability of the pressed juice of the fresh plant in two commercial preparations was halted in 1986.

Daily Dosage: Juice from the fresh plant used orally and as an inhalant: 50 to 60 drops 5 times daily p.o.; 25 drops with 1 ml physiological NaCl in a cold atomizer. Injection solution: initial dose is 2 ml ampule daily for 14 days. Maintenance dose: 1 ampule every second to third day I.M.

LITERATURE

Blaschek W, Hänsel R, Keller K, Reichling J, Rimpler G, Schneider G (Eds), Hagers Handbuch der Pharmazeutischen Praxis. Folgebände 1 und 2. Drogen A-Z. Springer. Berlin, Heidelberg 1998.

Veratrum album

See White Hellebore

Veratrum luteum

See False Unicorn Root

Veratrum viride

See American Hellebore

Verbascum densiflorum

See Mullein

Verbena officinalis

See Vervain

Veronica beccabunga

See Brooklime

Veronica officinalis

See Speedwell

Vervain

Verbena officinalis

DESCRIPTION

Medicinal Parts: The medicinal parts are the dried aerial parts collected during the flowering season, the fresh, flowering herb, the flowers and the whole fresh plant.

Flower and Fruit: The small flowers are pale lilac and arranged in thin paniculate spikes. The calyx is fused to a short, 5-tipped tube. The corolla has a 5-tipped, bent tube and a bilabiate margin. The mouth of the tube is closed by a cross of hairs. There are 4 stamens and 1 ovary, which breaks up into four, 1-seeded mericarps. These are oblong-cylindrical, 1.5 to 2 mm long, warty on the inside, reticulately grooved and light brown on the outside. The seeds are grooved on the inside and have very little endosperm.

Leaves, Stem and Root: The true variety is an annual or biennial to perennial with a fusiform, branched, whitish root. The stem is erect, rigid, quadrangular and branched above. The leaves are opposite, dull green, ovate-oblong and have a short broad petiole. They are deeply divided in 3 with notched, crenate tips. They are wrinkled and roughly bristled.

Habitat: The plant is probably indigenous to the Mediterranean region. It is cultivated worldwide, but mainly in eastern Europe.

Production: Verbena herb consists of the above-ground parts of Verbena officinalis. The herb is predominantly cultivated in eastern Europe. It is collected in the wild and harvested in southeastern Europe. After being cut, the drug is hung in bunches to dry.

Note: Improper drying leads to hydrolytic decomposition of verbenalin.

Not to be Confused With: Lippiae triphyllae folium

Other Names: Enchanter's Plant, Herb of the Cross, Juno's Tears, Pigeon's Grass, Pigeonweed, Simpler's Joy, Herb of Grace

ACTIONS AND PHARMACOLOGY

COMPOUNDS

Iridoide monoterpenes (0.2-0.5%): including among others verbenalin (cornin, 0.15%), hastatoside (0.08%), dihydroverbenalin (0.01%)

Flavonoids: including among others luteolin, scutellarin and 6-hydroxy-luteolin glycosides, artemitin, sorbifolin, pedalitin, nepetin (eupafolin)

Caffeic acid derivatives: verbascoside 0.8%), eucovoside, martynoside

EFFECTS

The amaroid-like affect of the iridoid glycosides explains its use as an astringent. The drug is weakly anti-edemic, analgesic, cytotoxic and antitumoral. The verbenalin has antitussive, secretolytic, and lactation-promoting properties.

INDICATIONS AND USAGE

Unproven Uses: Preparations of Vervain are used for diseases and ailments of the oral and pharyngeal mucosa, such as sore throat, and for diseases of the respiratory tract, such as coughs, asthma and whooping cough.

In addition, the drug is used internally for pain, cramps, fatigue, nervous disorders, digestive disorders, liver and gallbladder diseases, jaundice, kidney and urinary tract complaints, menopausal complaints and irregular menstruation. It is also used to promote lactation and to treat rheumatic diseases, gout, metabolic disorders, chlorosis and edema. The drug is used externally as a gargle for cold symptoms and for diseases of the oral and pharyngeal cavity.

Vervain is also used for antipruritic treatment of skin diseases and minor topical burns (in France) and for arthritis, rheumatism, dislocations and contusions.

Chinese Medicine: The herb is used for edema, chronic malaria, dysmenorrhea and carbuncles.

Homeopathic Uses: The herb is used for bruising and cerebral convulsions.

CONTRAINDICATIONS

Vervain should not be used during pregnancy.

PRECAUTIONS AND ADVERSE REACTIONS

No health hazards or side effects are known in conjunction with the proper administration of designated therapeutic dosages.

DOSAGE

Mode of Administration: Vervain is available as whole, cut and powdered drug for internal and external use.

Preparation: The ratio for the liquid extract is 1:1 in 25% ethanol; the tincture should be mixed with 40% ethanol. An infusion is prepared by adding 5 to 20 gm drug to 1 liter water.

Daily Dosage: For the liquid extract, take 2 to 4 ml daily. For the tincture, take 5 to 10 ml up to 3 times per day. For the infusion, take 2 to 4 gm up to 3 times per day.

Chinese Medicine Dosage: The daily dose is 4.5 to 9 gm of the drug.

Homeopathic Dosage: 5 to 10 drops, 1 tablet or 5 to 10 globules 1 to 3 times daily; parenterally: 1 ml injection solution sc twice weekly (HAB34).

Storage: Vervain must be stored in a dry environment to avoid hydrolytic decomposition of verbenalin.

LITERATURE

Carnat A et al., PM 61:490. 1995.

Inouye H et al., (1974) Planta Med 25:285.

McIlroy RJ, In: The Plant Glycosides, Arnold, London 1951.

Reynaud J et al., Pharm Acta Helv 67:216. 1992.

Weber R, Dissertation Marburg. 1995.

Yip L, Pei S, Hudson JB, Towers GHN, Screening of medicinal plants from Yunnan Province in southwest China for antiviral activity. In: ETH 34:1-6. 1991.

Further information in:

Hänsel R, Keller K, Rimpler H, Schneider G (Hrsg.), Hagers Handbuch der Pharmazeutischen Praxis, 5. Aufl., Bde 4-6 (Drogen): Springer Verlag Berlin, Heidelberg, New York, 1992-1994.

Madaus G, Lehrbuch der Biologischen Arzneimittel, Bde 1-3, Nachdruck, Georg Olms Verlag Hildesheim 1979.

Wagner H, Wiesenauer M, Phytotherapie. Phytopharmaka und pflanzliche Homöopathika, Fischer-Verlag, Stuttgart, Jena, New York 1995.

Wichtl M (Hrsg.), Teedrogen, 4. Aufl., Wiss. Verlagsges. Stuttgart 1997.

Viburnum prunifolium

See Black Haw

Vicia faba

See Broad Bean

Vinca minor

See Periwinkle

Viola odorata

See Sweet Violet

Viola tricolor

See Heartsease

Virola

Virola theiodora

DESCRIPTION

Medicinal Parts: The medicinal part of the plant is the bark.

Flower and Fruit: The flowers are in panicles. The male inflorescence has numerous flowers and is brown, gold-yellow and pubescent. The female flowers are either single or in clusters of 2 to 10 flowers. They are fused and have 3 to 5 stamens. The ovary develops from only 1 carpel with 1 ovule. The fruit is orbicular-oval, 10 to 20 mm long and 8 to 15 mm wide.

Leaves, Stem and Root: Virola theiodora is a diclinous tree that grows up to 23 m high. The leaves are alternate, 9 to 35 cm long and 4 to 12 cm wide; the lamina is simple, elongate to wide oval, acute, entire and paper-like. The trunk is approximately 0.5 m thick and cylindrical with a smooth, brown-speckled bark with gray spots.

Characteristics: The flowers have sharply astringent fragrance.

Habitat: Amazon region

Production: Virola bark is the dried bark of Virola theiodora.

There are various methods of production. Either the bark is scraped off, dried over a fire and powdered, or the outer bark is peeled off before sunrise and the inner bark with the resin is scraped off and cooked to a syrup. The syrup is pulverized after drying in the sun.

ACTIONS AND PHARMACOLOGY

COMPOUNDS

Tryptamine derivatives: particularly N,N-dimethyl tryptamine, 5-methoxy-NN-dimethyl tryptamine (5-MeO-DMT)

EFFECTS

Due to its psychotropic and narcotic-hallucinogenic characteristics (tryptamine alkaloids), the drug is chiefly used in the form of a snuff powder in connection with ritual and religious ceremonies. The resin is also administered topically to yeast infections of the skin and for the promotion of the healing of wounds.

INDICATIONS AND USAGE

Unproven Uses: Virola is used for skin disease and fungal skin diseases, to speed the healing of wounds, and to clean infected wounds (South America).

PRECAUTIONS AND ADVERSE REACTIONS

The drug is not used as a medication. The drug has a psychomimetic effect when administered through the nasal mucous membrane.

OVERDOSAGE

Signs of poisoning include nausea, increased irritability, numbness in the limbs, coordination disorders and hallucinations, among others. The tryptamine derivatives are resorbed only to a very limited extent following oral administration.

DOSAGE

Preparation: There is no information in the literature.

LITERATURE

de Smet PA, A multidisciplinary overview of intoxicating snuff rituals in the Western Hemisphere. J Ethnopharmacol, 13:3-49, 1985 Mar.

Hänsel R, Keller K, Rimpler H, Schneider G (Ed), Hagers Handbuch der Pharmazeutischen Praxis, 5. Aufl., Bde 4 - 6 (Drogen), Springer Verlag Berlin, Heidelberg, New York, 1992-1994.

MacRae WD, Towers GH, Justicia pectoralis: a study of the basis for its use as a hallucinogenic snuff ingredient. J Ethnopharmacol, 12:93-111, 1984 Oct.

MacRae WD, Towers GH, Phytochemical investigation of Virola peruviana, a new hallucinogenic plant. J Pharm Sci, 12:1561-3, 1973 Sep.

McKenna DJ, Towers GH, Abbott FS, Alkaloids in certain species of Virola and other South American plants of ethnopharmacologic interest. Acta Chem Scand, 12:903-16, 1969.

McKenna DJ, Towers GH, Abbott FS, Monoamine oxidase inhibitors in South American hallucinogenic plants. Part 2: Constituents of orally-active Myristicaceous hallucinogens. J Ethnopharmacol, 12:179-211, 1984 Nov.

Plotkin MJ, Schultes RE, Virola: a promising genus for ethnopharmacological investigation. J Psychoactive Drugs, 22:357-61, 1990 Jul-Sep.

Virola theiodora

See Virola

Viscum album

See European Mistletoe

Vitex agnus-castus

See Chaste Tree

Vitis vinifera

See Grape

Wafer Ash

Ptelea trifoliata

DESCRIPTION

Medicinal Parts: The medicinal parts are the leaves, the young bark and the root bark. The plant is also used in homeopathic medicine.

Flower and Fruit: The small, greenish-white flowers are in loose, terminal cymes and are dioecious. The 4- to 5-sepalled calyx and the 4 to 5 petals are downy on the outside. There are 4 to 5 stamens whose filaments are hairy at the base. The compressed ovary has a short style and stigma which is divided in two. The fruit is circular and winged with a broad, greenish-white, later ochre-colored margin.

Leaves, Stem and Root: The plant is a bush or small tree up to 4 m high with glabrous, smooth, dark or red-brown branches. The younger branches, leaves and petiols are downy. The leaves are large, 3-lobed, lanceolate narrowing to both ends, entire, dark green above, lighter beneath and covered with numerous fine glandular spots.

Characteristics: The flowers are pleasantly perfumed and the fruit is bitter-tangy.

Habitat: The plant is indigenous to Eastern North America and is cultivated in Europe as an ornamental bush.

Production: Wafer Ash is the root-bark of Ptelea trifoliata.

Other Names: Pickaway Anise, Prairie Grub, Scubby Trefoil, and Stinking Prairie Bush, Swamp Dogwood, Hop Tree, Three-Leafed, Wingseed

ACTIONS AND PHARMACOLOGY

COMPOUNDS

Furoquinoline alkaloids: including kokusaginine, skimmianine (beta-fagarine), ptelein, dictamnine, and maculosidine

Furanocoumarins: including isopimpinellin, marmesin, and phellopterin

EFFECTS

Wafer Ash is antimicrobial. The alkaloid content acts against microbes; pteleatinium chloride acts against *mycobacterium tuberculosis* and yeast fungus.

INDICATIONS AND USAGE

Unproven Uses: Wafer Ash is used for stomach complaints, gallstones, and rheumatism. It's root bark is used as a tonic.

PRECAUTIONS AND ADVERSE REACTIONS

No health hazards or side effects are known in conjunction with the proper administration of designated therapeutic dosages. The plant could trigger phototoxicosis through skin contact, possibly also through internal ingestion of larger quantities.

DOSAGE

Mode of Administration: Wafer Ash is available as an extract.

LITERATURE

Kern W, List PH, Hörhammer L (Hrsg.), Hagers Handbuch der Pharmazeutischen Praxis, 4. Aufl., Bde. 1-8, Springer Verlag Berlin, Heidelberg, New York, 1969.

Roth L, Daunderer M, Kormann K, Giftpflanzen, Pflanzengifte, 4. Aufl., Ecomed Fachverlag Landsberg Lech 1993.

Wahoo

Euonymus species

DESCRIPTION

Medicinal Parts: The medicinal parts are the trunk and root bark and the fruit.

Flower and Fruit: The flowers are yellowish-green, small and flat in double cymes with few blossoms. There are 4 sepals, 4 petals, 4 stamens and 4 styles on a glandular disc, which surrounds the ovary. The fruit is a 4-lobed, obtuse, pink capsule which bursts open at the tip showing the seeds covered in an orange-yellow skin.

Leaves, Stem and Root: The plant is an unwieldy shrub up to 3 m high with green rectangular young branches. The older branches are light gray. The leaves are opposite, oblong-lanceolate or elliptical, acuminate, finely serrate and glabrous.

Characteristics: The seeds are poisonous.

Habitat: The plant grows in the Eastern and Central U.S. and Canada.

Production: Wahoo root bark is the bark of the root and young branches of Euonymus atropurpureus. Wahoo fruit is the fruit of Euonymus europaeus.

Other Names: Burning Bush, Fusanum, Fusoria, Gadrose, Gatten, Gatter, Indian Arrowroot, Pigwood, Prickwood, Skewerwood, and Spindle Tree

ACTIONS AND PHARMACOLOGY

COMPOUNDS: WAHOO ROOT BARK (EUONYMUS ATROPURPUREUS)

Cardioactive steroids (cardenolides) in the root: including euatroside, euatromonoside

COMPOUNDS: WAHOO FRUIT (EUONYMUS EUROPAEUS)

Cardioactive steroids (cardenolides) in the seeds: including evonoside, evobioside, evomonoside, evolonoside, glucoevonoloside, glucoevonogenin

Alkaloids: polyester from a sesquiterpene polyol with pyrridine carbon acids (for example, evonine)

Peptide alkaloids: including frangula amine, franganin, frangufolin

1-benzyl-tetrahydro-isoquinoline alkaloids

Purine alkaloids: caffeine, theobromine

EFFECTS: WAHOO ROOT BARK AND FRUIT

The drug is reported to be a laxative and a choleretic. Larger doses have an effect on the heart.

INDICATIONS AND USAGE

Unproven Uses: In the past, the drug was used as a cholagogue, laxative, diuretic and tonic, and for dyspepsia. Today, it is used in homeopathy.

PRECAUTIONS AND ADVERSE REACTIONS

Poisonings caused by the berries have been recorded. Thirty-six berries of Euonymus europaeus are said to be enough to kill a person. After a latency period of several hours, intestinal colic, severe, sometimes bloody diarrhea, elevation of body temperature, shortness of breath and circulatory disorders with signs of collapse occur. Often there is elevation of cerebrospinal pressure with increasing stupor that may progress unconsciousness. The first measures to be taken with poisonings are gastric lavage, intestinal emptying, the instillation of activated charcoal and shock prophylaxis (which includes quiet, heat and the possible administration of a plasma volume expander). All other measures depend on the symptoms. For loss of potassium, careful replenishment of potassium should be undertaken. Lidocaine can be administered for ventricular extrasystole; atropine for partial atrioventricular block. For elimination of the glycosides hemoperfusion is possible, as is the administration of cholestyramine to interrupt enterohepatic circulation. Intubation and oxygen respiration may also be necessary in cases of asphyxiation.

DOSAGE

Mode of Administration: Wahoo root bark and fruit are not recommended for use, as the drug is considered too dangerous.

LITERATURE

Bishay DW et al., PH 12:693. 1973.

Bliss CA, Ramstad E, J Am Pharm Assoc 46:423. 1957.

Brüning R, Wagner H, PH 17:1821. 1978.

Kislichenko SG et al., Khim Prir Soedin 386. 1969.

Kislichenko SG et al., Khim Prir Soedin 193 et 241. 1967.

Tschesche R, Wirtz S, Snatzke G, Chem Ber 88:1619. 1955.

Further information in:

Frohne D, Pfänder HJ, Giftpflanzen - Ein Handbuch für Apotheker, Toxikologen und Biologen, 4. Aufl., Wiss. Verlagsges. mbH Stuttgart 1997.

Gazzinelli RT, Romanha AJ, Fontes G, Chiari E, Gazzinelli G, Brenner Z, Distribution of carbohydrates recognized by the lectins Euonymus europaeus and concanavalin A in monoxenic and heteroxenic trypanosomatids. J Protozool, 38:320-5, Jul-Aug, 1991.

Kern W, List PH, Hörhammer L (Hrsg.), Hagers Handbuch der Pharmazeutischen Praxis, 4. Aufl., Bde. 1-8, Springer Verlag Berlin, Heidelberg, New York, 1969.

Lewin L, Gifte und Vergiftungen, 6. Aufl., Nachdruck, Haug Verlag, Heidelberg 1992.

Madaus G, Lehrbuch der Biologischen Arzneimittel, Bde 1-3, Nachdruck, Georg Olms Verlag Hildesheim 1979.

Nickrent DL, Franchina CR, Phylogenetic relationships of the Santalales and relatives. J Mol Evol, 26:294-301. Oct, 1990.

Roth L, Daunderer M, Kormann K, Giftpflanzen, Pflanzengifte, 4. Aufl., Ecomed Fachverlag Landsberg Lech 1993.

Roussel F, Dalion J, Wissocq JC, Cytotoxic cardenolides from woods of Euonymus alata. Chem Pharm Bull (Tokyo), 26:615-7. Mar, 1996.

Roussel F, Dalion J, Wissocq JC, Euonymus europaeus lectin as an endothelial and epithelial marker in canine tissues. Lab Anim, 26:114-21. Apr, 1992.

Roussel F, Dalion J, Wissocq JC, Lectin binding defines and differentiates M-cells in mouse small intestine and caecum. Histochem Cell Biol, 26:161-8. Aug, 1995

Roussel F, Dalion J, Wissocq JC, Occupational wood-dust sensitivity from Euonymus europaeus (spindle tree) and investigation of cross reactivity between E.e. wood and Artemisia vulgaris pollen (mugwort). Allergy, 26:186-90. Apr, 1991.

Teuscher E, Biogene Arzneimittel, 5. Aufl., Wiss. Verlagsges. mbH Stuttgart 1997.

Wang W, Wang J, Zhao D, Liu H, Zhou W, Chen K, Comparison of Spatholobus suberectus Dum Euonymus alatus (Thunb.) Sieb. and Eupolyphaga sinensis Walker on regulation of plasma lipid. Chung Kuo Chung Yao Tsa Chih, 38:299-301 320, 1991 May

Wallflower

Cheiranthus cheiri

DESCRIPTION

Medicinal Parts: The medicinal parts are the dried flowers, the dried ripe seeds and the fresh aerial parts of the erect plant before flowering.

Flower and Fruit: The flowers are golden yellow to orange-yellow in dense racemes on 10 to 14 cm long, pubescent, erect stems. The sepals are 9 to 11 mm long, linear-lanceolate, with a membranous border. The stigma is curled back. The fruit is a pod, which has no beak but has distinct ribs. The seeds are arranged in 1 row, are 3 mm long, oblong, narrowly winged and light brown.

Leaves, Stem and Root: The plant grows from about 30 to 70 cm. The stems are woody below and semi-shrub-like with gray-appressed hairs and thick foliage above. The leaves are lanceolate with revolute tip, short-petioled, entire-margined and hairy.

Characteristics: The plant has a pleasant fragrance.

Habitat: The plant is probably only indigenous to the eastern Mediterranean region, but is cultivated today in Europe, northern Africa, western Asia, Japan and New Zealand.

Production: Wallflower can be obtained from commercial growers (cultivated regions).

Other Names: Gillyflower, Wallstock-Gillofer, Giroflier, Handflower, Keiri, Beeflower

ACTIONS AND PHARMACOLOGY

COMPOUNDS

Cardioactive steroid glycosides (cardenolids): in particularly high concentration in the seeds (0.5%), including cheirotoxin, erysimoside, glucoerysimoside, cheiroside A

Glucosinolates: glucocheiroline, glucoiberin, which yield the isothiocyanates cheiroline and iberin

Fatty oil (in the seeds)

EFFECTS

The drug has cardiac effects similar to digitaloid drugs, due to the cardenolide glycosides. Its application for constipation is plausible because of the inhibition of Na^+ and H_2O absorption and the stimulating effect on the smooth muscles of the gastrointestinal tract.

INDICATIONS AND USAGE

Unproven Uses: Wallflower is used for cardiac insufficiency, as a laxative and to encourage menstruation.

Homeopathic Uses: The herb is used for wisdom tooth pain.

PRECAUTIONS AND ADVERSE REACTIONS

No health hazards or side effects are known in conjunction with the proper administration of designated therapeutic dosages.

OVERDOSAGE

For possible symptoms of overdose and treatment of poisonings see *Digitalis folium*. Despite the strong efficacy of the drug's cardioactive steroid glycosides in parenteral application, serious poisoning is not expected due to the presumably low resorption rate following oral administration.

DOSAGE

Mode of Administration: Wallflower is used internally in drops and an infusion as well as in some combination preparations.

Preparation: To make an infusion from the flowers, mix 2 to 3 gm of drug per 100 ml of water.

Daily Dosage: Drink 3 to 4 cups of the infusion daily.

LITERATURE

Belokon VF, Makarevich IF, Khim Prir Soedin 424. 1980.

Makarevich IF, Belokon VF, Khim Prir Soedin 662. 1975.

Moore IA, Tamm C, Reichstein T, Helv Chim Acta 37:755. 1954.

Schwarz H, Katz A, Reichstein T, Pharm Acta Helv 21:250. 1946.

Wagner P, Ber Dtsch Chem Ges 41:4467. 1908.

Further information in:

Hänsel R, Keller K, Rimpler H, Schneider G (Hrsg.), Hagers Handbuch der Pharmazeutischen Praxis, 5. Aufl., Bde 4-6 (Drogen): Springer Verlag Berlin, Heidelberg, New York, 1992-1994.

Madaus G, Lehrbuch der Biologischen Arzneimittel, Bde 1-3, Nachdruck, Georg Olms Verlag Hildesheim 1979.

Roth L, Daunderer M, Kormann K, Giftpflanzen, Pflanzengifte, 4. Aufl., Ecomed Fachverlag Landsberg Lech 1993.

Teuscher E, Lindequist U, Biogene Gifte - Biologie, Chemie, Pharmakologie, 2. Aufl., Fischer Verlag Stuttgart 1994.

Walnut

Juglans regia

DESCRIPTION

Medicinal Parts: The medicinal parts are the feathery leaflets without the rachis and the green fruit shells.

Flower and Fruit: The flowers are green and appear before the leaves. They are monoecious. The male flowers are 10 cm long, sessile, globular-cylindrical, limp, hanging catkins. The female flowers are in groups of 1 to 3 at the tip of annual growth. They are greenish with a glandular pubescent calyx and 2 large, curved, warty, reddish stigmas. The fruit is globular or oblong-globular with a smooth, green, white-spotted outer shell and a wooden, wrinkled inner shell.

Leaves, Stem and Root: The plant grows to 25 m and has a broad, loose-branched crown. The bark is smooth and ash gray at first; later dark and fissured. The leaves are large, long petioled, odd-pinnate with 7 to 9 oblong or ovate, entire-margined leaflets. The leaflets are spotted with glands when young. The terminal leaflet is the largest and is petiolate.

Characteristics: The leaves are aromatic when rubbed. The taste is bitter.

Habitat: The walnut is indigenous to the Middle East and Iran. Today, it is cultivated in many regions.

Production: Walnut leaf consists of the dried leaf of Juglans regia.

Other Names: English Walnut, Caucasion Walnut, Circassian Walnut, Persian Walnut

ACTIONS AND PHARMACOLOGY

COMPOUNDS

Tannins (galloylglucose, ellagitannins)

Naphthalene derivatives: The fresh leaves and the fruit peels contain 1,4,5- trihydroxynaphthalene-4-beta-D-glucoside, which is transformed into juglone through bruising or drying. Juglone polymerizes readily into yellow or brown products (that stain the skin), so there can be hardly any juglone present in the drug itself.

Flavonoids: including, among others, hyperoside, quercitrin

EFFECTS

Walnut is astringent and fungistatic. The juglone content in the walnut hulls has been linked to mutagenic action. The topical use of walnut hulls has been linked to cancer of the tongue and leukoplakia of the lips. The main active principles are the tannins and juglon. There is an astringent effect because of the tannins. The antifungal effect comes from the juglon content and the essential oil.

INDICATIONS AND USAGE

Approved by Commission E:

- Inflammation of the skin
- Excessive perspiration

Unproven Uses: Externally, Walnut is used for mild, superficial inflammation of the skin and excessive perspiration. Internally, the drug is used for gastrointestinal catarrh and as an anthelmintic (so-called blood purifier).

Chinese Medicine: In China, Walnut is used to treat asthma, lumbago, beriberi, impotence and constipation.

Indian Medicine: In India, Walnut is used for alternating rheumatic complaints, and the oil of the seeds is used for tapeworms. The seeds are said to have an aphrodisiac effect and are also used for dysentery and colic.

PRECAUTIONS AND ADVERSE REACTIONS

No health hazards or side effects are known in conjunction with the proper administration of designated therapeutic dosages.

DOSAGE

Mode of Administration: Comminuted drug for decoctions and other galenic preparations for external use.

Preparation: To prepare a decoction, soak 2 teaspoonfuls of drug in 1 cup of water, boil and strain. An infusion is prepared by using 1.5 gm of finely cut drug, soaked in cold water, brought to simmer and strained after 3 to 5 minutes.

Daily Dosage: The average daily dose for external use is 3 to 6 gm of drug.

LITERATURE

Hegnauer R, Chemotaxonomie der Pflanzen, Bde 1-11, Birkhäuser Verlag Basel, Boston, Berlin 1962-1997.

Madaus G, Lehrbuch der Biologischen Arzneimittel, Bde 1-3, Nachdruck, Georg Olms Verlag Hildesheim 1979.

Nahrstedt A et al., (1981) Planta Med 42(4):313.

Teuscher E, Lindequist U, Biogene Gifte - Biologie, Chemie, Pharmakologie, 2. Aufl., Fischer Verlag Stuttgart 1994.

Teuscher E, Biogene Arzneimittel, 5. Aufl., Wiss. Verlagsges. Stuttgart 1997.

Thomson RH, Naturally Occuring Quinones, 2nd Ed., Academic Press, New York, 1971.

Wagner H, Wiesenauer M, Phytotherapie. Phytopharmaka und pflanzliche Homöopathika, Fischer-Verlag, Stuttgart, Jena, New York 1995.

Willuhn G, Pflanzliche Dermatika. Eine kritische Übersicht.. In: DAZ 132(37):1873. 1992.

Water Avens

Geum rivale

DESCRIPTION

Medicinal Parts: The medicinal parts are the dried, underground parts of the plant, the fresh, flowering plant and the roots.

Flower and Fruit: The flowering peduncle usually sprouts singly from the axils of the rosette leaves, rarely from the ends of the stems. It is often tinged red-brown and is downy. The flowers and subinflorescences are on long, dense and glandular-haired pedicles. The 5 sepals are red-brown. The 5 petals are pale yellow and tinged dirty pink. The flower remains attached long after flowering. The carpel axis is stemmed and villous, and stretches when mature. The fruit is hooked at the tip.

Leaves, Stem and Root: The plant is a 30 to 100 cm high semi-rosette shrub with the primary root replaced by adventitious roots. The rhizome is simple, thick, cylindrical and crooked with a terminal rosette. The rosette leaves are long-petioled, irregularly lyre-shaped and pinnate. The upper surface is glandular and hairy. The underside is heavily ciliated along the veins.

Habitat: The plant is found in Europe, temperate Asia and North America.

Production: Water Avens root is the root of Geum rivale.

Other Names: Cure All, Water Flower, Indian Chocolate, Chocolate Root, Throat Root, Water Chisch

ACTIONS AND PHARMACOLOGY

COMPOUNDS: IN THE FRESHLY HARVESTED RHIZOME

Gein (eugenol vicianoside): transformed into eugenol through drying or cutting into small pieces

Tannins

COMPOUNDS: IN THE DRIED RHIZOME AND ROOT

Volatile oil (traces): chief component eugenol

Tannins (15-20%)

EFFECTS

See Geum urbanum; overall, Water Avens has very weak action.

INDICATIONS AND USAGE

Unproven Uses: Uses are the same as for Geum urbanum.

PRECAUTIONS AND ADVERSE REACTIONS

Health risks or side effects following the proper administration of designated therapeutic dosages are not recorded.

DOSAGE

No information is available.

LITERATURE

Hänsel R, Keller K, Rimpler H, Schneider G (Hrsg.), Hagers Handbuch der Pharmazeutischen Praxis, 5. Aufl., Bde 4-6 (Drogen). Springer Verlag Berlin, Heidelberg, New York, 1992-1994.

Hegnauer R, Pharm Weekblad 87:641-646. 1952.

Madaus G, Lehrbuch der Biologischen Arzneimittel, Bde 1-3, Nachdruck, Georg Olms Verlag Hildesheim 1979.

Water Dock

Rumex aquaticus

DESCRIPTION

Medicinal Parts: The medicinal parts are the dried roots.

Flower and Fruit: The inflorescence is a large, dense panicle. The pedicles are filiform and up to 2.5 times as long as the capsules. The capsules are 6 to 8 mm long, ovate-triangular, more or less acute, longer than wide and entire-margined.

Leaves, Stem and Root: The herb is perennial and has an erect 100 to 200 cm high stem. The leaves are 7.5 to 10 cm wide with curly margins. The basal leaves are triangular, acute, deeply cordate at the base and 1.5 to 2.5 times as long as they are wide. The petiole is at least as long as the leaf blade. The rhizome is dark brown to blackish on the outside and porous.

Habitat: The plant is common in Europe.

Production: The root material is sliced and then dried in the shade.

ACTIONS AND PHARMACOLOGY

COMPOUNDS

Oxalates: oxalic acid, calcium oxalate

Tannins

Anthracene derivatives: including anthranoids

EFFECTS

The active agents are quercitrin, protein, fat, starch, essential oil and tannin. The herb acts as an aid to digestion.

INDICATIONS AND USAGE

Unproven Uses: Water Dock is used for blood purification and constipation. The powdered form is also useful for cleaning the teeth or for mouth ulcers. It is used externally for sores and scorbutic conditions.

PRECAUTIONS AND ADVERSE REACTIONS

No health hazards or side effects are known in conjunction with the proper administration of designated therapeutic dosages.

OVERDOSAGE

Oxalate poisonings are conceivable, but only with the consumption of very large quantities of the leaves as salad.

DOSAGE

Mode of Administration: The drug is used internally and externally as a liquid extract or as a powder. Use of the herb went out of favor during the 18th century.

LITERATURE

Grznar K, Rada K, Farmaceut Obzor 47:195. 1978.

Kern W, List PH, Hörhammer L (Hrsg.), Hagers Handbuch der Pharmazeutischen Praxis, 4. Aufl., Bde. 1-8: Springer Verlag Berlin, Heidelberg, New York, 1969.

Sharma M et al., Indian J Chem Sect B 15B:544. 1977.

Water Dropwort

Oenanthe crocata

DESCRIPTION

Medicinal Parts: The medicinal part is the rhizome.

Flower and Fruit: The flowers are in terminal umbels. The flowering shoots are longer than the 10 to 40 pedicled rays, which do not thicken in the fruiting phase. The cylindrical fruit is 4 to 6 mm long.

Leaves, Stem and Root: The plant is a branched, stout perennial up to 150 cm high. The roots are fleshy and pale yellow. They have obovoid or ellipsoid tubers close to the point of attachment to the stem. The stems are hollow, striate and grooved. The basal leaves are 3- to 4-pinnate. The lobes of the basal leaves are ovate to suborbicular, cuneate at base. The lobed, crenate, cauline leaves are 2- to 3-pinnate and almost sessile. The lobes of the cauline leaves are ovate to linear, and the segments are closer and sharper than the basal leaves.

Characteristics: The plant is extremely poisonous.

Habitat: The plant grows around ditches and ponds in the U.S., and parts of Europe, excluding Scandinavia, Holland, Germany, Russia, Turkey and Greece.

Production: Water Dropwort is the root of Oenanthe crocata, which is collected in the wild.

Other Names: Hemlock, Dead Men's Fingers, Horsebane, Dead Tongue, Five-Fingered Root, Water Lovage

ACTIONS AND PHARMACOLOGY

COMPOUNDS

Polyynes: including among others the highly toxic oenanthotoxin as well as oenanthetol, oenanthetone, dihydrooenanthotoxin

EFFECTS

The pharmacologically active substances of the root drug are the toxic oenanthotoxin and the less toxic polyacetylenes oenanthetol and oenantheton. Oenanthotoxin caused an irreversible inhibition of loading transfer and sodium inflow at the nerve fibers of frogs.

INDICATIONS AND USAGE

Unproven Uses: Water Dropwort was formerly used in the treatment of epilepsy, but this use can no longer be recommended.

Homeopathic Uses: Homeopathic uses include epilepsy and cerebral convulsions.

PRECAUTIONS AND ADVERSE REACTIONS

Use of the drug can no longer be recommended because of its severe toxicity, due to the oenanthotoxin content.

OVERDOSAGE

Symptoms of poisoning include a burning sensation in the mouth and nose, dizziness, weakness, chill, mild twitching and speech disorders. Higher dosages may produce tonic-colonic spasms, temporarily slowed cardiac activity, unconsciousness, bloody foam at the mouth and death through respiratory failure.

Following gastrointestinal emptying (inducement of vomiting, gastric lavage with burgundy-colored potassium permanganate solution and sodium sulfate), and the administration of activated charcoal, the therapy for poisonings consists of treating spasms with thiobarbiturates (diazepam is said to be less effective); hemodialysis or hemperfusion have been applied successfully.

DOSAGE

Mode of Administration: The drug is obsolete except in homeopathy.

Homeopathic Dosage: Adult dosages are 5 drops, 1 tablet or 10 globules every 30 to 60 minutes (acute) or 1 to 3 times daily (chronic); from D4 parenterally: 1 to 2 ml sc i.v., i. m. acute, 3 times daily; chronic: once a day. Children up to 6 years old are given a maximum of half the adult dose; children up to 12 are given a maximum of two-thirds the adult dose (HAB34).

LITERATURE

Anet E, Lythgoe B, Silk MH, Tripett S, The chemistry of oenanthotoxin and cicutoxin. In: Chem Ind 31:757. 1952.

Bohlmann F, Rode KM, Polyacetylenic compounds: CXVII. Polyynes of Oenanthe crocata. In: Chem Ber 101(4):1163-1175. 1968.

Grindy HF, Howarth F, Pharmacological studies on hemlock water dropwort. In: Brit J Pharmacol 11:225-30. 1956.

Mitchell MJ, Routledge PA, Hemlock water dropwort poisoning - a review. In: Clin Toxicol 12(4):417-426. 1978.

Further information in:

Frohne D, Pfänder HJ, Giftpflanzen - Ein Handbuch für Apotheker, Toxikologen und Biologen, 4. Aufl., Wiss. Verlags-Ges. Stuttgart 1997.

Kern W, List PH, Hörhammer L (Hrsg.), Hagers Handbuch der Pharmazeutischen Praxis, 4. Aufl., Bde. 1-8, Springer Verlag Berlin, Heidelberg, New York, 1969.

Lewin L, Gifte und Vergiftungen, 6. Aufl., Nachdruck, Haug Verlag, Heidelberg 1992.

Madaus G, Lehrbuch der Biologischen Arzneimittel, Bde 1-3, Nachdruck, Georg Olms Verlag Hildesheim 1979.

Roth L, Daunderer M, Kormann K, Giftpflanzen, Pflanzengifte, 4. Aufl., Ecomed Fachverlag Landsberg Lech 1993.

Teuscher E, Lindequist U, Biogene Gifte - Biologie, Chemie, Pharmakologie, 2. Aufl., Fischer Verlag Stuttgart 1994.

Water Fennel

Oenanthe aquatica

DESCRIPTION

Medicinal Parts: The medicinal parts of the plant are the ripe seeds.

Flower and Fruit: The flowers are white and grow in many-rayed compound umbels opposite the leaves. They have no involucre but there is a small epicalyx. The calyx is distinct with an irregular corolla and petals that have a distinct border. The calyx narrows at the base and has an involute tip. The style is long. The fruit is 5 mm long, 1.5 mm wide, with 5 broad obtuse ribs.

Leaves, Stem and Root: The plant grows from 30 to 120 cm high. The stem is angularly branched, hollow and soft. The lower end of the 3 cm thick stem, which grows underwater, has long roots at the nodes. When the stem end reaches above water, is grows to only 6 mm thick. The leaves are double pinnate, pinnatifid to pinnatisect with splayed leaflets, which are often turned backward and have lanceolate, deeply indented-serrate tips. The underwater leaves have a thread-like tip.

Habitat: Found near ponds and ditches in both the U.S. and Europe.

Production: Water Fennel fruit are the ripe seeds of Oenanthe aquatica, which are collected in the wild.

Not to be Confused With: Mistaken identity can occur with Cicuta virosa, Sium latifolium or Perculanum palustre.

Other Names: Water Dropwort, Horsebane

ACTIONS AND PHARMACOLOGY

COMPOUNDS

Volatile oil (1-2.5%): including among others (+)-beta-phellandrene, dillapiol, myristicin, 1-nonen-3-ol (androle), volatile polyynes, undecen-4-ole, camphene, isopropyl cyclohexene-2-ole-

Polyynes: including among others all-trans-pentadeca-2,8,10-trien-4,6-diin-12-on

Fatty oil (20%)

Lignans: including arctigenin, matairesinol, dimethyl matairesinol, secoisolariciresinol

EFFECTS

The drug's expectorant and antitussive effects are probably due to the essential oil. The active agents are the essential and fatty oil, resin, wax, galacton, and mannan and rubber substances. There is no further information available.

INDICATIONS AND USAGE

Unproven Uses: Water Fennel is used in folk medicine as an expectorant and for the relief of coughs due to inflammation of the bronchial mucus membranes or asthma and suppurating or festering inflammation of the lungs, as well as a diuretic and carminative.

Homeopathic Uses: Inflammation of the respiratory tract and breast pain in nursing mothers are considered indications for use in homeopathy.

PRECAUTIONS AND ADVERSE REACTIONS

No health hazards or side effects are known in conjunction with the proper administration of designated therapeutic dosages.

DOSAGE

Mode of Administration: Ground, as an extract and as a tea.

Preparation: A tincture is prepared using the drug in a 1:5 ratio with 70% ethanol (m/m)

Daily Dosage: The recommended daily dose is 4 to 5 g drug.

Homeopathic Dosage: Adult dosage is 5 drops, 1 tablet or 10 globules every 30 to 60 minutes (acute) or 1 to 3 times daily (chronic); from D4 parenterally: 1 to 2 ml sc i.v., i.m. acute, 3 times daily; chronic: once a day. Children up to 6 years are given half the dose, children up to 12 are given a maximum of two-thirds the adult dosage (HAB1).

LITERATURE

Hegnauer R, Chemotaxonomie der Pflanzen, Bde 1-11, Birkhäuser Verlag Basel, Boston, Berlin 1962-1997.

Kern W, List PH, Hörhammer L (Hrsg.), Hagers Handbuch der Pharmazeutischen Praxis, 4. Aufl., Bde. 1-8, Springer Verlag Berlin, Heidelberg, New York, 1969.

Madaus G, Lehrbuch der Biologischen Arzneimittel, Bde 1-3, Nachdruck, Georg Olms Verlag Hildesheim 1979.

Ram AS, Devi HM, (1983) Indian J Bot 6(1):21.

Roth L, Daunderer M, Kormann K, Giftpflanzen, Pflanzengifte, 4. Aufl., Ecomed Fachverlag Landsberg Lech 1993.

Wagner H, Wiesenauer M, Phytotherapie. Phytopharmaka und pflanzliche Homöopathika, Fischer-Verlag, Stuttgart, Jena, New York 1995.

Water Germander

Teucrium scordium

DESCRIPTION

Medicinal Parts: The medicinal parts are the herb harvested during or shortly before the flowering season and the fresh flowering herb.

Flower and Fruit: The flowers are light red, 8 to 10 mm long, with short pedicles. They are in inconspicuous clusters in 1 to 4 blossomed cymes between bracts, which are longer than the flowers. The calyx has 5 tips and is campanulate-tubular with a touch violet. The tips of the deeply divided upper lip lie on the lower lip in such a way as to make it appear 5-lobed. After flowering, the head drops. There are 4 stamens. The nutlets are 1 mm long and punctate-reticulate.

Leaves, Stem and Root: The plant is a perennial, downy herb smelling of garlic. The rhizome creeps in mud and produces overground runners, which immediately turn into leaves and flower shoots. The stems are unbranched or branched, erect, round and villous with soft-hairs. The leaves are sessile, oblong-oval and crossed opposite.

Characteristics: The plant has a garlic-like odor and a bitter taste.

Habitat: The plant is indigenous to most of Europe as far as northern Africa and central Asia.

Production: Water Germander is the aerial part of Teucrium scordium. It is picked during or shortly before flowering.

ACTIONS AND PHARMACOLOGY

COMPOUNDS

Diterpenes: including among others, 6,20-bisdeacetylteupyreinidin, 6-deacetylteupyreinidin, 2beta, 6beta-dihydroxyteuscordin, 2beta,6beta-dihydroxyteuscordin, dihydroteugin, teuflidin, teucrin E, teugin, 2-keto-19-hydroxyteuscordin

EFFECTS

See other Teucrium species.

INDICATIONS AND USAGE

Unproven Uses: The herb is used for the treatment of festering and inflamed wounds, bronchial ailments, diarrhea, fever, hemorrhoids, and intestinal parasites.

PRECAUTIONS AND ADVERSE REACTIONS

No health hazards or side effects are known in conjunction with the proper administration of designated therapeutic dosages.

DOSAGE

Mode of Administration: Water Germander is used internally and externally.

Daily Dosage: Four teaspoonfuls of the herb (7.2 gm) is taken daily as an infusion. The same preparation can be used internally or externally.

LITERATURE

Fikenscher LH, Hegnauer R, Plant Med Phytother 3(3):183.

Hänsel R, Keller K, Rimpler H, Schneider G (Hrsg.), Hagers Handbuch der Pharmazeutischen Praxis, 5. Aufl., Bde 4-6 (Drogen): Springer Verlag Berlin, Heidelberg, New York, 1992-1994.

Madaus G, Lehrbuch der Biologischen Arzneimittel, Bde 1-3, Nachdruck, Georg Olms Verlag Hildesheim 1979.

Papanov G, Malakov PY, (1981) Z Naturforsch (B)36:112.

Papanov GY et al., PH 24:297-299. 1985.

Singh S et al., Fitoterapia 63:555. 1992.

Watercress

Nasturtium officinale

TRADE NAMES

Watercress (available from numerous manufacturers and as combination product)

DESCRIPTION

Medicinal Parts: The medicinal parts are the aerial parts collected during the flowering season and the entire flowering plant.

Flower and Fruit: On the leading and side shoots there are terminal, raceme-like inflorescences, which are slightly umbelliferous and consist of small, white, solitary flowers. The 4 white sepals are 2 to 3 mm long and glabrous. The 4 white petals are 2.5 to 5 mm long and turn lilac. There are 2 to 4 stamens with yellow anthers and filaments, which also turn lilac. The fruit is 13 to 18 mm long, with a glabrous pod on an 8 to 12 cm stem. The seeds are flat, ovate, 1 mm long, 0.8 to 0.9 mm wide and roughly reticulate. There are about 25 sections on each seed surface.

Leaves, Stem and Root: The plant is a perennial that grows from 25 to 90 cm and has creeping runners. The stem is angular, hollow, decumbent, rooting and branched. The somewhat fleshy leaves are alternate, usually odd-pinnate, lyrate and petiolate. They remain grass-green in winter. They have broad-elliptical, entire-margined or sweeping-crenate leaflets and roundish, broadly cordate terminal leaflets.

Characteristics: The plant has a radish-like taste and smells tangy when rubbed.

Habitat: The plant is found almost all over the world and is cultivated in many regions.

Production: Watercress consists of the fresh or dried above-ground parts of Nasturtium officinale. The fresh herb is collected in the wild and dried in shady, well-aired conditions.

Not to be Confused With: Berula erecta or Cardamine amara

Other Names: Indian Cress

ACTIONS AND PHARMACOLOGY

COMPOUNDS

Glucosinolates in the fresh, unbruised plant (0.9% of fresh weight): chief components gluconasturtiin (80%), which releases in the course of cell destruction the mustard oil phenyl ethyl isothiocyanate, from which 3-phenyl propionitrile, among other substances, spontaneously arises; additionally glucotropaeolin (yielding benzyl isothiocyanate), as well as 7-methyl thioheptyl glucosinolate, 8-methyl thiooctyl glucosinolate

Flavonoids

Vitamin C (80 mg/100 gm)

EFFECTS

Watercress has antibiotic, antitumoral and diuretic actions. The diuretic effect is probably due to the mustard oil content. As an amaroid drug, it stimulates appetite and digestion.

INDICATIONS AND USAGE

Approved by Commission E:

- Cough/bronchitis

Unproven Uses: Internally, the plant is used for catarrh of the respiratory tract, as an appetite stimulant and for digestion complaints. Externally, a decoction of the leaves in poultices and compresses is used for arthritis.

Homeopathic Uses: Watercress is used to treat irritation of the efferent urinary tract.

CONTRAINDICATIONS

Contraindications include stomach or intestinal ulcers and inflammatory renal diseases.

PRECAUTIONS AND ADVERSE REACTIONS

General: No health hazards or side effects are known in conjunction with the proper administration of designated therapeutic dosages. The intake of large quantities of the freshly harvested plant (e.g., in salad) could lead to gastrointestinal complaints due to the mucous membrane-irritating effect of the mustard oil.

Pediatric Use: The drug should not be administered to children under 4 years old.

Pregnancy: The drug should not be used during pregnancy.

DOSAGE

Mode of Administration: The comminuted herb, freshly pressed juice, as well as other galenic preparations of the plant, are for internal use.

How Supplied:

Capsules — 500 mg

Preparation: To make a tea, pour 150 ml boiling water over 2 gm drug (1 to 2 teaspoonfuls), cover for 10 to 15 minutes and strain.

Daily Dosage: The daily dosage is 2 to 3 cups of the tea before meals, 4 to 6 gm of the dried herb, 20 to 30 gm of the fresh herb or 60 to 150 gm of freshly pressed juice. Externally, the drug is applied as a poultice or a compress.

Homeopathic Dosage: 5 drops, 1 tablet or 10 globules every 30 to 60 minutes (acute) or 1 to 3 times daily (chronic); parenterally: 1 to 2 ml sc, acute, 3 times daily; chronic: once a day (HAB1).

LITERATURE

Hänsel R, Keller K, Rimpler H, Schneider G (Hrsg.), Hagers Handbuch der Pharmazeutischen Praxis, 5. Aufl., Bde 4-6 (Drogen), Springer Verlag Berlin, Heidelberg, New York, 1992-1994.

MacLeod AJ, Islam R, J Sci Food Agric 26:1545-1550. 1975.

Madaus G, Lehrbuch der Biologischen Arzneimittel, Bde 1-3, Nachdruck, Georg Olms Verlag Hildesheim 1979.

Spence RMM, Tucknott OG, PH 22:2521-2523. 1993.

Wichtl M (Hrsg.), Teedrogen, 4. Aufl., Wiss. Verlagsges. Stuttgart 1997.

Wheat

Triticum aestivum

DESCRIPTION

Medicinal Parts: The medicinal parts are the fruit wall, seed shell and outer layers of the endosperm.

Flower and Fruit: The inflorescence is a 4 to 18 cm long, more or less 4-sided and double-rowed awnless spike (occasionally with an awn up to 16 cm long). The spikelet has 2 to 6 flowers, 2 to 4 of which are sterile. Each spikelet has 2 glumes at the base, is approximately 10 mm long, blunt, keeled at the tip with a blunt or acute tooth. The flowers are surrounded by 2 bracts; the first is bulbous and coriaceous, the second smaller and membranous. There are 3 stamens and an ovary with 2 feather-like styles. The fruit is a yellowish, reddish or brownish orbicular to elongate oval caryopse.

Leaves, Stem and Root: The herb grows up to 1.5 m high. The leaves are arranged in two rows, are parallel-veined and 5 to 15 mm wide. The leaf base clasps the stem, the ligule is short with a ciliate eyelet. The stem is thin-walled, hollow and glabrous at the nodes.

Habitat: Asia, North America and Europe

Production: Wheat bran is the fruit wall, seed shell and outer layers of the endosperm of Triticum aestivum. Wheat germ oil is the fatty oil derived from cold-pressing the embryo of Triticum aestivum in a filter press.

Not to be Confused With: Wheat bran is sometimes confused with rye bran; wheat germ oil with other oils such as sesame oil.

Other Names: Wheat Bran, Wheat Germ Oil

ACTIONS AND PHARMACOLOGY

COMPOUNDS: WHEAT BRAN

Polysaccharides

Glucans: starch (15 to 20%), cellulose (30 %)

Heteroglycans (10%): complex arabinoxylans, to some extent water-soluble

Fatty oil (2%)

Phospholipids (1%)

Glycolipids (0.5%): particularly acyldigalactosyl glycerols

Steroids (0.3%): sterol esters

Proteins (20%)

Lignin

Alkyl resorcinols (0.1 to 0.2%): chiefly with C21- or C17-side chains

EFFECTS: WHEAT BRAN

Wheat bran is laxative in effect through expanding polysaccharides, which, through an increased level of fullness pressure, stimulate intestinal peristalsis and markedly shorten the transition time. At the same time, a measurable bonding of bile acids and their elimination from the enterohepatic circulation takes place. In addition, a significant reduction of postprandial lipid levels is exhibited. The topical application of the drug as a bath additive for injured or irritated skin (due to the carbohydrates and proteins it contains) leads to milieu changes in the epidermis and thus to a reconstitution of the callous layer.

COMPOUNDS: WHEAT GERM OIL

Fatty oil: triacylglycerols (60 to 75%), diacylglycerols (to 4%): chief fatty acids linoleic acid (50 to 65%), oleic acid (15 to 22%), palmitic acid (7 to 18%), linolenic acid (5 to 8%)

Phospholipids (9 to 14%)

Glycolipids (0 to 2%): particularly acyldigalaktosyl glycerols

Free fatty acids (1 to 2%)

Steroids: sterol esters (2.5 to 3%), particularly those of beta-sitosterol and campesterol

Tocopherols (vitamin E, 0.2 to 0.3%): particularly alpha-tocopherol (share 60 to 70%), as well as beta-tocopherol, gamma-tocopherol, alpha-tocotrienol, beta-tocotrienol

Carotinoids (0.15 to 0.25%)

EFFECTS: WHEAT GERM OIL

Wheat germ oil protects and nurtures the skin, is a laxative and reduces lipids. It is a valuable dietetic because of the high level of polyunsaturated fatty acids and vitamin E.

INDICATIONS AND USAGE

WHEAT BRAN

Unproven Uses: Folk medicine internal uses include constipation. Externally, bran has been used for itching and inflammatory dermatoses (as a bran bath).

Chinese Medicine: Used to treat spontaneous night sweats.

Indian Medicine: Flatulence, constipation, itching and menorrhagia are considered to be indications for use in Indian medicine. Efficacy for constipation and dermatoses seems plausible, but efficacy for the other indications has not been sufficiently proven.

WHEAT GERM OIL

Unproven Uses: Used as a dietary agent because of the high level of polyunsaturated fatty acids and vitamin E.

PRECAUTIONS AND ADVERSE REACTIONS

WHEAT BRAN AND WHEAT GERM OIL

No health hazards are known in conjunction with the proper administration of designated therapeutic dosages.

DOSAGE

WHEAT BRAN

Mode of Administration: Whole drug preparations are for internal and external use.

Daily Dosage: As a laxative, the dose is 15 to 40 g 1 to 2 times daily, taken with meals and plenty of liquid. For a full/partial bath: minimum 0.34 g aqueous extract to 1 L water

Chinese Medicine Daily Dosage: 9 to 15 g drug

WHEAT GERM OIL

Mode of Administration: Soft gelcaps or oil for internal and external use.

Storage: Store tightly sealed in a cool place.

LITERATURE

Blaschek W, Hänsel R, Keller K, Reichling J, Rimpler G, Schneider G, (Eds) Hagers Handbuch der Pharmazeutischen Praxis. Folgebände 1 und 2. Drogen A-Z. Springer. Berlin, Heidelberg 1998.

Goff DJ, Kull FJ, The inhibition of human salivary alpha-amylase by type II alpha-amylase inhibitor from Triticum aestivum is competitive, slow and tight-binding. J Enzyme Inhib, 252:163-70, 1995.

White Bryony

Bryonia alba

DESCRIPTION

Medicinal Parts: The medicinal part is the root.

Flower and Fruit: The plant is monoecious, occasionally dioecious. The male flowers are in long-peduncled racemes, which are 10 to 12 mm wide and shed easily. The female flowers are in short-stemmed umbel-like clusters. The sepals are almost as long as the corolla. The 5-petaled corolla is yellowish-white and has green veins. The 3 styles are almost completely free. The stigmas are glabrous. The 2 fused, inferior ovaries are 3-valved. The fruit is a 1- to 2-seeded, thin-skinned, 7 to 8 mm thick, globose black berry.

Leaves, Stem and Root: White Bryony is an extremely fast-growing perennial. It has a thick, tuberous root. The root is fleshy, wrinkled horizontally, yellowish-gray on the outside and white and slimy on the inside. The grooved, angular stems are climbing, branched and have long internodes and simple screw-like climbers. They grow up to 4 m long. The leaves are short-petioled, broadly cordate, pentagonal to 5-lobed and covered with short bristles on both sides.

Characteristics: The root is bitter and spicy. The plant is categorized as extremely poisonous.

Habitat: Indigenous from northeastern and southeastern Europe and also Iran.

Production: Bryonia root consists of the dried taproot of Bryonia alba, which is cultivated.

Other Names: Devil's Turnip, English Mandrake, Ladies' Seal, Tamus, Tetterberry, Wild Hops, Wild Nep, Wild Vine, Wood Vine

ACTIONS AND PHARMACOLOGY

COMPOUNDS

Cucurbitacins: including cucurbitacins B, D, E, I, J, K, L, 23,24-dihydro-cucurbitacins, 1,2,23,24-tetrahydrocucurbitacins, 22-deoxycucurbitacins and bryodulcigenin; cucurbitacin glycosides, including bryonin, elaterinide, bryonosid, bryodulcigenin, cucurbitacin glycosides

Triterpenes with unusual structure: for example, bryonolic acid

Steroids: including sterols like C-4- and/or C-24-methylated or ethylated cholest-7-en-3-beta-oles

Polyhydroxy fatty acids: including 9,12,13-trihydroxy-octadeca-10 (E)-15(Z)-dienic acid.

Lectins

EFFECTS

The mainly glycosidically bonded cucurbitanes contained in the drug have a strong toxic and cytotoxic effect; in topical application they are irritating to the skin and mucous membrane. Various aqueous extracts of the drug display an antitumoral effect in animal tests. The resin is a drastic purgative. The methanol extracts have a strong hypoglycemic affect. Use of the drug as an emetic and purgative has become obsolete because of the toxicity.

INDICATIONS AND USAGE

Unproven Uses: Because of its strong purgative and emetic effect, use of the drug cannot be recommended. Bryonia root has been used as a laxative, emetic and diuretic in the treatment of various disorders of the gastrointestinal tract and respiratory tract and for rheumatic disorders. It has also been used prophylactically and therapeutically for metabolic disorders, liver disease, and acute and chronic infectious disease.

PRECAUTIONS AND ADVERSE REACTIONS

The drug is highly toxic when freshly harvested. The toxicity of the drug declines rapidly with dehydration and storage because of the instability of the cucurbitacins. Due to the cucurbitacin content, the drug has a severely irritating effect on skin and mucous membranes. Contact between skin and the juice of the plant can lead to rash, infection, blister formation and necroses.

OVERDOSAGE

The intake of toxic dosages can lead to vomiting, bloody diarrhea, colic, kidney irritation, anuria, collapse, spasms, paralysis and, under certain conditions, to death. Following gastric lavage, the treatment for poisonings should proceed symptomatically. Consumption of 40 berries is presumed fatal for an adult; 15 for a child.

DOSAGE

Mode of Administration: Since the efficacy of Bryonia preparations for the claimed applications is not documented, and since the use of it as a drastic laxative and emetic is obsolete, a therapeutic administration cannot be justified because of the risks involved.

Bryonia is found occasionally in some pharmaceutical preparations.

Preparation: A decoction is prepared by adding 0.5 to 1 g drug to 1 cup water.

Daily Dosage: Dosage of the powder is 0.3 to 0.5 g as an emetic and purgative.

LITERATURE

Hylands PJ, Mansour ESS, PH 21(11):2703-2707. 1982.

Konopa J et al., (1974) Arzneim Forsch 24(10), 1554.

Oobayashi K, Yoshikawa K, Arihara S, Structural revision of Bryonoside and structure elucidation of minor saponins from Bryonia dioica. In: PH 31:943-946. 1992.

Panossian AG et al., (1983) Planta Med 47(1), 17-25.

Pohlmann J, The cucurbitacins in Bryonia alba and Bryonia dioica. In: PH 14(7):1587-1589. 1980.

Suganda AG et al., (1983) J Nat Prod 46(5), 626.

Vartanian GS et al., (1984) Byull Eksp Biol Med 97(3), 295.

Further information in:

Frohne D, Pfänder HJ, Giftpflanzen - Ein Handbuch für Apotheker, Toxikologen und Biologen, 4. Aufl., Wiss. Verlags-Ges Stuttgart 1997.

Hänsel R, Keller K, Rimpler H, Schneider G (Hrsg.), Hagers Handbuch der Pharmazeutischen Praxis, 5. Aufl., Bde 4-6 (Drogen), Springer Verlag Berlin, Heidelberg, New York, 1992-1994.

Lewin L, Gifte und Vergiftungen, 6. Aufl., Nachdruck, Haug Verlag, Heidelberg 1992.

Madaus G, Lehrbuch der Biologischen Arzneimittel, Bde 1-3, Nachdruck, Georg Olms Verlag Hildesheim 1979.

Roth L, Daunderer M, Kormann K, Giftpflanzen, Pflanzengifte, 4. Aufl., Ecomed Fachverlag Landsberg Lech 1993.

Steinegger E, Hänsel R, Pharmakognosie, 5. Aufl., Springer Verlag Heidelberg 1992.

Teuscher E, Lindequist U, Biogene Gifte - Biologie, Chemie, Pharmakologie, 2. Aufl., Fischer Verlag Stuttgart 1994.

Teuscher E, Biogene Arzneimittel, 5. Aufl., Wiss. Verlagsges. Stuttgart 1997.

Wagner H, Wiesenauer M, Phytotherapie. Phytopharmaka und pflanzliche Homöopathika, Fischer-Verlag, Stuttgart, Jena, New York 1995.

White Fir

Abies alba

DESCRIPTION

Medicinal Parts: The medicinal part of the trees is the timber of the Fir.

Flower and Fruit: The ovules are in pairs on the upper surface of the seed scales, in axils of the spirally arranged covering scales, which are in turn fused into cones. The cones are 10 to 16 cm long and 3 to 5 cm thick, with protruding surface scales that are green and tinged brown-red before ripening. The stamens are arranged like catkins. The fruit is diclinous, monoecious. The seeds are long-winged on one side.

Leaves, Stem and Root: The tree grows up to 50 m and occasionally up to 75 m tall. The needles are 1 to 3 cm long, 1.8 to 2.3 mm wide. The needles are dark green on the upper surface with two white stripes on the lower surface. They are divided with a blunt apex indented at the tip. The trunk is initially grayish, later scaly.

Habitat: White Fir is found in the Balkan countries. It originated from former Yugoslavia, Bulgaria, Poland, Romania and Albania.

Production: The essential oil of White Fir is extracted from the needles and branch tips by aqueous steam distillation for 5 to 6 hours.

Not to be Confused With: May occur with turpentine oils, cone oils, fir needle oils, camphors, bornyl acetate and various Pinaceae oils.

Other Names: Common Silver Fir, Swiss Pine

ACTIONS AND PHARMACOLOGY

COMPOUNDS

Limonene (25 to 55%)

Alpha-pinene (6 to 35%)

Camphene (9 to 20%)

Bornyl acetate (2 to 10%)

Santene (2 to 3%)

Tricyclene (1.0 to 2.5%): including among others beta-pinene, beta-phellandrene and delta3-carene

EFFECTS

The essential oil has secretolytic and mildly antiseptic effects on the bronchial mucous membrane area and hyperemic effects on the skin. The constituents' camphene, limonene and alpha-pinene are responsible for the strong expectorate effect connected with its inhalation.

INDICATIONS AND USAGE

Approved by Commision E:

- Neuralgia
- Rheumatism

Unproven Uses: Internally, the drug is used for catarrh of the respiratory tract. Externally, it can be used for nervous unrest and neuralgic pain. It can also be used for sprains, strains, contusions, bruising and as a prophylactic treatment for bedsores.

CONTRAINDICATIONS

The plant is contraindicated for conditions like bronchial asthma, other obstructive bronchial diseases and whooping cough. Whole-body baths involving the essential oil should only be undertaken in consultation with a physician in the presence of larger skin injuries, severe feverish or infectious diseases, cardiac insufficiency or hypertonia. Inhalation is to be avoided when the patient suffers from acute infections of the respiratory passages.

PRECAUTIONS AND ADVERSE REACTIONS

No health hazards are known in conjunction with the proper administration of designated therapeutic dosages. Bronchial spasms could become worse following administration of the drug.

OVERDOSAGE

Poisonings are possible in connection with overdose and large-area external administration, including injuries to the kidneys and the CNS. The use of outdated essential oils with unsaturated terpene carbohydrates could lead to severe irritation of the skin and mucous membranes.

Severe poisonings are possible following the ingestion of very large doses, leading to nausea, vomiting, reddening of the face, salivation, throat soreness, thirst, diarrhea, intestinal colic, dyspnea, dizziness, staggering walk, twitching, stranguria, dysuria, hematuria, albuminuria and skin efflorescence. It should be followed with gastric lavage with sodium sulfate solutions, intestinal emptying through administration of sodium sulfate, instillation of paraffin oil and medicinal charcoal, and shock prophylaxis (suitable body position, quiet, warmth).

The treatment for poisonings consists of the treatment of spasms with diazepam (I.V.), electrolyte substitution and the countering of any acidosis imbalance that may appear through sodium bicarbonate infusions. In the event of shock, plasma volume expanders should be infused. Monitoring of kidney function is necessary. Intubation and oxygen respiration may also be required.

DOSAGE

Mode of Administration: Liquid preparations for internal and external use.

Daily Dosage:

Drops — 4 drops, 3 times daily in water or with sugar

Inhalation — add a few drops to hot water; and inhale several times daily

Lotion — rub into the affected parts

Storage: Keep sealed tightly and protected from light.

LITERATURE

Aronow WS, Starling L, Etienne F, D'Alba P, Edwards M, Lee NH, Parungao RF, Sales FF, Risk factors for atherothrombotic brain infarction in persons over 62 years of age in a long-term healthcare facility. J Am Geriatr Soc, 35:1-3, 1987 Jan.

Faure-Raynaud M, Determination of the chitinolytic activity of 'Abies alba Mill. litter microorganisms: bacteria and yeasts (author's transl) Ann Microbiol (Paris), 132B:267-79, 1981 Sep-Oct.

Faure-Raynaud M, Study of volatile oil from Abies alba Miller. I. Study of raw material Acta Pol Pharm, 132B:71-7, 1970.

Faure-Raynaud M, Study of volatile oil from sprigs of Abies alba Miller. II. Study of monoterpene fractions of oil, Acta Pol Pharm, 132B:155-62, 1970.

Faure-Raynaud M, Study of volatile oil of fir branches Abies alba Miller. 3. Study of non-monoterpene fraction and gas chromatography of oil, Acta Pol Pharm, 132B:301-5, 1970.

Hänsel R, Keller K, Rimpler H, Schneider G (Ed) Hagers Handbuch der Pharmazeutischen Praxis. 5. Aufl., Bde 4 - 6 (Drogen), Springer Verlag Berlin, Heidelberg, New York, 1992-1994.

White Hellebore

Veratrum album

DESCRIPTION

Medicinal Parts: The medicinal parts are the rhizome and root.

Flower and Fruit: The flowers are in racemes forming a 30 to 60 cm long panicle. The pedicles are much shorter than the flowers. The yellowish-white flowers consist of 6 similar tepals, which are oblong-lanceolate, acute, denticulate and broadly splayed. There are 6 stamens, which are shorter than the perigone, and 3 styles. The fruit is capsule-like.

Leaves, Stem and Root: The plant is roughly 60 to 120 cm high. The rhizome is short, cylindrical and stunted. It has numerous, long, thick and fleshy root fibers. The round, cane-like, glabrous stem is almost completely surrounded by the tight sheaths of the basal leaves. The basal leaves are whorled, broad, elliptical to linear-lanceolate and heavily ribbed.

Habitat: The plant is found from Lapland to Italy but not on the British Isles.

Production: White Hellebore root-stock is the rhizome of Veratrum album.

ACTIONS AND PHARMACOLOGY

COMPOUNDS

Steroid alkaloids (mixture is referred to as veratrine, 0.8-2.5%): C-nor-D-homo-sterane type-including protoverine, protoveratrines A and B, germerine, jervine, protoverine, veratroyl zygadenine

Solidane type-including isorubijervine, rubijervine

EFFECTS

Internally, the drug reduces blood pressure and heart rate, inhibits respiration in higher doses, and has an aconitine-like effect on the conductor system. Externally, the drug causes severe irritation to the skin, including numbing and poisoning through absorption.

INDICATIONS AND USAGE

Unproven Uses: Internally, White Hellebore is used for the treatment of vomiting, cramps, diarrhea, cholera, bradycardia and Graves' disease. Externally, the drug is used for neuralgia, rheumatism, joint pain and gout pain.

Homeopathic Uses: White Hellebore is used for neuralgia, infections, diarrhea, low blood pressure and as a stimulant.

PRECAUTIONS AND ADVERSE REACTIONS

The drug is severely toxic and has numerous severe side effects, even at therapeutic dosages. It is no longer administered in allopathic medicine for that reason. The veratrum alkaloids severely irritate mucous membranes. By inhibiting inactivation of sodium ion channels, the resorption of alkaloids has a paralyzing effect on numerous excitable cells, particularly those governing cardiac activity.

OVERDOSAGE

The first symptoms of poisoning are sneezing, lacrimation, salivation, vomiting, diarrhea, a burning sensation in the mouth and pharyngeal cavity, and inability to swallow. Then, following resorption, paresthesia, vertigo, possible blindness, paralysis of the limbs, mild convulsions, lowering of cardiac frequency, cardiac arrhythmias and hypotension occur. Death occurs either through systolic cardiac arrest or through asphyxiation. The lethal dosage is between 10 and 20 mg of the alkaloid mixture, corresponding to 1 to 2 gm of the drug. The alkaloids can be absorbed through uninjured skin.

Treatment of poisoning consists of gastrointestinal emptying (inducement of vomiting, gastric lavage with burgundy-colored potassium permanganate solution, sodium sulphate), administration of activated charcoal and shock prophylaxis (appropriate body position, quiet, warmth). Thereafter, spasms should be treated with diazepam or barbiturates (i.v.), bradycardia should be treated with atropine, hypotension should be treated with peripherally active circulatory medications, electrolyte substitution should be employed, and possible cases of acidosis should be treated with sodium bicarbonate infusions. Intubation and oxygen respiration may also be necessary.

DOSAGE

Mode of Administration: The drug is used in powders, tinctures and homeopathic dilutions for internal use; preparations made with fatty oils are used externally.

Preparation: Mix 5 gm drug with 10 gm lanolin and 20 gm fat for topical application.

Daily Dosage: Internally, the drug is administered as 0.02 to 0.1 gm of powder or 20 to 60 drops of tincture. Externally, the drug is applied as a poultice or compress.

Homeopathic Dosage: 5 drops, 1 tablet or 10 globules every 30 to 60 minutes (acute) and 1 to 3 times daily (chronic); parenterally: 1 to 2 ml s.c., acute: 3 times daily; chronic: once a day (HAB34). The globules are from D2; all others are from D4.

LITERATURE

Atta-Ur-Rahman, Ali RA, Choudhary MI, New steroidal alkaloids from rhizomes of Veratrum album. In: JNP 55:565-570. 1992.

Atta-Ur-Rahmann, Ali RA, Gilani A, Choudhary MI, ASftab K, Sener B, Turkz S, Isolation of antihypertensive alkaloids from rhizomes of Veratrum album. In: PM 59(6):569. 1993.

Atta-Ur-Rahman et al., Alkaloids from Veratrum album. In: PH 30(1):368. 1991.

Brossi, Buch. In: Brossi A, Cordell GA (Eds), The Alkaloids. Vol. 41. Academic Press, 1250 Sixth Avenue, San Diego, CA 92101. 1992.

Festa M, Andreetto B, Ballaris MA, Panio A, Piervittori R, A case of Veratrum poisoning. Minerva Anestesiol, 62:195-6, 1996 May.

Fogh A, Kulling P, Wickstrom E, Veratrum alkaloids in sneezing-powder a potential danger. J Toxicol Clin Toxicol, 20:175-9, 1983 Apr.

Garnier R, Carlier P, Hoffelt J, Savidan A, Acute dietary poisoning by white hellebore (Veratrum album L.). Clinical and analytical data. A propos of 5 cases. Ann Med Interne (Paris), 136:125-8, 1985.

Hruby K, Lenz K, Krausler J, Veratrum album poisoning (author's transl). Wien Klin Wochenschr, 93:517-9, 1981 Sep 4.

Jaspersen-Schib R, Theus L, Guirguis-Oeschger M, Gossweiler B, Meier-Abt PJ, Serious plant poisonings in Switzerland 1966-1994. Case analysis from the Swiss Toxicology Information Center. Schweiz Med Wochenschr, 60:1085-98, 1996 Jun 22.

Marinov A, Koev P, Mirchev N, Electrocardiographic studies of patients with acute hellebore (Veratrum album) poisoning. Vutr Boles, 26:36-9, 1987.

Further information in:

Frohne D, Pfänder HJ, Giftpflanzen - Ein Handbuch für Apotheker, Toxikologen und Biologen, 4. Aufl., Wiss. Verlags-Ges. Stuttgart 1997.

Kern W, List PH, Hörhammer L (Hrsg.), Hagers Handbuch der Pharmazeutischen Praxis, 4. Aufl., Bde. 1-8: Springer Verlag Berlin, Heidelberg, New York, 1969.

Lewin L, Gifte und Vergiftungen, 6. Aufl., Nachdruck, Haug Verlag, Heidelberg 1992.

Madaus G, Lehrbuch der Biologischen Arzneimittel, Bde 1-3, Nachdruck, Georg Olms Verlag Hildesheim 1979.

Roth L, Daunderer M, Kormann K, Giftpflanzen, Pflanzengifte, 4. Aufl., Ecomed Fachverlag Landsberg Lech 1993.

Teuscher E, Lindequist U, Biogene Gifte - Biologie, Chemie, Pharmakologie, 2. Aufl., Fischer Verlag Stuttgart 1994.

Teuscher E, Biogene Arzneimittel, 5. Aufl., Wiss. Verlagsges. Stuttgart 1997.

Wagner H, Wiesenauer M, Phytotherapie. Phytopharmaka und pflanzliche Homöopathika, Fischer-Verlag, Stuttgart, Jena, New York 1995.

White Lily

Lilium candidum

DESCRIPTION

Medicinal Parts: The medicinal part is the fresh and dried bulb.

Flower and Fruit: The inflorescence has 5 to 20 blossoms. The flowers are white, occasionally striped crimson or spotted and very fragrant. They are on erect pedicles, the lower ones nodding. The tepals are obtuse, the anthers yellow. The style is as long as the sepals. The fruit is obovate and is seldom developed.

Leaves, Stem and Root: The plant is perennial, 60 to 150 cm high. It has a broad, ovate, scaled and yellow bulb. The stem is rigid, erect and leafy. The leaves are oblong to linear-lanceolate and glabrous. The leaves survive winter, as does the rest of the plant, which is hardy. The bulb consists of imbricate, fleshy, lanceolate and bent scales, which are 3.25 cm long and 2.5 cm wide at the broadest point.

Characteristics: The bulbs are odorless and have a mildly bitter and unpleasant flavor.

Habitat: The plant is indigenous to Mediterranean regions and is cultivated in many other regions.

Production: Baurenlilien (Farmer's Lily) root is the subterranean part (onion) of Lilium candidum.

Other Names: Meadow Lily, Madonna Lily

ACTIONS AND PHARMACOLOGY

COMPOUNDS

Flavonoids: including isorhamnetin glycosides

Gamma-methylene glutamic acid

Soluble polysaccharides: glucomannans

Starch

Tuliposide

The constituents of the drug have not been investigated extensively.

EFFECTS

The plant has astringent, anti-inflammatory, pain reliever, diuretic and expectorant properties.

INDICATIONS AND USAGE

Unproven Uses: Internally for gynecological disorders and externally for ulcers, inflammation, furuncles, finger ulcers, reddened skin, burns and injuries.

PRECAUTIONS AND ADVERSE REACTIONS

No health hazards or side effects are known in conjunction with the proper administration of designated therapeutic dosages.

DOSAGE

Mode of Administration: An infusion made from the ground drug is used internally. The drug is also used externally as a wet compress (paste).

Daily Dosage: Apply a thick paste, made from fresh or cooked onions, in the middle of a compress or poultice, to the affected area. This should be done several times during the day.

LITERATURE

Delaveau P et al., (1980) Planta Med 40:49.

Kern W, List PH, Hörhammer L (Hrsg.), Hagers Handbuch der Pharmazeutischen Praxis, 4. Aufl., Bde. 1-8, Springer Verlag Berlin, Heidelberg, New York, 1969.

Masterova I et al., (1987) Phytochemistry 26(6):1844.

Nagy E et al., (1984) Z Naturforsch 39B(12):1813.

White Mustard

Sinapis alba

DESCRIPTION

Medicinal Parts: The medicinal parts are the dried seeds.

Flower and Fruit: The flowers form an umbelliferous-racemous inflorescence. The flowers are on 3 to 7 mm long, stiff-haired pedicles. When in bloom the 4 narrow, obtuse sepals lie horizontal. There are 3 green, ovate nectaries at the base of the stamens. The fruit is a 2 to 4 cm long bristly pod, divided into two chambers. Each chamber contains two to three 2.5 mm thick seeds. The chamber ends as a large curled lip. The seeds vary from brown to white and are arranged in opposite rows.

Leaves, Stem and Root: Sinapis alba is an annual plant. The lower part of the plant is covered in stiff, single hairs. The thin root is yellow to white and branched. The root produces a 30 to 60 cm high, erect, grooved and branched stem. The leaves are 4 to 10 cm long, petiolate, lyrate, pinnatifid to pinnatesect and always have 2 to 3 indented-dentate lobed pinna.

Habitat: The plant has been introduced and naturalized in all of Europe and in Siberia, east Asia and America. The areas of cultivation are western and northern Europe and the northern U.S.

Production: White Mustard seed consists of the ripe, dried seed of Sinapis alba.

Not to be Confused With: Other Sinapis or Brassica species. Artificial colorings such as butter yellow or turmeric may be added.

Other Names: Mustard

ACTIONS AND PHARMACOLOGY

COMPOUNDS

Glucosinolates: chiefly sinalbin (p-hydroxybenzylglucosinolates, 2.5%), grinding the seeds into powder and then rubbing with warm water (not with hot water — enzymes would be destroyed), as well as chewing, releases the non-volatile mustard oil p-hydroxybenzyl isothiocyanate

Fatty oil (20-35%)

Proteins (40%)

Phenyl propane derivatives: including among others sinapine (choline ester of sinapic acid, 1.5%)

EFFECTS

The p-hydroxybenzyl mustard oil that results from fermentation of sinalbin is bacteriostatic, irritating to the skin and hyperemic (as an additive in 35° to 40° C baths).

INDICATIONS AND USAGE

Approved by Commission E:

- Common cold
- Cough/bronchitis
- Rheumatism

Unproven Uses: Externally, White Mustard is used in poultices for congestion of the respiratory tract, for topical hyperemization of the skin as well as for segment therapy of chronic degenerative diseases affecting the joints and soft tissue. Mustard baths are used in the treatment of paralytic symptoms.

In folk medicine, Mustard is used to clear the voice. It is also used in Mustard plasters and poultices as a counter-irritant. Mustard is used in footbaths, and for the treatment of paralytic symptoms in the form of Mustard baths.

Chinese Medicine: In China, White Mustard is used to treat painfully swollen ribs and chest, coughs, vomiting, regurgitation, ulcerous swelling and rheumatic pains.

Homeopathic Uses: Sinapis alba is used to treat inflammation of the gastrointestinal tract and the respiratory tract.

CONTRAINDICATIONS

White Mustard is contraindicated in gastrointestinal ulcers and inflammatory kidney diseases. The drug should not be given to children under 6 years of age.

PRECAUTIONS AND ADVERSE REACTIONS

General: No health hazards or side effects are known in conjunction with the proper administration of designated therapeutic dosages. The danger of nerve damage exists with long-term intake. Long-term external application carries the danger of skin injury. The drug possesses minimal potential for sensitization (possible cause of food allergies).

Pediatric Use: White Mustard preparations should not be used in children under 6 years of age.

OVERDOSAGE

Gastrointestinal complaints could appear following the intake of large quantities, due to the mucous membrane-irritating effect of the Mustard oil.

DOSAGE

Mode of Administration: The drug is used internally as well as externally. Ground or powdered seeds are used for poultices.

Preparation: To prepare an external foot bath, 20 to 30 gm of the Mustard flour in 1 liter of water is used. To prepare a Mustard bath, 150 gm of the Mustard flour in a pouch is used in the bathwater.

Daily Dosage: The average daily dose of the drug is 60 to 240 gm. To brighten and clear the voice, Mustard flour is stirred with honey and formed into balls. 1 to 2 are taken orally on an empty stomach.

For external use, just prior to application, mix 50 to 70 gm of the powdered seeds with warm water to prepare a poultice. The poultice is applied for 10 to 15 minutes for adults and for 5 to 10 minutes for children, except for those with sensitive skin where the usage should be shortened. Treatment should not exceed 2 weeks.

Homeopathic Dosage: 5 drops, 1 tablet or 10 globules every 30 to 60 minutes (acute) or 1 to 3 times daily (chronic); parenterally: 1 to 2 ml sc, acute: 3 times daily; chronic: once a day (HAB34)

Storage: The drug must be protected from light and moisture.

LITERATURE

Josefsson E, J Sci Food Agric 21:94. 1970.

Kerber E et al., Angew Bot 55:457. 1981.

Kjaer A, Rubinstein K, Acta Chem Scand 4:1276. 1953.

Further information in:

Frohne D, Pfänder HJ, Giftpflanzen - Ein Handbuch für Apotheker, Toxikologen und Biologen, 4. Aufl., Wiss. Verlags-Ges. Stuttgart 1997.

Hänsel R, Keller K, Rimpler H, Schneider G (Hrsg.), Hagers Handbuch der Pharmazeutischen Praxis, 5. Aufl., Bde 4-6 (Drogen): Springer Verlag Berlin, Heidelberg, New York, 1992-1994.

Steinegger E, Hänsel R, Pharmakognosie, 5. Aufl., Springer Verlag Heidelberg 1992.

Teuscher E, Lindequist U, Biogene Gifte - Biologie, Chemie, Pharmakologie, 2. Aufl., Fischer Verlag Stuttgart 1994.

Teuscher E, Biogene Arzneimittel, 5. Aufl., Wiss. Verlagsges. Stuttgart 1997.

White Nettle

Lamium album

DESCRIPTION

Medicinal Parts: The medicinal parts are the flowers and leaves.

Flower and Fruit: The white, fairly large bilabiate flowers are in axillary false whorls of 6 to 16 flowers. The campanulate calyx is green and has 5 tips. The tube of the corolla is bent like a knee and the upper lip is curved like a helmet with a ciliate margin. The lower lip is gordate. The tube has 1 large and 1 small tip at the edge. There are 2 long and 2 short stamens under the upper lip. The calyx remains after flowering and protects the small nut. When the nut is ripe, slight pressure is sufficient to fling out the seeds.

Leaves, Stem and Root: The plant is 30 to 50 cm high with an underground creeping stem from which the aerial stems grow. These are erect, quadrangular, grooved, hollow and noded. The leaves are crossed opposite, petiolate, ovate to cordate, acuminate and serrate. The plant has no nettle hairs. The plant is similar to the stinging nettle but has a different stem.

Characteristics: The flowers have a weak honey-like fragrance and a slimy-sweet taste.

Habitat: The plant is common in Europe and central and northern Asia.

Production: White Nettle flower consists of the dried petal with attached stamens of Lamium album as well as its preparations.

Other Names: Blind Nettle, Dumb Nettle, Dead Nettle, Deaf Nettle, Bee Nettle, Archangel, Stingless Nettle, White Archangel

ACTIONS AND PHARMACOLOGY

COMPOUNDS

Iridoide monoterpenes: including among others lamalbide, caryoptoside, alboside A and B

Triterpene saponins

Caffeic acid derivatives: including among others rosmaric acid, chlorogenic acid

Flavonoids: including among others kaempferol glycosides

Mucilages

EFFECTS

Because of the mucins and saponins the drug is expectorant. It is astringent because of the tannins.

INDICATIONS AND USAGE

Approved by Commission E:

- Inflammation of the skin
- Cough/bronchitis
- Inflammation of the mouth and pharynx

Unproven Uses:

Internally — catarrh of the upper respiratory passages, gastrointestinal disorders such as gastritis, sensation of bloating and flatulence.

Externally — mild inflammation of the mucous membranes of the mouth and throat, non-specific fluor albus (leukorrhea) mild, superficial inflammation of the skin. In folk medicine used for climacteric complaints and complaints of the urogenital tract.

Chinese Medicine: In Chinese medicine, White Nettle is used for fractures, carbuncles, lumbago and inflammation of wounds.

PRECAUTIONS AND ADVERSE REACTIONS

No health hazards or side effects are known in conjunction with the proper administration of designated therapeutic dosages.

DOSAGE

Mode of Administration: Comminuted drug for infusions and other galenic preparations for internal applications, rinses, baths and moist compresses; occasionally used as a constituent of sedative teas and bronchial teas.

Preparation:

Infusion — Pour one cup of water over 1 gm drug, leave to draw for 5 minutes and strain.

Extract for poultices — Scald 50 gm of flowers with 500 ml of water, draw for 5 minutes and strain.

Daily Dosage: For internal use, the average daily dose is 3 gm drug. For external use, 5 gm drug is added to a bath.

LITERATURE

Damtoft S, Iridoid glucosides from Lamium album. In: PH 31(1):175. 1992.

Gora J et al., Chemical comparative studies of the herb and flowers of Lamium album L. In: Acta Pol Pharm 40(3):389-393. 1983.

Kern W, List PH, Hörhammer L (Hrsg.), Hagers Handbuch der Pharmazeutischen Praxis, 4. Aufl., Bde. 1-8, Springer Verlag Berlin, Heidelberg, New York, 1969.

Kooiman P, (1972) Acta Bot Neerl 21(4)417.

Madaus G, Lehrbuch der Biologischen Arzneimittel, Bde 1-3, Nachdruck, Georg Olms Verlag Hildesheim 1979.

Skrypczak L et al., Phenylpropanoid esters and flavonoids in taxonomy of Lamium species. In: PM 61(Abstracts of 43rd Ann Congr):70. 1995.

Wichtl M (Hrsg.), Teedrogen, 4. Aufl., Wiss. Verlagsges. Stuttgart 1997.

White Willow

Salix species

TRADE NAMES

Alcohol Free White Willow Bark, Standardized White Willow Bark, Wild Countryside White Willow

DESCRIPTION

Medicinal Parts: The medicinal part is the bark. Salix nigra is American Willow.

Flower and Fruit: The male flowers are yellow and the female green. They are dioecious and appear at the same time as the leaves on leafy stems in erect catkins. The male catkins are densely blossomed and cylindrical, up to 6.5 cm by 1 cm and have 2 stamens. The female catkins are cylindrical, 4.5 cm by 7 mm. The seeds have a tuft of hair.

Leaves, Stem and Root: Silver Willow is a 6 to 18 m high tree or bush with fissured gray bark. The leaves are short-petioled, lanceolate, acuminate and become cuneate at the base. They are finely serrate, silky-haired tomentose underneath and blue-green matte.

Characteristics: The annual twigs are not easy to break off at the base.

Habitat: The plant is indigenous to central and southern Europe.

Production: White Willow bark consists of the bark of the young, 2 to 3 year old branches harvested during early spring of Salix alba, Salix purpurea, Salix fragilis and other comparable Salix species.

Other Names: Willow, Salicin Willow, Withe Withy, Black Willow, Cartkins Willow, Pussywillow

ACTIONS AND PHARMACOLOGY

COMPOUNDS

Glycosides and esters yielding salicylic acid (1.5-12%): salicin (0.1-2%), salicortin (0.01-11%) and salicin derivatives acylated to the glucose residue (up to 6%, including, among others, fragilin, populin)

Tannins (8-20%)

Flavonoids

EFFECTS

The efficacy of the drug is due mainly to the proportion of salicin present. After splitting of the acyl residue, the salicin glycosides convert to salicin, the precursor of salicylic acid. Salicylic acid is antipyretic, antiphlogistic and analgesic. White Willow bark is the phytotherapeutic precursor to acetylsalicylic acid (aspirin).

The salicin component is responsible for the anti-inflammatory and antipyretic effects. The tannin content has astringent properties on mucous membranes.

INDICATIONS AND USAGE

Approved by Commission E:

- Rheumatism
- Pain

Salicin is useful in diseases accompanied by fever, rheumatic ailments, headaches and pain caused by inflammation.

CONTRAINDICATIONS

Willow Bark is contraindicated in patients that have a hypersensitivity to salicylates. Salicylates should not be used in children with flu-like symptoms due to the association of salicylates with Reyes Syndrome.

PRECAUTIONS AND ADVERSE REACTIONS

General: No health hazards are known in conjunction with the proper administration of designated therapeutic dosages. Stomach complaints could occur as a side effect due to the tannin content.

Drug Interactions: Due to the salicin component, caution should be exercised when used in combination with salicylates and other non-steroidal anti-inflammatory drugs. There are reports that salicylate decreased serum naproxen concentrations markedly and increased serum naproxen clearance by as much as 56% (Furst, 1987).

Though there are no reports of interactions with drugs that affect blood clotting times, and some studies suggest that thrombocyte inhibition is unlikely. Anti-platelet medications and any medication that prolongs the PT time should not be used with Willow Bark (Wichtl & Bisset, 1994).

Alcohol and barbiturates may mask the symptoms of salicylate overdosage and may enhance the toxicity of salicylates.

There have been reports of metabolic acidosis in children with normal renal and hepatic function that were treated with salicylates and carbonic anhydrase inhibitors for joint pain and glaucoma. This combination should be avoided (Cowan, 1984).

Disease Interactions: Patients with an active gastric or duodenal ulcer should avoid Willow Bark preparations. Hemophiliacs or anyone with a bleeding disorder should not use Willow Bark. Willow Bark should be avoided in asthmatics and diabetics.

Pregnancy: Salicylates should be avoided during pregnancy.

Nursing Mothers: Salicylates have been associated with rashes in breast-fed infants; use is not recommended.

DOSAGE

Mode of Administration: Liquid and solid preparations for internal use. Combinations with diaphoretic drugs could be considered. Drug extracts are contained in some standardized preparations of analgesics/antirheumatics, hypnotics/sedatives, and gastrointestinal remedies.

Preparation: To prepare an infusion, use 2 to 3 gm of finely cut or coarsely powdered drug in cold water, boil, allow to steep for 5 minutes, then strain.

Daily Dosage: Average daily dose corresponding to 60-120 mg total salicin.

Infusion—1 cup 3 to 5 times daily. (1 teaspoonful = 1.5 gm drug)

Liquid Extract—(1:1 in 25% alcohol) 1 to 3 ml 3 times daily.

LITERATURE

Amling R, Phytotherapeutika in der Neurologie. In: ZPT 12(1):9. 1991.

Anonym, Phytotherapie:Pflanzliche Antirheumatika - was bringen sie? In: DAZ 136(45):4012-4015. 1996.

Cowan, RA, Hartnell G, Lowdell C, Baird I, Leak A, Metabolic acidosis induced by carbonic anhydrase inhibitors and salicylates in patients with normal renal function. In: Br Med J (Clin Res Ed) 289(6441):347-8, Aug 11, 1984.

Furst DE, Sarkissian E, Blocka K et al., Serum concentrations of salicylate and naproxen during concurrent therapy in patients with rheumatoid arthritis. In: Arthritis Rheum 30(10):1157-61, Oct, 1987.

Kreymeier J, Rheumatherapie mit Phytopharmaka. In: DAZ 137(8):611-613. 1997.

Meier B, Pflanzliche versus synthetische Arzneimittel. In: ZPT 10(6):182. 1989.

Meier B, Liebi M, Salicinhaltige Arzneimittel. Überlegungen zu Wirksamkeit und Unbedenklichkeit. In: (2):50. 1990.

Meier B et al., DAZ 125:341. 1985.

Meier B et al., DAZ 127:2401. 1987.

Meier B et al., ZPT 11:50. 1990.

Meier R et al., A chemotaxonomic survey of phenolic compounds in swiss willow species. In: PM 58(7)98. 1992.

Nichols-Orians CM et al., PH 31:2180. 1992.

Schmid B, Heide L, The use of Salicis cortex in rheumatic disease: phytotherapie with known mode of action? In: PM 61(Abstracts of 43rd Ann Congr):94. 1995.

Schmid B, Heide L, Wirksamkeit und Verträglichkeit von Weidenrinde bei Arthrose: Design und Durchführung einer klinischen Studie. In: PUZ 26(1):33, Jahrestagung der DPhG, Berlin, 1996. 1997.

Shao Y et al., PM 55:617. 1989.

Thieme H, PM 13:431. 1965.

Thieme H, PA 20:570. 1965.

Further information in:

Kern W, List PH, Hörhammer L (Hrsg.), Hagers Handbuch der Pharmazeutischen Praxis, 4. Aufl., Bde 1-8: Springer Verlag Berlin, Heidelberg, New York, 1969.

Madaus G, Lehrbuch der Biologischen Arzneimittel, Bde 1-3, Nachdruck, Georg Olms Verlag Hildesheim 1979.

Schulz R, Hänsel R, Rationale Phytotherapie, Springer Verlag Heidelberg 1996.

Steinegger E, Hänsel R, Pharmakognosie, 5. Aufl., Springer Verlag Heidelberg 1992.

Teuscher E, Biogene Arzneimittel, 5. Aufl., Wiss. Verlagsges. Stuttgart 1997.

Wagner H, Wiesenauer M, Phytotherapie. Phytopharmaka und pflanzliche Homöopathika, Fischer-Verlag, Stuttgart, Jena, New York 1995.

Wichtl M (Hrsg.), Teedrogen, 4. Aufl., Wiss. Verlagsges. Stuttgart 1997.

Wild Carrot

Daucus carota

DESCRIPTION

Medicinal Parts: The medicinal part is the root.

Flower and Fruit: The flowers are in compact, terminal umbels or flattened, compound capitula. The peduncle divides in ray-like fashion from one particular point. Each ray divides and forms further umbels with white flowers. The outer flowers are irregular and larger than the others. The florets are small. When in bloom, the flower head is flattened or slightly convex. When they are ripe, the flowers draw together to form a cup-like structure. The double achaenes are formed in the fruit umbel. They are slightly flattened and have numerous bristles arranged in 5 rows.

Leaves, Stem and Root: The Wild Carrot is a biennial, 30 cm to 1 m high cultivated plant with a fusiform, usually red root and numerous pinnate, segmented, hairy leaves. In the second year, the plant produces a branched, angular stem with alternate jointed leaves, which terminates in the flowering umbels.

Habitat: Now found in its cultivated form all over the world.

Production: Wild Carrots are the roots of Daucus carota. The ripe roots are harvested.

Other Names: Carrot, Bird's Neat, Birds' Nest, Bees' Nest, Queen Anne's Lace, Philtron

ACTIONS AND PHARMACOLOGY

COMPOUNDS

Carotinoids: including alpha-, beta-, gamma-, zeta-carotene, lycopene

Volatile oil (very little): including among others p-cymene, limonene, dipenten, geraniol, alpha- and beta- caryophyllene

Polyynes: including falcarinol (carotatoxin)

Mono and oligosaccharides: glucose, saccharose

EFFECTS

Wild Carrot has anthelmintic and antimicrobial activity. It is also a mild vermifuge. The essential oil has an initially stimulating, followed by a paralyzing, effect on worms. In controlled animal tests, a temporary reduction of arterial blood pressure was observed. The pectin content is probably responsible for the severe constipating effect of the Carrot. The essential oil has a mild bactericidal effect, especially on gram-positive bacteria. The drug has a positive effect on visual acuity and scotopic (twilight) vision, as well as being a mild diuretic.

INDICATIONS AND USAGE

Unproven Uses: The Wild Carrot is an unreliable adjuvant in the treatment of oxyuriasis. It is a useful drug in pediatrics for tonsillitis, nutritional disorders and as a dietary agent for digestive disorders. It is also used in medicinal preparations for dermatological conditions such as photodermatosis and pigment anomalies. It is used in teas for intestinal parasites.

PRECAUTIONS AND ADVERSE REACTIONS

Health risks or side effects following the proper administration of designated therapeutic dosages are not recorded. The drug has a low potential for sensitization through skin contact.

DOSAGE

Mode of Administration: The drug is taken in a ground form or consumed as a juice or vegetable. It is found in ready-made medicinal preparations.

Preparation: The Carrot is finely grated and made into a juice or syrup.

LITERATURE

Gupta KR, Niranjan GS, (1982) Planta Med 46:240.

Hausen B, Allergiepflanzen, Pflanzenallergene, ecomed Verlagsgesellsch. mbH, Landsberg 1988.

Harborne JB, In: The Biology and Chemistry of the Umbelliferae, Ed. VN Heywood, Academic Press, London, 1971.

Kern W, List PH, Hörhammer L (Hrsg.), Hagers Handbuch der Pharmazeutischen Praxis, 4. Aufl., Bde 1-8, Springer Verlag Berlin, Heidelberg, New York, 1969.

Leung AY, Encyclopedia of Common Natural Ingredients Used in Food Drugs and Cosmetics, John Wiley & Sons Inc., New York 1980.

Ram AS, Devi HM, (1983) Indian J Bot 6(1):21.

Wild Cherry

Prunus serotina

DESCRIPTION

Medicinal Parts: The medicinal part is the inner tree bark, which has an almond-like smell, which dissipates on drying.

Flower and Fruit: The racemes are 6 to 15 cm long with about 30 flowers. The perianth remains when the fruit ripens. The 3 to 4 tepals are denticulate and creamy white. The fruit is 8 mm across, depressed-globose and purple-black. The endocarp is smooth.

Leaves, Stem and Root: Wild Cherry is a deciduous tree up to 20 m high with aromatic bark. The leaves are obovate to elliptical-oblong, acute, finely serrate with flattened, with forwardly directed teeth. The leaves are dark, glossy green above, paler and slightly pubescent beneath.

Habitat: Prunus serotina originates from North America but is cultivated in Europe.

Production: Wild Cherry bark is the bark of Prunus serotina.

Other Names: Wild Black Cherry, Virginian Prune, Black Choke, Choke Cherry, Rum Cherry

ACTIONS AND PHARMACOLOGY

COMPOUNDS

Cyanogenic glycosides: prunasin yielding 0.05 to 0.15%, 5 to 15 mg HCN/100 g

Tannins

EFFECTS

Wild Cherry bark is an astringent, antitussive, and sedative.

INDICATIONS AND USAGE

Unproven Uses: Wild Cherry bark is used for coughs, bronchitis and whooping cough, also used in the treatment of nervous digestive disorders and diarrhea.

PRECAUTIONS AND ADVERSE REACTIONS

No health hazards or side effects are known in conjunction with the proper administration of designated therapeutic dosages. Cyanide poisonings from the drug are unlikely, due to both its low cyanogenic glycoside content and the lack of incitement to ingest it.

DOSAGE

Mode of Administration: Wild Cherry bark is available as syrup or tincture for internal use and also available in commercial compounded preparations.

LITERATURE

Frohne D, Pfänder HJ, Giftpflanzen - Ein Handbuch für Apotheker, Toxikologen und Biologen, 4. Aufl., Wiss. Verlags-Ges. Stuttgart 1997.

Kern W, List PH, Hörhammer L (Hrsg.), Hagers Handbuch der Pharmazeutischen Praxis, 4. Aufl., Bde. 1-8, Springer Verlag Berlin, Heidelberg, New York, 1969.

Leung AY, Encyclopedia of Common Natural Ingredients Used in Food, Drugs and Cosmetics, John Wiley & Sons Inc., New York 1980.

Roth L, Daunderer M, Kormann K, Giftpflanzen, Pflanzengifte, 4. Aufl., Ecomed Fachverlag Landsberg Lech 1993.

Wild Daisy

Bellis perennis

DESCRIPTION

Medicinal Parts: The medicinal part is the whole flowering plant.

Flower and Fruit: The flower heads are usually found singly at the end of the sharply angular stem. The flower is small- to medium-sized and heterogamous. The epicalyx is semi-spherical to bell-shaped. The sepals of the epicalyx are more or less double-rowed. The receptacle is conical and glabrous when bearing fruit. The 1- to 2-rowed female ray flowers are linguiform, white, pink, purple or bluish and distinctly longer than the epicalyx. The disc flowers are androgynous, tubular and 5-tipped. The achenes are obovate, very flattened, ribless, and have side veins. The flower has no pappus but may have short, brittle bristles.

Leaves, Stem and Root: Wild Daisy is a 10- to 15-cm high perennial plant that has basal leaves in rosettes or alternate leaves at the lower part of the stem; its roots are short and cylindrical. The rosette leaves are circular to spatulate or heart-shaped, dentate and occasionally entire-margined with a single rib; they have vertical hairs on both sides.

Habitat: The plant is distributed from Portugal to the Moscow region and Asia Minor. It is also found from Great Britain to Ireland and southern Scandinavia, and as far south as the Mediterranean, with the exception of the Balearic Islands and the islands of Sardinia, Sicily, Crete and Cyprus.

Production: The capitula and short stems of the plant are picked and dried in either the sun or shade.

Other Names: Bruisewort

ACTIONS AND PHARMACOLOGY

COMPOUNDS

Triterpene saponins (2.7%): bisdemosides of the bayogenin-ic and polygalic acid (the latter acylated)

Polyynes: including trans-lachnophyllum ester

Flavonoids: including cosmosiin

EFFECTS

The drug acts as an astringent, reduces mucous production, and also has anti-inflammatory and fever-reducing effects, possibly due to the triterpene saponin content.

INDICATIONS AND USAGE

Unproven Uses: Wild Daisy is used as an expectorant and for easing diarrhea and gastrointestinal catarrh. It is also used for treating wounds, skin diseases, coughs and bronchitis, disorders of the liver and kidneys, and inflammation.

Homeopathic Uses: Wild Daisy is used for bruises, bleeding, muscular pain (after injuries), purulent skin diseases and rheumatism.

PRECAUTIONS AND ADVERSE REACTIONS

No health hazards or side effects are known in conjunction with the proper administration of designated therapeutic dosages.

DOSAGE

Mode of Administration: The drug is used topically—as an extract, in teas and in poultices of pressed leaves—for the treatment of skin diseases. A decoction can be used for wound poultices.

Preparation: An infusion or cold extract is prepared by adding 2 teaspoonfuls of drug to 2 cups of water, then allowing it to draw for 20 minutes. A decoction is made from the green leaves.

Daily Dosage: The daily dose of the infusion is 2 to 4 cups per day.

Homeopathic Dosage: 5 to 10 drops, 1 tablet or 5 to 10 globules 1 to 3 times daily; parenterally: 1 ml sc injection solution twice weekly; ointments: 1 to 2 times daily (HAB1).

LITERATURE

Avato P, Vitali C, Tava A, New acetylenic compounds from Bellis perennis L. and their antimicrobial activity. In: PM 61(Abstracts of 43rd Ann Congr):49. 1995.

Hänsel R, Keller K, Rimpler H, Schneider G (Hrsg.), Hagers Handbuch der Pharmazeutischen Praxis, 5. Aufl., Bde 4-6 (Drogen): Springer Verlag Berlin, Heidelberg, New York, 1992-1994.

Madaus G, Lehrbuch der Biologischen Arzneimittel, Bde 1-3, Nachdruck, Georg Olms Verlag Hildesheim 1979.

Schöpke T, Wray V, Hiller K, Triterpenoid saponins of plants of the Asteraeae tribe (Asteraceae). In: PM 59(7)

Schöpke Th et al., Saponin composition of the Bellis genus and related species. In: PM 61(Abstracts of 43rd Ann Congr):68. 1995.

Wagner H, Wiesenauer M, Phytotherapie. Phytopharmaka und pflanzliche Homöopathika, Fischer-Verlag, Stuttgart, Jena, New York 1995.

Willigmann I et al., Antimycotic compounds from different Bellis perennis varieties. In: PM 58(Suppl.7)36. 1993.

Wild Indigo

Baptisia tinctoria

TRADE NAMES:

Health From The Sun Wild Indigo Fresh Root Liquid, Nature's Answer Alcohol Free Wild Indigo Root Liquid

DESCRIPTION

Medicinal Parts: The medicinal part of the plant is the root.

Flower and Fruit: The flowers are terminal and axillary in 7 to 10 cm long, lightly flowered racemes. The pedicles are 3 to 5 cm long. The calyx is 4 to 5 mm long and glabrous but has a slight fringe. The corolla is yellow. The standard is circular with convoluted sides and is slightly shorter than the oblong wings. The 10 stamens are freestanding. The ovary is stemmed, elliptoid, drawn together at the style and stigma, and is glabrous. The fruit is a blue-black, ovoid, slightly swollen pod, 7 to 15 mm long, with a sharp tip. The seeds are yellowish-brown, kidney-shaped and 2 mm long.

Leaves, Stem and Root: The shrug is many-branched and grows to 1 m high with woody rootstock and knotty branches. The stem is 1 to 3 mm thick, round, slightly grooved and glabrous. The alternating leaves are trifoliate and have a 1 to 3 mm long petiole. The stipules are small and arrow-shaped, and drop early. The leaflets are 1 to 4 cm long, and 0.6 to 1 cm wide, ovate, almost sessile and entire-margined. They are wedge-shaped at the base and rounded at the tip. The distinct midrib on the lower surface is pubescent. The leaves are brittle. The roots vary in diameter from 0.2 to 1.5 cm. The outer surface is brownish, vertically wrinkled and grooved. It is also warty due to root fibers sticking to the surface. The tissue is solid and fibrous. The transverse fracture shows a thick bark and whitish wood with concentric rings.

Characteristics: The taste is bitter and acrid; the odor is faint. The leaves yield an indigo dye; the wood a red dye.

Habitat: Wild Indigo is indigenous to southern Canada and the eastern and northeastern U.S.

Production: Wild indigo root is the underground part of Baptisia tinctoria, which is collected and dried in autumn from plants growing in the wild.

Not to be Confused With: Wild Indigo can be confused or adulterated with the root of Baptisia australis (false blue indigo) and Baptisia alba.

Other Names: Horse-Fly Weed, Indigo Broom, Rattlebush

ACTIONS AND PHARMACOLOGY

COMPOUNDS

Water-soluble polysaccharide: in particular arabinogalactans

Glycoproteins

Quinolizidine alkaloids: including cytisine, N-methyl cytisine, anagyrine, sparteine

Isoflavonoids: formononetin baptigenin, pseudobaptigenin, (-)-maackiain, formononetin and their glycosides baptisin, pseudobaptisin, trifolirhizin

Hydroxycumarins: including scopoletine

EFFECTS

The ethanol extract has had a significantly positive effect on the phagocytosis of human erythrocytes. It has also been found to raise the leukocyte count and to improve the endogenous defense reaction. Wild Indigo has a mild estrogenic effect. In animal experimentation, the polysaccharide and glycoprotein fraction contained in the drug demonstrated an immune-stimulating effect. Changes in mice included an increase of phagocytosis activity of Kupffer's cells; a significant, dose-dependent stimulation of lymphocytes; and release of interleukin-1 macrophages.

INDICATIONS AND USAGE

Unproven Uses: Wild Indigo root is used for septic and typhoid cases with prostration and fever, such as diphtheria, influenza, malaria, septic angina and typhus. It is used internally for infections of the upper respiratory tract, the common head cold, tonsillitis, stomatitis, throat and mouth inflammation of the mucous membranes (catarrh), fever, lymphadenitis and furunculosis. It is used externally as an ointment for painless ulcers, inflamed nipples, and as a douche for leucorrhea. The efficacy of the drug has not been proven. Native America Indians traditionally have used the root to make a tea to treat fever, scarlet fever, typhoid and pharyngitis and externally as an ointment for sores. Water in which the root has been soaked is used to clean open and inflamed wounds. Canadian Indians used the plant for treating gonorrhea and disease of the kidneys and as an expectorant.

Homeopathic Uses: Uses in homeopathy include severe febrile infections, states of confusion and blood poisoning.

CONTRAINDICATIONS

Use of the drug is contraindicated during pregnancy.

PRECAUTIONS AND ADVERSE REACTIONS

No health hazards or side effects are known in conjunction with the proper administration of designated therapeutic dosages.

OVERDOSAGE

Only very high dosages (for example, 30 g of the drug) lead to signs of poisoning (vomiting, diarrhea, gastrointestinal complaints, spasms), due to the quinolizidine alkaloid content.

DOSAGE

Mode of Administration: Wild Indigo is not common as a drug, but is found in combination preparations; taken internally as a tea and tincture; and used externally as an ointment.

How Supplied:

Drops

Injection solutions

Liquid — 1:1 and 1:2, with and without alcohol.

Suppositories

Tablets

Preparation: To prepare an ointment, use 1 part liquid extract to 8 parts ointment base. A tincture may be prepared using the liquid extract in 60% alcohol 1:1.

Daily Dosage: Dosage for a single dose is 0.5 g to 1 g of the dried drug as decoction, to be taken 3 times daily.

Homeopathic Dosage: 5 to 10 drops, 1 tablet or 5 to 10 globules 1 to 3 times daily or 1 ml injection solution twice weekly sc (HAB34).

LITERATURE

Beuscher H, Kopanski L, Modulation of the immune response by polymeric substances from Baptisia tinctoria and Echinacea angustifolia. In: Pharm Weekblad Sci Ed. 9:229. 1987.

Beuscher N, Beuscher HU, Bodinet C, Enhanced Release of Interleukin-1 from Mouse Macrophages by Glykoproteins and Polysaccharides from Baptisia tinctoria and Echinacea Species. In: PM, Abstracts of the 37th Annual Congress on Medicinal Plant Research Braunschwe.

Beuscher N, Bodinet C, Willigmann I, Harnischfeger G, Biologiocal activity of Baptisia tinctoria extracts. In: Inst. für Angew. Botanik der Univ. Hamburg, Angewandte Botanik, Berichte 6, 46-61. 1997.

Beuscher N, Kopanski L, Erwein C, Modulation der Immunantwort durch polymere Substanzen aus Baptisia tinctoria und Echinacea purpurea. In: Adv in the Biosc 68:329. 1987.

Beuscher N, Kopanski L, Stimulation der Immunantwort durch Inhaltsstoffe aus Baptisia tinctoria. In: PM 1985:381-384. 1985.

Beuscher N, Scheit KH, Bodinet C, Egert D, Modulation der körpereigenen Immunabwehr durch polymere Substanzen aus Baptisia tinctoria und Echinacea purpurea. In: Immunotherapeutic prospects of infectious diseases, Hrsg. Masihi KN, Lange W. Springer, Heidel.

Beuscher N, Scheit KH, Bodinet C, Kopanski L, Immunologisch aktive Glykoproteine aus Baptisia tinctoria. In: PM 55:358-363. 1989.

Bodinet C, Beuscher N, Kopanski L, Purification of Immunologically Active Glycoproteins from Baptisia tinctoria Roots by Affinity Chromatography and Isoelectric Focussing. In: PM, Abstracts of the 37th Annual Congress on Medicinal Plant Research Braunschwe.

Harnischfeger, Buch, Harnischfeger G, Stolze H, Bewährte Pflanzendrogen in Wissenschaft und Medizin, Notabene-Verlag, Bad Homburg. 1983.

Vömel T, Arzneim-Forsch 35:1437-1439. 1985.

Vömel T, Der Einfluβ eines pflanzlichen Immunstimulans auf die Phagozytose von Erythrozyten durch das retikulohistiozytäre System der isolierte perfundierten Rattenleber. In: Arzneim Forsch 35(II): 1437-1439. 1985.

Wagner H, Proksch A, Riess-Mauer I, Vollmar A, Odenthal S, Stuppner H, Jurcic K, LeTurdu M, Fang JN, Arzneim-Forsch 35: 1069-10750. 1985.

Further information in:

Hänsel R, Keller K, Rimpler H, Schneider G (Hrsg.), Hagers Handbuch der Pharmazeutischen Praxis, 5. Aufl., Bde 4-6 (Drogen), Springer Verlag Berlin, Heidelberg, New York, 1992-1994.

Madaus G, Lehrbuch der Biologischen Arzneimittel, Bde 1-3, Nachdruck, Georg Olms Verlag Hildesheim 1979.

Roth L, Daunderer M, Kormann K, Giftpflanzen, Pflanzengifte, 4. Aufl., Ecomed Fachverlag Landsberg Lech 1993

Steinegger E, Hänsel R, Pharmakognosie, 5. Aufl., Springer Verlag Heidelberg 1992.

Teuscher E, Biogene Arzneimittel, 5. Aufl., Wiss. Verlagsges. Stuttgart 1997.

Wagner H, Wiesenauer M, Phytotherapie. Phytopharmaka und pflanzliche Homöopathika, Fischer-Verlag, Stuttgart, Jena, New York 1995.

Wild Mint

Mentha aquatica

DESCRIPTION

Medicinal Parts: The medicinal part is the dried leaf.

Flower and Fruit: The flowers are in 2 to 3 dense false axillary whorls with inconspicuous bracts. The upper ones are fused into a terminal, globular or ovate capitulum. The calyx is tubular, with 13 ribs and glabrous inside. The tips are awl-shaped to triangular. The pedicles are pubescent. The corolla is violet with a ring of hair in the tube. The fruit is hard with an ovoid, light brown nutlet.

Leaves, Stem and Root: Wild Mint is a perennial, 20 to 80 cm high plant with a branched underground rhizome and an erect stem with alternate sessile curly leaves. The stem is branched in the upper half and terminates in spikes of blue flowers. The leaves are ovate and serrated.

Characteristics: The whole plant smells of caraway. The plant is a result of many cross-breedings in gardens and fields.

Habitat: The plant grows in Europe, northern Africa and western Asia. In has been introduced to America, Australia and Madiera.

Production: Wild Mint is the aerial part of Mentha aquatica. The drug is derived from the dried leaves.

Other Names: Water Mint, Marsh Mint, Hairy Mint

ACTIONS AND PHARMACOLOGY

COMPOUNDS

Volatile oil: chief components - menthofurane, beta-caryophyllene, 1,8-cineole, germacren D, limonene, viridiflorol, a chemotype contains isopinocamphone as chief constituent (according to older references, also linalool, linalyl acetate, cineole, menthone)

Tannins

EFFECTS

The drug is an astringent and a stimulant.

INDICATIONS AND USAGE

Unproven Uses: Water Mint is used for diarrhea and dysmenorrhea.

PRECAUTIONS AND ADVERSE REACTIONS

No health hazards or side effects are known in conjunction with the proper administration of designated therapeutic dosages.

DOSAGE

Mode of Administration: Ground drug is used as an infusion.

Preparation: Add approximately 30 gm of the drug to 500 ml of water.

Daily Dosage: As a daily dose, drink a wineglassful during the course of the day.

LITERATURE

Hänsel R, Keller K, Rimpler H, Schneider G (Hrsg.), Hagers Handbuch der Pharmazeutischen Praxis, 5. Aufl., Bde 4-6 (Drogen), Springer Verlag Berlin, Heidelberg, New York, 1992-1994.

Wild Radish

Raphanus raphanistrum

DESCRIPTION

Medicinal Parts: The medicinal part is the fresh plant before flowering.

Flower and Fruit: The flowers are bright yellow, sometimes white with violet veins. The form of the flower corresponds to that of the Cruciferae. The calyx is erect. The pods are cylindrical with vertical grooves between which the seeds are tied (like a string of pearls). The pods fall apart at these points.

Leaves, Stem and Root: The leaves are petiolate and lyrate, the upper ones are lanceolate. The leaves and lower part of the stem are stiff-haired.

Habitat: The plant has been cultivated for a very long time and is grown in all parts of the world, especially in temperate regions.

Production: Wild Radish is the fresh plant of Raphanus raphanistrum before flowering.

Other Names: Jointed-Podded Charlock

ACTIONS AND PHARMACOLOGY

COMPOUNDS

Glucosinolates in the freshly harvested, unbruised plant: chief component glucoputranjivine, which yields isopropyl mustard oil as the cells are destroyed.

EFFECTS

No information is available.

INDICATIONS AND USAGE

Unproven Uses: Wild Radish is used for skin conditions and stomach disorders.

PRECAUTIONS AND ADVERSE REACTIONS

No health hazards or side effects are known in conjunction with the proper administration of designated therapeutic dosages. Administration of high dosages of the freshly harvested plant can lead to mucous membrane irritation of the gastrointestinal tract.

DOSAGE

Mode of Administration: Wild Radish is administered ground and as an alcoholic extract.

LITERATURE

Kern W, List PH, Hörhammer L (Hrsg.), Hagers Handbuch der Pharmazeutischen Praxis, 4. Aufl., Bde. 1-8: Springer Verlag Berlin, Heidelberg, New York, 1969.

Wild Service Tree

Sorbus torminalis

DESCRIPTION

Medicinal Parts: The medicinal parts are the ripe fruit. It is always the fruit that is used in the various preparations.

Flower and Fruit: The flowers are in erect, loose umbelliferous panicles on loosely tomentose, later glabrous pedicles. The petals are white and the anthers light yellow. The false fruit is orbicular-oblong and 1.5 cm long. The fruit is initially reddish-yellow, later brown and speckled. The 4 seeds are oblong, deltoid, 7 mm long and dark red-brown.

Leaves, Stem and Root: The plant is at times a small tree, but may sometimes grow up to 22 m tall tree with a widely domed crown. The bark is dark brown or gray. It is cracked into scaly plates to fairly high up. The older branches are glabrous, gray-brown, glossy and angular with lighter lenticles. The younger branches are loosely tomentose, greenish, later reddish-brown. The buds are broad ovoid and glabrous with shiny green scales. The buds are brown at the edge and loosely pubescent or glabrous. The leaves have 5 cm long, thin, downy, loosely tomentose petioles, which are fresh green. The petioles turn blood-red in autumn.

Habitat: The plant is common in northern temperate zones. It is cultivated in many regions.

Production: Wild Service Tree berries are the fruits of Sorbus torminalis.

Other Names: Wild Sorvice, Ash

ACTIONS AND PHARMACOLOGY

COMPOUNDS

Sugar alcohols: sorbitol

The fruits do not contain parasorboside, in contrast to those of Sorbus aucuparia.

The drug has not been fully researched.

EFFECTS

No information is available.

INDICATIONS AND USAGE

See Mountain Ash Berry (Sorbus aucuparia).

PRECAUTIONS AND ADVERSE REACTIONS

No health hazards or side effects are known in conjunction with the proper administration of designated therapeutic dosages.

DOSAGE

Mode of Administration: See Mountain Ash Berry (Sorbus aucuparia).

LITERATURE

There is no literature available.

Wild Thyme

Thymus serpyllum

DESCRIPTION

Medicinal Parts: The medicinal parts are the steamed distillation of the dried aerial parts, the aerial shoots collecting during the flowering season and dried, the fresh aerial parts of the flowering plant and the whole plant.

Flower and Fruit: The inflorescence is globular to very elongated, often interrupted in false whorls, which are separate from each other. The calyx is tubular-campanualte with 10 distinct ribs. The 3 tips of the upper lip are short and ciliate. The 2 lower tips are awl-shaped, longer than the upper tips and ciliate. The corolla is 3 to 6 cm long with a short tube. It is light to dark purple, occasionally white.

Leaves, Stem and Root: The plant is a slightly woody subshrub that grows from 10 to 30 cm high. The flowering stems are erect. The non-flowering stems are decumbent, round, or mildly quadrangular, pubescent all around and rooting at all points. The leaves are small, linear or elliptical and obtuse. The leaves are also flat, narrowing to the petiole, ciliate at the base, glabrous or rough-haired with protruding nerves.

Characteristics: The odor is aromatic.

Habitat: The plant is found in all temperate regions of Eurasia.

Production: Wild thyme consists of the dried, flowering, above-ground parts of Thymus serpyllum.

Not to be Confused With: Herba Thymi (thymian)

Other Names: Mother of Thyme, Serpyllum, Shepherd's Thyme

ACTIONS AND PHARMACOLOGY

COMPOUNDS

Volatile oil (0.2-0.6%): as a collective species, Thymus serpyllum (over 20 subspecies) encompasses a large number of chemical strains with different volatile oil make-up; chief component is usually carvacrol, further containing, among others, borneol, isobutyl acetate, caryophyllene, 1,8-cineole, citral, citronellal, citronellol, p-cymene, geraniol, geranyl acetate, linalool, linalyl acetate, alpha-pinene, gamma-terpinene, alpha-terpineol, terpinyl acetate and thymol

Flavonoids: including among others scutellarenine-7-O-glucoside-4-O-rhamnoside

Caffeic acid derivatives: in particular rosmarinic acid (2.3%)

EFFECTS

In animal experiments, an antihormonal and thyroid hormone-like effect on the pituitary has been demonstrated. The herbs efficacy for treating conditions of the upper respiratory tract is due to the presence of the aromatic and spicy smelling essential oil.

INDICATIONS AND USAGE

Approved by Commission E:

- Cough
- Bronchitis

Unproven Uses: The herb is used internally for catarrhs of the upper respiratory tract, kidney and bladder disorders, and as a stomachic, carminative, and expectorant. It is also used internally for dysmenorrhea, colic-like pain, and whooping cough. The herb is used externally in herbal cures, baths (especially for respiratory tract conditions), and alcoholic extracts, as well as in embrocations for rheumatic disorders and sprains.

Chinese Medicine: The herb is used for vomiting, diarrhea, flatulence, coughs, toothache, itching and general pain syndrome.

PRECAUTIONS AND ADVERSE REACTIONS

No health hazards or side effects are known in conjunction with the proper administration of designated therapeutic dosages.

DOSAGE

Mode of Administration: Wild Thyme is administered as a comminuted drug for infusions, teas, and other preparations internally. The drug is a component of various standardized preparations of antitussives. Alcoholic extracts of the herb are contained in cough drops.

Preparation: To make an infusion, pour boiling water over 1.5 to 2 gm finely cut drug, steep for 10 minutes, then strain (1 teaspoonful = 1.4 gm drug). For a liquid extract, use a ratio of 1:1 with either 45% ethanol or 20% ethanol. For a tincture, use a ratio of 1:10 with 70% ethanol. To make a bath, add 1 gm drug (or equivalent of 0.004 gm Wild Thyme oil) to 1 liter water, filter, then add to bath water.

Daily Dosage: The average daily dosage is 4 to 6 gm of herb. As a stomachic, drink one cup of tea before meals. Other daily dosages are as follows: powder: take 2 gm drug mixed with honey; infusion: single dose, 0.6 to 4 gm, 2 to 3 cups per day; liquid extract: single dose, 0.4 to 4 ml 3 times daily; liquid extract: daily dose, 5 to 15 gm (1 gm or 30 drops).

Storage: Protect from light.

LITERATURE

Adzet T et al., PM, Suppl. 1980:52. 1980.

Hänsel R, Keller K, Rimpler H, Schneider G (Hrsg.), Hagers Handbuch der Pharmazeutischen Praxis, 5. Aufl., Bde 4-6 (Drogen): Springer Verlag Berlin, Heidelberg, New York, 1992-1994.

Länger R et al., Sci Pharm 63:325. 1995.

Madaus G, Lehrbuch der Biologischen Arzneimittel, Bde 1-3, Nachdruck, Georg Olms Verlag Hildesheim 1979.

Steinegger E, Hänsel R, Pharmakognosie, 5. Aufl., Springer Verlag Heidelberg 1992.

Teuscher E, Biogene Arzneimittel, 5. Aufl., Wiss. Verlagsges. Stuttgart 1997.

Wichtl M (Hrsg.), Teedrogen, 4. Aufl., Wiss. Verlagsges. Stuttgart 1997.

Wild Turnip

Brassica rapa

DESCRIPTION

Medicinal Parts: The medicinal part of the plant is the root.

Flower and Fruit: The flowers are in racemes. There are 4 almost horizontally splayed sepals. The 4 petals are yellow, 11 to 14 mm long, approximately 1.5 times as long as the calyx, with an orbicular-elliptical plate. There are 2 short and 4 long stamens. The 4-carpeled ovary is superior and fused. The fruit is a 4.5 to 6.5 cm long, dehiscent pod opening on 2 sides, with a septum and 15 to 25 seeds. The seeds are globose and reticulate with a diameter of approximately 1.5 to 3 mm.

Leaves, Stem and Root: Turnip is an annual or biennial herb, and grows up to 0.8 m high. The leaves are alternate, grass-green, with a slight bluish bloom and always bristly pubescent. The lower ones are petiolate, pinnatisect with a not-very-large terminal lobe; the middle and upper ones are sessile, simple, dentate or entire. The stem of the larger plants is branched. The root is thin and spindle-shaped.

Habitat: Europe, North Africa, U.S.

Production: The seeds are cold-pressed and then refined. Rapeseed oil is the cold-pressed and refined oil from the ripe seeds of Brassica napus and Brassica rapa.

Other Names: Field Mustard, Oilseed Turnip, Turnip Rape, Turnip Greens, Chinese Cabbage

Not to be Confused With: Rapeseed oil may be adulterated with resins and mineral oil. Sinapis arvensis is a permitted substitute.

ACTIONS AND PHARMACOLOGY

COMPOUNDS

Fatty oil: chief fatty acids: oleic acid (45 to 65%), linoleic acid (18 to 32%), linolenic acid (10%), including as well palmitic acid, stearic acid, eicosanoic acid, behenic acid;

varieties with high erucic acid content (40 to 50%) are no longer cultivated (reduction of the erucic acid content in the Common Market countries to below 5%)

Sterols: beta-sitosterol, campesterol, brassicasterol, estered to some extent

EFFECTS

Rapeseed oil, when ingested in high dosages over an extended period of time, is cardiotoxic. The drug is chiefly used as a substitute for olive oil and in the manufacture of salves and liniments.

INDICATIONS AND USAGE

No medicinal indications

PRECAUTIONS AND ADVERSE REACTIONS:

No health hazards are known in conjunction with the proper administration of designated therapeutic dosages of the oil, which is low on erucic acid.

DOSAGE

Storage: Store in the dark, in well-filled containers.

LITERATURE

Hänsel R, Keller K, Rimpler H, Schneider G (Ed), Hagers Handbuch der Pharmazeutischen Praxis, 5. Aufl., Bde 4 - 6 (Drogen), Springer Verlag Berlin, Heidelberg, New York, 1992-1994.

Inamori Y, Muro C, Sajima E, Katagiri M, Okamoto Y, Tanaka H, Sakagami Y, Tsujibo H, Biological activity of purpurogallin. Biosci Biotechnol Biochem, 61:890-2, 1997 May.

Wild Yam

Dioscorea villosa

TRADE NAMES

Wild Yam Extract, Mexican Wild Yam Power, Wild Yam, Wild Yam Root & Rhizome Extract, Wild Yam Root (available from numerous manufacturers and as a combination product)

DESCRIPTION

Medicinal Parts: The medicinal part is the dried rhizome with the roots.

Flower and Fruit: The plant has small greenish-yellow flowers. The male flowers are in drooping panicles; the female ones in drooping spicate racemes.

Leaves, Stem and Root: Dioscorea villosa is a perennial vine. It has a pale brown, cylindrical, twisted, tuberous rhizome and a thin, woolly, reddish-brown stem that measures up to 12 m long. The leaves are broadly ovate, usually alternating, cordate and 6 to 14 cm long. The upper surface of the leaves is glabrous and they are pubescent beneath. The fracture is short and hard.

Characteristics: The taste is insipid at first, then acrid. The leaves are odorless.

Habitat: The plant is indigenous to the Southern U.S. and Canada. It is now widely cultivated in many parts of the world in tropical, subtropical and temperate regions.

Production: Wild Yam root is the root and rhizome of Dioscorea villosa.

Other Names: China Root, Colic Root, Devil's Bones, Rheumatism Root, Yuma

ACTIONS AND PHARMACOLOGY

COMPOUNDS

Saponins: including dioscin (aglycone diosgenin)

Isoquinuclidine alkaloids: including dioscorin

Pyrridinal alkaloids: including dioscorine

EFFECTS

Wild Yam has an antispasmodic, and a mild diaphoretic effect. The root of the plant is used as a precursor for manufacturing progesterone and estrogen. Though the diosgenin componant has been promoted as a ''natural progesterone,'' diosgenin does not have any progesterone-like effects. The body does not convert diosgenin into estrogen or any other steroid.

Anti-Inflammatory Effect:

In the rat model, diosgenin has been found to decrease the intestinal inflammation that accompanies indomethacin use (Yamada et al, 1997).

Biliary Cholesterol Elimination Effect:

Diosgenin has been shown to markedly increase the biliary output of cholesterol and lipid lamellar structures in the rat model. Diosgenin also has a cytoprotective effect on the rat liver that is subjected to obstructive cholestasis (Accatino et al, 1998).

Estrogenic Effect:

Diosgenin has been found to have an estrogenic effect on mouse mammary epithelium. Ovariectomized mice that received diosgenin (sc) at dosage levels between 20 and 40 mg/kg for 15 days had significant increases in mammary development scores. When administered estrogen and diosgenin, an augmentation of the estrogenic effect was recorded (Aradhana et al, 1992).

INDICATIONS AND USAGE

Unproven Uses: Wild Yam is used for rheumatic conditions, gallbladder colic, dysmenorrhea and cramps.

Wild Yam is used industrially as an active agent in the half-synthesis of steroid hormones and for the manufacture of homeopathic preparations.

PRECAUTIONS AND ADVERSE REACTIONS

General: Health risks or side effects following the proper administration of designated therapeutic dosages are not recorded.

Drug Interactions: There is evidence that the diosgenin componant of Wild Yam may decrease the anti-inflammatory effect of indomethacin by increasing the elimination constant and reducing plasma levels of indomethacin (Yamada et al, 1997). Wild Yam may have an additive estrogenic effect when administered with estrogen containing drugs.

OVERDOSAGE

Poisoning is conceivable with overdosages because of the picrotoxin-like effect of dioscorin (see Cocculi fructus).

DOSAGE

Mode of Administration: Liquid extract.

How Supplied:

Capsules—200 mg, 400 mg, 505 mg, 535 mg

Liquid—1:1; 1:2; 250 mg/ml

LITERATURE

Hegnauer R, Chemotaxonomie der Pflanzen, Bde 1-11, Birkhäuser Verlag Basel, Boston, Berlin 1962-1997.

Kern W, List PH, Hörhammer L (Hrsg.), Hagers Handbuch der Pharmazeutischen Praxis, 4. Aufl., Bde 1-8, Springer Verlag Berlin, Heidelberg, New York, 1969.

Madaus G, Lehrbuch der Biologischen Arzneimittel, Bde 1-3, Nachdruck, Georg Olms Verlag Hildesheim 1979.

Willow Herb

Epilobium species

DESCRIPTION

Medicinal Parts: The medicinal parts are the herb and the roots of the drug containing Epilobium varieties.

Flower and Fruit: The flowers are arranged in long clusters of crimson flowers. The receptacle extends over the ovary. There are 4 sepals that are often colored and 8 stamens. The petals are purple to pink seldom white or yellow. The style is erect or curved downwards. The stigma is capitual or club-like and has 4 grooves or is divided into 4. The fruit is long, linear capsule-like, quadrangular, 4-valved and opens with 4 bending valves. The seeds are numerous and smooth or they may be covered in tiny warts with a white, often short-stemmed, tuft of hair.

Leaves, Stem and Root: The species includes perennial herbs and occasionally up to 2 m high sub-shrubs with underground creeping rhizomes. The stems are erect, glabrous or covered with simple hairs or glandular hairs. The leaves are entire-margined or dentate. They are alternate or opposite and in whorls of 3, which are flat or occasionally with a turned-back border.

Habitat: The plant is found all over Europe, Asia, Africa and America, Australia, Tasmania and New Zealand.

Production: Willow Herb is the aerial part of Epilobium parviflorum and other small-blossomed Willow Herbs. The herb is dried in the open air in the shade.

Other Names: Blood Vine, Blooming Sally, Rose Bay Willow Herb, Willow-Herb

ACTIONS AND PHARMACOLOGY

COMPOUNDS: ANGUSTIFOLIUM VARIETY

Flavonoids: in particular myricitrin, isoquercitrin, quercitrin, guaiaverin, quercetin-3-O-beta-D-glucuronide

Palmitate

Steroids: in particular beta-sitosterol and its ester, including among others beta-sitosterol caproate

Tannins

COMPOUNDS: HIRSUTUM VARIETY

Flavonoids: in particular guaiaverin, hyperoside, myricitrin, quercetin-3-O-beta-D-glucuronide,quercetin-3-O-alpha-L-arabinofuranoside

Steroids: in particular beta-sitosterol

Tannins

COMPOUNDS: PARVIFLORUM VARIETY

Flavonoids: in particular guaiaverin, quercetin-3-O-beta-D-glucuronide, quercitrin

Palmitate

Steroids: in particular beta-sitosterol and its ester, including among others beta-sitosterol caproate

Tannins

EFFECTS

Willow Herb is reported to have antiphlogistic and antiexudative effects. A watery infusion revealed a significant inhibitory effect on edema in rat paws. The methanol infusion had a distinctly weaker effect.

Antimicrobial effects have also been demonstrated. A suspension of the fresh drug in ethanol stunts the growth of the bacteria of *Pseudomonas pyocyanea.* Tincture and the liquid extract showed anti-microbial effect against *Candida albicans*, *Staphylococcus albus* and *Staphylococcus aureus.*

The dried residue of a maceration, which is fixed on filter paper, shows a weak effect against *Bacillus subtilis, Escherichia coli, Mycobacterium smegmatis, Shigella flexneri, Shigella sonnei* and *Staphylococcus aureus*. An extra fraction of the drug (insufficiently chemically defined) showed a tumor-inhibiting effect on transplanted tumors in mice and rats. The drug was helpful in treating benign prostate hyperplasia and certain micturition disorders.

INDICATIONS AND USAGE

Unproven Uses: Willow Herb is used internally for micturition problems associated with prostatic hyperplasia (Stages I to II), and for gastrointestinal disorders and mucous membrane lesions of the mouth. Native Americans use the drug for rectal bleeding; the Chinese use it for menstrual disorders. The watery extract is used externally to improve the healing of wounds.

PRECAUTIONS AND ADVERSE REACTIONS

Health risks or side effects following the proper administration of designated therapeutic dosages are not recorded.

DOSAGE

Mode of Administration: The drug is not available as a ready made medicinal preparation; only as a tea, watery extract or as a vegetable.

LITERATURE

Ducrey B et al., Inhibition of 5alpha-Reduktase and aromatase by ellagitannins oenothein A and eonothein B from Epilobium species. In: PM 63(2):111-114. 1997.

Hänsel R, Keller K, Rimpler H, Schneider G (Hrsg.), Hagers Handbuch der Pharmazeutischen Praxis, 5. Aufl., Bde 4-6 (Drogen), Springer Verlag Berlin, Heidelberg, New York, 1992-1994.

Hiemann A, Mayr K, Sci Pharm 53:39. 1985.

Hiermann A, Sci Pharm 63:135. 1995.

Lesuisse D et al., Determination of Oenothein B as the active 5-alpha-reductase-inhibiting principles of the folk medicine Epilobium parvifloruam. In: JNP 59(5):490-492. 1996.

Slacanin I et al., J Chromatogr 557:391. 1991.

Wichtl M (Hrsg.), Teedrogen, 4. Aufl., Wiss. Verlagsges. Stuttgart 1997.

Winter Cherry

Physalis alkekengi

DESCRIPTION

Medicinal Parts: The medicinal parts are the ripe fruit and the leaves.

Flower and Fruit: The whitish, long-pedicled flowers are solitary and nodding. The calyx is fused and 5-tipped. The corolla is fused with a slightly 5-tipped margin. There are 5 stamens and 1 superior ovary. The fruit is a cherry-sized, globular, scarlet berry, enclosed in the swollen, orange-red calyx. It contains numerous flat, reniform seeds.

Leaves, Stem and Root: The plant is a perennial and grows from 30 to 60 cm. The stems are erect or ascending and angular with opposite, long-petioled, entire-margined leaves.

Characteristics: Winter Cherry has a lantern-like, enlarged calyx when the fruit is ripe.

Habitat: The plant is indigenous to central and southern Europe, China and Indochina and is naturalized in the U.S.

Production: Winter Cherry fruits are the ripe fruits of Physalis alkekengi.

Other Names: Cape Gooseberry, Coqueret, Strawberry Tomato

ACTIONS AND PHARMACOLOGY

COMPOUNDS

Whitasteroids: among others physalines A-C, F, L-O

Carotinoids: including zeaxanthine dipalmitic acid ester (red)

EFFECTS

No information is available.

INDICATIONS AND USAGE

Unproven Uses: Winter Cherry is used as a diuretic in kidney and bladder conditions and in the treatment of gout and rheumatism.

PRECAUTIONS AND ADVERSE REACTIONS

The ripe fruit is edible, but unripe fruit can cause poisoning in animals.

DOSAGE

Mode of Administration: The drug is administered in a ground form and as an extract.

LITERATURE

Christen P, Pharm Acta Helv 61:242. 1986.

Dornberger K, Untersuchungen über potentiell antineoplastisch wirksame Inhaltsstoffe von Physalis alkekengi L. var. franchettii MAST. In: PA 41:265. 1986.

Frohne D, Pfänder HJ, Giftpflanzen - Ein Handbuch für Apotheker, Toxikologen und Biologen, 4. Aufl., Wiss. Verlags-Ges Stuttgart 1997.

Jana M, Raynaud J, (1971) Plant Med Phytother 5:301.

Kawai M et al., PH 26:3313. 1987.

Kawai M, Matsuura T, (1970) Tetrahedron 26:1743.

Kern W, List PH, Hörhammer L (Hrsg.), Hagers Handbuch der Pharmazeutischen Praxis, 4. Aufl., Bde. 1-8, Springer Verlag Berlin, Heidelberg, New York, 1969.

Madaus G, Lehrbuch der Biologischen Arzneimittel, Bde 1-3, Nachdruck, Georg Olms Verlag Hildesheim 1979.

Teuscher E, Lindequist U, Biogene Gifte - Biologie, Chemie, Pharmakologie, 2. Aufl., Fischer Verlag Stuttgart 1994.

Vessal M, Mehrani HA, Omrani GH, Effects of an aqueous extract of Physalis alkekengi fruit on estrus cycle, reproduction and uterine craetive kinase BB-isoenzyme in rats. In: ETH 34(1):69-78. 1991.

Völksen W, Zur Kenntnis der Inhaltsstoffe und arzneilichen Verwendung einiger Physalisarten - Ph. alkekengi, Ph. franchettii, Ph. peruviana. In: DAZ 117(30):1199-1203. 1977.

Yamaguchi H et al., (1974) Yakugaku Zasshi 94:1115.

Winter's Bark

Drimys winteri

DESCRIPTION

Medicinal Parts: The medicinal part is the dried bark of the trunk and larger branches.

Flower and Fruit: The flowers are solitary or in umbels and often in clusters at the tips of the branches. They are fragrant and white. The sepals are membranous, broadly ovate to reniform. The 4 to 14 petals are also membranous, oblong to narrow-ovate. The 15 to 40 stamens are in 2 to 4 rows. The 2 to 10 carpels are free, ovate or elliptical. There are 9 to 18 ovules on a short seed stalk. The fruit is berry-like, black to violet, fleshy and usually contains 2 or 3 seeds.

Leaves, Stem and Root: The plant is an evergreen tree or shrub, with brownish or gray wrinkled branches. The bark is a romatic and smooth. The leaf blade is coriaceous, oblong-ovate to elliptical, with a somewhat revolute margin. The undersurface is usually punctate.

Characteristics: Winter's Bark has an astringent taste and mild smell.

Habitat: The plant is found from central Chile to Cape Horn and in neighboring Argentina.

Production: Genuine Winter's Bark is the bark of Drimys winteri. The bark is collected from the dried trunk or produced from the stronger branches. It is collected in uncultivated regions.

Not to be Confused With: The drug is often confused with Cortex Canellae albae and with the bark of Cinnamodendron corticosum.

Other Names: Pepper Bark, Winter's Cinnamon, Wintera Aromatica, Wintera

ACTIONS AND PHARMACOLOGY

COMPOUNDS

Sesquiterpenes: including drimenol, drimenin, confertifoline, polygodial, isodrimenine, winterin, valdiviolide, fuegin, futranolide, cryptomeridiol, 1beta-p-cumaroyloxypolygodial, a trimeric sesquiterpene lactone

Volatile oil: chief components eugenol, caryophyllene, 1,8-cineol, pinenes

EFFECTS

The drug has carminative, stomachic, and tonic effects due to the sesquiterpenes (bitter effect) and tannins.

INDICATIONS AND USAGE

Unproven Uses: In South America, the drug is used for toothache, as a stomachic and for dermatitis. Other uses include digestive disorders, flatulence and colic.

PRECAUTIONS AND ADVERSE REACTIONS

Health risks or side effects following the proper administration of designated therapeutic dosages are not recorded.

DOSAGE

Mode of Administration: As an infusion and domestic herb.

LITERATURE

Hänsel R, Keller K, Rimpler H, Schneider G (Hrsg.), Hagers Handbuch der Pharmazeutischen Praxis, 5. Aufl., Bde 4-6 (Drogen): Springer Verlag Berlin, Heidelberg, New York, 1992-1994.

Hegnauer R, Chemotaxonomie der Pflanzen, Bde 1-11, Birkhäuser Verlag Basel, Boston, Berlin 1962-1997.

Morton JF, An Atlas of Medicinal Plants of Middle America, Charles C. Thomas USA 1981.

Wintergreen

Gaultheria procumbens

DESCRIPTION

Medicinal Parts: The medicinal parts of the plant are the leaves and the oil extracted from them, as well as the fruit.

Flower and Fruit: The 7.5 mm long, solitary, hanging flowers grow from the base of the leaves. They are white or pale pink and campanulate. The fruit is the enlarged calyx. The scarlet berries are dull red and about 0.5 cm in diameter when dried. They are fleshy, globular, bilocular, and contain numerous whitish, ovoid, flattened seeds.

Leaves, Stem and Root: Gaultheria procumbens is a bushy evergreen plant with procumbent stems and upright rigid branches up to 15 cm high. It grows best under trees and shrubs. The branches bear clusters of leaves at their tips. The leaves are coriaceous, oval, 3 to 5 cm long, glabrous and glossy above, paler beneath, long and solitary.

Characteristics: Wintergreen has an aromatic odor; the taste of the whole plant is astringent.

Habitat: Gaultheria procumbens is indigenous to the northern United States and Canada.

Production: Wintergreen leaves are the leaves of Gaultheria procumbens.

Other Names: Canada Tea, Checkerberry, Deerberry, Ground Berry, Hillberry, Mountain Tea, Partridge Berry, Spiceberry, Wax Cluster, Boxberry, Teaberry

ACTIONS AND PHARMACOLOGY

COMPOUNDS: FRESHLY HARVESTED PLANT

Monotropitoside (Gaultherin): changing into methyl salicylate when the plant is dried

COMPOUNDS: DRIED PLANT

Volatile oil: chief component methyl salicylate (96-98%), in addition to oenanthic alcohol (n-heptan-1-ol) and its ester (which contributes to the odor of the volatile oil)

EFFECTS

The essential oil has a rubefacient effect.

INDICATIONS AND USAGE

Unproven Uses: Wintergreen was previously used as a carminative, tonic, antiseptic and aromatic. The drug was also used for neuralgia (particularly sciatica), gastralgias, pleurisy, pleurodynia (especially for medium stage pain), ovarialgia, orchitis, epidydimitis, diaphragmitis, uratic arthritis and dysmenorrhea. Folk medicine indications also include asthma and use of wintergreen as an antiseptic. The drug is administered externally in the treatment of rheumatoid arthritis and related conditions.

PRECAUTIONS AND ADVERSE REACTIONS

Health risks or side effects following the proper administration of designated therapeutic dosages are not recorded. The drug and its volatile oil can, however, trigger contact allergies.

OVERDOSAGE

Signs of poisoning such as severe stomach and kidney irritation appear with overdosages of the drug. Fatal poisonings can occur through oral and percutaneous administration of the pure volatile oil, often following are signs of central nervous system distress, lung edema and collapse. Poisonings with fatal results have been observed following the oral intake of as little as 4 to 6 g of the volatile oil.

DOSAGE

The drug is seldom used today. The active ingredient, methyl salicylate, is produced synthetically at a lower cost. Methyl salicylate is a constituent of liniments and bath additives.

LITERATURE

Friedrich H, Krüger, N, (1974) Planta Med 26:327.

Frohne D, Pfänder HJ, Giftpflanzen - Ein Handbuch für Apotheker, Toxikologen und Biologen, 4. Aufl., Wiss. Verlagsges. mbH Stuttgart 1997.

Kern W, List PH, Hörhammer L (Hrsg.), Hagers Handbuch der Pharmazeutischen Praxis, 4. Aufl., Bde. 1-8, Springer Verlag Berlin, Heidelberg, New York, 1969.

Leung AY, Encyclopedia of Common Natural Ingredients Used in Food Drugs and Cosmetics, John Wiley & Sons Inc., New York 1980.

Lewin L, Gifte und Vergiftungen, 6. Aufl., Nachdruck, Haug Verlag, Heidelberg 1992.

Madaus G, Lehrbuch der Biologischen Arzneimittel, Bde 1-3, Nachdruck, Georg Olms Verlag Hildesheim 1979.

Roth L, Daunderer M, Kormann K, Giftpflanzen, Pflanzengifte, 4. Aufl., Ecomed Fachverlag Landsberg Lech 1993.

Steinegger E, Hänsel R, Pharmakognosie, 5. Aufl., Springer Verlag Heidelberg 1992.

Witch Hazel

Hamamelis virginiana

TRADE NAMES

Witch Hazel (available from numerous manufacturers), Witch Hazel Leaf

DESCRIPTION

Medicinal Parts: The medicinal parts are the plant's hamamelis water, which is distilled from various plant parts; the bark; the fresh and dried leaves; the fresh bark of the roots and branches; and the dried bark of the trunk and branches.

Flower and Fruit: The androgynous and unisexual flowers grow in light to golden yellow, short-stemmed clusters on the trees before the leaves come out. The inflorescence is a small, head-like spike in the axils of the dropping leaves, with 5 to 8 flowers. The 4 sepals are ovate or triangular, curved outward, yellow-brown to brown on the inside. The petals are bright yellow, long, narrow-linear, rolled to a spiral in the bud and crushed like tissue paper when open. The ovary is villous, bivalvular with 2 anatropic ovules. Fertilization takes place during the spring that follows 5 to 7 months after pollination. The fruit capsule is woody, ovate, sectioned and divided, hazelnut-like, 12 to 15 mm long and thickly pubescent. It bursts so dramatically in autumn that the 2 dark seeds are projected up to 4 m away from the plant.

Leaves, Stem and Root: The plant is a tree-like deciduous bush that typically grows 2 to 3 m high (but sometimes reaches heights up to 10 m) with a trunk diameter of 40 cm. The bark is thin, brown on the outside, reddish on the inside. The older branches are bushy, divided and silver-gray to gray-brown. The younger branches are yellowish-brown with hairs. The alternate leaves have stipules. The leaf margin is roughly crenate, bluntly indented to irregularly sweeping.

Habitat: Witch Hazel originated in the deciduous forests of Atlantic North America. The tree is common in European gardens and parks, and is also cultivated in subtropical countries.

Production: Witch Hazel leaf is obtained from the leaves of Hamamelis virginiana, which are collected in autumn and dried rapidly. Witch Hazel bark is the dried bark of the trunk and branches of Hamamelis virginiana.

Not to be Confused With: Witch Hazel is sometimes confused with Hazelnut bark, to which it bears a resemblance. Confusion can arise between Witch Hazel leaves and the leaves of Corylus avellana (hazelnut leaves), which are sometimes substituted as an adulteration.

Other Names: Hamamelis, Hazel Nut, Snapping Hazel, Spotted Alder, Striped Alder, Tobacco Wood, Winterbloom

ACTIONS AND PHARMACOLOGY

COMPOUNDS: WITCH HAZEL BARK

Tannins (up to 12%): including hamamelitannin, monogalloyl hamameloses

Catechins: including (+)-catechin, (+)-gallocatechin, (-)-epicatechin gallate(III), (-)-epigallocatechin gallate(III)

Oligomeric procyanidins

EFFECTS: WITCH HAZEL BARK

Witch Hazel bark is astringent, anti-inflammatory and locally hemostatic.

COMPOUNDS: WITCH HAZEL LEAF

Tannins (5%): including hamamelitannin

Catechins: including (+)-catechin, (+)-gallocatechin, (-)-epicatechin gallate(III), (-)-epigallocatechin gallate(III)

Oligomeric procyanidins

Volatile oil (0.01 to 0.5%): steam distillate, consisting chiefly of aliphatic carbonyl compounds, for example hex-2-en-1-ale, 6-methyl-hepta-3,5-dien-2-one aliphatic alcohols, aliphatic esters

Flavonoids: including quercitrin, isoquercitrin

EFFECTS: WITCH HAZEL LEAF

The tannins and tannin elements have an astringent, anti-inflammatory and locally hemostatic effect.

INDICATIONS AND USAGE

Approved by Commission E:

- Hemorrhoids
- Inflammation of the mouth and pharynx (leaf only)
- Inflammation of the skin
- Venous conditions
- Wounds and burns

Unproven Uses: Witch Hazel leaf and bark are used internally in folk medicine for non-specific diarrheic ailments (such as inflammation of the mucous membrane of the large intestine and colon), hematemesis, hemoptysis and also for menstrual complaints. Efficacy in the treatment of diarrhea seems plausible because of the tannin content. Witch Hazel is used externally for minor injuries of the skin, localized inflamed swelling of the skin and mucous membranes, hemorrhoids and varicose veins. It is also used in folk medicine for inflammation of the mucosa of the colon, hematemesis and hemoptysis.

Homeopathic Use: Applications for use of Witch Hazel bark in homeopathy include hemorrhoids, varicose veins, skin inflammation and bleeding of the mucous membranes.

PRECAUTIONS AND ADVERSE REACTIONS

Health risks following the proper administration of designated therapeutic dosages are not recorded. If taken internally, the tannin content of the drug can lead to digestive complaints. Liver damage is conceivable following long-term administration, but rare.

DOSAGE

WITCH HAZEL BARK

Mode of Administration: Witch Hazel Bark is available as comminuted drug or extract for internal and external use as galenic preparations. A steam distillate of the fresh leaves and bark is used for internal and external application.

How Supplied: Forms of commercial pharmaceutical preparations include: cream; gel; ointment; suppositories.

Preparation: Various formulations of Witch Hazel are prepared as follows:

External—aqueous steam distillate (Witch Hazel water) undiluted, or diluted 1:3 with water.

For poultices—20 to 30% in semi-solid preparations.

Extract preparations—semi-solid and liquid preparations, corresponding to 5 to 10% drug.

Compresses and rinses—decoctions of 5 to 10 g of herb per cup (250 ml) of water.

Ointment/gel—5 g Witch Hazel extract in 100 g ointment base.

Suppositories—Use 0.1 to 1 g drug.

Daily Dosage: Suppositories can be used 1 to 3 times a day.

Homeopathic Dosage: 5 drops, 1 tablet or 10 globules every 30 to 60 minutes (acute) or 1 to 3 times daily (chronic); parenterally: 1 to 2 ml sc acute, 3 times daily; chronic: once a day, suppositories 2 to 3 times per day and ointment 1 to 2 times daily (acute and chronic); for the external application, 1 dessertspoonful to be mixed with 250 ml water and then used as a wash or poultice (HAB1).

Storage: Store Witch Hazel bark protected from exposure to light.

WITCH HAZEL LEAF

Mode of Administration: Witch hazel leaf is available as comminuted drug or extract for internal and external use as galenic preparations. A steam distillate of the fresh leaves and bark is used for internal and external applications.

How Supplied:

Liquid —1:1 liquid

Preparation:

Liquid extract—1:1 with 45% ethanol (PF X).

Stabilized liquid extract—100 g of leaf powder are moistened with 45 g 1:2 90% ethanol:water and subsequently percolated with 540 g 1:2 90% ethanol:water. Separation into 85 g forerun and the residue, which is evaporated until dry. The dried substance is dissolved with 15 g ethanol:water and is then mixed with the forerun. This solution is kept for 8 days at 2 to 8° C and then filtered at the same temperature. Tea: pour 150 ml boiling water over 2 to 3 g drug and strain after 10 minutes.

Daily Dosage:

Decoction—250 ml water with 5 to 10 g drug for washes or poultices; 2 to 3 g to 150 ml water as a gargle solution.

Suppositories—0.1 to 1 g drug/supp. 3 times daily.

Tea—1 cup 2 to 3 times daily between meals.

Liquid extract—2 to 4 ml 3 times daily.

Storage: Protect Witch Hazel leaf from light and moisture when stored.

LITERATURE

WITCH HAZEL BARK

Bernard P et al. J Pharm Belg 26:661

Dorsch W., Neues über antientzündliche Drogen. Z Phytother 14: 26. 1993.

Erdelmeier CAJ et al, Antiviral and antiphlogistic activities of Hamamelis virginiana bark. Planta Med 62: 241-245. 1996.

Friedrich H, Krüger N, Planta Med 25: 138. 1974.

Haberland C, Kolodziej H, Novel galloylhamamelose from Hamamelis virginiana. Planta Med 5908. 1993.

Hänsel R, Keller K, Rimpler H, Schneider G (Ed), Hagers Handbuch der Pharmazeutischen Praxis, 5. Aufl., Bde 4 - 6 (Drogen), Springer Verlag Berlin, Heidelberg, New York, 1992-1994.

Hartisch C et al., Dual inhibitory activities of tannins from Hamamelis virginiana and related polyphenols on 5-lipoxygenase and Lyso-PAF: Acetyl-CoA-Acetyltransferase. Planta Med 63: 106-110.

Hartisch C et al., Proanthocyanidin pattern in Hamamelis virginiana. Planta Med 62 (Abstracts of the 44th Ann Congress of GA) 119. 1996.

Hartisch C et al., Study on the localisation and composition of the volatile fraction of Hamamelis virginiana. Planta Med 62 (Abstracts of the 44th Ann Congress of GA) 133. 1996.

Knoch HG, Hämorrhoiden I. Grades, Wirksamkeit einer Salbe auf pflanzlicher Basis. Münch Med Wschr 31/32: 481-484. 1991

Korting HC, Schäfer-Korting M, Hart H et al., Anti-inflammatory activity of hamamelis distillate applied topically to the skin. Influence of vehicle and dose. Eur J Clin Pharmacol 44 315-318: 1993.

Laux P, Oschmann R, Die Zaubernuβ - Hamamelis virginiana L. Z Phytother 14: 155-166. 1993.

Leung AY, Encyclopedia of Common Natural Ingredients Used in Food Drugs and Cosmetics, John Wiley & Sons Inc. New York 1980.

Madaus G, Lehrbuch der Biologischen Arzneimittel, Bde 1-3, Nachdruck, Georg Olms Verlag Hildesheim 1979.

Mennet-von Eiff M, Meier B, Phytotherapie in der Dermatologie. Z Phytother 16: 201-210. 1995.

Messerschmidt W, Arch Pharm 300: 550. 1967.

Messerschmidt W, Arzneim Forsch 18: 1618. 1968,

Schulz R, Hänsel R, Rationale Phytotherapie. Springer Verlag Heidelberg 1996.

Sorkin B, Hametum-Salbe, eine kortikoidfreie antiinflammatorische Salbe. Phys Med Rehab 21: 53-57. 1980.

Steinegger E, Hänsel R, Pharmakognosie, 5. Aufl., Springer Verlag Heidelberg 1992.

Teuscher E, Biogene Arzneimittel. 5. Aufl., Wiss. Verlagsgesellschaft Stuttgart 1997.

Wagner H, Wiesenauer M, Phytotherapie. Phytopharmaka und pflanzliche Homöopathika. Fischer-Verlag, Stuttgart, Jena, New York 1995.

Wichtl M (Ed), Teedrogen, 4. Aufl., Wiss. Verlagsges. Stuttgart 1997.

WITCH HAZEL LEAF

Bernard P et al., J Pharm Belg 26: 661.

Dorsch W, Neues über antientzündliche Drogen. Z Phytother 14: 26. 1993.

Erdelmeier CAJ et al., Antiviral and antiphlogistic activities of Hamamelis virginiana bark. Planta Med 62: 241-245. 1996.

Friedrich H, Krüger N, Planta Med 25: 138. 1974.

Haberland C, Kolodziej H, Novel galloylhamamelose from Hamamelis virginiana. Planta Med 59: A608. 1993.

Hänsel R, Keller K, Rimpler H, Schneider G (Ed), Hagers Handbuch der Pharmazeutischen Praxis, 5. Aufl., Bde 4 - 6 (Drogen), Springer Verlag Berlin, Heidelberg, New York, 1992-1994.

Hartisch C et al., Dual inhibitory activities of tannins from Hamamelis virginiana and related polyphenols on 5-lipoxygenase and Lyso-PAF: Acetyl-CoA-Acetyltransferase. Planta Med 63: 106-110. 1997.

Hartisch C et al., Proanthocyanidin pattern in Hamamelis virginiana. Planta Med 62 (Abstracts of the 44th Ann Congress of GA) 119. 1996.

Hartisch C et al., Study on the localisation and composition ot the volatile fraction of Hamamelis virginiana. Planta Med 62 (Abstracts of the 44th Ann Congress of GA) 133.1996.

Knoch HG, Hämorrhoiden I. Grades, Wirksamkeit einer Salbe auf pflanzlicher Basis. Münch Med Wschr 31/32: 481-484. 1991.

Korting HC, Schäfer-Korting M, Hart H et al., Anti-inflammatory activity of hamamelis distillate applied topically to the skin. Influence of vehicle and dose. Eur J Clin Pharmacol 44: 315-318: 1993.

Laux P, Oschmann R, Die Zaubernuβ - Hamamelis virginiana L. Z Phytother 14: 155-166. 1993.

Leung AY, Encyclopedia of Common Natural Ingredients Used in Food Drugs and Cosmetics, John Wiley & Sons Inc. New York 1980.

Madaus G, Lehrbuch der Biologischen Arzneimittel, Bde 1-3, Nachdruck, Georg Olms Verlag Hildesheim 1979.

Mennet-von Eiff M, Meier B, Phytotherapie in der Dermatologie. Z Phytother 16 (1995), 201-210

Messerschmidt W, Arch Pharm 300: 550. 1967.

Messerschmidt W, Arzneim Forsch 18: 1618. 1968.

Schulz R, Hänsel R, Rationale Phytotherapie. Springer Verlag Heidelberg 1996.

Sorkin B, Hametum-Salbe, eine kortikoidfreie antiinflammatorische Salbe. Phys Med Rehab 21: 53-57. 1980.

Steinegger E, Hänsel R, Pharmakognosie, 5. Aufl., Springer Verlag Heidelberg 1992.

Teuscher E, Biogene Arzneimittel. 5. Aufl., Wiss. Verlagsgesellschaft Stuttgart 1997.

Wagner H, Wiesenauer M, Phytotherapie. Phytopharmaka und pflanzliche Homöopathika. Fischer-Verlag, Stuttgart, Jena, New York 1995.

Wichtl M (Ed), Teedrogen, 4. Aufl., Wiss. Verlagsges. Stuttgart 1997.

Wood Anemone

Anemone nemorosa

DESCRIPTION

Medicinal Parts: The medicinal parts are the fresh plant gathered shortly before the flowers open and the dried aerial parts of the plant.

Flower and Fruit: The white flowers are solitary and located at the end of a long stem. The stem is erect when in flower, white to reddish-violet, and has a diameter of 1.5 to 4 cm. The usually 6 (but possibly 5 to 9) bracts are oblong-ovate, entire-margined and glabrous. The flowers have numerous yellow stamens. The 10 to 20 carpels are oblong with a short curved beak. They are downy and 4 to 5 mm long. The fruit is a drooping compound with a roughly haired fruitlet.

Leaves, Stem and Root: Anemone nemorosa is a perennial plant, 6 to 30 cm high with a horizontally creeping, yellow to dark brown, roundish rhizome. The stems are usually solitary, erect, glabrous or sparsely pubescent. There is usually a long-stemmed basal leaf. The leaf is tri-pinnate and pinnatifid-serrate. The first row of pinna are stemmed and have horizontal pinna sections, each with 1 pinna of the second level. There are cauline rosettes of 3 leaf-like bracts, which have a 2-cm long petiole. The bracts do not generally have axillary buds, and are palmate and pinnatifid-serrate.

Habitat: The plant is spread almost all over Europe as far as the Volga region except in the Mediterranean and northern Lapland.

Production: Wood Anemone is the aerial part of Anemone nemorosa, collected shortly before the flowers open.

Other Names: Pasque Flower, Crowfoot, Wind Flower, Smell Fox

ACTIONS AND PHARMACOLOGY

COMPOUNDS

Protoanemonine-forming agents (yielding approximately 300 mcg protoanemonine per gram of fresh weight): presumably, the glycoside ranunculin, which changes enzymatically when the plant is cut into small pieces (and probably also when it is dried) into the pungent, volatile protoanemonine that quickly dimerizes to anemonine; when dried, the plant is not capable of protoanemonine formation

EFFECTS

No information is available.

INDICATIONS AND USAGE

Unproven Uses: The drug is used for stomach pains, delayed menstruation, gout, whooping cough and asthma.

PRECAUTIONS AND ADVERSE REACTIONS

No health hazards or side effects are known in conjunction with the proper administration of designated therapeutic dosages.

Prolonged skin contact with the freshly harvested plant can lead to slow-healing blisters and cauterizations due to the formation of protoanemonine, which is severely irritating to skin and mucous membranes. If taken internally, severe irritation to the gastrointestinal tract and urinary drainage passages, as well as colic and diarrhea, are possible.

Symptomatic treatment for external contact should consist of irrigation with diluted potassium permanganate solution followed by mucilage.

OVERDOSAGE

In case of internal contact, administer gastric lavage followed by activated charcoal. Death by asphyxiation following the intake of large quantities of protoanemonine-forming plants has been observed in animal experiments. The ingestion of 30 freshly harvested plants is considered the fatal level for humans.

DOSAGE

Mode of Administration: The drug can be found in dilute homeopathic preparations of the mother tincture.

LITERATURE

Bonora A et al., PH 26:2277. 1987.

Frohne D, Pfänder HJ, Giftpflanzen - Ein Handbuch für Apotheker, Toxikologen und Biologen, 4. Aufl., Wiss. Verlags-Ges Stuttgart 1997.

Hänsel R, Keller K, Rimpler H, Schneider G (Hrsg.), Hagers Handbuch der Pharmazeutischen Praxis, 5. Aufl., Bde 4-6 (Drogen): Springer Verlag Berlin, Heidelberg, New York, 1992-1994.

Lewin L, Gifte und Vergiftungen, 6. Aufl., Nachdruck, Haug Verlag, Heidelberg 1992.

Madaus G, Lehrbuch der Biologischen Arzneimittel, Bde 1-3, Nachdruck, Georg Olms Verlag Hildesheim 1979.

Roth L, Daunderer M, Kormann K, Giftpflanzen, Pflanzengifte, 4. Aufl., Ecomed Fachverlag Landsberg Lech 1993.

Ruijgrok HWL, PM 11:338-347. 1963.

Teuscher E, Lindequist U, Biogene Gifte - Biologie, Chemie, Pharmakologie, 2. Aufl., Fischer Verlag Stuttgart 1994.

Wood Betony

Betonica officinalis

TRADE NAMES

Wood Betony Herb Liquid

DESCRIPTION

Medicinal Parts: The medicinal part is the herb, including the basal leaves.

Flower and Fruit: The flowers are crimson and labiate in terminal, spike-like, irregular formation. The calyx, with 5 even, triangular tips, has long ciliate hairs and is shorter than the corolla tube. The corolla is curled downward, and the white tube has no ring of hair. The upper lip is erect, and the lower lip is 3-lobed with a broad middle lobe. There are 4 stamens.

Leaves, Stem and Root: The plant grows to a height of about 30 to 100 cm. The stem is erect, unbranched, quadrangular, bristly-haired and usually only has 2 distal pairs of leaves. The basal leaves are rosette-like. The leaves are elongate-ovate with a cordate base and crenate. The lower ones are larger and long-petioled, and the upper ones are smaller and shorter.

Habitat: The plant grows in Europe.

Production: Wood Betony is the flowering plant of Betonica officinalis collected from June to August at flowering time. The herb, including the basal leaves, is collected and dried in the shade at a maximum temperature of 40° C.

Not to be Confused With: Stachys alpina

Other Names: Betony, Bishopswort

ACTIONS AND PHARMACOLOGY

COMPOUNDS

Betaine: including betonicine [(-)-oxystachydrine), (-)- stachydrine), ((+)oxystachydrine]

Caffeic acid derivatives: including chlorogenic acid, isochlorogenic acid, rosemary acid iridoid glycosides

Diterpene lactone

Iridoids: iridoid glycosides, including harpagide

Flavonoids

EFFECTS

The drug is said to act as a tranquilizer, a disinfectant and an astringent. It contains glycosides with hypotensive characteristics.

INDICATIONS AND USAGE

Unproven Uses: Wood Betony is an astringent. As an expectorant, it is used for coughs, bronchitis and asthma. It is contained in combination preparations as a sedative and for the treatment of neuralgia and anxiety. In folk medicine, it is used as an antidiarrheal agent, a carmative, and a sedative, and for catarrh, lung catarrh, heartburn, gout, nervousness, bladder and kidney stones, and inflammation of the bladder.

Homeopathic Uses: Betonica officinalis is used in homeopathy for asthma and general states of debility.

PRECAUTIONS AND ADVERSE REACTIONS

No health hazards or side effects are known in conjunction with the proper administration of designated therapeutic dosages.

DOSAGE

Mode of Administration: The herb is used topically, as an extract and an infusion. The fresh leaves are also used.

Daily Dosage: The infusion can be taken daily. The total daily dosage of the powder is 1 to 2 gm, to be taken in 3 separate doses. The fresh leaves may be boiled and used for wounds and swelling.

LITERATURE

Hoppe HA, (1975-1987) Drogenkunde, 8. Aufl., Bde 1-3, W. de Gruyter Verlag, Berlin, New York.

Kern W, List PH, Hörhammer L (Hrsg.), Hagers Handbuch der Pharmazeutischen Praxis, 4. Aufl., Bde. 1-8, Springer Verlag Berlin, Heidelberg, New York, 1969.

Madaus G, Lehrbuch der Biologischen Arzneimittel, Bde 1-3, Nachdruck, Georg Olms Verlag Hildesheim 1979.

Wood Sage

Teucrium scorodonia

DESCRIPTION

Medicinal Parts: The medicinal parts are the herb, the fresh aerial parts of the flowering plant and the whole flowering plant.

Flower and Fruit: The flowers are approximately 1 cm long, pale yellow or greenish-yellow. They are solitary or in pairs on short pedicles in one-side-inclined, terminal racemes. The calyx of the labiate flower is tubular-campanulate and bilabiate with an undivided upper and a 4-tipped lower lip. The stamens are pubescent and the anthers are violet. The nutlet is round, about 2mm long, and almost smooth.

Leaves, Stem and Root: The plant is erect, 30 to 60 cm high and has far-reaching runners. The stem is erect, paniculate-branched above, quadrangular and soft-pubescent. The leaves are petiolate, opposite, wrinkled, ovate or oblong, unevenly crenate and have a shallowly cordate base.

Characteristics: The plant smells faintly of leeks when being dried.

Habitat: The plant is common to large parts of western and central Europe including the Mediterranean region. It is rarely found in eastern Europe and Scandinavia but it has naturalized there.

Production: Wood Sage is the aerial part of Teucrium scorodonia.

Other Names: Ambroise, Garlic Sage, Hind Heal, Large-Leaved Germander

ACTIONS AND PHARMACOLOGY

COMPOUNDS

Volatile oil (0.3%): containing among others, alloaromadendrene, aristolene, beta-caryophyllene, alpha-caryophyllene (humulene), spathulenone, caryophyllene epoxide

Iridoide monoterpenes: including among others, acetyl harpagide, reptoside

Diterpenes: the spectrum varies greatly according to strain, including among others teuscorodal, teuscorodin, teuscorodol, teuscorodonin, teuflin, teuscorolide, teupolin I

Flavonoids: including among others, cirsiliol, cirsimaritin, luteolin

EFFECTS

The expectorant effect attributed to the drug may be due to the amaroids and the essential oil. See other Teucrium species for the toxic effect.

INDICATIONS AND USAGE

Unproven Uses: Wood Sage is used for the treatment of tuberculosis, chronic bronchial catarrh, inflammation of mucous membranes of the nose and throat, spasms, hypertension, wounds and liver disorders.

Homeopathic Uses: The herb is used for chronic inflammation of the respiratory tract.

PRECAUTIONS AND ADVERSE REACTIONS

No health hazards or side effects are known in conjunction with the proper administration of designated therapeutic dosages.

DOSAGE

Mode of Administration: Wood Sage is obsolete as a drug in most countries, but it can be found as cut drug in capsules and drops.

Preparation: To treat bronchitis, a tea is made using 2 teaspoons of herb per cup.

LITERATURE

Bruno M et al., (1985) Phytochemistry 24(11):2597.

Fikenscher LH, Hegnauer R, Plant Med Phytother 3(3):183.

Hänsel R, Keller K, Rimpler H, Schneider G (Hrsg.), Hagers Handbuch der Pharmazeutischen Praxis, 5. Aufl., Bde 4-6 (Drogen): Springer Verlag Berlin, Heidelberg, New York, 1992-1994.

Madaus G, Lehrbuch der Biologischen Arzneimittel, Bde 1-3, Nachdruck, Georg Olms Verlag Hildesheim 1979.

Marco JL et al., Phytochemistry 21(10):2567.

Marco JL et al., PH 21:2567. 1982.

Marco JL et al., PH 22:727-731. 1983.

Velasco-Negueruela A et al., PH 29:1165-1169. 1990.

Wagner H, Wiesenauer M, Phytotherapie. Phytopharmaka und pflanzliche Homöopathika, Fischer-Verlag, Stuttgart, Jena, New York 1995.

Wood Sorrel

Oxalis acetosella

DESCRIPTION

Medicinal Parts: The medicinal part is the fresh flowering plant with the root.

Flower and Fruit: The solitary flower is white or reddish-white and red-veined with yellow spots. The pedicle is longer than the leaves. There are 5 sepals and 5 petals, 10 stamens and 1 ovary with 5 styles. The fruit is an ovate capsule. It is pentangular, tearing open in long slits when ripe, thus freeing the seeds.

Leaves, Stem and Root: The plant grows to a height of between 5 and 12 cm tall. The leaves are basal, tender, long-petioled and trifoliate. The leaflets are broad, obovate-cordate, downy and often tinged red underneath. The stem is leafless apart from bracts above the middle, which are fused at the base.

Characteristics: The plant has a pleasant, rather sour odor.

Habitat: The plant is commonly found in woods and forests throughout Europe.

Production: Wood Sorrel is the aerial part of Oxalis acetosella, which is harvested while the plant is in blossom.

Other Names: Cuckoo Bread, Cuckowes Meat, Fairy Bells, Green Sauce, Hallelujah, Shamrock, Sour Trefoil, Stickwort, Stubwort, Surelle, Three-Leaved Grass, Wood Sour

ACTIONS AND PHARMACOLOGY

COMPOUNDS

Oxalic acid (0.3-1.25%): especially present as potassium salt

EFFECTS

The drug, including the green parts of the plant, contains clover acid that, in small amounts, affects gallbladder activity by acting as a diuretic. The fresh plant provides a substantial source of vitamin C.

INDICATIONS AND USAGE

Unproven Uses: Wood Sorrel is no longer used as a remedy, but previously was used for liver and digestive disorders. Also, in the past, the fresh leaves were used to treat scurvy, wounds and inflammation of the gums.

PRECAUTIONS AND ADVERSE REACTIONS

No health hazards or side effects are known in conjunction with the proper administration of designated therapeutic dosages.

OVERDOSAGE

Oxalic acid poisonings could occur only through the ingestion of very large quantities of the leaves, for example as in salad. The poisonings mentioned in older scientific literature seem dubious.

DOSAGE

Mode of Administration: Ground and as an extract. Wood Sorrel is no longer used as a remedy.

LITERATURE

Kern W, List PH, Hörhammer L (Hrsg.), Hagers Handbuch der Pharmazeutischen Praxis, 4. Aufl., Bde. 1-8, Springer Verlag Berlin, Heidelberg, New York, 1969.

Madaus G, Lehrbuch der Biologischen Arzneimittel, Bde 1-3, Nachdruck, Georg Olms Verlag Hildesheim 1979.

Roth L, Daunderer M, Kormann K, Giftpflanzen, Pflanzengifte, 4. Aufl., Ecomed Fachverlag Landsberg Lech 1993.

Teuscher E, Lindequist U, Biogene Gifte - Biologie, Chemie, Pharmakologie, 2. Aufl., Fischer Verlag Stuttgart 1994.

Tosto DS, Hopp HE, Sequence analysis of the 5.8S ribosomal DNA and internal transcribed spacers (ITS1 and ITS2) from five species of the Oxalis tuberosa alliance. DNA Seq, 6:361-4, 1996.

Tschesche R, Struckmeyer K, (1976) Chem Ber. 109:2901.

Wormseed

Artemisia cina

DESCRIPTION

Medicinal Parts: The medicinal parts are closed flower-buds, that have not yet blossomed.

Flower and Fruit: The numerous flower heads are about 2 mm long with a diameter of 1.5 mm. They are ovoid and greenish-yellow when fresh, later brownish-green. They contain three to five minute, tubular, androgynous florets with a slim, cylindrical and glabrous receptacle. The epicalyces have numerous oblong-obtuse, imbricate scales.

Leaves, Stem and Root: Artemisia cina is an evergreen, perennial semi-shrub, 30 to 60 cm high with many slim sprouting stems. The gnarled rhizome produces numerous leaf and flower branches. The stems are smooth and woody and the leaves pinnatifid on the non-flowering branches. The leaves on the flowering branches are small and entire-margined.

Characteristics: The odor is aromatic and the taste bitter.

Habitat: The plant is indigenous to Iran, Turkestan and the Kirghizin Steppes around Buchara.

Production: Wormwood flowers are the inflorescent buds of Artemisia cina (occasionally incorrectly called Wormseed), which are cultivated and gathered in the wild.

Not to be Confused With: Refined mustard flour

Other Names: Levant, Santonica, Sea Wormwood

ACTIONS AND PHARMACOLOGY

COMPOUNDS

Sesquiterpene lactones: especially alpha-santonin, in addition to artemisin and beta-santonin

EFFECTS

The anthelmintic and antipyretic effect of the drug can be attributed to its alpha-santonin content. The drug acts as a vermifuge action for ascarids, including intestinal parasitic worms, whose muscles are paralyzed by the santonin. The worms are then forced into the large intestine where they are removed by means of a laxative. In rats, the rectal temperature was lowered during fevers that had been induced by brewer's yeast injections. This leads to the speculation that santonin effects body temperature in a similar manner to dopamine.

INDICATIONS AND USAGE

Unproven Uses: The drug is used for ascarid and oxyuris infestations.

Homeopathic Uses: Uses in homeopathy include fevers, tendency to convulsions and worms.

PRECAUTIONS AND ADVERSE REACTIONS

Even with the therapeutic dose there is a danger of poisoning. Side effects may resemble those of the alpha-santonins: kidney irritation, gastroenteritis, stupor, visual disorders (xanthopsia), muscle twitching and epileptiform spasms. Administration in allopathic dosages is to be avoided.

OVERDOSAGE

Deadly poisonings following the intake of less than 10 g of the drug are known.

DOSAGE

Preparation: Wormwood is considered completely obsolete as a drug, occasionally available as a powder for use when more modern antithelmintic agents fail. Symptoms of poisoning are possible even in therapeutic dosages.

Daily Dosage: The drug is always used in combination with a laxative. The average single dose is 0.025 g for adults. For children, take the child's age in years, and double this amount in milligrams of the drug. According to the Austrian pharmacopoeia, the single dose is 1 to 2 g. The powder is administered in the morning and followed later by castor oil or sodium sulfate. The remedy is repeated on the following day.

Homeopathic Dosage: 5 to 10 drops, 1 tablet, 5 to 10 globules, 1 to 3 times a day or 1 ml injection solution twice weekly sc (HAB34).

LITERATURE

Frohne D, Pfänder HJ: Giftpflanzen - Ein Handbuch für Apotheker, Toxikologen und Biologen, 4. Aufl., Wiss. Verlagsges. mbH Stuttgart 1997.

Hänsel R, Keller K, Rimpler H, Schneider G (Hrsg.), Hagers Handbuch der Pharmazeutischen Praxis, 5. Aufl., Bde 4-6 (Drogen): Springer Verlag Berlin, Heidelberg, New York, 1992-1994.

Lewin L, Gifte und Vergiftungen, 6. Aufl., Nachdruck, Haug Verlag, Heidelberg 1992.

Madaus G, Lehrbuch der Biologischen Arzneimittel, Bde 1-3, Nachdruck, Georg Olms Verlag Hildesheim 1979.

Roth L, Daunderer M, Kormann K, Giftpflanzen, Pflanzengifte, 4. Aufl., Ecomed Fachverlag Landsberg Lech 1993.

Teuscher E, Lindequist U, Biogene Gifte - Biologie, Chemie, Pharmakologie, 2. Aufl., Fischer Verlag Stuttgart 1994.

Teuscher E, Biogene Arzneimittel, 5. Aufl., Wiss. Verlagsges. mbH Stuttgart 1997.

Wormseed Oil

Chenopodium ambrosioides

DESCRIPTION

Medicinal Parts: The plant's medicinal parts are the seeds and the herb, including the flowers.

Flower and Fruit: The numerous small flowers are yellowish-green and form small racemes or roundish spikes in the axils of the apical leaves. The calyx is divided into 5; the lobes are ovate and pointed. There are 5 stamens. The ovary has small, oblong, stemmed glands at the tip. The angular fruit is enclosed in the calyx. The small seeds are achaenes, smooth and black.

Leaves, Stem and Root: The plant is an annual that grows to about 1 m in height with a branched, reddish stem. The stem is covered in alternate-linear to lanceolate leaves.

Characteristics: The whole plant gives off a pleasant fragrance. The oil is dangerously explosive.

Habitat: Wormseed originated in Mexico and South America but has spread to the eastern U.S.

Production: Wormseed Oil is the seed oil of Chenopodium ambrosioides.

Other Names: Mexican Tea, American Wormseed, Jesuit's Tea

ACTIONS AND PHARMACOLOGY

COMPOUNDS

Ascaridiole (chief constituent - up to 80%): including, according to variety and breed, p-cymene, L-pinocarvone, alpha-pinenes and/or alpha-terpenes, limonene. The combination creates a volatile, explosive oil.

EFFECTS

Wormseed Oil acts as an anthelmintic that causes flight and defensive reactions in worms. This is due to the main constituent of the terpene fraction, which is ascaridole, a monoterpene. This constituent is highly toxic.

INDICATIONS AND USAGE

Unproven Uses: Although considered obsolete as a drug, Wormseed Oil is used against roundworms and hookworms, if other, more modern anthelmintic drugs fail. The leaves and seeds have long been used in South American medicine as a vermifuge, stimulant, anti-asthmatic and abortifacient for cramps, paralysis and asthmatic complaints.

Chinese Medicine: The Chinese have used Wormseed Oil for rheumatism of the joints, metrorrhagia, eczema and bites.

PRECAUTIONS AND ADVERSE REACTIONS

Even the administration of therapeutic dosages can lead to disorders of the central nervous system, including spasms, signs of paralysis, Pachymeningitis haemorrhagica. Damage to the Nervus cochlearis is frequent, leading to buzzing in the ears and hearing impairment (sometimes lasting for years). In addition, the oil is dangerously explosive.

OVERDOSAGE

Cases of death have been observed following intake of 10 mg of the oil by adults, and much less for children. For that reason, an administration in allopathic dosages is to be avoided.

DOSAGE

Mode of Administration: Wormseed Oil is obsolete as a drug. In clinically described cases, which are exceptional, it can be used in combination with a fast-acting and powerful purgative.

Daily Dosage: Typical adult daily dosage is 20 drops taken in the morning on an empty stomach. Two hours later, a purgative is taken. Pediatric dosage is two single doses of drops taken one hour apart. Each dose has one drop per year of the child's age.

LITERATURE

Bombardelli E et al., (1976) Fitoterapia 47:3.

Chan, EH et al., (Eds), Advances in Chinese Medicinal Materials Research, World Scientific Pub. Co. Singapore 1985.

Gupta GS, Behari M, (1972) J Ind Chem Soc 49:317.

Leung AY, Encyclopedia of Common Natural Ingredients Used in Food Drugs and Cosmetics, John Wiley & Sons Inc., New York 1980.

Lewin L, Gifte und Vergiftungen, 6. Aufl., Nachdruck, Haug Verlag, Heidelberg 1992.

Madaus G, Lehrbuch der Biologischen Arzneimittel, Bde 1-3, Nachdruck, Georg Olms Verlag Hildesheim 1979.

Roth L, Daunderer M, Kormann K, Giftpflanzen, Pflanzengifte, 4. Aufl., Ecomed Fachverlag Landsberg Lech 1993.

Wormwood

Artemisia absinthium

DESCRIPTION

Medicinal Parts: The medicinal parts are the aerial shoots and leaves of the plant.

Flower and Fruit: The numerous flower heads are short-stemmed and hang in a many-flowered panicle. The capitula are small, globular, inclined and nearly as long as their 3 to 4 mm width. The bracts are gray, silky-pubescent with a rounded tip. The outer bracts are linear-oblong and pubescent, while the inner ones are ovate, obtuse, broad and have a transparent, membranous margin. The receptacle is rough-haired. The flowers are yellow and fertile. The disc florets are androgynous; the ray florets are female with an extending style stem. The fruit is about 1.5 mm long.

Leaves, Stem and Root: This semi-shrub grows from 60 to 120 cm in height with a woody, hardy rosette and a high-branch bearing stem. The stem is usually erect and leafy. The alternate, long-petioled leaves are silky pubescent on both sides. The lower leaves are abrupt pinnate and the upper ones simple. The leaf tips are lanceolate to linear-lanceolate, obtuse to acuminate and 2 to 3 mm wide.

Characteristics: The plant has an aromatic odor and a very bitter taste.

Habitat: Wormwood grows in Europe, northern Africa, parts of Asia, and North and South America.

Production: Wormwood consists of the fresh or dried upper shoots and leaves, the fresh or dried basal leaves, or a mixture of the aerial plant parts from Artemisia absinthium, that is harvested during flowering season from cultivated or wild plants.

Other Names: Green Ginger, Absinthe

ACTIONS AND PHARMACOLOGY

COMPOUNDS

Volatile oil: with a high level (varies a great deal among different strains) of (+)-thujone, cis-epoxy ocimene, trans-sabinyl acetate or chrysanthenyl acetate

Sesquiterpene bitter principles: including absinthine, anabsinthine, artabsine and matricine

EFFECTS

The cholagogic, digestive, appetite-stimulating and wound-healing effects ascribed to the drug are attributed to the essential oils and amaroids. A significant increase of alpha-amylase, liapse, bilirubin and cholesterol has been observed during the 70 to 100 minutes during which patients with liver disorders were given a suspension of 20 mg extract in 10 ml water via a duodenal probe. In rabbits, fever induced through yeast injection was reduced by using an esophageal probe to administer diverse fractions of the drug. In vitro, a watery extract of the whole drug is supposed to retard the growth of *Plasmodium falciparum.* The essential oil of the drug may possess an antimicrobial effect. The drug also stimulates the bitter receptors in the taste buds of the tongue. When bitter agents are introduced into the mouth, they trigger a reflexive increase of stomach secretion with higher acid concentration.

INDICATIONS AND USAGE

Approved by Commission E:

- Loss of appetite
- Dyspeptic complaints
- Liver and gallbladder complaints

Unproven Uses: In folk medicine, wormwood preparations are used internally for gastric insufficiency, intestinal atonia, gastritis, stomachache, liver disorders, bloating, anemia, irregular menstruation, intermittent fever, loss of appetite and worm infestation. Externally, the drug is applied for poorly healing wounds, ulcers, skin blotches and insect bites. Efficacy in the above-mentioned popular uses is insufficiently documented.

PRECAUTIONS AND ADVERSE REACTIONS

General: Due to the drug's thujone content, the internal administration of large doses can lead to vomiting, stomach and intestinal cramps, headache, dizziness and disturbances of the central nervous system. Continuous use is not advisable. The use of volatile oils and spirituous extracts from the drug for the manufacture of alcoholic drinks is forbidden in many countries because of possible injuries to health.

Drug Interactions: The thujone componant may lower the seizure threshold. Caution must be exercised when administering this herb to patients that have a predisposition to seizures. Drugs that are used to control seizures may have decreased effectiveness. Wormwood preparations should not be administered in conjunction with drugs that are known to lower the seizure threshold.

DOSAGE

Mode of Administration: Comminuted herb is used for infusions and decoctions. Powdered herb, extracts and tinctures in liquid or solid forms are used for oral administration. Combination with other bitters or aromatics is common.

Preparation: To prepare an infusion, pour 150 ml boiling water over 1/2 teaspoonful of the drug, strain after 10 minutes. A decoction is prepared by adding 1 handful of drug to 1 liter of boiling water for 5 minutes. To prepare a tea, use 1 g drug in 1 cup water.

Daily Dose: The total daily dose is 3 to 5 g of the herb as an aqueous extract. Internal dose of the infusion is 1 cup freshly prepared tea taken 30 minutes before each meal. The tincture dosage is 10 to 30 drops in sufficient water taken 3 times daily. The liquid extract dosage is 1 to 2 ml taken 3 times daily.

Externally, a decoction is used for healing of wounds and insect bites.

Storage: Wormwood must be kept in sealed containers and protected from light.

LITERATURE

Akhmedov IS et al., (1970) Khim Prir Soedin 6:691.

Akhmedov IS et al., (Artabin, a new lactone from Artemisia absinthium). In: Khim Prid Soed 5:622. 1970.

Baumann IC et al., (1975) Z Allg Med 51 (17):784.

Beauhaire J et al., (1981) Tetrahedron Letters 22 (24):2269.

Beauhaire J, Fourrey JL, (1982) J Chem Soc Perk Trans: 861.

Del Castillo J et al., (1975) Nature 253:365.

Dermanovic S et al., (1976): 87.

Greger H, Hofer O, New unsymmetrically substituted tetrahydrofuran lignans from Artemisia absinthium. In: Tetrahedron 36(24):3551. 1980.

Greger H, (1978) Phytochemistry 17:806.

Hoffman B, Herrmann K, (1982) Z Lebensm Unters Forsch 174 (3):211.

Kasimov Ah Z et al., (Anabsin-a new diguaianolide from Artemisia absinthium). In: Khim Prid Soed 4:495. 1979.

Kasymov SZ et al., (1979) Khim Prir Soed 5:658.

Kennedy AI et al., Volatile oils from normal and transformed roots of Artemisia absinthium. In: PH 32:1449. 1993.

Kinloch JD, (1971) Practitioner 206:44.

Lemberkovics E et al., Some phytochemical characteristics of essential oil of Artemisia absinthium L. In: Herba hung 21(3):197-215. 1982.

Marles RJ, Kaminski J, Arnason JT, Pazos-Sanou L, Heptinstall S, Fischer NH, Crompton CW, Kindack DG, A bioassay for inhibition of serotonin release from bovine platelets. In: JNP 55:1044-1056. 1992.

Rucker G, Manns D, Wilbert S, Peroxides as constituents of plants. 10. Homoditerpene peroxides from Artemisia-absinthium. In: PH:31(1):340. 1992.

Schneider Von G, Mielke B, (1979) Deutsch Apoth Ztg 119 (25):977.

Stahl E, Gerard D, (1983) Z Lebensm Unters Forsch 176 (1):1.

Swiatek L, Dombrowicz E, (1984) Farm Pol 40 (2):729.

Vostrowski O et al., (1981) Z NaturForsch (C) 36 (5/6):369.

Vostrowski O et al., Über die Komponenten des ätherischen Öls aus Artemisia absinthium L.. In: Z Naturforsch 36(5/6):369. 1981.

Zafar MM, Hamdard ME, Hameed A, Screening of Artemisia absinthium for antimalarial effects on Plasmodium berghei in mice: Preliminary report. In: ETH 30(2):223. 1990.

Zakirov SK et al., (1976) Khim Prir Soedin 4:548.

Further information in:

Hänsel R, Keller K, Rimpler H, Schneider G (Hrsg.), Hagers Handbuch der Pharmazeutischen Praxis, 5. Aufl., Bde 4-6 (Drogen): Springer Verlag Berlin, Heidelberg, New York, 1992-1994.

Lewin L, Gifte und Vergiftungen, 6. Aufl., Nachdruck, Haug Verlag, Heidelberg 1992.

Madaus G, Lehrbuch der Biologischen Arzneimittel, Bde 1-3, Nachdruck, Georg Olms Verlag Hildesheim 1979.

Roth L, Daunderer M, Kormann K, Giftpflanzen, Pflanzengifte, 4. Aufl., Ecomed Fachverlag Landsberg Lech 1993.

Schulz R, Hänsel R, Rationale Phytotherapie, Springer Verlag Heidelberg 1996.

Steinegger E, Hänsel R, Pharmakognosie, 5. Aufl., Springer Verlag Heidelberg 1992.

Teuscher E, Lindequist U, Biogene Gifte - Biologie, Chemie, Pharmakologie, 2. Aufl., Fischer Verlag Stuttgart 1994.

Teuscher E, Biogene Arzneimittel, 5. Aufl., Wiss. Verlagsges. Stuttgart 1997.

Wagner H, Wiesenauer M, Phytotherapie. Phytopharmaka und pflanzliche Homöopathika, Fischer-Verlag, Stuttgart, Jena, New York 1995.

Wichtl M (Hrsg.), Teedrogen, 4. Aufl., Wiss. Verlagsges. Stuttgart 1997.

Wormwood Grass

Spigelia anthelmia

DESCRIPTION

Medicinal Parts: The whole fresh plant, the juice prepared from the fresh plant and the dried leaves are used medicinally.

Flower and Fruit: The inflorescences are terminal or axillary, 5 to 12 cm long spikes turned to one side. They are often involute. The flowers in the axils of the bracts are sessile. The flowers are radial and their structures are in fives. The sepals are free, linear-lanceolate and 2 to 5 mm long. The 5 petals are fused with a 6.5 to 15 mm long, lilac, pink or white, funnel-shaped corolla. There are 5 stamens and a 2-chambered ovary. The fruit is a capsule approximately 5 mm long and 5 mm wide. The seeds are 2 to 3 mm long, elliptical or ovoid, dark brown and warty.

Leaves, Stem and Root: The herb grows upright to a height of up to 60 cm. The leaves are opposite and, because of short internodes, appear to be in whorls. They are 4 to 18 cm long, 2 to 6 cm wide, very short petiolate, simple, entire, ovate-lanceolate to elongate-ovate and long acuminate. The stipules are fused, membranous, broad and triangular. The stem and lateral branches are almost leafless, usually terminating in a 4-leafed whorl.

Habitat: Spigelia anthelmia is indigenous to North, Central and South America.

Production: Wormwood Grass herb is the dried aerial part of Spigelia anthelmia, which is collected in the wild and cultivated in tropical and subtropical regions of America.

Other Names: Annual Wormwood Grass, American Wormwood Grass, Pink Root, Demerara Pinkroot

ACTIONS AND PHARMACOLOGY

COMPOUNDS

Flavonoids: including hyperoside, quercetin-di-O-glucoside, quercetin-O-rhamnoglucoside

Phenol carboxylic acids: vanillic acid, dihydroxy benzoic acid, caffeic acid

Caffeic acid derivatives: chlorogenic acid

Amines: isoquinoline

Monoterpene alkaloids: actinidine

EFFECTS

The choline esters contained in the drug are possibly hypertensive in effect. Depending upon the dosage level, isoquinoline is positively inotropic in effect on isolated gerbil hearts. The experimental results in this area require further testing. The vermifugal action mechanism credited to the drug has not yet been proven. The isoquinoline found in the drug is not present at levels required for protoplasma-destroying effect.

INDICATIONS AND USAGE

Unproven Uses: Traditional folk medicine has included use for worm infestation.

Homeopathic Uses: Homeopathic uses include angina pectoris, neuralgia and headache, acute carditis and worm infestation.

PRECAUTIONS AND ADVERSE REACTIONS

General: The drug is considered to be severely poisonous. Animal poisonings were described in older literature sources, as was deliberate use to poison humans. The toxin is said to be a non-volatile alkaloid. Human consumption of large quantities of the drug is said to lead to vomiting, myositis, dyspnea and spasms.

Homeopathic Precautions: No health hazards are known in conjunction with the proper administration of designated homeopathic dosages.

DOSAGE

How Supplied: Whole and cut drug.

Daily Dosage: The literature has no information.

LITERATURE

Achenbach H, H bner H, Vierling W, Brandt W, Reiter M, Spiganthine, the cardioactive principle of Spigelia anthelmia. J Nat Prod, 58:1092-6, 1995 Jul.

Hänsel R, Keller K, Rimpler H, Schneider G (Ed), Hagers Handbuch der Pharmazeutischen Praxis, 5. Aufl., Bde 4 - 6 (Drogen), Springer Verlag Berlin, Heidelberg, New York, 1992-1994.

Wagner H, Seegert K, Gupta MP, Avella ME, Solis P, Cardiotonic active principles from Spigelia anthelmia. Planta Med, 378-81, 1986 Oct.

Woundwort

Stachys palustris

DESCRIPTION

Medicinal Parts: The medicinal part is the fresh and dried herb.

Flower and Fruit: The closely sessile flowers have very small bracteoles. They are arranged in false whorls of 6 florets joined in groups of 10 to 20 into a spike. The calyx is tubular-campanulate, violet-tinged with awned tips. The corolla is dull violet and the style pink. The nutlet is globular, 2 mm long, lightly striped and glossy dark brown.

Leaves, Stem and Root: The plant is a perennial, with long runners and barrel-like white swellings between the nodes. The shoots are usually loose and have partly appressed, partly patent silky hairs. They are pubescent or almost glabrous and almost odorless. The stems are erect or ascendent from the ground, 30 to 60 cm high, simple or branched, tough, usually with pubescent edges. The internodes are 2 to 10 cm long. The leaves are sessile or very short-petioled, usually clasping, ribbed, matte green and loosely appressed pubescent on both surfaces.

Habitat: The plant is common in Europe.

Production: Woundwort is the aerial part of Stachys palustris or Stachys sylvatica.

Not to be Confused With: S. palustris is Marsh Woundwort and S. sylvatica is Hedge Woundwort. Several other plants have the name Woundwort, among them, Prunella vulgaris and Achillea millefolium.

Other Names: Marsh Stachys

ACTIONS AND PHARMACOLOGY

COMPOUNDS

Iridoide monoterpenes

Betaines: (-)- and (+)stachydrine

Flavonoids: including among others palustrin

EFFECTS

Woundwort is said to be a disinfectant, an antispasmodic and a cure for wounds.

INDICATIONS AND USAGE

Unproven Uses: The herb is used externally for the treatment of wounds and internally for abdominal pain, cramps, dizziness, fever, gout and menstrual disorders.

PRECAUTIONS AND ADVERSE REACTIONS

No health hazards or side effects are known in conjunction with the proper administration of designated therapeutic dosages.

DOSAGE

Mode of Administration: As an extract or poultice for external application.

LITERATURE

Barberan FAT, (1986) Fitoterapia 57(2):67.

Hegnauer R, Chemotaxonomie der Pflanzen, Bde 1-11: Birkhäuser Verlag Basel, Boston, Berlin 1962-1997.

Kern W, List PH, Hörhammer L (Hrsg.), Hagers Handbuch der Pharmazeutischen Praxis, 4. Aufl., Bde 1-8: Springer Verlag Berlin, Heidelberg, New York, 1969.

Kooiman P, (1972) Acta Bot Neerl. 21(4):417.

Miller FM, Chow LM, (1954) J Am Chem Soc 76:1353

Xysmalobium undulatum

See Uzara

Yage

Banisteriopsis caapi

DESCRIPTION

Medicinal Parts: The medicinal part of the plant is the bark.

Flower and Fruit: The inflorescence is multi-flowered. The flowers are 10 to 15 mm wide with pale pink petals. Their structures are arranged in fives. The fruit, which resembles that of the maple, is up to 4 mm long and 0.4 mm wide. Each of the 3 schizocarps has an 18 to 42 mm long and 8 to 22 mm wide wing.

Leaves and Stem: Banisteriopsis caapi is a hardy tree. The leaves are opposite, 8 to 18 cm long, 3.5 to 8 cm wide, ovate and entire. The stem is woody with a brown, smooth bark.

Habitat: The plant is native to jungle areas of the Amazon basin.

Production: Yage bark is the dried or fresh trunk bark of Banisteriopsis caapi.

Other Names: Ayahuasca, Vine of the Souls

ACTIONS AND PHARMACOLOGY

COMPOUNDS

Indole alkaloids (beta-carboline type): particularly harmine (0.5 to 5.9%), harmaline (0.5 to 3.8%), tetrahydroharmine (0.3 to 3.3%), harmol (0.05 to 1.2%), harmalol (up to 0.4%)

Pyridine alkaloids: shinunine, dihydroshinunine

EFFECTS

The alkaloid-containing drug is psychotropic and hallucinogenic in effect, due to the harmine and harmaline it contains (pronounced MAO-inhibition in vitro and in animal experiments). Lower dosages bring on euphoric states in humans, while higher dosages have hallucinogenic effects.

INDICATIONS AND USAGE

Unproven Uses: The plant contains psychoactive substances, which intensify dreams and experiences.

PRECAUTIONS AND ADVERSE REACTIONS

The drug is not in medicinal use. Extracts of the drug (ayahuasca, 5 mg alkaloids/ml), ingested orally in low doses, have hallucinogenic and euphoric effects. These effects are primarily due to monoamine oxidase inhibition; later the effect becomes sedative.

OVERDOSAGE

The intake of higher dosages (corresponding to levels starting at approximately 0.3 gm alkaloids) leads to vomiting, nausea, ringing of the ears and tendency to collapse.

DOSAGE

Mode of Administration: Fresh or dried herb powder and liquid preparations for internal use.

Preparation: The fresh or dried cut bark is macerated for several hours resulting in a bitter syrup, which is then consumed in small amounts. In addition, some of the bark is pulverized, mixed with water and then consumed in larger amounts. The juice can be kept for up to 6 months in tightly sealed containers.

LITERATURE

McKenna DJ, Towers GH, Abbott F, Monoamine oxidase inhibitors in South American hallucinogenic plants: tryptamine and beta-carboline constituents of ayahuasca. J Ethnopharmacol, 10:195-223, 1984 Apr.

McKenna DJ, Towers GH, Abbott F, Relationship between occurrence of tremor/convulsion and level of beta-carbolines in the brain after administration of beta-carbolines into mice. Pharmacol Biochem Behav, 10:-SO-,-SI-.

McKenna DJ, Towers GH, Abbott F, Ritual and medicinal plants of the Ese'ejas of the Amazonian rainforest (Madre de Dios, Peru). J Ethnopharmacol, 10:45-51, 1996 May.

Yarrow

Achillea millefolium

TRADE NAMES

Yarrow Flowers, Yarrow Extract, Alcohol-Free Yarrow Flowers

DESCRIPTION

Medicinal Parts: The dried flower clusters and above-ground parts of the herb are used medicinally.

Flower and Fruit: The plant has white, pink or purple composite flowers in dense cymes with small capitula. The bracts are imbricate, long, thorn-tipped and taper to a point. There are 5 white female florets. The disc florets are tubular, yellowish-white and androgynous. The fruit is 1.5 to 2 mm long.

Leaves, Stem and Root: Achillea millefolium are 0.1 to 1.5 m high plants with hardy, horizontal rhizomes, which grow from underground runners. The stem is simple, erect and hairy. The leaves are lanceolate and multi-pinnate with short acute tips.

Habitat: The numerous subspecies of the Achillea millefolium group are found in various regions. They mainly grow in regions of eastern, southeastern and central Europe, as well as on the southern edge of the Alps from Switzerland to the Balkans.

Production: Yarrow herb consists of the fresh or dried, above-ground parts of Achillea millefolium, harvested at flowering season. Yarrow flower consists of the dried inflorescence of Achillea millefolium.

Other Names: Band Man's Plaything, Bloodwort, Carpenter's Weed, Devil's Nettle, Devil's Plaything, Milfoil, Nose Bleed, Old Man's Pepper, Sanguinary, Soldier's Woundwort, Staunchweed, Thousand Weed, Yarroway, Thousand Seal, Noble Yarrow, Knight's Milfoil

ACTIONS AND PHARMACOLOGY

COMPOUNDS

Volatile oil (0.2-1.0%): chief components (rendered through steam distillation) are chamazulene (blue, 6-19%, maximum 40%), camphor (up to 20%), beta-pinene (up to 23%), 1,8-cineole (up to 10%), caryophyllene (up to 10%), alpha-pinene (up to 5%), isoartemisiaketon (up to 8%). The composition depends greatly on the variety, and the volatile oil of some strains is free of chamazulene.

Sesquiterpene lactones: Mainly guaianolides including, achillicin, 8-alpha-angeloyloxy-10-epi-artabsin, 2,3-dihydro-desacetoxy-matricin, alpha-peroxyachifolide. There are also germacranolides such as millefoild and 3-oxaguaianolides. Some sesquiterpenes are transformed through steam distillation into chamazulene (proazulenes).

Polyynes: including pontica epoxide

Alkamids: including tetradeca-4,6-diin-10,12-dien acetyl isobutylamides

Flavonoids: including apigenine-7-O-glucoside, luteolin-7-O-glucoside, rutin

Betaine: including L-stachydrine, L-hydrostachydrine (betonicine)

EFFECTS

The herb has a cholagogue (stimulates the flow of bile) effect due to the guaianolide and germacranolide content. The flavonoid content exerts a spasmolytic effect, while the proazulene fraction has an anti-edema and anti-inflammatory effect. The effect probably results from the interaction of various structured bonds with the chamazulene and flavonoids. The plant has similar effects to those observed in Chamomile flowers, since some of their components are identical.

INDICATIONS AND USAGE

Approved by Commission E:

- Loss of appetite
- Dyspeptic complaints
- Liver and gallbladder complaints

Unproven Uses: Externally, the herb is used as a sitz bath for painful, cramp-like conditions of psychosomatic origin in the lower part of the female pelvis. Yarrow is also used externally as a palliative treatment for liver disorders and for the healing of wounds. In folk medicine, it is used for bleeding hemorrhoids, menstrual complaints, and as a bath for the removal of perspiration. It is contained in other cholagogic preparations and biliary tract therapeutic agents. It is also used as an adjuvant in preparations for many other indications such as laxatives, cough treatments, gynecological agents, cardiac agents and preparations for varicose veins.

Homeopathic Uses: Achillea millefolium is used in varicose veins, arterial bleeding, convulsions.

CONTRAINDICATIONS

Contraindications include allergy to Yarrow and other composites.

PRECAUTIONS AND ADVERSE REACTIONS

No health hazards or side effects are known in conjunction with the proper administration of designated therapeutic dosages. The drug possesses a weak to medium-severe potential for sensitization resulting in contact dermatitis. The main compound responsible for the sensitization is a sespuiterpene lactone, alpha-peroxyachfolid (Hausen, 1991; Rucker, 1991).

Pregnancy: The drug is not to be used during pregnancy.

DOSAGE

How Supplied:

Capsules — 340mg, 350 mg

Liquid — 1:1, 250 mg/ml

Mode of Administration: As a comminuted drug for teas and other galenical preparations for internal use and for sitz baths. The pressed juice of fresh plants is used internally. The drug is contained in standardized preparations of cholagogic and gallbladder therapeutics and as an adjunct in many other preparations, such as laxatives, antitussives, gynecological products, cardiac remedies and preparations for varicose veins.

Preparation: To make a tea, place 2 gm of finely cut drug in boiling water, cover, leave to steep for 10 to 15 minutes, and then strain. For sitz baths, use 100 gm Yarrow per 20 liters of water.

Daily Dosage:

Infusion — 4.5 gm Yarrow herb or 3 gm Yarrow flowers.

Tea — A cup of freshly made tea to be drunk 3 to 4 times daily between meals.

External application — 100 gm Yarrow to be drawn in 1 to 2 liter of water for 20 minutes and added to the bath water.

Homeopathic Dosage: 5 to 10 drops 1 to 3 times daily; 1 tablet or 5 to 10 globules; injection solution 1 ml 1/week sc (HAB1).

Storage: The herb must be protected from light and moisture. The essential oil should not be stored in synthetic containers.

LITERATURE

Chandler RF et al., (1982) Econ Bot 36 (2): 203.

Cuong BN et al., (1979) Phytochemistry 18: 331.

Czygan FC, Das ätherische Öl der Schafgarbe. In: DAZ 134(3):228. 1994.

Czygan FC, Schafgarbe: Alte Heilpflanze neu untersucht. In: PZ 139(6):439. 1994.

Falk AJ et al., (1974) Lloydia 37: 598.

Falk AJ et al., (1975) J Pharm Sci 64: 1838.

Kastner U et al., Anti-edematous activity of sesquiterepene lactones from different taxa of the Achillea millefolium group. In: PM 59(7)69. 1993.

Kastner U, Glasl S, Jurenitsch J, Achillea millefolium - ein Gallentherapeuticum. In: ZPT 16(1):34-36. 1995.

Kastner U, Glasl S, Jurentisch J, Kubelka W, Isolation and structure elucidation of the main proazulenes of the cultivar Achillea collina ''Proa''. In: PM 58(7)18. 1992.

Kastner U, Jurenitsch J, Lehner S, Baumann A, Robien W, Kubelka W, The major proazulenes from Achillea collina BECKER: a revision of structure. In: Pharm Pharmacol Letters 1(1):27. 1991.

Müller-Jakic B et al., In vitro inhibition of cyclooxygenase and 5-lipoxygenase by alkamides from Echinacea and Achillea species. In: PM 60:37. 1994.

Ochir G, Budesinsky M, Motl O, 3-Oxa-guaianolides from Achillea-millefolium. In: PH 30(12):4163. 1991.

Orth M, van den Berg T, Czygan FC, Die Schafgarbe - Achillea millefolium L. In: ZPT 15(3):176-182. 1994.

Schmidt M, Phytotherapie: Pflanzliche Gallenwegstherapeutika. In: DAZ 135(8):680-682. 1995.

Smolenski SJ et al., (1967) Lloydia 30: 144.

Verzár-Petri G et al., (1979) Herba Hung. 18 (2): 83.

Further information in:

Hänsel R, Keller K, Rimpler H, Schneider G (Hrsg.), Hagers Handbuch der Pharmazeutischen Praxis, 5. Aufl., Bde 4-6 (Drogen), Springer Verlag Berlin, Heidelberg, New York, 1992-1994.

Hausen B, Allergiepflanzen, Pflanzenallergene, ecomed Verlagsgesellsch. mbH, Landsberg 1988.

Madaus G, Lehrbuch der Biologischen Arzneimittel, Bde 1-3, Nachdruck, Georg Olms Verlag Hildesheim 1979.

Schulz R, Hänsel R, Rationale Phytotherapie, Springer Verlag Heidelberg 1996.

Steinegger E, Hänsel R, Pharmakognosie, 5. Aufl., Springer Verlag Heidelberg 1992.

Teuscher E, Lindequist U, Biogene Gifte - Biologie, Chemie, Pharmakologie, 2. Aufl., Fischer Verlag Stuttgart 1994.

Teuscher E, Biogene Arzneimittel, 5. Aufl., Wiss. Verlagsges. Stuttgart 1997.

Wagner H, Wiesenauer M, Phytotherapie. Phytopharmaka und pflanzliche Homöopathika, Fischer-Verlag, Stuttgart, Jena, New York 1995.

Wichtl M (Hrsg.), Teedrogen, 4. Aufl., Wiss. Verlagsges. Stuttgart 1997.

Yellow Dock

Rumex crispus

TRADE NAMES

Yellow Dock (available from a number of manufacturers), Yellowdock, Alcohol Free Yellow Dock, Yellow Dock Root, Wild Countryside Yellow Dock Root

DESCRIPTION

Medicinal Parts: The medicinal parts are the fresh and dried roots.

Flower and Fruit: The green androgynous flowers are in panicles. The inner tips of the perigone are entire-margined, orbicular or ovate. When the fruit ripens they are slightly longer than wide. Otherwise the flower is the same as R. acetosa in that there is a 6-tepalled perigone. The inner tepals are longer than the outer ones and grow closer together. When the fruit ripens they are usually red-tinged, membranous, entire-margined and have a downward curved, scale-like welt at the base. The outer 3 tips are revolute. There are 6 stamens and 3 styles with paintbrush-like stigmas. The fruit is a triangular, brown-black nut, which is enclosed by the wing-like enlarged inner tepal.

Leaves, Stem and Root: The plant is about 100 cm high and has a carrot-like rhizome. The roots are 20 to 30 cm long, about 1.25 cm thick, fleshy and are not usually branched. The roots are rusty brown on the outside, whitish on the inside and have a relatively thick bark. The stems are angular, grooved and usually branched from the base up. The lower leaves are large and have flat petioles. They are supported at the base or almost cordate, lanceolate acute, undate-curly at the margins and alternate. The upper leaves are smaller and narrow-lanceolate.

Habitat: The plant is indigenous to Europe and Africa, but grows wild in many regions of the world.

Production: Yellow Dock root is the fresh root harvested in spring from Rumex acetosa.

Other Names: Curled Dock

ACTIONS AND PHARMACOLOGY

COMPOUNDS

Oxalates: oxalic acid, calcium oxalate

Tannins (3-6%)

Flavonoids: including among others, quercitrin

Anthracene derivatives (0.9-2.5%): anthranoids, aglycones physcion, chryosphanol, emodin, aloe-emodin, rhein, their glucosides

Naphthalene derivatives: neopodin 8-glucoside, lapodin

EFFECTS

No documentation is available, but laxative, alterative and mildly tonic characteristics have been attributed to Rumex crispus.

INDICATIONS AND USAGE

Unproven Uses: Yellow Dock is used for acute and chronic inflammation of the nasal passages and respiratory tract. It is also used as an adjuvant in antibacterial therapy. The plant has traditionally been used like the Red Dock (R. aquatica) for its similar properties, in decoctions for scurvy and other skin eruptions, and as a 'blood cleanser.' It is also used as an astringent for hemorrhoids and pulmonary bleeding. It has been used as a remedy for jaundice and a tonic for the stomach.

Homeopathic Uses: Uses in homeopathy include inflammation of the mucous membranes of the respiratory tract, asthmatic conditions, tracheal cough and morning diarrhea.

PRECAUTIONS AND ADVERSE REACTIONS

No health hazards or side effects are known in conjunction with the proper administration of designated therapeutic dosages. However, mucus membrane irritation, accompanied by vomiting is possible following intake of the fresh rhizome, due to its anthrone content. The anthrones are oxidized to anthraquinones after dehydration and storage.

OVERDOSAGE

Oxalate poisonings are conceivable primarily with the consumption of numerous leaves eaten as salad. One case of death following consumption of a soup made from the leaves of the curled Yellow Dock has been described (see Frohne).

DOSAGE

Mode of Administration: Preparations are available in ground form or as an extract.

How Supplied:

Capsules — 500 mg, 505 mg

Liquid — 1:1

LITERATURE

Fairbairn JW, El Muhtadi FJ, (1972) Phytochemistry 11:263.

Frohne D, Pfänder HJ, Giftpflanzen - Ein Handbuch für Apotheker, Toxikologen und Biologen, 4. Aufl., Wiss. Verlags-Ges. Stuttgart 1997.

Grznar K, Rada K, Farmaceut Obzor 47:195. 1978

Kern W, List PH, Hörhammer L (Hrsg.), Hagers Handbuch der Pharmazeutischen Praxis, 4. Aufl., Bde. 1-8: Springer Verlag Berlin, Heidelberg, New York, 1969.

Madaus G, Lehrbuch der Biologischen Arzneimittel, Bde 1-3, Nachdruck, Georg Olms Verlag Hildesheim 1979.

Midiwo JO, Runkunga GM, (1985) Phytochemistry 24(6):1390.

Morton JF, An Atlas of Medicinal Plants of Middle America, Charles C Thomas Pub. USA 1981.

Sharma M et al., Indian J Chem Sect B 15B:544. 1977.

Teuscher E, Lindequist U, Biogene Gifte - Biologie, Chemie, Pharmakologie, 2. Aufl., Fischer Verlag Stuttgart 1994.

Koukol J, Dugger WM Jr, Anthocyanin formation as a response to ozone and smog treatment in Rumex crispus, L. Plant Physiol, 42:1023-4, Jul 1967.

Yellow Gentian

Gentiana lutea

DESCRIPTION

Medicinal Parts: The medicinal parts of the plant are the dried or fresh underground plant organs.

Flower and Fruit: The flowers are yellow, terminal, pedicled and axillary in cyme-like false whorls. The calyx is deeply divided in 2. The corolla is rotate and divided almost to the base into 5 or 6 lanceolate tips. There are 5 stamens with 8 mm long anthers and 1 superior ovary. The fruit is 6 cm long and capsule shaped. The numerous seeds are flat, oblong or round, with a membranous edge.

Leaves, Stem and Root: Yellow Gentian is a completely glabrous perennial plant that grows to 140 cm high. The rhizome has a number of heads, and the top of the rhizome can attain the thickness of an arm. The main root is a taproot, which grows up to 1 m long. The stem is round, unbranched, hollow and grooved in the upper region to finger thickness. The leaves are elliptical, bluish-green, have strongly curved ribs and grow up to 30 cm long and 15 cm wide.

Characteristics: The drug has a weak, sweetish odor. It tastes metallic/sweet at first, then bitter.

Habitat: The plant is indigenous to the mountainous regions of central and southern European, and cultivated in many other regions.

Production: The roots are collected from spring through October, cleaned and swiftly dried. Extended, slower drying causes the roots to ferment. The roots become brittle through drying, swollen and spongy through contact with moisture.

Not to be Confused With: The roots of Rumex alpinus or Gentiana asclepiadea

Other Names: Bitter Root, Bitterwort, Gentian Root, Pale Gentian

ACTIONS AND PHARMACOLOGY

COMPOUNDS

Iridoide monoterpenes (bitter principles): amarogentin (determines the value), gentiopricroside, swertiamarine, sweroside

Monosaccharides/Oligosaccharides: saccharose, gentianose (somewhat bitter), gentiobiose (bitter)

Pyrridine alkaloids

Xanthone derivatives (colored yellow): including gentisin, gentisein, isogentisin, 1,3,7-trimethoxyxanthone

Volatile oil (traces)

EFFECTS

The essential active principles are the bitter substances contained in the herb. These bring about a reflex stimulation of the taste receptors, leading to increased secretion of saliva and the digestive juices. Gentian root is therefore considered to be not simply a pure bitter, but also a roborant and tonic. There is also a possible cholagogic effect, although it is not clear if the mode of action is sensory-reflexive. In addition, a fungistatic effect has been proven for the gentian extract.

INDICATIONS AND USAGE

Approved by Commission E:

- Dyspeptic complaints
- Loss of appetite

Unproven Uses: Folk medicine uses of the drug include as a tonic and in teas to stimulate bile secretion and alleviate loss of appetite, fullness and flatulence.

Homeopathic Uses: Yellow Gentian is used in homeopathy for digestive disorders.

CONTRAINDICATIONS

The drug's stimulation of gastric juice secretion rules out its administration in the presence of stomach or duodenal ulcers.

PRECAUTIONS AND ADVERSE REACTIONS

Health risks or side effects following the proper administration of designated therapeutic dosages are not recorded.

DOSAGE

Mode of Administration: Comminuted drug and dried extracts for infusions and teas. Forms of commercial pharmaceutical preparations include digestives, drops and coated tablets.

Preparation: Tea is prepared by pouring boiling water over 1/2 teaspoon of the drug (1 to 2 g) and allowing it to steep for 5 to 10 minutes. The tea may be sweetened with honey to alleviate the bitter taste. Decoctions are made using 1 g of the drug to 1 cup boiled water.

Daily Dosage: The average single dose is 1 g of the drug; daily dose is 2 to 4 g. The average daily dose of tincture is 1 to 4 ml 3 times daily. Liquid extract: 2 to 4 g; root: 2 to 4 g. A one-cup dose of cold or lukewarm tea is taken several times a day, including 1/2 hour before meals.

Homeopathic Dosage: 5 drops, 1 tablet or 10 globules every 30 to 60 minutes (acute) or 1 to 3 times daily (chronic); parenterally: 1 to 2 ml sc acute, 3 times daily: chronic: once a day (HAB1)

Storage: The drug must be stored away from light sources.

LITERATURE

Chialva F et al., Z Lebensm Unters Forsch 182:212. 1986.

Hayashi T, Yamagishi T, PH 27:3696. 1988.

Schultze J, Dissertation T.U. München. 1980.

Wagner H, Münzing-Vasirian K, DAZ 115:1233. 1975.

Further information in:

Hänsel R, Keller K, Rimpler H, Schneider G (Hrsg.), Hagers Handbuch der Pharmazeutischen Praxis, 5. Aufl., Bde 4-6 (Drogen), Springer Verlag Berlin, Heidelberg, New York, 1992-1994.

Madaus G, Lehrbuch der Biologischen Arzneimittel, Bde 1-3, Nachdruck, Georg Olms Verlag Hildesheim 1979.

Schulz R, Hänsel R, Rationale Phytotherapie, Springer Verlag Heidelberg 1996.

Steinegger E, Hänsel R, Pharmakognosie, 5. Aufl., Springer Verlag Heidelberg 1992.

Teuscher E, Biogene Arzneimittel, 5. Aufl., Wiss. Verlagsges. mbH Stuttgart 1997.

Wagner H, Wiesenauer M, Phytotherapie. Phytopharmaka und pflanzliche Homöopathika, Fischer-Verlag, Stuttgart, Jena, New York 1995.

Wichtl M (Hrsg.), Teedrogen, 4. Aufl., Wiss. Verlagsges. Stuttgart 1997.

Yellow Jessamine

Gelsemium sempervirens

DESCRIPTION

Medicinal Parts: The medicinal part of the plant is the dried rhizome with the roots.

Flower and Fruit: Yellow, strongly perfumed, 2.5 to 4 cm, funnel-shaped, long flowers grow in axillary or terminal cymes of 2 to 5 blooms. The fruit consists of 2 separable, connected pods containing numerous flat-winged seeds.

Leaves, Stem and Root: The plant is a perennial evergreen vine on a tortuous, smooth root with a thin bark and woody center, showing broad medullary rays. The stem is slender, woody and up to 6 m high. The leaves are opposite, lanceolate to ovate-lanceolate, short-stemmed, entire-margined, 2.5 to 10 cm long, dark green above and paler green beneath.

Habitat: The plant is indigenous to southern North America, along the coast from Virginia to Florida and Mexico.

Production: Gelsemium root consists of the rhizome and roots of Gelsemium sempervirens.

Not to be Confused With: The plant should not be confused with yellow flowering Jasmine (Jasminum odoratissimum), which is also called True Yellow Jasmine or Gelsemium.

Other Names: Gelsemin, Woodbine, Yellow Jasmine, False Jasmin

ACTIONS AND PHARMACOLOGY

COMPOUNDS

Indole alkaloids: main alkaloid gelsemin, including among others 21-oxygelsemine, gelsemicin, gelsidin, gelsevirin, sempervirin

Hydroxycoumarins: including scopoletine (gelseminic acid) , fabiatrin

Anthracene derivatives: emodin monomethyl ether

Volatile oil

EFFECTS

In animal tests, the following effects on the autonomic nervous system have been documented: inhibition of cholinesterase; cardiac-circulatory effects (vasodilatory, hypotensive); a bronchodilatory effect on respiration; an effect on the smooth muscle; and an analgesic effect, as well as mydriasis on rabbits' eyes.

INDICATIONS AND USAGE

Unproven Uses: The drug is used for neuralgia, headache, gastric disorders, nervous stomach, feelings of fullness and heartburn.

CONTRAINDICATIONS

Particular dangers are associated with administration of the drug in the presence of cardiac weakness.

PRECAUTIONS AND ADVERSE REACTIONS

Health risks following the proper administration of designated therapeutic dosages are not recorded. The following side effects could appear: heaviness of the eyelids, inhibition of movement of the eyeball, double vision, hypocyclosis, dryness of the mouth and vomiting. Particular dangers lie with administration in the presence of cardiac weakness.

OVERDOSAGE

Poisonings through overdosages, sometimes with fatal outcome, are possible. Extracts corresponding to approximately 0.5 g of the drug can kill a child, 2 to 3 g can be fatal for an adult. Initial side effects can include heaviness of the eyelids, inhibition of movement of the eyeball, double vision, hypocyclosis, dryness of the mouth, swallowing difficulties or vomiting. They may progress to symptoms of poisoning that can include headache, dizziness, loss of speech ability, vision weakness or double vision, pupil enlargement, trembling of the limbs, paralysis or stiffening of the muscles, cyanosis, shortness of breath and coma.

The therapy for poisonings, following stomach emptying (gastric lavage with burgundy-colored potassium permanganate solution), consists of prophylaxis for shock, diazepam for spasms, electrolyte replenishment and sodium bicarbonate infusions for any acidosis that may arise. Intubation and oxygen respiration may also be necessary.

DOSAGE

Medicinal preparations are obsolete. Yellow Jessamine is currently used in homeopathic dilutions only.

LITERATURE

Frohne D, Pfänder HJ, Giftpflanzen - Ein Handbuch für Apotheker, Toxikologen und Biologen,

4. Aufl., Wiss. Verlagsges. mbH Stuttgart 1997.

Jensen SR et al., (1987) Phytochemistry 26(6):1725.

Kern W, List PH, Hörhammer L (Hrsg.), Hagers Handbuch der Pharmazeutischen Praxis, 4. Aufl., Bde 1-8, Springer Verlag Berlin, Heidelberg, New York, 1969.

Leung AY, Encyclopedia of Common Natural Ingredients Used in Food Drugs and Cosmetics, John Wiley & Sons Inc., New York 1980.

Lewin L, Gifte und Vergiftungen, 6. Aufl., Nachdruck, Haug Verlag, Heidelberg 1992.

Madaus G, Lehrbuch der Biologischen Arzneimittel, Bde 1-3, Nachdruck, Georg Olms Verlag Hildesheim 1979.

Roth L, Daunderer M, Kormann K, Giftpflanzen, Pflanzengifte, 4. Aufl., Ecomed Fachverlag Landsberg Lech 1993.

Wagner H, Wiesenauer M, Phytotherapie. Phytopharmaka und pflanzliche Homöopathika, Fischer-Verlag, Stuttgart, Jena, New York 1995.

Wenkert E et al., (1971) Experientia 28:377.

Yellow Lupin

Lupinus luteus

DESCRIPTION

Medicinal Parts: The medicinal parts are the seeds and the aerial parts of the plant.

Flower and Fruit: The terminal flowers are almost sessile. They are arranged in numerous, distinct whorls. They have dropping, silky-haired bracts. The corolla is bright yellow with a blunted boat-shaped tip. The fruit is an oblong-lanceolate, 5 to 7 cm by 1 cm, densely pubescent pod with nodes. It contains 4 to 7 yellowish, reddish-white, black or dark violet marbled seeds 5.5 to 6.5 mm long.

Leaves, Stem and Root: The plant is an annual with up to a 1 m long taproot, which contains numerous lateral roots. The stem is light green and pubescent with numerous side shoots. The 5 to 10 leaves are oblong-obovate to lanceolate, 4 to 8 cm long, acuminate and pubescent on both sides.

Habitat: The plant is indigenous to Europe, Asia, and North and South America.

Production: Lupin herb and seeds are the aerial part and seeds of Lupinus luteus and other Lupinus species.

ACTIONS AND PHARMACOLOGY

COMPOUNDS: IN THE FOLIAGE

Quinolizidine alkaloids (0.6-1.6%): sparteine (55-70%), lupinine (20-30%), p-cumaroyllupinine (10%); in cultivated strains (sweet lupins), alkaloid content is 0.01-0.8%

COMPOUNDS: IN THE SEEDS

Quinolizidine alkaloid (0.4-3.3%): lupinine (60%), sparteine (30%); in some cultivated strains, gramine; in cultivated strains (sweet lupins), alkaloid content is less than 0.1%

Fatty oil (4-6%)

Carbohydrates: including stachyose (6%)

Proteins (36-48%)

EFFECTS

There has been no research on the effects of the drug; however, an anthelmintic effect has been established for the constituents lupinin and benzolylupinin.

INDICATIONS AND USAGE

Unproven Uses: Yellow Lupin is used externally for ulcers. It is used internally for urinary tract disorders and worm infestation.

PRECAUTIONS AND ADVERSE REACTIONS

See Overdosage section.

OVERDOSAGE

Symptoms of poisoning include salivation, swallowing difficulties, vomiting, diarrhea, headaches, hypocyclosis, double vision, cardiac rhythm disorders and prickling sensation in the extremities. In cases of severe poisoning, symptoms include ascending paralysis and possible death through respiratory failure within a few hours. The intake of a single seed of a bitter lupin is said to be toxic for a child. In one case, a small child died following intake of several seeds. The intake of more than one pod of the plant or 10 seeds by an adult is said to trigger vomiting and should be treated with administration of activated charcoal. Following gastrointestinal emptying (inducement of vomiting, gastric lavage with burgundy-colored potassium permanganate solution, sodium sulfate) and installation of activated charcoal, the therapy for severe poisonings consists of electrolyte substitution, treating possible cases of acidosis with sodium bicarbonate infusions, and administering orciprenaline or lidocaine for cardiac rhythm disorders. In case of shock, plasma volume expanders should be administered. Intubation and oxygen respiration may also be necessary.

The lupinosis seen in animals is caused by mycotoxins that are formed from the fungus *Phomopsis leptostromiformis*, which can live as an endophyte in lupins.

DOSAGE

Mode of Administration: The drug is used internally as an infusion, and externally in poultices.

LITERATURE

Frohne D, Pfänder HJ, Giftpflanzen - Ein Handbuch für Apotheker, Toxikologen und Biologen, 4. Aufl., Wiss. Verlags-Ges Stuttgart 1997.

Kern W, List PH, Hörhammer L (Hrsg.), Hagers Handbuch der Pharmazeutischen Praxis, 4. Aufl., Bde 1-8, Springer Verlag Berlin, Heidelberg, New York, 1969.

Lewin L, Gifte und Vergiftungen, 6. Aufl., Nachdruck, Haug Verlag, Heidelberg 1992.

Plakhota VA, Berezyuk NK, Oleinik GV, Boiko VP, Poisoning of animals with lupins. In: Veterinariya, Moscow, USSR, No. 8, 79-81. 1966.

Roth L, Daunderer M, Kormann K, Giftpflanzen, Pflanzengifte, 4. Aufl., Ecomed Fachverlag Landsberg Lech 1993.

Schmeller Th et al., Binding of quinolizidine alkaloids to nicotinic and muscarinic acetylcholine receptors. In: JNP 57(9):1316-1319. 1994.

Seeger R, Lupanin und Anagyrin. In: DAZ 133(17):35. 1993.

Teuscher E, Lindequist U, Biogene Gifte - Biologie, Chemie, Pharmakologie, 2. Aufl., Fischer Verlag Stuttgart 1994.

Yellow Toadflax

Linaria vulgaris

DESCRIPTION

Medicinal Parts: The medicinal part is the fresh or dried herb.

Flower and Fruit: The flowers are in terminal dense racemes. They are sulfur yellow and remain closed until a bee gains entry. The calyx is only fused at the base and is 5-tipped. The corolla has a long sharp spur and is bilabiate with orange edges. There are 2 large and 2 small stamens and 1 superior ovary. The fruit is an orbicular, dry capsule with some chambers, which open when ripe, flinging out the seeds. The seeds are flattened and are in the middle of a circular wing.

Leaves, Stem and Root: A number of slim, glabrous, erect, simple stems 30 to 60 cm high grow from a perennial creeping root. The numerous leaves are alternate, sessile, very long and narrow. The leaves and stems are pale blue and completely glabrous.

Habitat: The plant is indigenous to the northern hemisphere and the southwest U.S.

Production: True Toadflax is the flowering herb of Linaria vulgaris.

Other Names: Fluellin, Pattens and Clogs, Flaxweed, Ramsted, Snapdragon, Churnstaff, Dragon-Bushes, Brideweed, Toadpipe, Yellow Rod, Larkspur Lion's Mouth, Devil's Ribbon, Eggs and Collops, Devil's Head, Pedlar's Basket, Gallwort, Rabbits, Doggies, Calves' Snout, Eggs and Bacon, Buttered Haycocks, Monkey Flower, Butter and Eggs, Pennywort

ACTIONS AND PHARMACOLOGY

COMPOUNDS

Iridoide monoterpenes: chief component - antirrhinoside

Flavonoids: including among others linarin, pectolinarin, linariin (pectolinarigenin-7-rhamnoglucoside- acetate)

Aurones: including among others aureusin, bracteatin-6-O-glucoside

Quinazoline alkaloids: peganine (vasicin)

EFFECTS

The main active agents are the flavon glycosides linarin and pectolinarin, pectin, phytosterol, tannic acid and vitamin C.

The drug is anti-inflammatory. Diaphoretic and diuretic effects have been documented.

INDICATIONS AND USAGE

Unproven Uses: Yellow Toadflax is used internally to aid digestion problems and urinary tract disorders.

Externally, the herb is used for hemorrhoids, ablution of festering wounds, skin rashes and ulcus cruris.

PRECAUTIONS AND ADVERSE REACTIONS

No health hazards or side effects are known in conjunction with the proper administration of designated therapeutic dosages.

DOSAGE

Mode of Administration: The powdered form and the extract are used as a diuretic and a mild laxative (tea). Externally the herb is used in poultices.

Preparation: Tea infusion is prepared from 1 to 2 teaspoonfuls of the drug and 2 to 4 cups of boiling water left to draw for 18 minutes.

Daily Dosage: Drink the tea during the course of the day.

LITERATURE

Hegnauer R, Chemotaxonomie der Pflanzen, Bde 1-11, Birkhäuser Verlag Basel, Boston, Berlin 1962-1997.

Ilieva E et al., 5-O-Allosylantirrinoside from Linaria species. In: PH 32:1068. 1993.

Kern W, List PH, Hörhammer L (Hrsg.), Hagers Handbuch der Pharmazeutischen Praxis, 4. Aufl., Bde. 1-8, Springer Verlag Berlin, Heidelberg, New York, 1969.

Madaus G, Lehrbuch der Biologischen Arzneimittel, Bde 1-3, Nachdruck, Georg Olms Verlag Hildesheim 1979.

Yerba Santa

Eriodictyon californicum

TRADE NAMES

Yerba Santa Resin-Rich Leaf (available from numerous manufacturers and as combination product)

DESCRIPTION

Medicinal Parts: The medicinal parts are the dried leaves.

Flower and Fruit: The flowers are tubular to funnel-shaped, lavender or white and clustered at the top of the plant. The calyx is ciliate. The fruit is a small, oval, grayish-brown seed capsule containing shriveled, almost black seeds.

Leaves, Stem and Root: The plant is a 2.5 m high, sticky, evergreen shrub, with woody rhizomes. The trunk is smooth and usually branched near the ground. It is completely covered in sticky resin. The leaves are up to 15 cm long and about 2 cm broad. They are thick, coriaceous, glabrous, greenish white, lanceolate and irregularly dentate at the margins. The upper surface appears to be varnished with resin, the lower surface is reticulate and tomentose.

Characteristics: The taste is balsamic and the odor, pleasant and aromatic.

Habitat: The plant grows in California, Oregon and parts of Mexico.

Production: Yerba Santa is the aerial part of Eriodictyon californicum.

Other Names: Bear's Weed, Consumptive's Weed, Eriodictyon, Gum Bush, Holy Herb, Mountain Balm, Sacred Herb, Tarweed

ACTIONS AND PHARMACOLOGY

COMPOUNDS

Flavonoids: including eriodictyonin, eriodictyol, chrysoeriodictyol, xanthoeriodictyol

Resinous substances: made up of flavonone and flavone aglycones

Volatile oil (very little)

Tannins

EFFECTS

Yerba Santa is mildly diuretic and masks bitter tastes.

INDICATIONS AND USAGE

Unproven Uses: The drug is used as a constituent of antiasthmatic treatments and application by brush (painted on) to counteract bitter tastes.

PRECAUTIONS AND ADVERSE REACTIONS

Health risks or side effects following the proper administration of designated therapeutic dosages are not recorded.

DOSAGE

Mode of Administration: As an additive to mask bitter flavors and for painting on as Tinctura Eriodictyonis.

How Supplied:

Liquid — 1:5

LITERATURE

Johnson ND, Biochem Syst Ecol 11:211. 1983.

Kern W, List PH, Hörhammer L (Hrsg.), Hagers Handbuch der Pharmazeutischen Praxis, 4. Aufl., Bde 1-8, Springer Verlag Berlin, Heidelberg, New York, 1969.

Liu YL, Ho DK, Cassady JM, Isolation of potential cancer chemopreventive agents from Eriodictyon californicum. In: JNP 55(3):357-363. 1992.

Yew

Taxus baccata

DESCRIPTION

Medicinal Parts: The medicinal parts are the fresh leaves, the branch twig tips, and the branches.

Flower and Fruit: The flowers are inconspicuous and dioecious. The male florets appear in autumn in yellowish catkins in the axils of the annual needle. The female florets, with only 1 pistil, are on short pedicles, which have scale-like high leaves. The hard, pea-sized, dark-brown seed is surrounded by a crimson, pulpy, beaker-shaped, sweet and edible aril.

Leaves, Stem and Root: The Yew may be a bush or small tree approximately 17 m high with a trunk diameter of over 1 m. The trunk has red-brown bark. The numerous branches are crowded and evergreen. The needles are 2 to 3 cm long, arranged in double rows, soft and acute. They are glossy dark green above, have a distinct midrib, and are lighter green beneath, matte, with no resin.

Characteristics: Yew is poisonous.

Habitat: The plant is common in large areas of Europe as far as Anatolia and Sicily.

Production: Yew leaves are the needles of Taxus baccata.

Other Names: Chinwood

ACTIONS AND PHARMACOLOGY

COMPOUNDS

Diterpene esters of the taxane-type (mixture is known as taxine, 0.6-2.0%): including among others, taxine A, taxine B, taxol

Flavonoids: including among others, sciadopytisin, ginkgetin, sequoia flavone (biflavonoids)

EFFECTS

In animal experiments, the taxin, a mixture of different ester alkaloids, leads to an improvement in cardiac metabolism. The motility-inhibiting effect may be attributable to the biflavonoid fraction. In higher doses the drug is cardiotoxic and can cause tachycardiac arrhythmia leading to diastolic cardiac arrest.

INDICATIONS AND USAGE

Unproven Uses: The cooked Yew leaves are used to promote menstruation; to treat diphtheria, epilepsy, tapeworm, and tonsillitis; and as an abortifacient. The plants are highly toxic and their use is not recommended.

Homeopathic Uses: The drug is used for poor digestion and skin pustules.

CONTRAINDICATIONS

The drug is considered an abortifacient and therefore should not be used during pregnancy.

PRECAUTIONS AND ADVERSE REACTIONS

General: The drug is severely toxic: 50-100 gm Yew needles (fresh weight) are fatal for an adult. The red seed coat of the berries—although not the green seed—is free of toxic taxane derivatives.

Use in Pregnancy: The drug is used as an abortifacient.

OVERDOSAGE

Symptoms of poisoning include queasiness, vomiting, severe abdominal pain, and feelings of vertigo, followed later by unconsciousness, mydriasis, reddening of the lips, tachycardia, and superficial breathing. Death results from asphyxiation and diastolic cardiac arrest.

Following gastrointestinal emptying, (inducement of vomiting, gastric lavage with burgundy-colored potassium permanganate solution, sodium sulphate), and use of activated charcoal, treatment for poisonings consists of treating spasms with diazepam or barbital (i.v.). In case of shock, plasma volume expanders should be infused. The administration of lidocaine has proven effective in cardiac rhythm disorders. Monitoring of kidney function, blood coagulation and liver values is necessary. Intubation and oxygen respiration may also be necessary.

DOSAGE

Mode of Administration: Yew is used in homeopathic dilutions of the mother tincture.

Homeopathic Dosage: 5 drops, 1 tablet or 10 globules, every 30 to 60 minutes (acute) or 1 to 3 times daily (chronic); parenterally: 1 to 2 ml sc, acute: 3 times daily; chronic: once a day (HAB1).

Storage: The mother tincture should be protected from light.

LITERATURE

Hoc S, Onkologie: Taxol, ein pflanzliches Zytostatikum. In: DAZ 133(26):2400. 1993.

Hof-Mussler S, Eiben-Zytostatikum Taxol bei Ovarialkarzinom. In: DAZ 133(1):42. 1993.

Jenniskens LHD, Identification of six taxine alkaloids from Taxus baccata needles. In: JNP 59(2):117-123. 1996.

Kelsey RG, Vance NC, Taxol and cephalomannine concentrations in the foliage and bark of shade-grown and sun-exposed Taxus baccata trees. In: JNP 55:912-917. 1992.

Kingston DGI, Sorties and surprises: unexpected reactions of taxol. In: PM 62, Abstracts of the 44th Ann Congress of GA, 5. 1996.

Kongreβbericht, Taxol in der onkologischen Therapie. In: ZPT 15(2):114. 1994.

Kubitschek J, Eibenwirkstoff gegen Malaria. In: PZ 140(8):684. 1995.

Ma W et al., New bioactive taxoids from cell cultures of Taxus baccata. In: JNP 57(1):116. 1994.

Mujumdar RB et al., (1972) Ind J Chem 10:677.

Poupat Ch et al., Noveau taxoide basique isolé des feuilles D'if, Taxus baccata: La 2-désacétyltaxine A. In: JNP 57(10):1468-1469. 1994.

Schneider B, Taxol, ein Arzneistoff der Eibe. In: DAZ 134(36):3389. 1994.

Vanek T et al., Study of the influence of year season on taxanes content in Taxus baccata bark. In: PM 59(7)99. 1993.

Vidensek N, Lim P, Campbell A, Carlson C, Taxol content in bark, wood, root, leaf, twig and seedling from several Taxus species. In: JNP 53:1609-1610. 1994.

Vohora Kumar, (1971) Planta Med 20:100.

Wasielewski S, Taxol, ein Zytostatikum aus der pazifischen Eibe. In: UPTA 7(12):914. 1993.

Further information in:

Frohne D, Pfänder HJ, Giftpflanzen - Ein Handbuch für Apotheker, Toxikologen und Biologen, 4. Aufl., Wiss. Verlags-Ges. Stuttgart 1997.

Hänsel R, Keller K, Rimpler H, Schneider G (Hrsg.), Hagers Handbuch der Pharmazeutischen Praxis, 5. Aufl., Bde 4-6 (Drogen): Springer Verlag Berlin, Heidelberg, New York, 1992-1994.

Lewin L, Gifte und Vergiftungen, 6. Aufl., Nachdruck, Haug Verlag, Heidelberg 1992.

Madaus G, Lehrbuch der Biologischen Arzneimittel, Bde 1-3, Nachdruck, Georg Olms Verlag Hildesheim 1979.

Roth L, Daunderer M, Kormann K, Giftpflanzen, Pflanzengifte, 4. Aufl., Ecomed Fachverlag Landsberg Lech 1993.

Teuscher E, Lindequist U, Biogene Gifte - Biologie, Chemie, Pharmakologie, 2. Aufl., Fischer Verlag Stuttgart 1994.

Teuscher E, Biogene Arzneimittel, 5. Aufl., Wiss. Verlagsges. Stuttgart 1997.

Yohimbe Bark

Pausinystalia yohimbe

TRADE NAMES

Yohimbe, Yohimbe Super Potent, Yohimbized 1000, Yocon Tablets, Actibine, Aphrobine, Testomar, Yohimex, Super Yohimbe Plus, Yohimbe Power Max 1500, Yohimbe Power Max for Women, Yohimbe Power Max 2000.

DESCRIPTION

Medicinal Parts: The medicinal part is the bark.

Flower and Fruit: The inflorescence consists of racemes of yellow blooms.

Leaves, Stem and Root: The evergreen tree grows up to 30 m in height. The bark is gray-brown, fissured and split, and is often spotted. The inner fracture is reddish brown and grooved. The leaves are oblong or elliptical.

Characteristics: The taste is bitter, and the plant is odorless.

Habitat: The plant grows in the jungles of west Africa, Cameroon, Congo and Gabon.

Production: Yohimbe bark consists of the dried bark of the trunk and/or branches of Pausinystalia yohimbe.

ACTIONS AND PHARMACOLOGY

COMPOUNDS

Indole alkaloids (2.7-5.9%): including among others yohimbine (quebrachine) and its stereoisomers alpha-yohimbine (rauwolscine), beta-yohimbine, and allo-yohimbine. Including also, ajamalicine, dihydroyohimbine, corynantheine, dihydrocorynantheine, corynanthine (rauhimbin)

Tannins

EFFECTS

Alpha 2-adrenergic Antagonist/Norepinephrine Release: Rauwolscine is a selective alpha 2-adrenergic receptor antagonist. Yohimbine increases plasma norepinephrine (NE) levels by stimulating the rate of norepinephrine release from sympathetic nerves (alpha 2-adrenergic antagonist) (Murburg, 1991). Plasma concentrations of 3-methoxy-4-hydroxyphenylglycol (MHPG), the major central nervous system metabolite of NE, also increases with yohimbine (Piletz, 1998). Central noradrenergic stimulation of yohimbine results in the enhancement of recall and recognition of emotional material (O'Carroll, 1999).

Analgesic Effects: Yohimbine significantly enhanced the overall analgesic effect of morphine with postoperative dental pain (Gear, 1995).

Clonidine Antagonism: Traditionally, yohimbine was thought to reverse the therapeutic effects of clonidine. One study demonstrated yohimbine reversed sedation and shortened the duration of analgesia associated with clonidine administered postoperatively. There was no effect on hypotension and bradycardia related to clonidine administration with yohimbine (Liu, 1993).

Epinephrine Effects: Yohimbine causes an increase in epinephrine release from the adrenals and results in a dose-dependent increase in plasma epinephrine (Murburg, 1991).

Improves Sexual Function: Because of the alpha-2 adrenergic blockade, the drug may be an effective treatment for sexual side effects, such as decrease libido and decreased sexual response, caused by selective serotonin reuptake inhibitors (Jacobsen, 1992; Hollander, 1992). There was no therapeutic response to yohimbine in women with hypoactive sexual desire (Piletz, 1998).

Cardiovascular/Pressor Effects: Yohimbine given in moderate doses increases systolic blood pressure in patients with orthostatic hypotension due to primary autonomic failure (Jordan, 1998). Yohimbine-induced enhancement of sympathetic tone in patients with neurally mediated syncope improves orthostatic tolerance (Mosqueda-Garcia, 1998).

Salivary Effects: Yohimbine (18 mg daily) increases salivary flow in patients treated with psychotropic drugs (tricyclic antidepressants or neuroleptics) suffering from xerostomia (Bagheri, 1997).

Miscellaneous Effects: Through enhancing inhibitory sympathetic input, yohimbine attenuates increases in colonic tone (Bharucha, 1997).

CLINICAL TRIALS

Non-organic Erectile Dysfunction

A double-blind, placebo-controlled clinical trial was conducted to determine the safety and efficacy of yohimbine hydrochloride in the treatment of nonorganic erectile dysfunction. Eighty-three patients were included in the intention-to-treat analysis. Yohimbine (10 mg three times daily) was administered orally for eight weeks. Subjective criteria included improvement in sexual desire, sexual satisfaction, frequency of sexual contacts, and quality of erection (penile rigidity) during sexual contact or intercourse. Objective criteria were based on improvement in penile rigidity determined by use of polysomnography in the sleep laboratory. Yohimbine was overall significantly more effective than placebo for response rate and was well tolerated (Vogt, 1970.

Mixed-type Erectile Dysfunction

The effect of yohimbine hydrochloride was evaluated in the treatment of mixed-type impotence. A randomized, double-blind, placebo-controlled, crossover trial included 29 patients administered either yohimbine hydrochloride 36 mg daily or placebo. The two groups received therapy for 25 days, then a washout period of 14 days, and finally, a switch of treatment groups for an additional 25 days. Positive clinical results were seen in 44% and 48% of patients in the yohimbine and placebo groups, respectively, with no significant difference between the groups (Kunelius, 1997).

Pressor Effects with Autonomic Failure

In 35 patients with severe orthostatic hypotension due to multiple system atrophy or pure autonomic failure, the effect was determined on seated systolic blood pressure (SBP) of placebo, phenylpropanolamine (12.5 mg and 25 mg), yohimbine (5.4 mg), indomethacin (50 mg), ibuprofen (600 mg), caffeine (250 mg), and methylphenidate (5 mg). The pressor response was significant for phenylpropanolamine, yohimbine, and indomethacin compared with placebo. In a subgroup of patients, the pressor effect was confirmed of phenylpropanolamine, yohimbine, and indomethacin corresponding to a significant increase in standing SBP. The pressor responses to ibuprofen, caffeine, and methylphenidate were not significantly different from placebo, and phenylpropanolamine and midodrine exerted similar pressor responses (Jordan, 1998).

INDICATIONS AND USAGE

FDA Approved Indications: Yohimbine Hydrochloride is indicated as a sympatholytic and mydriatic. Impotence has been successfully treated with Yohimbine in male patients with vascular or diabetic origins and psychogenic origins.

Unproven Uses: Yohimbe bark is used as an aphrodisiac, and for debility and exhaustion.

CONTRAINDICATIONS

Yohimbe bark is contraindicated in liver and kidney diseases.

PRECAUTIONS AND ADVERSE REACTIONS

General: Side effects that can appear include anxiety states, elevated blood pressure, exanthema, nausea, insomnia, tachycardia, tremor, and vomiting.

Posttraumatic Stress Disorder (PTSD): Yohimbine was reported to exacerbate anxiety/panic and PTSD-specific symptoms after oral ingestion of the drug (Southwick, 1999). Patients with PTSD consists of 2 subgroups, one with a sensitized noradrenergic system, and the other with a sensitized serotonergic system, and is why yohimbine-induced panic attacks occur in different patients (Southwick, 1997).

Hypertension: Yohimbine induced a significant increase in diastolic pressure, but only in hypertensive patients due to an alpha 2-adrenoreceptor desensitization or an alteration in the balance of alpha-adrenoreceptors in human hypertension (Musso, 1995).

Auditory Effects: The drug has been associated with a transient impairment in auditory sensory gating (Adler, 1994).

Salivation: Yohimbine significantly increases salivary flow in patients treated with psychotropic drugs (tricyclic antidepressants or neuroleptics) suffering from xerostomia (Bagheri, 1997).

Panic Disorder: Patients with agoraphobia with panic attacks had greater autonomic anxiety symptoms, increase in SBP and cortisol responses to yohimbine than healthy patients. Yohimbine also induced panic episodes in these patients (Gurguis, 1997).

Parkinson's Disease: Patients with Parkinson's Disease have demonstrated a vulnerability to yohimbine-induced somatic symptoms such as panic attacks (Richard, 1999).

Drug Interactions:

Naltrexone — Clinically used naltrexone doses alter sensitivity to yohimbine, and potentiates the drug's side effects, such as nervousness (Rosen, 1999).

Anti-hypertensive Medications — Because of the increase in diastolic pressure in hypertensive patients, caution should be taken with concomitant use of anti-hypertensive medications (Musso, 1995).

Ethanol — Intoxicating and anxiogenic effects of acute ethanol administration may be associated with increase norepinephrine turnover when administered concomitantly with yohimbine (McDougle, 1995).

OTC stimulants — These may have alpha-1 adrenergic receptor activity to potentiate hypertension when yohimbine is given concomitantly.

Morphine — The overall analgesic effect of morphine was significantly enhanced in the presence of yohimbine in one study (Gear, 1995).

OVERDOSAGE

Overdosage leads to salivation, mydriasis, evacuation, hypotension and disorders of the cardiac impulse-conducting system with negative-inotropic effect. Death occurs through cardiac failure.

Treatment of overdosage includes gastrointestinal emptying (inducement of vomiting, gastric lavage with burgundy-colored potassium permanganate solution, sodium sulfate) and administration of activated charcoal. For cardiac rhythm disorders, treat with lidocaine; possibly using physostigmine for its anticholinergic effect and electrolyte substitution. For cases of acidosis, treat with sodium bicarbonate infusions. In case of shock, plasma volume expanders should be infused.

DOSAGE

How Supplied:

Capsule — 500 mg

Liquid — 1000mg/ml

Tablet — 5.4 mg, 800 mg

Daily Dosage:

Erectile Dysfunction — Yohimbine hydrochloride was effective for nonorganic erectile dysfunction administered as 30 mg daily (10 mg three times daily). Given up to 30 mg daily and 36 mg daily, yohimbine, showed no effect for mixed-type impotence and erectile problems (Kunelius, 1997; Rowland, 1997). For erectile impotence, yohimbine 5.4 mg (1 tablet) three times daily is recommended, and if side effects of nausea, dizziness or nervousness are reported, reduce to one-half tablet three times daily. Gradually increase to 1 tablet three times daily and therapy should not exceed 10 weeks (Prod Info Yocon®, 1985).

Xerostomia Treatment — Yohimbine 6 mg three times daily has been effective for increasing salivary flow in patients treated with psychotropic drugs suffering from xerostomia (Bagheri, 1997).

LITERATURE

Adler LE; Hoffer L; Nagamoto HT et al. Yohimbine impairs P50 auditory sensory gating in normal subjects. Neuropsychopharmacology 1994 Jul;10(4):249-57.

Bagheri H; Schmitt L; Berlan M; Montastruc JL. A comparative study of the effects of yohimbine and anetholtrithione on salivary secretion in depressed patients treated with psychotropic drugs. Eur J Clin Pharmacol 1997;52(5):339-42.

Bharucha AE; Novak V; Camilleri M et al. Alpha 2-adrenergic modulation of colonic tone during hyperventilation. Am J Physiol 1997 Nov;273(5 Pt 1):G1135-40.

Buffum J, (1982) J Psychoactive Drugs 17:131.

Clark JT et al., Science 225:847.

Gear RW; Gordon NC; Heller PH; Levine JD. Enhancement of morphine analgesia by the alpha 2-adrenergic antagonist yohimbine. Neuroscience 1995 May;66(1):5-8.

Gurguis GN; Vitton BJ; Uhde TW. Behavioral, sympathetic and adrenocortical responses to yohimbine in panic disorder patients and normal controls. Psychiatry Res 1997 Jun 16;71(1):27-39.

Hollander E; McCarley A. Yohimbine treatment of sexual side effects induced by serotonin reuptake blockers. J Clin Psychiatry 1992 Jun;53(6):207-9.

Jordan J; Shannon JR; Biaggioni I et al. Contrasting actions of pressor agents in severe autonomic failure. Am J Med 1998 Aug;105(2):116-24.

Kunelius P; Hakkinen J; Lukkarinen O. Is high-dose yohimbine hydrochloride effective in the treatment of mixed-type impotence? A prospective, randomized, controlled double-blind crossover study. Urology 1997 Mar;49(3):441-4.

Liu N; Bonnet F; Delaunay L et al. Partial reversal of the effects of extradural clonidine by oral yohimbine in postoperative patients. Br J Anaesth 1993 May;70(5):515-8.

McDougle CJ; Krystal JH; Price LH et al. Noradrenergic response to acute ethanol administration in healthy subjects: comparison with intravenous yohimbine. Psychopharmacology (Berl) 1995 Mar;118(2):127-35.

Mosqueda-Garcia R; Fernandez-Violante R; Tank J et al. Yohimbine in neurally mediated syncope. Pathophysiological implications. J Clin Invest 1998 Nov 15;102(10):1824-30.

Murburg MM; Villacres EC; Ko GN; Veith RC. Effects of yohimbine on human sympathetic nervous system function. J Clin Endocrinol Metab 1991 Oct;73(4):861-5.

Musso NR; Vergassola C; Pende A; Lotti G. Yohimbine effects on blood pressure and plasma catecholamines in human hypertension. Am J Hypertens 1995 Jun;8(6):565-71.

Piletz JE; Segraves KB; Feng YZ et al. Plasma MHPG response to yohimbine treatment in women with hypoactive sexual desire. J Sex Marital Ther 1998 Jan-Mar;24(1):43-54.

Product Information Yocon® (yohimbine hydrochloride tablets). Glenwood, Tenafly, NJ, USA, 1985.

Richard IH; Szegethy E; Lichter D et al. Parkinson's disease: a preliminary study of yohimbine challenge in patients with anxiety. Clin Neuropharmacol 1999 May-Jun;22(3):172-5.

Rosen MI; Kosten TR; Kreek MJ. The effects of naltrexone maintenance on the response to yohimbine in healthy volunteers. Biol Psychiatry 1999 Jun 15;45(12):1636-45.

Rowland DL; Kallan K; Slob AK. Yohimbine, erectile capacity, and sexual response in men. Arch Sex Behav 1997 Feb;26(1):49-62.

Southwick SM; Morgan CA 3rd; Charney DS; High JR. Yohimbine use in a natural setting: effects on posttraumatic stress disorder. Biol Psychiatry 1999 Aug 1;46(3):442-4.

Southwick SM; Krystal JH; Bremner JD et al. Noradrenergic and serotonergic function in posttraumatic stress disorder. Arch Gen Psychiatry 1997 Aug;54(8):749-58.

Vogt HJ; Brandl P; Kockott G et al. Double-blind, placebo-controlled safety and efficacy trial with yohimbine hydrochloride in the treatment of nonorganic erectile dysfunction. Int J Impot Res 1997 Sep;9(3):155-61.

Further information in:

Kern W, List PH, Hörhammer L (Hrsg.), Hagers Handbuch der Pharmazeutischen Praxis, 4. Aufl., Bde. 1-8: Springer Verlag Berlin, Heidelberg, New York, 1969.

Lewin L, Gifte und Vergiftungen, 6. Aufl., Nachdruck, Haug Verlag, Heidelberg 1992.

Madaus G, Lehrbuch der Biologischen Arzneimittel, Bde 1-3, Nachdruck, Georg Olms Verlag Hildesheim 1979.

O'Carroll RE; Drysdale E; Cahill L et al. Stimulation of the noradrenergic system enhances and blockade reduces memory for emotional material in man. Psychol Med 1999 Sep;29(5):1083-8.

Roth L, Daunderer M, Kormann K, Giftpflanzen, Pflanzengifte, 4. Aufl., Ecomed Fachverlag Landsberg Lech 1993.

Southwick SM, Morgan CA 3rd, Charney DS, High JR. Yohimbine use in a natural setting: effects on posttraumatic stress disorder. VA CT Healthcare System, Psychiatry Service 116A, West Haven 06516, USA.

Steinegger E, Hänsel R, Pharmakognosie, 5. Aufl., Springer Verlag Heidelberg 1992.

Teuscher E, Biogene Arzneimittel, 5. Aufl., Wiss. Verlagsges. Stuttgart 1997.

Wagner H, Wiesenauer M, Phytotherapie. Phytopharmaka und pflanzliche Homöopathika, Fischer-Verlag, Stuttgart, Jena, New York, 1995.

Yucca filamentosa

See Adam's Needle

Zanthoxylum americanum

See Northern Prickly Ash

Zea mays

See Corn Silk

Zedoary

Curcuma zedoaria

TRADE NAMES

Turmeric Power, Turmeric Whole Rhizome, Turmeric Extract (available from numerous manufacturers and as a combination product)

DESCRIPTION

Medicinal Parts: The medicinal part is the dried tuberous part of the rhizome, cut in transverse slices or in longitudinal quarters.

Flower and Fruit: The inflorescences are on 5 to 15 cm long, obtuse and silky involucre bracts. The spike-like inflorescences are 7.5 to 12.5 cm long and 5 to 7.5 cm wide. The bracts bearing the flowers are ovate with revolute tips, pale green with a reddish border, densely punctuated with glands. There are more or less stiff hairs on the surface, in particular at the tip. The bracts at the tip of the inflorescence are 5 cm long, initially white, then pink to crimson. The flowers are pale yellow. The calyx is 8 mm long, obtuse and 3-tipped. The tips of the corolla are broadly triangular and pale pink at the extreme tips. The labellum is light yellow, fluorescent yellow in the center with very slightly reddish tinged borders at the lower part. The ovary is 4 to 5 mm long and very weakly pubescent. The fruit is an ovate, thin, smooth and irregularly opening capsule. The elliptical seeds have a white aril.

Leaves, Stem and Root: Curcuma zedoaria is a perennial, erect and leafy plant. The rhizome has a grayish outer surface and is ovate to pear-shaped, thick and palmately branched downwards. It is whitish-yellow, with numerous thin roots, and it has a strong smell of camphor. The roots are partially thickened to ovate, white tubers. The leaves, in groups of 4 and 6 on the rhizome, are up to 1 m long. The 20 to 60 cm long and 8 to 10 cm wide leaf blade is oblong-ovate, glabrous, and has a purple mark in the middle of the leaf.

Characteristics: The taste is bitter. The smell is like camphor and is reminiscent of cardamom and ginger.

Habitat: The plant is indigenous to northeast India and is also found in the Moluccas, the Philippines and New Guinea.

Production: Zedoary rhizome consists of the dried rhizome of Curcuma zedoaria and its preparations. After the root tubers have been harvested they are washed, cut and dried.

Other Names: Turmeric

ACTIONS AND PHARMACOLOGY

COMPOUNDS

Volatile oil (1.0-1.5%): chief components zingiberene, 1,8-cineole, D-camphor, D-camphene, D-borneol, alpha-pinene, also including among others curcumol, zederone, curcumeneol, curculone, furanodienone, isofuranodienone

Curcuminoids: curcumin, desmethoxycurcumin, bisdesmethoxycurcumin

Starch (50%)

EFFECTS

Main active principles: essential oil, tannins, mucilage, small-grained starch. In animal tests, the drug has a choleretic, mildly antacid and spasmolytic effect, as well as increasing intestinal transit time. The ethanol extract (main active principle p-methoxy cinnamic acid ethyl ester) is a strong fungicide. An anti-tumoral effect has also been proven.

INDICATIONS AND USAGE

Unproven Uses: Zedoary is used as a stomachic for digestive debility, colic and spasms (stomachic, carminative). In folk medicine, it is also used as a remedy for nervous diseases.

Indian Medicine: In India, the drug is used for loss of appetite, tuberculosis, wounds, leukodermia, fever, bronchitis and asthma.

PRECAUTIONS AND ADVERSE REACTIONS

General: No health hazards or side effects are known in conjunction with the proper administration of designated therapeutic dosages.

Pregnancy: Not to be used during pregnancy.

DOSAGE

Mode of Administration: Zeodary is available as solid and liquid dosage forms for oral intake.

How Supplied: Capsules: 300 mg, 450 mg; liquid: 1:4.

Preparation: Extracts of the drug are contained in numerous combination preparations for gastrointestinal indications and as cholagogues. To prepare an infusion, pour boiling water over 1 to 1.5 gm of comminuted or powdered drug, or put in cold water and strain after 3 to 5 minutes (1 teaspoonful = 3 gm of drug).

Daily Dosage: Drink 1 cup as an aromatic bitter at meals.

LITERATURE

Gupta SK et al., Lloydia 39:218-222. 1976.

Hänsel R, Keller K, Rimpler H, Schneider G (Hrsg.), Hagers Handbuch der Pharmazeutischen Praxis, 5. Aufl., Bde 4-6 (Drogen): Springer Verlag Berlin, Heidelberg, New York, 1992-1994.

Hikino H et al., (1970) Chem Pharm Bull 18:752.

Kuronayagi M, Natori S, Yakugaku Zasshi 90:1467-1470. 1970.

Latif MA et al., Br J Nutr 41:57. 1979.

Matthes HWD et al., (1980) Phytochemistry 19:2643.

Shiobara Y et al., (1985) Phytochemistry 24(11):2629.

Zingiber officinale

See Ginger

Zyzyphus jujube

See Jujube

Glossary

AB-DDR Minister für Gesundheitswesen der DDR (1987). Arzneibuch der DDR. 2nd Ed. Akademie-Verlag, Berlin.

abortifacient A drug or chemical that induces abortion.

achene A small 1-seeded fruit which has a pericarp attached to the seed at only one point.

acuminate Pointed or to taper to a slender point.

adaptogen A preparation that acts to strengthen the body and increase resistance to disease.

alterative Any drug used to favorably alter the course of an ailment and to restore health. To improve the excretion of wastes from the circulatory system.

amarum Bitters.

androgynous In botany, flowers with stamen and pistil in the same bunch.

annual A plant that completes its growth cycle in one year.

anthelmintic An agent or drug that is destructive to worms.

anther The part of the stamen that contains pollen.

antiphlogistic An agent that prevents or counteracts inflammation and fever.

antisialagogue An agent that prevents or counteracts the formation or flow of saliva.

Arg 66 6 Farmacopea Argentina 1966.

autumnalis In botany, referring to producing, gathering or harvesting in the autumn.

Belg IV Pharmacopée Belge IV (1930) + Suppl. to 1953, F. & N. Dantinne, Strée.

Belg V Pharmacopée Belge V (1962-1968), Vols. 1-3 + Suppl.

Belg VI Pharmacopée Belge VI (1982), J. Duculot-Gembloux.

BfArM German Federal Health Agency.

BHP 83 British Herbal Medicine Association (1983), British Herbal Pharmacopoeia. Megaron Press. Bournemouth.

BHP 90 British Herbal Medicine Association (1990), British Herbal Pharmacopoeia.

bitter An alcoholic liquid prepared by maceration or distillation of a bitter herb or herb part that is often used to improve appetite or digestion.

blood purification Removal of undesirable agents from the blood.

BP 68 British Pharmacopoeia XI (1968) + Suppl. 1971, The Pharmaceutical Press, London.

BP 88 British Pharmacopoeia XLI (1988), Her Majesty's Stationary Office, London.

BPC 79 The Pharmaceutical Codex (1979), The Pharmaceutical Press, London.

BPC XX British Pharmaceutical Codex X (1973) [IX (1986), VIII (1963), VII (1959) VI (1954), V (1949), IV (1934)].

bracteole A small leaf arising from the floral axis.

Brasil 1 Farmacopeia dos Estados Unidos do Brasil (1926).

Brasil 2 Farmacopeia dos Estados Unidos do Brasil (1959).

Brasil 3 Farmacopeia dos Estados Unidos do Brasil (1976).

brightening agent A substance added to the active constituents.

C1 10 parts mother tincture and 90 parts ethanol.

C2 (C3, C4, ...) C2 is 1 part C1 and 99 parts ethanol (the dilutions continue in a 1:99 fashion, each starting with the previous dilution as the 1 part fraction and adding 99 parts).

calculosis The condition or formation of calculi.

calyx The outer set of floral leaves consisting of fused or separate sepals.

campanulate Shaped like a bell.

capitulum A rounded or flattened cluster of sessile flowers.

capsule A closed container that contains seeds or spores.

carminative An aid to relieve gas from the alimentary canal. An agent that acts to relieve colic.

carpel A small pistil or seed vessel comprising the innermost whorl of a flower.

cataplasm A poultice or soft external application.

catarrh An inflammation of the air passages usually involving the nose, throat, or lungs.

catkin An ament or cattail-like spicate inflorescence bearing scaly bracts.

cauline Growing on the upper portion of a stem.

CF 49 Codex Francais = Pharmacopoea Gallica = Pharmacopée Francaise VII (1949).

ChinPIX The Pharmacopoeia Commission of PRC (1988), Pharmacopeia of the People's Medical Publishing House, Beijing.

cholagogue An agent that stimulates the flow of bile from the gallbladder to the duodenum.

choleretic An agent that stimulates the production of bile by the liver.

climacteric The syndrome of physical and psychic changes that occur during the transition to menopause.

comminuted To break or crush into small pieces.

Commission E Indications relating to the Commission E monographed as published by the German Federal Health Agency (BfArM).

cordate A heart-shaped leaf.

coriaceous Tough, strong, and leather-like.

corolla The inner set of floral leaves that consist of separate or fused leaves.

cortex In botany, the bark of a tree or the rind of a fruit.

cotyledon A seed leaf, or the first set of leaves from the embryo in seed plants.

crenate In reference to leaf structure, having a margin cut into rounded scallops.

CsL 2 Pharmacopoea Bohemoslovenica II (1954) + Suppl.

CsL 3 Pharmacopoea Bohemoslovenica III (1970) + Suppl. (1976).

cyme An inflorescence where the axes always end in a single flower.

D1 (2, 3, 4 ....) Mother tincture.

D2 1 part mother tincture and 9 parts ethanol.

D3 (D4, D5, ...) D3 is 1 part D2 and 9 parts ethanol (the dilutions continue in a 1:9 fashion, each starting with the previous dilution as the 1 part fraction and adding 9 parts).

DAB Deutsches Arzneibuch (German Pharmacopoeia).

DAB 10 Deutsches Arzneibuch 10. Ed. (1991), Deutscher Apotheker, Verlag, Govi-Verlag GmbH, Frankfurt/Main.

DAB 1998 Deutsches Arzneibuch 1998. Deutscher Apotheker Verlag, Govi-Verlag GmbH, Frankfurt/Main.

DAB 6 Deutsches Arzneibuch 6. Ed. (1926) + Suppl., R. V. Deckers Verlag, G. Schenck, Berlin.

DAB 7 Deutsches Arzneibuch 7. Ed. (1968) + Suppl., Deutscher Apotheker Verlag, Stuttgart, Govi-Verlag GmbH, Frankfurt/Main.

DAB 9 Deutsches Arzneibuch 9. Ed. (1986), Wissenschaftliche Verlagsgesellschaft, Stuttgart, Govi-Verlag GmbH, Frankfurt/Main.

DAC 79 Arbeitsgemeinschaft der Berufsvertretungen Deutscher Apotheker (Eds.) (1979), Deutscher Arzneimittel-Codex (und Ergänzungslieferungen), Govi-Verlag, Pharmazeutischer Verlag, Frankfurt/Main, Deutscher ApothekerVerlag, Stuttgart.

DAC 86 Bundesvereinigung Deutscher Apothekerverbände (1986), Deutscher Arzneimittel-Codex 1986 mit Ergänzungen, Deutscher Apotheker Verlag, Stuttgart, Govi-Verlag, Frankfurt/Main.

Dan IX Pharmacopoea Danica IX (1948) + Suppl.

deciduous A tree that sheds its leaves at the end of the growing season.

decoction A liquid substance prepared by boiling plant parts in water or some other liquid for a period of time.

decumbent A plant, stem, or shoot that lays on the ground but terminates with an ascending apex.

dentate Tooth-like projections on the margin of a leaf.

dessertspoonful A unit of measure equal to about 2½ fluidrams.

diaphoretic An agent that causes sweating or excessive perspiration.

dioecious In botany, when a plant has either a stamen or a pistil on each flower.

downy Covered with soft hairs.

dromotropic An effect on nerve fiber conduction.

dropsy An abnormal accumulation of fluid in body tissues or cavities usually related to an underlying disease.

drupe A one-seeded fruit; as in olive or peach.

EB 6 Ergänzungsbuch zum Deutschen Arzneibuch, 6. Ausg. (1941), Dr. Hans Hösel, Deutscher Apotheker Verlag, Berlin.

Egypt 84 Egyptian Pharmacopoeia 1984.

embrocation An external medication applied as a liniment or other liquid form.

emmenagogue A substance that renews or stimulates the menstrual flow.

endosperm The albumin of the seed.

epicalyx An external accessory calyx located outside the true calyx of the flower.

eructation The act of belching.

ESCOP European Scientific Cooperation on Phytotherapy, Elburg, Holland.

exocarp The outer wall of a fruit covering.

extraction The portion of a plant that is removed by solvents and used in drug preparations in solid or liquid form.

febrifuge An agent that counteracts fever; an antipyretic.

floret A little flower; one of the small individual flowers that form a cluster or head.

flos Flower.

fluidextract A hydroalcoholic preparation of a botanical drug where 1 ml of the preparation contains 1 gm of the standard botanical.

folium The leaf of a plant.

fructus Fruit.

furuncle A boil or sore caused by bacterial infection of the subcutaneous tissue.

galenic preparation Medications prepared from plants as opposed to refined chemicals.

glabrous Having a smooth surface; without hair or down.

globular Spherical.

globule A small round pill of compressed sucrose that has been saturated with an alcoholic tincture of a specified homeopathic dilution (commonly 1:100).

HAB 1 Homöopathisches Arzneibuch, 1. Ed. (1978), 1.-4. Suppl. (1985), Deutscher Apotheker Verlag, Stuttgart, Govi-Verlag, Frankfurt/Main.

HAB 34 Homöopathisches Arzneibuch (1934), Verlag Dr. Willmar Schwabe, Berlin Helv V Pharmacopoea Helvetica V (1933) + Suppl.

hastate Plant leaves with a triangular shape with the base coming together on each side into an acute lobe.

Helv VI Pharmacopoea Helvetica VI (1971) + Suppl., Eidgenössische Drucksachen- und Materialzentrale, Bern.

Helv VII Pharmacopoea Helvetica VII (1987), Eidgenössische Drucksachen- und Materialzentrale, Bern.

hilum The scar on a seed which indicates its point of attachment.

Hisp IX Farmacopea Oficial Espanola IX (1954).

homeopathic Substances that are administered in minute amounts with the theory that substances that may cause or mimic a disease in larger amounts can be used to treat or prevent disease if given in small amounts.

HPUS 78 Homoeopathic Pharmacopeia of the United States VIII (1978) mit Supplement A (1982).

HPUS 88 Homoeopathic Pharmacopoeia of the United States/Revision Service (1988).

Hung VII Lang B (Eds.) (1986) Pharmacopea Hungarica VII, Akademiai kiado, Budapest.

imbricate Overlapping flower petals; as in the bud.

indehiscent A fruit or grain that doesn't open spontaneously when ripe.

IndP 66 Ministry of Health (1966), Pharmacopoeia of India II, The manager of publications, Delhi.

IndP 85 Ministry of Health & Family Welfare (1985), Pharmacopoeia of India III, Publications & Information Directorate (CSIR), New Dehli.

IndPC 53 Mukerji B (1953), The Indian Pharmaceutical Codex, Council of Scientific & Industrial Research, New Dehli.

induration The process of hardening.

inflorescence The mode of disposition of flowers or the act of flowering. The spatial arrangement of flowers along the axis.

infusion The process of steeping or soaking plant matter in a liquid to extract its medicinal properties without boiling.

involucre A ring or rosette of bracts that surround the base of a flower cluster.

Ital 6 Farmacopea Ufficiale del Regno d'Italia VI (1940), Istituto poligrafico dello stato, Rom.

Ital 7 Farmacopea Ufficiale della Repubblica Italiana VII (1965), Istituto poligrafico dello stato P.V., Rom.

Ital 8 Farmacopea Ufficiale della Repubblica Italiana VIII (1972), Vols. 1-3, Istituto poligrafico dello stato P.F., Rom.

Ital 9 Farmacopea Ufficiale della Repubblica Italiane IX (1985), Instituto poligrafico e zecca dello stato, Rom.

Jap XI The Pharmacopeia of Japan 11th Edition (1986), The Society of Japanese Pharmacopoeia, Jakuji Nippo, Ltd., Tokyo.

Jug IV Pharmacopoea Jugoslavica IV (1984).

KomE Kommission E Monogr. d. BfArM (ehem. Bundesgesundheitsamt - Fed. Health Agency) publ. in Bundesanzeiger (German Federal Gazette) Mar 28.

labiate A lip-like part of a plant; like a calyx or corolla.

lanceolate Lance-like or spear shaped; often referring to a long, tapering leaf.

lignum Woody tissue.

maceration The softening of a solid preparation by soaking in a liquid.

meteorism The presence of gas in the intestine or stomach.

monoecious Having stamens and pistils in separate blossoms on the same plant.

mucilage 1. A viscid substance in a plant consisting of a gum dissolved in the juice of the plant. 2. A soothing application made from plant gums.

muscarinic An effect characterized by contraction of smooth muscle, excessive salivation and perspiration, abdominal colic and excessive bronchial secretion.

Ned 5 Nederlande Pharmacopee V (1926).

Ned 6 Nederlandse Pharmacopee VI (1958), Staatsdrukkerij - en uitgeverijbedrijf, 's-Gravenhage.

Ned 9 Nederlandse Pharmacopee IX (1983-87), staatsuitgeverij,'s-Gravenhage.

NF XV National Formulary XV

Nord 63 Pharmacopoea Nordica, Editio Danica III (1963), Nyt Nordisk Forlag Arnold Busck, Kopenhagen.

Norv V Pharmacopoea Novegica V (1939).

nutlet The stone in a drupe.

NYHA New York Heart Association.

ÖAB 81 Österreichisches Arzneibuch (1981), Vols 1-2, Österreichische Staatsdruckerei, Wien.

ÖAB 9 Österreichisches Arzneibuch 9. Ed. (1960), Vols. 1-2, Österreichische Staatsdruckerei, Wien.

ÖAB 90 Österreichisches Arzneibuch (1990) und 1. Suppl., Verlag der Österreichischen Staatsdruckerei, Wien.

obstipation Persistent or intractable constipation.

panicle A loose, multiple flower cluster usually formed from numerous branches.

pedicel The stalk that supports a single flower in an inflorescence of flowers arranged upon a common peduncle.

peduncle A stalk that bears a flower or flower cluster.

percolation A liquid containing the soluble portion of a drug that has been filtered or separated from the plant matter.

perennial A plant that grows for three or more years.

perianth The external envelope of a flower which does not include the calyx and corolla if they are distinguishable.

pericarp The wall of the ripened ovary of a flower containing the germ of the fruit.

petal One of the leaves of the corolla.

petiolate The footstalk of a leaf.

PF IX Pharmacopée Francaise IX (1973).

PF VIII Pharmacopée Francaise = Codex Francaise VIII (1965).

PF X La Commission Nationale de Pharmacopée (1988), Pharmacopée Francaise X. L'Adrapharm, Paris, + Suppl.

PhEur Euroäisches Arzneibuch, 2. Ed.

Pl Ed I/1 Pharmacopoea Internationalis I (1955), Internationales Arzneibuch, Vol. 1, Wissenschaftliche Verlagsgesellschaft mbH, Stuttgart.

pinnate Compound leaves or leaflets that have a feather-like arrangement with leaves arranged on both sides of a common axis.

pinnatisect Cleft pinnately or almost to the midrib.

pistil The seed-bearing organ of flowering plants consisting of the ovary and the stigma; usually with a style.

plaster A viscous substance that is spread on linen or cloth and applied to a part of the body for healing purposes.

Pol IV Farmakopea Polska IV (1965).

Portug 35 Pharmacopeia Portuguesa (1935).

Portug 46 Farmacopeia Portuguesa VI (1946) + Suppl. 1961, 1967.

poultice A soft, moist mass of plant parts that are wrapped in muslin or gauze and applied warm or hot to the skin.

pubescent In botany, having a fuzzy surface; covered with soft fine short hairs.

raceme An inflorescence where flowers are borne on stalks at an almost equal distance apart along an elongated axis that continues to grow with flowers opening in succession from below.

radix The root of a plant.

reniform When describing a leaf, kidney or bean shaped.

resin An amorphous, solid or semi-solid substance produced by plants usually as a result of terpene oxidation.

reticulate Veins, fibers, or lines crossing like a network across the surface of a leaf.

rhizome An underground stem.

roborant A tonic or substance that gives strength.

Rom IX Farmacopeea Romana, Editia A, IX-A (1976), Editura medicala.

Ross 10 Gosudarstwiennaja Farmakopoea X SSSR, National Pharmakopoea Nr. 10 der UdSSR.

Ross 9 Gosudarstwiennaja Farmakopoea IX SSSR, National Pharmakopoea Nr. 9 der UdSSR.

runners A plant that spreads or forms by means of runners.

scape A flower stalk or peduncle arising from the surface or below the ground.

schizocarp A dry fruit that splits at maturity into several one-seeded carpels.

scrofulous Having an ulcerous or diseased appearance on the surface.

secretagogue An agent that promotes secretion.

secretolytic To inhibit or dry secretions.

semen A seed or seed-like fruit.

sepal One of the modified leaves comprising a calyx; usually positioned outside and surrounding the carpels.

serrate Having notched, teeth-like protrusions along the margin of a leaf that point toward the apex.

sessile Attached directly to the base of a main stem or branch without the aid of an intervening stalk.

stamen The organ of the flower that comprises the anther and filament and gives rise to the male gamete.

stipule A stalk.

stomachic An agent that promotes digestion and improves appetite.

subshrub A perennial plant which has woody stems with the exception of the terminal portion of new growth, which drops off annually.

sudorific Causing or inducing sweat.

tendril The portion of a stem, leaf, or stipule that modified into a slender, spiral-shaped, touch-sensitive specialized appendage, which acts as an anchor to aid in the plants ability to climb.

tepal Any of the modified leaves that combine to make up the perianth.

testa The hard outer coating of a seed; the exocarp.

tincture An alcoholic or hydroalcoholic mixture prepared from plant parts.

tomentose Covered with densely matted hairs.

tonic A medication used to fortify and provide increased vigor.

turiones A shoot or sprout which develops from a bud on a subterranean rootstock.

umbel Numerous flower stalks arising from the same point at the apex of the main stalk and terminating at equal distance from the joining point.

undulate A wavy formation at the margin of a leaf, or bending in a gradual curve.

USP 23-NF 18 United States Pharmacopeial Convention (1995), The United States Pharmacopeia USP 23-NF 18 + Suppl. 1-7.

USP XIX United States Pharmacopeial Convention (1975), The United States Pharmacopeia USP XIX.

USP XX United States Pharmacopeial Convention (1980), The United States.

USP XXI United States Pharmacopeial Convention (1985), The United States Pharmacopeia USP XXI-NF XVI.

USP XXII United States Pharmacopeial Convention (1989), The United States Pharmacopeia USP XXII-NF XVII.

villous Having long, soft hairs.

vulnery A preparation applied externally.

wineglassful A measure equal to four fluidounces.

Poison Control Centers

Many of the centers listed below are certified by the American Association of Poison Control Centers. Certified centers are marked by an asterisk after the name. Each has to meet certain criteria. It must, for example, serve a large geographic area; it must be open 24 hours a day and provide direct-dial or toll-free access; it must be supervised by a medical director; and it must have registered pharmacists or nurses available to answer questions from the public.

The centers have a wide variety of toxicology resources, including a computerized database of some 750,000 substances maintained by MICROMEDEX, INC., an affiliate of PDR. Staff members are trained to resolve toxic situations in the home of the caller, though hospital referrals are given in some instances. The centers also offer a range of educational services to both the public and healthcare professionals. In some states, these larger centers exist side by side with smaller centers offering a more limited range of services.

Within each state, centers are listed alphabetically by city. Telephone numbers designated "TTY" are teletype lines for the hearing-impaired. "TDD" numbers reach a telecommunication device for the deaf.

ALABAMA

BIRMINGHAM
Regional Poison Control Center,
The Children's Hospital of Alabama (*)
1600 7th Ave. South
Birmingham, AL 35233-1711
Business: 205-939-9720
Emergency: 205-933-4050
205-939-9201
800-292-6678(AL)
Fax: 205-939-9245

TUSCALOOSA
Alabama Poison Center, Tuscaloosa (*)
2503 Phoenix Dr.
Tuscaloosa, AL 35405
Business: 205-345-0600
Emergency: 205-345-0600
800-462-0800(AL)
Fax: 205-759-7994

ALASKA

ANCHORAGE
Anchorage Poison Control Center,
Providence Hospital
P.O. Box 196604
3200 Providence Dr.
Anchorage, AK 99519-6604
Business: 907-562-2211
ext. 3633
Emergency: 907-261-3193
800-478-3193(AK)
Fax: 907-261-3645

FAIRBANKS
Fairbanks Poison Control Center
1650 Cowles St.
Fairbanks, AK 99701
Business: 907-456-7182
Emergency: 907-456-7182
Fax: 907-458-5553

ARIZONA

PHOENIX
Samaritan Regional Poison Center (*)
Good Samaritan Regional Medical Center
Ancillary-1
1111 East McDowell Rd.
Phoenix, AZ 85006
Business: 602-495-4884
Emergency: 602-253-3334
800-362-0101(AZ)
Fax: 602-256-7579

TUCSON
Arizona Poison and Drug Information Center (*)
Arizona Health Sciences Center
1501 North Campbell Ave.
Room. 1156
Tucson, AZ 85724
Emergency: 520-626-6016
800-362-0101(AZ)
Fax: 520-626-2720

ARKANSAS

LITTLE ROCK
Arkansas Poison and
Drug Information Center,
College of Pharmacy - UAMS
4301 West Markham St.
Slot 522
Little Rock, AR 72205
Business: 501-661-6161
Emergency: 800-376-4766(AR)
TDD/TTY: 800-641-3805

CALIFORNIA

FRESNO
California Poison Control System-Fresno/Madera (*)
Valley Children's Hospital
9300 Valley Children's Place
Madera, CA 93638-8762
Emergency: 800-876-4766(CA)

SACRAMENTO
California Poison Control System-Sacramento (*)
UCDMC-HSF Room 1024
2315 Stockton Blvd.
Sacramento, CA 95817
Business: 916-734-3415
Emergency: 800-876-4766(CA)
Fax: 916-734-7796

SAN DIEGO
California Poison Control System-San Diego (*)
UCSD Medical Center
200 West Arbor Dr.
San Diego, CA 92103-8925
Emergency: 800-876-4766(CA)

SAN FRANCISCO
California Poison Control System-San Francisco
San Francisco General Hospital
1001 Potrero Ave., Room E86
San Francisco, CA 94110
Emergency: 800-876-4766(CA)

COLORADO

DENVER
Rocky Mountain Poison and Drug Center (*)
8802 East 9th Ave.
Denver, CO 80220-6800
Business: 303-739-1100
Emergency: 303-739-1123
800-332-3073(CO)
Fax: 303-739-1119

CONNECTICUT

FARMINGTON
Connecticut Regional
Poison Control Center (*)
University of Connecticut Health Center
263 Farmington Ave.
Farmington, CT 06030-5365
Business: 860-679-3456
Emergency: 800-343-2722(CT)
Fax: 860-679-1623

DELAWARE

PHILADELPHIA, PA
The Poison Control Center (*)
3535 Market St.
Suite 985
Philadelphia, PA 19104-3309
Emergency: 800-722-7112(PA)
215-386-2100

DISTRICT OF COLUMBIA

WASHINGTON, DC
National Capital Poison Center (*)
3201 New Mexico Ave., NW
Suite 310
Washington, DC 20016
Business: 202-362-3867
Emergency: 202-625-3333
TTY: 202-362-8563
Fax: 202-362-8377

FLORIDA

JACKSONVILLE
Florida Poison Information Center-Jacksonville (*)
University Medical Center
University of Florida Health Science
Center-Jacksonville
655 W. 8th St.
Jacksonville, FL 32209
Emergency: 904-549-4480
800-282-3171(FL)
Fax: 904-549-4063

MIAMI

Florida Poison Information Center-Miami (*)
University of Miami,
School of Medicine
Department of Pediatrics
P.O. Box 016960 (R-131)
Miami, FL 33101
Emergency: 305-585-5253
800-282-3171(FL)
Fax: 305-242-9762

TAMPA

Florida Poison Information Center-Tampa (*)
Tampa General Hospital
P.O. Box 1289
Tampa, FL 33601
Emergency: 813-253-4444
(Tampa)
800-282-3171(FL)
Fax: 813-253-4443

GEORGIA

ATLANTA

Georgia Poison Center (*)
Hughes Spalding Children's Hospital,
Grady Health System
80 Butler St., SE
P.O. Box 26066
Atlanta, GA 30335-3801
Emergency: 404-616-9000
800-282-5846(GA)
TDD: 404-616-9287
Fax: 404-616-6657

HAWAII

HONOLULU

Hawaii Poison Center
1319 Punahou St.
Honolulu, HI 96826
Emergency: 808-941-4411
Fax: 808-535-7922

IDAHO

(DENVER, CO)

Rocky Mountain Poison & Drug Center (*)
8802 E. 9th Ave.
Denver, CO 80220-6800
Emergency: 800-860-0620(ID)
303-739-1123

ILLINOIS

CHICAGO

Illinois Poison Center (*)
222 South Riverside Plaza
Suite 1900
Chicago, IL 60606
Business: 312-906-6136
Emergency: 800-942-5969(IL)
Fax: 312-803-5400

URBANA

ASPCA/National Animal Poison Control Center (*)
1717 S. Philo Rd., Suite 36
Urbana, IL 61802
Business: 217-337-5030
Emergency: 888-426-4435
Fax: 217-337-0599

INDIANA

INDIANAPOLIS

Indiana Poison Center (*)
Methodist Hospital of Indiana
I-65 at 21st St.
Indianapolis, IN 46206-1367
Emergency: 317-929-2323
800-382-9097(IN)
Fax: 317-929-2337

IOWA

IOWA CITY

Poison Control Center
The University of Iowa Hospitals & Clinics
Dept. of Pharmaceutical Care, CC101 GH
200 Hawkins Dr.
Iowa City, IA 52242
Emergency: 800-272-6477(IA)

SIOUX CITY

Iowa Poison Center
2720 Stone Park Blvd.
Sioux City, IA 51104
Business: 712-277-2222
Emergency: 800-352-2222(IA)
Fax: 712-279-7852

KANSAS

KANSAS CITY

Mid-America Poison Control Center,
University of Kansas Medical Center
3901 Rainbow Blvd.
Room B-400
Kansas City, KS 66160-7231
Business & 913-588-6633
Emergency: 800-332-6633(KS)
TDD: 913-588-6639
Fax: 913-588-2350

TOPEKA

Stormont-Vail Regional Medical Center
Emergency Department
1500 S.W. 10th
Topeka, KS 66604-1353
Business: 785-354-6000
Emergency: 785-354-6100
Fax: 785-354-5004

KENTUCKY

LOUISVILLE

Kentucky Regional Poison Center (*)
Medical Towers South
Suite 572
234 E. Gray St.
Louisville, KY 40202
Business: 502-629-7264
Emergency: 502-589-8222
Fax: 502-629-7277

LOUISIANA

MONROE

Louisiana Drug and Poison Information Center (*)
Northeast Louisiana University School of Pharmacy
Sugar Hall
Monroe, LA 71209-6430
Business: 318-342-1710
Emergency: 800-256-9822(LA)
Fax: 318-342-1744

MAINE

PORTLAND

Maine Poison Control Center
Maine Medical Center
22 Bramhall St.
Portland, ME 04102
Business: 207-871-2950
Emergency: 800-442-6305(ME)
Fax: 207-871-6226

MARYLAND

BALTIMORE

Maryland Poison Center (*)
University of Maryland at Baltimore
School of Pharmacy
20 North Pine St., PH 230
Baltimore, MD 21201
Business: 410-706-7604
Emergency: 410-706-7701
800-492-2414(MD)
TDD: 410-706-1858
Fax: 410-706-7184

MASSACHUSETTS

BOSTON

Massachusetts Poison Control System (*)
300 Longwood Ave.
Boston, MA 02115
Emergency: 617-232-2120
800-682-9211(MA)
Fax: 617-738-0032

MICHIGAN

DETROIT

Poison Control Center (*)
Children's Hospital of Michigan
4160 John R. Harper Prof.Office Bldg.
Suite 616
Detroit, MI 48201
Business: 313-745-5335
Emergency: 313-745-5711
800-764-7661(MI)
TDD/TTY: 800-356-3232
Fax: 313-745-5493

GRAND RAPIDS

Spectrum Health Regional Poison Center (*)
1840 Wealthy SE
Grand Rapids, MI 49506-2968
Business: 616-774-5329
Emergency: 800-764-7661(MI)
TDD/TTY: 800-356-3232
Fax: 616-774-7204

MINNESOTA

MINNEAPOLIS

Hennepin Regional Poison Center (*)
Hennepin County Medical Center
701 Park Ave.
Minneapolis, MN 55415
Business: 612-347-3144
Emergency: 800-764-7661
(MN, SD)
612-347-3141
TTY: 612-904-4691
Fax: 612-904-4289

MISSISSIPPI

HATTIESBURG

Poison Center,
Forrest General Hospital
P. O. Box 16389
400 South 28th Ave.
Hattiesburg, MS 39404
Emergency: 601-288-2100
601-288-2197
601-288-2199
Fax: 601-288-2125

JACKSON

Mississippi Regional Poison Control Center,
University of Mississippi Medical Center
2500 North State St.
Jackson, MS 39216
Business: 601-984-1675
Emergency: 601-354-7660
Fax: 601-984-1676

MISSOURI

KANSAS CITY

Poison Control Center,
Children's Mercy Hospital
2401 Gillham Rd.
Kansas City, MO 64108-4619
Business: 816-234-3053
Emergency: 816-234-3430
Fax: 816-234-3421

ST. LOUIS

Cardinal Glennon Children's Hospital
Regional Poison Center (*)
1465 South Grand Blvd.
St. Louis, MO 63104
Emergency: 800-366-8888(MO)
314-772-5200
Fax: 314-577-5355

MONTANA

(DENVER, CO)

Rocky Mountain Poison and Drug Center (*)
8802 East 9th Ave.
Denver, CO 80220-6800
Emergency: 800-525-5042(MT)
303-739-1123
Fax: 303-739-1119

NEBRASKA

OMAHA

The Poison Center (*)
Children's Hospital
8301 Dodge St.
Omaha, NE 68114
Emergency: 402-354-5555 (Omaha)
800-955-9119 (NE & WY)

NEVADA

(DENVER, CO)

Rocky Mountain Poison and Drug Center (*)
8802 East 9th Ave.
Denver, CO 80220-6800
Emergency: 800-446-6179(NV)
303-739-1123
Fax: 303-739-1119

NEW HAMPSHIRE

LEBANON

New Hampshire Poison Information Center, Dartmouth-Hitchcock Medical Center
1 Medical Center Dr.
Lebanon, NH 03756
Emergency: 603-650-8000 (ask for Poison Center)
800-562-8236(NH)
Fax: 603-650-8986

NEW JERSEY

NEWARK

New Jersey Poison Information and Education System (*)
201 Lyons Ave.
Newark, NJ 07112
Business: 973-926-7443
Emergency: 800-764-7661(NJ)
Fax: 973-705-8098

NEW MEXICO

ALBUQUERQUE

New Mexico Poison and Drug Information Center (*)
University of New Mexico
Health Sciences Library, Room 125
Albuquerque, NM 87131-1076
Emergency: 505-272-2222
800-432-6866(NM)
Fax: 505-277-5892

NEW YORK

BUFFALO

Western New York Regional Poison Control Center (*) Children's Hospital of Buffalo
219 Bryant St.
Buffalo, NY 14222
Business: 716-878-7657
Emergency: 716-878-7654
800-888-7655 (NY Western Regions Only)

MINEOLA

Long Island Regional Poison Control Center (*)
Winthrop University Hospital
259 First St.
Mineola, NY 11501
Emergency: 516-542-2323
516-663-2650
TDD: 516-747-3323 (Nassau)
516-924-8811 (Suffolk)
Fax: 516-739-2070

NEW YORK

New York City Poison Control Center (*)
NYC Dept. of Health
455 First Ave., Room 123
Box 81
New York, NY 10016
Business: 212-447-8154
Emergency: 800-210-3985
212-340-4494
212-POISONS
212-VENENOS (Spanish)
TDD: 212-689-9014
Fax: 212-447-8223

ROCHESTER

Finger Lakes Regional Poison and Drug Information Center (*)
University of Rochester Medical Center
601 Elmwood Ave.
Box 321
Rochester, NY 14642
Business: 716-273-4155
Emergency: 716-275-3232
800-333-0542(NY)
TTY: 716-273-3854
Fax: 716-244-1677

SLEEPY HOLLOW

Hudson Valley Regional Poison Center (*)
Phelps Memorial Hospital Center
701 N. Broadway
Sleepy Hollow, NY 10591
Emergency: 914-366-3030
800-336-6997(NY)
Fax: 914-353-1050

SYRACUSE

Central New York Poison Control Center (*)
SUNY Health Science Center
750 East Adams St.
Syracuse, NY 13210
Business: 315-464-7073
Emergency: 315-476-4766
800-252-5655(NY)
Fax: 315-464-7077

NORTH CAROLINA

CHARLOTTE

Carolinas Poison Center (*)
Carolinas Medical Center
5000 Airport Center Pkwy.
Suite B
P.O. Box 32861
Charlotte, NC 28208
Business: 704-355-3054
Emergency: 704-355-4000
800-848-6946(NC)

NORTH DAKOTA

FARGO

North Dakota Poison Information Center, Meritcare Medical Center
720 North 4th St.
Fargo, ND 58122
Business: 701-234-6062
Emergency: 701-234-5575
800-732-2200 (ND, MN, SD)
Fax: 701-234-5090

OHIO

CINCINNATI

Cincinnati Drug & Poison Information Center and Regional Poison Control System (*)
2368 Victory Pkwy.
Suite 300
Cincinnati, OH 45206
Emergency: 513-558-5111
800-872-5111(OH)
Fax: 513-558-5301

CLEVELAND

Greater Cleveland Poison Control Center
11100 Euclid Ave.
Cleveland, OH 44106-6010
Emergency: 216-231-4455
888-231-4455(OH)
Fax: 216-844-3242

COLUMBUS

Central Ohio Poison Center (*)
700 Children's Dr.
Room L032
Columbus, OH 43205-2696
Business: 614-722-2635
Emergency: 614-228-1323
800-682-7625(OH)
800-762-0727 (Dayton only)
TTY: 614-222-2272
Fax: 614-221-2672

TOLEDO

Poison Information Center of NW Ohio, Medical College of Ohio Hospital
3000 Arlington Ave.
Toledo, OH 43614
Business: 419-383-3897
Emergency: 419-383-3897
800-589-3897(OH)
Fax: 419-383-6066

OKLAHOMA

OKLAHOMA CITY

Oklahoma Poison Control Center, University of Oklahoma and Children's Hospital of Oklahoma
940 Northeast 13th St.
Room 3512
Oklahoma City, OK 73104
Business: 405-271-5454
Emergency: 800-764-7661(OK)
TDD: 405-271-1122
Fax: 405-271-1816

OREGON

PORTLAND

Oregon Poison Center (*)
Oregon Health Sciences University
3181 S.W. Sam Jackson Park Rd.
Portland, OR 97201
Emergency: 503-494-8968
800-452-7165(OR)
Fax: 503-494-4980

PENNSYLVANIA

HERSHEY

Central Pennsylvania Poison Center (*)
University Hospital
Milton S. Hershey Medical Center
MC H043, P.O. Box 850
500 University Dr.
Hershey, PA 17033-0850
Emergency: 800-521-6110(PA)
717-531-6111
Fax: 717-531-6932

PHILADELPHIA

The Poison Control Center (*)
3535 Market St., Suite 985
Philadelphia, PA 19104-3309
Business: 215-590-2003
Emergency: 215-386-2100
800-722-7112(PA)
Fax: 215-590-4419

PITTSBURGH

Pittsburgh Poison Center (*)
Children's Hospital of Pittsburgh
3705 Fifth Ave.
Pittsburgh, PA 15213
Business: 412-692-5600
Emergency: 412-681-6669
Fax: 412-692-7497

PUERTO RICO

SANTURCE

San Jorge Children's Hospital Poison Center
258 San Jorge St.
Santurce, PR 00912
Emergency: 787-726-5674

RHODE ISLAND

PROVIDENCE

Lifespan Poison Center (*)
Rhode Island Hospital
593 Eddy St.
Providence, RI 02903
Emergency: 401-444-5727
Fax: 401-444-8062

SOUTH CAROLINA

COLUMBIA

Palmetto Poison Center,
College of Pharmacy,
University of South Carolina
Columbia, SC 29208
Business: 803-777-7909
Emergency: 803-777-1117
800-922-1117(SC)
Fax: 803-777-6127

SOUTH DAKOTA

(FARGO, ND)

North Dakota Poison Information Center
Meritcare Medical Center
720 North 4th St.
Fargo, ND 58122
Business: 701-234-6062
Emergency: 701-234-5575
800-732-2200
(SD, MN, ND)
Fax: 701-234-5090

(MINNEAPOLIS, MN)

Hennepin Regional Poison Center (*)
Hennepin County Medical Center
701 Park Ave.
Minneapolis, MN 55415
Business: 612-347-3144
Emergency: 800-764-7661
(MN, SD)
612-347-3141
TTY: 612-904-4691

TENNESSEE

MEMPHIS

Southern Poison Center
875 Monroe Ave.
Suite 104
Memphis, TN 38163
Business: 901-448-6800
Emergency: 901-528-6048
800-288-9999(TN)
Fax: 901-448-5419

NASHVILLE

Middle Tennessee Poison Center (*)
The Center for Clinical Toxicology,
Vanderbilt University Medical Center
1161 21st Ave. South
501 Oxford House
Nashville, TN 37232-4632
Business: 615-936-0760
Emergency: 615-936-2034
800-288-9999(TN)
TDD: 615-936-2047
Fax: 615-936-2046

TEXAS

AMARILLO

Texas Panhandle Poison Center
Northwest Texas Hospital
1501 S. Coulter Dr.
Amarillo, TX 79106
Emergency: 806-354-1000
800-764-7661(TX)

DALLAS

North Texas Poison Center (*)
5201 Harry Hines Blvd.
P.O. Box 35926
Dallas, TX 75235
Business: 214-590-6625
Emergency: 800-764-7661(TX)
Fax: 214-590-5008

EL PASO

West Texas Regional Poison Center (*)
Thomason Hospital
4815 Alameda Ave.
El Paso, TX 79905
Emergency: 800-764-7661(TX)

GALVESTON

Southeast Texas Poison Center (*)
The University of Texas
Medical Branch
301 University Ave.
Galveston, TX 77555-1175
Business: 409-766-4403
Emergency: 800-764-7661(TX)
Fax: 409-772-3917

SAN ANTONIO

South Texas Poison Center(*)
The University of Texas Health Sciences Center
7703 Floyd Curl Dr., MC 7849
San Antonio, TX 78229-3900
Emergency: 210-567-5762
800-764-7661(TX)
Fax: 210-567-5718

TEMPLE

Central Texas Poison Center (*)
Scott & White Memorial Hospital
2401 South 31st St.
Temple, TX 76508
Business: 254-724-4636
Emergency: 800-764-7661(TX)
254-724-7401
Fax: 254-724-1731

UTAH

SALT LAKE CITY

Utah Poison Control Center (*)
410 Chipeta Way
Suite 230
Salt Lake City, UT 84108
Emergency: 801-581-2151
800-456-7707(UT)
Fax: 801-581-4199

VERMONT

BURLINGTON

Vermont Poison Center,
Fletcher Allen Health Care
111 Colchester Ave.
Burlington, VT 05401
Business: 802-656-2721
Emergency: 802-658-3456
877-658-3456
(toll-free)
Fax: 802-656-4802

VIRGINIA

CHARLOTTESVILLE

Blue Ridge Poison Center (*)
University of Virginia Health System
Box 437
Charlottesville, VA 22908
Emergency: 804-924-5543
800-451-1428(VA)
Fax: 804-971-8657

RICHMOND

Virginia Poison Center (*)
Virginia Commonwealth University
P.O. Box 980522
Richmond, VA 23298-0522
Emergency: 800-552-6337(VA)
804-828-9123
Fax: 804-828-5291

WASHINGTON

SEATTLE

Washington Poison Center (*)
155 NE 100th St.
Suite 400
Seattle, WA 98125-8012
Business: 206-517-2351
Emergency: 206-526-2121
800-732-6985(WA)
TDD: 800-572-0638
206-517-2394
Fax: 206-526-8490

WEST VIRGINIA

CHARLESTON

West Virginia Poison Center (*)
3110 MacCorkle Ave. SE
Charleston, WV 25304
Business: 304-347-1212
Emergency: 304-348-4211
800-642-3625(WV)
Fax: 304-348-9560

WISCONSIN

MADISON

Poison Control Center,
University of Wisconsin Hospital and Clinics
600 Highland Ave.
F6-133
Madison, WI 53792
Business: 608-262-7537
Emergency: 608-262-3702
800-815-8855(WI)

MILWAUKEE

Children's Hospital Poison Center,
Children's Hospital of Wisconsin
9000 W. Wisconsin Ave.
P.O. Box 1997
Milwaukee, WI 53201
Business: 414-266-2000
Emergency: 414-266-2222
800-815-8855(WI)
Fax: 414-266-2820

Wyoming

OMAHA, NE

The Poison Center (*)
Children's Hospital
8301 Dodge St.
Omaha, NE 68114
Emergency: 402-354-5555
(Omaha)
800-955-9119
(WY, NE)

pharmacological and clinical trials, both in-house and in close cooperation with internationally recognized Universities or CROs.

IV. Regulatory Affairs, Patents, Proprietary Technologies

1. Our "regulatory affairs" department is experienced in the worldwide regulation of botanical products. We are actively involved in the international botanical legislation process.
Complete registration dossiers including expert reports are developed in-house, as are IND applications, claim substantiations, etc.

2. Patent protection and proprietary technologies for botanicals are an area of special expertise for us. We work closely with experienced product development companies to achieve a clear product differentiation including patent protection or development of proprietary technologies.
This starts with the seed material and plant specific SOPs for growth and harvesting, and continues through the extraction process and refinement including all possibilities for specific indication/use patents for botanical products.

V. Strategic and Marketing Support

Based on our knowledge of the present and future market trends, critical issues, and potential technologies, we develop strategies for companies that are already active in the herbal market as well as for those who wish to enter the international market.

VI. International Alliances and Technology Transfer

Our strong position within the worldwide pharmaceutical and herbal industry gives us the framework to support companies developing new technologies or products, companies looking for or offering new products, and companies interested in mergers and acquisitions. A special strength is our strong base in Europe and the USA to support the exchange of product information and the establishment of cooperatives, joint ventures, or the search for mergers and acquisitions.

Please feel free to contact us for detailed information about your specific needs:

US-Office:

PhytoPharm US, Inc.
Institute for Phytopharmaceutica
292 Fernwood Avenue
Edison, New Jersey 08837

Phone: 732-346-0488
Fax: 732-346-0442
E-mail: info@phytonet.com
Web site: www.phytonet.com

European Office:

PhytoPharm Consulting
Institute for Phytopharmaceutica
Waldseeweg 6
D-13467 Berlin
Germany

Phone: +49 30 405 999 -70
Fax: +49 30 405 999 -61
E-mail: info@phytopharm.org
Web site: www.phytonet.com

Joerg Gruenwald, Ph.D., President
Christof Jaenicke, MD, CEO
Thomas Brendler, BA, Senior Vice Presiden
Scientific Media
Elke Langner, Ph.D., Senior Vice President
Regulatory Affairs/Medical Writing
Stefan Spiess, MA, Senior Vice President
R&D Strategies and Implementation

Internet:
If you are interested in further details concerning our company, or in other subjects in the botanical field, consult our web page
www.phytonet.com
This web site includes more than 500 botanical links, which may be of interest to you.

Our Staff:
PhytoPharm Consulting is staffed by 20 dedicated, well-trained herbal experts: physicians, botanists, pharmacists, chemists, food chemists, and herbal practitioners with a combined business experience of over 150 years.

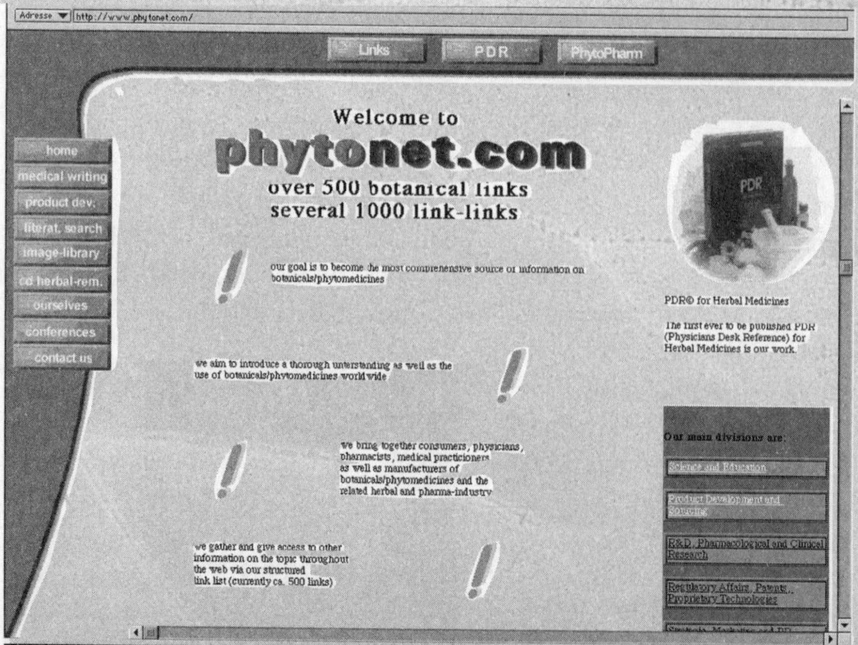

www.phytonet.com